ADAMS' LAMENESS IN HORSES

FIFTH EDITION

ADAMS' LAMENESS IN HORSES

FIFTH EDITION

TED S. STASHAK, DVM, MS

Diplomate American College of Veterinary Surgeons
Professor of Surgery
Head, Equine Services
Department of Clinical Sciences
College of Veterinary Medicine and Biomedical Sciences
Colorado State University
Fort Collins, Colorado

LIPPINCOTT WILLIAMS & WILKINS
A **Wolters Kluwer** Company
Philadelphia • Baltimore • New York • London
Buenos Aires • Hong Kong • Sydney • Tokyo

Editor: David Troy
Managing Editor: Dana Battaglia
Marketing Manager: Chris Kushner
Production Editor: Bill Cady
Designer: Armen Kojoyian
Compositor: Maryland Composition
Printer: R. R. Donnelley & Sons

Printed in the United States of America
First Edition, 1962
Second Edition, 1966
Third Edition, 1974
Fourth Edition, 1987

Library of Congress Cataloging-in-Publication Data

Adams' lameness in horses / [edited by] Ted S. Stashak.—5th ed.
     p. cm.
   Fourth ed. (1987) entered under O.R. Adams.
   Includes bibliographical references and index.
   ISBN 0-683-07981-6
     1. Lameness in horses. 2. Horseshoeing. I. Adams, O. R. (Ora Robert). Adams'
Lameness in horses.

SF959.L25 A3 1998
636.1′089758—dc21
                                                            98-007679

01 02 03 04 05
1 2 3 4 5 6 7 8 9 10

To my wife, Gloria, and my children, Angela, Stephanie, and Ryan, for their love, support, and understanding

To my parents for their support and guidance and to the memory of Dr. O. R. Adams

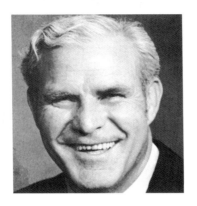

O. R. ADAMS

PREFACE TO THE FIFTH EDITION

First and foremost, I want to extend my sincere thanks to the veterinary profession, veterinary students, students in related equine science programs, paraprofessionals in the equine industry, and horse owners throughout the world for their wide acceptance of the fourth edition of *Adams' Lameness in Horses.* The many favorable comments I received throughout the years have, to a large degree, provided me with the impetus to embark on the much-needed revision of the fourth edition. That being said, it pleases me to provide the veterinary profession and persons in equine-related fields with the extensively revised fifth edition of *Adams' Lameness in Horses.* As with the fourth edition, the changes are substantial, including the addition of new authors, the reorganization of material, and the reduction in the number of chapters from 14 to 9. As with the other editions, the fifth edition is designed to appeal to a wide audience in equine-related fields.

Chapter 1 has been revised to provide the reader with an updated version of the functional anatomy of the equine locomotor system. The latest information regarding the dermal microcirculation of the foot and the anatomy of various joint capsules and their distribution has been added with detailed illustrations to support the discussion. As usual, Dr. Kainer's attention to detail provides a complete reference for the various regions of the musculoskeletal system. I would like to thank Dr. Robert Bowker for his contributions to this chapter.

Chapter 2 has changed considerably and covers a discussion of conformation and locomotion. The part on conformation has been extensively revised and updated with as much reference material as possible in hopes of providing objective data from which to draw conclusions. Additionally, the discussion of normal movement, movement abnormalities, and factors that affect move-ment, which expands on the material from Chapter 13, "Natural and Artificial Gaits," from the fourth edition, has also been included. Cherry Hill's co-authorship has provided much needed insight from a certified (carded by the U.S. breed associations) equine judge's standpoint. Cherry's background as a professional horse trainer and instructor has also added a practical perspective that I believe will appeal to veterinarians and horsemen alike.

Chapter 3 is presented in the same format as in the previous edition, with the addition of new material to make it as current as possible. Most of the anecdotal material has been removed except where personal experience was interjected to provide another perspective. Many new illustrations have been added to facilitate the discussion.

Chapter 4, the imaging chapter, has been completely updated and includes two new parts, one on ultrasound and one on nuclear medicine. The discussion of these two imaging modalities, used extensively for lameness diagnosis, has greatly increased the amount of material presented. Chapter 4 is divided into three parts. Part I, authored by Dr. Richard Park, provides an updated discussion of radiography in the diagnosis of equine lameness. This is followed by Part II, a comprehensive discussion by Dr. Robert Wrigley on the usefulness of ultrasound in lameness diagnosis. This part's many illustrations provide a useful and clear understanding of the anatomy being imaged. In Part III, Dr. Phillip Steyn provides a comprehensive discussion and presentation of illustrations on the value of nuclear medicine in the diagnosis of equine lameness. I would like to thank Dr. Richard Park for his leadership role in the development of this chapter.

Chapter 5 has also been completely updated with the addition of a new first author, Dr. Kate Savage, with Dr.

Lewis acting as second author. This chapter provides the most current information regarding the role that nutrition plays in musculoskeletal development and disease.

Chapter 6 has also been completely revised and updated. With the departure of my colleague, Dr. Simon Turner, from the clinical arena to research, Dr. Gary Baxter has taken over as the first author of this chapter, with Dr. Turner serving as second author. A significant addition to this chapter is a comprehensive and practical discussion of the emergency ("first aid") management of equine fracture patients for transport and/or treatment. Many illustrations have been added to support the discussion.

Chapter 7 has been extensively revised by Dr. Wayne McIlwraith. The addition of much research material to this chapter provides the reader with the most current information on the etiopathogenesis, diagnosis, and treatment of the various causes of joint disease and related structures. Many new illustrations have been added to augment the discussion of these various entities.

Chapter 8 has been extensively revised and greatly expanded, with the addition of new diseases. Dr. Alicia Bertone has updated discussion on the diseases associated with the fetlock region, including the metacarpus and carpus. Dr. Ken Sullins has updated discussion on the diseases of the hindlimb up to the coxofemeral joint. Dr. Dean Hendrickson has revised discussion on the diseases associated with the pelvis, back, and axial skeleton. The addition of these authors has greatly improved my ability to provide the reader with the most comprehensive and current discussion of the various diseases that cause lameness. As with the fourth edition, Chapter 8 concludes with discussion of "wobbler syndrome" and the various diseases of the spinal cord that can produce locomotor disorders that appear similar clinically. Dr. Alan Nixon has completely revised this section and, of note, has added a comprehensive discussion of the most current information on the diagnosis and treatment of equine protozoal myeloencephalitis (EPM).

Chapter 9 has been completely reorganized and updated and is presented in an entirely different format from that presented in the fourth edition. It incorporates information from Chapters 10 to 12 of the fourth edition. The addition of Cherry Hill, Richard Klimesh, and Gene Ovnicek as co-authors has greatly improved the presentation of this material, which should make this chapter most useful to all who read it. (Chapter 14, "Methods of Therapy," from the fourth edition has been eliminated, since most of this material is covered throughout the fifth edition for specific lesions or diseases and because many other texts cover the topic more completely than I possibly could in one chapter.)

With the expansion of the literature pertaining to lameness diagnosis and the recognition of new diseases, the reader will soon recognize that the reference lists have expanded in all portions of the text. In all cases the authors tried to include reference material from journals and text sources other than those of English-speaking countries. This was difficult at times, since frequently only summaries and abstracts were written in English.

I am grateful and indebted to Mark Goldstein for his untiring efforts and the many tasks he performed to make the fifth edition possible. Mark scanned the entire fourth edition onto computer. This unfortunately had to be done because the majority of the fourth edition text was lost in the archives of computer services. Following scanning, Mark proofread the material word for word, including checking superscripts and reference formatting. This had to be done, since the accuracy of the scanner at that time was only about 70%. Mark also did all the literature searches for the entire text and copied and organized the literature for distribution to contributing authors. Additionally, Mark combined new and old references for the fifth edition and added their numbered callouts in the text. Mark, thanks for your loyal and untiring effort; without you it would have been very difficult to complete the fifth edition.

The addition of numerous illustrations and photographs represents a tremendous time commitment and effort on behalf of the Computer-Assisted Teaching Service laboratory at Colorado State University. For the majority of the new illustrations I am deeply indebted to Jenger Smith for her skill and expertise in producing these fine illustrations for the fifth edition. Her desire to produce the best possible image and her untiring efforts are most appreciated. Additionally, I am grateful to Gale Mueller from Visible Productions for the excellent illustrations she made for Chapters 1, 3, and 7.

I am grateful to my colleagues, Drs. Baxter, Hendrickson, McIlwraith, and Trotter, including referring practitioners, for allowing me the courtesy of using some of their case material as examples. I also acknowledge the contribution of my colleagues and the surgical residents who have contributed to the care and treatment of some of the cases presented in this text. A special thanks is extended to the many practitioners who have referred cases that have been used in this text. Without their continued support, the accumulation of the case material would not have been possible. Additionally, I am grateful to the technicians who provided support in the care of these patients.

Dana Battaglia, Managing Editor, and the entire staff at Lippincott Williams & Wilkins have been most patient and helpful in the preparation of the fifth edition. I am grateful for their support and guidance. I also wish to thank Carroll Cann, former veterinary editor for Lippincott Williams & Wilkins, who provided early encouragement for this edition.

I hope the new fifth edition meets all the expectations and needs of those who read it. As always, I look forward to your cooperation in making corrections and suggested revisions for future editions.

Fort Collins, Colorado   TED S. STASHAK

PREFACE TO THE FOURTH EDITION

When I was contacted by Mr. George Mundorff, Executive Editor for Lea & Febiger, regarding the possibility of revising the third edition of "Lameness in Horses" by Dr. O. R. Adams, I was excited but naive to the task at hand. Dr. Adams had, in his previous three editions, established the state of the art of lameness diagnosis and treatment, presenting it in a unique manner that appealed to veterinarians, horse owners and trainers, and farriers. Without a doubt, he defined and directly influenced the course of this subject more than any other individual during this time. I was truly fortunate to train under him during my internship and surgical residency at Colorado State University. His never-ending thirst for knowledge, his humor, his friendship, and his love of the veterinary profession have inspired me throughout this endeavor. I only hope that I have served his memory well and that he would be proud of this fourth edition.

After considerable discussion with Lea & Febiger and the assurance of Mrs. Nancy Adams, Dr. Adams' widow, I embarked on the revision with some basic changes in format in mind. These included the addition of new authors, changes in chapter sequence and presentation, the addition of new chapters and deletion of some old ones, and the transition from a monograph to a reference text. Because I wanted the fourth edition to represent the school where Dr. Adams attended and taught, I selected mostly authors from our faculty on the basis of their expertise and their ability to provide a broad base of opinion for the reader.

With the idea of approaching the discussion of lameness as one would approach a lameness examination itself, I changed the sequence of presentation. Using the newest accepted nomenclature, Chapter 1 deals with the functional anatomy of the equine locomotor system and represents a complete revision of Chapter 2 in the previous edition. Dr. Kainer starts with the forelimb, advancing from the foot up the limb, describing the regional anatomy of each site. The hindlimb is covered in similar fashion. The nomenclature may be confusing initially to older graduates of American veterinary schools, but recent graduates as well as foreign veterinarians will be well versed in this terminology. We felt it was time to make this transition since the new nomenclature has been in use for at least 4 years. (Older terms are included parenthetically.)

Following a format similar to the previous edition, Chapter 2 deals with the relationship between conformation and lameness. I have eliminated "The Examination for Soundness," which was Chapter 3 in the previous edition, because it discussed many topics unrelated to lameness and, simply, because the subject of soundness is so comprehensive it could be covered in a separate text. The present Chapter 3 deals with the diagnosis of lameness. After defining lameness and establishing how to determine which limb is lame, the description of the physical examination begins at the foot of the forelimb and proceeds upward. Emphasis is placed on recognition of problems peculiar to the region examined. Following this is a description and illustration of perineural and intrasynovial anesthesia.

The next logical step in the diagnosis of lameness is radiology, which is discussed in Chapter 4. This chapter is comprehensive; nothing like it has been published elsewhere. The format of the text and illustrations should answer any question the reader may have regarding the techniques for taking radiographs and interpreting them. The artwork beautifully illustrates the different structures seen on various radiographic views, and the illustrations are labeled so that anatomic sites are easily identified.

Chapters 5 through 7 are new. Discussing the role of nutrition in musculoskeletal development and disease, Chapter 5 illustrates a unique approach not used elsewhere. Dr. Lewis provides a comprehensive review of specific nutritional disorders, their causes, and their treatment for all phases of growth and development in the foal, during pregnancy and lactation in the mare, and during maintenance of the working horse. This information will benefit both the horseman and the veterinarian. Chapter 6, by Dr. Turner, starts with a brief review of endochondral ossification and then discusses the diseases associated with bones and muscles and their treatment. In Chapter 7, Dr. McIlwraith describes the developmental anatomy of joints and related structures, disease processes, clinical signs, and treatments. Both of these chapters present in-depth reviews, with major emphasis on the pathogenesis and pathobiology of the diseases. They are heavily referenced, and will be of major interest to the veterinary profession.

Representing a complete revision of Chapter 8, "Lameness" updates the reader on new diseases as well as new findings and treatment for previously recognized entities. Unlike past editions, this material is heavily referenced. Information regarding the prevalence of the disease within various breeds according to sex and age introduces each subject. The format of the chapter has been changed to start with diseases relating to the foot region and then proceeding upward anatomically, consistent with the way most equine practitioners approach a systematic examination. Specific diseases of each region are discussed separately. This chapter, though referenced heavily and written technically, should be of interest to the horseman as well as the veterinary profession. I am particularly grateful to Dr. Alan Nixon for his thorough and comprehensive review of the diagnosis and treatment of the "wobbler's syndrome" in horses. His presentation is clear and well illustrated, giving the reader the confidence to differentiate among the diseases that cause this syndrome.

Chapters 9 through 12 were written primarily for the horseman and farrier, though they will also be of interest to the veterinarian, particularly the equine practitioner. I have updated these chapters with new information, as well as listing what the horseman should look for when the horse is properly trimmed and shod. Chapter 13, "Natural and Artificial Gaits," is essentially unchanged. Chapter 14, "Methods of Therapy," has been updated, and includes an extensive revision of different methods of external coaptation. This chapter is primarily directed toward the veterinary profession, though the horse owner will obtain insight into why different treatments are selected.

With the explosion of literature pertaining to musculoskeletal disease in the horse and the demands put on authors and editors alike, it became obvious that a transition from a monograph to a reference text was timely. To this end the authors have attempted to provide the latest information. As with any large text, however, authors and editors alike feel somewhat frustrated because at the time of publication some of this information will be out of date. With few exceptions, we stopped referencing material published in 1985. Occasionally publications in 1985 changed the presentation of the materials so much that it could not be denied and therefore was included.

I am grateful to Dr. Robert Kainer, Professor of Anatomy and author of the first chapter, for taking the time to review and advise me on the nomenclature used in this book. A special thanks is extended to Dr. A. S. Turner for his review and comments on Chapter 8. The fine contributions of all the authors is sincerely appreciated. I want to thank Dr. Robert Perce (California) and Mr. Richard Klimesh (farrier, Colorado) for their advice on the chapters dealing with trimming and shoeing horses.

The addition of many new illustrations and photographs represents a tremendous time commitment and effort on behalf of the Office of Biomedical Media at Colorado State University. For the illustrations, I am indebted to Mr. Tom McCracken and Mr. John Dougherty for their expertise and the cooperation they have given me. For the photographs I am grateful to Mr. Al Kilminster and Mr. David Clack, for their expertise, cooperation, and commitment to excellence. For the design of the book cover I thank Mr. Dave Carlson.

Most of the manuscript was typed by Mrs. Helen Acevedo. Her cooperation and patience with the many revisions necessary to complete this text are gratefully appreciated.

I am also grateful to my many colleagues who took the time to personally reveal their thoughts regarding certain topics. A special thanks is extended to the following: Dr. Joerg Auer (Texas), Dr. Peter Haynes (Louisiana), Dr. Larry Bramlage (Ohio), Dr. Joe Foerner (Illinois), Dr. Dallas Goble (Tennessee), Dr. Robert Baker (Southern California), Dr. Robert Copelan (Kentucky) and Dr. Scott Leith (deceased, Southern California).

Mr. Christian C. Febiger Spahr Jr., Veterinary Editor, Mr. George Mundorff, Executive Editor, Mr. Tom Colaiezzi, Production Manager, Ms. Constance Marino, and Mrs. Dorothy Di Rienzi, Manager of Copy Editors, and the entire staff at Lea & Febiger have been most helpful in the preparation of this book. I am grateful for their support and guidance.

I hope this book will be useful to all who read it. I hope to receive your cooperation in making corrections and suggested additions for further revisions.

Fort Collins, Colorado   Ted S. Stashak

CONTRIBUTORS

GARY M. BAXTER, VMD, MS

Diplomate American College of Veterinary Surgeons, Professor of Surgery, Assistant Department Head, Department of Clinical Sciences, College of Veterinary Medicine and Biomedical Sciences, Colorado State University, Fort Collins, Colorado

ALICIA L. BERTONE, DVM, PhD

Diplomate American College of Veterinary Surgeons, Professor of Equine Orthopedic Surgery, Department of Veterinary Clinical Sciences, College of Veterinary Medicine, The Ohio State University, Columbus, Ohio

DEAN A. HENDRICKSON, DVM, MS

Diplomate American College of Veterinary Surgeons, Associate Professor of Surgery, Department of Clinical Sciences, College of Veterinary Medicine and Biomedical Sciences, Colorado State University, Fort Collins, Colorado

CHERRY HILL, BS AN SCI

Livermore, Colorado

ROBERT A. KAINER, DVM, MS

Professor Emeritus Anatomy and Neurobiology, College of Veterinary Medicine and Biomedical Sciences, Colorado State University, Fort Collins, Colorado

RICHARD KLIMESH, CJF, RJF

Livermore, Colorado

LON D. LEWIS, DVM, PhD

Topeka, Kansas

C. WAYNE MCILWRAITH, BVSc, MS, PhD, DrMedVet(hc), DSc, FRCVS

Diplomate American College of Veterinary Surgeons, Diplomate European College of Veterinary Surgeons, Professor of Surgery, Director of Orthopaedic Research Center, College of Veterinary Medicine and Biomedical Sciences, Colorado State University, Fort Collins, Colorado

ALAN J. NIXON, BVSc, MS

Diplomate American College of Veterinary Surgeons, Professor of Surgery, Director, Comparative Orthopaedics Laboratory, Department of Clinical Sciences, College of Veterinary Medicine, Cornell University, Ithaca, New York

GENE OVNICEK

Colorado Springs, Colorado

RICHARD D. PARK, DVM, PhD

Diplomate American College of Veterinary Radiology, Professor, Department of Radiological Health Sciences, Head, Diagnostic Imaging, Veterinary Teaching Hospital, Colorado State University, Fort Collins, Colorado

CATHERINE J. SAVAGE, BVSc, PhD

Diplomate American College of Veterinary Internal Medicine, Arrabi Equine Internal Medicine, LLC, Aldie, Virginia

TED S. STASHAK, DVM, MS

Diplomate American College of Veterinary Surgeons, Professor of Surgery, Head, Equine Services, Department of Clinical Sciences, College of Veterinary Medicine and Biomedical Sciences, Colorado State University, Fort Collins, Colorado

PHILLIP F. STEYN, BVSc, MRCVS

Diplomate American College of Veterinary Radiology, Associate Professor, Department of Radiological Health Sciences, Head, Nuclear Medicine, Veterinary Teaching Hospital, Colorado State University, Fort Collins, Colorado

KENNETH E. SULLINS, DVM, MS

Diplomate American College of Veterinary Surgeons, Associate Professor of Surgery, Marion DuPont Scott Equine Medical Center, VA-MD Regional College of Veterinary Medicine, Leesburg, Virginia

A. SIMON TURNER, BVSc, MS

Diplomate American College of Veterinary Surgeons, Professor, Department of Clinical Sciences, College of Veterinary Medicine and Biomedical Sciences, Colorado State University, Fort Collins, Colorado

ROBERT H. WRIGLEY, BVSc, MS, DVR, MRCVS

Diplomate American College of Radiology, Diplomate European College of Veterinary Diagnostic Imaging, Professor, Department of Radiological Health Sciences, Head, Ultrasound Lab, Veterinary Teaching Hospital, College of Veterinary Medicine and Biomedical Sciences, Colorado State University, Fort Collins, Colorado

CONTENTS

Functional Anatomy of Equine Locomotor Organs

ROBERT A. KAINER

ANATOMIC NOMENCLATURE AND USAGE

Through the efforts of nomenclature committees, informative and logical names for parts of the horse's body (as well as positional and directional terms) have evolved, and are found in the *Nomina Anatomica Veterinaria* (N.A.V.).[32] Some older terminology is still acceptable. For example, while thoracic limb and pelvic limb are preferred anatomic designations, forelimb and hindlimb are commonly used. Navicular bone for distal sesamoid bone, coffin joint for distal interphalangeal joint, pastern joint for proximal interphalangeal joint, and fetlock joint for metacarpophalangeal joint are acceptable synonyms. It behooves one to be familiar with many of the older terms. But some have become archaic and even add to the confusion in communicating structural concepts. There are a few common departures from N.A.V. terminology: while some anatomists agree with the N.A.V. in considering the corium to be part of the hoof and the cartilage attached to the distal phalanx to be the cartilage of the hoof (ungual cartilage),[41,42,43] others maintain that the hoof is solely epidermal and that the cartilage of the distal phalanx is just that.[14,18,44] The term, sagittal, indicates a proximodistal, dorsopalmar (dorsoplantar) middle plane through the equine digit. A parasagittal plane is parallel to the sagittal plane. Axial means toward the axis of the digit (essentially synonymous with sagittal); abaxial, away from the digit. In this book acceptable synonyms will be indicated parenthetically, and the two terms may be used interchangeably.

In Figure 1.1 note that positional adjectives end in -al. When the terms are used as positional adverbs, the suffix -ally is substituted. When used as directional adverbs (those indicating direction from a given point), the suffix -ad is substituted. For example, a structure is located distally; another structure extends or courses distad. With the exception of the eye, the terms anterior and posterior are not applicable to quadrupeds. Cranial and caudal apply to the limbs proximal to the antebrachiocarpal (radiocarpal) joint and the tarsocrural (tibiotarsal) joint. Distal to these joints, dorsal and palmar (on the forelimb) or dorsal and plantar (on the hindlimb) are

the correct terms. The adjective, solar, is used to designate structures on the palmar (plantar) surface of the distal phalanx and the ground surface of the hoof.

THORACIC LIMB

Digit and Fetlock

The foot and pastern make up the equine digit, a region including the distal (third), middle (second), and proximal (first) phalanges and associated structures (Fig. 1.2). The fetlock consists of the metacarpophalangeal (fetlock) joint and the structures surrounding it. Since the digits and fetlocks of the thoracic limb and the pelvic limb are similar in most respects, consider the following descriptions to pertain to both limbs unless otherwise indicated. Where the term, palmar, is used the term, plantar, is implied. Such terms as metacarpophalangeal and metatarsophalangeal are obvious counterparts.

Foot

The foot consists of the epidermal hoof and all it encloses: the connective tissue corium (dermis), digital cushion, distal phalanx (coffin bone, since it is enclosed as in a coffin), most of the cartilages of the distal phalanx, distal interphalangeal (coffin) joint, distal extremity of the middle phalanx (short pastern bone), distal sesamoid (navicular) bone, bursa podotrochlearis (navicular bursa), several ligaments, tendons of insertion of the common digital extensor and deep digital flexor muscles, blood vessels, and nerves. Skin between the heels is also part of the foot. Cartilages of the distal phalanx are palpable where they project under the skin proximal to the coronet.

The hoof is continuous with the epidermis at the coronet. Here the dermis of the skin is continuous with the dermis (corium or pododerm) subjacent to the hoof. Regions of the corium correspond to the parts of the hoof under which they are located: perioplic corium, coronary corium, laminar (lamellar) corium, corium of the frog (cuneate corium), and corium of the sole.

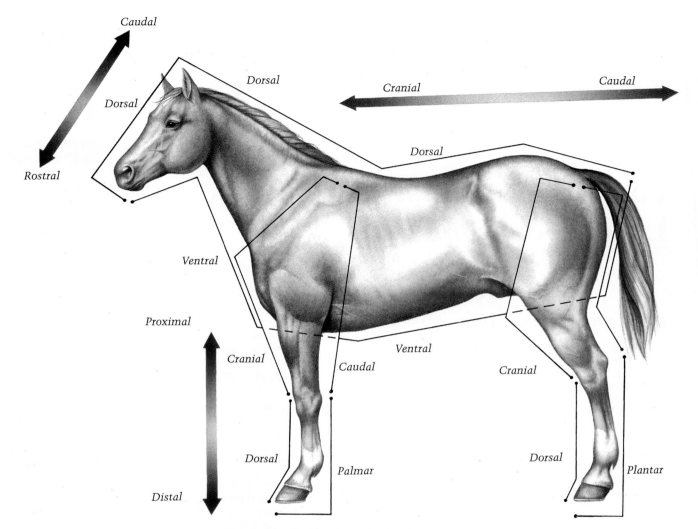

Figure 1.1   Positional and directional terms.

Grossly definitive parts of the hoof protect underlying structures of the foot and initiate dissipation of concussive forces when the hoof strikes the ground. Examination of the ground surface of the hoof reveals the sole, frog, heels, bars, and ground surface of the wall (Fig. 1.3). The ground surface of the forefoot is normally larger than that of the hindfoot, reflecting the shape of the distal surface of the enclosed distal phalanx (coffin bone).

The hoof wall extends from the ground proximad to the coronary border where the soft white horn of the periople joins the epidermis of the skin at the coronet. Regions of the wall are the dorsal toe, the medial and lateral quarters, and the rounded heels continuing palmarad from the quarters (Figs. 1.3 and 1.4). From the thick toe the wall becomes progressively thinner and more elastic toward the heels, where it thickens again at the junction of the bars (the "buttress" of the hoof). The wall usually curves more widely on the lateral side, and the lateral angle is less steep than the medial angle. Ranges for the angle of the toe between the dorsal surface of the hoof wall and the ground surface of the hoof vary

widely.[1,18] For example, a range of 48 to 60° was measured on the hooves of the forefeet in a series of common riding horses (Wright C, unpublished data, 1983). In the ideal digit, the dorsal surface of the hoof wall and the dorsal surface of the pastern should be parallel, reflecting the axial alignment of the subjacent phalanges. In most horses, the parallel alignment of dorsal surfaces of the foredigit is achieved when the hooves are trimmed between 50 and 54°.[1]

The highly vascular and innervated dense collagenous connective tissue of the coronary corium (dermis) extends elongated, distally directed papillae. Laminar (lamellar) corium forms a series of laminae that interdigitate with epidermal laminae of the stratum internum of the hoof wall. Shorter papillae extend from the perioplic, solar, and cuneate (frog) coria. The corium provides sensation, as well as nourishment and attachment for the overlying stratified squamous epithelium making up the ungual epidermis (Latin, *ungula,* hoof).

In the coronary region, the stratum basale of the ungual epidermis is a single layer of proliferating columnar keratinocytes lying upon and between long dermal papil-

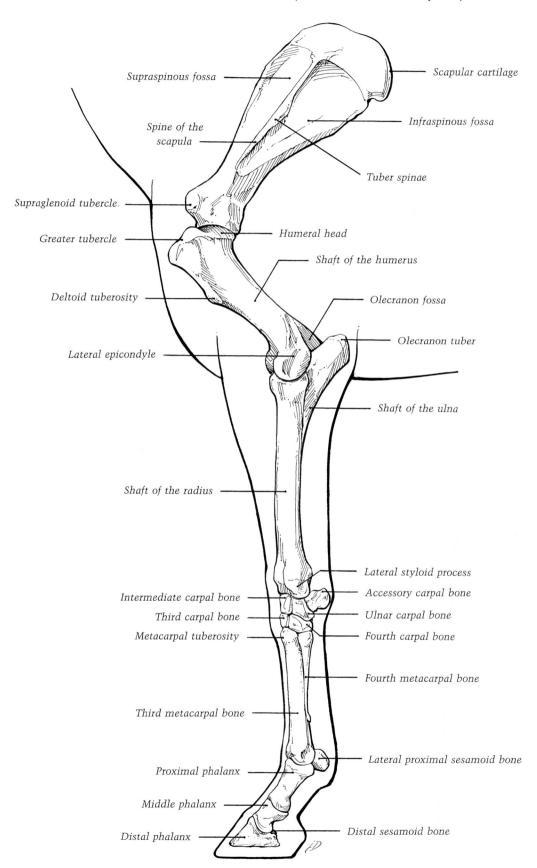

Supraspinous fossa

Scapular cartilage

Spine of the scapula

Infraspinous fossa

Tuber spinae

Supraglenoid tubercle

Humeral head

Greater tubercle

Shaft of the humerus

Deltoid tuberosity

Olecranon fossa

Olecranon tuber

Lateral epicondyle

Shaft of the ulna

Shaft of the radius

Lateral styloid process

Accessory carpal bone

Intermediate carpal bone

Ulnar carpal bone

Third carpal bone

Fourth carpal bone

Metacarpal tuberosity

Fourth metacarpal bone

Third metacarpal bone

Lateral proximal sesamoid bone

Proximal phalanx

Middle phalanx

Distal phalanx

Distal sesamoid bone

Figure 1.2 Bones of left equine thoracic limb. Lateral view.

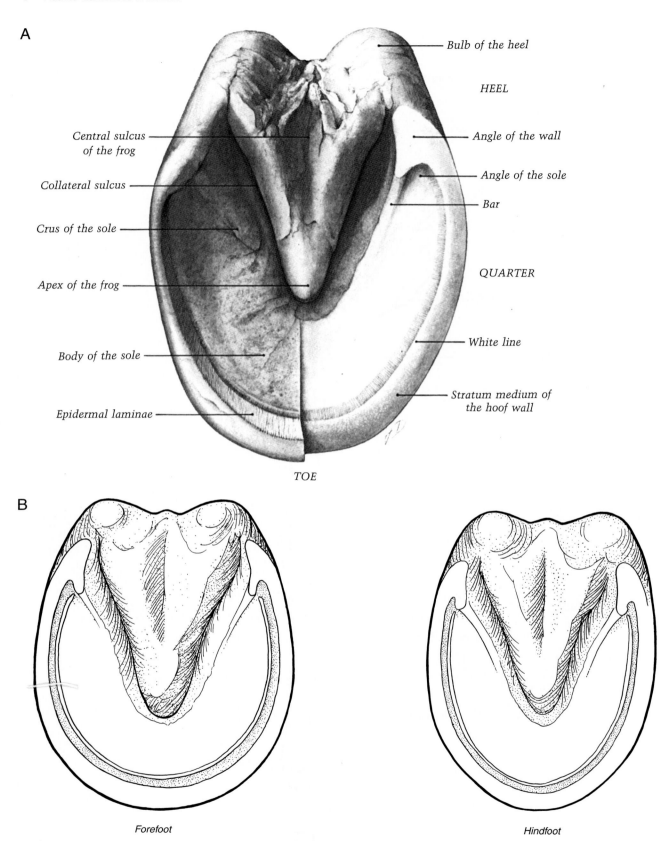

A

Bulb of the heel

HEEL

Central sulcus
of the frog

Angle of the wall

Angle of the sole

Collateral sulcus

Bar

Crus of the sole

Apex of the frog

QUARTER

White line

Body of the sole

Stratum medium of
the hoof wall

Epidermal laminae

TOE

B

Forefoot

Hindfoot

Figure 1.3   A. Topography of the ground (solar) surface of the hoof. The right half has been trimmed to emphasize the formation of the white line by the epidermal laminae. B. Comparison of normal size and shape of the ground surface of the forefoot and hindfoot.

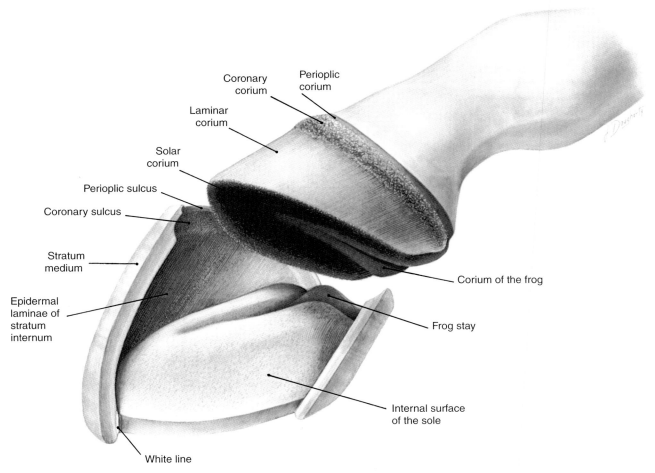

Coronary
corium

Perioplic
corium

Laminar
corium

Solar
corium

Perioplic sulcus

Coronary sulcus

Stratum
medium

Epidermal
laminae of
stratum
internum

Corium of the frog

Frog stay

Internal surface
of the sole

White line

Figure 1.4   Dissected view of relationships of the hoof to underlying regions of the corium (dermis).

lae. This proliferation forces cells distad into the wide stratum medium of the hoof wall, forming tubular and intertubular epidermis that undergoes cornification.[2] A few layers of polyhedral cells joined by desmosomes make up a region corresponding to the stratum spinosum of cutaneous epidermis. The rest of the ungual epidermis is a stratum corneum of anucleate, squamous keratinocytes. The following sequence of events in cornification of the hoof walls leads to apoptosis of keratinocytes, resulting in the dead but functional cells of the stratum corneum:[21]

1. In the stratum basale—early keratin synthesis
2. In the stratum spinosum—keratin synthesis, intermediate-filament formation, and assembly into cytoskeleton by intermediate-filament–associated proteins
3. In the stratum corneum—keratinocytes made rigid by cross-linking cell-envelope proteins; secretion of a lipid in which mature keratinocytes are embedded

Fine, proximodistal, parallel lines visible on the smooth surface of the wall are caused by the vertical orientation of the horn tubules resulting from cornifica-

tion of the ungual epidermis (Fig. 1.5). Differential growth rates from the coronary border toward the ground account for the smooth ridges parallel to the coronary border.

Most of the ungual epidermis, the horny stratum corneum, is devoid of nerve endings; it is the "insensitive" part of the foot. However, a few sensory nerve endings from nerves in the corium penetrate between cells of the stratum basale of the epidermis. In addition to many sensory nerve endings, the corium contains sympathetic motor endings to blood vessels.

Three layers make up the hoof wall: the stratum externum (stratum tectorium), stratum medium, and stratum internum (stratum lamellatum) (Fig. 1.5). The superficial stratum externum is a thin layer of horn extending distad from the periople a variable distance that decreases with age. The bulk of the wall is a stratum medium consisting of horn tubules and intertubular horn. Horn tubules are generated by the stratum basale of the coronary epidermis covering the long papillae of the coronary corium.[2] Intertubular horn is formed in between the projections. The relationship of the coronary papillae to the epidermis can be clarified by examining the coronary groove of the hoof into which the coro-

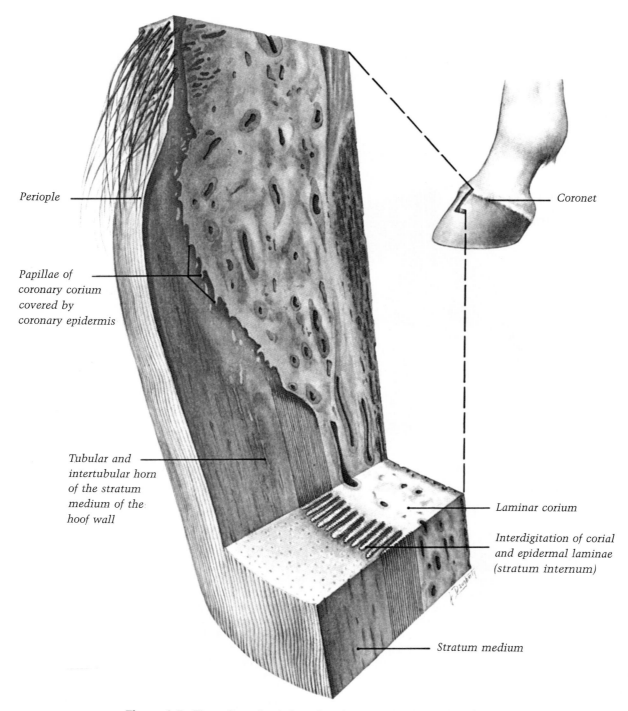

Periople

Papillae of coronary corium covered by coronary epidermis

Tubular and intertubular horn of the stratum medium of the hoof wall

Coronet

Laminar corium

Interdigitation of corial and epidermal laminae (stratum internum)

Stratum medium

Figure 1.5 Three-dimensional dissection of coronary region of the hoof wall.

nary corium fits. Fine pits that accommodate the papillae can be seen in the coronary groove.

Distal to the coronary groove, some 600 primary epidermal laminae (lamellae) of the stratum internum interleave with the primary dermal laminae of the laminar (lamellar) corium (Figs. 1.4 and 1.5). Approximately 100 microscopic secondary laminae branch at an angle from each primary lamina, further binding the hoof and co-

rium together (Fig. 1.6). Some confusion exists concerning the terms "insensitive" and "sensitive" laminae. In the strictest sense, the keratinized parts of the primary epidermal laminae are insensitive; the stratum basale, which includes all of the secondary epidermal laminae, and the laminar corium are "sensitive." The terms epidermal and dermal (or corial) are far more accurate adjectives.[47]

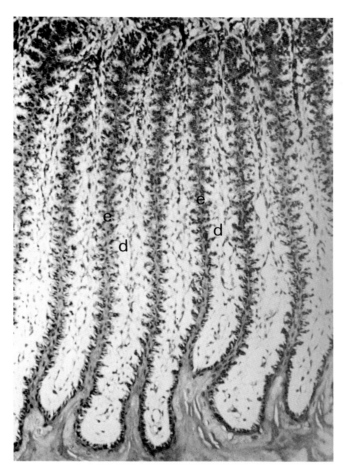

Figure 1.6 Photomicrograph of a field from a cross section of an equine fetal hoof (×40). Interdigitations of primary epidermal laminae (e) and dermal (corial) laminae (d) can be seen. Notice the small secondary laminae.

A relationship similar to that between the coronary epidermis and coronary corium exists between the perioplic epidermis and the perioplic corium at the coronary border. Softer, white horn immediately distal to the cutaneous epidermis constitutes the periople, an encircling band that expands to form the covering of the bulbs of the heels.

While the medial side of the hoof has a slightly steeper angle than the lateral side, the hoof wall should be as symmetrical as possible from side to side and from coronet to solar border. Not all otherwise normal hooves have the desired symmetry. In the normally worn wall of an unshod hoof, the toe is worn down dorsally. The concave sole should be thick enough to shed excess horn. The frog should be prominent and should clear the ground by approximately 12 mm.[15]

Growth of the hoof wall is primarily from the basal layer of the coronary epidermis toward the ground. Whereas most of the laminar epidermis nominally keratinizes minimally, primary laminae keratinize as the mass moves distad.[16] Trauma or inflammation of the region will stimulate greater keratinization, i.e., production of horn. The laminar epidermis over terminal projections of the laminar corium keratinizes more heavily, forming

pigmented horn and filling the spaces between the distal ends of the epidermal laminae. Ultrastructural studies indicate that progressive keratinization does not occur in cells of secondary epidermal laminae of the stratum internum and that, during growth of the hoof, primary epidermal laminae move past the secondary epidermal laminae by breaking desmosomes between the two cell populations.[28] Submicroscopic, peglike dermal projections increase the surface of attachment of the dermis (corium) and epidermis of the hoof.[47] This configuration and the blending of the laminar corium with the periosteum of the distal phalanx suspend and support the bone, aiding in the dissipation of concussion and the movement of blood.

The growth of the wall progresses at the rate of approximately 6 mm per month, taking from 9 to 12 months for the toe to grow out. The wall grows more slowly in a cold environment. Growth is also slower in a dry environment, when adequate moisture is not present in the wall. The hoof wall grows evenly distal to the coronary epidermis, so that the youngest portion of the wall is at the heel. Since this is the youngest part of the wall, it is also the most elastic, aiding in heel expansion during concussion.

Stratum medium may be pigmented or nonpigmented. Contrary to popular belief, pigmented hooves are no stronger than nonpigmented hooves. There is no difference in the stress-strain behavior or ultimate strength properties of pigmented and nonpigmented equine hooves.[26] It has also been demonstrated that pigmentation has no effect on fracture toughness of hoof keratin.[3] Water content of the hoof significantly affects its mechanical properties. In the natural hydration gradient in the hoof wall, the moisture content decreases from within outward, i.e., deep to superficial.[28] Very dry or extremely hydrated hoof wall is more likely to crack than normally hydrated hoof wall. A normally hydrated hoof is better able to absorb energy.[4]

The slightly concave sole should not bear weight on its ground surface except near its junction with the white line, but it bears internal weight transmitted from the solar surface of the distal phalanx through the solar corium. That portion of the sole at the angle formed by the wall and the bars is the angle of the sole. Two crura extend from the body of the sole to the angles. In the unworn, untrimmed hoof wall, insensitive laminae are seen on the internal surface as the wall extends distad to the plane of the sole (Fig. 1.3). When the wall is trimmed, the white line (white zone) of nonpigmented horn of the internal wall and pigmented horn over terminal papillae is evident where it blends with the horn of the sole. The sensitive corium is immediately internal to the white line that serves as a landmark for determining the position and angle for driving horseshoe nails.[15]

The sole's horn tubules are oriented vertically, conforming to the direction of the papillae of the solar corium. Intertubular horn binds the tubules together. The relationship of the solar epithelium to the solar corium is responsible for this configuration (Fig. 1.7). Near the ground the horn tubules curl, accounting for the self-limiting growth of the sole, and cause shedding from the superficial part. Approximately one-third of the sole is water.[45]

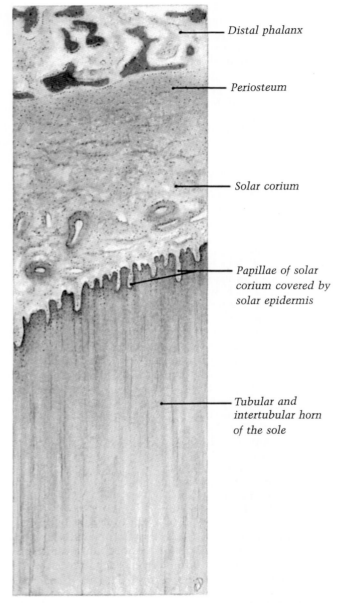

Distal phalanx

Periosteum

Solar corium

Papillae of solar
corium covered by
solar epidermis

Tubular and
intertubular horn
of the sole

Figure 1.7 Histologic relationships of periosteum, corium, and horn of the sole.

The frog (cuneus ungulae) is a wedge-shaped mass of keratinized stratified squamous epithelium, rendered softer than other parts of the hoof by a 50% water content.[45] Apocrine glands, spherical masses of tubules in the corium of the frog, extend ducts that deliver secretions to the surface of the frog.[48] The ground surface of the frog presents a dorsal apex and central sulcus enclosed by two crura. The proximally projecting frog stay contacts the digital cushion. Paracuneal (collateral) sulci separate the crura of the frog from the bars and the sole. The palmar aspect of the frog blends into the bulbs of the heels. Papillae of the corium of the frog are slightly longer than those of the solar corium.

The dense, white, fibrous connective tissue of the corium is rich in elastic fibers, highly vascular, and well

supplied with nerves. The arterial supply is from numerous branches radiating outward from the terminal arch in small canals extending from the solar (semilunar) canal in the distal phalanx, and from the dorsal and palmar branches of the distal phalanx from the digital arteries (Fig. 1.15).

The coronary and perioplic coria and the stratum basale of the coronary and perioplic epidermis constitute the coronary band. Deep to the coronary band, the subcutis is modified into the highly elastic coronary cushion. The coronary band and cushion form the bulging mass that fits into the coronary groove of the hoof. Part of the coronary venous plexus is within the coronary cushion. The plexus receives blood from the dorsal venous plexus in the laminar corium.

Where the corium is adjacent to the distal phalanx, it blends with the bone's periosteum, serving (particularly in the laminar region) to connect the hoof to the bone.

The medial and lateral cartilages of the distal phalanx (ungual cartilages) lie under the corium of the hoof and the skin, covered on their abaxial surfaces by the coronary venous plexus. Roughly rhomboid in shape, they extend proximad from each palmar process of the bone proximal to the coronary border of the hoof where they may be palpated. The cartilages are concave on their axial surfaces, convex on their abaxial surfaces, and thicker distally where they attach to the bone. Toward the heels, they curve toward one another. Each cartilage is perforated in its palmar half by several foramina for the passage of branches connecting the palmar venous plexus with the coronary venous plexus.

Five ligaments stabilize each cartilage of the distal phalanx (Figs. 1.8 and 1.10):

1. A short, prominent ligament extends from the dorsal surface of the middle phalanx to the dorsal part of the cartilage.
2. A poorly defined elastic band extends from the side of the proximal phalanx to the proximal border of the cartilage, and also detaches a branch to the digital cushion.
3. Several short fibers attach the distal part of the cartilage to the distal phalanx.
4. A ligament extends from the dorsal aspect of the cartilage to the termination of the tendon of insertion of the common digital extensor muscle. The dorsal part of each cartilage also serves as part of the distal attachment for the respective collateral ligament of the coffin joint.
5. An extension of the collateral sesamoidean ligament attaches the end of the navicular bone to the cartilage of the distal phalanx.

The ungual cartilages (cartilages of the distal phalanx) are hyaline cartilage in young horses and fibrocartilage in middle-aged animals. In older horses, the cartilages tend to ossify, forming "sidebones." Examination of parasagittal, transverse, and coronal sections of feet from different breeds of light horses has revealed the following basic structure and variations in the composition of the ungual cartilages:[9] An axial projection extends from each ungual cartilage into the substance of the digital cushion towards the axis (midline) of the foot. This fibrocartilaginous and/or fibrous connective tissue pro-

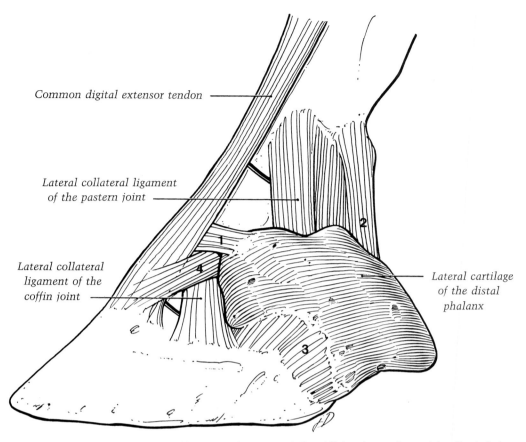

Figure 1.8   Four chondrocompedal ligaments (1, 2, 3, and 4) stabilizing the cartilage of the distal phalanx.

jection overlies the keratinized epidermis of the ipsilateral bar and attaches along the semilunar line of the distal phalanx, sending fibrous attachments to the deep digital flexor tendon and the distal sesamoid bone. From the axial projection, elastic connective tissue, bundles of collagenous fibers, or both extend toward the axis of the foot through the tissues of the digital cushion to fuse with fiber bundles from the axial projection of the contralateral ungual cartilage. In forefeet with thicker ungual cartilages, axial projections of fibrocartilage interconnect at the axis of the foot, tending to form a layer distal to the digital cushion. The palmar (plantar) aspect of the vertical part of the ungual cartilage is thinner. Ungual cartilages are thinner in the hindfeet, and axial projections do not meet and interconnect in these feet. Whereas the thickness of the ungual cartilages and number of vascular channels within the cartilage vary, proximodistal orientation of the vessels and venovenous anastomoses are common features. Sensory nerve fibers are present in association with the vessels.

The digital cushion, a highly modified subcutis, fills in between the ungual cartilages. Histologic composition of the digital cushion varies widely among individual horses and different breeds. In feet with thin ungual cartilages, the digital cushion consists mainly of adipose and elastic connective tissues; in feet with thicker ungual cartilages, it consists predominantly of fibrous connective tissue and islands of fibrocartilage or hyaline cartilage with minimal elastic connective tissue and adipose tissue.

Digital cushions in forefeet contain more fibrous connective tissue and cartilage than digital cushions in hindfeet.[9] Only a few blood vessels ramify in the digital cushion. Superficially, it contacts the corium of the frog and thus encloses the frog stay (Fig. 1.9). Dorsoproximally the digital cushion connects with the distal digital anular ligament. The apex of the wedge-shaped digital cushion is attached to the deep digital flexor tendon as the latter expands to its insertion on the semilunar line on the solar surface of the distal phalanx. The base of the digital cushion bulges into the bulbs of the heels, which are separated superficially by a central shallow groove. The structure and relationships of the digital cushion indicate its anticoncussive function.

As the deep digital flexor tendon courses to its insertion on the distal phalanx, it is bound down by the distal digital anular ligament, a sheet of deep fascia supporting the terminal part of the tendon and sweeping proximad to attach on each side of the proximal phalanx (Fig. 1.13). The tendon passes over the complementary fibrocartilage (middle scutum), a fibrocartilaginous plate extending from the proximal extremity of the palmar surface of the middle phalanx. Then the tendon gives off two secondary attachments to the distal aspect of the palmar surface of the bone (Fig. 1.10). Continuing distad toward its primary attachment on the flexor surface of the distal phalanx, the deep digital flexor tendon passes over the navicular bursa (bursa podotrochlearis manus) interposed between the tendon and the fibrocartilagi-

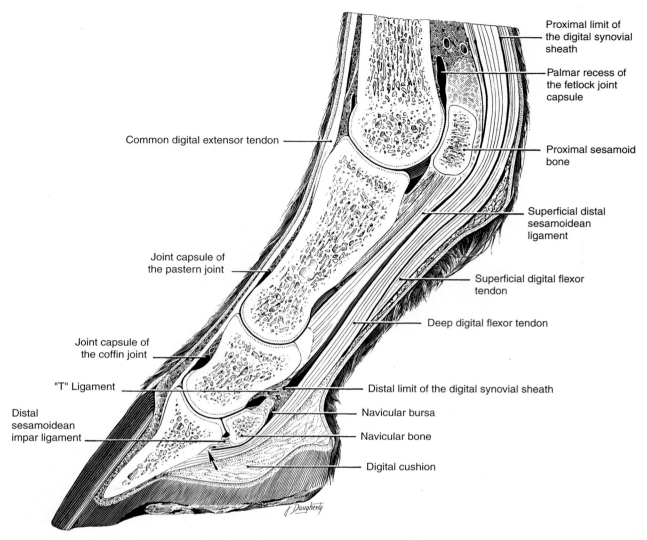

Common digital extensor tendon

Joint capsule of
the pastern joint

Joint capsule of
the coffin joint

"T" Ligament

Distal
sesamoidean
impar ligament

Proximal limit of
the digital synovial
sheath

Palmar recess of
the fetlock joint
capsule

Proximal sesamoid
bone

Superficial distal
sesamoidean
ligament

Superficial digital flexor
tendon

Deep digital flexor tendon

Distal limit of the digital synovial sheath

Navicular bursa

Navicular bone

Digital cushion

Figure 1.9   Parasagittal section of equine fetlock and digit, showing intersection of distal sesamoidean impar ligament and deep digital flexor tendon (arrow).

nous distal scutum covering the flexor surface of the na-vicular bone. Here the tendon is cushioned as its direc-tion is changed. From the exterior, the location of the navicular bursa may be approximated deep to the middle third of the frog on a plane parallel to the coronet over the quarters of the hoof wall.

The proximal border of the boat-shaped navicular bone (distal sesamoid bone) presents a groove containing foramina for the passage of small vessels and nerves. The distal border of the bone has a small, elongated facet that articulates with the distal phalanx. Several variously enlarged, foramina-containing cones lie in an elongated depression palmar to the facet (Fig. 1.11). Two concave areas on the main articular surface of the navicular bone contact the distal articular surface of the middle phalanx. The navicular bone is supported in this position by three ligaments making up the navicular suspensory appara-tus. A collateral sesamoidean (suspensory navicular) lig-ament arises from the distal end of the proximal phalanx on each side between and partially blending with the

lateral palmar ligament of the pastern joint and the ex-tensor branch of the suspensory ligament (Figs. 1.10 and 1.13). The two collateral sesamoidean ligaments sweep obliquely distad, each ligament crossing the pastern joint, attaching in a groove on the side of the middle phalanx, and then giving off a branch that joins the end of the navicular bone to the cartilage of the distal pha-lanx and the angle of the bone. Each collateral sesa-moidean ligament terminates by attaching to the proxi-mal border of the navicular bone and joining with the contralateral ligament. Distally, the navicular bone is stabilized by the distal sesamoidean impar ligament, a fibrous sheet extending from the distal border of the bone to intersect with the deep digital flexor tendon just before the tendon inserts on the flexor surface of the distal phalanx (Fig. 1.9).[8]

The distal articular surface of the middle phalanx, the articular surface of the distal phalanx, and the two articular surfaces of the navicular bone form the coffin joint, a ginglymus of limited action. Short collateral liga-

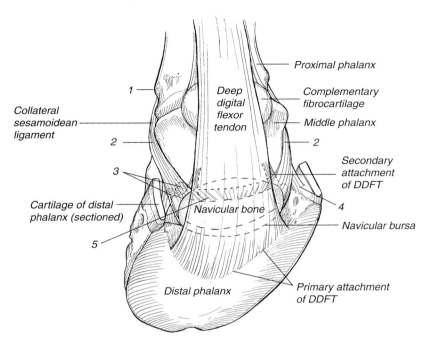

Collateral
sesamoidean
ligament

Proximal phalanx

Deep
digital
flexor
tendon

Complementary
fibrocartilage

Middle phalanx

Secondary
attachment
of DDFT

Cartilage of distal
phalanx (sectioned)

Navicular bone

Navicular bursa

Distal phalanx

Primary attachment
of DDFT

Figure 1.10   Attachments of deep digital flexor tendon (DDFT) and collateral sesamoidean ligaments (CSL). Semidiagrammatic illustration based on personal communication with Dr. R. M. Bowker, Michigan State University. (1) Attachment of CSL to proximal phalanx; (2) attachment of CSL to middle phalanx; (3) abaxial outpocketings of palmar pouch of the synovial cavity of the distal interphalangeal joint; (4) attachment of CSL to cartilage of the distal phalanx; (5) attachment of medial and lateral CSLs to navicular bone.

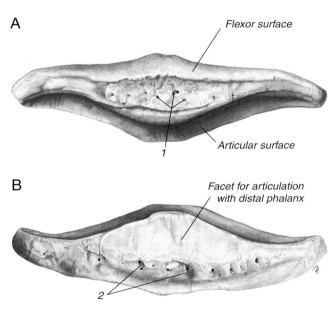

A

Flexor surface

Articular surface

B

Facet for articulation
with distal phalanx

Figure 1.11   Distal sesamoid (navicular) bone. A. Proximal view. B. Distal view. (1) foramina; (2) fossae.

ments arise from the distal end of the middle phalanx, pass distad deep to the cartilages of the distal phalanx, and terminate on either side of the extensor process and the dorsal part of each cartilage.

Examination of sagittal, parasagittal, and coronal sections of distal interphalangeal joints injected with polymer plastic has provided the following description of the joint's synovial membrane.[6] A dorsal pouch extends proximad on the dorsal surface of the middle phalanx under the common digital extensor tendon to a level near the pastern joint. The palmar extent of the synovial membrane is divided into a complex proximal palmar pouch and a distal palmar pouch. On each side, the proximal palmar pouch forms cranial and caudal abaxial compartments that wrap around the respective dorsal and palmar surfaces of the distal end of each collateral sesamoidean ligament (Figs. 1.10 and 1.12). Proximally, the cranial compartment protrudes between and around the two secondary branches of the deep digital flexor tendon. The cranial compartment is continuous with the caudal compartment around the proximal surface of the collateral sesamoidean ligament. A narrow sheet from the cranial compartment extends along the palmar surface of the middle phalanx. The caudal compartment is adjacent to a neurovascular bundle that courses toward the distal phalanx. The distal palmar pouch forms a thin extension between the articulation of the navicular bone and the distal phalanx. Distally, this pouch's synovial membrane surrounds the distal sesamoidean impar ligament on each side where the distal interphalangeal joint is closely associated with the neurovascular bundle that will enter the distal phalanx. Although a direct connection between the distal interphalangeal joint and the navicular bursa is rare, passive diffusion of injected dye and anesthetic occurs.[7]

The tendon of insertion of the common digital extensor muscle terminates on the extensor process of the distal phalanx, receiving a ligament from each cartilage of the distal phalanx as it inserts.

Pastern

Deep to the skin and superficial fascia on the palmar aspect of the pastern, the proximal digital anular ligament adheres to the superficial digital flexor tendon and extends to the medial and lateral borders of the proximal phalanx (long pastern bone). This fibrous band of deep fascia covers the superficial digital flexor as it bifurcates

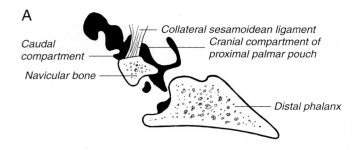

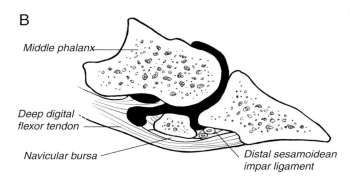

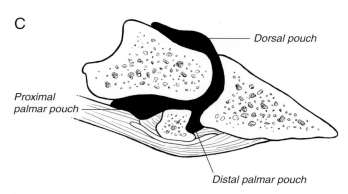

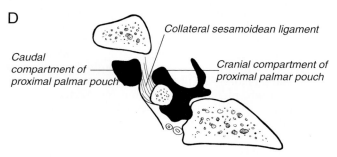

Figure 1.12 Drawings of sections of corrosion casts of polymer plastic injected into the distal interphalangeal joint. A. Superficial parasagittal section. B. Deeper parasagittal section. C. Approximate sagittal section. D. Contralateral superficial parasagittal section. (Redrawn from Bowker RM, Linder K, Van Wulfen KK, et al. An anatomical study of the distal interphalangeal joint of the adult horse: its relationship to the navicular suspensory ligaments, sensory nerves and neurovascular bundle. Equine Vet J 1997;29:126.)

and aids in binding down the deep digital flexor tendon as well.

Two distinct ligaments of the ergot diverge distodorsad from beneath the horny ergot on the palmar skin of the fetlock. Each ligament descends obliquely just under the skin superficial to the proximal digital anular ligament, the terminal branch of the superficial digital flexor tendon, and the respective digital artery and palmar digital nerve, finally widening and connecting with the distal digital anular ligament. Its dense structure and glistening surface distinguish a ligament of the ergot from a digital nerve (Fig. 1.19).

The tendon of insertion of the superficial digital flexor muscle terminates by bifurcating into two branches that insert on the distal extremity of the proximal phalanx and the proximal extremity of the middle phalanx just palmar to the collateral ligaments of the proximal interphalangeal (pastern) joint (Fig. 1.13). The tendon of insertion of the deep digital flexor muscle descends between the two branches of the superficial digital flexor tendon. A digital synovial sheath enfolds both tendons, including both branches of the superficial digital flexor tendon and continuing around the deep digital flexor tendon as far as the T ligament (Fig. 1.9). The latter is a fibrous partition attaching to the middle of the palmar surface of the middle phalanx.

Deep to the digital flexor tendons three distal sesamoidean ligaments extend distad from the bases of the two proximal sesamoid bones. The superficial straight sesamoidean ligament attaches distally to the fibrocartilaginous plate on the proximal extremity of the palmar surface of the middle phalanx; the triangular middle (oblique) sesamoidean ligament attaches distally to a rough area on the palmar surface of the proximal phalanx; and the pair of deep cruciate ligaments cross, each attaching distally to the contralateral eminence on the proximal extremity of the proximal phalanx (Fig. 1.13).

A short sesamoidean ligament extends either laterad or mediad from the dorsal aspect of the base of each proximal sesamoid bone to the palmar edge of the articular surface of the proximal phalanx (Fig. 1.13).

A ligamentous extensor branch of the suspensory ligament (interosseus medius muscle) passes from the abaxial surface of the respective proximal sesamoid bone dorsodistad obliquely across each side of the proximal phalanx to the dorsal surface where each branch joins the tendon of insertion of the common digital extensor muscle near the distal extremity of the proximal phalanx. An elongated bursa under each extensor branch is extensive enough to be considered a synovial sheath.[18]

In the dorsal aspect of the pastern, the tendon of the common digital extensor muscle inserts partially on the middorsal aspect of the proximal extremities of the proximal and middle phalanges on its way to a final insertion on the extensor process of the distal phalanx. A bursa often occurs under the common digital extensor tendon near its union with the extensor branches of the suspensory ligament. The tendon of the lateral digital extensor muscle inserts lateral to the partial insertion of the common digital extensor tendon on the proximal middorsal surface of the proximal phalanx.

The proximal interphalangeal (pastern) joint is formed by two convex areas on the distal extremity of the proximal phalanx and two shallow concave areas

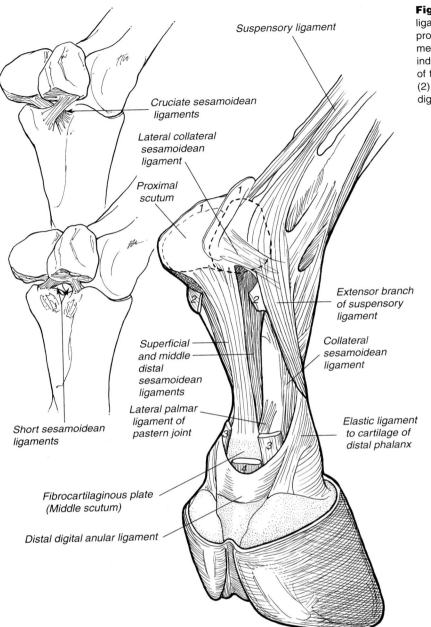

Figure 1.13   Dissections of sesamoidean ligaments. Dashed lines indicate positions of the proximal sesamoid bones embedded in the metacarpointersesamoidean ligament. Numbers indicate cut stumps of the palmar anular ligament of the fetlock (1), proximal digital anular ligament (2), superficial digital flexor tendon (3), and deep digital flexor tendon (4).

expanded by a palmar fibrocartilaginous plate (Fig. 1.13) on the proximal extremity of the middle phalanx.

Bones of the pastern joint are held together by two short collateral ligaments and four palmar ligaments. The collateral ligaments joining the distal extremity of the proximal phalanx with the proximal extremity of the middle phalanx are oriented vertically between the eminences on the bones rather than parallel to the axis of the digit. A central pair of palmar ligaments extends from the triangular rough surface on the proximal phalanx to the palmar margin of the proximal extremity of the middle phalanx; medial and lateral palmar ligaments

pass from the center of the borders of the proximal phalanx to the palmar surface of the proximal extremity of the middle phalanx. The central ligaments blend somewhat with the branches of the superficial digital flexor tendon and the straight sesamoidean ligament, and they may be difficult to discern in their entirety.

The joint capsule of the pastern joint blends with the deep surface of the common digital extensor tendon dorsally where it is accessible for arthrocentesis (Fig. 1.9). It also blends with the collateral ligaments. The palmar aspect of the capsule extends slightly proximad against the terminal branches of the superficial digital flexor tendon and the straight sesamoidean ligament, subdividing the capsule into medial and lateral pouches that are accessible for arthrocentesis.

Fetlock

The fetlock of the thoracic limb is the expanded region around the metacarpophalangeal (fetlock) joint. On the palmar aspect of the fetlock, the horny ergot is a prominent cutaneous feature. Its dermal base gives origin to the two distally diverging ligaments of the ergot.

Deep to the skin and superficial fascia, the superficial transverse metacarpal ligament (palmar anular ligament of the fetlock) binds the digital flexor tendons and their enclosing digital synovial sheath in the sesamoid groove. The palmar anular ligament fuses lightly with the superficial digital flexor tendon and blends on the palmar border of each proximal sesamoid bone with the attachment of the collateral ligament of the proximal sesamoid bone. Distally, the palmar of the fetlock blends with the proximal digital anular ligament.

The sesamoid groove is formed by the fibrocartilage of the metacarpointersesamoidean ligament covering the flexor surfaces of the proximal sesamoid bones. The groove contains the digital flexor tendons. Immediately proximal to the canal formed by the palmar anular ligament of the fetlock and the sesamoid groove, the deep digital flexor tendon penetrates through a circular opening in the superficial digital flexor tendon, the manica flexoria.

The common and lateral digital extensor tendons pass over the dorsal aspect of the fetlock joint, where a bursa is interposed between each tendon and the underlying joint. Small but common subcutaneous bursae may occur on the palmar surface of the fetlock joint and on the lateral aspect of the joint just proximal to the extensor branch of the suspensory ligament.[33]

The distal extremity of the third metacarpal bone, the proximal extremity of the proximal phalanx, the two proximal sesamoid bones, and the extensive fibrocartilaginous metacarpointersesamoidean ligament in which the proximal sesamoids are embedded form the metacarpophalangeal (fetlock) joint. A somewhat cylindrical articular surface on the third metacarpal bone is divided into unequal parts by a sagittal ridge, and this surface fits into an accommodating depression formed by the proximal phalanx, the proximal sesamoid bones, and the metacarpointersesamoidean ligament. The latter has a proximal groove into which the sagittal ridge on the third metacarpal bone fits.

Collateral ligaments of the fetlock joint extend distad from the eminence and depression on each side of the third metacarpal bone. The superficial part of each ligament attaches distally to the edge of the articular surface of the proximal phalanx; the shorter, stouter, deep part of the ligament attaches to the abaxial surface of the adjacent proximal sesamoid and the proximal phalanx.

The palmar part of the fetlock joint capsule is thicker and more voluminous than the dorsal part. A continuous bursa deep to the digital flexor tendons at the distal extremity of the third metacarpal bone lies against the thickened capsule, and may communicate with the joint cavity.[17] A palmar recess (pouch) of the fetlock joint capsule extends proximad between the third metacarpal bone and the suspensory ligament. This pouch is palpable and even visible when the joint is inflamed, distending the palmar recess with synovial fluid. The joint capsule is reinforced on each side by the collateral ligaments, and dorsally by fascia attaching to the common digital extensor tendon.

Support for the fetlock and stabilization during locomotion are rendered by its suspensory apparatus, a part of the stay apparatus. The suspensory apparatus of the fetlock includes the suspensory ligament (interosseus medius muscle) and its extensor branches to the common digital extensor tendon and the distal sesamoidean ligaments extending from the bases of the proximal sesamoid bones distal to the proximal or middle phalanges. The proximal sesamoids embedded in the metacarpointersesamoidean ligament may be thought of as being intercalated in this ligamentous continuum.

Blood Vessels of the Digit and Fetlock

ARTERIAL SUPPLY

The arterial supply to the digit and fetlock of the thoracic limb is derived principally from the medial palmar artery (common palmar digital artery II), which divides in the distal quarter of the metacarpus between the digital flexor tendons and the suspensory ligament into the medial and lateral digital arteries. An anastomotic branch from the distal deep palmar arch unites with the initial part of the lateral digital artery (palmar branch of the median artery) to form the superficial palmar arch. Branches from this arch supply the fetlock joint (Fig. 1.22). Each digital artery becomes superficial on the proximal part of the fetlock covered by superficial fascia. The artery emerges palmar to its satellite vein between the ipsilateral palmar digital nerve and its dorsal branch (Figs. 1.19 and 1.20). As each digital artery courses distad over the swelling of the fetlock, it gives off branches to the fetlock joint, digital extensor and flexor tendons, digital synovial sheath, ligaments, fascia, and skin.

At the middle of the proximal phalanx, a short artery of the proximal phalanx divides immediately into dorsal and palmar branches of the proximal phalanx. An arterial circle is formed around the proximal phalanx by anastomoses of the dorsal and palmar branches, thus providing an arterial supply to this bone and adjacent structures (Fig. 1.14). The palmar branch extends between the proximal phalanx and the digital flexor tendons and joins the contralateral vessel between the straight and oblique sesamoidean ligaments. The dorsal branch anastomoses with the contralateral vessel deep to the common digital extensor tendon.

Near the level of the proximal interphalangeal joint, a prominent bulbar artery (artery of the digital cushion) arises from each digital artery and descends to bifurcate into axial and abaxial branches. The axial branch courses to the cuneate corium toward the apex of the frog, eventually uniting with the contralateral vessel. The abaxial branch sends branches to the digital cushion, palmar part of the cuneate corium, laminar corium of the heel and bar, and palmar parts of the perioplic and coronary coria. Next, a small coronal artery detaches from the digital artery or the bulbar artery. Branches from the coronal artery supply the heel and perioplic corium, anastomosing with fine branches from the dorsal artery of the middle phalanx. A lateral trunk from the coronal artery that supplies the corium of the heel and quarter has been described,[43] but in a sequential angiographic study there was no evidence of arterial flow from the coronary corium distad to the laminar corium.[10]

The dorsal branch of the middle phalanx is detached from each digital artery just below the middle of the middle phalanx, and anastomoses with the contralateral branch deep to the common digital extensor tendon to form a coronary arterial circle (Fig. 1.14). This vascular complex supplies branches to the distal interphalangeal joint, common digital extensor tendon, perioplic and coronary coria, fascia, and skin.

The two contralateral palmar branches of the middle phalanx arise opposite the dorsal arteries. These vessels course inward parallel to the proximal border of the distal sesamoid bone in association with the palmar surface of the middle phalanx, joining to complete an arterial circle around the middle phalanx. A collateral arch projects dorsad from the conjoined vessels supplemented by small branches from the digital arteries.[22] Branches from the conjoined palmar branches of the middle phalanx supply an anastomotic proximal navicular plexus providing several small arteries to foramina along the proximal border of the distal sesamoid bone.[11,22] The bone receives approximately one-third of its blood supply from this plexus.

Within the foot opposite each extremity of the navicular bone, an artery to the dermal laminae of the heel arising from the digital artery has been noted on radiographic angiograms.[10,19] At the level of the palmar process of the distal phalanx, the digital artery detaches the dorsal branch of the distal phalanx and then continues distad to the terminal arch (Fig. 1.14). Before passing through the notch or foramen in the palmar process, the dorsal branch of the distal phalanx gives off a small artery supplying branches to the digital cushion and corium of the frog. Following passage through the notch or foramen in the palmar process, the dorsal branch of the distal phalanx bifurcates on the dorsal surface of the distal phalanx. One branch supplies the laminar corium of the heels and quarters. The other courses dorsad in the parietal sulcus of the distal phalanx to supply the laminar corium of the toe, eventually branching to join the palmar part of the marginal artery of the sole and branches of the coronal artery. The termination of the dorsal branch of the distal phalanx joins with a vessel coming through the distal phalanx from the terminal arch in the solar canal.

Immediately distal to each extremity of the distal sesamoid bone, the ipsilateral digital artery gives off one to three small arteries that supply a total of three to six branches entering the distal border of the bone adjacent to the extremity (Fig. 1.14). The lateral and medial digital arteries follow the solar grooves in the distal phalanx. Each artery detaches branches to the distal navicular plexus in the distal sesamoidean impar ligament. Six to nine distal navicular arteries from the plexus enter the distal sesamoid bone through the distal border, anastomosing to form cones in the osseous foramina. Arterioles radiating from the cones supply the distal two-thirds of the distal sesamoid bone.[22]

Microscopic examination of sections from the distal part of the distal sesamoidean impar ligament reveal loose, collagenous connective tissue septa containing vascular channels and neural networks penetrating between dense, collagenous connective tissue bundles. Arteriovenous complexes are observed within the intersection of the distal sesamoidean impar ligament and the deep digital flexor tendon. This vascular arrangement does not occur within the deep digital flexor tendon at the level of the distal scutum on the distal sesamoid bone.[8]

Each digital artery enters a solar foramen and anastomoses with the contralateral artery to form the terminal arch within the solar (semilunar) canal of the distal phalanx (Figs. 1.14 and 1.15). Branches from the terminal arch course through the bone, four or five of them emerging through middorsal foramina on the parietal surface to supply the proximal part of the laminar corium; eight to ten vessels emerge through foramina near the solar border of the bone and anastomose to form the prominent marginal artery of the sole. The latter vessel supplies the solar and cuneate coria.

The arterial network of the corium has been divided arbitrarily into three regions with independent blood supplies:

1. Dorsal coronary corium
2. Palmar part of the coronary corium and laminar corium
3. Dorsal laminar corium and solar corium[18]

Other regions are supplied by several arteries. Sequential angiographic studies indicate that blood flow within dermal laminae is from distal to proximal.[10]

Branches of the digital arteries in the hindfoot are essentially the same as in the forefoot except for the blood supply to the distal sesamoid bone. In 50% of hindfeet examined in a definitive study, the collateral arch from the plantar branches of the middle phalanx supplied the primary arteries to the proximal navicular network.[22]

DERMAL MICROCIRCULATION OF THE FOOT

A scanning electron microscopic study revealed the following vascular patterns in the dermal microcirculation of the foot, with emphasis on the distribution of arteriovenous anastomoses (Fig. 1.16).[35] Axial arteries branching from parietal arteries enter dermal laminae between pairs of axial veins. Interconnecting branches join adjacent axial arteries and proximodistally oriented abaxial arteries. Anastomosing laminar veins drain the capillary network. In addition, numerous arteriovenous anastomoses occur in the laminar circulation (Fig. 1.17), with the largest and longest located near the origins of axial arteries. Dermal papillae of the periople, coronary band, distal laminae, frog, and sole each contain a central artery and vein ensheathed by a network of fine capillaries. Arteriovenous anastomoses occur at the base of each dermal papilla and between the central artery and vein.

Two functions have been suggested for these arteriovenous anastomoses.[35] The large number of arteriovenous anastomoses in dermal laminae may prevent cold-induced tissue damage by their periodic vasodilation. This would permit warm blood to bypass the capillary bed and enter the digits quickly to maintain temperatures above the freezing point. Another proposed function

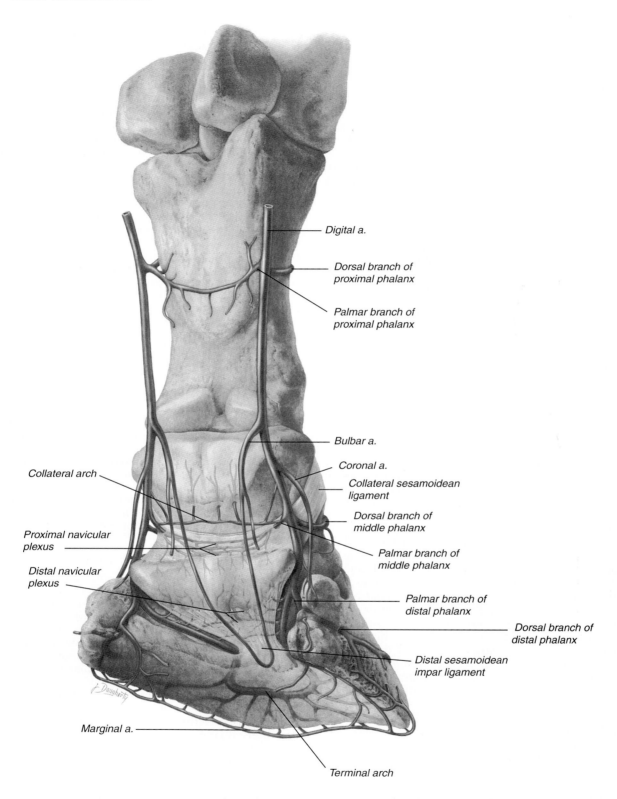

Figure 1.14 Arterial supply to digit of the forelimb with emphasis on branches supplying the distal sesamoid bone and distal phalanx.

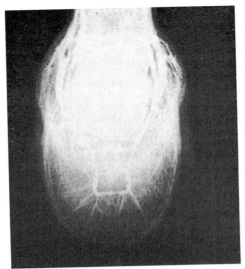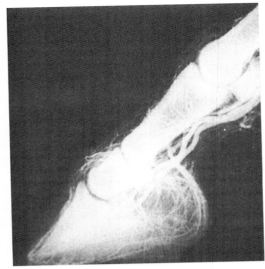

Figure 1.15   Angiograms of the foot following intra-arterial injection of radio-opaque medium into the medial palmar artery.

considers arteriovenous anastomoses safety valves that help offset the large pressure changes that occur within the hoof capsule during galloping and jumping. The possible role of arteriovenous anastomoses in the pathophysiology of laminitis is discussed in Chapter 8.

VENOUS DRAINAGE OF THE FOOT

Venous drainage from the laminar corium begins with parietal veins from the laminar circulation continuing into the parietal venous plexus and, proximally, into the coronary venous plexus. Central veins from dermal papillae in the perioplic and coronary coria drain toward the coronary venous plexus; central veins from dermal papillae in the solar and cuneate coria drain into the palmar venous plexus.

The following description is abstracted from a study of the extrinsic and intrinsic veins of the equine hoof wall.[30] Some terminology has been changed (Fig. 1.18).

Two parallel veins in the solar canal of the distal phalanx drain a deep venous network. As the parallel veins emerge from each solar foramen, the vein abaxial to the digital artery receives small satellite veins to the arterial branches supplying the proximal and distal navicular plexuses. The parallel veins come together at the level of the distal sesamoid bone to form the contralateral terminal veins. Each terminal vein joins with branches of an inner venous plexus to form a digital vein. The digital vein receives the following veins: an anastomosis with the contralateral digital vein that, in turn, receives branches from the distal sesamoid bone; the coronary vein draining the subcoronary vein and the coronary plexus; the independent superficial vein; and the large bulbar vein (palmar foot vein) carrying blood from the superficial region of the heel.

The inner venous plexus receives tributaries from the solar venous plexus, the parietal venous plexus, and occasionally from a large branch passing through each cartilage of the distal phalanx. Connecting veins from the bulbar vein join the inner venous plexus, paracuneal vein, and veins from the deep heel region.

The coronary venous plexus consists of a superficial plexus of short collecting veins of large caliber in the coronary and perioplic coria, and a deeper plexus of long collecting veins coming from the proximal laminar corium. The coronary venous plexus drains mainly into the conjoined coronary veins and their branches, the subcoronary veins, and palmarly into the independent superficial vein and bulbar vein.

The palmar venous plexus consists of a bilevel solar venous plexus and a cuneate venous plexus. The extensive solar venous plexus is drained through several potential routes: the marginal vein of the sole, branches of the bulbar vein, the paracuneal vein, and the inner venous plexus. Anastomosing veins connecting the palmar and coronary plexuses pass through foramina in each cartilage of the distal phalanx.[47]

The greater part of blood in the foot is drained by veins located in the palmar aspect of the foot. Whereas most of the veins of the foot are valveless, valves are present in the tributaries of the coronary and subcoronary veins and in the bulbar veins and their branches. Thus, the flow of blood may take different routes with the weight-bearing force essential to its proximal flow.

Nerves of the Digit and Fetlock

As they descend to the proximal swelling of the fetlock, the medial and lateral palmar nerves supply small branches to the fetlock and the flexor tendons, then continue as the medial and lateral palmar digital nerves. Each immediately gives off a dorsal branch (Figs. 1.19 and 1.20). The corresponding digital artery emerges between the dorsal branch and the palmar continuation of the nerve. The dorsal branch courses distad between the digital vein and artery. Midway down the pastern the nerve branches, the main part continuing dorsad superficial to the palmar digital vein. In approximately one-third of the cases, an intermediate branch arises from the dorsal aspect of the palmar digital nerve.[31] The dorsal and intermediate branches supply sensory and vaso-

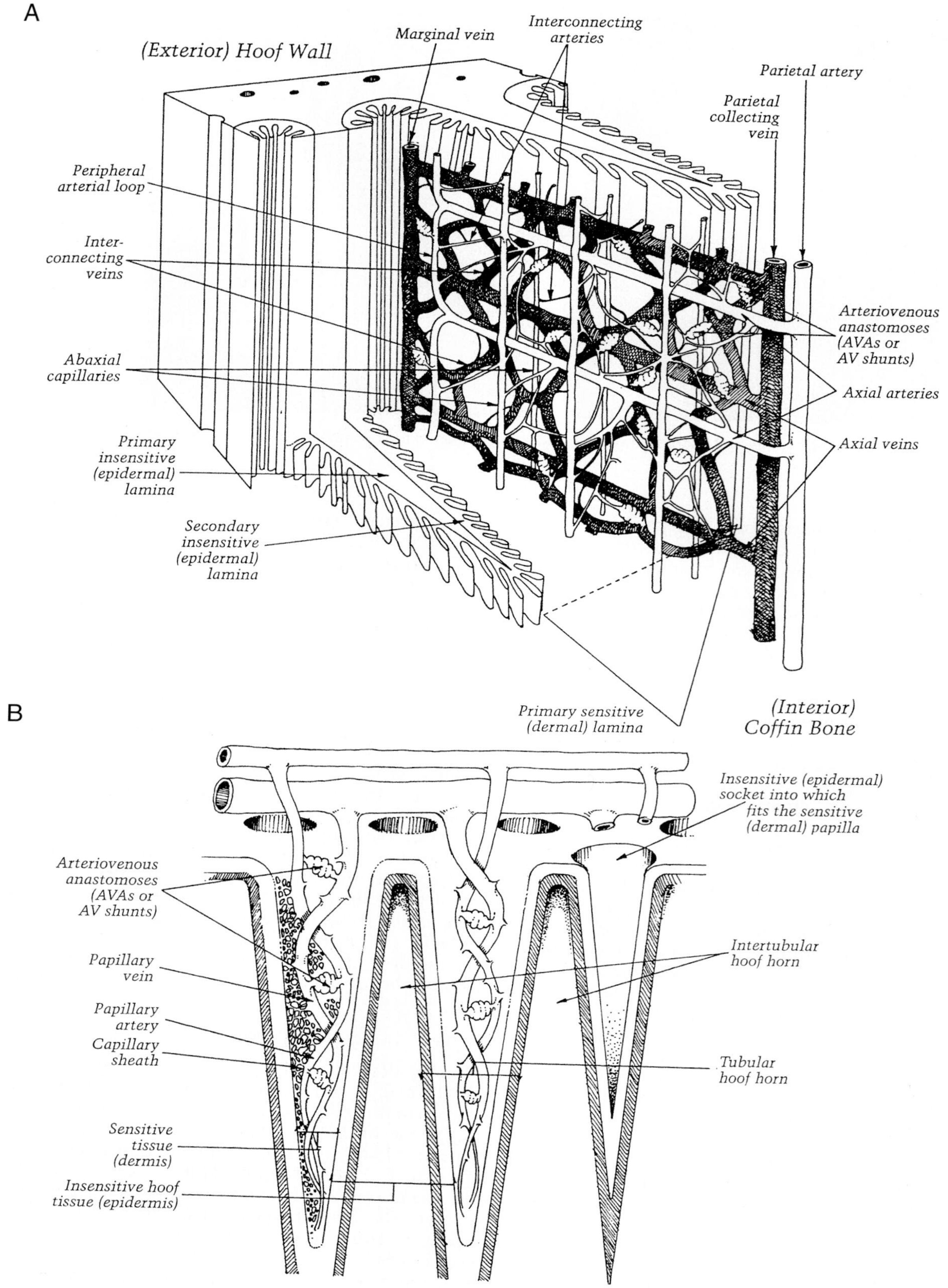

Figure 1.16 Schematic diagrams of the microcirculation of (A) digital dermal laminae and (B) digital dermal papillae. (Reprinted with permission from Pollitt CC, Molyneux GS. A scanning electron microscopical study of the dermal microcirculation of the equine foot. Equine Vet J 1990;22:79.)

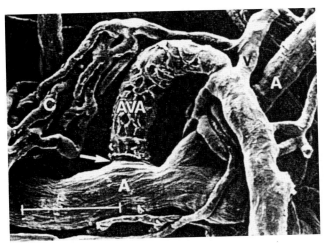

Figure 1.17 Scanning electron micrograph of a corrosion cast of laminar dermal vessels with an arteriovenous anastomosis (AVA) between an artery (A) and a vein (V). At the arterial end of the AVA there is a sphincter-like ring (arrow). A venous side arm close to the AVA leads to a venular-capillary network (C). (bar = 100 μ). (Reprinted with permission from Pollitt CC, Molyneux GS. A scanning electron microscopical study of the dermal microcirculation of the equine foot. Equine Vet J 1990;22:79.)

motor innervation to the skin of the fetlock, dorsal part of the fetlock joint, dorsal parts of the interphalangeal joints, coronary corium and dorsal parts of the laminar and solar coria, and dorsal part of the cartilage of the distal phalanx.

The main continuation of the palmar digital nerve descends palmar and parallel to the ipsilateral digital artery. The nerve and artery lie deep to the ligament of the ergot as it descends obliquely across the lateral aspect of the pastern. The ligament then passes deep to the digital vein to spread out toward its attachment on the distal digital anular ligament. A branch may arise from the lateral palmar nerve and perforate the lateral ligament of the ergot (Fig. 1.20).

The palmar continuations of the palmar digital nerves supply the fetlock joint capsule and then descend to supply the palmar structures of the digit: skin, pastern joint capsule, digital synovial sheath and flexor tendons, distal sesamoidean ligaments, coffin joint capsule, navicular bone and its ligaments, navicular bursa, palmar part of the cartilage of the distal phalanx, part of the laminar corium, coria of the sole and frog, and the digital cushion.

A fine terminal branch of each palmar nerve and an accompanying small artery constitute a neurovascular bundle that descends adjacent to the synovial membrane of the distal interphalangeal joint to enter the distal phalanx.[6]

Further cutaneous innervation of the fetlock is supplied by terminal branches of the medial cutaneous antebrachial nerve dorsomedially and the dorsal branch of

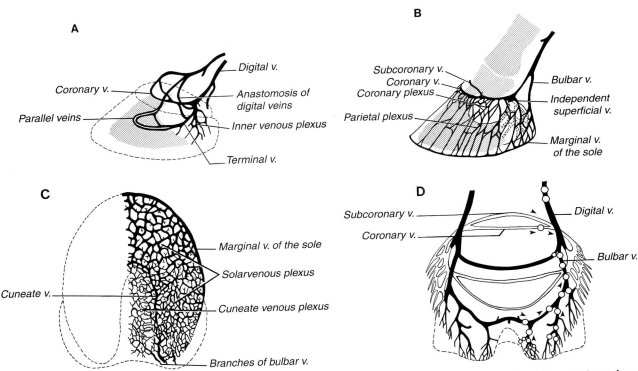

Figure 1.18 Venous drainage of the equine foot. A. Mostly deep veins. B. Major veins of the laminar corium. C. Palmar venous plexus. D. Valves in the superficial veins. Circles = valve locations. Arrowheads = direction of blood flow. (Redrawn from Mishra PC, Leach DH. Extrinsic and intrinsic veins of the equine hoof wall. J Anat 1983;136:543.)

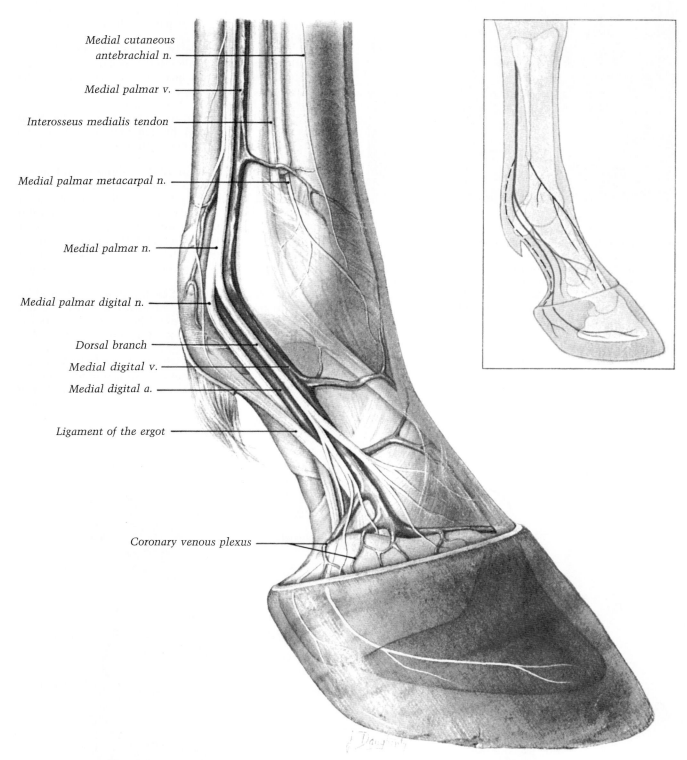

Medial cutaneous
antebrachial n.

Medial palmar v.

Interosseus medialis tendon

Medial palmar metacarpal n.

Medial palmar n.

Medial palmar digital n.

Dorsal branch

Medial digital v.

Medial digital a.

Ligament of the ergot

Coronary venous plexus

Figure 1.19 Medial aspect of distal metacarpus, fetlock, and digit. Skin and superficial fascia are removed. Inset: schematic of the distribution of major nerves indicating variant branches (dashed lines).

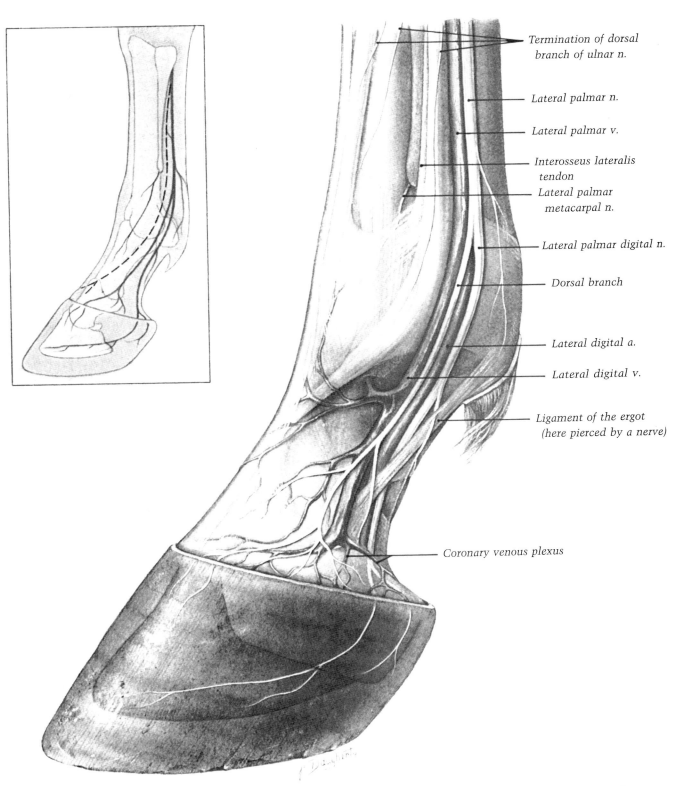

Termination of dorsal
branch of ulnar n.

Lateral palmar n.

Lateral palmar v.

Interosseus lateralis
tendon

Lateral palmar
metacarpal n.

Lateral palmar digital n.

Dorsal branch

Lateral digital a.

Lateral digital v.

Ligament of the ergot
(here pierced by a nerve)

Coronary venous plexus

Figure 1.20   Lateral aspect of distal metacarpus, fetlock, and digit. Skin and superficial fascia are removed. Inset: schematic of the distribution of major nerves indicating variant branches (dashed lines).

the ulnar nerve dorsolaterally. After supplying branches to the fetlock joint capsule, the medial and lateral palmar metacarpal nerves emerge immediately distal to the distal extremity of the respective small metacarpal bone, and ramify in the superficial fascia of the pastern. It has been reported that, in some instances, a terminal branch from the medial palmar metacarpal nerve descends to the coronary band (Fig. 1.19).[24,34] While their fields overlap, there is no communication between the palmar metacarpal nerves and the dorsal branches of the palmar digital nerves.[40] An occasional variant, a palmarly directed branch from the medial palmar nerve in the distal metacarpus, courses palmad to the medial palmar digital nerve, reaching the digital cushion (Fig. 1.19). Another variant branch may arise from the lateral palmar nerve in the proximal metacarpus, cross over the fetlock, and extend obliquely to the coronary band (Fig. 1.20).

Electrophysiologic studies confirm that stimuli on the medial half of the digit and fetlock of a forelimb are mediated by the median nerve; stimuli on the lateral half are mediated by the median and ulnar nerves.[5]

Although direct communication between the distal interphalangeal joint and the navicular bursa is rare, indirect communication via diffusion of molecules has been demonstrated.[7] Dye injected experimentally into the distal interphalangeal joint diffused into the navicular bursa and also stained the synovial coverings of the collateral sesamoidean ligaments and the distal sesamoidean impar ligament and medullary cavity of the navicular bone. Peptide immunocytochemistry and silver/gold axonal impregnation have identified sensory nerves superficially on the dorsal and palmar parts of the collateral sesamoidean ligaments, the distal sesamoidean impar ligament, and in periarticular connective tissues.[6] In consideration of these observations, it is suggested that an injection of anesthetic into the distal interphalangeal joint desensitizes not only joint surfaces but also much of the navicular suspensory apparatus, navicular bone, and proximal intramedullary portions of the distal phalanx.

Pacinian corpuscles are present within the corium of the frog and coronet.[29] They also occur in the bulbs of the heels and along each neurovascular bundle descending in the loose connective tissue across the interphalangeal joints and on to the distal phalanx.[6] The locations of these mechanoreceptors may be significant in mediating proprioception from the foot when it is in motion and as it impacts the ground.

Functions of the Digit and Fetlock

In the standing position, essentially in extension, the fetlock and digit are supported by the suspensory apparatus of the fetlock (interosseus muscle, intersesamoidean ligament, and distal sesamoidean ligaments), the digital flexor and extensor tendons, and the collateral ligaments of the joints. The forelimbs support more weight (60 to 65% of the total) than the hindlimbs, owing to the body's center of gravity being at a locus where a dorsal plane through the shoulder joint, a transverse plane through the fifteenth thoracic vertebra, and the median plane intersect.[40] On the forelimb the dorsal articular angle of the fetlock is about 140°. The angle of the toe varies widely—from 48 to 60° in one series of

measurements (Wright C, unpublished data, 1983). Medially and laterally the angle increases toward the heels, with a slightly steeper angle on the medial side. The slopes of the pastern and foot are ideally in parallel alignment.[1] This pastern-foot axis is usually the same as the slope of the shoulder.

The locomotor functions of the digit and fetlock include the flexion essential to movement, extension when the foot is off the ground, the diminution of concussion when the hoof contacts the ground, and the recovery from extension.

During flexion of the fetlock and digit, most of the movement is in the fetlock; the least amount of movement is in the pastern joint; and movement in the coffin joint is intermediate. Although the pastern joint is a ginglymus, providing only limited flexion and extension, manipulation can cause transverse flexion and some axial rotation when the joint is flexed.

Contraction of the common and lateral digital extensor muscles brings the bones and joints of the digit into alignment just before the hoof strikes the ground.

When the unshod hoof contacts the ground, the heels strike first, followed in sequence by the ground surface of the quarters and toe. After the heels strike the ground, there is a drop in force that may be attributed to the heel strike being followed by the quarters and then the toe.[38] Expansion of the heels is facilitated by the elasticity of the hoof wall, which becomes thinner from toe to heels. Most of the impact is sustained by the hoof wall, and compression of the wall creates tension on the interlocking epidermal and dermal laminae and, hence, to the periosteum of the distal phalanx. Axial compressive force is transmitted through the phalanges. The concave sole does not support much force and it is depressed slightly by the pressure of the distal phalanx, causing expansion of the quarters. The position of the bars minimizes expansion of the sole. Descent of the coffin joint occurs as the navicular bone gives in a distopalmar direction, stretching its collateral (suspensory) and distal sesamoidean impar ligaments and pushing against the navicular bursa and tendon of the deep digital flexor muscle. Forces acting on the distal phalanx are indicated in Figure 1.21. Magnitude and direction of the forces may change with limb position and loading state.[27] Concussion is further dissipated by pressure from the frog being transmitted to the digital cushion and the cartilages of the distal phalanx.

Lateral expansion of the hoof and cartilages of the distal phalanx compresses the venous plexuses of the foot, forcing blood proximad into the digital veins. The hydraulic shock absorption by the blood within the vessels augments the direct cushioning by the frog and digital cushion and the resiliency of the hoof wall.

During concussion, the four palmar ligaments of the pastern joint, the straight sesamoidean ligament, and the tendon of the deep digital flexor muscle provide the tension necessary to prevent overextension of the joint. Tension of the contracting superficial digital flexor muscle tightens against its tendon's insertions on the distal end of the proximal phalanx and proximal end of the middle phalanx, preventing the pastern joint from buckling.

The suspensory apparatus of the fetlock and the digital flexor tendons ensure that overextension of the fetlock joint, i.e., decreasing the dorsal articular angle, is

A

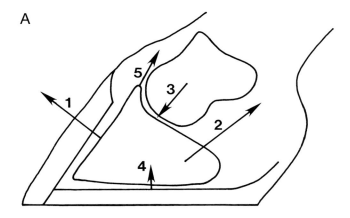

B

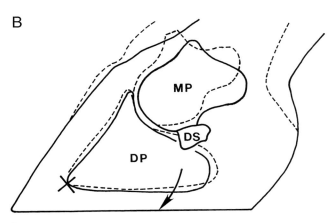

Figure 1.21   A. Diagram of forces acting on the distal phalanx. (1) Forces from laminae of wall; (2) tensile force from deep digital flexor tendon; (3) compressive force from middle phalanx; (4) compressive force from sole; (5) tensile forces from extensor branches of suspensory ligament joining the common (or long) digital extensor tendon. B. Positional changes in the middle phalanx (MP), distal phalanx (DP), distal sesamoid bone (DS), and hoof wall resulting from weight bearing. X = axis about which the distal phalanx rotates; arrow indicates direction of rotation. Dotted line = before loading; solid line = after loading. (Redrawn from Leach D. Biomechanical considerations in raising and lowering the heel. Proc Am Assoc Equine Pract 1983;33.)

minimal when the hoof strikes the ground. Yet at the gallop, when all of the horse's weight is on one forelimb momentarily, the palmar aspect of the fetlock comes very close to the ground. During this descent of the fetlock, the coffin joint is flexed by the deep digital flexor tendon.

Metacarpus

The equine metacarpus consists of the large third metacarpal (cannon) bone and the second (medial) and fourth (lateral) small metacarpal bones (splint bones) and the structures associated with them. The three-sided shaft of each small metacarpal bone is united (splinted,

if you will) on the rough side by an interosseous ligament to the large metacarpal bone. The cortex under the rounded dorsal surfaces of the metacarpal bones is thicker than the cortex under their concave palmar surfaces. Length and curvature of the shafts and the prominence of the free distal extremities ("buttons") of the small metacarpal bones are variable. The proximal extremities of the metacarpal bones articulate with the distal row of carpal bones; the second metacarpal articulates with the second and third carpals; the third metacarpal articulates with the second, third, and fourth carpals; and the fourth metacarpal articulates with the fourth carpal bone.

Dorsal Aspect

The skin, fascia, and digital extensor tendons on the dorsal aspect of the metacarpus receive their blood supply from small medial and lateral dorsal metacarpal arteries originating from the dorsal carpal rete and descending between the large metacarpal bone and the respective medial or lateral metacarpal bone. Innervation to this region is furnished by the medial cutaneous antebrachial nerve (Figs. 1.19 and 1.24) and the dorsal branch of the ulnar nerve (Figs. 1.22 and 1.27). Deep to the skin the main tendon of the common digital extensor muscle inclines proximolaterad from its central position at the fetlock across the dorsal surface of the third metacarpal bone. Proximally, the main tendon and the accompanying tendon of the radial head of the common digital extensor muscle lie lateral to the attachment of the tendon of the extensor carpi radialis muscle on the prominent metacarpal tuberosity of the third metacarpal bone (Fig. 1.24). The tendon of the lateral digital extensor muscle is lateral to the common extensor tendon, and the small radial tendon of the latter usually joins the lateral digital extensor tendon. Occasionally the radial tendon pursues an independent course to the fetlock. A strong fibrous band from the accessory carpal bone reinforces the lateral digital extensor tendon as it angles dorsad in its descent from the lateral aspect of the carpus (Fig. 1.27).

Medial and Lateral Aspects

From the medial digital vein at the fetlock, the medial palmar vein continues proximad in the subcutaneous fascia on the medial aspect of the metacarpus. In the distal half of the metacarpus, the vein is related palmarly to the medial palmar nerve (Fig. 1.19); in the proximal half, the large medial palmar (common digital) artery is palmar to the vein (Fig. 1.22). A similar relationship exists on the lateral side, except that the very small lateral palmar artery does not intervene appreciably between the satellite vein and nerve. At the middle of the metacarpus, the medial palmar nerve detaches a communicating branch that angles distolaterad in the subcutaneous fascia across the digital flexor tendons to join the lateral palmar nerve distal to the middle of the metacarpus. The medial palmar nerve does not give off cutaneous branches proximal to the communicating branch.[13] The palmar nerves supply the digital flexor tendons and the skin over them. The palmar nerves are related to the

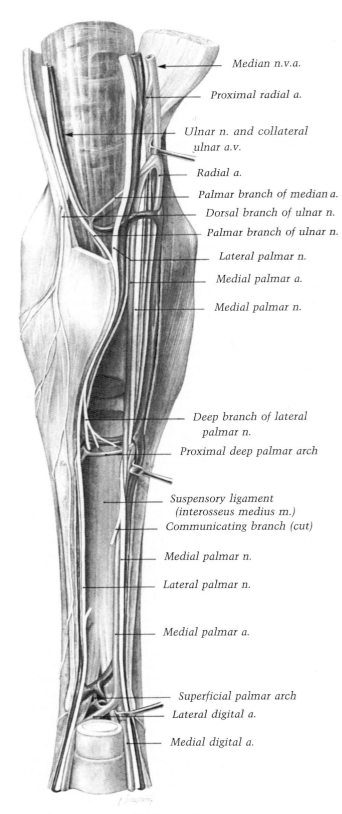

Median n.v.a.

Proximal radial a.

Ulnar n. and collateral ulnar a.v.

Radial a.

Palmar branch of median a.

Dorsal branch of ulnar n.

Palmar branch of ulnar n.

Lateral palmar n.

Medial palmar a.

Medial palmar n.

Deep branch of lateral palmar n.

Proximal deep palmar arch

Suspensory ligament (interosseus medius m.)

Communicating branch (cut)

Medial palmar n.

Lateral palmar n.

Medial palmar a.

Superficial palmar arch

Lateral digital a.

Medial digital a.

Figure 1.22 Caudal view of left carpus and metacarpus; most of the digital flexor tendons have been removed.

dorsal border of the deep digital flexor tendon and to the edges of the suspensory ligament. Branches from the dorsal branch of the ulnar nerve ramify in the fascia and skin of the lateral aspect of the metacarpus. Branches from the medial cutaneous antebrachial nerve supply the medial and dorsal skin of the metacarpus, with the large dorsal branch reaching the skin over the dorsomedial aspect of the fetlock.

Palmar Aspect

The superficial digital flexor tendon is deep to the skin and subcutaneous fascia throughout the length of the metacarpus, related superficially to the communicating nerve branch. Dorsally, it is intimately related to the fascial covering of the deep digital flexor tendon. The latter, in turn, lies against the palmar surface of the suspensory ligament (M. interosseus medius, middle or third interosseous muscle). The carpal synovial sheath extends distad to enclose both digital flexor tendons as far as the middle of the metacarpus. At this level, the deep digital flexor tendon is joined by its accessory ligament (carpal check ligament or "inferior" check ligament), the distal continuation of the palmar carpal ligament (Fig. 1.36). Two fibrous slips, the medial and lateral lumbricales muscles, originate from either side of the deep digital flexor tendon and insert under the ergot. The digital synovial sheath around the digital flexor tendons extends proximad into the distal fourth of the metacarpus (Fig. 1.9).

The metacarpal groove, formed by the palmar surface of the third metacarpal bone and the axial surfaces of the second and fourth metacarpal bones, contains the suspensory ligament and the diminutive interosseus medialis and lateralis muscles. The suspensory ligament arises from the distal row of carpal bones and the proximal end of the third metacarpal bone (Fig. 1.23). It is broad, relatively flat, and shorter than the suspensory ligament of the hindlimb. Variable amounts of striated muscle fibers within the mainly collagenous suspensory ligament are organized into two longitudinal bundles within the proximal part and body of the ligament, i.e., interosseus medius muscle.[50] The content of muscle fibers is 40% greater in the suspensory ligament of Standardbred horses than in Thoroughbred horses. In Standardbreds, the content of muscle fibers is significantly greater in the suspensory ligament of the hindlimb; in Thoroughbreds, the content is slightly greater in the forelimb ligament, but the content diminishes when Thoroughbreds are in training.[50] A central depression in the dorsal (deep) surface of the proximal part of the ligament accommodates a slight elevation of the palmar surface of the third metacarpal bone, the thicker edges of the ligament giving the appearance of a bipartite origin. In the distal fourth of the metacarpus, the suspensory ligament bifurcates into two divergent extensor branches (Fig. 1.22). Each extensor branch crosses the abaxial surface of proximal sesamoid bone and extends across the abaxial aspect of the proximal phalanx, where it contacts the origin of the ipsilateral collateral sesamoidean ligament. It continues on to join the tendon of the common digital extensor muscle on the dorsal surface of the proximal phalanx (Fig. 1.13). Two small interossei muscles originate on the respective small metacarpal bones with fine, strong tendons ending in the fascia of the fetlock.

branches to the interosseus muscles, perforates the suspensory ligament, and then divides into the medial and lateral palmar metacarpal nerves. After sending branches to the fetlock joint capsule, each palmar metacarpal nerve emerges distal to the distal extremity (the "button") of the respective small metacarpal bone to ramify in the fascia and skin of the pastern (Fig. 1.19).

The palmar metacarpal arteries originate from the proximal deep palmar arch (subcarpal arch), an anastomotic complex formed by the termination of the radial artery passing over the interosseus medialis muscle to join the smaller palmar branch of the median artery (Fig. 1.22). Part of the arch lies between the accessory ligament of the deep digital flexor tendon and the suspensory ligament; a smaller, inconstant transverse branch lies deep to the suspensory ligament on the third metacarpal bone. Another contribution to this vascular complex may be provided by a prominent branch from the medial palmar artery, which branches to anastomose with the radial artery and the medial palmar metacarpal artery (Fig. 1.23). The medial palmar metacarpal artery supplies a nutrient artery to the third metacarpal bone and then often detaches a middle palmar metacarpal artery. Small branches from the medial and lateral palmar metacarpal arteries extend through interosseous spaces to join the medial and lateral dorsal metacarpal arteries. In the distal fourth of the metacarpus, the medial and lateral palmar metacarpal arteries join to form the distal deep palmar arch. A branch from this arch to the lateral digital artery is termed the superficial palmar arch.

A single, large, palmar metacarpal vein courses proximad to join the venous deep palmar arch. The vascular patterns described above are subject to variations, but the variations are of no clinical significance.

Carpus

The carpal region includes the carpal bones (radial, intermediate, ulnar, and accessory in the proximal row; first, second, third, and fourth in the distal row), the distal extremity of the radius (and fused ulna), the proximal extremities of the three metacarpal bones, and the structures adjacent to these osseous components.

Dorsal Aspect

In the skin on the dorsal aspect of the carpus a vascular network, the rete carpi dorsale, is formed by branches from the cranial interosseus, transverse cubital, and radial arteries. Medial and lateral cutaneous antebrachial nerves supply branches to the medial and dorsal aspects of the carpus. Tendon sheaths of the extensor carpi radialis, extensor carpi obliquus (abductor digiti I longus), and the common digital extensor muscles are enclosed in fibrous passages through the deep fascia and then through the extensor retinaculum. The tendon sheaths of the common digital and oblique carpal extensor tendons extend from the carpometacarpal articulation proximad to a point 6 to 8 cm proximal to the carpus (Fig. 1.24).

A subtendinous bursa lies between the ensheathed tendon of the extensor carpi obliquus muscle and the medial collateral ligament of the carpus, facilitating the proximal excursion of the tendon during flexion.[39] In

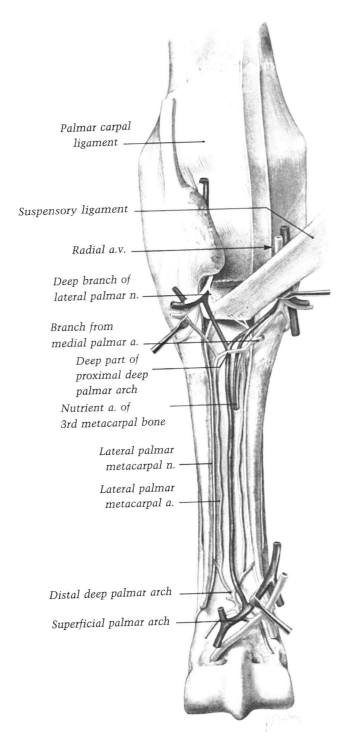

Palmar carpal ligament

Suspensory ligament

Radial a.v.

Deep branch of lateral palmar n.

Branch from medial palmar a.

Deep part of proximal deep palmar arch

Nutrient a. of 3rd metacarpal bone

Lateral palmar metacarpal n.

Lateral palmar metacarpal a.

Distal deep palmar arch

Superficial palmar arch

Figure 1.23 Deep dissection of caudal aspects of left carpus and metacarpus with the medial palmar artery removed.

Medial and lateral palmar metacarpal nerves and satellite vessels lie in the grooves formed by the third metacarpal bone with the respective small metacarpal bones (Fig. 1.23). The two nerves originate from the deep branch of the lateral palmar nerve which supplies

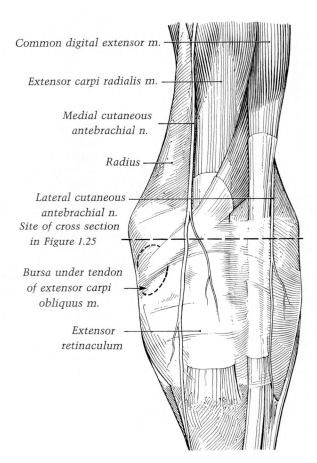

Common digital extensor m.

Extensor carpi radialis m.

Medial cutaneous
antebrachial n.

Radius

Lateral cutaneous
antebrachial n.
Site of cross section
in Figure 1.25

Bursa under tendon
of extensor carpi
obliquus m.

Extensor
retinaculum

Figure 1.24 Dorsal view of left carpus.

most colts younger than two years, the bursa is a separate synovial structure; in older horses it communicates with the adjacent tendon sheath. A small tendon from the radial head of the common digital extensor muscle occupies the same synovial sheath as the main tendon; the small tendon may angle palmarad to join the tendon of the lateral digital extensor muscle, or it may pursue a course between the main extensor tendons to the fetlock. The tendon sheath of the extensor carpi radialis muscle terminates at the middle of the carpus, and then the tendon becomes adherent to the retinaculum as it extends to its insertion on the metacarpal tuberosity.

Deeply the extensor retinaculum serves as the dorsal part of the common fibrous joint capsule of the carpal joints—the antebrachiocarpal (radiocarpal), midcarpal, intercarpal, and carpometacarpal joints (Figs. 1.25 and 1.26). The extensor retinaculum attaches to the radius, the dorsal intercarpal and dorsal carpometacarpal ligaments, the carpal bones, and the third metacarpal bone. Laterally and medially it blends with the collateral ligaments of the carpus.

Branches from the cranial interosseous artery supply the superficial structures of the lateral aspect of the carpal region. The proximal radial and lateral palmar arteries supply deeper structures. The dorsal branch of the ulnar nerve emerges between the tendon of insertion of

the flexor carpi ulnaris muscle and the short tendon of the ulnaris lateralis, or between the short and long tendons of the latter muscle (Figs. 1.22 and 1.27). As it courses distad, the nerve supplies branches to the fascia and skin of the dorsal and lateral aspects of the carpus.

Lateral Aspect

The lateral collateral carpal ligament extends distad from its attachment on the styloid process of the radius, immediately distal to the groove for the tendon of the lateral digital extensor muscle (Fig. 1.28). The superficial part of the ligament attaches distally on the fourth metacarpal bone and partly on the third metacarpal bone. A canal between the superficial part and the deep part of the ligament provides passage for the tendon of the lateral digital extensor muscle and its synovial sheath. The deep part of the ligament attaches on the ulnar carpal bone.

Palmar to the lateral collateral carpal ligament, four ligaments support the accessory carpal bone. These ligaments, named according to their attachments, are (from proximal to distal) the accessorioulnar, accessoriocarpoulnar, accessorioquartal, and accessoriometacarpal ligaments (Fig. 1.28). Tendons of two muscles are associated with the accessory carpal bone. The short tendon of the ulnaris lateralis muscle attaches to the proximal border and lateral surface of the bone; the muscle's long tendon, enclosed in a synovial sheath, passes through a groove on the bone's lateral surface and then continues distad to insert on the proximal extremity of the fourth metacarpal bone (Fig. 1.27). Proximally, a palmarolateral pouch of the antebrachiocarpal joint capsule is interposed between the long tendon of the ulnaris lateralis and the lateral styloid process of the radius. The single tendon of the flexor carpi ulnaris muscle attaches to the proximal border of the accessory carpal bone, blending palmarly with the flexor retinaculum. A fibrous band from the accessory carpal bone attaches to the lateral digital extensor tendon.

Medial Aspect

On the medial side of the carpus the skin and fascia receive blood from branches of the radial artery. Innervation is supplied by the medial cutaneous antebrachial nerve.

The medial collateral carpal ligament extends from the medial styloid process of the radius and widens distally to attach to the proximal ends of the second and third metacarpal bones. Bundles of fibers also attach to the radial, second, and third carpal bones (Fig. 1.29). Palmarly the ligament joins the flexor retinaculum. At this juncture a canal is formed that accommodates the passage of the tendon of the flexor carpi radialis muscle and its synovial sheath as the tendon pursues its course to the proximal extremity of the second metacarpal bone. The inconstant first carpal bone may be embedded in the palmar part of the medial collateral carpal ligament adjacent to the second carpal bone.

Palmar Aspect

The flexor retinaculum is a fibrous band extending from the medial collateral ligament, distal end of the

Figure 1.25 Cross section immediately proximal to left antebrachiocarpal joint.

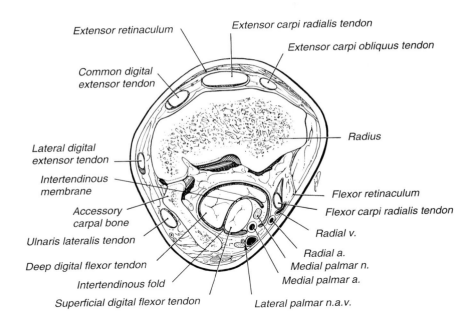

Figure 1.26 Palmaromedial view of exposed left carpal synovial sheath and relationships of major tendons and ligaments. Flexor retinaculum cut and reflected. SDFT = superficial digital flexor tendon; DDFT = deep digital flexor tendon.

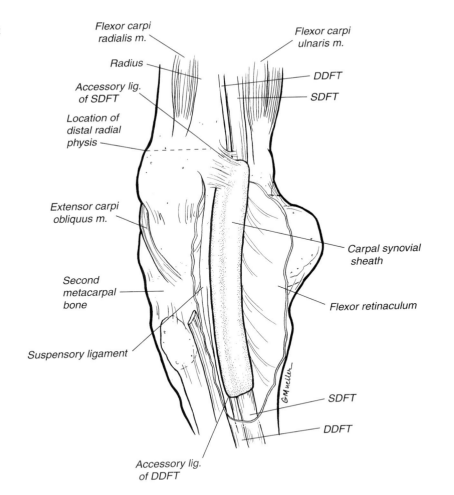

radius, radial and second carpal bones, and proximal end of the second metacarpal bone laterad to the accessory carpal bone and the accessorioquartal and accessoriometacarpal ligaments. By bridging the carpal groove, the flexor retinaculum forms the mediopalmar wall of the carpal canal. It blends proximally with the caudal antebrachial fascia; distally, with the palmar metacarpal fascia. Proximally, the fan-shaped accessory ligament (radial check or "superior" check ligament) of the superficial digital flexor tendon completes the medial wall of the carpal canal. The lateral wall is formed by the accessory carpal bone and its two distal ligaments. The palmar carpal ligament forms the smooth dorsal wall, its deep surface serving as the palmar part of the common fibrous capsule of the carpal joints. It attaches to the three palmar radiocarpal, three palmar intercarpal, and four carpometacarpal ligaments as well as the carpal bones. Distally, the palmar carpal ligament gives origin to the accessory ligament (carpal check or "inferior" check lig-

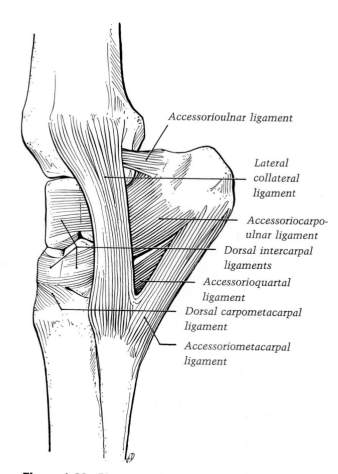

Figure 1.28   Dissection of carpal ligaments. Lateral view.

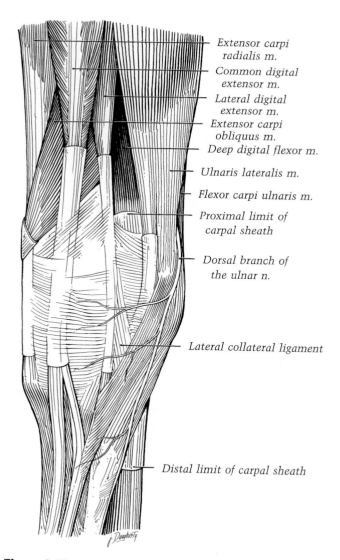

Figure 1.27   Lateral view of left distal forearm, carpus, and proximal metacarpus.

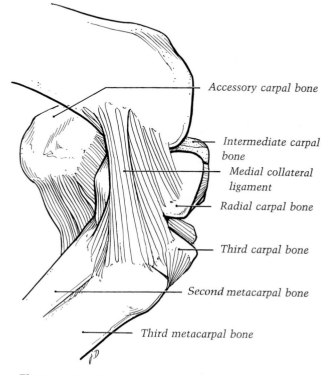

Figure 1.29   Dissection of carpal ligaments. Medial view.

ament) of the deep digital flexor tendon, which joins the tendon at approximately the middle of the metacarpus.

The carpal canal (Fig. 1.25) contains the following structures: the superficial and deep digital flexor tendons enclosed in the carpal synovial sheath; the medial palmar nerve and medial palmar (median) artery medial to the tendons; and the lateral palmar nerve, artery, and vein crossing obliquely along the medial face of the accessory carpal bone to arrive at the deep part of the flexor retinaculum. Medial to the carpal canal, the tendon of the flexor carpi radialis muscle enclosed in its tendon sheath descends to its attachment on the proximal part of the second metacarpal bone. The radial artery and vein lie palmar to the tendon embedded in the flexor retinaculum.

The carpal synovial sheath enclosing the digital flexor tendons extends from a level 8 to 10 cm proximal to the antebrachiocarpal joint distad, to near the middle of the metacarpus (Fig. 1.26). Under the caudal antebrachial fascia, fibers from the accessory ligament of the superficial digital flexor tendon blend into the medial aspect of the wide proximal end of the carpal sheath. The distal end is covered by the palmar metacarpal fascia. An intertendinous fold of the carpal sheath indents between the lateral aspects of the digital flexor tendons. At the level of the distal radial physis, an elongated aperture penetrates the fold. Between the tendons, an intertendinous membrane attaches to the palmaromedial surface of the deep digital flexor tendon and the dorsomedial surface of the superficial digital flexor tendon, dividing the carpal synovial sheath into lateral and medial compartments.[46]

In the forearm proximal to the carpus, the palmar branch of the median and collateral ulnar arteries anastomose deep to the flexor carpi ulnaris muscle to form the lateral palmar artery (Fig. 1.22). The vascular network of the deep palmar carpal region, the rete carpi palmare, is supplied by small branches from the palmar branch of the median and proximal radial arteries. The lateral palmar artery continues distad to near the proximal end of the fourth metacarpal bone, where it concurs with the radial artery in forming the proximal deep palmar (subcarpal) arch. Dorsal arches from the radial artery (also a terminal branch of the median artery) extend around the medial aspect of the carpus to contribute to the dorsal carpal rete.

Carpal Joints

The articular surface of the radius in the antebrachiocarpal (radiocarpal) joint is essentially concavoconvex craniocaudally as it opposes the reciprocal articular surfaces of the radial, intermediate, and ulnar carpal bones. Caudal facets on the radius and ulnar carpal bone articulate with the accessory carpal bone, a bone that does not bear direct weight. The distal articular surface of the proximal row of carpal bones is convexoconcave dorsopalmarly, accommodating the reciprocal surfaces of the second, third, and fourth carpal bones in the middle carpal joint. The articular surfaces in the carpometacarpal joint between the distal row of carpal bones and the second, third, and fourth metacarpal bones are more or less flattened with reciprocal facets and ridges. An inconstant, pea-sized first carpal bone may be present embedded in the distal part of the medial collateral ligament.

Intercarpal joints are plane joints between adjacent carpal bones in the same row held in place by intercarpal ligaments.

An extensive antebrachiocarpal synovial sac deep to the common fibrous joint capsule sends extensions between the carpal bones of the proximal row as far as the intercarpal ligaments permit and also encompasses the joints formed by the accessory carpal bone. A palmorolateral pouch extends from the antebrachiocarpal sac out between the long tendon of the ulnaris lateralis muscle and the lateral styloid process of the radius. The middle carpal synovial sac communicates with the small carpometacarpal sac between the third and fourth carpal bones.[18]

The antebrachiocarpal and middle carpal joints act as ginglymi. The antebrachiocarpal joint is flexed 90 to 100° and the middle carpal joint 45° by the action of the flexor carpi radialis and ulnaris lateralis muscles.[14] The joints are extended by the extensor carpi radialis and extensor carpi obliquus (abductor digiti I longus) muscles. The carpometacarpal joint is a plane joint with minimal movement. The flattened, dorsal parts of the articular areas of the carpal bones and the palmar carpal ligament uniting the palmar aspects of the carpal ones serve to prevent hyperextension of the carpal joints.

Further stability is given to the extended carpus dorsally by the tendon of the extensor carpi radialis muscle and palmarly by the tendoligamentous support of the "check ligaments" and the digital flexor tendons. The accessory (radial check) ligament (really the radial head) of the superficial digital flexor is a fan-shaped, flat, fibrous band originating on a ridge on the caudomedial aspect of the distal part of the radius. It joins the tendon of the humeral head under the proximal part of the flexor retinaculum (Fig. 1.36) and contributes to the medial wall of the carpal canal. The accessory (carpal check) ligament of the deep digital flexor continues distad from the palmar carpal ligament to join the main tendon near the middle of the metacarpus.

Antebrachium

The antebrachium (forearm) includes the radius and ulna and the muscles, vessels, nerves, and skin surrounding the bones. The prominent muscle belly of the extensor carpi radialis muscle bulges under the skin on the cranial aspect. A horny cutaneous structure, the chestnut, is present on the medial skin of the distal third of the forearm. The chestnut is considered a vestige of the first digit.

Superficial Nerves and Vessels

There is extensive overlapping among adjacent sensory cutaneous branches of the axillary, radial, musculocutaneous, and ulnar nerves in the forearm.[5] The axillary nerve detaches brachial cutaneous branches to the lateral aspect of the arm and terminates as the cranial cutaneous antebrachial nerve, crossing the insertion of the cleidobrachialis muscle and coursing distad in the fascia over the extensor carpi radialis muscle.

The lateral cutaneous antebrachial nerve is detached from the superficial branch of the radial nerve as the latter runs between the extensor carpi radialis and the lateral head of the triceps brachii (Fig. 1.33). In its subcutaneous course, the lateral cutaneous antebrachial nerve descends to supply the skin on the craniolateral distal part of the forearm. Terminal branches often course to the carpus and proximal metacarpus (Fig. 1.24).

The medial cutaneous antebrachial nerve continues laterodistad from the musculocutaneous nerve, coursing in the subcutis over the terminal part of the biceps brachii muscle and then along the deep face of the muscle's long tendon, the lacertus fibrosus, which blends with the antebrachial fascia and continues into the tendon of the extensor carpi radialis muscle. The nerve is readily palpable through the skin as it crosses the cranial edge and then the medial surface of the lacertus fibrosus, where it divides into two main branches (Fig. 1.30). The larger branch accompanies the accessory cephalic vein ascending from the rete carpi dorsale. The nerve continues distad on the dorsomedial aspect of the carpus and metacarpus to the fetlock. The smaller branch accompanies the cephalic vein as the vein continues proximad from the medial palmar vein between the flexor carpi radialis muscle and the radius and then courses obliquely across the medial surface of the radius, where the bone is subcutaneous. This branch of the nerve is sensory to the skin as far as the medial aspect of the carpus. Whereas the medial cutaneous antebrachial nerve is primarily sensory, it also supplies motor fibers to the pectoralis transversus muscle.

Ascending over the cranial edge of the pectoralis transversus, the cephalic vein gains the lateral pectoral groove between the pectoralis descendens and cleidobrachialis muscles. A small artery, the deltoid branch of the superficial cervical artery, accompanies the cephalic vein in the groove. Under cover of the cutaneus colli muscle, the cephalic vein empties into the jugular vein or occasionally into the subclavian vein. The accessory cephalic vein joins the cephalic vein after the latter detaches the median cubital vein (Fig. 1.30). The median cubital vein courses proximocaudad over the short medial attachment of the biceps brachii to the radius, and then passes over the median nerve and brachial artery to join the brachial vein in the distal fourth of the arm covered by the pectoralis ascendens (deep pectoral) muscle. Midway in its course the median cubital vein may receive a large branch emerging from between the radius and the flexor carpi radialis muscle.

The caudal cutaneous antebrachial nerve (from the ulnar nerve) emerges through the terminal part of the pectoralis transversus and ramifies in the superficial fascia on the caudal aspect of the forearm.

Fascia and Muscles

Beneath the skin and superficial antebrachial fascia (to which the pectoralis transversus muscle is attached) the thick, deep antebrachial fascia invests all of the muscles of the forearm. It provides for insertion of the tensor fasciae antebrachii muscle medially, the cleidobrachialis muscle laterally, and the biceps brachii muscle cranially by means of the lacertus fibrosus. The deep fascia merges with the periosteum on the medial surface of the radius, and attaches to the collateral ligaments and bony prominences at the elbow. Extensor muscles are invested more

tightly than the flexor muscles. An intermuscular septum extends from the deep fascia between the common and lateral digital extensors. Another septum extends between the common digital extensor and extensor carpi radialis muscles, and a third septum lies between the radial and ulnar carpal flexors.

EXTENSOR MUSCLES

Four muscles make up the extensor group of the antebrachium. The lateral digital extensor muscle lies under the deep fascia against the radius and ulna between the ulnaris lateralis caudally and the larger common digital extensor muscle belly cranially (Fig. 1.31). Whereas the lateral digital extensor originates from the radius, ulna, lateral collateral ligament of the elbow joint, and the intermuscular septum from the deep fascia, most of the common digital extensor muscle (the humeral head) originates from the radial fossa and adjacent rough area of the humerus, with additional attachments to the ulna, deep fascia, lateral aspect of the radius, and the lateral collateral ligament. A small tendon from the radial head of the muscle accompanies the main tendon as the two tendons enter the synovial sheath above the carpus.

The extensor carpi radialis is the largest of the extensor muscles of the antebrachium. It attaches proximally to the lateral epicondyle and radial fossa of the humerus along with the tendon of origin of the common digital extensor. It also attaches to the elbow joint capsule, the deep fascia, and the septum between the two muscles. The extensive tendon traversing the extensor carpi radialis blends with the deep fascia of the forearm after the fascia receives the lacertus fibrosus (long tendon of the biceps brachii muscle) (Fig. 1.30). A tendon lies across the tendon of insertion of the extensor carpi radialis. This obliquely placed tendon is that of the smallest muscle of the extensor group, the extensor carpi obliquus muscle (abductor digiti I longus), which originates on the lateral surface of the distal half of the radius. In its oblique course the muscle is at first deep to the common digital extensor. Then its tendon crosses the tendon of the extensor carpi radialis superficially. The tendon sheath of the tendon of insertion is adherent to the extensor retinaculum as the tendon angles over the carpus toward its insertion on the head of the second metacarpal bone. On the medial aspect of the carpus, the tendon and its sheath are related deeply to a bursa that usually communicates with the tendon sheath in older horses.[39]

The common digital extensor tendon, enclosed in its tendon sheath, occupies its respective groove on the distal extremity of the radius.

FLEXOR MUSCLES

The flexor carpi radialis muscle is related to the mediocaudal surface of the radius (Figs. 1.30 and 1.34), extending distad from the medial epicondyle of the humerus to the proximal extremity of the second metacarpal bone. Caudal and partially deep to the preceding muscle, the flexor carpi ulnaris muscle is formed by an ulnar head from the olecranon and a humeral head from the medial epicondyle and extends to the accessory carpal bone. The next muscle belly caudal to the flexor carpi ulnaris is that of the ulnaris lateralis muscle, which originates on the lateral epicondyle of the humerus caudal to

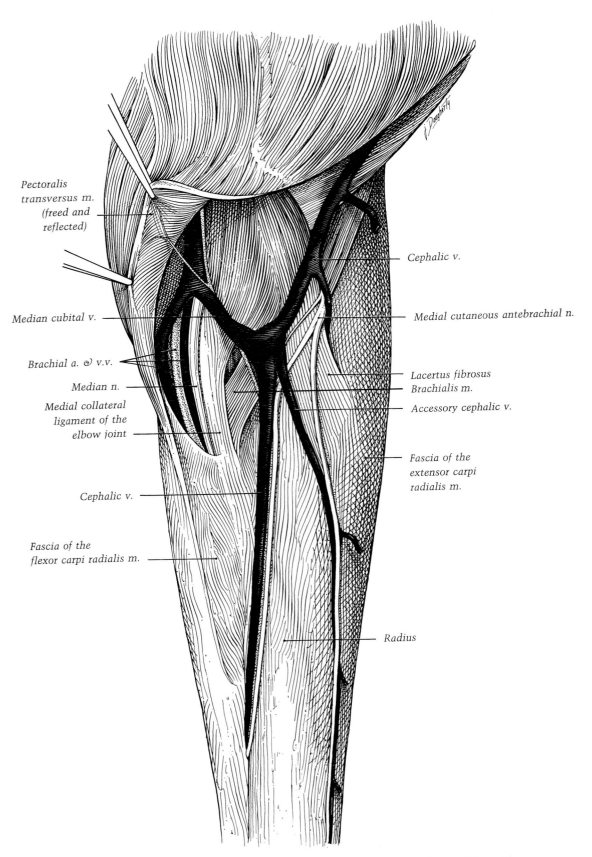

Figure 1.30 Caudomedial view of a superficial dissection of left elbow and forearm.

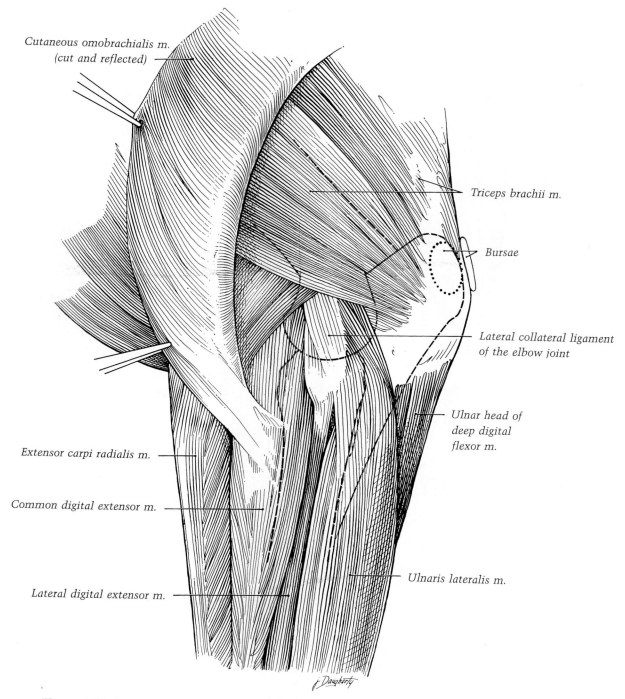

Cutaneous omobrachialis m.
(cut and reflected)

Triceps brachii m.

Bursae

Lateral collateral ligament
of the elbow joint

Ulnar head of
deep digital
flexor m.

Extensor carpi radialis m.

Common digital extensor m.

Ulnaris lateralis m.

Lateral digital extensor m.

Figure 1.31   Lateral view of left elbow. Distal extremity of humerus, proximal extremity of radius, and the ulna are indicated by dashed lines.

the lateral collateral ligament of the elbow joint. The muscle extends distad to insert on the proximal and lateral aspects of the accessory carpal bone and, by means of a longer, sheathed tendon, to the proximal end of the fourth metacarpal bone. Over the elbow joint, a synovial sheath lies deep to the first part of the muscle. The synovial sheath opens into the elbow joint cavity. The preced-

ing three muscles flex the carpal joints and extend the elbow joint, even though the ulnaris lateralis is morphologically an extensor of the carpal joint and supplied by the radial nerve.

The humeral head of the superficial digital flexor muscle originates from the medial epicondyle of the humerus and then lies deep to the ulnar head of the deep digital flexor (which is quite superficial as it originates from the medial surface of the olecranon) and the flexor carpi ulnaris. The muscle belly of the superficial digital flexor lies flat against the large, partially subdivided head of the deep digital flexor muscle. Under the proximal part of the flexor retinaculum, the tendon of the humeral head of the superficial digital flexor is joined by a flat, wide fibrous band, the accessory ligament (radial head of the muscle), which comes from its attachment on a ridge on the mediocaudal surface of the distal half of the radius (Fig. 1.36).

The long, distinct tendon of the ulnar head of the deep digital flexor muscle joins the main tendon of the large humeral head proximal to the antebrachiocarpal joint, just before the combined tendon becomes enclosed with the tendon of the superficial digital flexor in the carpal synovial sheath. When present, the tendon of the small radial head of the deep digital flexor also joins the main tendon at this level. The inconstant radial head takes origin from the middle half of the caudal surface of the radius and adjacent surface of the ulna deep to the humeral head. As the humeral head descends from its origin on the medial epicondyle of the humerus, a synovial pouch from the elbow joint capsule protrudes distad beneath the muscle.

Nerves and Deep Vessels

The deep branch of the radial nerve descends over the flexor surface of the elbow and supplies branches to the extensor muscles of the forearm and the ulnaris lateralis.

Accompanied by the collateral ulnar artery and vein, the ulnar nerve crosses the medial epicondyle of the humerus, descends obliquely distocaudad across the medial head of the triceps brachii muscle and the elbow, and then runs between the ulnar head of the flexor carpi ulnaris and the ulnar head of the deep digital flexor. The ulnar nerve gives branches to these two muscles and the superficial digital flexor. From this level the nerve pursues a distal course under the deep antebrachial fascia on the ulnar head of the deep digital flexor, and then on the superficial surface of the superficial digital flexor muscle. The ulnar nerve continues distad between the latter and the ulnaris lateralis, and finally between the ulnaris lateralis and flexor carpi ulnaris muscles as they near their insertions. Here the ulnar nerve divides into its palmar and dorsal branches.

Distal to the elbow the median nerve lies along the caudal border of the long part of the medial collateral ligament of the elbow joint. It lies against the cranial brachial vein cranial to the brachial artery (Fig. 1.30). This relationship continues distally after the brachial artery gives off the common interosseous artery and becomes the median artery. In the proximal part of the forearm, the median nerve supplies branches to the flexor carpi radialis muscle, the humeral and radial heads of the deep digital flexor muscle, and the periosteum of the radius and ulna. At about the middle of the forearm, the median nerve divides into the medial and lateral palmar nerves, which remain together in a common sheath before separating in the distal fourth of the forearm. The medial palmar nerve descends into the carpal canal; the lateral palmar nerve is joined by the palmar branch of

the ulnar nerve and descends within the flexor retinaculum (Fig. 1.22).

The common interosseous artery gives off a small caudal interosseous artery, then passes through the interosseous space, supplying nutrient arteries to the radius and ulna. The cranial interosseous artery is the main continuation of the common interosseous. Together with the transverse cubital artery, the cranial interosseous provides branches to the cranial and medial aspects of the forearm.

Distal to the origin of the common interosseous artery, the brachial artery continues as the median artery between the flexor carpi radialis muscle and the caudomedial surface of the radius. In the distal part of the forearm, the median artery angles caudad and detaches the proximal radial artery, a small vessel that courses distad on the radius to the palmar aspect of the carpus. The median artery terminates at the distal end of the forearm by bifurcating into the large medial palmar artery (common palmar digital artery II), the much smaller lateral palmar artery (palmar branch of the median artery or common palmar digital artery III), and, medially, the radial artery.

Two median veins accompany the median artery and nerve: a proximal continuation of the lateral palmar vein, which ascends caudal to the artery, and a vein formed by radicles from the caudal antebrachial muscles, which ascends cranial to the artery.

Radioulnar Relationships

The interosseous ligament of the forearm attaches the shaft of a foal's ulna to the radius distal and proximal to the interosseous space. Ossification of the ligament distal to the space occurs in the young horse, but the proximal part of the ligament persists until it becomes ossified in very old horses.[18] Proximal to the interosseous space, a radioulnar ligament extends from the borders of the ulna to the caudal aspect of the radius, stabilizing the proximal radioulnar joint.

Cubital (Elbow) Joint

Muscles adjacent to the equine cubital joint include two principal flexors: the biceps brachii and the brachialis (aided by the extensor carpi radialis and common digital extensor muscles) and three principal extensors: the tensor fasciae antebrachii, triceps brachii, and the anconeus (assisted by the flexors of the carpus and digit).

Cranially the terminal part of the biceps brachii muscle crosses the joint, its long tendon of insertion (the lacertus fibrosus) joining the deep fascia of the extensor carpi radialis and its short tendon attaching to the radial tuberosity and medial collateral ligament of the cubital joint (Fig. 1.34). The terminal part of the brachialis muscle, curving around from its location in the musculospiral groove of the humerus, passes between the biceps brachii and extensor carpi radialis muscles to attach to the medial border of the radius under the long part of the medial collateral ligament of the elbow joint (Fig. 1.30). The medial collateral ligament represents the pronator teres muscle in the horse. A bursa is situated between the tendon and the collateral ligament.[33]

Over the medial aspect of the elbow joint deep to the cranial part of the superficially located pectoralis transversus muscle, the median nerve, cranial brachial vein, brachial artery, and caudal brachial vein lie caudal to the medial collateral ligament of the elbow joint (Fig. 1.30). The short part of the collateral ligament is deep and attaches to the radial tuberosity. Proximocaudal to the joint the collateral ulnar artery and vein, the ulnar nerve, and its cutaneous branch (caudal cutaneous antebrachial nerve) cross obliquely between the medial head of the triceps brachii and tensor fasciae antebrachii muscles.

All three principal extensors of the cubital joint insert on the olecranon tuberosity of the ulna. A subcutaneous bursa may cover the caudal aspect of the olecranon tuberosity; deeply a subtendinous bursa lies under the tendon of insertion of the long head of the massive triceps brachii muscle[33] (Fig. 1.31). The medially located tensor fasciae antebrachii muscle also inserts on and acts to tense the deep antebrachial fascia. Deep to the triceps brachii the small anconeus muscle originates from the caudal surface of the humerus, covers the olecranon fossa, and attaches to the elbow joint capsule, acting to elevate it when the joint is extended.

Laterally the cubital joint is covered by the distal part of the omobrachialis muscle. A short, stout lateral collateral ligament extends from the lateral tuberosity of the radius to the lateral epicondyle of the humerus. Deep fascia covers muscular attachments, anchors to bony prominences, and attaches to the lateral collateral ligament. Bands of fascia extend deeply, blending with the cranial part of the joint capsule. Caudally the joint capsule becomes thinner as it extends into the olecranon fossa deep to adipose tissue and the anconeus muscle. The joint capsule is adherent to the anconeus muscle and tendons of surrounding muscles. Extensions of the synovial lining of the joint project distad under the origins of the ulnaris lateralis and the digital flexor muscles and into the radioulnar articulation. The cubital joint is supplied by branches from the transverse cubital artery cranially and a branch from the collateral ulnar artery caudally.

A fovea on the head and a ridge on the proximal extremity of the radius and the trochlear notch of the ulna articulate with the trochlea of the humerus, forming a ginglymus. The cranial articular angle is approximately 150° with a range of movement up to 60°. In flexion the forearm is carried laterad on account of the slightly oblique axis of movement of the elbow joint.[18]

Arm and Shoulder

The arm is the region around the humerus. The shoulder includes the shoulder joint (scapulohumeral joint) and the region around the scapula that blends dorsally into the withers. Whereas the superficial fascia of the shoulder continues around to the medial side as the subscapular fascia, the heavy deep fascia closely invests the underlying muscles and sends intermuscular septa in to attach to the spine and borders of the scapula. Within the superficial fascia over the lateral aspect of the shoulder and arm, the cutaneous omobrachialis muscle covers the deep fascia over the lateral musculature and extends as far distad as the cubital joint (Fig. 1.31). The muscle is innervated by the intercostobrachial nerve. Cutaneous sensation in this region is also mediated by brachial branches of the axillary and radial nerves. Superficial blood vessels are branches of the caudal circumflex humeral vessels.

The cleidobrachialis muscle (of the brachiocephalicus) covers the craniolateral aspect of the shoulder joint and associated structures on the way to its insertion on the deltoid tuberosity, the humeral crest, and the fascia of the arm (Fig. 1.32). When the head and neck are fixed, this muscle acts as an extensor of the shoulder joint, drawing the forelimb craniad. By means of the fascia of the arm it also acts to extend the elbow joint.

Muscles Substituting for Shoulder Joint Ligaments

Cranially the heavy, partly cartilaginous tendon of the biceps brachii muscle originates on the supraglenoid tubercle of the scapula and occupies the intertuberal groove of the humerus. A tendinous band from the pectoralis ascendens muscle extends from the lesser tubercle to the greater tubercle, serving to bind down the tendon of the biceps brachii. An intertuberal bursa lies under the tendon and extends around its sides. Fascial sheaths of the muscle attach to the humeral tubercles. A tendinous intersection extends distad through the muscle. In addition to flexing the elbow, the biceps brachii fixes the elbow and shoulder in the standing position. The musculocutaneous nerve supplies the biceps brachii. The supraspinatus muscle, which arises from the supraspinous fossa, the spine, and cartilage of the scapula, divides distally to attach to the greater and lesser tubercles of the humerus, serving with the bicipital tendon to stabilize the shoulder joint cranially.

Laterally the infraspinatus muscle extends distad from the scapular cartilage and infraspinous fossa to insert on the caudal eminence of the greater tubercle and on a triangular area on the distal part of the tubercle distal to the insertion of the supraspinatus (Fig. 1.33). The partly cartilaginous tendon is protected from the underlying caudal eminence by adipose tissue and a constant synovial bursa that may communicate with the shoulder joint cavity. The tendon is the main lateral support of the shoulder joint. It is assisted by the teres minor, a smaller, flat muscle arising from the infraspinous fossa, the caudal border, and a small tubercle on the distal extremity of the scapula and inserting proximal to and on the deltoid tuberosity (Fig. 1.33). The lateral insertion of the supraspinatus muscle also lends lateral support.

The supraspinatus muscle extends the shoulder joint; the teres minor muscle flexes the joint and, together with the infraspinatus, abducts the arm. The infraspinatus also rotates the arm laterad. The supraspinatus and infraspinatus muscles are supplied by the suprascapular nerve, which reaches the supraspinous fossa by passing out between the subscapularis and supraspinatus muscles and then going around the distal fourth of the cranial border of the scapula. The nerve continues proximocaudad into the infraspinous fossa where it ends by sending branches to the infraspinatus.

The subscapularis muscle supports the shoulder joint medially. This adductor of the arm originates in the sub-

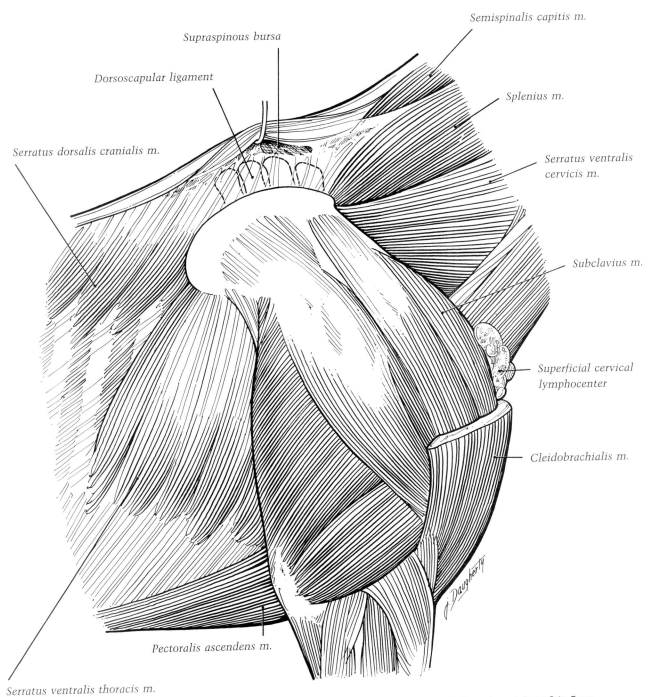

Figure 1.32 Dissection of right shoulder and dorsoscapular ligament. Spines of thoracic vertebrae 2 to 5 are outlined by dashed lines.

scapular fossa of the scapula and inserts on the caudal eminence of the lesser tubercle of the humerus. Caudal support to the joint is rendered by the long head of the triceps brachii, the only head of this muscle originating from the scapula.

Flexor Muscles of the Shoulder Joint

In addition to the long head of the triceps brachii muscle, four muscles flex the shoulder joint: laterally, the deltoideus and teres minor (which also abduct the arm); medially, the teres major and coracobrachialis (which also adduct the arm), and the latissimus dorsi. The first three muscles are innervated by branches from the axillary nerve; the coracobrachialis, by the musculocutaneous nerve; and the latissimus dorsi, by the thoracodorsal nerve.

The deltoideus muscle originates from the proximal part of the caudal border of the scapula and the scapular

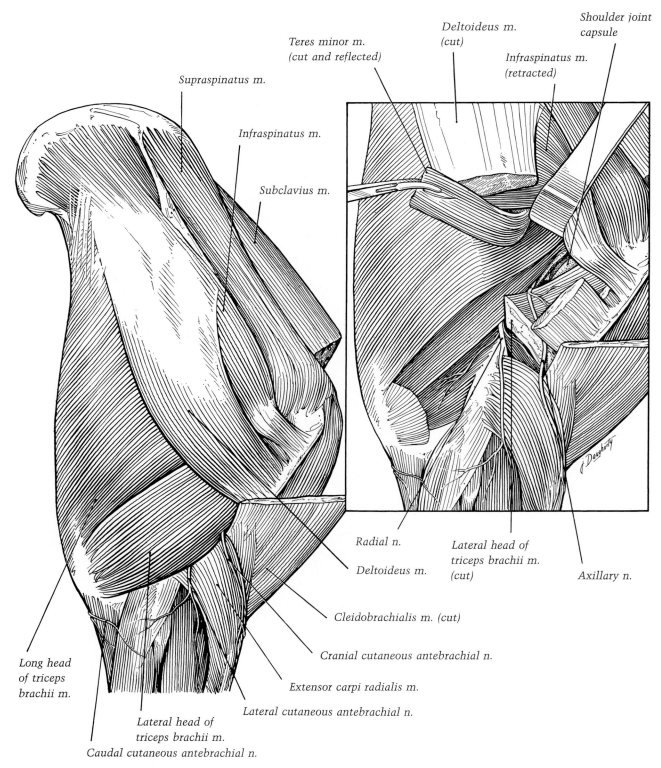

Supraspinatus m.

Teres minor m. (cut and reflected)

Deltoideus m. (cut)

Shoulder joint capsule

Infraspinatus m.

Infraspinatus m. (retracted)

Subclavius m.

Radial n.

Lateral head of triceps brachii m. (cut)

Axillary n.

Deltoideus m.

Cleidobrachialis m. (cut)

Cranial cutaneous antebrachial n.

Extensor carpi radialis m.

Lateral cutaneous antebrachial n.

Long head of triceps brachii m.

Lateral head of triceps brachii m.

Caudal cutaneous antebrachial n.

Figure 1.33   Lateral aspect of right shoulder. Inset: deeper dissection exposing shoulder joint.

spine via the aponeurosis investing the infraspinatus (Fig. 1.33). The muscle lies in a groove on the lateral surface of the triceps brachii and partly on the infraspinatus and teres minor muscles as it extends distad to attach to the deltoid tuberosity of the humerus and the brachial fascia.

The teres major muscle extends from the caudal angle and nearby caudal border of the scapula across the medial surface of the triceps brachii to the teres tuberosity of the humerus, where it inserts with the latissimus dorsi muscle (Fig. 1.34).

The coracoid process of the scapula gives origin to the coracobrachialis muscle, which crosses the medial aspect of the shoulder joint and proximal arm to attach to the humerus just proximal to the teres tuberosity and on the middle of the cranial surface of the bone. A bursa is interposed between the tendon of origin of the coracobrachialis and the tendon of insertion of the subscapularis muscle.

From the subscapular fascia adjacent to the shoulder joint the thin omohyoideus muscle ascends the neck obliquely to insert on the basihyoid bone. This muscle is not concerned with movement of the shoulder but acts to retract the hyoid bone and tongue.

Shoulder Joint

The shoulder joint may be approached surgically by freeing and retracting the cranial edge of the deltoideus muscle to visualize the underlying teres minor muscle. The tendon of insertion of the teres minor may be transected near its attachment on the humerus, and the muscle is dissected free and reflected dorsad to expose the shoulder joint (Fig. 1.33).

The fibrous part of the ample joint capsule of the shoulder joint attaches up to 2 cm away from the margins of the articular surfaces. Two elastic glenohumeral ligaments reinforce the joint capsule as they diverge from the supraglenoid tubercle to the humeral tuberosities. A very small articularis humeri muscle lies on the flexion surface of the joint capsule. The muscle extends from the caudal part of the scapula proximal to the rim of the glenoid cavity passing through the origin of the brachialis muscle to terminate on the caudal surface of the humerus just distal to the head. Innervated by the axillary nerve, the articularis humeri tenses the joint capsule during flexion of the shoulder joint.

Within the shoulder joint, the articular surface of the humeral head has approximately twice the area of the glenoid cavity of the scapula, even with the small extension afforded by the glenoid lip around the rim. The articular configuration of this spheroidal (ball-and-socket) joint and the support of the surrounding muscles give great stability to the joint. Major movements are flexion and extension. While standing, the caudal angle of the shoulder joint is 120 to 130°. The angle increases to approximately 145° in extension and decreases to 80° in flexion.[18] Muscles around the joint restrict abduction and adduction. Rotation is very limited.

Shoulder Girdle

The equine shoulder girdle is muscular and ligamentous. Component parts of the shoulder girdle connect the shoulder, arm, and forearm to the trunk, neck, and head.

MUSCLES

Beneath the skin over the scapular region the broad, triangular, flat trapezius muscle covers parts of eight underlying muscles. The cervical part of the trapezius arises by a thin aponeurosis from most of the funiculus nuchae and inserts on the scapular spine and fascia of the shoulder and arm. The muscle's ventral edge is connected closely to the omotransversarius muscle by cervical fascia. The aponeurosis of the thoracic part of the trapezius takes origin from the supraspinous ligament from the third to the tenth thoracic vertebrae, and the muscle inserts on the tuber spinae of the scapula. An aponeurosis joins the two parts of the trapezius. Innervated by the accessory nerve and dorsal branches of adjacent thoracic nerves, the trapezius muscle elevates the shoulder and draws it either craniad or caudad, depending on the activity of the cervical or thoracic parts, respectively.

Deep to the trapezius, the rhomboideus cervicis originates from the funiculus nuchae, and the rhomboideus thoracis originates from the superficial surface of the dorsal part of the dorsoscapular ligament. Both parts of the rhomboideus muscle insert on the medial side of the scapular cartilage (Fig. 1.34). A fascial sheath around the rhomboideus cervicis separates it from adjacent structures. This muscle pair is innervated by the sixth and seventh cervical nerves and dorsal branches of nerves adjacent to the rhomboideus thoracis. The rhomboideus draws the scapula dorsocraniad, and when the limb is stationary, the cervical part helps to raise the neck.

The widest muscle of the shoulder girdle, the latissimus dorsi, has roughly the shape of a right triangle with the altitude of the triangle taking origin through a broad aponeurosis from the thoracolumbar fascia. Thin at first, the muscle becomes thicker as it dips medial to the long head of the triceps brachii to converge on a flat, common tendon of insertion with the teres major muscle (Fig. 1.34). As the tendon of insertion passes to its attachment on the teres tuberosity of the humerus, it is attached lightly to the thin tendon of the cutaneus trunci muscle, passing to that muscle's insertion on the lesser tubercle of the humerus. The common tendon of the latissimus dorsi and teres major muscles also gives origin to the cranial portion of the tensor fasciae antebrachii.

From within outward, the muscles contributing most substantially to this attachment of the thoracic limb (a synsarcosis) to the trunk and neck are the serratus ventralis, the four pectoral muscles, the brachiocephalicus, and the omotransversarius. The serratus ventralis cervicis extends from the transverse processes of the last four cervical vertebrae to the cranial facies serrata on the medial surface of the scapula and adjacent scapular cartilage; the serratus ventralis thoracis converges dorsad from the lateral surfaces of the first eight or nine ribs to the caudal facies serrata of the scapula and adjacent scapular cartilage. Elastic lamellae from the ventral part of the dorsoscapular ligament are interspersed through the attachments of the serratus ventralis on the scapula (Fig. 1.34). The two parts of the muscle and the contralateral serratus ventralis form a support suspending the thorax between the thoracic limbs. When both muscles

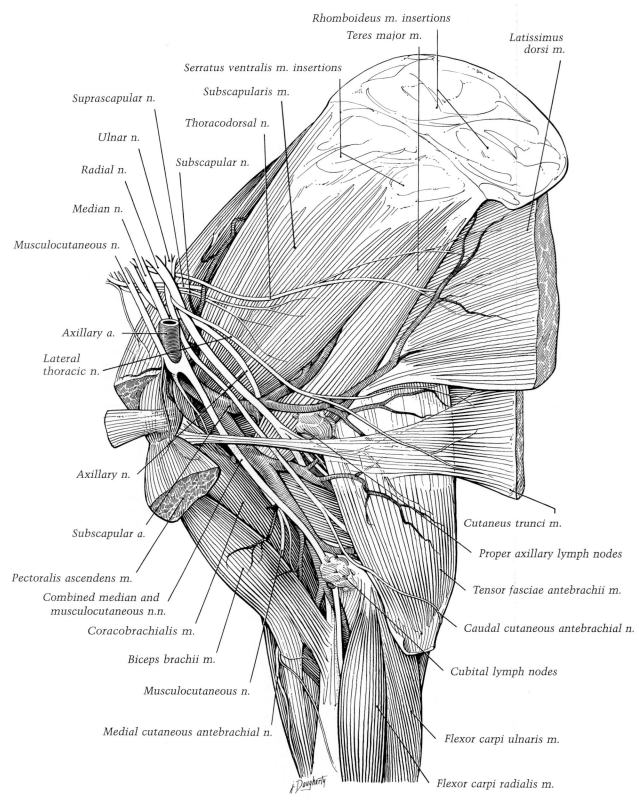

Figure 1.34   Medial dissection of left shoulder, arm, and proximal forearm. Veins excluded.

contract, they elevate the thorax; acting independently, each serratus ventralis shifts the trunk's weight to the ipsilateral limb. During locomotion the cervical part of the muscle draws the dorsal border of the scapula craniad; the thoracic part draws the scapula caudad. When the limb is fixed, the serratus cervicis extends the neck or pulls it laterad. The long thoracic nerve and branches from the fifth to the eighth cervical nerves supply the serratus ventralis muscle.

All four pectoral muscles attach to the sternum. There are two superficial pectoral muscles: 1) the pectoralis descendens muscle descends from the cartilage of the manubrium sterni to the deltoid tuberosity and the crest of the humerus and the brachial fascia, and 2) the pectoralis transversus muscle extends from the ventral part of the sternum between the first to the sixth sternebrae to the superficial fascia of the medial aspect of the antebrachium and to the humeral crest. The largest pectoral muscle, the pectoralis ascendens (deep pectoral) muscle (Fig. 1.32), ascends from its attachments (the xiphoid cartilage, the ventral part of the sternum, the fourth to ninth costal cartilages, and the abdominal tunic) to the cranial parts of the lesser and greater humeral tubercles and the tendon of origin of the coracobrachialis muscle. The band from the lesser tubercle to the greater tubercle helps to stabilize the underlying tendon of the biceps brachii muscle. The fourth pectoral muscle, the subclavius, comes from the first four costal cartilages and the cranial half of the sternum and ends in an aponeurosis over the dorsal part of the supraspinatus muscle and the scapular fascia (Figs. 1.32 and 1.33).

The superficial pectoral muscles adduct the thoracic limb and tense the antebrachial fascia. The pectoralis ascendens and subclavius also adduct the limb, and if the limb is fixed in the advanced position, they pull the trunk craniad. Cranial and caudal pectoral nerves (with musculocutaneous and intercostal nerves contributing to the cranial pectoral nerves) supply these muscles.

As has been noted, the cleidobrachialis part of the brachiocephalicus muscle extends from the tendinous clavicular intersection to the arm. The cleidomastoideus part of the muscle lies between the tendinous intersection and its attachments to the mastoid process and nuchal crest, partly overlapping the omotransversarius muscle dorsally. The omotransversarius originates from the wing of the atlas and the transverse processes of the second, third, and fourth cervical vertebrae and inserts on the humeral crest and fascia of the shoulder and arm. As it passes along the dorsal border of the brachiocephalicus on its way to the point of the shoulder, the omotransversarius covers parts of the omohyoideus, serratus ventralis cervicis, subclavius, and biceps brachii muscles. The dorsal branch of the accessory nerve passes through the cranial part of the omotransversarius and then between that muscle and the trapezius.

DORSOSCAPULAR LIGAMENT

Further attachment of the shoulder to the trunk is afforded by a thickened, superficial lamina of the thoracolumbar fascia, the dorsoscapular ligament. It consists of two histologically distinct parts.[17] A collagenous part attaches to the third, fourth, and fifth thoracic spines under the flattened part of the nuchal ligament subjacent

to the supraspinous bursa. This part of the dorsoscapular ligament passes ventrad, ultimately attaching to the medial surface of the rhomboideus thoracis muscle. As it curves laterad under the muscle, the collagenous part changes to an elastic part. A horizontal lamina of the elastic part forms the ventral sheath of the rhomboideus thoracis muscle. Several vertical laminae project from the ventral aspect of the horizontal lamina, surrounding bundles of the serratus ventralis muscle that insert on the scapula (Fig. 1.35).

In this region, three other laminae detach from the thoracolumbar fascia. A superficial lamina gives origin to the splenius and serratus dorsalis cranialis muscles; an intermediate lamina passes between the iliocostalis thoracis and longissimus thoracis muscles; a deep lamina passes between the longissimus thoracis and spinalis thoracis muscles to attach to the transverse processes of the first several thoracic vertebrae. The semispinalis capitis muscle attaches to the deep lamina. Exudate spreading from septic supraspinous bursitis would be contained by an intact dorsoscapular ligament until the infection would possibly penetrate the ligament and invade deeper structures.

Nerves and Vessels

The medial aspect of the arm and shoulder contains the large vessels and nerves supplying the thoracic limb (Fig. 1.34). Suprascapular vessels accompany the suprascapular nerve, passing laterad between the cranial edges of the subscapularis and suprascapularis muscles. A fibrous connective tissue band covers the nerve as it passes around the cranial border of the scapula. The median nerve descends medial to the axillary artery, forming an axillary loop distal to the artery by uniting with a large detachment from the musculocutaneous nerve. Proximal branches from the musculocutaneous nerve supply the coracobrachialis and biceps brachii muscles. Distal to the axillary loop, the median and musculocutaneous nerves are contained in a common sheath. They swing craniad and course distad cranial to the brachial vein and medial to the brachial artery. In the middle of the arm the musculocutaneous nerve divides into a distal branch supplying the brachialis muscle and the medial cutaneous antebrachial nerve that spirals around the biceps brachii to that muscle's lacertus fibrosus. The median nerve crosses back over the brachial artery and descends caudal to it.

The axillary nerve traverses the medial surface of the subscapularis muscle and, together with the large subscapular vessels (from the axillary vessels), the nerve passes laterad between the subscapularis and teres major muscles. As the axillary nerve continues its course, it is accompanied by the caudal circumflex humeral artery, a branch of the subscapular artery.

Two nerves in this region course caudad more or less parallel to one another: the thoracodorsal nerve to the latissimus dorsi muscle, and the lateral thoracic nerve, which distributes branches to the cutaneous muscles and skin. Thoracodorsal vessels from the subscapular vessels follow the thoracodorsal nerve. A prominent superficial thoracic vein and smaller satellite artery from the thoracodorsal vessels accompany the lateral thoracic nerve.

A

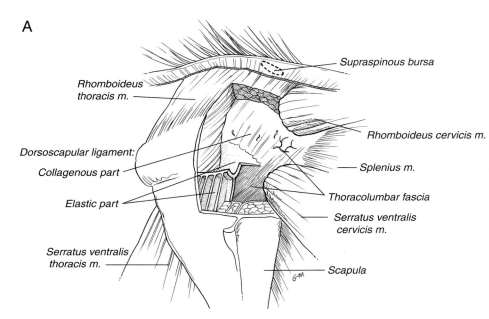

Rhomboideus thoracis m.

Dorsoscapular ligament:

Collagenous part

Elastic part

Serratus ventralis thoracis m.

Supraspinous bursa

Rhomboideus cervicis m.

Splenius m.

Thoracolumbar fascia

Serratus ventralis cervicis m.

Scapula

Figure 1.35 A. Craniolateral view of dorsoscapular ligament. The elastic part is associated with the rhomboideus thoracis and serratus ventralis muscles. B. Cross section of right dorsoscapular ligament. Notice the proximity of the ligament to the supraspinous bursa and the blending of the collagenous part of the ligament with the thoracolumbar fascia. (Reprinted with permission from Garrett PD. Anatomy of the dorsoscapular ligaments of horses. J Am Vet Assoc 1990;196:446.)

B

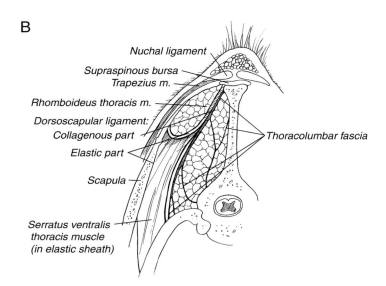

Nuchal ligament

Supraspinous bursa
Trapezius m.

Rhomboideus thoracis m.

Dorsoscapular ligament:
Collagenous part

Elastic part

Scapula

Serratus ventralis thoracis muscle (in elastic sheath)

Thoracolumbar fascia

The large radial nerve and smaller ulnar nerve descend distocaudad close to each other medial to the subscapular artery, then lateral to the external thoracic vein, and finally caudal to the brachial vein. After supplying a branch to the tensor fasciae antebrachii muscle, the radial nerve plunges laterad between the teres major and medial and long heads of the triceps brachii muscle to the musculospiral groove of the humerus, lying against the caudal aspect of the brachialis muscle. In the groove it gives off lateral cutaneous branches to the caudodistal aspect of the arm, and then supplies branches to the triceps brachii and anconeus muscles. Just proximal to the flexor surface of the elbow joint, the radial nerve divides into deep and superficial branches. The deep branch divides into branches supplying the ulnaris lateralis muscle and the extensor muscles of the carpus and digit. The superficial branch courses laterad between the lateral head of the triceps brachii and the extensor carpi radialis muscles accompanied by the transverse cubital artery. The lateral cutaneous antebrachial nerve is detached and courses through the distal edge of the lateral head of the triceps brachii to supply sensory innervation to the fascia and skin of the lateral aspect of the forearm (Fig. 1.33).

Leaving its position between the axillary artery and vein adjacent to the radial nerve, the ulnar nerve crosses the vein and angles caudodistad to the middle of the arm. At the cranial edge of the tensor fasciae antebrachii muscle, the ulnar nerve detaches the caudal cutaneous antebrachial nerve that courses caudodistad across the medial surface of the muscle (Fig. 1.34). The main trunk of the ulnar nerve continues its course by passing between the tensor fasciae antebrachii and the medial head of the triceps brachii accompanied by the collateral ulnar vessels. The nerve and vessels then cross the medial epicondyle of the humerus.

The short axillary vessels give off four branches: the suprascapular, external thoracic, subscapular, and cranial circumflex humeral vessels. The origin and distribution of the external thoracic vessels are most variable. They may arise from vessels adjacent to the axillary vessels. Branches of the subscapular vessels are the thoracodorsal, caudal circumflex humeral, and circumflex scapular vessels. A lateral branch of the circumflex scapular artery gives off the nutrient artery of the scapula.

After giving off the cranial circumflex humeral vessels, the axillary vessels continue as the brachial artery and vein. As they descend the arm they detach the deep brachial vessels caudally and then, on opposite sides, the collateral ulnar vessels caudally and the bicipital vessels cranially (Fig. 1.34). The transverse cubital vessels are given off cranially and pass distolateral under the biceps brachii and brachialis muscles to the cranial aspect of the cubital joint. The nutrient artery of the humerus may come from the first part of the collateral ulnar artery, or it may arise from the brachial artery.

Blood is supplied to the medial and cranial muscles of the shoulder by branches from the costocervical trunk, deep cervical artery, and superficial cervical artery. The latter vessel sends a prescapular branch through the superficial cervical lymphocenter and a deltoid branch that courses across the subclavius muscle to course eventually in the lateral pectoral groove with the cephalic vein.

Lymphatic Drainage

Cubital and proper axillary lymph nodes and the axillary lymph nodes of the first rib make up the axillary lymphocenter.

Lymphatic vessels from structures distal to the elbow are afferent to the cubital lymph nodes, a group of several small nodes of varying sizes located just proximal to the cubital joint, medial to the brachial vessels and median nerve, caudal to the biceps brachii, and cranial to the tensor fasciae antebrachii muscle (Fig. 1.34). Efferent vessels from the cubital lymph nodes end as afferent vessels to the proper axillary lymph nodes, an aggregate of many small lymph nodes on the medial surface of the teres major muscle adjacent to the origin of the subscapular artery. Other lymphatic vessels afferent to the proper axillary lymph nodes come from the muscles of the arm and shoulder and from the skin over this region, and from the adjacent ventrolateral trunk. Efferent vessels from the proper axillary lymph nodes carry lymph to the several small axillary lymph nodes of the first rib. From these nodes efferents go to the nearby caudal deep cervical lymph nodes.

Lymphatic vessels from the skin of the entire thoracic limb, neck, and dorsolateral trunk, several muscles of the shoulder, arm, and forearm, and the phalangeal, carpal, and shoulder joints are afferent to the lymph nodes of the superficial cervical lymphocenter on the cranial border of the subclavius muscle (Fig. 1.32), complementing the lymphatic drainage afforded by the numerous lymph nodes of the three groups making up the axillary lymphocenter. Efferent lymphatic vessels from the superficial cervical lymph nodes terminate in the caudal deep cervical lymph nodes or by entering the common jugular vein.[18]

Stay Apparatus of the Thoracic Limb

In the standing position, interacting muscles, tendons, and ligaments making up the stay apparatus of the thoracic limb fix the alignment of the bones of the manus, suspend the fetlock, lock the carpus, and stabilize the elbow and shoulder joints. This complex of structures functions almost entirely as a passive, automatic, force-resisting system.[38] It permits the horse to stand (and sleep) with a minimum of muscular activity. The following paragraphs detail the functional structures of the stay apparatus (Fig. 1.36).

The four palmar ligaments stretched tightly across the pastern joint, the straight distal sesamoidean ligament attached to the complementary cartilage of the middle phalanx, and the deep digital flexor tendon stabilize the pastern joint and prevent its overextension. Under tension in the standing position, the superficial digital flexor tendon forestalls flexion by exerting palmar force on the joint.

The suspensory apparatus of the fetlock is a ligamentous continuum extending from the proximal end of the third metacarpal bone to the proximal and middle phalanges. It consists of the suspensory ligament (M. interosseus medius), metacarpointersesamoidean ligament and the embedded proximal sesamoid bones, and the distal sesamoidean ligaments. The superficial and deep digital flexor tendons and their accessory (check) ligaments act as a functional unit because of the intimate fascial binding of the tendons.[38] They assist the suspensory apparatus of the fetlock in suspending the fetlock and preventing excessive overextension of the metacarpophalangeal joint and collapse of the fetlock during weight bearing, especially on impact.[12] Disruption of the suspensory ligament alters its support of the fetlock, resulting in sinking or hyperextension of the fetlock.[50] The dorsally positioned common digital extensor tendon contributes to stabilizing the fetlock and digit.

Stabilization of the carpus is provided by the configuration of the joint surfaces of the carpal bones, the palmar carpal ligament, and the collateral ligaments. Palmarly, the digital flexor tendons bridging the carpus in the carpal canal between their respective accessory ligaments and, dorsally, the extensor tendons, principally the extensor carpi radialis tendon attaching to the metacarpal tuberosity, lend further stability to the carpus.

A certain amount of muscle tone prevails in all "resting" muscles of the limb. The superficial and deep digital flexor muscles apparently serve as prestiffeners and dampers throughout the support phase, being most significant during loading of the limb.[38] Tension exerted by the long head of the triceps brachii muscle is essential to prevention of flexion of the cubital joint and collapse of the forelimb.[36] Flexion of the cubital joint is further limited by the muscle belly and fibrous components of the superficial digital flexor muscle descending from its attachment of the medial epicondyle of the humerus.[12] Collateral ligaments and the radial tendon of the biceps brachii muscle help stabilize the cubital joint.

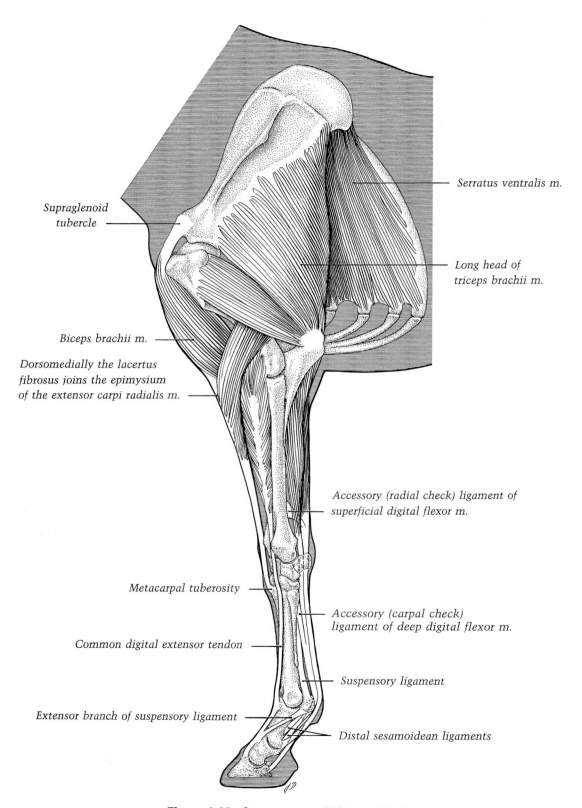

Supraglenoid
tubercle

Biceps brachii m.

Dorsomedially the lacertus
fibrosus joins the epimysium
of the extensor carpi radialis m.

Metacarpal tuberosity

Common digital extensor tendon

Extensor branch of suspensory ligament

Serratus ventralis m.

Long head of
triceps brachii m.

Accessory (radial check) ligament of
superficial digital flexor m.

Accessory (carpal check)
ligament of deep digital flexor m.

Suspensory ligament

Distal sesamoidean ligaments

Figure 1.36   Stay apparatus of left thoracic limb.

A tendinous continuum extending from the supraglenoid tubercle to the metacarpal tuberosity is formed by the main tendon of the biceps brachii muscle and its superficial tendon (lacertus fibrosus), which joins the tendon of the extensor carpi radialis muscle. This complex prevents flexion of the shoulder joint caused by the weight of the trunk via the scapular attachments of the serratus ventralis muscle and the dorsoscapular ligament. Additionally, the tendon of the extensor carpi radialis opposes flexion of the carpus.

Growth Plate (Physeal) Closure

Several investigators have reported on closure times for the growth plates (physes or epiphyseal cartilages) of the bones in equine limbs.[18] Table 1.1 summarizes the ranges of reported closure times based on examination of radiographs and gross and microscopic specimens.

PELVIC LIMB

Digit and Fetlock

The hindfoot is somewhat smaller than the forefoot, reflecting the shape of the contained distal phalanx. The plantar processes of this bone are closer together and not as well developed; the plantar surface is more concave. It has been commonly reported that, compared to the forehoof, the angle of the toe of the hindhoof is slightly greater, in one study ranging from 52 to 62° with an average 55.4° (Wright C, unpublished data, 1983). To achieve parallelism between the dorsal surface of the hoof wall and the dorsal surface of the pastern in the hind digits of most horses, it is recommended that the hooves be trimmed between 53 and 57°.[1] Within the hind pastern, the middle phalanx is narrower and longer and the proximal phalanx somewhat shorter than their counterparts in the thoracic limb (Fig. 1.37).

The long digital extensor muscle's tendon attaches to the dorsal surfaces of the proximal and middle phalanges and the extensor process of the distal phalanx, but the tendon of the lateral digital extensor usually does not attach to the proximal phalanx as it does in the thoracic

Table 1.1 RANGES OF GROWTH PLATE (PHYSEAL) CLOSURE TIMES IN EQUINE THORACIC LIMBS[18]

Scapula		Third metacarpal bone	
Proximal*	36 + mo.	Proximal	Before birth
Distal	9–18 mos.	Distal	6–18 mos.
Humerus		Proximal phalanx	
Proximal	26–42 mos.	Proximal	6–15 mos.
Distal	11–34 mos.	Distal	Before birth to 1 mo.
Radius		Middle phalanx	
Proximal	11–25 mos.	Proximal	6–15 mos.
Distal	22–42 mos.	Distal	Before birth to 1 wk.
Ulna		Distal phalanx	
Proximal	27–42 mos.	Proximal	Before birth
Distal	2–12 mos. (some up to 4 yrs.)		

* Ossification center

limb. Digital flexor tendons, tendon sheaths, and bursae of the hind digit are not remarkably different. The suspensory apparatus of the fetlock and the configuration of the fetlock (metatarsophalangeal) joint are much the same as in the thoracic limb, except that the dorsal articular angle of the fetlock is approximately 5° greater at 145°.

Blood Vessels and Nerves of the Hind Digit and Fetlock

The principal blood supply to the fetlock and digit of the pelvic limb is derived from the distal perforating branch (the continuation of dorsal metatarsal artery III), which supplies branches to the distal deep plantar arch and then bifurcates into medial and lateral digital arteries in the distoplantar region of the metatarsus. A small secondary supply is contributed by the medial and lateral plantar arteries that join the digital arteries to form the superficial plantar arch just proximal to the enlargement of the fetlock (Fig. 1.38). Distributing branches of the digital arteries form a pattern similar to that in the thoracic limb except for the blood supply to the navicular bone. In contrast to all arteries of the proximal anastomotic network originating from palmar arterial branches of the middle phalanx, in the pelvic limb the origin of the primary arteries is split between the plantar arterial branches of the middle phalanx and those of the collateral arch. More significantly, a greater number of vessels enter the distal border of the navicular bone from the distal anastomotic network in the hindfoot than enter the same region in the forefoot.[22]

Venous drainage of the digit of the pelvic limb is similar to that of the forelimb. The medial digital vein carries blood to the plantar common digital vein II; the lateral digital vein carries blood to the plantar common digital vein III.

The pattern of distribution of the sensory plantar digital and plantar metatarsal nerves in the fetlock and digit of the pelvic limb is similar to the pattern of the counterpart nerves in the thoracic limb. But some differences exist. The dorsal branch of each plantar digital nerve is given off more distally than the corresponding branch in the pastern of the forelimb. Medial and lateral dorsal metatarsal nerves (from the deep peroneal nerve) course distad subcutaneously parallel and dorsal to the medial and lateral plantar metatarsal nerves (Figs. 1.38 and 1.39). The lateral plantar metatarsal nerve is the shortest of these four nerves, extending distad over the fetlock to the lateral aspect of the pastern. The medial plantar metatarsal nerve may reach the coronet; both dorsal metatarsal nerves continue into the laminar corium.[23] Communications may exist between the dorsal and plantar metatarsal nerves. Terminal small branches of the saphenous nerve (medially), the superficial peroneal nerve (dorsally and laterally), and the caudal cutaneous sural nerve (dorsolaterally) complete the sensory innervation to the skin of the fetlock.

Metatarsus

The equine metatarsus is about 16% longer than the corresponding metacarpus, and the third (large) metatar-

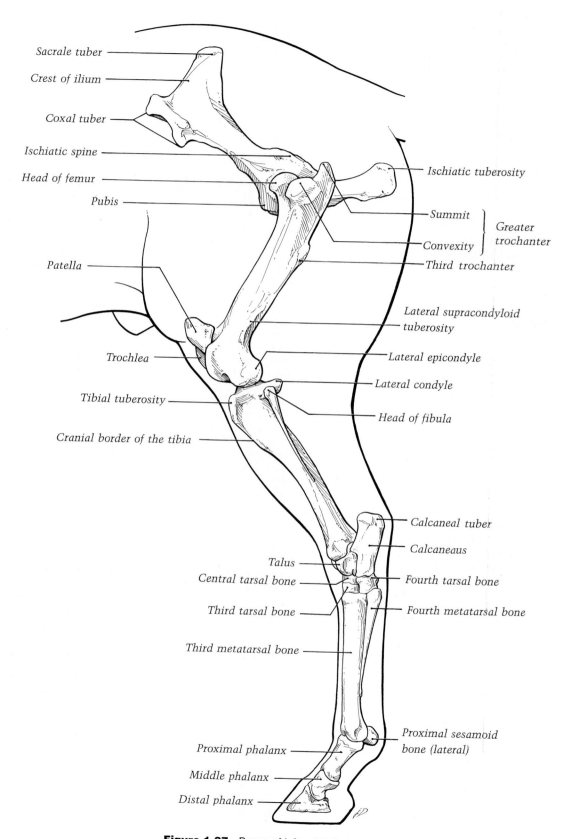

Sacrale tuber
Crest of ilium
Coxal tuber
Ischiatic spine
Head of femur
Pubis
Patella
Trochlea
Tibial tuberosity
Cranial border of the tibia
Talus
Central tarsal bone
Third tarsal bone
Third metatarsal bone
Proximal phalanx
Middle phalanx
Distal phalanx

Ischiatic tuberosity
Summit ⎱ Greater
Convexity ⎰ trochanter
Third trochanter
Lateral supracondyloid
tuberosity
Lateral epicondyle
Lateral condyle
Head of fibula
Calcaneal tuber
Calcaneaus
Fourth tarsal bone
Fourth metatarsal bone
Proximal sesamoid
bone (lateral)

Figure 1.37   Bones of left pelvic limb. Lateral view.

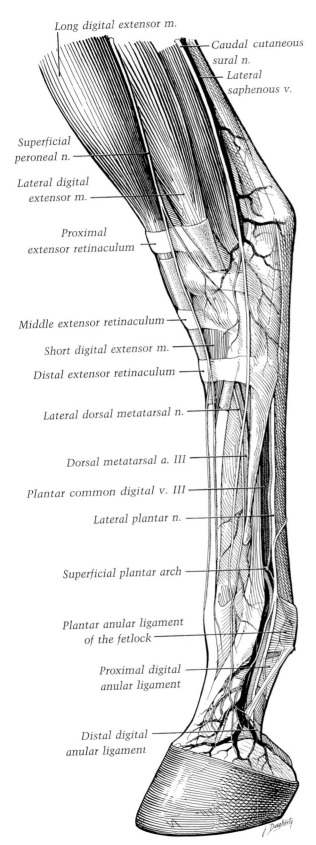

Long digital extensor m.

Caudal cutaneous sural n.

Lateral saphenous v.

Superficial peroneal n.

Lateral digital extensor m.

Proximal extensor retinaculum

Middle extensor retinaculum

Short digital extensor m.

Distal extensor retinaculum

Lateral dorsal metatarsal n.

Dorsal metatarsal a. III

Plantar common digital v. III

Lateral plantar n.

Superficial plantar arch

Plantar anular ligament of the fetlock

Proximal digital anular ligament

Distal digital anular ligament

Figure 1.38 Lateral view of left distal crus and pes. Skin and some of the fascia have been removed.

sal bone is more rounded than the third metacarpal bone. The fourth metatarsal bone, particularly its proximal extremity, is larger than the second metatarsal bone.

Dorsal Aspect

Three superficial nerves supply sensory innervation to the skin of the dorsal, lateral, and medial aspects of the metatarsus. Dorsally and laterally the two terminal branches of the superficial peroneal nerve descend as far as the fetlock. The terminal branch of the caudal cutaneous sural nerve descends obliquely from the lateral aspect of the hock to course over the dorsolateral part of the third metatarsal bone, where it terminates in the skin of the fetlock. The terminal branch of the saphenous nerve supplies the medial skin of the metatarsus down to the fetlock.

The dorsal common digital vein II (great metatarsal vein) ascends from a venous arch proximal to the proximal sesamoid bones as the proximal continuation of the medial digital vein. At first, the dorsal common digital vein II lies along the medial border of the suspensory ligament, then in a groove on the proximal part of the dorsal surface of the third metatarsal bone to the hock, where it continues into the cranial branch of the medial saphenous vein (Fig. 1.39). The dorsal metatarsal vein II (middle metatarsal vein) is more central, lying medial to the long digital extensor tendon and continuing proximad to join the cranial branch of the medial saphenous vein or, alternatively, the dorsal pedal vein.

A small dorsal metatarsal artery II carries blood distad from the dorsal tarsal rete, coursing in the groove between the second and third metatarsal bones.

The tendon of the long digital extensor muscle extends the length of the metatarsus on the dorsal surface of the third metatarsal bone beneath the skin and fascia. At the proximal third of the metatarsus, the long digital extensor tendon is joined by the tendon of the lateral digital extensor muscle. Rarely, the tendon of the lateral digital extensor courses separately to the proximal phalanx. The angle formed by the conjoined long and lateral digital extensor tendons is occupied by the thin, triangular extensor digitorum brevis (short digital extensor) muscle. The short digital extensor originates on the lateral collateral ligament of the hock, the lateral tendon of the peroneus tertius muscle, and the middle extensor retinaculum. It inserts on the two large digital extensor tendons with which the short extensor acts. The short digital extensor is related deeply to the termination of the deep peroneal nerve as it bifurcates into the medial (II) and lateral (III) dorsal metatarsal nerves, the dorsal metatarsal artery III, and the distal part of the hock joint capsule; the dorsal metatarsal nerves send motor branches to the muscle. All digital extensor muscles are bound down by the distal extensor retinaculum in the proximal third of the metatarsus (Fig. 1.38).

Emerging under the distal edge of the distal extensor retinaculum, the large dorsal metatarsal artery III (great metatarsal artery) pursues an oblique course distad to lie in the dorsolateral groove between the third and fourth metatarsal bones. The artery is accompanied by a very small satellite vein and the lateral dorsal metatarsal nerve that lies along the dorsal surface of the artery. The terminal branch of the caudal cutaneous sural nerve crosses

Figure 1.39 Medial view of left distal crus and pes. Skin and some of the fascia have been removed.

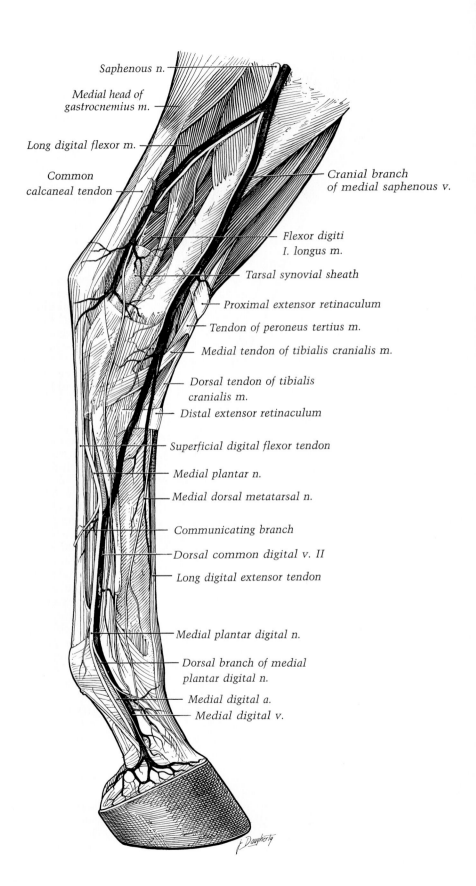

Saphenous n.

Medial head of gastrocnemius m.

Long digital flexor m.

Common calcaneal tendon

Cranial branch of medial saphenous v.

Flexor digiti I. longus m.

Tarsal synovial sheath

Proximal extensor retinaculum

Tendon of peroneus tertius m.

Medial tendon of tibialis cranialis m.

Dorsal tendon of tibialis cranialis m.

Distal extensor retinaculum

Superficial digital flexor tendon

Medial plantar n.

Medial dorsal metatarsal n.

Communicating branch

Dorsal common digital v. II

Long digital extensor tendon

Medial plantar digital n.

Dorsal branch of medial plantar digital n.

Medial digital a.

Medial digital v.

j. Daugherty

superficial to the dorsal metatarsal artery III (Fig. 1.38). Distally the artery passes between the third and fourth metatarsal bones, continuing deeply as the distal perforating branch. The distal perforating branch sends branches to the distal deep plantar arch, and then divides into medial and lateral digital arteries adjacent to the plantar aspect of the third metatarsal bone in the distal fourth of the metatarsus. The lateral dorsal metatarsal nerve remains superficial, courses dorsodistad to the fetlock, and descends in the dorsal fascia of the pastern, eventually terminating in the laminar corium.

The slightly larger medial dorsal metatarsal nerve supplies sensory fibers to the hock joint capsule and a motor branch to the short digital extensor muscle. The nerve emerges under the medial edge of the long digital extensor tendon, and then courses obliquely between the tendon and the second metatarsal bone to be distributed distally in the same manner as the lateral dorsal metatarsal nerve (Fig. 1.39).

Lateral and Medial Aspects

The lateral and medial plantar nerves lie plantar to their satellite veins and arteries along the respective lateral or medial border of the deep digital flexor tendon (Figs. 1.38 and 1.39). These nerves supply the lateral, medial, and plantar structures of the metatarsus. The lateral plantar nerve emerges between the two digital flexor tendons to reach their lateral borders. The nerve is heavily covered by fibrous connective tissue, and here it detaches its deep branch, the parent trunk of the deeply located lateral and medial plantar metatarsal nerves that pursue courses homologous to the palmar metacarpal nerves in the forelimb. At about the midmetatarsus, the medial plantar nerve gives off the communicating branch that angles laterodistad across the superficial digital flexor tendon to join the lateral plantar nerve in the distal fourth of the metatarsus. The communicating branch is generally smaller than its counterpart in the metacarpus, and it may be absent.

On each side the small medial and lateral plantar arteries course down to the distal end of the metatarsus, where they send branches to the respective digital arteries, forming the superficial plantar arch. The proximal deep plantar arch is supplied mainly by the proximal perforating branch from the dorsal pedal artery with minor contributing branches from the plantar arteries.

Plantar Aspect

The superficial digital flexor tendon is similar to the corresponding tendon in the metacarpus except that its lateral border is thicker.[12] The deep digital flexor muscle's principal tendon is intimately related to the dorsomedial aspect of the superficial digital flexor tendon. In the proximal third of the metatarsus, the principal tendon is joined by the tendon of the long digital flexor muscle (the medial head of the deep digital flexor muscle). A weakly developed, slender accessory ligament (subtarsal or "inferior" check ligament) arises from the plantar aspect of the fibrous joint capsule of the hock. Longer than its counterpart in the forelimb, it joins the deep digital flexor tendon near the middle of the metatarsus. This accessory ligament may be absent in horses,

and it is usually absent in donkeys, mules, and ponies.[18] The deep digital flexor tendon perforates the manica flexoria, a sleeve formed by the superficial digital flexor tendon at the level of the metatarsophalangeal joint.

The suspensory ligament (middle or third interosseous muscle) takes origin from a large area on the proximal aspect of the third metatarsal bone and a smaller attachment on the distal row of tarsal bones. Lying within the metatarsal groove deep to the deep digital flexor tendon, the suspensory ligament of the hindlimb is relatively thinner, more rounded and longer than the ligament of the forelimb. In some horses, e.g., Standardbreds, the suspensory ligament of the hindlimb contains more muscle than the suspensory ligament of the forelimb.[50] The two extensor branches pursue courses similar to those in the forelimb. Small medial (second) and lateral (fourth) interossei and lumbricales muscles are present in the metatarsus.

The medial and lateral plantar metatarsal arteries course distad under the suspensory ligament to the distal deep plantar arch. Their distribution is similar to the distribution of the palmar metacarpal arteries. Satellite veins accompany the arteries. The dorsal common digital vein II lies along the deep digital flexor tendon in the distal half of the metatarsus, then deviates across the medial surface of the third metatarsal bone to ascend across the tarsus as the cranial branch of the saphenous vein.

Tarsus (Hock)

The bones of the tarsus include the talus; calcaneus; and the central, first and second fused, and third and fourth tarsal bones (Fig. 1.34). Proximally the trochlea of the talus articulates with the cochlear surface of the tibia in the tarsocrural (tibiotarsal) joint; distally the distal row of tarsal bones and the three metatarsal bones articulate in the tarsometatarsal joint. Extensive collateral ligaments span the latter two joints and the intertarsal joints. Blood vessels, nerves, and the tendons of digital and crural muscles traverse and/or attach to the tarsus.

Dorsal Aspect

In the superficial fascia, the large cranial branch of the medial saphenous vein continues proximad from the dorsal common digital vein II. It crosses the mediodorsal aspect of the tarsus, lying upon the dorsomedial pouch of the tarsocrural joint capsule (Figs. 1.40 and 1.42). An anastomotic branch joins the medial saphenous vein with the deeper cranial tibial vein just proximal to the tarsocrural joint. The cranial tibial vein is the proximal continuation of the dorsal pedal vein. The superficial peroneal nerve lies in the fascia lateral and parallel to the tendon of the long digital extensor muscle. A fibrous loop (the middle extensor retinaculum) leaves the lateral tendon of insertion of the peroneus (fibularis) tertius muscle, wraps around the long digital extensor tendon and its sheath, and attaches to the calcaneus. The thick dorsal part of the tarsal fascia joins the long digital extensor tendon just distal to the tarsometatarsal joint. The tendon's synovial sheath extends from the level of the

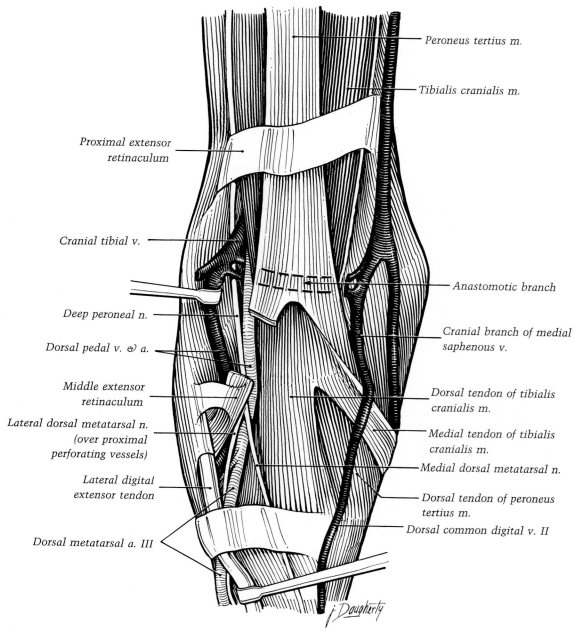

Peroneus tertius m.

Tibialis cranialis m.

Proximal extensor retinaculum

Cranial tibial v.

Anastomotic branch

Deep peroneal n.

Cranial branch of medial saphenous v.

Dorsal pedal v. & a.

Middle extensor retinaculum

Dorsal tendon of tibialis cranialis m.

Lateral dorsal metatarsal n. (over proximal perforating vessels)

Medial tendon of tibialis cranialis m.

Medial dorsal metatarsal n.

Lateral digital extensor tendon

Dorsal tendon of peroneus tertius m.

Dorsal common digital v. II

Dorsal metatarsal a. III

Figure 1.40 Dorsal dissection of right tarsus. The long digital extensor and short digital extensor muscles have been removed. The lateral tendon of the peroneus tertius muscle is sectioned. Notice its junction with the middle extensor retinaculum.

lateral tibial malleolus distad nearly to the junction of the tendon with the tendon of the lateral digital extensor muscle (Fig. 1.38). The long digital extensor tendon is located just lateral to the palpable medial ridge of the trochlea of the talus. The proximal part of the extensor digitorum brevis muscle covers the tarsal joint capsule, the lateral tarsal artery (which supplies the muscle), the dorsal pedal artery continuing into the dorsal metatarsal artery III, and the termination of the deep peroneal nerve as it bifurcates into the two dorsal metatarsal nerves (Fig. 1.40).

As it crosses the dorsal surface of the tarsocrural joint and onto the tarsus, the tendon of the peroneus tertius

muscle is superficial to the tendon of the tibialis cranialis muscle (Figs. 1.40, 1.41, 1.42, and 1.43). Then the tendon of the peroneus tertius forms a sleevelike cleft through which the tendon of the tibialis cranialis and its synovial sheath pass. The latter tendon then bifurcates into a dorsal tendon, which inserts on the large metatarsal bone, and a medial (cunean) tendon, which angles mediodistad under the superficial layer of the long medial collateral ligament of the hock to insert on the first tarsal bone. A large bursa is interposed between the cunean tendon and the long medial collateral ligament.

After forming the cleft that admits passage of the tibialis cranialis tendon, the peroneus tertius divides into

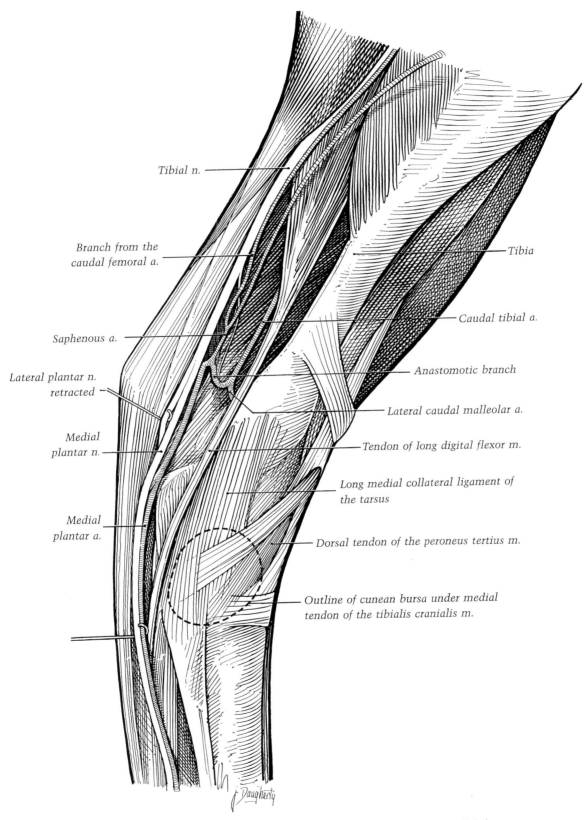

Tibial n.

Branch from the
caudal femoral a.

Saphenous a.

Lateral plantar n.
retracted

Medial
plantar n.

Medial
plantar a.

Tibia

Caudal tibial a.

Anastomotic branch

Lateral caudal malleolar a.

Tendon of long digital flexor m.

Long medial collateral ligament of
the tarsus

Dorsal tendon of the peroneus tertius m.

Outline of cunean bursa under medial
tendon of the tibialis cranialis m.

Daugherty

Figure 1.41   Dissection of left distal crus, tarsus, and metatarsus. Medial view.

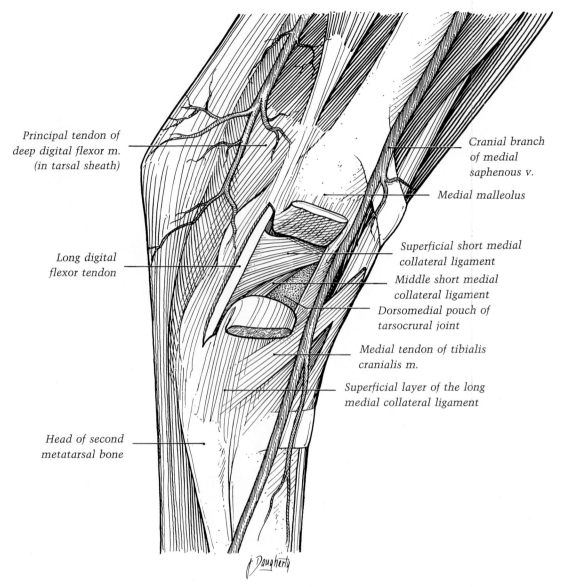

Principal tendon of
deep digital flexor m.
(in tarsal sheath)

Long digital
flexor tendon

Head of second
metatarsal bone

Cranial branch
of medial
saphenous v.

Medial malleolus

Superficial short medial
collateral ligament

Middle short medial
collateral ligament

Dorsomedial pouch of
tarsocrural joint

Medial tendon of tibialis
cranialis m.

Superficial layer of the long
medial collateral ligament

Figure 1.42   Medial view of left tarsus. The long medial collateral ligament has been cut and reflected. The
sheath of the long digital flexor tendon has been opened.

two tendons. The dorsal tendon passes under the cunean
tendon and inserts on the third tarsal bone and the third
metatarsal bone medial to the dorsal tendon of the tibialis cranialis muscle (Fig. 1.40). The lateral tendon of the
peroneus tertius extends distad deep to the long digital
extensor tendon, blends with the middle extensor retinaculum, and continues laterad distal to the lateral ridge
of the trochlea of the talus. The lateral tendon then bifurcates and inserts on the calcaneus and the fourth tarsal
bone (Fig. 1.46).

The main blood supply to the pes (tarsus, metatarsus,
and digit), the cranial tibial artery, continues as the dorsal pedal artery at the level of the tarsocrural joint (Fig.
1.40). Small branches from the dorsal pedal artery form
the dorsal tarsal rete in the tarsal fascia. Medial and
lateral tarsal arteries are small vessels arising from the

dorsal pedal artery and supplying their respective sides
of the tarsus. Before continuing as the dorsal metatarsal
artery III, the dorsal pedal artery gives off the proximal
perforating branch (a. tarsea perforans) which traverses
the vascular canal formed by the central, third, and
fourth tarsal bones. This branch supplies the proximal
deep plantar arch. Satellite veins accompany the arteries.

Lateral Aspect

Innervation to the lateral aspect of the tarsus is provided by branches from the caudal cutaneous sural nerve
as it courses superficial to the calcaneus, and from the
more dorsally located superficial peroneal nerve (Fig.
1.38).

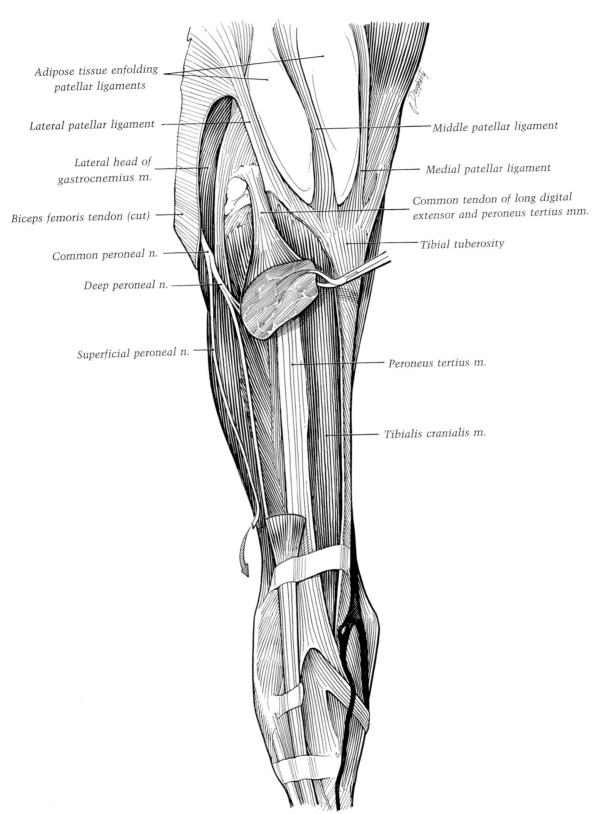

Adipose tissue enfolding
patellar ligaments

Lateral patellar ligament

Lateral head of
gastrocnemius m.

Biceps femoris tendon (cut)

Common peroneal n.

Deep peroneal n.

Superficial peroneal n.

Middle patellar ligament

Medial patellar ligament

Common tendon of long digital
extensor and peroneus tertius mm.

Tibial tuberosity

Peroneus tertius m.

Tibialis cranialis m.

Figure 1.43 Dorsal view of a dissection of right stifle, crus, and
tarsus. The long digital extensor muscle belly has been removed.

The terminal section of the superficial peroneal nerve (arrow) has
been removed with the fascia.

Surrounded by its tendon sheath, the tendon of the lateral digital extensor muscle is bound by a fibrous band in a groove in the lateral malleolus of the tibia. It then traverses a passage through the long lateral collateral ligament of the tarsus as the tendon angles dorsodistad. A synovial sheath enfolds the tendon from just proximal to the lateral malleolus to halfway between the edge of the distal extensor retinaculum and the tendon's junction with the long digital extensor tendon. Plantar to the lateral extensor tendon, the lateroplantar pouch of the tarsocrural joint capsule protrudes between the lateral malleolus and the calcaneus.

Medial Aspect

A horny chestnut, the presumed vestige of the first digit, is located in the skin on the distomedial aspect of the tarsus. Branches from the cranial and caudal branches of the saphenous nerve and from the tibial nerve supply sensory innervation to the medial aspect of the tarsus. The large cranial branch of the medial saphenous vein courses subcutaneously in a distoproximal direction, superficial to the dorsomedial pouch of the tarsocrural joint capsule (Fig. 1.33). At the level of the medial malleolus of the tibia, it sends an anastomotic branch deeply to the cranial tibial vein. The caudal branch of the medial saphenous vein receives blood from branches in the medial and plantar regions of the hock.

A palpable feature of the medial aspect of the hock is the medial (cunean) tendon of the tibialis cranialis muscle as it goes to its insertion on the first tarsal bone. The bursa between the cunean tendon and the distal part of the long medial collateral ligament of the tarsus is not normally palpable (Fig. 1.41). The tendon of the long digital flexor (medial head of the deep digital flexor muscle) passes through a fascial tunnel plantar to the medial collateral ligament. A synovial sheath surrounds the tendon from the distal fourth of the tibia to the tendon's junction with the main tendon of the muscle. A compartment of the tarsocrural joint capsule, the medioplantar pouch, is located a short distance plantar to the long digital flexor tendon and proximal to the sustentaculum tali of the calcaneus at the level of the medial malleolus.

The tarsal fascia thickens into a flexor retinaculum, bridging the groove on the sustentaculum tali of the calcaneus to form the tarsal (flexor) canal containing the principal tendon of the deep digital flexor muscle (Fig. 1.42). The tendon's synovial sheath, the tarsal sheath, extends from a level proximal to the medial malleolus to the proximal fourth of the metatarsus (Fig. 1.39). After joining the anastomotic branch of the caudal tibial artery just proximal to the tarsus, the now enlarged saphenous artery (really a common trunk of the two vessels) continues distad with the tendon (Fig. 1.41). The trunk bifurcates into medial and lateral plantar arteries. Medial and lateral plantar nerves from the tibial nerve in the distal crural region also accompany the principal deep digital flexor tendon, lying lateral to the tendon in the tarsal canal (Fig. 1.41). At the level of the tarsometatarsal joint, the medial plantar nerve and artery cross obliquely over the plantar surface of the deep digital flexor tendon to the tendon's medial border.

Plantar Aspect

In the distal third of the crus, the tendon of the superficial digital flexor muscle curls around the medial side of the tendon of the gastrocnemius muscle to become superficial as the tendons approach the calcaneal tuber (Fig. 1.39). The superficial digital flexor tendon flattens, and is joined by the flat tarsal tendons of the biceps femoris and semitendinosus muscles. This tendinous complex attaches to the point and sides of the calcaneal tuber. The tendon proper of the superficial digital flexor then narrows and continues distad superficial to the long plantar ligament. The calcaneal tendon of the gastrocnemius lies deep (dorsal) to the superficial digital flexor at the hock, and inserts on the plantar surface of the calcaneal tuber. An elongated bursa is interposed between the two tendons just above the tarsus. A smaller bursa is present between the superficial digital flexor tendon and the calcaneal tuber. These two bursae usually communicate across the lateral surface of the gastrocnemius tendon.[41] An inconstant subcutaneous bursa may develop over the superficial digital flexor at the level of the calcaneal tuber.

Dorsolateral to the superficial digital flexor, the long plantar ligament is attached to the plantar surface of the calcaneus, terminating distally on the fourth tarsal bone and the proximal extremity of the fourth metatarsal bone (Fig. 1.45).

Tarsal Joint (Hock Joint)

The principal component of the composite tarsal joint is the tarsocrural joint, a ginglymus based on the shape of the articular surfaces or a snap joint based on the snapping movement of the joint into or out of extension. Deep grooves on the cochlear articular surface of the distal end of the tibia articulate with the doubly extensive surface of the trochlea of the talus at an angle of 12 to 15° dorsolateral to the limb's sagittal plane.[18] The interarticular and tarsometatarsal joints are plane joints capable of only a small amount of gliding movement.

A long collateral ligament and three short collateral ligaments bind each side of the equine hock.[49] The long lateral collateral ligament, oval in cross section, extends from the lateral malleolus of the tibia caudal to the groove for the tendon of the lateral digital extensor. It attaches distally to the calcaneus, fourth tarsal bone, talus, and the third and fourth metatarsal bones (Figs. 1.44 and 1.45). The fascial tunnel for the tendon of the lateral digital extensor muscle blends into the dorsal border of the long lateral collateral ligament. In the foal this tunnel is a structure separate from the long lateral collateral ligament.[49] The three short lateral collateral ligaments are fused proximally where they attach to the lateral malleolus, cranial to the groove for the lateral digital extensor tendon. The superficial component, its fibers spiraling 180°, attaches distoplantarly to both the talus and calcaneus, whereas the middle and deep short lateral collateral ligaments attach solely on the lateral surface of the talus (Fig. 1.45).

The long medial collateral ligament of the hock has less well-defined borders than its lateral counterpart. [49] From its proximal attachment on the medial tibial malle-

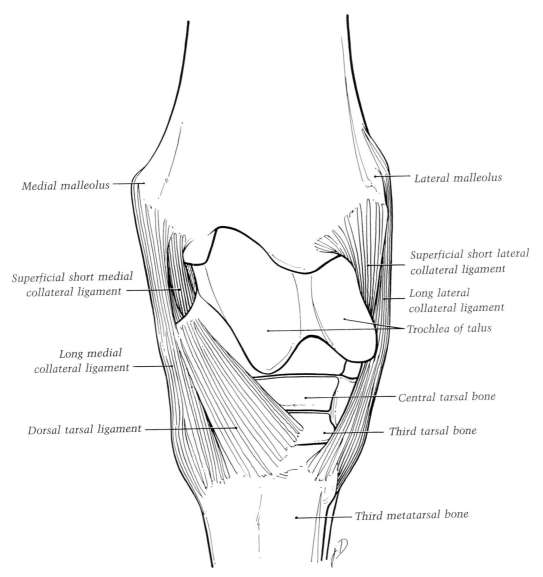

Figure 1.44 Dorsal view of tarsal ligaments. Right tarsus.

olus cranial to the groove for the long digital flexor muscle, the long medial collateral ligament extends distad and divides into two layers along its dorsal border on a plane with the proximal edge of the cunean bursa (Figs. 1.42 and 1.44). The superficial layer goes over the medial (cunean) tendon of the tibialis cranialis muscle and attaches to the fused first and second tarsal bones and the proximal ends of the second and third metatarsal bones just distal to the distal edge of the cunean bursa. The deep layer attaches distally to the distal tuberosity of the talus and the central and third tarsal bones. The plantar edge of the ligament attaches to the deep fascia over the sustentaculum tali and the interosseous ligament between the second and third metatarsal bones. Fascia from the plantar edges of the long medial collateral ligament and superficial short medial collateral ligament combines with fascia covering the sustentaculum tali to form the tunnel for the long digital flexor tendon.

The flat superficial short medial collateral ligament extends from the medial tibial malleolus to the tuberosities of the talus and the ridge between them (Fig. 1.42). The middle short medial collateral ligament extends obliquely from the medial tibial malleolus to the sustentaculum tali and central tarsal bone. It lies on the medial surface of the talus between the two tuberosities, varying in position during movement of the joints. The smallest component, the deep short medial collateral ligament, courses from the distal edge of the medial tibial malleolus obliquely to the ridge between the two tuberosities of the talus.

A dorsal tarsal ligament fans out distad from the distal tuberosity of the talus and attaches to the central and third tarsal bones and the proximal extremities of the second and third metatarsal bones (Fig. 1.44). A plantar tarsal ligament attaches to the plantar surface of the calcaneus and fourth tarsal bone and the fourth metatarsal

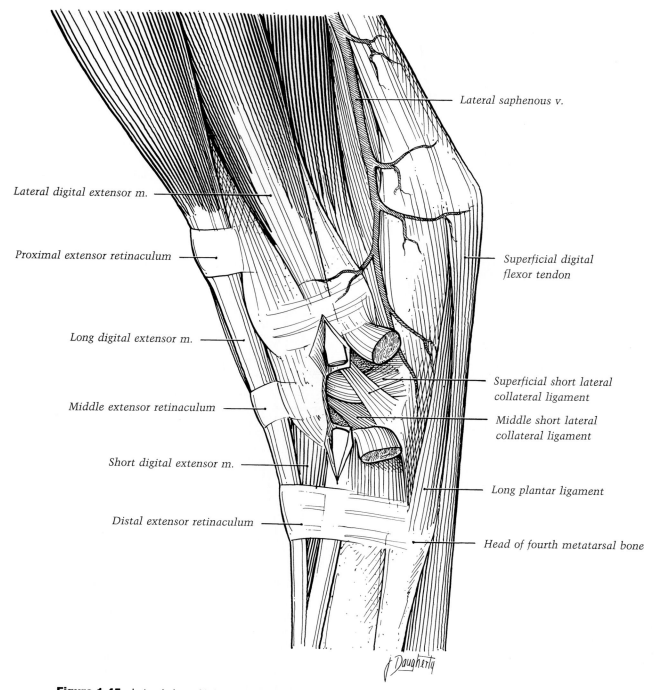

Lateral saphenous v.

Lateral digital extensor m.

Proximal extensor retinaculum

Superficial digital flexor tendon

Long digital extensor m.

Superficial short lateral collateral ligament

Middle short lateral collateral ligament

Middle extensor retinaculum

Short digital extensor m.

Long plantar ligament

Distal extensor retinaculum

Head of fourth metatarsal bone

Figure 1.45 Lateral view of left tarsus. The long lateral collateral ligament has been cut and reflected. A section of the lateral digital extensor tendon has been removed.

bone. Smaller, less distinct ligaments join contiguous tarsal bones.

The ligaments blend deeply with the common fibrous joint capsule of the tarsal joints. The joint capsule is thinnest dorsally and thickest in its plantar and distal parts. Cartilage in the capsule covering the flexor groove of the sustentaculum tali provides a smooth surface for the contained deep digital flexor tendon. Distally the accessory (subtarsal or "inferior" check) ligament of the

deep digital flexor tendon takes origin from the fibrous joint capsule.

Three pouches can protrude from the large tarsocrural synovial sac where it is not bound down by ligaments: the dorsomedial (largest), medioplantar, and lateroplantar pouches. The intertarsal joints formed by the talus and calcaneus proximally, and the central and fourth tarsal bones distally, are lined by the proximal intertarsal sac that communicates with the larger tarsocrural sac. The distal intertarsal sac provides synovial fluid for the joints between the central tarsal and contiguous bones distally and on each side. Except for hocks with fused central and third tarsal bones, communications may exist between the distal intertarsal and tarsometatarsal joints. In 8.3 to 23.8% of cases studied (depending on the technique employed), communications have been demonstrated.[42] Injected materials move through the space between the third tarsal and the fused first and second tarsal bones. The tarsometatarsal joint and joints formed by the third tarsal with the bones on each side are lined by the tarsometatarsal sac.[18]

Movements of the Tarsocrural Joint

The tarsocrural joint is flexed by contraction of the tibialis cranialis muscle and the passive pull of the tendinous peroneus tertius muscle. Contraction of the gastrocnemius, biceps femoris, and semitendinosus muscles and the passive pull of the tendinous superficial digital flexor muscle extend the joint. By virtue of its attachments in the extensor fossa of the femur proximally, and on the lateral aspect of the tarsus and dorsal surface of the third metatarsal bone distally, the peroneus tertius passively flexes the tarsocrural joint when the femorotibial joint is flexed. The superficial digital flexor muscle originates in the supracondyloid fossa of the femur and inserts first on the calcaneal tuber. This part of the superficial digital flexor serves to passively extend the tarsocrural joint when the femorotibial joint is extended. The two tendinous, passively functioning muscles constitute the reciprocal apparatus (Fig. 1.46).

In the standing position, the dorsal articular angle of the hock is around 150°.[18] During flexion of the tarsocrural joint, the pes is directed slightly laterad, owing to the configuration of the joint. Approximately one-third of the distance from the point of maximum extension to the point of maximum flexion, a snapping motion occurs influenced through tension exerted by the three short medial collateral ligaments.[49]

Crus (Leg or Gaskin)

The crus or true leg is the region of the hindlimb containing the tibia and fibula. Thus it extends from the tarsocrural joint to the femorotibial joint. The transversely flattened proximal end of the fibula articulates with the lateral condyle of the tibia. Distally the fibula narrows to a free end, terminating in the distal one-half to two-thirds of the crus as a thin ligament (Figs. 1.37 and 1.46). An interosseous ligament occupies the space between the two bones. The cranial tibial vessels pass through the proximal part of the ligament.

Beneath the skin and superficial fascia a heavy crural fascia invests the entire leg region. The superficial layer of the deep crural fascia is continuous with the femoral fascia; the middle layer is continuous with tendons descending from the thigh. In several places the two layers are inseparable. The crural fascia blends with the medial and lateral patellar ligaments and attaches to the cranial and medial surfaces of the tibia in the middle of the leg. Caudally the crural fascia forms the combined flat tarsal tendons of the biceps femoris and semitendinosus muscles that attach with the superficial digital flexor tendon to the calcaneal tuber. Under the two common fasciae, a deeper layer covers the muscles of the leg. Laterally an intermuscular septum passes between the long digital extensor and lateral digital extensor muscles; another septum passes between the lateral digital extensor and the deep digital flexor muscles.

Cranial Aspect

The belly of the long digital extensor muscle is a prominent structure beneath the skin on the craniolateral aspect of the crus. It originates in common with the peroneus tertius muscle from the extensor fossa of the femur, the common tendon descending through the extensor sulcus of the tibia. The long digital extensor muscle is related deeply to the tendinous peroneus tertius and the fleshy tibialis cranialis muscles, and caudally to the lateral digital extensor muscle from which it is separated by the distinct intermuscular septum. The superficial peroneal nerve courses distad in the groove between the digital extensor muscles, and angles craniad toward the hock. Deeply, the deep peroneal nerve courses distad between the two muscles on the cranial surface of the intermuscular septum. At its origin the nerve sends branches to the digital extensor muscles and the peroneus tertius and tibialis cranialis muscles (Figs. 1.43 and 1.47).

Deep to and intimately associated with the peroneus tertius, the tibialis cranialis muscle covers the craniolateral surface of the tibia, originating from the bone's tuberosity, lateral condyle, and lateral border and from the crural fascia (Fig. 1.43). After it passes through the interosseous space (between the tibia and fibula), the cranial tibial artery courses distad on the tibia deep to the tibialis cranialis muscle accompanied by two satellite veins.

Lateral Aspect

The caudal cutaneous sural nerve is derived principally from the tibial nerve (Fig. 1.48). In company with the lateral saphenous vein, which empties proximally into the caudal femoral vein, the caudal cutaneous sural nerve courses across both heads of the gastrocnemius muscle. The nerve and vein then descend under the crural fascia and tarsal tendon of the biceps femoris muscle to the distal third of the crus, where the nerve penetrates the crural fascia and divides into several branches, one of which courses distad over the hock to the metatarsus (Fig. 1.38). The tibial tendon of the biceps femoris muscle sweeps across the proximal third of the lateral aspect of the crus to attach to the cranial border of the tibia. The tarsal tendon of the muscle extends to the calcaneal tuber. Deep to the terminal part of the middle belly of the biceps femoris, the common peroneal nerve crosses the lateral surface of the lateral head of the gastrocnemius muscle and divides into superficial and deep peroneal nerves (Fig. 1.47). Caudal to the two branches of the peroneal nerve, the lateral digital extensor muscle extends distad from its origins on the fibula, interosseus ligament, lateral surface of the tibia, and the lateral collateral ligament of the femorotibial joint. The lateral part of the deep belly (flexor digit I longus) of the deep digital

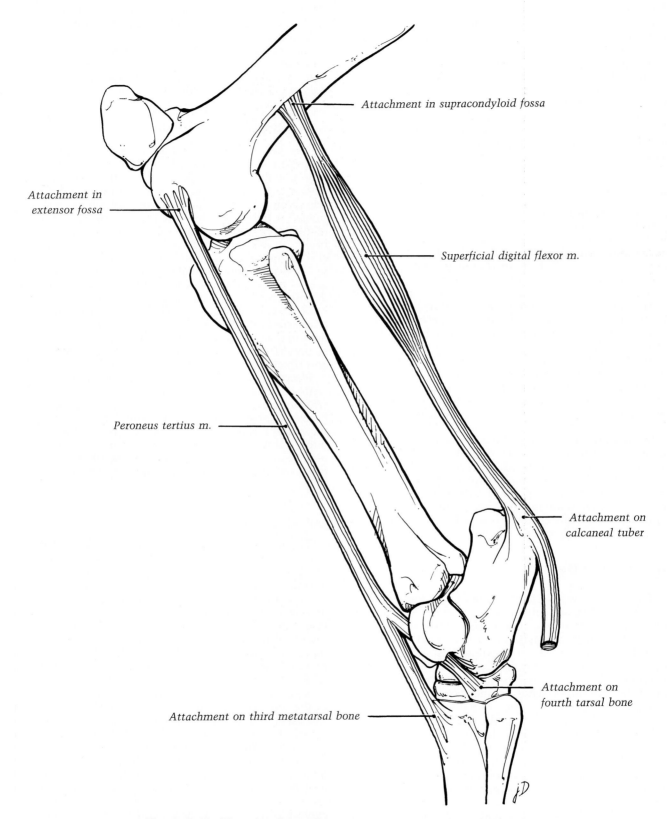

Attachment in supracondyloid fossa

Attachment in
extensor fossa

Superficial digital flexor m.

Peroneus tertius m.

Attachment on
calcaneal tuber

Attachment on
fourth tarsal bone

Attachment on third metatarsal bone

Figure 1.46   Dissection of the reciprocal apparatus. Lateral view, left hindlimb.

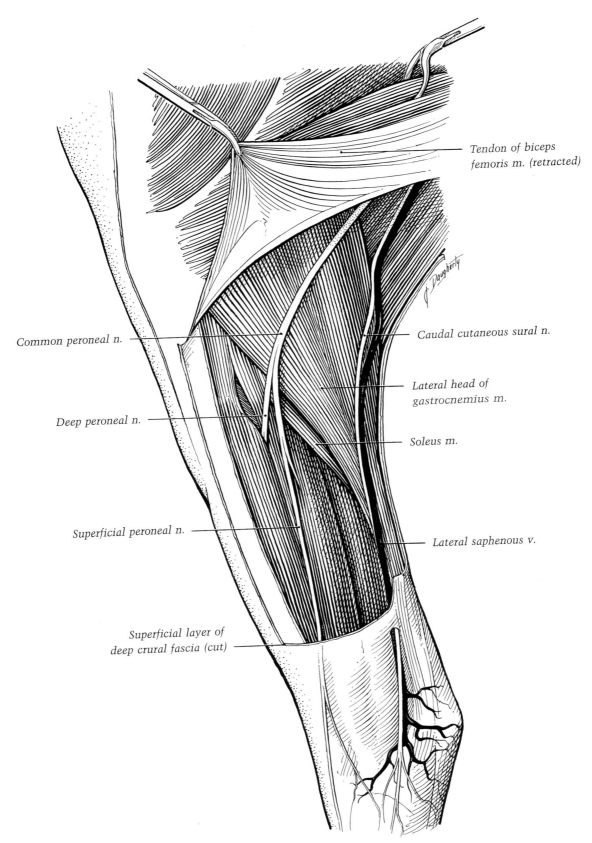

Tendon of biceps
femoris m. (retracted)

Common peroneal n.

Caudal cutaneous sural n.

Lateral head of
gastrocnemius m.

Deep peroneal n.

Soleus m.

Superficial peroneal n.

Lateral saphenous v.

Superficial layer of
deep crural fascia (cut)

Figure 1.47   Superficial dissection of lateral aspect of left stifle, crus, and tarsus.

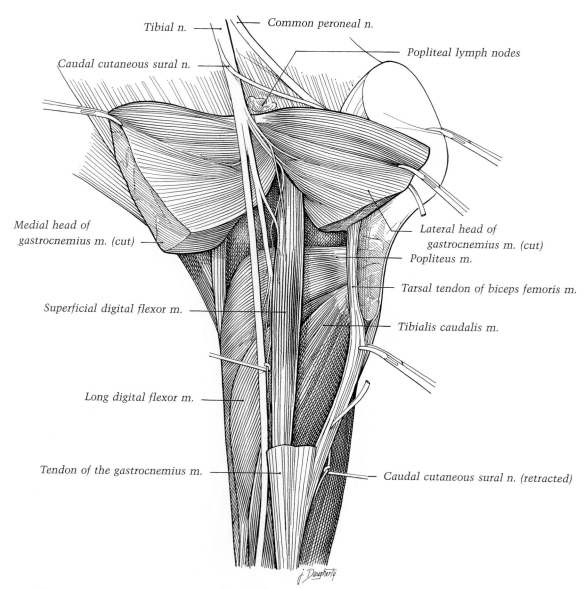

Figure 1.48 Dissection of caudal aspect of right stifle and crus, revealing distribution of the tibial nerve.

flexor muscle lies caudal to the belly of the lateral digital extensor.

The lateral head of the gastrocnemius originates on the lateral supracondyloid tuberosity of the femur. Under the common crural fascia in the proximal half of the crus, the small soleus muscle extends from its origin on the fibula along the lateral aspect of the gastrocnemius muscle to join the gastrocnemius tendon (Fig. 1.47).

Medial Aspect

Throughout most of its length, the medial surface of the tibia is subcutaneous (Fig. 1.39). Sensation is provided to the medial and cranial aspects of the crus by numerous branches of the saphenous nerve ramifying in the superficial fascia. The distal continuation of the nerve follows the prominent cranial branch of the medial saphenous vein that angles obliquely across the medial surface of the tibia. Accompanied by the saphenous artery, the smaller caudal branch of the medial saphenous vein crosses medial to the belly of the long digital flexor muscle and joins the cranial branch of the vein superficial to the tibial attachment of the semitendinosus muscle.

Deep to the crural fascia and caudal to the caudal branch of the medial saphenous vein, the tibial nerve descends with branches of the caudal femoral vessels. The tibial nerve is enclosed in its own fascial compartment, bifurcating about a hand's breadth proximal to the level of the point of the calcaneal tuber into the medial and lateral plantar nerves. These nerves continue in close apposition distad to the tarsus, where they pursue their independent courses.

The caudal tibial vessels lie deep to the tendon of the long digital flexor as it angles distad. Distal to this relationship, the anastomosis between the caudal tibial and saphenous vessels is located medial to the principal tendon of the deep digital flexor muscle. Proximally, the medial head of the gastrocnemius muscle lies under the tendon of the semitendinosus. Then the tendon of the gastrocnemius begins to wrap around the tendon of the superficial digital flexor.

Caudal Aspect

Descending from their origins on the supracondyloid tuberosities of the femur, the two heads of the gastrocnemius enclose the round, mostly tendinous superficial digital flexor. The tendon of the latter wraps medially from deep to superficial around the gastrocnemius tendon. Deeply, the deep digital flexor muscle's three heads originate from the lateral condyle of the tibia, the interosseous ligament, the fibula, and the caudal surface of the tibia (Figs. 1.48 and 1.49). The long digital flexor muscle angles from lateral to medial in a groove between the popliteus muscle proximally and the flexor digiti I longus (the deep head) distally. The tibialis caudalis (superficial head) is continuous deeply with the deep head. In the distal third of the crus, the flat tendon of the superficial head joins the larger tendon of the deep head, whereas the tendon of the medial head (long digital flexor) pursues its course over the medial aspect of the hock to join the principal tendon in the metatarsus.

Stifle (Genu)

The stifle is the region including the stifle (genual) joint (femorotibial joint plus the femoropatellar joint) and surrounding structures.

Cranial Aspect

Cutaneous innervation of the cranial aspect of the stifle is provided by terminal branches of the lateral cutaneous femoral nerve and lateral branch of the iliohypogastric nerve.

Deep to the skin three patellar ligaments descend from the patella, converging to their attachments on the tibial tuberosity. An extensive pad of adipose tissue is interposed between the ligaments and the joint capsule of the femoropatellar joint (Fig. 1.43). The adipose tissue enfolds the ligaments, wrapping around their sides. The space between the medial and middle patellar ligaments is greater than the space between middle and lateral ligaments. This difference reflects the origin of the medial patellar ligament. The parapatellar fibrocartilage is a large mass extending mediad from the patella in such a manner that its continuation, the medial patellar ligament, courses proximal and then medial to the medial ridge of the trochlea on the femur. The medial patellar ligament, now thinner than the other two patellar ligaments, attaches to the tibial tuberosity medial to the groove. As it descends from the patella to the groove in the tibial tuberosity, two bursae lie under the middle patellar ligament. One lies between the proximal part of the ligament and the apex of the patella, and the other

between the ligament and the proximal part of the groove. Swinging in mediad from the lateral aspect of the cranial surface of the patella, the lateral patellar ligament serves as an attachment for a tendon from the biceps femoris muscle and then for the fascia lata just before the ligament attaches to the lateral aspect of the tibial tuberosity. The tendon from the biceps femoris continues on to the cranial surface of the patella.

The base, cranial surface, and medial border of the patella, and the parapatellar fibrocartilage and femoropatellar joint capsule, serve as attachments for the insertions of the quadriceps femoris muscle.

Lateral Aspect

Beneath the skin, the terminal parts of the three divisions of the biceps femoris muscle (Fig. 1.50) and, caudally, the semitendinosus muscle (Fig. 1.51) dominate the lateral aspect of the stifle region. The tendon from the cranial division of the biceps femoris inserts on the lateral patellar ligament and the patella, and the tendon from the middle division of the muscle sweeps craniodistad to the cranial border of the tibia. Cranially, the fascia lata extends distad, attaching to the lateral patellar ligament (Fig. 1.52).

Superficial innervation is supplied to this region by branches from several nerves: lateral branches of the iliohypogastric and ilioinguinal nerves; the lateral cutaneous sural nerve originating from the common peroneal nerve and passing out between the middle and caudal divisions of the biceps femoris; the caudal cutaneous sural nerve (from the tibial nerve); and terminal branches of the caudal cutaneous femoral nerve (from the caudal gluteal nerve).

Reflection of the distal part of the biceps femoris muscle reveals the following (Fig. 1.50): The lateral femoropatellar ligament extends obliquely from the lateral epicondyle of the femur to the lateral border of the patella. The lateral surface of the lateral head of the gastrocnemius muscle is crossed by the common peroneal nerve and, further caudad, by the caudal cutaneous sural nerve and the lateral saphenous vein carrying blood to the caudal femoral vein. As it extends from the lateral epicondyle of the femur to the head of the fibula, the thick lateral collateral ligament of the femorotibial joint covers the tendon of origin of the popliteus muscle that also originates from the lateral epicondyle. A pouch from the lateral femorotibial joint capsule lies beneath the tendon. A common tendon of the long digital extensor and peroneus tertius muscles takes origin from the extensor fossa in the distal surface of the lateral epicondyle of the femur. The tendon is cushioned as it extends distad by an elongated pouch from the lateral femorotibial joint capsule.

Caudal Aspect

Under the skin and fascia on the caudal aspect of the stifle (supplied by branches of the caudal femoral nerve) the caudal part of the biceps femoris muscle covers the lateral head of the gastrocnemius. The tibial tendon of the biceps femoris extends to the cranial border of the tibia, its tarsal tendon continuing distad (Fig. 1.53). The semitendinosus muscle sweeps from lateral to medial on the way to its insertion on the cranial border of the tibia

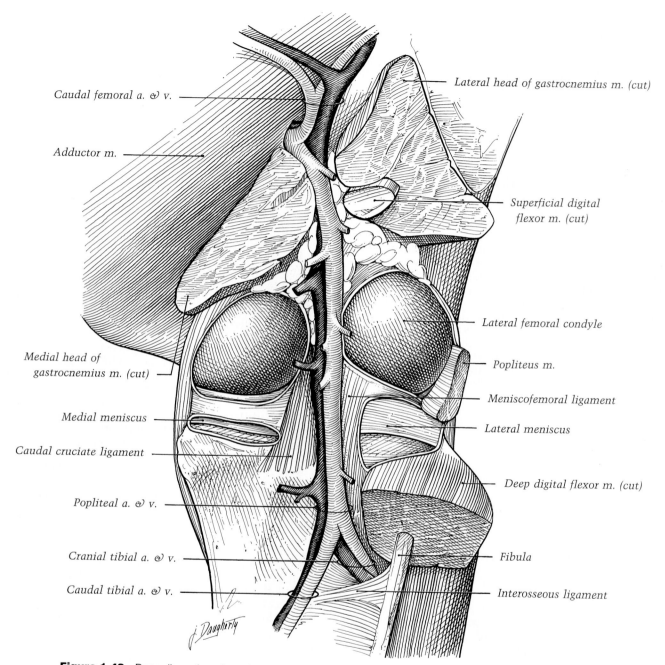

Caudal femoral a. & v.

Adductor m.

Medial head of
gastrocnemius m. (cut)

Medial meniscus

Caudal cruciate ligament

Popliteal a. & v.

Cranial tibial a. & v.

Caudal tibial a. & v.

Lateral head of gastrocnemius m. (cut)

Superficial digital
flexor m. (cut)

Lateral femoral condyle

Popliteus m.

Meniscofemoral ligament

Lateral meniscus

Deep digital flexor m. (cut)

Fibula

Interosseous ligament

Figure 1.49 Deep dissection of caudal aspect of right stifle. Joint capsule of the femorotibial joint has been opened.

and distad toward its tarsal insertion, covering the medial head of the gastrocnemius. The tendons of the
smaller medial head and larger lateral head of the gastrocnemius combine. At first, the tendon is related deeply
to the tendon of the superficial digital flexor muscle.

Separation of the two heads of the gastrocnemius
muscle reveals the cordlike superficial digital flexor muscle that arises in the supracondyloid fossa of the femur
between the two heads, its initial part enfolded by the
lateral head. After detaching the caudal cutaneous sural

nerve, the tibial nerve descends between the two heads of
the gastrocnemius along the medial side of the superficial
digital flexor. Branches from the tibial nerve supply the
gastrocnemius, soleus, superficial digital flexor, deep
digital flexor, and popliteus muscles (Fig. 1.48). The femoral artery and vein terminate by giving off the caudal
femoral vessels and continuing as the popliteal vessels
that descend between the two heads of the gastrocnemius
and cross the caudal surface of the stifle joint (Fig. 1.49).
Distal to the joint, the popliteal vessels divide into cranial

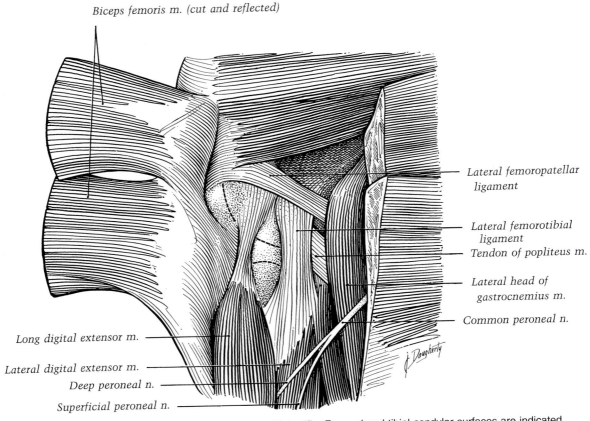

Biceps femoris m. (cut and reflected)

Lateral femoropatellar ligament

Lateral femorotibial ligament

Tendon of popliteus m.

Lateral head of gastrocnemius m.

Common peroneal n.

Long digital extensor m.

Lateral digital extensor m.

Deep peroneal n.

Superficial peroneal n.

Figure 1.50 Deep dissection of lateral aspect of left stifle. Femoral and tibial condylar surfaces are indicated by dashed lines.

and caudal tibial vessels. The larger cranial vessels, the main blood supply to the pes, deviate laterad into the interosseous space between the tibia and fibula; the smaller caudal tibial vessels continue distad between the tibia and the popliteus muscle.

The triangular popliteus muscle extends mediodistad from its origin on the lateral epicondyle of the femur (Fig. 1.48). The tendon of origin passes under the lateral collateral ligament of the stifle joint cushioned deeply by an extension of the lateral pouch of the femorotibial joint capsule (Fig. 1.50). The popliteus spreads out and inserts on the medial part of the caudal surface of the tibia proximal to the popliteal line, contacting the long digital flexor muscle.

Medial Aspect

Skin and fascia on the medial aspect of the stifle are supplied by the saphenous and lateral cutaneous femoral nerves. The region is crossed by the saphenous vein, artery, and nerve. Deep to the skin and fascia cranially, the vastus medialis of the quadriceps femoris muscle attaches to the parapatellar fibrocartilage, medial border of the patella, and medial patellar ligament. The straplike sartorius muscle attaches to the medial patellar ligament and the tibial tuberosity. Caudal to the sartorius, the wide gracilis muscle also attaches to the medial patellar ligament and to the medial collateral ligament of the femorotibial joint and the crural fascia (Fig. 1.51).

A thinner medial collateral ligament of the femorotibial joint reaches from the medial epicondyle of the femur to just distal to the margin of the medial tibial condyle, detaching fibers to the medial meniscus (Fig. 1.51). The adductor muscle inserts on the ligament and the medial epicondyle. The medial femoropatellar ligament is also thinner than its lateral counterpart, blending with the femoropatellar joint capsule as the ligament extends from the femur proximal to the medial epicondyle to the parapatellar fibrocartilage.

Stifle Joint

Overall the two joints of the stifle, the femoropatellar and femorotibial joints, form a ginglymus.

Femoropatellar Joint

The patella is essentially a sesamoid bone intercalated in the termination of the quadriceps femoris muscle, with the three patellar ligaments making up the tendon of insertion. As indicated previously, thin femoropatellar ligaments lend some collateral stability to the patella.

A thin, voluminous joint capsule attaches peripheral to the edge of the femoral trochlea, whereas the patellar attachment is close to the edge of the patellar articular surface. A proximal pouch from the joint capsule protrudes proximad under a mass of adipose tissue and the

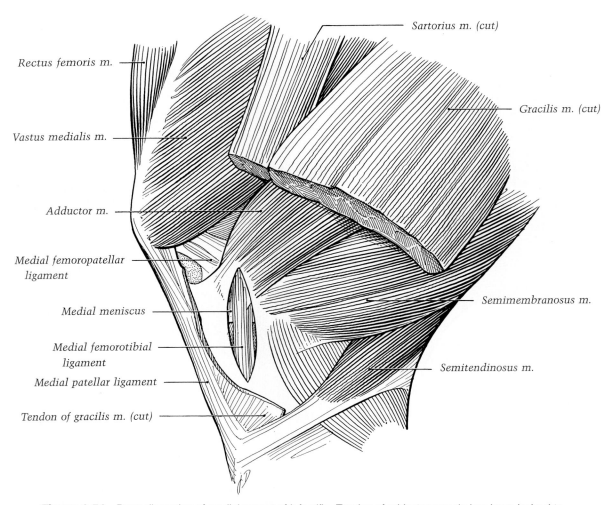

Rectus femoris m.

Vastus medialis m.

Adductor m.

Medial femoropatellar
ligament

Medial meniscus

Medial femorotibial
ligament

Medial patellar ligament

Tendon of gracilis m. (cut)

Sartorius m. (cut)

Gracilis m. (cut)

Semimembranosus m.

Semitendinosus m.

Figure 1.51 Deep dissection of medial aspect of left stifle. Tendon of adductor muscle has been incised to reveal medial femorotibial ligament.

distal part of the quadriceps femoris muscle. The distal extremity of the femoropatellar joint capsule contacts the femorotibial joint capsule. The vastus intermedius of the quadriceps femoris attaches, in part, to the femoropatellar joint capsule, acting to tense the capsule during extension of the femoropatellar joint.

Even with the medial extension of the parapatellar fibrocartilage and a smaller lateral cartilaginous band, the articular surface of the patella is much smaller than the trochlear surface of the femur. The larger gliding surface of the trochlea accommodates the proximal-distal movements of the patella. A wide groove separates the larger medial ridge of the trochlea from the smaller, slightly more distal lateral ridge, the two ridges deviating slightly laterad. Articular cartilage covers all of the large, rounded medial ridge that expands proximally; the cartilage covering the more regularly rounded lateral ridge extends only part way over the lateral surface. Contact between the patella and trochlea changes as the patella moves proximad on its larger gliding surface during flexion of the stifle joint. The patella rolls on to its narrow distal articular surface (resting surface) as the parapatel-

lar fibrocartilage maintains its tight relationship over the trochlea's medial ridge as a result of tension exerted by the medial patellar ligament. The narrow craniodorsal surface of the proximal part of the trochlea may be termed its resting surface.[41]

Femorotibial Joint

The femorotibial joint is complex, with the cranial and caudal cruciate ligaments lying between the joint capsule's medial and lateral synovial sacs. Two fibrocartilaginous menisci intervene partially between the femoral and tibial articular surfaces, thus partially subdividing each sac. The joint capsule extends distad from a line about 1 cm from the proximal edge of the articular cartilage of the medial femoral condyle and closer to the articular cartilage of the lateral condyle, attaching to the peripheral borders of the menisci and then to the edges of the articular surfaces of the tibial condyles. The fibrous part of the joint capsule is thick caudally, thin cranially. It also attaches to the cruciate ligaments. From the lateral sac, one extension encloses the tendon of ori-

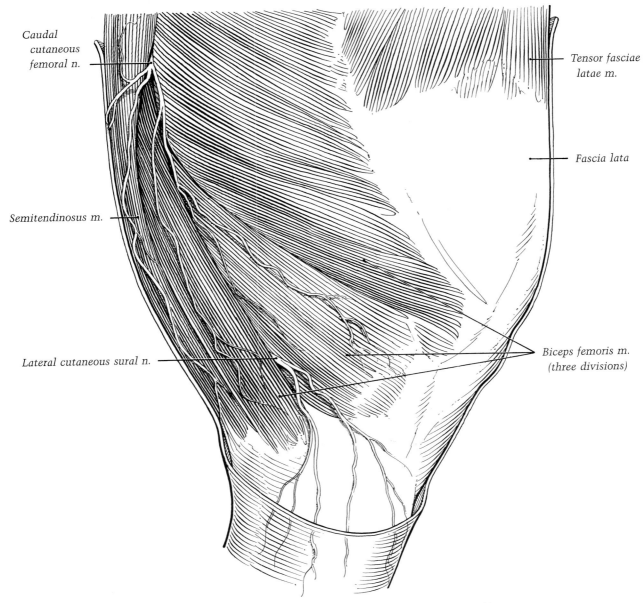

Caudal cutaneous femoral n.

Tensor fasciae latae m.

Fascia lata

Semitendinosus m.

Biceps femoris m. (three divisions)

Lateral cutaneous sural n.

Figure 1.52 Lateral view of right stifle and thigh, deep to the skin.

gin of the popliteus muscle and another pouches distad under the common tendon of origin of the long digital extensor and peroneus tertius muscles.

In a study of communications between the femoropatellar and femorotibial joints, anatomical communication between the femoropatellar joint sac and the medial sac of the femorotibial joint was demonstrated in 65% of 46 stifles examined.[37] Communication existed between the femoropatellar joint sac and both the medial and lateral sacs of the femorotibial joint in 17.5% of the joints examined, but there was no communication between the femoropatellar joint sac and either sac of the femorotibial joint in 17.5%. Anatomical communications between joints of the two stifles were bilaterally symmetrical. Functional communication indicated by

dye penetration was present in 74% of 19 horses in which anatomical communication existed. This study suggests that, when performing intra-articular anesthesia, each synovial sac needs to be injected separately to ensure that anesthesia of the appropriate synovial sac is obtained.[37] The narrow, partially covered opening from the femoropatellar sac into the medial sac of the femorotibial joint is 10 to 15 mm long; the opening into the lateral sac is smaller.

The two fibrocartilaginous menisci are somewhat crescent-shaped, being thicker peripherally and thinner along the concave edge. Their proximal surfaces are concave to accommodate the convexity of the femoral condyles. Distally they conform to the peripheral parts of the articular surfaces of the tibial condyles. Cranial and

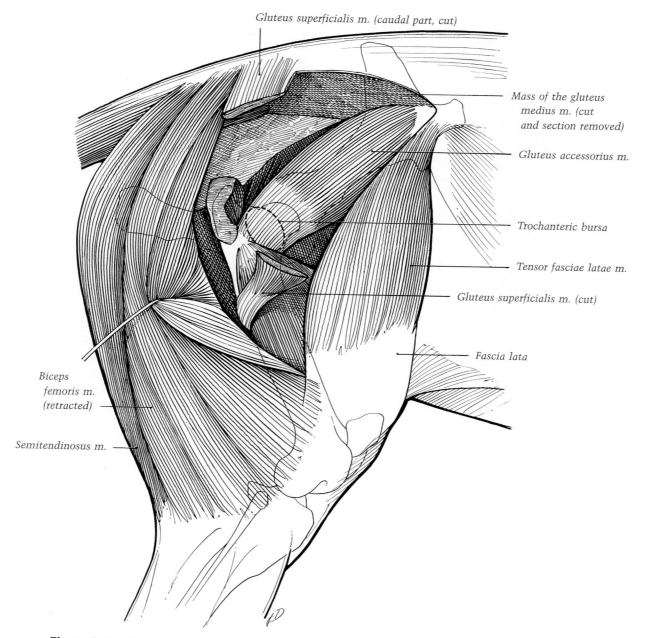

Gluteus superficialis m. (caudal part, cut)

Mass of the gluteus medius m. (cut and section removed)

Gluteus accessorius m.

Trochanteric bursa

Tensor fasciae latae m.

Gluteus superficialis m. (cut)

Fascia lata

Biceps femoris m. (retracted)

Semitendinosus m.

Figure 1.53 Dissection of right thigh and hip. Most of the gluteus superficialis and gluteus medius muscles have been removed. Lateral view.

caudal ligaments attach each meniscus to the tibia, and a meniscofemoral ligament attaches the caudal aspect of the lateral meniscus to the caudal surface of the intercondyloid fossa of the femur (Fig. 1.49).

In addition to the support rendered by medial and lateral collateral ligaments, the femur and tibia are joined by two cruciate ligaments that cross one another in the intercondyloid space between the two synovial sacs of the femorotibial joint. The caudal (or medial) cruciate ligament, the larger of the two, extends distocaudad from the cranial surface of the intercondyloid fossa to the popliteal notch of the tibia, crossing the medial aspect of the cranial (or lateral) cruciate ligament. Extending

distocraniad from the lateral wall of the intercondyloid fossa, the cranial cruciate ligament attaches to a central fossa in the tibial spine between the articular surfaces of the condyles.

The stifle is supplied principally by branches of the descending genicular artery that originates from the femoral artery and descends toward the medial aspect of the stifle joint deep to the sartorius and vastus medialis muscles.

Movements of the Stifle Joint

In the standing position with resting surfaces of the patella and trochlea in apposition, the caudal angle of the stifle joint is around 150°.[18] The quadriceps femoris muscle is relatively relaxed in this position. Extension of the stifle joint through action of the quadriceps femoris, tensor fasciae latae, and cranial division of the biceps femoris muscles (plus passive traction exerted by the peroneus tertius) is limited by tension from the collateral and cruciate ligaments. There is minimal lateral rotation of the crus during full extension. Flexion of the joint by the semitendinosus, middle division of the biceps femoris, popliteus, and gastrocnemius muscles, plus passive traction exerted by the superficial digital flexor, is limited only by the caudal muscle masses. During flexion the crus is rotated slightly mediad, and the femoral condyles and menisci move slightly caudad on the tibial condyles with somewhat more movement on the lateral surfaces.

When a horse shifts its weight more to one hindlimb, that limb flexes slightly as the contralateral relaxed limb is brought to rest on the toe. The pelvis is tilted so that the hip of the supporting limb is higher. The stifle on the supporting limb is locked in position owing to a slight medial rotation of the patella as the medial patellar ligament and parapatellar cartilage slip farther caudad on the proximal part of the medial trochlear ridge. This action moves the medial patellar ligament to a position about twice as far from the cranial surface of the medial trochlear ridge as it was initially. A binding loop is thus completed with the middle patellar ligament. The locked position achieved by this configuration together with the support rendered by the other components of the stay apparatus minimizes muscular activity in the supporting limb while the relaxed contralateral hindlimb is resting. When the position is shifted, the patella snaps off the proximal part of the medial trochlear ridge.

Thigh and Hip

Extending from the hip to the stifle, the thigh includes the femur (femoral bone) and the structures around it. The region adjacent to and the muscles acting upon the coxal joint make up the hip (coxa).

Lateral Aspect

Cutaneous innervation is supplied to the lateral aspect of the thigh and hip by the lateral branches of the iliohypogastric and ilioinguinal nerves, the caudal cutaneous femoral nerve, and the dorsal branches of the lumbar and sacral nerves.[20]

From caudal to cranial the superficial muscles of the lateral thigh and hip are the semitendinosus, biceps femoris, gluteus superficialis, gluteus medius, and tensor fasciae latae. Both the semitendinosus and biceps femoris have ischiatic tuberal and vertebral origins. The semitendinosus attaches to the first and second caudal vertebrae and fascia of the tail, and the biceps femoris attaches to the dorsal sacroiliac ligament and the gluteal and tail fasciae. A prominent longitudinal groove marks the site of the intermuscular septum between the semitendinosus and the biceps femoris muscles.

The strong gluteal fascia gives origin to and unites the long caudal head and the cranial head of the gluteus superficialis muscle. Attachment is also provided by the coxal tuber and adjacent ilium, and by the intermuscular sep-

tum between the cranial head and the tensor fasciae latae muscle. The two heads of the gluteus superficialis muscle unite in a flat tendon that attaches to the trochanter tertius of the femur. Extending caudad from the aponeurosis of the longissimus lumborum muscle, the large gluteus medius (middle gluteal) muscle forms most of the mass of the rump. The gluteus medius muscle also takes origin from the gluteal surface of the ilium, the coxal tuber and sacral tuber, the sacrotuberal and dorsal sacroiliac ligaments, and the gluteal fascia. Distally the muscle attaches to the summit of the greater trochanter (trochanter major), a crest distal to the greater trochanter, and the lateral greater surface of the intertrochanteric crest.

The tensor fasciae latae muscle arises from the coxal tuber and fans out distally to insert into the fascia lata. An intermuscular septum attaches the caudal part of the muscle to the cranial head of the gluteus superficialis. The fascia lata (which is also tensed by the biceps femoris) attaches to the patella and the lateral and middle patellar ligaments (Fig. 1.52). The intermuscular septum between the biceps femoris and semitendinosus, the septa between the three divisions of the biceps femoris, and a septum between the biceps femoris and vastus lateralis all arise from the fascia lata.

Deeply on the lateral aspect of the hip, the smaller deep part of the gluteus medius (the gluteus accessorius) has a distinct flat tendon that plays over the convexity of the greater trochanter on its way to attach on the crest distal to the trochanter. The large trochanteric bursa lies between the tendon and the cartilage covering the convexity (Fig. 1.53). The small gluteus profundus (deep gluteal) muscle is deep to the caudal part of the gluteus medius, arising from the ischiatic spine and body of the ilium and attaching on the medial edge of the convexity of the greater trochanter (Fig. 1.54). This muscle covers the hip (coxal) joint and parts of the articularis coxae and rectus femoris muscles. A bursa is commonly present under the tendon of insertion of the gluteus profundus.[33]

The main head of the small, fusiform articularis coxae muscle arises from the ilium proximal to the lateral tendon of the rectus femoris, and a second head often takes origin between the lateral and medial tendons of the rectus femoris (Fig. 1.54). The articularis coxae extends over the lateral aspect of the hip joint to attach on the cranial surface of the femur. The muscle detaches fibers to the capsule of the hip joint.

On the caudal side of the proximal part of the femur the gemelli, external obturator, and internal obturator muscles come from their respective origins on the ischium, pubis, ilium, and wing of the sacrum to insert in the trochanteric fossa. The quadratus femoris muscle extends from the ventral aspect of the ischium to a line on the femur near the distal part of the lesser trochanter (trochanter minor).

A broad sheet of dense white fibrous connective tissue, the sacrotuberal ligament, forms most of the lateral wall of the pelvic cavity, attaching dorsally to the sacrum and first two caudal vertebrae and ventrally to the ischiatic spine and ischiatic tuber. The ventral edge of the sacrotuberal ligament completes the tissue-occluded lesser ischiatic foramen and the cranial edge completes the greater ischiatic foramen. The dorsal sacroiliac ligament has two parts: a bandlike part extending from the sacral tuber to the summits of the sacral spines, and a triangular part oc-

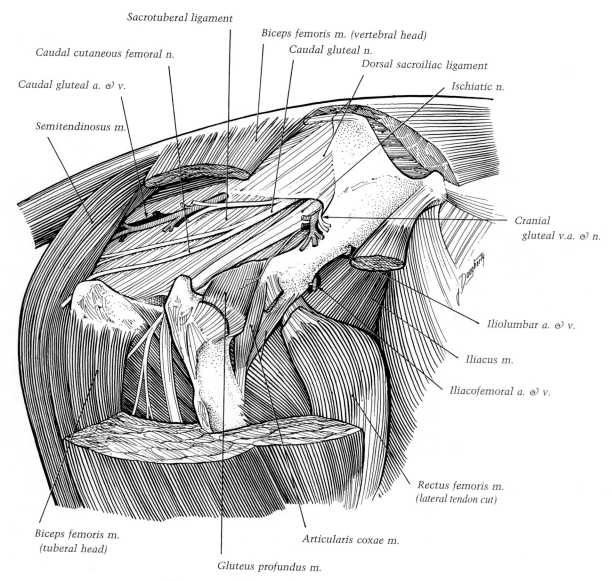

Sacrotuberal ligament

Biceps femoris m. (vertebral head)

Caudal cutaneous femoral n.

Caudal gluteal n.

Dorsal sacroiliac ligament

Caudal gluteal a. & v.

Ischiatic n.

Semitendinosus m.

Cranial gluteal v.a. & n.

Iliolumbar a. & v.

Iliacus m.

Iliacofemoral a. & v.

Rectus femoris m. (lateral tendon cut)

Biceps femoris m. (tuberal head)

Articularis coxae m.

Gluteus profundus m.

Figure 1.54 Deep dissection of right hip. Lateral view.

cupying the space between the sacral tuber and adjacent ilium and the lateral border of the sacrum and blending ventrally with the sacrotuberal ligament.

Branches of the cranial gluteal vessels and the cranial gluteal nerve come through the greater ischiatic foramen to supply the gluteal muscles, the tensor fasciae latae, and the articularis coxae. The caudal gluteal vessels and nerve perforate the sacrotuberal ligament dorsal to the ischiatic nerve. The caudal gluteal nerve divides into two trunks. The dorsal trunk supplies branches to the biceps femoris, gluteus medius, and long head of the gluteus superficialis, and after supplying a branch to the semitendinosus, the ventral trunk continues as the caudal cutaneous femoral nerve. The latter nerve goes through the biceps femoris and then outward between the biceps femoris and semitendinosus to branch subcutaneously over the lateral and caudal surfaces of the thigh and hip. Muscles in this region are supplied by branches from the cau-

dal gluteal vessels, the caudal gluteal artery also forming anastomoses with the medial circumflex femoral, caudal femoral, and obturator arteries. In this region the internal pudendal artery courses on the deep face and within the sacrotuberal ligament. Iliolumbar vessels (from the cranial gluteal vessels) course laterad between the iliacus muscle and the ilium, supplying branches to the iliopsoas and longissimus lumborum muscles. The vessels then go around the lateral border of the ilium and supply branches to the gluteus medius and tensor fasciae latae. The large, flat ischiatic (sciatic) nerve passes through the greater ischiatic foramen and courses ventrocaudad on the sacrotuberal ligament and then on the origin of the gluteus profundus. Turning distad, the ischiatic nerve passes over the gemelli, the tendon of the internal obturator, and the quadratus femoris, supplying branches to these muscles. A large branch is detached from the deep side of the nerve. This branch supplies branches to the semimembranosus and the tuberal heads of the biceps femoris and semitendinosus, and adductor medially, and to the biceps femoris laterally. After giving off the common peroneal nerve, the ischiatic nerve continues distad as the tibial nerve that passes between the two heads of the gastrocnemius muscle.

Medial Aspect

Cutaneous innervation to the medial aspect of the thigh is supplied by the lateral cutaneous femoral nerve; medial branches of the iliohypogastric, ilioinguinal, and genitofemoral nerves; and branches from the caudal cutaneous femoral and saphenous nerves.[20]

Accompanied by the small saphenous artery and the saphenous nerve, the large medial saphenous vein pursues a subcutaneous course cranioproximad on the cranial part of the gracilis muscle, then in between the gracilis and sartorius muscles to join the femoral vein in the femoral canal. Beneath the medial femoral fascia the broad gracilis muscle covers most of the medial aspect of the thigh. It attaches proximally to the symphysial (prepubic) tendon, adjacent surface of the pubis, accessory femoral ligament, and middle of the symphysis pelvis. The muscle belly ends distally by joining a wide thin tendon of insertion. A narrow sartorius muscle takes origin from the tendon of the psoas minor muscle and iliac fascia and descends toward its insertion in the stifle, which blends with the tendon of the gracilis.

Deep to the gracilis lies the cylindrical pectineus muscle. It attaches proximally to the cranial border of the pubis, the symphysial tendon, and accessory femoral ligament. Distally the pectineus attaches to the medial border of the femur adjacent to the entrance of the nutrient artery (from the femoral or caudal femoral artery) into the nutrient foramen. The femoral canal is delimited caudally by the pectineus, cranially by the sartorius, laterally by the vastus medialis and iliopsoas (combined iliacus and psoas major muscles), and medially by the femoral fascia and cranial edge of the gracilis. The canal contains the femoral artery and vein, the saphenous nerve (from the femoral nerve) and an elongated group of several lymph nodes of the deep inguinal lymphocenter embedded in adipose tissue. Within the canal the saphenous nerve detaches a motor branch to the sartorius muscle (Fig. 1.55).

Caudal to the pectineus and vastus medialis the thick, roughly prismatic adductor muscle extends from the ventral surface of the ischium and pubis and the origin of the gracilis muscle to the caudal surface of the femur, the medial femoral epicondyle, and the medial collateral ligament of the femorotibial joint. The obturator nerve comes through the cranial part of the obturator foramen and external obturator muscle and branches to supply the external obturator, adductor, pectineus, and gracilis muscles (see Fig. 1.55). Branches from the obturator artery (from the cranial gluteal artery) supply the muscles in this region.

Cranial Aspect

The quadriceps femoris, articularis coxae, and sartorius muscles are in the cranial part of the thigh and hip. The articularis coxae may also be viewed laterally; the sartorius, medially. In addition, the iliacus muscle crosses the cranial aspect of the hip where the muscle encloses the psoas major. Combined, they are termed the iliopsoas. The two muscles join in a common tendon that inserts on the lesser trochanter. The psoas major arises from the last two ribs and the lumbar transverse processes; the iliacus comes from the wing of the sacrum, ventral sacroiliac ligaments, sacropelvic surface of the ilium, and tendon of the psoas minor muscle.

Three heads of the quadriceps femoris muscle (the vastus lateralis, vastus intermedius, and vastus medialis) take origin from the shaft of the femur. The fourth head, the rectus femoris, originates from two tendons, one arising from a medial depression on the ilium craniodorsal to the acetabulum, and one from a lateral depression (Fig. 1.54). A constantly occurring bursa is located under the lateral tendon.[33] All four heads of the quadriceps femoris attach to the patella. Bursae occur commonly under the insertions of the rectus femoris, vastus lateralis, and vastus medialis.

The femoral nerve passes between the psoas minor (a small muscle extending from the lumbar vertebral bodies to the ilium) and the psoas major, then between the iliopsoas and sartorius muscles. It supplies branches to the iliopsoas (which also receives innervation from lumbar nerves) and to all heads of the quadriceps femoris.

Caudal Aspect of the Thigh

Innervation to the caudal skin of the thigh and hip is provided principally by the caudal cutaneous femoral nerve. The caudal rectal nerve supplies a small part dorsally. Deep to the skin and fascia, the main muscle mass is that of the semimembranosus. The semitendinosus and the caudal division of the biceps femoris relate to it laterally; the gracilis, medially. The long head of the semimembranosus attaches to the caudal border of the sacrotuberal ligament. The thicker short head attaches to the ventral part of the ischiatic tuber. The thick, roughly three-sided belly of the semimembranosus ends on a flat tendon that attaches to the medial femoral epicondyle.

Blood Supply to the Thigh

Before the external iliac artery passes through the femoral ring to continue as the femoral artery, it gives off the deep femoral artery. This vessel courses between the sartorius and iliopsoas muscles and then between the latter muscle and the pectineus. After supplying small branches to the deep inguinal lymphocenter, the deep femoral artery gives off the large pudendoepigastric trunk. The trunk divides into the cranially directed caudal epigastric artery and the external pudendal artery. Beyond the pudendoepigastric trunk, the deep femoral artery continues caudad ventral to the pubis as the medial circumflex femoral artery. The medial circumflex femoral artery supplies the iliopsoas, pectineus, external obturator muscles, the adductor (through which it passes), and the semimembranosus (where its branches end). Branches are also supplied to the deep inguinal lymphocenter and the gracilis and quadratus femoris muscles. Homonymous veins accompany the arteries.

The femoral artery courses distad through the femoral canal related caudally to the femoral vein and cranially to the saphenous nerve (Fig. 1.55). Within the canal the

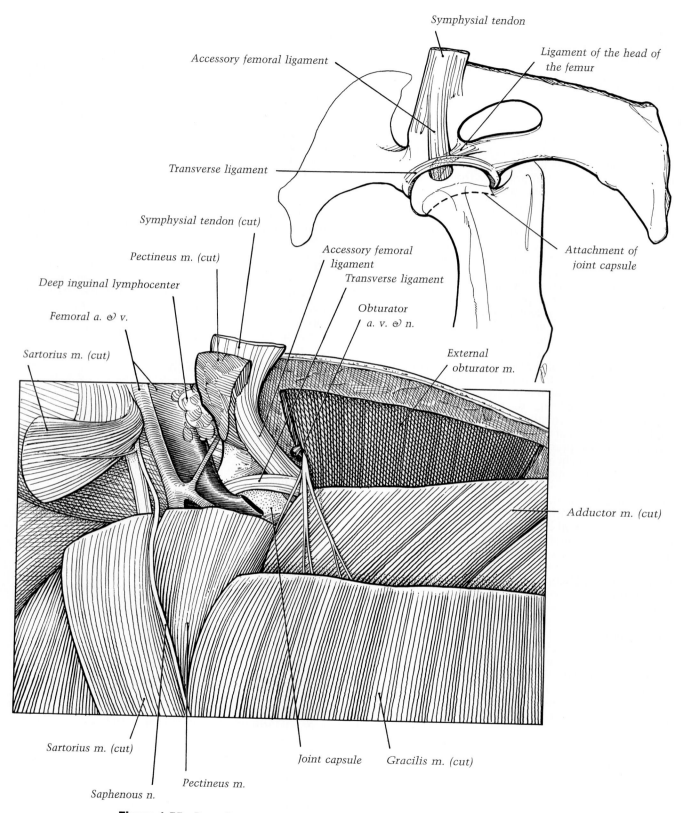

Figure 1.55 Deep dissection of right hip. Ventromedial view of ligaments of the hip joint.

femoral artery gives off the lateral circumflex femoral artery. This artery passes craniodistad between the sartorius and iliopsoas muscles and then enters the quadriceps femoris, passing between the vastus medialis and rectus femoris.

The femoral artery directly supplies branches to muscles in this region. At the distal end of the femoral canal, the saphenous artery leaves the femoral artery and passes out between the gracilis and sartorius muscles. This subcutaneous artery courses caudodistad, related caudally to the much larger medial saphenous vein. The saphenous nerve accompanies the vessels as they course caudodistad over the tendon of the gracilis. At the level of the tendon of insertion of the semitendinosus, the saphenous artery and medial saphenous vein each divide into cranial and caudal branches. In its course the saphenous artery supplies the sartorius, gracilis, and adductor muscles as well as fascia and skin.

The next branch of the femoral artery is the nutrient artery of the femur. Then the large descending genicular artery is detached from the cranial wall of the femoral artery. In the distal third of the thigh, the descending genicular artery courses distocraniad between the sartorius and vastus medialis and adductor, supplying these muscles and terminating in branches to structures of the stifle, including the femoropatellar and femorotibial joints.

From its caudal wall the termination of the femoral artery gives off its last branch, the caudal femoral artery, and continues between the medial and lateral heads of the gastrocnemius as the popliteal artery (Fig. 1.49). The caudal femoral artery pursues a short course caudad, giving off muscular branches to the superficial digital flexor and gastrocnemius. A branch runs distad to the crus, where it joins a branch of the caudal tibial artery. Then the caudal femoral artery divides into an ascending branch and a descending branch. The ascending branch courses proximad between the semimembranosus and adductor, supplying these muscles and sending branches to the lateral head of the gastrocnemius, vastus lateralis, biceps femoris, and semitendinosus muscles. The descending branch of the caudal femoral artery runs distocaudad over the lateral head of the gastrocnemius in company with the lateral saphenous vein. Then the artery changes direction and passes proximad between the semitendinosus and the biceps femoris supplying them and the small lymph nodes of the popliteal lymphocenter. A branch may also course proximad adjacent to the ischiatic nerve and anastomose with a branch from the obturator artery. A distally coursing branch supplies branches to both heads of the gastrocnemius and the superficial digital flexor and continues distad to join the saphenous artery (Fig. 1.41).

Hip (Coxal) Joint

The acetabulum of the os coxae (hip bone) is formed where the ilium, ischium, and pubis meet. The lunate surface of the acetabulum, a cotyloid cavity containing a deep nonarticular fossa, articulates with the head of the femur. The radius of curvature of the acetabulum is slightly greater than that of the femoral head. A fibrocartilaginous rim, the labrum acetabulare, increases the bony margin of the acetabulum. The transverse acetabular ligament continues from the labrum across the medially located acetabular notch, binding two ligaments as they emerge from the fovea capitis of the femoral head

(Fig. 1.55). The shorter ligament of the head of the femur comes from the narrow apex of the fovea and attaches in the pubic groove. The thick accessory femoral ligament arises from the wider, peripheral part of the fovea and passes out through the acetabular notch in a medial-cranial-ventral direction to be in the pubic groove. After giving partial origin to the gracilis and pectineus muscles, the accessory femoral ligament blends into the symphysial (prepubic) tendon. Among domestic animals, the accessory femoral ligament is peculiar to equids.

In an average-sized horse the volume of the spacious hip joint is around 50 mL.[51] The joint capsule attaches to the labrum acetabulare and on the neck of the femur a few millimeters from the margin of the femoral head (Fig. 1.55). Within the joint the synovial membrane wraps around the ligaments. An outpocketing of the synovial membrane passes out through the acetabular notch to lie between the accessory femoral ligament and the pubic groove. A small pouch also lies under the ligament of the head of the femur. The fibrous joint capsule is reinforced laterally and cranially by thick tracts of collagenous fibers. It is intimately attached to the epimysium of the external obturator and deep gluteal muscles. Adipose tissue covers the capsule dorsally. The articularis coxae muscle is related to the lateral aspect of the hip joint, detaching some fibers to the joint capsule. During flexion of the coxal joint, the articularis coxae can serve to tense the joint capsule.

Movements of the Coxal Joint

Whereas the coxal joint is a ball-and-socket joint (enarthrosis) capable of very limited rotation, the principal movements are flexion and extension. In equids, abduction of the thigh is restricted by the ligament of the head of the femur and the accessory femoral ligament. Adduction is checked by the attachments of the gluteal muscles on the femur. In the normal standing position, the caudolateral part of the head of the femur lies outside the acetabulum. The coxal joint is slightly flexed in this position, the cranial angle being around 115°.[18] The range of motion between extreme flexion and extension is only 60°.[51]

Flexor muscles of the hip joint are the gluteus superficialis, tensor fasciae latae, rectus femoris, iliopsoas, sartorius, and pectineus. Extensor muscles of the hip joint are the gluteus medius, biceps femoris, semitendinosus, semimembranosus, adductor, and quadratus femoris. Muscles adducting the thigh include the gracilis, sartorius, adductor, pectineus, quadratus femoris, and external obturator. Slight abduction is exerted on the thigh by all three gluteal muscles. The thigh is rotated laterad by the iliopsoas, external and internal obturators, and the gemelli. Medial rotation is accomplished through the combined action of the adductor and gluteus profundus muscles.

Sacroiliac Joint

Since it is provided with a joint capsule and since the roughened articular surfaces of the sacrum and ilium are covered with a minimal layer of hyaline cartilage, the nearly immovable sacroiliac joint is a synovial (diarthrodial) joint (Fig. 1.56). However, the joint cavity is just a slit, and it may be crossed by bands of dense white fibrous connective tissue.[18] As the animal ages, the apposed surfaces become even rougher. The joint is stabi-

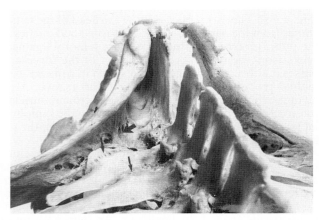

Figure 1.56 Photograph of sacroiliac joint (large arrow) and intertransverse joints (small arrows) in an osteologic preparation. Dorsocranial view.

lized by the surrounding strong fibrous bands of the ventral sacroiliac ligament.

Symphysis Pelvis

The medial borders of pubis and ischium from each side meet ventrally at the symphysis pelvis. In the young animal fibrocartilage joins the bones. Later in life a synostosis is formed as the cartilage ossifies in a cranial to caudal sequence.

Lymphatic Drainage

Two lymphocenters are involved in the lymphatic drainage of the pelvic limb. The popliteal lymphocenter consists of a few small deep popliteal lymph nodes embedded in adipose tissue between the biceps femoris and semitendinosus muscles adjacent to the tibial nerve just before the nerve plunges distad between the two heads of the gastrocnemius muscle (Fig. 1.49). They may be absent. The popliteal lymph nodes receive afferent lymphatic vessels from the pelvic limb distal to the lymphocenter. Efferent lymphatic vessels course proximad to the deep inguinal lymphocenter in the femoral canal.

Table 1.2 RANGES OF GROWTH PLATE (PHYSEAL) CLOSURE TIMES IN EQUINE PELVIC LIMBS[17]

Ilium, ischium, pubis	10–12 mos.
Secondary centers for crest, tuber coxae, ischiatic tuber and acetabular part of pubis	4½–5 yrs.
Femur	
Proximal	36–42 mos.
Distal	22–42 mos.
Tibia	
Proximal	36–42 mos.
Distal	17–24 mos.
Fibula	
Proximal	3½ yrs.
Distal (lateral malleolus of tibia)	3–24 mos.
Calcaneus	19–36 mos.

(Growth plate closure times for bones distal to the tarsus are similar to those distal to the carpus.)

In addition to receiving lymphatic vessels from the popliteal lymphocenter, the numerous lymph nodes of the deep inguinal lymphocenter (Fig. 1.55) receive afferent vessels from the caudal abdominal wall and superficial inguinal lymph nodes. Efferent vessels from the deep inguinal lymphocenter are afferent to the medial iliac lymph nodes.

Stay Apparatus of the Pelvic Limb (Fig. 1.57)

The quadriceps femoris muscle and the tensor fasciae latae act to pull the patella, parapatellar cartilage, and medial patellar ligament proximad to the locked position over the medial trochlear ridge of the femur when the limb is positioned to bear the weight of the caudal part of the trunk and the hip. Through the restraint of the components of the reciprocal apparatus (cranially, the peroneus tertius from the femur to the lateral tarsus and proximal metatarsus and, caudally, the superficial digital flexor from the femur to the calcaneal tuber) the tarsus is locked correspondingly. Minimal muscular activity assures continuation of this locked configuration, preventing flexion of the stifle and tarsocrural joints. Distal to the hock the digital flexor tendons support the pes plantarly, the superficial digital flexor extending distad from the calcaneal tuber and, in the midmetatarsus, the deep digital flexor usually receiving the accessory (subtarsal check) ligament of the deep digital flexor tendon from the thick plantar part of the tarsal fibrous joint capsule. Prevention of overextension of the fetlock joint during the fixed, resting position is accomplished through the support rendered by the digital flexor tendons on the way to their digital attachments, the two extensor branches of the suspensory ligament extending from the proximal sesamoid bones to the long digital extensor tendon, and the sesamoidean ligaments, particularly the three distal sesamoidean ligaments.

Growth Plate (Physeal) Closure

Table 1.2 summarizes the ranges of reported closure times for the growth plates (physes or epiphyseal cartilages) of bones in the pelvic limb.[18]

AXIAL CONTRIBUTORS TO LOCOMOTION

Hypaxial muscles of the trunk (the psoas minor, quadratus lumborum, and the four abdominal muscles on each side) act to flex the vertebral column during the gallop. Epaxial muscles of the trunk and neck (from lateral to medial, the iliocostalis system, the longissimus system, and the transversospinalis system) are extensors of the vertebral column. Acting unilaterally, the hypaxial and epaxial muscles are responsible for lateral movement of the trunk and neck.

Excluding the atlantoaxial joint (a trochoid joint), the joints of the vertebral column all permit flexion, extension, lateral flexion, and even limited rotation. Whereas these movements are limited at each joint, taken as a whole, the movement is fairly extensive. Intervertebral discs of fibrocartilage (with a peripheral anulus fibrosus

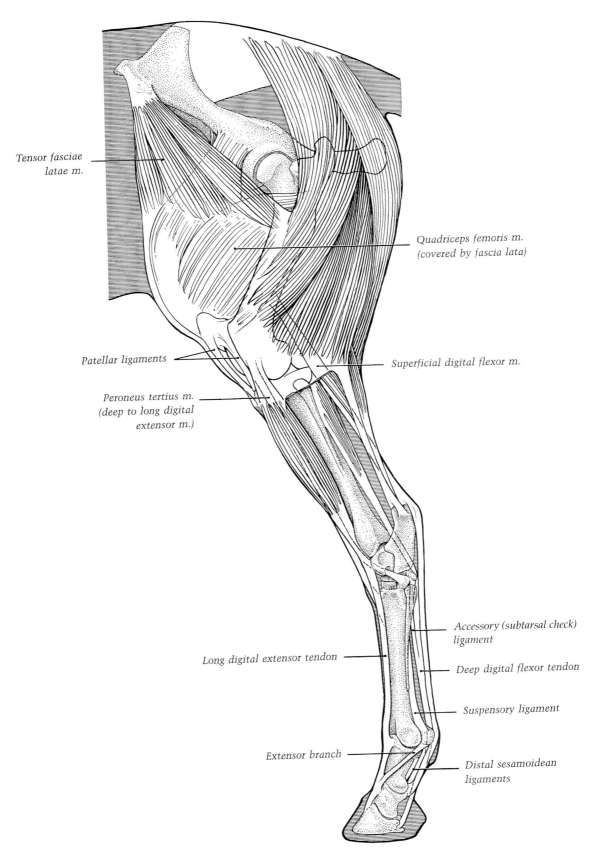

Tensor fasciae
latae m.

Quadriceps femoris m.
(covered by fascia lata)

Patellar ligaments

Superficial digital flexor m.

Peroneus tertius m.
(deep to long digital
extensor m.)

Accessory (subtarsal check)
ligament

Long digital extensor tendon

Deep digital flexor tendon

Suspensory ligament

Extensor branch

Distal sesamoidean
ligaments

Figure 1.57   Stay apparatus of left pelvic limb.

and a central nucleus pulposus) are interposed between adjacent vertebral bodies. These are termed symphysial joints. Joint cavities exist between the last cervical and first thoracic vertebral bodies and between the last lumbar and first sacral vertebral bodies.[18] Support is rendered to the vertebral column by the continuous dorsal and ventral longitudinal ligaments on their respective surfaces of the vertebral bodies. In the cervical region the dorsal longitudinal ligament is poorly developed and blends with the periosteum. Intercapital ligaments between the heads of contralateral ribs bind down intervertebral discs in the thoracic region of the vertebral column. Articulations between articular processes on vertebral arches are true joints—arthrodial in the cervical and thoracic regions, and trochoid in the lumbar region. True joints also exist between the transverse processes of the fifth and sixth lumbar vertebrae and between the transverse processes of the sixth lumbar vertebra and the wings of the sacrum (see Fig. 1.56).

References

1. Balch O, White K, Butler D. Factors involved in the balancing of equine hooves. J Am Vet Med Assoc 1991;198:1980.
2. Banks WJ. Applied Veterinary Histology. 3rd ed. St. Louis, MO: Mosby-Year Book, 1993.
3. Bertram JEM, Gosline JM. Fracture toughness design in horse hoof. J Exp Biol 1986;125:29.
4. Bertram JEA, Gosline JM. Functional design of horse hoof keratin: The modulation of mechanical properties through hydration effects. J Exp Biol 1987;130:121.
5. Blythe LL, Kitchell RL. Electrophysiologic studies of the thoracic limb of the horse. Am J Vet Res 1982;43:1511.
6. Bowker RM, Linder K, Van Wulfen KK, et al. An anatomical study of the distal interphalangeal joint in the horse: Its relationship to the navicular suspensory ligaments, sensory nerves and neurovascular bundle. Equine Vet J 1997;29:126.
7. Bowker RM, Rockershouser SJ, Vex KB, et al. Immunocytochemical and dye distribution studies of nerves potentially desensitized by injections into the distal interphalangeal joint or navicular bursa of horses. J Am Vet Med Assoc 1993;203:1708.
8. Bowker RM, Van Wulfen KK. Microanatomy of the intersection of the distal sesamoidean impar ligament and the deep digital flexor tendon: a preliminary report. Pferdeheilkunde 1996;12:623.
9. Bowker RM, Van Wulfen KK, Springer SE, Linder KE. Functional anatomy of the cartilage of the distal phalanx and digital cushion in the equine foot and a hemodynamic flow hypothesis of energy dissipation. Am J Vet Res 1998;59:961.
10. Colles CM, Garner HE, Coffman JR. The blood supply of the horse's foot. Proc Am Assoc Equine Pract 1979;385.
11. Colles CM, Hickman J. The arterial supply of the navicular bone and its variation in navicular disease. Equine Vet J 1977;9:150.
12. Denoix JM. Functional anatomy of tendons and ligaments in the distal limbs (manus and pes). Vet Clin North Am Equine Pract 1994;10:273.
13. Derksen FG. Diagnostic local anesthesia of the equine front limb. Equine Pract 1980;2:41.
14. Dyce KM, Sack WO, Wensing CJG. Textbook of Veterinary Anatomy. Philadelphia: WB Saunders, 1987.
15. Emery L, Miller J, Van Hoosen N. Horseshoeing Theory and Foot Care. Philadelphia: Lea & Febiger, 1977.
16. Ernst RR. Die Bedeutung der Wandepidermis (Hyponychium) des Pferdehufes fur die Hornbildung. Acta Anat 1954;22:15.
17. Garrett PD. Anatomy of the dorsoscapular ligament of horses. J Am Vet Med Assoc 1990;196:446.
18. Getty R. Sisson and Grossman's The Anatomy of the Domestic Animals, Vol 1. 5th ed. Philadelphia: WB Saunders, 1975.
19. Goetz TE. Anatomic, hoof and shoeing considerations for the treatment of laminitis in horses. J Am Vet Med Assoc 1987;190:1323.
20. Grau H. Die Hautinnervation an den Gliedmassen des Pferdes. Arch Wochenschr Prakt Tierheilk 1935;69:96.
21. Grosenbaugh DA, Hood DM. Practical equine hoof wall biochemistry. Equine Pract 1993;15:8.
22. James PT, Kemler AG, Smallwood JE. The arterial supply to the distal sesamoid bones of the equine thoracic and pelvic limbs. J Vert Orthoped 1983;2:38.
23. Koch T. Die Nervenversorgung der Hinterzehe des Pferdes. Berl Munch Tierarztl Wochenschr 1939;28:440.
24. Koch T. P Uber die Nervenversorgung der Gliedmassenspitzen des Pferdes. Tierarztl Rundschau 1938;44:333.
25. Krolling O, Grau H. Lehrbuch der Histologie und vergleichenden mikroskopischen Anatomie der Haustiere. 10th ed. Berlin: P. Parey, 1960.
26. Landeau LJ, Barnett DJ, Batterman SC. Mechanical properties of equine hooves. Am J Vet Res 1983;44:100.
27. Leach D. Biomechanical considerations in raising and lowering the heel. Proc Am Assoc Equine Pract 1983;33.
28. Leach DH, Oliphant LW. Ultrastructure of equine hoof wall secondary epidermal lamellae. Am J Vet Res 1983;44:1561.
29. Mettam AE. On the development and histology of (1) the hoof wall and subjacent soft structures of the horse's foot, and (2) the structure of the frog, with a description of the sweat glands and some nerve-endings found therein. Veterinarian 1896;69:85.
30. Mishra PC, Leach DH. Extrinsic and intrinsic veins of the equine hoof wall. J Anat 1983;136:543.
31. Nilsson SA. Bidrag till kannedomen om fotens innervation hos hast. (Engl. summary). Skandinavisk Veterinar-Tidskrift 1948;38:401.
32. Nomina Anatomica Veterinaria. World Association of Veterinary Anatomists. 3rd ed. 1983.
33. Ottaway CA, Worden AN. Bursae and tendon sheaths of the horse. Vet Rec 1940;52:477.
34. Pohlmeyer K, Redecker R. Die fur die Klinik bedeutsamen Nerven an dem Gliedemassen des Pferdes einschliesslich moglicher Varianten. Deutsche Tierarztl Wochenschr 1974;81:501.
35. Pollitt CC, Molyneux GS. A scanning electron microscopical study of the dermal microcirculation of the equine foot. Equine Vet J 1990;22:79.
36. Preuss F, Eggers H. Zur Radialishlahmung des Pferdes. Tierarztl Umschau 1951;6:435.
37. Reeves MJ, Trotter GW, Kainer RA. Anatomical and functional communications between synovial sacs of the equine stifle joint. Equine Vet J 1991;23:215.
38. Rooney JR, Quddus MA, Kingsbury HB. A laboratory investigation of the function of the stay apparatus of the equine foreleg. J Emu Med Surg 1978;2:173.
39. Sack WO. Subtendinous bursa on the medial aspect of the equine carpus. J Am Vet Med Assoc 1976;165:315.
40. Sack WO. Nerve distribution in the metacarpus and front digit of the horse. J Am Vet Med Assoc 1975;167:298.
41. Sack WO, Habel RE. Rooney's Guide to the Dissection of the Horse. Ithaca, NY: Veterinary Textbooks, 1977.
42. Sack WO, Orsini PG. Distal intertarsal and tarsometatarsal joints in the horse: Communication and injection sites. J Am Vet Med Assoc 1981;179:355.
43. Schummer A, Wilkens H, Vollmerhaus B, et al. Nickel, Schummer and Seiferle's The Anatomy of the Domestic Animals, Vol 3. New York: Springer-Verlag, 1981.
44. Smallwood JE. A Guided Tour of Veterinary Anatomy. Philadelphia: WB Saunders, 1992.
45. Smith F. A Manual of Veterinary Physiology. 4th ed. London: Bailliere, Tindall and Cox, 1912.
46. Southwood LL, Stashak TS, Kainer RA. Tenoscopic anatomy of the equine carpal flexor synovial sheath. Vet Surg 1998;27:150.
47. Stump JE. Anatomy of the normal equine foot, including microscopic features of the laminar region. J Am Vet Med Assoc 1967;151:1588.
48. Talukdar AJ, Calhoun ML, Stinson AW. Sweat glands of the horse: A histologic study. Am J Vet Res 1970;31:2179.
49. Updike SJ. Functional anatomy of the equine tarsocrural collateral ligaments. Am J Vet Res 1984;45:867.
50. Wilson DA, Baker GJ, Pijanowski GJ, et al. Composition and morphologic features of the interosseous muscle in Standardbreds and Thoroughbreds. Am J Vet Res 1991;52:133.
51. Zietzschmann D, Ackernecht E, Grau H. Ellenberger and Baum's Handbuch der vergliechenden Anatomie der Haustiere. 18th ed. Berlin: Springer-Verlag, 1977.

Conformation and Movement

TED S. STASHAK AND CHERRY HILL

To develop an appreciation of lameness and gait defects, it is important to have an understanding of conformation and movement. While many lamenesses occur in the lower limbs, the causative factors may be located in the upper limbs or body; therefore, overall conformation must be considered. Certain conformation traits can predispose to lameness, and these should be eliminated through responsible breeding. Understanding the relationship between conformation, movement, and lameness is essential for making wise breeding decisions and devising sound management and training programs.

CONFORMATION

Conformation refers to the physical appearance and outline of a horse as dictated primarily by bone and muscle structures.[21] It is impractical to set a single standard of perfection or to specifically define *ideal* or *normal* conformation, because the guidelines would depend on the classification, type, breed, and intended use of the horse. Therefore, a conformation evaluation must relate to function.[1,6]

When conformational discrepancies are identified, it is important to differentiate between "blemishes" and "unsoundnesses." Blemishes are scars and irregularities that do not affect the serviceability of the horse. Unsoundnesses cause a horse to be lame or otherwise unserviceable. Superficial scars from old wire cuts, small focal muscle (atrophies), and white spots from old injuries are considered blemishes if they do not affect the horse's soundness. Examples of unsoundnesses include but are not limited to blindness, parrot mouth, defective hearing, heaves, roaring, cryptorchidism, sterility, and lameness caused from such conditions as navicular syndrome, wounds, ring bone, spavin, and bowed tendons.

TYPES AND BREEDS

Horses are classified as draft horses, light horses, or ponies. Classifications are further divided by type (Fig. 2.1) according to overall body style and conformation and the work for which the horse is best suited. Light (riding and driving) horses can be described as one of six types: pleasure horse, hunter, stock horse, sport horse, animated (show) horse, and racehorse.

Pleasure horses have comfortable gaits, are conformed (designed) for ease of riding, and are typified by smooth movement in any breed. Hunters move with a long, low (horizontal) stride, are suited to cross-country riding and negotiating hunter fences, and are typified by the American Thoroughbred. Stock horses are well muscled, agile, and quick, are suited to working cattle, and are typified by the American Quarter Horse. The sport horse can be one of two types: a large, athletic horse suited for one or all of the disciplines of eventing (dressage, cross-country, and jumping) and typified by the European warmbloods; or a small, lean, tough horse suited for endurance events and typified by the Arabian. The animated (show) horse is one with highly cadenced, flashy gaits (usually with a high degree of flexion), is suited mainly for the showring, and is typified by the American Saddlebred. The racehorse is lean in relation to height, with a deep but not round barrel, and is typified by the racing Thoroughbred.

A "breed" is a group of horses with common ancestry and usually strong conformational similarities. In most cases, a horse must come from approved breeding stock to be registered with a particular breed. If a horse is not eligible for registration, it is considered a "grade" or "crossbred" horse.

Several breeds can have similar makeup and be of the same type. For example, most Quarter Horses, Paint Horses, and Appaloosas are considered to be stock horse types. Some breeds contain individuals of different types within the breed. American Thoroughbreds can be of the race, hunter, or sport horse type.

METHOD OF EVALUATION

Although breed characteristics vary greatly, the process of evaluating any horse is similar. First, a general assessment of the horse's four functional sections is made, giving each section approximately equal importance. (Wildly colored horses and those with dramatic limb markings can result in visual distortions and inaccurate conclusions.) The horse's conformational compo-

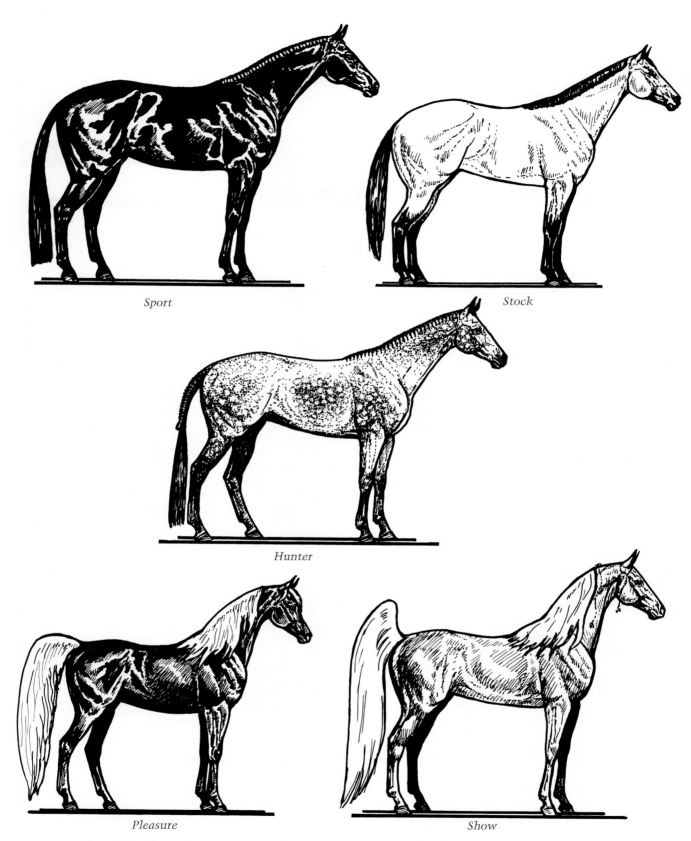

Sport

Stock

Hunter

Pleasure

Show

Figure 2.1   Types of horses: sport, stock, hunter, pleasure, show. (Reprinted with permission from Hill C. From the Center of the Ring. Pownal, VT: Garden Way Publishing, 1988.)

nents are then evaluated in detail. The horse is viewed in a systematic fashion and the observations are summarized.

Systematic Conformation Evaluation

Evaluation begins by viewing the horse from the near (left) side in profile, and assessing balance by comparing the forehand (head, neck, and forelimbs) to the hindquarters (hindlimbs and croup). When viewing the horse in profile, attention must be paid to the curvature and proportions of the topline. The horse should be observed from poll to tail and down to the gaskin. Then the attachment of the appendicular skeleton (limbs) to the axial skeleton (head and trunk) is observed. Limb angles are evaluated.

From the front of the horse, the limbs and hooves are evaluated for straightness and symmetry. The depth and length of the muscles in the forearm and chest are observed. The head, eyes, nostrils, and ears are evaluated, and the teeth are examined.

Then, from the off (right) side, the evaluation of the balance, topline, and limb angles is confirmed or modified.

The hindquarters are observed from directly behind. The tail, the straightness and symmetry of the back, the croup, the point of hip and buttock, and the limbs are evaluated. Observation should be made slowly from the poll to the tail, because this is the best vantage point for evaluating back muscling, alignment of the vertebral column, and (provided the horse is standing square) left-to-right symmetry. The observer's position may need to be elevated if the horse is tall. The spring (width and curve) of rib is also best observed from the rear.

The observer then makes another entire circle around the horse, this time stopping at each quadrant to look diagonally across the center of the horse. From the rear of the horse, the observer steps to the left hind and looks toward the right front. This angle will often reveal abnormalities in the limbs and hooves that were missed during the side, front, and rear examinations. The horse is then viewed from the left front toward the right hind and from the right front toward the left hind. The revolution is completed at the right hind looking toward the left front. Finally, from the near side, the whole horse is viewed once again in profile.

While looking at a horse, it is helpful to obtain an overall sense of the correctness of each of the four functional sections: the head and neck, the forelimbs, the trunk (barrel), and the hindlimbs.

Head and Neck

The vital senses are located in the head, so it should be correct and functional. The neck acts as a lever to help regulate the horse's balance while moving; therefore, it should be long and flexible, with a slight convex curve to its topline.[6]

Forelimbs

The forelimbs support approximately 60 to 65% of the horse's body weight, so they should be well muscled and conformed normally.[1]

Trunk (Barrel)

The midsection houses the vital organs; therefore, the horse must be adequate in the heart girth and must have good width (spring) to the ribs. The back should be well muscled and strong so that the horse is able to carry the weight of its internal organs and the rider and saddle.

Hindlimbs

The hindlimbs are the source of power for propulsion and stopping. The hindlimb muscling should be appropriate for type, breed, and use. The croup and points of the hip and buttock should be symmetric, and the limbs should be straight and sound.

CONFORMATION COMPONENTS

Balance

A well-balanced horse has a better chance of moving efficiently, thereby experiencing less stress. Balance refers to the relationship between the forehand and hindquarters, between the limbs and the body, and between the right and the left sides of the body (Figs. 2.2 through 2.4).

The center of gravity is a theoretical point in the horse's body around which the mass of the horse is equally distributed. At a standstill, the center of gravity is located at the point of intersection of a vertical line dropped from the highest point of the withers and a line from the point of the shoulder to the point of the buttock. This usually is a spot just behind the xiphoid and two-thirds the distance down from the topline of the back. (Fig. 2.4).

Although the center of gravity remains relatively constant when a well-balanced horse moves, most horses must learn to rebalance their weight (and that of the rider and tack) when ridden. To simply pick up a front foot to step forward, the horse must shift its weight toward the rear. How far the weight must shift to the hindquarters depends on the horse's conformation, the position of the rider, the gait, the degree of collection, and the style of the performance. The higher the degree of collection, the more the horse steps under the center of gravity with the hindlimbs.

If the forehand is proportionately larger than the hindquarters, especially if it is associated with a downhill topline, the horse's center of gravity tends to shift forward. This causes the horse to travel heavy on its front end, setting the stage for increased concussion, stress, and lameness. When the forehand and hindquarters are balanced and the withers are level with or higher than the level of the croup, the horse's center of gravity is located more toward the rear. Such a horse can carry more weight with its hindquarters, thus moving in balance and exhibiting a lighter, freer motion with the forehand than the horse with withers lower than the croup.

When evaluating young horses, the growth spurts that result in a temporarily uneven topline should be taken into consideration. Generally horses approach level at 3 years of age. However, 2-year-olds that show an extremely downhill configuration should be suspect. Even

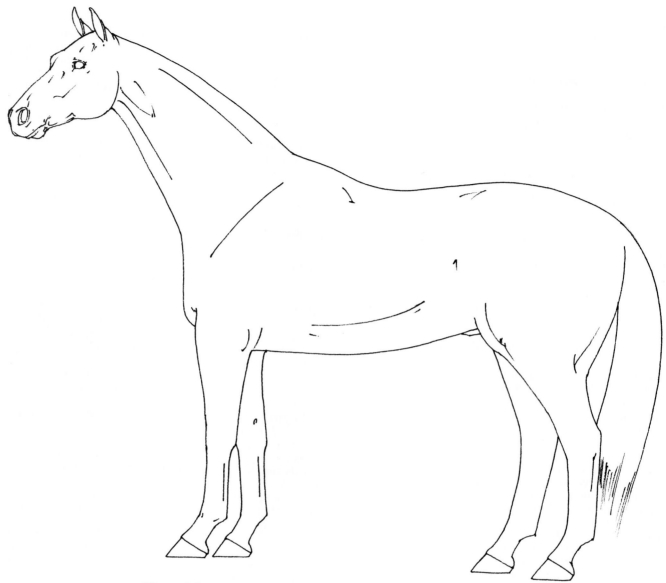

Figure 2.2   Normal horse. The body and limbs should be well proportioned.

if a horse's topline is level, if the forehand is excessively heavily muscled in comparison to the hindquarters, the horse is probably going to travel heavy on the forehand and have difficulty moving forward freely.

A balanced horse has approximately equal lower limb length and depth of body. The lower limb length (chest floor to the ground) should be equal to the distance from the chest floor to the top of the withers (Fig. 2.4). Proportionately shorter lower limbs are associated with a choppy stride. The horse's height or overall limb length (point of withers to ground) should approximate the length of the horse's body (the point of the shoulder to the point of buttock) (Fig. 2.4). A horse with a body that is a great deal longer than its height often experiences difficulty in synchronization and coordination of movement. A horse with limbs proportionately longer than the body may be predisposed to forging, overreaching, and other gait defects.

Overall, the right side of the horse should be symmetric to the left side.

Proportions and Curvature of the Topline

The ratio of the topline's components, the curvature of the topline, the strength of loin (longissimus dorsi muscles in the lumbar region), the sharpness of withers, the slope to the croup, and the length of the underline in relation to the length of back all affect a horse's movement.

The neck is measured from the poll to the highest point of the withers (Fig. 2.4). The back measurement is taken from the withers to the caudal extent of the loin located in front of the pelvis. The hip length is measured from the caudal loin to the point of buttock (Figs. 2.4 and 2.5).

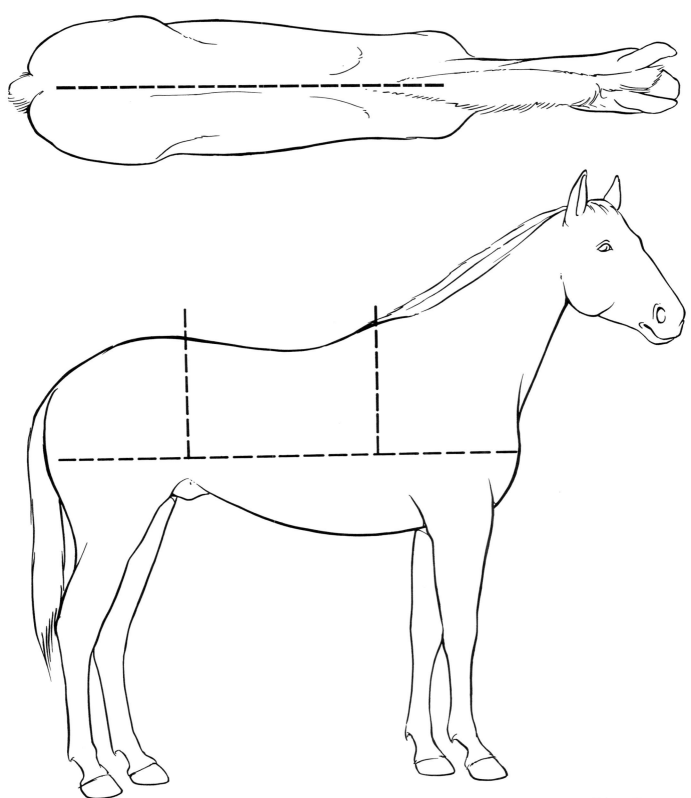

Figure 2.3   Top. Axial alignment is evaluated. A line drawn from the center of the withers through the center of the back roughly divides the body into two equal halves. Bottom. Balance is evaluated by dividing the body into three equal parts.

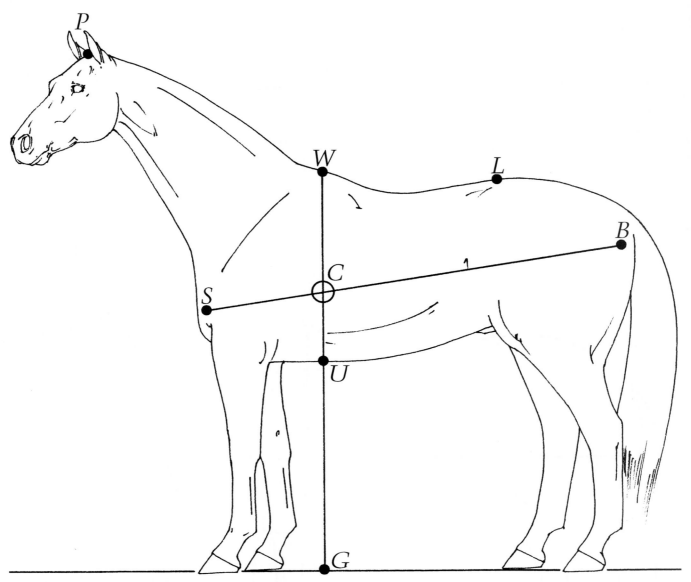

Figure 2.4 Proportions. P, poll; W, highest point of withers; L, caudal loin; B, point of buttock; S, point of shoulder; C, center of gravity; U, underline, G, ground; WU, depth of body; UG, lower limb length; WG, height and overall limb length; SB, length of body; PW, length of neck; WL, length of back; LB, length of hip. (Reprinted with permission from Hill C, Klimesh R. Maximum Hoof Power. North Pomfret, VT: Trafalgar Square Publishing, 2000.)

A neck that is shorter than the back tends to decrease a horse's overall flexibility and balance. A back that is very much longer than the neck tends to hollow. A very short hip, in relation to the neck or back, is associated with lack of propulsion and often a downhill configuration. A general rule of thumb is that the neck length should be greater than or equal to the back length and that the hip should be at least two-thirds the length of the back (Fig. 2.4).

The neck should have a graceful shape that rises up out of the withers, not dipping ventrad (downward) in front of the withers. The shape of the neck is determined by the "S" shape formed by the seven cervical vertebrae. A longer, flatter (more horizontal) attachment of the upper cervical vertebrae (C1–C2) at the poll results in a

cleaner, more flexible throat latch. If the upper cervical vertebrae form a short, straight attachment to the skull, it results in a thick throat latch and a hammerhead appearance. The attachment of the lower neck (caudal cervical region) should be short and shallow and should attach relatively high on the horse's chest. The thickest point in the neck is at the ventral limits. Ewe-necked horses have necks that have a long, ventral curve and that appear to attach low on the chest. The attachment of the neck muscles to the shoulders should be smooth. Prominent depressions in the muscles in front of the shoulders are undesirable.

The dorsal (upper) neck length (poll to withers) should be twice the ventral (lower) neck length (throat latch to chest). This is dictated to a large degree by the

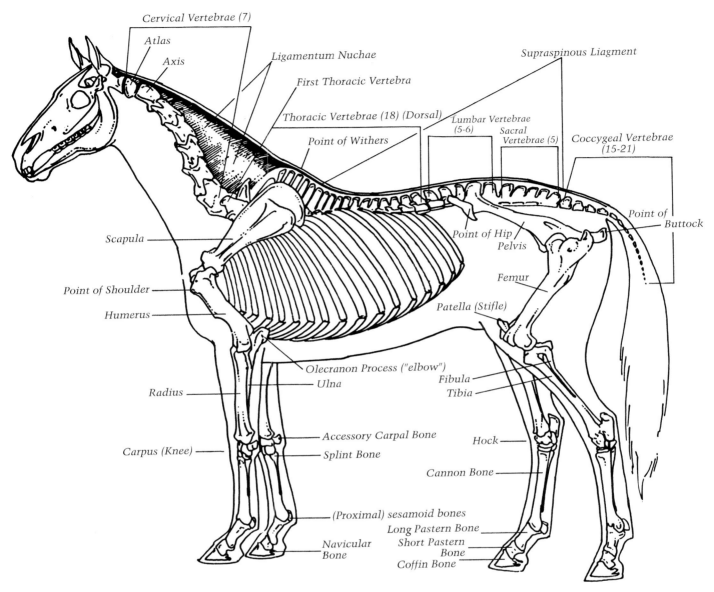

Figure 2.5 Equine skeleton. (Reprinted with permission from Hill C. Making Not Breaking. Ossining, NY: Breakthrough Publications, 1992.)

slope of the shoulder. A horse with a steep shoulder has an undesirable ratio (approaching 1:1) between the dorsal neck length and ventral neck length.

The back should look like it has a natural place for a saddle, beginning with prominent withers located above or behind the heart girth. The withers should blend gradually into the back, ending ideally at about the midpoint of the back. The withers provide a place for the neck and forearm muscles and the ligamentum nuchae to anchor; the neck muscles should attach at the highest point of the withers. There should not be a prominent dip in the muscles in front of or behind the withers.

The withers also act as a fulcrum. As a horse lowers and extends its neck, the back rises. Low (mutton) withers limit a horse's ability to raise its back. A horse with a well-sloped shoulder usually has correctly placed with-

ers. The heart girth should be deep, which provides adequate room for the heart and lungs.

The longissimus muscles that run along the spine should be flat and appear strong, rather than sloped and weak. The back muscles aid in counteracting the gravitational pull from the weight of the horse's internal organs as well as support the rider's weight.

The loin is located along the lumbar vertebrae from the last thoracic vertebrae to the lumbosacral junction (Fig. 2.5). The loin should be well muscled and relatively short. Horses termed "long-backed" often have an acceptable back length but a long, weak loin. A horse with a weak and/or long loin and loose coupling (flanks) tends to have a hollow back. (The coupling is the area behind the ribs and in front of a vertical line dropped from the point of hip.) A horse that chronically hollows its back may be predisposed to focal lumbar myofacial pain, pinched nerves, or vertebral damage.

The loin and the coupling transfer the motion of the hindquarters up through the back and forward to the forehand; therefore, they must be strong and well connected. A short, heavily muscled loin has great potential strength, power, and durability but may lack the flexibility of a more moderately muscled loin. A lumpy appearance in the loin may indicate abnormal alignment (subluxations) of the vertebrae.

The croup is measured from the lumbosacral junction to the tail head (Fig. 2.5). The croup should be fairly long, as this is associated with a good length to the hip and a desirable forward-placement of lumbosacral articulation.

The topline (the back) should be short in relation to the underline. Such a combination indicates strength plus desirable length of stride.

Head

The head should appear symmetrical and functional. Adequate cranial space is necessary. The length from the ear to the eye should be at least one-third the distance from the ear to the nostril. The width between the eyes should be a similar distance as that from the ear to the eye. A wide-open throat latch permits an adequate airway during flexion; a narrow throat latch is often associated with a ewe-neck attachment. Eyes set off to the side of the head allow the horse to have a panoramic view.[6] The eye should be prominent without bulging. Prominence refers to the bony orbit, not a protruding eyeball. The expression of the eye should indicate a quiet, tractable temperament.

The muzzle can be trim, but if it is too small, the nostrils may be pinched. There may also be inadequate space for the incisor teeth, resulting in dental misalignments. The width of the cheek bones indicates the space for molar teeth; adequate room is required for sideways grinding of food. The shape of the nasal bone and forehead is largely a matter of breed and personal preference.

Quality

Quality is depicted by "flat" cannon (third metacarpal/metatarsal) bones, clean (unswollen) joints, sharply defined (refined) features, smooth muscling, overall blending of parts, and a fine, smooth hair coat. "Flat" bone is a misnomer because the cannon bone is round. "Flat" refers to well-defined tendons that stand out cleanly behind the cannon bone and give the impression, when viewed from the side, that the cannon bone is flat.

Substance

"Substance" describes the thickness, depth, and breadth of bone, muscle, and other tissues. Muscle substance is described by type of muscle, thickness of muscle, length of muscles, and position of attachment. Other substance factors include weight and height of the horse, size of the hooves, depth of the heart girth and flank, and spring of rib.

"Spring of rib," which is best viewed from the rear, refers to the curve of the ribs. In addition to providing room for the heart, lungs, and digestive tract, a well-sprung rib cage provides a natural, comfortable place for a rider's legs. A slab-sided horse with a shallow heart girth is difficult to sit upon properly; an extremely wide-barreled horse can be stressful to the rider's legs.

"Substance of bone" refers to adequacy of the bone to weight ratio. Traditionally, the circumference around the cannon bone just below the carpus (knee) serves as the measurement for substance of bone. For riding horses, an adequate ratio is approximately 0.7 inches of bone for every 100 lb. of body weight. Using that rule, a 1200-lb. horse should have an 8.4-inch cannon bone.

Correctness of Angles and Structures

The correct alignment of the skeletal components provides the framework for muscular attachments. The length and slope of the shoulder, arm, forearm, croup, hip, stifle, and pasterns should be moderate and should work well together. There should be a straight alignment of bones when viewed from the front and rear, large clean joints, high-quality hoof horn, adequate height and width of heel, concave sole, and adequate size hoof.

Forelimbs

CRANIAL VIEW

Both forelimbs should appear to be of equal length and size, and should appear to bear equal weight. A line dropped from the point of the shoulder (middle of the scapulohumeral joint) to the ground should bisect the limb. The toes should point forward, and the feet should be as far apart on the ground as the limbs are at their origin in the chest (Fig. 2.6). The shoulder should be well muscled without being heavy and coarse.

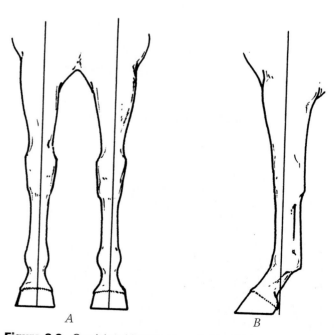

Figure 2.6 Cranial and lateral views of normal forelimbs. A. Line dropped from the point of the shoulder joint bisects the limb. B. Line from the tuber spinae of the scapula bisects the limb as far as the fetlock and drops at the heel.

The manner in which the shoulder blade and arm (humerus) are conformed and attach to the chest dictates, to a large degree, the alignment of the lower limbs. Whether the toes point in or out is often a result of upper limb structures. This is the reason it is dangerous, in many cases, to attempt to alter a limb's structure and alignment through radical hoof adjustments. It is important to be sure the horse is standing square when assessing the lower limbs.

The medial-lateral slope of the humerus is evaluated by finding the left point of shoulder and a spot in front of the left point of elbow. The same is done on the right side. The four points are then connected visually. If the resulting box is square, the humerus lies in an ideal position for straight lower limbs and straight travel. If the bottom of the box is wider, the horse may toe-in and travel with loose elbows and paddle. If the bottom of the box is narrower, the horse will probably toe-out, have tight elbows, and wing in.

The muscles of the forearm (antebrachium) should go all the way to the knee, ending in a gradual taper rather than ending abruptly a few inches above the knee. It is generally believed that this will allow the horse to use its front limbs in a smooth, sweeping, forward motion. The pectoral muscles should also reach far down onto the limb. The pectoral and the forearm muscles help a horse to move its limbs laterally and medially as well as to elevate the forelimb. It is the belief of some horsemen that the combination of long forearms and short cannon bones on horses is conducive to speed.[19]

The carpal joints should be balanced, and should not deviate toward or away from one another. The cannon bone should be centered under the carpus and not to the lateral side (Bench knees). Deviations from a straight limb will cause strain on the collateral support structures and asymmetric loading (compression) of the hinge joints in the forelimb.

Lateral View

Limbs, when viewed from the side, should exhibit a composite of moderate angles so that shock absorption is efficient (Fig. 2.7). The shoulder angle is measured along the spine of the scapula, from the point of the shoulder to the point of the withers. The shorter and straighter the shoulder, the shorter and quicker the stride is, the more stress and concussion is transmitted to the limb, and thus the greater is the risk of developing lameness.[15,22] Retrospective studies in dressage horses and show jumpers showed that a more horizontal scapula was related to a higher level of performance.[14,18] Also important is the angle the shoulder makes with the arm, which should be at least 90° but is most often > 100°. Horses with a more horizontal scapula or a more flexed shoulder joint show more maximal extension of the elbow joint relative to the angle at initial ground contact. This prolongs the stance phase.[3] It is also known that good gait and collection of performance horses is associated with longer stance duration in the forelimbs.[4,16]

The length of the humerus, from the point of the shoulder to the point of elbows, also affects stride length. A long humerus is associated with a long, reaching stride and good lateral ability; a short humerus is related to a short, choppy stride and poor lateral ability. The steeper the angle of the humerus, generally, the higher the action; the closer the angle is to horizontal, the lower the action. The scapulohumeral (shoulder) joint is supported entirely by the muscles and tendons surrounding it. This purely muscular support allows the joint freedom of movement during flight, which is in keeping with its ball-and-socket arrangement. Because this muscle support is so important, a horse should have well-developed muscles in this region.

The angle formed by the humerus and radius and ulna at the elbow joint should be between 120 and 150°. Together with a horizontal scapula, a more flexed elbow results in a longer stance duration, which improves gait quality by increasing collection in the forelimbs.[4,16] Straighter conformation (lesser angulation) at this joint results in a short, choppy gait and increased concussion on the distal limb. The radius and ulna should be of sufficient length to provide good muscular function.

Ideally, the limb should form a straight column from the elbow joint to the fetlock. This conformation will disseminate the axial compression forces to all bony surfaces equally. If the bones are out of alignment, axial compressive forces become focused on one side and tensional forces are created opposite to it, resulting in increased stress and strain.

The carpus (knee) is a compound joint that is interposed between two long bones. Its major functions include: 1) flexion, 2) absorption of concussion, and 3) extension. Flexion primarily occurs at the antebrachiocarpal and midcarpal joint spaces. Concussion is absorbed by all three carpal joints, and extension is developed by a locking mechanism that occurs while the horse is weight-bearing and in the extension phase of the stride. Because of this requirement it is important that the carpal bones be in good axial alignment with the radius and ulna and the third metacarpal (cannon) bone. They also should be of sufficient size to support the force brought to bear on them. Since flexion and extension are an important function of the carpus, the muscles of the forearm should be well developed to support these functions. The carpus should appear straight and not deviate forward or backward (Fig. 2.8). The region just distal to the carpus should not be cut in on the dorsal surface (cut out under the knees) or cut in on the palmar surface (tied in knees).

Fetlock joints should be large enough and angled to allow free movement. Back et al. (1994) found that a more extended fetlock joint resulted in more maximal extension, which correlated with a good gait in the forelimbs. He also found that a straighter hindlimb fetlock joint angle was related to a longer stride and swing duration.[4] Adams (1974) stated that the angle between the third metacarpal (cannon) bone and the proximal (first) phalanx is about 125 to 135°.[1] However, in a study done on Swedish Warmblood horses it was found that the mean front fetlock angle was 146 to 155° and the mean hind fetlock angle was 153 to 161°.[14]

The normal mean fore pastern and foot angle is 54°.[7,8] Exceptionally long, sloping pasterns can result in increased strain to flexor support structures of the fetlock and phalanges. Short, upright pasterns deliver greater concussive stresses to the fetlock, phalangeal joints, and foot. The hoof should be appropriate for the

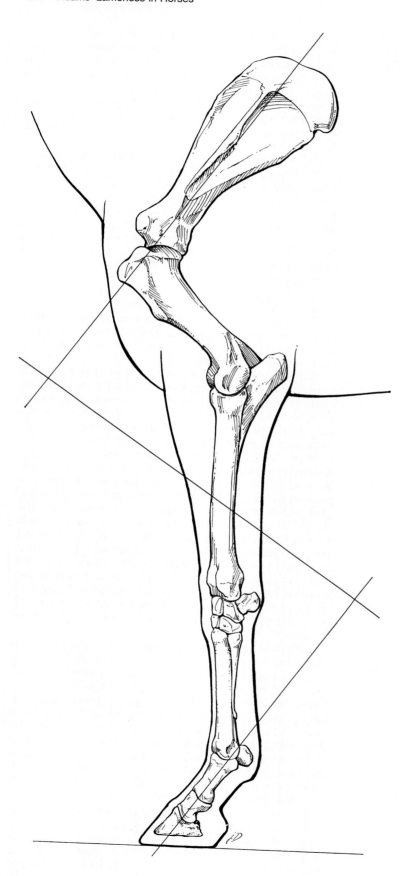

Figure 2.7   The angle of the shoulder joint usually influences the angle of the pastern.

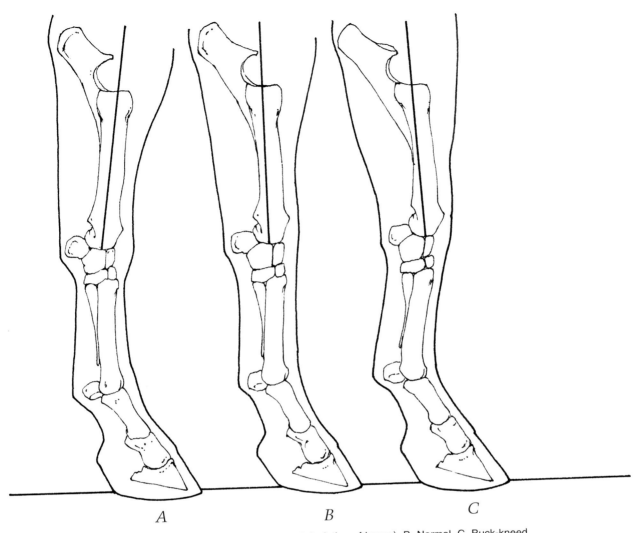

Figure 2.8   A. Calf-kneed (backward deviation of knees). B. Normal. C. Buck-kneed (forward deviation of knees).

size of the horse, well shaped, and symmetric. It should have high-quality hoof horn, adequate height and width of heel, concave sole, and an adequately sized hoof. Normally trimmed hooves impact the ground heel first (40% of the time) or flat footed (60% of the time).[8] One study documented that lower hoof angles predisposed racehorses to musculoskeletal injury.[19]

Faults in Conformation of the Forelimbs

BASE-NARROW (Fig. 2.9)

In base-narrow conformation, the distance between the center lines of the feet at their placement on the ground is less than the distance between the center lines of the limbs at their origin in the chest when viewed from the front. This is found most often in horses having large chests and well-developed pectoral muscles, such as the Quarter Horse. This conformation may be accompanied by a toe-in (pigeon-toed) or toe-out (splay-footed) conformation.

Base-narrow conformation inherently causes the horse to bear more weight on the outside of the foot than on the inside. Consequently, whether the foot toes-in or toes-out, the outside of the foot and limb is subjected to more stresses.

BASE-WIDE (Fig. 2.10)

In base-wide conformation, the distance between the center lines of the feet on the ground is greater than the distance between the center lines of the limbs at their origin in the chest when viewed from the front. This condition is found most commonly in narrow-chested horses such as the American Saddlebred and the Tennessee Walking Horse. In base-wide conformation, the horse is often affected with a toe-out (splay-footed) position of the feet. Base-wide, toe-out conformation usually causes winging to the inside (Figs. 2.11B and 2.12).

Base-wide conformation forces the horse to bear more weight on the inside of the foot than the outside of the foot. Because the weight is distributed in this fashion,

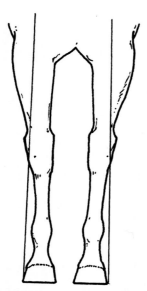

Figure 2.9   Base-narrow. Note that the distance between the center lines of the limbs at their origin is greater than the distance between the center lines of the feet on the ground.

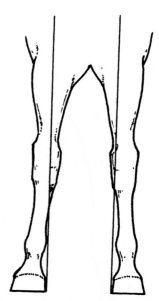

Figure 2.10   Base-wide conformation. Note that the distance between the center lines of the feet is wider than the distance between the center lines of the limbs at the chest.

Figure 2.11   How toe-in and toe-out affects foot path. A. Normal foot path. B. Foot path of a horse with toe-out conformation. C. Foot path of a horse with toe-in conformation.

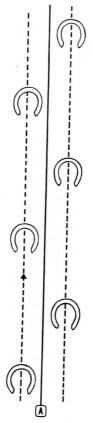
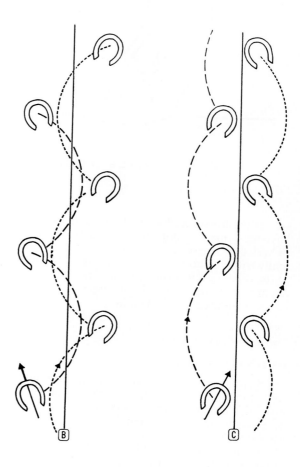

(see Chapter 9). If an angular limb deformity is contributing to the problem, surgery may be helpful within the first six weeks after birth. When the affected horse moves, it tends to paddle with the feet (Figs. 2.11C and 2.15). This is an outward deviation of the foot during flight. The foot breaks over the outside toe and lands on the outside wall. If a horse toes-in, it will usually paddle whether it is base-narrow or base-wide. If the pastern and foot deviate inward from the fetlock down (varus deformity), the horse may carry the foot to the inside instead of the outside. This complication of base-narrow, toe-in conformation can cause interference, especially at the fetlock region. One study documenting variations in conformation in Swedish Warmblood horses found a

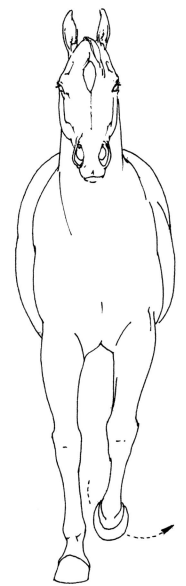

Figure 2.12 Winging, which may cause interference, is caused by a toe-out position of the feet.

the horse will usually land on the inside of the foot, a situation opposite to that seen in base-narrow conformation. Consequently, the inside of the limb takes the most stress in base-wide conformation.

TOE-IN OR PIGEON-TOED (Figs. 2.13 and 2.14)

Toe-in is the position of the feet in which the toes point toward one another when viewed from the front. It is congenital, and the limb may be crooked as high as its origin at the chest or as low as the fetlock down.[1] It is usually accompanied by a base-narrow conformation but rarely is present when the horse is base-wide. In the young foal, the condition may be partially corrected by proper trimming of the hooves, and young horses may be correctively shod to prevent a worsening of the condition

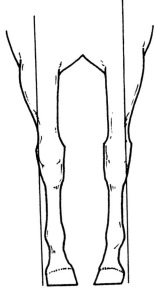

Figure 2.13 Base-narrow, toe-in conformation.

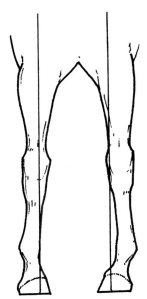

Figure 2.14 Base-wide, toe-in position of feet.

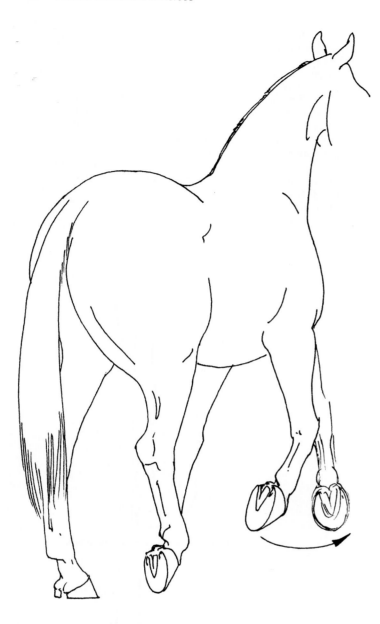

Figure 2.15   Paddling at the pace. This accompanies toe-in conformation.

50% frequency of mild toe-in conformation in elite sport horses, indicating minor deviations do not impair soundness or performance.[14]

TOE-OUT OR SPLAY-FOOTED (Figs. 2.16 and 2.17)

In toe-out or splay-footed position, when viewed from the front, the toes point away from one another. The condition is usually congenital and is usually caused by limbs that are crooked from their origin down. In some cases, however, the condition is aggravated by a rotation at the fetlock. It may be accompanied by either base-wide or base-narrow conformation. As with a toe-in conformation, it may be controlled or partially corrected by corrective trimming or corrective shoeing in the foal. If an angular limb deformity is contributing to the problem, surgery may be helpful at a very young age. The flight of the foot goes through an inner arc when advancing and may cause interference with the opposite fore-

limb (Figs. 2.11B and 2.12). A horse that toes-out will usually wing to the inside, whether it is base-narrow or base-wide. When a toe-out attitude of the feet coincides with base-narrow conformation, limb interference and plaiting (Fig. 2.18A) are more likely. One study done in Swedish Warmblood horses found < 5% toe-out conformation.[14]

BASE-NARROW, TOE-IN CONFORMATION (Fig. 2.13)

Base-narrow, toe-in conformation causes excessive strain on the lateral collateral support structures of carpus, fetlock, and phalangeal joints. Base-narrow, toe-in conformation usually causes paddling (Figs. 2.11C and 2.15). This is a common type of conformational abnormality.

BASE-NARROW, TOE-OUT CONFORMATION (Fig. 2.16)

Base-narrow, toe-out conformation is one of the worst types of conformation in the forelimb. Horses hav-

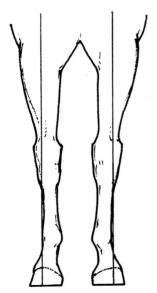

Figure 2.16 Base-narrow, toe-out conformation.

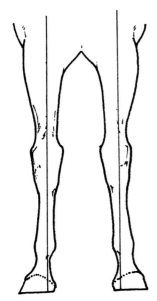

Figure 2.17 Base-wide, toe-out position of the feet.

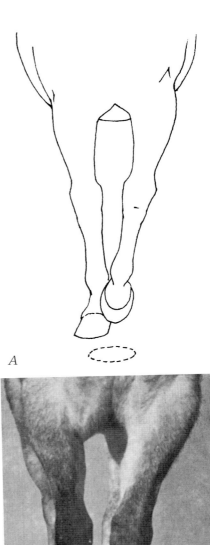

ing this conformation can seldom handle heavy work. The closely placed feet, combined with a tendency to wing inwardly from the toe-out position, commonly cause limb interference. The base-narrow attitude of the limb places the weight on the outside wall, as with base-narrow, toe-in conformation. The hoof breaks over the inside toe, swings inward, and lands on the outside wall. This causes great strain on the limb below the fetlock. Plaiting (Fig. 2.18A) may be evident. One should study the foot closely in flight before making any corrections (Fig. 2.18B). Corrective shoeing is discussed in Chapter 9.

BASE-WIDE, TOE-OUT CONFORMATION (Fig. 2.17)

When a horse is base-wide, the feet usually toe-out. The base-wide conformation places the greatest stress on

Figure 2.18 A. Plaiting. Plaiting is most often found in a horse with base-narrow, toe-out conformation. After the foot travels an inward arc, it lands more or less directly in front of the opposite forefoot. In some cases, this leads to stumbling as a result of interference. B. Base-narrow, toe-out conformation. Note left forefoot landing on the outside wall, typical of this type of conformation. There is also a degree of plaiting.

the inside of the limb. This means that there is greater stress on the medial collateral support structures of the fetlock and phalangeal joints. With this conformation, the foot usually breaks over the inside toe, deviates (wings) to the inside, and lands on the inside hoof wall. Blemishes on the medial aspect of the cannon bone, medial splints, and fracture of the medial splint bone occur with this conformation because of interference.

BASE-WIDE, TOE-IN CONFORMATION (Fig. 2.14)

This type of conformation is unusual. The base-wide attitude of the limbs places the greatest stress on the inside of the limb, similar to the base-wide, toe-out conformation. In most cases, a horse affected with base-wide, toe-in conformation will paddle to the outside even though it breaks over the inside toe and lands on the inside wall.

There is always the possibility that other conformational abnormalities of the limb, especially from the fetlock down, may change the path of the foot so it does not correspond to the above descriptions. These abnormalities include twisting of the fetlock so that the base-narrow, toe-in horse actually wings to the inside. Since these variations are rare and because they all cannot be listed, there will be no discussion of them here.

PLAITING (Fig. 2.18A)

Some horses, especially those with base-narrow, toe-out conformation, tend to place one forefoot directly in front of the other. This is an undesirable characteristic, because it can produce interference and stumbling resulting from an advancing forelimb hitting the one placed in front of it.

PALMAR (BACKWARD) DEVIATION OF THE CARPUS (HYPEREXTENDED KNEES, CALF KNEES, OR SHEEP KNEES) (Fig. 2.19)

Backward deviation of the carpus (back at the knee) is a weak conformation, and the limbs seldom remain sound under heavy work. The weight of the horse descends through the misaligned limb to end behind the hoof. This conformation places increased stress on the palmar carpal, radial check, and the proximal middle and distal accessory carpal bone ligaments. It also increases compression on the dorsal aspect of the carpal bones. It is believed that this conformation makes horses working at speed more susceptible to carpal chip frac-

Figure 2.19 A. Calf-kneed. B. Normal. C. Buck-kneed.

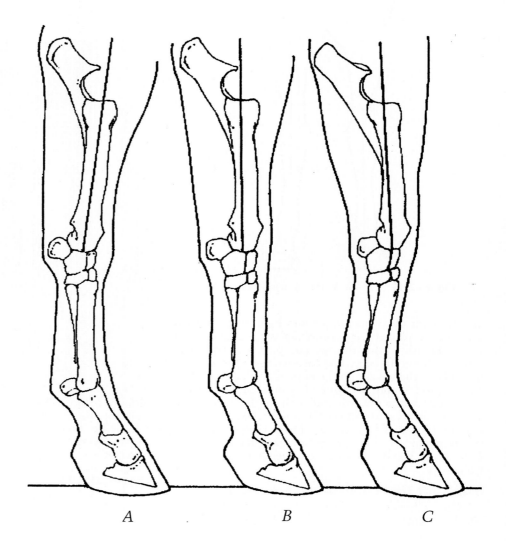

A   *B*   *C*

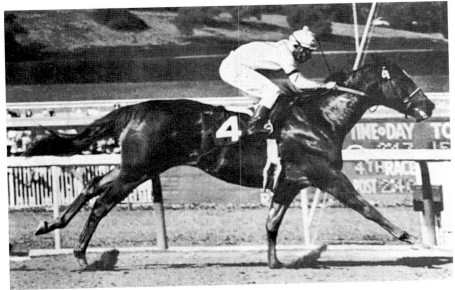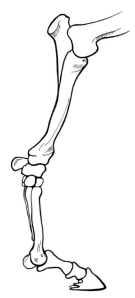

Figure 2.20   Photograph of a Thoroughbred near the finish of a race. Note the backward deviation of the carpus, predisposing to chip fracture of the carpal bones. If a horse has a backward deviation of the carpus before limb fatigue forces it into this position there is even greater possibility of carpal fracture. (Courtesy of Dr. W. Berkley.)

tures (Fig. 2.20). Interestingly, in a limited study done on 21 Thoroughbred racehorses with carpal chip fractures, they were not significantly more hyperextended at the carpus than 10 normal racehorses with normal carpi.[5] Therefore, the hyperextended carpus conformation is not the only reason carpal chip fractures develop. Additionally, it was felt that alteration in, or injury to, the palmar soft tissue support structures might be the reason for this carpal conformation and therefore it is not entirely a result of genetic influence.[5]

DORSAL (FORWARD) DEVIATION OF THE CARPUS (BUCKED KNEES OR KNEE SPRUNG) (Fig. 2.19)

This condition may also be called "goat knees" or "over in the knees." It is generally believed that the conformation is less severe than the calf-knee condition. However, severe dorsal deviation may be more dangerous for the rider, because the horse's knees are on the verge of buckling forward. Forward deviation of the carpus may be caused by contraction of the carpal flexors (i.e., ulnaris lateralis, flexor carpi ulnaris, and flexor carpi radialis). Extra strain may be placed on the extensor carpi radialis and the suspensory ligament. The condition is often present at birth, but if it is not severe, it usually disappears by 3 months of age. Congenital forms are nearly always bilateral and may be accompanied by a knuckling of the fetlocks. One study documenting the variations in conformation in Swedish Warmblood horses found considerably more elite sport horses were "buck-kneed" than "calf-kneed," while the reverse was true in riding school horses.[14]

MEDIAL DEVIATION OF THE CARPUS (KNOCK KNEES, CARPUS VALGUS, OR KNEE-NARROW CONFORMATION) (Fig. 2.21B)

Medial angular deviation of the carpus can result from abnormalities of the distal metaphysis, physis

(growth plate), and epiphysis of the radius, from abnormal development and alignment of the carpal bones and small metacarpal bones, or from carpal joint laxity. As a result of this deviation, an increased tensional strain is placed on the medial collateral ligaments of the carpus with increased compression on the lateral (concave) surface of the carpus. Varying degrees of stresses are also transmitted to the joints proximal and distal to the carpus. Usually, varying degrees of outward rotation of the cannon bone, fetlock, and foot accompany this entity. Carpus valgus (slight inward rotation of the limbs) of 5 to 7° associated with asynchronous growth of the distal radial metaphysis is common in foals and weanlings. This condition usually corrects itself with maturity.

LATERAL DEVIATION OF THE CARPUS (BOWLEGS, CARPUS VARUS, OR BANDY-LEGGED CONFORMATION) (Fig. 2.21A)

Carpus varus is an outward deviation of the carpus when viewed from the front of the horse. It may be accompanied by a base-narrow, toe-in conformation. This condition causes increased tension on the lateral surface of the carpus, and an increased compression on the medial surface of the carpus and carpal bones.

OPEN KNEES

The term "open knees" refers to an irregular profile of the carpal region when viewed from the side (Fig. 2.22). This irregularity gives the impression that the carpal joints are not fully apposed. This conformation is usually found in young horses (1 to 3 years of age) before full maturity, and is often accompanied by physitis. As the horse matures, the joints usually become more pleasing in appearance. Some people regard this as a weak conformation subject to carpal injury. However, on radiographic exam, this irregularity does not reveal outstanding changes.

Figure 2.21 Examples of poor conformation. Compare with Figure 2.6A. A. Bowlegs. B. Knock-knees.

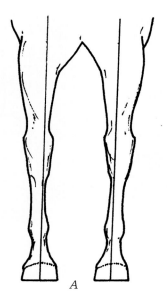
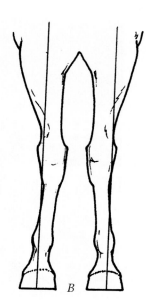

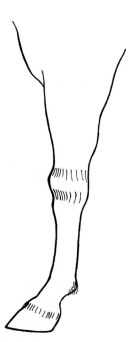
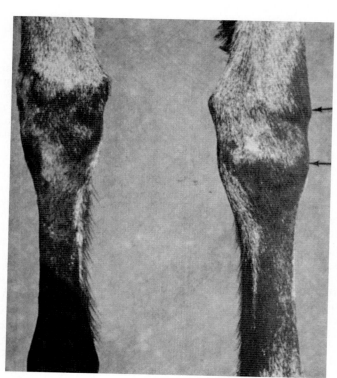

Figure 2.22 Open knees. This term refers to the irregular profile of the carpal joints when viewed from the side, which is caused by the enlarged distal physis of the radius and enlargement in the area of the carpometacarpal joint.

BENCH KNEES (OFFSET KNEES) (Fig. 2.23)

Bench knee is a conformation in which the cannon bone is offset to the lateral side and does not follow a straight line from the radius. It is evident when the limbs are viewed from the front. It is congenital in origin, and is considered a weak conformation. Since the medial splint bone normally supports more weight than the lateral splint bone, it is believed that there is even more direct weight-bearing on the medial splint bone in benched-kneed horses. This would cause more stresses on the in-terosseous ligament, increasing the possibility of splints. In a study documenting the conformational abnormalities in 356 Warmblood horses, > 50% were bench-kneed.[14] The combination of bench knees and carpus valgus is common.

TIED-IN KNEES (Fig. 2.24B)

Viewed from the side, the flexor tendons appear to be too close to the cannon bone just below the carpus. This is considered undesirable and appears to inhibit free

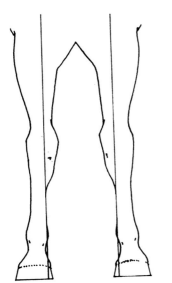

Figure 2.23   Offset knees (bench knees). Note that the cannon bones are set too far laterally.

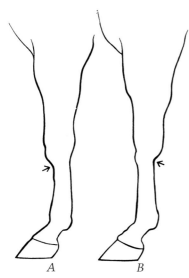

Figure 2.24   Examples of poor conformation. A. Cut out under the knees, as indicated by arrow. B. Tied-in knees, as indicated by arrow.

movement. A heavy fetlock may give the appearance of tied-in knees, even though the condition is not actually present.

Cut Out Under the Knees (Fig. 2.24A)

Viewed from the side, this condition causes a "cut out" appearance just below the carpus on the dorsal surface of the cannon bone. It is believed to be a fundamentally weak conformation, because the cannon bone does not line up with the carpal bones dorsally.

Standing Under in Front (Fig. 2.25A)

This is a deviation in which the entire forelimb from the elbow down is placed too far back to be perpendicu-

lar to the body, and too far under the body when the animal is viewed from the side. This stance may occur in certain diseases and may not be a conformational fault.

With this conformation, the base of support is shortened, the forelimbs become overloaded, the cranial phase of the stride is shortened and the arc of foot flight is low. All of this may predispose the horse to stumbling.

Camped in Front (Fig. 2.25B)

This is a condition opposite to that described above. The entire forelimb, from the body to the ground, is too far forward when viewed from the side. This limb attitude may be present in certain conditions, such as bilateral navicular syndrome and laminitis.

Short Upright Pastern (Fig. 2.26B)

A short upright pastern is believed to increase concussion on the fetlock joint, the phalangeal joints, and the navicular (distal sesamoid) bone.[1] A horse with this conformation may be predisposed to traumatic arthritis of the fetlock and phalangeal joints and navicular syndrome. This type of conformation is often associated with a base-narrow, toe-in conformation, and is most often present in the horse with short limbs and a powerful body and limb musculature. Additionally, a straight shoulder usually accompanies this type of conformation.

Long Sloping Pastern (Fig. 2.27)

A long sloping pastern is one characterized by a normal or subnormal angulation of the forefoot ($\leq 45°$) with a pastern that is too long for the length of the limb. This type of conformation is believed to predispose a horse to injury of the flexor tendons, sesamoid bones, and the suspensory ligament.

Long Upright Pastern (Fig. 2.26C)

With a long upright pastern, concussion to the fetlock and phalanges is increased, because the anticoncussion

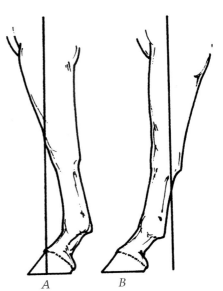

Figure 2.25   Examples of poor conformation. A. Standing under in front. B. Camped in front.

Figure 2.26   Examples of pastern conformation. A. A normal angulation of hoof and pastern. B. A short upright pastern predisposing to injuries of the fetlock joint, ringbone of the pastern joint, and navicular disease. C. Long upright pastern predisposes to injuries of the fetlock joint and navicular bone. This type of conformation does not seem to predispose to ringbone as often as does B.

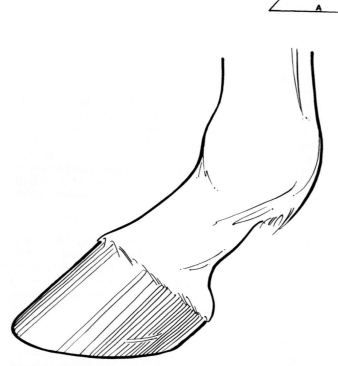

Figure 2.27   Example of a long sloping pastern. The foot and pastern axes are less than normal ($<45°$ in front or $<50°$ behind).

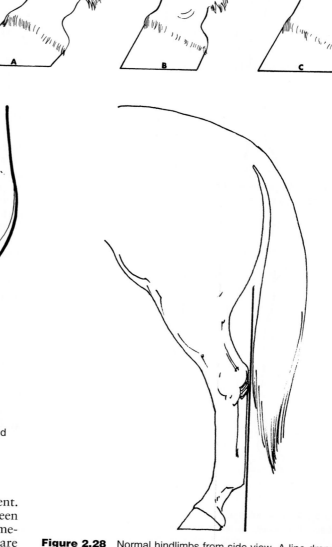

Figure 2.28   Normal hindlimbs from side view. A line dropped from the point of buttock (tuber ischii) follows the cannon.

mechanism of a normally sloping pastern is not present. Traumatic arthritis and navicular syndrome may be seen with this type of conformation, and both types of lameness may be present at the same time.[1] The stresses are very similar to those found in the short upright pastern (Fig. 2.26B), but reportedly the trauma to the pastern region is not as severe.[1]

The Hindlimbs

The bone structure and muscling of the hindlimb should be appropriate for the intended use. Endurance horses are characterized by longer, flatter muscles; stock horses are characterized by shorter, thicker muscles. All-around horses have moderate muscling.

LATERAL VIEW

Limbs, when viewed from the side, should exhibit a composite of moderate angles, so that shock absorption will be efficient (Fig. 2.28). A line from the point of buttock to the ground should touch the hock and end slightly behind the bulbs of the heels. A hindlimb in front of this line is often standing under (Fig. 2.29) or sickle-hocked (Fig. 2.30); a hindlimb behind this line is often post-legged (Fig. 2.31) or camped out (Fig. 2.32).

The hindquarter should be symmetric and well connected to the barrel and the lower limb. The gluteals should tie well forward into the back. The hamstrings should tie down low into the Achilles tendon of the hock.

The relationship of the length of the bones, the angles of the joints, and the overall height of the hindlimb will

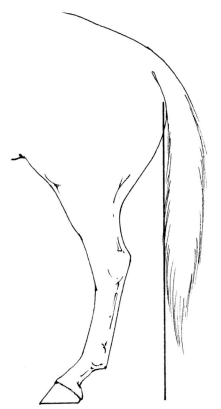

Figure 2.29   Standing under behind. Compare with Figure 2.28.

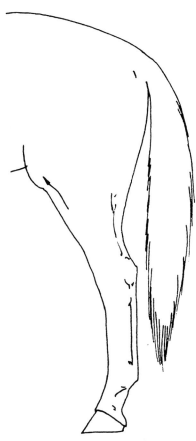

Figure 2.31   Post-legged too straight behind. There is too little angulation of the hock and stifle joints.

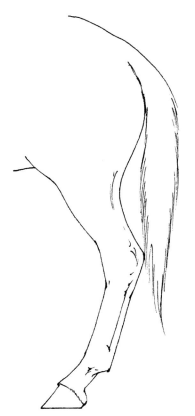

Figure 2.30   Sickle hocks. Note the excessive angle of the hock joints. Compare with Figure 2.28.

dictate the type of action and the amount of power produced. The length and slope to the pelvis (croup) are measured from the point of hip to the point of buttock. A flat, level croup is associated with hindlimb action that occurs *behind* the hindquarters rather than underneath it. A "goose rump" is a very steep croup that places the hindlimbs so far under the horse's belly that structural problems may occur because of the overangulation. Somewhere in between these is ideal. Generally, a more flexed hip results in a more protracted position of the hindlimb at stance phase and in a more horizontal femur during the swing phase. This results in the horse keeping its hindlimbs more under the body, which is important for collection in dressage and lift off in show jumpers.[16] A short femur is associated with the short, rapid stride characteristic of a sprinter. A long femur results in a longer stride with more reach. High hocks are associated with snappy hock action and a difficulty getting the hocks under the body. Low hocks tend to have a smoother hock action and the horse usually has an easier time getting the hocks under the body. The gaskin length (stifle to hock) should be shorter than the femur length (buttock to stifle). A gaskin longer than the femur tends to be associated with cow hocks and sickle hocks.

Hindlimbs with less angulation (open angles and straighter hindlimbs when viewed from the side) have a

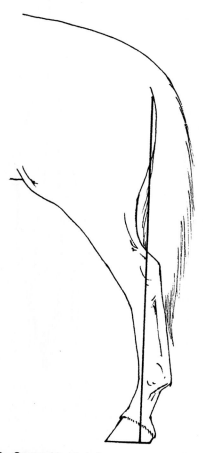

Figure 2.32 Camped behind. Compare with Figure 2.28.

shorter overall limb length and produce efficient movement suitable for hunters or racehorses. Generally, hindlimbs with more angulation (closed joints) have a longer overall limb length and produce a more vertical, folding action necessary for the collection characteristic of a high-level dressage horse. If the overall limb length is too long, it can be associated with either camped-out or sickle-hocked conformation. No matter what the hindlimb conformation is at rest, however, the connection to the loin and operation in motion are most important. An exception to this is that Holmstrom found in his study of elite horses that they had larger (straighter) hock angles than other groups of horses.[14] Back et al., 1996, reported that straighter hock joints were related to longer strides and swing duration and to an increased range of tarsal motion. This caused maximal protraction and retraction, which improved gait quality.[3] Magnuson et al., 1985, found a positive relationship between large hock angles and soundness in the Standardbred trotters.[20] The normal mean pastern angle for the hindlimbs is 55°.[7,8]

CAUDAL VIEW

From the rear, both hindlimbs should appear to be symmetric, to be of the same length, and to bear equal weight (Fig. 2.33). A left-to-right symmetry should be evident between the peaks of the croup (tuber sacrale),

the points of the hip, the points of the buttock, and the midline position of the tail. In one study done in Standardbred trotters, they found that hindquarter asymmetry (tuber sacrale at unequal heights) and associated factors had a negative effect on performance[12] (Fig. 2.34). The widest point of the hindquarters should be the width at the stifles. A line dropped from the point of the buttock to the ground will essentially bisect the limb, but hindlimbs are not designed to point absolutely straight forward. It is necessary and normal for the stifles to point slightly outward in order to clear the horse's belly. This causes the points of the hocks to face slightly inward and the toes to point outward to the same degree. The rounder the belly and/or the shorter the loin and coupling, the more the stifles must point out and the points of the hocks will appear to point inward. The more the horse is slab-sided and/or longer coupled, the more straight ahead the stifles and hocks can point. When the cannon bone faces outward, the horse is often cow-hocked (Fig. 2.35); when cannon bones face inward the horse is bowlegged (Fig. 2.36).

Increased stress on the hock and fetlock joints can occur when the hocks point absolutely straight ahead and the hooves toe-out. The hindfeet should be as far apart on the ground as the limbs are at their origin in the hip.

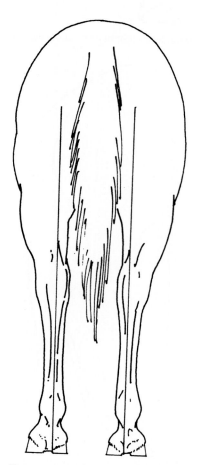

Figure 2.33 Normal hindlimbs. A line dropped from the point of the buttock (tuber ischii) bisects the limb.

required for good performance in advanced classes. In one study done on elite Swedish Warmblood sport horses, none of the show jumpers and only one of the dressage horses were "sickle hocked."[14]

EXCESSIVELY STRAIGHT LIMBS OR "STRAIGHT BEHIND" (Fig. 2.31)

When viewed from the side, there is very little angle between the tibia and femur, and the hock is excessively straight. This is believed to predispose the horse to bog spavin and upward fixation of the patella. Generally, the pastern conformation will also be too straight. One study, however, documented that straighter hock angles resulted in a longer stride and swing duration and an increase in hock joint action (protraction and retraction), which improved gait quality.[14]

CAMPED BEHIND (Fig. 2.32)

"Camped behind" means that the entire limb is placed too far caudally when viewed from the side. A perpendicular line dropped from the point of the buttock would hit at the toe, or halfway between the toe and heel. This condition is often associated with upright pasterns behind.

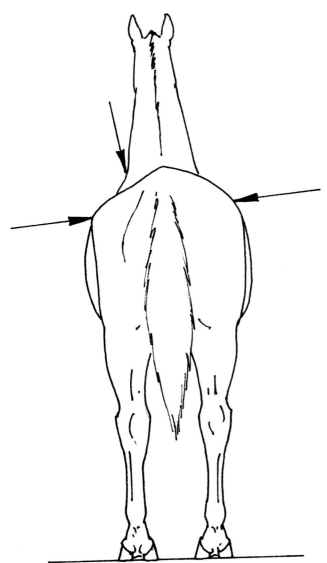

Figure 2.34   Illustrates asymmetry between peaks of the croup, points of the hip, and points of the buttock.

Faults in Conformation of the Hindlimbs

STANDING UNDER BEHIND (Fig. 2.29)

Viewed from the side, the entire limb is placed too far forward to be perpendicular to the body, or sickle hocks are present. A perpendicular line drawn from the point of buttock (tuber ischii) would strike the ground well behind the limb.

EXCESSIVE ANGULATION OF THE HOCK (SICKLE HOCKS, SMALL HOCK ANGLES) (Fig. 2.30)

When viewed from the side, the angle of the hock is decreased ($\leq 53°$) so that the horse is standing under from the hock down. Hock angles $< 53°$ are considered sickle.[15] This places the hock under a greater stress and predisposes the soft tissue support structures on the planter hock region to strain. Small hock angles may also impair a horse's ability to attain the level of collection

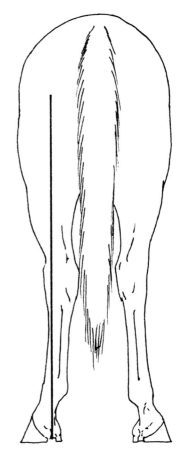

Figure 2.35   Cow hocks accompanied by base-wide conformation. Such horses are usually base-narrow as far as the hocks, but base-wide from the hocks down. Compare with Figure 2.33.

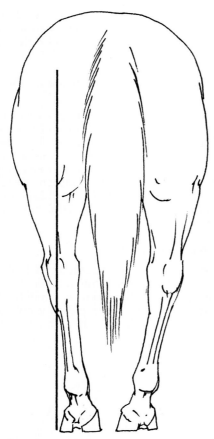

Figure 2.36 Base-narrow behind. This is often accompanied by "bowlegs," as shown. Compare with Figure 2.33.

BASE-WIDE (Fig. 2.35)

Base-wide means that when viewed from behind, the distance between the center lines of the feet at their placement on the ground is greater than the distance between the center lines of the limbs in the thigh region. Base-wide conformation is not as frequent in the hindlimbs as in the forelimbs. The most common form of base-wide conformation is associated with cow hocks.

MEDIAL DEVIATION OF THE HOCK (COW HOCKS OR TARSUS VALGUS) (Fig. 2.35)

"Cow-hocked" means that the limbs are base-narrow to the hock and base-wide from the hock to the feet. Cow-hocked conformation is a common defect. The hocks are too close, pointing toward one another, and the feet are widely separated. Viewed laterally, the horse may be sickle-hocked. Cow-hocked is believed to be one of the worst hindlimb conformations there is, because the excessive stress on the hock joint may cause bone spavin. A combination of sickle hocks and cow hocks is observed commonly in western performance horses.

BASE-NARROW (Fig. 2.36)

Base-narrow conformation of the hindlimbs means that when the animal is viewed from behind, the distance between the center lines of the feet is less than the dis-

tance between the center lines of the limbs in the thigh region. This is most common in heavily muscled horses. It causes excessive strain on the lateral aspect of the limb. The feet may toe-in or have straight toes. Base-narrow conformation is often accompanied by "bowlegs" or a condition in which the hocks are too far apart. The limbs may appear fairly straight to the hock and then deviate inward. Most of the horse's weight is placed on the outside edges of the hooves. The hocks may bow outward during movement. When a horse has good conformation in front and is base-narrow behind, many types of interference can occur between the forelimbs and hindlimbs.

BASE-NARROW FROM FETLOCKS DOWN

This conformation places stress on the lateral collateral ligaments of the fetlock and phalangeal regions.

Conformation of the Foot

Hoof anatomy and conformation are also discussed in Chapters 1 and 9.

THE FOREFOOT (Fig. 2.37)

Ideally, the forefoot should be round and wide in the heels, and the size and shape of the heels should correspond to the size and shape of the toe. The bars should be well developed. The wall should be thickest at the toe, and should thin gradually toward the heels; the inside wall should be slightly straighter than the outside wall.

The sole should be slightly concave medial to lateral and front to back, but an excessive concavity is evidence of a chronic foot disease. There should be no primary contact between the ground and the sole, as it is not a weight-bearing structure.

The mean foot and pastern axis in the forefoot is 54°.[7,8] The angle of the heel should correspond to the angle of the toe, and there should be no defects in the wall. The foot should show that the animal is breaking squarely over the center of the toe and not over the medial or lateral portion of the toe. The wall should show that it is wearing evenly.

The frog should be large and well developed with a good cleft. It should have normal consistency and elastic-

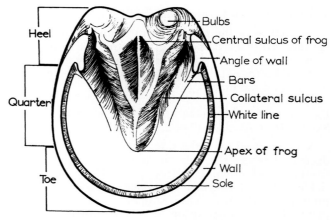

Figure 2.37 Normal forefoot showing structures.

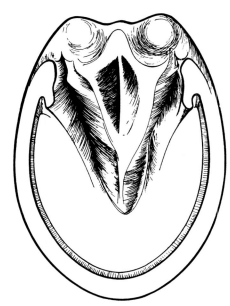

Figure 2.38 Normal hindfoot. Compare with Figure 2.37. The toe of the hindfoot is more pointed than that of the forefoot.

ity, and should be dry and soft. It should divide the sole into two nearly equal halves, and the apex should point to the center of the toe. Unequal size of the two halves may indicate a base-wide or base-narrow conformation.

THE HINDFOOT (Fig. 2.38)

The hindfoot should present a more pointed appearance at the toe than does the forefoot. It should show evidence of breaking straight over the toe, and the frog should divide the sole into equal halves. The mean foot and pastern axis in the hindfoot is 55°, and there should be no defects in the wall.[7,8] The walls should show normal wear on the medial and lateral sides, and the sole should be slightly concave medial to lateral and front to back. The sole of the hindfoot is normally more concave than that of the forefoot.

Abnormal Conformation of the Foot

FLAT FEET

A flat foot lacks the natural concavity in the sole; it is not a normal condition in light horses but is present in some draft breeds. Flat feet may be heritable and are much more common in the forefeet than in the hind. A horse with this condition may land on the heels in order to avoid pressure on the soles. Sole bruising and the lameness that results are common sequelae of flat feet. No remedy will cure a flat foot, but corrective shoeing can help prevent aggravation of the condition.

CONTRACTED FOOT OR CONTRACTED HEELS (Fig. 2.39)

Contracted foot is a condition in which the foot is narrower than normal. This is especially true of the back half of the foot. This condition is much more common in the front feet than in the hind feet, and it may be

unilateral or bilateral. Hoof contraction can occur rapidly, particularly in heels with long toe-low heel conformation resulting in a hoof angle < 45°.[13] Local or coronary contraction of the foot is a contraction at the heels confined to the horn immediately below that occupied by the coronary cushion. This term merely reflects an arbitrary subdivision of contracted foot.

One should bear in mind that certain breeds of horses normally have a foot that more closely approaches an oval than a circle in form. A narrow foot is not necessarily a contracted foot, and donkeys and mules normally have a foot shape that would be called contracted on a horse. Foot contraction may be present in the Tennessee Walking Horse and American Saddlebred when these horses are used for show because the hoof wall is allowed to grow excessively long.

UNILATERAL CONTRACTED FOOT

In some horses, a unilateral contraction of one forefoot is present. This may be congenital or developmental, and it is not known whether this abnormality tends to be inheritable. The contracted foot may or may not eventually show lameness, but it should be regarded as an undesirable feature. A small foot on one side may also indicate a chronic lameness, and can be associated with a clubbed foot.

BULL-NOSED FOOT (Fig. 2.40)

A foot that has a dubbed toe is called a "bull-nosed foot."

BUTTRESS FOOT (Fig. 2.41)

"Buttress foot" is a swelling on the dorsal surface of the hoof wall at the coronary band. This swelling may be from a low ringbone or the result of a fracture of the extensor process of the distal phalanx (coffin bone). A conical deformity of the toe from the coronary band to

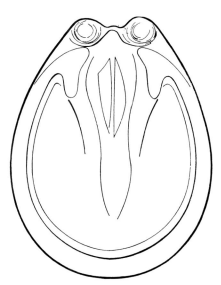

Figure 2.39 Contracted foot. Note narrowing of the heels and quarters. Compare with Figure 2.37.

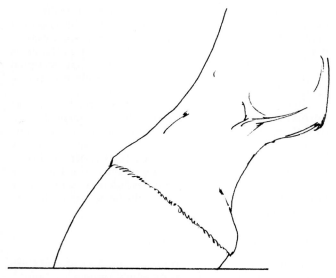

Figure 2.40   Bull-nosed foot.

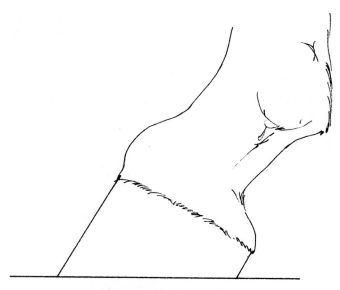

Figure 2.41   Buttress foot.

the ground surface (a result of deformed hoof growth) is caused by chronic swelling at the coronary band.

THIN WALLS AND SOLE

Thin walls and sole accompany one another and are heritable. The conformation of the foot may appear normal, but the hoof wall either wears away too rapidly or does not grow fast enough to avoid the effects of sole pressure. This condition is especially noticeable at the heels, where the foot axis may be broken by the tendency of the heel to be too low.

CLUB FOOT

A "club foot" is one that has a foot axis of 60° or more. When a club foot is unilateral, it may be the result

of some injury that has prevented proper use of the foot or may be caused by a flexural deformity involving the deep digital flexor tendon. It may be heritable or developmental.

COON-FOOTED (Fig. 2.42)

The pastern of the coon-footed horse slopes more than the dorsal surface of the hoof wall. In other words, the foot and pastern axis is broken forward at the coronary band. It may occur in either the forefeet or hindfeet, and it may cause strain on the flexor support structures and on the common digital extensor tendon.

MOVEMENT

Movement is composed of a horse's travel and action. Although the lower limbs are the focal point of evaluation, movement is a combined effort of the horse's entire body. "Travel" refers to the flight of a single hoof in relation to the other limbs, and is often viewed from the front or rear. "Action" takes into account joint flexion, stride length, suspension, and other qualities. It is usually assessed from a side view.

The Natural Gaits

The "walk" is a four-beat gait (Fig. 2.43) that should have a very even rhythm as the feet land and take off in the following sequence: left hind, left fore, right hind, right fore. A horse that is rushing at the walk might either jig or prance (impure gaits composed of half walking, half trotting) or might develop a pacey walk. The "pace" (Fig. 2.44) is a two-beat lateral gait in which the two right limbs rise and land alternately with the two left limbs. Although the pace is a viable gait for a Standardbred racehorse, a pacey walk is considered an impure gait for most riding horses because the even four-beat pattern of the walk is broken.

The "trot" is a two-beat diagonal gait (Fig. 2.45). Traditionally, the trot refers to an English gait with a moderate to great degree of impulsion. The right fore and left hind rise and fall together alternately with the

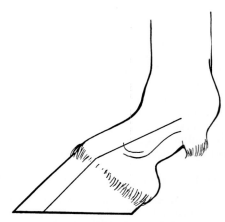

Figure 2.42   Broken angle between hoof and pastern axis (coon-footed). The foot axis is steeper than the pastern axis.

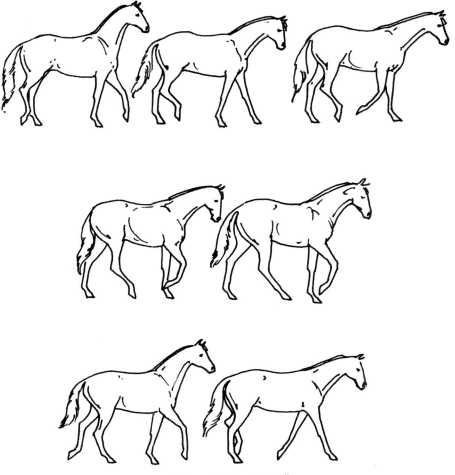

Figure 2.43   The walk.

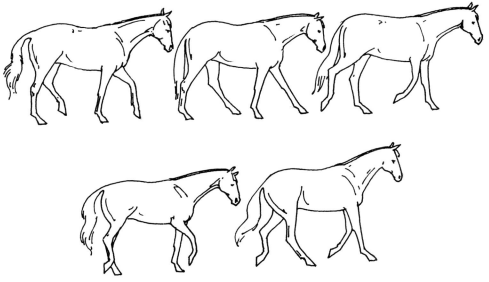

Figure 2.44   The pace.

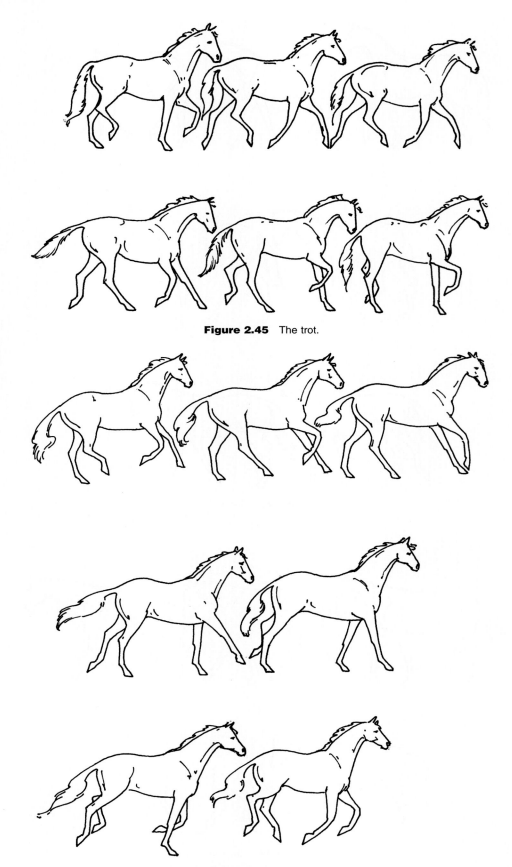

Figure 2.45   The trot.

Figure 2.46   The canter, right lead.

opposite diagonal pair (left fore and right hind). Often, the trot is a horse's steadiest and most rhythmic gait. The (western) jog is a shorter-strided trot with less impulsion. If a horse is jogged too slow, the gait becomes impure as the diagonal pairs break and the horse essentially walks behind and trots in front.

The "canter" or "lope" (Fig. 2.46) is a three-beat gait with the following sequence: one hindlimb, then the other hindlimb simultaneously with its diagonal forelimb, and finally the remaining forelimb. If a horse is on the right lead, the initiating hind will be the left hind, the diagonal pair will be the right hind (sometimes referred to as the supporting hind) and the left fore, and the final beat will occur when the leading forelimb (the right fore) lands. Then there is a moment of suspension as the horse gathers its limbs up underneath itself to get organized for the next cycle. When observing a horse on the right lead from the side, it is evident that the right limbs will reach farther forward than the left limbs. A change of lead (Fig. 2.47) should occur during the moment of suspension so that the horse can change both front and hind simultaneously.

The "gallop" or run is a four-beat variation of the canter (Fig. 2.48). With increased impulsion and length of stride, the diagonal pair breaks, resulting in four beats. The footfall sequence of a right lead gallop is left hind, right hind, left fore, and right fore. As in the canter, the right limbs will reach farther forward than the left limbs when the horse is in the right lead. There is a more marked suspension at the gallop than at the canter.

The "back," performed in its correct form, is a two-beat diagonal gait in reverse. The left hind and right fore are lifted and placed down together, alternating with the right hind and left fore.

The Phases of a Stride

The five phases of a horse's stride are landing, loading, stance, breakover, and swing (Figs. 2.49, 2.50, and 2.51).

Landing (Fig. 2.49). The hoof touches the ground, and the limb begins to receive the impact of the body's weight.

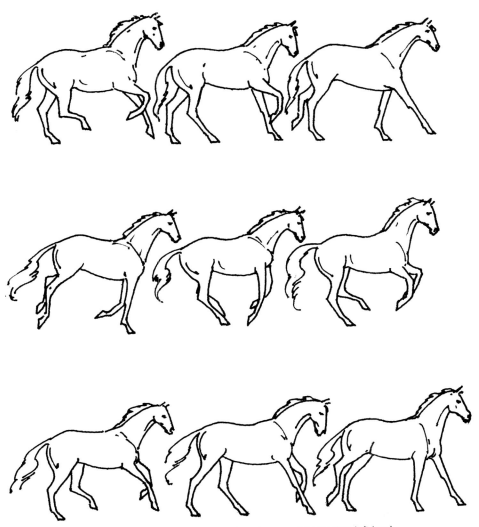

Figure 2.47 Canter with flying change, right lead to left lead.

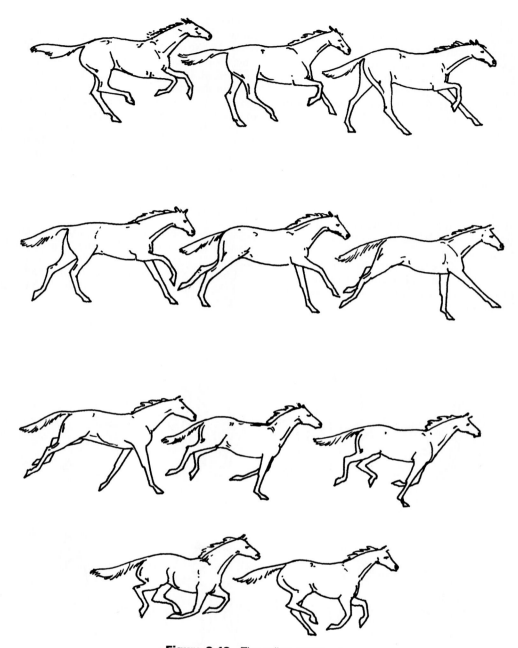

Figure 2.48 The gallop, right lead.

Loading (Fig. 2.49). The body moves forward, and the horse's center of gravity passes over the hoof. Usually, this is when the fetlock descends (extends) to its lowest point, sometimes resulting in an almost horizontal pastern.

Stance (Fig. 2.50). The fetlock rises to a configuration comparable to the horse's stance at rest. The transition between the loading phase and the stance phase is very stressful to the internal structures of the hoof and lower limb. The horse's center of gravity moves ahead of the hoof. The flexor apparatus lifts the weight of the horse

and rider and the fetlock begins to move upward. The pastern straightens and the limb begins pushing up off the ground.

Breakover (Fig. 2.50). Breakover is the phase when the hoof leaves the ground. It starts when the heels lift and the hoof begins to pivot at the toe. The knee (or hock) relaxes and begins to flex. Breakover is measured from the time the heels leave the ground to the time the toe leaves the ground. The deep digital flexor tendon (assisted by the suspensory ligament) is still stretched just prior to the beginning of breakover, to counteract

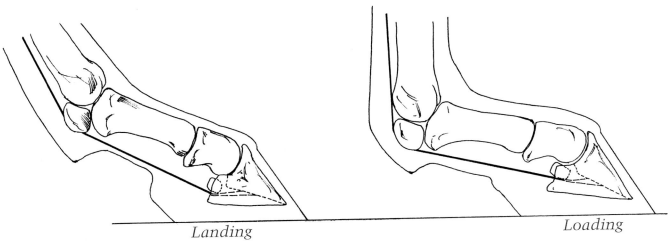

Landing   *Loading*

Figure 2.49 Phases of the stride: landing, loading. (Reprinted with permission from Hill C, Klimesh R. Maximum Hoof Power. North Pomfret, VT: Trafalgar Square Publishing, 2000.)

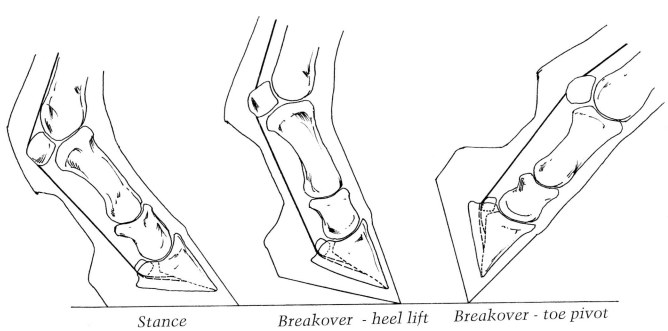

Stance   *Breakover - heel lift*   *Breakover - toe pivot*

Figure 2.50 Phases of the stride: stance, breakover-heel lift, breakover-toe pivot. (Reprinted with permission from Hill C, Klimesh R. Maximum Hoof Power. North Pomfret, VT: Trafalgar Square Publishing, 2000.)

the downward pressure of the weight of the horse's body.

Swing (Fig. 2.51). The limb moves through the air and straightens out in preparation for landing.

Stride Length

For years, it was believed that leaving the toe of a hoof long would increase a horse's stride length, thereby contributing to a smooth and efficient stride and fewer strides over a given distance. In the past, racehorses, showring hunters, and jumpers have mistakenly been shod with long toes and low heels to create a supposedly advantageous acute hoof angle. Research has shown that, contrary to popular opinion, horses with long toes and an acute hoof angle do not take longer strides.[9–11] Long toes (often accompanied by low, run-under heels) put the pivot point of the hoof farther forward than normal. The long toe acts as a lever arm during breakover, making it more difficult for the heels to rotate around the toe; consequently, tension in the deep digital flexor tendon may be prolonged and/or exaggerated. Additionally, the navicular ligaments, which stabilize the navicular bone and which are already stretched to the maxi-

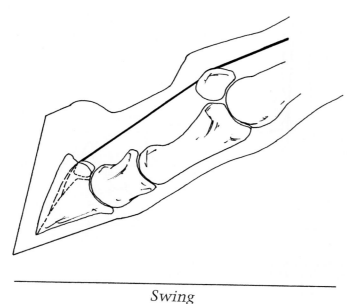

Swing

Figure 2.51 Phases of the stride: swing. (Reprinted with permission from Hill C, Klimesh R. Maximum Hoof Power. North Pomfret, VT: Trafalgar Square Publishing, 2000.)

mum at the beginning of breakover in a normal hoof, are stressed excessively during the breakover of a hoof with an acute angle. The delayed breakover allows the mass of the horse's body to move farther forward over the horse's limbs before the limbs leave the ground.

Research has shown that the arc of hoof flight was not significantly changed by trimming (Fig. 2.52).[10] However, the approach to the loading phase and the landing phase were affected. With a normally trimmed hoof, the toe of the hoof elevated slightly prior to landing as the hoof prepared for a heel-first or flat-foot impact. The hoof with an acute angle approached the ground toe-first, often landing with the toe impacting first. Such stabbing into the ground with the toes resulted in a broken, jarring motion rather than smooth action. Additionally, when the front feet were trimmed normally and the hind toes were long, the hind feet left the ground significantly later than their diagonal forefeet. However, the hindlimbs compensated for the delay in breakover by moving through the air more rapidly so that they could catch up and land at the same time as their corresponding diagonal forefeet. This caused an unevenness in the gait; the horse was first delayed behind and then hurried the movement of the hindlimbs to catch up.

Research has also disproved the popular theory that long toes in the hind may make a horse reach farther forward.[10] On the contrary, rather than the hindlimbs reaching farther forward, the horse's mass moves further ahead of the weight-bearing limbs before they leave the ground. This tends to put the cycle of the forelimb movement further under the horse, thereby lessening the potential for (hindquarter) engagement.

Top

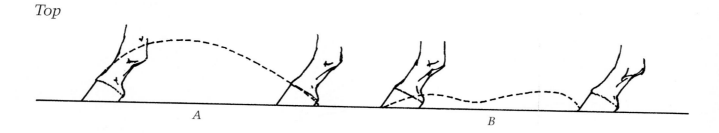

A

B

Bottom

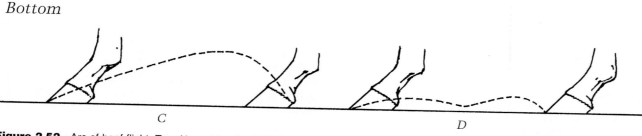

C

D

Figure 2.52 Arc of hoof flight. Top. Normal hoof and pastern angle. A. Proposed arc of foot flight. B. Actual arc of foot flight. Bottom. Long toe, low heel, acute hoof angle. C. Proposed arc of foot flight. D. Actual arc of foot flight shown by recent research.

Normal Movement

The straight foot flight pattern that is used as a basis when referring to deviations has often been termed "ideal." The fact is that such a foot flight is ideal only for a horse with ideal body and limb conformation. Horses with structural imperfections (virtually all horses) will have individual ideal foot flight patterns that compensate for imperfections; such individual patterns may not be "textbook pretty," but may well be functional. Instead of thinking of the straight foot flight as ideal, think of it as "standard" so that, rather than representing a goal to strive for, the term indicates a baseline for comparison.

The standard for forelimb movement starts with a straight bony column and a series of hinge joints all symmetrically conformed and working in a true forward-backward plane. Add to this a balanced hoof, and the result should be a straight foot flight.

Because hindlimbs nearly always turn out to some degree, the standard foot flight for the hindlimb will be different than for the front limb. Depending on the conformation of the hindquarters, this turning out of the limb facilitates a freer working of the stifle. The bone structure of a heavily muscled horse may, by genetic design, turn out in order to allow more drive and reach with the hindlimbs. This would also counteract the inward pull characteristic of a horse with heavy inside gaskin muscles.

Movement Abnormalities

"Gait defects" are movement abnormalities that consistently occur during regular work.

FORGING

Forging is a gait defect that is commonly heard when a horse is trotting. Forging (Figs. 2.53 and 2.54) occurs

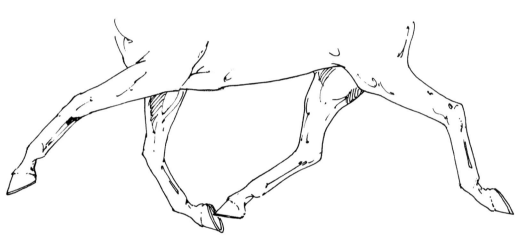

Figure 2.53   Forging at the trot, hind foot and front foot on same side make contact.

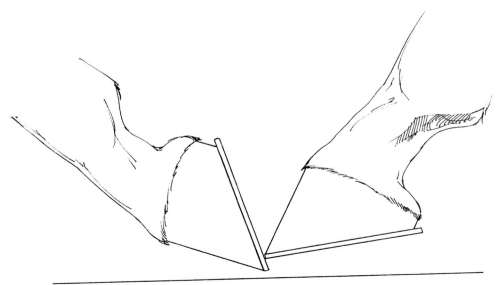

Figure 2.54   Forging close-up. (Reprinted with permission from Hill C, Klimesh R. Maximum Hoof Power. North Pomfret, VT: Trafalgar Square Publishing, 2000.)

when a hind foot contacts a front foot on the same side. Frequently, contact is made when the hind foot is gliding in for a landing and the front foot is beginning its swing phase. If the front foot is delayed in its breakover, the hind foot may arrive before the forefoot has a chance to get out of the way. As the fore fetlock begins flexing, the toe of the front shoe may swing back and slap the toe of the landing hind shoe. This creates a characteristic "clicking" as the shod horse trots, or a dull "thwacking" if the horse is barefoot.

Forging is related to overreaching. Forging customarily refers to the contact made between shoes or hooves. A horse can receive sole bruises from a single blow or repeated tapping. Overreaching (Fig. 2.55) usually indicates that a front shoe has been pulled off by a hind, or that the hind has injured some part of the forelimb such as the heel bulb, coronary band, or even the fetlock or flexor tendons. A horse that forges or overreaches may be more prone to stumble or fall, especially at the moment when the shoe is stepped on or pulled off. If the conditions that cause a horse to forge are ignored or unintentionally perpetuated, the stride imbalances may progress to overreaching.

Forging and overreaching are indications that the horse's movement is out of balance. Balance is customarily discussed in terms of dorsal-palmar (DP) balance, left-right (LR) balance, and medial-lateral (ML) balance.

DP balance can refer to the relationship between the front and rear of the horse's entire body as well as to the relationship between the toe and heel of the hoof. LR balance refers to the relationship between the left and right sides of the horse's body. There are inherent discrepancies in LR balance in most horses. ML balance is often used to describe the relationship between the two halves of a limb or hoof when viewed from the front or rear. Each limb and hoof is evaluated individually for ML balance. The most graphic examples of ML imbalance are seen in the knees, hocks, fetlocks, and hooves. These imbalances are implicated as causes of gait defects such as winging in and paddling. Although LR and ML imbalances can complicate a forging horse's problems,

forging and overreaching are mainly attributed to DP imbalances. Other movement abnormalities include cross firing (Fig. 2.56) and scalping (Fig. 2.57).

CAUSES OF FORGING.   A horse's balance during movement is affected by many factors: conformation, condition, energy level, mental attitude, footing, level of training, gait or maneuver being performed, proficiency of rider, and shoeing. All of these factors affect breakover, but the theoretical discussion of breakover deals with the function of one limb at a time. To correct forging, the timing and direction of breakover of all of the hooves must be coordinated so that the limbs work in harmony and avoid collision.

LATERAL GAIT DEFECTS

A lateral gait defect is one that involves a regularly occurring, abnormal sideways swing of a limb. Some lateral gait defects result in actual physical contact with an opposite limb; others do not. Paddling or dishing, often seen with bowlegged, toed-in, or wide-chested and base-narrow horses, is a swinging out of the limb from the midline so that contact rarely results. In contrast, interfering is frequently associated with narrow-chested and/or toed-out horses. Such chest conformation places the limbs closer together, and the toed-out hoof predisposes the horse to winging, i.e., swinging the limb toward the midline during flight. As one limb swings inward, it passes the opposite limb, which usually is in a weight-bearing position. It is at this moment that contact might occur. The higher up the limb the turned-out deviation is located, the greater the torque that is imparted to the limb and the worse the winging-in will likely be. Swinging in of the limb, often called "brushing," is commonly referred to as "interfering" when contact between the two limbs is made.

Interfering occurs rarely at the walk. It appears most commonly at the trot and the other two-beat diagonal gait, backing up. The speed and energy level with which a horse moves its limbs has an effect on its tendency to

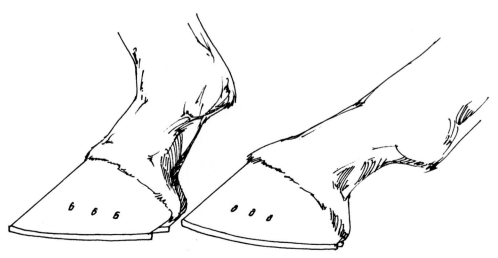

Figure 2.55 Overreaching close up. Overreaching or "grabbing" can occur when the front feet are delayed in breakover.

(Reprinted with permission from Hill C, Klimesh R. Maximum Hoof Power. North Pomfret, VT: Trafalgar Square Publishing, 2000.)

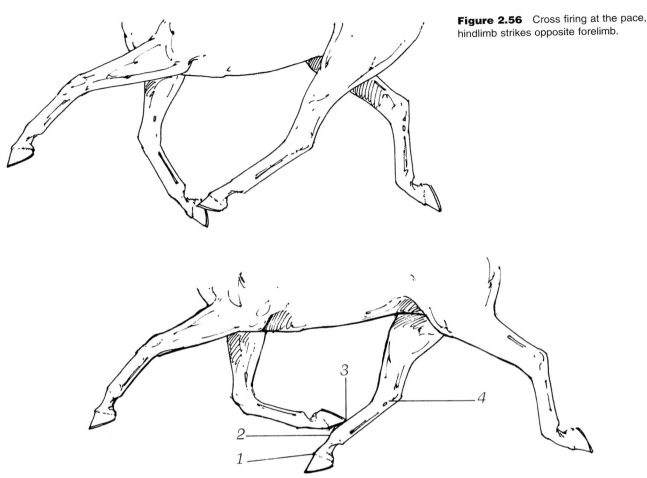

Figure 2.56 Cross firing at the pace, hindlimb strikes opposite forelimb.

Figure 2.57 Various forms of hindlimb contact at the trot. 1, scalping; 2, speedy cutting; 3, shin hitting; 4, hock hitting.

interfere. One horse may interfere at a jog but not at the extended trot; another horse may move with adequate clearance at the jog but not at an energetic trot. Similarly, one horse performing a quiet rein back might place its limbs carefully, but if it were asked to speed up the back in a reining pattern, its limbs might swing from side to side and collide. Another horse may work its limbs with piston-like precision while backing quickly and straight but might exhibit an altered foot flight if asked to slow down.

Interference can occur from the knee to the hoof of the front limbs, and usually from the fetlock to the hoof of the hindlimbs. If a horse does not wear protective boots, the first signs of interference may be pain, heat, or swelling in the area of contact. The problem may escalate to include missing hair, bruises, cuts, lesions, chronic sores, and perhaps underlying bone damage.

Protective boots should be used, examined, and cleaned after each workout, and points of contact noted. However, just because contact was made with a boot or leg wrap does not mean that contact would have been made without the protective gear, because the thickness of the boot may be the safe tolerance in which the un-booted horse would work. Rather than take a chance of injury, however, it is best to use protective boots on all

young horses and older horses with interference tendencies.

A horse sometimes will show reluctance to perform certain maneuvers that have caused it to hit itself in the past. The horse may try to avoid circular or lateral work by stiffening the back and working with short hopping strides with the hindlimbs. With a reining horse, interference problems in the front limbs may make it reluctant to add speed to its turnaround.

Factors That Affect Movement

There are many elements that affect a horse's movement. When lameness is a concern, the factors that are traditionally considered are lower limb conformation, pain, and shoeing. However, other factors should be considered because, in many cases, understanding the whole picture will result in a better treatment program and ultimately a more effective plan for lameness prevention.

CONFORMATION

There are no absolutes when it comes to predicting whether a horse will paddle, wing-in, or travel straight. Generalizations related to stance, breed, or type are frequently proved wrong. Lateral gait defects can affect a pair of limbs or a single limb. Conformational components include (in the front limb, for example) shoulder to rib cage attachment; width of chest; width at knees, fetlock, and hoof; and straightness of forearm, cannon, and pastern regions.

The abnormal development of a joint (particularly the carpal and fetlock joints) can also cause a limb to exhibit a lateral gait defect. Normally, the fetlock and carpal joints work in a hingelike fashion, backward and forward in a straight line, parallel to the horse's midline. An abnormally developed joint tends to hinge in a swivel-like motion at an angle to the horse's midline. This arc causes the limb to deviate in flight.

Many factors influence how close a horse's front and hind feet come together when it is moving: the relationship between the height at the wither and the height at the hip; the amount of muscling and the width of the chest and hips; the length, proportion, and shape of the topline components; the relationship between the length of the topline and the length of the underline; and, perhaps, most commonly, the relationship between the length of the underline and the length of the limbs. Horses with short backs and long limbs, and especially those with short forelimbs and long hindlimbs, are the most likely to have contact between forelimbs and hindlimbs.

Pain

Even if a horse shows all of the conformational traits that theoretically add up to straight travel, if it experiences pain in a portion of its body, it may break all of the conformation rules as it attempts to use its limbs in a manner that creates the least stress and pain. An injury or soreness in a limb or an associated structure can cause a horse to protect one portion of the limb when landing, subsequently altering the arc of the foot's flight. For example, if the horse is sore in the navicular region of the front feet, instead of landing heel first and rolling forward, he may land toe first, which will shorten the stride.

When a horse has pain in a part of the body other than the hooves or limbs, its balance during movement may be negatively altered as it compensates for the soreness. Back soreness can mimic a lower limb lameness and alter foot flight. A variety of other factors can cause the horse to carry its body in a stiff or crooked fashion (e.g., muscle cramping, or poor-fitting tack). Sometimes, the stiffness or pain is subtle but just enough to prevent the horse from tracking straight.

Imbalance

Gait defects often occur simply because the horse is trying to keep its balance. It is attempting to keep its limbs under its center of mass. Basically, there are three forces at work when a horse moves: the vertical force of the weight of the horse and rider, the horizontal force of the horse moving forward, and the swinging or side-to-side motion of the horse at various gaits. Exactly where under its body a horse places its limbs is determined in large part by the interaction of these three forces and the direction of their composite. A barefoot horse moving free in a pasture rarely interferes. It is when a horse carries a rider and is asked to perform in collected

and extended frames at both faster and slower speeds that interfering occurs.

A rider can make a horse move well or poorly. Rider proficiency will determine how the horse distributes its weight (from front to rear and from side to side), how the horse changes the speed or the length of a stride within a gait, and how the horse adapts the stride when turning, stopping, and performing such maneuvers as lead changes. Inadequate riding skills exaggerate the deficiencies in a horse's conformation and way of going. Because no horse moves perfectly at all times, it takes a knowledgeable and competent rider to compensate for a horse's shortcomings. A rider's balance and condition, as well as talent, coordination, and skill at choosing and applying the aids, greatly affect a horse's coordination. A horse must be warmed up in a progressive manner before being given more difficult work.

Inexperienced riders often ask a cold or poorly conditioned horse to do three things at once (such as come to a hard stop from a thundering gallop, make a sharp turn, and lope off in the opposite direction) without properly preparing the horse or helping it perform in a balanced fashion. When a horse is asked to do something it is not physically ready to do (such as a flying lead change, a deep stop, a fast burst out of the roping box, any kind of lateral work, a tight landing after a jump, or a sharp turn), it can easily overreach or interfere.

An unskilled rider can easily throw off a horse's balance formula. Inexperienced riders often commit one or more of these imbalance errors: sit off to one side of the saddle, often with a collapsed rib cage; ride with one stirrup longer; ride with a twisted pelvis; lean one shoulder lower than the other; hold one shoulder farther back than the other; or sit with a tilted head. All of these postures can alter the horse's composite center of mass and can cause the horse to make adjustments in order to stay balanced. Riders that let their horses ramble on in long, unbalanced frames, heavy on the forehand, also seem to have more forging problems. Some horses are able to compensate for an imbalanced rider without forging or interfering and others are not.

Some horses simply have an imbalanced way of going. Certain horses are uncoordinated, inattentive, and sloppy, whereas others move precisely, gracefully, and balanced. Training, conditioning, and conscientious shoeing can improve a poor mover's tendencies; but some horses, no matter how talented the rider and farrier, will consistently move in an imbalanced fashion.

Shoeing

Recent but improper shoeing can be responsible for gait defects. If a farrier's shoeing style is the "long-toe, low-heel," a horse is set up to forge and possibly interfere. When a horse is overdue for a reset, even if it was shod by a world-class farrier 8 weeks previously, its hooves have probably grown so out of balance that it could easily exhibit gait abnormalities. Sometimes, just going a week past the horse's needs can adversely alter the gait synchronization.

Footing

The surface the horse is worked on will directly affect its movement. Traction on dirt occurs when the horse's weight descends through the bone columns of the limbs, causing the hooves to drop 0.5 inch or more into the ground at the same time the soil is cupped upward toward the sole. This happens whether a horse is barefoot or shod. Shoes basically extend the hoof wall, creating a potentially deeper cup to the bottom of the hoof, therefore increasing traction potential in dirt or soft footing.

Ideal arena footing is light and does not stay compressed, so some dirt falls out of the hoof readily with every stride. During the work of a very active horse, dirt literally flies out of the shoes; but a placid horse may not move its limbs energetically enough to release some dirt with each stride. In dry arenas, the moderate amount of dirt in the shoe comes in contact with the dirt of the arena and results in good traction. However, if conditions are damp to wet and the footing is heavy, the hooves may pack and mound, thereby decreasing stability and traction. Packed dirt left in for prolonged periods of time creates constant pressure on the sole and can cause sole and frog bruises. Therefore, for work in soft, wet, and/or deep footing, it is important for shoes to be self-cleaning: they should allow mud, manure, or snow to move out at the base of the frog. This will ensure that the horse has an open sole and maximum traction potential for each stride.

Heavy footing (sand, mud, snow, long grass) generally delays front foot breakover. If a horse must be worked on footing it is unaccustomed to, protective boots may be helpful. Bell boots and scalping boots may prevent injury to the heels and coronary bands. Overreach boots provide protection to the tendons.

TRACTION

In some instances, a horse requires greater traction than would be provided by a standard shoe. Generally, the wider the web of the shoe, the less traction the shoe provides. The extreme is the sliding plate, which can be over 1 inch wide and allows the horse to "float" over the ground surface. Optimum traction can increase horse and rider safety, increase a horse's feeling of security so it will stride normally, and help a horse to maintain its balance in unstable footing such as mud, ice, snow, or rock.

Permanent calks, those driven into the shoe, forged into the shoe, or brazed or welded onto the shoe, provide good traction. However, such calks cannot be changed between shoeings and may lose their effectiveness as they wear down.

Removable screw-in calks (studs) may be the best answer when performance requirements or footing are constantly changing. Event riders can use large studs for the cross-country phase of competition and take them out or replace them with smaller studs for dressage and stadium jumping.

Jar calks (either rectangular or triangular pieces of steel) can be brazed on the shoes to prevent sideways slipping while allowing the hoof to slide forward on landing. They are usually applied at the heels and set in the direction of travel, not parallel to the sides of the shoe. However, if the goal is to decrease both sideways and forward/backward slipping, the jar calks can be placed parallel to the sides of the shoe.

Toe grabs, as the name implies, are placed on the front of the shoe. They are commonly used on racehorses to improve traction. One study documenting the effects of toe grabs on Thoroughbred racehorses found that toe grabs were associated with increased odds of fatal appendicular musculoskeletal injury and, specifically, suspensory ligament failure.[17] Increasing the height of the toe grabs also was associated with increased odds of injury. Conversely, horses shod with rim shoes appeared to have a decreased risk of injury.[17]

Before additional traction devices are considered, the horse must be fit and in working condition. A conditioning program should be designed to strengthen the ligaments, muscles, and tendons via progressive, regulated stretching and exercise. Adding traction to an unconditioned horse may result in injured ligaments and tendons.

CONDITION, LEVEL OF FITNESS

A horse's level of fitness as well as energy level affects its movement. In general, a horse has 15 minutes of peak performance, whether in a daily work session or at a competition. The horse may be either approaching that peak period or coming away from it. A rider must know how to properly warm up a horse to establish the most natural and efficient way of going for that horse; then the rider must assist (and not hinder) the horse in working in a balanced frame during the peak period. Finally, a rider must know how to gradually let the horse come down from its peak. A horse predisposed to forging or overreaching may likely do so if it is allowed to dawdle around on the forehand during the warm-up, if the bridle reins are pulled up suddenly and the horse is put to work when it is "cold," if contact is "thrown away" all at once or engagement is allowed to slip away during work, or if the horse is allowed to fall on its forehand immediately following the completion of its peak performance.

If a rider asks too much in relation to a horse's current physical capabilities or fitness level, the horse, commonly, will attempt to adapt while complying. If overworked, many horses will continue moving forward but will modify stride to minimize fatigue and discomfort to flexor muscles and tendons. One study done on kinematics of unmounted and mounted horses at a walk before and after treadmill exercise concluded that strenuous workload significantly influenced kinematics even at a walk, although each horse kept its characteristic gait pattern.[11,23] When a tired horse adjusts the timing of the various phases of its stride, it can result in gait defects. If the hindquarters have not been properly conditioned and strengthened, a horse will rely heavily on the forehand for both propulsion and support. This makes it even harder for the already heavily weighted forehand to get out of the way of the incoming hindfeet.

Poor condition or fatigue will often cause a horse to fling its limbs aimlessly; the horse does not have the muscle strength or energy necessary to project its limbs in a controlled fashion. In some cases, when a lazy horse moves slowly at a trot, it may move sloppily and carelessly, causing it to interfere occasionally. Requiring such a horse to move out with more energy may smooth out gait defects. This situation can be interpreted as an exception to the general rule that an increase in speed usually brings an increase in the potential to interfere. The amount of weight that a horse is carrying can also exaggerate its lateral limb movements. An overweight horse or heavy rider may cause more side-to-side sway, which will alter the net force of forward movement.

AGE AND STAGE OF DEVELOPMENT

A study looking at longitudinal development of equine locomotion from foal to adult concluded that there appears to be a high similarity and a good correlation between foal and adult locomotor variable, thereby enabling an accurate prediction of adult kinematics from those recorded at foal age.[2]

However, young horses that do not have fully developed muscles may lack the width of chest, stifle, or hip that will prevent them from interfering once they are adults. The relationship between the inside (axial) and outside (abaxial) muscles also can affect how the limb swings. A horse with heavy outside gaskin muscling and (in comparison) light inside gaskin muscling, especially if its hindlimbs toe-out, will tend to have trouble keeping its limbs under its body during a stop. This can be a major problem for a stock horse. There simply is not enough inside gaskin muscle power to counteract the outward rotation of the limb during the stop. To complicate things, this type of limb tends to wing inward during forward movement, so interference might occur.

TRAINING

One of the main causes of intermittent gait defects is asking a horse to perform something beyond its level of training. One of the first goals of training is to teach a horse to track straight. Until a horse learns to strongly and decisively step up underneath itself, its travel is often wobbly and inconsistent. Working on circles and lateral maneuvers before a horse is balanced and supple can cause it to make missteps and interfere. Asking a horse to perform advanced movements like the passage, canter pirouette, or turnaround before the horse is physically developed and trained can increase the possibility of interference. These movements are characterized by either higher action, greater speed, or a greater degree of joint flexion, all of which tend to increase rotational forces of the limb and the possibility of interference. Gait defects tend to surface with an increase in speed within a gait as well as the extension of a stride within a gait.

TACK

Poor-fitting saddles can be a cause of back pain and subsequently poor movement. If the tree is too narrow, it can cause pinching of the nerves and muscular pain. If the tree is too wide, it can cause the weight of the saddle and rider to be borne directly by the vertebrae.

OTHER FACTORS

Many other factors can cause a horse to move in an irregular fashion. Some mares move with extreme stiffness and tension during their estrous cycle. A horse with

---

Terms Associated With Movement

Action   the style of the movement, including joint flexion, stride length, and suspension; usually viewed from the side.

Asymmetry   a difference between two body parts or an alteration in the synchronization of a gait; when a horse is performing asymmetrically, it is often said to be "off."

Balance   the harmonious, precise, coordinated form of a horse's movement as reflected by equal distribution of weight from left to right and an appropriate amount of weight carried by the hindquarters.

Breakover   the moment between the stance and swing phases as the heel lifts and the hoof pivots over the toe.

Cadence   see "Rhythm."

Collection   a shortening of stride within a gait, without a decrease in tempo; brought about by a shift of the center of gravity rearward; usually accompanied by an overall body elevation and an increase in joint flexion.

Directness   trueness of travel, the straightness of the line in which the hoof (limb) is carried forward.

Evenness   balance, symmetry, and synchronization of the steps within a gait in terms of weight bearing and timing.

Extension   a lengthening of stride within a gait, without an increase in tempo; brought about by a driving force from behind and a reaching in front; usually accompanied by a horizontal floating called "suspension."

Gait   an orderly footfall pattern such as the walk, trot, or canter.

Height   the degree of elevation of arc of the stride, viewed from the side.

Impulsion   thrust, the manner in which the horse's weight is settled and released from the supporting structures of the limb in the act of carrying the horse forward.

Overtrack   "tracking up"—the horse's hind feet step on or ahead of the front prints.

Pace   the variations within the gaits such as working trot, extended trot, collected trot; a goal (in dressage) is that the tempos should remain the same for the various paces within a gait. Pace also refers to a specific two-beat lateral gait exhibited by some Standardbreds and other horses.

Power   propelling, balancing, and sometimes pulling forces.

Rapidity   promptness, quickness; the time consumed in taking a single stride.

Regularity   the cadence, the rhythmical precision with which each stride is taken in turn.

Relaxation   absence of excess muscular tension.

Rhythm   the cadence of the footfall within a gait, taking into account timing (number of beats) and accent.

Sprain   injury to a ligament when a joint is carried through an abnormal range of motion.

Step   a single beat of a gait; a step may involve one or more limbs. In the walk, there are four individual steps. In the trot, there are two steps, and each involves two limbs.

Stiffness   inability (pain or lack of condition) or unwillingness (bad attitude) to flex and extend the muscles or joints.

Strain   injury (usually to muscle and/or tendon) from overuse or improper use of strength.

Stride, length of   the distance from the point of breaking over to the point of next contact with the ground of the same hoof; a full sequence of steps in a particular gait.

Suppleness   flexibility.

Suspension   the horizontal floating that occurs when a limb is extended and the body continues moving forward; also refers to the moment at the canter and gallop when all limbs are flexed or curled up, reorganizing for the next stride.

Tempo   the rate of movement, the rate of stride repetition; a faster tempo results in more strides per minute.

Travel   the path of the hoof (limb) flight in relation to the midline of the horse and the other limbs; usually viewed from the front or rear.

Defects in Travel

Paddling   the foot is thrown *outward* in flight, but the foot often lands *inside* the normal track; often associated with wide and/or toed-in conformation.

Winging   the foot swings *inward* in flight but often lands *outside* the normal track; often associated with narrow and/or toed-out conformation; dangerous because it can result in interfering.

Plaiting   also called rope-walking. The horse places one foot directly in front of the other; dangerous because of stumbling and tripping; associated with narrow, toed-out conformation.

Interfering   striking a limb with the opposite limb; associated with toed-out, base-narrow conformation; results in tripping, wounds.

Forging   hitting the sole or the shoe of the forefoot with the toe of the hindfoot on the same side; associated with sickle-hocked or short-backed/long-limbed conformation; a tired, young, or unconditioned horse; one that needs its shoes reset; or one with long toes.

Overreaching   hitting the heel of the forefoot with the hindfoot on the same side before the forefoot has left the ground; also called "grabbing"; often results in lost shoes.

dental problems often carries its head and neck in an unnatural position, which affects its movement. A sour, balky, or otherwise ill-tempered animal moves with characteristic resistance.

Encourage the horse owner to be involved in analyzing his/her horse's problem. Begin with an objective assessment of the horse's conformation, and then watch and listen to the horse as it is led and ridden on a smooth, level surface in a straight line at a walk and trot. View the horse from the front and the rear. Using a video camera with a high-speed shutter, videotape the horse's limbs and hooves moving at various forward gaits and backing. Play the tape in slow motion or in single-frame advance, and you will be able to see precisely when and where contact occurs or is most likely to occur. You can also note how the hoof lands and breaks over, which is critical information in formulating treatment.

References

1. Adams OR. Lameness in Horses. 3rd ed. Philadelphia: Lea & Febiger, 1974.
2. Back W, Schamhardt HC, Barnveld A. Longitudinal developement of equine locomotion from foal to adult. Proc Am Assoc Equine Pract 1995;41:146.
3. Back W, Schamhardt HC, Barnveld A. The influence of conformation on fore and hind limb kinematics of trotting Dutch Warmblood horses. Pferdeheilkunde 1996;12:647–650.
4. Back W, Barneveld A, Bruin G, et al. Kinematic detection of superior gait quality in young trotting warmbloods. Vet Q 1994;16:S91–S96.
5. Barr ARS. Carpal conformation in relation to carpal chip fractures. Vet Rec 1994;134:646.
6. Beeman GM. Correlation of defects in conformation to pathology in the horse. Proc Am Assoc Equine Pract 1983;19:177.
7. Bushe T, Turner TA, Poulos PW, et al. The effects of hoof angle on coffin, pastern and fetlock joint angles. Proc Am Assoc Equine Pract 1987;33:729.
8. Clayton HM. No foot – no horse. Anvil 1987;13:32.
9. Clayton HM. New research in hoof angles. Western Coll Vet Med Suppl 1988; Jan.
10. Clayton HM. The effect of an acute hoof wall angulation on the stride kinematics of trotting horses. Equine Vet J Suppl 1990; June: 86.
11. Clayton HM. Comparison of the stride kinematics of the collected, working, medium, and extended trot in the horses. Equine Vet J 1994;26:230.
12. Dalin G, Magnuson LE, Thafvelin BC. Retrospective study of hind quarter asymmetry in Standardbred trotter and its correlation with performance. Equine Vet J 1985;17:292–296.
13. Glade MJ, Salzman RA. Effects of hoof angle on hoof growth and contraction in the horse. J Equine Vet Sci 1985;5:45.
14. Holmstrom M, Magnuson LE, Philipssen J. Variations in conformation of Swedish Warmblood horses and conformational characteristics of elite sport horses. Equine Vet J 1990;22:186–193.
15. Holmstrom M, Phillippsson J. Relationship between conformation, performance and heath in 4-year-old Swedish Warmblood riding horses. Livestock Production Sci 1993;33:293.
16. Holmstrom M, Fredricson I, Drevemo S. Biokinamatic effects of collection on trotting gaits in the dressage horse. Equine Vet J 1995; 27:281.
17. Kane AJ, Stover MS, Gardner IA, et al. Toe and rim shoes as possible risk factors for catastrophic injury of Thoroughbred racehorses. Proc Am Assoc Equine Pract 1996;42:286.
18. Konen EPC, Velduizen AE, Brascamp EW. Genetic parameters of linear scored conformation traits and their relation to dressage and showjumping performance in the Dutch Warmblood riding horse population. Livestock Production Sci 1995;43:85.
19. Kobluk CN, Robinson A, Gordon BG, et al. The effect of conformation and shoeing: A cohort study of 95 thoroughbred racehorses. Proc Am Assoc Equine Pract 1990;36:259.
20. Magusson LE, Thafvelin B. Studies on the conformation and related traits of Standardbred trotters in Sweden. IV: Relationship between conformation and soundness of Standard trotters. Thesis SLU Skara ISBN91–576–2315–5.
21. Mawdsley A, Kelly EP, Smith FH, et al. Linear assessment of the Thoroughbred horse: An approach to conformation evaluation. Equine Vet J 1996;28:461–467.
22. Slade LM, Grau RB, Barbalace RC. Influence of conformation on concussive forces. In: Proceedings. 4th Equine Nutrition and Physiology Symposium, Pomona, CA, 1975;131–134.
23. Sloet van Oldruitenborgh-Oosterban MM, Barnveld A, Schamhardt HC. Kinematics of unmounted and mounted horses at a walk before and after treadmill exercise. Pferdeheilkunde 1996;12: 651–655.

Examination for Lameness

TED S. STASHAK

Lameness is an indication of a structural or functional disorder in one or more limbs or the back that is evident while the horse is standing or in movement.[1,55] Lameness can be caused by trauma, congenital or acquired anomalies, infection, metabolic disturbances, circulatory and nervous disorders, and any combination of these. The diagnosis of lameness requires a detailed knowledge of anatomy, an understanding of kinematics, and an appreciation for geometric design and resultant forces.

The examiner must also be able to differentiate between lameness resulting from painful and nonpainful alterations in gait, often referred to as "mechanical lameness," and lameness resulting from neurologic (nervous system) dysfunction.[1,4] To make this differentiation, a complete history (including signalment and use) is taken. The horse is then observed at rest and at exercise to identify the limb or limbs involved. Next, the examiner palpates and performs manipulation to identify the region of pain. Note that veterinarians often palpate the limbs, digital pulses, back, and neck and perform the hoof tester examination before exercising the horse. Diagnostic anesthesia and imaging may follow to clarify the location of pain, the problem, and the extent of injury. Blood samples may also be taken for laboratory analysis.

CLASSIFICATION OF LAMENESS

Lameness can be classified into one of four types:

1. *Supporting limb lameness* is apparent when the foot first contacts the ground or when the limb is supporting weight (stance phase). It is considered to be caused by injury to bones, joints, soft tissue support structures (e.g., ligaments and flexor tendons), motor nerves, or the foot.
2. *Swinging limb lameness* is evident when the limb is in motion. It is considered to be caused by pathologic changes involving joints, muscles, tendons (primarily extensors), tendon sheaths, or bursas.
3. *Mixed lameness* is seen when the limb is moving (swing phase) and when it is supporting weight (stance phase). It can involve any combination of the structures affected in swinging or supporting limb

lameness. By observing the gait from a distance, the examiner can determine whether the lameness is supporting limb, swinging limb, or mixed. Some conditions that produce supporting limb lameness may cause the horse to alter the movement of the limb to protect the foot when it lands. This could be mistaken for a swinging limb lameness.

4. *Complementary or compensatory lameness* occurs when pain in a limb causes uneven distribution of weight on another limb or limbs. This can produce lameness in a previously sound limb. It is common to have a complementary lameness in a forelimb (or hindlimb) as a result of lameness in the opposite forelimb (or hindlimb).[55] In addition, lameness in a hindlimb can result in lameness in the opposite forelimb (e.g., left rear and right front). This occurs most frequently in horses that are required to work off their hindlimbs (e.g., cutting or dressage).

Even minor changes in weight bearing can produce complementary lameness at high speeds, especially over long distances. The feet, suspensory ligament, sesamoid bones, hocks, and flexor tendons seem to be affected most commonly. However, horses that fracture both carpi in identical places may have shifted their weight unevenly after one carpus becomes sore or one carpal bone is fractured.

Complementary lameness in the same limb usually results when excess stress occurs to an otherwise healthy structure and the horse attempts to protect the painful region in that limb. For example, a horse with navicular syndrome often lands toe first. This constant landing on the toe can cause bruising of the toe, which can result in pedal osteitis (inflammation of the coffin bone).

Character of the Stride

The character of the stride of a limb is also important to the diagnosis of lameness. When observing the stride, note the following characteristics:

1. *Phases of the stride.* The stride consists of a cranial phase and a caudal phase (Fig. 3.1). The cranial

113

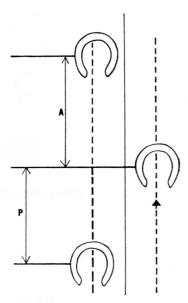

Figure 3.1 Phases of a stride. The cranial phase of the stride (A) is the half of the stride in front of the print of the opposite foot. The caudal phase of the stride (P) is the half of the stride in back of the print of the opposite foot.

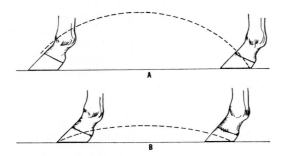

Figure 3.2 A. Normal arc of foot flight. B. Low arc of foot flight caused by lack of flexion in either the forelimbs or the hindlimbs.

phase of the stride is in front of the footprint of the opposite limb, and the caudal phase is behind it. With lameness, the cranial or caudal phase may be shortened. If the cranial phase is shortened, the caudal phase may undergo compensatory lengthening.

Alterations in the phase of the stride are best viewed from the side. Potential causes for a shortened cranial phase include navicular syndrome, chip fractures in joints, degenerative joint disease, trauma to the extensor tendons, shoulder problems, gonitis, and bone spavin. Some causes of a shortened caudal phase include palmar and plantar digital anular ligament desmitis, tendinitis (inflammation of a tendon), and tendosynovitis (inflammation of a tendon and its sheath) of the flexor tendons.

2. *Arc of foot flight.* The arc of foot flight is changed when there is pain anywhere in the limb (Fig. 3.2). The arc of one foot is compared with that of the opposite member when viewed from the side. In some cases, the arc is changed in both forefeet (bilateral navicular syndrome, laminitis) or in both hind-

feet (bilateral bone spavin). In the hindlimb, the arc may be changed enough to cause the toe to drag when the limb is advanced (bone spavin, gonitis) because of reduced flexion of the hock or stifle joints. In some types of lameness, the horse will over-flex the lame limb while leaving the sound limb as close to the ground as possible; thus the sound limb has a decreased height of the foot flight arc.

Most horses exhibiting a lowered foot flight arc also show an alteration in their phase of stride. To note subtle alterations in the hoof flight arc of the hindlimb, it is sometimes helpful to observe the horse from the rear to compare the extent and duration that the horse presents the surfaces of the sole of both feet to the observer. Generally, the less sole seen, the lower the arc of foot flight.

3. *Path of the foot in flight.* If the foot travels inward, it may cause an interference problem (e.g., trauma to a medial sesamoid or splint bone, painful lesions of the knee). When the foot travels in an outward path (paddling), no special problem usually results. If paddling does develop, however, it may be a sign of bilateral carpal pain.

4. *How the foot lands.* When a painful condition is present in the foot, the horse will usually indicate the pain by placing its weight opposite to the pain. For example, in a nail puncture at the toe, the weight is placed on the heel. If the lesion is in the lateral portion of the sole, the weight is carried on the medial side of the foot, and if the lesion is in the medial portion of the sole, the weight is carried on the lateral side of the foot.

5. *Joint extension.* The degree of extension of the fetlock (how close the back of the fetlock approaches the ground) during weight bearing is a sensitive indicator of how much weight the horse is willing to bear on that limb. Reduction in fetlock extension during weight bearing usually indicates the lame limb. This sign can be observed at a walk or a trot.

6. *Joint flexion angles.* Joint flexion angles are best viewed from the side and may be associated with alterations in the hoof flight arc and phase of stride. One limb is compared to the other, and the degree of flexion is assessed. In some cases, the horse compensates with an increased flexion of the unaffected limb. In others, it may reduce the flexion angle in the unaffected limb.

7. *Symmetry and duration of gluteal use.* To identify hindlimb lameness, it is helpful to observe the horse from the rear to compare the symmetry and duration of gluteal use and to correlate these findings with alterations in the character of the stride viewed from the side (for details, see the section on the hindlimbs in this chapter).

Other Lameness Factors

Most lamenesses are found in the forelimb, and approximately three lamenesses will be seen in the forelimb to every lameness in the hindlimb. The reason for this increased occurrence is because the forelimbs carry 60 to 65% of the horse's weight and are thus subject to much greater concussion than the hindlimbs (the hindlimbs propel the limbs, whereas the forelimbs receive the shock of landing). However, breed and use are important considerations. Standardbred racehorses have a higher percentage of hindlimb lameness than do other breeds, which is believed to be the result of their balanced gait characteristics. And horses used for performance events such as dressage, cutting, and reining, which place greater stress on the hindquarters, have a higher incidence of hindlimb lameness than do other breeds. In the hindlimb, most lamenesses occur in the hock and stifle. Table 3.1 lists lamenesses and their associated activities. Although there is considerable overlap, the common lameness associated with the type of work should be suspected first.

It is believed that at least 95% of lameness in the forelimb occurs from the knee down. Therefore, if the lameness is in the forelimb, eliminate all common lamenesses that affect the distal portion of the limb before considering other lameness, unless some other condition is obvious. In the hindlimb, approximately 80% of lamenesses are seen in the hock or stifle. Therefore, if the lameness is the hindlimb, conduct a preliminary examination of the foot and lower limb and then give primary consideration to the hock and stifle. In difficult cases, diagnostic anesthesia can be helpful.

There are other factors to consider as the cause of lameness. Horses that are improperly or irregularly shod may become lame.[43] Shoeing should be considered as a complementary aid to the way the horse moves; if not properly done, shoeing can produce lameness, especially at high speeds. The surface on which the horse works may be a contributing factor in lameness. Surfaces that are too soft, too hard, slippery, or rocky may aggravate conformational imperfections or may be the outright

Table 3.1 LAMENESSES AND THEIR GENERALLY ASSOCIATED ACTIVITIES

Event	Movement	Lameness
Dressage	Sitting trot	Back
	Weight carried rearward	Hip
	Increased joint flexion	Early hock arthritis → bone spavin
	Great impulsion	Gonitis
	Collection; extension	Fetlock arthritis (synovitis/capsulitis)
Reining	Deep, sliding stops	Hamstring tear → fibrotic myopathy
	Fast spins	Early hock arthritis → bone spavin
	Rollbacks	p2 fracture, hind
Cutting	Balancing and turning on hindquarters with power and torque	Front bruised soles
	Lateral driving with forelimbs	p1 and p2 fractures
		Early hock arthritis → bone spavin
		Gonitis
Roping	Explosive bursts	p2 and p3 fractures
	Hard stops and abrupt change in direction	Bone spavin
		Navicular syndrome
TB and QH racing	Young horses	Bucked shins
	Top speed	Fatigue fractures
	Footing stresses	Bowed tendons
	Fatigue	Carpitis
		Carpal chip and slab fractures
		Suspensory ligament injuries
		Fetlock arthritis and chip fractures
		Sesamoid fractures
SB racing	Extended and fast pacing and trotting	Same as TB and QH racing
		Hock and stifle problems
		Cunean tendinitis
Barrel racing, pole bending	Speed with turning	Fetlock arthritis (synovitis/capsulitis)
	Torque and twist	p3 fractures
		Navicular syndrome
		Ringbone
		Ligament sprain
Show ring	Repetitive circular and arena work (often on hard footing)	Navicular syndrome
		Sprain trauma to fetlock and phalanges
Jumping, eventing	Fetlock hyperextension landing after jump	Navicular syndrome
	Cross-country footing	Bowed tendon
		Ligament sprain
Endurance	Long miles	Bowed tendons
	Often hard or rocky footing	Pedal osteitis
	Fatigue	Hoof injuries
		Sole bruises
		Fatigue fractures
Inactivity	Lack of movement	Laminitis
	Poor blood flow	
	Overweight	
Confinement	Overexuberance	Trauma injuries
	Sudden outbursts	

p1, long pastern; p2, short pastern; p3, coffin bone; TB, Thoroughbred; QH, Quarter Horse; SB, Standardbred.

cause of lameness. Improper conditioning resulting in muscle fatigue is believed to be a common cause of performance-related injuries. The age of a horse is often a factor in predisposition to lameness. Because of the emphasis on racing and showing 2-year-olds, many lamenesses are produced in these horses that may not occur in older, more mature horses.

SIGNALMENT AND USE

Patient age and use are important considerations. For example, an aged crossbred horse used for ranch work, occasional rodeo performance, and trail riding will have a higher incidence of problems associated with the forefeet, low-motion joints (e.g., pasterns and distal tarsal joints), and ligaments. In contrast, a racehorse most often presents with lameness associated with high-motion joints (e.g., carpus and fetlock), sprain or strain of flexor support structures, and stress-related fractures. Horses used for competitive trail or endurance riding sustain a higher incidence of sprain and strain injuries and stress-related fractures to the phalanges. Young horses beginning training may suffer from developmental orthopedic-related lameness problems.

HISTORY (ANAMNESIS)

A detailed medical history should be obtained on every horse. Records should include specific information regarding the duration and intensity of the lameness, the symptoms, the activity immediately preceding the lameness, and any previous treatments or therapies employed. The following questions should be answered:

1. *How long has the horse been lame?* If lameness has been present for a month or more, it is considered a chronic condition and permanent structural changes may have taken place that render complete recovery unlikely. Therefore, the prognosis is usually guarded. Generally, a young horse has a better chance for recovery from a chronic condition than has a mature horse.
2. *Has the horse been rested or exercised during the lameness period?* Horses that have been rested may not exhibit the lameness that was seen while the horse was in training.
3. *Has the lameness worsened, stayed the same, or improved?* Horses that have shown a marked improvement in the lameness will usually have a better prognosis than horses that have remained static or have worsened.
4. *What caused the lameness?* The owner may have removed a nail from the foot or may have seen the injury occur. If so, the owner's description should include the character of the lameness at the time it was first noticed. If the lameness was acute initially, this may indicate a condition such as a fractured distal phalanx; if the lameness developed insidiously, extension of a subsolar abscess resulting in osteomyelitis of the distal phalanx may be the cause.
5. *Does the horse warm out of the lameness?* If so, sore muscles or arthritic joints (such as bone spavin) may be involved.

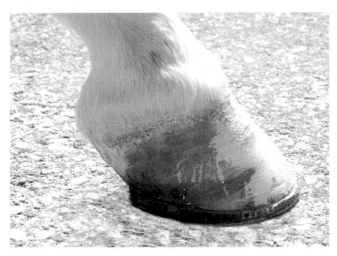

Figure 3.3 The horse presented with a history of stumbling. Note how long the hoof is.

6. *Does the horse stumble?* Stumbling may be the result of some interference with the synergistic action of the flexor and extensor muscles. It may be caused by pain, a neurologic disorder (spinal ataxia), or simply feet that are too long (Fig. 3.3).
7. *What treatment was given and was it helpful?* The answers may help in the prognosis of the case. If the horse received recommended therapy for an appropriate period with no results, the prognosis is guarded. It is important to record the names and dosages of drugs used. It is also important to know if the horse was treated with nonsteroidal anti-inflammatory drugs (NSAIDs) or with parenteral or intrasynovial anti-inflammatory agents, because these drugs may mask symptoms of lameness and give a false impression of recovery.
8. *When was the horse shod?* Sometimes the feet are trimmed too short or a nail is driven into or near sensitive tissue. If the feet have been trimmed too short, usually more than one foot is involved in the lameness. A hoof tester examination often identifies diffuse pain. If a nail has been driven into or close to sensitive tissue, the lameness will involve one limb, and hoof tester sensitivity is usually focal to the site of penetration. If the nail was driven into sensitive tissue, signs of infection may not be evident for several days. If the nail did not enter sensitive tissue but is near it, lameness from pressure on the sensitive tissue may result. This is commonly called a "close nail," and the pressure will not be relieved until the nail is pulled (see Chapter 9 for more information).

PROCEDURES FOR EXAMINATION

Visual Examination

At Rest

A careful visual examination is made with the horse standing squarely on a flat surface at rest.[4,39] This should be done at a distance and then up close, with the horse viewed from all directions. From a distance, the body type is characterized (stocky vs. slender), conformation is noted, and body condition and alterations in posture, weight shifting, and pointing are also noted.

In the normal attitude, the forelimbs bear equal weight and are opposite each other. With bilateral forelimb involvement, the weight may be shifted from one foot to the other or both limbs may be placed too far out in front, called "camped in front." In the hindlimbs, it is normal for the horse to shift the weight from one limb to the other. If the horse consistently rests one hindlimb and refuses to bear weight on it for a length of time or cannot be forced to bear weight on it at all, lameness in that hindlimb should be considered.

At close observation, each limb and muscle group is observed and compared to its opposing member for symmetry. Feet are observed for abnormal wear, hoof cracks, imbalance, size, and heel bulb contraction (Fig. 3.3). All joints and tendons and their sheaths are visually inspected for swelling and the muscles of the limbs, back, and rump are observed for swelling and atrophy. Comparing one side to the other is most important.

Each abnormal finding should be ruled out as a cause of lameness during the exercise and palpation examination. For the forelimbs, the limb with the narrowest (smallest) foot and highest heel with varying degrees of extensor muscle atrophy is usually the lame or lamer (if the problem is bilateral) limb (Fig. 3.4). The foot is smaller because of the chronic alteration in weight bearing, and muscle atrophy results from a reluctance to extend that limb, which would commit it to longer period of weight bearing. For the hindlimb, atrophy of the middle gluteal and/or gracilis muscles usually indicates the lame limb (Fig. 3.5). Generally, if one tuber sacrale is higher than the other ("hunter's bump") and/or the pelvis appears tilted, the horse will not have a symmetric gait.

At Exercise

The characteristics of the gait of all limbs should be observed from a distance. In most cases, it is best to observe the forelimbs first, followed by observation of the hindlimbs. Once the examiner is able to observe all limbs at once and then each limb individually, the diagnosis of lameness is simplified. Usually, a horse is observed at exercise with shoes on; in some cases, however, it is helpful to view the horse in motion without shoes.

The main objective in exercising the horse is to identify the limb or limbs involved and the degree of lameness and incoordination in movement. To do this, the horse is observed at a walk and trot in a straight line and then while lunging in circles. Sometimes, it is helpful to observe the horse under tack or at high speed on a treadmill. Examination includes watching the horse from the front, side, and rear. In general, forelimb lamenesses are best viewed from the front and side, and hindlimb lamenesses

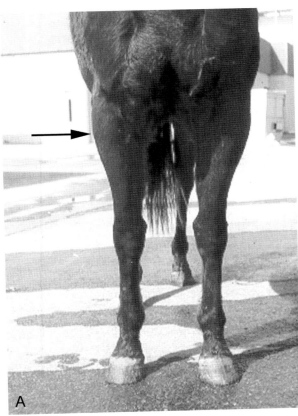

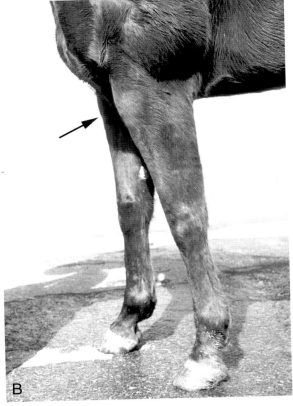

Figure 3.4   A. Cranial view of extensor muscle atrophy of the right forelimb (arrow). Note that the right foot is smaller than the left.

B. Lateral view of the same horse. Note that the heel height is higher in the right forefoot than the left forefoot.

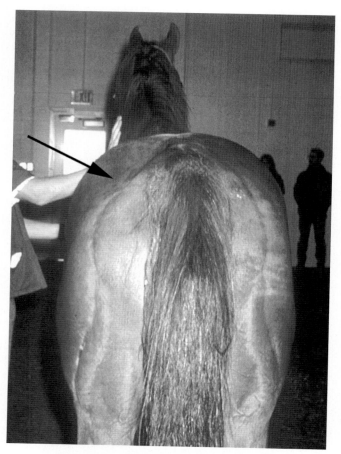

Figure 3.5   Gluteus muscle atrophy (arrow).

are best observed from the side and rear. What the examiner is looking for is head nodding, gait asymmetry, alterations in height of the foot flight arc, alterations in foot flight, phase of stride, joint flexion angle, foot placement, degree of fetlock extension with weight bearing, action of shoulder muscles, and symmetry in gluteal rise and use. To visualize these gait changes, it is best to look at the horse from a distance. The action of all four limbs is observed first, then the limb in question is isolated and looked at closely, and finally attention is shifted to the opposite limb for comparison. To detect subtle gait changes, it may necessary to shift visually from one limb to the other or to jog alongside or behind the horse for better comparison.

How to Handle the Horse

The handler plays an important role in lameness examination. In general, horses should be held loosely with their heads centered on line with their bodies and exercised at a constant speed in a straight line as slowly as practical (Fig. 3.6). If the head and neck are allowed to sway from one side to the other, an asymmetric gait will be created. If the handler holds the horse too tightly, subtle head nodding is difficult to observe. Fast trotting or cantering makes it more difficult to focus in on limb movement, but sometimes it may be helpful in identifying a neurologic deficit, since more coordination is re-

quired for movement at speed. In addition, the handler should not look at the horse and should be far enough in front of the horse's limbs so as not to obscure the examiner's view (Fig. 3.7).

Circling a horse at a trot accentuates low-grade lameness, usually on the inside limb. This can be done by having the handler jog in a circle or, preferably, by lunging the horse in a circle. The horse should be relaxed at a trot, starting with a large circle, which gradually gets smaller. A smaller circle will sometimes reveal lameness not seen in a larger circle. The handler should avoid giving the horse voice commands or attempt to train the horse while circling. Horses with bilateral forelimb lameness not seen at a trot in a straight line will often begin to show lameness on the inside limb. This will be manifested, when the lame limb contacts the ground, by head and neck lifting, splinting the shoulder muscles in anticipation of weight bearing, and placing the head and neck to the outside of the circle to unweight the lame limb. In some cases, the horse will attempt to make a square out of the circle or, when circled to the lame side, will act up or stop periodically. If the lameness persists or is exaggerated when the limb is on the outside of the circle, high suspensory ligament desmitis, collateral ligament injury, medial carpal problems, medial splint bone problems, or medial sesamoid bone problems should be considered. Circling usually accentuates hindlimb lameness when the limb is on the inside of the circle. A more delayed protraction of the limb, a shorter cranial phase of the stride, and a greater degree of unweighting of the limb (hip roll and lack of extension of the fetlock) will be seen. A toe drag may also become more apparent.

If the horse is flighty or apprehensive, the examination can be facilitated by the administration of 15 to 20 mg of acepromazine maleate intravenously to a 1000-lb (450-kg) horse.[4] Wait 15 to 20 minutes after the injection before resuming the examination. The tranquilization allows the horse to relax, making the lameness more apparent. This is particularly true for painful conditions that alter the gait. If the horse is unbroken, it can be encouraged to move in a round pen without the assistance of a handler. To examine a foal, the dam can be exercised, and the foal observed as it follows the mare.

Selection of Surfaces

In most cases, the evaluation of lameness is best carried out on a hard, level surface. A hard surface provides more concussion than a softer surface, and it affords the examiner the opportunity to listen to, as well as to visualize, foot placement. Usually, there is an obvious difference in the horse's landing between the unsound and sound foot. The unsound foot makes less noise because less weight is taken on that foot, whereas the sound foot makes a louder noise because it is bearing more weight. This is true for both forelimbs and hindlimbs. Foot placement also is best observed on hard surfaces, because softer surfaces tend to envelop the foot, making placement more difficult to see.

Because hard surfaces typically do not apply sole and frog pressure, horses with suspected foot problems can be exercised on dirt, turf, or gravel (short distance) surfaces to accentuate the lameness. This is particularly true of horses with chronic symmetric conditions involving

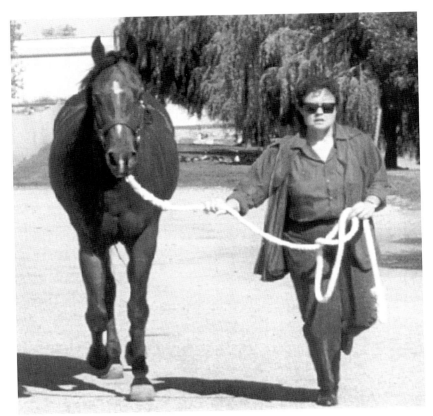

Figure 3.6   A handler properly exercising a horse at a trot.

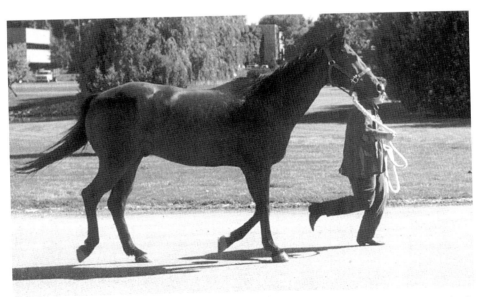

Figure 3.7   The handler is well out in front of the horse and does not obscure the examiner's view.

the feet. When exercised on asphalt, they may travel with a stilted, shuffling-like gait but appear comfortable. When exercised on gravel, bilateral lameness becomes quite evident.

THE FORELIMBS

As a result of lameness in a forelimb, the head will drop when the sound foot lands and will rise when weight is placed on the unsound foot or limb. If the lameness is not evident at the walk, it usually will be at the trot; this is because there is only one other supporting foot on the ground (Table 3.2). In addition, splinting of the caudal neck and shoulder muscles in anticipation of weight bearing on that limb will be seen.

When the horse is at the trot, be cautious not to confuse a left hind lameness with a left fore lameness or a right hind lameness with a right fore lameness. This can happen when a hindlimb is lame at the trot, because the horse will often land more solidly on the sound opposite forelimb. For example, if a left hindlimb is lame at the trot, the horse will lower its head when the left hindlimb and right forelimb land, taking more weight on the right forelimb (see the section on hindlimbs in this chapter). On a hard surface, this gives the impression that the horse is yielding on the left forelimb, indicating lameness in that limb.

Occasionally, a situation arises in which left hindlimb lameness is confused with right forelimb lameness. This usually occurs when there is little or no head nodding at the trot. The sound diagonals (right hind and left fore) contact the ground with such force that it appears that the horse is protecting the right forelimb. The confusion commonly arises when watching the horse from the side. Watching the horse from behind reveals the hip asymmetry typical of hindlimb lameness. Head movement may also be absent in bilateral involvement of the limbs or with mild lameness.

In the normal gait, the heel is lifted first when the limb is advanced. When the foot lands, the hoof should land flat or the heel should hit just before the toe. Selective weight bearing and alteration in the phases of stride may be observed when pain involves one region of the foot. If pain is present in the lateral portion of the foot, the weight will be taken medially. In general, pain in the toe region will cause a shortened caudal phase of the stride, whereas involvement of the heel region will cause a shortened cranial phase of the stride.

The arc that the foot makes in flight should be observed (Fig. 3.2). If it is too low in the forelimb, there

may be interference with flexion of the shoulder, knee, or fetlock, resulting from pain or mechanical injury. Fixation of these joints will reduce the arc of the foot flight, limit the cranial phase of the stride, and lengthen the caudal phase. When the shoulder is involved, the scapulohumeral joint usually remains semifixed during progression (swing phase), and the head may show marked lifting and be pulled toward the unaffected side. When both forefeet are involved, the gait often appears unanimated (stilted or stiff), giving the false impression of shoulder involvement.

If interference of the limbs is suspected but cannot be seen, the hoof walls can be coated with chalk; the contact will leave a mark of chalk on the limb. This can be done for both the forelimbs and the hindlimbs. Although chalking the hooves will work, a better approach is to use a video camera, which will identify interference as well as foot flight.

The forms of limb contact are defined as follows (Fig. 3.8; see also Chapter 2):

1. *Brushing.* A general term for light striking, especially as in interfering.

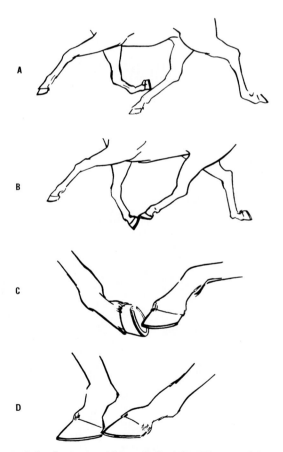

Figure 3.8 Contact problems. A. Scalping: The toe of the forefoot hits the dorsal surface of the pastern or metatarsal region of the hindlimb on the same side. B. Cross firing: Contact is made between the inside of the toe of the hindfoot and the inside of the forefoot on the opposite side. This occurs in pacers. C. Forging: The toe of the hindfoot hits the bottom of the forefoot on the same side. D. Overreaching can cause pulling of the front shoe.

Table 3.2 HEAD MOVEMENT AT A TROT WITH SUPPORTING LIMB LAMENESS[a]

Lame Limb[b]	Head Down When These Limbs Land	Head Up When These Limbs Land
Right front	Left front, right hind	Right front, left hind
Left front	Right front, left hind	Left front, right hind
Right hind	Left front, right hind	Right front, left hind
Left hind	Right front, left hind	Left front, right hind

[a]Although not absolute, the movements are true in many cases.
[b]Note the potential confusion between right front and right hind lameness and left front and left hind lameness when head movement with the horse at a trot is used as the indicator.

2. *Cross firing.* Generally confined to pacers, it consists of contact on the inside of the diagonal forefoot and hindfoot and commonly involves the inside of the hindfoot hitting the inside quarter of the diagonal forefoot.

3. *Elbow hitting.* Occurring when the horse hits the elbow with the shoe of the same limb, it is rare except in horses with weighted shoes.

4. *Forging.* The toe of the hindfoot hits the sole or shoe of the forefoot on the same side, usually on the heel. Depending on when forging occurs, it may also be described as the front sole or shoe slapping the toe of the hindfoot as it comes gliding in for a landing.

5. *Knee hitting.* High interference, generally seen in Standardbred horses.

6. *Interfering.* Occurring in both the forefoot and the hindfoot, it is a striking, anywhere between the coronary band and the cannon, by the opposite foot that is in motion.

7. *Overreaching.* The toe of the hindfoot catches the forefoot on the same side, usually on the heel. The hindfoot advances more quickly than in forging, stepping on the heel of the forefoot. The toe of the hindfoot may step on the show of the forefoot on the same side and cause shoe pulling.

8. *Scalping.* The toe of the forefoot hits the hairline at the coronary band or above on the hindfoot of the same side and may hit the dorsal (front) face of the pastern or cannon bone. Generally, this is a fault of the trotting horse.

9. *Speedy cutting.* Difficult to determine because it apparently has no positive definition, it may be the same as cross firing or may mean that the outside wall of the hindfoot comes up and strikes the medial aspect of the forelimb on the same side. Thus it can be considered any type of limb interference at the fast gaits.

Contact problems can occur in well-shod horses with good conformation as a result of the type of work they are performing. For instance, in barrel racing, cutting, pole bending, and reining, the horse's weight is suddenly shifted and the horse may be off balance, resulting in uncoordinated movement and contact.

THE HINDLIMBS

In observing movement of the hindlimbs, the arc of the foot flight is best viewed from the side (Fig. 3.2). Involvement of the hock and stifle joints generally reduces the arc of the foot flight and thus shortens the cranial phase of the stride with a compensating lengthening of the caudal phase. Because of the reciprocal apparatus of the hock and stifle, incomplete flexion is characteristic of involvement of both joints. The toe may be worn excessively (dubbed off) with involvement of the hock or stifle (Fig. 3.9). Although head and neck movements can be observed from the rear, they are best viewed from the side with the horse at the trot. With mild hindlimb lameness, abnormal movements of the head and neck may not be evident. In moderate to severe lameness, the head and neck will rise as the unaffected hindlimb contacts the ground and will lower when the affected hindlimb contacts the ground (Table 3.2). In severe cases, the horse not only will lower its head and neck but also will

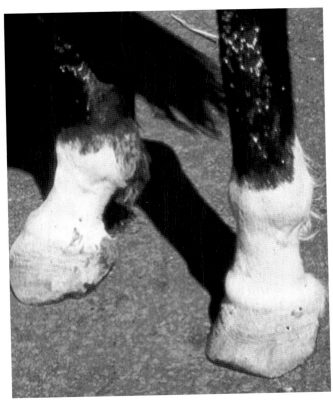

Figure 3.9 Excessive toe wear of both hindlimbs.

extend its head. The lowering of the head and neck while the affected hindlimb is in the weight-bearing phase at a trot serves to reduce the weight placed on the affected hindlimb when it contacts the ground.

The symmetry of gluteal rise and the duration of gluteal use (movement of the croup) are evaluated from the rear. The rise is evident during the swing phase of the stride; the use is evident during the support (stance) phase of the stride. This observation is best made on a level surface so that the examiner can see the uppermost excursion of the gluteal muscles. A symmetric gluteal rise as the hindlimbs are brought forward indicates that both limbs are swinging symmetrically and subsequently are elevated to the same height. On the other hand, the duration of gluteal use is a function of weight bearing with subsequent contraction of the gluteal muscles as the limb moves from cranial to caudal during weight bearing (support/stance phase of the stride). In the painful situation, most horses attempt to get off the hindlimb quickly, and the gluteal muscle contraction is shortened, which leads to a shortened duration of gluteal use and a subsequent hip "roll" or "drop off." Following this, there is a rapid elevation of the hip and gluteals recognized as a "hip hike" or "upward flick" on the affected side. May and Wyn-Jones[38] documented head and hip movement in 13 horses suffering hindlimb lameness at various sites. They examined the horses from the rear, using tuber coxae (hip) markers and a video camera. Hip and croup heights were measured at four points in stride. It was found that the hip marker on the lame side was highest at the point of initial weight bearing but dropped rapidly during weight bearing until the limb left the ground. The lame limb was then rapidly elevated during the swing phase. Despite the rapid elevation and the end of stride (swing phase)—recognized as an upward flick of the hip marker—the affected hip was often not elevated above the hip on the sound side (6 cases were elevated; 7 cases were not). In fact, the midpoint of the vertical displacement for each hip marker was lower in the lame limb in all 13 cases. The croup (gluteal rise) was always higher when the lame limb started to bear weight; this was difficult to see, however, when the lameness was slight. In all cases, the head dropped when the lame hindlimb contacted the ground. I recognize three situations in regard to gluteal rise and use:

1. *Depressed gluteal rise and decreased use.* Usually seen in horses that are in pain during the swing phase of the stride, this gait often involves structures above the stifle. Along with muscle atrophy, this gait is commonly seen with problems involving the hip region.
2. *Symmetric gluteal rise but decreased gluteal use.* Usually seen in horses with subtle hindlimb lameness, this gait is not commonly seen with head nodding, and only subtle changes in the height of the foot flight arc, phase of stride, and flexion angles may be observed.
3. *Rapid, increased gluteal rise ("hip hike" or "upward flick") and decreased gluteal use.* Usually seen in horses that are in considerable pain during the support phase of the stride, the affected limb is brought up rapidly. Varying degrees of head nodding will be seen, and the height of the foot flight arc, phase of stride, and flexion angles are usually altered.

Grading the Lameness

The degree of lameness should be recorded. Although categorizing lameness as mild, moderate, or severe may suffice, a more objective approach using a grading system is recommended. A lameness grading system is beneficial because it not only defines the degree of lameness but also makes record keeping easier and provides the examiner with an objective reference to assess improvement at reevaluation. The lameness grading system of the American Association of Equine Practitioners (AAEP) is outlined in Table 3.3.[67]

Table 3.3 AAEP LAMENESS GRADING SYSTEM

Grade	Description
0	Lameness not perceptible under any circumstances
1	Lameness difficult to observe; not consistently apparent regardless of circumstances (e.g., weight carrying, circling, inclines, hard surface)
2	Lameness difficult to observe at a walk or trot in a straight line; consistently apparent under some circumstances (e.g., weight carrying, circling, inclines, hard surface)
3	Lameness consistently observable at a trot under all circumstances
4	Lameness obvious; marked nodding, hitching, and/or shortened stride
5	Lameness obvious; minimal weight bearing in motion or rest; inability to move

Examination by Palpation and Manipulation

After observing the animal at exercise, make a close visual examination, including palpation of the limbs; or inspect and palpate the horse before watching it exercise. In either case, a systematic method of palpation should be followed so nothing is overlooked. Therefore, start at the foot and palpate the entire limb.

Examination of the Forelimb

FOOT

The size and shape of the foot on the lame limb should be compared with the size and shape of the foot on the opposite limb. The examiner is looking for asymmetry in foot size, abnormal hoof wear, ring formation and heel bulb contraction, shearing of the heels and quarters, hoof wall cracks, swellings that are primarily associated with the coronet, and foot imbalances.[1,43]

Asymmetry in foot size may be a result of trauma, lack of weight bearing leading to contraction, and congenital or developmental defects. In general, the limb with the smallest foot is usually the lame limb.

Hoof wall ring formation can be unilateral (resulting from trauma) or bilateral (resulting from selenium toxicosis, laminitis, or generalized systemic disease). Ring formation is not always associated with lameness (Fig. 3.10).

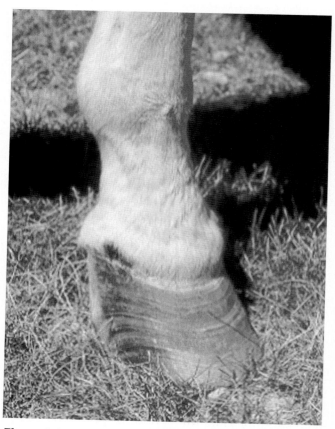

Figure 3.10 Hoof wall ring formation in a horse that is not lame.

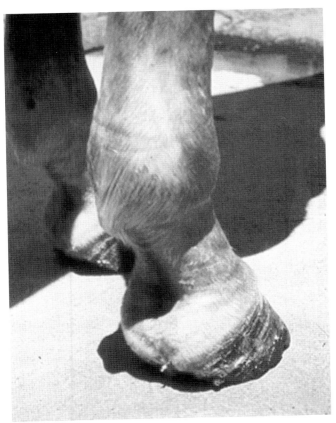

Figure 3.11   Heel bulb contraction. Note how close together the heel bulbs are.

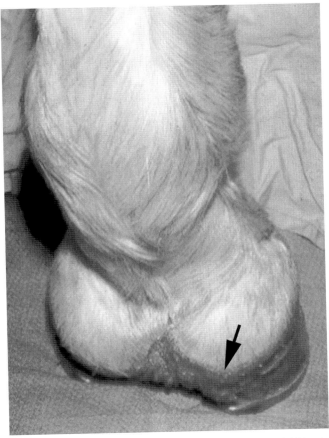

Figure 3.12   Proximal displacement (shearing) of the right heel (arrow).

Heel bulb contraction is often misunderstood. It usually results from decreased weight bearing of the affected limb and is a symptom rather than the cause of the lameness (Fig. 3.11). Visual examination of heel bulb contraction is best performed by the examiner standing or squatting near the flank and looking at both right and left heel bulbs at once. An objective assessment can be made by checking the heel bulb spacing with finger measurements. Asymmetry in the heel bulb height (sheared heels) is recorded (Fig. 3.12). This is most frequently associated with improper trimming and shoeing.[43]

Hoof wall cracks may be associated with lameness but must be ruled out with a hoof tester examination and, in some cases, nerve blocks.

Swellings at the coronet can result from superficial scar formation from wire cuts or constant bruising during exercise, keratoma, dermatitis, or deeper involvement (e.g., gravel and quittor).

Foot imbalances can either be dorsopalmar, lateral medial, or a combination of the two (Fig. 3.13). These imbalances often alter the shape of the hoof wall and can result in abnormal stresses applied to the foot and other support structures.

After superficially cleaning the sole, note abnormal wear, collapsed heels, heel bulb contraction, and frog atrophy (Fig. 3.14). Heel bulbs that are closer than normal are consistent with any condition that has resulted in decreased weight bearing by that limb or improper trimming and shoeing. In chronic cases, there may be

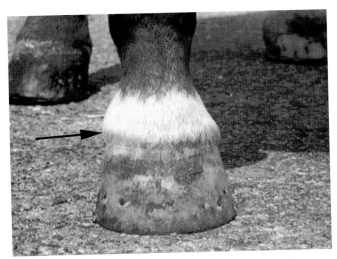

Figure 3.13   Lateral medial hoof imbalance. Note that the medial coronet band (arrow) is higher than the lateral coronet band.

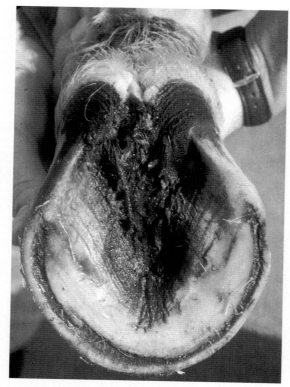

Figure 3.14   Frog atrophy and heel bulb contraction.

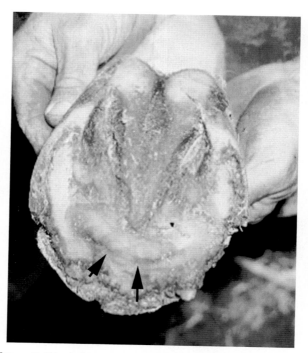

Figure 3.15   A dropped sole and a crescent-shaped crack (arrows) in the sole, indicating rotation and penetration of the distal phalanx.

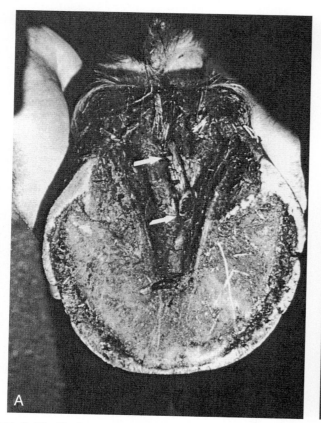

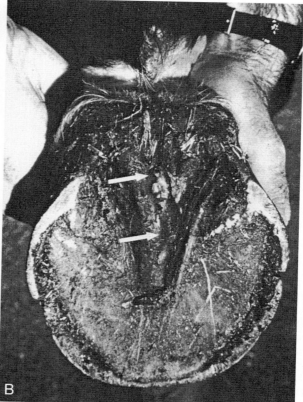

Figure 3.16   The horse presented with a history of hindlimb lameness of 3 weeks' duration. A. Examination of the ground surface of the hoof revealed a piece of wood buried in the frog (arrows). B. Frog after the wood was removed. Note that the sensitive corium is exposed (arrows).

some frog atrophy associated with the heel bulb contraction.

Observe the shape of the sole. A slightly concave shape is normal. Some horses are flatfooted and, therefore, predisposed to sole bruising. Convexity dorsal to the apex of the frog ("dropped soles" in front of the frog) is considered abnormal and may be associated with rotation of the distal phalanx (coffin bone) (Fig. 3.15). If the foot has not been trimmed recently, it may be done at this time. During trimming, look for any discoloration of the sole and/or a white line. Sometimes, the cause of the lameness may be identified, such as a stick or nail wedged in the frog (Fig. 3.16) or pus exuding from a small hole in the sole or white line (Fig. 3.17). The clefts of the frog may have to be opened if the frog is excessively overgrown and any indications of thrush are noted.

Next, the examiner applies a hoof tester, in a systematic manner, to the entire sole and frog region and hoof wall (Fig. 3.18). When applied properly, this instrument allows the examiner to palpate the hoof. For a sensitive horse, the examiner may need to use a gentle application at first, followed by firmer pressure. The examiner is trying to identify and localize hoof sensitivity. Although this sounds simple, it requires experience.

The arm of the hoof tester that is applied to the hoof wall needs to be continually checked so pressure is not

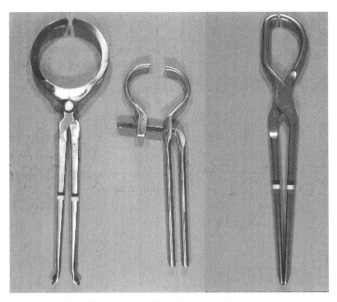

Figure 3.18 Three types of hoof testers. The left tester is made by GE Forge and Tool Works (Grover Beach, CA); the middle tester is a Ryding Hoof Tester made by Jorgenson Labs (Loveland, CO); and the right tester is made by Kane Enterprises (Sioux Falls, SD).

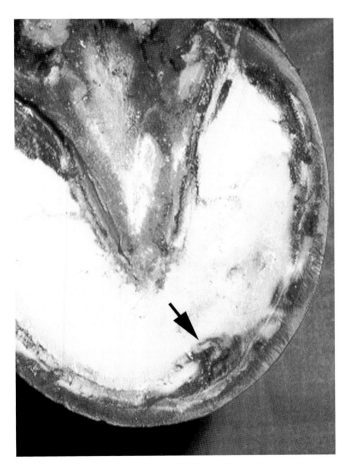

Figure 3.17 A defect in the white line with pus draining from a tract (arrow).

being applied to the coronet band. I prefer to begin at the lateral or medial angle of the sole and continue the examination by applying hoof tester pressure every 2 to 3 cm until the entire surface of the sole has been checked. Next, I apply pressure to the frog (caudal, central, and cranial). Then, I use the hoof tester on the hoof wall at the heels. Finally, I apply the tester diagonally from the medial heel to the dorsolateral hoof and from the lateral heel to the dorsolateral hoof. The diagonal application is probably most useful for horses with pads.

If sensitivity is encountered, it is absolutely necessary to confirm that the examiner has revealed true sensitivity resulting from pain and not just a whimsical reaction by the horse. True sensitivity is identified by repeated intermittent hoof tester pressure that results in persistent (nonfatigable) reflexive withdrawal (flexing the shoulder). Obviously, different amounts of hoof tester pressure are applied to elicit a response, depending on sole thickness and the painfulness of the condition. Hoof tester responses should be compared with those obtained from the opposite foot.

In general, diffuse sole sensitivity indicates a sagittal fracture of the distal phalanx, diffuse pododermatitis, diffuse pedal osteitis, or sometimes laminitis. More localized hoof tester sensitivity is obtained with corns, sole bruising, nonarticular fractures of the distal phalanx, puncture wounds, close or hot nail, localized subsolar abscesses, or gravel. Hoof tester sensitivity over the central third of the frog usually indicates navicular syndrome and/or sheared heels and quarters (Fig. 3.19). Although sensitivity from other locations in the frog may result from a puncture, a sensitive cranial portion may indicate pain emanating from the attachment of the deep digital flexor tendon to the distal phalanx. Any other region of sensitivity associated with cracks or abnormal

Figure 3.19 Hoof tester applied over the central third of the frog of the left forefoot to produce direct pressure over the navicular region.

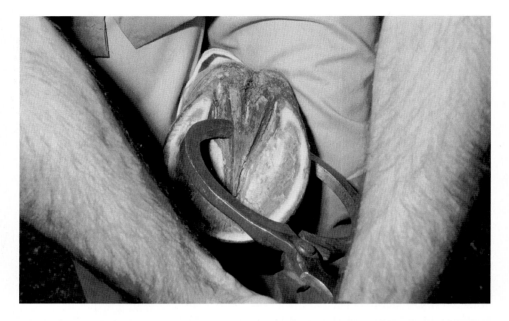

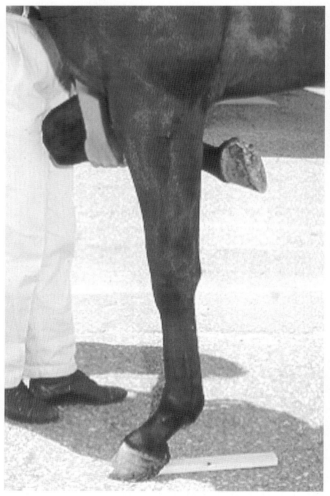

Figure 3.20 A piece of wood is placed under the frog to provide selective pressure.

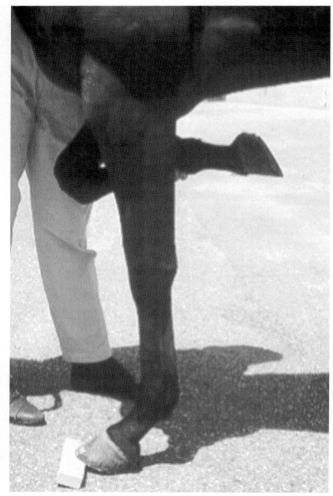

Figure 3.21 A piece of wood is placed under the toe to elevate it.

discolorations of the sole should be thoroughly explored with a hoof knife until normal tissue is seen.

Additional tests can be used if navicular syndrome is suspected.[69] One test is performed by placing a wedge underneath the frog of the affected foot while the opposite limb is held up (Fig. 3.20). This is done for 1 minute, after which it is trotted off. An increase in lameness indicates a positive test. In a second test, the toe is forced into an elevated position relative to the heel by placing a wedge or some other object under the toe (Fig. 3.21). This increases the tension on the deep digital flexor tendon, causing an increase in pressure on the navicular bone. The opposite limb is elevated for 1 minute, after which the horse is trotted off. An increase in lameness should make the examiner suspicious of navicular syndrome or heel soreness.

A hoof tester or a hammer can also be used to strike (percuss) the hoof wall. If this is painful, laminitis or gravel may be the problem. If a hollow sound is heard over the dorsal hoof wall, there is probably a separation between the sensitive and insensitive laminae (e.g., white line disease or incomplete avulsion of hoof wall). The hoof wall is checked for cracks that may extend into the sensitive laminae (they are most common in the toe and quarter), uneven wear, and excessive dryness. Dishing (concavity) of the dorsal part (front) of the hoof wall indicates a prior rotation of the distal phalanx or a flexural deformity involving the deep digital flexor tendon (Fig. 3.22).

The coronary band is palpated for heat, swelling, and pain on pressure. A generalized increase in the temperature of the coronary band of both limbs is consistent with laminitis, whereas selective swelling with or without pain on deep palpation just dorsal and proximal to the coronary band indicates distal interphalangeal (coffin) joint effusion (Fig. 3.23).[16] Firm, often nonpainful swelling in this region may also indicate a low ringbone. Point swelling and pain with or without drainage at the coronet

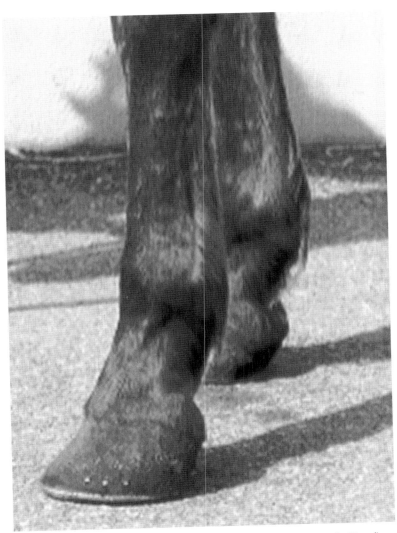

Figure 3.22 An upright pastern and dishing of the dorsal hoof wall associated with a flexural deformity.

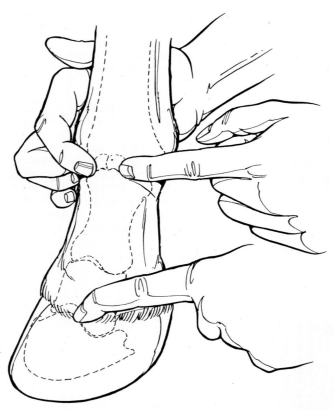

Figure 3.23   Lower finger marks the site of swelling and pain associated with fracture of the extensor process. Upper fingers are applied over the dorsal surface of the fetlock to identify synovial distension and thickening of the joint capsule.

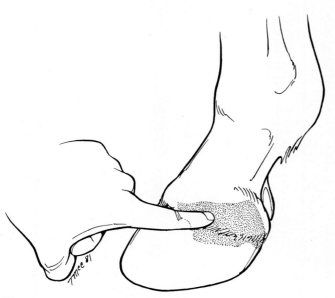

Figure 3.24   Finger marks area in which gravel and/or quittor occurs. Heat, pain, and swelling are palpated, and drainage of purulent material is common in the affected animal.

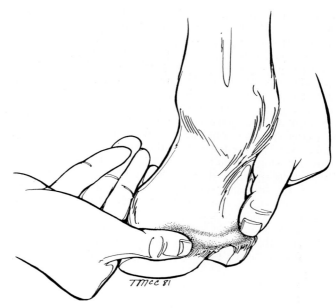

Figure 3.25   Palpation of the heel bulbs to identify heat, pain, and swelling that may be associated with subsolar abscesses.

in the midquarter region may indicate "gravel" (abscess in the white line) (Fig. 3.24). If the heat and swelling are more diffuse, "quittor" (infection of the collateral cartilage of the distal phalanx) should be considered. Calcification of the cartilage of the distal phalanx generally causes firm and nonpainful swelling.

Heat, pain, and swelling with or without drainage of one of the heel bulbs is consistent with a subsolar abscess (Fig. 3.25). Most penetrating wounds that do not involve the white line or navicular bursa and that develop into an abscess eventually break out in the heel bulb region. In situations in which a small puncture hole in the sole has been identified, hoof tester pressure adjacent to the hole not only will cause pain but also often will be sufficient to force pus out of the hole, which is diagnostic for subsolar abscess.

PASTERN

The dorsal (front) medial and lateral surfaces of the proximal interphalangeal (pastern) joint are palpated for enlargement and a slight increase in temperature, which may indicate ringbone (Fig. 3.26). If there is any question as to whether there is an enlargement, the opposite pastern is palpated. It is not uncommon, however, for the lateral to medial dimensions of one pastern to be slightly larger than the dimensions of its opposite member.

Holding the limb off the ground, deeply palpate the distal sesamoidean ligaments and flexor tendons (superficial and deep digital flexors) for pain (Fig. 3.27). Pay particular attention to the lateral and medial branches of the superficial digital flexor tendon. Desmitis and tendinitis or tendosynovitis of the deep digital flexor tendon are identified by swelling and sometimes pain in this region (Fig. 3.28). Deep palpation of the lateral and medial eminences (wings) of the middle phalanx may elicit pain if a fracture is present. With the hands placed on the hoof wall, rotate the phalangeal joints. Pain can be elic-

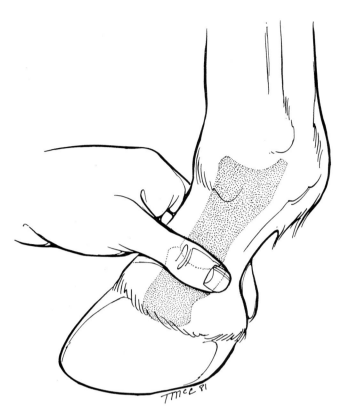

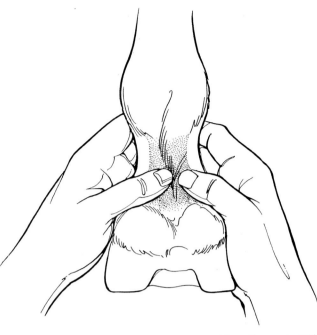

Figure 3.27   Palpation of the distal sesamoidean ligaments and superficial digital and deep digital flexor tendons on the palmar aspect of the pastern.

Figure 3.26   Palpation of the pastern. Thickening in this region often indicates ringbone.

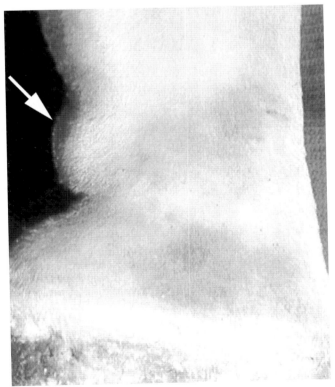

Figure 3.28   Lateral view of the pastern region of a horse with tendinitis of the deep digital flexor tendon and swelling of the digital sheath (arrow).

ited with degenerative joint disease (high and low articular ringbone) and with proximal and middle phalangeal fractures.

The collateral ligaments are stressed laterally and medially by placing one hand lateral or medial over the pastern joint and using the other hand to pull the foot toward that side (Fig. 3.29). This bending force creates increased tension on the collateral ligament of the phalangeal joints. Pain may signal a sprain or fracture or nonarticular ringbone (high or low).

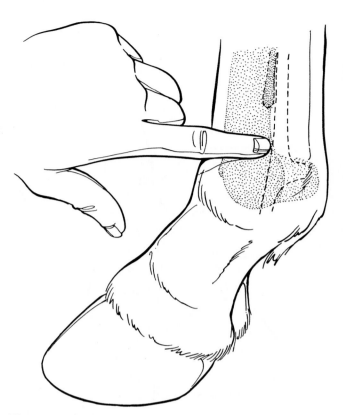

Figure 3.30 Finger marks the palmar recesses of the fetlock joint capsule. Distension at this site results from synovial effusion (also called windpuffs).

FETLOCK

The dorsal aspect and palmar/plantar reflection (recess) of the metacarpophalangeal joint are palpated for thickening and swelling, which may indicate an idiopathic synovitis ("windpuffs"), chronic proliferative synovitis/capsulitis, chip fracture of the proximal phalanx, or articular fracture (Figs. 3.23 and 3.30). Pressure is then applied to the lateral and medial branches of the suspensory ligament just above their attachments to the proximal sesamoid bones. Pain here may indicate desmitis, sesamoiditis, or apical chip fractures of the sesamoid. The superficial and deep digital flexor tendon and sheath are palpated for heat, pain, and swelling (Fig. 3.31), which may signal tendinitis and synovitis or tendosynovitis. Some distension of the digital flexor tendon sheaths of all four limbs is not uncommon in performance horses. This often is referred to as "windpuffs." The anular ligament is palpated for constriction.

Holding the limb off the ground, apply finger pressure to the basilar, body, and apical portions of the proximal sesamoid bones (Fig. 3.32). Sensitivity and pain may indicate a sesamoid fracture or desmitis of the suspensory ligament. Rotate the fetlock and check the collateral ligaments in a manner similar to that used to check the pastern joint (Fig. 3.29). Pain associated with this type of manipulation could indicate the same entities that are associated with the pastern.

Next, examine the fetlock joint to assess for pain and range of motion. This is done by extending the carpus

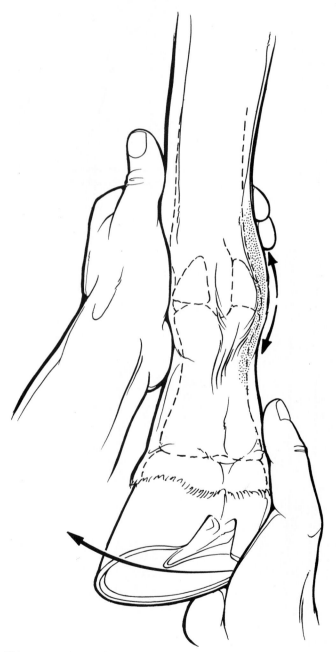

Figure 3.29 Tension is applied to the collateral ligament supporting the fetlock and interphalangeal joints (pastern and coffin) to identify sprain trauma.

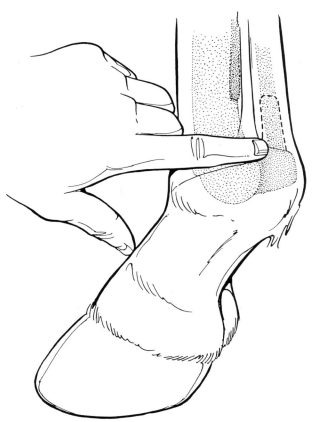

Figure 3.31   Palpation of the digital synovial sheath around the superficial and deep digital flexor tendons. Synovial distension of this sheath is referred to as windpuffs.

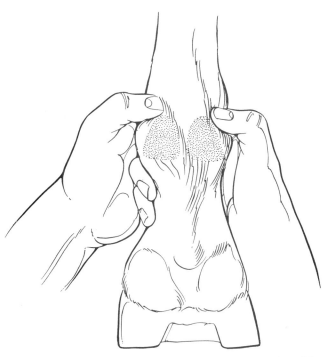

Figure 3.32   Digital pressure applied to the apical portion of the proximal sesamoid bones located on the palmar aspect of the fetlock. Pain over this site may indicate apical fracture of the sesamoids or desmitis of the branches of the suspensory ligament. The midbody and basilar regions are also palpated.

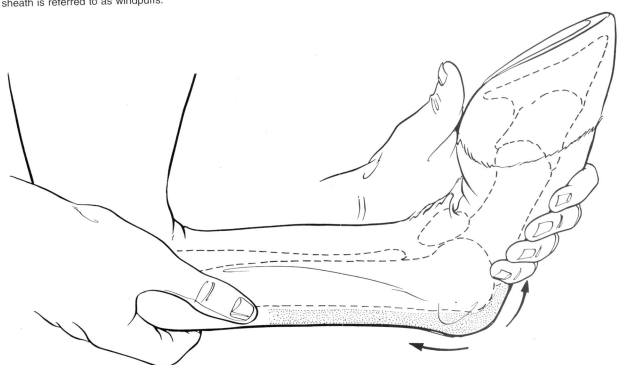

Figure 3.33   Fetlock flexion test, which is performed by extending the carpus and flexing the fetlock joint. Note that one hand is placed on the dorsal pastern to create fetlock flexion. The fetlock is flexed for 30 seconds, and lameness is evaluated. A positive test suggests problems within the fetlock joint.

as much as possible and flexing the fetlock. Notice that one hand is placed on the pastern (Fig. 3.33). This technique flexes the fetlock joint separately. If painful, a flexion test is performed by holding the fetlock in this position for 30 seconds, after which the horse is trotted off and observed for lameness. If no lameness is seen, the phalangeal joints and the fetlock joint are flexed by extending the carpus and applying hand pressure at the toe region (Fig. 3.34). This is done for 30 seconds, after which the horse is trotted off and observed for lameness. If the manipulation elicits pain, the examiner should be suspicious of involvement in either the coffin or the pastern joint, of sprain to soft tissue support structures in this region, or of desmitis of the anular ligament or suspensory ligament.[16,18,45] Any positive signs should be checked against the opposite limb.

One study evaluated the force applied by different examiners when conducting the fetlock and phalangeal flexion test in normal horses.[73] The authors found that the force varied considerably and was frequently too high. Thus it was recommended that the fetlock flexion test be performed with a calibrated measuring device (Flextest; Krypton Electronic Engineering N.V., Research Park, Interleuvenlaan 86, 3001 Leuven, Belgium) to standardize the examination and that a force of 100 N be applied for 1 minute.

METACARPUS

The extensor tendons on the dorsal surface of the cannon bone (third metacarpal bone) are palpated for swelling and pain and manipulated with the thumb and forefinger to identify adhesions. This is particularly important if a history of trauma to the dorsal surface of the cannon bone is obtained, reduced flexion of the fetlock is noted during exercise, and the fetlock flexion test is positive. Laceration involving the dorsal surface of the cannon bone will often involve the extensor tendons and periosteum, resulting in adhesive scar formation to the bone (Fig. 3.35). Selective heat, pain, and swelling over the dorsal middle third of the cannon bone may indicate dorsal metacarpal disease (bucked shins) (Fig. 3.36).

The entire length of each small (second and fourth) metacarpal bone (splint bone) is palpated. This is first done with the animal standing, after which the limb is elevated with the fetlock flexed. The palmar and axial surfaces of the splint bone can be palpated by pushing the suspensory ligament toward the opposite side (Fig. 3.37). Heat, pain, and swelling may indicate a fracture or a condition referred to as "splints" if the proximal second metacarpal bone is involved. Splint fractures most commonly involve the medial splint bone of the forelimb and the lateral splint bone of the hindlimb. A chronic splint bone fracture associated with excessive

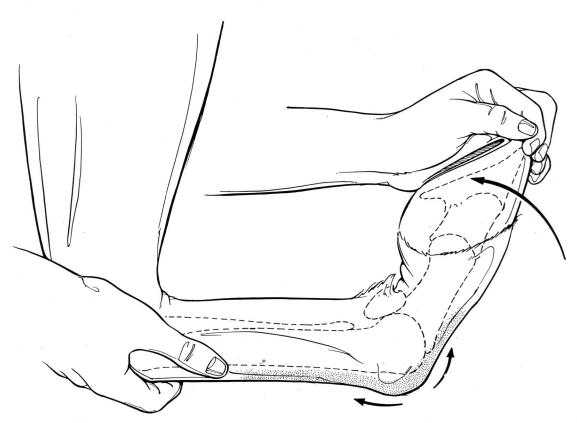

Figure 3.34   Flexing of the interphalangeal (pastern and coffin) and fetlock joints. A painful response implicates any one of the joint spaces.

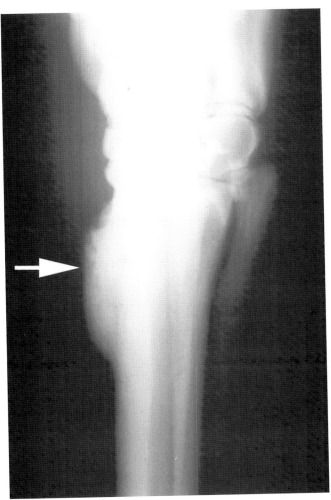

Figure 3.35 An extensive laceration to the dorsal aspect of the metatarsus transected the long digital extensor tendon and damaged the periosteum, resulting in an adhesive scar to the proliferative bone (arrow).

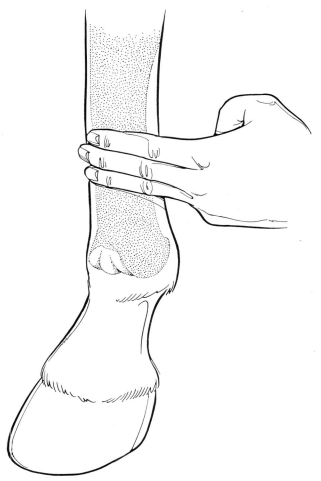

Figure 3.36 Palpation over the dorsal middle third of the large metacarpal bone to identify heat, pain, and swelling associated with the bucked-shin complex (dorsal metacarpal disease).

swelling and pain, which presents as a history of recurrent drainage, usually indicates a bone sequestrum. It is not uncommon to palpate nonpainful enlargements of the splint bones. These presumably represent sites of previous trauma.

SUSPENSORY LIGAMENT

The suspensory ligament (interosseus medius muscle) lies just palmar to the metacarpal bones in the metacarpal groove. It should be palpated with the limb weight bearing and with the limb flexed. Deep palpation is used to identify swelling and pain.[18,45] Damage to this structure often occurs in the distal third of the metacarpus associated with the suspensory ligament branches. However, desmitis may be associated with a splint fracture that is healing by callus formation anywhere along its length. With the limb held in a flexed position, the proximal attachment of the suspensory ligament to the cannon bone is palpated. (Fig. 3.38). Alternatively, one hand can

be used to apply pressure to this region. This is done by placing the palm of the hand on the dorsal metacarpus and wrapping the fingers around the medial side to apply pressure to the proximal palmar metacarpal region (Fig. 3.39). Most horses react initially by withdrawing (flexing) the limb. With constant pressure, however, this response fatigues. Painful withdrawal that persists may indicate a desmitis of the origin of the suspensory ligament with or without avulsion fracture, carpal check ligament desmitis, or a fissure fracture of the proximal palmar metacarpus.[9,18,45,50,57]

CARPAL (INFERIOR) CHECK LIGAMENT

The carpal check ligament (accessory ligament of the deep digital flexor) originates from the palmar carpal ligaments and attaches in a cuplike manner to the deep digital flexor tendon at about the middle of the metacarpus. A painful, inflammatory process of the carpal check ligament picked up by digital examination is referred to as "check ligament desmitis."

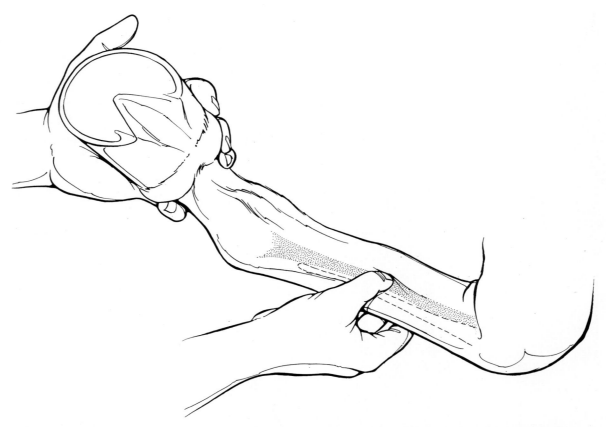

Figure 3.37 Palpation of the medial (axial) surfaces of the small metacarpal bones. The fetlock is flexed to relax the suspensory ligament so that the medial surfaces of the small metacarpal bones can be palpated.

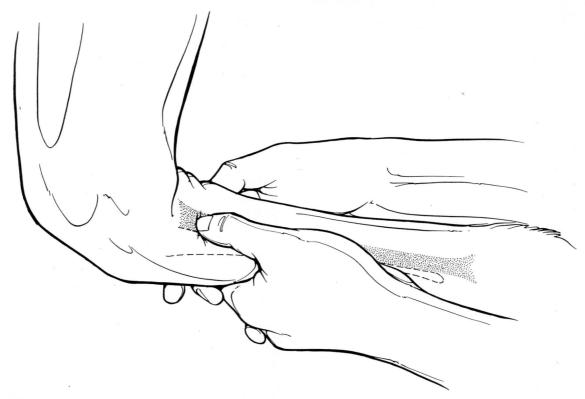

Figure 3.38 Palpation of the origin of the suspensory ligament as it arises from the proximal palmar surface of the large metacarpal bone and distal row of carpal bones. A painful response may indicate sprain trauma and/or avulsion fracture.

FLEXOR TENDONS

The superficial and deep digital flexor tendons are located palmar to the suspensory ligament and are intimately associated with each other. The proximal third (associated with the carpus) and distal third (associated with the fetlock) of the flexors are encased in tendon sheaths, whereas the central third is covered by a paratendon only. Each region is palpated carefully for pain, swelling, and heat. The degrees of tension are assessed if a flexure deformity is present. Palpation is first performed during weight bearing. After this, the dorsal aspect of the limb is held in one hand with the fetlock flexed, and an attempt is made to roll or separate the superficial flexor tendons off the deep digital flexor tendons with the thumb and forefinger (Fig. 3.40). In their normal state, they can be easily separated and differentiated. In a pathologic state, they cannot be separated because of some degree of adhesion between the two and/or of thickening. Damage to these structures results in a tendinitis or tendosynovitis.

CARPUS

The carpus is visualized for swelling on the dorsal and palmar surfaces. Point swelling associated with the antebrachiocarpal and middle carpal joints that occurs medial to the extensor carpi radialis tendon usually indicates chip fractures. More diffuse swelling of these joints may indicate synovitis/capsulitis, articular slab fracture, degenerative joint disease, or proliferative exostosis (carpitis). The synovial sheaths of the extensor tendons overlying the carpus may also be distended, indicating synovitis, tendosynovitis, and/or rupture, particularly of the common digital extensor tendon in foals (Fig. 3.41). A diffuse fluctuant swelling over the dorsal surface of the carpus is consistent with acute hematoma/seroma or chronic hygroma (Fig. 3.42). Swelling of the palmar carpal canal may signal accessory carpal bone fracture, ten-

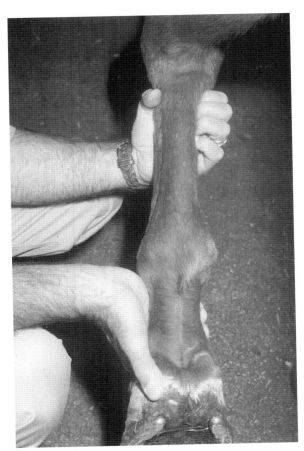

Figure 3.39 Digital pressure applied to the suspensory ligament in the proximal palmar metacarpal region of the left forelimb.

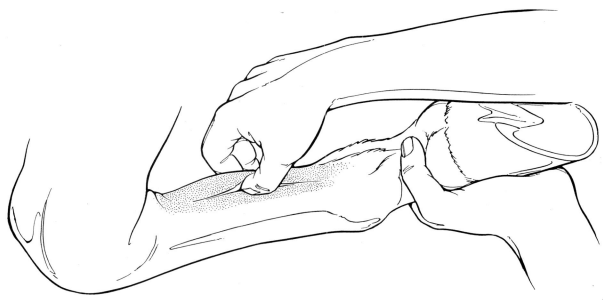

Figure 3.40 Palpation of the flexor tendons with the fetlock flexed so that the superficial and deep digital flexor tendons can be separated. If they cannot be separated easily, it is most likely that adhesions have formed and a bowed tendon is present.

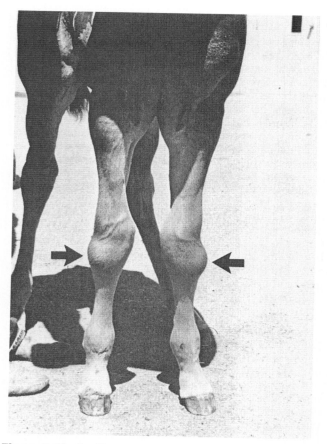

Figure 3.41 Swelling over the dorsal surface of the carpus, typical of rupture of the common digital extensor tendon in foals (arrows).

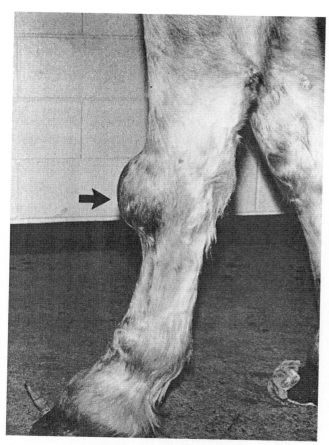

Figure 3.42 Swelling over the dorsal surface of the carpus, typical of hygroma (arrow).

dosynovitis (carpal tunnel syndrome),[37] or osteochondroma formation of the caudal distal aspect of the radius (Fig. 3.43).

Palpation of the carpal joints and bones, including the accessory carpal bone, is best done with the carpus flexed. The degree of carpal flexion can be evaluated first. In most cases, when the carpus is flexed in the normal horse, the flexor surface of the metacarpal region can approximate that of the forearm (Fig. 3.44). When severe lameness associated with diffuse joint swelling exists, the flexion must be performed slowly. Rapid flexion in the presence of severely painful conditions, such as slab fractures of the third carpal bone, may result in the horse rearing and injuring itself or the examiner. A reduced degree of flexion with pain is consistent with acute synovitis/capsulitis, chip or slab fractures, and desmitis of the proximal attachment of the suspensory ligament. Reduction in carpal flexion without pain is consistent with chronic degenerative joint disease and proliferative exostosis.

After flexion, the carpus can be rotated by swinging the metacarpus laterad and mediad (Figs. 3.45 and 3.46). With the carpus held in flexion, the individual carpal bones can be evaluated by deep digital pressure along the dorsal articular surfaces (Fig. 3.47). While the carpus is still flexed, the accessory carpal bone is manipulated, and with the tension of the ulnaris lateralis and flexor

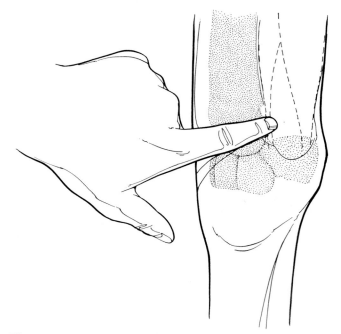

Figure 3.43 Finger marks the carpal canal. Distension can be associated with tendosynovitis, a fractured accessory carpal bone, or osteochondroma of the distal radius. Carpal tunnel syndrome may also be present.

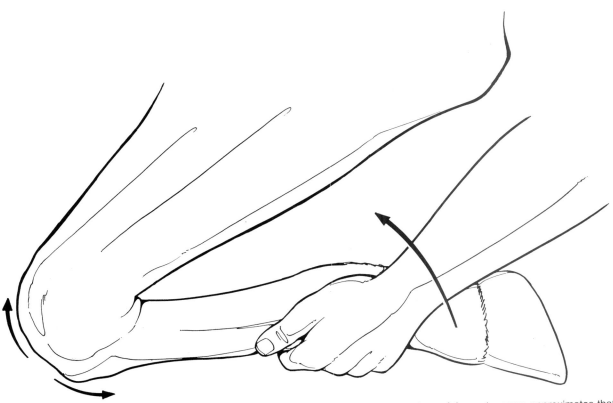

Figure 3.44   Flex the carpus to identify a painful response. Do this slowly in horses suspected of having slab fracture of the carpal bones and acute painful synovitis/capsulitis. In the normal horse, the flexor surface of the metacarpus approximates that of the forearm.

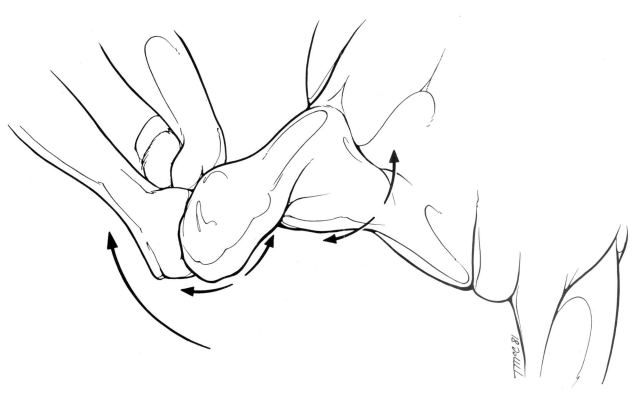

Figure 3.45   Abduction of the elbow joint and carpus places stress on the medial support structures. Pain may indicate strain or sprain trauma.

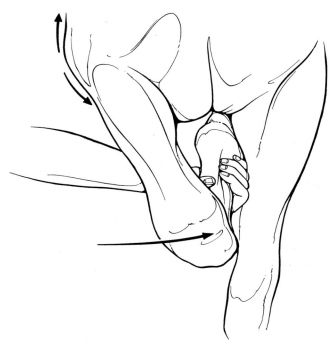

Figure 3.46 Adduction of the elbow joint and carpus places stress on the lateral support structures. Pain may indicate strain or sprain trauma.

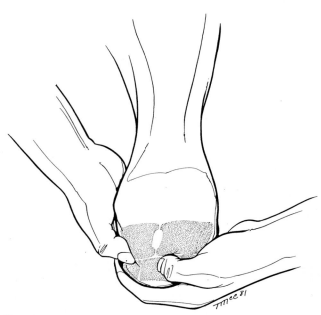

Figure 3.47 The dorsal articular margins of the carpal bones can be palpated after the carpus is flexed. Pain may signal a carpal chip and/or acute synovitis/capsulitis.

carpi ulnaris reduced, a fracture of the accessory carpal bone is palpated (Fig. 3.48). In some cases, osteochondroma formation on the caudodistal aspect of the radius may also be noted, depending on the degree of synovitis present. The carpus is then held flexed for 30 seconds,

after which the horse is jogged and observed for increased lameness.

FOREARM (ANTEBRACHIUM)

The soft tissues between the carpus and elbow are evaluated for inflammation. When severe inflammation is present and a puncture wound is suspected but no drainage or wound is seen, it may be helpful to clip the hair over the region. A firm swelling associated with the flexor muscles may be consistent with a myositis or a fibrotic or ossifying myopathy of these structures. The distal aspect of the radius is palpated for swelling and pain.

ELBOW

The soft tissues surrounding the elbow joint (cubital joint) are palpated. A firm, usually nonpainful but fluctuant swelling at the point of the elbow is consistent with elbow hygroma (olecranon bursitis). If increased swelling and an inability to extend the limb (dropped elbow) are present, a fracture of the olecranon process is likely (Fig. 3.49). When the olecranon fracture has not separated, palpation of the caudal aspect of the olecranon will reveal some degree of swelling and pain with digital pressure. In addition, carefully elevating the limb into extension will often cause pain (Fig. 3.50).

The collateral ligaments, the humerus, and proximal radius can be stressed by abducting and adducting the elbow (Figs. 3.45 and 3.46). This is not selective, since the carpal and shoulder joints are also manipulated. With a fracture, crepitation with increased pain may be observed. *A word of caution:* This test should be performed gently when a fracture is suspected. If a fractured humerus is suspected, placing a stethoscope to this region may help the examiner identify crepitation. The axilla is also palpated for swelling.

SHOULDER

The soft tissues around the shoulder (scapulohumeral) joint are observed and palpated for swelling or atrophy (Fig. 3.51). Particular attention should be paid to the bicipital bursa region, with deep digital palpation performed in an attempt to elicit pain (Fig. 3.52). The muscle and tendon are grasped and pulled laterad. If pain is elicited, bicipital bursitis and biceps tendinitis may be present. Another test to evaluate this region is to flex the shoulder joint by placing one hand on the olecranon process and pulling the limb caudad (Fig. 3.53). The position is maintained for 1 minute; then the horse is trotted and the degree of lameness is evaluated. Young horses exhibiting an obvious shoulder lameness at exercise and evidencing variable degrees of pain on manipulation may be suffering from osteochondrosis of the shoulder joint.[46] Degenerative change within the shoulder joint and fractures of the scapula and proximal humerus will be painful on manipulation. Elevation of the limb as described for the elbow joint will result in a painful response, particularly if there is a fracture or a lesion within the joint (Fig. 3.50). The limb can be held in this position for 1 minute, after which lameness is evaluated. Another test to evaluate the shoulder region is done by placing one arm over the midline at the withers and the

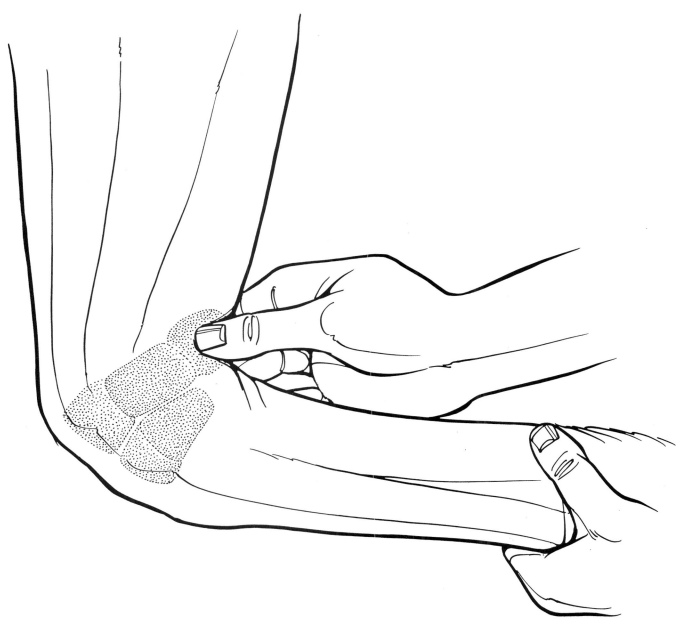

Figure 3.48 Palpation of the accessory carpal bones to identify a fracture. This is best done with the carpus flexed to decrease the tensional influence created by the tendinous insertions of the ulnaris lateralis and flexor carpi ulnaris muscles.

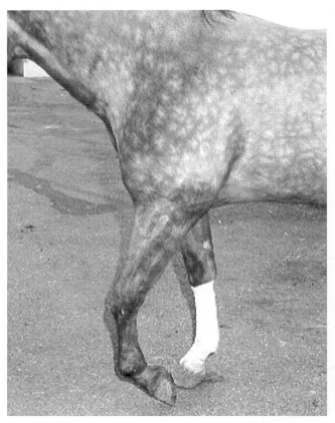

Figure 3.49 A dropped elbow associated with a fracture of the olecranon process.

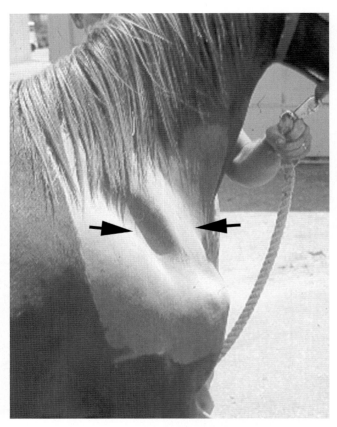

Figure 3.51 Muscle atrophy (arrows) associated with suprascapular nerve paralysis (Sweeney shoulder).

Figure 3.50 Elevating the limb into extension to flex the elbow joint extends the shoulder joint and increases the tension of the triceps brachii tendon as it inserts on the olecranon process. Pain may indicate a nondistracted fracture of the olecranon process or problems within the shoulder joint (e.g., osteochondrosis, fractured scapula).

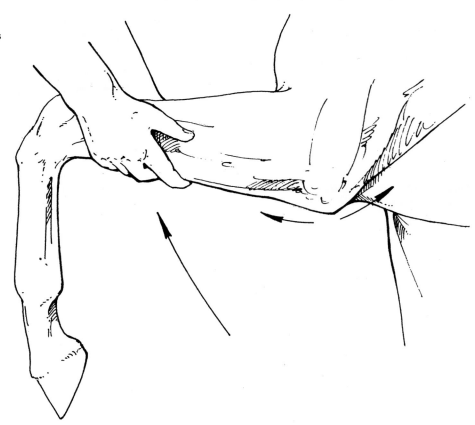

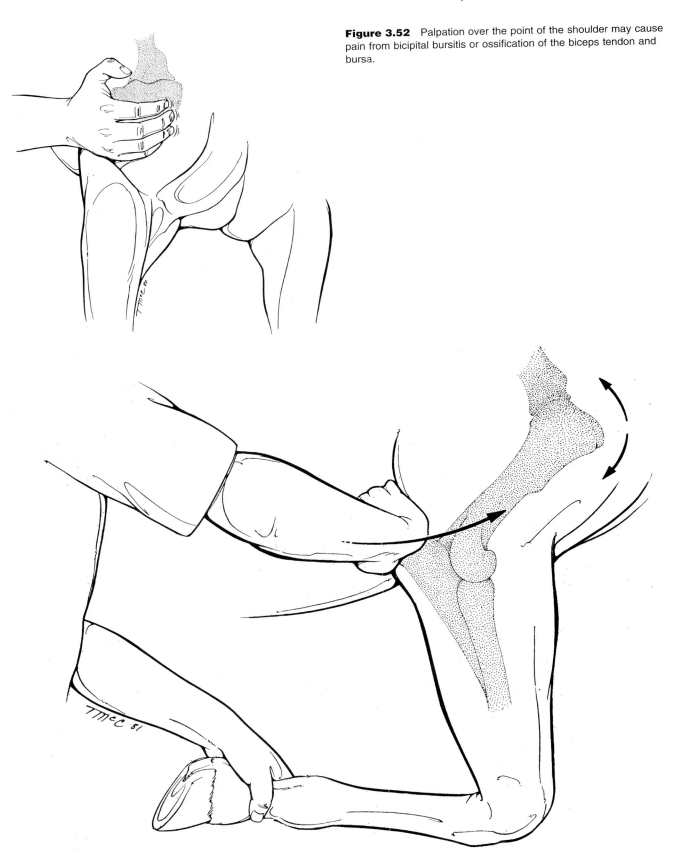

Figure 3.52 Palpation over the point of the shoulder may cause pain from bicipital bursitis or ossification of the biceps tendon and bursa.

Figure 3.53 A test that flexes the shoulder and increases the tension on the biceps tendon to produce pressure on the bicipital bursa. Reluctance in the horse suggests bicipital bursitis or fracture of the supraglenoid tuberosity. To use as a flexion test, hold this position for 1 minute.

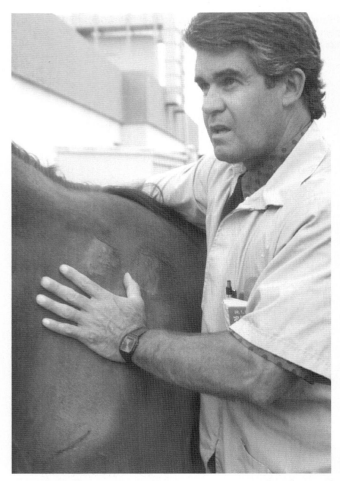

Figure 3.54 Hand position for evaluating the shoulder region.

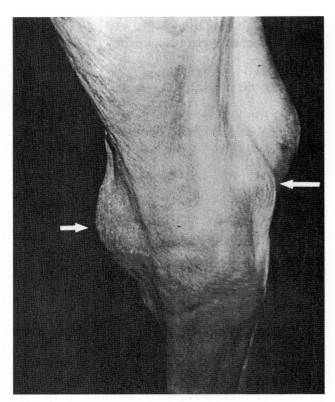

Figure 3.55 Synovial swelling of the medial and lateral pouches of the tarsocrural joint capsule in a horse with bog spavin (arrows).

other hand over the distal third of the scapula. The hand overlying the distal scapula is rapidly forced axially and then released (Fig. 3.54). If a painful response is elicited, the shoulder joint may be implicated.

SCAPULA

The infraspinatus and supraspinatus muscles are observed for atrophy, which is consistent with suprascapular nerve paralysis (Sweeney shoulder) (Fig. 3.51), and for swelling, which is consistent with external trauma. Deep palpation and manipulation in conjunction with a stethoscopic examination at the swollen site may define a fracture. Extension or flexion and abduction or adduction of the shoulder joint will elicit pain.

Examination of the Hindlimb

The hindlimbs are examined in the same manner as the forelimbs up to the hock joint.

TARSUS (HOCK)

The tarsus is observed and palpated for 1) tarsocrural joint distension (synovitis, bog spavin), 2) thickening of

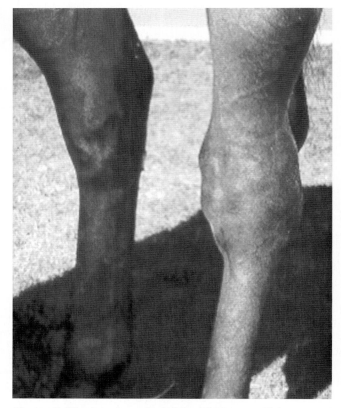

Figure 3.56 An enlargement of the left tarsocrural joint associated with capsulitis.

the fibrous joint capsule (capsulitis), 3) bone proliferation of the distal tarsal joints (bone spavin), 4) distension of the tarsal sheath (thorough-pin), 5) inflammation of the long plantar ligament or superficial flexor tendon (curb), 6) luxation of the superficial digital flexor tendon, 7) capped hock, and 8) subtendinous bursal effusion (bursitis). Cunean bursitis and tarsitis of the distal tarsal joints are not identified until flexion or pressure tests and intrasynovial anesthesia are performed.[22,23]

Generally, there are three types of soft tissue swelling associated with the tarsus. The first is felt as a fluid distension of the tarsocrural joint. It results from synovitis and is referred to as "bog spavin." Synovitis can occur alone or in conjunction with osteochondritis dissecans and/or interarticular chip fractures. Most frequently, the synovial effusion can be easily compressed from the dorsal medial pouch to distend the plantar-lateral reflection of the joint capsule and vice versa (Fig. 3.55).

The second type of swelling (capsulitis) is a palpable firm distension of the tarsocrural joint capsule. It is usually difficult to compress the synovial fluid from one

pouch to the other (Fig. 3.56). The firmness results from an extension of the synovial inflammation or direct inflammation of the fibrous layer of the joint capsule (capsulitis). Chronic synovitis resulting from degenerative joint disease, chronic interarticular fractures, and sprain trauma to the fibrous joint capsule may be the cause. If the lameness is severe, chronic septic arthritis should be considered.

The third type of swelling is a firm, diffuse swelling of the entire tarsal joint region (Fig. 3.57). Usually, it is a result of severe sprain to the fibrous joint capsule and the surrounding ligamentous support structures.

The distal tarsal joint region (distal intertarsal and tarsometatarsal joints) is palpated on the medial side (Fig. 3.58). In the normal horse, there is a smooth contour that tapers to the distal tarsal bones as they join the proximal metatarsus. This is easily visualized from the rear and palpated from the side. If this region appears boxy and/or firm with nonpainful, thickened projections (Fig. 3.59), the examiner should be suspicious of degenerative joint disease of the distal intertarsal and/or the

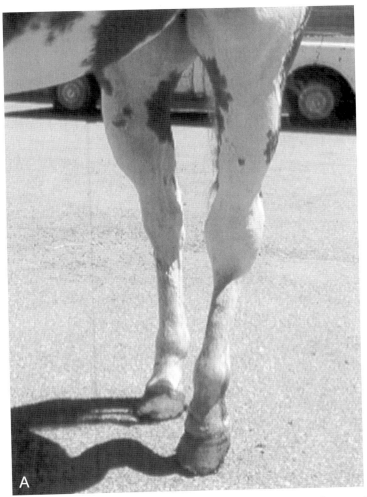

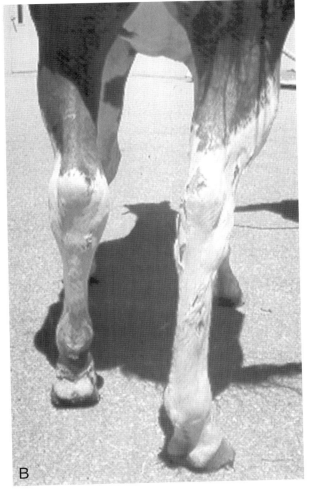

Figure 3.57 Diffuse swelling of the left hock region associated with severe sprain and tearing of the medial collateral ligament. A. Cranial view. B. Caudal view. On palpation, the tissues associated with the hock felt firm, and when pressure was applied to the medial aspect of the hock, pain was elicited.

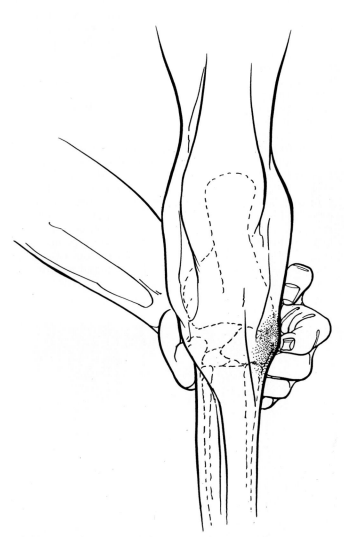

Figure 3.58 Palpation over the distal tarsal joints on the medial side of the tarsus. Firm swelling located is this area gives the hock a boxy appearance in cases of bone spavin.

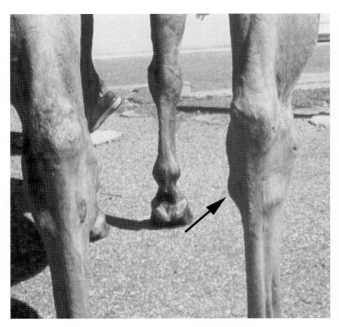

Figure 3.59 Swelling on the medial side of the distal hock region (arrow), often a sign of bone spavin.

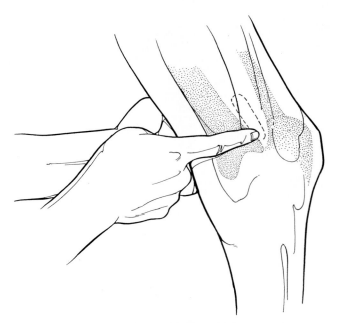

Figure 3.60 Finger marks site where tendosynovitis of the tarsal sheath and deep digital flexor tendon occurs. When distended, it is referred to as thorough-pin.

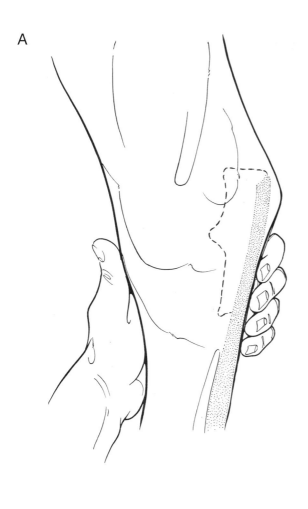

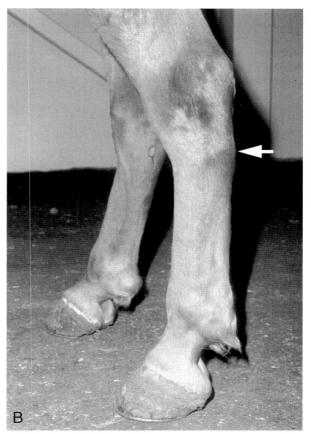

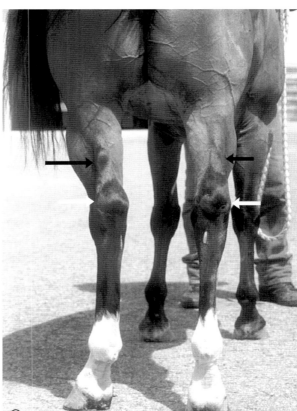

Figure 3.61   A. Palpation of the long plantar ligament over the plantar surface of the calcaneous. Swelling here is referred to as a curb. Foals that have a curby appearance may have collapse of the central and third tarsal bones. B. Note the swelling on the plantar aspect of the hock (arrow). C. Bilateral lateral displacement of the superficial digital flexor tendons (SDFTs). Black arrows, lateral displacement of the SDFTs proximal to the hock; white arrows, lateral displacement of the SDFTs at the point of the hock.

tarsometatarsal joints (bone spavin). The Churchill pressure test can be applied at this time. With the index and middle fingers, firm pressure is applied to the plantar aspect of the proximal end (head) of the medial small second metatarsal (splint) bone. The test is considered positive and specific for hock pain (lameness) if the horse flexes and abducts the limb.[11]

The tendon sheath of the deep digital flexor tendon is visualized and palpated for swelling. Swelling in this area is a result of synovitis or tendosynovitis of the tarsal sheath and tendon ("thorough-pin") (Fig. 3.60). The plantar aspect of the os calcis is palpated for inflammation of the plantar ligament ("curb") (Fig. 3.61A), tendinitis of the superficial flexor tendon (Fig. 3.61B), displacement of the superficial digital flexor tendon (Fig. 3.61C), and a fluid swelling at its proximal limits, which is referred to as the "capped" hock. The subtendinous bursa are visualized and palpated for swelling (Fig. 3.62). Distension of the bursa usually represents a cosmetic blemish and is not a cause of lameness.

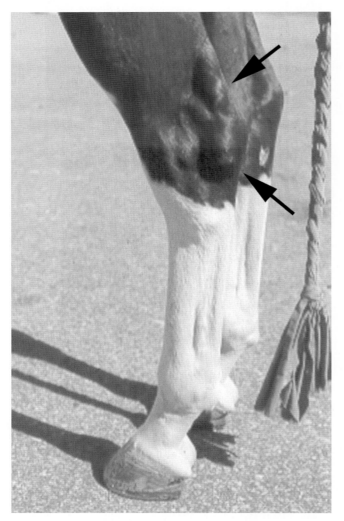

Figure 3.62 Swelling of the subtendinous bursa at the plantar aspect of the hock (arrows).

In most cases, palpation of the rest of the hindlimb is continued; but for the sake of continuity, the hock flexion test (spavin test) will be discussed now. The examiner should place the hands on the plantar surface of the distal third of the metatarsus, specifically avoiding the sesamoid bones, then elevate the limb to flex the hock (Fig. 3.63). Both hand placement and grip pressure are important. This test should not be run by holding the foot with the pastern and fetlock in a flexed position or by holding the pastern or sesamoid bone region. The examiner should hold the limb with a loose grip. A firm grip may cause sufficient pressure to the flexor tendon and suspensory ligaments to elicit withdrawal or result in a positive test. Alternatively, the tip of the toe can be held so the pastern and fetlock joints are extended and the hock is flexed (Fig. 3.64). It is often beneficial to flex the tarsus gradually to its fullest extent over a 15-second period. This allows a sensitive or painful horse to accommodate to the flexion. If the horse tends to lean away from the examiner, it is helpful to place the horse adjacent to a solid support (e.g., wall or fence) or to have an assistant provide counterbalance pressure to the tuber coxae of the opposite hip.

Once the tarsus is in full flexion, it is held in that position for 1 to 1½ minutes. If the horse forces the limb into extension, it is best to start the test over again. As the end of the flexion test period nears, the handler should obtain a loose grasp on the lead shank. This is important because the person performing the flexion test should initiate the horse's movement. If the handler attempts to do this, the horse will often balk, either standing still or backing up, which reduces the effectiveness of the test. Ideally, the flexion test is performed in an area where the horse can be jogged away in a straight line. The examiner initiates the movement by a gentle swat on the rump, which most horses accept well. If the horse is swatted too hard, it may break into a gallop, negating the test. The first few steps the horse takes after this test are often the most important.

A positive hock flexion test is indicated by an increase in the asymmetry in the gluteal use and often a more pronounced decrease in the height of foot flight arc and a shortened cranial phase of the stride. For nonpalpable inflammatory diseases of the distal tarsal joints (tarsitis and bursitis), the increase in lameness may be evidenced only for the first 3 to 10 steps, after which the horse assumes its original gait.[22,23] More prolonged lameness results from degenerative joint disease (bone spavin), incomplete tibial fractures, intraarticular fractures, severe sprain, and synovitis/capsulitis. Not all horses with osteochondritis dissecans exhibit increased lameness after the hock flexion test.

If there is any question regarding the validity of the flexion test, it should be rerun. Two of the most common errors in performing this test are not obtaining full tarsal flexion and spooking the horse so that it balks at the onset of the test instead of jogging off at a smooth pace. Because the hip, stifle, fetlock, and phalangeal joints are flexed, this test cannot be considered definitive for the tarsal joints alone. Thus it is recommended that the other joints be examined before the hock flexion test is performed. Furthermore, the Churchill pressure test (described earlier) is believed to be more specific for hock lameness.[11]

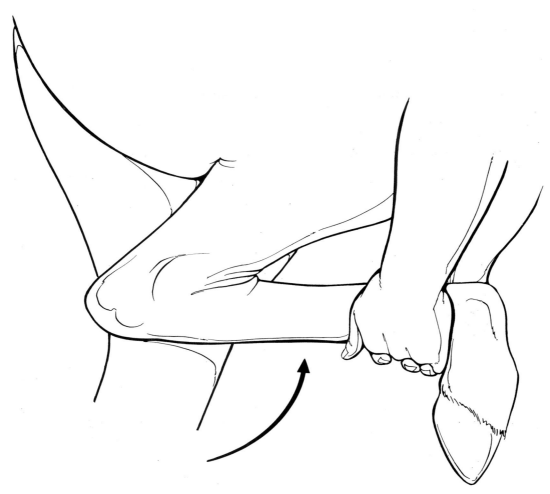

Figure 3.63 Hock flexion (spavin) test. The hindlimb is flexed so the metatarsus is approximately parallel to the ground surface. It is held in this position for 1 to 1½ minutes, and the horse is observed for increased lameness. Increased lameness is considered a positive test but is not pathognomonic for spavin because the stifle and fetlock joints are also flexed.

In addition, an attempt can be made to extend the hock joint if clinical signs consistent with rupture of the peroneus tertius muscle are noted during exercise. With the stifle flexed, the hock is extended to reveal the characteristic dimpling of the gastrocnemius tendon (Fig. 3.65).

Tibia

The tibial region should be observed from all angles for swelling and then palpated. Swelling in the caudal tibial region may indicate myositis of the semimembranous and semitendinous muscles (Fig. 3.66) or gastrocnemius tendinitis (Fig. 3.67). Inflammation associated with the distal medial epicondyle region could be associated with a fracture or sprain to the medial collateral ligament. Swelling and pain with deep digital palpation of the distal third of the tibia, associated with proximal tibial pain and severe lameness and a positive spavin test, should alert the examiner to the possibility of an incomplete tibial fracture. A complete fracture of the tibia is associated with a non-weight-bearing lameness, severe swelling, and crepitation on palpation and manipulation. The limb may also appear shortened as a result of bone fragment overriding. Swelling and angular deformity of the limb associated with the tibia are common findings (Fig. 3.68). The semimembranosus and semitendinosus muscles are palpated for any evidence of pain and swelling, which indicate myositis (hamstring pull), and for firm scarring, which signals either fibrotic or ossifying myopathy. The gastrocnemius tendon is palpated for swelling and pain.

Stifle

The stifle is observed for swelling and/or atrophy of the associated muscle groups. Distension of the femoropatellar joint is best seen from the lateral view (Fig. 3.69). Distension of the medial femorotibial joint can be seen

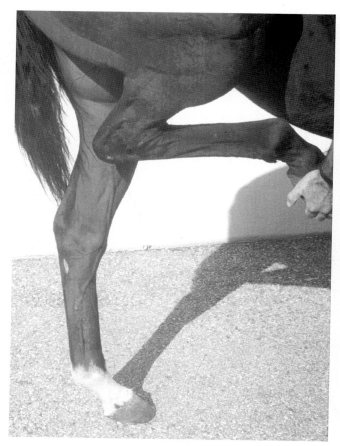

Figure 3.64   The toe of the hoof is held to extend the fetlock and phalanges, and the hock is flexed.

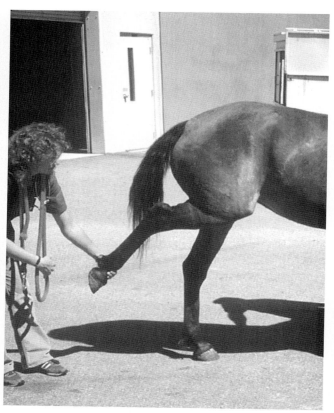

Figure 3.65   Ruptured peroneus tertius. Note the flexed stifle, extended hock, and dimpling on the caudal aspect of the gastrocnemius tendon.

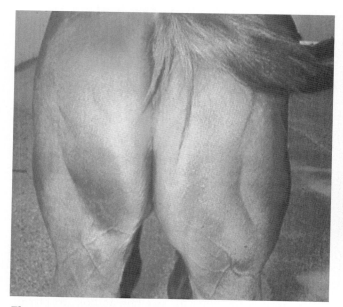

Figure 3.66   Caudal view showing swelling of the muscles of the right hindlimb.

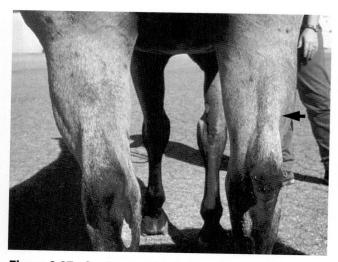

Figure 3.67   Swelling associated with the gastrocnemius tendon (arrow).

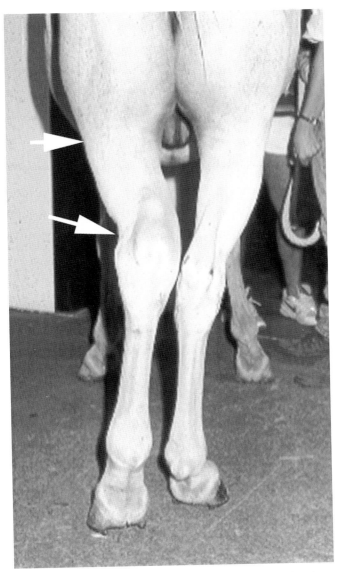

Figure 3.68 Swelling and angular deformity of the tibial region (arrows). This horse had a comminuted tibial fracture.

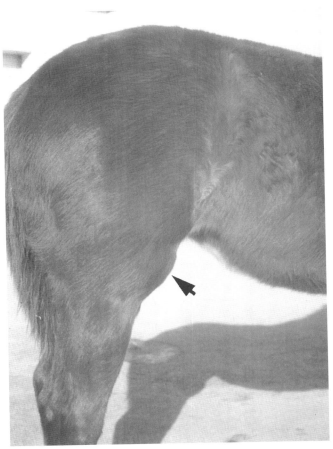

Figure 3.69 Lateral view of the right hindlimb showing distension of the femoropatellar joint pouch (arrow).

from the cranial view (Fig. 3.70). Fairly diffuse swelling may indicate medial collateral ligament injury (Fig. 3.71).

Next, the three distal patellar ligaments are palpated deeply for desmitis, and the medial patellar ligament is checked for scarring, which indicates a previous desmotomy. The femoropatellar joint pouch is palpated for fluid distension and capsulitis (gonitis). Synovitis/capsulitis in the femoropatellar pouch indicates pathology within the femoropatellar joint or in the medial femorotibial joint. Results of the examination are compared with those of the opposite limb. In general, the greater the fluid distension and the thicker the joint capsule, the more severe the pathology. Mild distension and capsulitis are normal for horses that are in active training. Excessive fluid distension of the femoropatellar pouch, which is associated with marked capsulitis, suggests cruciate ligament desmitis or rupture, meniscal damage,

medial collateral ligament sprain and/or rupture, intra-articular fracture, degenerative joint disease, and osteochondritis dissecans of the trochlea. The patella should be palpated for peripatellar inflammation and pain, crepitation, and displacement.

Manipulation tests of the stifle include the patellar displacement test, stifle flexion test, and cruciate test. The examiner should also evaluate the medial collateral ligament.

The patellar displacement test is performed with the base of the patella held between thumb and forefinger. The patella is then displaced proximad (upward) and laterad (outward) in an attempt to engage the medial patellar ligament over the medial trochlea. Most horses object to this manipulation and will attempt to flex the stifle to prevent the forced upward displacement of the patella. Sometimes they attempt to kick. To prevent this, I find it helpful to grasp the tail in one hand to force the horse into weight bearing on the limb that is being examined. It may help to place the opposite side of the horse against a solid object so it cannot withdraw to that side. If the patella is easily displaced upward with apparent locking, the horse is walked off and its reaction is observed. With complete upward fixation, the horse will be unable to flex its stifle and will drag its limb behind in extension (Fig. 3.72). If the patella is easily placed proximad and does not lock—and crepitation

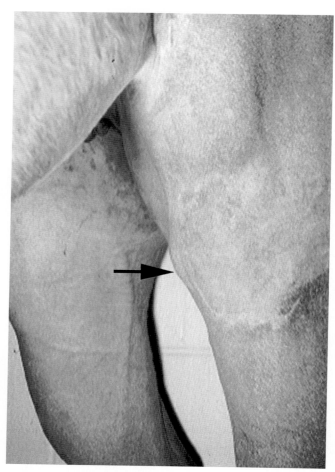

Figure 3.70 Cranial view illustrating swelling of the medial femorotibial joint (arrow).

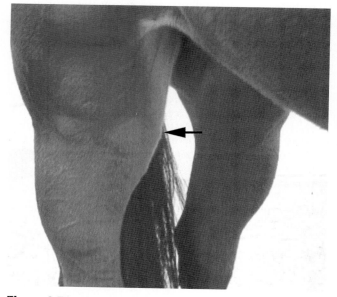

Figure 3.71 Extensive swelling on the medial side of the stifle joint (arrow), caused by an injury to the medial collateral ligament.

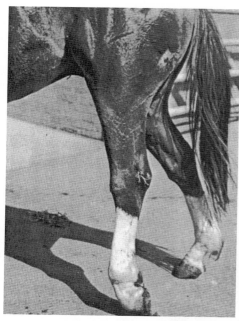

Figure 3.72 Typical attitude of upward fixation of the patella. Extension of the stifle and hock joints and flexion of the fetlock joint are evident.

and femoropatellar capsule distension are present and there is increased toe wear—partial upward fixation of the patella should be considered. In some cases, repeated dorsal displacement of the patella 8 to 10 times will result in an increased lameness in the affected limb.

The stifle flexion test is performed by grasping the distal tibia and pulling the limb backward and upward until maximal stifle flexion is achieved (Fig. 3.73). The limb is held in this position for 1 minute, after which the horse is trotted off. Generally, this test is done before the hock flexion test.

The cruciate test can be run in one of two ways. For the first method, the examiner stands behind the horse with arms brought around the limb and the hands clasped together at the proximal end of the tibia (Fig. 3.74). The examiner's knees or knee should be in close contact with the plantar aspect of the calcaneus, and the examiner's toe should be placed between the bulbs of the heels. This position stabilizes the limb. Then the examiner pulls the tibia sharply caudad and releases it to go craniad, feeling for looseness and crepitation, which may indicate cruciate ligament damage. If the caudal cruciate ligament is ruptured, the looseness and crepitation are felt when the tibia is pulled caudad, whereas if a cranial cruciate ligament is ruptured, the looseness is felt as a sliding movement in a cranial direction (cranial drawer sign). In many cases, the only thing that is felt with this test is a generalized looseness, and it is difficult to identify in what phase (caudal or cranial) it is felt. In the normal horse, of course, no joint laxity is appreciated. This test is not routinely conducted on all horses; it is conducted only on those horses that are lame enough, with localizing signs to the stifle, to indicate the possibility of a cranial cruciate ligament rupture.

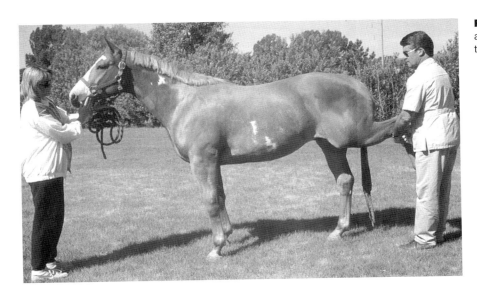

Figure 3.73 The distal tibia is grasped and elevated to perform the stifle flexion test.

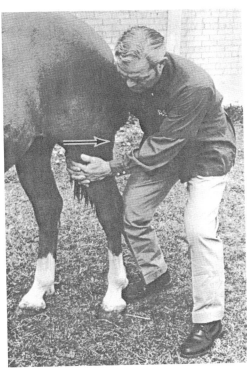

Figure 3.74 First method for cruciate test. The examiner places his knee behind the point of the hock and jerks the proximal part of the tibia caudad (arrow). Any looseness or crepitation felt when the tibia moves caudad or slides forward indicates rupture of the cranial ligament and possibly the caudal cruciate ligament. No movement between the tibia and femur can be produced in the normal horse.

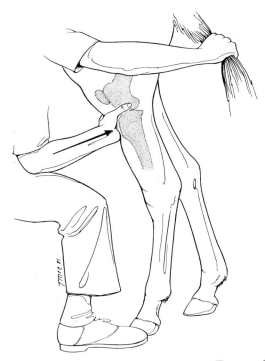

Figure 3.75 Second method for cruciate test. The examiner stands cranial to the stifle. One hand is placed on the proximal tibia and forces it caudally (arrow) and releases it craniad for 20 to 25 times. During this manipulation, the horse's tail is pulled to the side of the examiner to force the horse into weight bearing. With cruciate rupture, joint laxity is associated with severe pain. With sprain trauma of the cranial cruciate ligament, increased lameness will be observed at exercise.

For the second method of the cruciate test, the examiner stands cranial to the affected limb and places one hand on the proximal tibial tuberosity. The examiner then pushes caudad as quickly and forcibly as possible and lets go. The other hand pulls the tail to that side to force the horse into weight bearing. The caudal and rebound forces cause stress to the cranial and caudal cruciate ligaments (Fig. 3.75). This is done 20 to 25 times, after which the horse is trotted off and the degree of lameness is observed. An assistant, if present, can help to hold up the forelimb on the same side as the affected hindlimb. An increase in lameness may indicate a

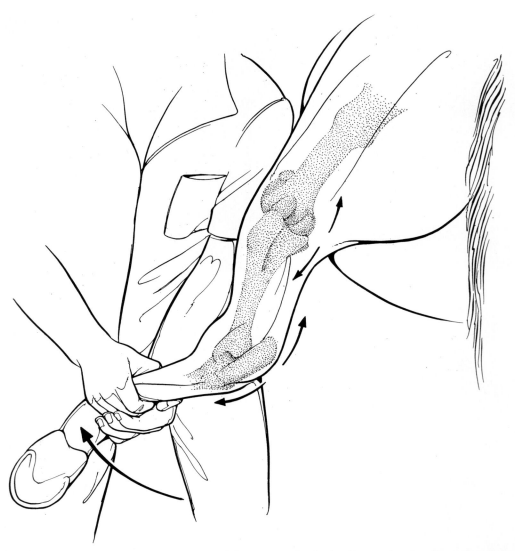

Figure 3.76 Test to stress the medial collateral ligaments of the hock and stifle. Alternatively, one hand can be placed on the medial aspect of the distal end of the tibia to stress the medial collateral ligament of the femorotibial joint more selectively. The examiner's shoulder can be placed over the middle of the tibia and both hands on the distal metatarsus to create selective tension on the medial collateral ligament of the hock. A painful response may indicate sprain trauma.

sprained cruciate ligament; degenerative joint disease, interarticular fracture, and medial meniscal damage, however, cannot be ruled out.[22]

The medial collateral ligament test is performed by placing the shoulder over the lateral aspect of the femorotibial joint and abducting the distal limb (Fig. 3.76). This test can be performed in two ways. In cases of medial collateral ligament rupture, the test usually elicits enough pain to cause the horse to fall to the opposite side. In cases of ligament sprain, the limb is abducted 5 to 10 times, after which the horse is trotted off and the degree of lameness is noted. Medial meniscus damage associated with rupture of the cranial cruciate ligament and rupture of the medial collateral ligament usually causes a grade 4 to 5 lameness. The lateral collateral ligament is tested by forcing the limb mediad. Because the coxofemoral joint is also being manipulated, pain from this region will also elicit a positive response to this test.

FEMUR

The muscles surrounding the femur are examined for swelling and/or atrophy (Fig. 3.77). The femoral artery is palpated for the quality of pulsations on the medial side of the thigh in the groove between the sartorius muscle cranially and the pectineus muscle caudally. If the pulse is weak or nonexistent, thrombosis of the iliac artery may be the cause. Pressure can be applied to the greater trochanter; if pain is elicited, middle gluteal muscle strain or trochanteric bursitis (whirlbone disease) should be suspected.[11] Standardbred horses evidencing pain in this region may also have hock or stifle problems.[22] Complete fractures of the femur result in non-

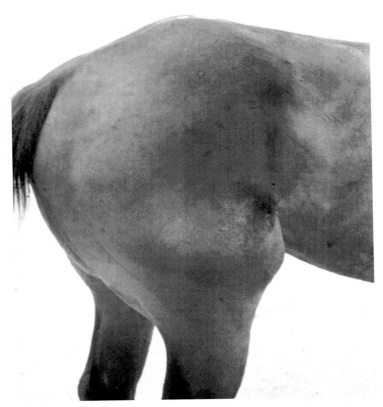

Figure 3.77 Neurogenic atrophy of the vastus lateralis muscle.

weight-bearing lameness associated with swelling and limb shortening resulting from overriding of the fracture (Fig. 3.78).

When it is difficult to discern crepitation by palpation, try placing a stethoscope over the region of the suspected fracture to pick up any audible crepitation. Femoral neck fractures can be particularly difficult to diagnose. If the horse is examined shortly after the fracture has occurred, the swelling will be localized to the hip region, and the hip joint can be rotated more easily. As time passes, the swelling migrates distad and is observed on the medial side of the thigh, giving the impression that the distal femoral region is involved.

Hip

The hip is examined for asymmetry and atrophy of associated muscle groups. The examiner can estimate the location of the greater trochanter of the femur in relationship to the other structures by using finger-hand measurements; checking the distance from the tuber ischiadicum to the greater trochanter and from the tuber sacrale to the greater trochanter. Luxation of the hip causes a disparity in these measurements. Because the head of the femur usually luxates cranial and dorsal to the acetabulum, the distance between the tuber ischiadicum and greater trochanter will be increased, whereas the distance between the tuber sacrale and the greater trochanter will be decreased, compared with the opposite side. At a walk, a stifle-out, hock-in, toe-out gait is frequently observed, with an apparent shortening of the limb length evidenced by the horse stepping down to the

affected limb (Fig. 3.79). From the side, the affected limb will appear to be straighter than the contralateral limb. On manipulation, the limb cannot be rotated craniomediad. When the round ligament is ruptured without coxofemoral luxation, the horse will still walk with the stifle-out, hock-in, and toe-out appearance, but the measurements from the greater trochanter will not be greatly affected and the limb length will appear normal. With the metatarsus held in the hand, the examiner can manipulate the coxofemoral joint into extension, flexion, and abduction. Furthermore, the hip can be intermittently flexed and, with a stethoscope, auscultated at the same time to identify any crepitation. If crepitation is present, the examiner should be suspicious of a femoral neck and/or acetabular fracture with non-weight-bearing lameness and/or degenerative joint disease. The sounds heard on one side should be compared with those heard on the other. Auscultation over the coxofemoral joint can be done while the horse is being walked. However, it is important to interpret only the sounds that emanate from this region when the foot is off the ground in flight as being abnormal. Myriad sounds are heard as the horse places the foot on the ground and progresses through weight bearing to lift off. These sounds are difficult to interpret. Perceived abnormal sounds should be compared with sounds from the opposite side. Fracture of the acetabulum, if suspected, may be diagnosed by examination of the region per rectum. For degenerative conditions of the hip, limb abduction is often painful, and repeated limb abduction will usually exacerbate the lameness.

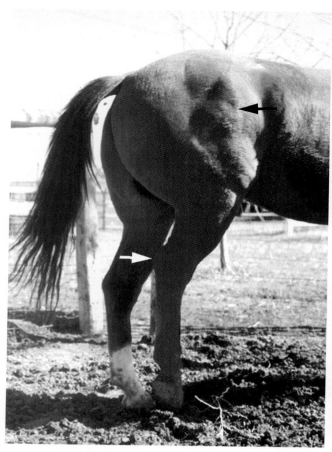

Figure 3.78 Fractured femur. Note the swelling of the thigh muscles (black arrow) and the location of the point of the hock (white arrow). The injured limb appears shorter than the unaffected limb.

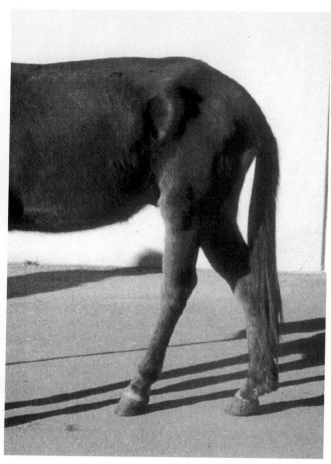

Figure 3.79 A luxated hip. Note the shortened limb and the stifle-out, hock-in, and toe-out appearance.

PELVIS

The pelvis is examined externally. First, the symmetry of the tuber coxae, the tuber ischiadicum, and tuber sacrale on each side is checked. Asymmetry in the tuber coxae or tuber ischiadicum should make the examiner suspect fracture of these prominences. Asymmetry of the tuber sacrale (hunter's bump) may indicate a sacroiliac problem. If a mare shows swelling in the perivaginal tissues and edema of the vaginal mucosa, the examiner should consider a symphyseal fracture of the pubis. This can be confirmed in the mare by a vaginal examination in conjunction with manipulation of the hindlimb by an assistant. If present, crepitation and separation of the pubis can be palpated. Fractures of the ileum and acetabulum can also be picked up by rectal examination (covered in greater detail later).

Examination of the Back

First, the horse's back is observed for contour from the side and for axial alignment from the rear (Figs. 3.80 and 3.81). Next, the tips of the dorsal spinous processes are palpated for axial alignment, protrusion or depression, and interspinous distance (Fig. 3.82). Malalign-

ment of these processes may indicate fracture and luxation or subluxation or overlapping of the dorsal spinous processes (Fig. 3.83).

Then, the horse's reaction to gentle running of the fingertips of both hands down the back from the withers to the base of the tail is assessed. Thin-skinned, hypersensitive horses will cringe when this is done; but if the horse does not respond dramatically, the reaction should not be considered clinically significant. Any muscle swelling, atrophy, or asymmetry is noted. After this, firmer pressure is applied to the dorsal epaxial muscles in the same manner as before (Fig. 3.84). Most horses respond to pressure in the lumbar region by ventroflexing their backs. After a few repeated applications of hand pressure, however, the response fatigues and withdrawal is less prominent. For horses that appear sensitive (painful), a gradual increase in finger-applied pressure is indicated. Back sensitivity that continues with minimal reduction in response should be considered clinically significant. As with any of these tests, each animal responds somewhat differently; therefore, the assessment requires clinical experience. In some cases, tightening rather than withdrawal of the longissimus dorsi muscle is felt. This usually signifies that the horse is attempting to fix the vertebral column because ventroflexion and withdrawal from pressure is painful. Finally, fingertip

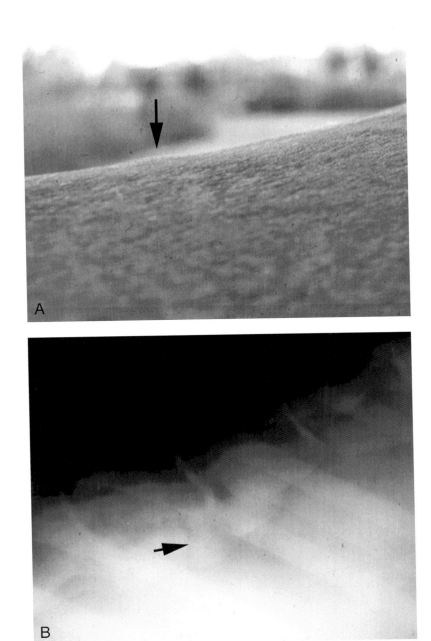

Figure 3.80 A. Lateral view of swelling (arrow) in the thoracic region. B. Vertebral body changes (arrow) can be seen on the radiograph.

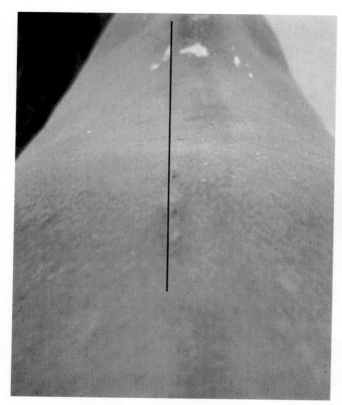

Figure 3.81 Dorsal view of deviation of the spine (line).

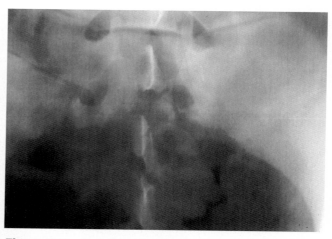

Figure 3.83 Deviation of the dorsal spinous process seen on the dorsal-ventral view radiograph.

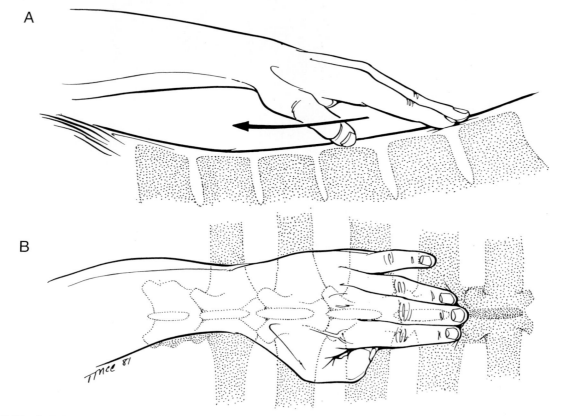

Figure 3.82 A. Palpation of the summits of the dorsal spinous processes to identify depressions or protrusions that may indicate subluxation or fracture. B. Palpation of the axial alignment of the dorsal spinous processes.

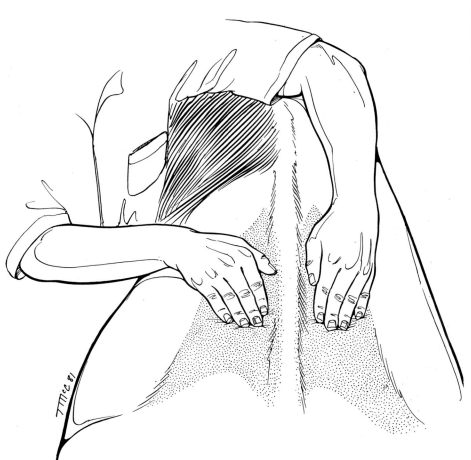

Figure 3.84 Firm pressure applied to the back muscles along their entire length, from the withers to the tuber sacrale, to identify a painful response. Note that the fingers are held flat.

pressure is applied to the epaxial muscles lateral to the dorsal spinous processes and the response is observed (Fig. 3.85).

FLEXION AND MANIPULATION TESTS

Flexion and manipulation tests allow the examiner to gain an appreciation of the horse's willingness to ventroflex, dorsiflex, and lateralflex its thoracic and lumbar vertebrae.[32] Assessment of the horse's ability to ventroflex the back is obtained by pinching the muscles in the thoracolumbar region. For dorsiflexion of the back, either the horse is pinched over the croup, or a blunt instrument is run over this region (Fig. 3.86). This is done to create a dorsal arching of the thoracolumbar region and a coupling under of the croup region. Lateral flexion is assessed by firm stroking of the lateral thoracolumbar region. This procedure is performed on both sides with a blunt instrument (Fig. 3.87). Reluctance to flex, associated with muscle tightening and back rigidity, often indicates a problem in the thoracolumbar region. In some instances, the pain can be localized by selective finger pressure. For a definitive identification of the location and cause, nuclear scintigraphy and/or radiographs of the region should be done. Tail elevation usually causes the horse to couple under behind. With damage to the sacrococcygeal region, however, the dorsal lifting of the tail may result in a camping out behind. Radiographic examination of this region can be definitive.

Examination of the Neck

The neck is visually examined for contour from the side and for axial alignment from the front and rear. Excessive ventral arching of the neck in the midcervical region is seen in some cases of cervical vertebral malformation (CVM). A straight (extended) poll can be seen with atlantooccipital and atlantoaxial malformations. Axial deviations of the neck are most commonly the result of a development problem (e.g., hemivertebrae) or trauma. Splinting and spastic contraction of the neck muscles with or without signs of spinal ataxia are consistent with vertebral fracture. Generally, these horses are in great pain.

Palpation is done to identify muscle atrophy or swelling and to document the alignment of the vertebrae. Muscle atrophy is most often observed in the caudal neck region dorsal to the cervical vertebrae. The atrophy may be symmetric or asymmetric (affecting one side). Causes for muscle atrophy include CVM, arthritic articular facets, and equine protozoal myelopathy. Lateral or ventral swelling of the neck is generally a sign of trauma and/or infection. The transverse processes of the vertebrae are palpated for alignment and symmetry.

The neck should be flexed laterally and ventrally and extended to assess flexibility, range of motion, and pain. Lateral flexing can be done by pulling the horse's head by the halter to one side, then to the other. Alternatively, lateral neck flexion can be encouraged by holding a car-

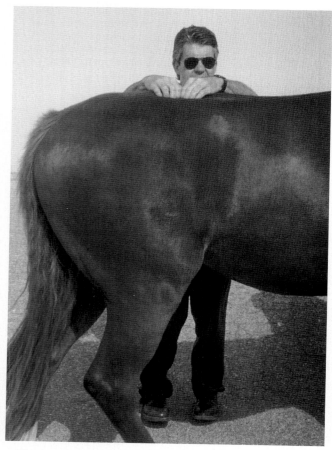

Figure 3.85   Digital pressure applied to the epaxial muscles.

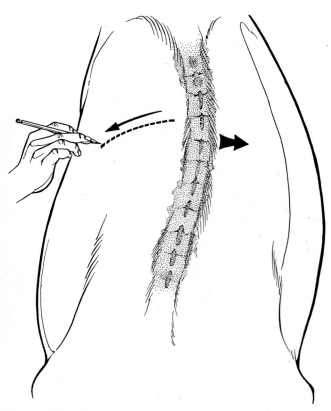

Figure 3.87   Test lateral flexion by stroking the lateral lumbar and thoracic area with a blunt object, such as a ballpoint pen. Normal horses are usually quite expressive and flex readily.

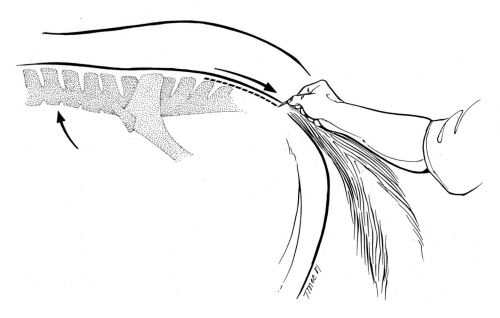

Figure 3.86   A blunt instrument such as a ballpoint pen is run over the croup to create dorsiflexion in the back region. Reluctance to dorsiflex may indicate a problem of either the soft tissues or the vertebral column associated with the back region.

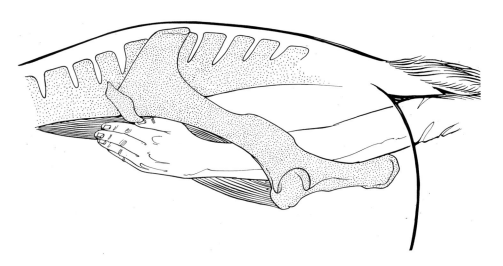

Figure 3.88 Lateral view of rectal examination showing palpation of the iliopsoas muscles just cranial to the pelvic brim.

rot or apple at the horse's shoulder. Most horses can lateral flex their neck enough that the muzzle almost contacts the craniolateral shoulder region. Ventroflexion is assessed by feeding the horse at ground level, and extension is evaluated by elevating the head and neck. Resistance to neck movement in any direction may be a result of pain or extensive degenerative changes in the articular facets.

Rectal Examination

The rectal examination can be an important part of the lameness evaluation, particularly if myositis, fractured vertebrae, thrombosis of the iliac arteries, or pelvic fracture is suspected. The horse is first examined while it is standing still. The examination begins in a cranial to caudal direction. Pressure is applied to the iliopsoas muscle located cranial to the pelvic brim (Fig. 3.88). If pain is elicited, with the horse assuming a splinted (muscular fixing) position, local myopathy or fracture of the lumbar vertebrae should be suspected. In some cases of fracture, there will be ventral swelling associated with the lesion.

Next, the aorta is checked for pulsation. If a strong pulse is not present in one of the iliac arteries, thrombosis should be suspected. Conformation of iliac thrombosis can be obtained with ultrasound examination per rectum and/or flow phase nuclear scintigraphy.

Then, symmetry of the palpable pelvis is checked by comparing one side with the other (Fig. 3.89). An obvious asymmetry will be seen with displaced ileal fractures. If a hairline pelvic fracture is present, manipulation of the limbs may cause crepitation or result in enough separation of the fragments so that the break can be felt digitally.

Lastly, the ventral aspect of the sacral vertebral bodies is checked for alignment and for any depression or protrusion into the pelvic canal, which may indicate fracture or subluxation. If any question exists, the examination continues first with the horse being rocked from side to side by alternate pressure applied to each tuber coxae. In some cases, it is beneficial to walk the horse while performing the rectal examination.

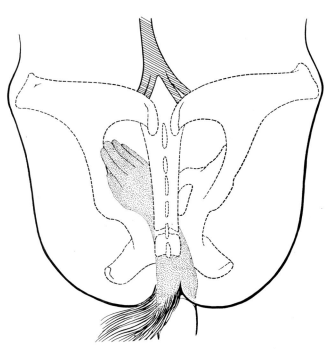

Figure 3.89 Dorsal view of rectal examination showing evaluation of the symmetry of the pelvis. One side is compared with the other. The pelvis is also palpated for crepitation while the horse is swayed from side to side while standing or during movement.

Sway Response

The horse is checked for weakness in the hindlimbs that may indicate ataxia (wobbler syndrome). The horse can either be pushed from one side to the other or be pulled by its tail (Fig. 3.90). Normal horses resist this pressure or pull effectively. Ataxic horses, on the other hand, appear relatively weak and do very little to resist swaying from one side to the other.

Special Considerations

Hyperthermia (heat) is best checked by touching the area with the back of the hand and comparing this with

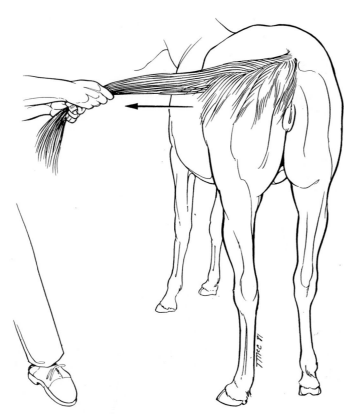

Figure 3.90 Pulling the tail to check the horse's response. Normal horses resist this, whereas ataxic horses ("wobblers") can be pulled toward the examiner with at least some degree of ease.

the opposite limb. Keep in mind that an area that has been clipped will feel warmer than an unclipped area, and the sun's rays on one limb will make it feel warmer than the other limb.

Crepitation without pain may be produced in normal joints, and there is more movement (laxity) on manipulation of the proximal interphalangeal (pastern) and distal interphalangeal (coffin) joints of some horses than in others. The examiner should always compare the lame limb with the opposite limb to determine if abnormalities are present.

If similar regions on both limbs appear painful to pressure, it must be determined whether this is truly a painful response or the horse is reacting because it is nervous. Young untrained horses are more difficult to examine than horses that are well trained, and some mature horses have nervous temperaments that hamper examination procedures. Thus, some allowances should be made for nervousness or fear. Tranquilization may be necessary, or at least helpful, for conducting a thorough examination.

Local Anesthesia

Local anesthesia is commonly used to confirm or identify the site or sites of pain when obvious pathology does not exist.[1,10,14,15,21,24,26,30,31,36,42,47,71,74] It is also useful to prove a diagnosis to the horse's owner who is suspi-

cious of another site of pain causing the lameness. Local anesthesia may be accomplished by perineural infiltration (nerve block), field block (ring block), direct infiltration of a sensitive region, or intrasynovial injection (joint capsules, bursa, and sheaths). Perineural infiltration and field blocks are used to localize the source of pain causing lameness to a specific region and, therefore, must be performed in a systematic manner, starting with the distal (lower) extremity and progressing proximad (upward). Direct infiltration and intrasynovial anesthesia are used to identify the involvement of a specific structure.[10]

Once the region of pain has been identified and the lameness has been improved or eliminated by anesthesia, diagnostic imaging (radiographic, ultrasonographic, or scintigraphic examination) of that region should follow. It has been estimated that difficulties in interpretation of the results of diagnostic anesthesia occur in approximately 5% of cases, and the reasons for the difficulties are poorly understood.[17,64]

For direct infiltration or perineural anesthesia, the site should be scrubbed with 4- by 4-inch gauzes soaked in alcohol until clean. The horse may be clipped when the hair is unusually long or soiled. Although it has been shown that clipping the horse is not necessary for intrasynovial anesthesia, if the site is properly scrubbed for injection,[28,28a] unless the owner and/or trainer requests that the hair not be clippped, I still clip the hair over the site to be injected.

In all cases, because of residual tissue irritation, the least amount of local anesthetic should be used. Since the injection site needs to be palpated for perineural or direct infiltration before needle placement, the hands should be cleansed before injection. In all cases of intrasynovial anesthesia, the use of sterile gloves is recommended. It is also recommended that sterile needles and syringes be handled by the sterile-gloved hand and that a new, unused bottle of local anesthetic be used.

When performing local anesthesia, the horse should be haltered and restrained by an attendant who is standing on the same side of the horse. For intrasynovial anesthesia, a twitch is usually applied so that there will be minimal limb movement during the insertion of the needle and injection of the anesthetic. When using local anesthesia for the hindlimb, the practitioner should always be in a position so that minimal bodily harm will result if rapid movement occurs. In most cases, the needle is inserted rapidly and the syringe is applied just tight enough to prevent loss of local anesthetic solution when injection pressure develops.

The most frequently used local anesthetics are 2% lidocaine hydrochloride (Xylocaine hydrochloride) and 2% mepivacaine hydrochloride (Carbocaine). These solutions are potent, rapidly effective, and irritating, so minimal amounts should be used. Because mepivacaine is longer lasting and less irritating than lidocaine, it is my choice in most cases.[61] Although 2% procaine hydrochloride can be used, it is not as effective as other local anesthetic drugs. Also, procaine has no topical effect and, therefore, is of no value for intrasynovial injections for the diagnosis of lameness. The use of local anesthetics containing epinephrine should be avoided because of the potential to cause skin necrosis over the site of injection. Marcaine, a long-acting local anesthetic, may be used in some cases.

Perineural Anesthesia

When the lame limb has been identified but, after manipulation, the practitioner is either not sure of the exact region affected or is suspicious of several areas causing pain in the limb, perineural anesthesia and field blocks may be of help. Even if a suspicious region is identified, it is often useful to anesthetize the region to be absolutely sure that all the lameness is emanating from that region. It is not uncommon to find several regions on one limb or to find that other limbs may be contributing to the overall lameness problem. In these cases, local anesthesia will allow the examiner to interpret the percentage that each region is contributing to the lameness.

To properly interpret perineural anesthesia, the examiner must have a thorough knowledge of the neuroanatomy of the involved region and a good understanding of the limitations of perineural anesthesia and field blocks. In most cases, perineural anesthesia is applied in a stepwise manner, starting from the distalmost peripheral part of the limb and progressing proximad. The more distal the nerve, the more specific the region anesthetized.

Field blocks (ring blocks) can be used in conjunction with perineural anesthesia to regionalize the pain. They are not needed in most cases, however. The most useful of the field blocks is the pastern ring block, which will block out the entire region distal to the block. It was once believed that field blocks were necessary because some skin sensations persisted distal to the block.[14] With a clearer understanding of neuroanatomy, however, it has been recognized that all deep structures are anesthetized with perineural anesthesia distal to its application. The only exception is when an aberrant nerve supply exists. Also, since the nerves distribute from palmar and plantar locations and distribute distad obliquely to the dorsal surface, the examiner can be more specific with a field block at the pastern region.

Traditionally, the effectiveness of perineural anesthesia and field blocks has been evaluated by checking the skin sensation distal to the point of injection. With experience, however, most clinicians have realized that this is not always reliable and that some horses will retain skin sensation but do not feel pain to manipulation tests that previously caused pain (such as hoof tester examination, deep palpation, and flexion). Furthermore, lameness at exercise is no longer present. Therefore, it is recommended that all these approaches be used before finally deciding whether perineural anesthesia or field blocks are successful. Skin sensation is checked with a blunt object, such as a ballpoint pen; instead of jabbing it, apply it gently at first and then increase the pressure. Most horses are receptive to this technique, particularly those that are not totally anesthetized. Alternatively hemostats can be applied to the skin. Perineural anesthesia and field blocks are performed in a similar manner in both forelimbs and hindlimbs distal to the carpus and tarsus, because, with some exceptions, the neuroanatomy is similar.

THE FORELIMB

PALMAR DIGITAL NERVE BLOCK. The medial and lateral palmar digital nerves are located just palmar to their respective artery and vein and lie along the dorsal border of the superficial digital flexor tendon proximal to the pastern joint and along the deep digital flexor tendon distal to the pastern joint. The injection is usually done with the foot elevated. Some examiners prefer to stand with their backs toward the animal's rear end while holding the hoof between their knees. Others prefer holding the pastern with one hand while injecting with the other and assume either a lateral or a frontal position in relation to the limb. The palmar digital nerves are anesthetized just distal to the cartilages of the distal phalanx (Fig. 3.91). Blocking the nerves at this location alleviates the chances of the dorsal branches of the palmar digital nerves also becoming anesthetized.

A ⅝-inch (1.58-cm) 25-gauge needle is inserted into the subcutaneous tissue, and 1.0 to 1.5 mL of local anesthetic solution are injected perineurally. Care is taken not to enter the digital sheath, which lies deep to the nerve. If the pressure required to inject the anesthetic solution is excessive, the needle is retracted slightly and redirected. Because there are several tissue planes, it is advisable to inject a small amount of local anesthetic as the needle is being withdrawn.

Clinically important structures that are desensitized by bilateral digital nerve blocks are listed in Table 3.4. Recently, it has been shown that the coffin joint is desensitized following the injection of the medial and lateral palmar digital nerves at the level of the heel with 3 mL of local anesthetic.[35a] After 5 to 10 minutes, the block is checked by testing skin and deep sensation between the heel bulb. If skin sensation is gone, the examiner can be assured that the significant structures listed in Table 3.4 have been desensitized. If a question exists, apply hoof testers or deep digital pressure to the painful region. If the block is complete, there should be no response to hoof tester pressure. If the block is done above the

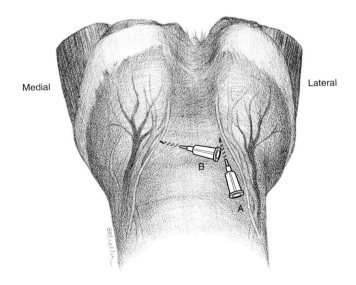

Medial   Lateral

Figure 3.91 Injection sites for the palmar digital nerves below the level of the collateral cartilages on the right forelimb. In this case, the right hand is used to inject both nerves. *A*, the needle is inserted parallel to the lateral palmar digital nerve; *B*, the needle enters just off midline and is inserted in the subcutaneous tissues to approximate the medial palmar nerve.

Table 3.4 SIGNIFICANT STRUCTURES DESENSITIZED BY THE MEDIAL AND LATERAL PALMAR DIGITAL NERVE BLOCKS

Navicular bone (distal sesamoid bone)
Navicular bursa (podotrochlear bursa)
Distal straight, oblique, and cruciate ligaments (distal sesamoidean ligaments)
Distal superficial flexor and deep digital flexor tendons and sheaths
Digital cushion
Corium of the frog
Corium of the sole
Palmar aspect of the phalangeal joints (all of the coffin joint in some cases)
Palmar third and solar aspect of the distal phalanx

collateral cartilages, it is advisable to evaluate the limitations of desensitization by checking skin sensation on the dorsal region of the pastern.

Once the block has been assessed, the horse is exercised in a manner similar to that which led to the original signs of lameness. In cases of navicular syndrome, the lameness will often shift to the opposite forelimb. In general, other conditions affecting this region, such as wing fractures of the distal phalanx, subsolar abscess, pedal osteitis, and gravel, are unilateral, and the lameness should be greatly reduced or eliminated.

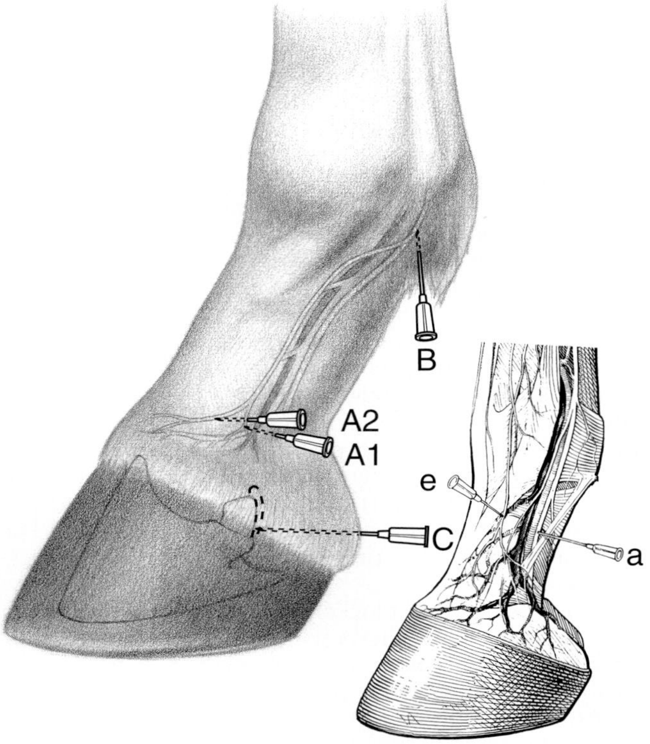

Figure 3.92 Injection sites for local anesthesia. *A1* and *A2*, sites for pastern field (ring) block; *B*, site for digital nerve block at the base of the proximal sesamoid bones; *C*, site for the navicular bursa. Inset. *a*, plantar digital nerve; *e*, lateral and medial dorsal metatarsal nerves from the deep peroneal.

Pastern Field Block (Ring Block of the Pastern). If after the palmar digital nerve block the horse is still lame, a pastern field (ring) block can be performed just above the cartilages of the distal phalanx (Fig.3.92). Three to 5 mL of anesthetic are injected subcutaneously laterally and medially, extending from the respective palmar digital nerves dorsad to just about the level of the medial and lateral collateral ligaments. This will anesthetize the dorsal branches of the palmar digital nerve. This block can be performed with the limb in a full weight-bearing position or while the foot is off the ground. These nerves supply all the deep structures distal to the blocks. The pastern field block will also anesthetize some terminal branches of the medial and lateral palmar metacarpal nerves. The subcutaneous tissue on the palmar surface of the flexor tendon should also be infused with 2 to 3 mL of local anesthetic. Alternatively, the palmar digital nerve block at the base of the proximal sesamoid bones can accomplish the same thing (Fig. 3.92).

Palmar Digital Nerve Block at the Proximal Sesamoid Bones (Abaxial Sesamoid Block). The digital artery, digital vein, and palmar digital nerve are easily palpated at the abaxial surface of the proximal sesamoid bone. Elevate the limb by holding the fetlock in the palm of the hand and identify the digital vein, artery, and nerve. The palmar digital nerve is isolated by rolling it away from the artery and vein with the thumb or forefinger. A ⅝-inch (1.58-cm) 25-gauge needle is used to inject 2 to 3 mL of anesthetic perineurally. Anesthesia of the palmar digital nerves lateral and medial to this level desensitizes all deep structures distal to it.[25] The block is tested 5 to 10 minutes after injection.

The block is evaluated via the same techniques that were described for the palmar digital nerve block. It is common to find that skin sensation still exists over the dorsal surface of the phalanges. This does not mean that the phalanges and all the deep structures are not desensitized, however. The skin sensation is derived from the medial and lateral palmar metacarpal nerves.[14,58]

Most veterinarians familiar with this block prefer it to the pastern field block because it is easier and quicker and requires less anesthetic. One criticism of the block is that it desensitizes a larger region (including the fetlock joint in some cases) than the low pastern field block, which is performed just above the collateral cartilages of the distal phalanx. For this reason, when no radiographic lesions can be identified, it might be beneficial to perform the field block at a later time. This will be more definitive for identifying lesions of the foot and middle phalangeal region.

An alternative to this block is the abaxial sesamoid block, which can be performed at the base of the proximal sesamoid bones (Fig. 3.92, site *B*). Because this site is more distal, it reduces the risk of blocking out the fetlock joint.

Low Palmar Nerve and Palmar Metacarpal Nerve Blocks (Low Four-Point Block or Four-Point Block Above the Fetlock). The next step in localizing a lameness that has not responded to the previous nerve blocks is to block the palmar nerves and palmar metacarpal nerves at the level of the distal end of the second and

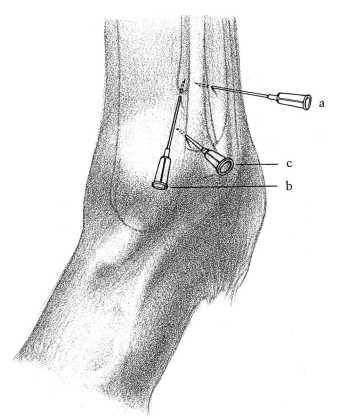

Figure 3.93 Low four-point block. *a*, site for palmar nerve block at the level of the distal end of the small metacarpal bones; *b*, site for palmar metacarpal nerve block at the distal end of the small metacarpal bones; *c*, site for intrasynovial anesthesia of the fetlock joint (needle enters the palmar or plantar recess of the joint capsule).

Table 3.5   SIGNIFICANT STRUCTURES DESENSITIZED BY BLOCKING THE PALMAR DIGITAL NERVE AT THE BASE OF THE PROXIMAL SESAMOIDS

All three phalanges
Proximal and distal interphalangeal joints
Lamellar corium and corium of the sole
Dorsal branches of the suspensory and distal sesamoidean ligaments
Digital extensor tendon and flexor tendons

a non-weight-bearing position. Anesthesia of these four nerves will effectively desensitize the deep structures of the fetlock region (Table 3.5). Some skin sensation may be present over the dorsal surface of the fetlock joint as a result of the sensory supply from the medial cutaneous antebrachial distribution.[58] A ring block at this level will remove only skin sensation. Evaluation of the effectiveness of these blocks should include skin sensation distal to it, fetlock flexion if previously painful, and exercise. If the horse improves, diagnostic imaging of the fetlock region should follow.

PROXIMAL PALMAR METACARPAL ANALGESIA

Proximal palmar metacarpal analgesia can be accomplished by 1) high palmar and palmar metacarpal nerve blocks, 2) a lateral palmar nerve block at the level of the middle carpal joint, and 3) a direct infiltration of the origin of the suspensory ligament.

HIGH PALMAR AND PALMAR METACARPAL NERVE BLOCKS (HIGH FOUR-POINT BLOCK). Regional anesthesia of the proximal palmar metacarpal region can be achieved with the high palmar nerve block performed below the level of the carpus and above the communicating branches of the palmar nerves in the groove between the suspensory ligament and the deep digital flexor tendon. The nerves lie under heavy fascia, palmar to the vein and artery, and rest against the dorsal, lateral, and medial aspects of the deep digital flexor tendon. This block is performed while the horse is standing. A ⅝-inch (1.58-cm) 25-gauge needle is inserted through the heavy fascia and comes to rest in close approximation to the nerve (Figs. 3.94, sites *a* and *b* and 3.95, sites *A1* and *A2*). Then 3 mL of local anesthetic are deposited. This is repeated on the opposite side.

The high four-point block will not completely desensitize the deep structures of the metacarpus.[14] The medial and lateral palmar metacarpal nerves innervate the interosseous ligaments of the second and fourth metacarpal bones, the interosseous lateralis and medialis muscles, and the suspensory ligament (interosseus muscle).[14,58] The palmar metacarpal nerves run parallel and axial to the second and fourth (small) metacarpal bones, and each can be desensitized by infiltration of 3 mL of local anesthetic injected between the third metacarpal bone, suspensory ligament, and the second and fourth metacarpal bones, respectively (Fig. 3.95, sites *B1* and *B2*). These four nerve blocks will effectively desensitize the deep structures of the metacarpus, except for the proximal part of the suspensory ligament. Horses that become sound after this block warrant diagnostic imaging of the metacarpal region.

fourth metacarpal bones (Fig. 3.93, sites *a* and *b*). The lateral and medial palmar nerves lie between the suspensory ligament and the deep digital flexor tendon. Because they assume a vein-artery-nerve relationship, these nerves are located closer to the deep digital flexor tendon and lie on its dorsal edge. The nerves are relatively deep but can be reached in most cases with a ⅝-inch (1.58-cm) 25-gauge needle, after which 3 mL of local anesthetic are deposited. Again, it is advisable to deposit a small amount of local anesthetic as the needle is being retracted.

This block alone does not completely desensitize the fetlock joint. Two additional nerves, the medial and lateral palmar metacarpal nerves, innervate the deep structures of the fetlock.[14,27,58] These nerves course parallel and axial to the second and fourth metacarpal bones and are not usually blocked by a field (ring) block at this level. A ⅝-inch (1.58-cm) 25-gauge needle is used to inject 3 mL of anesthetic around these nerves as they emerge distal to the ends of the second and fourth metacarpal bones (Fig. 3.93, site *b*). The nerves are superficial at this point and are easily desensitized.

Both the palmar and palmar metacarpal nerve blocks can be performed while the horse is bearing full weight or its limb is being supported by the examiner's hand in

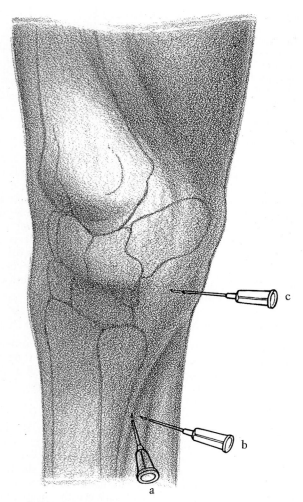

Figure 3.94 High four-point block. *a* and *b*, needle positioned lateral and medial to block the palmar nerves; *c*, needle positioned for perineural anesthesia of the lateral palmar nerve. The site for blocking the palmar metacarpal nerves is not shown; the nerves lie in the palmar groove adjacent to the lateral and medial small metacarpal bones.

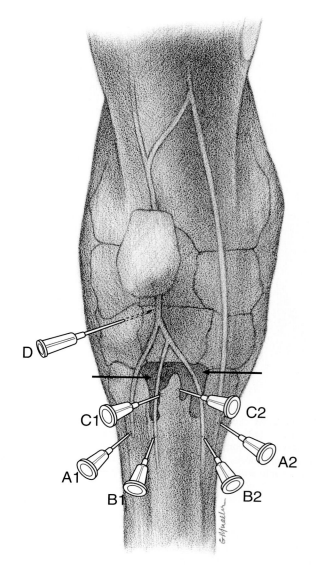

Figure 3.95 Palmar view of the carpometacarpal region of the left forelimb showing the synovial outpouchings of the carpometacarpal joint (arrows). *A1* and *A2*, sites for injection of the palmar nerves; *B1* and *B2*, sites for injection of the palmar metacarpal nerves; *C1* and *C2*, sites for direct infiltration of the origin of the suspensory ligament; *D*, site for injection of lateral palmar nerve.

LATERAL PALMAR NERVE BLOCK AT THE LEVEL OF THE MIDDLE CARPAL JOINT. The lateral palmar nerve originates at a variable distance proximal to the carpus and represents a continuation of the median nerve plus the palmar branch of the ulnar nerve. The lateral palmar nerve courses in a dorsolateral direction distal to the accessory carpal bone and runs along the palmar-distal aspect of the accessory metacarpal ligament (Fig. 3.95, site *D*). At the proximal end of fourth metacarpal bone, the lateral palmar nerve gives off its deep branch, which detaches branches to the origin of the suspensory ligament and divides into the lateral and medial palmar metacarpal nerves (Fig. 3.95, sites *B1* and *B2*).

The lateral palmar nerve is anesthetized with 5 mL of local anesthetic administered through a 1-inch (2.5-cm) 22-gauge needle midway between the distal border of the accessory carpal bone and the proximal end of fourth metacarpal bone on the palmar border of the accessory metacarpal ligament (Figs. 3.94, site *c*, and 3.95, site *D*).

The needle must penetrate the 2- to 3-mm-thick flexor retinaculum of the carpus at this point.[74] If this block is used in conjunction with the high medial palmar nerve block just distal to the carpus, the deep and superficial structures distal to it will be desensitized, including the proximal end of the second and fourth metacarpal bones and the origin of the suspensory ligament.

DIRECT INFILTRATION OF THE ORIGIN OF THE SUSPENSORY LIGAMENT. The origin of the suspensory ligament can be desensitized by direct infiltration (Fig. 3.95, sites *C1* and *C2*). The limb is held with the carpus flexed and the fetlock extended. A 1-inch (2.5-cm), 22-gauge needle is inserted between the attachments of the suspensory ligament and the carpal check ligament. The needle is directed toward the origin of the suspensory ligament, and 6 mL of anesthetic are injected. Both lateral and medial sides are blocked in the same manner.

One study documented that distopalmar outpouchings of the carpometacarpal joint are in close proximity to the proximal attachment of the suspensory ligament and the palmar metacarpal nerves in the proximal metacarpal region.[20] These outpouchings are located axial to the small metacarpal bones and extend a mean distance of 1 inch (2.5 cm) (Fig. 3.95, arrows). It was conjectured that deep injections at these sites could result in desensitization of the carpometacarpal joint and middle carpal joints.[57] If this occurred, it would lead to an incorrect assumption about the site of the lameness.[21]

The three techniques for proximal palmar metacarpal analgesia described above have been evaluated for the frequency of inadvertent injection of the carpometacarpal.[21] Of the three techniques, blocking the lateral palmar nerve distal to the accessory carpal bone at the level of the middle carpal joint resulted in significantly less (0%) inadvertent injections into the carpometacarpal joint. This is my preferred approach, and I rarely find it necessary to block the medial palmar nerve. Skin sensation is not useful for evaluating the effect of the block.

ULNAR, MEDIAN, AND MEDIAL CUTANEOUS ANTEBRACHIAL NERVE BLOCKS. Perineural anesthesia is most frequently used for blocks up to the level of the carpus. Above this region, intrasynovial anesthesia is usually used. The entire manus (carpus, metacarpus, and digit) can be anesthetized, however, by blocking the ulnar, median, and medial cutaneous antebrachial nerves. This procedure can be used to localize a lameness in the shoulder and elbow when other blocks have failed. In most cases, the examiner should be able to localize the site of lameness without the use of these blocks.

The ulnar nerve is blocked approximately 10 cm above the accessory carpal bone on the caudal aspect of the forearm (Fig. 3.96, site C). Careful palpation will reveal a groove between the flexor carpi ulnaris and ulnaris lateralis muscles. A 1.5-inch (3.8-cm) 20-gauge needle is inserted through the skin and fascia to the nerve. Although the depth of this nerve will vary, it is usually about 1 to 1.5 cm below the skin surface. Using at least 10 mL of local anesthetic, the examiner can block both superficially and deeply in this region, which usually ensures success. Since the palmar branch of the ulnar nerve gives rise to the lateral palmar and palmar metacarpal nerves, anesthesia desensitizes the lateral skin of the forelimb distal to the injection site down to the fetlock. Furthermore, the accessory carpal bone, surrounding structures, palmar carpal region, carpal canal, proximal metacarpus, and suspensory ligament are partially blocked by this technique.

The median nerve is blocked on the caudal aspect of the radius, cranial to the origin of the flexor carpi radialis muscle (Fig. 3.96). The site for injection is located approximately 5 cm distal to the elbow joint, where the distal edge of the pectoralis descenders muscle inserts in the fascia of the forearm. At this point, the nerve is superficial and lies directly on the caudal surface of the radius. A 1.5-inch (3.8-cm) 20-gauge needle is inserted

obliquely through the skin and fascia to a depth of 2.5 to 3.8 cm. The needle should be kept as close to the radius as possible so the median artery and vein, which lie caudal to the nerve, are not punctured.[25] Ten and 20 mL of anesthetic are injected. Blocking this nerve alone accomplishes little more than a medial and lateral palmar nerve block. Blocking the median nerve in conjunction with the ulnar nerve, however, will effectively anesthetize the most important areas of lameness distal to the blocks.

The two branches of the medial cutaneous antebrachial nerve are blocked on the medial aspect of the forearm halfway between the elbow and the carpus, just cranial to the cephalic vein (Fig. 3.96, inset site b2) and just cranial to the accessory cephalic vein (Fig. 3.96, inset site b1). The nerve is usually just below the skin; however, its location can vary. It is best to block the subcutaneous tissues both cranial and caudal to the cephalic vein. A 1-inch (2.5-cm) 22-gauge needle is used to deposit 5 mL of anesthetic solution. Alternatively, the medial cutaneous antebrachial nerve may be blocked as it crosses the lacertus fibrosus before it branches (Fig. 3.96, inset site b). Horses that become sound after these nerves are blocked warrant a thorough radiographic examination of the carpus and associated structures.

THE HINDLIMB

If visual observation and manipulative procedures isolate the lameness to one hindlimb, perineural anesthesia can be used to localize the area of pain. Because the neuroanatomy of the limb below the tarsus is somewhat similar to that of the forelimb below the carpus, the techniques for perineural anesthesia are also similar. One difference in the neuroanatomy is that lateral and medial dorsal metatarsal nerves from the deep peroneal (fibular) nerve course over the dorsolateral and dorsomedial surfaces of the third metatarsal bone and digits (Fig. 3.92, inset site e). Because of this, it is recommended that additional anesthetic solution be injected dorsally for plantar digital nerve blocks at the pastern and proximal (abaxial) sesamoid bones and for the low and high four-point plantar nerve blocks.

Anesthesia of the dorsal metatarsal nerves is accomplished by injecting 2 to 3 mL of local anesthetic subcutaneously, lateral and medial to the long digital extensor tendon. A ⅝-inch (1.58-cm) 25-gauge needle is used. Blocking these dorsal metatarsal nerves will effectively anesthetize all structures distal to the block (see the neuroanatomy section in Chapter 1).

Local anesthesia proximal to (above) the metatarsus is most frequently accomplished by intrasynovial injection of the various joints and bursas. Perineural anesthesia of the tibial and peroneal nerves can be used, however, to desensitize the tarsal region. The tibial and peroneal nerve blocks can also be used to determine if the pain from a severe lameness without clinical findings is located proximal or distal to the hock region. Horses exhibiting subtle lameness are generally not good candidates for tibial and peroneal anesthesia because blocking the peroneal nerve affects the horse's ability to extend the digit, making the interpretation of the results difficult.[10]

For work on the hindlimb, proper restraint and body positioning are important to prevent bodily harm. In

Figure 3.96 Forelimb blocks. *A*, site for median nerve block; *B*, site for medial cutaneous antebrachial nerve block; *C*, site for perineural anesthesia of the ulnar nerve. Inset. *a*, site for median nerve block; *b*, site for medial cutaneous antebrachial nerve block as nerve crosses the lacertus fibrosus, which blocks both the cranial (b_1) and the caudal (b_2) branches.

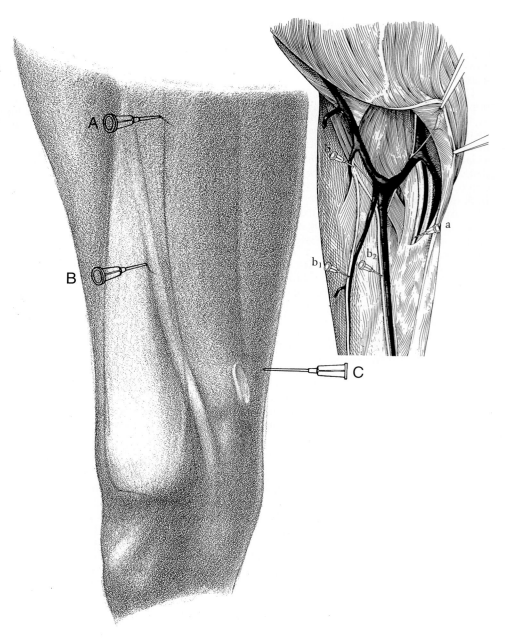

most cases, a twitch is applied, and the handler should be standing on the same side as the veterinarian. I routinely begin diagnostic nerve blocks at the base of the proximal sesamoid bones unless I am not sure of foot involvement. Then I will begin with the plantar digital nerve block in the distal pastern region. The plantar digital nerve blocks at the level of the pastern and proximal sesamoid bones are best done with the limb extended behind the horse. The limb is held in a position similar to that when performing a fetlock and phalangeal flexion test or applying a horseshoe. The point of the hock is held fast by cradling it with the inside of the arm and axilla. This position reduces the ability of the horse to withdraw the limb to kick. Nerve blocks done proximal to the basic sesamoid block are usually performed while standing close to the

horse and with the horse's limb on the ground. If the horse is prone to kicking, the limb can be held fast by grasping the foot, after which the limb is brought forward (similar to performing a spavin test) to perform the injection.[10]

PROXIMAL PLANTAR METATARSAL ANALGESIA. Diagnostic anesthesia of the proximal plantar metatarsal region can be accomplished by perineural analgesia of the plantar and plantar metatarsal nerves or by direct infiltration of the origin of the suspensory ligament.[19] However, it is recommended that both blocks be done for best results. To accomplish this, a 1.5-inch (3.8-cm) 20-gauge needle is inserted between the fourth metatarsal bone and the superficial digital flexor tendon and directed dorsally toward the midline. Six mL of local anesthetic are injected into the region of the origin of the suspensory ligament. Usually, minimal injection resistance is encountered. As the needle is withdrawn, 3 mL more of anesthetic are injected around the lateral plantar nerve, which gives rise to the plantar metatarsal nerves.[10] This block may occasionally alleviate pain within the tarsal sheath, and extension into the tarsometatarsal joint is probably infrequent.[10,19] The fact that local anesthetic sometimes does enter these synovial spaces highlights the need for careful skin preparation before this block is performed.[19]

TIBIAL NERVE. The tibial nerve may be blocked in conjunction with the deep and superficial peroneal nerves or common peroneal nerve to desensitize the hock region and structures distal to it. The site for injection of the tibial nerve is approximately 10 cm above the point of the hock on the medial aspect of the limb, between the Achilles tendon and the deep flexor tendon (Fig. 3.97A). When the horse is bearing weight on the limb, the nerve lies close to the caudal edge of the deep flexor tendon. The nerve can be palpated by unweighting and firmly grasping the limb cranial to the Achilles tendon with the thumb and forefinger. The nerve is felt as a structure approximately 6 mm in diameter just caudal to the deep flexor tendon. Depending on the horse's temperament, tranquilization may be necessary; and in most cases, a twitch is used.

The nerve may be blocked by either standing on the lateral side of the limb to be blocked or by standing on the lateral aspect of the limb opposite the one to be blocked. In the latter case, the examiner must reach across the horse to insert the needle. The method selected depends on the horse's disposition and personal preference. An area approximately 10 cm above the point of the hock is prepared for injection. A ⅝-inch (1.58-cm) 25-gauge needle is directed through the skin over the nerve, and 1.5 to 2.0 mL of local anesthetic are injected intradermally and subcutaneously. This makes it easier for passage of the 1.5-inch (3.8-cm) 20-gauge needle through the skin. When it is obvious that the needle has penetrated the fascia enclosing the nerve, 15 to 20 mL of local anesthetic are injected; the needle should be moved superficially and deeply and caudally and cranially until the region is adequately infused. Blocking the tibial nerve provides anesthesia to the plantar tarsus, metatarsus, distal Achilles tendon, calcaneus, and most of the foot.[10]

DEEP AND SUPERFICIAL PERONEAL (FIBULAR) NERVES. The deep and superficial peroneal nerves are usually blocked in conjunction with the tibial nerve for diagnosis of hock lameness or as a "screening" block to determine whether the pain causing the lameness is proximal or distal to the hock. The location of injection is just distal to the most prominent portions of the muscle bellies of the lateral digital extensor and the long digital extensor in the groove formed between these two muscles. This site is usually about 10 cm above the point of the hock on the lateral aspect of the limb (Fig. 3.97B). The deep peroneal nerve lies near the lateral edge of the cranial tibial muscle close to the tibia. The superficial peroneal nerve lies slightly caudal and more superficial to the septum of the two extensor muscles. The groove between these two

muscles is identified and prepared for injection. A twitch for restraint is often used.

A ⅝-inch (1.58-cm) 25-gauge needle is inserted through the skin in the groove between the two muscles, and 1.5 to 2.0 mL of local anesthetic are injected intradermally and subcutaneously to ease the passage of a larger needle. After this, a 1.5-inch (3.8-cm) 20-gauge needle is passed through the intradermal bleb in a slightly caudal direction. It is inserted until the needle point is close to the lateral edge of the cranial tibial muscle. To block the deep peroneal nerve, 10 to 15 mL of local anesthetic are injected on the deep edges of the two extensor muscles and the lateral border of the cranial tibial muscle, close to the tibia. The needle is then retracted, and another 10 to 15 mL of local anesthetic are injected more superficially, with the needle being moved cranially and caudally to be sure that the superficial peroneal nerve is blocked. The depth of the superficial peroneal nerve can vary, so the injection should include a region 0.6 to at least 2.5 cm deep.

COMMON PERONEAL (FIBULAR) NERVE. An alternative to blocking the superficial and deep peroneal nerves separately is to block the common peroneal nerve proximal to its division.[10] This can be accomplished by blocking the nerve near the origin of the long digital extensor tendon. The nerve can be palpated at this point, and it is anesthetized by using a 1.5-inch (3.8-cm) 20-gauge needle to inject 20 mL of anesthetic solution.

Because blocking the peroneal nerve, particularly the common trunk, affects the ability of the horse to extend the limb, care should be taken to avoid injuring the horse during the lameness evaluation. Applying a lower limb bandage will protect the fetlock from injury if the horse knuckles over, and placing the horse in confinement until motor function returns is recommended.[10]

FIELD BLOCKS (RING BLOCKS)

Field blocks were commonly performed with palmar digital nerve blocks just above the pastern joint, low palmar nerve blocks at the level of the distal end of the second and fourth metacarpal/metatarsal bones, and high palmar and palmar metacarpal/metatarsal blocks just below the carpus and tarsus. With a better understanding of the neuroanatomy of the structures desensitized with perineural anesthesia, however, there appears to be little need for them. Field blocks may be beneficial for an auxiliary nerve supply that is not desensitized with perineural infiltration and for a low pastern ring block, which is more definitive for foot and pastern joint problems than for perineural anesthesia of the palmar digital nerve at the base of the sesamoid.[14]

Direct Infiltration of Sensitive Areas

Direct infiltration anesthesia can be used anywhere a sensitive area is identified. It is most often used at insertions of ligaments and tendons (e.g., the proximal interosseous muscle) and/or at bony prominences (e.g., splints or swellings). The region is infused directly with local anesthetic. This approach allows the examiner to be more definitive regarding a painful region's contribution to the lameness. The amount of local anesthetic adminis-

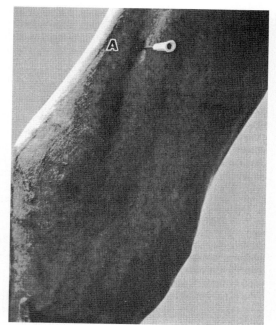
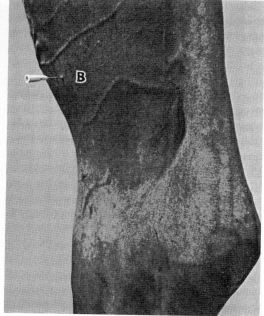
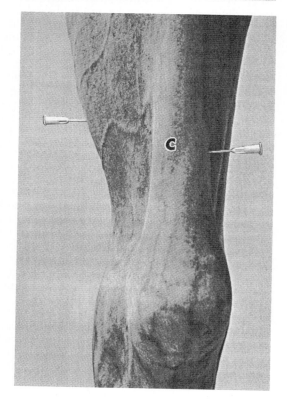

Figure 3.97 Blocking the caudal tibial and deep peroneal nerves. A. A 1.5-inch (3.8-cm) 18-gauge needle over the caudal tibial nerve on the medial aspect of the left hindlimb. B. A 2-inch (5-cm) 18-gauge needle between the long and lateral extensors of the left hindlimb. This is the site for blocking the deep peroneal nerve. C. Caudal view showing the sites—approximately 4 inches (10 cm) above the point of the hock—for the blocks described in panels A and B.

tered depends on the location and dimensions of the area involved.

Intrasynovial Anesthesia

The use of intrasynovial anesthesia plays an important role in the diagnosis of equine lameness.[1,26,30,31,36,42,44,56,68] It is indicated when specific synovial structures (e.g., joint capsules, tendon sheaths, or bursae) are thought to be the cause of the lameness. In many instances, intrasynovial anesthesia below the carpus and hock is done after nerve blocks have localized the pain to a region but imaging has not identified a specific abnormality. If this is the case, the veterinarian must wait 1½ to 2 hours for sensation to return before the affect of intrasynovial anesthesia can be evaluated.[47]

In a practice in which there is a high incidence of joint problems (e.g., racehorses) or when clinical findings indicate joint or tendon sheath involvement, intrasynovial anesthesia may be performed first. If the block is effective and eliminates the pain, it suggests that intrasynovial treatment with an anti-inflammatory may be useful. Because of this, some veterinarians prefer combining an anti-inflammatory (e.g., corticosteroid) with the local anesthetic to avoid a second arthrocentesis. Although this practice is common, the interaction of the local anesthetic and a corticosteroid is not completely understood.[68]

Intrasynovial anesthesia is also commonly performed in synovial structures above the proximal end of the metacarpus and metatarsus. Furthermore, it is more specific than perineural anesthesia because if the lameness is blocked out, it isolates the pain to a specific synovial site and usually eliminates the need to consider perisynovial structures. An exception to this is when regional nerves lie close to a synovial outpouching. Such is the case when intrasynovial anesthesia of the coffin joint anesthetizes the nerves supplying the navicular ligaments and bone at the bottom of the foot.[6–8,15,62a] Another example is when intrasynovial anesthesia of the middle and carpometacarpal joints results in analgesia of the proximal palmar metacarpal region (proximal attachment of the suspensory ligament).[20] In addition, it has been shown that there can be passive diffusion of a local anesthetic to a site somewhat remote from the synovial cavity. Such is the case when local anesthetic is injected into the coffin joint; the local anesthetic desensitizes the navicular bursa.[33,51] Nerves that lie close to the site of intrasynovial injection may be inadvertently desensitized. For example, when a local anesthetic is injected into the tarsometatarsal joint, the lateral plantar nerve may be desensitized.[19] Also, performing intrasynovial anesthesia of the digital sheath from the lateral approach may anesthetize the lateral palmar/plantar nerve.

If the examiner is unfamiliar with the anatomic landmarks for intrasynovial injection, it is helpful to review the relevant anatomy first and then practice on a cadaver. This will increase confidence and proficiency in performing the injection techniques. A more stringent preparation of the injection site is required for intrasynovial anesthesia than for perineural anesthesia. Although no appreciable difference has been noted in bacteria-forming units in clipped and haired skin after 5 minutes of preparation with povidone iodine scrub followed by an alcohol rinse,[28] I still clip the hair overlying the site in most instances. Generally, a 2.5- by 2.5-cm area is clipped. Clipping the hair also has the advantage of marking the site where the injection is to be done. The skin preparation is done aseptically, taking at least 5 to 7 minutes to accomplish. In a retrospective study done on 192 horses that presented with septic arthritis/tenosynovitis, approximately 22% developed the infection as a result of intrasynovial injection.[62] This is a higher incidence than I experience in my practice, in which intrasynovial injection is commonly done and postinjection infection is rare.

To perform intrasynovial anesthesia, a clean, uncluttered, quiet environment is ideal. An experienced helper makes the procedure much easier and safer. Proper restraint of the horse is required to prevent injury to personnel involved and to the articular cartilage and to reduce the chances of rapid movement causing needle breakage. The methods employed to restrain a horse largely depend on the animal's disposition. Usually, a lead shank or a twitch properly applied by an experienced person will suffice. Be sure always to keep in mind that the handler and any observer become your assumed responsibility.[44] Horses that are excitable and difficult to manage may require a small dose of tranquilizer to help control them. In addition, after appropriate preparation, injection of 1 to 3 mL of local anesthetic with a 22- or 25-gauge needle into the structures superficial to the joint capsule will reduce the objection to intrasynovial injection with a larger-gauge needle.

Careful palpation of important anatomic landmarks is done prior to injection to increase success on the first attempt. It is also recommended that sterile gloves be worn, which not only allows the examiner to palpate the landmarks without the risk of contamination of the injection site but also allows handling of the needle shaft, providing greater control for needle insertion. The arthropuncture should be done carefully yet rapidly. Once the needle has penetrated the joint capsule, synovial fluid may be observed draining from the needle hub. If this is the case, the synovial fluid is allowed to run freely until its ejection pressure is reduced to a slow drip or an amount equal to that being injected is removed. The syringe is then inserted on the finger-stabilized needle hub, and the anesthetic is injected as rapidly as possible.

If synovial fluid is not observed, the veterinarian can apply a 3-mL syringe to the needle to create negative pressure. If synovial fluid is not retrieved with aspiration, it does not mean that the arthropuncture was not successful. To confirm correct needle placement in this case, inject a small amount of sterile solution; if there is little or no plunger pressure, the joint was entered.

Mepivacaine is my choice for intrasynovial anesthesia because there is some evidence that it is less irritating than lidocaine after intraarticular injection.[13] The joints of the forelimbs and hindlimbs where intrasynovial anesthesia is used are listed in Table 3.6.

A period of 10 to 30 minutes is allowed to pass before the block is evaluated. Evaluation of the effectiveness of the block should include repeating the exercise that resulted in the lameness and repeating the manipulative test that made the examiner suspicious that this region was involved. Remember that structures superficial to the joint capsule (tendons, ligaments, and the intracapsular subchondral bone) may retain their sensitivity.[1] In a study documenting the onset and duration of intraarticu-

Table 3.6 JOINTS OF THE FORELIMBS AND HINDLIMBS WHERE INTRASYNOVIAL ANESTHESIA IS USED

Both limbs
  Interphalangeal joints (pastern and coffin joints)
  Fetlock joint
    Metacarpophalangeal joint (forelimb)
    Metatarsophalangeal joint (hindlimb)
Forelimbs
  Carpal joint (knee)
  Cubital joint (elbow)
  Scapulohumeral joint (shoulder)
Hindlimbs
  Tarsal joint (hock)
  Femorotibial joint (lateral and medial) and femoropatellar (stifle)
  Coxofemoral joint (hip)
  Sacroiliac joint (rarely)

Table 3.7 TENDON SHEATHS AND BURSAE WHERE INTRASYNOVIAL ANESTHESIA IS USED

Forelimb
  Bicipital bursa
  Carpal synovial sheath
  Digital synovial sheath (metacarpo/metatarsophalangeal region)

lar mepivacaine in the horse, Andreen et al.[3] found that lameness induced by injection of *Escherichia coli* endotoxin in the middle carpal joint was not apparent after 5 minutes; this lasted for 55 minutes.

Intrasynovial anesthesia of tendon sheaths and bursae is used less frequently but performed in a manner similar to that of intrasynovial anesthesia of joints. The tendon sheaths and bursae commonly injected are listed in Table 3.7.

THE FORELIMB

PODOTROCHLEAR (NAVICULAR) BURSA. In light of several studies that document diffusion of local anesthetic into the navicular bursa from injection into the coffin joint, it is questionable whether injection directly into the navicular bursa is warranted.[6–8,15,33,55] For completeness, however, the techniques will be covered.

The navicular bursa can be entered in one of three ways. The injection can be made from the palmar aspect of the foot at a point centered between the heel bulbs at the base of the digital fossa. First, 1 mL of local anesthetic is deposited in the subcutaneous tissue with a ⅝-inch (1.58-cm) 25-gauge needle at this site. After 1 to 2 minutes, a 1.5-inch (3.8-cm) 20-gauge needle is introduced at the same site and advanced dorsad on the midline and parallel to the sole until bone is encountered (Fig. 3.92, site C). At this point, the bursa has been penetrated. The needle is then withdrawn slightly, and 2 to 3 mL of local anesthetic are injected.[9,41,46,50]

In another approach, a 1.5-inch (3.8-cm) 20-gauge needle is inserted at the lowest part of the depression between the heel bulbs. The needle is directed dorsally toward the coronet band and inserted to a depth of approximately 1 cm before the navicular bone is contacted.[26,61]

In the third approach, the navicular bursa is entered from the lateral side (abaxial position) just proximal to the collateral cartilage of the distal phalanx. A 1.5-inch (3.8-cm) 20-gauge needle is directed distally toward the opposite heel between the middle phalanx and deep digital flexor tendon.[26]

Because it easy to pass the needle proximal to the navicular bone and enter the coffin joint, radiographic or fluoroscopic documentation of the needle's location is recommended in all cases before the injection is done.[8,26]

DISTAL INTERPHALANGEAL (COFFIN) JOINT. The distal interphalangeal (DIP) joint can be entered in one of three ways. The most familiar site of injection is on the dorsal surface of the digit, 1 cm above the coronet and 1.5 cm lateral to the midline. A 1- to 1.5-inch (2.5- to 3.8-cm) 20-gauge needle is inserted from a vertical position and directed distad, mediad toward the center of the foot at an angle, and 90° to the bottom of the foot to enter the

coffin joint capsule at the edge of the extensor process (Fig. 3.98, site A). I prefer this approach; others prefer to enter the joint via a dorsal midline approach[44,68] (Figs. 3.98, site B, and 3.99, site A).

If there is some question about entry into the joint, the practitioner can direct the needle at a more acute angle to the skin and insert until the needle contacts the distal end of the middle phalanx. The needle is then "walked" distally until the joint is penetrated.[68]

I prefer to perform these injections while the horse is standing; others prefer to inject the joint when it is flexed in a non-weight-bearing position.[24] This can be done by picking the limb up, pulling it forward, and resting the sole on the knee. A total of 5 mL of local anesthetic is injected.

Difficulties associated with the approach include mild hemorrhage and patient movement. Hemorrhage comes from penetration of the coronary vascular plexus. This

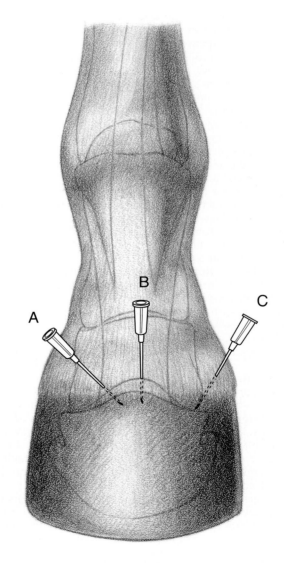

Figure 3.98 Dorsal view of the injection sites for the coffin joint. *A*, dorsal lateral approach; *B*, dorsal approach; *C*, lateral approach.

of the limbs had contrast exclusively in the DIP joint, 20% had contrast in the digital sheath, and 5% had contrast in the subcutaneous tissues.

Another approach is palmar (plantar).[24] The needle is inserted slightly proximal to the deepest depression of the fossa above the heel bulbs and is directed dorsal and distal to a point midway between the coronet and toe. The position is proximal to the site for injection of the navicular bursa (Fig. 3.99, site C).

Several studies have documented that injection of the coffin joint with a local anesthetic is not selective and will cause analgesia of the suspensory and impar ligaments of the navicular bone and the navicular bursa.[6–8,15,33,51] One study found that injection of the coffin joint caused at least partial, and often complete, analgesia of the sole dorsal to the apex of the frog.[62b] Another study found that anesthesia of the coffin joint was more effective in alleviating solar pain at the tow region than at the heel region.[62a] Both the time after administration of anesthetic and the volume also affected the degree of the solar analgesia. The analgesic effect increased with time, and 10 mL of anesthetic was more effective than 6 mL in alleviating pain.

PROXIMAL INTERPHALANGEAL (PASTERN) JOINT. There are three approaches—two dorsal and one palmar/plantar (palmaroproximal)—to arthrocentesis of the pastern joint. Five mL of anesthetic solution are injected.

One dorsal site of injection is on the midline approximately 0.5 cm dorsal to an imaginary line drawn from the medial and lateral eminences of the proximal end of the middle phalanx. A 1.5-inch (3.8-cm) 20-gauge needle is directed slightly distad and mediad to enter the joint capsule underneath the extensor tendon (Figs. 3.100, site A, and 3.101, site A).

Another site is dorsolateral. The injection can be done while the horse is standing or in a non-weight-bearing position with the limb extended and the sole supported on the knee (my preference). It is accomplished by identifying the palpable condylar eminence of the distolateral proximal phalanx. A 1.5-inch (3.8-cm) 20-gauge needle is inserted parallel to the ground surface and directed underneath the edge of the extensor tendon to enter the joint (Figs. 3.100, site B, and 3.101, site B).

The palmaroproximal approach is accomplished in the non-weight-bearing position. A 1.5-inch (3.8-cm) 20-gauge needle is inserted into the distinct and palpable V-shaped depression formed by the palmar aspect of the proximal phalanx dorsally, the distal eminence of the proximal phalanx distally, and the lateral branch of the superficial digital flexor tendon as it inserts on the palmaroproximal eminence of the middle phalanx palmaro-distally[40] (Figs. 3.100, site C, and 3.101, site C). My experience with this technique, although limited, has been favorable.

METACARPOPHALANGEAL AND METATARSOPHALANGEAL (FETLOCK) JOINTS. There are several approaches to arthrocentesis of the fetlock joint. Arthrocentesis of the palmar or plantar recesses (reflections) of the joint capsule can be done with a 1-inch (2.5-cm) 20-gauge needle. The boundaries for the palmar recess of the fetlock joint are the apical border of the proximal sesamoid distally, the distal ends of the lateral splint bone proximally, the

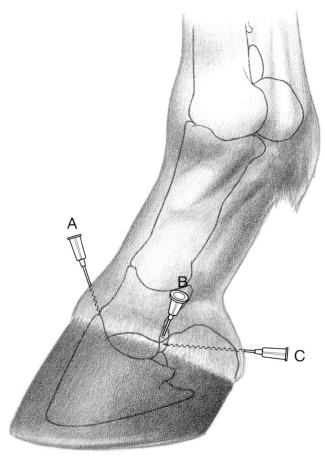

Figure 3.99 Lateral view of the injection sites for the coffin joint. *A*, dorsal approach; *B*, lateral approach; *C*, palmar approach.

can be avoided to a large degree by directing the needle distad at 90° to the sole. Proper restraint is required to prevent the horse's movement. In addition, a small amount of local anesthetic may be injected with a ⅝-inch (1.58-cm) 25-gauge needle to desensitize the skin and subcutaneous tissue (wait 2 to 3 minutes) prior to inserting the 20-gauge needle.

An alternative lateral approach can be done while the horse is weight bearing or with the limb held in a non-weight-bearing position.[44] The site for injection is bounded distally by a depression in the proximal border of the lateral collateral (ungular) cartilage of the distal phalanx and proximodorsally by the palmar border of the middle phalanx (Fig. 3.99, site B). A 1.5-inch (3.8-cm) 20-gauge needle is used (Fig. 3.98, site C). The needle is directed at a 45° angle to the ground and toward the medial weight-bearing hoof surface.[72] The depth of penetration is 1 to 1.5 inches. Horses generally accept this approach readily.

One study of 8 cadavers and 12 living horses evaluated the specificity of the two injection techniques (dorsal and lateral approaches) for entering the DIP joint.[72] The authors found that contrast material entered the DIP joint in 100% of the cases injected via the dorsal approach and in 85% of the cases injected via the lateral approach. Note that with the lateral approach, only 65%

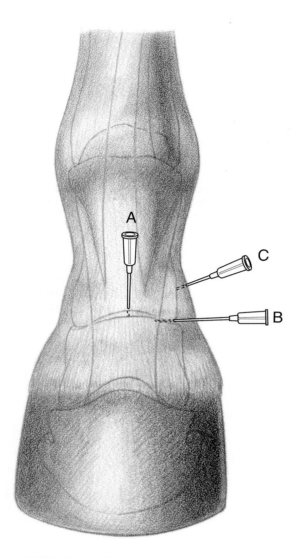

Figure 3.100 Dorsal view of injection sites for the pastern joint. *A*, dorsal approach; *B*, dorsal lateral approach; *C*, palmaroproximal approach.

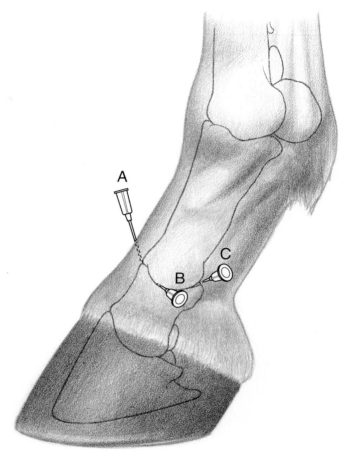

Figure 3.101 Lateral view of injection sites for the pastern joint. *A*, dorsal; *B*, dorsal lateral approach; *C*, palmaroproximal approach.

third metacarpal/metatarsal bone dorsally, and the suspensory ligament palmarly or plantarly (Fig. 3.102, site *A*). When the palmar (plantar) recesses (pouches) are injected, it is best to have the horse bearing full weight; this increases the distension of the joint capsule, making it easier to identify. The needle is centered over the recess and inserted from lateral to medial and directed distally at a 45° angle to the long axis of the limb until the synovial membrane is penetrated. In the normal horse, the palmar recess appears as a depression, and attempts to retrieve synovial fluid or inject substances may be difficult. The disadvantages of this approach are the possibility of blood contaminating the synovial fluid sample, because the highly vascular synovial membrane is penetrated and the prominent highly mobile synovial villi can plug the needle, interfering with synovial fluid aspiration.[30,41]

Arthrocentesis through the lateral collateral sesamoidean ligament can be done to obtain a hemorrhage-free synovial fluid sample. The fetlock is flexed to increase the space between the articular surfaces of the proximal sesamoid bone and the distal end of metacarpus/metatarsus. A 1-inch (2.5-cm) 20-gauge needle is inserted at 90° through the proximal limits of the collateral ligament[41] (Fig. 3.103). This is the approach I prefer for the hindlimb.

Alternatively, arthrocentesis of the fetlock joint can be done at the dorsal distal end of the proximal sesamoid bone. The site for arthrocentesis is located in the palpable depression of the distodorsal aspect of the proximal sesamoid bone and the proximopalmar or plantar eminence of the proximal phalanx. The landmarks are the distal aspect of the proximal sesamoid bone and the collateral sesamoidean ligament proximally, the proximal palmar/plantar eminence of the proximal phalanx distally, and the digital vein, artery, and nerve palmarly/plantarly. A 1.5-inch (3.8-cm) 20-gauge needle is inserted in the depression and directed slightly dorsad (10 to 20°) and proximad (10°) until the joint is entered (Fig. 3.102, site *B*). To avoid penetration of the digital sheath, the needle must be inserted dorsal to the palmar digital artery, vein, and nerve. The advantages to this approach are that the landmarks are easily palpated, synovial fluid is easy to obtain, the procedure can be done while the

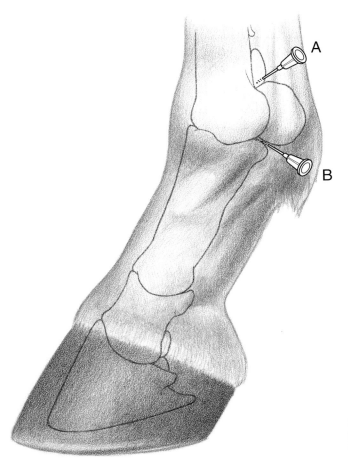

Figure 3.102 Lateral view of injection sites for the fetlock joint. *A*, site for the palmar/plantar recess; *B*, site for the dorsal distal end of the proximal sesamoid bone.

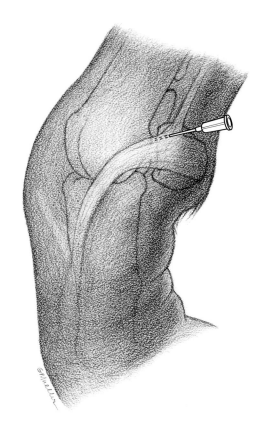

Figure 3.103 Lateral view of the injection site for the flexed fetlock joint. The site is through the collateral sesamoidean ligament.

horse is standing, and most horses readily tolerate the procedure.[65] This is the approach I prefer for the forelimb.

Another site for injection of the fetlock joint is located dorsally. The sole of the foot is placed on the knee, which provides a moderate degree of flexion of the fetlock. The needle is then inserted proximal to the proximodorsal limits of the proximal phalanx in an oblique manner, either lateral or medial to the extensor tendons, to enter the joint (Fig. 3.104). This approach generally causes greater discomfort than the other techniques. A total of 5 to 7 mL of anesthetic is injected.

DIGITAL FLEXOR TENDON SHEATH. There are several approaches for synoviocentesis of the digital flexor tendon sheath. Penetration of the proximolateral pouch can be done by using a 1-inch (2.5-cm) 20-gauge needle. The needle is inserted 1 cm proximal to the palmar/plantar anular ligament and 1 cm palmar/plantar to the lateral branch of the suspensory ligament and directed slightly distad until the sheath is penetrated. Alternatively, the sheath can be entered axial to the midbody of the proximal sesamoid bone.[28a] To accomplish this, the fetlock joint is flexed to approximately 225°, and a 1-inch (2.5-cm) 20-gauge needle is inserted 3 mm axial to the palpa-

ble border of the midbody of the lateral proximal sesamoid bone. The needle is directed, at an angle of 45° to the sagittal plane, to a depth of approximately 1.5 to 2 cm.

CARPAL JOINTS. Arthrocentesis of the antebrachiocarpal (radiocarpal) and middle (intercarpal) carpal joints can be accomplished easily by using one of two approaches. Because the carpometacarpal and middle carpal joints communicate, anesthetics injected into the middle carpal joint will also desensitize the carpometacarpal joint. Furthermore, because the carpometacarpal has palmar pouches that extend palmarodistal, adjacent to the origin of the suspensory ligament (Fig. 3.95), anesthetic injected into the middle carpal joint will desensitize the proximal suspensory ligament and proximal palmar metacarpal region.[20,21]

One report identified a failure of intraarticular anesthesia of the antebrachiocarpal to abolish lameness associated with chip fracture of the distal radius.[64] Nuclear medicine was used to identify the region of inflammation, and radiography was used to document the fracture. Proposed reasons for failure of intraarticular anesthesia to abolish the lameness included the following: Intact cartilage found at arthroscopy could provide a physical barrier to the penetration of the local anesthetic, and innervation to the subchondral bone via the nutrient

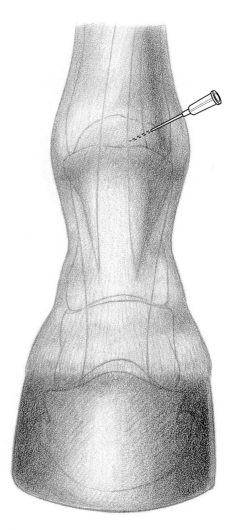

Figure 3.104 Dorsal view of the injection site for the dorsal approach to the fetlock joint.

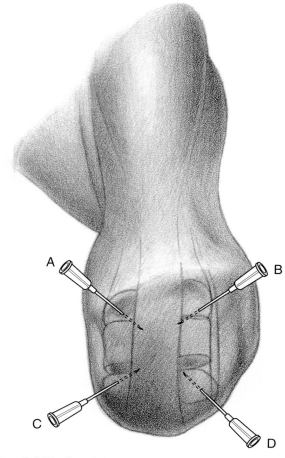

Figure 3.105 Dorsal view of the injection sites for the carpus. Needles can enter the antebrachiocarpal joint (*A* and *B*) or middle carpal joint (*C* and *D*) either lateral (*B* and *D*) or medial (*A* and *C*) to the extensor carpi radialis tendon. When the lateral site is chosen, the lateral digital extensor tendon must be avoided.

foramen nerve supply may not be reached by the local anesthetic.

With a dorsal approach, the antebrachiocarpal and middle carpal joints can be injected, with the carpus held in a flexed position to open the carpal joints. The site for injection is located in the depression either lateral or medial to the extensor carpi radialis tendon (Fig. 3.105, sites *A* and *B*). If the lateral approach is selected, the common digital extensor tendon must be avoided. The injection is made with a 1-inch (2.5-cm) 20-gauge needle. Because the surfaces of the carpal bones are at an angle, it is advisable to direct the needle slightly proximad to avoid needle penetration of the articular cartilage. After removing liberal quantities of synovial fluid, 5 to 7 mL of anesthetic are injected.

Alternatively, a palmarolateral approach with the limb bearing weight can be used for arthrocentesis of both joints. The landmarks for arthrocentesis of the ante-brachiocarpal joint are the palmarolateral aspect of the radius, proximolateral aspect of the accessory carpal bone, and palmarolateral aspect of the ulnar carpal

bone[34,44,68] (Fig. 3.106, site *A*). A 1-inch (2.5-cm) 20-gauge needle is inserted in this palpable depression at 90° to the long axis of the limb, and the needle is directed dorsomedially.

Another palmarolateral approach to the antebrachio-carpal joint is at the midaccessory carpal bone level between the palpable tendons of the ulnaris lateralis and the lateral digital extensor. The needle is inserted in the space between the distal lateral aspect of the radius (vestigial ulna) and the proximal lateral aspect of the ulnar carpal bone.[44] The palmarolateral approach to the middle carpal joint can be used if the joint is distended (Fig. 3.106, site *B*). With distension, the joint capsule is superficial and protrudes palmar and lateral to the ulnar and fourth carpal bones. Injection into this site is done while the horse is standing. A 1-inch (2.5-cm) 20-gauge needle is used. After liberal amounts of synovial fluid are retrieved, 5 to 7 mL of local anesthetic are injected.[68]

ELBOW JOINT. There are three approaches to the elbow joint. In the cranial approach, arthrocentesis is done cranial to the lateral collateral ligament either while the horse is standing[31] or while the limb is flexed and not bearing weight.[36] The lateral collateral ligament extends across the joint from the lateral epicondyle of the humerus to the lateral tuberosity of the radius. Both of these bony landmarks are easily palpated. The site for injection is two-thirds the distance distal, measured from the lateral epicondyle of the humerus to the lateral tuberosity of the radius (Fig. 3.107, site *A*). A 1.5-inch (3.8-cm) 20-gauge needle is inserted at a 90° angle to the skin just cranial to the lateral collateral ligament, to a depth of 1 inch.[31,44]

With the cranial approach, it is important to verify that the anesthetic is being injected into the joint and not into the periarticular tissues cranial to the joint. If the anesthetic is injected outside the joint in this location, it can anesthetize the distal branches of the radial nerve and cause temporary paralysis of the extensor carpi radialis and common digital extensor muscles. This is a problem, because the horse will not be able to lock its carpus in extension and the lameness examination will have to be discontinued until sensation returns. If this occurs, a polyvinylchloride (PVC) pipe bandage splint can be applied to the caudal aspect of the limb from the elbow to the ground until the block wears off.[36]

Another site for arthrocentesis of the elbow joint is just caudal to the lateral collateral ligament. The same landmarks are used as described for the cranial approach, and a 1.5-inch (3.8-cm) 20-gauge needle is inserted at 90° to the skin. In this location, the needle enters the bursa of the ulnaris lateralis muscle, which is thought to communicate with the elbow joint. One study, however, found communication between the bursa and the joint in only 9 of 24 (37.5%) joints examined.[60] Because of this, I prefer to place the needle more caudal in the palpable depression formed by the caudal epicondyle of

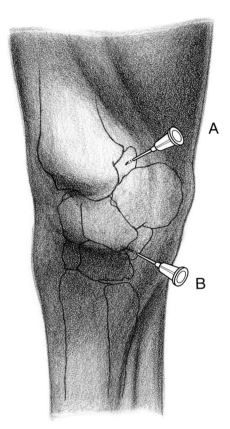

Figure 3.106 Lateral view of the palmarolateral injection sites for the carpal joints. *A*, site for the antebrachiocarpal joint; *B*, site for injection for the middle carpal joint.

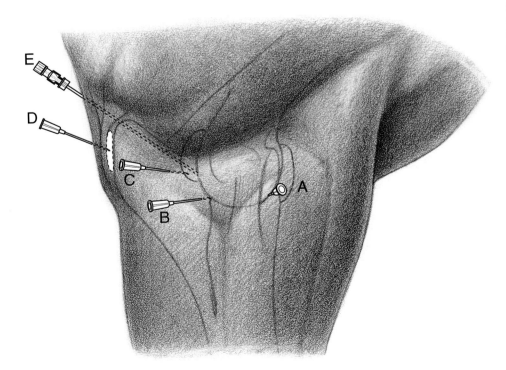

Figure 3.107 Lateral view of injection sites for the elbow joint and bursa. *A*, cranial approach; *B*, caudal to the collateral ligament in the palpable notch; *C*, caudolateral approach, with a 1.5-inch 20-gauge needle used; *D*, caudolateral approach, with a 3.5-inch spinal needle used; *E*, site for the olecranon bursa.

the humerus, the caudal proximal tuberosity of the radius, and the olecranon process (Fig. 3.107, site *B*). A 1.5-inch (3.8-cm) 20-gauge needle is inserted at a 90° angle to the skin.

An alternative site for arthrocentesis of the elbow joint is caudolateral.[31,60] In one approach, the palpable V-shaped depression in the regional musculature 2.4 to 3.2 inches (6 to 8 cm) cranial and slightly distal to the proximal lateral eminence of the olecranon process is the site for arthrocentesis. A 1.5-inch (3.8-cm) 20-gauge needle is inserted at approximately a 45° angle to the skin and is directed craniad and mediad to enter the large caudolateral joint pouch (Fig. 3.107, site *C*).

The caudolateral joint pouch can also be entered from a more proximal site. The landmarks are the lateral supracondylar crest of the distal humerus and the most proximal point of the olecranon process.[31] A 3.5-inch (8.9-cm) 18- to 20-gauge spinal needle is inserted one-third the measured distance caudal from the supracondylar eminence to the olecranon and 1 cm proximal to this imaginary line. The needle is directed distomedially at a 45° angle to the long axis of the limb. The needle penetrates the triceps muscle before entering the caudolateral joint pouch.[31]

Another approach (my preference) is to insert a 3.5-inch (8.9-cm) 18- to 20-gauge needle 3 cm distal to the proximal limits of the olecranon process and 2 cm cranial to the palpable lateral eminence. The needle is directed distad and follows the shaft of the olecranon process to enter the caudolateral joint capsule (Fig. 3.107, site *D*).

OLECRANON BURSA. The olecranon bursa can be injected with a 1.5-inch (3.8-cm) 18- to 20-gauge needle, as shown in Figure 3.107, site *E*. Three to 5 mL of anesthetic are injected. This block is rarely done.[1]

SCAPULOHUMERAL (SHOULDER) JOINT. The site for arthrocentesis of the shoulder joint is located in the notch formed between the cranial and caudal prominences of the lateral tuberosity of the humerus. The caudal prominence is the most easily palpated, and with deep finger pressure exerted, a notch (depression) 3.5 to 4 cm cranial to the caudal prominence can be palpated. This notch is not as readily palpable in heavily muscled horses. A 3.5-inch (8.9-cm) 18-gauge spinal needle is inserted into this notch and directed in a horizontal plane caudomediad at a 45° angle to the body. The joint capsule is entered at a depth of 5 to 7 cm. Synovial fluid can usually be aspirated, and 10 to 20 mL of anesthetic are injected (Fig. 3.108, site *A*).

A complication associated with intrasynovial anesthesia of the shoulder joint is temporary anesthesia of the suprascapular nerve and paralysis of the infraspinatus and supraspinatus muscles. This can occur if local anesthetic either diffuses out from the arthropuncture site or if the local anesthetic is injected outside the joint capsule. For this reason, some veterinarians prefer to use only 10 mL of local anesthetic to block the joint, hoping that the lower volume will be less likely to involve the suprascapular nerve.[36]

An alternative site for arthrocentesis is located just proximal to the caudolateral tuberosity 1 to 1.5 cm cranial to the infraspinatus tendon. A 3.5-inch (8.9-cm) 18-

Figure 3.108 Lateral view of injection sites for the shoulder region. *A*, site for the shoulder joint; *B*, site for the bicipital bursa.

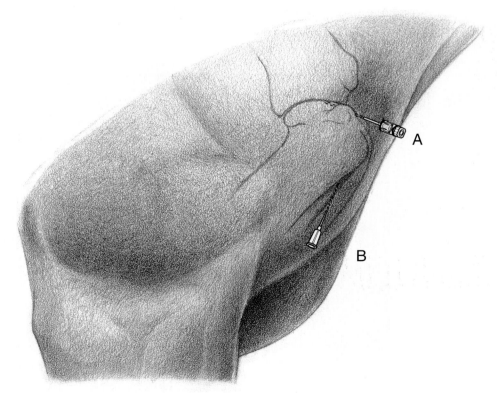

gauge needle is directed at 90° to the skin, slightly distad and mediad, until the joint is penetrated.

BICIPITAL BURSA. The cranial prominence of the lateral tuberosity of the humerus is palpated as was done for the shoulder joint. The site of injection is 3.5 cm distal and 7 cm caudal to this prominence. A 3.5-inch (8.9-cm)18-gauge spinal needle is inserted and directed mediad and proximad for a depth of 3.5 to 5.0 cm. The side of the needle shaft should contact bone.

Alternatively, the distal aspect of the deltoid tuberosity can be palpated and used as a landmark. At 4 cm proximal to this site, a 3.5-inch (8.9-cm) 18-gauge spinal needle is directed proximomediad to enter the bursa. Aspiration of fluid is usually possible.[26] Five to 10 mL of anesthetic are injected (Fig. 3.108, site *B*).

THE HINDLIMB

The injection sites for intrasynovial anesthesia of the joints below the tarsus are the same as for the forelimb.

TARSAL (HOCK) JOINTS. Four synovial sacs are associated with the tarsal joints: tarsocrural (tibiotarsal), proximal intertarsal, distal intertarsal, and tarsometatarsal. Numerous studies have been done to determine the consistency of communication between these joints. The tarsocrural and proximal intertarsal joints communicate consistently and, for intraarticular injection purposes, are considered to be one joint. For the distal intertarsal and tarsometatarsal joints, reports of communication vary from 8 to 38%.[5,19,35] It has also been determined that the proximal and distal intertarsal joints and the proximal and tarsometatarsal joints occasionally communicate, which could confuse interpretation of intraarticular anesthesia.[35] Because of these findings, it is recommended that the two distal tarsal joints be injected separately to ensure that the joints are blocked.

The tarsocrural sac is the largest joint space and communicates with the proximal intertarsal joint. A 1-inch (2.5-cm) 20-gauge needle is used to penetrate it at its dorsomedial aspect just distal and dorsal to the medial malleolus of the tibia and plantar to the cranial branch of the medial saphenous vein (Fig. 3.109, site *A*). If synovial effusion is present, the needle is advanced until fluid flows readily from the needle. If synovial effusion is not present, the needle is carefully advanced until the nonarticular surface of the talus is contacted.[68] Generally, 20 mL of local anesthetic are injected, which will desensitize the tarsocrural and the proximal intertarsal joints.

The site for injection of the distal intertarsal joint is on the medial surface of the tarsus. An imaginary line can be drawn between the palpable distal tubercle of the talus and the space between second and third metatarsal bones at their proximal limits.[59] A small depression is often felt just distal to the cunean tendon along this imaginary line. A ⅝-inch (1.58-cm) 25-gauge or a 1-inch (2.5-cm) 22-gauge needle is directed perpendicular to the long axis of the limb and slightly caudal to enter the joint space between the combined first and second tarsal bones and the third and central tarsal bones. The needle is advanced to about 0.5 inch (1.25 cm), and 5 mL of local anesthetic are injected[59] (Fig. 3.109, site *B*).

The tarsometatarsal joint is best approached from the plantarolateral aspect of the tarsus. The site for injection

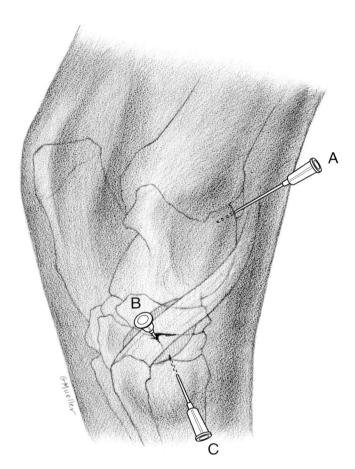

Figure 3.109 Medial view of injection sites for the tarsal joints. *A*, site for the tarsocrural joint; *B*, site for the distal intertarsal joint; *C*, site for the cunean bursa.

is the proximal head of the fourth metatarsal bone. A 1- to 1.5-inch (2.5- to 3.8-cm) 20- or 22-gauge needle is inserted 0.5 to 1 cm proximal to the fourth metatarsal bone and is directed in a dorsal and slightly distomedial direction to enter the space between the fourth metatarsal and the fourth tarsal bone[42,68] (Fig. 3.110). One study investigating injection techniques of the equine tarsus found that contrast injected into the tarsometatarsal joint from the plantarolateral approach extended around the tendons of the tibialis cranialis and fibularis tertius in 18 of 20 limbs injected and that some contrast entered the tarsal sheath in 7 of 20 limbs.[19]

An alternative, but more difficult, approach to the tarsometatarsal joint is similar to that used to inject the distal intertarsal joint. The site for injection is approximately 0.5 inch distal to the medial approach for the distal intertarsal joint. A ⅝-inch (1.58-cm) 25-gauge needle is used. Five mL of local anesthetic are injected.

CUNEAN BURSA. The cunean bursa is located on the medial surface of the hock and lies between the medial collateral ligament and the medial branch of the tibialis cranialis (cunean) tendon. A 1-inch (2.5-cm) 22-gauge needle is inserted under the distal border of the cunean tendon, and 5 to 7 mL of local anesthesia are injected[22,23] (Fig. 3.109, site *C*).

GENUAL (STIFLE) JOINT. The stifle joint is made up of three synovial compartments: femoropatellar, lateral femorotibial, and medial femorotibial synovial sacs. Contrast studies have shown that the frequency of communication between the femoropatellar and medial femorotibial joints is 60 to 65%.[54,70] The communication, however, is not reliable and appears to depend on the direction of flow of the injectable agent, amount of joint inflammation, and anatomic variation. Communication between the femoropatellar and medial femorotibial joints is observed more frequently when the medial femorotibial joint is injected than when the femoropatellar joint is injected. Communication between the femoropatellar and lateral femorotibial joints occurs rarely, and communication between the lateral and medial femorotibial joints has not been observed.[33] With inflammation it is likely that these openings become occluded. To ensure accurate distribution of the local anesthetic, each synovial compartment should be injected separately.[56]

The femoropatellar joint is the largest of the compartments and can be entered in one of three ways. It can be easily entered either lateral or medial to the middle patellar ligament. A 3.5-inch (8.9-cm) 18-gauge needle is inserted approximately 3 cm proximal to the tibial crest and is directed dorsad underneath the patella in the trochlear grove (Fig. 3.111, site *A*). For this approach to be successful, the limb should be in a partial weight-bearing (slightly flexed) position.

The femoropatellar joint can also be entered just distal to the apex of the patella on either side of the middle patellar ligament[68] (Fig 3.112, site *a*). A 1.5-inch (3.8-

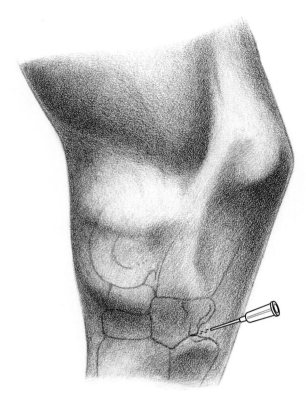

Figure 3.110 Lateral view of the injection site for the tarsometatarsal joint.

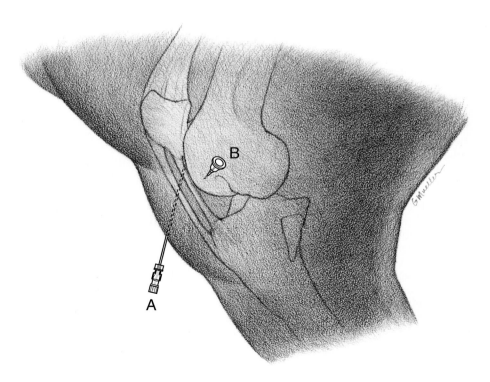

Figure 3.111 Lateral view of injection sites for the femoropatellar (stifle) joint. *A*, site for femoropatellar joint, with a 3.5-inch spinal needle used; *B*, site for the lateral approach.

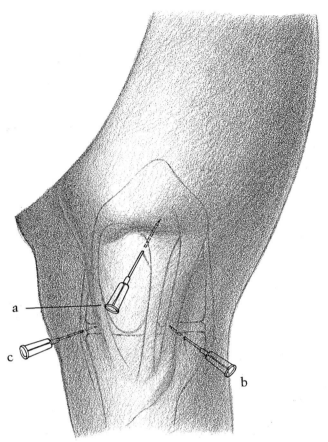

Figure 3.112 Cranial view of the injection sites for the stifle joint. *a*, needle inserted medial to the middle patellar ligament to enter the femoropatellar joint capsule; *b*, needle positioned just caudal to the lateral patellar ligament to enter the lateral sac of the femorotibial joint capsule; *c*, needle positioned to enter the medial sac of the femorotibial joint capsule.

cm) 18-gauge needle is directed at right angles to the skin. The joint capsule is superficial at this location, and the needle is advanced until the articular surface is contacted. This approach can be done with the horse bearing full weight. In cases in which obvious joint capsule distension exists, synovial fluid can be drained or aspirated. On the other hand, when the capsule is not distended, little fluid can be retrieved. Joint penetration is ensured when there is little resistance to injection.

The femoropatellar joint can also be entered via a lateral approach[29] (Fig 3.111, site *B*), which can be done with the horse weight bearing. The lateral cul-de-sac of the femoropatellar joint pouch is palpated caudal to the lateral trochlea and the lateral patellar ligament, approximately 5 cm proximal to the lateral condyle of the tibia. A 1.5-inch (3.8-cm) 18-gauge needle is inserted into the recess, perpendicular to the long axis of the femur, until the nonarticular portion of the lateral trochlea is contacted. The needle is withdrawn 1 to 2 mm before injection. Synovial fluid can be retrieved in most cases, and the approach is usually well tolerated. Generally, 20 mL of anesthetic solution are injected.

The site for injection of the medial femorotibial joint is located in the space between the medial patellar and

medial collateral ligaments (Fig. 3.112, site *c*).[16] The veterinarian may approach this joint for arthrocentesis from the same side or from the opposite side and reach under the horse's belly to visualize the injection site directly (my preference). A 1.5-inch (3.8-cm) 18- to 20-gauge needle is inserted between the ligaments, 1 cm proximal to the tibia and directed perpendicular to the long axis of the limb in a slightly cranial direction. The medial meniscus will be contacted (penetrated) if the needle is directed lateral or caudolateral or if it is inserted too close to the proximal tibia.[31,68]

An alternative site for injection is cranial and just proximal to the tibia in a space between the medial and middle patellar ligaments. A 3.5-inch (8.9-cm) 18-gauge needle is inserted from cranial to caudal to a depth of 4 to 6 cm. Then 20 mL of local anesthetic solution are injected.

The site for injection of the lateral femorotibial joint is just caudal to the edge of the lateral patellar ligament (Fig. 3.112, site *b*). The horse will have to be pulled into weight bearing to palpate the ligament. A 1.5-inch (3.8-cm) 18- to 20-gauge needle is inserted 1 cm proximal to the tibia at right angles to the long axis of the femur and directed from lateral to medial to enter the joint.

An alterative approach is to insert the needle just proximal to the tibia in the space between the lateral collateral ligament of the femorotibial joint and the tendon of origin of the long digital extensor tendon. The needle is inserted slowly until the joint capsule is entered. Deeper insertion will result in penetration of the meniscus and a painful response.

A third approach is to inject the large diverticulum beneath the long digital extensor tendon at the proximolateral limits of the tibia. This diverticulum is in direct communication with the lateral femorotibial joint.

A fourth approach is cranial and just proximal to the tibia in the space between the middle and lateral patellar ligaments. A 3.5-inch (8.9-cm) 18-gauge needle is inserted from cranial to caudal to enter the joint. Generally, 20 mL of local anesthetic solution are injected.

All three joints can be injected from one site with a 3.5-inch (8.9-cm) 18-gauge spinal needle. The site for injection is cranial between the lateral and middle patellar ligaments, 1.5 cm proximal to the tibia. First, a 1-inch (2.5-cm) 22-gauge needle with 3 mL of local anesthetic is used to block the skin and subcutaneous tissues. Then, a 3.5-inch (8.9-cm) 18-gauge spinal needle is inserted and directed toward the medial femorotibial joint; 20 mL of local anesthetic are injected (Fig 3.113, site *A*). The needle is then withdrawn to the subcutaneous tissue and redirected to the lateral femorotibial joint; another 20 mL of anesthetic are injected (Fig. 3.113, site *B*). The needle is again withdrawn to the subcutaneous tissue and redirected proximal under the patella in the trochlear groove (Fig. 3.113, site *C*); the stifle must be slightly flexed to accomplish this. Another 20 mL of anesthetic are injected.

TROCHANTERIC BURSA. The trochanteric bursa is located beneath the tendon of insertion of the gluteus accessorius (middle gluteal muscle) on the cranial portion of the greater trochanter of the femur. The bursa covers the majority of the greater trochanter, which is covered with cartilage. The site for injection is the most proximal as-

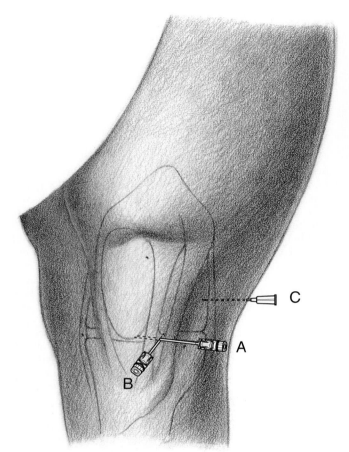

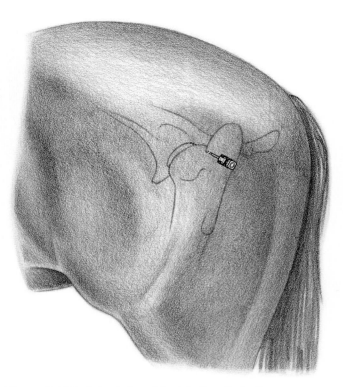

Figure 3.114 Lateral view of the injection site for the coxofemoral joint. The needle is inserted in the trochanteric notch, directed at a 45° angle with the long axis until the coxofemoral joint is penetrated.

Figure 3.113 Dorsal view of the injection sites for the stifle joint. *A*, site for the medial femorotibial joint, with a spinal needle used; *B*, site for the lateral femorotibial joint, with a spinal needle used; *C*, lateral approach to the femoropatellar joint.

pect of the palpable bony eminence of the cranial summit of the greater trochanter. A 1.5-inch (3.8-cm) 18-gauge needle is usually all that is needed, although a longer needle may sometimes be required for larger Warmblood horses.[26]

The needle is inserted and directed horizontally at right angles to the sagittal plane until bone is encountered. Seven to 10 mL of anesthetic are injected. Because the bursa lies directly lateral over the cranial portion of the cartilage-covered trochanter major under the tendon of the gluteus medius, an alternate method whereby the needle is directed mediad through the middle gluteal muscle directly over the bursa toward the trochanter can be employed. Anesthetic injection is made when the needle contacts bone.

COXOFEMORAL (HIP) JOINT. The coxofemoral joint is one of the most difficult joints to inject.[36,41] This is particularly true in a heavily muscled horse. The horse should be standing squarely and be restrained within stocks. Mild sedation is often advised because any movement of the horse during the injection procedure may lead to bending or breaking of the needle. At the proximal end

of the femur, the most prominent bony landmark that can be palpated laterally is the greater trochanter. The trochanter is located about three-fourths the distance between the tuber coxae and the tuber ischii and is divided into the greater (caudal) and lesser (cranial) protuberances, with the trochanteric notch between them. Deep palpation in a relaxed patient will usually allow identification of the protuberances, but the cranial part can be difficult to feel in heavily muscled horses. When the protuberances cannot be palpated, attempts to inject the joint should be avoided.

The site for injection is located at the caudal aspect of the lesser protuberance and 1 cm dorsal to it. A small bleb of local anesthetic is injected subcutaneously over the injection site. A 6-inch (15.2-cm) 16-to 18-gauge spinal needle is inserted in the site and directed in a horizontal plane slightly cranial and slightly distal. Be sure the needle stays close to the femoral neck. As the needle approaches full penetration, i.e., 11 to 12.5 cm, firm fibrous tissue is felt just before entry into the joint capsule. Synovial fluid is retrieved, and 10 to 15 mL of anesthetic are injected (Figs. 3.114 and 3.115).

Diagnostic Imaging

Imaging techniques commonly used in making a diagnosis, formulating a prognosis, and evaluating the progress of healing include radiography, ultrasonography, and nuclear medicine (scintigraphy). These modali-

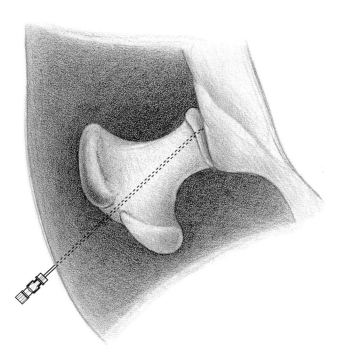

Figure 3.115 Overhead view of the injection site for the coxofemoral joint. The needle is inserted just caudal to the greater trochanter and directed at a 45° angle to enter the joint.

ties are available at most referral facilities. Thermography is also available at some centers, but it is still not widely used. Computed tomography has shown great promise for imaging the head, neck, and distal extremities. Unfortunately, a special table is required to image horses over 300 pounds. Magnetic resonance imaging has also shown great promise as a method of imaging the extremities. Presently, it is being used as a research tool for horses. Portable units are currently being evaluated (for more information, see Chapter 4).

Angiography

Angiography is a technique whereby radio-opaque material is injected into an artery or vein to evaluate blood-flow patterns to the musculoskeletal or other organ systems. The distribution of the dye is monitored by single, serial, or fluoroscopic radiography. This technique allows identification of anatomic alterations and their causes.[63] Horses are most frequently put under general anesthesia, and the most accessible artery is identified. After aseptic preparation of the area over the vessel, the vessel is catheterized either by percutaneous puncture or after surgical cutdown. Then, 20 mL (for a 450-kg horse) of angiographic contrast material is injected over a 2- to 3-second period. Radiographs are taken 2 to 4 seconds after injection is complete.[8] This technique may be of value in diagnosing alterations in blood supply to the horse's limb resulting from trauma (wire cuts) and laminitis.

Infrared Thermometer

A portable infrared thermometer that allows the examiner to conveniently record the body surface tempera-

ture of the horse is available. It converts the infrared radiation energy to electrical signals that are amplified and displayed on a temperature dial.[48,49] Temperature measurements are obtained by aiming the instrument tip at the area of interest and simply pulling the trigger. Although this appeared to have some appeal when it was first introduced, the instrument is not commonly used.

Arthroscopy

The value of and technique for arthroscopy are discussed in Chapter 7.

Gait and Force Analysis

Telemetric Strain Measurements

In vivo telemetric strain measurements can be made by surgically implanting an electrical-resistance strain gauge on the surface of a bone, tendon, or ligament. From this, strain measurements are recorded with a wireless telemetric system.[66] The technique allows the investigator to evaluate a horse's movement at fast gaits and during progression over various obstacles. This technique has provided important information regarding the pathogenesis of fractures and the best orientation for application of internal fixation devices for fracture repair. It has also been useful for documenting strain magnitudes applied to tendons and ligaments during movement.

The strain gauges have also been applied to the outer surface of hoof walls to directly evaluate the hoof wall elasticity and indirectly evaluate the amount of compression.[12] Telemetry has also been employed with ergometric measurements of joint flexion angles. In this case, electrogoniometers (Elgons) are centered over the joint to be evaluated and then taped into position. The technique is used most frequently in research facilities and has little practical value for the practicing veterinarian.

Cinematography and Videography

Cinematography with a high-speed camera and high-speed videography can be used to record the horse's movement at various gaits.[12,52,53] Anatomic landmarks are usually identified on the limb, and the horse is exercised either on a level surface over a known distance or over obstacles. The high-speed camera can be arranged perpendicular to the course so that the field of view covers the entire course. Additional cameras can be placed at the beginning and end of the course to record movements, providing a three-dimensional analysis. Or the camera can be mounted on a camera car that moves with the horse.

For gait analysis, a maximum speed of 500 frames/second is adequate.[12] The analysis consists of plotting the position of each marked anatomic site for each frame through a complete stride. With this, the stride length and rate, height of foot flight arc, limb displacement, range of motion, acceleration, and linear and angular velocities can be determined.[52] The advantage of high-speed videography is immediate viewing.

Electrogoniometric Analysis

An electrogoniometer (Elgon) is used to measure the variation in joint angles during locomotion, providing a permanent record (goniogram). The Elgons are attached to the limbs, and flexion and extension movements are recorded as upward and downward displacements. This technique has been used to evaluate the movements of normal and pathologic joints quantitatively and qualitatively; if performed properly, it is accurate to within 1° of movement.[2,52,53]

Elgons are centered and fixed in place by taping them over the center of the joint to be evaluated; the wire leads are attached to the saddle. An oscillographic recording can be obtained from extension leads from the saddle to the recorder or by an FM telemetric method. A major advantage of telemetric measurement is that it allows for unrestricted movement of the horse while recording.

The advantages of electrogoniometry are the simultaneous recordings of joint movement, amplitude, stride, angular velocity, acceleration, and total stride time. The disadvantages are that without telemetry, electrogoniometry is limited to evaluation at a walk and a trot and that when Elgons are positioned above the carpus and hock, errors in recording can result from skin movement. Goniograms are somewhat difficult to interpret and do not allow direct visualization of the horse during movement. A combination of electrogoniometry and cinematography has been used successfully for evaluation of subtle lameness.

Hoof Force Measurements

Hoof force measurements can be made with force plates placed in the ground or with instrumented shoes.[12,52] The force transducer in common use consists of force plates that are embedded in the ground. As the hoof strikes these force plates, the deformation caused by the weight is converted to strain measurements. Strain is recorded as a percent of body weight in vertical, cranial, caudal, horizontal, lateral, and medial directions. Vertical forces result from the body weight during the support phase of the stride. Lateral and medial strain forces result from hoof impact, rotary motion of the limb, and direction of travel. The disadvantages include infrequent hoof strikes, insufficient resiliency, and slow speed of response. In addition, some horses avoid striking the plate even when the surface is camouflaged. Several instruments have been developed to overcome the disadvantages of the force plates.

References

1. Adams OR. Lameness in Horses. 3rd ed. Philadelphia: Lea & Febiger, 1974.
2. Adrian M, et al. Electrogoniometric analysis of equine metacarpophalangeal joint lameness. Am J Vet Res 1977;38:431.
3. Andreen DS, Trumble TN, Caron JP, et al. Onset and duration of intra-articular mepivacaine in the horse. Proc Am Assoc Equine Pract 1994;40:151.
4. Beeman GM. The clinical diagnosis of lameness. Cont Educ 1988;10:209.
5. Bell BTL, et al. In vivo investigation of communication between the distal intertarsal and tarsometatarsal joints in horses and ponies. Vet Surg 1993;22:289–292.
6. Bowker RM, Linder K, Van Wulfen KK, et al. Distribution of local anesthetics injected into the distal interphalangeal joint and podotrochlear bursa: An experimental study. Pferdehilkunde 1996;12:609–612.
7. Bowker RM, Rockershouser SJ, Vex KB, et al. Immunocytochemical and dye distribution studies of nerves potentially desensitized by injections into the distal interphalangeal joint or the navicular bursa of horses. J Am Vet Med Assoc 1993;203:1708–1714.
8. Bowker RM, Van Wulfen KK, Grentz DJ. Nonselectivity of local anesthetics injected into the distal interphalangeal joint and navicular bursa. Proc Am Assoc Equine Pract 1995;41:240–242.
9. Bramlage LR, Gabel AA, Hackett RP. Avulsion fractures of the origin of the suspensory ligament in the horse. J Am Vet Med Assoc 1980;176:1004.
10. Carter GK, Hogan PM. Use of diagnostic nerve blocks in lameness evaluation. Proc Am Assoc Equine Pract 1996;42:26–32.
11. Churchill EA. The methodology of diagnosis of hind leg lameness. Proc Am Assoc Equine Pract 1979;25:297–304.
12. Clayton HM. Locomotion. In: Jones WE, Ed. Equine Sports Medicine. 1st ed. Philadelphia: Lea & Febiger, 1989;49–163.
13. Day TK, Skarda RT. The pharmacology of local anesthetics. Vet Clin North Am Equine Pract 1991;7:489.
14. Derksen EJ. Diagnostic local anesthesia of the equine front limb. Equine Pract 1980;2:41.
15. Dyson S. Comparison of responses to analgesia of the navicular bursa and intra-articular analgesia of the distal interphalangeal joint in 102 horses. Proc Am Assoc Equine Pract 1995;41:234–239.
16. Dyson S. Lameness due to pain associated with the distal interphalangeal joint: 45 cases. Equine Vet J 1991;23:128–135.
17. Dyson S. Problems associated with the interpretation of the results of regional and intraarticular anesthesia of the horse. Vet Rec 1986;118:419–422.
18. Dyson S. Suspensory ligament desmitis. Vet Clin North Am 1995;11:177–214.
19. Dyson S, Romero JM. An investigation of injection techniques for local analgesia of the equine distal tarsus and proximal metatarsus. Equine Vet J 1993;25:30–35.
20. Ford TS, et al. Communication and boundaries of the middle carpal and carpometacarpal joints in horses. Am J Vet Res 1988;49:2161–2164.
21. Ford TS, Ross MW, Orsini PG. A comparison of methods of proximal palmar metacarpal analgesia in horses. Vet Surg 1989;18:146–150.
22. Gabel AA. Diagnosis, relative incidence, and probable cause of cunean tendon bursitis-tarsitis of Standardbred horses. J Am Vet Med Assoc 1979;175:1079–1085.
23. Gabel AA. Lameness caused by inflammation of the distal hock. Vet Clin North Am Large Anim Pract 1982;2:101.
24. Goodman NL, Baker BK. Lameness diagnosis and treatment in the Quarter Horse racehorse. Vet Clin North Am 1990;6:85–108.
25. Goshal NG. Nervous system. In: Getty R, Ed. Anatomy of Domestic Animals. 5th ed. Philadelphia: WB Saunders, 1975;665–668.
26. Grant BD. Bursal injections. Proc Am Assoc Equine Pract 1996;42:64–68.
27. Gray BW, et al. Clinical approach to determine the contribution of the palmar and palmar metacarpal nerves to the innervation of the equine fetlock joint. Am J Vet Res 1980;41:940.
28. Hague BR, Honnas CM, Simpson RB, Peloso JG. Evaluation of skin bacterial flora before and after aseptic preparation of clipped and nonclipped arthrocentesis sites. Proc Am Assoc Equine Pract 1995;41:54–55.
28a. Hassel DM, Stover SM, Yarbrough TB, et al: Palmar-plantar axial sesamoidean approach to the digital flexor sheath in horses. J Am Vet Med Assoc 2000;217–1343–1347.
29. Hendrickson DA, Nixon AJ. A lateral approach for synovial fluid aspiration and joint injection of the femoropatellar joint of the horse. Equine Vet J 1992;24:397–398.
30. Hogan PH, Honnas CM, Carter KG. Arthrocentesis and joint injection techniques in horses: Articulations of the lower limb. Vet Med 1996;91:1111–1118.
31. Hogan PM, Honnas CM, Carter GK. Arthrocentesis and joint injection techniques in horses: Articulations of the upper limb. Vet Med 1997;38:70–74.
32. Jeffcott LB. Diagnosis of back problems in the horse. Cont Educ 1981;3:134.

33. Keegan KG, Wilson DA, Kreeger JM, et al. Local distribution of mepivacaine after distal interphalangeal joint injection in horses. Am J Vet Res 1996;57:422–426.

34. Kiely RG, McMullan W. Lateral arthrocentesis of the equine carpus. Equine Pract 1987;9:22–24.

35. Kraus-Hansen AE, Jann HW, Kerr DV, et al. Arthrographic analysis of communication between the tarsometatarsal and distal intertarsal joints of the horse. Vet Surg 1992;21:139–144.

35a. Lane Easter J, Watkins JP, Stephens SL, et al: Effects of regional anesthesia on experimentally induced coffin joint synovitis. Am Assoc Equine Pract 2000;46:214–216.

36. Lewis RD. Techniques for arthrocentesis of equine shoulder, elbow, stifle and hip joints. Proc Am Assoc Equine Pract 1996;42:55–63.

37. Mackey-Smith MP, et al. Carpal canal syndrome in horses. J Am Vet Med Assoc 1972;160:93.

38. May SA, Wyn-Jones G. Identification of hindleg lameness. Equine Vet J 1987;19:185–188.

39. Merriam JG. Hind limb lameness in the dressage horse. Proc Am Assoc Equine Pract 1986;32:669–676.

40. Miller SM, Stover SM. Palmaroproximal approach for arthrocentesis of the proximal interphalangeal joint in the horse. Equine Vet J 1996;28:376–380.

41. Misheff MM, Stover SM. A comparison of two techniques for arthrocentesis of the meta carpophalangeal joint. Equine Vet J 1991;23:273–276.

42. Moyer W. A Guide to Equine Joint Injections. Lawrenceville, NY: Veterinary Learning Systems, 1993.

43. Moyer W, Anderson JP. Sheared heels: Diagnosis and treatment. J Am Vet Med Assoc 1975;166:53.

44. Moyer W, Carter GK. Techniques to facilitate intra-articular injection of equine joints. Proc Am Assoc Equine Pract 1996;42:48–54.

45. Moyer W, Ford TS, Ross MW. Proximal suspensory desmitis. Proc Am Assoc Equine Pract 1988;34:409.

46. Nyack B, et al. Osteochondrosis of the shoulder joint of the horse. Cornell Vet 1981;71:149.

47. Nyrop KA, Coffman JR, DeBowes RM, Booth LC. The roll of diagnostic nerve blocks in the equine lameness examination. Cont Educ 1983;12:669–676.

48. Palmer SE. Use of the infrared thermometer as a means of measuring limb surface temperature in the horse. Am J Vet Res 1981;42:105.

49. Palmer SE. Use of the portable infrared thermometer in equine practice. Proc Am Assoc Equine Pract 1980;26:327.

50. Pleasant RS, Baker JB, Muhlbauer MC, et al. Stress reaction and stress fractures of the proximal palmar aspect of the third metacarpal bone in horses: 58 cases (1980–1990). J Am Vet Med Assoc 1992;201:1918–1923.

51. Pleasant RS, Moll HD, Leg WB, et al. Intra-articular anesthesia of the distal interphalangeal joint alleviates lameness associated with the navicular bursa in horses. Vet Surg 1997;26:137–140.

52. Ratzlaff MH. Cinematography, electrogoniometry, thermography and dynamography. In: Mansmann RA, McAllister EJ, Eds. Equine Medicine and Surgery. 3rd ed. Santa Barbara, CA: American Veterinary Publications, 1982;954.

53. Ratzlaff MH, et al. Evaluation of equine locomotion using electrogoniometry and cinematography: Research and clinical application. Proc Am Assoc Equine Pract 1979;25:381.

54. Reeves M, Trotter GW, Kainer R. Anatomic and functional communications between the synovial sacs of the equine stifle joint. Equine Vet J 1991;23;215–218.

55. Rooney JR. Biomechanics of Lameness in Horses. Baltimore: Williams & Wilkins, 1969.

56. Rose RJ, Frauenfelder HC. Arthrocentesis in the horse. Equine Vet J 1982;14:173.

57. Ross M, Ford T, Orsini P. Incomplete longitudinal fracture of the proximal palmar cortex of the metacarpal bone in horses. Vet Surg 1988;17:82–86.

58. Sack WO. Nerve distribution in the metacarpus and front digit of the horse. J Am Vet Med Assoc 1975;167:298.

59. Sack WO, Orsini PG. Distal intertarsal and tarsometatarsal joints in the horse: Communication and injection sites. J Am Vet Med Assoc 1981;179:355.

60. Sams AE, Honnas CM, Sack WO, Ford TS. Communication of the ulnaris lateralis bursa with the equine elbow joint and evaluation of caudal arthrocentesis. Equine Vet J 1993;25:130–133.

61. Schmotzer WB, Timm KI. Local anesthetic techniques for diagnosis of lameness. Vet Clin North Am 1990;6:705–728.

62. Schneider RK, Bramlage LR, Moore LM, et al. A retrospective study of 192 horses affected with septic arthritis/tenosynovitis. Equine Vet J 1992;24:436–442.

62a. Schumacher JI, Schramme M, Schumacher JO, et al: The effect of volume of local anesthetic administered into the coffin joint on solar toe or heel pain. Am Assoc Equine Pract 2000;46:27–28.

62b. Schumacher JO, Schramme M, Schumacher JI, et al: Abolition of lameness caused by experimentally induced solar pain in horses after analgesia of the distal interphalangeal joint. Am Assoc Equine Pract 1999;45:193–194.

63. Scott EA, Sandier GA, Shires MH. Angiography as a diagnostic technique in the equine. J Equine Med Surg 1978;2:270.

64. Shepherd MC, Pilsworth RC. Failure of intra-articular anaesthesia of the antebrachiocarpal joint to abolish lameness associated with chip fracture of the distal radius. Equine Vet J 1993;25:458–461.

65. Southwood LL, Baxter GM, Fehr JE. How to perform arthrocentesis of the fetlock joint by using a distal palmar (plantar) approach. Proc Am Assoc Equine Pract 1997;43:151–53.

66. Summer Smith G, et al. Telemetric measurements of strain in the metacarpus of the horse: A pilot study. Am J Vet Res 1977;38:1675.

67. Swanson TD. Guide for Veterinary Service and Judging of Equestrian Events. 3rd ed. Golden, CO: American Association of Equine Practitioners, 1984.

68. Trotter GW, McIlwraith CW. Clinical features and diagnosis of equine joint disease. In: McIlwraith CW, Trotter GW. Eds. Joint Disease in the Horse. Philadelphia: WB Saunders, 1996;125–134.

69. Turner T. Diagnosis and treatment of navicular disease in horses. Vet Clin North Am 1989;5:131–143.

70. Vacek JR, et al. Communication between the femoropatellar and medial and lateral femorotibial joints in horses. Am J Vet Res 1992;53:1431–1434.

71. Van Pelt RW. Intra-articular injection of the equine stifle for therapeutic and diagnostic purposes. J Am Vet Med Assoc 1965;147:490.

72. Vazquez de Mercado R, Stover SM, Taylor KT, et al. Lateral approach for arthrocentesis of the distal interphalangeal joint in horses. J Am Vet Med Assoc 1998;212:1413–1418.

73. Verschooten F, Verbeeck J. Flexion test of the metacarpophalangeal and interphalangeal joints and flexion angle of the metacarpophalangeal joint in sound horses. Equine Vet J 1997;29:50–54.

74. Wheat JD, Jones K. Selected techniques of regional anesthesia: Symposium on equine anesthesia. Vet Clin North Am Large Anim Pract 1981;3:223.

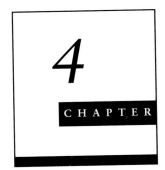

Equine Diagnostic Imaging

RICHARD D. PARK, ROBERT H. WRIGLEY, AND
PHILLIP F. STEYN

Imaging is an important diagnostic tool for identifying the cause, location, extent, and severity of lesions that cause lameness. The information obtained from imaging should always be incorporated with physical findings, history, and laboratory results to arrive at a final clinical diagnosis. The number of imaging modalities has increased in recent years. In addition to radiography, ultrasound and nuclear scintigraphy provide substantial contributions to lameness diagnosis. Thermography is used to a lesser extent, and computed radiography, computed tomography (CT), and magnetic resonance imaging (MRI) offer the potential for more accurate and detailed diagnoses. Because of the number and variety of imaging modalities available, a basic knowledge of the attributes and respective role of each imaging modality in lameness diagnosis is essential for effective and efficient clinical use.

This chapter presents the basic principles of diagnostic imaging modalities, including equipment. Radiation safety, special radiographic examinations (contrast studies), and interpretation principles for each diagnostic imaging modality are discussed. Routine diagnostic imaging examinations and normal imaging anatomy of the equine extremities are illustrated for radiology, ultrasound, and nuclear scintigraphy.

Part I

RADIOLOGY

Richard D. Park

Radiology has evolved into an acceptable and routine procedure for assisting the veterinarian in equine lameness diagnosis, prognosis, and treatment. Although it is an important diagnostic aid, it should be used in conjunction with an accurate history, physical examination, other imaging modalities, and diagnostic tests. The veterinarian must be familiar with x-ray machines, examination techniques, accessory equipment, darkroom equipment and procedures, radiation safety, normal radiographic anatomy, and basic radiographic interpretation principles to perform diagnostic radiographic studies. Too often, knowledge of these basic tools is overlooked, resulting in inferior radiographic examinations. Poor-quality radiographs may result in erroneous diagnoses and conclusions. The axiom "no radiograph is better than a poor-quality radiograph" is true in equine radiology.

Radiographs are part of the permanent case record and, as such, are the property of the veterinarian. Radiographs should be properly identified and filed for future reference and retrieval. They may be needed for comparison with future examinations or documentation for medical-legal purposes.

EQUIPMENT

A knowledge of x-ray equipment is necessary for obtaining quality radiographs safely. Since the equipment is relatively expensive, proper care and maintenance should be followed to ensure a long equipment life. An x-ray machine, accessory x-ray equipment, and darkroom equipment are needed; and the clinician must practice radiation safety procedures to make a quality radiograph.

X-Ray Machines

An x-ray machine is the most expensive and complex piece of equipment needed for equine radiography. A detailed discussion of the theory and physics of the x-ray machine is not attempted here; the reader is referred to several excellent references for such material.[7,15,36]

The x-ray machine's settings may be changed to vary the exposure. Milliamperage (mA), exposure time, and kilovoltage potential (kVp) can be changed on the control panel (Fig. 4.1). Milliamperage is the tube current and refers to the quantity of electrons flowing per second

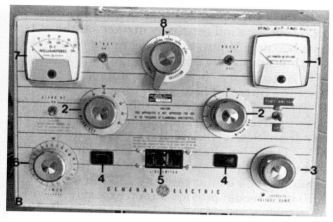

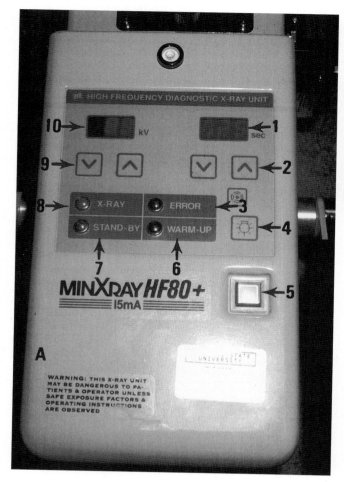

Figure 4.1 A. Control panel for a 30-mA portable x-ray machine. 1, exposure time indicator; 2, exposure time adjustment buttons; 3, error indicator; 4, collimator lamp "on" switch; 5, main power switch; 6, warm-up indicator; 7, standby indicator; 8, x-ray indicator; 9, kilovolt adjustment buttons; 10, kilovolt indicator. B. Control panel for a 200-mA mobile x-ray machine. 1, line voltage meter; 2, kilovoltage potential selectors; 3, line voltage compensation knob; 4, indicator lights; 5, "on-off" switch; 6, exposure time selector; 7, milliamperage exposure meter; 8, milliamperage selector.

in the x-ray tube. Ultimately, it determines the quantity of x-rays emitted from the x-ray tube.

Exposure time is an important variable in equine radiology. Because of problems related to animal and cassette movement, exposure time should be 0.1 second or less, if possible, for equine limb examinations. Electronic timers permit accurate timing when the exposure is less than 0.1 second and are recommended. For equine radiology, an electronic timer with a two-step exposure button is desirable.[47] The first step warms the x-ray tube filament; the second step is when the exposure is made. The two-step exposure button prolongs the x-ray tube life.

Because exposure time (in seconds) multiplied by the milliamperage equals milliamperage-seconds (mAs), radiation exposure is directly related to milliamperage-seconds.

$$0.1 \text{ second} \times 10 \text{ mA} = 1 \text{ mAs}$$
$$0.1 \text{ second} \times 15 \text{ mA} = 1.5 \text{ mAs}$$
$$0.2 \text{ second} \times 10 \text{ mA} = 2 \text{ mAs}$$

Kilovoltage determines the energy of x-rays being produced. Kilovoltage potential should range from 70 to 90 for equine limb radiographs on mature horses when a portable x-ray machine is used. A 10% increase or decrease in kilovoltage potential effectively doubles or halves the radiation exposure.

The focal spot-film distance (FFD) is the distance from the x-ray tube focal spot to the x-ray film. The focal spot location is usually marked on the outside tube housing; if not, the approximate center of the tube housing can be used for its location. A constant FFD is necessary to minimize improper exposures, since the intensity of x-rays that expose the film is inversely proportional to the square of the FFD. A small difference in the FFD can, therefore, dramatically change the exposure on the x-ray film. For example, if the FFD were changed from 36 to 40 inches, the exposure from the x-ray machine would have to be increased by 23% to maintain a constant film exposure. In other words, if 10 mAs provided a good exposure at an FFD of 36 inches, 12.3 mAs would be required at 40 inches.

Some method of measuring the FFD before each exposure should be employed (Figs. 4.2 and 4.3). Such things as a lightweight metal bar or a small rope can be used for fast FFD measurement. More elaborate measuring devices with converging light beams at the correctly set FFD may also be used. The FFD for equine limb radiography should be between 36 and 40 inches (85 and 100 cm) and no less than 24 inches (60 cm). When the FFD is less than 24 inches, the object is magnified and spatial resolution is reduced. FFDs greater than 40 inches may be used if exposure times are not excessively long.

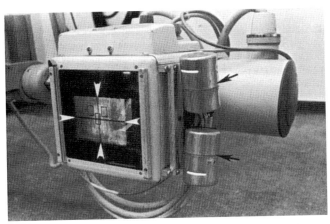

Figure 4.2 Adjustable light-beam collimator. The primary beam is limited by adjustable leaves in the collimator. A light source within the collimator defines the limits of the primary beam (white arrows). A double light source within the canisters on the side of the collimator provides a converging double line on the cassette to position the x-ray tube at the correct FFD (black arrows).

Collimation is the process of limiting or restricting the primary x-ray beam to the size of the x-ray cassette being used. Collimating the primary beam is a safety practice that must be monitored for each exposure and must be reset if the cassette size changes. Limiting the size of the primary x-ray beam is a major factor in reducing scatter radiation, which keeps radiation exposure to personnel as low as possible.[70] Fixed cylinders or cones and adjustable light-beam collimators are available (Fig. 4.2). The disadvantage of fixed primary beam restrictors is that they do not conform to different cassette sizes. Adjustable light-beam collimation is recommended for equine radiography. Adjustable collimators can be affixed to most x-ray machines. They come with an internal light source, preferably 40 W or greater,[47] so the limits of the primary x-ray beam are projected on the x-ray cassette as visible light.

The type of x-ray machine best suited for equine practice depends on the type of practice: out-of-hospital vs. in-hospital. The features of the x-ray machine must be matched to fit different practice situations. Some compromises or trade-offs have to be made, e.g., less milliamperage or kilovoltage potential for more portability. An ideal x-ray machine for equine radiography has the following features: 1) easily and quietly movable, with a tube head that can extend to the floor or ground surface; 2) adjustable milliamperage and kilovoltage potential settings; 3) an electronic, two-step timer capable of accu-

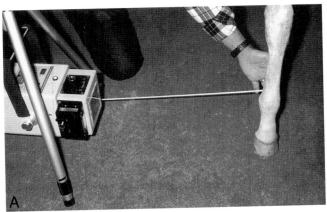

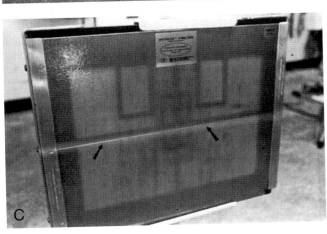

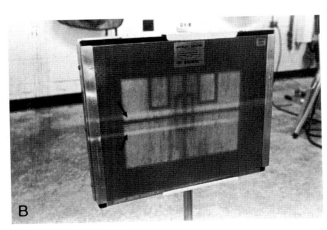

Figure 4.3 Methods of measuring FFD. A. Some portable x-ray machines come with a built-in measuring tape. B and C. Other machines use a converging light-bar system. When the cassette is not at the preset FFD, a double light bar, projected from the canisters (see Fig. 4.2), is present (B, arrows). When the cassette is at the preset FFD, a single light bar is seen (C, arrows).

rate exposure times of 0.1 second or faster; 4) some form of tube head support so that handholding the x-ray tube during the exposure is not necessary; 5) line voltage compensator and compensation meter; 6) primary x-ray beam restrictor (the preferred system is an adjustable light-beam collimator); and 7) free of radiation or electrical hazards.

Types of x-ray machines available for equine radiography are portable, mobile, and fixed (ceiling suspended) (Fig. 4.4). These machines differ in size and capacity from small portable 15-mA machines to large fixed 800-mA machines.

Portable x-ray machines are best suited for out-of-hospital locations. They are lightweight (30 to 55 lb) and can be easily stored for transport. Even though portable machines are lightweight and easily moved, for radiation safety purposes they should be used with a stand or other mechanical support system. Impediments for using x-ray tube stands include cost, incompatibility with the machine, and lack of field versatility. A two-legged stand

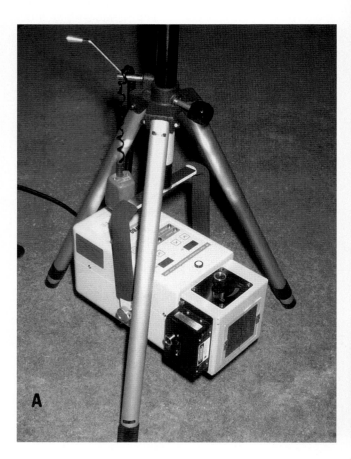

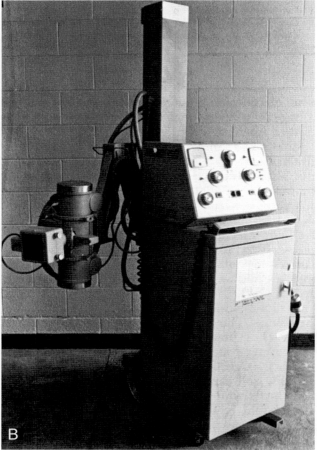

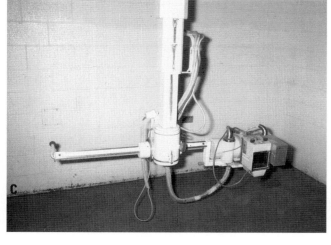

Figure 4.4 Types of x-ray machines used in equine radiography. A. Portable 30-mA, 90-kVp machine on a tripod stand. B. Mobile 200-mA machine. C. Fixed or ceiling-suspended 1000-mA machine with a 3-m telescoping crane that extends to the floor. The exposure capabilities and mobility of each type of x-ray machine determines how and where they may be most effectively used.

system is the most adaptable to the variety of conditions encountered in the field.[25] The maximum milliamperage on portable x-ray machines is between 10 and 40 mA, and the kilovoltage potential varies between 50 and 100 kVp. Milliamperage and kilovoltage potential settings on portable x-ray machines are usually interdependent, e.g., 10 mA at 80 kVp and 20 mA at 60 kVp. Desirable control settings on a portable x-ray machine are multiple kilovoltage potential settings and multiple time settings. Time setting increments should be 50% or less below 0.5 second.[47]

High-frequency transformers that reduce the exposure time are available for portable x-ray machines. They are equivalent to a three-phase, 12-pulse x-ray generator and provide a 40 to 50% increase in exposure compared with a full-wave rectified machine. The practical application is to reduce the exposure time and still obtain an adequate exposure for a diagnostic radiograph. A line voltage compensator is also desirable for portable x-ray machines. It is especially important in farm situations, where the line voltage may fluctuate with the simultaneous use of other electrical equipment and can compensate for a line voltage drop when a long electrical extension cord is used.

Mobile x-ray machines are best suited for in-hospital radiography. They can be moved easily and quietly, although they are not as easily moved as portable machines. Mobile x-ray machines generally have a milliamperage range between 100 and 200 mA. The x-ray tube should be movable in the vertical plane to extend to the floor. Sometimes, mechanical modifications must be made to provide the necessary degree of x-ray tube travel. Timers on mobile x-ray machines usually have exposure times as fast as 1/60th or 1/120th of a second.

Fixed x-ray machines are usually suspended from the ceiling. They are limited to use within a single room. These machines can be coupled with large transformer systems that are capable of providing high milliamperage (800 to 1000 mA). Ceiling-suspended tubes are easily movable and can be locked into position by magnetic locks while the x-ray exposure is made. The tube should be capable of extending to the floor. X-ray machines with high milliamperage capability have fast exposure times, eliminating most motion artifacts when radiographing equine limbs.

Accessory X-Ray Equipment

Accessory x-ray equipment for equine limb examinations have special requirements. Good-quality, well-maintained accessory equipment is necessary to ensure that quality radiographic examinations are performed safely. Accessory equipment consists of x-ray film, x-ray cassettes, intensifying screens, grids, markers and film-marking systems, cassette holders, positioning aids, and x-ray viewing devices. Most accessory equipment is available commercially, but because of the unique requirements of equine radiology, some equipment—such as cassette holders and positioning aids—may have to be manufactured locally.

Film

Both screen and nonscreen x-ray film are available. Nonscreen film is used with a cardboard holder or comes individually wrapped in a protective paper envelope. Nonscreen film has excellent spatial resolution and good exposure latitude but requires high exposure settings to obtain a diagnostic radiograph; therefore, it is not recommended for equine radiography. Such high exposures cause unnecessary radiation exposure to personnel and can increase the probability of motion artifacts.

Single-emulsion film with a single fine or detail-intensifying screen may be used to maintain excellent spatial resolution but decrease the exposure necessary with nonscreen film. The exposure needed with single-emulsion film and a single detail screen is still considerably more than that needed with double-emulsion film and two intensifying screens. With the single-emulsion, single intensifying screen system, the trade-off is higher exposure for better spatial resolution.

Double-emulsion film is used with two x-ray intensifying screens. The x-ray exposure necessary to obtain diagnostic radiographs is significantly lower with this system than with a nonscreen film or a single-emulsion, single intensifying screen system. Several different brands and types of films are available commercially. In general, wide-latitude film is most desirable for radiography of equine extremities. This film allows for greater variation in x-ray machine exposure to obtain an acceptable film and has a wider film contrast latitude than other film has. The wider film contrast latitude provides better visualization of soft tissue structures and bone on the same film.

Cassettes

Cassettes used for equine radiography should be strong and durable. The hinges and latches should be sturdy and easily movable, and the foam or felt backing should seal the cassette to prevent light leaks that would cause light fog on the film.

Cassette sizes most convenient for equine limb examinations are 8 by 10 inches (20 by 25 cm), 11 by 14 inches (27.5 by 35 cm), and 7 by 17 inches (17.5 by 42.5 cm). The 8- by 10-inch cassettes are sufficient for most examinations. The 11- by 14-inch cassettes are most convenient for tarsal, stifle, elbow, and shoulder examinations; and the 7- by 17-inch cassettes work well for metacarpal and metatarsal studies and for evaluating angular limb deformities in young animals.

The useful life of cassettes is prolonged with proper care. Rough handling of cassettes should be avoided when possible. The outside surface should be kept free of blood, water, or other staining materials. When working in extremely dusty or dirty areas, it may help to enclose the cassette in a small plastic bag to prevent the accumulation of dust, dirt, and debris from entering the cassette when opened.

Intensifying Screens

Poor technical quality radiographs are frequently the result of old or poor-quality intensifying screens. An understanding of intensifying screens is therefore important to improve quality. The basic function of intensifying screens is to convert x-ray energy into a visible light pattern that contains the same information as the original x-ray beam. In the conversion process, the latent image is intensified, which makes possible a properly exposed film with 10 to 40 times less x-ray exposure than would be necessary if intensifying screens were not used.

Image quality is adversely affected when screens are damaged, old, or not in uniform contact with the x-ray film. Intensifying screens should be evaluated by visually inspecting the screens, determining the screen's exposure efficiency, and checking the film-screen contact. The screen surface should be free of scratches, marks, and discoloration. This can be determined by visually inspecting the screens and making a trial exposure. The exposure consistency from cassette to cassette should be determined by using an aluminum step wedge. A consistent exposure should be made on each cassette, with the aluminum step wedge placed on the front cassette surface (Fig. 4.5). The number of steps visualized on each film should not vary by more than one. Determining exposure consistency is particularly important when buying used screens, as screens will lose efficiency with age. Screens with different exposure efficiencies result in variable film densities from the same x-ray exposure settings.

Film-screen contact should be evaluated by making an exposure with a fine wire mesh screen or paper clips placed on the front surface of the cassette (Fig. 4.6). Areas with poor spatial resolution (blurry) on the exposed film indicate poor film-screen contact.

Maintenance of intensifying screens is important for prolonging screen life. A regular cleaning schedule should be established, and a commercial screen-cleaning solution or distilled water should be used. Other types of cleaning solutions and nondistilled water may chemically degrade or otherwise ruin the screen.

To quickly identify dirty screens, number the screens on their edge and place the same number on the outside of the cassette. Unexposed spots on the film that are caused by foreign material on the screen can be discovered and immediately removed from the cassette if the numbering identification system is used. Properly maintained screens will last longer and provide better-quality radiographs than will unmaintained screens.

Although calcium tungstate screens have been used, rare earth screens are recommended for equine radiography. Several brands with different speed combinations are available (Table 4.1). Rare earth screens are faster—some as much as 12 times faster—than calcium tungstate screens with comparable spatial resolution. The following are some advantages of rare earth intensifying screens:[24]

- Exposure to personnel can be decreased 40 to 60%, depending on the screen speed used.
- Diagnostic capabilities of low-milliamperage x-ray machines can be increased (e.g., a 30-mA machine may have the potential of a 60- to 80-mA machine). This is particularly important in equine radiography, since low-milliamperage, portable x-ray machines are used extensively.
- Workload on x-ray generators and tubes can be reduced, which prolongs the life of the x-ray tube and machine and thus reduces costs.
- Exposure time can be decreased or shortened, which reduces motion artifacts that occur frequently in equine radiography.

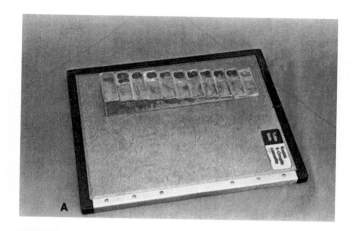

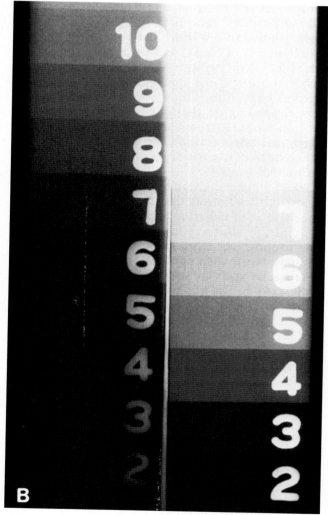

Figure 4.5 Testing x-ray screen efficiency. A. An aluminum step wedge is placed on the front of the cassette and radiographed to check consistency between x-ray screens. B. Two step-wedge radiographs made with the same x-ray exposure factors. The difference in the number of steps visualized indicates a difference in screen speed (efficiency). The difference in efficiency between these two screens means that the exposure factors on the x-ray machine need to be adjusted to obtain comparable radiographic studies.

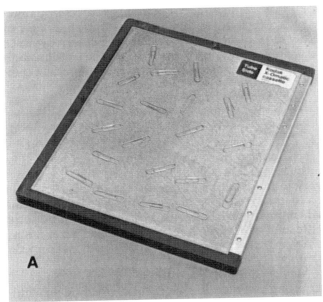

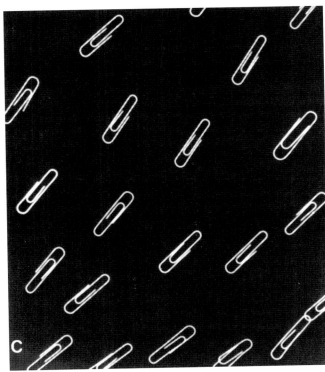

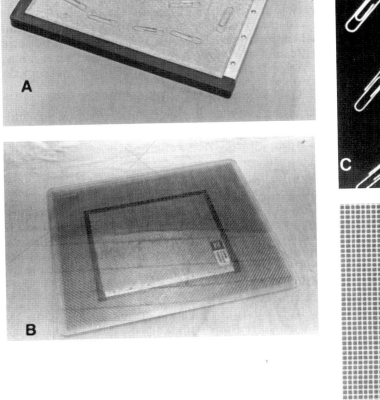

Figure 4.6   Two methods for determining film-screen contact. A. Paper clips placed on the front surface of an x-ray cassette. B. Wire mesh screen placed over the front surface of an x-ray cassette. C and D. Radiographs of paper clips (C) or wire mesh (D) on the front surface of an x-ray cassette. The borders of the paper clips and the wire mesh screen are well defined throughout the radiographs, indicating good film-screen contact.

Table 4.1 RARE EARTH INTENSIFYING SCREEN AND FILM COMBINATIONS

Screen (Manufacturer)	Film	Relative Speed
Trimax (3M)		
2	XDA	100–125
6/12	XDA	400
6/12	XM	800
12	XDA	600
12	XM	1200
Lanex (Kodak)		
Fine	T-Mat L	75–100
Regular	Ortho L	400
Regular	Ortho H	800
Fast	T-Mat L	600
Quanta (DuPont)		
Detail	Cornex 4L	100
Fast detail	Cornex 4L	400
III	Cornex 4L	800

- A smaller focal spot, which increases spatial resolution, can be used with machines that have more than one focal spot.
- Different speed screens are available, providing examination flexibility.

The screen speed can be matched with the power potential of the x-ray machine being used and the part being examined. Factors to consider when purchasing intensifying screens are cost, screen speed, image quality,[55] examination area, type (power) of x-ray machine, and radiation safety for personnel. Screen speed and spatial resolution have an inverse relationship, i.e., fast screens have decreased spatial resolution, whereas slow screens have increased spatial resolution. Fast screens require less exposure from the x-ray machine for a properly exposed film, but the film may appear grainy because of quantum mottle. The combination of film and screen determines the relative system speed, i.e., the film-screen speed.

When matched correctly, rare earth screen and film combinations provide tremendous advantages for the examination of equine extremities (Table 4.1). With portable x-ray machines, a medium-speed combination (400 to 600) is recommended for routine examination of the extremities distal to the antebrachial carpal and the tarsocural joints. A slow-speed combination (100) may be used for the occasional view that requires higher spatial resolution, e.g., navicular bone or distal phalanx. A high-speed combination (800) may be used for examinations proximal to the antebrachial carpal and the tarsocural joints. With mobile or fixed x-ray machines, a slow-speed combination (100) may be used for examination of the extremities distal to the antebrachial carpal and tarsocural joints, and medium-speed combinations (400 to 600) may be used proximal to these joints.

Grids

A radiographic grid is a thin wafer consisting of lead foil strips separated by x-ray-transparent spacers. Grids differ by grid ratio, lines per inch, and pattern. Grid ratio is the height of the lead foil strips relative to the width between strips and may vary from 5:1 to 16:1. Lines per inch is the number of lead foil strips per inch. The more lines per inch, the less apparent the lines are on the exposed x-ray film. Grid patterns differ depending on the longitudinal orientation of the lead strips and can be linear, linear focused, and cross-hatched. The clinician must consider these variables when purchasing a grid for use in equine radiography.

Grids are generally used to decrease the amount of scattered radiation that exposes the x-ray film. Since scattered radiation exposes film from several directions, it has the effect of decreasing details and "fogging" the film. A fogged film has a gray or flat appearance and little contrast.

Stationary grids are the most common grids used in equine radiography (Fig. 4.7). The grid may be placed over the front of the cassette or may be fixed permanently in the cassette holder or cassette. Examination of areas more than 12 cm thick is best performed with a grid; this usually includes the limbs proximal to the carpus and tarsus. A grid is desirable for the caudocranial view of the stifle but may not be necessary for the lateromedial view. A grid may also be helpful for foot examinations when the x-ray cassette is positioned under the foot and in a cassette tunnel that has a thick protecting cover between the horse's foot and x-ray cassette.

A nonfocused linear grid with a 6:1 ratio and more than 100 lines per inch is adequate for equine limb examinations. A smaller ratio and/or fewer lines per inch may be used with less powerful x-ray machines to facilitate a decrease in exposure time.

The advantages of using a grid are increased film detail and contrast, which improve the diagnostic quality of the film. The disadvantages of a grid are cost, increased radiation exposure to personnel, and the need for more precise centering of the x-ray beam and positioning of the grid to prevent grid cutoff. Increased radiation exposure is particularly important in equine radiography for which low-output x-ray machines are extensively used. The grid must be perpendicular to the x-ray beam; and if a focused grid is used, the center of the x-ray beam must be aligned with the center of the grid. Improper positioning results in grid cutoff and a nondiagnostic radiograph.

Film Markers and Marking Systems

Adequate, legible film marking is necessary but often overlooked in equine radiography. Proper identification procedures are necessary for follow-up comparative examinations and for accurately documenting when, where, what, and by whom the examination was performed. Such documentation on the film in a proper, permanent fashion may also be needed for medical-legal purposes.

Radiographs should be identified with the veterinarian's name and/or hospital or the place where the radiograph was made, the date, and the animal's name or number. The view and anatomic part examined should also be recorded at the time the film is exposed.

Acceptable methods of film labeling include lead-impregnated tape, lead letters and/or numbers, and a photoflash marking system (Fig. 4.8). Adhesive tape and coins are not acceptable methods of marking radiographs.

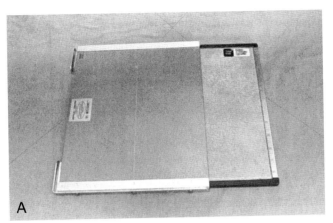

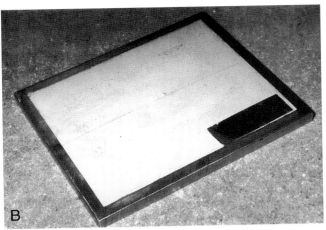

Figure 4.7 A. Stationary grid that slides over the top of the cassette for examination of thick areas, such as the stifle, shoulder, elbow, and pelvis. B. Grid cassette. The grid is built into the front surface of the cassette and is not visible or removable.

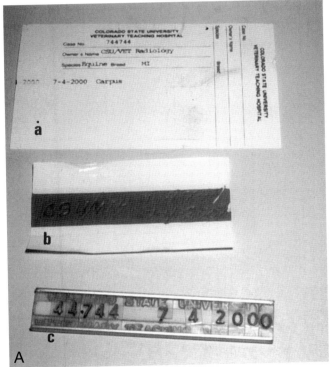

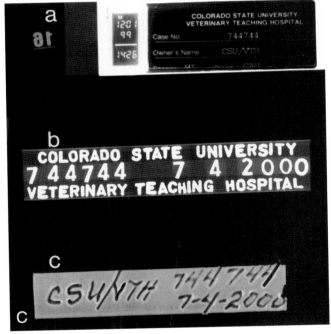

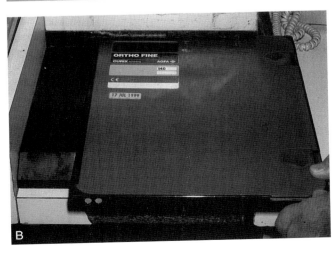

Figure 4.8 A. Labeling systems for film and patient identification, including a card for a photoflash marking system (a), lead tape (b), and lead letters (c). B. Photoflash film identification marker system. C. Radiographs of photoflash marker (a), lead letters (b), and lead tape (c).

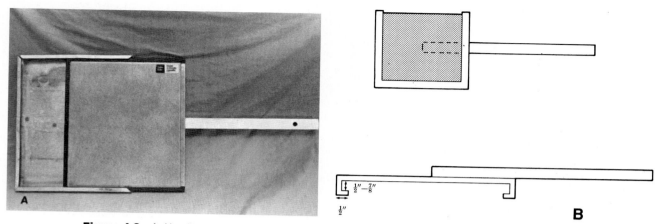

Figure 4.9 A. Handle cassette holder with x-ray cassette partially inserted into it. B. Line diagram and dimensions of a handle cassette holder.

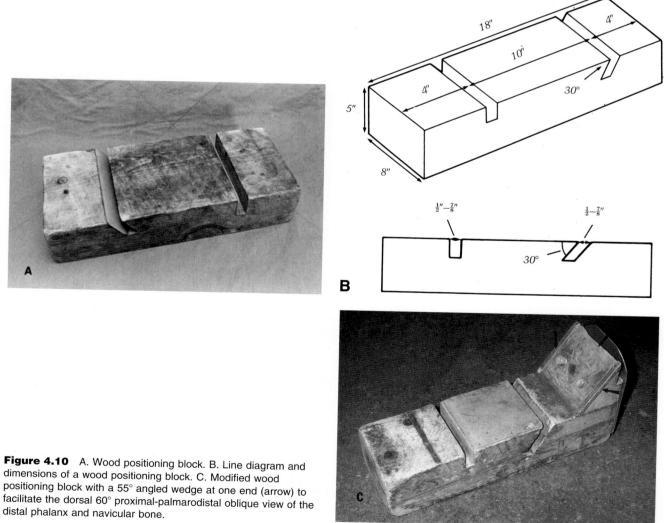

Figure 4.10 A. Wood positioning block. B. Line diagram and dimensions of a wood positioning block. C. Modified wood positioning block with a 55° angled wedge at one end (arrow) to facilitate the dorsal 60° proximal-palmarodistal oblique view of the distal phalanx and navicular bone.

A permanent aluminum plate containing the veterinarian's name and other information can be used with lead-impregnated tape and lead letters. These plates are placed on the front of the cassette before the radiograph is made and provide legible figures on the radiograph. Without the aluminum plate, the figures on the lead-impregnated tape may not be legible.

The photoflash marking system requires a permanent lead blocker impregnated in the corner of the x-ray cassette. This area is exposed with identification information that is written or typed on a card placed in the photoflash machine.

The part examined and the x-ray view used should also be labeled with lead letters or other available lead markers.[50] The part examined should be labeled left (L) or right (R) for all examinations and labeled fore or hind distal to the carpus and tarsus. Regardless of the system used, the essential information must be on the x-ray film in clear legible form.

Cassette Holders and Positioning Aids

Cassette holders and positioning blocks are necessary for radiation safety purposes and to facilitate consistent views or projections of an examined part. Cassette holders and blocks enable personnel who hold the cassette to position their hands away from the primary x-ray beam, even though they are wearing lead-impregnated gloves. For equine limb examinations, a handled cassette holder, a cassette holder (tunnel) for weight-bearing foot studies, and a positioning block are necessary.

A handled cassette holder for limb examinations may be made from aluminum or wood (Fig. 4.9). One wood block with two grooves in the top can be used for phalangeal and navicular examinations (Fig. 4.10). A 55° wedge may be added to one end of the block to accommodate an upright foot examination, and a metal strip may be recessed into the flat surface to mark the plane of the sole (Fig. 4.10C). A cassette holder (tunnel) can be used for weight-bearing studies of the feet and navicular bone (Fig. 4.11). The cassette holder protects the cassette from damage caused by direct weight bearing by the horse. Lead may be added to the underside of the holder to prevent back-scattered radiation from fogging the film (Fig. 4.11C). Cassette holders that have thick (more than 0.25-inch) Plexiglas fronts may produce excess scatter radiation and, therefore, require a grid to obtain an acceptable radiograph of the navicular bone.

These positioning aids allow routine examinations of the limb to be performed in a safe, consistent manner.

Viewing Devices

The entire x-ray examination will have been done in vain if the x-ray film cannot be adequately viewed or is read with poor illumination. Good-quality x-ray viewers and a bright light are necessary equipment. They should be placed in an area where external light can be subdued. Each properly exposed film should be inspected with a bright light (Fig. 4.12), which may reveal soft tissue structures and subtle bone changes not apparent with regular x-ray viewers.

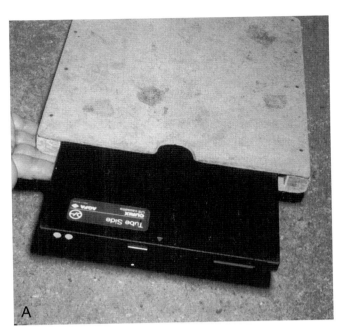

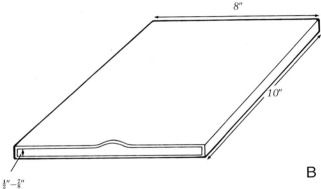

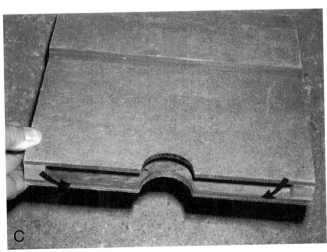

Figure 4.11 A. Weight-bearing cassette holder with the cassette partially inserted into the holder. B. Line diagram and dimensions of a weight-bearing cassette holder. C. A 1-mm-thick piece of lead can be added to the bottom of the cassette holder (arrows) to stop radiation backscatter from the ground to the x-ray film. Radiation backscatter will produce background film fog and decrease the image quality.

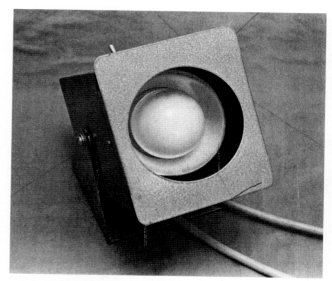

Figure 4.12 Bright light for viewing high-exposure (dark) areas on an x-ray film.

Darkroom Equipment

Basic darkroom equipment, film processing, and developing and fixing solution properties have been covered elsewhere and are not discussed in detail here.[36]

Poor-quality radiographs are frequently the result of inconsistent darkroom techniques and procedures. Inconsistency results from not using necessary darkroom equipment and procedures and from not following a system of solution management. The most often neglected darkroom equipment includes good-quality processing tanks that have circulating water bath capability with a mixing valve for water temperature control, a timer, and a thermometer (Fig. 4.13). If used properly, these three pieces of equipment will control the time and temperature of the film processing (Table 4.2).[67] The film manufacturer should be consulted for specific time and temperature recommendations for the film being used.

In addition to the darkroom equipment listed above, a system of solution management should be used. Solution management ensures active developing and fixing solutions and decreases the number of poorly developed and fixed radiographs. Several management systems exist.

The replenishing method is a simple system that works well:

1. Place the films directly into the water bath from the developing and fixing solutions. Do not allow the solutions to drip from the film back into the developing or fixing solutions.
2. When the level of solution in a tank drops, add developing or fixing replenishment solution to the appropriate tank to bring the solution to the original level.
3. Replace the solutions and clean the tanks at approximately 3-month intervals. The specific interval depends on the number of films processed.

Another system is the comparison film strip method:

1. Develop a film strip when the solutions are first placed in the tanks.

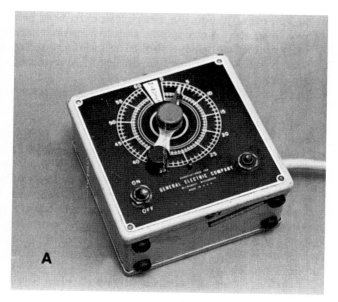

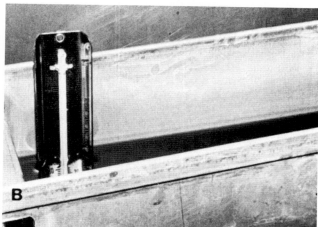

Figure 4.13 Timer (A) and thermometer (B) are necessary for establishing accurate settings for proper x-ray film processing.

Table 4.2 TYPICAL TIME AND TEMPERATURE SETTINGS FOR X-RAY FILM PROCESSING[a]

Temperature °F (°C)	Developing Time (Minutes)
60 (15.5)	8.5
65 (18.5)	6.0
68 (20.0)	5.0
70 (21.0)	4.5
75 (24.0)	3.5

[a] Consult the film manufacturer for specific recommendations.

2. At regular intervals, expose and process a test strip in exactly the same manner as the original film strip.
3. Compare the test strip to the original strip. When the test strip is noticeably lighter than the original strip, change the solutions.

Automatic film processors are available and recommended when economically feasible. They add consis-

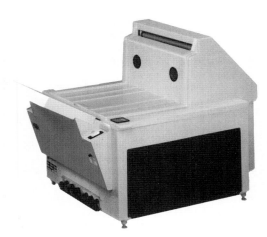

Figure 4.14 Countertop automatic film processor.

tency to film processing, increase film quality, and decrease the time spent in processing film. Because of the convenience, speed, and quality of films obtained, the number of radiographic examinations performed in a practice usually increases. Compare the convenience, purchase price, and maintenance and operation costs of an automatic processor to those of processing film manually before deciding to buy an automatic processor.

Countertop film processors are also available (Fig. 4.14). These require little or no structural building modifications for installation and need only a cold water outlet and a 110-volt electrical connection. They are less expensive than large stationary models. Most countertop models accept all sizes of film and require only a slightly longer time for film processing. Automatic film processors are recommended when the caseload and circumstances justify their use.

RADIATION SAFETY

Radiation safety has become more important in equine practice as the use of radiology has increased. Safe radiation procedures are often not followed because of insufficient knowledge of biologic radiation effects, lack of awareness of radiation safety principles, inadequate radiation safety equipment, and/or neglect of radiation safety practices because these practices require too much time and effort. None of these reasons justifies the unsafe use of radiation.

Veterinarians in equine practice may receive low doses of radiation over long periods of time. Because the clinician's extremities (hands, eyes, and feet) are the most common body parts to be exposed to radiation, they are subject to chronic radiation injury. Chronic radiation injury may be manifest as skin ridge flattening on fingertips, ridging of fingernails, or, in severe cases, skin carcinomas. Such changes may result from not routinely following safe radiation procedures.

The general principles of radiation safety are 1) keeping personnel as far away from the radiation source (x-ray tube) as possible, 2) using protective barriers, 3) re-

ducing x-ray exposure factors, and 4) using a radiation-monitoring system.

Keeping personnel as far away from the x-ray source as possible can be accomplished by having nonessential personnel leave the immediate area, using cassette holders and positioning blocks, providing tranquilization or general anesthesia when needed,[1] using an x-ray tube stand or support, and having a 1- to 2-meter-long cord connected to the exposure button. No part of the body should be exposed to the primary x-ray beam.

Protective barriers should always be used. Walls and lead screens are good protective barriers to use when practical. Adequate wall thickness in a new or remodeled facility should be determined by consulting with a health physicist. The personnel subject to the greatest exposure when performing equine examinations are those holding the horse's limb or cassette holder and those holding the halter.[1] Therefore, if personnel must be near the animal when the x-ray examination is performed, they should wear lead aprons and gloves. Periodically aprons and gloves should be radiographed to check for cracks and holes in the lead-impregnated lining (Fig. 4.15).

Fast film-screen combinations and a decreased FFD can be used to reduce x-ray exposure factors. As mentioned, for good-quality films, the FFD should not be less than 24 inches and preferably not less than 36 inches.

A radiation-monitoring system should be used by all radiology personnel. These systems not only provide safety guidance but also protect against possible legal

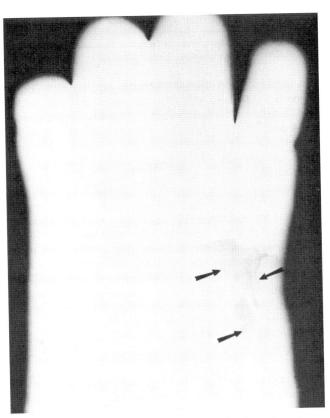

Figure 4.15 Radiograph of a lead glove, showing a lucent area (arrows) that represents a defect or hole in the lead lining.

implications. Film-badge monitoring systems and service can be purchased from commercial sources.

Equipment necessary for safely operating an x-ray machine includes cassette holders, lead aprons and gloves, aluminum filters, and an adjustable light-beam collimator. Cassette holders eliminate the need to hand-hold cassettes, increasing the distance between hands and the x-ray beam. The cassette holder should be durable and lightweight. As discussed, several designs for cassette holders are available (Figs. 4.9 to 4.11).[52]

Lead aprons and gloves should be worn by everyone assisting with the x-ray examination. Protective gear should have at least 0.5-mm lead equivalent. Lead aprons and gloves provide adequate protection from secondary and scattered radiation but not from primary radiation. The life of lead aprons and gloves can be prolonged by hanging them up when they are not in use. This prevents cracks or holes forming from improper care (Fig. 4.15).

Primary beam filtration should be at least 2.5-mm aluminum. The filtration should be added at the x-ray tube port. Filtration makes the x-ray beam more energetic (hardens) and reduces the amount of less energetic (soft) radiation. This has the effect of decreasing the amount of scattered radiation to surrounding personnel.

An x-ray beam-limiting device or collimator (Fig. 4.2) is one of the most important, yet overlooked, pieces of radiation safety equipment. The size of the primary x-ray beam is a major factor in determining radiation dose to the hands.[70] Several beam-limiting devices are available. Fixed-size cones and cylinders and adjustable light-beam collimators limit the primary x-ray beam. Adjustable light-beam collimators have the advantage of limiting the primary x-ray beam to the exact cassette size, regardless of the FFD. The light also assists alignment of the primary x-ray beam with the cassette. Every x-ray machine should have a primary beam-limiting device. An adjustable light-beam collimator is highly recommended.

In summary, the following safety measures should be observed[52,65,70]:

- Never handhold the x-ray cassette during an exposure. Cassette holders or general anesthesia should be used so that cassettes do not have to be handheld.
- All personnel not needed for assistance with the x-ray examination should leave the immediate area.
- Lead gloves and aprons should be worn by all individuals assisting with the x-ray examination.
- A primary x-ray beam-restricting device should be used, preferably an adjustable light-beam collimator.
- Primary beam filtration equivalent to 2.5-mm aluminum should be used.
- Rotate personnel responsible for holding the cassette, if possible; avoid routinely using the same person for this job.
- Do not allow anyone under 18 years of age or anyone who is pregnant to assist with an x-ray examination.
- Appropriate-speed rare earth screens are recommended.
- Consistent x-ray exposures and darkroom techniques should be used. Repeat exposures require unnecessary radiation exposure to personnel.
- A radiation-monitoring system should be used.

The veterinarian in charge is responsible for the radiation safety practices used by his or her employees. Providing necessary radiation safety equipment and following these rules should keep exposure levels below the limits recommended by the National Council on Radiation Protection.[38]

TECHNIQUE CHARTS

A technique chart should be formulated for each x-ray machine, because no two machines have exactly the same exposure characteristics (Fig. 4.16). A technique chart ensures consistent exposure factors from each x-ray machine's settings, decreasing the number of repeat radiographs, thus reducing radiation exposure to personnel and the wasting of x-ray film.

Several variables should be kept constant when a technique chart is being formulated: the FFD, film-processing conditions, line voltage, type of intensifying screen, type of x-ray film, type of collimation, and the amount of primary beam filtration. If these variables are changed, indicated settings from the chart may no longer be valid.

The following general rules and principles should be observed when a technique chart for equine limb examinations is being formulated: 1) the exposure times should be as fast as possible to limit motion artifacts on the radiograph, and 2) the kilovoltage potential range should be between 70 and 90 kVp for most examinations but may be higher when mobile or fixed x-ray machines are used.

Manipulation of exposure factors on the x-ray machine is often necessary when a technique chart is being formulated and used. To double or halve the x-ray exposure by changing the milliamperage-seconds, simply double or halve either the milliamperage or time. To double or halve the x-ray exposure by changing the kilovoltage potential, simply add or subtract approximately 10% from the original kilovoltage potential.

Equivalent Exposures

80 kVp	15 mA	0.1 second	1.5 mAs
90 kVp	15 mA	0.05 second	0.75 mAs
70 kVp	30 mA	0.1 second	3.0 mAs
70 kVp	15 mA	0.2 second	3.0 mAs

A technique chart may be formulated with or without a grid. A grid is usually not used and not necessary in most extremity examinations because of insufficient part thickness. If a grid is used, exposure factors must be increased; the amount of increase depends on the grid type, grid ratio, and lines per inch.

A trial exposure should be made on each part to find the most suitable exposure. For example, for the fetlock (metacarpophalangeal joint), foot (distal phalanges), metacarpus, and metatarsus, a baseline exposure with a FFD of 30 inches (75 cm) and exposure settings of 2.0 mAs and 70 kVp with a 400-speed rare earth film-screen combination and no grid may be used. The baseline exposure should be slightly higher for tarsal and carpal studies and decreased by half for dorsopalmar-plantar studies of the distal phalanx.

HF100 EQUINE TECHNIQUE CHART*

X-ray Unit: MinXray, Inc. **Model *HF100***
Screen/Film Combination: Sterling Ultravision Rapid Screens/Ultravision L Film/400 Speed Combination
Focal Film Distance (FFD): As Specified (Adjust Exposure Time If Using Different FFD)

	Thk, cm	FFD, in	kV	mA	Time, sec	mAs
P3						
Lateral	16	40	68	20.0	0.05	1.0
D65P-PD view	11	40	62	20.0	0.05	1.0
DP	11	40	70	20.0	0.05	1.0
Navicular						
Lateral	11	40	68	20.0	0.05	1.0
D65P-PD (cone)	11	40	68	20.0	0.07	1.4
Flexor	N/A	16	65	20.0	0.04	0.8
Fetlock						
Lateral	11	40	68	20.0	0.05	1.0
Oblique	8	40	70	20.0	0.05	1.0
D15P-PD	9	40	72	20.0	0.05	1.0
Carpus						
Lateral	10	40	72	20.0	0.05	1.0
Oblique	9	40	74	20.0	0.05	1.0
DP	12	40	78	20.0	0.04	0.8
Skyline	N/A	31	74	20.0	0.05	1.0
Tarsus						
Lateral	10	40	72	20.0	0.05	1.0
Oblique	10	40	72	20.0	0.05	1.0
DP	13	40	92	20.0	0.04	0.8
Stifle						
Lateral	24	40	78	20.0	0.08	1.6
CC	26	40	96	20.0	0.10	2.0
Skull						
Lateral (Nasal)	16	40	80	20.0	0.08	1.6
Lateral (Teeth)	16	40	80	20.0	0.12	2.4
Lateral (Guttural Pouch)	16	40	88	20.0	0.13	2.6

* These are recommended starting techniques. Final results depend upon many factors. Please note examples of adjustments that follow.

Adjustments in kV for Variations in Thickness:

40-80 kV - Add or subtract 2kV for each 1cm increase or decrease in thickness
80-100kV - Add or subtract 3kV for each 1cm increase or decrease in thickness

Adjustments in Time for Variations in Film Density:

If films are too dark (overexposed), decrease time.
If films are too light (underexposed), increase time.

Developed At:

THE UNIVERSITY OF TENNESSEE
COLLEGE OF VETERINARY MEDICINE
KNOXVILLE, TN

UT

Radiology Section

Figure 4.16 Technique chart for equine examinations. (Reprinted with permission from The University of Tennessee College of Veterinary Medicine, Knoxville, TN.)

Three trial exposures should be made on each part: the baseline exposure, an exposure half the baseline, and an exposure twice the baseline. If all three exposures are too light (underexposed) or too dark (overexposed), the baseline exposure should be adjusted to compensate and the three exposures should be repeated. A good-quality film should eventually be made with one trial film darker and one trial film lighter. A good-quality film should show soft tissue as well as bone without the use of a bright light, and bone trabeculae should be identifiable. Once a good exposure is made for a given part, it should be recorded on the technique chart. With additional work, the chart can be refined to include more-specific exposure information for each view (Table 4.3).

The technique chart should be established for an average-sized horse. For smaller and larger horses, the expo-

sure factors will have to be adjusted to produce acceptable radiographs.

CONTRAST EXAMINATIONS

A contrast radiographic examination consists of using contrast material to better define suspicious lesions detected clinically or radiographically but not distinctly seen on survey radiographs. Triiodinated contrast material is most useful for contrast examinations in lame horses. Positive-contrast agents are commercially available in an injectable form (Table 4.4). The use of negative-contrast agents (gas) has been reported[2] but has not found wide, routine acceptance. Although the number and kinds of contrast examinations for equine lameness

Table 4.3 EXAMPLE TECHNIQUE CHART FOR CARPUS

Trial exposures
  Good trial exposure: 70 kVp, 1.5 mAs
  More film contrast (black and white): 60 kVp, 3.0 mAs
  Less film contrast (more gray shades): 80 kVp, 0.75 mAs
Refinements per view[a]
  Dorsopalmar (DPa): 70 kVp, 1.5 mAs
  Dorsolateral-palmaromedial oblique (D45L-PaMO): 70 kVp, 1.5 mAs
  Dorsomedial-palmarolateral oblique (D45M-PaMO): 70 kVp, 1.5 mAs
  Lateromedial (LM): 75 kVp, 1.5 mAs
  Flexed lateromedial (flexed LM): 75 kVp, 1.5 mAs

[a] If more or less film contrast is desired, adjust the kilovoltage potential and milliamperage-seconds.

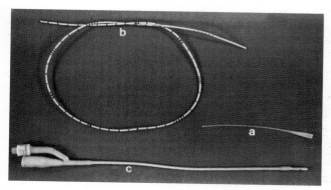

Figure 4.17 Catheters for draining tract injections. a, Tom-Cat Catheter (Sherwood Medical, St. Louis, MO); b, male uretheral catheter; c, Foley catheter. The Foley catheter has an inflatable cuff for internal occlusion of the draining tract, which prevents reflux of contrast material onto the external surface.

Table 4.4 ORGANIC IODIDE CONTRAST MATERIAL

Brand Name	Generic Name	Manufacturer
Hypaque sodium 20%	20% Diatrizoate Na	Nycomed[a]
Hypaque sodium 25%	25% Diatrizoate Na	Nycomed
Hypaque sodium 50%	50% Diatrizoate Na	Nycomed
Hypaque meglumine 60%	60% Diatrizoate meglumine	Nycomed
Omnipaque[b]	Iohexol	Nycomed
Reno-DIP	30% Diatrizoate meglumine	Bracco[c]
Renocal-76	66% Diatrizoate meglumine and 10% Diatrizoate Na	Bracco
Reno—30 and 60	30% and 60% Diatrizoate meglumine	Bracco
Renovist	35% Diatrizoate Na and 10% Diatrizoate Na	Bracco
Isovue[b] 200, 250, 300, and 370	41%, 51%, 61%, and 76% Iopamidol	Bracco

[a] Nycomed Inc, 90 Park Avenue, New York, NY.
[b] Nonionic contrast medium.
[c] Bracco Diagnostics, Princeton, NJ 08543.

diagnosis are limited, when indicated and used properly, they can add invaluable information. Procedures most commonly used are injection of a draining tract (sinography or fistulography), arthrography, tendonography, and myelography.[66,69]

Fistulography or Sinography

Fistulograms provide valuable diagnostic information when chronic draining tracts or recent traumatic puncture wounds are present. Survey radiographs of the area should be made first. If the source or cause of the draining tract or puncture wound is not clearly identified on the survey radiographs, a fistulogram can be performed to obtain additional diagnostic data.[11,14,28,32]

The technique consists of injecting undiluted water-soluble triiodinated contrast material into the draining tract as aseptically as possible. Water-soluble contrast material is used because it is less viscous and penetrates chronic draining tracts more easily than does oil-based contrast material. Because it is less viscous, it has the disadvantage of draining from the tract after injection. This can be overcome by using an inflatable, cuffed (Foley) catheter in the tract or inserting a small polyethylene tube some distance into the tract before injecting the material (Fig. 4.17). Filling is best accomplished if

the contrast material is injected under pressure; thus some form of occlusion of the tract opening is necessary.

When the distal extremity is being examined, it is important to flex and extend the region slowly. This will allow a tract that may be closed while the horse is standing to open up, permitting the contrast to enter the tract. The volume needed for injection is not consistent, and when fistulograms are being performed, the injection of an insufficient volume is a common error.[28] Contrast material should be injected until back pressure is felt on the syringe plunger or external leakage is observed. A single radiograph can also be made to determine if an adequate volume of contrast material was injected. After contrast material has been injected to delineate the entire tract, orthogonal radiographic views should be made for complete evaluation. Any contrast material that leaks onto the skin surface should be removed before radiographs are made.

A fistulogram may demonstrate 1) the extent and direction of the tract to aid in surgical exploration, 2) communication with underlying soft tissue structures (e.g., tendon sheaths or synovial joints), 3) osseous involvement (e.g., sequestra or osteomyelitis associated with surgical implants), and 4) filling defects (which appear radiolucent because of displacement of contrast material).[14] Filling defects may be caused by fibrous reaction

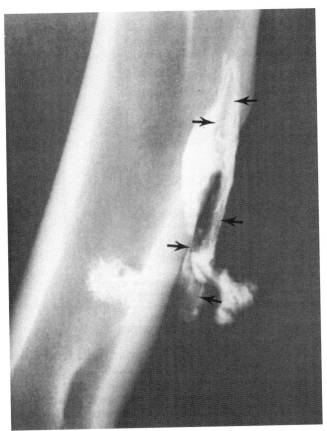

Figure 4.18 Mediolateral (ML) view of the femur after injection of contrast material into an externally draining tract. A wood foreign body is outlined by the contrast material (arrows). Note the filling defects (radiolucent areas) with sharply demarcated borders.

within the tract or by foreign bodies. Fibrous tissues generally have irregular borders, whereas foreign bodies, such as wood splinters, have sharp, straight borders (Fig. 4.18). Small foreign bodies may not be identifiable on a fistulogram because of the overlying opacity of the contrast material. In such cases, ultrasound imaging may provide additional diagnostic information.[11]

Arthrography

Arthrography is a relatively safe and simple procedure for examining equine joints.[10,12,39,71] Clinical indications include selected cases with chronic joint distension, with or without lameness. Arthrography provides diagnostic information when a more complete evaluation of suspected articular cartilage, subchondral bone, and synovial membrane lesions is needed. It is a valuable technique for determining the location of periarticular opacities (ossification or mineralization) within soft tissue (intracapsular or extracapsular). Arthrography provides important diagnostic data complementary to other imaging modalities; the need for arthrography will likely decrease, however, as other imaging modalities become more readily available (e.g., arthroscopy, ultrasonography, and MRI).

The arthrographic technique consists of injecting a local anesthetic agent in the overlying soft tissue before

aseptic joint centesis is performed. Synovial fluid can be withdrawn if joint capsule distension is present, but this is not necessary before contrast material injection. Three types of arthrography can be performed: negative (gas), positive (iodinated contrast material), and double contrast (combination of gas and iodinated contrast medium).

Negative-contrast arthrography can be performed with air, carbon dioxide, or nitrous oxide. It can be used to identify the location of opacities (intracapsular or extracapsular). Because of its limited diagnostic value, however, it is not recommended for equine arthrography.

Positive-contrast arthrography is performed by injecting triiodinated water-soluble contrast material intraarticularly (300 to 350 mg/mL). Between 5 and 20 mL of contrast material should be used, depending on the joint and animal's size.

The joint should then be flexed and extended briefly to mix the contrast material with the synovial fluid, and the films should be exposed immediately. A delay of more than 5 minutes may result in a nondiagnostic arthrogram because of contrast material resorption from the joint and dilution by fluid drawn into the joint as a result of the higher intraarticular osmotic pressure created by the contrast material. The contrast material borders will appear indistinct when this occurs.

Nonionic contrast materials, such as iohexol and iopamidol (Table 4.4), have greater opacification over time than ionic contrast material.[10] Newer, dimer contrast materials remain opacified longer with less inflammatory reaction than ionic or nonionic materials.[64] Radiographic exposure can be optimized with iodine-containing contrast material by setting the kilovoltage potential in the range of 75 to 80.[26] This range takes advantage of the photoelectric absorption of iodine, producing more contrast in the arthrogram.

Double-contrast arthrograms are performed by aseptically injecting gas intraarticularly until the joint distends. Then positive-contrast material is injected to equal 10% of the injected gas volume.[10] Double-contrast arthrography is most beneficial in larger joints, such as the stifle, and is good for identifying minor abnormalities of articular cartilage and outlining the synovial membrane surface.[10,39] Double-contrast arthrography is not recommended for smaller joints, e.g., the metacarpophalangeal joint, because gas bubbles are often present, creating pseudofilling defects and masking lesions that may be present.[10]

Arthrography helps detect fractures and/or fissuring in articular cartilage, the outline and integrity of the joint capsule, and the presence of cartilage and mineralized joint bodies. Cartilage fissuring and fragmentation, such as occurs with osteochondrosis, is best identified with positive-contrast arthrography, as the contrast material fills cartilage defects or infiltrates beneath the articular cartilage (Fig. 4.19). The extent of an osteochondrosis lesion and communication of a subchondral cyst with the joint are also best demonstrated with positive-contrast arthrography.[39]

Joint capsule proliferation, tears, hernias, and abnormal communications are best diagnosed with positive-contrast arthrography. Proliferative synovitis produces an irregular border on the contrast margins and may produce small filling defects that extend into the contrast

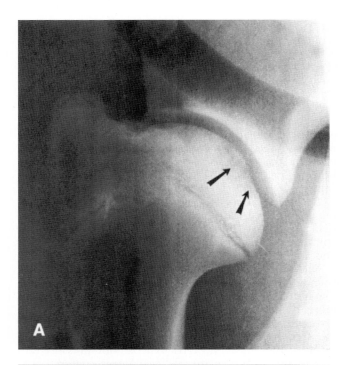

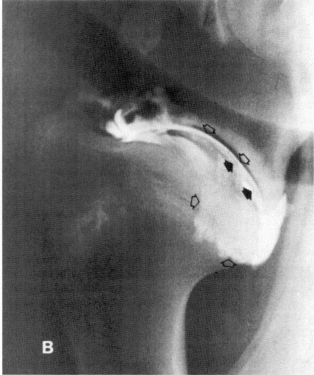

Figure 4.19 A. Mediolateral (ML) view of the shoulder, showing a large subchondral lucent region in the humeral head (arrows). There is a flattened area on the articular surface but no definite subchondral bone fracture or fragmentation. B. Shoulder arthrogram showing contrast material outlining the shoulder joint (open arrows) and dissecting beneath loose articular cartilage and subchondral bone fragments (solid arrows). The radiographic and arthrographic findings indicate osteochondritis desiccans of the humeral head.

material. Abnormal communications are easily seen, since tendon sheaths and bursa fill simultaneously with the joint (Fig. 4.20). Tears or perforations in the joint capsule are identified as contrast extravasates into surrounding soft tissue.

Free joint bodies can be identified with all three arthrographic techniques. Free joint bodies, whether opaque or nonopaque, produce lucent filling defects when surrounded by positive contrast, and both are opaque when surrounded by air.

Tendonography

Tendonography is a technique that consists of injecting positive-contrast material, negative-contrast (gas) material, or both into a tendon sheath or bursa to outline the sheath and outside surfaces of the tendons. Tendonography has been used most extensively to outline ligaments and tendons on the palmar/plantar aspect of the distal third metacarpal and metatarsal regions but can be used in any tendon sheath or bursa.[2,3,12,19,20,66,69]

For positive-contrast tendonography, 10 to 20 mL of positive contrast material is injected into the tendon sheath or fluid-filled swelling. A 25% iodine concentration is recommended to lessen the inflammatory reaction caused by more concentrated iodine solutions.[19] Double-contrast studies can be performed by injecting 5 mL of contrast material and then injecting gas to distend the sheath or bursa.[12] Gas tendonograms have also been described for the digital sheath. For negative-contrast (gas) tendonography, gas is injected in the digital sheath, between the superficial and deep digital flexor tendons, and subcutaneously.[8,69] Normal anatomy and variations of the tendon sheaths in the horse limb have been documented and demonstrated.[19]

Tenosynovitis, desmitis of the palmar and plantar annular ligaments, and intersynovial communications with bursae or joint capsules can be diagnosed with contrast studies of the tendon sheaths and bursae.[8,12,20,66] In cases of chronic tenosynovitis or bursitis, filling defects project into the contrast material from the synovial surface.[12,20] Thickening of the flexor tendons is thought to indicate tendinitis.[8] Ultrasonography is superior for demonstrating tendon pathology; but contrast studies are more effective for demonstrating synovial herniations and intersynovial communications[12] and should be used if such pathology is suspected clinically.

Myelography

Myelography in the horse is used to substantiate cervical spinal cord compression suspected from a neurologic and/or radiographic examination. It also serves to identify the location, extent, and type of compressive lesion present, which is necessary for determining the prognosis and indication for surgical intervention.

A survey radiographic examination is performed by making neutral lateral radiographs centered on the cranial, midcervical, and caudal cervical regions. Observed radiographic changes include malalignment in the midcervical area that is accentuated on the flexed lateral view

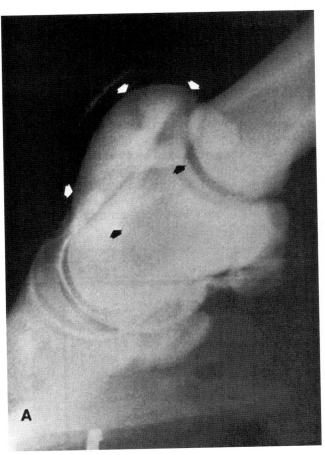

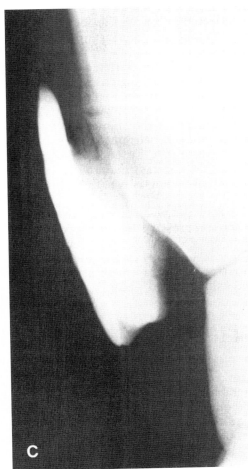

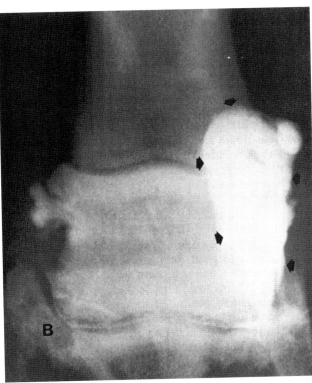

Figure 4.20   Lateromedial (LM) (A) and dorsoproximal-distopalmar (D30Pr-DiPaO) (B) views of the foot. Contrast material was injected into a fluctuant soft tissue swelling. Note the cul-de-sac (joint capsule herniation) filled with contrast material (*arrows*) and communicating with the distal interphalangeal joint. C. Lateromedial (LM) view of the carpus after injection of contrast material into a fluctuant, fluid-filled swelling. Note the supracarpal bursa in the soft tissue cranial to the distal radius with no communication to other carpal structures.

(Fig. 4.21), dorsal flaring of the caudal vertebral epiphysis into the spinal canal, abnormal ossification patterns, bony proliferation on the articular facets, and ventral extension of the cranial margin of the dorsal lamina[35,40] (Fig. 4.22). The accuracy of predicting a

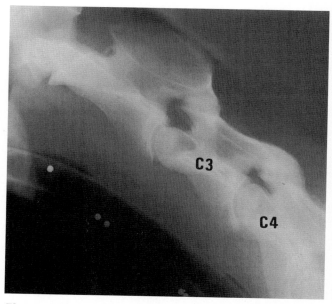

Figure 4.21 Lateral survey radiograph of the cervical spine, showing a possible dynamic cervical stenosis. A mild kyphotic malalignment is present between C3 and C4.

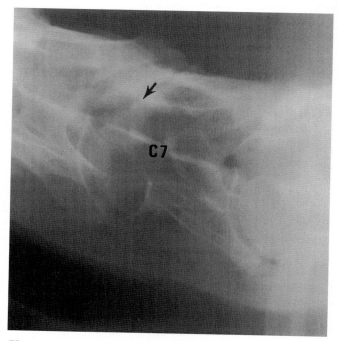

Figure 4.22 Lateral cervical view at the level of C6–7, showing bony proliferation around the articular facets, sclerosis of the rostral dorsal lamina of C7 (arrow), and narrowing of the spinal canal at the rostral aspect of C7.

compressive lesion from survey radiographs compared with myelography has been reported to be only 40% in all areas of the cervical spine except at C3–4, where there was a 70% predictive rate.[44] Sagittal ratio values appear to be a more accurate method than using only the midsagittal diameter for predicting cervical stenosis from survey radiographs.[58,59] The sagittal ratio value is the midsagittal diameter (measured in the conventional manner) divided by the width of the corresponding vertebral body at the widest point on the cranial aspect of the vertebra.[35]

Myelography with nonionic, water-soluble contrast material has proven to be an acceptable and safe diagnostic procedure in the horse (Table 4.4).[4,5,29,33,41] Iohexol and iopamidol are nonionic contrast agents that have relatively few side effects.[29,33,68] With the horse under general anesthesia and in the lateral recumbent position, its head is elevated, and approximately 40 mL iopamidol 300 or 370 mg iodine/mL or iohexol 300 or 350 mg iodine/mL is injected into the subarachnoid space at the cisterna magna.[5,33] Iohexol may produce slightly less of an inflammatory reaction than iopamidol produces,[5] but both contrast agents are relatively safe for myelography in the horse. The higher concentration contrast material provides better contrast in larger horses.

Lateral cervical radiographs centered over the cranial, midcervical, and caudal cervical regions are made with the spine in a neutral position. A flexed lateral view is then made in the midcervical region, and an extended lateral view is made in the caudal cervical region. The contrast material can be visualized via ventrodorsal radiographs over the cranial and midcervical regions, but because of thickness of the body area, it is usually not possible to visualize the contrast material in the caudal cervical region of the adult horse.

On a normal myelogram study, several variations need to be noted and not confused with extradural lesions. On neutral lateral radiographs, there are areas of some degree of elevation of the ventral contrast column at each intervertebral disk. On flexed lateral radiographs, there is also narrowing of the dorsal subarachnoid space, most frequently at C3–4 and C4–5, and the ventral column at these locations appears as a thin line. On extended lateral views, the dorsal column does not narrow, and the ventral column is increased in width.

Most lesions detected via cervical myelograms in the horse are compressive lesions from cervical stenoses, either bony or ligamentous, or the result of vertebral instability (Fig. 4.23). These lesions may cause substantial narrowing, obliteration, or displacement of the contrast column.[34] The most common sites of compression, in order of decreasing frequency, are reported to be C3–4, C6–7, C5–6, and C4–5.[44] Significant compressive lesions have been determined by a 50% or more reduction of the dorsal column compared with the thickness of the subarachnoid space cranial to the narrowing[41] and narrowing of the dorsal and ventral columns by more than 50% in diametrically opposed sites.[35,44] Other systems for determining significant spinal cord compression have also been proposed.[58,59] Misinterpre-

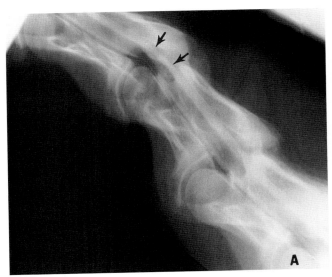

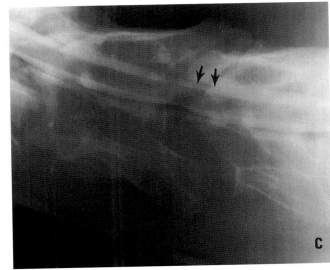

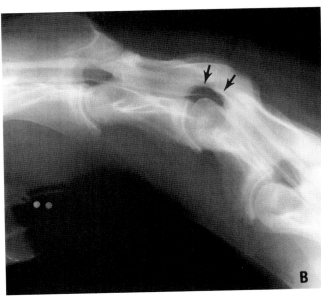

Figure 4.23 A. Lateral myelogram of the cervical region, showing contrast material in the subarachnoid space and narrowing of the ventral column at C3–4. No narrowing of the dorsal column (arrows) or significant spinal cord compression is present. B. Flexed lateral myelogram of the cervical region, showing ventral and dorsal (arrows) contrast columns narrowed by more than 50% and a narrowed spinal cord, suggesting dynamic cervical stenosis. C. Lateral myelogram of the cervical region at the level of C6–7, showing a static stenosis of the spinal canal on the rostral aspect of C7 with narrowing of the dorsal contrast column by at least 50% (arrows).

tation of myelograms can occur with suboptimal technique or when the lesion is lateralized and only lateral radiographic views are made.

PRINCIPLES OF RADIOGRAPHIC INTERPRETATION

There are three basic steps to radiographic interpretation: 1) evaluating the film and quality of the examination, 2) reading the radiograph, and 3) formulating a radiographic impression, diagnosis, and/or prognosis. Film quality should be evaluated by checking film exposure, labeling, collimation, and positioning. This is an important step because poor-quality radiographs result in missed or improperly diagnosed conditions. A prop-

erly exposed radiograph should have enough film contrast latitude to allow observation of bone and soft tissue outlines, and the film detail should be sufficient to demonstrate bone trabeculae.

Positioning should be evaluated by inspecting joint space and bone alignment. Poorly positioned studies may result from the horse standing with the limb not perpendicular to the ground, the cassette not parallel with the limb, or the x-ray tube not perpendicular to the x-ray cassette or the part being examined.

A thorough radiographic examination should be done on each part for which pathology is expected from the physical examination. The routine examination may consist of two to eight views, depending on the part examined. Sometimes, additional views are needed to better define and demonstrate suspected lesions.

The second step in radiographic interpretation is reading the radiograph. If the clinician is in a hurry to make a diagnosis, this step may be overlooked or cut short, resulting in interpretational errors. A systematic, thorough inspection of the entire film should be done so that nothing is missed. Identifying radiographic abnormalities requires a knowledge of both radiographic anatomy and radiographic signs of disease. Without a knowledge of either, a correct radiographic interpretation is usually not made.

The third step is formulating a radiographic impression, diagnosis, or differential diagnosis. A knowledge of disease pathophysiology and its relationship to radiographic signs is necessary for this step. Finally, the radiographic diagnosis should be integrated with other diagnostic information, such as history, physical examination, and perineural anesthesia results, to arrive at a final diagnosis.

If these basic steps of radiographic interpretation are not followed, the clinician may reach erroneous conclusions, leading to a faulty impression, diagnosis, and/or prognosis.

Radiology of Soft Tissue Structures

Soft tissue changes may be primary pathologic changes, secondary to more serious bone changes, or an incidental finding of no clinical significance. A bright light is helpful for evaluating soft tissue structures radiographically. Fascial planes, tendons, ligaments, and some portions of joint capsules may be seen because of adipose tissue (fat) within and around these structures. Fat is less opaque and appears slightly darker than muscle, skin, tendons, or ligaments on a radiograph (Fig. 4.24). Soft tissue structures should be evaluated for swelling, mineralized opacities, and free gas (radiolucencies).

Swelling

Soft tissue swelling in the equine extremity is usually caused by inflammation from infection or trauma. The soft tissue swelling may be localized or diffuse. Localized swelling may be identified radiographically within or around joints, tendons, or muscles (Fig. 4.24). Radiographic signs of soft tissue swelling include an increased soft tissue prominence, displacement of fat bodies (adipose tissue) around the joint capsule or tendon sheaths, and mottling or obliteration of adipose tissue in fascial planes around muscles, joint capsules, or tendons.

Mineralization

Soft tissue mineralization in equine limbs may be dystrophic or metastatic. Dystrophic mineralization is most frequent and is present in damaged tissues after physical, chemical, or thermal trauma (Fig. 4.25). Hematomas, necrotic, and postinflammatory foci and cartilaginous areas are frequent sites of dystrophic mineralization. Calcinosis circumscripta is a form of dystrophic mineralization and is most frequently seen periarticular in the horse. Metastatic mineralization occurs in primarily normal soft tissue from a disturbance in calcium and phosphorus metabolism but is seldom observed in the horse.

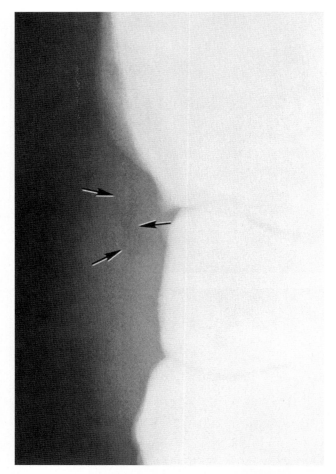

Figure 4.24 Lateromedial (LM) view showing the carpal fat pads (adipose tissue bodies) as slightly lucent structures in the dorsal soft tissues of the carpus (arrows). They are slightly displaced from the dorsal aspect of the antebrachiocarpal (radiocarpal) joint, indicating joint capsule distension. Most of the soft tissue swelling is dorsal to the fat pads, suggesting extracapsular soft tissue swelling.

Radiographic signs of soft tissue mineralization include an amorphous radiopacity within soft tissue structures, absence of trabecular or cortical bone within the radiopacity, indistinct borders with dystrophic mineralization, and well-defined and distinct borders. A round "cauliflower-shaped" appearance is usually present with calcinosis circumscripta.

Gas

Gas may be present in the soft tissue structures of equine limbs as a result of traumatic lacerations, puncture wounds, needle centesis, or gas-producing bacterial organisms (Fig. 4.26). Radiographic signs of soft tissue emphysema include radiolucent regions within soft tissue structures (the radiolucencies should be differentiated from fat) and a focal accumulation of gas with an air-fluid level that occurs with abscesses.

Soft tissue gas can be identified radiographically in subcutaneous tissue, in muscle fascial planes, in intra-

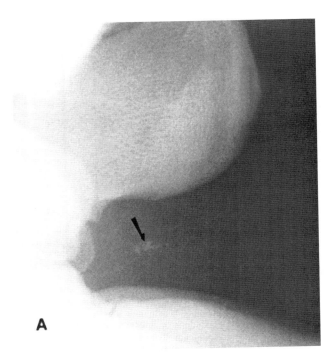

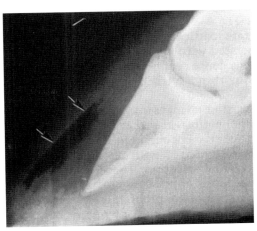

Figure 4.26 Lateromedial (LM) view of the foot, showing soft tissue gas as a large radiolucent area (*arrows*) on the dorsal aspect of the foot.

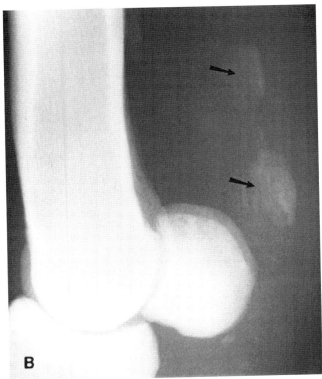

Figure 4.25 A. Flexed lateromedial (flexed LM) view of the carpus, showing a small region of soft tissue mineralization on the palmar aspect of the middle carpal joint (arrow). This pattern of mineralization is commonly seen as a result of corticosteroid injections. B. Lateromedial (LM) view of the metacarpophalangeal joint, showing dystrophic mineralization within the superficial digital flexor tendon and/or digital sheath (arrows).

muscular tissues, and within the joint. Localization of soft tissue gas is important diagnostically and prognostically: Gas within muscle tissue occurs with a gas phlegmon; intraarticular gas may be associated with the "vacuum phenomenon" when a joint is flexed (of no clinical significance); or an air-fluid level within soft tissue may be diagnostic of an abscess.

Radiology of Bone

A knowledge of normal radiographic anatomy and basic bone response patterns is essential for evaluating bone structures radiographically in equine limbs. If the veterinarian is not familiar with physeal closure and ossification times of both epiphyses and apophyses in immature animals, he or she can easily look them up in anatomy textbooks. The clinician should be familiar with the normal shape of bones and the location and appearance of protuberances and fossae in mature animals; this information is available from standard references.

Fundamental Patterns of Bone Response

Bone is limited in its response to disease; therefore, the number of bone changes identified on radiographs is limited.[17] Basic radiographic changes that may be seen in equine bones are new bone production (adjacent to the cortex or sclerosis within the cortex), localized areas of bone lysis, generalized increased bone density, and generalized decreased bone density. To formulate a correct diagnosis, the clinician should note fundamental bone response patterns and distribution within bones and any associated soft tissue changes on equine limb radiographs.

Periosteal Reactions

The periosteum is stimulated when elevated by hemorrhage, pus, edema, or infiltrating neoplastic cells. In

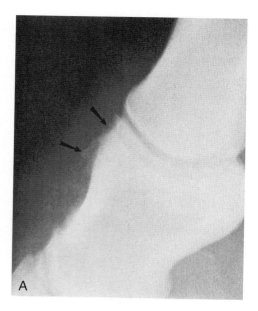
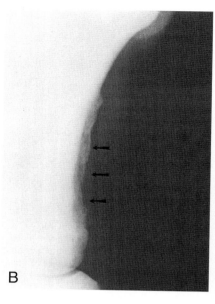

Figure 4.27 A. Lateromedial (LM) view of the phalanges, showing an irregular active periosteal reaction (*arrows*) in the region where the common digital extensor tendon and joint capsule attach. B. Dorsomedial-palmarolateral oblique (DM-PaLO) view of the proximal phalanx, showing smooth, inactive periosteal reaction (arrows) where the middle distal sesamoidean ligament attaches.

the horse, direct trauma, extension of soft tissue infections, and avulsion of ligaments, tendons, and/or joint capsules are most frequently associated with periosteal new bone production.

Periosteal bone production may be acute or chronic (Fig. 4.27). Acute periosteal bone production has an irregular, indistinct border and may be continuous or interrupted, laminated or spiculated. Acute periosteal reaction is usually active. Chronic periosteal bone production has a smooth, well-defined border; is solid; and often blends with the adjacent cortex. This type of periosteal reaction is usually inactive and often indicates a healed process, such as a healed fracture or previous active periosteal bone production that has changed to a chronic, probably inactive stage.

Cortical Changes

Cortical changes that can be identified radiographically consist of defects, erosion, lysis, and changes in thickness. Cortical defects seen most frequently in equine extremities are caused by fractures. Fractures must be differentiated from nutrient foramina, physeal lines, and edge enhancement shadows caused by superimposed bones (Fig. 4.28).

Cortical lysis is usually caused by infection and typically has a punctate pattern. A sequestrum may also be associated with a focal area of cortical lysis (Fig. 4.29). In such cases, a dense sequestered piece of bone can be identified surrounded by a lytic zone, which, in turn, is surrounded by bone sclerosis, producing an involucrum.

Cortical erosion changes can extend from either the endosteal or the periosteal surface. In the horse, they are most frequently encountered adjacent to the periosteal surface. Erosive changes with an irregular border usually result from infiltration into the bone and are most often caused by infectious processes. Cortical erosive areas with a smooth border are the result of pressure erosion (Fig. 4.30), such as that seen with proliferative synovitis

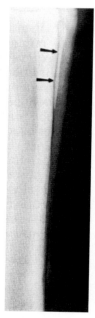

Figure 4.28 Dorsomedial-plantarolateral oblique (DM-PILO) view of the metatarsus, showing edge enhancement simulating a fracture (arrows) where the cortices of the metatarsal bones are superimposed.

in the metacarpophalangeal and metatarsophalangeal joints.

Changes in the cortical width are usually increases caused by increased weight bearing. Such changes in cortical width are frequently present with valgus or varus limb abnormalities (Fig. 4.31).

Generalized bone density changes are almost always decreased. Decreased bone density is seen secondary to disuse of the limb or distal to a fracture. The osteopenia

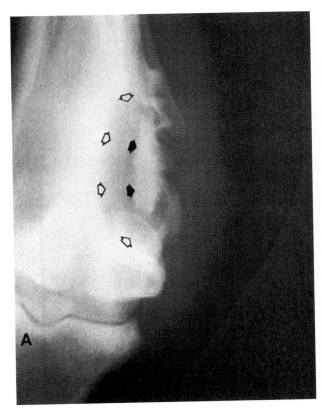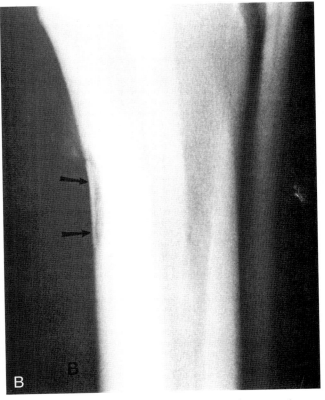

Figure 4.29 A. Dorsolateral-palmaromedial oblique (DL-PaMO) view of the distal third metacarpal bone, showing a large opaque sequestrum (solid arrows) within an involucrum (open arrows). Sclerotic bone forms the walls of the involucrum, and smooth periosteal new bone production is external to the sequestrum. B. Dorsolateral-plantaromedial oblique (DL-PIMO) view of the metatarsus, showing a longitudinal cortical fracture on the third metatarsal bone (arrows).

that develops in these limbs can be recognized radiographically as a coarse primary trabecular pattern with thin cortices (Fig. 4.32). There appear to be few, if any, reported conditions in the horse that cause generalized increased bone density.

Radiographic Signs (Bone Response Patterns) With Osteomyelitis

Osteomyelitis in equine limbs may be hematogenous in origin, resulting from penetrating wounds or open fractures. The region affected depends on the source and route of infection. Both acute and chronic osteomyelitis can be identified radiographically (Figs. 4.29 and 4.33).[17] It generally takes 7 to 10 days after clinical signs of acute osteomyelitis are observed before the earliest detectable radiographic bone changes occur.

Since osteomyelitis can affect any bone in an equine limb and must be differentiated from other focal bone lesions, it will be used to illustrate the use of radiographic signs or bone response patterns to arrive at a radiographic diagnosis. Identifying radiographic signs requires close inspection of the radiograph and is an important step in accurately establishing a specific or differential diagnosis.

The following are radiographic signs manifested by acute osteomyelitis:

- Soft tissue swelling adjacent to the bone. This swelling is manifested by mottling and obliteration of adipose tissue in fascial planes.
- Periosteal new bone production. This new bone has an irregular, indistinct border and parallels the bone cortices. Subtle areas of subperiosteal bone lysis may be seen in association with the acute periosteal bone reaction. These changes are not usually seen until 7 to 10 days after clinical signs of the disease have been observed. As the disease progresses, the periosteal bone production parallels the cortex and spreads proximal and distal from the original infection site.
- Punctate cortical lysis. The lysis is observed as small round lucent areas, 2 to 3 mm in size, within cortical bone. These changes usually develop at least 2 to 3 weeks after the initial infectious insult and are usually seen in association with acute periosteal bone production.
- Areas of bone lysis within the physis, metaphysis, or epiphysis with little or no bone response. The lysis occurs with septicemic osteomyelitis in young animals.

Chronic osteomyelitis may have the following radiographic changes:

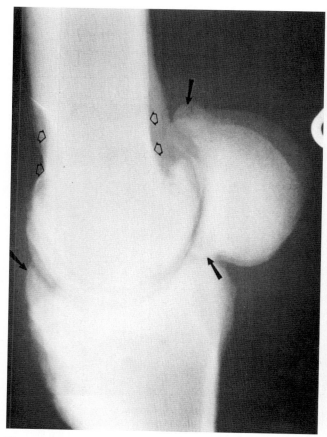

Figure 4.30 Flexed lateromedial (flexed LM) view of the metacarpophalangeal joint, showing changes that indicate chronic degenerative joint disease. Note the osteophytes on the joint margin of the dorsal proximal first phalanx and the proximal sesamoid bones (solid arrows). Smooth cortical reabsorption (open arrows) is caused by chronic synovial proliferation in the proximal palmar and dorsal joint pouches.

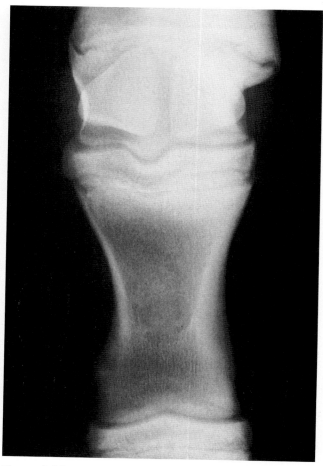

Figure 4.31 Dorsopalmar (DPa) view of the metacarpophalangeal joint, showing a thick cortex on the medial side of the proximal phalanx as a result of a varus deformity and increased weight bearing through the medial cortex.

- Large cortical defects, some of which may be as large as 1 cm in size
- Localized increased bone densities (sclerosis), which are produced within the host bone, e.g., thick cortices, and in which a sequestrum sometimes may be identified within the sclerotic and lytic bone patterns
- Periosteal bone production, which is usually abundant with a well-defined, irregular or smooth border

It is often impossible to determine radiographically if the chronic osteomyelitis is active or inactive. This diagnosis is probably best determined by physical examination, clinical signs, or other imaging techniques, such as nuclear scintigraphy.

Radiology of Synovial Joints

Radiographic evaluation of joints in the equine limb is an important part of the diagnostic workup for lameness and encompasses evaluation of several joint struc-tures or areas, including soft tissue structures (both intra-capsular and extracapsular), joint margins, subchondral bone, the "joint space," ligament, tendon, and joint cap-sule attachment areas, and joint alignment (Fig. 4.34).

Normal Joint Structures

The joint capsule and periarticular soft tissue struc-tures should not be distended. Fat bodies and adipose tissue within muscle fascial planes can be identified around some normal joints. Visibility and location of adipose tissue may change with swelling, inflammation, or joint capsule distension. The normal location and the presence of fat bodies vary depending on the joint and animal being examined.

Joint margins are bony regions at the edge of articular cartilage that also coincide with the edge of the subchon-dral bone. Articular cartilage, the periosteum, and the joint capsule meet in this region. In the normal joint, the margins are smooth and blend with the surrounding

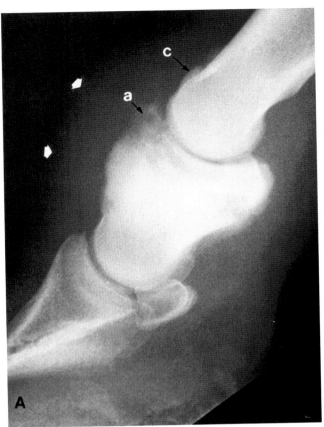 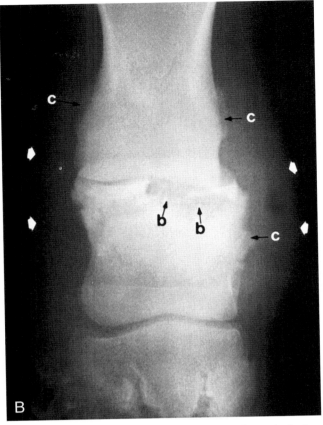

Figure 4.32 Lateromedial (LM) (A) and dorsopalmar (DPa) (B) views of the phalanges, showing changes compatible with septic arthritis, namely, periarticular soft tissue swelling (white arrows), marginal lysis (a), subchondral bone lysis (b), and active periosteal bone reaction (c). Osteoporosis can be seen in the navicular bone and distal phalanx in panel A as a prominent trabecular bone pattern produced by the remaining primary trabeculae and the pencil-line-thin subchondral and cortical bone.

bone structures. Subchondral bone is a dense, compact bony zone 1 to 3 mm in width and adjacent to the articular cartilage. The subchondral bone surface adjacent to the articular cartilage is smooth and even.

The so-called "joint space" as seen on a radiograph is not an actual space but is composed of articular cartilage with a thin layer of synovial fluid between the opposing cartilaginous surfaces. It appears black on a radiograph, compared with the adjacent white subchondral bone. The joint space should be of even thickness throughout a specific joint, but thickness differs from joint to joint, e.g., the distal interphalangeal joint space is wider than the proximal interphalangeal joint space, which is wider than the metacarpophalangeal joint space.

Ligaments, tendons, and the joint capsule, which attach periarticularly, add stability to the joint. The attachment areas vary with the joint and may be located at different distances both proximal and distal to the joint margins. It is important to know regions of insertion for ligaments and tendons around specific joints.

The normal subchondral bone surfaces should align evenly. Positional changes of the horse or of the x-ray tube when the radiograph is made may make a normal joint appear slightly malaligned.

Radiographic Changes Associated With Joint Disease

The radiographic examination is helpful for evaluating the type and extent of joint disease. The radiographic manifestations of joint disease occur in the soft tissue and bone structures and may develop before or after clinical signs of the disease. The bone changes follow clinical signs in septic arthritis and may precede or follow clinical manifestations with degenerative joint disease.

Soft tissue changes that may be observed radiographically are periarticular soft tissue swelling, joint capsule distension, and mineralization. The location of fat bodies (adipose tissue masses) and adipose tissue in fascial planes can be used to evaluate periarticular swelling and joint capsule distension. Periarticular mineralization may be associated with numerous causes but is predominantly seen in the horse after corticosteroid injections or blunt soft tissue trauma.

Marginal joint changes consist of periarticular osteophyte formation and bone lysis (see Figs. 4.30 and 4.32). Marginal periarticular osteophytes are usually associated with degenerative joint disease, whereas marginal bone lysis is most often seen with septic arthritis. In early

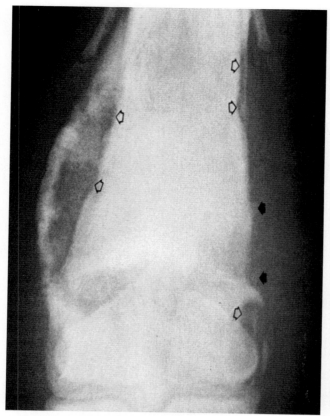

Figure 4.33 Dorsopalmar (DPa) view of the metacarpophalangeal joint, showing active periosteal reaction (solid arrows), cortical lysis (open arrows), and soft tissue swelling around the distal third metacarpal bone. These changes are compatible with acute, active osteomyelitis.

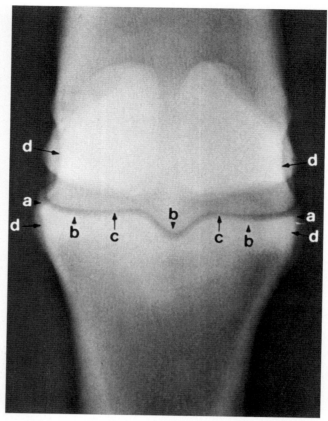

Figure 4.34 Dorsoproximal-distopalmar oblique (D30Pr-DiPaO) view of the metacarpophalangeal joint, showing the structures that should be evaluated around a joint, namely, periarticular soft tissue (a), joint margins (b), subchondral bone (c), the "joint space" (articular cartilage) (d), areas for ligament and tendon attachment, and general joint alignment.

stages, marginal changes may be subtle, but with advanced or more severe disease, the changes are easily identified.

Subchondral bone changes consist of sclerosis, lysis, and fragmentation (Figs. 4.32, 4.35, and 4.36). Subchondral bone sclerosis may be present with degenerative joint disease, although it seems to be recognized radiographically in only the more pronounced or longstanding cases. Subchondral bone lysis can have a local or general distribution within the joint and may be seen in association with subchondral bone fragments. Subchondral bone lysis may be present with septic arthritis, degenerative joint disease, osteochondrosis, or "traumatic arthritis." Localized or general subchondral lytic patterns with irregular, indistinct margins are associated with septic arthritis. Localized, well-defined lytic lesions are seen with osteochondrosis, which may develop into subchondral cystlike lesions. Focal subchondral lytic areas associated with bone fragments are seen with osteochondritis dissecans and traumatic arthritis lesions from chronic microfractures in the subchondral bone. Traumatic arthritis lesions are usually seen on the dorsal surfaces of joints and are caused by hyperextension trauma.

The joint space width may be increased or decreased. An increased width may be associated with joint effusion, although in weight-bearing studies, this is seldom apparent. An increased joint space associated with subchondral bone lysis can be seen with extensive septic arthritis. A decreased joint space, either general or localized within the joint, is associated with cartilaginous erosion and degeneration and occurs predominately with degenerative joint disease (Fig. 4.35).

Periarticular enthesiophytes are usually associated with joint capsule, ligament, or tendon damage or avulsion from their bony attachments (Fig. 4.35). The enthesiophytes (periosteal new bone production) are irregular in the acute stages, which distinguishes them from marginal periarticular osteophytes, and occur at tendinous and ligamentous attachment areas.

Alignment abnormalities may consist of subluxation or luxation of a joint or may simply result in an abnormal degree of flexion or extension of a joint in a resting position. Abnormal joint alignment may be associated with ligament laxity and/or injury, tendon injury or contracture, abnormal bone growth, i.e., angular limb deformities in foals, and healed malaligned fractures.

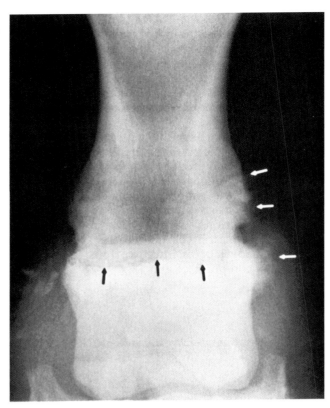

Figure 4.35 Dorsopalmar (DPa) view of the proximal interphalangeal joint, showing radiographic signs compatible with degenerative joint disease. Note the joint space narrowing (black arrows) from articular cartilage degeneration and erosion and subchondral bone sclerosis. The active periarticular periosteal bone reaction (white arrows) is a result of tendon, ligament, and joint capsule avulsion and tearing.

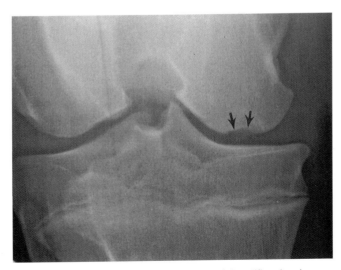

Figure 4.36 Caudocranial (CaCr) view of the stifle, showing a subchondral defect (arrows) in the medial femoral condyle that is compatible with osteochondrosis.

Chronic alignment abnormalities predispose the joint to degenerative joint disease from abnormal weight bearing and stress distribution through the joint.

Radiographic Changes With Specific Joint Conditions

Degenerative joint disease (osteoarthrosis) is a secondary condition in the horse (Fig. 4.35). The severity of radiographic changes usually correlates with the severity and/or duration of the disease process. The following are radiographic changes seen in the horse, listed in order from most common to least common:

- Marginal periarticular osteophytes
- Narrowed joint space, which may involve all or only part of the joint; distinct, smooth borders remain on the subchondral bone adjacent to the articular cartilage
- Subchondral bone sclerosis
- Subchondral bone cysts, which occur infrequently as sequelae to degenerative joint disease

Septic arthritis may be hematogenous in origin or result from extension of an adjacent osteomyelitis or cellulitis (Fig. 4.32). The following are radiographic signs of septic arthritis:

- Periarticular soft tissue swelling and joint capsule distension
- Marginal bone lysis, which may occur early in the disease
- Subchondral bone destruction, which may be an extension from or occur without the marginal lysis
- Periosteal reactions, which may be adjacent to the joint but are generally distributed around the joint; when septic arthritis has occurred from extension of an adjacent osteomyelitis or cellulitis, the periosteal reaction may precede the intraarticular changes

Osteochondrosis is associated with regions of high predilection in specific joints, which should be observed when diagnosing the condition. It is caused by defective osteochondral development, which usually involves subchondral bone (Fig. 4.36). The following are radiographic changes present with osteochondrosis:

- Flattening of the subchondral bone surface
- Localized subchondral bone defect (lysis)
- Subchondral bone fragments (dissecans)
- Secondary degenerative joint disease changes that may also be present
- Subchondral cystlike lesions that may develop secondary to osteochondrosis

Traumatic osteochondrosis or traumatic joint disease also manifests with subchondral bone lysis. These lesions must be differentiated from true osteochondrosis lesions. Areas of predilection for traumatic joint disease are the metacarpophalangeal joints (Fig. 4.37) and carpus (Fig. 4.38). Traumatic osteochondrosis develops from increased weight bearing and stress on a joint surface, resulting in bone sclerosis and eventual microfractures, which lead to subchondral bone lysis. Traumatic joint disease may also develop after hyperextension injury in

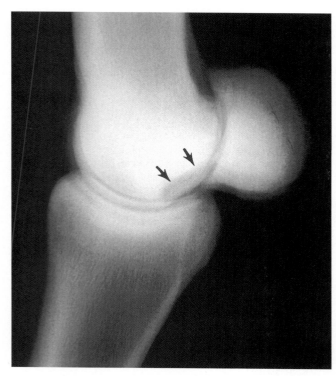

Figure 4.37 Traumatic osteochondrosis on the distal palmar surface of the third metacarpal bone (arrows).

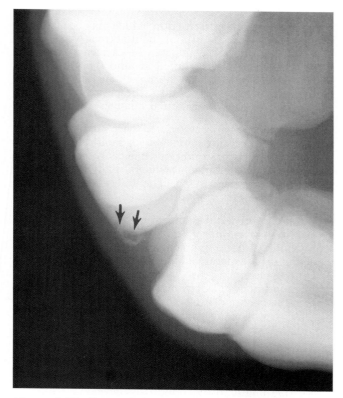

Figure 4.38 Traumatic degenerative joint disease from hyperextension of the carpus, visible as subchondral bone lysis and small bone fragments on the distal articular margin of the radial carpal bone (arrows).

joints such as the carpus, producing microfractures, subchondral bone lysis, and small subchondral bone fragments. The following are signs of traumatic joint disease:

- Focal subchondral bone lysis with indistinct borders
- Subchondral bone sclerosis
- Bone fragments, which may be adjacent to the subchondral bone lysis

Systematic use of the radiographic signs of bone and joint disease discussed in this chapter provide the basis for correct, consistent radiographic diagnoses. Without close observation of the radiograph for these changes, missed or incorrect diagnoses will be made.

NORMAL RADIOGRAPHIC ANATOMY

Recognition of normal radiographic anatomy and variations of normal in the mature and immature horse is essential in equine radiology. Erroneous diagnoses or misdiagnoses may result if normal anatomy is not known. The normal radiographic anatomy of horse extremities is presented for reference in the following pages.

Nomenclature of labeling radiographic views of equine limbs has been confusing.[53] Several systems have been used or proposed for use.[18,54] The system used here is that proposed by the Nomenclature Committee of the American College of Veterinary Radiology,[54] which uses proper veterinary anatomic directional terms[21] and describes the direction in which the central x-ray beam penetrates the body part of interest, from the point of entrance to the point of exit (Fig. 4.39). The standard abbreviation for the view is given in parentheses in the figure legends.

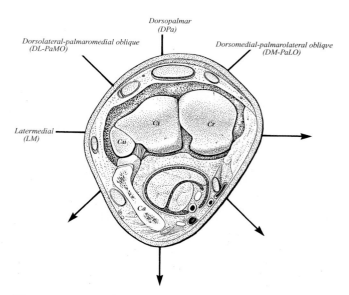

Figure 4.39 Cross-sectional diagram at the level of the proximal row of carpal bones demonstrating the nomenclature and method for labeling radiographic views. Cr, radial carpal bone; Ci, intermediate carpal bone; Cu, ulnar carpal bone; Ca, accessory carpal bone.

Normal Radiographic Anatomy for Equine Lameness Examination

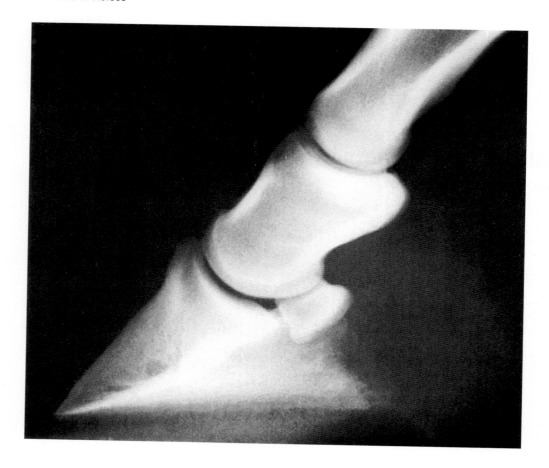

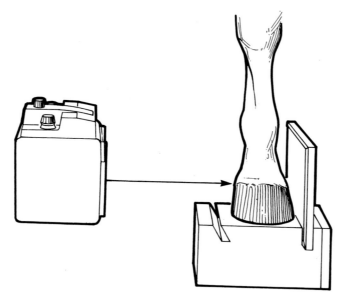

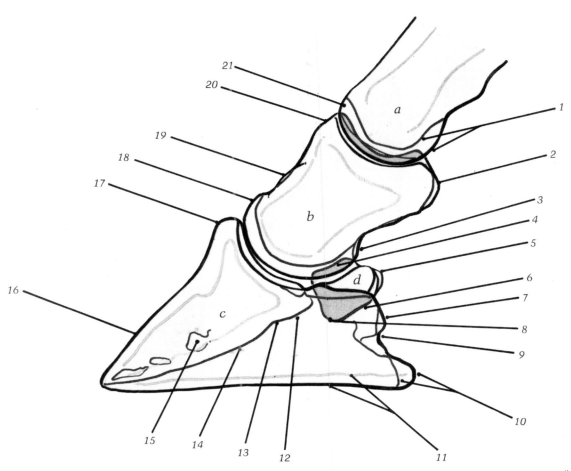

Figure 4.40   Lateromedial (LM) view of the distal phalanges and navicular bone. a, proximal phalanx; b, middle phalanx; c, distal phalanx; d, navicular bone.

1. Palmar aspect of the medial and lateral condyles on the distal extremity of the proximal phalanx.
2. Transverse bony prominence on the proximopalmar aspect of the middle phalanx.
3. Superimposed medial and lateral condyles on the distopalmar aspect of the middle phalanx.
4. Articular surface of the navicular bone.
5. Proximal border of the navicular bone.
6. Flexor cortex and surface of the navicular bone; the medullary cavity (spongiosa) is the less opaque area in the center of the navicular bone.
7. Superimposed medial and lateral proximal parts of the palmar process on the distal phalanx. The size of this palmar process varies depending on the mineralization and ossification of the collateral cartilages. The palmar process also superimposes over the navicular bone, sometimes creating confusing opacities.
8. Distal border of the navicular bone, the border of which may appear as a distinct ridge or may blend with the contour of the navicular bone. Slight obliquity on the lateromedial view alters the navicular bone's apparent shape.
9. Palmar process incisure.
10. Superimposed distal parts of the medial and lateral palmar processes on the distal phalanx.

11. Medial and lateral distal (solar) borders of the distal phalanx. On oblique projections, these borders may be separated farther.
12. Flexor surface of the distal phalanx, where the deep digital flexor attaches.
13. Semilunar line on the solar surface of the distal phalanx.
14. Opaque line representing the bone cortex on the concave solar surface of the distal phalanx.
15. Solar canal of the distal phalanx on end. This canal makes a semicircular loop in the distal phalanx, and its visibility depends on its size and the x-ray beam angle.
16. Dorsal surface of the distal phalanx.
17. Extensor process of the distal phalanx, which may have a single, double-humped, or pointed appearance. The surface should always be smooth.
18. Dorsal extent of the distal articular surface on the middle phalanx. The slight projection on the articular margin should not be mistaken for an osteophyte.
19. Eminences for collateral ligament attachments from the distal interphalangeal joint. They may be prominent or small, but their surface should be smooth; they should not be mistaken for periosteal bone production.
20. Extensor process of the middle phalanx.
21. Distal dorsal articular surface of the proximal phalanx.

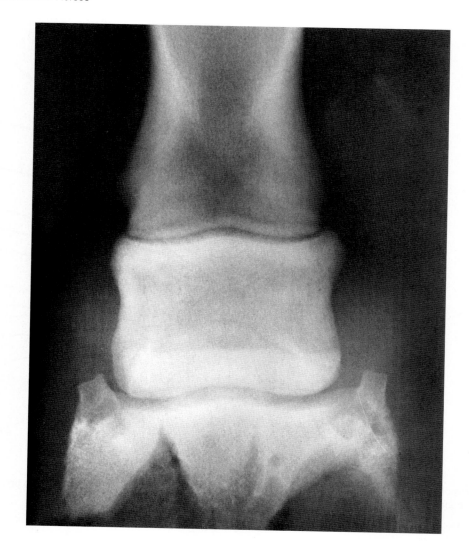

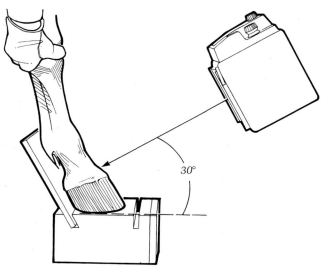

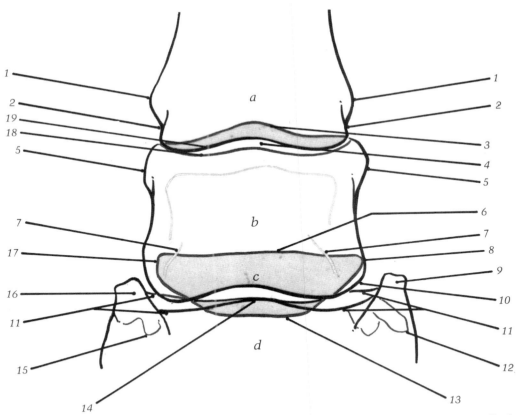

Figure 4.41   Dorsoproximal-palmarodistal oblique (D30Pr-PaDiO) view of the distal phalanges and navicular bone (foot). a, proximal phalanx; b, middle phalanx; c, navicular bone (distal sesamoid bone); d, distal phalanx.

1. Medial and lateral eminences on the distal extremity of the middle phalanx for attachment of collateral ligaments.
2. Medial and lateral depressions for attachment of collateral ligaments.
3. Proximal palmar border of the middle phalanx.
4. Articular cartilage thickness in the proximal interphalangeal joint space, which is approximately half the thickness of the articular cartilage in the distal interphalangeal joint.
5. Medial and lateral eminences for ligamentous and tendinous attachments on the proximal palmar aspect of the middle phalanx.
6. Proximal border of the navicular bone, which is seen with the least amount of distortion on this view. It should be straight, smooth, and distinct.
7. Dorsal eminences on the medial and lateral aspects of the middle phalanx for attachment of the collateral ligaments of the distal interphalangeal joint.
8. Medial extremity of the navicular bone, which is slightly more rounded in appearance than the lateral extremity.
9. Proximal part of the medial palmar process on the distal phalanx.
10. Medial aspect of the distal articular surface on the middle phalanx.
11. Proximal articular surface of the distal phalanx; palmar and dorsal borders.
12. Fossa on the palmar medial surface of the distal phalanx.
13. Distal palmar border of the navicular bone, which cannot be adequately evaluated on this view because of superimposition over the distal interphalangeal joint.
14. Extensor process for the distal phalanx.
15. Fossa on palmar lateral surface of the distal phalanx.
16. Proximal part of the lateral palmar process, the size of which depends on the extent of ossification in the cartilages of the distal phalanx. Separate ossification centers may occur in this region and should not be mistaken for fracture fragments.
17. Lateral extremity of the navicular bone, which has a sharper angled appearance than the medial extremity.
18. Proximal articular surface (articular fovea) of the middle phalanx.
19. Distal articular surface of the proximal phalanx.

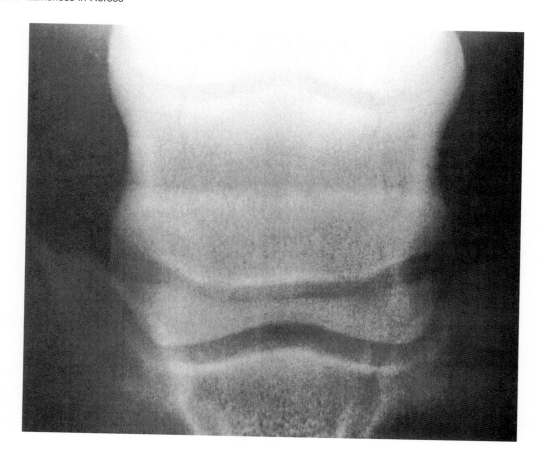

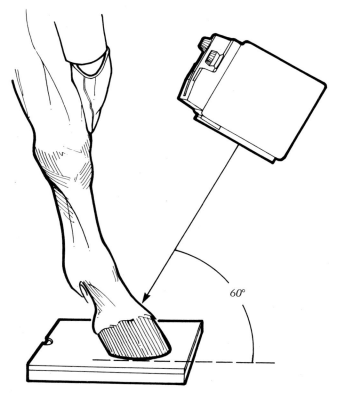

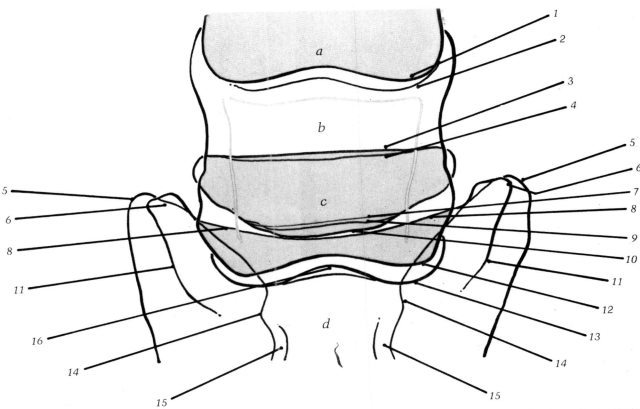

Figure 4.42 Palmarodistal oblique (D60Pr-PaDiO) view of the distal phalanx and navicular bone (foot). This view is used extensively for evaluating the navicular bone. Position and exposure are critical for optimal visualization. a, proximal phalanx; b, middle phalanx; c, navicular bone (distal sesamoid bone); d, distal phalanx.

1. Distal articular surface of the proximal phalanx.
2. Proximal articular surface of the middle phalanx.
3. Proximal border of the flexor surface on the navicular bone.
4. Proximal border of the articular surface on the navicular bone, which often looks indistinct and slightly irregular on this view because of the projection angle of the x-ray beam.
5. Distal part of the medial and lateral palmar processes.
6. Proximal part of the medial and lateral palmar processes.
7. Groove on the distal navicular bone between the flexor and articular margins. Vascular foramina are in this groove.
8. Palmar articular margin of the distal phalanx.
9. Distal margin on the navicular bone.
10. Distal margin of the flexor surface on the navicular bone.
11. Medial and lateral parietal sulci on the distal phalanx.
12. Distal articular surface of the middle phalanx.
13. Articular border of the distal phalanx.
14. Medial and lateral solar grooves on the solar surface of the distal phalanx.
15. Solar canal.
16. Extensor process of the distal phalanx.

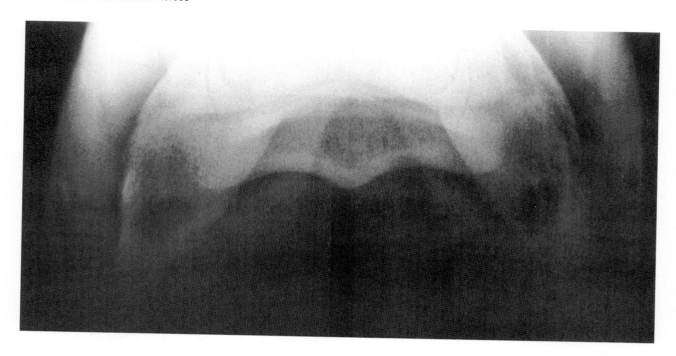

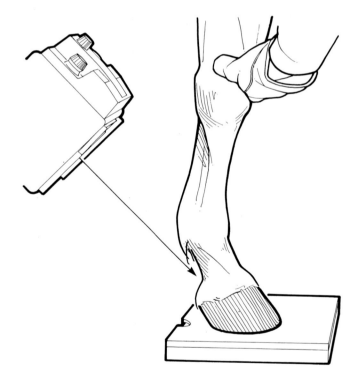

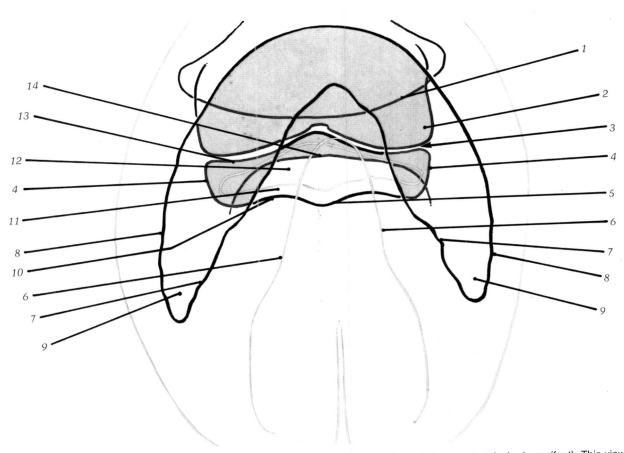

Figure 4.43   Palmaroproximal-palmarodistal oblique (Pa45Pr-PaDiO) view of the distal phalanx and navicular bone (foot). This view shows the navicular bone with minimal superimposition over other bones. The angle of the x-ray beam and exposures are critical for eliminating projection artifacts, e.g., lack of good cortical and medullary cavity definition or superimposition of the distal phalanx over the navicular bone.

1. Palmar border of the middle phalanx.
2. Distal medial condyle of the middle phalanx.
3. Articulation between the navicular bone and the middle phalanx.
4. Medial and lateral extremities of the navicular bone.
5. Central eminence on the flexor surface of the navicular bone.
6. Collateral (paracureal) sulci of the frog.
7. Semilunar line on the solar surface of the distal phalanx.

8. Medial and lateral aspects of the solar border of the distal phalanx.
9. Distal part of the medial and lateral palmar processes.
10. Flexor surface of the navicular bone.
11. Cortical bone on the flexor surface of the navicular bone.
12. Medullary (spongiosa) cavity of the navicular bone.
13. Articular surface of the navicular bone.
14. Palmar articular border of the distal phalanx.

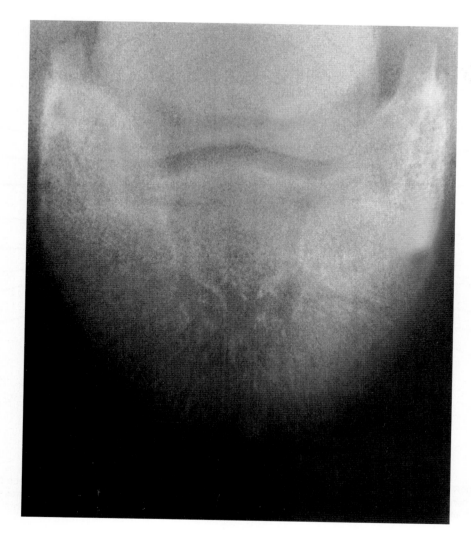

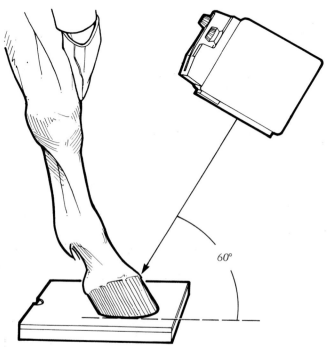

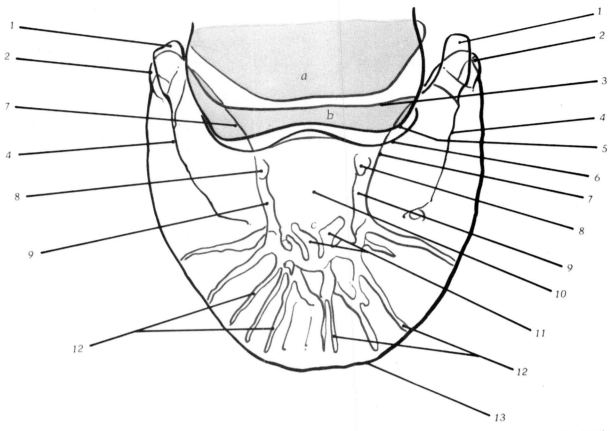

Figure 4.44 Dorsoproximal-palmarodistal oblique (D60Pr-PaDiO) view of the distal phalanx (foot). The x-ray beam for this view is centered at the coronet, and the exposure is half that necessary for visualizing the navicular bone. a, navicular bone (distal sesamoid bone); b, middle phalanx; c, distal phalanx.

1. Proximal part of the medial and lateral palmar processes.
2. Distal part of the medial and lateral palmar processes.
3. Palmar articular margin of the distal phalanx.
4. Medial and lateral parietal sulci of the distal phalanx.
5. Distal articular surface of the middle phalanx.
6. Proximal dorsal margin of the articular surface of the distal phalanx.
7. Borders of the medial and lateral solar grooves.
8. Medial and lateral solar foramina.
9. Solar canal, the width and distinctness of which are variable in normal distal phalanges.
10. Flexor surface of the distal phalanx, where the deep digital flexor tendon attaches.

11. Vascular canals in the region of the solar canal.
12. Peripheral vascular canals. The vascular canals may be of variable width in normal distal phalanges. The peripheral solar border of the distal phalanx should be relatively smooth and symmetrical, although a slightly irregular peripheral border may be considered normal in older animals.
13. Distal solar margin of the distal phalanx. The normal distal border of the distal phalanx may be convex or have some degree of concavity. A middistal notch, when present, is the crena marginis solaris.

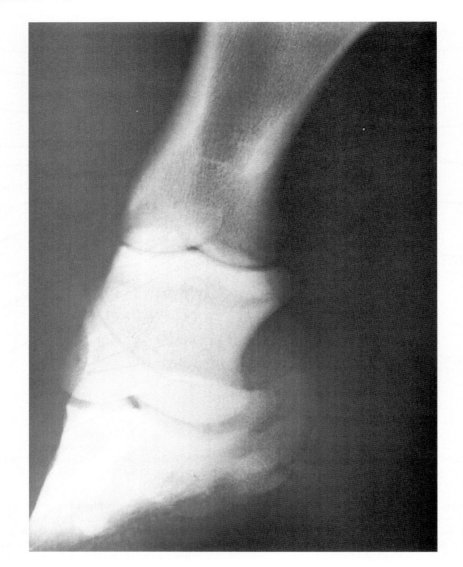

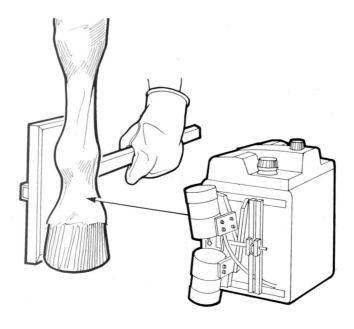

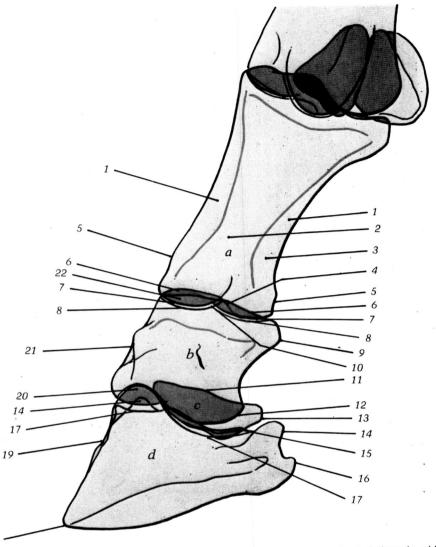

Figure 4.45   Dorsomedial-palmarolateral oblique (D35M-PaLO) view of the phalanges. a, proximal phalanx; b, middle phalanx; c, navicular bone; d, distal phalanx.

1. Mediopalmar and dorsolateral cortices of the proximal phalanx.
2. Medullary cavity of the proximal phalanx, which can sometimes be distinctly seen as a 2- to 3-cm lucency in the center of the proximal phalanx.
3. Surface for attachment of the middle (oblique) distal sesamoidean ligament.
4. Sagittal ridge on the proximal articular surface of the middle phalanx.
5. Eminences for attachment of the medial and lateral collateral ligaments of the proximal interphalangeal joint on the distal aspect of the proximal phalanx.
6. Palmar border of the articular fovea on the base of the middle phalanx.
7. Medial and lateral condyles on the distal aspect of the proximal phalanx.
8. Articular fovea on the base of the middle phalanx.
9. Medial proximal eminence for attachment of the medial collateral ligament and the medial branch of the tendon of the superficial digital flexor on the middle phalanx.
10. Sagittal ridge between the fovea on the base of the middle phalanx.

11. Proximal border of the navicular bone.
12. Distal medial condyle of the middle phalanx.
13. Medial extremity of the navicular bone.
14. Proximal part of the medial palmar process of the distal phalanx.
15. Palmar border of the articular surface on the distal phalanx.
16. Distal part of the medial palmar process of the distal phalanx.
17. Medial and lateral aspects of the coronary border of the articular surface on the distal phalanx.
18. Solar border of the distal phalanx.
19. Depression and bony prominence on the lateral parietal surface of the distal phalanx for lateral collateral ligament attachment. The bony prominence has a smooth surface and should not be mistaken for bone production.
20. Extensor process of the distal phalanx.
21. Eminence on the dorsal surface of the middle phalanx for collateral ligament attachment, which has a smooth surface and should not be mistaken for periosteal bone production.
22. Dorsolateral articular border on the middle phalanx.

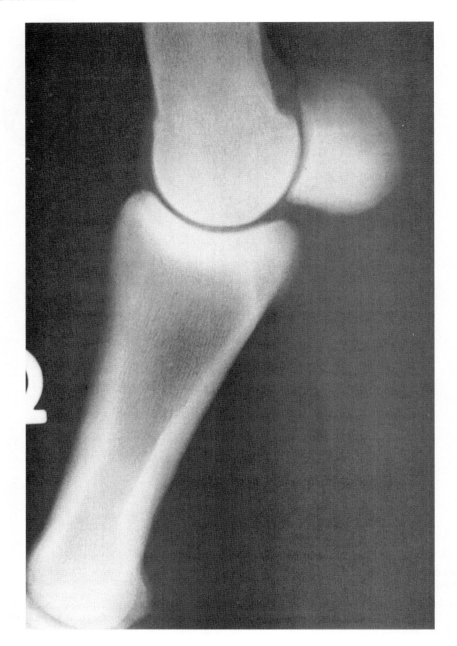

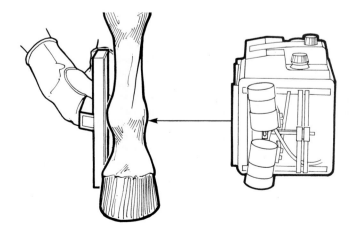

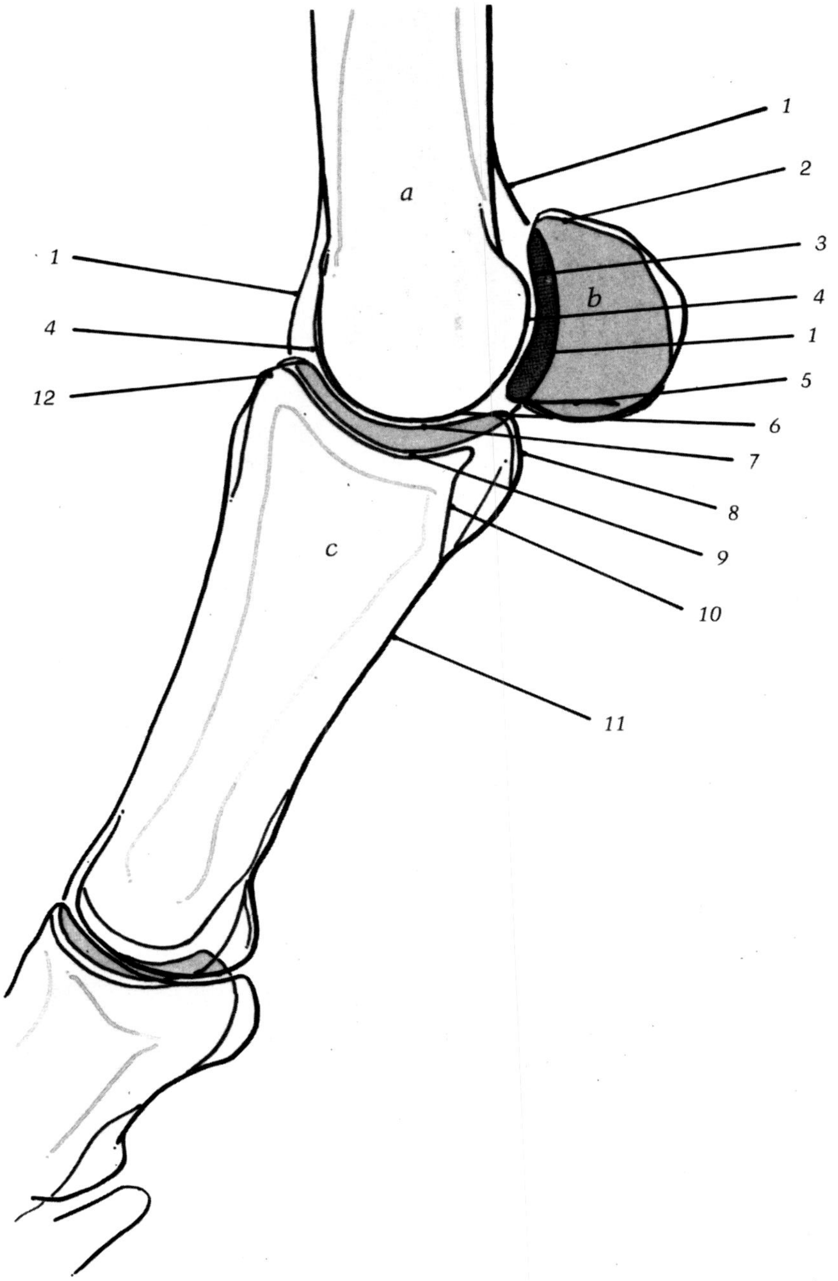

Figure 4.46 Lateromedial (LM) view of the metacarpophalangeal joint. a, third metacarpophalangeal bone; b, proximal sesamoid bones; c, proximal phalanx.

1. Sagittal ridge on the distal extremity of the third metacarpal bone.
2. Apex of the superimposed proximal sesamoid bones.
3. Articular surface of the proximal sesamoid bones.
4. Articular surface of the superimposed medial and lateral condyles of the third metacarpal bone.
5. Superimposed base of the proximal sesamoid bones.
6. Transverse ridge on the distal articular surface of the third metacarpal bone, which divides the distal metacarpal articular surface into dorsal and palmar areas. It varies in size and visibility.
7. Superimposed medial and lateral articular fovea of the proximal phalanx.
8. Superimposed medial and lateral tuberosities on the proximal caudal aspect of the proximal phalanx for ligamentous attachment.
9. Sagittal groove on the proximal articular surface of the proximal phalanx, which articulates with the sagittal ridge of the third metacarpal bone.
10. Midpalmar surface of the proximal phalanx located between the lateral and medial tuberosities.
11. Palmar surface of the proximal phalanx, where the middle (oblique) distal sesamoidean ligament attaches.
12. Superimposed medial and lateral bony eminences for attachment of the extensor tendon on the proximal phalanx.

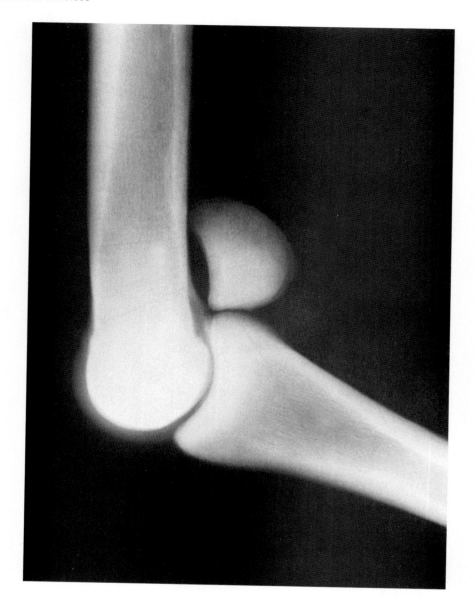

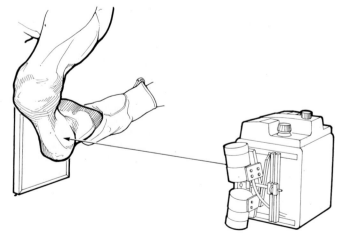

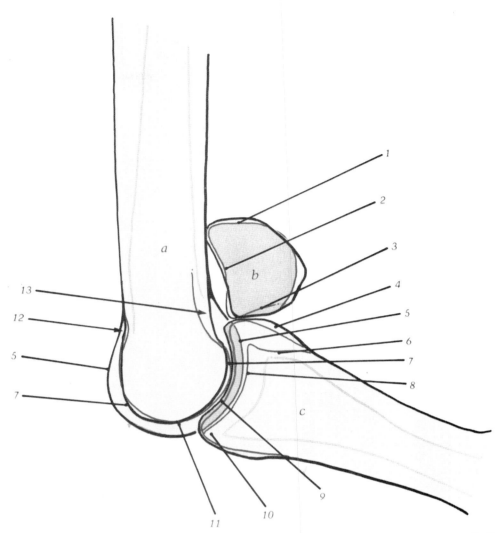

Figure 4.47   Flexed lateromedial (flexed LM) view of the metacarpophalangeal joint. This view allows the most effective evaluation of the articular surface of the sesamoid bones, offers good visualization of small articular basilar sesamoid fractures and changes, and provides a distinct view of the proximal tuberosities. Furthermore, the dorsal articular surface of the third metacarpal bone can be evaluated without superimposition of the proximal phalanx. a, third metacarpal bone; b, proximal sesamoid bones; c, proximal phalanx.

1. Apex of the superimposed proximal sesamoid bones.
2. Superimposed articular surfaces of the proximal sesamoid bones.
3. Bases of the superimposed proximal sesamoid bones.
4. Superimposed medial and lateral tuberosities on the proximal caudal aspect of the proximal phalanx, where ligamentous attachments occur.
5. Sagittal ridge on the distal articular surface of the third metacarpal bone; the dorsal and palmar aspects are labeled.
6. Midpalmar surface of the proximal phalanx, located between the medial and lateral tuberosities.
7. Palmar and dorsal aspects of the superimposed medial and lateral condyles of the third metacarpal bone.
8. Sagittal groove on the proximal articular surface of the

proximal phalanx, which articulates with the sagittal ridge on the distal third metacarpal bone.
9. Superimposed fovea (articular surface) of the proximal extremity of the proximal phalanx.
10. Superimposed medial and lateral parts of the extensor eminence of the proximal phalanx.
11. Transverse ridge on the distal articular surface of the third metacarpal bone, which separates the distal articular surface of the third metacarpal bone into dorsal and palmar parts.
12. Bony depression where the proximal dorsal recess from the metacarpophalangeal joint is located.
13. Bony depression where the proximal palmar recess from the metacarpophalangeal joint is located.

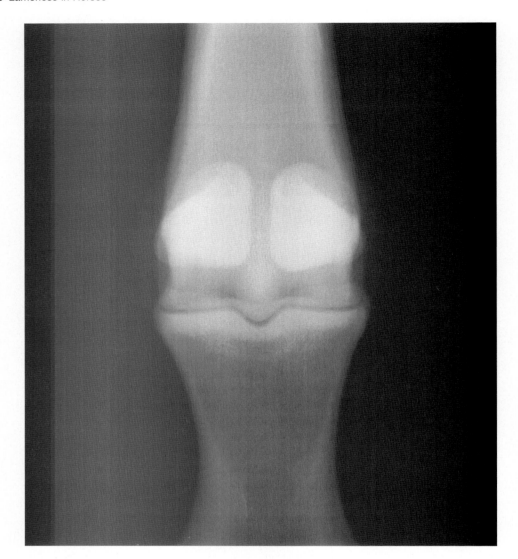

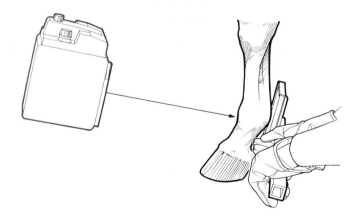

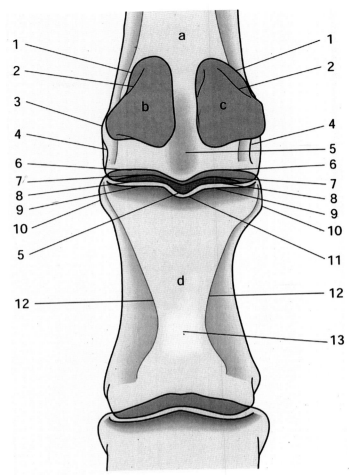

Figure 4.48 Dorsoproximal-palmarodistal (D30Pr-PaDi) view of the metacarpophalangeal joint. a, third metacarpal bone; b, lateral proximal sesamoid bone; c, medial proximal sesamoid bone; d, proximal phalanx.

1. Peripheral abaxial margins of the proximal sesamoid bones. The peripheral margin of the medial proximal sesamoid bone is more convex than that of the lateral proximal sesamoid bone.
2. Abaxial margin of the articular surfaces of the medial and lateral proximal sesamoid bones.
3. Eminence for attachment of the lateral collateral ligament.
4. Depression on the medial and lateral aspects of the third metacarpal bone, where collateral ligaments attach.
5. Sagittal ridge on the distal articular surface of the third metacarpal bone.
6. Medial and lateral palmar margins of the articular fovea on the proximal extremity of the proximal phalanx.
7. Medial and lateral dorsal margins of the articular fovea on the proximal extremity of the proximal phalanx.
8. Medial and lateral condyles (articular surface) of the third metacarpal bone.
9. Articular fovea on the proximal extremity of the proximal phalanx.
10. Medial and lateral palmar tuberosities on the proximal extremity of the proximal phalanx for ligament attachment.
11. Sagittal groove on the proximal articular surface of the proximal phalanx.
12. Bony ridges on the palmar surface of the proximal phalanx for attachment of the middle (oblique) distal sesamoidean ligament.
13. Medullary cavity in the proximal phalanx.

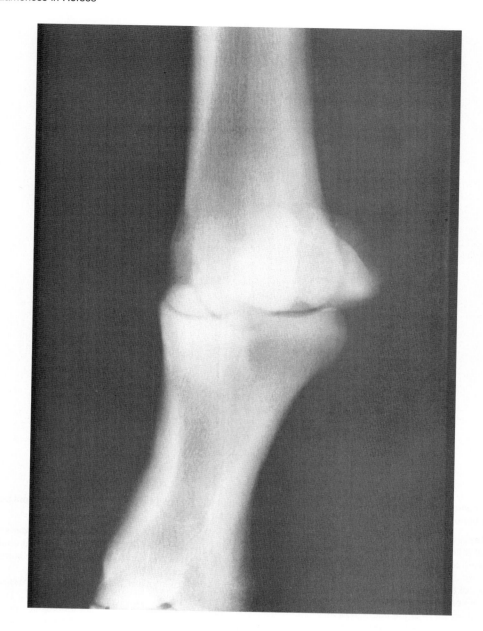

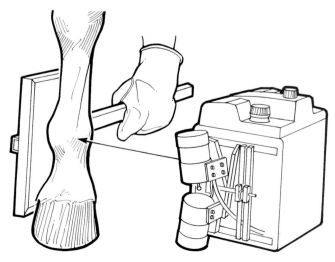

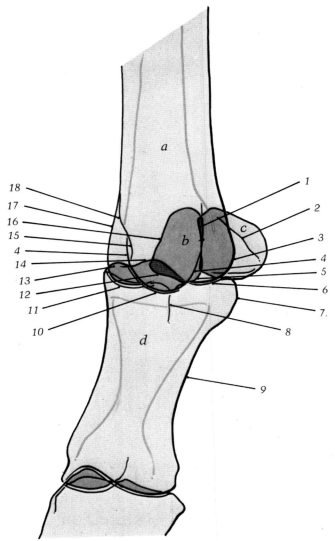

Figure 4.49   Dorsolateral-palmaromedial oblique (D45L-PaMO) view of the metacarpophalangeal joint. a, third metacarpal bone; b, medial proximal sesamoid bone; c, lateral proximal sesamoid bone; d, proximal phalanx.

1. Articular surface of the lateral proximal sesamoid bone.
2. The difference in radiographic opacity is caused by a difference in bone thickness on the lateral proximal sesamoid bone. The base and body are more opaque than the apex and peripheral border. The convex shape on the abaxial surface produces the distinct line between the two opacities.
3. Palmar surface of the lateral condyle distal aspect of the third metacarpal bone.
4. Palmar and dorsal aspects of the sagittal ridge on the distal third metacarpal bone.
5. Junction of the peripheral and basilar margins of the medial proximal sesamoid bone.
6. Lateral articular fovea of the proximal extremity of the proximal phalanx.
7,8. Lateral and medial tuberosities on the proximal palmar aspect of the proximal phalanx.
9. Lateral bony ridge for attachment of the middle (oblique) distal sesamoidean ligament.
10. Sagittal groove on the proximal articular surface of the proximal phalanx.
11. Medial articular fovea of the proximal extremity of the proximal phalanx.
12. Basilar margin of the medial proximal sesamoid bone.
13,14. Medial and lateral dorsal margins of the articular fovea on the proximal phalanx. Both margins are visible on correctly exposed and positioned oblique views of the metacarpophalangeal joint.
15. Depression (concave surface) for attachment of the medial collateral ligament on the distal third metacarpal bone. The visibility and distinctness of the concave line change on different projections. It may be more prominent on some examinations and not visible on others.
16. Abaxial articular margin of the medial proximal sesamoid bone.
17. Dorsal aspect of the medial condyle on the third metacarpal bone.
18. Eminence on the third metacarpal bone for attachment of the medial collateral ligament.

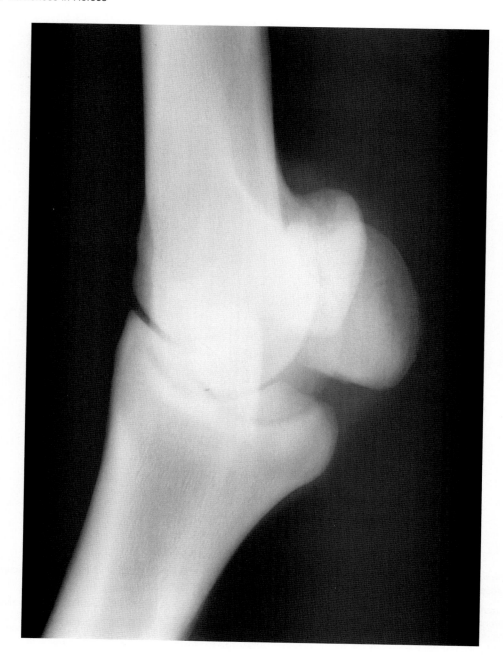

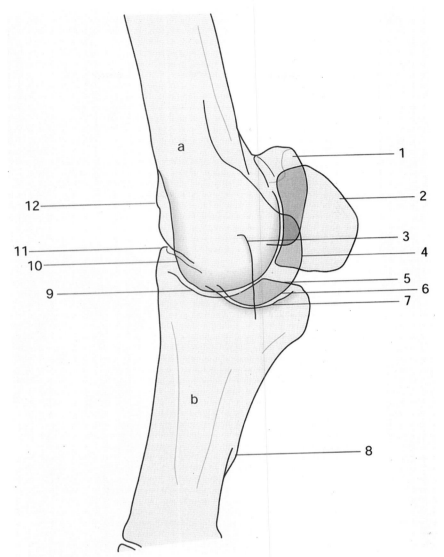

Figure 4.50   Lateroproximodorsal-mediodistopalmar oblique (L20Pr20D-MDiPaO) view of the fetlock. a, third metacarpal bone; b, proximal phalanx.

1. Medial proximal sesamoid bone.
2. Peripheral margin of the lateral proximal sesamoid bone.
3. Medial proximal palmar border of the proximal phalanx.
4. Lateral condyle of the third metacarpal bone.
5. Lateral palmar eminence of the proximal phalanx.
6. Lateral condyle (articular surface) of the third metacarpal bone.
7. Lateral articular fovea of the proximal phalanx.
8. Bony ridge for attachment of the middle (oblique) distal sesamiodean ligament.

9. Sagittal grove on the proximal articular surface of the proximal phalanx.
10. Distal surface of the sagittal ridge of the third metacarpal bone.
11. Medial articular margin of the articular fovea on the proximal phalanx.
12. Dorsal border of the medial condyle of the third metacarpal bone.

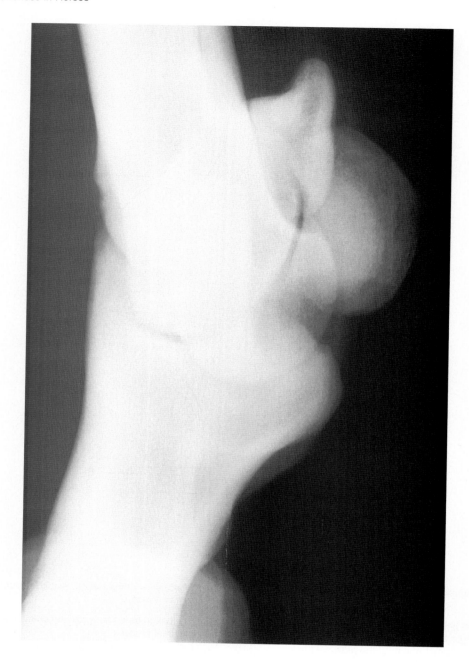

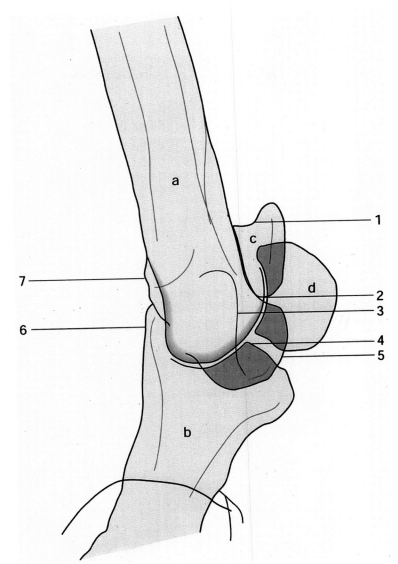

Figure 4.51 Lateroproximal-distomedial oblique (L45P-DiMO) view of the fetlock. a, third metacarpal bone; b, proximal phalanx; c, medial proximal sesamoid bone; d, lateral proximal sesamoid bone.

1. Abaxial surface of the medial proximal sesamoid bone.
2. Palmar surface of the sagittal ridge of the third metacarpal bone.
3. Medial proximal border of the proximal phalanx.
4. Lateral palmar eminence of the proximal phalanx.
5. Lateral condyle of the third metacarpal bone.
6. Proximal medial surface of the proximal phalanx.
7. Dorsal border of the medial condyle on the third metacarpal bone.

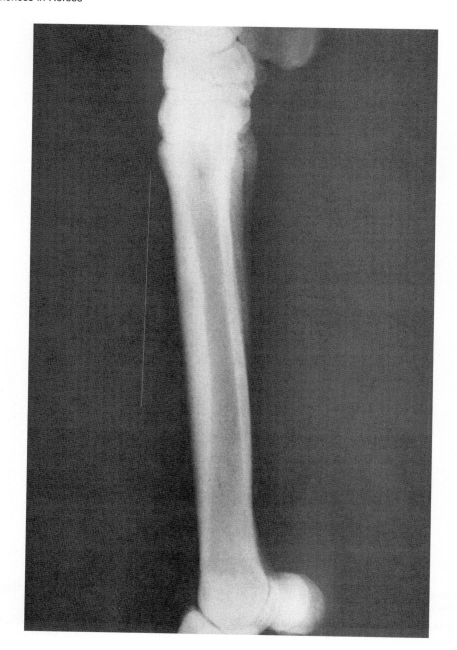

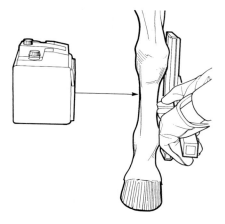

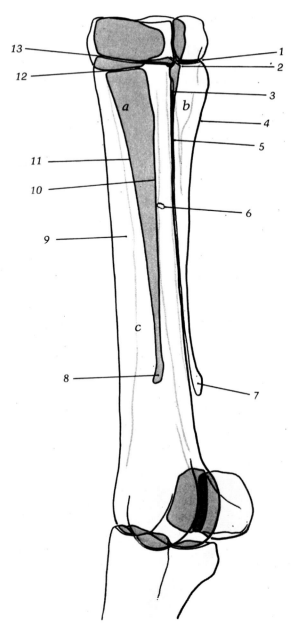

Figure 4.54   Dorsomedial-palmarolateral oblique (D55M-PaLO) view of the metacarpus. a, fourth metacarpal bone; b, second metacarpal bone; c, third metacarpal bone.

1. Articulation between the second carpal and the second metacarpal bone.
2. Proximal palmar medial angle of the third metacarpal bone.
3. Junction between the second and third metacarpal bones.
4,5. Palmar and dorsal borders, respectively, of the second metacarpal bone.
6. Nutrient foramen on the palmar surface of the third metacarpal bone.

7,8. Distal ends of the second and fourth metacarpal bones, respectively.
9. Dorsolateral cortex of the third metacarpal bone.
10,11. Palmar and dorsal surfaces, respectively, of the fourth metacarpal bone.
12. Articulation between the fourth carpal and the fourth metacarpal bone.
13. Articulation between the third carpal and the third metacarpal bone.

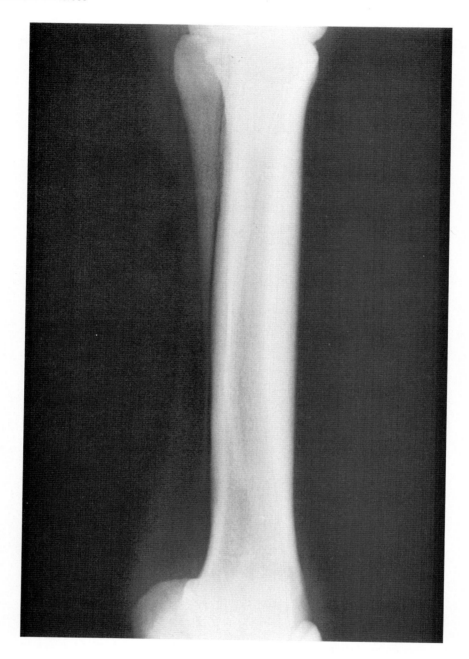

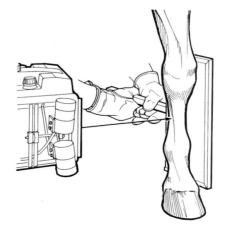

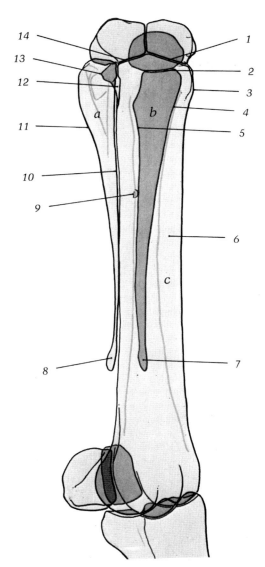

Figure 4.55 Dorsolateral-palmaromedial oblique (D55L-PaMO) view of the metacarpus. a, fourth metacarpal bone; b, second metacarpal bone; c, third metacarpal bone.

1. Articulation between the third carpal and the third metacarpal bone.
2. Articulation between the second carpal and the second metacarpal bone.
3. Metacarpal tuberosity on the dorsomedial surface of the proximal extremity of the third metacarpal bone.
4,5. Dorsal and palmar borders, respectively, of the second metacarpal bone.
6. Dorsomedial cortex of the third metacarpal bone. The dorsal cortex is normally thick, and the periosteal surface of the cortex should be straight and smooth.
7,8. Distal ends of the second and fourth metacarpal bones, respectively, which vary in size, shape, and position.

9. Nutrient foramen on the palmar surface of the third metacarpal bone, which may be prominent or not visualized, depending on its size and the projection.
10,11. Dorsal and palmar borders, respectively, of the fourth metacarpal bone.
12. Articulation between the third and fourth metacarpal bones, the visualization of which depends on the incident angle of the primary x-ray beam.
13. Proximal-palmar-lateral angle of the third metacarpal bone.
14. Articulation between the fourth carpal and the third metacarpal bone.

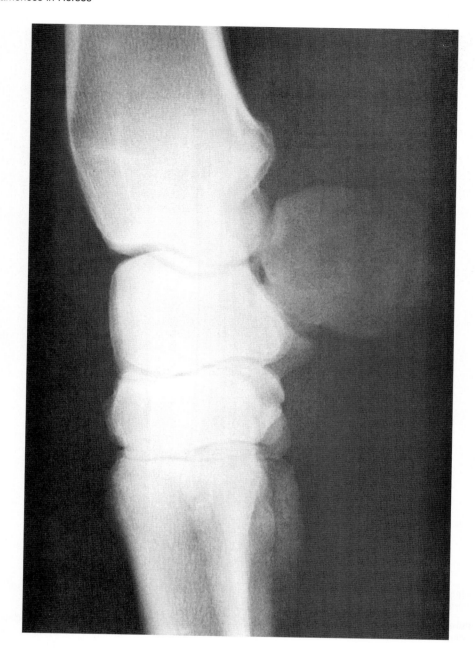

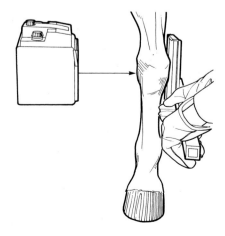

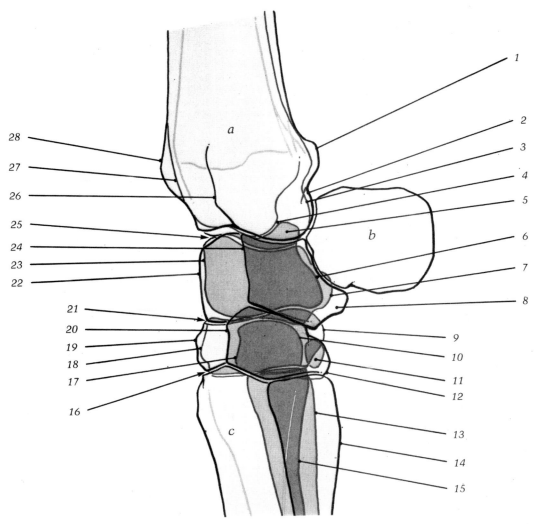

Figure 4.56   Lateromedial (LM) view of the carpus. The relative positions of the bony ridges of the distal cranial radius depend on the x-ray beam projection angle. a, radius; b, accessory carpal bone; c, third metacarpal bone.

1.   Transverse crest, which projects caudad from the closed distal radial physis.
2.   Lateral facet of the radial trochlea (lateral styloid process), which articulates with the ulnar carpal bone.
3.   Medial facet of the radial trochlea (medial styloid process), which articulates with the radial carpal bone.
4.   Intermediate facet of the radial trochlea, which articulates with the intermediate carpal bone.
5.   Tuberosity from the proximal palmar aspect of the intermediate carpal bone.
6–8.   Closely superimposed palmar borders of the intermediate, radial, and ulnar carpal bones, respectively. Their positions may change with slight changes in angulation of the x-ray tube or the horse's limb.
9,10,12.   Palmar borders of the third, second, and fourth carpal bones, respectively.
11.   First carpal bone, which sometimes is not present.
13–15.   Proximal palmar borders of the second, fourth, and third metacarpal bones, respectively.

16.   Carpometacarpal joint.
17,18,20.   Dorsal border of the second, third, and fourth carpal bones, respectively (distal row of carpal bones).
19.   Transverse ridge on the dorsal border of the third carpal bone, which projects with varying degrees of prominence in each horse.
21.   Midcarpal joint.
22–24.   Dorsal border of the radial, intermediate, and ulnar carpal bones, respectively (proximal row of carpal bones).
25.   Antebrachiocarpal (radiocarpal) joint.
26.   Lateral bony ridge of the distal cranial radius, adjacent to the common digital extensor tendon.
27.   Bony ridge of the distal cranial radius, adjacent to the medial border of the extensor carpi radialis tendon.
28.   Bony ridge of the distal cranial radius between the common digital extensor tendon and the extensor carpi radialis tendon.

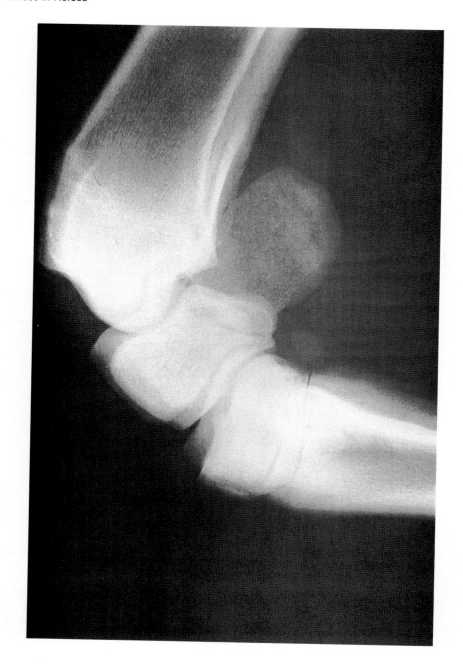

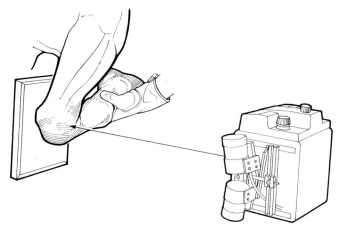

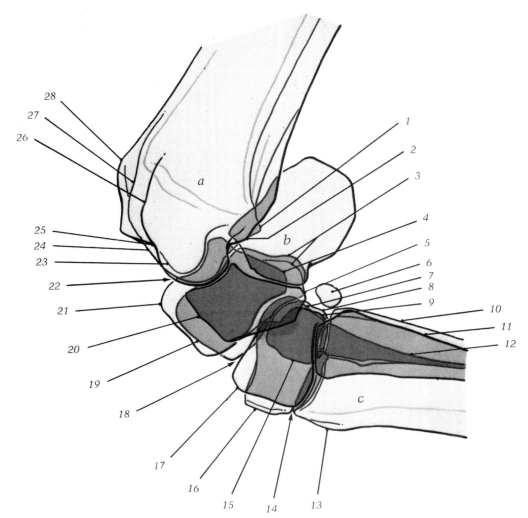

Figure 4.57 Flexed lateromedial (flexed LM) view of the carpus. The size and shape of the first and fifth carpal bones may vary, and sometimes the bones are absent. The palmar borders of the carpal and metacarpal bones are closely superimposed in this view, and their positions may vary slightly with x-ray tube angulation and/or the horse's limb position. Projection of the bony ridges and facets of the radial trochlea may vary with the position of the limb and the angle of the x-ray beam. a, radius; b, accessory carpal bone; c, third metacarpal bone.

1. Transverse crest, which projects from the caudal aspect of the closed distal radial physis.
2. Ridges produced by the caudal aspect of the medial (medial styloid process) and lateral (lateral styloid process) parts of the radial trochlea.
3–5. Palmar borders of the radial, intermediate, and ulnar carpal bones, respectively.
6. First carpal bone.
7–9. Palmar borders of the fourth, third, and second carpal bones, respectively.
10–12. Proximal palmar borders of the second, fourth, and third metacarpal bones, respectively.
13. Metacarpal tuberosity, which may vary in prominence.
14. Carpometacarpal joint. Numerous joint space lines are produced by the irregular contour of the bones forming this joint.
15–17. Dorsal borders of the second, third, and fourth carpal bones, respectively. The proximal dorsal aspect of the fourth carpal bone (17) projects proximal to the third carpal bone (16) on the flexed lateral view.

18. Middle carpal joint.
19–21. Dorsal borders of the radial, ulnar, and intermediate carpal bones, respectively. The dorsal borders of the radial (19) and intermediate (21) carpal bones are closely superimposed and may vary slightly. The intermediate carpal bone usually projects proximal to the radial carpal bone on the flexed lateral view.
22. Antebrachiocarpal (radiocarpal) joint.
23. Intermediate facet of the radial trochlea, which articulates with the intermediate carpal bone (21).
24,25. Medial and lateral borders, respectively, of the radial trochlea.
26. Lateral bony ridge adjacent to the lateral border of the common digital extensor tendon.
27. Bony ridge adjacent to the medial border of the extensor carpi radialis.
28. Bony ridge between the lateral digital extensor tendon and the extensor carpi radialis tendon.

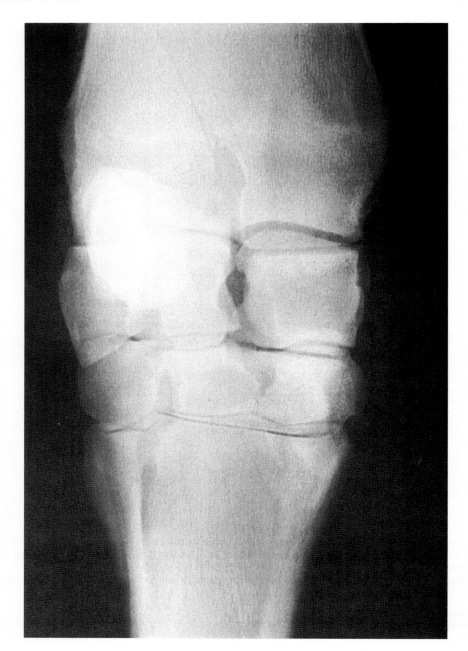

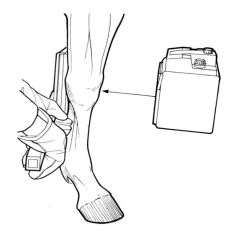

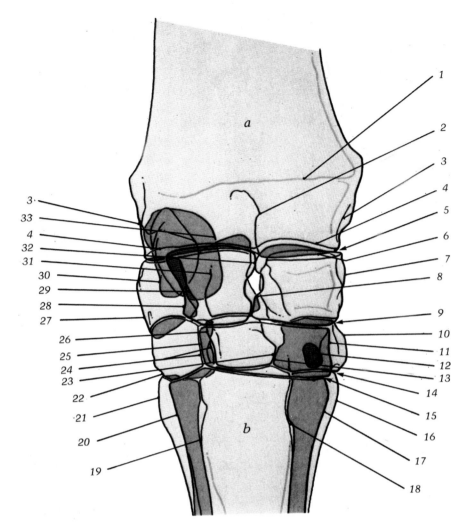

Figure 4.58 Dorsopalmar (DPa) view of the carpus. a, radius; b, third metacarpal bone.

1. Physeal scar in the distal extremity of the radius after physeal closure.
2. Caudolateral border of the medial facet (medial styloid process) on the radial trochlea.
3. Depressions in the medial and lateral styloid processes for attachment of medial and lateral collateral ligaments. Their appearances and apparent depths can change with a slight obliqueness of the limb.
4. Cranial articular margin on the distal radius.
5. Antebrachiocarpal (radiocarpal) joint.
6. Medial facet (medial styloid process) on the distal radial trochlea, which articulates with the radial carpal bone (7 and 8).
7,8. Medial and lateral borders, respectively, of the radial carpal bone.
9. Midcarpal joint. The different levels of the joint space are the result of many bones forming the articular surfaces and of slight angulation of the x-ray tube or position of the horse's limb.
10. Medial border of the second carpal bone.
11. Dorsomedial border of the third carpal bone.
12. First carpal bone superimposed over the second and third carpal bones.
13. Lateral border of the second carpal bone.
14,15. Palmar and dorsal aspects, respectively, of the carpometacarpal joint space.

16,17. Proximomedial borders of the second and third metacarpal bones, respectively.
18. Articulation between the second and third metacarpal bones.
19. Articulation between the third and fourth metacarpal bones.
20,21. The lateral borders of the third and fourth metacarpal bones, respectively.
22. Lateral border of the fourth carpal bone.
23. Medial border of the palmar process on the third carpal bone.
24. Medial border of the fourth carpal bone.
25. Dorsolateral border of the third carpal bone.
26. Lateral border of the palmar process on the third carpal bone.
27,28. Lateral borders of the ulnar and intermediate carpal bones, respectively.
29. Medial border of the ulnar carpal bone.
30. Lateral border of the accessory carpal bone.
31. Lateral border of the palmar tuberosity on the intermediate carpal bone.
32. Medial border of the intermediate carpal bone.
33. Concave medial surface of the accessory carpal bone.

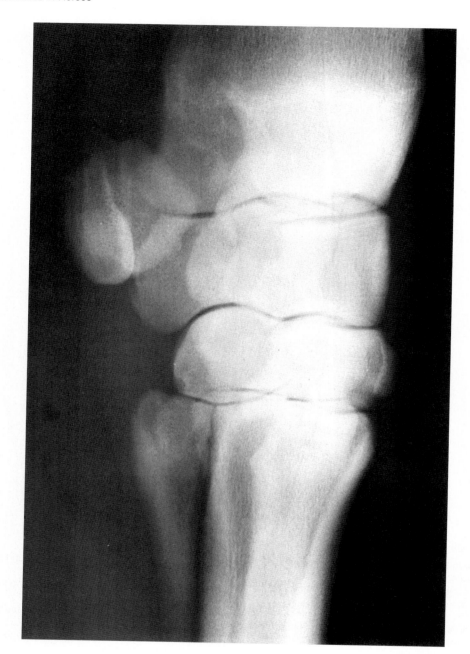

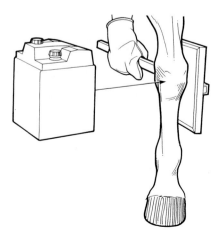

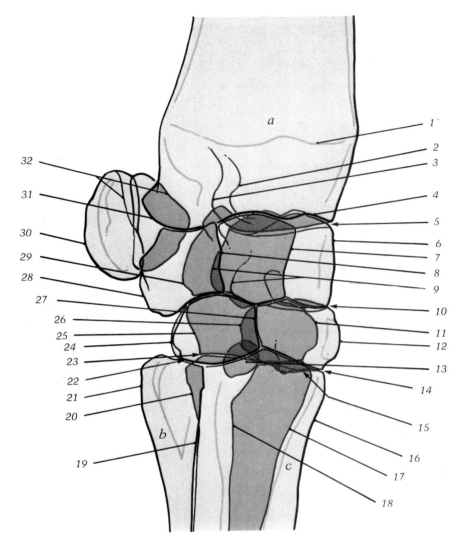

Figure 4.59 Dorsolateral-palmaromedial oblique (D45L-PaMO) view of the carpus. a, radius; b, fourth metacarpal bone; c, third metacarpal bone.

1. Physeal scar remaining after distal radial physeal closure.
2. Caudal aspect of the intermediate facet on the radial trochlea.
3. Caudal aspect of the medial facet (medial styloid process) on the radial trochlea.
4. Cranial articular margin on the radial trochlea.
5. Dorsomedial aspect of the antebrachiocarpal (radiocarpal) joint.
6–8. Dorsomedial borders of the radial, intermediate, and ulnar carpal bones, respectively.
9. Tubercles on the palmar surface of the radiocarpal bone.
10. Dorsomedial aspect of the midcarpal joint.
11. Dorsomedial border of the second carpal bone.
12. Transverse ridge on the dorsomedial border of the third carpal bone.
13. First carpal bone, which is difficult to see on this view because of superimposition.
14,15. Medial and dorsal aspects, respectively, of the carpometacarpal joint. The multiple joint spaces are associated with the carpometacarpal joint and vary in appearance on different projection angles.

16,17. Dorsomedial borders of the third and second metacarpal bones, respectively.
18. Palmarolateral border of the second metacarpal bone.
19. Dorsomedial border of the fourth metacarpal bone.
20, 21. Palmarolateral borders of the third and fourth metacarpal bones, respectively.
22. Palmarolateral aspect of the carpometacarpal joint between the fourth carpal bone and the third and fourth metacarpal bones.
23. Palmar aspect of the carpometacarpal joint between the third carpal and the third metacarpal bone.
24. Tubercle on the palmarolateral border of the fourth carpal bone.
25,26. Palmarolateral borders of the third and second carpal bones.
27. Dorsomedial border of the fourth carpal bone.
28–30. Palmarolateral borders of the ulnar, intermediate, and accessory carpal bones, respectively.
31. Lateral facet (lateral styloid process) on the radial trochlea.
32. Medial, concave surface of the accessory carpal bone.

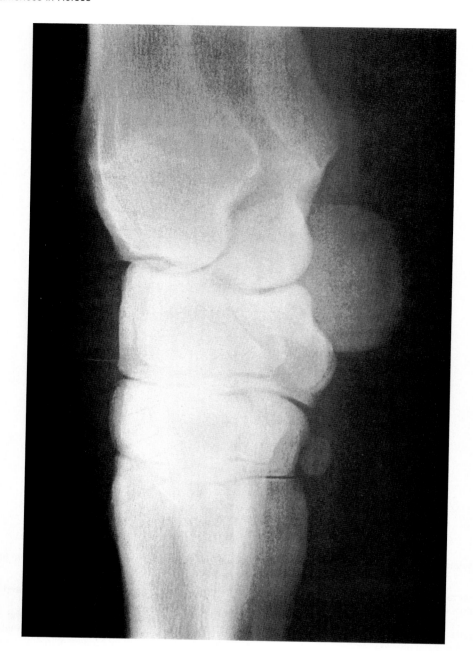

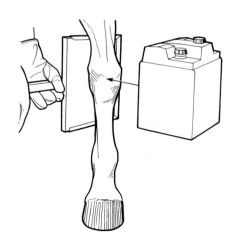

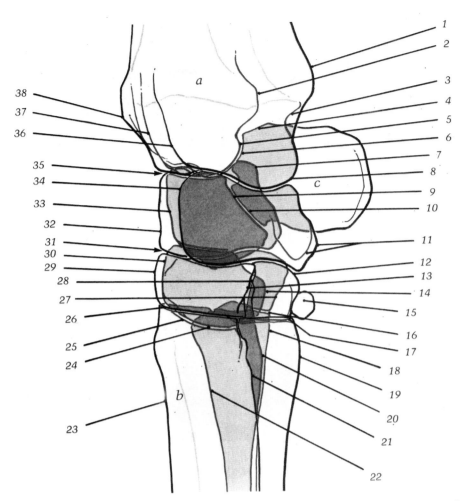

Figure 4.60 Dorsomedial-palmarolateral oblique (D30M-PaLO) view of the carpus. The relative positions of the bony ridges on the distocranial aspect of the radius change slightly with different x-ray beam projections. a, radius; b, third metacarpal bone; c, accessory carpal bone.

1. Bony projection from the mediocaudal surface of the radius.
2. Transverse crest proximal to the lateral facet (lateral styloid process) of the radial trochlea.
3. Indentation proximal to the medial facet (medial styloid process) of the radial trochlea.
4. Proximal border of the accessory carpal bone.
5. Caudal borders of the lateral and intermediate facets of the radial trochlea superimposed.
6. Proximal articular surface of the accessory carpal bone.
7. Palmaromedial border of the intermediate carpal bone.
8. Medial facet (medial styloid process) of the radial trochlea.
9. Palmaromedial border of the ulnar carpal bone.
10. Distal articular surface of the accessory carpal bone.
11–14. Palmaromedial borders of the radial, second, third, and fourth carpal bones, respectively.
15. First carpal bone.
16. Carpometacarpal articulation between the third carpal and the third metacarpal bone.
17. Carpometacarpal articulation between the second carpal and the second metacarpal bone.
18–20. Palmaromedial borders of the third, second, and fourth metacarpal bones, respectively.

21–23. Dorsolateral borders of the second, fourth, and third metacarpal bones, respectively.
24. Carpometacarpal articulation between the fourth carpal and the fourth metacarpal bone.
25. Carpometacarpal articulation between the fourth carpal and the third metacarpal bone.
26. Carpometacarpal articulation between the third carpal and the third metacarpal bone.
27. Palmaromedial border of the third carpal bone.
28–30. Dorsal borders of the second, third, and fourth metacarpal bones, respectively.
31. Dorsolateral aspect of the midcarpal joint.
32–34. Dorsal borders of the intermediate, ulnar, and radial carpal bones, respectively. The relative position and appearance of these borders may change with slight projection differences of the x-ray beam.
35. Antebrachiocarpal (radiocarpal) joint.
36. Bony ridge forming the medial border of the groove for the common digital extensor tendon.
37. Bony ridge along the lateral border of the extensor carpi radialis tendon.
38. Bony ridge between the grooves for the common digital extensor and extensor carpi radialis tendons.

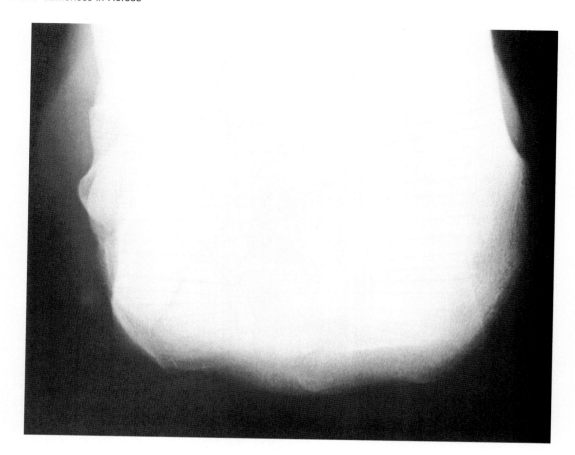

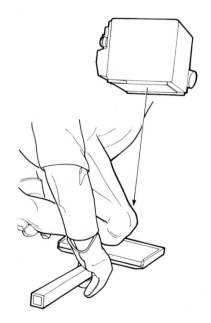

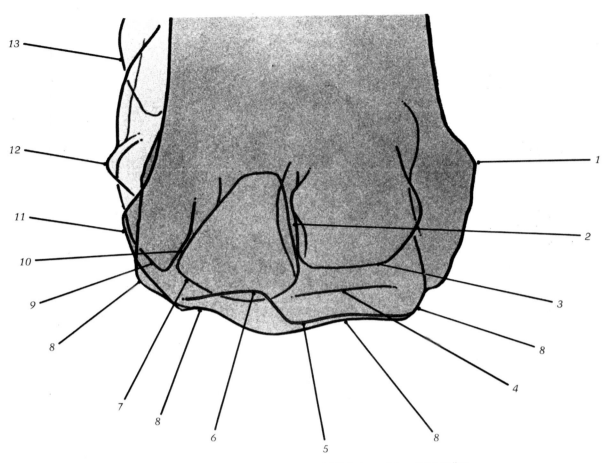

Figure 4.61 Flexed dorsoproximal-dorsodistal oblique (flexed D80Pr-DDiO) view of the distal radius.

1. Tuberosity on the distomedial aspect of the radius for attachment of the medial collateral ligament.
2. Junction between the radial and intermediate carpal bones.
3. Dorsal border of the radial carpal bone.
4. Dorsoproximal border of the radial carpal bone.
5. Medial facet (medial styloid process) of the radial trochlea.
6. Intermediate facet of the radial trochlea.
7. Dorsal border of the intermediate carpal bone.

8. Dorsal articular margin of the radial trochlea.
9. Dorsal border of the ulnar carpal bone.
10. Junction between the ulnar and intermediate carpal bones.
11. Tuberosity on the distal lateral radius for attachment of the lateral collateral ligament.
12. Lateral border of the accessory carpal bone.
13. Proximolateral border of the fourth metacarpal bone.

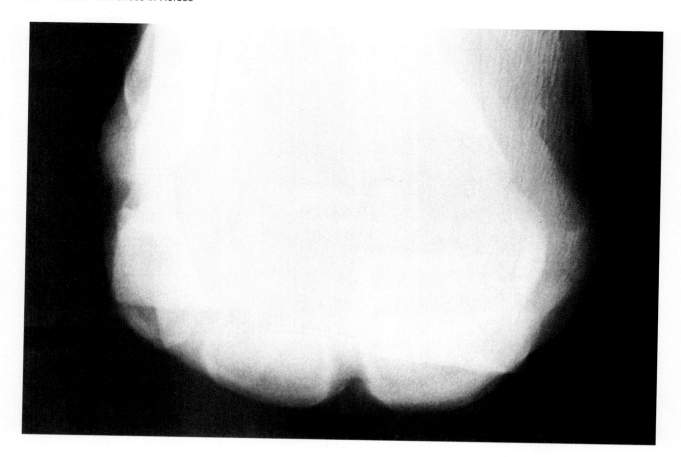

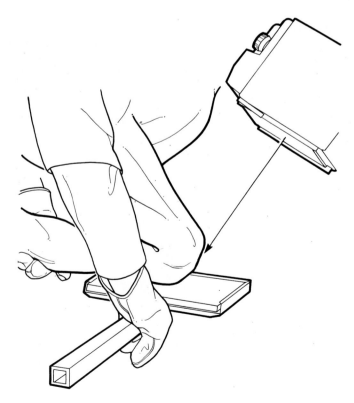

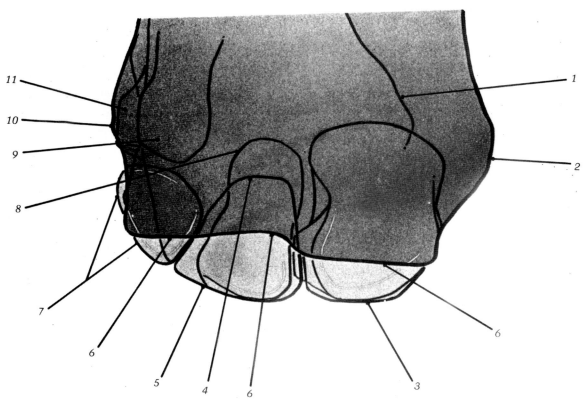

Figure 4.62 Flexed dorsoproximal-dorsodistal oblique (flexed D55Pr-DDiO) view of the proximal carpal bones. The position of the distal extremity of the radius relative to the proximal carpal bones varies with the position of the horse's limb and the angulation of the primary x-ray beam. Slight changes in either may cause different degrees of superimposition of the radius and carpal bones.

1. Medial border of the second metacarpal bone.
2. Tuberosity on the distomedial aspect of the radius for attachment of the medial collateral ligament.
3. Dorsal border of the radial carpal bone.
4. Proximopalmar border of the intermediate carpal bone.
5. Dorsal border of the intermediate carpal bone.
6. Radial trochlea.
7. Dorsolateral border of the ulnar carpal bone.
8. Palmarodistal border of the intermediate carpal bone.
9. Proximal aspect of the fourth metacarpal bone.
10. Lateral tuberosity on the distal extremity of the radius for attachment of the lateral collateral ligament.
11. Accessory carpal bone.

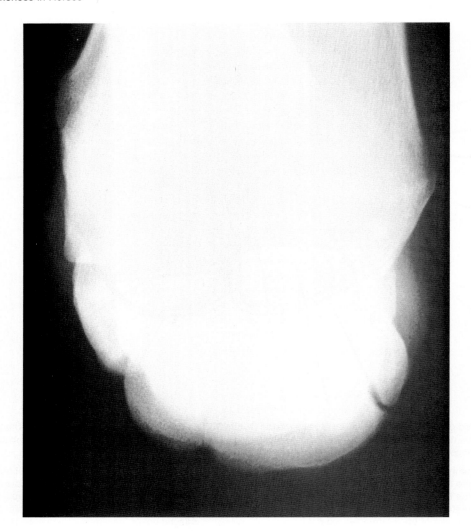

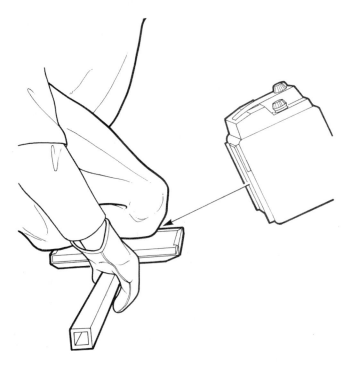

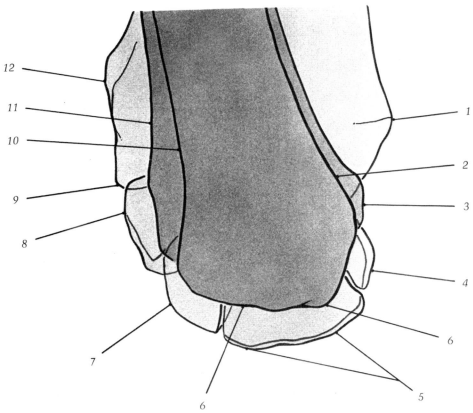

Figure 4.63 Flexed dorsoproximal-dorsodistal oblique (Flexed D30Pr-DDiO) view of the distal carpal bones. The apparent shape of the third carpal bone may be changed by x-ray tube angulation and the position of the horse's limb and may appear more elongated than shown here. The dorsal cortex and medullary cavity should be evident on the medial aspect of the normal third carpal bone if properly positioned.

1. Medial tuberosity on the distal radius for attachment of the medial collateral ligament.
2. Medial border of the third metacarpal bone.
3. Medial border of the second metacarpal bone.
4. Second carpal bone.
5. Dorsal border of the third carpal bone.
6. Superimposed dorsal border of the proximal carpal bones and the third metacarpal bone.
7. Fourth carpal bone.
8. Lateral border of the accessory carpal bone.
9. Lateral aspect (lateral styloid process) of the radial trochlea.
10. Lateral border of the third metacarpal bone.
11. Lateral border of the fourth metacarpal bone.
12. Lateral tuberosity on the distal extremity of the radius for attachment of the lateral collateral ligament.

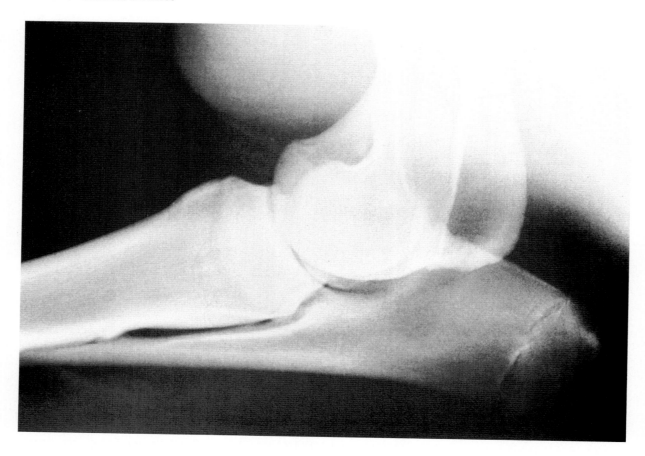

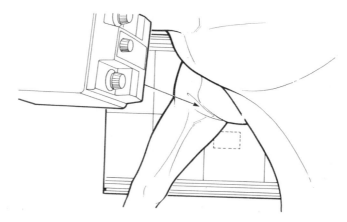

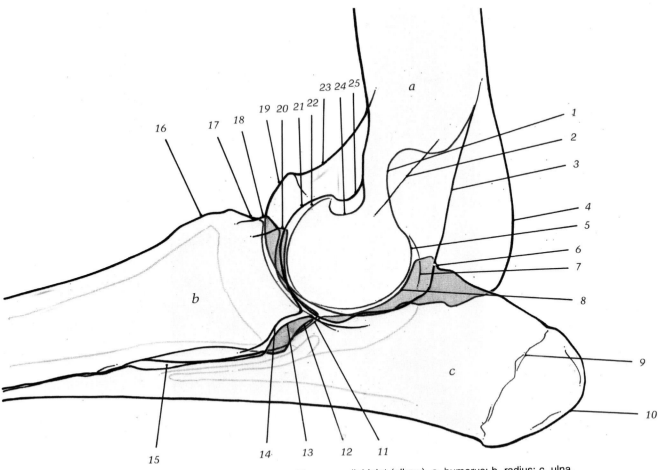

Figure 4.64 Mediolateral (ML) view of the humeroulnar and humeroradial joint (elbow). a, humerus; b, radius; c, ulna.

1. Floor of the olecranon fossa.
2. Lateral supracondylar crest on the distal extremity of the humerus.
3,4. Lateral and medial epicondyles of the distal humerus, respectively.
5. Sagittal trochlear groove on the medial humeral condyle.
6. Anconeal process of the ulna.
7. Articular surface of the trochlea (medial condyle) on the humerus.
8. Trochlear notch (ulnar articular surface).
9. Growth plate (physis) in the proximal ulna.
10. Olecranon tuberosity.
11. Medial aspect of the coronoid process of the ulna.
12. Middle caudal border of the radial head.

13. Lateral aspect of the coronoid process of the ulna.
14. Laterocaudal border of the radial head.
15. Interosseous space between the radius and ulna.
16. Radial tuberosity.
17. Craniomedial border of the radial head.
18. Midcranial border of the radial head.
19. Trochlea (medial condyle) of the humerus.
20. Cranial lateral border of the radial head.
21. Capitulum of the humerus.
22. Cranial surface (floor) of the sagittal groove on the trochlea of the humerus.
23. Medial border of the radial fossa.
24. Floor of the radial fossa.
25. Lateral border of the radial fossa.

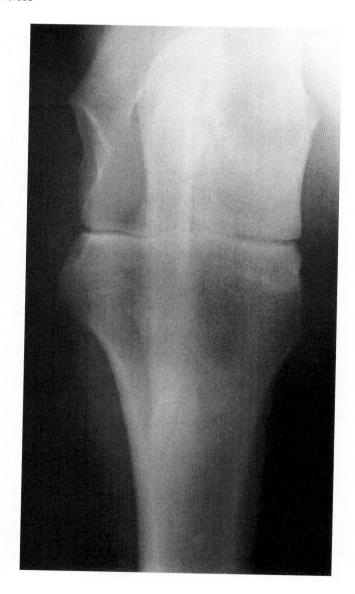

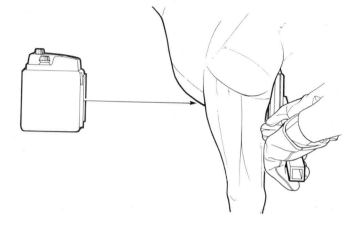

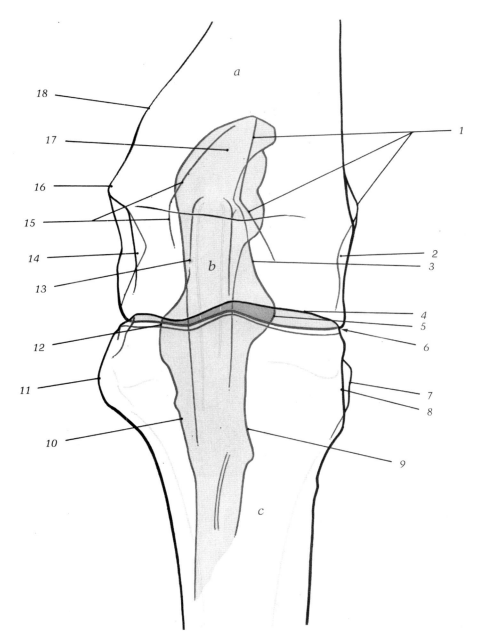

Figure 4.65 Craniocaudal (CrCa) view of the humeroulnar and humeroradial joint (elbow). a, humerus; b, ulna; c, radius.

1. Medial epicondyle of the humerus, which is large and superimposed over the distal extremity of the humerus except for a slight convex projection on the distal medial humerus where the medial collateral ligament attaches.
2. Depression on the distomedial aspect of the humerus.
3. Medial border of the trochlear notch on the ulna.
4. Caudal margin of the capitular fovea (proximal radial articulation).
5. Medial aspect of the coronoid process of the ulna.
6. Humeroradial articulations.
7. Radial tuberosity.
8. Medial tuberosity of the radius for collateral ligament attachment.

9,10. Medial and lateral borders of the ulna, respectively.
11. Lateral tuberosity of the radius for collateral ligament attachment.
12. Lateral aspect of the coronoid process of the ulna.
13. Lateral border of the trochlear notch on the ulna.
14. Depression for attachment of the lateral collateral ligament.
15. Lateral border of the olecranon fossa.
16. Lateral epicondyle of the humerus.
17. Olecranon tuberosity of the ulna.
18. Lateral supracondylar crest.

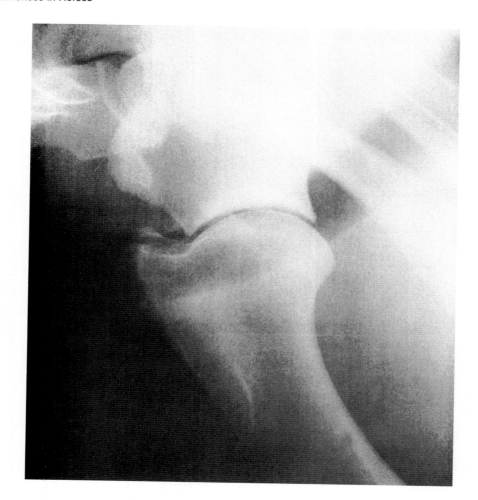

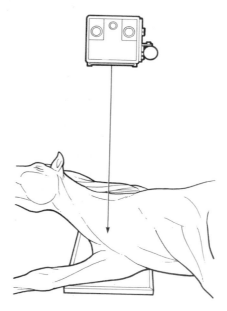

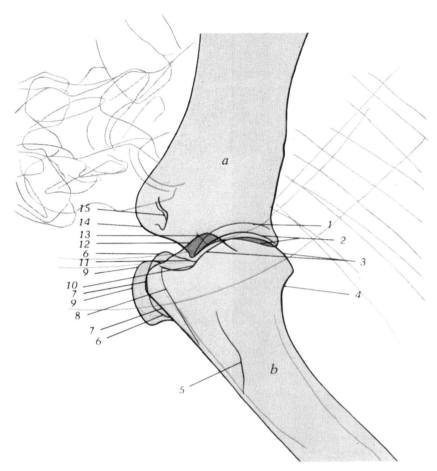

Figure 4.66 Mediolateral (ML) view of the scapulohumeral joint (shoulder). a, scapula; b, humerus.

1. Subchondral bone on the concave surface of the glenoid cavity.
2. Medial and lateral borders of the glenoid cavity.
3. Cranial and caudal borders of the humeral head.
4. Caudal border of the humeral neck.
5. Deltoid tuberosity superimposed on the humerus.
6. Proximal and distocranial borders of the lesser (medial) tubercle.
7. Cranial border of the greater (lateral) tubercle.
8. Floor of the intertuberal groove between the lateral and intermediate tubercles.
9. Intermediate tubercle.
10. Fossa between the tubercles and the humeral head.
11. Caudal part of the lesser (medial) tubercle.
12. Caudal part of the greater (lateral) tubercle.
13. Glenoid notch, which is more or less apparent, depending on the x-ray beam projection angle and development in the horse.
14. Supraglenoid tubercle.
15. Coracoid process.

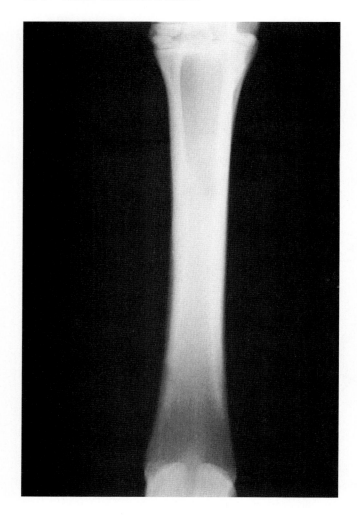

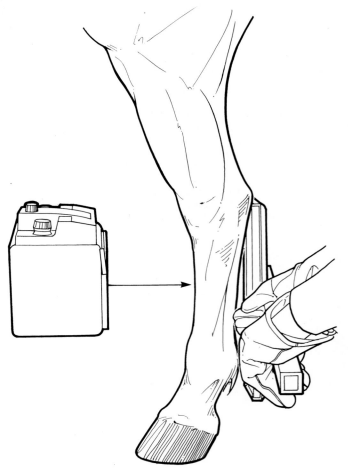

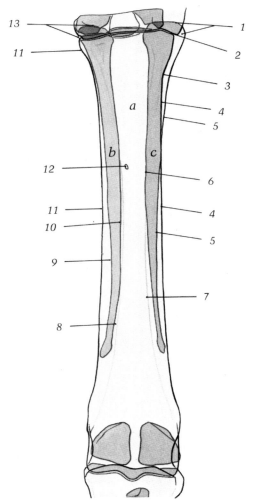

Figure 4.67   Dorsoplantar (DPI) view of the metatarsus. a, third metatarsal bone; b, second metatarsal bone; c, fourth metatarsal bone.

1.   Proximal extremity (base) of the fourth metatarsal bone, which is larger than the second metatarsal bone and is superimposed over the third and fourth tarsal bones.
2.   Articulation between the fourth tarsal and the third metatarsal bone.
3.   Lateral surface of the third metatarsal bone.
4.   Abaxial surface of the fourth metatarsal bone.
5.   Axial surface of the fourth metatarsal bone.
6.   Axial surface of the fourth metatarsal bone.
7.   Endosteal surface on the lateral cortex of the third metatarsal bone.

8.   Endosteal surface on the medial cortex of the third metatarsal bone.
9,10.   Abaxial and axial surfaces, respectively, of the second metatarsal bone.
11.   Medial surface of the third metatarsal bone.
12.   Nutrient foramen on the plantar surface of the third metatarsal bone.
13.   Proximal extremity (base) of the second metatarsal bone, which is superimposed over the fused first and second tarsal bones and the third tarsal bone.

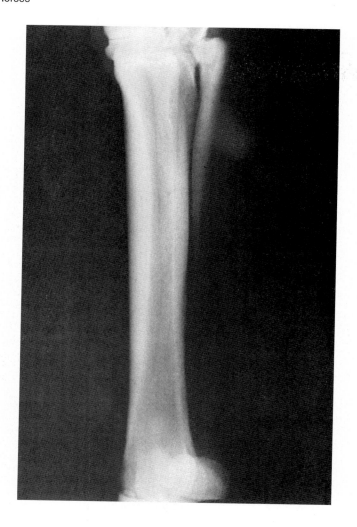

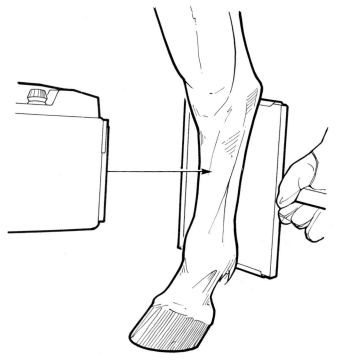

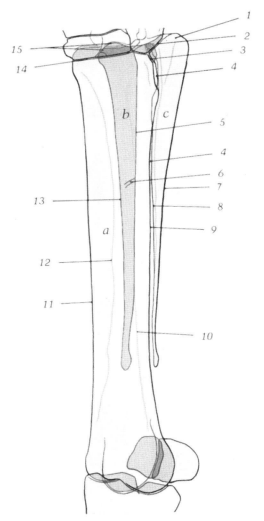

Figure 4.68 Dorsolateral-plantaromedial oblique (D45L-PIMO) view of the metatarsus. a, third metatarsal bone; b, second metatarsal bone; c, fourth metatarsal bone.

1. Proximal extremity (base) of fourth metatarsal bone.
2. Articulation between the fourth metatarsal and the fourth tarsal bone.
3. Articulation between the fourth and third metatarsal bones.
4. Interosseous space between the third and fourth metatarsal bones.
5. Plantarolateral border of second metatarsal bone.
6. Nutrient foramen on the plantar surface of third metatarsal bone.
7. Plantarolateral border of fourth metatarsal bone.
8. Dorsomedial border of fourth metatarsal bone.
9. Plantarolateral border of third metatarsal bone.
10. Endosteal surface on the plantarolateral cortex of third metatarsal bone.
11. Dorsomedial surface of third metatarsal bone.
12. Endosteal surface on the dorsomedial cortex of third metatarsal bone.
13. Dorsomedial surface of second metatarsal bone.
14. Articulation between the third tarsal and the third metatarsal bone.
15. Proximal extremity (base) of the second metatarsal bone superimposed over the distal tarsal bones.

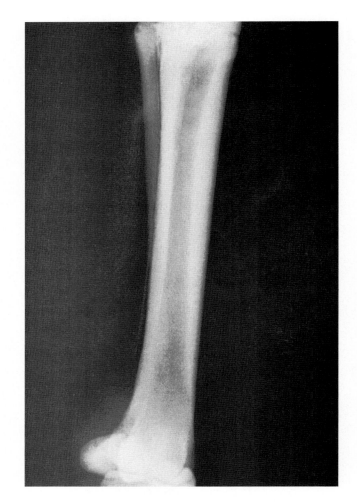

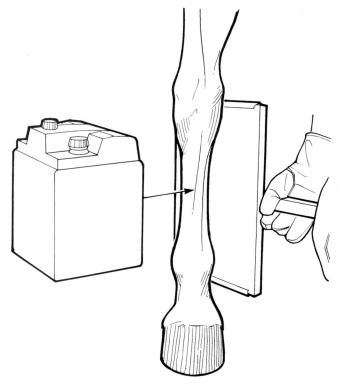

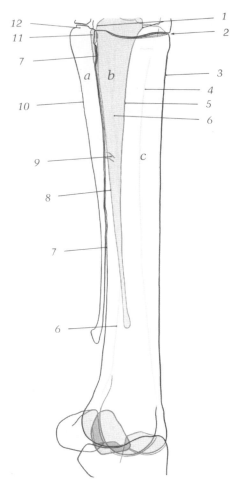

Figure 4.69   Dorsomedial-plantarolateral oblique (D45M-PILO) view of the metatarsus. a, second metatarsal bone; b, fourth metatarsal bone; c, third metatarsal bone.

1. Proximal extremity (base) of the fourth metatarsal bone.
2. Articulation between the third tarsal and the third metatarsal bone.
3. Dorsolateral surface of the third metatarsal bone.
4. Endosteal surface on the dorsolateral cortex of the third metatarsal bone.
5. Dorsolateral surface of the fourth metatarsal bone.
6. Endosteal surface on the plantar medial cortex of the third metatarsal bone.

7. Interosseous space between the second and third metatarsal bones.
8. Plantaromedial surface of the fourth metatarsal bone.
9. Nutrient foramen on the plantar surface of the third metatarsal bone.
10. Plantaromedial surface of the second metatarsal bone.
11. Articulation between the second and third metatarsal bones.
12. Proximal extremity (base) of the second metatarsal bone.

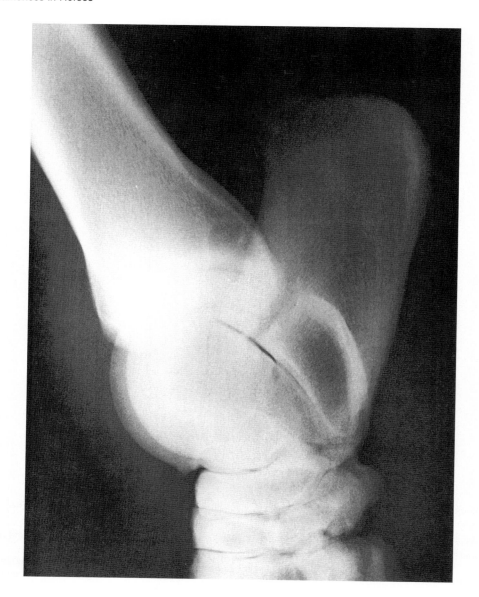

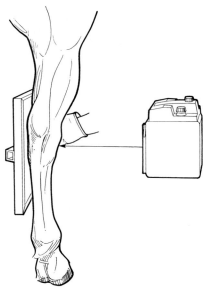

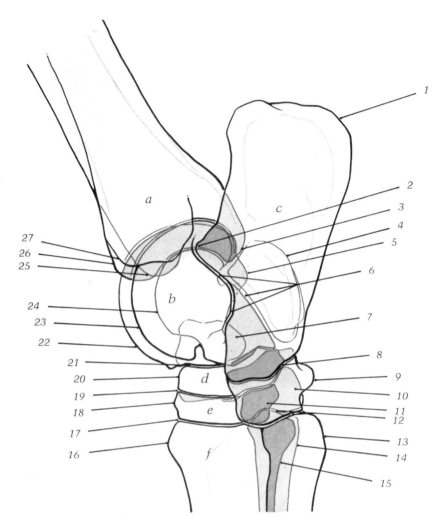

Figure 4.70 Lateromedial (LM) view of the tarsus. Depending on obliquity of the radiographic projection, the cranial borders of the malleoli and trochlear ridges may be in different relative positions. a, tibia; b, talus; c, calcaneus; d, central tarsal bone; e, third tarsal bone; f, third metatarsal bone.

1. Calcaneal tuber.
2. Coracoid process of the calcaneus.
3. Caudal intermediate part of the tibial cochlea.
4. Sustentaculum tall of the calcaneus.
5. Proximomedial tuberosity of the talus for ligamentous attachments (superficial short medial collateral ligament).
6. Articulation between the talus and the calcaneus. All of these joint surfaces may not be distinguishable on any one radiograph; they should not be mistaken for fractures.
7. Distomedial tuberosity of the talus for ligamentous attachment (dorsal tarsal ligament).
8. Articulation between the calcaneus and the fourth tarsal bone.
9. Plantar surface of the fourth tarsal bone.
10. Second tarsal bone. The first and second tarsal bones are fused and project as different densities because of superimposition.
11. First tarsal bone.
12. Plantar aspect of the tarsometatarsal articulations.
13. Plantar border of the fourth metatarsal bone. The fourth metatarsal bone is larger than the second metatarsal bone and projects on the plantar surface.

14,15. Plantar borders of the second and third metatarsal bones, respectively.
16. Dorsoproximal ridge on the third metatarsal bone for attachment of the tibialis cranialis.
17. Articulation between the third tarsal and the third metatarsal bone.
18. Dorsal border of the third tarsal bone.
19. Articulation between the third and central tarsal bones.
20. Dorsal border of the central tarsal bone.
21. Articulation between the central tarsal bone and the talus.
22. Medial trochlear ridge of the talus. The small bony projection on the distal part of the medial trochlear ridge is variable in size and shape and should not be mistaken for a periarticular osteophyte or any other bony abnormality.
23. Lateral trochlear ridge of the talus.
24. Depth of the trochlear groove between the trochlear ridge on the talus.

25,27. Distocranial borders of the medial and lateral tibial malleoli, respectively.
26. Cranial intermediate part of the tibial cochlea.

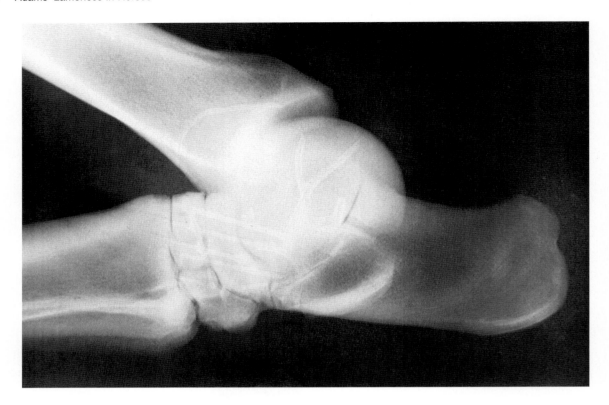

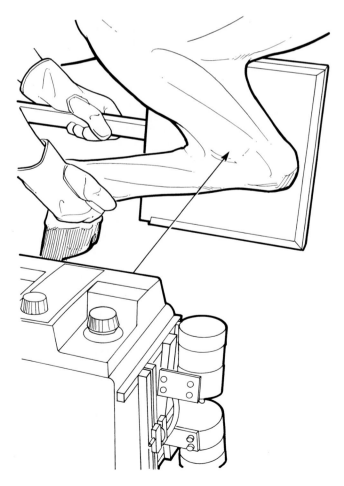

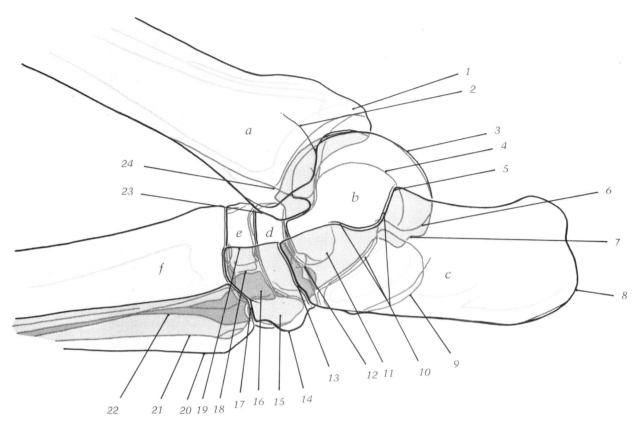

Figure 4.71   Flexed lateromedial (flexed LM) view of the tarsus. a, tibia; b, talus; c, calcaneus; d, central tarsal bone; e, third tarsal bone; f, third metatarsal bone.

1. Caudal intermediate part of the tibial cochlea.
2. Distocaudal border of the lateral tibial malleolus.
3. Superimposed medial and lateral trochlear ridges of the talus.
4. Depth of the trochlear groove between the trochlear ridges of the talus.
5. Coracoid process of the calcaneus.
6,7. Plantar borders of the lateral and medial trochlear ridges, respectively, on the talus.
8. Calcaneal tuber.
9. Sustentaculum tali.
10. Articulations between the talus and calcaneus, the visualization of which depends on the projection angle.
11. Distomedial tuberosity of the talus for ligamentous attachment (dorsal tarsal ligament).
12. Articulation between the talus and the central tarsal bone.
13. Articulation between the calcaneus and the fourth tarsal bone.

14. Plantar border of the fourth tarsal bone.
15. Second tarsal bone. The first and second tarsal bones are fused.
16. First tarsal bone.
17. Tarsometatarsal articulation.
18. Junction between the first and third tarsal bones, which is not always distinctly visible. Do not mistake the junction, when present, for a slab fracture.
19. Dorsal border of the fourth tarsal bone.
20–22. Plantar borders of the fourth, second, and third metatarsal bones, respectively. The superimposed plantar border of the third metatarsal bone and the dorsal borders of the second and fourth metatarsal bones may produce pseudolongitudinal fracture lines.
23. Cranial intermediate part of the tibial cochlea.
24. Cranial border of the medial tibial malleolus.

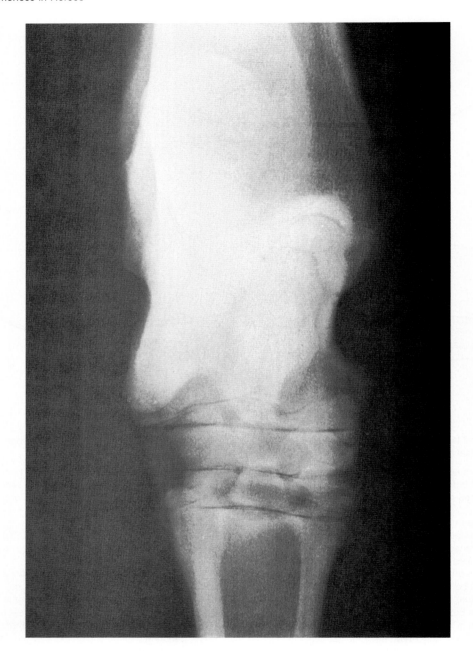

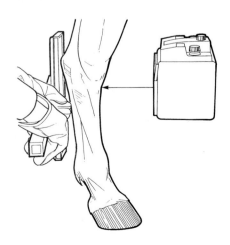

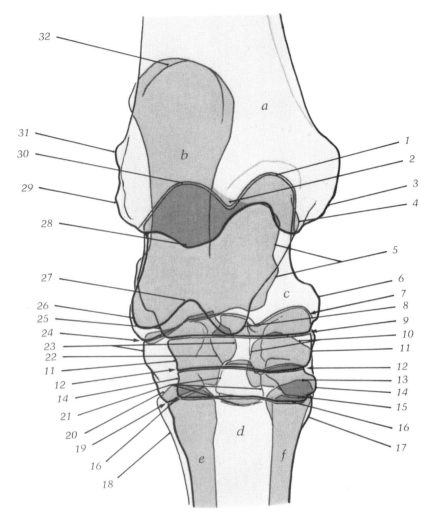

Figure 4.72 Dorsoplantar (DPI) view of the tarsus. The bones and joints of the tarsus are irregular and have complex shapes; thus, their appearance can vary with little change in projection angle. Because of this, careful observation is necessary when the tarsus is being evaluated radiographically. a, tibia; b, calcaneus; c, talus; d, third metatarsal bone; e, fourth metatarsal bone; f, second metatarsal bone.

1. Articulation between the medial trochlear ridge of the talus and the medial cochlear groove of the tibia (tarsocrural joint).
2. Intermediate ridge of the tibial cochlea.
3. Medial malleolus on the distal tibia, where the medial collateral ligaments attach.
4. Proximal medial tuberosity on the talus, where the superficial short medial collateral ligament attaches.
5. Sustentaculum tali.
6. Distal medial tuberosity on talus for ligamentous attachment.
7. Plantar medial aspect of the talocalcaneocentral (proximal intertarsal) joint.
8. Distomedial border of the medial trochlear ridge on the talus.
9. Dorsomedial aspect of the talocalcaneal central (proximal intertarsal) joint. The difference in position of the plantar and dorsal aspects of this joint is caused by the curved contour of the articular surfaces in the proximal intertarsal joint.
10. Medial and lateral borders of the second tarsal bone.
11. Medial and lateral borders of the central tarsal bone.
12. Articulation between the third and central tarsal bones (centrodistal or distal intertarsal joint).
13. Proximal border of the second metatarsal bone superimposed on the first and third tarsal bones.
14. Medial and lateral borders of the third tarsal bone.
15. Articulation between the second metatarsal and the fused first and second tarsal bones.
16. Medial and lateral aspects of the articulation between the third tarsal and the third metatarsal bone.
17. Proximomedial border of the second metatarsal bone.
18. Proximolateral border of the fourth metatarsal bone.
19. Articulation between the fourth tarsal and the fourth metatarsal bone (tarsometatarsal joint).
20. Proximal border of the fourth metatarsal bone superimposed over the fourth tarsal bone.
21. Bony prominence on the plantar surface of the third tarsal bone.
22. Prominence on the plantar surface of the central tarsal bone.
23. Lateral and medial borders of the fourth tarsal bone.
24. Articulation of the fourth tarsal bone and the calcaneus (calcaneoquartal or proximal intertarsal joint).
25. Distal lateral border of the talus.
26. Lateral trochlear ridge of the talus.
27. Groove between medial and lateral trochlear ridges on the talus.
28. Caudal aspect of the intermediate ridge on the tibial cochlea.
29. Cranial part of the lateral malleolus.
30. Articulation between the lateral trochlear ridge on the talus and the lateral tibial cochlear groove in the tarsocrural (tibiotarsal) joint.
31. Caudal part of the lateral malleolus.
32. Calcaneal tuber.

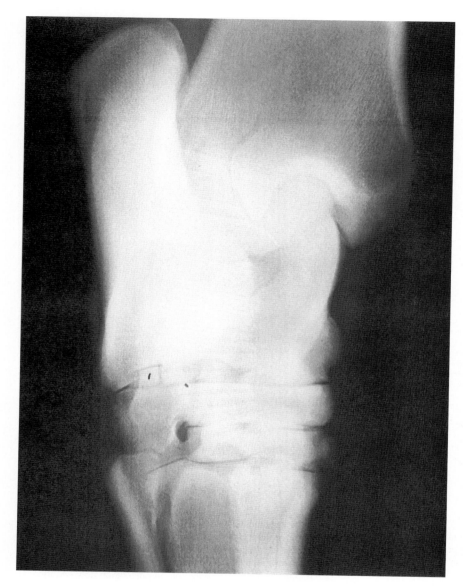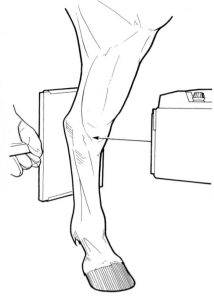

Figure 4.73 Dorsolateral-plantaromedial oblique (D35L-PlMO) view of the tarsus. a, tibia; b, calcaneus; c, talus; d, third metatarsal bone; e, fourth metatarsal bone; f, second metatarsal bone

1. Articulation between the medial trochlear ridge of the talus and the medial tibial cochlear groove in the tarsocrural (tibiotarsal) joint.
2. Medial malleolus.
3. Articulation between the intermediate ridge of the tibial cochlea and the groove in the trochlea tali in the tarsocrural joint.
4. Cranial aspect of the intermediate ridge on the tibial cochlea.
5. Caudal aspect of the intermediate ridge on the tibial cochlea.
6,7. Medial and lateral trochlear ridges, respectively, of the talus.
8. Dorsomedial border of the sustentaculum tali.
9. Distomedial tuberosity of the talus for ligamentous attachment.
10. Plantaromedial aspect of the talocalcaneocentral (proximal intertarsal) joint.
11. Dorsomedial aspect of the talocalcaneocentral (proximal intertarsal) joint.
12. Dorsomedial aspect of the articulation between the central and the third tarsal bone (centrodistal or distal intertarsal joint).
13. Medial and lateral borders of the fused first and second tarsal bones.
14. Prominent ridge for ligamentous attachment on the dorsomedial surface of the third tarsal bone.
15. Articulation between the fused first and second tarsal bones and the second metatarsal bone.
16. Dorsomedial aspect of the articulation between the third tarsal bone and the third metatarsal bone (tarsometatarsal joint).
17,18. Dorsomedial borders of the third and fourth metatarsal bones, respectively.
19. Plantarolateral border of the fourth metatarsal bone.
20. Interosseous space between the third and fourth metatarsal bones.

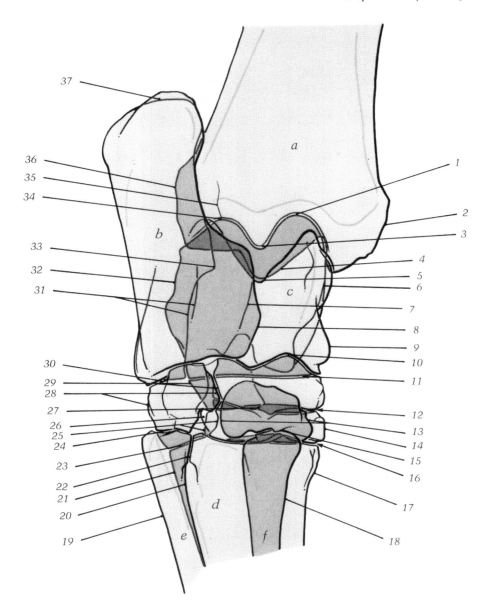

21. Lateral border of the third metatarsal bone dorsal to the fourth metatarsal bone.
22. Articulation between the third and fourth metatarsal bones.
23. Articulation between the fourth tarsal and the third metatarsal bone.
24. Articulation between the fourth tarsal and the fourth metatarsal bone.
25. Plantarolateral and plantaromedial borders of the third tarsal bone.
26. Vascular tarsal canal, which encloses the perforating tarsal artery and vein and a deep perineal nerve branch. It may be more or less apparent on this view, depending on the projection angle.
27. Nonarticular area between the central and the third tarsal bones. These nonarticular areas may simulate subchondral bone lysis and must be differentiated from disease by their location.

28. Plantarolateral and dorsomedial borders of the fourth tarsal bone.
29. Plantarolateral and plantaromedial borders of the central tarsal bone.
30. Articulation between the calcaneus and the fourth tarsal bone (calcaneoquarteral or proximal intertarsal joint).
31. Borders of the sinus tarsi, which is a space between the calcaneus and talus that appears as a more or less lucent region.
32. Plantarolateral border of the sustentaculum tali.
33. Coracoid process of the calcaneus.
34. Articulation between the lateral trochlear ridge of the talus and the lateral tibial cochlear groove in the tarsocrural joint (tibiotarsal joint).
35,36. Cranial and caudal parts, respectively, of the lateral malleolus.
37. Calcaneal tuber.

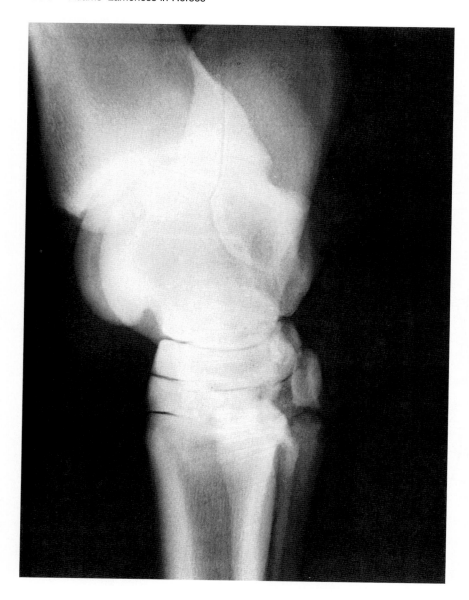

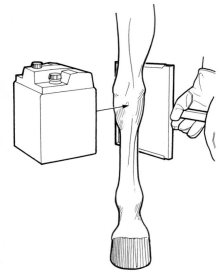

Figure 4.74 Dorsomedial-plantarolateral oblique (D55M-PILO) view of the tarsus. a, tibia; b, talus; c, calcaneus; d, third metatarsal bone.

1. Calcaneal tuber.
2. Articulation between the medial trochlear ridge of the talus and the medial tibial cochlear groove of the tarsocrural joint.
3. Articulation between the lateral trochlea of the talus and the lateral tibial cochlear groove of the tarsocrural joint.
4. Caudal aspect of the intermediate ridge of the tibial cochlea.
5. Proximomedial tuberosity of the talus.
6. Plantar borders of the talus superimposed on the calcaneus.
7. Plantar border of the sustentaculum tali.
8. Nonarticular depression between the talus and the central tarsal bone. These nonarticular depressions, which

appear more or less distinct, depending on the angle of x-ray beam projection, may simulate subchondral bone lysis.

9. Medial and lateral plantar borders of the central tarsal bone.
10. Plantar border of the fourth tarsal bone.
11. Plantar border of the fused first and second tarsal bones.
12. Area of nonarticular depressions between the central and third tarsal bones.
13. Junction between the fused first and second tarsal bones and the medial plantar border of the third tarsal bone.
14. Articulation between the fourth tarsal and the fourth metatarsal bone.
15. Articulation between the fused first and second tarsal bone and the second metatarsal bone.

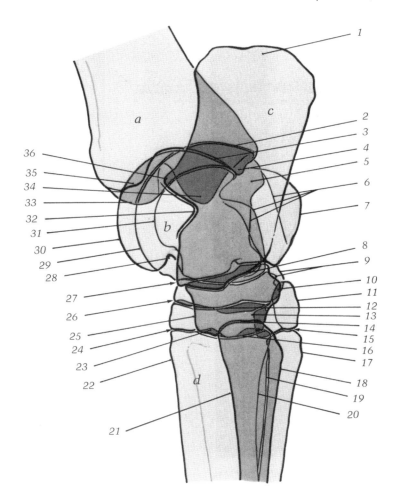

16. Articulation between the fourth tarsal bone and the third metatarsal bone.
17,18. Plantar borders of the second and fourth metatarsal bones, respectively.
19. Interosseous space between the second and third metatarsal bones.
20. Plantar border of the third metatarsal bone.
21,22. Dorsolateral borders of the fourth and third metatarsal bones, respectively.
23. Nonarticular depressions in the adjacent surface of the third tarsal and the third metatarsal bone.
24. Dorsolateral aspect of the articulation between the third tarsal and the third metatarsal bone (tarsometatarsal joint).
25. Dorsolateral border of the fourth tarsal bone.
26. Dorsolateral aspect of the articulation between the central and the third tarsal bone (centrodistal or distal intertarsal joint).
27. Dorsolateral aspect of the talocalcaneal central (proximal intertarsal) joint.

28. Notch at the distal aspect of the lateral trochlear ridge on the talus.
29,30. Medial and lateral trochlear ridges, respectively, of the talus.
31. Depth of the groove between the medial and lateral trochlear ridges on the talus.
32. Articulation between the talus and the calcaneus (talocalcaneal articulation), the visibility of which depends on the x-ray beam projection.
33. Cranial aspect of the intermediate ridge on the tibial cochlea.
34. Medial malleolus superimposed over the talus and calcaneus.
35. Lateral malleolus superimposed over the intermediate tibial cochlear ridge and the lateral trochlear ridge of the talus.
36. Coracoid process of the calcaneus.

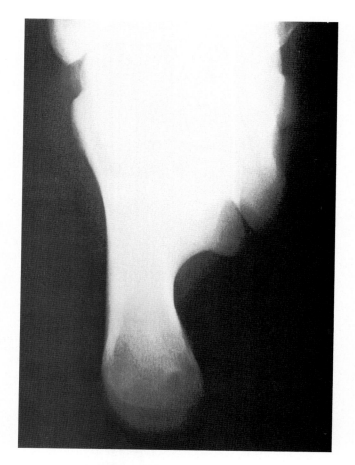

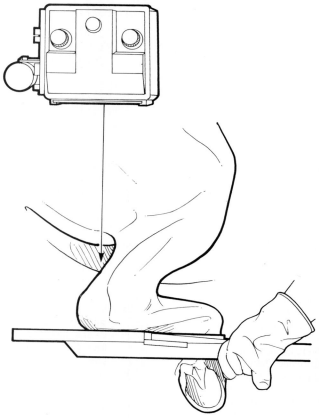

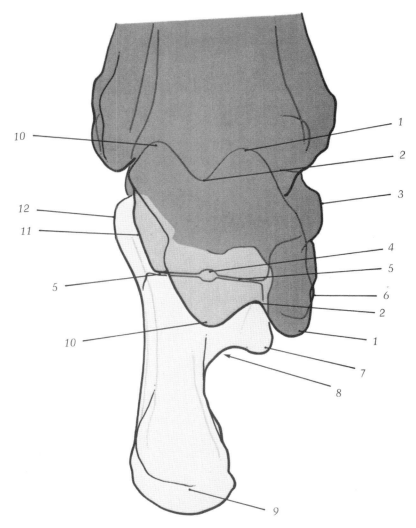

Figure 4.75 Flexed dorsoplantar (flexed DPI) view of the tarsus.

1. Medial trochlear ridge on the talus.
2. Groove between the medial and lateral trochlear ridges of the talus.
3. Distomedial tuberosity of the talus.
4. Nonarticular depressions between the talus and calcaneus. This opening communicates with the sinus tarsi.
5. Medial and lateral aspects of the articulation between the talus and calcaneus.

6. Proximomedial tuberosity of the talus.
7. Sustentaculum tali.
8. Tarsal groove for the deep digital flexor principal tendon.
9. Calcaneal tuber.
10. Lateral trochlear ridge on the talus.
11,12. Areas of attachment of the lateral collateral ligament on the talus and calcaneus, respectively.

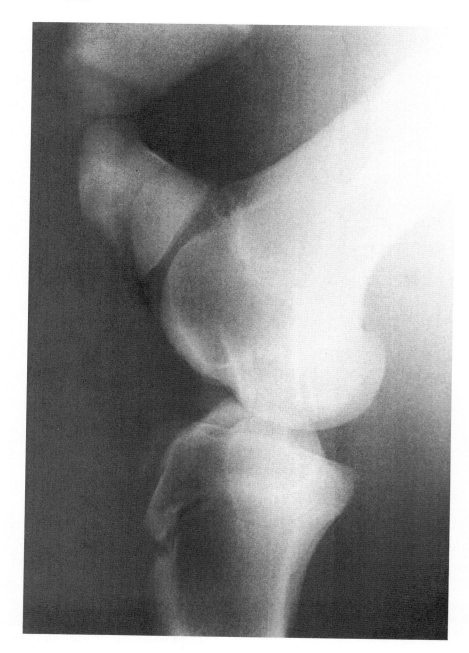

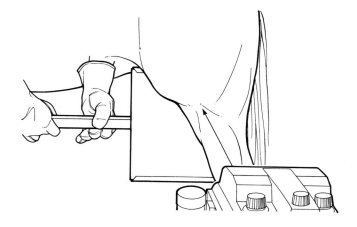

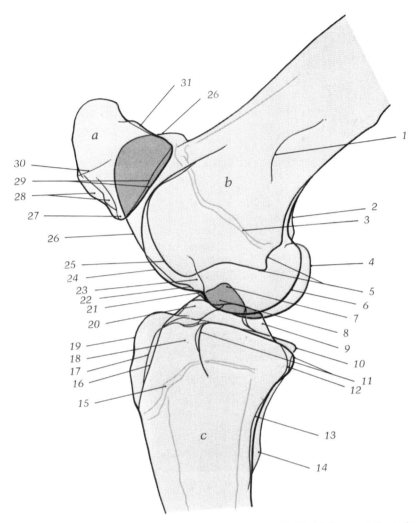

Figure 4.76   Lateromedial (LM) view of the femorotibial and femoropatellar joints (stifle joint). a, patella; b, femur; c, tibia.

1. Supracondyloid fossa.
2. Medial supracondyloid tuberosity.
3. Distal femoral growth plate.
4. Medial femoral condyle.
5. Intercondyloid fossa.
6. Lateral femoral condyle.
7. Medial tubercle on the intercondyloid eminence of the tibia.
8. Central intercondylar area.
9. Medial part of the articular surface on the lateral tibial condyle.
10. Medial tibial condyle.
11. Lateral tibial condyle.
12. Popliteal notch.
13. Concavity of the popliteal incisure.
14. Tubercle on the caudal medial surface of the tibia.
15. Growth plate on the proximal tibia.
16. Groove for the medial patellar ligament.
17. Medial part of the tibial tuberosity.
18. Extensor sulcus.
19. Lateral part of the tibial tuberosity.
20. Lateral tubercle on the intercondyloid eminence of the tibia.
21. Ridge connecting the lateral trochlear ridge and the lateral condyle on the femur.
22. Ridge connecting the medial trochlear ridge and the medial condyle on the femur.
23. Extensor fossa.
24. Lateral femoral trochlear ridge.
25. Compact bone in the femoral trochlea between the lateral and medial trochlear ridges.
26. Medial femoral trochlear ridge.
27. Apex of the patella.
28. Areas of ligamentous attachment on the cranial surface of the patella.
29. Articular surfaces of the patella.
30. Edge of the medial articular surface and medial border of the patella.
31. Base of the patella.

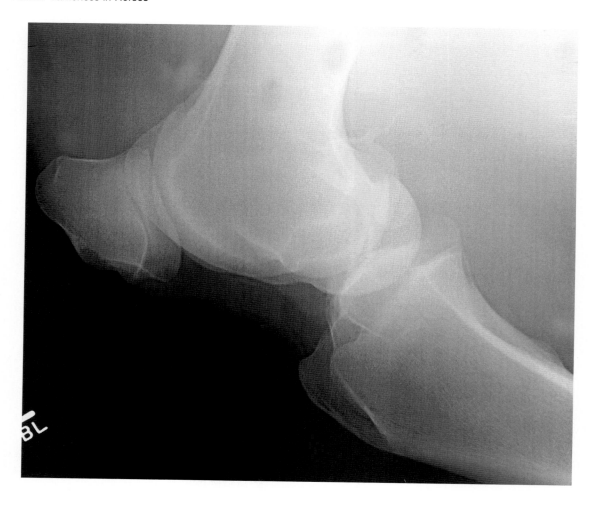

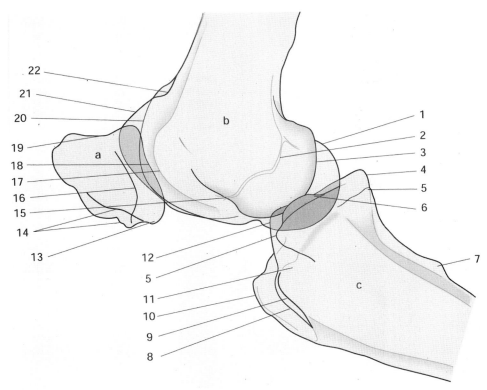

Figure 4.77   Flexed lateromedial (flexed LM) view of the femorotibial and femoropatellar joints (stifle). a, patella; b, femur; c, tibia.

1. Medial femoral condyle.
2. Intercondyloid fossa.
3. Lateral femoral condyle.
4. Lateral tibial condyle.
5. Medial tibial condyle.
6. Medial tubercle on the intercondyloid eminence of the tibia.
7. Tubercle on the caudal medial surface of the tibia.
8. Medial part of the tibial tuberosity.
9. Groove for the medial patellar ligament.
10. Lateral part of the tibial tuberosity.
11. Extensor sulcus.
12. Lateral tubercle on the intercondyloid eminence of the tibia.
13. Apex of the patella.
14. Areas for ligament attachment on the cranial surface of the patella.
15. Extensor fossa.
16. Medial aspect of the articular surface of the patella.
17. Subchondral bone in the femoral trochlea between the lateral and medial trochlear ridges.
18. Lateral aspect of the articular surface of the patella.
19. Base of the patella.
20. Lateral femoral trochlear ridge.
21. Medial femoral trochlear ridge.
22. Nonarticular fossa between the femoral trochlear ridges.

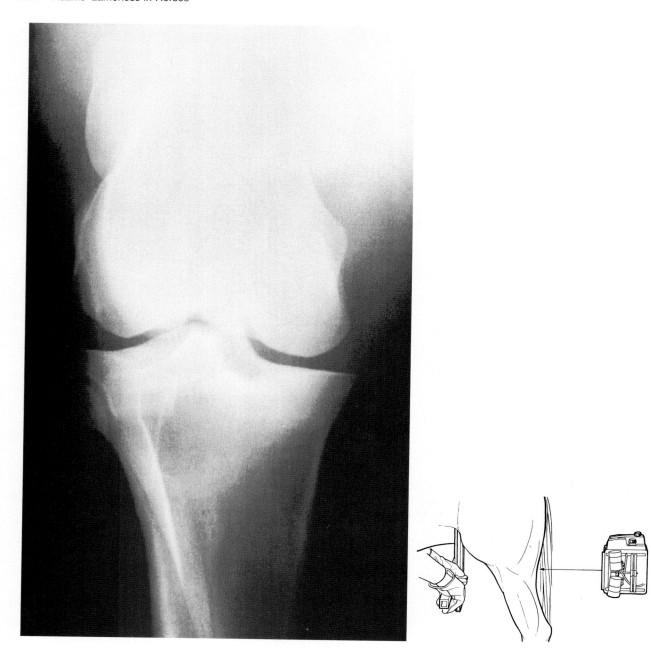

Figure 4.78 Caudocranial (CaCr) view of the femorotibial and femoropatellar joints (stifle). The entire patella may or may not be seen, depending on the x-ray exposure. The patella is normally located to the lateral side of the distal aspect of the femur. The fibula may be a complete bone (as here), but it is usually rudimentary with only the proximal part present or with one or two transverse lines that give the mistaken appearance of fractures. a, patella; b, femur; c, fibula; d, tibia.

1. Medial angle of the patella. A large cartilaginous process extends from the medial angle of the patella and is not visible radiographically.
2. Lateral border of the medial trochlear ridge on the distal femur, the visibility of which depends on the x-ray exposure.
3. Medial epicondyle for ligamentous attachment.
4. Medial and lateral borders of the medial femoral condyle.
5. Intercondyloid fossa on the caudal aspect of the distal femur.

6. Medial tubercle of the intercondylar eminence on the proximal tibia.
7. Lateral tubercle on the intercondylar eminence of the proximal tibia.
8. Central intercondylar area.
9. Cranial and caudal borders of the articular surface on the medial tibial condyle.
10. Medial tibial condyle.
11. Tubercle on the caudal medial tibial surface.
12. Muscular lines on the caudal tibial surface.

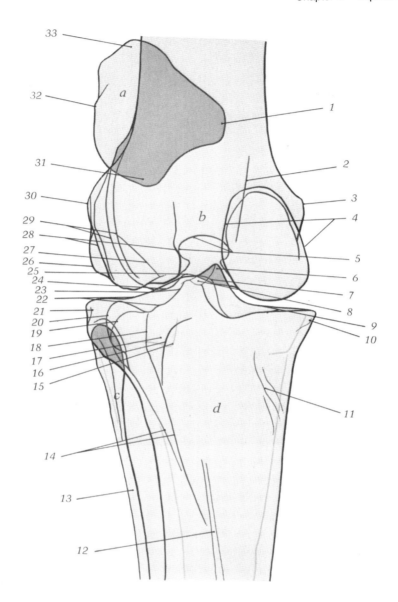

13. Fibula.
14. Tibial crest.
15. Bony margin of the extensor sulcus.
16. Medial part of the tibial tuberosity.
17. Groove between the medial and lateral parts of the tibial tuberosity for the medial patellar ligament.
18. Medial border of the lateral part of the tibial tuberosity.
19,21. Cranial and caudal aspects, respectively, of the lateral tibial condyle.
20. Lateral proximal border of the lateral part of the tibial tuberosity.
22. Cranial and caudal articular surfaces on the lateral tibial condyle.

23. Articular surface on the medial part of the lateral tibial condyle.
24. Distal aspect of the lateral trochlear ridge on the femur.
25. Distal aspect of the groove between the distal femoral trochlear ridges.
26. Lateral femoral epicondyle for ligamentous attachment.
27. Bony borders of the extensor fossa on the distal femur.
28. Lateral and medial borders of the lateral femoral condyle.
29. Lateral trochlear ridge on the distal extremity of the femur.
30. Proximolateral border of the lateral femoral condyle.
31. Apex of the patella.
32. Lateral angle and the patella.
33. Base of the patella.

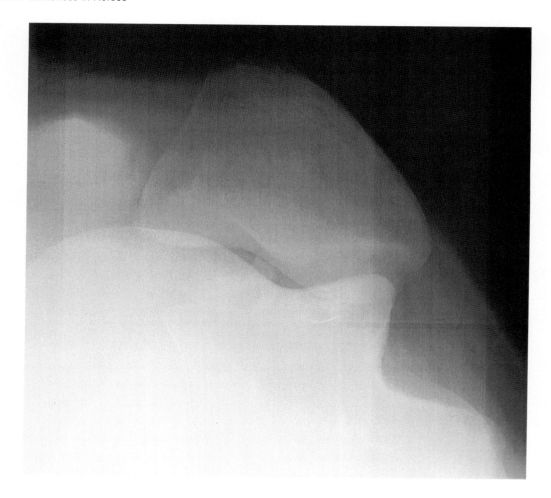

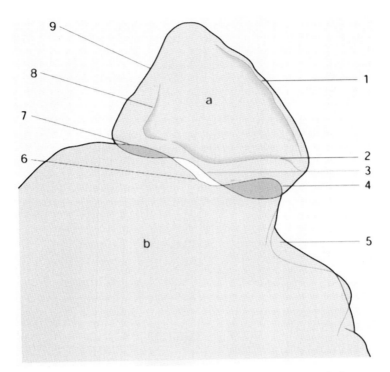

Figure 4.79　Cranioproximal-distal cranial oblique (CrPr-DiCrO) view of the patella. a, patella; b, femur.

1. Dorsal surface and area of ligament attachment on the patella.
2. Distal articular surface on the patella.
3. Proximal articular surface on the patella.
4. Lateral femoral trochlear ridge.
5. Extensor fossa.

6. Trochlear groove between the medial and lateral trochlear ridges.
7. Medial femoral trochlear ridge.
8. Distal medial border of the patella.
9. Proximal medial border of the patella.

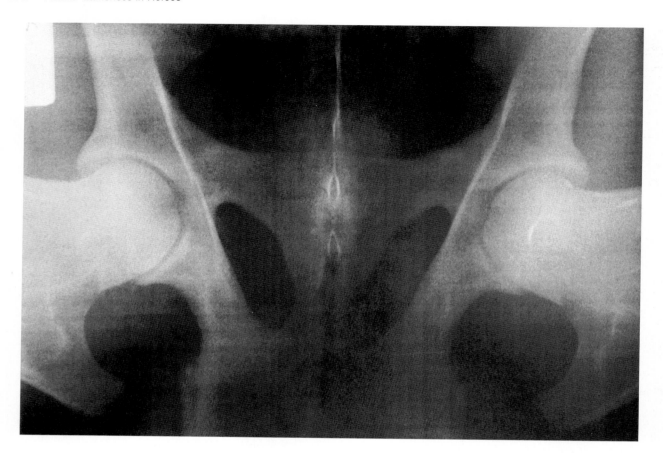

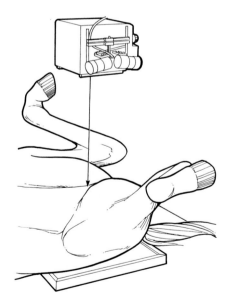

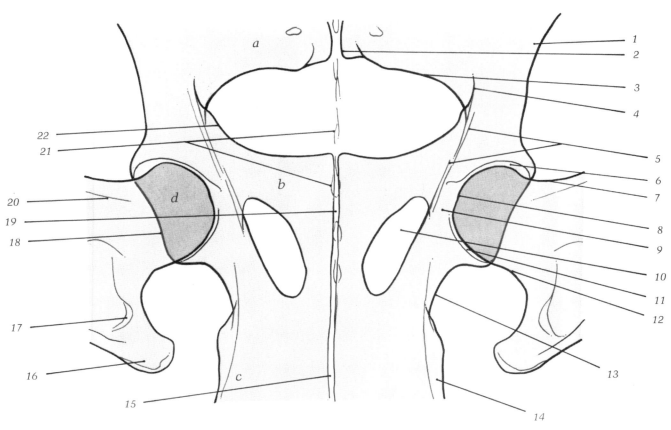

Figure 4.80   Ventrodorsal (VD) view of the pelvis. a, right ilium; b, right pubis; c, right ischium; d, right femoral head.

1. Body of the ilium.
2. Tuber sacrale. Fecal material in the large colon may be superimposed over the tuber sacrale and sacrum, compromising good radiographic evaluation of these structures.
3. Greater ischiatic notch on the dorsal border of the ilium.
4. Ventral border of the ilium.
5. Ischiatic spine.
6. Articulation between the cranial border of the acetabulum and the femoral head.
7. Medial border of the femoral neck.
8. Fovea capitis femoris, which is a flattened region on the femoral head, the visibility of which depends on the angulation and position during radiography.
9. Acetabular fossa. Because there is no articular cartilage or subchondral bone in the region of the acetabular fossa,

it appears as a break or defect in the articular surface of the acetabulum, but it is normal.
10. Obturator foramen.
11. Articulation between the caudal border of the acetabulum and the femoral head.
12. Lateral border of the femoral neck.
13. Lateral border of the ischium.
14. Ischiatic tuberosity.
15. Ischiatic symphysis.
16,17. Caudal and cranial parts, respectively, of the greater trochanter.
18. Dorsal rim of the acetabulum.
19. Pubic symphysis.
20. Lesser trochanter superimposed over the femur.
21. Dorsal spinous processes of the sacrum.
22. Cranial border of the pubis.

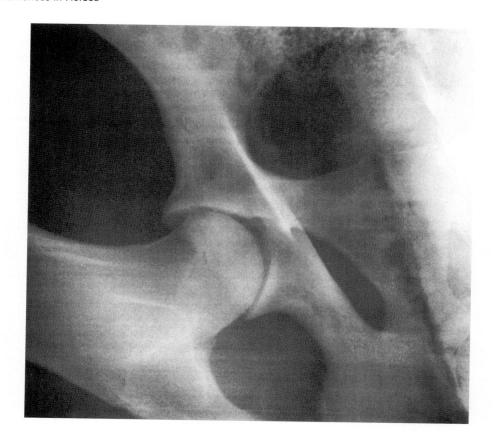

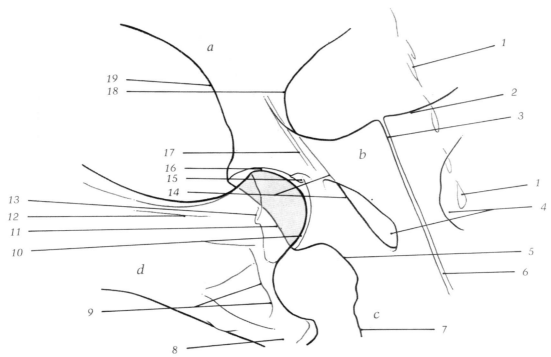

Figure 4.81   Ventromedial-dorsolateral oblique (V25M-DLO) view of the pelvis. a, ilium; b, pubis; c, ischium; d, femur.

1. Dorsal spinous process of the sacrum.
2. Cranial border of the pubis.
3. Pubic symphysis.
4. Obturator foramina.
5. Lateral border of the ischium.
6. Ischiatic symphysis.
7. Ischiatic tuberosity.
8,9. Caudal and cranial parts, respectively, of the greater trochanter.
10. Articulation between the caudal aspect of the acetabulum and the femoral head.
11. Dorsal acetabular rim.
12. Lesser trochanter superimposed over the femur.
13. Growth plate (physis) between the femoral head and the neck.
14. Medial dorsal border of the ischium.
15. Acetabular fossa.
16. Articulation between the cranial acetabulum and the femoral head.
17. Ischiatic spine on the dorsal border of the ischium.
18. Medial dorsal border of the ilium.
19. Lateral border of the ilium.

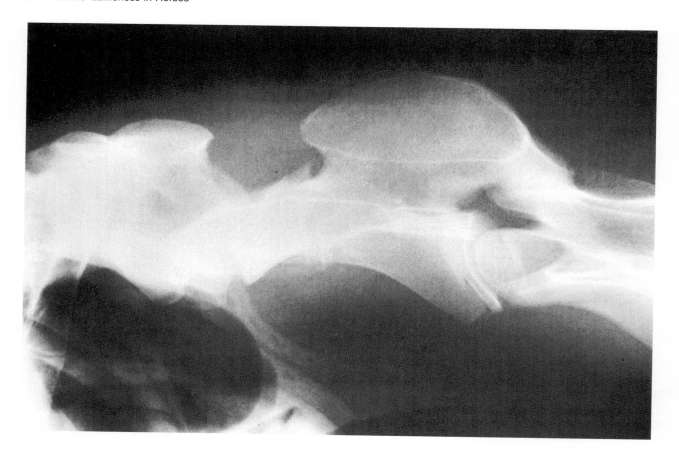

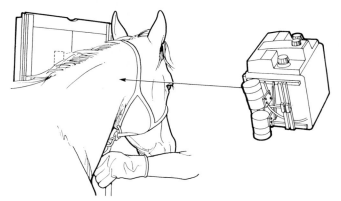

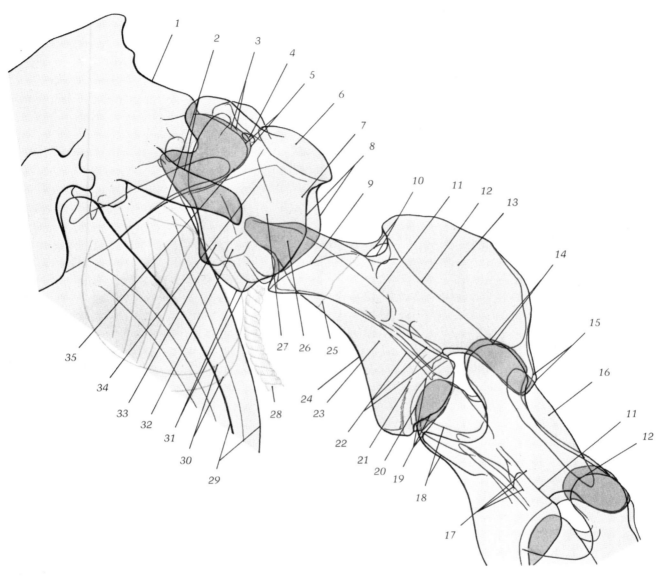

Figure 4.82 Right-to-left lateral (Rt-LeL) view of the cranial cervical vertebral column (C1 to C3).

1. Occipital bone.
2. Jugular process.
3. Dorsal surface of the right and left occipital condyles.
4. Right and left margins of the lateral foramen of the atlas.
5. Caudal borders of the occipital condyles (atlantooccipital articulation).
6. Dorsal tubercle of the atlas.
7. Atlas.
8. Caudal margins of the articular fovea.
9. Cranial articular process of the axis.
10. Margins of the lateral vertebral foramen.
11. Ventral margin of the vertebral canal.
12. Dorsal margin of the vertebral canal.
13. Dorsal spinous process of the axis.
14. Right and left cranial articular fovea of C3.
15. Caudal articular fovea of the atlas.
16. Dorsal spinous process of C3.
17. Base of the transverse processes of C3.
18. Transverse process of C3.

19. Concave margins of the caudal extremity of the axis.
20. Convex cranial extremity of C3.
21. Caudal growth plate of the axis.
22. Multiple linear opacities produced by the wide bases on the right and left transverse processes of the axis.
23. Axis.
24. Ventral border of the axis.
25. Cranial growth plate of the axis.
26. Dens of the axis.
27. Atlas.
28. Shadow produced by braided rope used for halter.
29. Right and left rami of the mandible.
30. Right and left ventral margins of the guttural pouches.
31. Right and left ventrocaudal margins of the axis.
32. Shadow caused by margins of the transverse foramen.
33. Base of the wings of the atlas.
34. Shadow formed by the concavity of the atlantal fossa.
35. Right and left caudal margins of the occipital condyles.

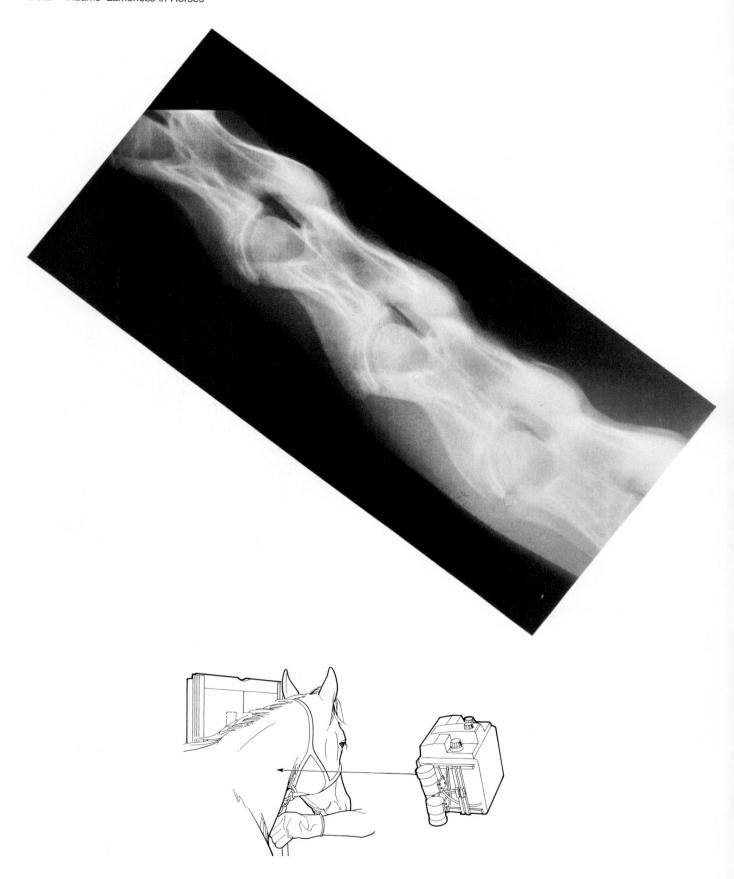

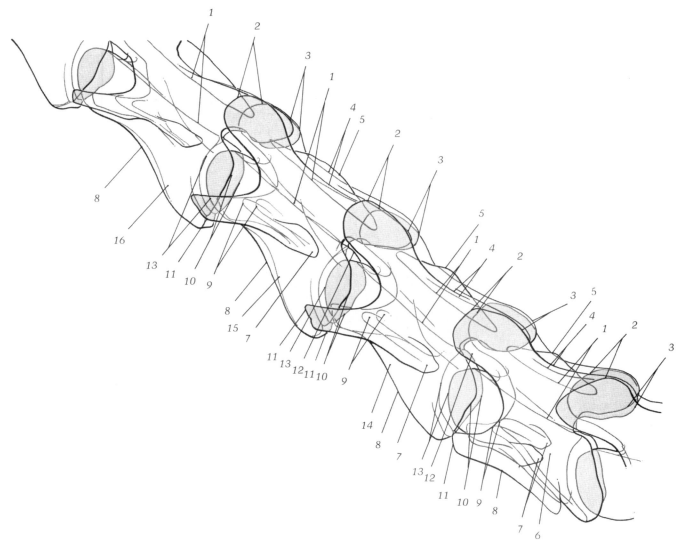

Figure 4.83 Right-to-left lateral (Rt-LeL) view of the midcervical spine (C3 to C6).

1. Dorsal and ventral borders of the vertebral canal.
2. Right and left cranial articular processes.
3. Right and left caudal articular processes.
4. Shadows formed by vertebral arches on either side of the spinous processes.
5. Dorsal spinous processes of C4, C5, and C6.
6. C6.
7. Bases of lateral transverse vertebral processes.
8. Ventral borders of the vertebrae.

9. Bases of the transverse processes, which also form the ventral and dorsal margins of transverse foramina.
10. Caudal extremities of the vertebrae.
11. Transverse processes.
12. Dorsal tuberculums.
13. Concave borders of the caudal extremities.
14. C5.
15. C4.
16. C3.

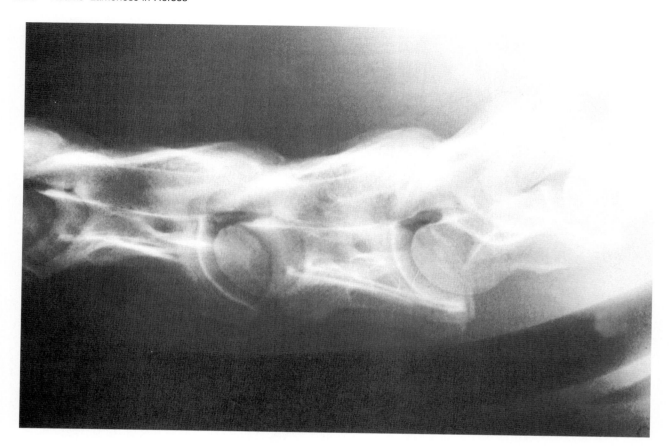

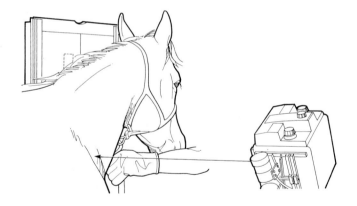

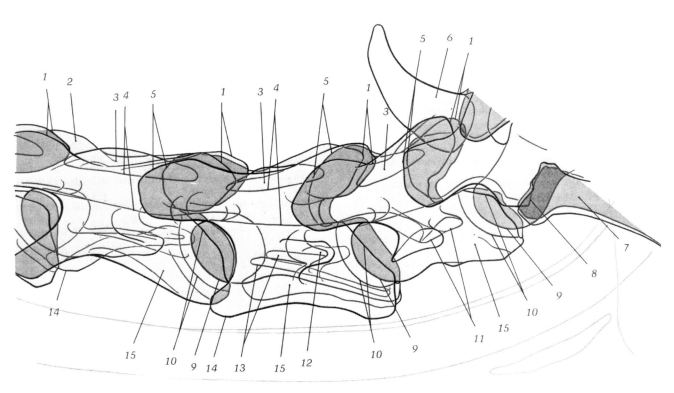

Figure 4.84   Right-to-left lateral (Rt-LeL) view of the caudal cervical spine (C5 to C7).

1. Caudal articular processes.
2. Vertebral lamina on either side of the spinous process.
3. Dorsal spinous processes and dorsal laminae.
4. Dorsal and ventral borders of the vertebral canal.
5. Cranial articular processes.
6. Dorsal spinous process of T1.
7. First rib.
8. Tubercle of the first rib.

9. Cranial extremities of the vertebrae.
10. Caudal extremities of the vertebrae.
11. Bases of the transverse processes.
12. Shadow of the transverse foramen.
13. Bases of transverse processes.
14. Cranial part of the transverse processes of C6 and C7.
15. C5, C6, and C7.

COMPUTED RADIOGRAPHY

Computed radiography is an imaging modality that produces a radiographic image from digital information. Although the result is a radiographic image similar to one obtained from conventional radiography, the equipment used to acquire and process the images is different. One process consists of using a storage phosphor-imaging plate made of europium-doped barium fluorohalide (BaFBr:Eu) instead of a conventional film-screen cassette. The storage phosphor plate is placed in a holding cassette and exposed to x-rays in the same manner as a conventional x-ray cassette (Fig. 4.85). The energy from the x-ray exposure is stored on the phosphor-imaging plate. After the plate is exposed, it is placed in a laser reader, which scans it with a laser beam. The stored energy is then released, detected, and digitized.

The digitized image can be viewed on a monitor and manipulated for improved interpretation. The density, latitude, and size of the image can be adjusted before the image is printed (hard copy). Because the image can be manipulated, both soft tissue structures and bone can be visualized from the same exposure. Improper exposures produced by minor to moderate exposure variations can be adjusted to produce an acceptable image.

The exposure dose per image can be reduced with digital radiography,[31] but as the exposure is decreased, the spatial resolution is also decreased. Therefore, the amount of exposure needed to obtain an acceptable image is not greatly reduced, compared with medium-speed rare earth film-screen systems.

One advantage of computed radiography is the ability to alter the imaging algorithm and produce improved edge enhancement and wide contrast latitude (Fig. 4.86). As with xeroradiography, the advantage of edge enhancement is that subtle margins, such as occur with hairline fractures or subtle periosteal reaction, are more easily identified. Spatial resolution, however, may not be as good with computed radiography as with film-screen radiography. Furthermore, a lucent halo may be produced on low-frequency edge-enhanced images (Fig. 4.87). The lucent halo is seen in areas where there is a transition between high and low tissue or material densities. The halo may appear as a pseudofracture, and when seen around metallic implants, the lytic zone may be confused with bone lysis.[16] The perimetallic bone halo may erroneously be diagnosed as an unstable implant or an infection.

The cost of equipment necessary to produce digital radiographs is relatively high, and the modality is technically complex. Improvements in and simplification of computed radiography will likely increase the use of this imaging modality.

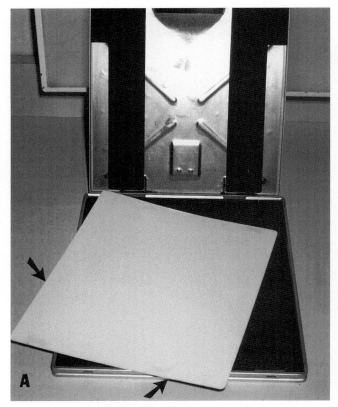
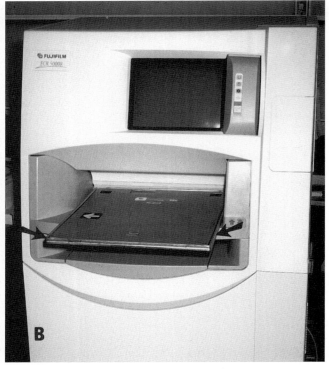

Figure 4.85 A. A computed radiographic plate (arrows) in an open cassette. B. The cassette (arrows) being inserted into the computed radiographic reader, where it will be scanned with a laser beam so a digitized image can be produced.

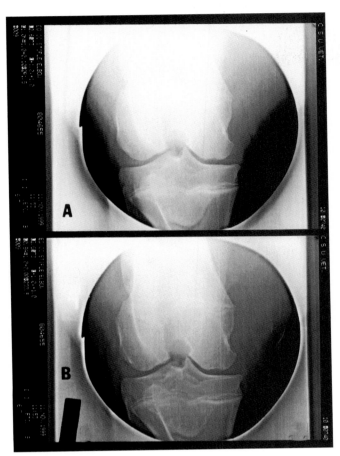

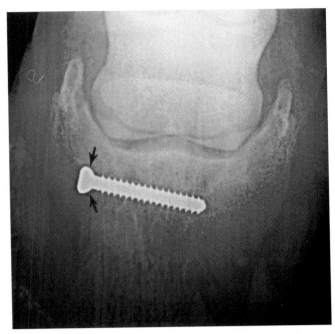

Figure 4.87 Dorsopalmar view computed radiograph of the distal phalanx, showing a black pseudohalo (arrows) around a metallic screw within the distal phalanx. The halo mimics bone lysis.

Figure 4.86 A. Caudocranial view computed radiograph of a stifle, produced with an algorithm similar to that of a regular film-screen radiograph. B. Caudocranial view of a stifle, produced with an algorithm that provides edge enhancement.

XERORADIOGRAPHY

Xeroradiography is a process in which an electrostatically charged selenium-coated aluminum plate is exposed by x-rays. The x-rays form a latent image on the plate by altering the electrostatic charges. The plate is then processed by exposing it to an aerosol of charged powder (toner). The charged toner particles are attracted to or repelled by the electrostatic charge on the plate. This image is transferred to plastic-coated paper by direct contact and then fused to the paper by heat.

Xeroradiography provides good resolution, wide contrast latitude, and excellent edge enhancement (Fig. 4.88). Edge enhancement on a xeroradiograph provides additional information to that found on conventional radiographs[43] and may provide a diagnosis in cases of hairline fractures that are not identified on conventional radiographs.

Xeroradiography is valuable when good image detail is needed and inherent contrast is poor.[3] It gives good visualization of soft tissue structures, possible foreign bodies in soft tissue, and good detail to subtle osseous lesions. Therefore, in cases in which a lesion may be sus-

pected clinically but not seen on routine radiographs, xeroradiography may provide the necessary information to make a diagnosis. The percentage of lameness cases in which xeroradiography provides vital information not present on routine radiographs has not been documented.

The limitations of xeroradiography are the cost of special processing equipment versus the amount of time in use, magnitude of radiation exposure to obtain a diagnostic study[3] (Xerox recommends a 125-kVp, 200-mA machine as a minimum), technical expertise to produce a good-quality film, and increased cost of film compared with radiographic film.

In summary, xeroradiography is not economical for most practice situations. Furthermore, although the image obtained is superior to conventional radiographs, the percentage of cases in which the technique is absolutely necessary for diagnosis has not been documented, although it is probably quite low.

COMPUTED TOMOGRAPHY

CT provides an adjunct examination to radiography in cases in which a three-dimensional image could add important information to help the clinician arrive at a diagnosis or decide on surgical intervention and treatment.[42] A CT scanner consists of an x-ray tube and sensors in a circular gantry, a table, an x-ray generator, a computer, a video monitor, and some form of recorder to reproduce the image on film (hard copy).

The image is made with x-rays while the x-ray tube travels 360° within the gantry. The gantry size limits

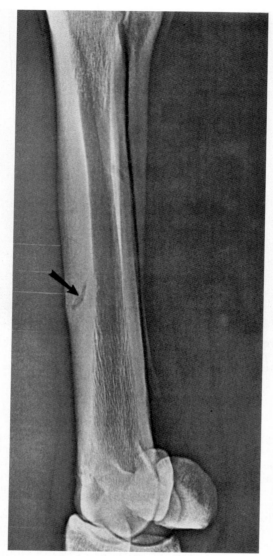

Figure 4.88   Dorsomedial-palmarolateral oblique (D45M-PaLO) view xeroradiograph of the metacarpal bone, showing a fracture through the dorsal lateral metacarpal cortex (arrow). (Courtesy of CF Reid, University of Pennsylvania, Philadelphia.)

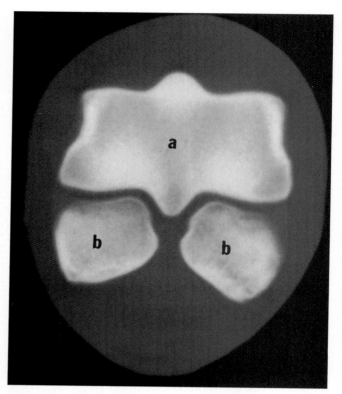

Figure 4.89   A 2-mm-thick CT image of the distal third metacarpal (a) and the proximal sesamoid bones (b) in transverse plane, with a bone window setting.

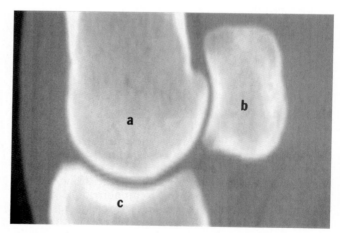

Figure 4.90   A 2-mm-thick, reformatted CT image of a fore fetlock in sagittal plane. a, third metacarpal bone; b, proximal sesamoid bone; c, proximal phalanx.

scans on a horse to the extremities distal to the level of the midradius and tibia. Cervical spine studies can be performed through the rostral and midcervical area. Scans of the caudal cervical spine are limited and depend on the size of the horse. A specially designed table that can accommodate the horse's size and weight is also necessary.

Direct images are acquired in a transverse (axial) plane at a specified image thickness, interval, and size, resulting in a three-dimensional image (Fig. 4.89). From the digital information acquired on the direct scan, images can be reformatted in any other desired plane (Fig. 4.90) or may be processed to provide a three-dimensional image.

The CT image has superior contrast resolution but inferior spatial resolution, compared with a radiograph.

The contrast level and width can be adjusted on CT images for better visualization of bone or soft tissue structures. For example, to optimize bone on the image, a wide window width (1500 to 2000 ct number) and relatively high window level (250 to 350 ct number) are used; and to optimize soft tissue structures within a limb, lower window levels (60 ct number) and widths (200 to 350 ct number) are used.

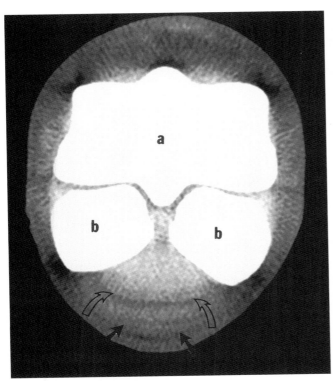

Figure 4.91 A 2-mm-thick CT image through the distal third metacarpal bone (a) and proximal sesamoid bones (b) in transverse plane, with a soft tissue window setting, which increases the opaqueness of the bones. The deep digital flexor tendon (open arrows) and superficial digital flexor tendon (solid arrows) can be seen.

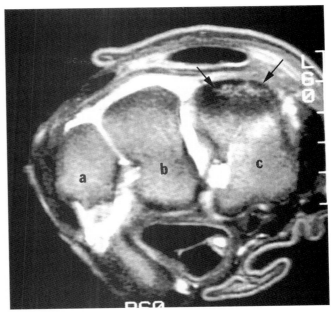

Figure 4.92 MRI study of the proximal row of carpal bones in transverse plane, using a proton-dense sequence. Note the traumatic arthritis (arrows) on the dorsal border of the radial carpal bone; normal marrow has been replaced with low-intensity bone sclerosis. a, ulnar carpal bone; b, intermediate carpal bone; c, radial carpal bone.

Subchondral, cortical, and trabecular bone structures can be evaluated with CT. Small soft tissue structures are often not defined well enough to demonstrate subtle pathology, such as small ligament injuries,[46] minor damage to tendons, cartilage erosion, and joint capsule changes. Larger soft tissue structures can be imaged and moderate to severe lesions can be observed (Fig. 4.91).

CT is helpful for defining complex intraarticular fractures, fractures not seen on radiographs,[42] stress-induced subchondral bone sclerosis, and other subchondral bone lesions, such as cysts or subtle defects. Complex intraarticular fractures can be better defined with CT because the images are produced in the third dimension and can be reformatted in other planes. Transverse CT images of cervical spine studies also add three-dimensional information to cervical radiographic studies, which are often confined to lateral views only; thus lateral compressive lesions on the spinal cord may be missed. In most cases, the CT examination is done after the radiographic examination; it adds data for a more accurate diagnosis and effective treatment plan.

MAGNETIC RESONANCE IMAGING

Magnetic resonance images are sectional images much the same as CT images. They are produced in machines similar in structure and configuration to CT scanners.

The images are proton images, mainly of hydrogen nuclei, with high-contrast resolution. MRI provides exceptionally good anatomic, pathoanatomic, and pathophysiologic information of intraarticular and periarticular structures (Fig. 4.92). MRI has the potential to provide information from images not available from any other imaging modality, including arthroscopy.

A MRI scanner consists of a strong magnet, transmit/receive radiofrequency coils, gradient magnets, a computer, a gantry, a table, and a video monitor. A detailed description of MRI scanners and the mechanism of image production may be found elsewhere,[13] but a simple description follows. Nuclei that have an asymmetric spinning charge are imaged, and the proton from the hydrogen nucleus is used to produce the image for most diagnostic studies. These spinning charged nuclei are aligned in the strong magnetic field of the scanner. The spinning aligned nuclei precess around an axis in the magnetic field much the same as a spinning top. A radiofrequency wave is used to bombard the precessing nucleus, tilting the precessing axis 90°. The signal from the precessing nucleus or proton then produces an electric signal in the radiofrequency receiver coil, which is transmitted to the computer for image construction. The signal for image construction is produced as the nuclei relax into their demagnetized states.

By varying the radiofrequency pulse, the time for protons to become magnetized before the radiofrequency pulse (TR), and the time after the radiofrequency pulse (TE), a clinician can produce different images with varying information. These images are termed T1-weighted, T2-weighted, and proton density images. By adjusting the magnetic gradient coils, the clinician is able to obtain direct sectional images in any plane.

T1-weighted images are used most often to evaluate joints and musculoskeletal structures, although T2-weighted images provide different tissue contrast and may offer valuable information in selected cases.[23,37] T2-weighted images are best for demonstrating lesions in periarticular muscles and synovial fluid. A knowledge of tissue intensities on T1- and T2-weighted images is necessary for interpreting the scans. On T1-weighted images, subcutaneous and fascial plane fat and bone marrow have the brightest signal (white), hyalin cartilage is less bright (white gray), and muscle is even less bright (gray white). Fluid, ligaments, tendons, and bone have little or no signal intensity (black).[37] Sometimes, synovial fluid produces a signal and can be seen (gray) adjacent to articular cartilage. On T2-weighted images, fluid has the highest intensity (white), followed by fat, bone marrow, and muscle in decreasing order of intensity. Ligaments, tendons, and bone have little or no signal intensity (black).[37]

MRI is an effective imaging modality for evaluating and detecting pathologic changes in articular cartilage, menisci, and periarticular bone marrow changes. Erosive cartilage changes, meniscal injuries, and alterations in periarticular bone marrow owing to stress-induced bone sclerosis or fluid accumulation secondary to infection or inflammation can be detected. Ligament, tendon, joint capsule, and muscle injury can also be diagnosed. Hyperintense and hypointense defects may be observed in injured ligaments, tendons, and muscle. With edema or fluid accumulation, the signal intensity is hyperintense on T2-weighted images and hypointense on T1-weighted images. Signal intensity of blood or hemorrhage changes over time. Acute hemorrhage is isointense with muscle on T1-weighted images and hyperintense on T2-weighted images. After 2 days, the signal on T1-weighted images is more intense, and in several days, the hemorrhage is hyperintense on both T1- and T2-weighted images.[37]

Most MRI studies of equine joints have been done on cadaver specimens. The normal magnetic resonance anatomy of the foot and fetlock[45] and pathologic conditions of the foot[22,51] and tendons[6] have been demonstrated via MRI. The equine extremity lends itself to imaging with smaller-sized magnets and surface receiver coils, if and when MRI is developed for use in the standing animal. Drawbacks to MRI of equine joints are no appropriate equipment configuration for in vivo imaging on the unanesthetized animal, high cost of equipment, including maintenance, and the complexity of imaging sequences needed to obtain a diagnostic examination. When these constraints are overcome, MRI of equine extremities will add a new dimension for in vivo diagnostic imaging in cases of equine lameness.

THERMOGRAPHY

Thermography is an imaging modality by which a visual image is produced from infrared radiation emitted from the skin surface. The infrared radiation is detected by a photon detector, converted to electrical impulses, and displayed on a television monitor (cathode ray tube)

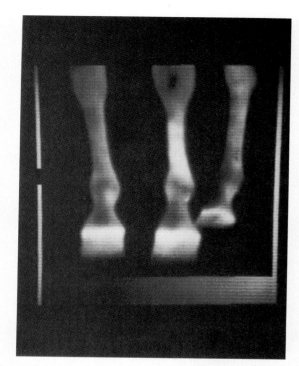

Figure 4.93 A normal thermogram of the bilateral forelimbs of a horse, showing warmer vascular areas (lighter areas). (Courtesy of RC Purohit, Auburn University, Auburn, AL.)

(Fig. 4.93). The image is displayed in colors (isotherms) that correspond to different temperatures on the skin surface. The skin surface temperature also reflects changes in circulation and temperature changes in deeper tissues.[62] A total of 10 isotherms are available, and the temperature sensitivity between isotherms is adjustable.

Normal thermographic patterns have been reported for the horse.[48] In general, hotter areas follow the normal vasculature. Thermographic patterns are bilaterally symmetric, with all four limbs having a similar pattern below the carpus and tarsus. Slight variations in normal patterns occur between horses.

The general clinical uses for thermography are 1) to define the extent of a lesion when a diagnosis has been made, 2) to localize a previously unidentified abnormal area, so further diagnostic tests can be performed, 3) to detect early lesions before they are clinically evident, and 4) to follow the healing process before the animal is returned to work or training.[48,49,63] Specific clinical conditions reported to be diagnosed with thermography are early subclinical osteoarthritis,[49,63] particularly in the tarsus, subsolar abscesses, laminitis, serous arthritis, tendinitis, and heel pain not associated with the navicular bone.[30,49,56,57,62] Temperature changes identified in the superficial digital flexor tendon may indicate multiple small subclinical fibrillary ruptures.[57] These changes may repair without progressing to a clinical syndrome and can be identified as much as 2 weeks before clinical signs of tendinitis are observed.[31] Muscle injury consisting of strain and inflammation has also been identified in the lumbar and pelvic areas and upper hindlimbs and forelimbs with thermography.[60–62]

Disadvantages and limitations of thermography are 1) the cost of the equipment,[48] 2) the low specificity for detection of chronic bone and joint lesions,[27] and 3) the nonspecificity of findings. An area of increased temperature on an animal's limb may be a normal thermographic variation, an inflammatory area on the skin surface, or a benign vascular abnormality. For a horse with lameness problems and a high skin temperature reading, differential diagnosis would most usually be between an inflammatory lesion and a normal thermographic variation. After an abnormal thermographic pattern has been detected, further tests using ultrasonography, radiography, and/or biopsy are necessary to provide a more specific diagnosis.[61] Because of the nonspecificity of thermographic changes, this method should be considered as a complementary procedure for diagnosis and a follow-up procedure for disease conditions that produce lameness.[9]

References

1. Ackerman N, Spencer CP, Hager DA, Poulos PW Jr. Radiation exposure during equine radiography. Vet Radiol 1988;29: 198–201.
2. Arnbjerg J. Contrast radiography of joints and tendon sheaths in the horse. Nord Vet Med 1969;21:318.
3. Barber DL. Imaging: Radiography-II. Vet Radiol 1981;22:149.
4. Beech J. Metrizamide myelography in the horse. J Am Vet Radiol Soc 1979;20:22.
5. Burbidge HM, Kannegieter N, Dickson LR, et al. Iohexol myelography in the horse. Equine Vet J 1989;21:347–350.
6. Crass JR, Genovese RL, Render JA, Bellon EM. Magnetic resonance, ultrasound and histopathologic correlation of acute and healing equine tendon injuries. Vet Radiol Ultrasound 1992;33: 206–216.
7. Curry TS, Dowder JE, Murry RC. Christensen's Physics of Diagnostic Radiology. Philadelphia: Lea & Febiger, 1990.
8. DeMoor A, Verschooten F. Tendonitis in the horse: Its radiographic diagnosis with air-tendograms. J Vet Radiol Soc 1978;19: 23.
9. Denoix JM, D'Esquermes S. Thermographic examination and documentation of locomotor injuries in the horse—preliminary results. Pratique Vet Equine 1995;27:189–196.
10. Dik KJ. Equine arthrography. Vet Radiol 1984;25:93–96.
11. Dik KJ. Fistulographie beim Pferd—retrospecktive Auswertung. Pferdeheilkunde 1987;3:255–261.
12. Dik KJ, Keg PR. The efficacy of contrast radiography to demonstrate "false thoroughpins" in five horses. Equine Vet J 1990;22: 223–225.
13. Edelman RR, Zlatkin MB, Hesselink JR. Clinical Magnetic Resonance Imaging. Philadelphia: WB Saunders, 1996.
14. Farrow C. Sinography in the horse. Proc Am Assoc Equine Pract 1987;505–521.
15. Gillette EL, Thrall DE, Lebel JL. Carlsons Radiography Radiology. Philadelphia: Lea & Febiger, 1977.
16. Glanski M, Oestmann JW, Kattapuram SV, et al. Digital radiography in bone and joint disease. In: Green RE, Oestmann JW, Eds. Computed Digital Radiography in Clinical Practice. New York: Thieme Medical Publishers, 1992;126.
17. Greenfield GB. Radiology of Bone Diseases. Philadelphia: JB Lippincott, 1975.
18. Habel RE, et al. Nomenclature for radiologic anatomy. J Am Vet Med Assoc 1963;142:38.
19. Hago BED, Vaughan LC. Radiographic anatomy of tendon sheaths and bursae in the horse. Equine Vet J 1986;18:102–106.
20. Hago BED, Vaughan LC. Use of contrast radiography in the investigation of tenosynovitis and bursitis in horses. Equine Vet J 1986; 18:375–382.
21. International Committee on Veterinary Anatomical Nomenclature. Vienna: Adoph Holzhausen's Successors, 1973.
22. Kaneps AJ, Koblik PD, Freeman DM, et al. A comparison of radiography, computed tomography, and magnetic resonance imaging for diagnosis of palmar process fractures in foals. Vet Radiol Ultrasound 1995;36:467–477.
23. Kang HS, Resnick D. MRI of the Extremities: An Anatomic Atlas. Philadelphia: WB Saunders, 1991.
24. Koblik PD, Hornof WJ, O'Brien TR. Rare earth intensifying screens for veterinary radiography. Vet Radiol 1980;21:224.
25. Koblik PD, Toal R. Portable veterinary x-ray support systems for field use. J Am Vet Med Assoc 1991;199:186–188.
26. Lamb CR. Contrast radiography of equine joints, tendon sheaths and draining tracts. Vet Clin North Am Equine Pract 1991;7: 241–257.
27. Lauk HD, Kimmich M. Comparison of scintigraphy and thermography in the horse. Pferdeheilkinde 1997;13:329–334.
28. Lundin CS, Clem MF, Debowes RM, Bertone AL. Diagnostic fistulography in horses. Comp Cont Educ Equine Pract 1988;10: 639–645.
29. Maclean AA, Jeffcott LB, Lavelle RB, Friend SCE. Use of iohexol for myelography in the horse. Equine Vet J 1988;20:286,290.
30. Marr C. Microwave thermography: A non-invasive technique for investigation of injury of the superficial flexor tendon in the horse. Equine Vet J 1992;24:269–273.
31. Masumitsu H, Shibata E. Application of computed radiography system for horses. I. Decrease of x-ray exposure and improvement of x-ray quality. II. Superimposed and subtracted image processings. Bull Equine Res Inst Jpn 1990;27:7–24.
32. May SA, Wyn-Jones G. Contrast radiography in the investigation of sinus tracts and abscess cavities in the horse. Equine Vet J 1987; 19:218–222.
33. May SA, Wyn-Jones G, Church S. Iopamidol myelography in the horse. Equine Vet J 1986;18:199–202.
34. Mayhew IG, Whitlock RH, DeLahunta A. Spinal cord disease in the horse. Cornell Vet 1978;68:44.
35. Moore BR, Reed SM. Equine spinal ataxia: Ancillary diagnostic tests. Proc Am Assoc Equine Pract 1993;39:107–122.
36. Morgan JP, Silverman S. Techniques of Veterinary Radiography. Ames, IA: Iowa State University Press, 1989.
37. Murphy W. Magnetic resonance imaging. In: Resnick D, Ed. Bone and Joint Imaging. Philadelphia: WB Saunders, 1989;120.
38. National Council on Radiation Protection and Measurement. Radiation Protection In Veterinary Medicine. Washington DC: National Council on Radiation Protection and Measurement, 1970.
39. Nixon AJ, Spencer CP. Arthrography of the equine shoulder joint. Equine Vet J 1990;22:107–113.
40. Nixon AJ, Stashak TS, Ingram JT. Diagnosis of cervical vertebral malformation in the horse. Proc Am Assoc Equine Pract 1983;28: 253–266.
41. Nyland TG, et al. Metrizamide myelography in the horse; clinical, radiographic and pathologic changes. Am J Vet Res 1980;41:201.
42. O'Callaghan M. The integration of radiography and alternative imaging methods in the diagnosis of equine orthopedic disease. Vet Clin North Am Equine Pract 1991;7:339–365.
43. Osterman FA, et al. Xeroradiography in veterinary radiology: A preliminary study. Vet Radiol 1975;16:143.
44. Papageorges M, Gavin PR, Sande RD, et al. Radiographic and myelographic examination of the cervical vertebral column in 306 ataxic horses. Vet Radiol 1987;28:53–59.
45. Park RD, Nelson TR, Hoopes PJ. Magnetic resonance imaging of the normal equine digit and metacarpophalangeal joint. Vet Radiol 1987;28:105–116.
46. Peterson PR, Bowman KF. Computed tomographic anatomy of the distal extremity of the horse. Vet Radiol 1988;29:147–156.
47. Phillips D. Radiology in your practice: Choosing the right equipment. Vet Med 1987;6:587–598.
48. Purohit CR. The diagnostic value of thermography in equine medicine. Proc Am Assoc Equine Pract 1987;26:317.
49. Purohit RC, McCoy MD. Thermography in the diagnosis of inflammatory processes in the horse. Am J Vet Res 1980;41:1167.
50. Reid CF. Radiographic film identification and positioning. Proc Am Assoc Equine Pract 1965;11:167.
51. Ruohoniemi M, Karkkainen M, Tervahartiala P. Evaluation of the variably ossified collateral cartilages of the distal phalanx and adjacent anatomic structures in the Finnhorse with computed tomography and magnetic resonance imaging. Vet Radiol Ultrasound 1997; 38:344–351.

52. Ryan GD, Deigle HJ. Safety in large animal radiography. J Am Vet Med Assoc 1969;155:898.
53. Smallwood JE, Shively MJ. Nomenclature for radiographic views of the limbs. Equine Pract 1979;1:41.
54. Smallwood JE, Shively MJ, Rendano VT, Habel RE. A standardized nomenclature for radiographic projections used in veterinary medicine. Vet Radiol 1985;26:2.
55. Spencer CP. Screen and film combination for equine radiography: An update. Proc Am Assoc Equine Pract 1978;24:271.
56. Stromberg B. Morphologic, thermographic and ^{133}Xe clearance studies on normal and diseased superficial digital flexor tendons in race horses. Equine Vet J 1973;5:156–161.
57. Stromberg B. The normal and diseased flexor tendon in racehorses. Acta Radiol 1972;319:295.
58. Tomizawa N, et al. Efficacy of the new radiographic measurement method for cervical vertebral instability in wobbling foals. J Vet Med Sci 1994;56:1119–1122.
59. Tomizawa N, et al. Relationships between radiography of cervical vertebra and histopathology of the cervical cord in wobbling 19 foals. J Vet Med Sci 1994;56:227–233.
60. Turner T. Hindlimb muscle strain as a cause of lameness in horses. Proc Am Assoc Equine Pract 1990;35:281–290.
61. Turner T. Thermography as an aid in the localization of upper hindlimb lameness. Pferdeheilkunde 1996;12:632–634.
62. Turner T. Use of thermography in lameness evaluation. Proc Am Assoc Equine Pract 1998;44:224–226.
63. Vaden M. Thermography: A technique for subclinical diagnosis of osteoarthritis. Am J Vet Res 1980;41:1175.
64. VanBree H, Van Rigssen B, Tshamala M, et al. Comparison of the nonionic contrast agents, iopromide and iotrolan, for positive-contrast arthrography of the scapulohumeral joints in dogs. Am J Vet Res 1992;53:1622–1626.
65. Vaughan LC. Symposium on equine radiology/radiography. I. Radiation protection and the equine practitioner. Equine Vet J 1970; 2:73.
66. Verschooten F, Picavet T-M. Desmitis of the fetlock annular ligament in the horse. Equine Vet J 1986;18:138–142.
67. Walker M. Radiological equipment and techniques. Proc Am Assoc Equine Pract 1978;24:267.
68. Widmer W. Iohexol and iopamidol: New contrast material for veterinary myelography. J Am Vet Med Assoc 1998;194:1714–1716.
69. Williams FL, Campbell DY. Tendon radiography in the horse. J Am Vet Med Assoc 1961;139:224–226.
70. Wood AKW, Robotham FPJ, Reynolds KM, et al. Radiation protection in equine radiography. Aust Vet J 1974;50:373–379.
71. Wright JD, Wood AKW. Arthrography of the equine tarsus: A comparison between iohexol and sodium and meglumine diatrizoate. Vet Radiol 1988;29:191.

Part II

ULTRASONOGRAPHY OF THE TENDONS, LIGAMENTS, AND JOINTS

Robert H. Wrigley

DIAGNOSTIC ULTRASOUND

Diagnostic ultrasound imaging of equine soft tissues began after the development of a gray-scale real-time scanner in the early 1980s. As the equipment became more portable and less expensive, ultrasound imaging of the equine reproductive tract was in widespread use by the mid-1980s. Imaging of equine tendons and ligaments became practical with the availability of high-frequency near-focused ultrasound transducers and high-resolution real-time display systems.[42,49] When high-resolution, 7-MHz, mechanical sector ultrasound scanners became available, the normal ultrasonographic anatomy of equine tendons, ligaments, and joints and clinical applications were described.[7,26,27,31–35,39,40,42,46,48,49,51–52,60–62] Continued technical improvements resulting in better near-field resolution, lower-cost portable ultrasound machines, and familiarity generated by ultrasonography of the reproductive organs have led to the widespread use of ultrasonography in the evaluation of soft tissues and joint injuries of lame horses.[7,26,27,31,35,39,40,46,52,61,62]

Ultrasound machines operate by producing pulses of ultrasound via intermittently energizing piezoelectric crystals mounted in a transducer. The same crystals then detect the returning echoes resulting from sound-reflecting interfaces. Ultrasound frequencies used for diagnostic ultrasonography range from 1 to 10 MHz; the range most commonly used for horses is 3 to 7 MHz. Higher-frequency sound is more rapidly attenuated by the body, so tissues deeper than 8 cm may not be imaged with 7 MHz. In higher-frequency transducers, the crystals are smaller, and the sound pulses are close together, leading to maximal resolution. This makes higher-frequency transducers (more than 5 MHz) most desirable for imaging superficial, fine-detailed structures such as tendons and ligaments. Lower-frequency transducers (e.g., 3 to 5 MHz) provide images of lower resolution but are able to display deeper anatomy.

Resolution of the display also depends partly on the width of the scanning sound beam. The sound beam size is controlled by the degree of focusing. The manufacturer routinely provides a focusing lens on the crystal surface. It is important to select transducers with a focal depth optimal for the structures of diagnostic interest. Transducers with multiple crystals may allow focus adjustment, so an appropriate focal depth can be selected to achieve optimum resolution of each patient.

Returning echoes generate electrical pulses that are electronically manipulated and displayed on a monitor by the ultrasound machine. B-mode images are generated when the echo intensity is distributed over a gray scale in which the brightness is proportional to the magnitude of each echo. Displays with a gray-scale range of 32 to 64 are adequate. The contrast of the image is determined by the contrast setting of the monitor and the dynamic range over which the signal information is displayed. High-contrast images are useful for defining the boundaries of fluid-containing structures. Lower-contrast images are more desirable for soft tissue display.

The depth (top to bottom location of each object) is determined by the time delay associated with the round trip travel time of the sound pulses. Echoes from deeper reflecting boundaries arrive later and are displayed at greater depths on the monitor. The other component of spatial orientation (left to right location) on the display may be established by tracking the coordinates of echoes as the crystal (mechanical sector transducers) is moved across the patient. Alternately, in an array of many small crystals, the display of each region on the monitor is generated from each appropriate crystal.

Controls routinely adjusted during the scan include the depth and brightness of the display. Depth also controls the size of the displayed images, so the dimensions of each structure must always be correlated to a reference centimeter scale. Gain controls (overall gain, near and far gain) need to be optimized frequently during the study to display the objects of interest at an optimum gray shade on the monitor.

Principles of Interpretation

Echoes are generated whenever the sound beam crosses a boundary between structures of differing acoustic impedance. Acoustic impedance depends on both the sound velocity and the density within a tissue. If the sound beam orientation is perpendicular to the acoustic boundary, echoes are reflected back toward the transducer. The greater the difference in acoustic impedance at the boundary, the greater the intensity of the returning echo. Highly reflective boundaries result in a bright display. If the sound beam is obliquely angled to a boundary, however, it is less bright. If few boundaries are present, the display is gray to black. When the sound beam traverses perpendicular boundaries separated by distances greater than the sound beam pulse length, the boundaries are consistently displayed by the ultrasound machine as echogenic (specular) reflectors. Boundaries closer together than the pulse length cause objects to summate together. Interaction of the sound beam with small, uneven interfaces causes scattering of the sound beam. The random realignment and interaction of the sound beam result in many weak echoes, which give rise to the gray, textured appearance of parenchymal organs.

A water-filled structure is displayed by ultrasound as a black (anechoic) region surrounded by an echogenic hyperechoic (bright) wall. If cells or crystals are suspended within the fluid, then variable amounts of scattered echoes are generated, resulting in a grayer (hypoechoic) appearance to the fluid (Fig. 4.94). Purulent fluids and suspended gas bubbles generate many echoes, so that some abscess cavities can become equally or more echogenic than the surrounding tissue.[56]

The acoustic impedance of a gas is greatly different from tissue. Air and other gases create loud echoes, which are displayed as hyperechoic regions (Fig 4.95). If the gas is contained in a cavity, repeating echoes occur because the sound is trapped in the highly reflective cavity. This effect (reverberation), combined with slower sound velocities in gases, leads to erroneous echoes being

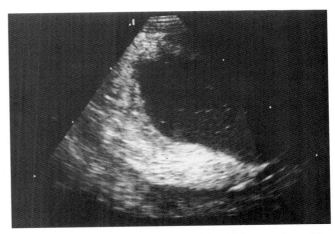

Figure 4.94 Transverse sonogram of the thigh, revealing a 12-cm, well-demarcated fluid accumulation in the region. Differential diagnosis would be focal abscess or chronic hematoma. Diagnosis of an abscess was made from cytology of a sample of fluid aspirate.

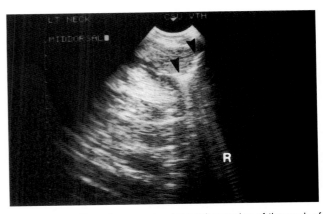

Figure 4.95 Dorsal sonogram of the left muscles of the neck of a horse that had developed a swelling 3 days after an intramuscular injection of Banamine. Ultrasonography reveals an abnormal hyperechoic focus (arrows) that generates far-field reverberation (R) associated with intramuscular gas. Culture of a sample of fluid aspirate revealed *Clostridium perfringens*, which was the source of the gas and myositis.

displayed on the monitor, which obscure the display of deeper tissues. Reverberation artifacts may be recognized by observing repeating equally spaced hyperechoic lines down the monitor (Fig. 4.95).

Alternately, the region below a gas-tissue interface begins as a more superficial hyperechoic area overlying an area that appears to fade to a black zone. The detection of these artifacts helps the clinician locate the site of the gas but precludes sonographic evaluation of tissues underneath the gas layers.

Similarly, the acoustic impedance difference at the surface of a calcified region is large. Bone surfaces are highly reflective and are displayed as bright hyperechoic lines (Figs. 4.96 and 4.97). This great difference in acoustic impedance essentially precludes display of tissue information deep to the bony surface. A distinct anechoic,

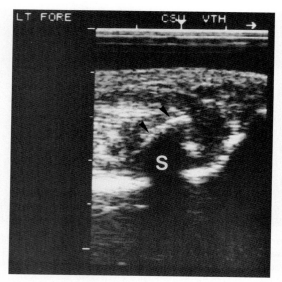

Figure 4.96 Longitudinal sonogram of a swollen medial branch of the suspensory ligament, showing a bony fragment that had avulsed from the surface of the proximal sesamoid. The fragment is identified by the hyperechoic line (arrows) generating far-field acoustic shadowing (S).

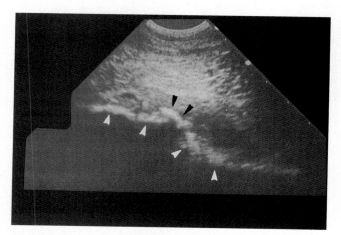

Figure 4.97 Longitudinal sonogram centered along the spine of the scapula of a horse that had received a penetrating wound to the region and subsequently developed a draining tract. Ultrasonography shows an irregular surface contour of the normally smooth spine of the scapula (white arrows), which seems elevated from the adjacent bones. This appearance is consistent with periostitis resulting from osteomyelitis. The fragment (black arrows) could be a detached bone fragment or an echogenic foreign body. The diagnosis of osteomyelitis and a bone sequestrum was confirmed by surgical exploration.

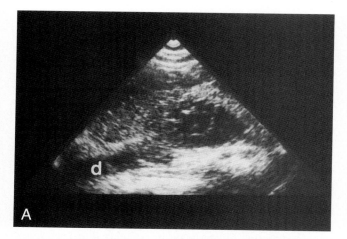

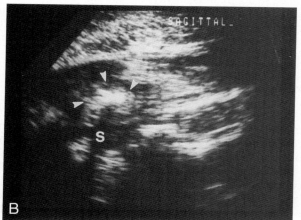

Figure 4.98 A. Sonogram of the axilla, showing a fluid-filled draining tract (d) extending caudally to a multiloculated fluid cavity. A piece of wood had been removed from the area several months earlier. B. Sonogram of the fluid compartment revealing a hyperechoic focus (arrows) with underlying acoustic shadow (S). Surgical exploration confirmed another piece of wood in the abscess cavity.

blacked-out region is displayed below bone and is described as an acoustic shadow artifact, which helps localize the surface of bones (Fig. 4.96). Areas of dystrophic calcification or foreign bodies in soft tissues are also displayed as hyperechoic reflections (Fig. 4.98B). When the calcified region or foreign body is of larger dimensions than the sound beam, acoustic shadows often occur, which help detection of such abnormalities.[25]

Normal soft tissues generate intermediate levels of echoes. Alignment of the ultrasound beam perpendicular to a fibrous tissue layer, such as a fascial plane, blood vessel wall, tendon, or ligament surface, leads to reproducible display of hyperechoic (specular) boundaries (Fig. 4.99). Boundaries aligned perpendicular to the ultrasound beam appear brightest. Other layers oriented obliquely to the incident sound beam are less bright or are not displayed at all. Reorientation of the transducer can help display the missing anatomy. The internal parenchyma of the organs generates a variable degree of scattered echoes, which fill in the regions between the specular echoes. In most parenchymal organs, the scattering is independent of scan angle. In organs in which the parenchymal structure is aligned in a linear fashion, however, echo intensity varies with beam angle. This marked angle-dependent echogenicity (anisotropy) is especially noticeable in equine tendons and ligaments.[43]

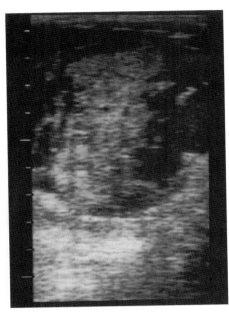

Figure 4.99 Sonogram of the right thigh 3 weeks after a suspected torn muscle, showing a large fluid accumulation caused by a hematoma.

Applications

Diagnostic ultrasound imaging of bones has limited use, because only the nearest surface is displayed as an echointense line. The bony anatomy routinely displayed on radiographs (cortices, medulla, and trabecula) is not imaged by ultrasonography. Larger discontinuities to bony surfaces, such as distracted fractures,[56] avulsed chips, and ossification defects resulting from osteochondrosis, may be identified by ultrasound imaging (Fig. 4.96). Practical applications include examination of the surfaces of bones of the pelvis (via transrectal and subcutaneous acoustic windows) and fractured ribs and long bones, such as the scapula, femur, and humerus. Chronic osteomyelitis may also be diagnosed after finding an abnormally irregular bone surface adjacent to a draining tract or an abscess (Fig. 4.97).[4,56]

Unlike radiography, ultrasonography is extremely sensitive to variations in the composition of soft tissues. Fluid, such as that in joints, bursa, blood vessels, and the reproductive tract, is readily detected and differentiated from the surrounding soft tissues. Walled-off abscesses are detected as encapsulated fluid pockets (Fig. 4.94).[1,30,36] The echogenicity of the contents of abscess cavities depends on the degree of cellularity/inspissation or gas formation. Abscess echogenicity most commonly ranges from anechoic to hypoechoic, compared with the adjacent soft tissue; an abscess can also be more echogenic than the surrounding tissue. Ballottement of echogenic abscesses gives the echoes a swirling appearance, aiding recognition of the fluid nature of the material.

If the abscess is secondary to a foreign body (Fig. 4.98), an additional hyperechoic object may be detected within the cavity. The foreign body may generate a far-field acoustic shadow when it is larger than the diameter of the ultrasound beam.[2,37] Unfortunately, the shadow-ing generated by gas and calcified structures can be confusingly similar in appearance. A radiographic examination of the region helps, as gas, metallic foreign bodies, and calcification are readily apparent. If no abnormalities are detected on the radiographs, the shadowing object in the abscess is most likely to be a foreign body (Fig. 4.98B).

Ultrasonography also helps in the evaluation of the course of a draining tract (Fig. 4.98A).[37] The soft tissues in the region should be imaged to locate possible abscess cavities or foreign bodies. Further delineation of the tract can be achieved by injecting sterile water or saline (being careful not to include air) to make the distended fluid-filled tract more visible. It may be possible to trace the tract to a foreign body or a bone surface, which may suggest the presence of osteomyelitis.[56]

Ultrasonography of a normal triceps muscle reveals echogenic striations separated by anechoic areas. The fascia dividing muscle bellies appears as echoic lines. Postanesthetic triceps myopathy results in an overall increase in echogenicity with loss of the normal striations.[58]

Injuries to muscle may result in hematomas, abscesses, and fibrosis. An acute or diffuse bleed may be difficult to locate via ultrasound because fresh clotted blood is initially echogenic.[3] After 3 to 4 days, hematoma formation results in anechoic loculated fluid. Unfortunately, the ultrasonographic appearance of organized hematomas (Fig. 4.99) and abscesses (Fig. 4.94) is similar. Once the fluid cavity has been located, needle aspiration and cytology can establish a diagnosis. Alternately, muscle injury may appear hyperechoic because of regions of abnormal fibrosis.[3] Chronic fibrotic myopathy of the semimembranosus and semitendinosus muscles can be detected as hyperechoic changes in the muscle tissue (Fig. 4.100).[13]

Tendon, ligament, and joint injuries commonly occur in equine athletes. Clinical evaluation may reveal lame-

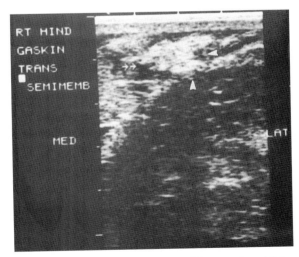

Figure 4.100 Transverse sonogram of the muscles of the thigh, showing hyperechoic tissue (arrows) in the semimembranosus muscle, caused by marked fibrotic myopathy. Compared with the adjacent fibrosis, the underlying muscle belly has the relatively hypoechoic appearance of normal muscle.

ness, local heat, swelling, and pain. Ultrasonography enables the evaluation of the size, shape, and relative echogenicity of each of the tendons and ligaments and of the surrounding tissues (bursa, tendon sheath, and synovial and subcutaneous tissues). The exact location, severity, and extent of the injury can be determined.[7,12,26,27,31–35, 39,40,42,46,48,49,51,52,60–62] This additional information helps the veterinarian develop the best therapeutic plan. Surgical intervention may be indicated, depending on the type, nature, and extent of the injury. Serial follow-up ultrasound imaging is useful for monitoring the healing process and customizing the exercise regime to maximize the likelihood of recovery.

Equipment

Veterinary ultrasound equipment represents a small segment of the medical imaging market, and so the veterinary practitioner has a limited choice of affordable equipment suitable for tendon imaging. A small portable machine is desirable, as it can be moved easily around horses and be carried to racetracks, training facilities, and horse farms (Fig. 4.101). High-resolution images are mandatory, since the tendons and ligaments are relatively small structures and it is important to detect even slight injuries. High-frequency transducers (about 7 MHz) are necessary for obtaining detailed images of tendons and ligaments (Fig. 4.102). Resolution also is dependent on using an ultrasound beam that is focused to a narrow width in the structures of most diagnostic interest. An ultrasound machine that allows the operator to select the depth of the focal plane is optimal because it allows the tendon or ligament of most interest to be examined in highest detail.

The initial descriptions of tendon ultrasonography were made with 7-MHz, mechanical sector transducers.[32–34,42,48,49,51] With these transducers, the crystal is rotated or rocked back and forth to create a pie-shaped (inverted V) scan. When such transducers are configured with only a single crystal, the focus is at a fixed depth.

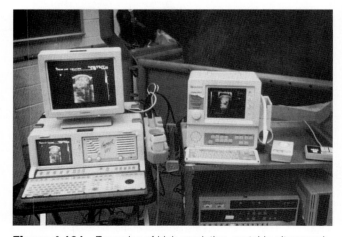

Figure 4.101 Examples of high-resolution, portable ultrasound machines. Multiple linear and convex array and mechanical sector transducers can be connected to the ultrasound machines. Focus depth and operating frequency are adjusted on the machine.

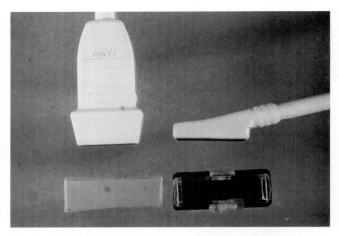

Figure 4.102 Linear array-type, 7.5-MHz transducers used for tendon imaging. Top left. An end fire-type transducer that can be operated at 10 or 7.5 MHz. Top right. A side fire-type transducer suitable for transrectal applications. Bottom right. Standoff attachment for the transducer just above is readily attached to the transducer with Velcro tape. Bottom left. An alternate, more difficult approach is to hold the standoff material between the transducer and the skin.

Imaging of structures below the skin, such as the superficial digital flexor tendon, is difficult, as the tendon is incompletely displayed in the narrow region of the sector image. The addition of an acoustic standoff (Fig. 4.102),[50] either built into the transducer or provided as a slip-on attachment,[67] greatly improves the superficial resolution. Such a system provides excellent images in a transverse plane. When a sector transducer is aligned to the long axis of a tendon, the scan angle varies along the long axis of the fibers. Directly below the transducer, the insonation angle is 90°, optimizing the return and detection of echoes. As the crystal moves to each side, fewer echoes return to the transducer, and the tendons or ligaments appear to have less echogenicity.

The development of affordable ultrasound machines that control arrays of stationary crystals (up to 128) has helped to overcome some of the limitations of mechanical sector transducers. Such arrays can be fabricated into a curved surface, creating a pie-shaped image, or can be arranged in a line, creating a rectangular image. Broader ranges of frequency are available, allowing a single transducer to be operated at about 7 MHz for tendon imaging and 5 MHz for imaging of deeper structures such as is necessary for deep-seated muscle abscesses and transrectal reproductive examinations. The effective focal plane is also adjustable, so the sonographer can select the optimal plane for the structures of interest. The near-field image is improved; and superior acoustic impedance matching of the crystal surface to patient tissues has been developed, which reduces the need for shaving the hair.

Accessory Equipment

Optimum imaging of the most superficial tissues can be problematic, as the structures may be hidden in the near-field artifact and be out of the focal plane. Acoustic standoff materials allow elevation of the ultrasound transducer from the skin while an air-free acoustic coupling path is being maintained. Soft standoff materials conform to the curved surface of the limb, enabling a wider field of view.[5] A 7-MHz sector transducer with a built-in soft-ended standoff is easy to use and provides excellent resolution of both superficial and deeper structures in a transverse plane. Less-expensive options include silicone and gel standoff pads and a removable standoff pad. Inexpensive gel pads can be cut to size and cupped between the fingers holding the transducer when imaging superficial structures. Attachable silicone pad standoffs are more convenient, although more expensive.[5] A thin strap (about 1 cm) of standoff pad, combined with a 7-MHz, high-resolution, adjustable-focus linear transducer, provides excellent tendon and ligament images (Fig. 4.102).

Image Records

A method of recording the ultrasound images is necessary for medical and legal reasons. Still (frozen) images can be photographed onto Polaroid or regular photographic film (by a video camera), printed out by a medical-grade printer, or digitized and stored on computer disk. The cost per paper print is low. An alternate approach is to make a videotape record of the examination.

IMAGING PROCEDURES AND PROTOCOLS

Facilities and Restraint

The restraint required while performing equine ultrasonography varies greatly with the procedure and temperament of the horse. A major concern is that an unrestrained horse may damage the expensive ultrasound machine. Furthermore, because the sonographer is working around the lower limbs and watching the monitor rather than the horse, he or she may react too late to an unexpected movement by the horse. Restraining the horse in stocks is ideal, and using appropriate levels of sedation should be considered. A combination of xylazine and butorphanol seems adequate in most cases. Because it is advantageous to watch the ultrasound image in a darkened environment, optimum scanning is achieved in stocks that have subdued lighting.

Patient Preparation

Ultrasound images cannot be obtained unless there is good acoustic coupling between the transducer and skin. Images are obtained after clipping the hair over the region of interest. When standoff material is used, optimum acoustic coupling occurs when the remaining hair stubble is shaved. Ultrasound acoustic coupling gel should be applied to the transducer and/or standoff surfaces and the clipped surfaces. Thick and sticky gel adheres best to the skin during the study. After completion of the examination, the gel should be washed from the skin and adjacent hair to prevent the possibility of a hypersensitivity reaction.

If for aesthetic reasons hair removal is unacceptable (e.g., with show animals), diagnostic images can be obtained as long as the hair coat is thin and liberal amounts of liquids are applied to the hair and skin before and during the study. It is best to identify, from the ultrasound machine manufacturer, which solutions (e.g., soapy water, diluted alcohol, hair conditioner, or mineral oil) will not damage the transducer.

Localization Techniques

Accurate localization and recording of the abnormalities are important for diagnosis and for allowing comparison on reexamination. The first described localization technique divided the length of the metacarpus into three anatomic zones (1 to 3) and then divided each zone into subsections (A to B or A to C) (with the length of each zone being the width of four fingers).[26] An alternate and more reproducible technique (my preference) is to reference scans to palpable bone landmarks (e.g., accessory carpal bone, calcaneus, or sesamoids). This can be readily achieved by attaching a tape measure to the side of the limb (Fig. 4.103), which also helps to document the length of a lesion.

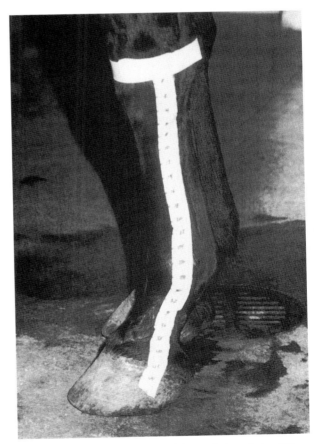

Figure 4.103 A convenient localizing technique is to write centimeter markings on a strip of adhesive bandage. Readily palpable points in this case include the distal border of the accessory carpal bone, the proximal sesamoids, and the tuber calcaneus.

Scanning Procedures

Ultrasound scanning should be performed in at least two right-angle planes. Transverse scans (made by aligning the ultrasound beam parallel to the ground) are useful for evaluating the cross-sectional size and echogenicity of the tendons and ligaments. Longitudinal scans (made by aligning the ultrasound beam vertically to the ground) establish the length and morphology of the tendon fibrils. Tendons and ligaments should be examined while under full weight-bearing tension. Relaxation of the flexor tendons results in a significant reduction in the mean gray scale of the tendon image,[44] resulting in hypoechoic artifacts that could be mistaken for injuries.

Transverse plane imaging is usually done first. After placing the transducer on the skin surface, it is important to align the ultrasound beam perpendicular to the long axis of the tendon or ligament. This can be achieved by slightly rocking the rear side of the transducer up and down and observing the relative echogenicity of the structures. The optimum angle of insonation is achieved when the image of the ligament or tendon is brightest. Once this angle has been established, then optimization of the machine settings should be checked. Machine contrast settings should be set to the full gray scale available on the ultrasound machine.

If the focus is adjustable, it should be moved to the depth of diagnostic interest. Near- and far-gain settings need to be balanced so that similar structures near the surface appear the same as they do in the deeper field. Also, the overall gain (brightness) of the image should be optimized for the surrounding environmental light conditions.

The transducer is then moved slowly proximal and distal so that the tendons and ligaments of interest are well displayed. The angle of insonation needs to be constantly reoptimized so that each structure can be visualized. Overall gain settings should be frequently adjusted to keep the image display optimized. Use firm digital pressure to push the transducer or standoff against the skin, and add more gel frequently. Firm digital pressure should not be used when synovial distension is being evaluated, as the pressure can result in collapse of fluid spaces. Scan slowly over regions of interest multiple times to allow full observation of the relative sizes, shapes, borders, relationships, and internal echogenicity of the tendons, ligaments, and surrounding structures.

After the structures are evaluated in a transverse plane, the transducer should be turned into a longitudinal plane with the image aligned so that the proximal end of the region is displayed on the left side of the monitor (distal to the right). After reoptimizing the imaging parameters, move the transducer slowly to the lateral and medial sides. The relative echogenicities and internal alignment of the tendons and ligaments can be compared. Lesions found on the transverse images must be reevaluated on the longitudinal plane. This establishes the length of the injury and the relative fiber alignment in the tendons and ligaments.

Ultrasonography of Normal Flexor Tendons and Accessory Ligaments

The figures discussed in the following text appear in the section, Normal Sonographic Anatomy for Equine Lameness Examinations, later in this chapter.

Forelimb

Figure 4.104 shows the major structures of the forelimb, and Table 4.5 provides linear measurements and cross-sectional area measurements.[6,59]

The flexor tendons proximal to the carpus (Fig. 4.105) are examined by placing the transducer on the medial aspect of the distal antebrachium just distal to the chestnut.[8,57] The superficial and medially located radial and median arteries and cephalic vessels should be identified, as they are useful landmarks. The tendon of the flexor carpi radialis is the most medially located tendon lying against the surface of the radius. This tendon and the median artery help locate the accessory ligament of the superficial digital flexor tendon.[10] The accessory ligament originates on the caudomedial aspect of the radius, 7 to 11 cm proximal to the antebrachiocarpal joint. The accessory ligament is homogenously echogenic and is located lateral to the tendon of the flexor carpi radialis, between the surface of the radius medial to the superficial digital flexor tendon and deep to the median vessels.[10] This fan-shaped fibrous band runs distocaudally, to attach to the medial side of the superficial digital flexor tendon.

The superficial digital flexor tendon arises from the musculotendinous junction of the superficial digital flexor muscle and blends with the accessory ligament to fuse into a round tendon just proximal to the carpus (Figs. 4.105 to 4.107).[8,57] The tendon runs through the carpal synovial sheath on the medial side of the carpal canal. The deep digital flexor tendon arises from three muscular bodies and appears just proximal to the carpus. Additional insertions occur from muscle bellies to the level of the carpus. In the carpal canal, the deep digital flexor tendon is triangular in shape and measures 0.9 to 1.1 cm in the dorsal to palmar direction and is located lateral to the adjacent superficial digital flexor tendon and medial to the accessory carpal bone.

The flexor tendons and accessory (check) ligament of the deep digital flexor tendon are best examined by placing the transducer on the palmar skin surface. A standoff pad helps obtain optimal images of the superficial digital flexor tendon. In the proximal metacarpal region, the superficial digital flexor tendon (Figs. 4.108 to 4.111, 4.117, and 4.118) is slightly to the medial side of the deep digital flexor tendon and becomes flattened into a half-moon shape. The lateral border is sharp, and the medial border is more rounded.[59] The transducer and standoff should have good contact on the lateral surface to ensure detection of smaller lateralized lesions. The superficial digital flexor tendon is slightly less echogenic (blacker) than the adjacent and rounded deep digital flexor tendon. The shape of the superficial digital flexor tendon gradually becomes flattened and more straplike proximal to the fetlock (Figs. 4.111 to 4.114 and 4.119). There, the superficial digital flexor tendon blends into

Table 4.5 ULTRASOUND MEASUREMENTS OF FORELIMB TENDONS AND LIGAMENTS

Zone	Distance From Accessory Carpal Bone (cm)	Superficial Digital Flexor Tendon Dimensions (cm)[a]		Superficial Digital Flexor Tendon Cross-Sectional Area (mm²)[b]			Deep Digital Flexor Tendon Dimensions (cm)[a]		Deep Digital Flexor Tendon Cross-Sectional Area (mm²)[b]			Ratio Cross-Sectional Area of Superficial Digital Flexor Tendon to Deep Digital Flexor Tendon (mm²)[b]		Accessory Ligament of Deep Digital Flexor Tendon Dimensions (cm)[a]		Suspensory Ligament Dimensions (cm)[a]	
		PD	LM	UHH	CTB	Ponies	PD	LM	UHH	CTB	Ponies	HH and TB	Ponies	PD	LM	PD	LM
1A	2.5	0.5–1.1	1.3–1.9	97–159	97–173	31–134	0.8–1.4	1.3–2.1	96–181	84–175	38–148	0.82–1.35	0.65–1.19	0.6–1.0	1.7–2.3	0.9–1.3	1.8–1.9
1B	7.5	0.5–1.1	1.4–1.9	90–156	90–169	34–120	0.6–1.5	1.3–1.9	69–136	65–128	29–101	1.09–1.66	0.81–1.72	0.5–1.0	1.4–2.0	0.8–1.3	1.5–2.1
2A	12.5	0.5–0.9	1.5–1.9	84–164	87–159	27–115	0.8–1.8	1.3–2.2	128–248	116–248	66–186	0.48–0.96	0.40–0.73			0.8–1.7	1.5–1.9
2B	17.5	0.4–0.9	1.8–2.5	93–158	77–177	28–115	0.9–1.4	1.5–2.4	113–250	118–225	60–166	0.50–1.06	0.45–0.83			0.8–1.1	0.9–1.3
3A				93–159	72–178	28–123			120–217	102–228	53–168	0.53–1.08	0.48–0.93			0.9–1.0	0.9–1.0
3B	22.5	0.5–0.6	2.3–2.5	91–176	81–194	36–128	0.9–1.1	1.9–2.3	124–232	113–229	57–168	0.57–1.11	0.52–1.00				
3C				110–190	100–192	34–130			171–277	150–276	75–223	0.53–0.88	0.37–0.78				

PD, palmar to dorsal measurement; LM, lateral to medial measurement; UHH, unconditioned heavy horses; HH, heavy horses; CTB, conditioned Thoroughbred horses; TB, Thoroughbreds.

[a] Anglo-Arabian-Andalusian crossbred horses more than 3 years old. Data from Cuesta IC, Riber C, Pinedo M, et al. Ultrasonographic measurement of palmar metacarpal tendon and ligament structures in the horse. Vet Radiol Ultrasound 1995;:131–136.

[b] Data from Smith RK, Jones R, Webbon PM. The cross-sectional areas of normal equine digital flexor tendons determined ultrasonographically. Equine Vet J 1994;26:460–465.

the manica flexoria, a fibrous ring that encircles the underlying deep digital flexor tendon.

Distal to the fetlock and palmar to the deep digital flexor tendon, the superficial digital flexor tendon becomes thinner and separates to form two echogenic branches that run beside the lateral and medial borders of the deep digital flexor tendon (Figs. 4.121 to 4.125). The branches are best detected by rocking the transducer away from midline and directing the sound beam somewhat lateral or medial in order to image the respective branch.[22] The superficial digital flexor tendon ends when two branches insert onto the scutum medium, a thick fibrocartilaginous structure attached to the proximopalmar aspect of the middle phalanx.[59]

At the level of the proximal metacarpus, the deep digital flexor tendon is rounded and located dorsal to the superficial digital flexor tendon (Figs. 4.108 to 4.114, 4.117 to 4.119).[8,57] The accessory ligament of the deep digital flexor tendon arises from the palmar ligamentous tissues of the carpus (Figs. 4.108 to 4.111 and 4.117 to 4.119).[6,44] In the proximal half of the metacarpus, the accessory ligament runs obliquely toward and attaches to the dorsal surface of the deep digital flexor tendon. After incorporating the accessory ligament, the deep digital flexor tendon becomes more oval and passes through the manica flexoria. At the level of the proximal phalanx, the deep digital flexor tendon may appear as two symmetrical bundles, the echogenicity of which depends on the scan angle (Figs. 4.121 to 4.125). The transducer should be rocked from side to side to evaluate the size and margins of the deep digital flexor tendon, which should be symmetrical and well defined.[22] The tendon continues distally, becoming flatter, until it disappears from view under the heel bulbs.

SYNOVIAL SHEATHS

The carpal synovial sheath encircles the superficial digital flexor tendon and deep digital flexor tendon in the carpal canal (Figs. 4.108, 4.109, and 4.117).[8] The synovial sheath extends distad for approximately one-third the length of the metacarpus. On ultrasonography, a small amount of fluid is frequently observed in the distal recess between the deep digital flexor tendon and the accessory ligament.

The digital synovial sheath begins in the distal metacarpus, 4 to 7 cm above the proximal sesamoid bones, and extends distad to the distal third of the middle phalanx (Figs. 4.113, 4.114, and 4.121 to 4.125).[8] The palmar border of the digital sheath blends with and is supported by the palmar anular ligament at the fetlock and the proximal digital anular ligament below the fetlock. The proximal recess of the digital sheath is located proximal to the manica flexoria in the distal fourth of the metacarpus.

Additional collateral recesses are located on the lateral and medial aspects of the pastern, between the flexor tendons and the distal sesamoidean ligaments. Fluid is frequently revealed by ultrasonography in the collateral recesses of normal horses.

SUSPENSORY LIGAMENT

The suspensory ligament runs along the palmar surface of the third metacarpal bone and between the second

and fourth metacarpal bones.[10,59] In the forelimb, the suspensory ligament originates, in part, from the palmar carpal ligament and the proximal end of the third metacarpal bone (Figs. 4.108 and 4.117). In the hindlimb, the suspensory ligament originates just below the tarsus. The body of the suspensory ligament along the proximal half of the metacarpal and/or metatarsal region should be examined with a deeper-focused transducer without a standoff pad (Figs. 4.108 to 4.110 and 4.117 and 4.118). The suspensory ligament has a less orderly ultrasonic appearance than the overlying ligaments and tendons because of the presence of some amount of residual muscle tissue.[66]

In one study of 350 normal horses, similar echogenicity and dimensions were found in the suspensory ligaments of both forelimbs in each horse.[21] Variable echogenicity, including well- or poorly defined, centrally located hypoechoic areas, however, were observed between horses. The fore suspensory ligaments were approximately rectangular in cross section, sometimes appearing with two heads that were separated by a less-echogenic band.[21] Standardbreds have more residual muscle tissue (14% of total area) than Thoroughbreds (10% of total area). Thoroughbred horses in training have significantly less residual muscle remaining in the suspensory ligament than similar nontrained horses have.[66]

At the level of the distal third of the metacarpus and/or metatarsus, the suspensory ligament divides into two branches (Fig. 4.111), each of which continues distad to attach onto the abaxial surfaces of the proximal sesamoid bones. The branches are best imaged by moving the transducer and standoff either dorsolaterally or dorsomedially, directly onto each respective branch (Figs. 4.112, 4.113, 4.115, 4.116, and 4.120). The medial branch is slightly larger than the lateral branch. Both branches are more echogenic than the body of suspensory ligament. Orderly longitudinally aligned fibers can be seen inserting onto the abaxial border of the proximal sesamoids (Fig. 4.120).

ACCESSORY LIGAMENT OF THE DEEP DIGITAL FLEXOR TENDON

The accessory ligament of the deep digital flexor tendon (carpal, distal, or inferior check ligament) is a distal continuation of the common palmar ligament (fascia) of the carpus (Figs. 4.108 to 4.111 and 4.117 to 4.119).[8,10] Proximally, the accessory ligament is rectangular and becomes progressively thinner as the ligament becomes adherent to the dorsal surface of the deep digital flexor tendon. Throughout its length in the middle third of the metacarpal region, the ligament is crescent shaped and molded to the dorsal surface of the deep digital flexor tendon (Figs. 4.109 to 4.111). The accessory ligament blends into the deep digital flexor tendon, ending just proximal to the distal extremities of the small metacarpal (splint) bones (Figs. 4.111, 4.118, and 4.119). The fibers of the accessory ligament are aligned in a slightly dorsal to palmar direction as the ligament runs toward the deep digital flexor tendon. This unparalleled alignment precludes simultaneous optimum insonation angles to both the accessory ligament and the deep digital flexor tendon.

Examination of the accessory ligament should be made while the limb is weight bearing, since reduced tension can produce a hypoechoic appearance.[8] The dense, compact fibrous nature of the ligament normally gives rise to a hyperechoic appearance. In most horses imaged optimally, the accessory ligament is more echogenic than are the flexor tendons (Figs. 4.108 to 4.111). Some variability exists, however, and if the insonation angle is made optimal for the flexor tendons, then the accessory ligament often appears less echogenic.[6,53] Ultrasound examination should be focused on the accessory ligament alone, and interpretation should be limited to insonation angles at which the ligament appears most echogenic.

DISTAL SESAMOIDEAN LIGAMENTS

The distal sesamoidean ligaments act as a functional distal continuation of the suspensory ligament.[8,57] All the ligaments arise from the base of the proximal sesamoids and intersesamoidean ligament. The intersesamoid ligament is readily observed between the proximal sesamoid bones during transverse scanning of the flexor tendons at the level of the fetlock joint (Fig. 4.114). The straight sesamoidean ligament is a thick echogenic band that inserts on the scrutum medium at the distal end of the middle phalanx (Figs. 4.121 to 4.125).[40] It is triangular in shape proximally—measuring 6 to 8 mm dorsal to palmar and 18 to 22 mm lateral to medial—and becomes more oval distally—measuring 7 to 9 mm by 14 to 18 mm (Figs. 4.121, 4.124, and 4.125).[53]

The oblique sesamoidean ligaments are observed as two thin triangular bands running on the palmar surface of the proximal phalanx adjacent to each side of the straight sesamoidean ligament (Fig. 4.121). The ligaments become progressively thinner as they insert on to the middle half of the proximal phalanx.[40] The short sesamoidean ligaments are difficult to differentiate from the deep portions of the proximal end of the oblique sesamoidean ligament.[53] The cruciate sesamoidean ligaments are thin and closely opposed to the dorsal surface of the straight sesamoidean ligament.

ANULAR LIGAMENTS

The palmar digital anular ligament attaches to the palmar border of the proximal sesamoid bones (Fig. 4.114). This strong ligament binds down the flexor tendons and, combined with the proximal sesamoid bones, forms a tunnel through which the flexor tendons cross the fetlock joint.[8] Since the ligament is difficult to detect with ultrasound, a practical approach is to measure the distance from the skin surface to the edge of fluid in the digital synovial sheath or to the surface of the superficial digital flexor tendon.[11,17] This measurement is made at the level of the apex of the proximal sesamoid bone. The skin and the ligament thickness in normal horses measure 3.6 mm and 0.7 mm, respectively.[17] In the absence of overlying scar tissue, measurements of 9.1 mm and 2.3 mm were associated with desmitis of the anular ligament.[17] When the anular ligament is thickened, transverse scans (best angled obliquely toward the sesamoids) may demonstrate a thickened hyperechoic ligament.

The proximal digital anular ligament is normally a thin fibrous tissue layer supporting the digital sheath distal to the fetlock (Figs. 4.121, 4.122, and 4.124). In normal horses, the ligament is not detected by ultrasound.[16] The combined thickness of the skin and ligament at the level of the middle of the proximal phalanx should not exceed 3 mm.

BLOOD VESSELS

The digital vessels, especially the veins, are observed on the lateral and medial sides of the metacarpus and/or metatarsus just superficial to the suspensory ligament (Figs. 4.111 and 4.112).[8,57] Branches at various locations are sometimes observed joining the two veins between the accessory ligament of the deep digital flexor tendon and the suspensory ligament. In the distal metacarpal and/or metatarsal region, the vessels lie beside the branches of the suspensory ligament (Fig. 4.115 and 4.116). The vessels become larger in size and prominent after injury to the tendons and ligaments.

Hindlimb

The tendons and ligaments distal to the midmetatarsal region appear similar to those of the forelimb. The tendons and ligaments of the tarsal canal and proximal metatarsus, however, differ greatly from those of the forelimb.

Examination of the flexor tendons and ligaments of the hindlimb begins on the plantar aspect of the tarsus. The gastrocnemius tendon can be located by finding its insertion onto the plantaroproximal end of the calcaneal tuberosity and tracing it proximad (Figs. 4.126 and 4.127).[24] The two bellies of the gastrocnemius muscle form a common tendon enfolding caudally the proximal portion of the superficial digital flexor tendon.[15] The combined tendons of the gastrocnemius and superficial digital flexor and contributions from the biceps femoris and semitendinous muscles form the Achilles tendon.[13] Proximal to the tarsus, the gastrocnemius tendon is rounded and then becomes progressively flattened and crescent shaped at its insertion on the calcaneal tuberosity. The proximal end of the gastrocnemius tendon has a patchy echogenicity because of the persistence of muscle tissue (Fig. 4.126). The echo pattern becomes more uniform as the gastrocnemius tendon becomes aligned cranial to the superficial digital flexor tendon.[24]

The superficial digital flexor tendon at the level of the distal tibia is located medial and deep to the gastrocnemius tendon (Fig. 4.127). The rounded superficial digital flexor tendon then crosses to lie superficially to the gastrocnemius tendon at the level of calcaneal tuberosity.[13] There the superficial digital flexor tendon becomes flattened (cranial to caudal) and wider than the underlying gastrocnemius tendon.[57] The calcaneal bursa lies between the two tendons and runs from the distal tibia to the midtarsus, usually communicating with the gastrocnemius bursa. An additional subcutaneous bursa may be observed overlying the superficial digital flexor tendon. A small amount of synovial fluid is normally observed in these bursae.

An additional thick fibrous structure, the plantar ligament, arises on the calcaneus distal to the insertion of the gastrocnemius tendon.[13,57] The plantar ligament is a thick band lying on the lateral plantar surface of the tarsal bones and extends distally to insert on the fourth tarsal and metatarsal bones (Fig. 4.128). The superficial digital flexor tendon is located superficial and medial to the plantar ligament.[57] As the superficial digital flexor tendon courses distad over the tarsus, the tendon becomes more semicircular and moves medially toward the deep digital flexor tendon.[13] By the proximal metatarsus, the tendon lies plantar and lateral to the deep digital flexor tendon (Fig. 4.129). The superficial digital flexor tendon assumes a comma shape, with the thicker portion lying lateral to deep digital flexor tendon and measuring 7 to 9 mm in the dorsal to palmar direction.[5] As in the forelimb, the tendon becomes thinner and wider by the midmetatarsal region and replicates the anatomy observed in the forelimb.[8]

The principal component of the deep digital flexor tendon forms at the distal end of the tibia. The round tendon runs in the tarsal groove, over the surface of the sustentaculum and medial to the tuberosity of the calcaneus (Fig. 4.128). The deep digital flexor tendon is held in place by the flexor retinaculum and is encircled by a synovial sheath. This tarsal sheath begins at the level of the distal tibia and extends to the proximal metatarsus.[57] The flexor tendons at the level of the proximal metatarsus are not as well aligned as in the forelimb. The superficial digital flexor tendon is more lateral and the deep digital flexor tendon is more medial to both the superficial digital flexor tendon and the suspensory ligament (Fig. 4.129). Deep digital flexor tendon has dimensions similar to those in the forelimb. The accessory ligament of the deep digital flexor is thinner and more variable in size (1 to 3 mm).[53]

Examination of the proximal suspensory ligament (Fig. 4.129) in the hindlimb is more difficult than is examination in the forelimb because of edge shadow artifacts resulting from the offset location of the overlying flexor tendons.[21] In Standardbreds, the muscle content is significantly greater in the hindlimb than in the forelimb. An opposite trend is found in Thoroughbreds[66]; the proximal end of the suspensory ligament is more rounded in the hindlimb than in the forelimb. Measurements of the proximal suspensory ligament are 1 to 2 mm larger in the hindlimb than in the forelimb. Measurements of the branches are usually equal to or 1 to 2 mm larger than those in the forelimb.[5]

Ultrasonography of Joints

Although radiology remains the primary diagnostic imaging technique for evaluating equine joints, ultrasonography can be used to evaluate cartilage thickness, differentiate between soft tissue thickening[41,63] and fluid distension, identify avulsed bone fragments, and evaluate periarticular ligaments.

Articular cartilage appears as a well-defined, thin hypoechoic line overlying a smooth appropriately shaped bone surface. Ultrasonography enables assessment of the cartilage thickness.[14,47] The cartilage is more obvious in foals than in adult horses because of its greater thickness.[47] Unfortunately, the curving and opposing nature of the bony surfaces prevent ultrasonographic display of the majority of articular cartilage. Additional areas of the articular surface may be examined, however, after flexing selected joints to allow greater exposure of the articular cartilage.[9,64]

Synovial fluid is difficult to detect, except in periarticular recesses. However, ultrasonography can readily reveal distension of periarticular joint recesses associated with joint effusion.[9] The clinician must be careful not to apply excessive scanning pressure because it may compress the joint sufficiently to squeeze out the synovial fluid, making it difficult to detect the abnormal synovial effusion.[9] Light scanning pressure is recommended. Effusion is relatively easily recognized in a severely distended joint because the elevated synovial fluid pressure makes the joint less likely to collapse. Ultrasonography can identify joint capsule thickening and reveal chronic proliferative synovitis.[41,63]

Ultrasonography is particularly useful for evaluating the major periarticular ligaments.[9,14,15,47] The larger collateral ligaments and patella ligaments are readily examined.[9,14,47] The collateral ligaments tend to have a more variable echogenicity because of the presence of spiral and crossed fibers, which result in a more heterogeneous echogenicity.[9] Examination of the contralateral joint is especially useful, since it helps establish the normal sonographic appearance of infrequently evaluated structures.

Carpus

The extensor carpi radialis tendon is imaged on the dorsal surface of the distal radius and courses distad across the medial aspect of the carpal bones to insert on the third metacarpal tuberosity.[64] In the transverse plane, the tendon appears as an oval to elliptical echogenic structure between 6 and 7 mm thick and 16 and 19 mm wide. The tendon flattens and widens as it crosses the carpus and is surrounded by a sheath containing minimal fluid. In the longitudinal plane, parallel linear fiber alignment can be seen. Deep to the tendon, less-echogenic fat pads are located on the surface of the antebrachiocarpal and middle carpal joints. The surfaces of the underlying carpal bones are seen as hyperechoic lines.[64] The radiointermediate ligament can be detected as a hypoechoic structure running between the radial and intermediate carpal bones.

The common digital extensor tendon begins on the distal surface of the radius, lateral to the extensor carpi radialis tendon and superficial to the hypoechoic extensor carpi obliquus muscle. In the transverse plane, the tendon begins as a triangular-shaped structure and then becomes oval and flattened as it runs distally across the carpus. At the level of the radius, the common digital extensor tendon measures between 4 and 5 mm thick and 16 and 18 mm wide. The tendon runs mainly over the surface of intermediate carpal bone and becomes more flattened in cross section as it runs distad over the third and fourth carpal bones. At the level of the metacarpus, the tendon measures between 3 and 4 mm thick and 12 and 14 mm wide and fuses with the lateral digital extensor tendon. In the longitudinal plane, parallel alignment of hyperechoic fibers, similar to that of the extensor carpi radialis tendon, is observed. Because of the presence of a synovial sheath, a thin anechoic line encircles the tendon.

The lateral digital extensor and extensor carpi obliquus tendons are much smaller structures and more difficult to evaluate than the extensor carpi radialis tendon because they are only 3 to 4 mm thick.[64] The collateral ligaments are not as easily located as are the extensor tendons.[64] The lateral collateral ligament can be traced along the lateral distal aspect of the radius and across the ulnar and fourth carpal bones. The lateral collateral ligament has a more heterogeneous echo pattern than the medial collateral ligament. The articular cartilage cannot be evaluated in a standing horse. If the carpus is held in a fully flexed position, the articular cartilage on the distal aspect of the radius can be observed as a smooth anechoic layer between two echogenic lines representing the soft tissue-cartilage and cartilage-bone interfaces.[64]

Fetlock

The dorsal aspect of the fetlock joint is readily accessible to ultrasound imaging.[9,41,63] The entire dorsal aspect of the fetlock can be examined in both longitudinal and transverse planes. If hypoechoic changes are seen on the dorsal joint capsule, repeat imaging should be performed with the limb in a flexed non-weight-bearing position, which tightens the joint capsule and causes artifactual hypoechoic areas to disappear.[9] The distal dorsal surface of the metacarpus and the proximal phalanx serve as useful landmarks. In the transverse plane, the intermediate sagittal ridge will be apparent at the level of the joint. The dorsal articular synovial capsule is a heterogeneous ill-defined hypoechoic area lying dorsal to the articular surface and deep to the overlying more echogenic extensor tendons. The thickness of a normal dorsal articular capsule ranges from 7 to 11 mm.[9]

Stifle

Ultrasonography is useful for evaluating the patellar ligaments, the articular cartilage of the femoral trochlea, the collateral ligaments, and the menisci.[9,14,47] The medial, middle, and lateral patellar ligaments should be evaluated in both cross-sectional and longitudinal planes.[9] The middle patellar ligament is easily identified, as it lies between the medial and lateral ridges of the femoral trochlear. The ligaments appear oval in cross section and are homogenously hyperechoic. The articular surface of the trochlear appears as a hypoechoic line located between the overlying hyperechoic synovial capsule and the underlying hyperechoic ossified subchondral bone.[9,14,47]

Meniscal imaging is performed by placing the transducer between the middle and either the lateral or the medial patellar ligament.[9] The medial meniscus is more readily imaged than the lateral meniscus. Lower-frequency (5-MHz) transducers may be required to image the more caudal aspects of the menisci.[9] The meniscus appears as a triangular-shaped hyperechoic structure located between the hyperechoic curving surfaces of the femoral condyles and the proximal end of the tibia.

Careful ultrasound beam orientation is necessary, as alignment off perpendicular to the abaxial border of the menisci leads to a partially hypoechoic appearance.[9] Such a change is also observed when there are meniscal injuries. When the transducer is placed between the medial collateral ligament and the medial patellar ligament, the longitudinal plane will reveal an anechoic synovial fluid filling the proximal recess of the medial femoral tibial joint.

The cruciate ligaments are not detected in the standing horse, as they are hidden behind the femoral condyles. If the stifle is flexed maximally, the cruciate ligaments may be detected as hypoechoic structures running through the surrounding hyperechoic fat pad. Unfortunately, horses afflicted with cruciate ligament injuries are often reluctant to adopt this stance, limiting clinical utility of this technique.[9]

Tarsus

On the medial aspect of the tarsus, the long collateral ligament can be observed arising from the medial tibial malleolus and extending to the distal tuberosity of the tibial tarsal bone and continuing across the small tarsal bones to insert on the second and third metatarsal bones.[15] The short collateral ligaments arise from the cranial medial surface of the tibial malleolus and descend obliquely plantarodistal under the long collateral ligament.[57] Collateral ligaments are readily detectable by ultrasound, but it is difficult to differentiate between the long and the short collateral ligaments. The long collateral ligaments tend to have a more organized linear structure, whereas the short collateral ligaments have a more heterogeneous echo texture.

Scanning on the dorsal medial aspect of the tarsus reveals the tendons of the peroneus tertius and tibialis cranialis running distal across the tarsus.[15] Scanning the dorsal surface of the tarsus between the medial collateral ligament and medial to the tendons demonstrates the cartilage and the trochlear ridges of the tibial tarsal bone.[15] In a normal horse, synovial fluid is not detected in the joint.

PRINCIPLES OF ULTRASOUND DIAGNOSIS

Tendons and Ligaments

In general, the sonographic detection of injury to a tendon (tendinitis) or a ligament (desmitis) is based on the observation of enlargement, altered shape, and a changed echo pattern (Fig. 4.130).[5,20,28,29,45,55] An injury to a tendon or ligament can often be detected by physical examination. Palpation helps locate the injured region. Concurrent surrounding soft tissue swelling, however, may make identifying the extent of the injury more difficult. Peritendinous swelling may be misinterpreted as a tendon injury. Ultrasonography is useful for determining the exact location and extent of the injury.[5,7,12,23,20,26-29,31-35,39-41,45,46,48,49,51,52,56,55,60-62]

The size and shape of each tendon and ligament must be evaluated. If during the examination the clinician is uncertain of a diagnosis, scanning at the same level on the contralateral limb often helps establish the normal size and appearance. Thorough evaluation of the structures in the region of palpable enlargement or pain needs to be done.

Determination of the cause of the enlargement must be made by evaluating the size of each structure by ultrasound.[6,59] In an acute injury, much of the enlargement can result from peritendinous or periligamentous edema and swelling. In an older injury, the enlargement more likely results from tendon or ligament swelling. Thus it is important to determine the clinical duration of the injury.

Serial ultrasound examinations should be made to reevaluate the injured structures during therapy.[29] The shape of each tendon and ligament should be carefully evaluated. Transverse scans are most useful. Knowledge of the shape of the normal tendons and ligaments aids in recognition of abnormalities.[7] Injuries to the thinner portions of tendons or ligaments make them appear abnormally rounded.

Border definition of the tendon or ligament should be evaluated.[7] Peritendinous edema or effusion next to a normal tendon will normally enhance the ultrasonic definition of the border. A hyperechoic injury extending to the border may be more difficult to detect, since it may blend with the adjacent normal structures.

Transverse scans allow measurement of the lateral to medial and dorsal to palmar and/or plantar dimensions of the injured structures by means of electronic calipers on the ultrasound machine.[6,59] The measurements can be repeated and compared on subsequent recheck examinations. Some ultrasound machines are able to calculate the size (cross-sectional area) after the sonographer electronically traces the margin of the structure object. This provides a better measurement of size changes than does a linear measurement and has been incorporated into a scoring system for superficial digital flexor tendon injuries.[28]

Altered echogenicity is frequently observed with tendinitis (Fig. 4.130) and desmitis. Great care needs to be taken to obtain scans while the structure is positioned in weight-bearing traction, with optimum sound transmission,[44] machine settings, and angle of insonation for each structure to obtain reproducible results. Fiber rupture reduces the echogenicity of the tendon or ligament. The resultant inflammation leads to variable degrees of hemorrhage, edema, and cellular inflammation. The resultant increased water content results in further reduction in echogenicity. The hypoechoic changes can be diffusely scattered throughout the injured area or localized to one region. Hemorrhage or tendon and/or ligament rupture can result in anechoic changes.

Grading of the echogenicity of the injured region helps the clinician rank the severity of the injury. Genovese et al.[26,28] described a system for ranking the severity of lesions to the superficial digital flexor tendon:

Type 0	Enlarged tendon without a change in echogenicity
Type 1	Injuries are slightly hypoechoic, although mostly echogenic
Type 2	Less echogenic, with approximately half of the lesion being hypoechoic and the other half being anechoic
Type 3	Mostly anechoic
Type 4	Anechoic

This ranking needs to be correlated with the time of onset of the injury, however. Ultrasonography of the superficial digital flexor tendon soon after an acute injury can sometimes be misleading.[29] Excess hemorrhage and edema in the tendon may give a false impression of a more severe lesion. On the other hand, injuries with little hemorrhage produce fewer changes in echogenicity,

making them difficult to detect until enzymatic degradation gives rise to a greater reduction of echogenicity. Reexamination of acute superficial digital flexor tendon injuries should be performed 3 to 4 weeks after the initial onset of lameness so that a more reliable evaluation of the degree of injury can be made.[29]

Recent focal injuries to the superficial digital flexor tendon typically result in focal hypoechoic to anechoic areas within the tendon (Figs. 4.130 and 4.131). Quantitative analysis of superficial digital flexor tendon injuries can be made by incorporating information from the cross-sectional area measurements and the subjective qualitative score of the lesion.[28] On transverse scans, the outer border of the superficial digital flexor tendon and the less-echogenic injured region are traced so that the percent cross-sectional area can be calculated. A severity rating is determined by multiplying the percent of the area of the injury by the qualitative scoring and a scaling factor of 0.025.[28] A lesion that encompasses 100% of the tendon with a qualitative score of 4 thus has a severity rating of 10. A lesion that involves 50% of the tendon with a qualitative score of 2 will have a severity rating of 2.5. Horses with superficial digital flexor tendinitis rated less than 2.3 have a 83% chance to return to the same or better level of preinjury athletic performance.[28] Lesions rated greater than 3.9 have a 57% chance to return to an equal level of performance. More severe lesions predispose the horse to reoccurrence of the tendinitis.

An alternate approach to a subjective grading scheme is computerized gray-scale analysis of the image.[45] The limited availability of such equipment has precluded widespread use and evaluation of such techniques.

As long as severe blistering has not been used, the hypoechoic peritendinous swelling and edema resolves in the early phase of tendon repair. As tendon healing proceeds, the tendon cross-sectional area may return to a more normal size, and the severity rating will improve (Fig. 4.130).[29] Longitudinal evaluation of fiber alignment aids in monitoring the healing of the tendon. A grading system has been developed from the subjective assessment of the fiber alignment in the maximally injured zone on the longitudinal scan[29]:

Score 0	76–100% of the tendon injury has aligned fibers
Score 1	51–75% of the tendon injury has aligned fibers
Score 2	26–50% of the tendon injury has aligned fibers
Score 3	0–25% of the tendon injury has aligned fibers

As tendon healing progresses, the newly formed collagen fibers tend to align longitudinally, resulting in a slowly improving score for the injured regions.[29] If scar tissue repairs the tendon injury, a more random fiber alignment may be observed in the longitudinal plane. In some horses, excessive fibrous scar tissue may lead to a patchy hyperechoic appearance. Calcification and bony metaplasia can also develop, resulting in hyperechoic shadowing foci being observed in the tendon (Fig. 4.131).[34,51]

In general, the sonographic diagnosis of ligament injury (desmitis) follows the same principles as those described for tendinitis.[5,7,18,19,55] Detection of desmitis in the body of the suspensory ligament is more difficult, however, because of the inherently more variable echo-genicity of the body of the suspensory ligament (Fig. 4.132).[19] Desmitis often leads to enlargement and rounding of the margins of the suspensory ligament. Size comparison of the suspensory ligament to the contralateral normal limb is often helpful.[19] Reduced definition of one or more borders may be observed, as the ligament is usually bilaterally symmetrical. In more severe injuries, a hypoechoic appearance may develop at the site of the injury.

Sometimes, clinical signs and pain on palpation to the suspensory ligament indicate a likely injury, although no abnormalities may be detected on the initial ultrasound study.[19] Repeat examination 2 to 4 weeks later may detect an injury, since some lesions become more hypoechoic. Radiographic abnormalities and nuclear scintigraphy help locate injury at the proximal attachment of the suspensory ligament, which could be missed by ultrasound examination.[19] Injuries to the distal branches of the suspensory ligament are more readily detected, since normal branches are more uniformly hyperechoic. Desmitis in the branches can be diagnosed by finding enlargement and a variable hypoechoic echogenicity. Also, adjacent edema and swelling are often present in the acute phase of the injury.

Tendon Sheaths

Tenosynovitis, inflammation of a tendon sheath, is readily detected via ultrasound by the discovery of excessive synovial fluid and/or tendon sheath thickening (Figs. 4.133 and 4.134).[5,7,17,23,54,65] Take care not to use excessive scanning pressure when evaluating tenosynovitis, because the synovial effusion can be squeezed out of the sheath under the examination site.[7] Evaluation of the echogenicity of the fluid is important, since the presence of abnormal echoes can indicate hemorrhage, fibrin, or sepsis within the tendon sheath.[23,55,56] In septic tenosynovitis, echogenic fibrin strands and cellular material can result in an echogenic effusion (Fig. 4.135).[55,56]

Chronic inflammation of the tendon sheath results in abnormal synovial membrane thickening of the tendon sheath,[7,17,23,54,65] making the wall of the sheath readily detectable by ultrasound (Fig. 4.134). A canal syndrome may develop, in which tendons are encircled by a distended or thickened synovial sheath.[38]

Chronic synovial membrane irritation and fibrinous and septic effusions may lead to the formation of adhesions between the enclosed tendons (Fig. 4.135). Sometimes, the adhesive bands are visible when they are surrounded by excessive synovial fluid. In other cases, the adhesions are difficult to detect unless ultrasonography is performed during dynamic flexion and extension of the part. Adhesions often reduce the mobility of the tendon. Careful evaluation of the encircled tendons is needed because the synovial sheath inflammation may be secondary to tendinitis. Such an observation leads to the diagnosis of tendosynovitis.

Joints

Normally, the joint capsule and synovial fluid are difficult to detect on ultrasound. Excessive joint effusion is readily detected, however, as the joint capsule is displaced away from the surface of the articular cartilage.[9] Abnormal echogenic fluid may be observed with traumatic arthritis, hemarthrosis, or septic arthritis. The normal synovial membrane is thin, less echogenic, and difficult to distinguish.[9] The synovial membrane thickens and becomes hyperechoic with chronic joint inflammation.[15,41,63] Evaluation of the ligament and bone surface near the insertion of the ligaments onto the epiphysis may reveal bony irregularity arising from chronic injuries. Hypertrophied synovial villi may be seen interdigitating into the synovial fluid.[15] Rupture of the synovial membrane is difficult to detect on ultrasound; contrast arthrography is a more reliable technique for evaluating this condition.[9]

Osteochondrosis of the femoral trochlear can be diagnosed by finding increased thickness of the cartilage and irregularities in the contour of the underlying subchondral bone.[9,47] Incomplete subchondral ossification results in irregular echogenicity of the subchondral bone as a result of partially ossified and degenerate cartilage in the area of osteochondrosis.

Detection of the thickened joint capsule and synovial tissues suggests inflammation in the joint. Proliferative synovitis, such as on the dorsal aspect of the fetlock joint, results in excessive thickening of hypoechoic tissue in the region.[9,42,63] Displaced osteochondral fragments may be seen as hyperechoic foci generating with far-field shadowing at the edges of the joint capsule.[9]

Normal Sonographic Anatomy for Equine Lameness Examinations

NORMAL SONOGRAMS OF THE FLEXOR TENDONS AND PALMAR LIGAMENTS OF THE FORELIMB

Transverse Scans

The following transverse view sonograms of the palmar flexor tendons and associated ligaments of a left forelimb were made with a 7.5-MHz linear array transducer and standoff pad. The scans were aligned with the medial side to the left on the images. The metacarpal region was divided into seven zones between the carpus and fetlock (Fig. 4.104). The superficial digital flexor tendon is present just below the skin surface as a relatively less echogenic band; the deep digital flexor tendon is more echogenic. The accessory ligament of the deep digital flexor tendon is most echogenic and is adjacent to the dorsal surface of the deep digital flexor tendon. The suspensory ligament lies against the hyperechoic surface of the third metacarpus. Linear (dorsal to palmar) measurements of each structure are provided in centimeters.

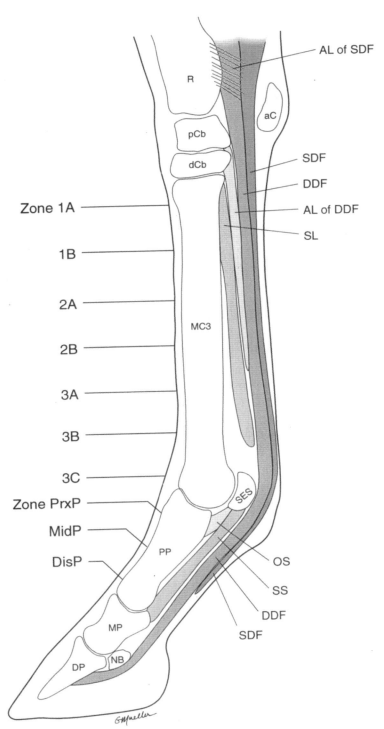

Figure 4.104   Major bones, flexor tendons, and associated ligaments of the forelimb. Representative ultrasound images and measurements were obtained at each zone (labeled at left).

AL of SDF: accessory ligament of superficial digital flexor tendon
R: radius
aC: accessory carpal bone
pCb: proximal row of carpal bones
dCb: distal row of carpal bones
SDF: superficial digital flexor tendon
DDF: deep digital flexor tendon
AL of DDF: accessory ligament of deep digital flexor tendon
SL: suspensory ligament
MC3: third metacarpal bone

SES: proximal sesamoid bones
OS: oblique sesamoidean ligament
SS: straight sesamoidean ligament
PP: proximal phalanx
MP: midphalanx
NB: navicular bone
DP: distal phalanx
PrxP: proximal end of the proximal phalanx
MidP: middle of the proximal phalanx
DisP: distal end of the proximal phalanx

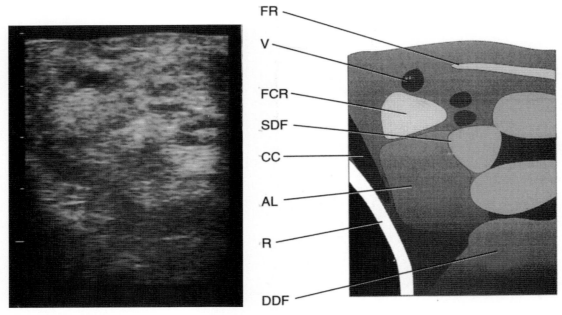

Figure 4.105 Transverse sonogram made with the transducer on the palmaromedial aspect of the antebrachium at the level of the chestnut. The tendon of the flexor carpi radialis (FCR) is seen deep to the cephalic vein (V). The palmar surface of the radius (R) helps locate the adjacent carpal sheath (CC). The accessory ligament (AL) of the superficial digital flexor tendon (SDF) is located just caudal to the radius and deep to the flexor carpi radialis tendon. The edge of the flexor retinaculum (FR) overlies the superficial digital flexor tendon. Both the superficial digital flexor tendon (SDF) and the adjacent deep digital flexor tendon (DDF) still contain muscle tissue, giving rise to a variably hypoechoic appearance.

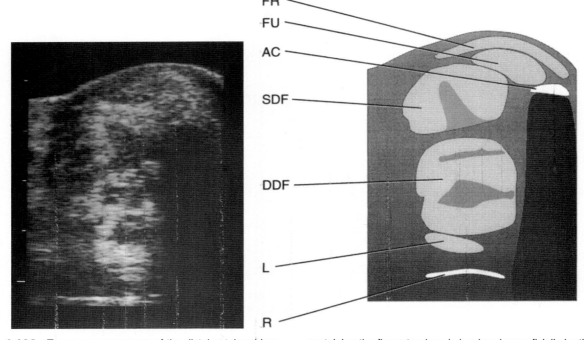

Figure 4.106 Transverse sonogram of the distal antebrachium at the level of the proximal border of the accessory carpal bone (AC). The superficial digital flexor tendon (SDF) and deep digital flexor tendon (DDF) have a variably patchy hypoechoic appearance because of residual muscle tissue. The carpal canal containing the flexor tendons is bordered superficially by the flexor retinaculum (FR) and dorsally by the palmar antebrachioradial ligaments (L) adjacent to the radius (R). The tendon of the flexor carpi ulnaris (FU) is seen palmar to the tip of the accessory carpal bone.

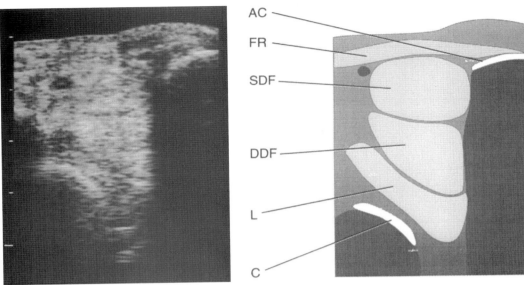

Figure 4.107 Transverse sonogram of the carpal canal. The accessory carpal bone (AC) forms the lateral border. The common palmar ligament (L) lies on the palmar surface of the radial and intermediate carpal bones (C) and adjacent to the deep digital flexor tendon (DDF). The flexor retinaculum (FR) borders the palmar surface of the superficial digital flexor tendon (SDF).

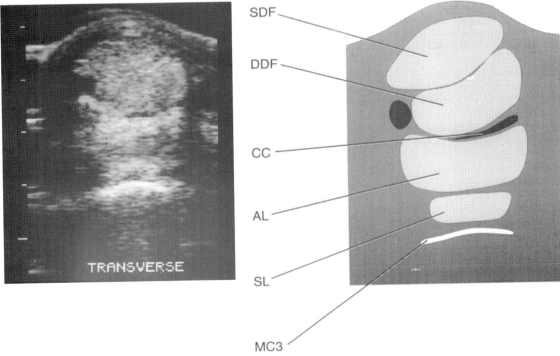

Figure 4.108 Transverse sonogram made just below the carpus (zone 1A). The superficial digital flexor tendon (SDF) and deep digital flexor tendon (DDF) are slightly offset and wedge shaped. Fluid is present in the carpal sheath (CC) between the deep digital flexor tendon and its accessory ligament (AL). The origin of the suspensory ligament (SL) lies adjacent to the third metacarpus (MC3).

SDF	DDF	AL	SL
0.9 cm	0.9 cm	0.6 cm	0.6 cm

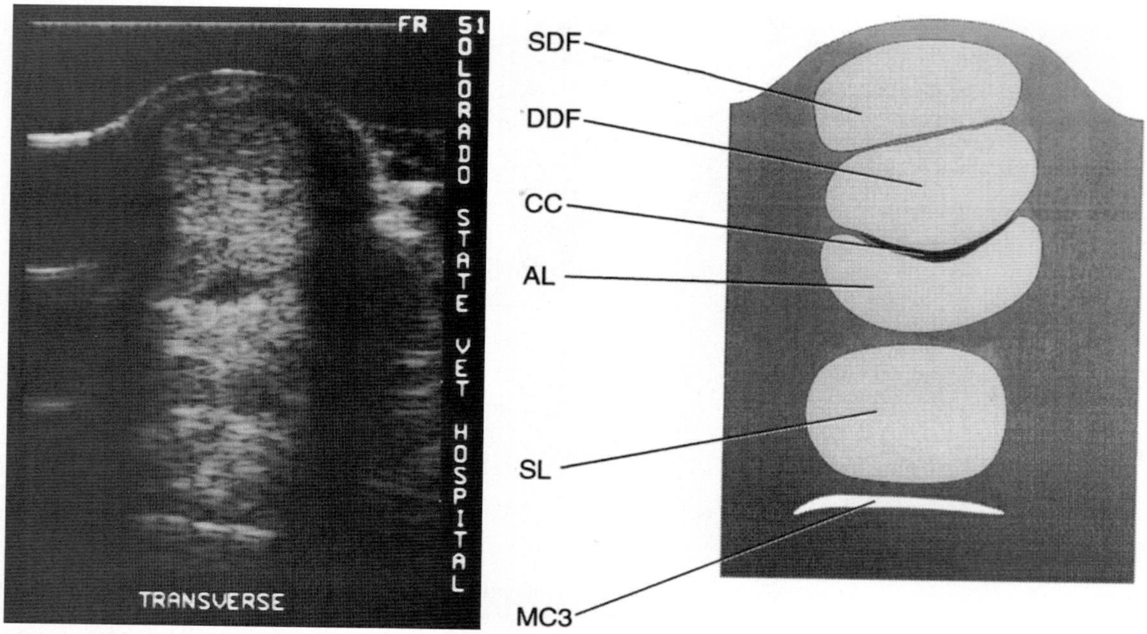

Figure 4.109 Transverse sonogram of the proximal third of the metacarpus (zone 1B). The accessory ligament (AL) is crescent shaped as it approaches the dorsal surface of the deep digital flexor tendon (DDF). A small amount of fluid is seen in the carpal sheath (CC). The body of the suspensory ligament (SL) is fully formed, and the third metacarpus (MC3) is just visible. SDF, superficial digital flexor tendon.

SDF	DDF	AL	SL
0.8 cm	0.9 cm	0.6 cm	0.7 cm

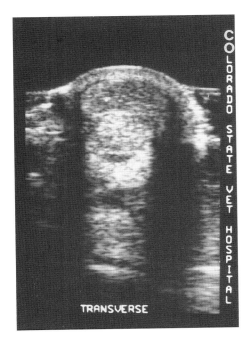

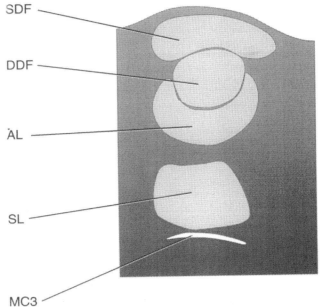

Figure 4.110 Transverse sonogram of the metacarpus just proximal to midway (zone 2A). The less-echogenic superficial digital flexor tendon (SDF) is somewhat flattened at this level. The more echogenic accessory ligament (AL) begins to blend into the dorsal surface of the deep digital flexor tendon (DDF). The body of the suspensory ligament (SL) has variable echogenicity and lies along the surface of the third metacarpus (MC3).

SDF	DDF	AL	SL
0.7 cm	0.8 cm	0.5 cm	0.9 cm

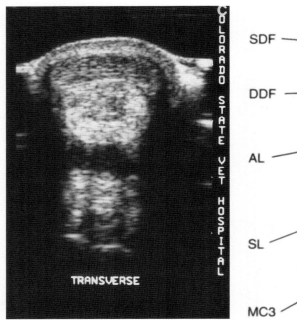

Figure 4.111 Transverse sonogram of the metacarpus just distal to midway (zone 2B). The more hypoechoic superficial digital flexor tendon (SDF) is straplike and elongated in the lateral to medial plane. The more echogenic accessory ligament (AL) is thinner and blends into the deep digital flexor tendon (DDF). The suspensory ligament (SL) has a mixed echogenicity and is widened just proximal to its bifurcation; the third metacarpus (MC3) is just visible.

SDF	DDF	AL	SL
0.5 cm	0.8 cm	0.4 cm	0.7 cm

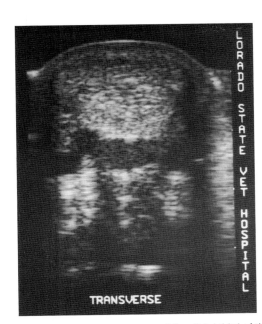

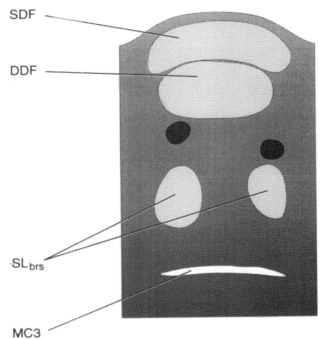

Figure 4.112 Transverse sonogram of the distal third of the metacarpus (zone 3A). The accessory ligament cannot be seen at this level. The suspensory ligament is divided, forming two branches (SL$_{brs}$). The hypoechoic area between the two suspensory ligament branches and the metacarpus represents the tissues of the palmar pouch of the fetlock. SDF, superficial digital flexor tendon; DDF, deep digital flexor tendon; MC3, third metacarpus.

SDF	DDF	SL Med Br	SL Lat Br
0.5 cm	0.9 cm	1.0 cm	0.9 cm

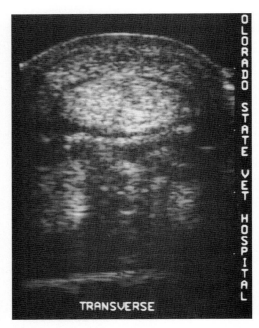

Figure 4.113 Transverse sonogram just proximal to the sesamoids (zone 3B). The strap-shaped superficial digital flexor tendon (SDF) and the digital sheath blends into the manica flexoria (M), a fibrous ring that encircles the deep digital flexor tendon (DDF). A small amount of fluid can be detected in the digital sheath (DS) around the deep digital flexor tendon. The relatively hypoechoic region between the deep digital flexor tendon, the third metacarpus (MC3), and the suspensory ligament branches (SLbrs) results from echoes generated by connective tissue in the region of the palmar pouch of the fetlock joint.

SDF	DDF	SL Med Br	SL Lat Br
0.5 cm	0.9 cm	1.0 cm	0.9 cm

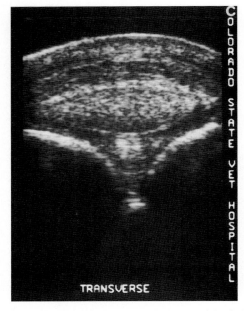
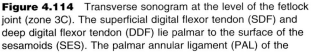
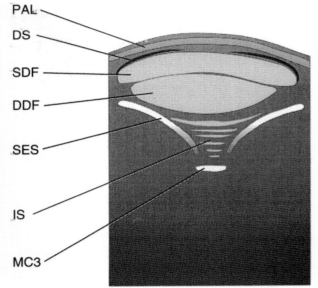

Figure 4.114 Transverse sonogram at the level of the fetlock joint (zone 3C). The superficial digital flexor tendon (SDF) and deep digital flexor tendon (DDF) lie palmar to the surface of the sesamoids (SES). The palmar annular ligament (PAL) of the fetlock is not a distinct structure but is seen as a hyperechoic band lying between the skin and subcutaneous tissues and the digital sheath (DS). The intersesamoidean ligament (IS) runs between the sesamoids; the third metacarpus (MC3) can be seen.

SDF	DDF	Skin to SDF
0.4 cm	0.8 cm	0.4 cm

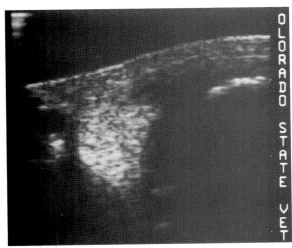

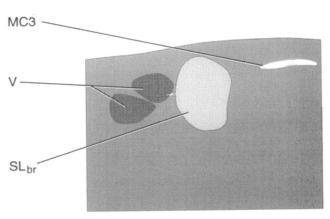

Figure 4.115 Transverse sonogram made by placing the transducer directly on the suspensory ligament branch just proximal to the fetlock at zone 3. The suspensory ligament branch (SL~br~) proximal to the fetlock is better visualized adjacent to the palmar vessels (V). The third metacarpus (MC3) can be seen.

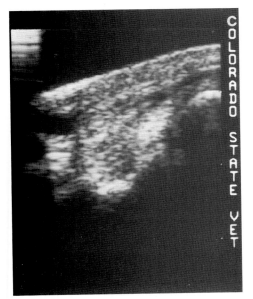

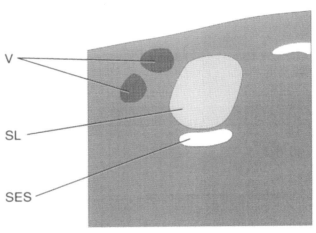

Figure 4.116 Transverse sonogram at the level of the proximal sesamoid. The suspensory ligament (SL) branch attaches to the proximal sesamoid (SES). The palmar vessels (V) can also be seen.

Longitudinal Scans

The following longitudinal sonograms of the palmar metacarpal flexor tendons and associated ligaments were made with a 7.5-MHz linear array transducer. The images were aligned with proximal to the left side and distal to the right side.

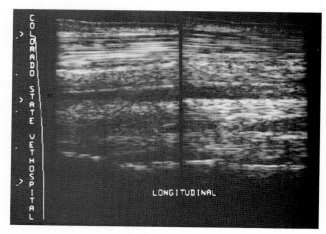 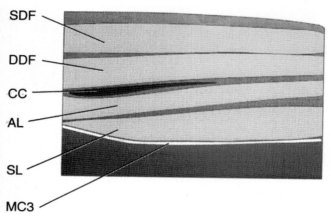

Figure 4.117 Dual longitudinal sonograms of zones 1A to 2A. The more hypoechoic superficial digital flexor tendon (SDF) is just under the skin. Fluid is present in the carpal sheath (CC) between the deep digital flexor tendon (DDF) and its accessory ligament (AL). The suspensory ligament (SL) originates along the proximal surface of the third metacarpus (MC3).

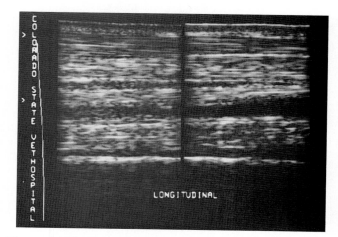 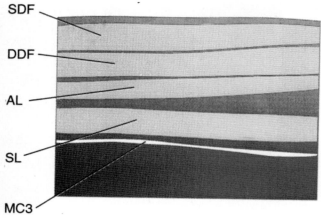

Figure 4.118 Dual longitudinal sonograms of zones 2A to 2B. The accessory ligament (AL) blends into the dorsal surface of the deep digital flexor tendon (DDF). The suspensory ligament (SL) appears as a distinct structure. SDF, superficial digital flexor tendon; MC3, third metacarpus.

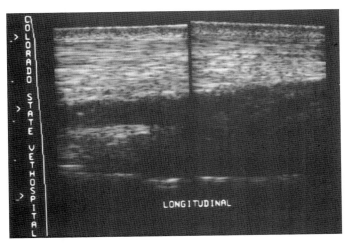

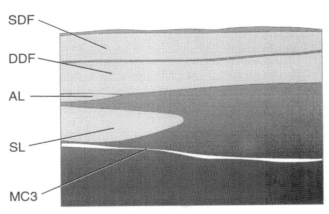

Figure 4.119 Dual stored longitudinal sonograms of zones 2B to 3B. At this level, the accessory ligament (AL) ends. The suspensory ligament (SL) appears to end as it splits into two branches that pass out of the scan plane. The thinner superficial digital flexor tendon (SDF) and deep digital flexor tendon (DDF) continue toward the fetlock. The less echogenic tissues of the palmar pouch lie between the tendons and the third metacarpus (MC3).

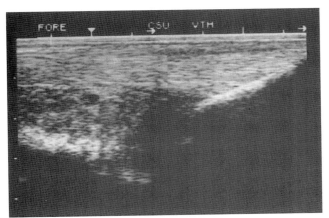

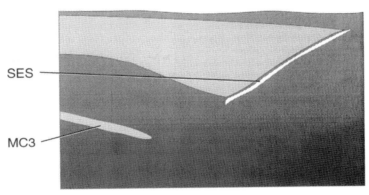

Figure 4.120 Dual stored longitudinal sonograms of zone 3, made by placing the transducer on the surface of the suspensory ligament branch. The longitudinal alignment of the ligament fibers is readily seen. Distally, the branch inserts onto the abaxial surface of the sesamoid bone (SES). MC3, third metacarpus.

NORMAL SONOGRAMS DISTAL TO THE FETLOCK

Transverse Scans

The following transverse sonograms of the tendons and ligaments along the palmar surface of the proximal phalanx were made with a 7.5-MHz linear array transducer and standoff pad.

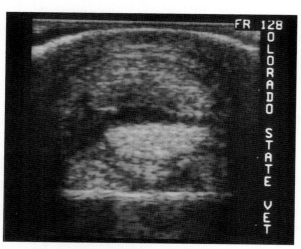

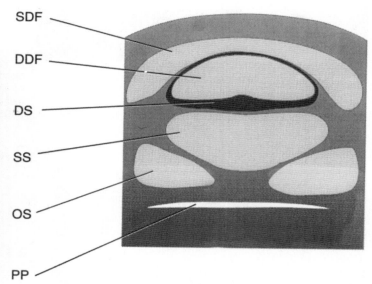

Figure 4.121 Transverse sonogram just below the ergot (proximal phalangeal zone). The superficial digital flexor tendon (SDF) is a thin band overlying the deep digital flexor tendon (DDF) and is surrounded by a synovial fluid in the digital sheath (DS). The proximal digital annular ligament lies below the skin and subcutaneous tissues and is palmar to the superficial digital flexor tendon, but it is not normally observed. The straight distal sesamoidean ligament (SS) is obvious. The two oblique sesamoidean ligaments (OS) lie adjacent to the surface of the proximal phalanx (PP).

SF	DDF	SS	OS	Skin to SDF
0.2 cm	0.7 cm	0.5 cm	0.4 cm	0.3 cm

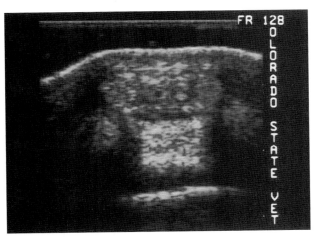

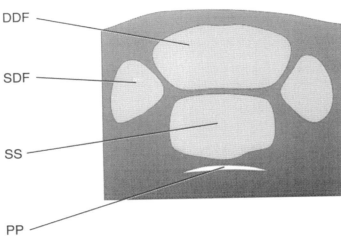

Figure 4.122 Transverse sonogram (middle phalangeal zone) proximal to the distal condyles of the proximal phalanx (PP). The superficial digital flexor tendon (SDF) is split into two branches.

The deep digital flexor tendon (DDF) is relatively flat. The straight sesamoidean ligament (SS) can still be seen at this level.

SDF	DDF	SS
0.7 cm	0.7 cm	0.7 cm

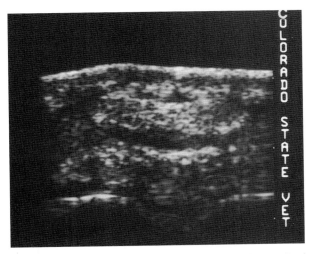

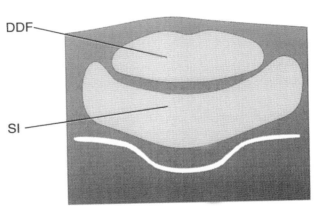

Figure 4.123 Transverse sonogram at the level of the proximal interphalangeal joint just proximal to the heel bulbs (distal phalangeal zone). Dorsal to the deep digital flexor tendon (DDF), the straight sesamoidean ligament and the branches of the

superficial digital flexor tendon coalesce with the scutum interomedialis (SI) fibrocartilage at the proximal end of the middle phalanx.

DDF
0.6 cm

Longitudinal Scans

The following longitudinal sonograms of the tendons and ligaments along the palmar surface of the proximal phalanx were made with a 7.5-MHz linear-array transducer with a standoff pad. The scans were aligned with the proximal to the left side and the distal to the right side of each image.

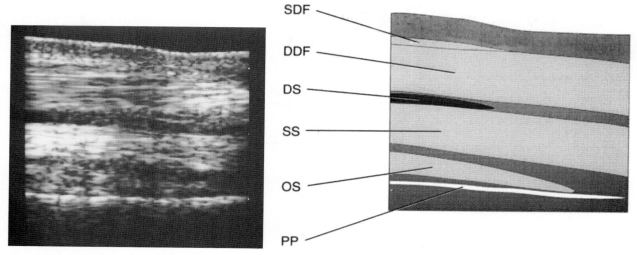

Figure 4.124 Longitudinal sonogram just distal to the ergot, showing the palmar surface of the proximal phalanx (PP) and the insertion of an oblique sesamoidean ligament (OS). The straight sesamoidean ligament (SS) is notably hyperechoic, and the deep digital flexor tendon (DDF) is less echogenic. A small amount of fluid may normally be observed in the distal end of the digital sheath (DS) between the deep digital flexor tendon and straight sesamoidean ligament. Only a thin section of the superficial digital flexor tendon (SDF) is detected proximally, as at this level the superficial digital flexor tendon is divided into two branches. The region of the proximal digital annular ligament is seen deep to the skin and subcutaneous tissues and palmar to the digital sheath adjacent to the superficial digital flexor tendon.

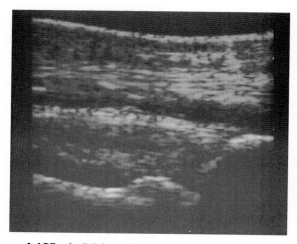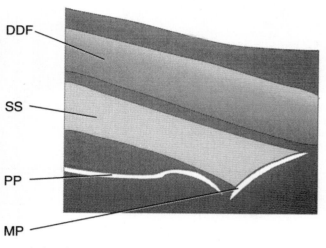

Figure 4.125 A slightly medially angled longitudinal sonogram ending at the proximal edge of the heel bulb. The conjunction of the straight sesamoidean ligament (SS) and scrutum interomedialis insert onto the proximal eminence of the middle phalanx (MP). The palmar surface of the medial condyle of the proximal phalanx (PP) is well demonstrated. The deep digital flexor tendon (DDF) continues distally.

NORMAL SONOGRAMS OF THE HINDLIMB

Transverse Scans

The following transverse sonogram of the tendons and ligaments adjacent to the tarsus were made with a 7.5-MHz linear-array transducer and standoff pad.

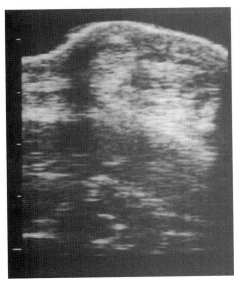

Figure 4.126   Transverse sonogram of the gastrocnemius tendon (G) 10 cm proximal to the calcaneus. The superficial digital flexor tendon (SDF) lies beside the gastrocnemius tendon.

At this level, a patchy hypoechoic echogenicity is seen in the gastrocnemius tendon, resulting from the presence of some residual muscle tissue.

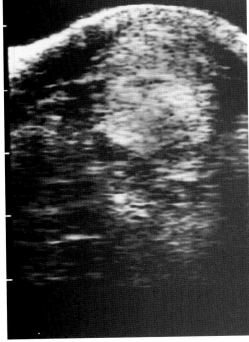

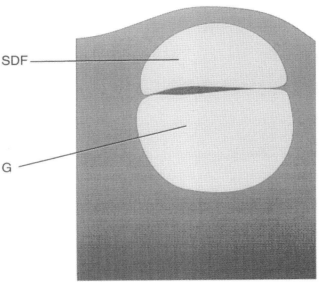

Figure 4.127   Transverse sonogram of the gastrocnemius tendon (G) just proximal to the calcaneus. At this level, the superficial digital flexor tendon (SDF) lies plantar to the gastrocnemius tendon, which is uniformly echogenic. A small amount of fluid is present in the calcaneal bursa lying between the two tendons.

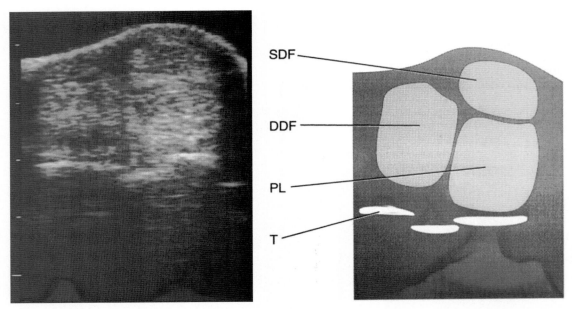

Figure 4.128 Transverse sonogram made midway along the plantar surface of the tarsus. The deep digital flexor tendon (DDF) lies to the medial side. The thick plantar ligament (PL) of the tarsus lies between the plantar surface of the tarsal bones (T) and the superficial digital flexor tendon (SDF).

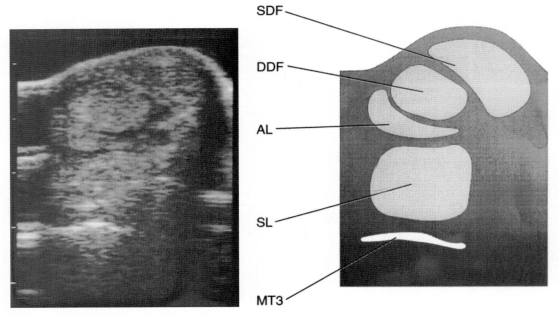

Figure 4.129 Transverse sonogram of the proximal metatarsus (zone A). The superficial digital flexor tendon (SDF) lies toward the lateral side. The accessory ligament (AL) of the deep digital flexor tendon (DDF) is thinner in the hindlimb. The suspensory ligament (SL) lies against the plantar surface of the third metatarsus (MT3).

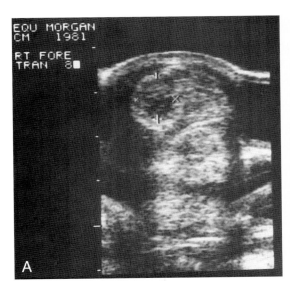

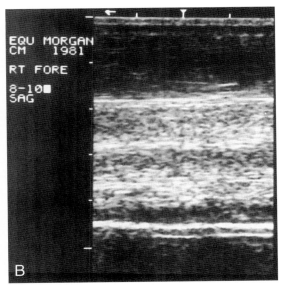

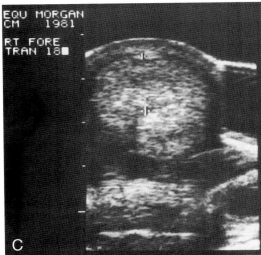

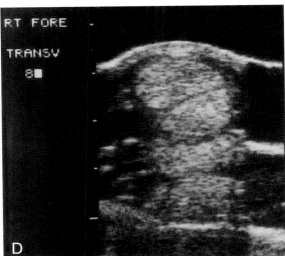

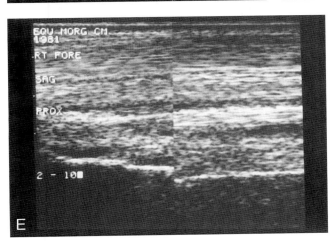

Figure 4.130   A. Transverse sonogram of the palmar tendons and ligaments of the right forelimb made 8 cm distal to the accessory carpal bone. Peritendinous swelling is evident below the skin. A focal hypoechoic to anechoic lesion of tendinitis (cursors) is seen in the medial side of the superficial digital flexor tendon. B. Longitudinal sonogram of the medial side of the superficial digital flexor tendon, showing the long axis view of the hypoechoic change caused by tendinitis of the superficial digital flexor tendon. C. Further examination of the tendons distally reveals enlargement of the superficial flexor tendon. At 18 cm distal to the accessory carpal bone, the transverse sonogram of the superficial digital flexor tendon shows enlargement with a more diffuse-type patchy change that may also be seen with acute tendinitis. D. Transverse sonogram taken 4 months later at 8 cm distal to the accessory carpal bone, showing resolution of the focal lesion in the superficial digital flexor tendon. A heterogeneous hyperechoic appearance remains in the thickened tendon. E. Follow-up longitudinal sonogram showing incomplete, though improved, tendon fiber formation throughout the region of the superficial digital flexor tendon injury.

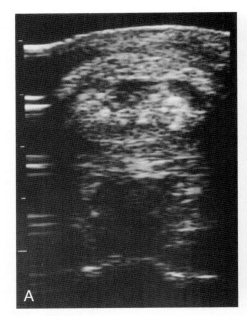

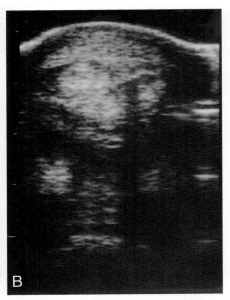

Figure 4.131 A. Transverse sonogram made 20 cm distal to the accessory carpal bone. A patchy, focal hypoechoic area of tendinitis was detected in the deep digital flexor tendon. B. Transverse sonogram taken 5 months later. Note an area of hypoechoic tendinitis has been replaced by a bright hyperechoic line generating far-field acoustic shadowing resulting from the formation of dystrophic calcification in the injured region of the tendon.

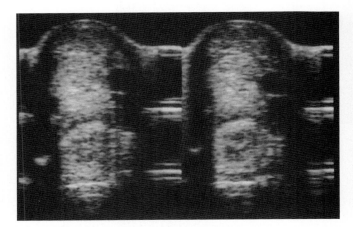

Figure 4.132 Transverse sonograms at 12 cm and 14 cm distal to the accessory carpal bone. The suspensory ligament is abnormally enlarged and hypoechoic as a result of desmitis.

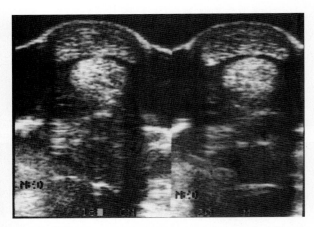

Figure 4.133 Transverse sonograms made at 18 and 20 cm distal to the accessory carpal bone, showing an anechoic separation between the superficial and deep digital flexor tendons, caused by excessive effusion of the digital sheath.

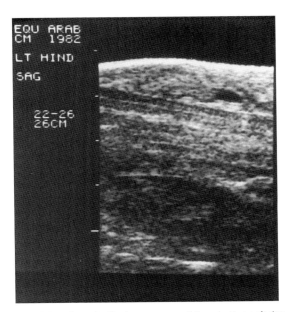

Figure 4.134 Longitudinal sonogram of the plantar soft tissue structures just proximal to the level of the proximal sesamoids. Excessive thickening is seen between the surface of the superficial digital flexor tendon and the skin. Irregular-shaped fluid pockets are also present in this region. The tissue and fluid are the result of chronic proliferative tenosynovitis.

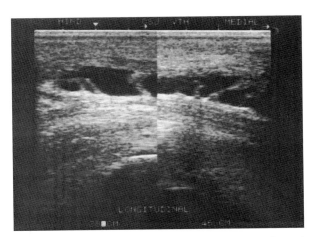

Figure 4.135 Longitudinal sonogram of the flexor tendons at the level of the fetlock. Marked fluid distension is seen in the digital sheath. Multiple fibrous adhesions are observed traversing the digital sheath. The distance between the skin and the fluid in the digital sheath is increased as a result of proliferative tenosynovitis. The adhesions and thickened digital sheath resulted from septic tenosynovitis.

References

1. Byars TD, Halley J. Uses of ultrasound in equine internal medicine. Vet Clin North Am Equine Pract 1986;2:253–258.
2. Cartee RE, Rumph PF. Ultrasonographic detection of fistulas tracts and foreign objects in muscles of horses. J Am Vet Med Assoc 1984;184:1127–1132.
3. Coelho JC, Sigel B, Ryva JC, et al. B mode sonography of blood clots. J Clin Ultrasound 1982;10:323–327.
4. Crass JR, van de Vegte GL, Harkavy LA. Tendon echogenicity: Ex vivo study. Radiology 1988;167:499–501.
5. Craychee TJ. Ultrasonographic evaluation of equine musculoskeletal injury. In: Nyland TG, Mattoon JS, Eds. Veterinary Diagnostic Ultrasound. Philadelphia: WB Saunders, 1996;265–304.
6. Cuesta I, Riber C, Pinedo JA, Castejon F. Ultrasonographic measurement of the palmar metacarpal tendon and ligament structures in the horse. Vet Radiol Ultrasound 1995;36:131–136.
7. Denoix JM. Diagnostic techniques for identification and documentation of tendon and ligament injuries. Vet Clin North Am Equine Pract 1994;10:365–407.
8. Denoix JM. Functional anatomy of tendons and ligaments in the distal limbs (manus and pes). Vet Clin North Am Equine Pract 1994;10:273–322.
9. Denoix JM. Ultrasonographic examination in the diagnosis of joint disease. In: McIlwraith CW, Trotter GW, Eds. Joint Disease in the Horse. Philadelphia: WB Saunders, 1996;165–202.
10. Denoix JM, Yousti S. Spontaneous injury of the accessory ligament of the superficial digital flexor tendon (proximal check ligament), a new ultrasonographic diagnosis. J Equine Vet Sci 1996;16:191–194.
11. Dik KJ. Ultrasonographic evaluation of fetlock annular ligament constriction in the horse. Equine Vet J 1991;23:285–288.
12. Dik KJ. Ultrasonography in the diagnosis of equine lameness. Vet Ann 1990;30:162–171.
13. Dik KJ. Ultrasonography of the equine crus. Vet Radiol Ultrasound 1993;34:28–34.
14. Dik KJ. Ultrasonography of the equine stifle. Equine Vet Educ 1995;7:154–160.
15. Dik KJ. Ultrasonography of the equine tarsus. Vet Radiol Ultrasound 1993;34:36–43.
16. Dik KJ, Burofka B, Stolk P. Ultrasonographic assessment of the proximal digital annular ligament in the equine forelimb. Equine Vet J 1994;26:59–64.
17. Dik KJ, Dyson SJ, Vail TB. Aseptic tenosynovitis of the digital flexor tendon sheath, fetlock and pastern annular ligament constriction. Vet Clin North Am Equine Pract 1995;11:151–162.
18. Dyson S. Desmitis of the accessory ligament of the deep digital flexor tendon: 27 cases (1986–1990). Equine Vet J 1991;23:438–444.
19. Dyson S. Proximal suspensory desmitis: Clinical, ultrasonographic and radiographic features. Equine Vet J 1991;23:25–31.
20. Dyson S. The use of ultrasonography for the assessment of tendon damage. Equine Vet Educ 1989;1:42–45.
21. Dyson SJ, Arthur RM, Palmer SE, Richardson D. Suspensory ligament desmitis. Vet Clin North Am Equine Pract 1994;11:177–215.
22. Dyson SJ, Denoix JM. Tendon, tendon sheath and ligament injuries in the pastern. Vet Clin North Am Equine Pract 1995;11:217–233.
23. Dyson SJ, Dik KJ. Conditions of tendon, tendon sheaths and ligaments. Vet Clin North Am Equine Pract 1995;11:315–318.
24. Dyson S, Kidd L. Five cases of gastrocnemius tendinitis in the horse. Equine Vet J 1991;24:351–356.
25. French DA, Pharr JW, Fretz PB. Removal of a retropharyngeal foreign body in a horse, with the aid of ultrasonography during surgery. J Am Vet Med Assoc 1989;194:1315–1316.
26. Genovese RL, Rantanen NW, Hauser ML, et al. Diagnostic ultrasonography of equine limbs. Vet Clin North Am Equine Pract 1986;2:145–226.
27. Genovese RL, Rantanen NW, Hauser ML, et al. The use of ultrasonography in the diagnosis and management of injuries to the equine limb. Comp Cont Educ Pract Vet 1987;9:945–957.
28. Genovese RL, Rantanen NW, Simpson BS, et al. Clinical experience with quantitative analysis of superficial digital flexor tendon injuries in Thoroughbred and Standardbred racehorses. Vet Clin North Am Equine Pract 1990;6:129–145.

29. Genovese RL, Reef VB, Longo KL, et al. Superficial digital flexor tendinitis—long term sonography and clinical study of racehorses. In: Proceedings. Dubai International Equine Symposium. Bonsall, CA: Matthew R. Rantanen Design, 1996;187–206.

30. Hager DA. The diagnosis of deep muscle abscesses using two-dimensional real time ultrasound. Proc Am Assoc Equine Pract 1986; 32:523–529.

31. Hauser ML. Ultrasonographic appearance and correlative anatomy of the soft tissues of the distal extremities in the horse. Vet Clin North Am Equine Pract 1986;2:127–144.

32. Hauser ML, Rantenan NW. Ultrasound appearance of the palmar metacarpal soft tissues of the horse. J Equine Vet Sci 1983;3:19–22.

33. Hauser ML, Rantanen NW, Genovese RL. Suspensory desmitis: Diagnosis using real-time ultrasound imaging. J Equine Vet Sci 1984;4:258–283.

34. Hauser ML, Rantanen NW, Modransky PD. Ultrasound examination of distal interphalangeal joint, navicular bursa, navicular bone and deep digital tendon. J Equine Vet Sci 1982;2:95–97.

35. Henry GA, Patton CS, Goble DO. Ultrasonographic evaluation of iatrogenic injuries of the equine accessory (carpal check) ligament and superficial digital flexor tendon. Vet Radiol 1986;27: 132–140.

36. Hutchinson JL, Traub J, Ingram J, et al. Cervical vertebral osteomyelitis, ophthitis and pachymeningitis in a horse. Equine Pract 1993;15:23–26.

37. Love NE, Nickels F. Ultrasonographic diagnosis of a deep muscle abscess in a horse. Radiol Ultrasound 1993;34:207–209.

38. Mackay-Smith M, Cushing L, Leslie J. "Carpal canal" syndrome in horses. J Am Vet Med Assoc 1972;160:993–997.

39. Marr CM, McMillan I, Boyd JS, et al. Ultrasonographic and histopathological findings in equine superficial digital flexor tendon injury. Equine Vet J 1993;25:23–29.

40. McClellan PD, Colby J. Ultrasonic structure of the pastern. J Equine Vet Sci 1986;6:99–101.

41. Modransky PD, Rantanen NW. Diagnostic ultrasound examination of the dorsal aspect of the equine metacarpophalangeal joint. Vet Radiol 1983;3:56–58.

42. Modransky PD, Rantanen NW, Hauser ML, et al. Diagnostic ultrasound examination of the dorsal aspect of the equine metacarpophalangeal joint. J Equine Vet Sci 1983;3:21–26.

43. Neuwirth LA, Selcer BA, Mahaffey MB. Equine tendon ultrasonography: Common artifacts. Equine Vet Educ 1991;3:149–152.

44. Nicoll RG, Wood AKW, Martin ICA. Ultrasonographic observations of the flexor tendons and ligaments of the metacarpal region of the horses. Am J Vet Res 1993;54:502–506.

45. Nicoll RG, Wood AKW, Rothwell TLW. Ultrasonographical and pathological studies of equine superficial digital flexor tendons: Initial observations, including tissue characterization by analysis of image grey scale, in a Thoroughbred gelding. Equine Vet J 1992; 24:318–320.

46. Palmer SE, Genovese RL, Lango KL, et al. Practical management of superficial digital flexor tendinitis in the performance horse. Vet Clin North Am Equine Pract 1994;10:425–439.

47. Penninck DG. Ultrasonography of the equine stifle. Vet Radiol 1990;31:293–298.

48. Pharr JW, Nyland TG. Sonography of the equine palmar metacarpal soft tissues. Vet Radiol 1984;25:265–273.

49. Rantanen NW. The use of diagnostic ultrasound in limb disorders of the horse: A preliminary report. J Equine Vet Sci 1982;2:62–64.

50. Rantanen NW. Ultrasound standoff techniques. J Equine Vet Sci 1990;10:17.

51. Rantanen NW, Genovese RL, Gaines R. The use of diagnostic ultrasound to detect structural damage to the soft tissues of the extremities of horses. J Equine Vet Sci 1983;3:134–135.

52. Rantanen NW, Hauser ML, Genovese RL. Superficial digital flexor tendinitis: Diagnosis using real-time ultrasound imaging. J Equine Vet Sci 1985;5:115–119.

53. Redding WR. Distal sesamoidean ligament injuries and desmitis of the accessory ligament of the deep digital flexor tendon. In: Proceedings. Dubai International Equine Symposium. Bonsall, CA: Matthew R. Rantanen Design, 1996;227–239.

54. Redding WR. Ultrasonographic imaging of the structures of the digital flexor tendon sheath. Comp Cont Educ Pract Vet 1991;13: 1824–1832.

55. Reef VB. Ultrasonic evaluation of tendons and ligaments. In: White NA, Moore JN, Eds. Current Practice in Equine Surgery. Philadelphia: JB Lippincott, 1990;425–435.

56. Reef VB. The use of diagnostic ultrasound in the horse. Ultrasound Q 1991;9:1–34.

57. Sisson S. Equine syndesmology. In: Getty R, Ed. Sisson and Grossman's Anatomy of Domestic Animals. Vol. 1. 5th ed. Philadelphia: WB Saunders, 1975;349–453.

58. Smith RK, Dyson SJ, Head MJ, Butson RJ. Ultrasonography of the equine triceps muscle before and after general anesthesia and in post anesthetic myelopathy. Equine Vet J 1996;28:311–319.

59. Smith RK, Jones R, Webbon PM. The cross-sectional areas of normal equine digital flexor tendons determined ultrasonographically. Equine Vet J 1994;26;460–465.

60. Spaulding K. Ultrasonic anatomy of the tendons and ligaments in the distal metacarpal-metatarsal region of the equine limb. Vet Radiol 1984;25:155–166.

61. Steyn PF, McIlwraith CW, Rawcliff N. The ultrasonographic examination of the palmar metacarpal tendons and ligaments of the equine digit. Equine Pract 1991;13:24–34.

62. Steyn PF, McIlwraith CW, Rawcliff N. The use of ultrasonographic examination in conditions affecting the palmar metacarpal soft tissues of the equine limb. Equine Pract 1991;13:8–17.

63. Steyn PF, Schmitz D. The sonographic diagnosis of chronic proliferative synovitis in the metacarpophalangeal joints of a horse. Vet Radiol 1989;30:125–127.

64. Tnibar M, Kaser-Hotz B, Auer J. Ultrasonography of the dorsal and lateral aspect of the equine carpus. Vet Radiol Ultrasound 1993;34:413–425.

65. Watrous B, Dutra F, Wagner P, et al. Villonodular synovitis of the palmar and plantar digital flexor tendon sheaths and the calcaneal bursa of the gastrocnemius tendon of the horse. Proc Am Assoc Equine Pract 1987;33:413–428.

66. Wilson D, Baker G, Pijanowski G, et al. Composition and morphologic features of the interosseous muscle in Standardbreds and Thoroughbreds. Am J Vet Res 1991;52:133–139.

67. Wood AKW, Newell WH, Borg RP. An ultrasonographic off-set system for examination of equine tendons and ligaments. J Vet Res 1991;52:1945–1947.

Part III

NUCLEAR MEDICINE

Phillip F. Steyn

Although radiography, ultrasound, computed tomography (CT), and magnetic resonance imaging (MRI) produce images that reveal anatomic detail, nuclear medicine techniques image the blood flow to bone and the function or the physiologic activity of bone. Nuclear medicine imaging is a sensitive tool that augments, but does not replace, the basic lameness examination.[5,13,18,22,26,28,38,40,42,49,50] Most academic institutions and several private clinics have nuclear medicine imaging facilities, making this modality within the reach of many equine practitioners in North America. This part of the chapter discusses the principles, techniques, indications for, and interpretations of nuclear medicine imaging in the evaluation of the musculoskeletal system of the horse.

PRINCIPLES

Nuclear medicine imaging, also known as scintigraphy, is based on the functional distribution of a radiopharmaceutical in the body. The radiopharmaceutical is made of a radionuclide, most commonly technetium-99m (^{99m}Tc), which is labeled to a pharmaceutical that determines the target tissue of the radiopharmaceutical in the body. Technetium-99m decays by emitting a 140-kEv γ-ray. A γ-ray is identical to an x-ray, except that it originates from the nucleus of an unstable atom (e.g., ^{99m}Tc) as the atom strives toward a more stable state. Nuclear medicine imaging can also be described as an emission imaging technique, since the image is made by γ-rays that are emitted by the ^{99m}Tc inside the horse. In contrast, radiography is considered a transmission imaging technique, since the x-rays that produce the image are transmitted through the patient.

Technetium-99m can be produced on site by using a molybdenum-99m generator or, when needed, can be ordered from a nuclear pharmacy. Technetium-99m has a relatively short natural half-life ($T_{1/2}$) of 6 hours, which means, for example, that 100 mCi of ^{99m}Tc will decay to 50 mCi in 6 hours or that an exposure rate of 4 mrem/hour will decrease to 2 mrem/hour in 6 hours. The effective $T_{1/2}$ of a radiopharmaceutical, however, is generally shorter than the natural $T_{1/2}$ because of biologic excretion of the tracer.

The pharmaceutical part of the radiopharmaceutical determines the distribution of the tracer radionuclide in the body. A variety of molecules and cells can be labeled. Red blood cells can be labeled for the evaluation of the circulating blood compartment, most commonly done to study cardiac function. The intravenous administration of ^{99m}Tc-pertechnetate (^{99m}TcO$_4$) is the most accurate scintigraphic technique for looking at the perfusion (blood flow) of soft tissue structures, such as the joints of the distal limbs.

White blood cells can be selectively labeled with ^{99m}Tc-hexamethylpropyleneamine oxime (^{99m}Tc-HMPAO) to look for areas of active inflammation.[4,30] Renal function can be studied by using ^{99m}Tc-diethylenetriamine pentaacetic acid (^{9m}Tc-DTPA), and quantitative hepatobiliary studies can be performed with ^{99m}Tc-disophenin. Functional lung ventilation studies have been described by using aerosolized ^{99m}Tc-DTPA; and lung perfusion, by using ^{9m}Tc-macroaggregates of albumin (MAA).[3,27]

Although each of these techniques uses ^{99m}Tc, the distribution of the radiopharmaceutical differs and is based on the biokinetics of the pharmaceutical or cell to which the ^{99m}Tc has been labeled.

Bone scans are done by using radiolabeled polyphosphonates, which have a high affinity for the calcium-hydroxyappetite molecules in bone. Images made at 2 to 4 hours postinjection reveal the uptake pattern in the bones. A predictable uptake pattern is seen in normal animals, and increased uptake is seen with increased blood flow or increased osteoblastic activity.[13] Either ^{99m}Tc-oxidronate (HDP) or ^{99m}Tc-methylene diphosphonate (MDP) are administered intravenously at a dose of about 0.35 mCi/kg body weight. ^{99m}Tc-HDP has the advantage of faster soft tissue clearance, thus allowing image acquisition to begin sooner after injection. A second advantage of ^{99m}Tc-HDP is improved visualization of bones surrounded by large amounts of muscle, e.g., the spine, pelvis, and hips.

An average 450-kg horse receives about 160 mCi of the radiolabel. The dose rate can be adjusted for age, i.e., increased by about 10% in older horses and decreased by about 10% in juveniles because of the difference in metabolic activity of bone tissue. Approximately 50% of the injected radiolabel is excreted in the urine, which results in the effective $T_{1/2}$ being shorter than the natural $T_{1/2}$.[35]

Although the classic nuclear medicine evaluation of the skeleton is the three-phase bone scan, I generally do only the soft tissue phase and the delayed phase. During the initial vascular phase, the radiopharmaceutical is in the blood vessels and has not yet diffused into the extracellular fluid; this phase lasts for 1 or 2 minutes after injection. The body region to be evaluated must be positioned in front of the gamma camera at the time of injection, and dynamic rapid-frame acquisition is made as the radiolabel perfuses the vasculature. Multiple images are acquired over the first few minutes, while the radiolabel is still within the vascular system. The vascular phase is used to compare the blood flow to, especially, the distal limbs; but it can also be used to document perfusion deficits elsewhere, e.g., occlusive thrombi in the distal aorta.

During the soft tissue phase, the radiopharmaceutical is distributed in the extracellular fluid, which occurs 3 to 10 minutes postinjection. This phase is used to evaluate blood flow to soft tissues. An increased signal is observed with hyperemia because of, for example, edema or inflammation. Increased radioactivity during the pool or soft tissue phase is best used in the distal limbs and has been associated with navicular syndrome and inflamed joints, e.g., degenerative changes of the sacroiliac joint. Early or intense bone uptake of the radiopharmaceutical (^{99m}Tc-HDP or ^{99m}Tc-MDP) can sometimes be seen as soon as 5 minutes after injection, especially in cases of intense delayed-phase bone uptake, e.g., with fractures or infectious processes. This can sometimes make the evaluation of soft tissues challenging, if not impossible.

The best scintigraphic technique for looking at only soft tissues, without any possibility of bone uptake, is to use intravenous ^{99m}TcO$_4$ (unlabeled to a pharmaceutical) and to make images as soon as radiopharmaceutical equilibrium in the extracellular space is achieved. A dose similar to that of the bone scanning agents is recommended.

The bone phase occurs several hours after injection, when approximately 50% of the radiopharmaceutical has attached to bone. The remainder of the tracer is excreted by the kidneys in the first one or two urine voids postinjection. The uptake pattern of normal bone is quite predictable and is described later in this chapter. The least uptake occurs in the diaphysis of long bones, and the most uptake occurs in juxtaphyseal and subchondral bone in normal subjects. Increased uptake by or near the joints during the delayed (bone) phase has been related to several conditions, including degenerative joint disease, various enthesopathies, periarticular bone sclerosis, and septic arthritis. Variations from the normal uptake pattern are discussed later in this chapter.

RADIATION SAFETY AND PROTECTION

Radiation detection equipment is used to find ^{99m}Tc traces that might have accidentally spilled and to detect the levels of radiation in a patient before releasing the patient back to the public. Geiger Muller survey instruments are used to survey areas and surfaces for spills (Fig. 4.136) and ion chambers are used to record the levels of radioactivity in patients (Fig. 4.137).

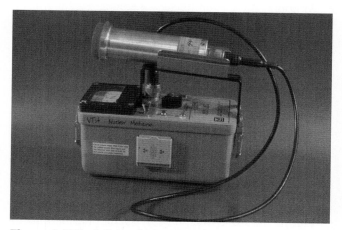

Figure 4.136 A Geiger Muller survey instrument is used to scan for radioactive spills and possible contamination.

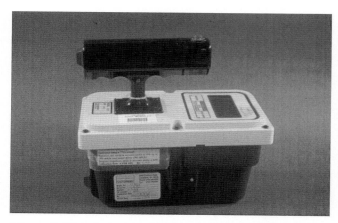

Figure 4.137 An ion chamber records the levels of radioactivity in patients, e.g., to determine whether they can be released. Acceptable radioactivity levels depend on state law but should be defined in the license description for each nuclear medicine clinic.

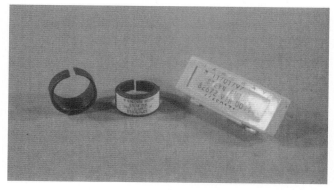

Figure 4.138 Film badges (personal dosimeters) should always be worn to monitor the total cumulative radiation dose. Finger (ring) thermoluminescent dosimeter film badges should be worn by personnel who prepare and inject the radiopharmaceutical.

The ALARA procedures and protocols as described by the local radiation safety officer should always be followed. ALARA means that the radiation dose to which you are exposed will be kept *"as low as reasonably achievable."* These procedures were developed to protect you, others, and the environment from unnecessary risks from radiation exposure. Film badges (personal dosimeters) should always be worn to monitor the total cumulative radiation dose. Finger (ring) thermoluminescent dosimeter film badges should be worn by personnel who prepare and inject the radiopharmaceutical (Fig. 4.138). Eating, drinking, or smoking while handling radioactive materials or a radioactive patient is not permitted.[48] Lead syringe shields are designed to help reduce the radiation dose to the fingers (Fig. 4.139). To achieve an even greater reduction in radiation exposure to the fingers, an indwelling jugular catheter with a short extension tube should be placed before the study is performed.

The nuclear medicine clinician should be conscious of two basic methods of exposure to ionizing radiation: internal contamination and external radiation. Care must be taken to avoid internal contamination through the accidental ingestion of the radionuclide. This most

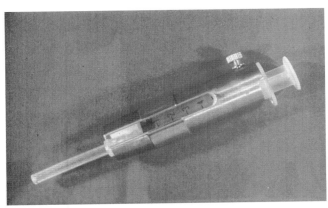

Figure 4.139 Lead syringe shields are designed to help reduce the radiation dose to the fingers.

commonly occurs by contamination of the hands and subsequent accidental ingestion, although absorption by the mucous membranes of the eyes and nose or inhalation can occur if, for example, the material is accidentally sprayed during injection. Direct injection via accidental hypodermic needlestick is a less likely, although possible, route of internal contamination. Latex gloves should always be worn when working with either radiopharmaceuticals or the radioactive patient. These gloves and other items used to treat the horse should be disposed of appropriately, as described by the local radiation safety officer.

External radiation exposure occurs when the clinician is in the immediate vicinity of the horse, such as when scanning. The three basic rules of radiation safety are time, distance, and shielding. Therefore, do not spend more time than necessary with the horse. Doubling the distance between you and the horse reduces your radiation exposure by a quarter. Similarly, standing just half that distance closer to the horse quadruples your exposure. Therefore, standing 1 meter away from the horse significantly reduces your radiation exposure. For example, if the exposure rate at the surface of a horse is 6.6 mrem/hour, it is only 1.3 mrem/hour at 1 meter away.

Syringe shields should be used to reduce the radiation dose to the fingers (Fig. 4.139). Personnel who scan horses on a frequent basis should consider wearing a lead apron and a lead thyroid shield (Fig. 4.140). Protective lead clothing reduces the radiation exposure dose by threefold to fourfold. For example, if the exposure at the surface of a horse is 6.6 mrem/hour, the exposure to a person wearing a lead apron (at skin surface) is only 1.5 mrem/hour. Thus, with this example, standing 1 meter away from the horse and wearing a lead apron reduces exposure to about 0.5 mrem/hour.

Appropriate radiation warning signs and patient handling procedures should be posted on the stall in which a radioactive horse has been housed. The horse is hospitalized until the radiation exposure at skin level is below the level specified by state law, usually between 1.0 and 5.0 mrem/hour. Survey meters, such as Geiger counters (Fig. 4.136) and ion chambers (Fig. 4.137), are used to monitor the work area for possible contamination and to monitor the horse for release. After the horse has been released, the stall is closed off for an additional 24 hours

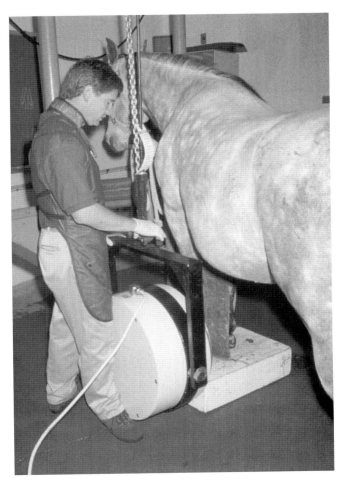

Figure 4.140 A lead apron and thyroid shield reduce the radiation dose to the clinician. Latex gloves prevent skin contamination, e.g., by radioactive urine.

before it is cleaned out. This allows the ^{99m}Tc that has been excreted via the urine to undergo four more natural half-lives, reducing the exposure to the workers even further (ALARA). Other precautionary steps, such as placing absorbent material (e.g., socks) in front of the stalls to prevent radioactive urine from leaking into the walkway, when indicated, should be considered (Fig. 4.141).

IMAGING EQUIPMENT

The gamma camera contains a collimator made of small holes in a lead plate that allow only perpendicular γ-rays through (Fig. 4.142). This reduces scatter, thereby improving image resolution. The γ-rays interact with a fluorescent crystal (a thallium-activated sodium iodide crystal is commonly used), which changes the γ-energy to light photons. The light photons interact with a photocathode, which generates electrons; and the electrons are amplified by an array of photomultiplier tubes. The x-y coordinates of the electrons are then recorded, and the image is reconstructed. Therefore, the image represents the geographic distribution of the radiopharmaceutical in the horse. Images are acquired in a 256×256 matrix,

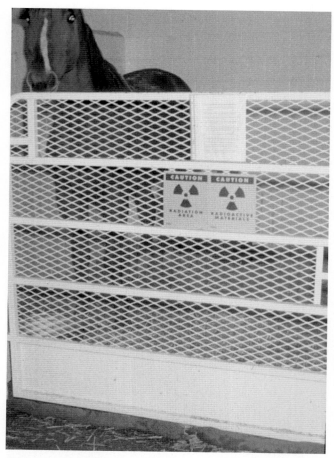

Figure 4.141 Horses should be housed in stalls approved by the radiation safety officer until skin levels reach the standards set by the state. Radioactive warning signs and patient handling procedures should be posted on the stall, and absorbent material such as socks can be used on the floor in front of the stall to absorb potentially radioactive urine.

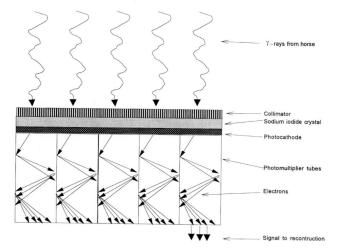

Figure 4.142 In the gamma camera, the γ-photons from the ^{99m}Tc in the horse are changed to light photons by the sodium iodide crystal and then to electrons by the photocathode. The electrons are amplified by the photomultiplier tubes, and the signal is used for image reconstruction by the computer.

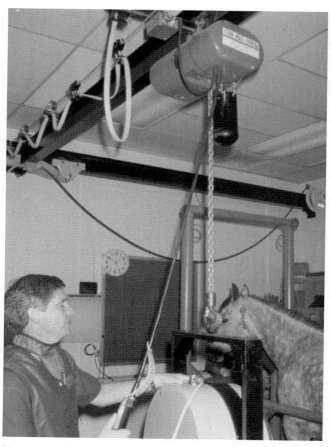

Figure 4.143 This gamma camera is suspended by a chain hoist from a track system, allowing it to be moved in all directions around the horse.

which optimizes image resolution but does not require excessive computer storage capabilities.

Various techniques have been devised to suspend the gamma camera, including forklifts, hydraulic systems, and track-and-hoist systems (Fig. 4.143).[36] The gamma camera and collimator weigh approximately 1500 lb (682 kg) and must be kept still for the acquisition time of 30 to 90 seconds. The gamma camera computer acquires the data, reconstructs the images, and sends the digitized images to the processing computer (Fig. 4.144).

The processing computer is usually dedicated to the nuclear medicine facility and is used for postprocessing the images and maintaining image storage (Fig. 4.145). Hard copies of nuclear medicine images can be made to x-ray-type film by using a multiformatter or a medical laser imager (Fig. 4.146). Paper printers are also used to produce color or black-and-white images. Interpretation reports should be generated as soon as possible and stored with the images as part of the medical record of each patient.

The equipment needed for a nuclear medicine imaging service consists of relatively high technology electronic instrumentation and must be maintained appropriately to ensure that optimal diagnostic images are acquired. Although the maintenance of the equipment is beyond the scope of this text, image quality and resolution can be affected by a number of factors, including 1) insufficient

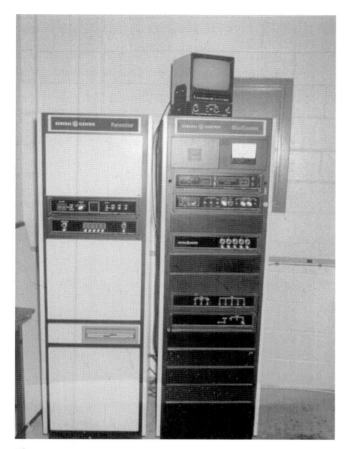

Figure 4.144 The gamma-camera computer reconstructs the acquired image, makes necessary digital adjustments to improve the basic image resolution, and then sends the image to the processing computer.

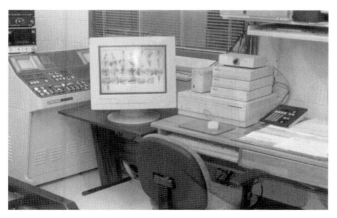

Figure 4.145 The processing computer processes the images and is used for digital image (soft copy) storage.

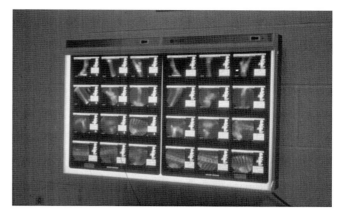

Figure 4.146 Nuclear medicine images can be processed on x-ray-type film by using technologies provided by either a multiformatter or a medical laser imager and examined on a view box.

Table 4.6   MINIMUM IMAGE ACQUISITION COUNTS

Body Region	Number of Counts × 1000
Foot	100–150
Carpus	100–150
Elbow	150–200
Shoulder	200–300
Hock	150–200
Stifle	150–200
Hip	200–300
Sacroiliac area	200–300
Spine	200–300
Soft tissue (pool) phase image	75–100

Image acquisition is determined by either the number of counts or the acquisition time. The number of counts per image is the most critical factor in terms of image quality. Although a minimum number of counts is needed for a diagnostic image, more counts will result in a superior image. Table 4.6 suggests minimum counts per image by body part. A longer image acquisition time is needed for more counts per image, although at some stage a long image acquisition time becomes impractical. I have found that most horses will stand still for about 60 seconds when sedated with intravenous butorphanol and detomidine, so I rarely acquire an image for less than 60 seconds. For example, if a 60-second image of the foot results in 250,000 counts, I acquire the image for 60 seconds and not for 30 seconds, which would have given a diagnostic image, albeit with less resolution.

The risk with limiting the acquisition to a certain number of counts (as opposed to time) is that if there is urine contamination under a foot, or another limb is in the field of view, or the urinary bladder is in the field of view, then the counts recorded by the acquisition computer will include these aberrant γ-rays, which do not contribute to image quality. In fact, they would reduce image quality by diminishing the number of γ-rays used for image reconstruction. Therefore, during scanning, it is better to use acquisition time rather than counts per image, given the premise that the number of counts is

counts (e.g., acquisition time too short, ^{99m}Tc dose too low, extravascular injection of radiopharmaceutical, camera not adequately peaked), 2) incorrect collimator, 3) inadequate correction floods, 4) motion of patient, camera, or both, and 5) incorrect position of the gamma camera. See your service company for other problems.

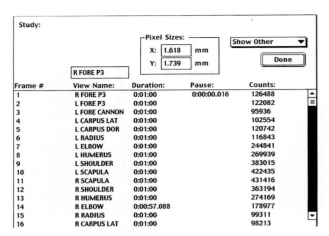

Figure 4.147 Acquisition data from a typical scintigraphic study showing the name, acquisition time, and number of counts for each view.

the more critical factor in image quality. The object is to have sufficient radioactivity in the skeletal system to acquire sufficient counts per image in an appropriate length of time. When using Table 4.6, remember that the more counts acquired per image, the better the image resolution.

Figure 4.147 shows the acquisition data from a typical case. I found that it takes the same amount of time to acquire sufficient data for a lateral foot image as to acquire nearly any other image. Therefore, I generally limit subsequent images to the time that was needed to acquire sufficient counts for a lateral foot image.

The use of a radionuclide scanner in equine scintigraphy has been described.[31,32] This technique does not produce images but, rather, collects the number of counts in specific areas via a single (handheld) probe counter. The counts are recorded and compared with counts on the contralateral side.

METHOD

The radiolabeled pharmaceutical, either ^{99m}Tc-MDP or ^{99m}Tc-HDP, is generally used at a dose of 0.35 mCi/kg. The radiolabel must be given intravenously, or a slow, continuous release of ^{99m}Tc will result in suboptimal images because of high levels of circulating radioactivity. Patient control is important; the horse must be immobile during the 60 seconds it generally takes to acquire the image. Chemical restraint is helpful; I use a combination of intravenous detomidine and butorphanol.

The tracer is given intravenously, and the blood flow (phase 1) images are acquired immediately, if required. Soft tissue (pool) phase images are acquired within the next 10 minutes. Soft tissue phase images must be limited to three or four, so they can be completed before significant bone uptake occurs. Delayed-phase images are acquired from 2 to 4 hours after injection.

If lumbar spine, pelvis, and stifle images are being acquired, furosemide is given intravenously 60 to 90 minutes before the delayed phase starts; this increases the chances of an empty bladder (^{99m}Tc-HDP in the urine obscures visualization of the stifles, lumbosacral junction, sacroiliac joints, and coxofemoral joints). Lateral

images of the limbs are made with the camera carefully positioned lateral to the region being imaged, which is not necessarily lateral to the horse. Dorsal views are generally made of the carpi. The orthogonal view (dorsal or plantar) of a lesion should always be attempted to help document the third dimension.

Lead sheets are used to shield out scatter radiation from the other limbs (Fig. 4.140). Lead should also be placed medial to the olecranon and stifle to shield out the sternum and the penis and urinary bladder, respectively. Be sure to overlap the views slightly, so that no area is left unscanned.

Wait 3 to 4 days after palmar digital nerve blocks and 14 days after low- and high-palmar nerve blocks before scanning, because this leads to increased tracer uptake in the soft tissue (pool) phase.[45] Similarly, wait about 7 days after any intraarticular analgesia before scanning.[44] Local nerve blocks (intraarticular or perineural) will not, however, affect bone uptake in the delayed phase.[6]

The following views are recommended for the full evaluation of the forelimbs: lateral foot (distal metacarpus, metacarpophalangeal joints, and phalanges), solar distal phalanx, lateral metacarpus, lateral and dorsal carpus, lateral radius, lateral elbow, lateral humerus, lateral shoulder, and lateral scapula.

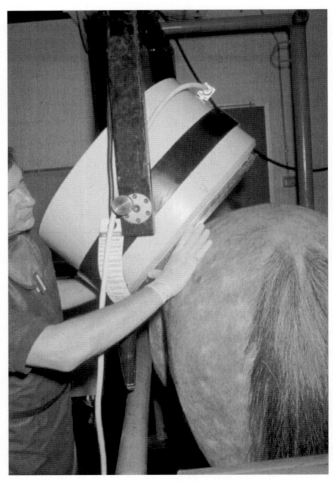

Figure 4.148 Camera positioned for the LDO view of the lumbosacral junction.

The following views are recommended for the full evaluation of the spine: right dorsal oblique (RDO) lumbosacral junction, RDO lumbar spine, RDO caudal thoracic spine, RDO cranial thoracic spine, left dorsal oblique (LDO) lumbosacral junction (Fig. 4.148), LDO lumbar spine, LDO caudal thoracic spine, LDO cranial

thoracic spine, dorsal pelvis (Fig. 4.149), caudal pelvis (tail on detector, TOD), RDO sacrum, and LDO sacrum. Lateral and dorsal views of the spine are less effective because of the great distance that the camera is from the vertebrae. They can, however, be included as orthogonal views when a lesion is found. A point source (e.g., the syringe and needle that was used for the ^{99m}Tc-HDP injection, sealed in a latex glove) can be placed along the dorsum of the back to localize the exact position of a lesion, which is then marked with a permanent marker.

The following views are recommended for the full evaluation of the hindlimbs: lateral foot, lateral cannon, lateral hock, lateral tibia, lateral stifle, lateral femur (Fig. 4.150), lateral hip, dorsal oblique hip, dorsal pelvis, caudal pelvis, and dorsal oblique sacrum. A plantar view of the hock should be made if increased uptake is seen on the lateral view.

Lateral views of the feet can be made by placing both forefeet (or both hindfeet) on a wooden box that is about 25 cm high (Fig 4.151). The top of the box should be strong enough to support a large horse (I use 1.5-inch, 3.75-cm, plywood). The gamma camera can then be lowered to acquire a lateral view. The same box can be used to acquire dorsal views of the forefeet by placing the feet at the front edge of the box and the gamma camera in front of the feet. An alternate system is to dig a pit into

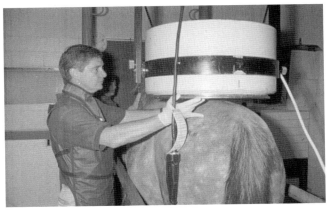
Figure 4.149 Camera positioned for the dorsal view of the pelvis, allowing good visualization of the sacroiliac joint region.

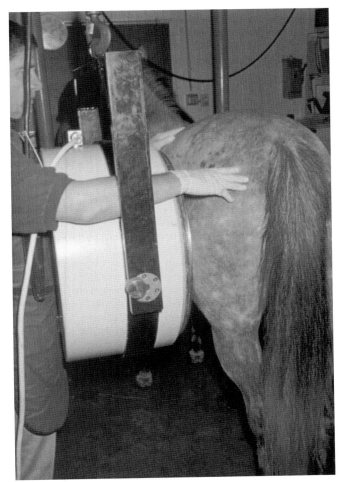
Figure 4.150 Camera positioned for the lateral view of the femur.

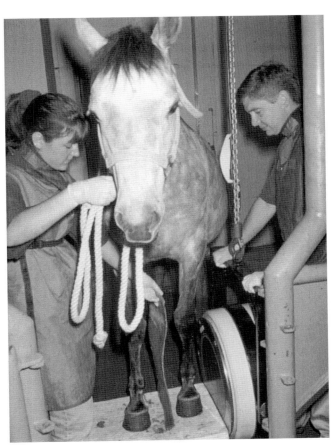
Figure 4.151 Camera positioned for the lateral view of the left forefoot. The horse is standing on a wooden box to allow the gamma camera to be moved far enough distally to image the foot, and lead shielding is used to block out the right forefoot.

which the gamma camera can be lowered. Although this might seem easier than positioning the horse on a box, the camera position is thus fixed and the horse must be moved to acquire images of each foot. Some clinics have constructed a ramp for the horse. The ramp takes up more space than the box. Furthermore, the horse cannot remain on the ramp for the entire scan because of upper vertical limits of both the camera suspension system and the camera operator.

The solar view of the foot has been shown to be more sensitive for the evaluation of the navicular bone than the lateral view.[11] The camera is positioned face up in front of the horse, with the surface of the camera at or just below the level of the carpus. Solar views of the feet are best made by stretching the forefoot out cranially and placing it on the camera face (Fig. 4.152). The collimator is protected from the foot by 6-mm Plexiglas, which is attached with Velcro. Be sure to move the horse's head away from the field of view to reduce scatter. The solar view of the hindfoot is done less frequently, but can be made by stretching the limb caudally, placing the foot on a wooden box, and positioning the camera behind it. An alternative method is to dig a pit in the floor and to place the camera in it faceup. Then cover the pit with appropriate material, and position the standing horse over the camera. Although it is easier to position the horse over the pit than to stretch the foot out forward and hold it on the camera, the standing view causes the superimposition of the pastern and fetlock over the navicular bone region.

The camera hoist system should be designed so that lateral, dorsal, and dorsal oblique views of the axial skeleton of even large horses are possible (Figs. 4.148 and 4.149).

INDICATIONS FOR NUCLEAR BONE SCANS IN HORSES

Vascular Phase (Phase 1)

Imaging the vascular phase is an excellent technique for determining blood flow to specific areas and is of particular importance for evaluating trauma to the distal extremities. The vascular phase can also help document thrombi to the internal iliac arteries.

Soft Tissue Phase (Phase 2)

Soft tissue (pool) phase images are important in cases of acute lameness because they allow the clinician to identify changes (especially increases) in blood flow to local areas. For example, these images reveal hyperemia of the synovium or joint capsule and at the proximal attachment of the suspensory ligament.[52] This is particularly important in the distal limb, although increased blood flow to the sacroiliac joint regions can also be seen. Focal areas of trauma can be evaluated for altered soft tissue perfusion. Sometimes, it is difficult to differentiate between early bone uptake by a lesion and increased blood flow to an area. Therefore, the more accurate soft tissue phase images are those done with $^{99m}TcO_4$ instead of a bone-seeking radiolabel.

Delayed Phase (Phase 3)

Delayed-phase images can help in the diagnostic workup of horses presenting with ill-defined lameness, multiple-cause lameness in the same limb or in different regions of the body, acute lameness of unknown origin, unblockable lameness, back pain, conditions affecting the spine (e.g., facet degenerative joint disease, impingement of dorsal processes, trauma),[2,41] sacroiliac and hip joint problems, dental disease,[20] fracture of the distal sesamoid (navicular) bone or distal phalanx,[9,49] and navicular disease.[11] These images are also used to follow up a known lesion (to check the progress of healing), to examine radiographically normal but painful joints (e.g., the metatarsophalangeal joint),[37] to determine bone viability, and to round out a prepurchase examination.

Soft tissue uptake in the muscles can be seen during the delayed phase in cases of rhabdomyolysis.[23] Scintigraphy is not considered particularly sensitive to changes associated with subchondral bone cysts.[39] The scintigraphic appearance of systemic conditions such as hypertrophic osteopathy has been described.[14]

THE NORMAL BONE SCAN

Vascular phase images are best viewed as a cine loop on the acquisition computer (the cine loop is a software application that allows the images to be viewed sequentially and in rapid order). A composite of vascular phase images can be generated and should show good perfusion. When the images of the distal limbs are being examined, it is best to have both limbs in view and to look for perfusion symmetry. Composite images of the distal

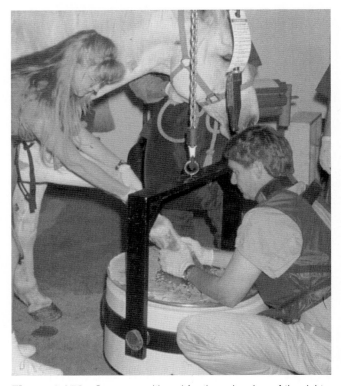

Figure 4.152 Camera positioned for the solar view of the right forefoot.

aorta should show the bifurcation of the aorta into the internal and external iliac arteries (Fig. 4.153).

Soft tissue (pool) phase images of the foot show some vascular activity, but the fetlock and pastern regions should have homogeneously smooth uptake (Fig. 4.154).

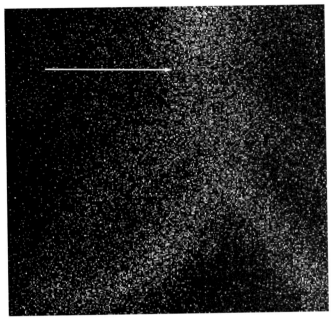

Figure 4.153 Composite image of the blood flow in the region of the distal aorta, showing the normal bifurcation of the aorta (arrow) into the internal and external iliac arteries.

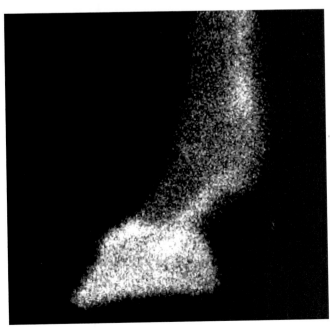

Figure 4.154 Soft tissue (pool) phase image of a normal left forefoot, showing vascular activity on the palmar aspects proximal and distal to the fetlock and in the area of the coronary band. Note that the fetlock and pastern regions have homogeneously smooth uptake.

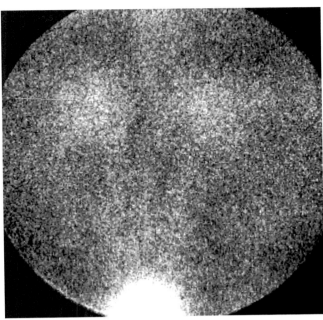

Figure 4.155 Soft tissue phase image of the dorsal pelvis region of a normal horse, showing symmetrical perfusion to the left (arrow) and right sacroiliac joint regions.

The palmar and plantar blood vessels are seen as distinct linear activity, and the coronet has increased activity resulting from a vascular plexus. In addition, the distal phalanx has a generous blood supply to the sensitive laminae, and increased activity is seen. Soft tissue phase images of the dorsal pelvis should show symmetrical perfusion to the left and right sacroiliac joint regions (Fig. 4.155).

Delayed-phase uptake in the phalangeal area of a normal horse is similar in the fetlock, pastern, and coffin joints (Fig. 4.156). Comparison of the relative radiopharmaceutical uptake of joints is best made within a foot or leg but not between opposite feet, although the relationship between two joints in one foot should be the same as the relationship between the same joints in the opposite limb. This allows an accurate comparison of regions in contralateral limbs even when the total uptake by the limbs is dissimilar.

Increased uptake in the dorsal and palmar/plantar cortex of the proximal phalanx is sometimes seen as an incidental finding in hunters and jumpers as a normal response to training (Fig. 4.157).[19] The solar view of the distal phalanx should not reveal superimposition of the other phalanges. The distal phalanx should have a smooth homogeneous uptake pattern, and the navicular bone should not be seen as a discrete structure (Fig. 4.158). The metacarpus and metatarsus (cannon bone) should show similar uptake between them and the small metacarpal and metatarsal (splint) bones and thus should not be distinguished separately (Fig. 4.159).

The carpus generally has more uptake than the diaphyses of the radius or the cannon, but it should be homogeneous in nature (Fig. 4.160). The distal radial physis shows increased uptake in growing foals, but it can be seen as a distinct area in horses up to 8 years old (Fig.

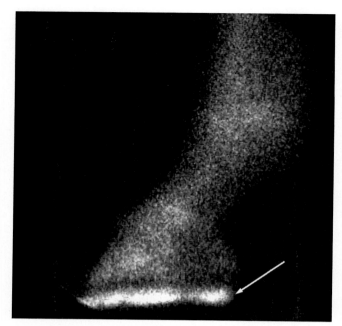

Figure 4.156 Delayed-phase image of the foot of a normal horse, showing similar or equal radiopharmaceutical uptake in the fetlock, pastern, and coffin joints. The proximal sesamoids and the distal cannon should have similar or equal uptake. Urine contamination (arrow) is seen on the sole of the hoof.

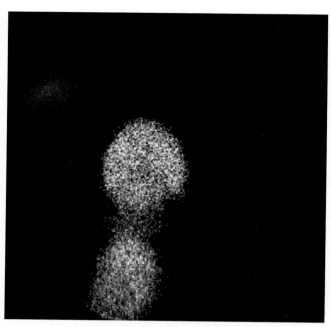

Figure 4.158 Solar view of a normal foot, showing the distal phalanx imaged without superimposition of the other phalanges. The navicular bone should not be seen as a separate entity.

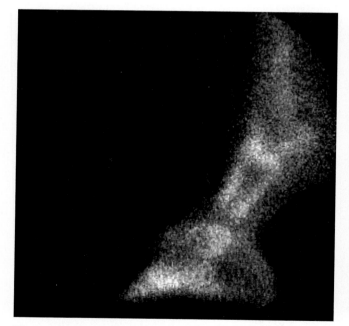

Figure 4.157 Increased uptake in the dorsal and palmar/plantar cortex of the proximal phalanx (arrow) is sometimes seen as an incidental finding in hunters and jumpers as a normal response to training.

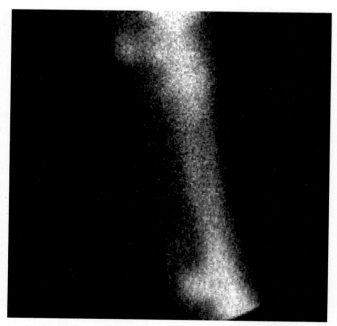

Figure 4.159 Lateral view of a normal right metacarpus (cannon) bone, showing similar uptake between the cannon bone and the small metacarpal/metatarsal (splint) bones.

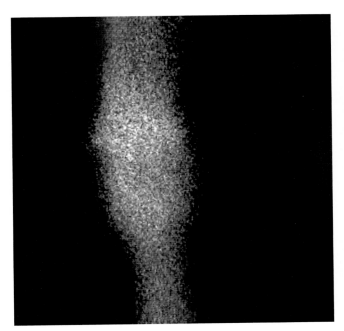

Figure 4.160 Dorsal view of a normal carpus, showing homogeneously more uptake in the carpus than in the adjacent radial and metacarpal diaphyses.

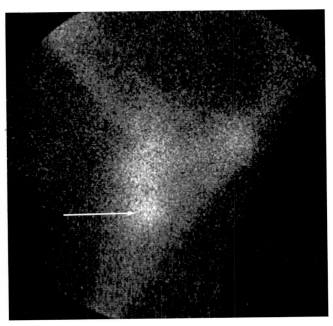

Figure 4.162 Lateral view of a normal elbow, showing the higher uptake pattern in the subchondral bone and the olecranon of the proximal ulna at the attachment of the triceps muscles. Increased uptake is often seen in the radioulnar joint of normal elbows (arrow).

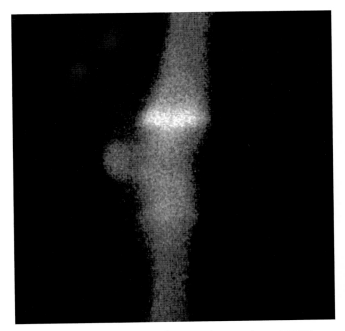

Figure 4.161 Lateral view of a normal carpus in a younger horse, showing increased uptake in the distal radial physis.

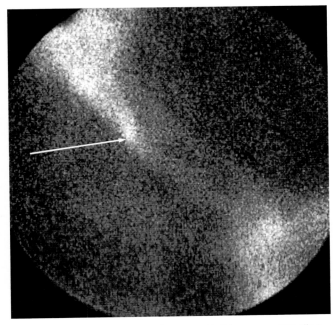

Figure 4.163 Lateral view of a normal left humerus, revealing the deltoid tuberosity (arrow), which is easily identified and can be used as an imaging landmark.

4.161). The physis will have closed radiographically, and growth is no longer occurring at that site, but there is still sufficient osteoblastic activity to differentiate the physis from the adjacent metaphysis and the epiphysis. Increased uptake is often seen in the radioulnar joint of normal elbows (Fig. 4.162).

The deltoid tuberosity is easily visualized on the cra-

nial cortex of the humerus (Fig. 4.163). The normal shoulder joint demonstrates increased uptake in the areas of the greater and lesser tubercles and the humeral head (Fig. 4.164). The glenoid cavity, however, should have less activity than the humeral head. The scapula

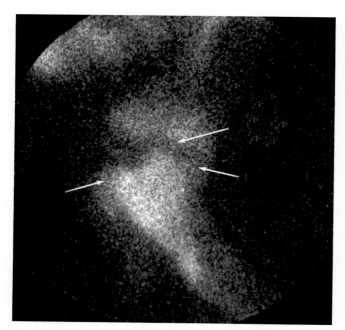

Figure 4.164 Lateral view of a normal left shoulder joint, demonstrating increased uptake in the areas of the greater and lesser tubercles and the humeral head. The deltoid tuberosity and the spine of the scapula can also be seen.

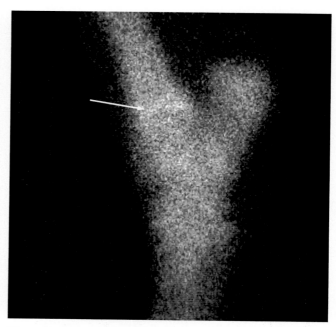

Figure 4.166 Lateral view of a normal left hock, showing more uptake in the subchondral bone than in the diaphyseal bone of the cannon or in the distal tibia.

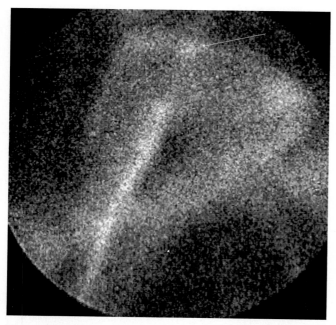

Figure 4.165 Lateral view of a normal left scapula, showing the spine of the scapula and a superimposition artifact (arrow) created by overlap between the scapula and dorsal spines of the withers.

should be easy to visualize, and in some cases the withers can be evaluated at the same time (Fig. 4.165). Superimposition artifact from the withers and thoracic spine often occurs on images of the scapula, creating an area of perceived increased uptake.

The lateral image of the hock should include the distal portion of the tibia and the proximal metatarsus (cannon bone) (Fig. 4.166). Tracer uptake in the bones of the hock is greater than that in the tibia and cannon bone but should always be homogeneous and smooth, with similar uptake in the tarsocrural, intertarsal, and tarsometatarsal joints. Increased uptake is often seen in the distal tibia at the level of the physis. When increased uptake (in the hock joint) is seen on the lateral view, a plantar view should be made to determine whether the lesion is medial or lateral.

Resolution of the cranial and caudal cortices of the tibia should be possible on the lateral view of the tibia (Fig. 4.167). The stifle shows similar uptake between the patella, trochlea, and condyles; slightly more uptake is noted in the proximal tibia, tibial crest, and head of the fibula (Fig. 4.168). The femur of smaller (shorter) horses can be evaluated on the lateral stifle and lateral hip images. In larger (taller) horses, however, a separate lateral femur image should be made (Fig 4.169). The third trochanter is an important landmark and should be seen. The cranial and caudal cortices should also be seen on the scintigrams.

Lateral images of the hip should identify the cranial and caudal portions of the greater trochanter and third trochanters (Fig. 4.170). Dorsal oblique views of the hip allow improved visualization of the femoral head and neck and the acetabular region (Fig. 4.171). The normal acetabulum should not be seen as a separate entity; i.e., the acetabulum should not have a signal greater than that of the ilium. Urine in the urinary bladder sometimes obscures visualization of the hip joint and can be mistaken for disease. Dorsal or caudal views of the hip region should be made to differentiate the urinary bladder (a midline structure) from the hip joints.

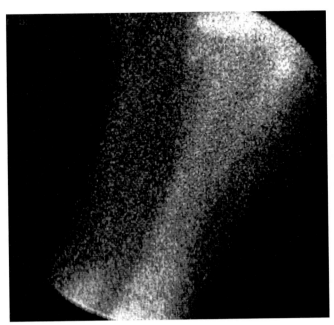

Figure 4.167 Lateral view of a normal right tibia, showing homogeneous uptake by the cranial and caudal cortices.

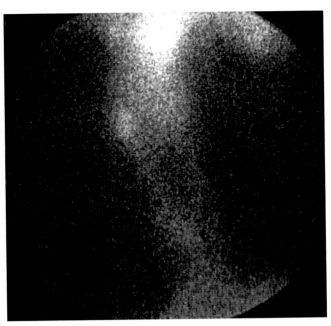

Figure 4.169 Lateral view of a normal right femur, showing a well-defined third trochanter. The greater trochanter is seen proximally.

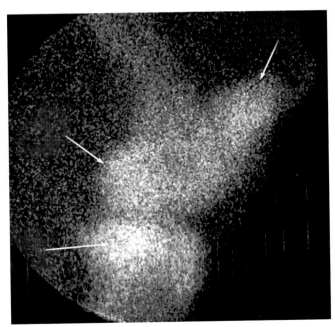

Figure 4.168 Lateral view of a normal right stifle, showing similar uptake by the patella, trochlea, and condyles and slightly more uptake in the proximal tibia, tibial crest, and head of the fibula.

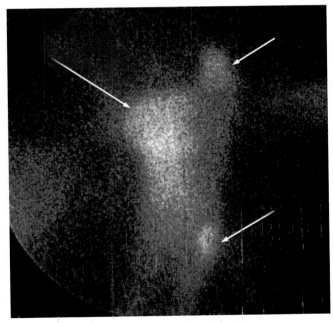

Figure 4.170 Lateral view of a normal left hip joint region, showing the cranial and caudal portions of the greater trochanter and third trochanter.

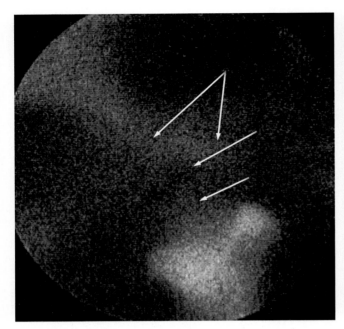

Figure 4.171 Dorsal oblique view of a normal left hip, which allows improved visualization of the femoral head and neck and the acetabular region.

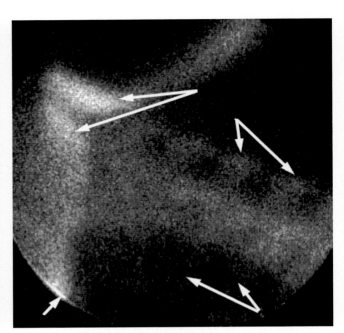

Figure 4.173 RDO view of the lumbosacral region of a normal horse, showing good resolution of the tubera sacrale, dorsal spines, and transverse processes. Refer to Figure 4.148 for gamma-camera orientation for the contralateral image. The edge of the tuber coxa is seen at the lower left aspect of the image.

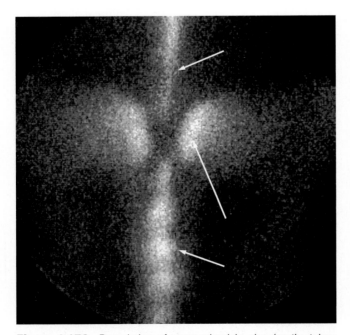

Figure 4.172 Dorsal view of a normal pelvis, showing the tuber sacrale and the sacroiliac joints. Note the symmetry between left and right.

The dorsal view of the pelvis is the best for the evaluation of the tuber sacrale and the sacroiliac joints; symmetry between left and right is considered normal (Fig. 4.172). Although the dorsum of L6 and L7 and the sacrum can also be seen on the dorsal view, the dorsal spinous processes are best evaluated on the dorsal oblique views. These views, made from the left and right sides,

are invaluable for the evaluation of the spine. For most horses, the thoracolumbar spines can be imaged in eight views (four from each side); make sure that sufficient overlap exists between views so that no part is excluded. I take the following dorsal oblique views from both sides: lumbosacral region, lumbar spine, caudal thoracic spine, and thoracic spine (Figs. 4.173 to 4.176). I also take a dorsal view if a lesion is found.

Resolution of the dorsal spines and the transverse processes should be possible in all but the largest of horses. The back muscles of horses that weigh more than 1500 lb (682 kg) can be so bulky that they reduce or attenuate the γ-signal enough to reduce the resolution of these structures. Adjacent spinal units should each have similar amounts of uptake. Be sure to evaluate the dorsal spines, articular facets, and transverse processes of the entire spine, including the sacrum and tail head (sacro-coccygeal region) (Fig. 4.177).

The caudal view of the pelvis, or the tail-on detector (TOD) view, is essential for the evaluation of the floor of the pelvis and the tubera ischii (Fig. 4.178). The camera is positioned directly behind the pelvis of the horse for the TOD view. Make sure that the gamma camera is equidistant from the left and right tuber ischiadicum during acquisition of this view or the closer tuber ischiadicum will appear to have more uptake than the other. Asymmetric uptake by the tuber ischiadicum is considered abnormal. Angling the camera dorsally (slope of the rump) should be done if the urinary bladder is interfering with the image. This will project the bladder above the tuber ischiadicum (Fig. 4.179).

The diaphyses of long bones have less uptake than other parts of the bones because of the relatively low

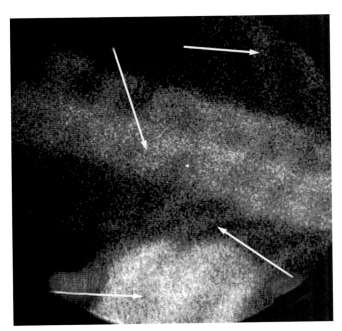

Figure 4.174 RDO view of the lumbar region of a normal horse, showing good resolution of the dorsal spines, transverse processes, right kidney, and caudal right ribs.

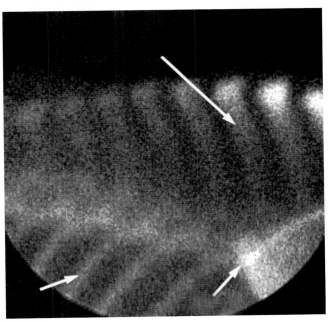

Figure 4.176 RDO view of the thoracic region of a normal horse, showing good resolution of the dorsal spines of the withers, the ribs, and the caudal angle of the right scapula.

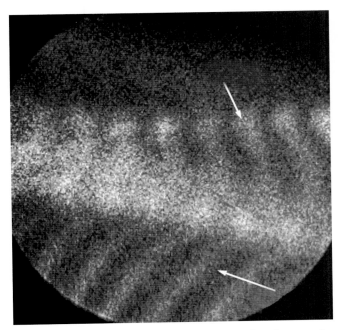

Figure 4.175 RDO view of the midthoracic region of a normal horse, showing good resolution of the dorsal spines and ribs. Note the upward slope of the base of the withers.

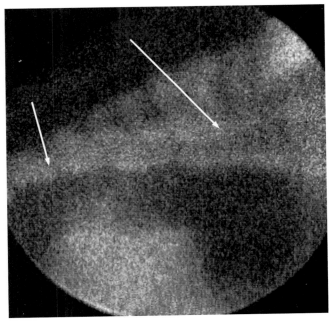

Figure 4.177 RDO view of the sacral region of a normal horse, showing good resolution of the dorsal spines of the sacrum and the proximal tail.

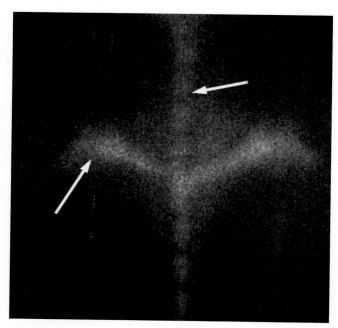

Figure 4.178 TOD view showing good visualization of the floor of the pelvis, especially the ischiatic tuberosities. The tail is seen as a midline structure. Note the bilateral symmetry.

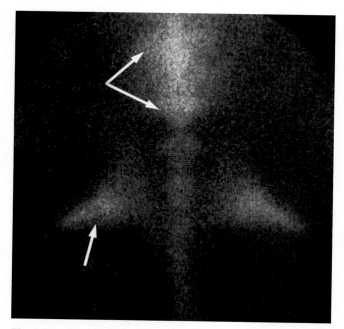

Figure 4.179 TOD view taken with the gamma camera angled to project the bladder away from the ischiatic tuberosities. Use this view when urine obscures visualization of the pelvic floor on the TOD view.

metabolism in the diaphyses of normal patients. The uptake should, however, be smoothly homogeneous with no focal areas of increased uptake. Contralateral imaging can be useful when evaluating borderline lesions. Physes, epiphyses, and apophyses demonstrate increased uptake because the bone tissue in these areas has increased metabolic rates.

Although the distribution of the radiopharmaceutical in the normal horse—young and old—is predictable, experience is necessary for interpreting bone scans. Comparing the relative uptake in opposite limbs or comparing images from horses of a similar age can assist the clinician in arriving at significant conclusions. It is important to look at relative uptake between structures on the same image and then compare it with the relative uptake between the same structures on the contralateral image. This compensates for times when, for example, an entire leg has less uptake than the opposite one. In these cases it is inappropriate to compare the uptake, for example, of the fetlock of the right with that of left foot. It is more accurate to evaluate the uptake ratio between the fetlock and the pastern region in one foot to the same ratio in the other foot. This reduces the risk of misinterpreting radiopharmaceutical uptake disparities that occur as natural phenomena or as image acquisition artifacts (e.g, camera-body-distance inequalities or collimator decentering). The comparison of relative uptake ratios should be used for images throughout the body. Generally, the more intense the uptake, the more severe the condition.

SCINTIGRAPHIC SIGNS OF DISEASE

Vascular Phase

Increased blood flow can be seen as a subacute or chronic response to trauma during the healing phase. Soft tissue imaging is useful for determining the amount of perfusion to the distal extremity and can thus help determine the best therapy and prognosis. The vascular phase is acquired by making 2-second images for 2 to 3 minutes directly after the intravenous injection of the tracer. It generally takes about 1 minute for the leading edge of the tracer to reach the distal limb. The images can be viewed either individually or as a composite image, or the data from the individual images can be displayed in the form of a graph.

Figure 4.180 presents the composite vascular phase image of the forelimbs of a horse 1 week after it had a near-degloving injury to the distal left fore cannon. After the intravenous administration of about 150 mCi $^{99m}TcO_4$, 90 images of 2 seconds each were acquired. The study was performed to determine if there was blood flow to the pastern region. The composite image shows increased blood flow to the distal cannon, where granulation tissue has already started to form. The pastern, however, shows more blood flow than that of the (normal) contralateral limb. This is believed to be the result of reflex hyperemia secondary to the healing process and is considered a positive sign, indicating that there is good blood flow to the foot. Figure 4.181 presents the data in graph form. The curve reflects the amount of radioactivity in the left and right pastern regions, determined

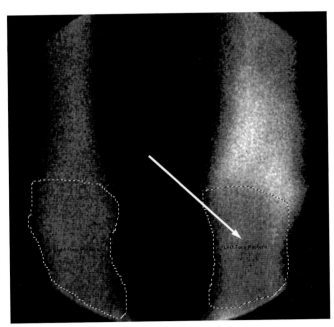

Figure 4.180 Composite vascular phase image of the bilateral pasterns of a horse 1 week after a near-degloving injury to the distal left fore cannon region, showing moderately increased blood flow to the left pastern region and markedly increased blood flow to the distal left cannon region.

by the region of interest that had been drawn around them. Each data point on the curve is one of the 90 images. Quantitation of the respective blood flow can be done by determining the area under the curve of each pastern and calculating the percentage of total flow. Empirical evaluation of the images is generally sufficient for most clinical cases.

Decreased blood flow to a region is often associated with nonviable bone or other tissue. Although seldom used, the vascular phase can be used to evaluate large sequestra.

Soft Tissue Phase

Increased activity in soft tissues is a good method of documenting increased blood flow to that region, e.g., joints with a joint synovitis and/or capsulitis. With fetlock joint capsulitis, for example, there is a region of increased tracer over the joint, compared with the distal cannon bone region and the proximal phalange (compare Fig. 4.182 with Fig. 4.154, which has normal uptake). The relationship between the fetlock and the adjacent regions is compared with the relationship between the same structures on the contralateral limb. Increased blood flow to the sacroiliac joint suggests sacroiliac joint capsulitis (compare Fig. 4.183 with Fig. 4.155, which has normal uptake); this increased uptake is sometimes seen in the delayed phase. Increased soft tissue phase uptake with a normal delayed-phase image is compatible with an acute degenerative condition, whereas increased uptake in both phases implies that the condition is probably chronic in nature. Soft tissue phase imaging of the

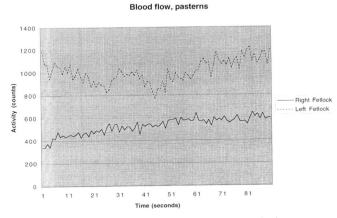

Figure 4.181 Graph of the data from the composite image shown in Figure 4.180, confirming that the left pastern has more blood flow than does the right one.

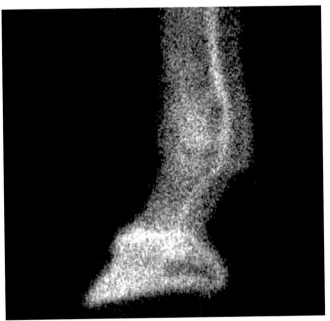

Figure 4.182 Soft tissue (pool) phase image of the left forefoot, showing increased blood flow to the fetlock region, which is suggestive of hyperemia associated with joint synovitis and/or capsulitis. Figure 4.154 provides the normal comparison.

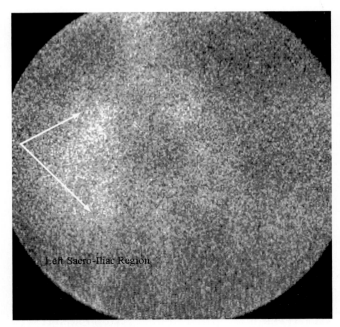

Figure 4.183 Soft tissue (pool) phase image of the dorsal pelvis, showing increased blood flow to the left sacroiliac region (arrows), suggesting hyperemia associated with joint synovitis and/ or capsulitis. Figure 4.155 provides the normal comparison.

navicular region often helps the clinician stage navicular syndrome; both lateral and solar views of the foot are acquired. Soft tissue phase imaging also helps with diagnosing desmitis or avulsion-type injuries of the proximal attachment of the suspensory ligament. These injuries are not necessarily evident on ultrasound or radiographic studies. Deep-lying regions (e.g., the coxofemoral joints) are difficult, if not impossible, to evaluate during soft tissue phase imaging because of the meager nature of the signal and the large amount of other tissues between the hip and the camera. These tissues make up several half-value layers (a layer of tissue that causes the signal to be reduced by half), which attenuate the beam significantly before it reaches the gamma camera.

Care must be taken not to overinterpret soft tissue phase images in instances in which severe increased uptake is also seen in the delayed-phase images; soft tissue phase "hot spots" in these cases often represent early bone uptake. For example, the soft tissue image shown in Figure 4.184A probably represents early bone uptake of the radiopharmaceutical by the proximal phalanx because of the intense uptake seen in that bone on the delayed-phase image (Fig. 4.184B). This horse had a fissure fracture of the first phalanx, which was also seen on radiographs (Fig. 4.184C).

Delayed Phase

Regions with increased blood flow and osteoblastic activity demonstrate increased uptake of the radiopharmaceutical in delayed-phase images. The severity or intensity of the increased uptake varies and is often associated with conditions such as fractures, stress fractures,

degenerative joint disease, enthesopathy, osteomyelitis, and neoplasia.

Distal phalanx fractures are generally easily seen because of the amount of osteoblastic activity that occurs with them, e.g., fissure margin fractures (Fig. 4.185).[10] Navicular disease is seen as increased uptake in lateral/ solar view delayed-phase images of the navicular bone region (Fig. 4.186).[46] The uptake might be subtle, because of the relatively small size of the navicular bone compared with the distal phalanx. The navicular should not be seen as a separate entity on normal scans. Laminitis results in moderate to severe radiopharmaceutical uptake in the distal aspect of the distal phalanx, seen on the lateral view and, especially, on the solar view (Fig. 4.187).

The amount of tracer uptake seen at a fracture site can help determine the type of fracture (pathologic versus traumatic) and the relative time of injury (acute versus chronic). Chronic and subacute fractures (older than 48 hours) have intense increased uptake because of the considerable osteoblastic activity that is occurring (Fig. 4.184B). Acute fractures have less radiopharmaceutical uptake because it takes approximately 24 hours for the osteoblastic activity at the injury site to be greater than that of the surrounding bone. In fact, acute traumatic fractures of less than 24 hours duration fail to show increased tracer uptake when compared with adjacent bone.

Figure 4.188 shows a delayed-phase image taken 48 hours after the horse experienced a comminuted fracture of the middle phalanx. Although mild increased uptake is seen, the fracture is best diagnosed because of the anatomic abnormality, not its physiologic peculiarity. Compare this figure with Figure 4.184B, which shows a chronic proximal phalangeal fracture with intense uptake and minimal anatomic displacement. Fracture uptake in humans can be expected at about 24 hours post-injury (although it takes longer in older patients) and generally lasts 6 to 12 months (again, longer in older patients).[43] The uptake by a fracture should decrease over time as fracture healing occurs. Figure 4.189 shows the delayed-phase image of a fractured right tuber ischiadicum of approximately 2 weeks duration, demonstrating both abnormal anatomy (ventral displacement of the fragment on the caudal view) and increased tracer uptake. Acetabular fractures are best seen on the dorsal oblique view of the hips, especially when compared with the contralateral joint (Fig. 4.190).

Stress fractures of the dorsal cortex of the metacarpal bone are most commonly seen in racing Thoroughbreds[12] and are often detected by nuclear medicine before they can be seen on radiographs (Fig 4.191). Stress fractures have also been diagnosed with scintigraphy at other sites, including the proximal palmar third metacarpal bone,[34] proximal caudolateral humerus, distal craniolateral humerus, midshaft radius, proximal lateral tibia, distal caudolateral tibia, midshaft tibia,[15] and tibia.[29] Fractures of the proximal radius, distal tibia, central tarsal bone, tibia, and ileum have also been described.[8,17,21,25,33]

Increased uptake can be seen in joints with degenerative joint disease. First, the uptake in the diseased joint must be compared with that in adjacent joints. Then, the uptake relationships are compared with those in the opposite limb for confirmation. Increased uptake during

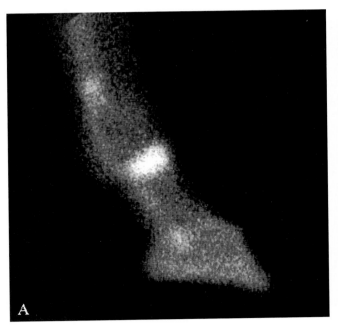

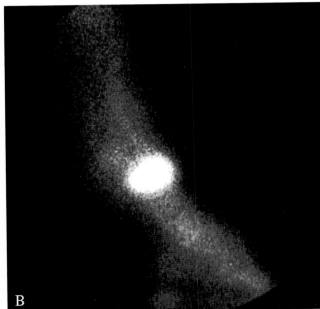

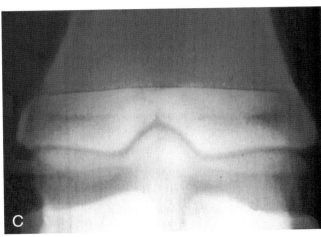

Figure 4.184   Right forefoot of a horse suffering from a chronic proximal first phalanx fracture. A. Soft tissue (pool) phase image showing marked increased blood flow to the proximal portion of the first phalanx. B. Delayed-phase image showing marked increased uptake by the proximal portion of the first phalanx. C. Radiograph showing a proximal first phalanx fracture. The increased uptake seen in the soft tissue image likely represents early radiopharmaceutical uptake by the bone, not just increased blood flow, because of the marked increased uptake seen in the delayed-phase image.

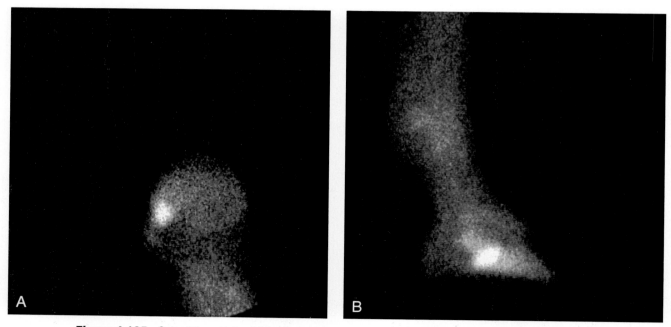

Figure 4.185 Solar (A) and lateral (B) delayed-phase images of a right fore distal phalanx with a marginal fracture.

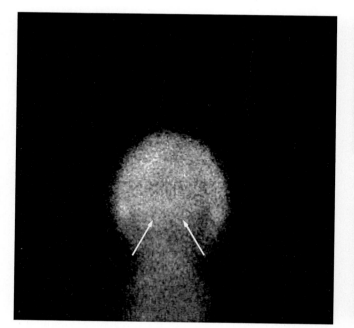

Figure 4.186 Solar delayed-phase image of the left fore distal phalanx, showing increased uptake in the navicular bone.

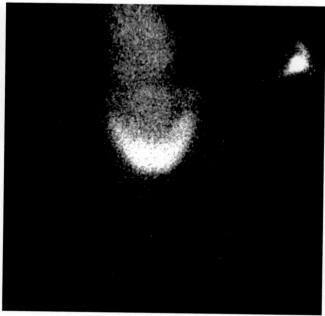

Figure 4.187 Solar delayed-phase image of the right hind distal phalanx, showing increased uptake along the distal portion, compatible with laminitis.

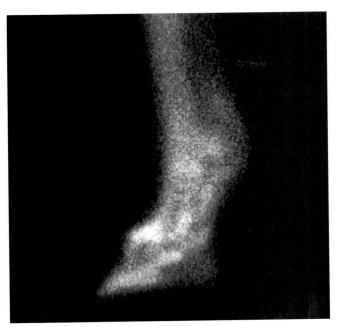

Figure 4.188 Delayed-phase image of a comminuted left fore middle phalangeal fracture 48 hours postinjury. Anatomic displacement is apparent, although tracer uptake is only mildly increased.

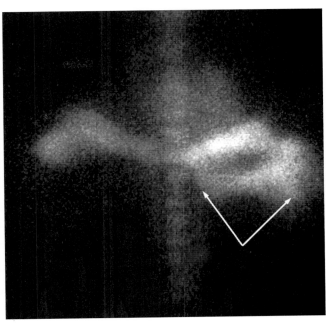

Figure 4.189 TOD delayed-phase image of a fractured right tuber ischiadicum (arrows) 2 weeks postinjury. Note both the anatomic abnormality and the severe increased tracer uptake.

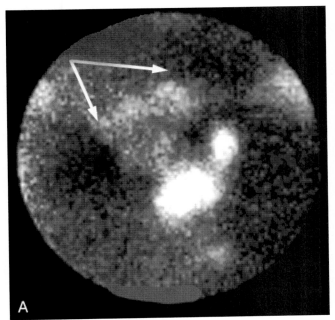

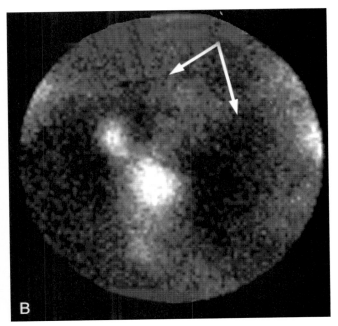

Figure 4.190 A. LDO delayed-phase image of an acetabular fracture of the left hip. B. RDO delayed-phase image of the normal contralateral (right) hip.

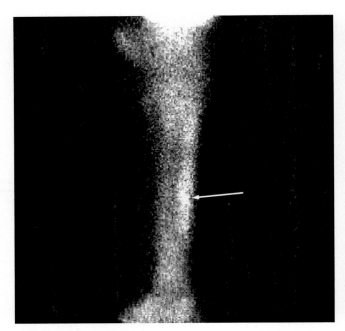

Figure 4.191 Delayed-phase image of the right fore cannon with stress fracture caused by dorsal metacarpal disease.

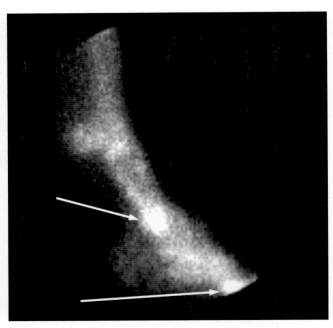

Figure 4.192 Delayed-phase image of the right forefoot, showing more uptake in the pastern joint than in the fetlock, which is compatible with degenerative joint disease of the pastern. Note the urine contamination on the sole.

the soft tissue phase is seen with synovitis and/or capsulitis; these joints do not necessarily have increased delayed-phase uptake or the radiographic changes seen with degenerative changes. Degenerative joint disease is commonly diagnosed in the pastern, fetlock, hock, stifle, and sacroiliac joints (Figs. 4.192 to 4.196).

Osteomyelitis has an intense uptake pattern because of increased blood flow and osteoblastic activity.[16,51] Figure 4.197 shows focal osteomyelitis on the greater tubercle of the right humerus. Radiographs documented the lesion, and a fine-needle aspirate confirmed a suppurative process. White blood cells can be labeled with ^{99m}Tc-HMPAO and reinjected to look for areas of inflammation.[30]

Degenerative changes in the spine are most commonly associated with overcrowding of the dorsal processes (kissing spines) and degenerative joint disease of the articular facets. The radiographic evaluation of the lumbar spine is especially difficult, if not impossible. Thus the scintigraphic evaluation of the spine is probably the best method for looking at the back (Fig. 4.198A). LDO and RDO views of the spine are ideal, although straight lateral and dorsal views are made if a lesion is found. Figure 4.198B shows the dorsal view of the lumbar region, which demonstrates increased uptake in the dorsal spinous process of the L2. These lesions are generally more easily visualized on the dorsal oblique view than on the dorsal view.

Enthesopathies show up as areas of increased radiopharmaceutical uptake and may be radiographically apparent lesions. A positive nuclear medicine scan reflects degenerative changes at the attachment of the joint capsule, ligaments, or tendons. Common sites for enthesopathies are the proximal sesamoids (sesamoiditis), where the suspensory ligament attaches to the abaxial surface; the proximal palmar/plantar region of the metacarpus or metatarsus (high suspensory ligament desmitis),

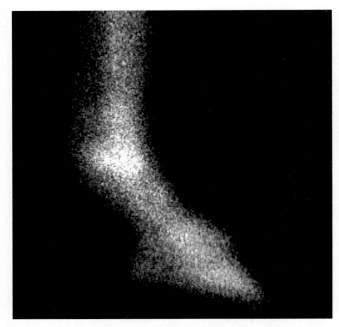

Figure 4.193 Delayed-phase image of the right forefoot, showing more uptake in the fetlock joint than in the pastern, which is compatible with degenerative joint disease of the fetlock.

where the suspensory ligament attaches proximally; and at the level of the tuber ischiadicum, where the caudal thigh muscles originate (Figs. 4.199 to 4.201). Increased uptake in the proximal region of the attachment of the small metacarpal bones to the third metacarpal bone may be evidence of enthesopathy of the interosseous liga-

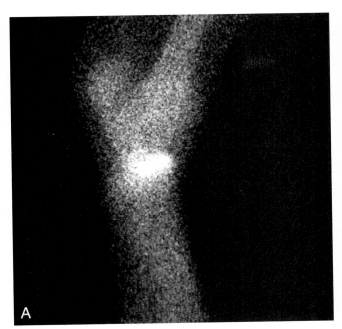

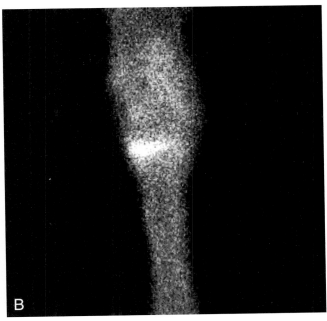

Figure 4.194 Lateral (A) and plantar (B, medial aspect) delayed-phase images of the right hock, showing severe increased uptake in the distal intertarsal and tarsometatarsal joints, which is compatible with degenerative joint disease of the hock.

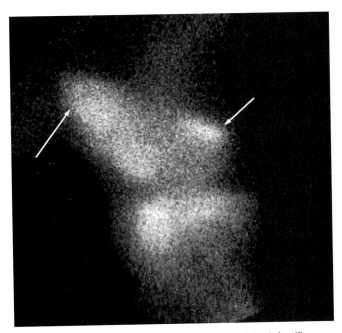

Figure 4.195 Lateral delayed-phase image of the left stifle, showing increased uptake by the femoral condyle.

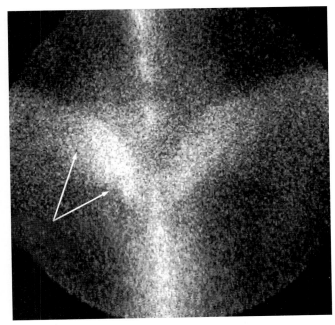

Figure 4.196 Delayed-phase image of the dorsal pelvis, showing increased tracer uptake in the left sacroiliac region (arrows), suggesting degenerative joint disease of the left sacroiliac joint. Figure 4.172 provides the normal comparison.

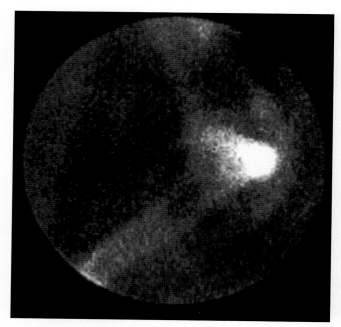

Figure 4.197 Delayed-phase image of the right humerus, showing focal severe increased radiopharmaceutical uptake in the greater tubercle, caused by a suppurative process.

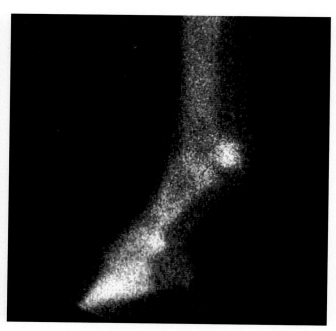

Figure 4.199 Lateral delayed-phase image of the left forefoot, showing increased uptake in the proximal sesamoid bones, which is consistent with sesamoiditis. The increased uptake in the pastern joint is suggestive of degenerative joint disease.

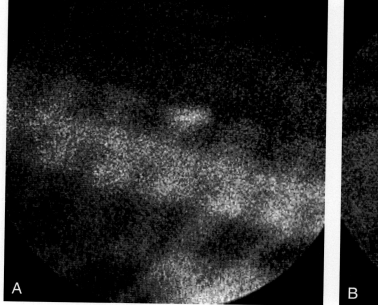

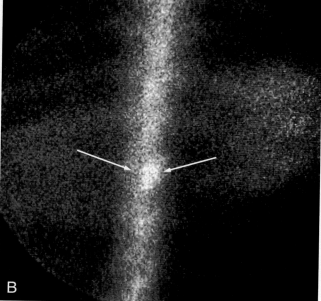

Figure 4.198 A. RDO delayed-phase image showing moderately increased uptake in the dorsal spine at L1 in a horse with chronic back pain. B. Dorsal delayed-phase image of the same lesion.

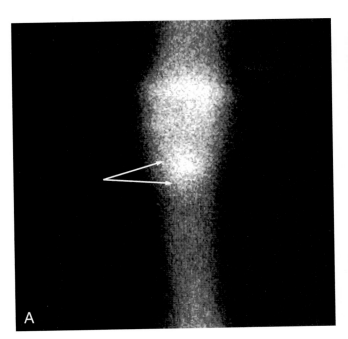

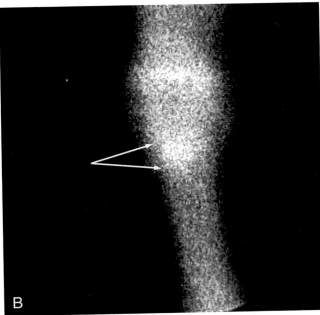

Figure 4.200 Dorsal soft tissue (pool) phase (A) and delayed-phase (B) images of the left fore carpus, showing increased uptake (arrows) at the proximal attachment of the suspensory ligament in a horse with high suspensory disease.

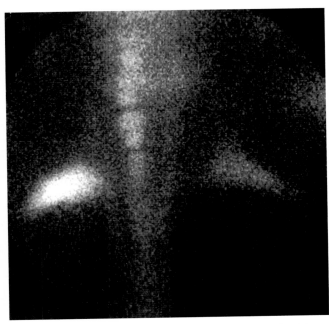

Figure 4.201 TOD delayed-phase image of the dorsal pelvis, showing increased uptake over the left tuber ischiadicum.

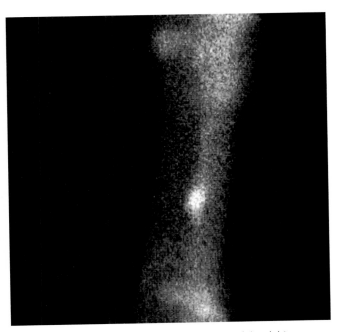

Figure 4.202 Lateral delayed-phase image of the right metacarpus, showing increased uptake by the splint bone.

ment (splints) or fracture of the splint bones (Fig 4.202). Similar scintigraphic changes can occur in the hindlimb.

In horses, direct trauma, often blunt in nature, can occur from a kick or trailer accident or can be self-inflicted from rapid movement (e.g., with interference).[41] The dorsal sacrum and/or tail head appears to be predisposed to trauma. Figure 4.203 is a scan from a horse that was thought to have received direct blows to the sacrum region, resulting in pain and increased uptake. Figure 4.204 is a scan from a horse suffering from

trauma of unknown origin that caused inflammatory changes in the sacrum. Figure 4.205 is a scan from a horse that had fallen from a bridge and landed on the tail head. Figure 4.206 is a scan from a horse that had been in a trailer accident. The horse presented with severe neurologic deficits that could be attributed to spinal trauma in the midthoracic region.

Metastatic spread of neoplasia to bone, rarely seen in horses, can result in localized uptake in multiple bones.

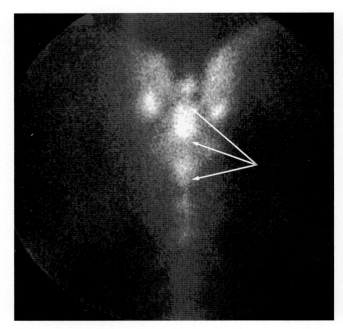

Figure 4.203 Dorsal delayed-phase image of the sacrum (arrows), showing increased uptake by the dorsal spines. Blunt trauma was suspected.

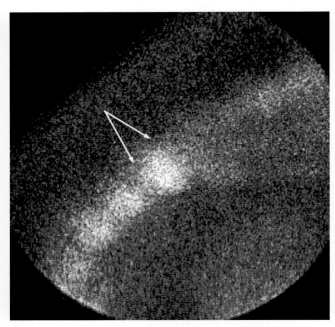

Figure 4.205 LDO delayed-phase image of the sacrum of a horse that had fallen from a bridge, landing on the tailhead. The image shows increased uptake by the dorsal spines (arrows). Figure 4.177 provides the normal comparison.

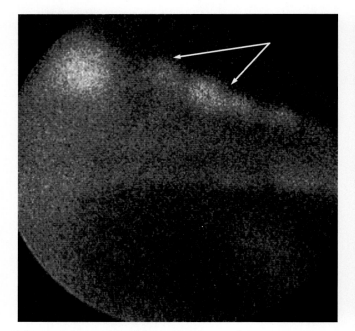

Figure 4.204 LDO delayed-phase image of the sacrum. The image shows increased uptake by the dorsal spines (arrows). Figure 4.177 provides the normal comparison.

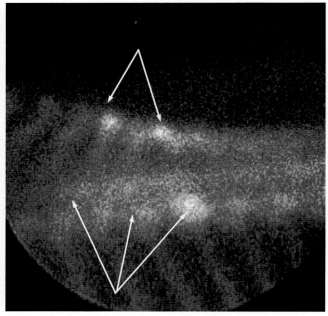

Figure 4.206 Left lateral delayed-phase image of the midthoracic region of a horse that had survived a trailer wreck, with neurologic deficits compatible with spinal cord compression at the sites showing increased uptake (arrows). Figure 4.175 provides the normal comparison.

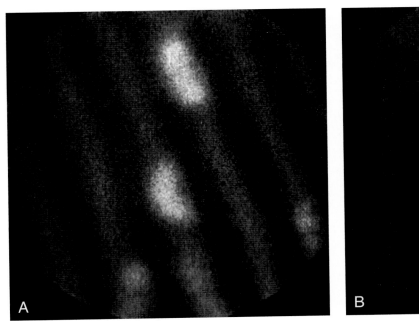
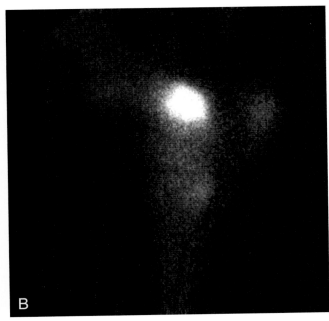

Figure 4.207   Delayed-phase image showing a metastatic intestinal adenocarcinoma, which resulted in severe focal increased uptake in (amongst others) the ribs (A) and distal left humerus (B).

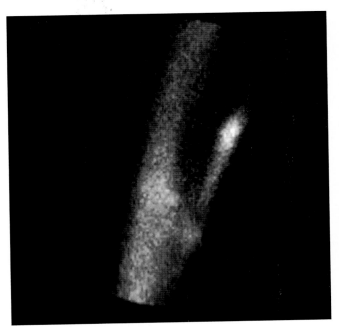

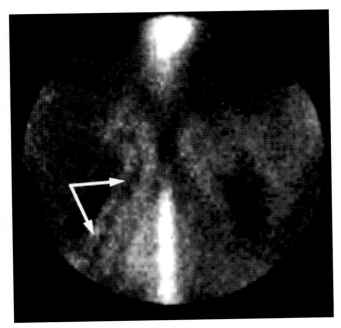

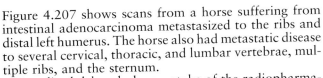

Figure 4.208   Lateral delayed-phase image of the left carpus, taken 3 weeks after an ulnar nerve block. Note the soft tissue uptake.

Figure 4.209   Dorsal delayed-phase image of the pelvis, showing linear uptake in the muscles (arrows) of a horse with rhabdomyolysis (tying-up syndrome).

Figure 4.207 shows scans from a horse suffering from intestinal adenocarcinoma metastasized to the ribs and distal left humerus. The horse also had metastatic disease to several cervical, thoracic, and lumbar vertebrae, multiple ribs, and the sternum.

Localized delayed-phase uptake of the radiopharmaceutical in soft tissues is not commonly seen but can occur with a variety of conditions, including regional anesthesia, rhabdomyolysis, and intramuscular injection of butorphanol.[13] In Figure 4.208, delayed-phase soft tissue uptake was seen 3 weeks after the horse received an ulnar nerve block.[1]

Rhabdomyolysis (tying-up syndrome) is seen as linear uptake patterns in the muscles (e.g., gluteals) on delayed-phase images. Figure 4.209 shows the typical scintigraphic appearance on a dorsal pelvis view, with linear

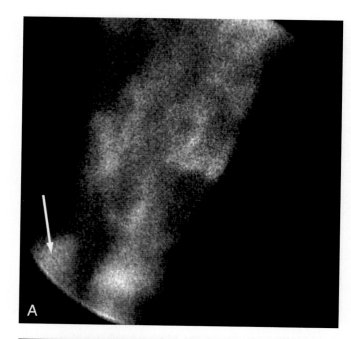

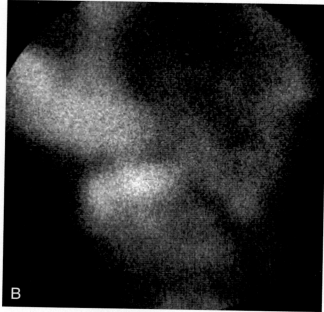

Figure 4.210 Lateral delayed-phase images of the left stifle (A) and proximal tibia (B) of a horse with rhabdomyolysis (tying-up syndrome), showing severe soft tissue uptake in the muscles over the tibia and caudal to the stifle, respectively.

uptake in the gluteal muscles. Figure 4.210 shows severe rhabdomyolysis, with severe uptake shown during the delayed phase in the muscles caudal to the left stifle and over the proximal left tibia.[7,24]

References

1. Allhands RV, Twardock AR, Boero MJ. Uptake of ^{99m}TcMDP in muscle associated with a peripheral nerve block. Vet Radiol 1987; 28:181–184.
2. Andrews FM, Matthews HK, Reed SM. The ancillary techniques and tests for diagnosing equine neurologic disease. Vet Med 1990; 85:1325–1330.
3. Berry CR, Daniel G, O'Callahan M. Pulmonary scintigraphy. In: Daniel G, Berry CR, eds. Handbook of Veterinary Nuclear Medicine. Raleigh, NC: North Carolina State University Press, 1996; 143–153.
4. Butson RJ, Webbon PM, Fairbairn SM. ^{99m}Tc-HMPAO labelled leukocytes and their biodistribution in the horse: A preliminary investigation. Equine Vet J 1995;27:313–315.
5. Chambers MD, Martinelli MJ, Baker GJ, et al. Nuclear medicine for diagnosis of lameness in horses. J Am Vet Med Assoc 1995; 206:792–796.
6. Gaughan EM, Wallace RJ, Kallfelz FA. Local anesthetics and nuclear medical bone images of the equine fore limb. Vet Surg 1990; 19:131–135.
7. Hornof WJ, Koblik PD. The scintigraphic detection of muscle damage. Equine Vet J 1991;23:327–328.
8. Johnson PJ, Allhands RV, Bake GJ, et al. Incomplete linear tibial fractures in two horses. J Am Vet Med Assoc 1988;192:522–524.
9. Kaser-Hotz B, Ueltschi G, Hess N. Navicular bone fracture in the pelvic limb in two horses. Vet Radiol 1991;32:283–285.
10. Keegan KG, Twardock AR, Losonsky JM, Baker GJ. Scintigraphic evaluation of fractures of the distal phalanx in horses: 27 cases (1979–1988). J Am Vet Med Assoc 1993;202:1993–1997.
11. Keegan KG, Wilson DA, Lattimer JC, et al. Scintigraphic evaluation of ^{99m}Tc-methylene diphosphonate uptake in the navicular area of horses with lameness isolated to the foot by anesthesia of the palmar digital nerves. Am J Vet Res 1996;57:415–421.
12. Koblik PD, Hornof WJ, Seeherman HJ. Scintigraphic appearance of stress-induced trauma of the dorsal cortex of the third metacarpal bone in racing Thoroughbred horses: 121 cases (1978–1986). J Am Vet Med Assoc 1988;192:390–395.
13. Lamb CR, Koblik PD, O'Callaghan MW, Mariner JC. Comparison of bone scintigraphy and radiography as aids in the evaluation of equine lameness: Retrospective analysis of 275 cases. Am Assoc Equine Pract 1989;34:34.
14. Long MT, Foreman JH, Wallig MA, et al. Hypertrophic osteopathy characterized by nuclear scintigraphy in a horse. Vet Radiol Ultrasound 1993;34:289–294.
15. Mackey VS, Trout DR, Meagher DM, Hornof WJ. Stress fractures of the humerus, radius, and tibia in horses. Clinical features and radiographic and/or scintigraphic appearance. Vet Radiol 1987; 28:26–33.
16. Markel MD, Madigan JE, Lichtensteiger CA, et al. Vertebral body osteomyelitis in the horse. J Am Vet Med Assoc 1986;188: 632–634.
17. Martin F, Herthel DJ. Central tarsal bone fractures in six horses: Report on the use of a cannulated compression bone screw. Equine Pract 1992;14:23–27.
18. Martinelli MJ, Chambers MD. Equine nuclear bone scintigraphy: Physiological principles and clinical application. Equine Vet Educ 1995;5:281–287.
19. Metcalf MR, Forrest LJ, Sellett LC. Scintigraphic pattern of ^{99m}Tc-MDP uptake in exercise induced proximal phalangeal trauma in horses. Vet Radiol 1990;31:17–21.
20. Metcalf MR, Tate LP, Sellett LC. Clinical use of ^{99m}Tc-MDP scintigraphy in the equine mandible and maxilla. Vet Radiol 1989;30: 80–87.
21. Metcalf MR, Tate LP, Sellett LC, Henry M. Radiographic and scintigraphic imaging of a proximal radial physeal injury in a young horse induced by olecranon fracture repair. Equine Vet J 1990;22: 56–59.
22. Morris E, Seeherman HJ. Clinical evaluation of poor performance in the racehorse: The results of 275 evaluations. Equine Vet J 1991; 23:169–174.
23. Morris E, Seeherman HJ, O'Callaghan MW, Blake-Caddel L. Scintigraphic identification of rhabdomyolysis in horses. Am Assoc Equine Pract 1992;37:315–325.
24. Morris E, Seeherman HJ, O'Callaghan MW, et al. Scintigraphic identification of skeletal muscle damage in horses 24 hours after strenuous exercise. Equine Vet J 1991;23:347–352.
25. Nelson A. Stress fractures of the hind limb in 2 Thoroughbreds. Equine Vet Educ 1994;6:245–248.
26. O'Callaghan MW. The integration of radiography and alternative imaging methods in the diagnosis of equine orthopedic disease. Vet Clin North Am Equine Pract 1991;7:339–364.

27. O'Callaghan MW, Hornof WJ, Fisher PE, Rabbe OG. Ventilation imaging in the horse with ^{99m}technetium-DTPA radioaerosol. Equine Vet J 1987;19:19–24.

28. O'Callaghan MW, Seeherman HJ, Blake-Caddel L. Scintigraphic screening of lameness and the benefits of combining imaging methods. Am Assoc Equine Pract 1992;37:301–314.

29. Peloso JG, Watkins JP, Keele SR, Morris EL. Bilateral stress fractures of the tibia in a racing American Quarter Horse. J Am Vet Med Assoc 1993;203:801–803.

30. Peters AM. Imaging infection and inflammation in veterinary practice. Equine Vet J 1995;27:242–244.

31. Pilsworth RC, Holmes MA, Blake-Caddel L. A low-cost, computer based scintigraphy system for use in lameness investigation in general practice. Am Assoc Equine Pract 1992;37:327–350.

32. Pilsworth RC, Holmes MA, Shepherd M. An improved method for the scintigraphic detection of acute bone damage to the equine pelvis by probe point counting. Vet Rec 1993;133:490–495.

33. Pilsworth RC, Shepherd MC, Herinckx BMB, Holmes MA. Fracture of the wing of the ilium, adjacent to the sacroiliac joint, in Thoroughbred racehorses. Equine Vet J 1994;26:94–99.

34. Pleasant RS, Baker GJ, Muhlbaue MC, et al. Stress reactions and stress fractures of the proximal palmar aspect of the third metacarpal bone in horses: 58 cases (1980–1990). J Am Vet Med Assoc 1992;201:1918–1923.

35. Riddolls LJ, Byford GG, McKee SL. Biological and imaging characteristics and radiation dose rates associated with the use of technetium-99-m-labelled imidodiphosphate in the horse. Can J Vet Res 1996;60:81–88.

36. Riddolls LJ, Willoughby RA, Dobson H. A method of mounting a gamma detector and yoke assembly for equine nuclear imaging. Vet Radiol 1991;32:78–81.

37. Ross MW, Nolan PM, Palmer JA, et al. The importance of the metatarsophalangeal joint in Standardbred lameness. Am Assoc Equine Pract 1992;37:741–756.

38. Seeherman HJ, Morris E, O'Callaghan MW. The use of sports medicine techniques in evaluating the problem equine athlete. Vet Clin North Am Equine Pract 1990;6:239–274.

39. Squire KRE, Fessler JF, Cantwell HD, Widmer WR. Enlarging bilateral femoral condylar bone cysts without scintigraphic uptake in a yearling foal. Vet Radiol Ultrasound 1992;33:109–113.

40. Steckel RR. The role of scintigraphy in the lameness evaluation. Vet Clin North Am Equine Pract 1991;7:207–239.

41. Steckel RR, Kraus-Hansen AE, Fackelman GE, et al. Scintigraphic diagnosis of thoracolumbar spinal disease in horses: A review of 50 cases. Am Assoc Equine Pract 1992;37:583–591.

42. Stewart M. Clinical applications of musculoskeletal scintigraphy in the horse. Aust Equine Vet 1994;12:71–75.

43. Taylor A Jr, Datz FL. Clinical Practise of Nuclear Medicine. New York: Churchill Livingstone, 1991;397.

44. Trout DR, Hornof WJ, Fisher PE. The effects on intra-articular anesthesia on soft tissue- and bone-phase scintigraphy in the horse. Vet Radiol 1991;32:251–255.

45. Trout DR, Hornof WJ, Liskey CC, Fisher PE. The effects of regional perineural anesthesia on soft tissue and bone phase scintigraphy in the horse. Vet Radiol 1991;32:140–144.

46. Trout DR, Hornof WJ, O'Brien TR. Reports of original studies. Soft tissue- and bone-phase scintigraphy for diagnosis of navicular disease in horses. J Am Vet Med Assoc 1991;198:73–77.

47. Twardock AR. Scintigraphy. Nuclear medicine scans complement x-rays as equine diagnostic tool. Large Anim Vet 1995;50(5):30–31.

48. Voute LC, Webbon PM, Whitelock R. Rules, regulations and safety aspects of scintigraphy. Equine Vet Educ 1995;7:169–172.

49. Wan PY, Tucker RL, Latimer FG. Scintigraphic diagnosis [fracture of the phalanx in a Quarter Horse]. Vet Radiol Ultrasound 1992;33:247–248.

50. Weaver MP. Twenty years of equine scintigraphy—a coming of age? Equine Vet J 1995;27:163–165.

51. Wisner ER, O'Brien TR, Pool RR, et al. Osteomyelitis of the axial border of the proximal sesamoid bones in seven horses. Equine Vet J 1991;23:383–389.

52. Young RL, O'Brien TR, Craychee TJ. Examination procedures for the diagnosis of suspensory desmitis in the horse. Am Assoc Equine Pract 1990;35:233–241.

Suggested Reading

Lamb CR. Non-skeletal distribution of bone-seeking radiopharmaceuticals. Vet Radiol 1990;31:246–253.

Twardock AR, Baker GJ, Chambers MD. The impact of nuclear medicine as a diagnostic procedure in equine practice. Comp Cont Educ Pract Vet 1991;13:1717–1719.

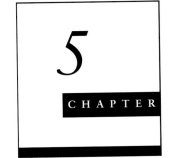

5

CHAPTER

The Role of Nutrition in Musculoskeletal Development and Disease

CATHERINE J. SAVAGE AND LON D. LEWIS

Since nutrition and exercise are important in the maintenance and development of healthy muscular and skeletal systems, deficiencies or excesses in these may cause or predispose these systems to disease. Accordingly, this chapter will emphasize the role that various nutrients and exercise play in the disease process. Diseases will be covered according to the time when they most commonly occur: 1) during the preparturient and postparturient periods, showing effects on the mare and nursing foal, 2) during growth, and 3) during maintenance or work.

In many instances, the only way to diagnose and correct nutritional imbalances is to evaluate the ration and water ingested. For ration evaluation and proper feeding procedures to prevent nutritional imbalances, the reader is referred to the National Research Council's (NRC's) *Nutrient Requirements of Horses*[67] and to Lewis.[59]

THE MARE AND FOAL

If the mare is not properly fed during pregnancy, the fetus will be deprived of nutrients important for its development and growth. In most cases, however, normal fetal development occurs unless the deficiency is sufficiently severe and prolonged that the mare's reserves are depleted. This usually would be evident by poor body condition and health of the mare. Generally, if the mare appears to be in good body condition, it is likely that the fetus is receiving the proper amount of nutrients (energy, protein, vitamins, and most minerals, etc.) for normal development. Exceptions may include deficient or excessive intake of selenium, vitamin A, iodine, or possibly manganese by the mare, which may affect the fetus yet have no observable effect on the mare. Dietary imbalances severe enough to be clinically observable in the mare may have a profound effect on the fetus, newborn, and nursing foal.

Inadequate Feed Intake

Inadequate feed intake sufficient to cause a thin mare may greatly decrease the mare's colostrum production and reproductive efficiency. Reduced colostrum production can occur secondary to inadequate dietary energy and/or protein. If colostral intake (i.e., passive transfer of maternal antibodies, cytokines, and other proteins) by the newborn foal is insufficient, then protection from infectious diseases will be compromised.

Since 80 to 90% of all food eaten is needed for supplying energy requirements, the major effect of inadequate feed intake is an energy deficiency. If the mare is thin at foaling and is not fed so that she reaches optimal body weight within the next several months, her reproductive efficiency may be greatly diminished.[41] In addition, a decrease in feed intake during the latter stages of pregnancy and early lactation in ponies and miniature horses may result in a syndrome of hyperlipidemia/hyperlipemia in the mare, which has a poor prognosis. Thoroughbred, Standardbred, Quarter Horse, and other full-sized horse mares are not at risk unless they have pituitary adenoma or concurrent azotemia.

Excess Feed Intake

When a pregnant mare engages in excess feed intake to the point of obesity, the results may be just as harmful as inadequate feed intake. The mare that is overweight at parturition may have trouble with the following: 1) foaling, because of the decreased muscle tone associated with the decreased physical activity that occurs with obesity, 2) producing sufficient quantities of colostrum and milk for the foal because of fat deposition in the mammary gland, and 3) conceiving and maintaining pregnancy.

Overly obese mares are poor breeders.[30] Obesity in mares has been reported to be one of the most common breeding problems observed at Thoroughbred brood mare farms.[27] If the mare is overweight at foaling, it will frequently lose weight during the first few months of lactation. It is reported that these mares frequently do not come into heat or conceive as readily as those that are maintaining or gaining weight during the initial stages of lactation.[30] A recent study concluded that the mare's reproductive efficiency is enhanced by having her at optimum body weight and condition at foaling and that feeding the mare sufficiently during lactation to maintain this condition is important.[41] If she is thin at foaling, she should be fed so that she gains weight during lactation. If she is overweight at foaling, she should be fed to maintain this weight until 90 days after conception, at which time digestible energy (DE) intake (e.g., grains, concentrates, sweet feeds) should be reduced as much as necessary to reach optimum body weight by the eighth month of pregnancy. Optimum body weight and condition are achieved when the ribs cannot be seen but can be felt without feeling any fat between the skin and ribs. A report of equine condition scoring is given by Carroll and Huntington.[13] Horse owners should avoid trying to reduce the mare's weight during either the first or last 3 months of pregnancy or early in lactation. Weight reduction during the first 3 months of pregnancy may result in fetal resorption,[41] while during the last 3 months of pregnancy, it may decrease colostral production and affect the fetus' birth weight. Weight reduction during lactation will decrease milk production. In addition, excessive feeding during the last 2 weeks of gestation should be avoided, since this practice has been associated with an increased incidence of cecal rupture.[118]

Protein Imbalances

Much of our knowledge regarding protein deficiencies during gestation is extrapolated from other species. Inadequate protein in the diet during pregnancy has been shown to decrease cerebral weight, protein content, and glial and neuron cell numbers in newborn mice.[66] A similar decrease in neuronal cell numbers in young rats was not corrected when they were offered adequate postnatal nutrition.[99] A severe protein deficiency during pregnancy has also been shown to decrease plasma thyroxine concentration, cause a 20 to 30% lower birth weight, and result in permanent stunting in newborn pigs.[1] Protein restriction in prenatal or early postnatal life may result in long-term impairment of thyroid hormone synthesis or release. The importance of thyroid hormone for normal growth has been established in many species; however, the issues of hypothyroidism are controversial in the horse. Inadequate protein in the mare's diet during pregnancy may induce hypothyroidism in the fetus, which could persist following birth. Hypothyroidism in the fetus will cause delays in normal prenatal and postnatal development. This may decrease birth weight and postnatal growth, resulting in permanent stunting. In addition, there may be a delay in the ossification of the cartilaginous cuboidal bones of the carpus and tarsus.[83] Ossification of these bones normally occurs between the last 6 to 8 weeks of gestation up to 33 days postgestation. Delayed ossification of the cuboidal bones,[2] owing to prematurity or a dietary protein-deficiency- or iodine-

deficiency-induced hypothyroidism, may result in severe angular limb deformities, especially carpal and tarsal valgus.[98] These deformities may be present at birth, but usually occur within the first few days of life, as weight bearing produces a "crush" or "collapse" syndrome. Premature birth is an important cause of cuboidal bone immaturity and resultant angular limb deformities.[98] Tarsal bone collapse has been reported in foals that are putatively hypothyroid.[83,98] The administration of thyroid hormone is controversial, but appeared beneficial in one case.[83]

A deficiency in protein intake during pregnancy sufficient to have a detrimental effect on the fetus or neonate generally also manifests as a poor body-condition score in the mare. The mare's appearance would be similar to that which would occur as a result of a dietary energy deficiency because of inadequate feed intake; however, a moderate dietary protein deficiency during lactation will usually decrease milk production without causing an observable effect on the mare. In one study, mares fed a diet containing 10.5% protein in the total ration dry matter, as compared to the 14% required, had decreased milk production by an average of 2.8 lb (i.e., 1.3 kg) per day during the first 3 months of lactation, even though the intake of energy-supplying nutrients and other nutrients was similar in both groups.[63] This resulted in 52 lb (23.6 kg) less gain and 1 inch (2.5 cm) less growth in height by the foals nursing the protein-deficient mares during this period.[63]

In contrast, excessive dietary protein intake during pregnancy and lactation anecdotally does not appear to have any detrimental or beneficial effect on the fetus or nursing foal. However, theoretically excessive amounts of protein may be metabolized so that excessive energy is available to the mare, which could be detrimental. If the protein is high in sulfur-containing amino acids, then a secondary calcium deficiency may be induced in the short term,[31] although horses appear able to acclimate to this.[94]

Effects on the Nursing Foal

If the foal is normal at birth and during the first weeks of life, yet musculoskeletal problems develop before 3 months of age, then five nutritional causes may exist: 1) inadequate milk intake, 2) excessive milk intake, 3) intake of milk containing inappropriate amounts of minerals, 4) early, incorrect introduction of high-energy creep feed, or 5) early, incorrect introduction of creep feed containing unsuitable amounts of minerals. It is difficult to assess milk production of mares, as udder size, udder development, and ability to strip milk from the teat are not necessarily reflective of the mare's milk production.

Inadequate milk intake is most commonly a result of inadequate milk production by the mare. Agalactia is more obvious than insidious poor milk production. Agalactia commonly occurs secondary to the mare's ingestion of endophyte-infested fescue grasses and hays, but sometimes may occur in maiden mares or mares that have been sick for another reason. Lactation greatly increases the mare's requirements for the nutrients excreted in milk. If the intake of those nutrients by the mare is inadequate, the amount of milk produced will decrease. Even though some mares on a nutritionally-deficient diet will use nutrients from their body to produce an adequate quantity of milk, the ability to do this is variable. Some mares receiving a deficient diet will maintain their own body weight and condition at the expense of milk production. Others, even on adequate diets, are just poor milk producers. A decrease in milk production, which can occur as a result of nearly any nutritional deficiency in the mare's diet, decreases the amount of milk available to the nursing foal. Without adequate quantities of milk, the foal's diet may be deficient in a number of nutrients, including energy. Owing to its dietary energy deficiency, the foal will consume additional amounts of solid food. Unfortunately, the solid food consumed by the foal frequently will not provide the high levels of nutrients needed. As a result, a number of nutritional deficiencies may occur depending on the type of feed ingested. Preventative measures should be taken to ensure that the mare is fed properly to produce enough milk so that, prior to two to three months of age, the foal needs to consume little solid food. If the mare fails to produce adequate milk, it is important to ensure that the foal is fed the correct amount and composition of milk replacer and/or solid creep feed.

If the milk contains the proper concentrations of calcium and phosphorus and yet skeletal problems occur in the foal that is receiving little other than the mare's milk, the mare may be producing more milk than the foal can tolerate or a copper deficiency may exist. The former may result in a loose, pasty stool, or possibly alterations in endochondral ossification. To correct this, the mare's feed intake should be reduced to decrease the mare's milk production, or if the foal is at least 2 months old, it should be weaned.

If the mare appears to be producing an adequate amount of milk, but musculoskeletal problems occur in the foal that is less than 2 to 3 months of age and consuming little other than mare's milk, then the mineral composition of the milk (e.g., calcium, phosphorus, copper) should be determined (Hamar D, personal communication, 1998, Diagnostic Laboratory, Colorado State University; Warren Analytical Laboratory, Greeley, CO). Occasionally a mare will produce adequate quantities of milk, but with improper amounts of calcium, phosphorus, or other nutrients. Mare's milk should contain at least 80 to 120 mg/dL of calcium, 45 to 90 mg/dL of phosphorus, and more calcium than phosphorus.[59] Mare's milk is low in copper, and copper levels do not increase despite supplementation of the mare. The typical level is 2 to 5 ppm (mg/kg), being highest early in lactation.[59] This is less than the amount that the NRC[67] and many researchers currently recommend.[53,48]

If the mare's milk does not contain the proper concentration of nutrients, particularly calcium or phosphorus, ensure that there is an adequate amount of these nutrients in the diet to meet the mare's requirements and then recheck the milk. Recognize that milk composition will change with the stage of lactation. However, if it still does not contain the proper concentrations of calcium and phosphorus, the foal should be weaned from the mare. If the foal is younger than five to six weeks of age, a mare's milk replacer should be fed until the foal is consuming 2 to 3 lb (approximately 1 kg)/day of milk replacer pellets. Two milk replacers commonly used at

the Colorado State University's Veterinary Teaching Hospital are: Mare's Match Milk Replacer (Land O' Lakes, Fort Dodge, IA) and Foal-Lac (Borden Chemical Company, Norfolk, VA). If these or other reputable equine milk replacers are not available, we prefer to use pasteurized goat's milk. Occasionally people elect to use milk replacers that have been formulated for other species (e.g., goat milk replacer)—if this is your choice, ascertain that no antimicrobials are present in the formulation, as their presence can lead to considerable gastrointestinal upset in foals. After 5 to 8 weeks of age, the foal does not need milk and can be fed as a weanling.[59]

Mineral Imbalances

Deficiencies or excesses of most of the minerals in the mare's diet have not been demonstrated to have an effect on prenatal or postnatal foal development. Selenium, iodine, and possibly manganese and copper are exceptions.[73,74] In contrast to a dietary energy or protein deficiency, dietary imbalances in iodine, manganese, and copper may have profound effects on the fetus or neonate without any observable effects on the dam. However, selenium deficiency or selenium toxicity may also have profound effects on the dam (see the section on selenium in this chapter).

Manganese Deficiency

A naturally occurring manganese deficiency has not been reported in the horse. Manganese deficiency is described here because of its effects on the skeletal systems of ruminants, swine, and poultry, and the similarity of some of these signs to those seen in horses for which the cause frequently is unidentified. A manganese deficiency in ruminants, swine, and poultry may cause any of the following: 1) sterility, 2) decreased libido, 3) delayed estrus, 4) decreased conception, 5) poor growth, 6) abortion or stillbirths, 7) the birth of weak neonates, and 8) the birth of neonates that may show incoordination or limb deformities (e.g., enlarged joints; knuckled pasterns; twisted forelimbs; and weak, shortened bones resulting in lameness, stiffness, joint pain, and a reluctance to move).[111]

Although the manganese requirement for the horse is unknown, 40 ppm in the total dry matter (DM) ration is considered adequate for all horses.[67] Most roughage contains more than this amount, but most cereal grains, excluding oats, do not.[59] Trace mineralized salt generally contains 0.28% (2800 ppm) manganese. One ounce (i.e., approximately 28 g) of trace mineralized salt, or 250 mg of $MnSO_4$, ingested daily will add about 80 mg of manganese to the diet, which is approximately equivalent to adding 8 ppm (i.e., 8 mg of manganese per kg of dry matter feed) to the diet.

A manganese concentration of less than 0.02 ppm in plasma or blood, 6 ppm in liver dry matter, or 4.5 ppm in kidney dry matter is indicative of a manganese deficiency in ruminants.[111] Although excessive manganese intake is known to be toxic to other animals, toxicity levels are not known in the horse. The NRC[67] suggests the maximum tolerable level of manganese for horses is 1000 ppm. Manganese toxicity does not appear to occur naturally, even with the ingestion of large amounts over a long period of time.

Selenium

Both selenium deficiency and toxicity may occur in horses under natural feeding regimens. Since selenium toxicity most commonly affects the mature horse rather than the foal, it is discussed under the section, In the Mature Horse for Maintenance or Work. However, excessive selenium ingestion by the mare during pregnancy may result in hoof deformities in the foal at birth.[49,85]

Selenium Deficiency

Conversely, selenium deficiency may become clinically apparent in foals at 1 to 60 days of age, but may occur up to 12 months of age and rarely affects mature horses.[121,21] The condition is usually termed "nutritional muscular dystrophy" or "white muscle disease." Most of the areas around the Great Lakes and the eastern and northwestern United States and much of Canada are low in selenium (Fig. 5.1). Forage and grain grown in these areas may contain less than 0.1 ppm of selenium. Consumption of such feeds for prolonged periods of time may result in a deficiency. Although maps of soil mineral composition are an excellent source of information, some mineral levels (e.g., selenium) may vary considerably within a small region. Therefore soil testing is essential if unexpected problems arise on a property, especially if clinical signs are seen in a number of animals. The NRC[67] recommends that horses require 0.1 ppm (mg/kg) of selenium in total rations on a dry matter basis, although 0.2 ppm is preferred by one of the authors.[59] The maximum tolerance level for selenium in the horse is currently 2 ppm.[67,59]

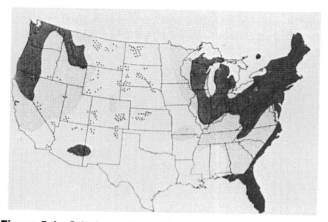

Figure 5.1 Selenium content of forages and grains by regional distribution in the United States. ■ Low, i.e., approximately 80% of all forage and grain contains less than 0.05 ppm. ▨ Variable, i.e., approximately 50% of all forage and grain contains more than 0.1 ppm. ☐ Adequate, i.e., 80% of all forage and grain contains more than 0.1 ppm. • Local areas where selenium accumulator plants contain more than 50 ppm. (Adapted from Kubota J, Allaway WH. J Dairy Sci 1975;58(10):1563.)

Selenium deficiency in the neonate occurs as a result of inadequate selenium intake by the dam during pregnancy or lactation. Mild deficiencies may decrease the foal's immune response to infectious diseases and decrease growth rate.[104] Severe selenium deficiencies cause muscle damage, resulting in stiffness, muscle pain, listlessness, and an increased release and plasma concentration of muscle enzymes (i.e., AST, CK, and LDH). In severe cases, myoglobin that is lost from damaged muscles is excreted in the urine (i.e., myoglobinuria), giving it a coffee-colored appearance. It is important to recognize that myoglobinuria may occur in all cases of selenium deficiency and in equine rhabdomyolysis syndrome (ERS) (see the section on ERS in this chapter), as this can potentially affect the kidneys and induce renal damage through prostaglandin-mediated injury. Both the skeletal and myocardial muscles may be involved. Young foals exhibit severe myocardial, diaphragmatic, and respiratory muscle involvement. These foals develop heart failure, respiratory distress, and pulmonary edema and frequently die within a few hours to days after the onset of clinical symptoms. Older foals may become recumbent, with tachycardia, tachypnea, and excess salivation. Muscular exertion may initiate the onset of symptoms. Another syndrome recognized in foals with selenium deficiency is dysphagia. Foals may present because milk has been noticed running from the nares after nursing. In these cases, no cleft palate will be found, and the foal's pharynx will appear endoscopically normal.

Lesions that may be observed on necropsy include pulmonary edema, a yellowish-brown discoloration of fat, and pallor and ischemic necrosis of the muscles. Pallor and necrosis are particularly noticeable on the muscles of the hindlimbs and neck, giving them a white appearance. Consequently, the condition is often called "white muscle disease." Histologically, there is widespread tissue lipoperoxidation, leading to hyaline degeneration and calcification of muscle fibers.[7]

Although much less common, a selenium deficiency in the mature horse may affect the muscles of mastication and/or those of the limbs, resulting in a stiff gait.[72,121] It has also been implicated in the equine rhabdomyositis syndrome (ERS) seen after strenuous exercise.

Selenium deficiencies may be treated or prevented in horses in selenium-deficient areas by 1) allowing free access to trace mineralized salt containing 30 ppm of selenium (with the expected daily consumption of trace mineralized salt being approximately 33 g, the horse ingests 1 mg of selenium), 2) feeding a total ration containing 0.1 to 0.5 ppm of selenium in its dry matter content, or 3) administering a selenium injection (e.g., E-SE, Schering-Plough Corp., Madison, NJ) intramuscularly as directed by the manufacturer. This product contains selenium (as sodium selenite) equivalent to 2.5 mg/mL and 50 mg (68 IU) of vitamin E. It should be remembered that vitamin E-selenium products have been associated with anaphylactic reactions in horses.

Even though clinical signs of selenium deficiency do not occur unless the ration contains less than 0.08 to 0.1 ppm, a ration containing levels of 0.5 ppm may be necessary to maintain optimal plasma selenium concentrations.[104] Amounts greater than this should not be added to the ration. Greater than 2 ppm in the ration is toxic,[67] and rations containing greater than 5 ppm are extremely detrimental to equine health.

In addition to feeding a selenium-containing salt or adding selenium to the pregnant mare's ration, the mare should be given a single selenium injection 3 weeks to 3 months prior to foaling, as a preventative to selenium deficiency in the foal. Selenium injections early in pregnancy may be teratogenic in sows.[117] Although this has not been observed in mares, selenium injections should be avoided in early pregnancy. Selenium supplementation to the lactating mare will increase milk selenium concentration and result in elevation of the nursing foal's plasma selenium concentration.[6] In areas in which selenium deficiency has occurred in foals, a selenium injection also may be given shortly after birth and every 2 to 3 months during the first 6 months of life.

Iodine Imbalances

Iodized and trace mineralized salts generally contain 70 ppm of iodine. Ingestion of 0.5 oz (i.e., approximately 14 to 15 g) daily of these salts provides all of the iodine needed by the horse (1 mg/horse per day[67,68]). An iodine deficiency will not occur if these products are available for the horse to consume (and it actually ingests it) or if 15 g is added to the horse's ration daily.

An iodine toxicity is more common than a deficiency. Five ppm of iodine in the horse's total ration dry matter, or greater than 40 mg of iodine intake per horse daily, will cause toxicity.[68] Seaweed and some seaweed- or kelp-containing products may contain high levels of iodine.[3,24,25] Iodine is also present in many commercial supplements, which, if fed in amounts greater than those recommended by the manufacturer, may cause toxicity. Other causes of iodine toxicity include 1) feeding the horse several iodine-containing products that will have a cumulative effect (unfortunately, horse owners often do not look at the ingredients on supplements, and ingredients frequently overlap), 2) adding greater than 7% iodized or trace-mineralized salts to the ration, and 3) ingestion of excessive amounts of organic iodine such as ethylenediaminedihydroiodide (EDDI). Even though EDDI is not commonly added to the horse's ration, it is frequently added to cattle and sheep rations to treat and prevent foot rot, respiratory disease, and "woody tongue" and "lumpy jaw" (i.e., actinobacillosis or actinomycosis, respectively). If horses are fed this ration, iodine toxicity occasionally may ensue, the signs of which include excessive lacrimation, scurfing of the skin, and loss of appetite. Ingestion of greater than 0.5 mg of EDDI per kg body weight per day is not generally harmful for short periods of time (1 to 2 weeks), but levels substantially below this may be detrimental if they are fed over a prolonged period.

Iodine toxicity not only increases susceptibility to infectious diseases, but it apparently decreases the response to treatment of these diseases. A reduction in antibody formation, lymphocyte mitosis, phagocytosis, and cell-mediated immunity occurs.[3] Since iodine is actively transported across the placenta and through nursing, excessive iodine intake by the mare during either pregnancy or lactation may result in thyroid gland hypertrophy (goiter) in the fetus or nursing foal.

Excesses or deficiencies of iodine intake may result in hypothyroidism, although in general clinical hypothyroidism is a controversial disorder in horses. Excess iodine inhibits the rate of iodide trapping and diminishes endocytosis of colloid from the thyroid gland follicles. Hence release of thyroid hormones from the colloid does not occur, thus resulting in hypothyroidism and a hypoplastic thyroid gland. Goiter has also been described in foals born to mares that have been excessively supplemented with iodine. With iodine deficiency there is an insufficient amount of iodine available for the synthesis of an adequate amount of the iodine-containing thyroid hormones, but excessive thyroglobulin (i.e., colloid) is manufactured because of excessive levels of thyroid stimulating hormone (TSH); consequently, both hypothyroidism and goiter may follow.

Hypothyroid foals from iodine deficiency or toxicity will be weak at birth, and generally die within the first few days of life if the iodine deficiency or excess continues following birth. Additionally, hypothyroidism is thought to alter ossification of the cuboidal bones of the carpus or tarsus, resulting in angular limb deformity; however, there is little documentation regarding iodine as a cause. This condition may be present at birth or develop in the first few days of life, as weight bearing increases the forces on these underdeveloped bones.

Hypomagnesemic and Hypocalcemic Tetany

Although relatively uncommon, tetany because of a fall in plasma calcium (Ca) and/or magnesium (Mg) concentration may occur in any horse. However, it occurs most commonly during lactation because of the additional, substantial amounts of calcium and lesser amounts of magnesium lost into the milk. When tetany results from hypomagnesemia, the condition is referred to as grass tetany. Tetany as a result of hypocalcemia is called lactation, stress, or transit tetany. Both hypocalcemia and hypomagnesemia result in muscle fasciculations, tachycardia, a stiff stilted gait, and reluctance to move. If severe, either condition may lead to recumbency and death, generally within a few hours after the onset of symptoms. Hypocalcemia is diagnosed infrequently in horses, and hypomagnesemia is a very uncommon diagnosis in horses. Other differential diagnoses to consider when a decreased calcium level is measured on equine plasma include 1) cantharidin toxicity (i.e., blister beetle intoxication secondary to a horse's ingestion of contaminated alfalfa hay; this will probably increase in prevalence in areas in the United States not previously affected, because of increased movement of hays around the country), 2) pancreatitis (which is rarely diagnosed antemortem in horses), and 3) acute renal failure. One must also remember that if the total calcium, rather than the ionized calcium fraction, is measured, then it must be corrected for the albumin status. To obtain the corrected calcium level in a hypoalbuminemic horse (e.g., a horse with diarrhea causing a protein-losing enteropathy), the measured albumin value should be subtracted from the mean albumin value (e.g., 3.35 g/dL is often used in horses), and the difference added back to the measured calcium concentration.

Hypocalcemia may occur in lactating mares as a result of calcium loss into the milk. The chances of this occurring are increased if the mare is on a calcium-deficient ration and is subjected to prolonged stress, such as inclement weather, disease, trauma, strenuous physical exertion, or transportation. This condition is prevented by ensuring that the ration meets or exceeds the lactating mare's calcium requirements of 0.5% in the total ration dry matter (i.e., approximately 50 g/day in a 450-kg [1000-lb] lactating mare) and by preventing prolonged stress. If a grass roughage is being consumed, an additional 60 to 90 g of limestone ($CaCO_3$) daily is generally needed.[59] If a legume roughage such as alfalfa is being consumed, no additional calcium is generally needed in the ration.

Hypocalcemic tetany is treated by administering a calcium-containing solution intravenously (e.g., 23% calcium gluconate). The safest method is to base the decision to treat on a corrected or ionized calcium plasma concentration. In rare cases in which it is elected to administer a bolus of calcium or calcium/magnesium (e.g., in cases in which hypomagnesemic tetany is suspected) solution, the solution should be given slowly while ausculting the heart. An increase in the amplitude of heart sounds and a decrease in heart rate indicate a favorable response. If arrhythmias or an increased heart rate occurs, solution administration should be stopped immediately, or heart block and death may occur. The safest way to treat hypocalcemia in horses is to place an intravenous jugular catheter and place 100 to 350 mL of 23% calcium gluconate solution into each of four 5-liter bags of isotonic fluids (e.g., Plasmalyte; Baxter, Overland Park, KS) for a total of 400 to 1400 mL of 23% calcium gluconate in 20 liters of isotonic fluid to make a hypertonic solution. These should be administered intravenously continuously over 5 to 6 hours. The plasma calcium, magnesium, and electrolytes should be rechecked. Even if the corrected calcium level is within the normal range, calcium-containing fluids may be safely maintained at a slow infusion rate for the next 24 hours (e.g., 80 to 100 mL of 23% calcium gluconate per 5-liter bag at an administration rate of approximately 1 to 3 liters/hour, IV). The horse should be encouraged to eat a ration of alfalfa hay (which is high in calcium) or one should ensure that an increased calcium supplement is provided.

Vitamin Deficiencies

Rarely is a vitamin deficiency recognized as the cause of musculoskeletal disease in the horse. Vitamin A deficiency is the vitamin imbalance most likely to occur. Vitamin A, like all of the fat-soluble vitamins (A, D, E, and K), is poorly transported across the placenta. As a result, regardless of the amount available to the mare, the foal is deficient in these vitamins at birth. The colostrum, however, contains adequate quantities of vitamins A and D to correct this deficiency and meet the foal's daily requirements. However, this is dependent on the foal receiving adequate quantities of colostrum, and the mare having ample quantities of these vitamins available to secrete into the colostrum. Bone remodeling is modulated by vitamin A in growing animals;[67] however, research in horses is minimal. Signs of vitamin A deficiency that may occur are not restricted to the musculoskeletal system, and night blindness (which is difficult to assess

in the horse), hyperkeratinization of the cornea and skin, poor growth, anorexia, weakness, increased rate of infections, reproductive disorders, and neurologic disease have been associated with hypovitaminosis A. To diagnose a vitamin A deficiency, plasma or hepatic (i.e., after hepatic biopsy) levels should be measured.[22] Owing to the paucity of equine data, only estimates have been made of vitamin A requirements in the horse by the NRC.[67] Currently, 2,000 to 3,000 IU vitamin A per kg dry matter is recommended with an upper tolerance limit of 16,000 IU/kg dry matter fed.[67]

Although vitamin D is included in most preparations containing vitamin A, it is not necessary to give vitamin D if the foal receives colostrum or milk or has access to 3 to 4 hours or more of sunlight daily. A substance produced in the body, 7-dehydrocholesterol, is converted by the sun's ultraviolet rays to previtamin D_3 (cholecalciferol). Conversion will even occur during cloudy overcast days, but not when sunlight shines through a glass windowpane. The glass filters out the ultraviolet rays. Cholecalciferol and related ingested forms of vitamin D are converted in the liver to 25-hydroxycholecalciferol, which is converted to the active form of vitamin D (1,25-dihydrocholecalciferol) in the kidney. Consequently, in renal failure the active form of vitamin D is not formed, and little of vitamin D's biologic effect occurs. Growing ponies that were deprived of both sunlight and a dietary source of vitamin D showed clinical signs of inappetance and decreased average daily gain, as well as decreased ash content, density, cross-sectional area, and breaking strength of the third metacarpal bones.[26]

Dietary supplementation of vitamin D is not necessary in horses having access to direct sunlight (even if cloudy) and to green or sun-cured forages. However, if excessive vitamin D is ingested because of supplementation, accumulation occurs as a result of its fat solubility, and may cause renal failure, cardiovascular compromise, and musculoskeletal alterations (predominantly because of calcification of the kidneys, cardiac musculature, and great vessels, and tendons and ligaments). Musculoskeletal problems in horses of various age groups, secondary to the administration of excessive quantities of vitamin A and D, are discussed later in this chapter.

Bacteria in the large intestine produce vitamin K. Like other fat-soluble vitamins, little crosses the placenta. However, soon after birth these bacteria colonize the foal's large intestine and produce ample quantities of vitamin K to meet the foal's requirements. Therefore deficiencies of vitamin K, other than those induced by vitamin K antagonists (rodenticides) have not been documented in the horse.

Vitamin E deficiency is discussed both previously and later in this chapter.

All B vitamins are produced by bacteria in the horse's intestinal tract, and are present in natural feeds in ample amounts to meet the horse's needs, unless there is interference with production or utilization.

Ample quantities of vitamin C are produced in the liver, and it is consequently not needed in the diet. The fetus and foal receive ample quantities of water-soluble vitamins B and C in utero, from the milk, from their own body, and from bacterial intestinal tract production. Vitamin C supplementation is used by some to enhance immunity, although its benefits for this or any other purpose have not been documented in the horse.

IN THE GROWING HORSE

The major nutritional imbalances that play a role in the development of musculoskeletal diseases in the growing horse are an excess of DE[87] and a deficiency of copper.[8,48,53] Excessive phosphorus caused development of osteochondrosis in foals; however, the level of phosphorus was not practically attainable[88] and is unlikely to occur in horses in the United States, Europe, Australia, or New Zealand. Other important factors may include a deficiency of digestible energy, a relative deficiency of calcium in comparison to phosphorus intake, a deficiency of calcium, an excess of calcium,[57] an excess of zinc and/or cadmium, and an excess or deficiency of vitamins D and A. The major effect of these nutritional imbalances is interference with endochondral ossification.[70,109]

Defects in endochondral ossification may result in 1) metaphyseal enlargement (i.e., physitis, physeal dysplasia), 2) osteochondrosis,[49,70,109] 3) cervical vertebral malformation ("wobbler syndrome"),[79] 4) cuboidal bone collapse, and 5) angular limb deformity (e.g., valgus or varus deformities).

Acquired flexural deformities (contracted flexor tendons) may sometimes be included in the category of developmental orthopedic disease (DOD),[15] although pathogenesis of these deformities appears to have little in common with defects in endochondral ossification.

Causes of Alterations in Endochondral Ossification

The major factors predisposing the growing animal to alterations in endochondral ossification are: 1) nutritional imbalances, 2) trauma to the metaphyseal growth plate or articular cartilage, and 3) genetic predisposition.

These three factors are interrelated, and there are many additional factors that affect each one. A combination of two or more of these factors may increase the incidence and severity of these conditions, although any one of them may be responsible. For example, if a growing animal is forced to bear an excessive amount of weight on a limb as a result of pain in the contralateral limb, the increased weight bearing may cause alterations in endochondral ossification and result in an angular limb deformity,[29,84] or may cause contracted tendons in the same painful limb. Conversely, nutritional imbalances may result in alterations in endochondral ossification regardless of the amount of trauma to the metaphyseal growth plate or articular cartilage.[86] Superimposition of one on the other may worsen the condition.

Nutritional Imbalances

Nutritional imbalances that may predispose the growing animal to alterations in endochondral ossification include: energy and phosphorus excesses; calcium, phosphorus, and copper deficiencies; or any combination of these nutritional imbalances.

Energy

Excessive dietary energy from an intake of large amounts of grain/concentrate is one of the major factors responsible for alterations in endochondral ossification. However, it is possible that defective endochondral ossification frequently attributed to excessive energy intake may be caused by inadequate levels of phosphorus, calcium, copper, or other minerals in the ration to support the rate of skeletal development permitted by the amount of energy and protein consumed. A lesser amount of energy or protein in the ration may simply mask the deficiency by slowing the growth rate. Thus, to prevent alterations in bone development, the ration must provide the nutrients necessary to support the rate of growth occurring. To accomplish this the growing horse should be properly fed.[59,67]

In several species, including the horse, excessive energy intake during growth has been shown to decrease bone specific gravity, cortical thickness, and ash content and result in osteochondrosis.[34,40,50,61,87,91] To prevent excessive energy-intake–induced alterations in endochondral ossification, it is recommended that the total concentrate intake be limited to 0.5 to 0.75 lb/100 lb body weight per day (i.e., 0.5 to 0.75 kg/100 kg per day) for nursing foals, 1.0 to 1.5 lb/100 lb body weight per day (i.e., 1.0 to 1.5 kg/100 kg per day) for weanlings, and 0.5 to 1.0 lb/100 lb body weight per day (i.e., 0.5 to 1.0 kg/100 kg per day) for yearlings. A good rule of thumb is to feed a *maximum* of 1 lb (i.e., 0.45 kg) of concentrate per day for each month of age up to a maximum of 7 lb (i.e., 3.2 kg) daily.

Extrapolation of work in dogs and pigs initially identified overnutrition or the feeding of specifically excessive digestible energy as a predisposing cause of osteochondrosis in the horse. Then Glade and others[32] fed young horses approximately 130% of the NRC recommendations for both digestible energy (using a predominantly carbohydrate source) and protein, and this appeared to induce lesions of both osteochondrosis and physitis. It was postulated that the cartilaginous lesions of horses fed excessive carbohydrate were mediated by endocrinologic alterations. Thyroxine is required for the maturation of chondrocytes and possibly for collagen and proteoglycan synthesis. Horses fed high carbohydrate diets could theoretically become temporarily hypothyroxemic in the postprandial period because of insulin's effect causing a rapid inactivation of thyroxine (T_4) and triiodothyronine (T_3). This could subsequently lead to adverse effects on the cartilage. However, if this were the only cause, then it would be expected that young horses fed high amounts of lipid (i.e., fat/oil) might be protected, and this is not the case.[87] Lipid diets do not induce the hypothyroxemia secondary to insulin alterations that carbohydrate feeding instigates.

Savage et al.[87] demonstrated that diets with approximately 128% NRC digestible energy recommendations, composed of both carbohydrate and corn oil components, were instrumental in the induction of osteochondrosis. Control foals in these experiments were fed a diet based on 100% of NRC requirements for weanlings growing at an average daily gain (ADG) of 0.65 to 0.85 kg/day. Only 1 of 12 control weanlings had a single osteochondrosis lesion, whereas all foals (18 of 18) fed excessive digestible energy had histologic lesions of osteochondrosis. Most (17 of 18) of these foals also had macroscopic lesions of osteochondrosis evident at autopsy. One theory is that feeding excessive digestible energy, either carbohydrate or fat/oil, may cause endocrinologic alterations especially of the local cartilaginous growth factors. There may also be selective activation of genes, causing a specific alteration in cartilage matrix phenotype. Another possible reason that foals fed excessive digestible energy may develop osteochondrosis is that copper absorption may be decreased or, when excessive fat is fed, the calcium absorption may be decreased, inducing a relative phosphorus excess.

Protein

Although alterations in endochondral ossification occur most commonly in the overfed horse, it may occur in the underfed horse as well. This may occur as a result of inadequate protein in the ration. Since protein constitutes 20% of the bone matrix,[44] inadequate dietary protein may interfere with proper bone growth and development. However, inadequate protein intake sufficient to interfere with endochondral ossification usually results in an extremely poor condition in the horse.

Feeding protein in excess of the animal's requirement does not increase the growth rate above that achieved when requirements are just met.[123] Feeding less protein than needed, however, decreases the growth rate. Therefore, increasing the protein content of a protein-deficient but energy-sufficient ration results in a faster growth rate. If the ration does not contain adequate minerals, such as calcium and phosphorus, to support a faster rate of growth, alterations in bone development may occur. This is the most likely explanation of the implications frequently made (but never confirmed) that excessive protein intake predisposes to or causes alterations in endochondral ossification. In fact researchers found no significant lesions of osteochondrosis in six foals fed excessive protein.[87] However, theories existed that the hypercalciuric effect of excessive protein caused diminished calcium and thus problems with endochondral ossification. Excessive protein intake may increase urinary calcium excretion, because if the protein consists of amino acids with an excessive proportion of sulfur-containing amino acids (e.g., methionine), then there may be a subsequent overload of the renal buffering capacity of sulfuric acid. The subsequent urofiltrate is therefore likely to be acidic, which may be responsible for inhibition of calcium and phosphorus reabsorption, consequently producing hypercalciuria and hyperphosphouria.[31] These results were unconfirmable when foals were fed various levels of protein; it was postulated that horses could acclimate to chronic excessive dietary protein, so that the inhibition of mineral reabsorption and subsequent loss of calcium and phosphorus into the urine is diminished.[94] It is recommended that the protein content of the growing horse's ration meet and not exceed by more than 2% its protein requirements (e.g., if 16% is required, it should not exceed 18%), which in the total ration dry matter is 18% for nursing foals, 16% for weanlings, 13% for yearlings, and 10% for 2-year-olds.[68] Feeding excessive protein is expensive and appears wasteful.

Calcium and Phosphorus

Adequate amounts of calcium and phosphorus must be available for the endochondral ossification of the cartilage. The diet must not only contain adequate amounts of calcium and phosphorus, but the animal must be able to absorb and utilize these nutrients. Phosphorus, bound to an organic substance such as phytate, is less available than phosphorus present in inorganic forms.[92,107] Cereal grains are high in phytate and their content increases with maturity.[37] Thus, the phosphorus present in cereal grains, wheat bran, and other concentrates is less available than the phosphorus present in roughages and minerals. The true digestibility of phosphorus present in most concentrates is 29 to 32%, in roughage it is 44 to 46%, and in inorganic minerals it is 58%.[92,97]

Calcium and phosphorus requirements for the horse assume that 55% of the calcium and 35% of the phosphorus will be absorbed.[68] Since the digestibility of calcium and phosphorus in the horse's total ration is generally higher than this, digestibility does not usually need to be considered in ensuring that the horse receives adequate amounts of calcium and phosphorus. However, several factors may decrease the efficiency of absorption.

Excess ingested phosphorus and oxalates bind cations such as calcium, decreasing their absorption.[37,92,97] Thus, even if adequate calcium is present in the ration, it is not absorbed, and a calcium deficiency may occur. The effect of excess dietary phosphorus is more important when the calcium content of the diet is low. In one study with 2-year old ponies, net deposits of skeletal calcium decreased by more than 50% in ponies fed a diet that just met their calcium requirements (0.4%) but contained excessive phosphorus (1.2%), as compared to another group of ponies fed a diet that contained the minimum amount of both calcium and phosphorus needed to meet requirements (0.4% calcium and 0.2% phosphorus).[95]

Excessive calcium in the diet has little effect on phosphorus absorption.[92,97] This is because calcium is absorbed primarily from the small intestine whereas phosphorus is absorbed from both the small and large intestines. Phosphorus ingested in excess competes with the calcium, preventing its absorption from the small intestine. However, since much of the excess calcium ingested is absorbed from the small intestine and excreted in the urine, it is not available to decrease phosphorus absorption from the large intestine. Thus, excessive dietary calcium is much less detrimental than excessive phosphorus. Schryver et al.[93] demonstrated that high calcium diets had little effect on the rate of calcium deposition in the skeletal ash. If quantities of both calcium and phosphorus in the ration are adequate to meet the animal's requirements, the amount of calcium with respect to phosphorus, or Ca:P ratio, in the ration of the mature horse can vary from 1:1 to 8:1, and in the growing horse from 1.1:1 to 4:1, without resulting in major problems.[88] However, as there may be substantial variation in the calcium and phosphorus content of feeds, a ratio of less than 1.2:1 is not recommended for any horse, and for the mature horse, a ratio of greater than 4:1 is not recommended. The calcium to phosphorus ratio favored by the authors is 1.3 to 1.5:1. If the amount of dietary calcium or phosphorus is insufficient to meet the growing horse's requirements, or if the amount of one mineral with respect to the other is outside of these ratios, alterations in endochondral ossification may occur.

Excessive dietary calcium can decrease the intestinal absorption of a number of trace minerals, such as zinc, manganese, and iron, and may cause a deficiency if the ration contains only marginal amounts of these minerals. This can occur from adding excessive amounts of calcium-containing minerals to the ration. Therefore, it is recommended that no more than 1% calcium from calcium-containing minerals be added to the horse's total dry ration. Excessive zinc, manganese, iron, and other minerals decrease calcium and phosphorus absorption as well.

In the 1980s it was postulated that foals could be fed excess DE safely if combined with excessive calcium, but this was later proven to be unfounded.[88] Krook and Maylin[57] proposed that diets excessive in calcium (i.e., alfalfa-based or highly supplemented rations), as are commonly found in the United States, were responsible for the induction of osteochondrosis and secondary fractures, through the initiation of hypercalcitoninism. This was believed to cause disturbances of chondrocytic maturation, disturbances in cartilage's replacement by bone, and finally osteosclerosis, which may have increased the likelihood of pathologic fracture. Thyroid parafollicular cell (C cell) hyperplasia has been documented in dogs fed excess calcium and also in fetal lambs whose dams had been fed excess calcium.[16] These researchers also showed that there was retarded cartilage differentiation in these fetal lambs, yet studies in foals fed excess calcium (i.e., 342% of the recommended NRC level for calcium) did not show significant numbers or severity of cartilage lesions.[88] Two of six foals fed high calcium in this study had histologic lesions of either the articular-epiphyseal cartilage complex or metaphyseal growth plates. One of these had only minor histologic metaphyseal growth plate lesions, which were observed at necropsy. The other foal had bilateral lesions of the distal third metatarsal bones, which were also documented on macroscopic examination at necropsy.[88]

Knight et al.[52] reported that farms feeding rations with the lowest calcium levels (as well as other nutritional aberrations) had the largest percentage of young horses with DOD. They recommended that growing horses be fed higher levels of calcium and phosphorus than recommended by NRC at that time. Diets containing excessive phosphorus or a low calcium to phosphorus ratio have been incriminated as a cause of DOD. A ratio of 1.3 to 1.5:1 is considered adequate and reasonable. Five of six weanling foals fed extremely high phosphorus levels (i.e., 388% of the NRC requirement for phosphorus) showed numerous severe lesions of osteochondrosis, yet no clinical signs of nutritional secondary hyperparathyroidism. Histomorphometrical studies of these foals revealed a significantly increased cortical bone porosity from wing of ilium bone biopsies, which supported the existence of subclinical nutritional secondary hyperparathyroidism. It is not clear what the initiating cause of the osteochondrosis was in these foals, but it is possible that the high concentration of phosphorus interfered with matrix vesicle function, and thus endochondral ossification, or that calcium absorption was

diminished. Osteochondrosis lesions in foals fed excessive phosphorus were severe, despite a diminished average daily weight gain (kg body weight per day) caused by diminished dietary intake related to an apparently unpalatable diet. This further strengthens the proposal that average daily weight gain is not solely responsible for disturbance of endochondral ossification in growth cartilages.

It is also possible that diets with excess phosphorus result in acidosis because of an excess of phosphate anions, which along with the chloride ions are normally buffered by cations (i.e., Ca^{2+} and Mg^{2+}). If the buffering capacity of the cations is surpassed, then acidemia may result. Acidemia may result in faulty bone mineralization since alkalinity promotes calcification, which is normally present in the hypertrophic zone as a result of the presence of carbonic anhydrase. This is supported by the increased incidence of tibial dyschondroplasia seen in broiler chickens fed excess phosphate and chloride ions.[60]

Trace Minerals

The trace minerals that may be involved in alterations in endochondral ossification are copper, zinc, and possibly manganese. Manganese imbalances were discussed previously in this chapter.

COPPER

Copper deficiency may cause lameness, stiffness, spontaneous fractures, enlarged joints, physitis, and contracted flexor tendons in ruminants.[111] However, copper deficiencies and toxicities have not been commonly documented in animals other than ruminants. Copper is an essential component of the enzyme, lysyl oxidase, which is essential for the cross-linking of collagen and elastin. Collagen type II is an integral component of cartilage matrix in the horse, and its cross-linkage is required for the development of normal cartilage matrix and cartilage's replacement by bone. Consequently, in foals DOD may be caused in part by diets deficient in copper.

Mature ponies probably only need 3.5 ppm copper in their ration dry matter;[17] however, the NRC[67] has a recommendation of 10 ppm (i.e., 10 mg/kg dry matter feed) for all classes of horses. Knight et al.[52] postulated that diets with excessive zinc or molybdenum could cause a secondary copper deficiency, as occurs in ruminants, but this has not been substantiated in the horse. However, selenium excess may increase the horse's dietary copper requirements (Ralston S, personal communication, 1997). Copper imbalances can be diagnosed by finding copper concentrations (in ppm in their tissue wet weight) significantly outside of the normal range of 0.7 to 2 in plasma, 3 to 15 in the hoof,[59] 0 to 16 in the liver, 4 to 13 in the renal cortex, or 1 to 5 in the pancreas.[36] Hair copper content of less than 8.5 ppm is suggestive, but does not confirm, the presence of a copper deficiency.[59]

Copper (Cu) deficiency has been incriminated as a cause of equine DOD, especially physitis and osteochondrosis. However, there is a great deal of controversy surrounding the subject, as disparate results have been obtained in a number of research projects.[8,48,53,73,74,87,88] In one study mares were either fed recommended (approximate NRC) or high concentrations of Cu daily through the last trimester of gestation and lactation, and their unweaned foals were given access to creep feeds with 15 or 55 ppm Cu, respectively.[53] No differences in the rate of growth were documented, yet foals born to dams on the recommended (approximate NRC) Cu diet and supplemented with only 15 ppm creep feed had an increase (albeit insignificant) in the incidence of the number of cartilage lesions. The NRC subcommittee did not consider the data conclusive, hence their recommendation remained 10 ppm Cu in the ration dry matter.

Diets containing 11.1 to 11.7 ppm Cu [87,88] and thus slightly higher than the NRC recommendations for all classes of horses but lower than the 40 to 50 ppm suggested for growing horses by Knight et al.[53] were not associated with an increased incidence of osteochondrosis in foals, provided the DE and phosphorus content were at the recommended levels. In an earlier study,[8] two diets were used to clarify the effects of Cu deficiency. One contained only 1.7 ppm (low Cu diet) and the other 14 ppm (adequate control Cu diet), which is similar to the NRC[67] recommendation. The salt-soluble collagen measurements, an indicator of defects in the collagen cross-linkage, in the foals fed 14 ppm Cu were normal, which contrasted with the greatly increased solubility in foals fed diets containing 1.7 ppm Cu.[8] However, in another study foals were fed either 7 ppm Cu (low Cu diet) or 30 ppm Cu (high copper diet).[48] The group fed the lower copper level had a higher incidence of macroscopic osteochondrosis. These changes were found predominantly in the cervical vertebrae, yet many sites commonly associated with lesions of osteochondrosis were not involved.[48] Pearce and co-workers found that foals did not appear to have significant lesions of osteochondrosis unless their dams were not supplemented with copper during late gestation.[73,74] Because milk copper is not altered in response to Cu supplementation of the dam during lactation (i.e., remains at approximately 2 to 4 ppm on a dry matter basis), Cu supplementation of the dam is probably most important during the last trimester of gestation, when the fetus is actively increasing its own hepatic stores of copper.

Horses are much more tolerant of low and high Cu levels compared to both sheep and cattle. Ponies have been shown to tolerate up to 791 ppm dietary Cu, although these ponies had decreased average daily weight gain and high liver Cu concentrations.[100] Since the maximum threshold for dietary Cu is so high, it appears that growing horses could easily tolerate dietary Cu levels of 15 to 40 ppm suggested by some,[48,52] and this may alleviate some of the signs of osteochondrosis seen in growing foals.

Zinc

A zinc deficiency has not been confirmed in horses on natural feeds at this time. An experimental deficiency was induced, but only when the zinc content of the ration was reduced to 4 ppm.[38] Natural feeds usually contain 4 to 12 times this amount of zinc. The NRC[67] recommendation for zinc in equine diets is 40 ppm on a dry matter basis.

A zinc-responsive osteodystrophy in foals has been reported.[42] Forty-two foals were given 200 mg of zinc per head per day, which increased the zinc content of their ration from 25 to 65 ppm, whereas 47 other foals on the same ration were not given any supplemental zinc. Some of the foals in both groups had osteodystrophy. It was reported that those given zinc appeared to improve more rapidly than those not given zinc.

Zinc toxicity may be caused by adding excessive zinc to the ration (greater than 200 to 500 ppm), grazing pasture forage contaminated with efflux from nearby smelters, or drinking water containing greater than 15 ppm of zinc. Excessive zinc may be released from galvanized surfaces when subjected to electrolysis, which occurs when galvanized water pipes and copper pipes are joined.[64,77]

Gunson et al.[36] and Kowalczyk et al.[55] found that foals pastured in the vicinity of a smelter had generalized cartilage lesions that appeared similar to osteochondrosis on a macroscopic basis. The surrounding environment and pasture had high levels of zinc and cadmium. Environmental exposure of pregnant pony mares and their foals to zinc and cadmium was evaluated. Only 2 of the 5 foals had signs of lameness, but all foals (5 of 5) had macroscopic lesions resembling osteochondrosis when euthanasia and necropsy were performed at ages of approximately 2 to 18 months. Histologic examination of cartilage from some of these foals showed superficial cartilage erosion rather than core lesions, which does not support a primary defect in endochondral ossification.

A zinc deficiency or excess may be present if zinc concentration in ppm in the tissue wet weight is significantly outside of the normal of 0.8 to 2 in the plasma, 0 to 50 in the liver or renal cortex, or 5 to 10 in the pancreas.[36,59] Pancreatic zinc content appears to be the most reliable indicator of zinc toxicosis.[59]

Vitamins

Vitamin E

Controversy about vitamin E deficiency in the growing horse exists. In recent years researchers have implicated diminished access to green forage as a cause of vitamin E deficiency and, consequently, equine degenerative myeloencephalopathy (EDM).[19] However, no specific musculoskeletal signs occur in this neurologic syndrome.

Trauma to Endochondral Ossification Centers

Trauma is another predisposing factor to alterations in endochondral ossification.[34,69] Weight, upright conformation, and exercise appear to play a role. The greater the body weight, the greater the force on bones and joints will be per cross-sectional area. Additionally, the greater the body weight, the smaller the ratio of the bones' articular-epiphyseal cartilage complex or metaphyseal physis to body weight is, which makes them more susceptible to trauma. Theoretically, horses with upright conformation also bear increased weight on the metaphyseal growth plate and articular-epiphyseal cartilage complex, which may result in alterations in endochondral ossification. Exercise may also be an important factor in increasing biomechanical trauma in foals that already have osteochondrosis, thus aggravating the lesion and increasing the chance of development of degenerative joint disease (i.e., osteoarthritis).

Growth and Conformation

Faster growing, larger, finer-boned breeds of horses with upright conformation, particularly those with short upright pasterns,[15] appear to be affected with DOD more frequently. DOD is seen less frequently in draft horses, presumably because they have larger bones and reach mature size more slowly. Also DOD is believed to occur less frequently in ponies, presumably because of their smaller body size. However, two reports identified lesions of osteochondrosis in two ponies.[88,105]

Controversy still exists on the effects of rapid growth on alteration of endochondral ossification and the appearance of DOD. The importance of this concept has been documented in numerous animal studies including horses,[45,61,71,106] dogs,[40,51,69] swine,[33,35,80] and cattle.[81] A rapid growth rate is promoted by 1) genetics, 2) high energy intake, and 3) stunting early in life followed by increased feeding for maximum growth, which results in a compensatory growth spurt.

In one study flexural deformities (contracted flexor tendons) developed in 4 of 6 foals whose food intake was restricted and who were later fed ad libitum, whereas none of the 6 foals that were continually fed ad libitum developed flexural deformities.[45] In other studies attempting to induce osteochondrosis or other forms of DOD, foals were fed excessive DE without increasing growth significantly compared to control foals, but the foals fed high amounts of DE had significantly more severe osteochondrosis lesions.[87]

High-energy diets do not simply manifest their effects through increases in growth rate and subsequent biomechanical trauma on the articular-epiphyseal cartilage complex. A number of studies have demonstrated an increase in DOD in foals fed excessive energy with no increased growth rate. This means that an increase in the weight per unit area of physeal cartilage (e.g., metaphyseal or articular-epiphyseal growth plates) is not the simple reason for lesions seen in foals that have grown quickly or to heavier than normal weights.

By 2 to 3 months of age, the foal's nutritional needs exceed that provided by the mare's milk. If additional quantities of a feed containing the nutrients needed are not fed, growth may be slowed during this period. Then, if following weaning, enough grain is fed to provide the energy necessary for rapid growth, a compensatory growth spurt will occur. Compensatory growth does appear to be problematic, and should be avoided if possible after illness or periods of feed deprivation.

Exercise

Exercise and its subsequent effects on the presence and severity of osteochondrosis lesions are controversial. A study using unexercised foals fed recommended DE

levels had a low incidence of osteochondrosis, while foals fed excessive energy during a low plane of exercise had numerous lesions (Bruin and Smolders, personal communication, 1990). Preliminary data found that exercise may play a role in decreasing the incidence of osteochondrosis when foals are fed excessive DE, but may increase the incidence of osteochondrosis in foals fed basal DE levels (Bruin and Smolders, personal communication, 1990). The results of the latter study are difficult to reconcile with current information on the induction of osteochondrosis. One explanation for the occurrence of osteochondral lesions in the exercised foals fed only basal DE may be that they already had minor lesions of osteochondrosis prior to exercise and these were biomechanically exacerbated. In contrast to findings by Savage et al.[87] and Bruin and Smolders (personal communication, 1990), another study found a trend towards an increased incidence of macroscopic lesions consistent with osteochondrosis in unexercised weanling foals fed 110% of NRC recommendations for DE and protein, compared to moderately exercised foals on this diet, or to moderately exercised foals that received 135% of NRC DE and protein recommendation (Leedle R, Raub R, Anderson K, Warren J, personal communication, 1995). However, no histologic evaluation was performed, and therefore interpretation is difficult.

In summary, results are somewhat conflicting and do not fit with a simple relationship between exercise and DE intake. Findings appear to indicate that increased exercise may be beneficial when high energy diets are consumed, but detrimental if lesions are already present. Unfortunately, usually it is not possible to determine when lesions first develop. Hence, the dilemma on the appropriate degree of exercise for foals on varying DE feeding regimens has not yet been resolved.

Genetic Predisposition

Genetic predisposition to alterations in endochondral ossification that is unrelated to growth rate, bone size, or conformation may be a factor in some cases. A genetic predisposition has been demonstrated in dogs,[69] swine,[35] and horses.[82] Eight foals with severe contracted flexor tendons resulting from a mutation in the sire have been reported.[47]

Some horses appear genetically predisposed to developing osteochondrosis. Numerous radiographic studies have yielded heritability scores between 0.24 and 0.32. Unfortunately, genetic studies currently rely on progeny testing using radiographic means. As lesions of osteochondrosis can be radiographically "silent," it is difficult to attest to the accuracy of the heritability scores. Presently there is insufficient evidence to mandate that stallions or mares with osteochondrosis lesions not be bred, although owners should be informed about the possibility of genetic influence.

Nutritional Management of Alterations in Endochondral Ossification

A feed analysis over a 24-hour period should be performed in order to assist in this decision. Generally energy intake is decreased, and copper, calcium, and phosphorus levels in the original diet and in the proposed diet should be scrutinized carefully. Often ad libitum grass hay and a small amount of grain (e.g., less than 0.5 kg/day) can be offered to weanlings with problems of DOD for a period of 3 to 6 weeks, in order to administer supplementary calcium, and possibly phosphorus and copper. However, although dietary copper levels of 15 to 25 ppm appear safe and rational, recent research does not demonstrate a decrease in DOD defects in foals directly supplemented with copper, unless their dams had been supplemented during gestation.[73]

IN THE MATURE HORSE FOR MAINTENANCE OR WORK

Nutritional deficiencies resulting from inadequate intake are less common in mature, nonpregnant, nonlactating, nonworking animals because of their lower nutrient requirements. Conversely, excessive feed intake resulting in obesity is most likely to occur during maintenance, when the animal's energy needs are lowest. Additionally, nutritional toxicities are just as likely to occur during maintenance as they are during any other time of life. A common cause for nutritional toxicities is the ingestion or administration of excessive quantities of specific nutrients or feeds high in those nutrients. These nutrients include vitamin A, vitamin D, phosphorus, selenium, iodine and iron (especially in supplements), and fluoride. Excessive intake of any of these nutrients may result in musculoskeletal diseases. In addition, during frequent strenuous or prolonged physical exertion, body electrolyte and acute energy deficiencies may occur because of excessive losses or utilization of these nutrients.

Water, Electrolyte, and Energy Deficits

Energy utilization may be increased 10- to 20-fold during physical exertion. Most of this energy is expelled as heat, which the animal must eliminate in order to avoid heat exhaustion. Because the majority of this heat is lost by the evaporation of sweat from the body surface, the greater the temperature, humidity, and energy utilized, the greater the volume of sweat and, as a result, the greater the loss of water and electrolytes there will be. A failure to replace these losses results in dehydration, electrolyte deficits, decreased circulation, and decreased sweating, which can result in fatigue or heat exhaustion. To prevent this, allow and encourage the horse to drink as frequently as possible during physical activity. However, when physical activity ceases and the horse is hot, it should be cooled by walking, and a rest period of 20 to 30 minutes should be given before allowing access to small volumes of water. After watering, hay and grain may be fed. Electrolyte supplements may be beneficial in some cases.

The major electrolytes lost during physical exertion are sodium, potassium, chloride, and calcium.[11,96] Loss of the first three electrolytes causes fatigue and muscle weakness, and decreases the thirst response to dehydration, so the horse may have little inclination to drink or eat. Dehydration and electrolyte deficits commonly occur in horses exhausted from prolonged or frequent physical exertion. To prevent this, water should be offered frequently and the electrolytes lost should be replaced. This may be done by giving the horse 2 oz (57 g) of a mixture of three parts "lite" salt (a 1:1 mixture of sodium chloride and potassium chloride) plus one part limestone. Since the body does not store these electrolytes, they should be given just before, during, and several times after physical exertion is completed. Electrolytes may be given through any means; however, if electrolytes are added to water, plain, nonsupplemented water must also be available. This is because some horses do not find electrolyte-supplemented water palatable and thus decrease total water intake, which is more harmful than any possible benefits that electrolyte consumption may provide. If electrolyte losses are small, little benefit is derived from electrolyte supplementation. However, if extensive electrolyte deficits occur, synchronous diaphragmatic flutter ("thumps"), hypocalcemic tetany, and prolonged postexercise fatigue may occur. These conditions may be prevented to a large degree by electrolyte supplementation.

Exhaustion and Postexercise Fatigue

Exhaustion generally occurs as a result of a body deficit in energy, water, and electrolytes. Affected animals appear obtunded and lethargic, often with little interest in food or water. Varying degrees of muscle energy depletion, hypochloremia, hypocalcemia, and electrolyte deficits may also be present and, therefore, may result in muscular cramping, colic, and synchronous diaphragmatic flutter. The dehydration and electrolyte deficits decrease or prevent sweating. If there is any sweat, it is generally sticky rather than watery. As a result, the body temperature increases because of the horse's inability to sweat. Although the pulse and respiratory rates of the exhausted and the nonexhausted horse are similar immediately following exercise, these parameters return to normal more quickly following exercise in the nonexhausted horse.[43] In the nonexhausted horse the pulse rate should fall to less than 55 beats/minute and the respiratory rate to less than 25 breaths/minute (unless there is an extremely high ambient temperature) after 20 to 30 minutes of rest.[43] Indications of exhaustion are 1) the rectal temperature does not fall to less than 102°F (39°C) within 10 minutes of rest and 2) after 20 to 30 minutes of rest the pulse rate is greater than 70 beats/minute and the respiratory rate is more than one-half pulse rate.[43] An exhausted horse will frequently demonstrate an increased packed cell volume and plasma protein concentration owing to dehydration, and an increase in muscle enzyme activities and phosphorus concentration in the plasma as a result of muscle exertion or damage. A metabolic alkalosis and hypochloremia from excessive chloride losses may be present. A white blood cell differential will indicate a typical stress response of a mature neutrophilia, lymphopenia, monocytosis (irregularly present), and eosinopenia (often present even in the normal horse).

Treatment of the exhausted horse may require the intravenous administration of 40 to 120 liters of fluids. Recommended initial treatment consists of 10 to 20 liters of isotonic electrolyte solution (e.g., Plasmalyte; 0.9%

saline) given intravenously, with additions of 20 mL of a 23% calcium gluconate solution per liter, 10 mEq of potassium chloride solution per liter, and 50 mL of a 50% glucose solution per liter. Hypertonic saline given intravenously is useful in the exhausted horse with signs of shock to increase circulating volume quickly. However, if hypertonic saline is utilized, it is imperative that it be followed by intravenous administration of a minimum of 20 liters of isotonic [or barely hypertonic (e.g., minor additions of calcium gluconate and potassium chloride)] fluids.

At the same time intravenous fluids are being administered, 4 to 8 liters of an oral nutrient-electrolyte fluid should be given by nasogastric tube. Few oral nutrient-electrolyte powders are made with the exhausted horse in mind. Calcium is often not included in calf scour powders, and these will usually have bicarbonate, lactate, or citrate in them (e.g., Biolyte, Upjohn, Kalamazoo, MI). An additional 3 to 6 liters of this fluid should be given orally every 3 to 4 hours as needed. Free choice water should also be allowed once the horse is cool. The horse should be moved as little as possible during treatment and should be rested for several weeks afterward. One to two ounces (i.e., approximately 28 to 60 g) of a non-iodized salt (i.e., sodium chloride) and "lite" salt (i.e., a 1:1 mixture of sodium chloride and potassium chloride) should be added to the grain/concentrate and fed twice a day for several days. Depending on the horse's muscle involvement, it may be beneficial to administer nonsteroidal anti-inflammatory drugs in conjunction with intravenous and nasogastric fluids.

Synchronous Diaphragmatic Flutter (Exhausted Horse Syndrome, Thumps)

Synchronous diaphragmatic flutter (SDF) results from electrolyte losses that occur during physical exertion or from hypocalcemic tetany or hypocalcemia secondary to blister beetle toxicosis. This syndrome is often seen in horses participating in competitive trail or endurance races or on long-distance rides. Typical biochemical abnormalities include hypoglycemia (especially in horses participating in endurance races), increased fatty acid concentrations, increased glycerol concentrations, hyponatremia, hypochloremia, hypokalemia, hypocalcemia, hypomagnesemia, and hyperphosphatemia. Minimal to modest elevations in blood lactate and creatine kinase (CK) may be observed; however, arterial pH rarely indicates acidemia, presumably because of compensation, which is possible during slower exercise. Indeed, alkalosis may develop more commonly, especially when there is a severe hypochloremia. Hemoconcentration is also commonly observed.

A decrease in the plasma calcium, chloride, and/or potassium concentration, or a body deficit of these electrolytes, is thought to increase the irritability of the phrenic nerves. As a result, the electrical activity occurring when the heart beats stimulates these nerves where they pass over the heart. As a result the diaphragm, which is stimulated by the phrenic nerves, contracts with each beat of the heart. This is usually observed as sudden bilateral, and occasionally unilateral, movement of the horse's flanks (and sometimes the hindlimbs) each time the heart beats (i.e., synchronous with the heart's con-

traction). This may occur during or following physical exertion, severe diarrhea, or colic or following prolonged surgery or anesthesia. Prevention and treatment include the replacement of the depleted electrolytes. If the condition is severe, 20 to 100 liters of an isotonic or slightly hypertonic [i.e., isotonic fluid supplemented with calcium (i.e., 10 to 20 mL 23% calcium gluconate per liter of solution), potassium chloride (i.e., 20 to 40 mEq potassium chloride per liter of intravenous fluids), and glucose (i.e., 20 to 40 mL of 50% dextrose per liter of intravenous fluids)] replacement fluid should be given intravenously over a 24-hour period. Fluids containing greater than 25 mEq/liter of bicarbonate, lactate, or acetate should be avoided, unless the presence of metabolic acidosis has been established through blood gas analysis, as metabolic alkalosis rather than acidosis may actually be present. As with cases of exhaustion with hyponatremia and hypochloremia, intravenous hypertonic saline administration followed by intravenous isotonic fluids may ameliorate the situation quickly. One liter of 5 to 7.5% saline (i.e., hypertonic) may be used followed by a minimum of 20 liters of isotonic fluids. As the chloride concentration has an impact on the acid-base status of a horse, correction of a hypochloremia may simultaneously improve or even correct metabolic alkalosis.

In less severe cases, electrolytes and glucose may be replaced orally, including via nasogastric intubation. Nasogastric intubation may be necessary, because ingestion (and thus amelioration of the condition) that is voluntary may be incomplete.

Hypocalcemic Tetany

Prolonged strenuous physical activity or stress from any cause results in a prolonged high level of secreted corticosteroids. Corticosteroids inhibit vitamin D activity and renal tubular resorption of calcium, resulting in increased calcium loss in the urine in some species. Inhibition of vitamin D activity decreases intestinal calcium absorption and parathyroid hormone mobilization of skeletal calcium. Extensive quantities of calcium can also be lost in sweat.[96] Thus, during strenuous physical activity there may be increased loss of calcium from the body, decreased calcium absorption, and decreased calcium mobilization from the bone. As a result of these factors, hypocalcemia and thus tetany may occur. A definitive diagnosis is made by identifying a decrease in plasma calcium concentration. More commonly, a presumptive diagnosis is made based on clinical signs, history, and response to treatment; however, therapy must be approached cautiously when the plasma calcium level is not known. The clinical symptoms and treatment of hypocalcemia are described later in this chapter, in the section titled, Hypocalcemic and Hypomagnesemic Tetany.

Equine Rhabdomyolysis Syndrome (ERS) (Exercise-Related Myopathy, Exertional Myopathy, Exertional Rhabdomyolysis, Myositis, "Monday Morning Disease," "Tying-up" Syndrome)

Many predisposing factors have been proposed as the cause of equine rhabdomyolysis syndrome (ERS); however, those that remain at the forefront include: 1) diet, 2) training regime and fitness, and 3) intensity of exercise.

Horses subjected to the stress of race training may undergo some degree of thyroid suppression. However, it has become apparent that racing animals usually demonstrate low concentrations of thyroxine (T_4), the inactive thyroid hormone, and this is not likely a reflection of glandular thyroid disease (Bayly W, personal communication, 1998). However, it has been postulated that myopathy may be related to hypothyroidism. This is extremely controversial, as there is currently no good method for assessing the thyroid status of a horse.[101] Transient postprandial hypothyroidism has been associated with feeding high levels of protein and energy,[32] and this may be associated with the development or exacerbation of ERS.

Common clinical manifestations of ERS include: 1) anxiety, 2) sweating, 3) tachycardia, 4) reluctance to walk, 5) lameness, 6) hardening of muscle groups (especially the gluteal muscles) with pain evident on palpation, 7) recumbency, and 8) myoglobinuria.

Increased creatine kinase (CK) and aspartate aminotransferase (AST) levels are commonly observed biochemical abnormalities. The CK is usually elevated initially, while the membrane-associated AST takes longer to elevate. The concentrations of these enzymes are thought to increase in the serum when myodegeneration occurs, and are not associated with simple sarcolemmal leakage from altered, abnormal permeability of the myocyte.[112]

The cause of ERS remains elusive. Early investigators[12] hypothesized that horses fed high levels of carbohydrate during rest would experience an increased accumulation of muscle glycogen, which underwent rapid glycogenolysis during exercise leading to lactic acidosis at the muscular level. More recently, investigators have not been able to confirm this. Valberg et al.[112] demonstrated that there is no evidence supporting the role of lactic acidosis in initiation of ERS; and Koterba and Carlson[54] showed that hypochloremia and, thus, alkalosis were the most common abnormalities.

Other possible pathogenic mechanisms for ERS include electrolyte deficiencies, especially sodium and potassium deficiency. Unfortunately, studies showing improvements in horses with ERS after dietary supplementation with sodium and potassium[39] were not corroborated by Hodgson (unpublished data).[46] Horses with ERS had lower muscle potassium levels on a dry weight basis than normal horses, yet red blood cell potassium concentration was no different between ERS horses and normal horses.[4] It is still not clear as to the exact role of electrolyte imbalances in ERS.

Another potential cause of ERS may be altered homeostasis of intracellular calcium induced by exercise, stress, and even diet. Research in other species supports this contention, in that muscle under conditions of sufficient exercise to cause muscular damage becomes refractory to maintenance of intracellular calcium concentrations. This appears to occur because of an inability of calcium channels to function: They remain open, thereby allowing the sarcolemma to leak calcium, overwhelming the mitochondrial capacity and leading to a progressive buildup of calcium in the myoplasm.[46] This may allow stimulation of calcium-activated proteases, which dam-

age and destroy intracellular organelles.[78] Relaxation times of muscles may also be lengthened.[5]

Muscle enzymes, such as AST, CK, and lactate dehydrogenase (LDH), and myoglobin and phosphorus concentrations in the blood may be elevated as a result of muscle damage. A mild hypochloremia and hypocalcemia are frequently present, but metabolic acidosis generally is not.[54] Myoglobin is excreted in the urine. If sufficient quantities are excreted, it gives the urine a coffee-colored appearance. In milder cases, myoglobinuria is not grossly evident but may be detected by using occult test reagent tablets or sticks. Myoglobin excretion may cause renal damage. The appearance of dark-colored urine or recumbency indicates a grave prognosis, and a large volume of intravenous fluids must be administered.

Affected animals should not be moved, since it will worsen the condition. Mild cases may recover with no treatment if they are not moved. If moved even a short distance, the condition may become severe, resulting in death regardless of the treatment given. Intravenous fluids (i.e., 6 liters/hour for the first 4 to 8 hours and then 2 to 4 liters/hour) should be administered to increase circulation and to diminish the chances of renal damage secondary to myoglobin-induced alterations, which may be secondary to prostaglandin alterations. Administration of a minimum of 20 liters of intravenous fluids containing potassium, sodium chloride, and calcium is routine, although it is rare for bicarbonate to be required. Practitioners without the luxury of biochemical analyses should avoid bicarbonate-containing fluids and instead should use isotonic to slightly hypertonic fluids containing sodium chloride, potassium, and calcium. Dimethyl sulfoxide (DMSO) is often utilized as a supplement to fluids in horses with ERS. It is used as an anti-inflammatory drug, as it may be able to scavenge oxygen free radicals. Its use is controversial, but anecdotal evidence suggests that it is useful at an appropriately low concentration (e.g., 500 mL of 90 to 99% DMSO split into 10 to 24 liters). It may be given intravenously or orally (via nasogastric tube) at a dose of 1g/kg body weight. Concentrations greater than 10% should not be utilized, because of the likelihood of hemolysis.

Nonsteroidal anti-inflammatory drugs (NSAIDs) to control pain and decrease inflammation, such as flunixin meglumine (Banamine), are often utilized at varying doses (e.g., flunixin meglumine: 0.5 mg/kg given intravenously two, three, or four times a day, up to 1 mg/kg given intravenously twice a day). It should be remembered that NSAIDs have been associated with renal papillary necrosis, and their use may compound the renal effects of myoglobin. Hence they should only be used with adequate volumes of fluids administered intravenously or via nasogastric tube.

Phenothiazine-derivative tranquilizers cause vasodilation, which is helpful; however, they should not be given until after adequate fluid therapy has been administered. Shock is frequently present in severe cases. Vasodilators given prior to the correction of shock by adequate fluid administration may exacerbate the hypotension and even cause death.

Phenytoin (i.e., diphenylhydantoin) may decrease the incidence of ERS, possibly through influencing sarcolemmal and sarcoplasmic reticulum function.[5] Although research shows that Verapamil (a calcium channel blocker) may assist in amelioration of signs and may even protect against the development of ERS, it has not been assessed in the horse.

Following recovery, an injection or oral supplementation of vitamin E and selenium is sometimes administered, although plasma vitamin E and serum selenium levels should be checked prior to this. Only hay and high fat feeds should be given for 2 to 14 days, and there should be no exercise nor any grain fed for 2 weeks. Return to normal exercise and feeding should be gradual and incremental. It appears helpful to divide feedings of concentrate into numerous, smaller feeds (e.g., divide total daily allowance into four, fairly evenly spaced feedings). A high-fat, low-starch diet appears to decrease postexercise CK in ERS horses (McKenzie EC, and Valberg SJ, personal communication, 2000). It is not known in horses whether administration of thiamine (500 mg/horse) and/or pantothenic acid (both of which are generally present in vitamin B complex solutions) is helpful, although in humans thiamine (vitamin B_1) has been shown to hasten lactic acid metabolism,[120] and pantothenic acid is necessary for aerobic metabolism and therefore may be helpful. However, there is no data currently supporting their utilization in the treatment of ERS.

On necropsy, affected muscles may show minimal gross changes or may appear swollen, hemorrhagic, or pale, with grayish-yellow streaks to a dark reddish-brown waxy-cooked appearance. Petechial hemorrhages are frequently present in the epicardium. The kidney cross section may show brownish discoloration with reddish streaks. Histologically there is hyaline degeneration and muscle fiber fragmentation, but little or no calcification or inflammation. Renal tubular nephrosis and congestion and pallor of central hepatic lobules may also be present.

Equine Polysaccharide Storage Disorder (Equine Polysaccharide Storage Myopathy)

A number of breeds of horses (including Quarter Horses,[114] Quarter Horse-related breeds,[113] Draft horses,[116] and draft horses including Belgian and Percheron draft horses[115]) have been identified as having polysaccharide storage myopathy syndrome, with clinical signs of repetitive exertional rhabdomyopathy. These horses appear to have an abnormal amount of polysaccharide (i.e., complex polysaccharide and glycogen) that appears to be metabolically unavailable, stored in their skeletal muscle. Researchers believed that this accumulation occurred because of a defect in the glycogen metabolic pathway, leading to improper use of carbohydrates for energy production. However, these horses have greater insulin sensitivity (putatively causing an increased GLUT4) and thus enhanced clearance of blood glucose into skeletal muscle, resulting in excessive glycogen storage (Valberg SJ, personal communication, 2000).

Treadmill studies conducted by Valberg et al.[114] on two affected horses demonstrated that their maximum achievable speed was lower than that of normal horses and that they had less oxygen consumption and less lac-

tate production. These investigators postulated that this was consistent with a syndrome that involves impairment of the glucose-1-P to pyruvate pathway, which would result in an insufficient amount of pyruvate for either oxidation or anaerobic conversion to lactate. If glycolysis is limited in exercising horses, their generation of muscle ATP is diminished, inducing painful contractions of skeletal musculature. It may be necessary to study larger numbers of horses to confirm these findings.

A whole blood sample (i.e., collected in an ethylenediaminetetraacetic acid [EDTA] blood tube) and a biopsy of the semitendinosus or semimembranosus muscles should be taken. The sample size of muscle should be approximately $3 \times 1 \times 1$ cm, and it should be incised in such a way that the long axis is parallel to the muscle fiber length and the short axis transects the muscle fiber direction. The biopsied material should be placed in a plastic bag/container (without being stretched) and shipped on dry ice via overnight express mail to Dr. S. Valberg at the College of Veterinary Medicine, University of Minnesota, St. Paul, MN. The whole blood sample must not be frozen, so a second package is usually necessary (Valberg S, personal communication, 1996). Muscle biopsies of affected horses reveal increased periodic acid Schiff (PAS) staining; vacuolization; and abnormal, non-bioavailable polysaccharide accumulation. The syndrome has only been recognized histologically in foals greater than 3 to 9 months of age, so suspect foals should be biopsied after this time. This is probably because an extended period of time is necessary to accumulate sufficient polysaccharide in cells.

Feeding regimes that may ameliorate the condition are a low-carbohydrate, high-lipid (i.e., fat/oil) diet, which may increase the oxidative capacity of skeletal musculature. If one can provide 20 to 25% of the total daily calorie requirements in the form of lipid (e.g., corn oil etc.), then it likely that the accumulation of complex polysaccharides will diminish. Adult horses weighing 500 kg (i.e., 1100 lb) need 16.4 Mcal (i.e., 69 MJ) DE per day for maintenance and 20.5 Mcal (i.e., 86 MJ) DE per day for light work.[67] Twenty-five percent of 16.4 to 20.5 Mcal is 4.1 to 5.1 Mcal. As corn oil provides approximately 0.0086 Mcal/mL, 475 to 600 mL of corn oil should be fed daily. A daily nutritional analysis for DE should be performed to ensure that the diet has sufficient lipid and carbohydrate. It should also be remembered that excess lipid may decrease calcium absorption, warranting additional calcium supplemention.

In reports to date, horses on this diet have shown clinical improvement, but draft horses have had an unexpected increase in serum CK and AST approximately 4 to 8 weeks after diet alteration implementation. Valentine et al.[116] proposed that this may follow increased necrosis of the polysaccharide-loaded muscle fiber segments, because these horses may have increased fatty acid utilization as a source of muscle energy.

Regular, gradual, and incrementally increasing exercise regimens are also imperative for control of clinical signs in horses diagnosed with this mypathy. Unexpected, intense exercise must be avoided to prevent a rapid increase in the muscle ATP requirements. Since glycolysis is limited in these horses, the rate of generation of muscle ATP is diminished, inducing the painful contractions of skeletal musculature and rhabdomyolysis.

Hyperkalemic Periodic Paralysis (HYPP)

The genetic defect causing hyperkalemic periodic paralysis (HYPP) is in the genes controlling the voltage-dependent sodium channel. It is an autosomal dominant trait in horses,[102] just as it is in humans. This syndrome occurs primarily in American Quarter Horses and those with this ancestry (i.e., American Paint Horses and Appaloosas). The mutation promoting this disease is found in bloodlines that were initiated by the stallion, "Impressive," who has since died.

Clinically the syndrome is typified by horses that have intermittent episodes of weakness, including facial muscle spasm, prolapse of the third eyelid (i.e., nictitating membrane), muscle spasms and/or fasciculations, sweating, stridor, and sometimes flaccid paralysis with recumbency. There is a wide variation in the severity of clinical signs, and these may vary with temperature, diet, exercise level, anesthesia, and stresses, including trailer rides. During an episode, serum potassium is usually elevated because of the sodium channel defect. A normal sodium channel allows rapid membrane depolarization during the initial phase of the skeletal muscle's action potential. However, defective sodium channels fail to inactivate, thus remaining open, allowing an excessive inward sodium current and persistent depolarization (i.e., increased depolarization and thus closer to threshold) of the skeletal muscle's cell membrane. Elevations of serum potassium during an episode may exacerbate the syndrome by inducing additional repetitive opening of the defective sodium channels, thus inducing increased depolarization of the muscle cell membrane, and causing severe clinical signs.

Acute episodes are usually treated by intravenous administration of potassium-free isotonic fluids, including 2.5 to 5% dextrose, 0.6 to 1.2% sodium bicarbonate, or solutions containing calcium gluconate. Dextrose and bicarbonate function by increasing the net movement of extracellular potassium into the cell. In rare instances insulin is also utilized to assist in the inward movement of potassium from the extracellular fluid spaces into the intracellular space. Calcium-containing solutions may function to stabilize the membrane potential of muscle cells; however, some veterinarians are concerned about induction of hypercalcemia in affected horses and will use only dextrose and/or bicarbonate solutions.

Long-term control of episodes may include 1) dietary management, 2) administration of the potassium-wasting diuretic and carbonic anhydrase inhibitor, acetazolamide (2 to 4 mg/kg given orally every 12 to 24 hours), and 3) administration of phenytoin, which affects both sodium and calcium channels.

The daily requirement of potassium for a 500-kg (i.e., 1100-lb) adult horse at maintenance is 25 g, yet the same sized horse performing intense work requires 50 g (i.e., the requirement has doubled). These amounts are provided by 0.2 to 0.4% potassium in the dietary dry matter. It is rare for Quarter Horses, Paints, and Appaloosas (i.e., those at potential risk of HYPP) to be performing at anything more than light or moderate work. This would increase the requirement of a 500-kg adult horse to 31 to 37 g of potassium. The aim of dietary management for horses with HYPP should be to diminish potassium intake to near these amounts. High-potassium feeds include alfalfa hay and grass, some grass hays (i.e., Bermuda grass hay, Kentucky bluegrass hay, fescue, ryegrass hay, and timothy hay), soybean meal, molasses, sweet feeds, and many vitamin and mineral supplements. In general, potassium levels are low in grains (0.3 to 0.5%), yet high in forages (1 to 3%), especially immature forages. Potassium requirements are increased in performance horses that have increased losses through sweating. Potassium levels in water are unlikely to be toxic, but high concentrations may decrease palatability, so water may not be the best choice as a carrier for potassium supplements.

Normokalemic Periodic Paralysis

Episodic paralysis in horses without associated peripheral serum hyperkalemia does not preclude the possibility of diagnosing hyperkalemic periodic paralysis.[103] This syndrome, normokalemic periodic paralysis, has not been definitively proven to occur in horses. Two horses have been described with such a syndrome, but the descriptions were made prior to the advent of the DNA-probe for testing whether the mutation affecting the sodium channel gene was present. In humans this variant of the disease syndrome is rare and not well described; however, because serum potassium may not be elevated unless veins draining affected muscle groups are directly sampled, it is considered a variant of hyperkalemic periodic paralysis. This means that, in general, if normokalemic variations are suspected, then dietary guidelines for horses with hyperkalemic periodic paralysis should be adhered to (see the section on Hyperkalemic Periodic Paralysis immediately preceding this section).

Equine Motor Neuron Disease

Vitamin E deficiency is thought to be the cause of the neurologic disease, equine motor neuron disease (EMND).[20] The vitamin E requirements currently recommended by the NRC[67] are 50 IU/kg dry matter for maintenance and 80 IU/kg dry matter for pregnancy, lactation, work, and growth, respectively. However, horses with EMND or EDM (see the section titled, In the Growing Horse, earlier in this chapter) have been fed up to 6000 IU of vitamin E per day without apparent ill effects. This amount is equivalent to approximately 600 IU/kg dry matter. Currently the maximum tolerance level recommended by the NRC[67] is 1000 IU/kg dry matter.

Nutritional Secondary Hyperparathyroidism (NSH) (Bran Disease, Big-Head, Miller's Disease, Fibrous Osteodystrophy, Osteodystrophia Fibrosa)

Hyperparathyroidism may be primary, pseudo, or secondary. Regardless of the cause, it results in a generalized osteodystrophy in the horse. Primary hyperparathyroidism is extremely rare in the horse. It occurs when there is excessive, uncontrolled secretion of parathyroid hormone (i.e., parathormone, PTH). The parathyroid gland may be histologically normal[28] or neoplastic. One of the authors (C.J.S.) has had only one horse diagnosed at necropsy with neoplasia of the parathyroid glands, resulting in primary hyperparathyroidism. The horse presented in an emaciated, catabolic state (presumed to be cancer cachexia) antemortem and had a greatly elevated serum calcium concentration. Pseudohyperparathyroidism is a result of the secretion of parathyroid-like substances from nonparathyroid gland tumors and has been diagnosed in the horse especially in association with lymphoma (lymphosarcoma), gastric squamous cell carcinoma, and mesothelioma. Both primary hyperparathyroidism and pseudohyperparathyroidism generally cause hypercalcemia.

In contrast, the plasma calcium concentration is usually normal or slightly decreased in secondary hyperparathyroidism. Secondary hyperparathyroidism is a compensatory response to hypocalcemia. It may be a result of nutritional imbalances and, possibly in the horse, the result of chronic renal disease. In most species, chronic renal disease results in phosphorus and parathyroid hormone retention and a decreased production of the active form of vitamin D. Plasma calcium concentration generally remains normal until late stages of the disease, when it may be decreased. In the horse, however, chronic renal disease usually results in hypercalcemia because of a decrease in urinary calcium excretion, and hypercalcemia inhibits parathyroid hormone secretion.

Nutritional secondary hyperparathyroidism (NSH) is called by a variety of names, including big-head (because of the enlarged facial and mandibular bones in severely affected horses), bran disease [because excessive bran (high in phosphorus) intake will cause NSH] or Miller's disease (because in previous years byproducts of the milling process were high in phosphorus and could induce NSH when fed to horses), and osteodystrophia fibrosa (because the resorbed bone is replaced by fibrous connective tissue). Nutritional secondary hyperparathyroidism occurs as a result of prolonged ingestion of a calcium-deficient ration, or a ration low in calcium with respect to substances that bind it and decrease its absorption. Excessive amounts of phosphorus and oxalates in the ration are most commonly responsible for decreasing calcium absorption, allowing a relative calcium deficiency, and causing NSH.[37,92,97,108,119] If hyperphosphatemia occurs, it may also decrease renal formation of active vitamin D (1,25-dihydroxycholecalciferol), thus decreasing intestinal calcium absorption, and diminishing the inhibitory effect of the 1,25-dihydroxycholecalciferol on parathyroid hormone.

A ration containing a Ca:P ratio of less than 0.8:1 for the growing horse or 0.5:1 for the mature horse may cause NSH. It is recommended that a Ca:P ratio of greater than 1:1 be maintained in the ration for all horses (e.g., 1.3 to 1.5:1 Ca:P). Bran contains approximately 1.3% phosphorus and 0.1% calcium, as compared to 0.3% calcium required in the mature horse's diet and 0.7% calcium required in the weanling's diet.[68] Thus, the intake of high amounts of bran results in a calcium deficiency and a low Ca:P ratio, resulting in NSH and giving rise to the name "bran disease." It is interesting that Savage et al.[88] fed excessive amounts of phosphorus [i.e., 388% of the phosphorus recommended by the

NRC[67]] combined with the NRC[67] recommendation for calcium to growing foals for 16 weeks, yet no macroscopic signs of NSH were observed. Wing of ilium bone biopsies were performed on these foals and compared to foals fed NRC[67] requirements (i.e., control foals). The foals fed excessive phosphorus had increased cortical bone porosity (p = 0.001), and there was a trend towards decreased cancellous bone volume.[89] More than 16 weeks of feeding diets likely to induce NSH may be required to induce the disease clinically; or the amount of calcium fed, despite the excessive phosphorus level, may have halted clinical progression in these foals.

Excessive amounts of oxalates may be present in some plants, e.g., *Setaria sphacelata*, *Panicum* (giant blue or green panic grass), *Paspalum* spp., *Sporobolus* spp., *Cenchrus ciliaris* (buffel grass), *Halogeton*, greasewood, beets, docks, and rhubarb leaves. Plants containing oxalates often have a red color to their leaves or stems. These plants may contain 1 to 2% oxalate and less than 0.3% calcium.[119] Adding 1% oxalate to a pony's diet containing 0.45% calcium has been shown to cause a decreased calcium absorption with no change in urinary calcium excretion, resulting in a negative calcium balance.[108] Thus, if the horse consistently eats sufficient quantities of these plants over an extended period of time, it may result in NSH. In addition, very rarely insoluble oxalate crystals may be deposited in the kidneys, resulting in kidney damage. However, renal manifestations of oxalate toxicity are not common in horses.[18]

Inadequate calcium intake or excessive ingestion of phosphorus (or oxalate), which decreases calcium absorption, will decrease the plasma calcium concentration. Reduced plasma calcium concentration stimulates parathyroid hormone secretion, which stimulates calcium and phosphorus mobilization from the bone, renal calcium reabsorption, and renal phosphorus excretion. Thus, the effect of an increase in parathyroid hormone secretion and a decrease in calcitonin secretion is to maintain a normal (or elevated) plasma calcium concentration and a normal (or decreased or increased) plasma phosphorus concentration at the expense of bone demineralization. Homeostatic mechanisms are very effective at maintaining the calcium and phosphorus serum levels, hence it is rare to observe increased serum calcium and decreased serum phosphorus concentrations. As bone minerals are mobilized, they are replaced by fibrous connective tissue, leading to the condition called osteodystrophia fibrosa. Fibrous deposition in the bone causes an enlargement in that region. Although the entire skeletal system is affected, it is most noticeable in the growing horse at the metaphyseal growth plate and may result in physitis, although this has not been confirmed experimentally. In the mature horse it is most noticeable in the facial bones, giving rise to the name "big-head." Immature horses are more likely to be severely affected because of their higher rate of bone turnover.[90]

Other clinical signs and extensive bone demineralization may occur prior to an observable enlargement of the metaphyses or facial bones. An insidious shifting-limb lameness and generalized bone and joint tenderness may occur. Radiographic changes include a decrease in bone density and mottling of the bone. Although demineralization is generalized, different degrees of demineralization may occur in various parts of the skeletal system.

It is rare to find two limbs that have the same degree of demineralization.[9] However, lameness may be present for several months before radiographic changes are evident.[56] To be radiographically detectable, 30 to 60% of the mineral content of the bone must be lost.[56] Later, enlargement of the facial bones and mandible usually occurs. This may result in the teeth becoming loose or falling out. Fractures of long bones and compression fractures of the vertebrae may occur. Plasma alkaline phosphatase levels are often increased.[10] Diagnosis must be based on an evaluation of the ration consumed,[59,67] as well as urinary fractional excretions of calcium and phosphorus. These, especially the fractional excretion of phosphorus, are invaluable in recognizing the syndrome, as they reflect the dietary intake of these minerals (i.e., expect a low-to-normal calcium fractional excretion and a high-to-normal phosphorus fractional excretion). Excessive serum concentration of intact parathyroid hormone is also indicative of NSH, especially in combination with dietary analysis, radiographic alterations, and low-to-normal serum/plasma calcium (total or ionized) and high-to-normal serum/plasma phosphorus.

Treatment is strictly dietary. The ration is corrected by increasing calcium and decreasing phosphorus intake to levels needed by the weanling (0.7% calcium and 0.5% phosphorus in the total ration dry matter[68]). Plants containing oxalates should also be restricted from the diet. One of the authors (C.J.S.) often uses a calcium to phosphorus ratio of 2:1 to 4:1 for a period of 6 to 12 weeks after diagnosis, before decreasing to the high side of recommended values. Lameness usually disappears within 6 weeks after the ration is corrected, unless fractures are present. Generally, little regression in the size of the enlarged bones of the skull will occur.[56] Younger horses have a greater chance of their enlarged facial bones diminishing in size because of their greater rate of bone remodeling, compared to adult horses.[90]

Vitamin D Imbalances

Vitamin D not only promotes intestinal calcium and phosphorus absorption and renal calcium reabsorption, but it is necessary for parathyroid hormone mobilization of calcium from the bone. Collectively, these actions assist in maintaining the normal plasma calcium and phosphorus concentrations necessary for the ossification of endochondral cartilage. Either an excess or a deficiency of vitamin D results in bone abnormalities.

Vitamin D_2 is present in sun-cured feeds. In addition, 7-dehydrocholesterol, which is synthesized in the body, is converted in the skin by ultraviolet rays from the sun to previtamin D_3. This conversion occurs even during cloudy, overcast days. It does not occur, however, when sunlight shines through glass, since glass filters out ultraviolet rays. Previtamin D_3 and vitamin D_2 are both converted to the active form in the kidney and are utilized by the horse. If the animal receives either sun-cured feeds or is outside 3 to 4 hours a day, a vitamin D deficiency will not occur. Horses that are stabled every day and never allowed access to direct sunlight for more than 1 hour should have 2500 to 5000 IU of vitamin D added to the ration daily; however, this is a very rare occurrence. This is the only situation in which vitamin D supplementation might be needed. Note that no amount of vitamin D will compensate for inadequate calcium or phosphorus or an improper Ca:P ratio in the diet. Dietary calcium and phosphorus imbalances in the horse's diet are much more common than vitamin D imbalances and can be diagnosed only by evaluating the horse's ration as described in Lewis[59] and by the NRC.[67]

Vitamin D Deficiency

A vitamin D deficiency is characterized by a lack of bone calcification, osteosclerosis, osteomalacia, and osteitis fibrosa.[26] It produces a highly stable cartilage matrix, which is uncalcified and difficult to resorb. The cartilage cells do not degenerate, but instead build up to produce a large, more nonresorbable matrix. This produces a palpable and observable broadening of the metaphyses. In severe or chronic cases, affected animals are reluctant to stand and do so with difficulty and pain.

Vitamin D Toxicity

Feeding greater than 22,000 to 50,000 IU of vitamin D daily for several months, or higher levels for a shorter period of time, may result in vitamin D toxicity.[110] The maximum tolerance level recommended by the NRC[67] is 2200 IU/kg dry matter feed. Ponies fed 3300 IU/kg of body weight daily died within 4 months. Severe signs of vitamin D toxicity occurred in horses fed 200,000 IU/day for several months and in horses given 2 injections weekly of 4,000,000 IU of vitamin D for 2 months.[65] Vitamin D toxicity may also occur from the ingestion of *Cestrum diurnum* (jasmine, wild jessamine, or king-of-the-day),[49] *Solanum malacoxylon*, or *llisetum flavescens* (golden or yellow oat grass).[75] *Cestrum* species is an ornamental plant found in subtropical areas of Texas, California, and Florida. These plants contain a substance similar to the active form of vitamin D.

Excessive vitamin D stimulates intestinal calcium absorption resulting in hypercalcemia, which inhibits normal osteocytic osteolysis.[14] Hypercalcemia decreases parathyroid hormone secretion and stimulates calcitonin secretion, which, in conjunction with the inhibition of osteocytic osteolysis, decreases bone resorption. The decrease in bone resorption results in osteopetrosis and hypophosphatemia. Higher levels of vitamin D cause further inhibition of osteocytes, possibly resulting in osteonecrosis. Osteonecrosis and vitamin D toxicity induce atrophy of osteoblasts, resulting in osteopenia and osteoclasis.[14] Inhibition of cartilage maturation and cessation of cell proliferation in the articular cartilage and metaphyseal growth plate decreases growth. Soft tissue calcinosis also may occur.

Clinical signs of vitamin D toxicity observed in the horse include: a chronic debilitation with decreased feed intake, decreased growth, or loss of body weight; polyuria; polydipsia; exostosis; generalized stiffness; pain with a reluctance to move, especially the first few steps; and sensitivity to palpation of tendons and suspensory ligaments.[58,65] The diagnosis is based on evidence of excessive vitamin D intake or administration, clinical signs, and hypercalcemia. Treatment is to prevent the administration of vitamin D.

Vitamin A Imbalances

Vitamin A may be inadequate in rations routinely fed to the horse. The precursor of vitamin A, beta-carotene, is present in all green forages at concentrations many times over the horse's requirements. However, its content in the forage decreases as the forage matures and when it is stored for a period of time. A rough approximation of the amount of beta-carotene present in forage is judged by the amount of green color. Unless forage is brown or yellow, it will contain more than enough beta-carotene to meet the horse's vitamin A requirements. In addition, the liver is able to store sufficient quantities of vitamin A to supply the animal's requirements for 3 to 6 months.

Both a deficiency and an excess of vitamin A can cause similar clinical syndromes. Ponies 4 to 9 months old that are fed rations providing less than 10 or greater than 1800 IU of vitamin A per lb of body weight daily gained 20 to 30% less weight, grew 43% less in height, had duller haircoats, and had lower packed cell volumes, fewer red blood cells, and lower plasma albumin concentrations than those receiving 18 IU of vitamin A per lb of body weight daily.[23]

A vitamin A deficiency has not been identified as a clinical cause of skeletal problems in the horse.[44] However, a severe vitamin A deficiency may lower the animal's resistance to infectious diseases such as pneumonia, diarrhea, and endometritis. Excessive lacrimation, night blindness, and photophobia are suggestive of a vitamin A deficiency. The hair may become rough, dry, dull, and brittle. In addition, there is poor muscle tone, severe depression, ataxia progressing to lateral recumbency with a failure to respond to external stimuli, and finally death.[23] In other species a severe vitamin A deficiency has been shown to decrease endochondral bone growth and cause abnormal bone remodeling.

Selenium Toxicity

Three selenium toxicity conditions occur: 1) acute toxicity from excessive selenium administration, 2) subacute toxicity called blind staggers, and 3) chronic toxicity called alkali or bobtail disease. In contrast to a selenium deficiency that most commonly affects the foal, selenium toxicity most commonly affects the adult.

Acute toxicity is caused by the ingestion of greater than 500 to 1000 ppm of selenium in the dry ration or 2 to 11 mg of selenium per kg body weight, or the administration of greater than 0.8 to 2 mg/kg parenterally. Acute selenium toxicity causes nervousness and fear initially and later depression, anorexia, diarrhea, fever, generalized muscular weakness resulting in ataxia, trembling, paresis, and respiratory distress. Respiratory distress is associated with pulmonary edema and results in cyanosis, coma, and death. Death occurs from several hours to several days after excessive selenium intake. There is no treatment for acute selenium toxicity.

Subacute and chronic selenium toxicity occur in all herbivores from the ingestion of plants containing greater than 2 to 5 ppm of selenium in their dry matter content. There are limited areas, particularly in the Rocky Mountains and Great Plains areas, which have selenium levels high enough in the soil to result in toxicity from the ingestion of plants grown on these soils. Any soil containing greater than 0.5 ppm selenium is potentially dangerous. Soil in some of these areas may contain 50 ppm. Early settlers to these areas called chronic selenium toxicity "alkali disease" because they saw the condition occurring in animals grazing plants growing on alkaline soils and believed the cause was the high salt content of the water in these semiarid regions. Selenium toxicity occurs more commonly on alkaline soils because selenium is taken up by the plants (i.e., accumulator plants) more readily as soil pH increases.

Subacute selenium toxicity ("blind staggers"), is caused by the ingestion of plants that accumulate selenium from the soil. There are two types of these plants: obligate selenium accumulators or indicator plants, and facultative or secondary selenium accumulators.[14,122] Indicator plants accumulate selenium at levels up to 100 times that present in other plants in the same area. They may contain levels as high as 10,000 ppm even on soils containing only moderate amounts of selenium. These plants require selenium for growth and are thus named obligate accumulators. Since they require selenium, they grow only on relatively high selenium-containing soils on which many other plants will not grow and are thus named selenium indicator plants. These plants include certain *Astragalus* spp. (milk vetches), *Aster xylorrhiza* (woody aster), *Oonopsis* (golden weed), and *Stanleya* (prince's plume). Their selenium content is highest during growth. These plants have a garlic-sulfur odor when their selenium content is high, and the odor increases when their leaves are rubbed together. Because they are relatively unpalatable, most animals will not eat them if ample quantities of other feed are available. As a result, these plants are not a common cause of selenium toxicity. However, like many poisonous plants, they are one of the first plants to become green in the spring. They may be eaten at that time by an animal looking for anything green and lush.

Facultative or secondary selenium accumulators do not require high selenium soils for growth, but when growing on seleniferous soils, they may accumulate levels up to 10 times that of nonaccumulator plants in the same area. These plants may contain from 25 to a few hundred ppm of selenium in their dry matter content. They include *Asters* or *Machaeranthera*, *Atriplex* (four-winged salt bush), *Agropyron* (wheat grass or blue stem), *Sideranthus*, *Gutierrezia sarothral* (broomweed, snakeweed, or matchweed), *Grindelia squarrosa* (gumweed), *Castilleja*, and *Comandra*. When grown where soil selenium content is not high, some of these plants are good feed. These plants and, less commonly, nonaccumulator or passive accumulator plants are often responsible for causing selenium toxicity. Most cultivated crops, plants, grains, and native grasses are passive accumulator or nonaccumulator plants when soil selenium content is high. They may contain from 1 to 30 ppm selenium in their dry matter content.

Blind staggers are caused by the ingestion of greater than 2 mg of selenium/kg of body weight. The minimum lethal dose of selenium for the horse is 3.3 mg/kg of body weight. These amounts of selenium intake are caused by eating indicator plants, often in a single feeding. However, they may be eaten over several days or weeks. Frequently, clinical signs are similar to those occurring with acute selenium toxicity. If signs of acute toxicity do not occur, the animal suffers impaired vision and wanders aimlessly, frequently in circles, often stumbling and showing signs of ataxia. Therefore, a common name for this condition is blind staggers. Anorexia and often a dark, watery diarrhea and pica occur. These signs are followed by any one or more of the following: 1) blindness, often with inflamed, swollen eyelids and a cloudy cornea, 2) respiratory distress, occasionally with a bloody froth from the nose, 3) an inability to swallow, 4) excess salivation and lacrimation, 5) teeth grinding, 6) colic, 7) recumbency, and 8) death from respiratory failure.

The course of the disease from onset to death is from a few hours to several days.

Chronic selenium toxicity is caused by the consumption of a ration containing 5 to 10 ppm selenium in its dry matter content or greater than 10 ppb in the water, resulting in a selenium intake of 0.5 to 2 mg of selenium per kg of body weight. This results in anorexia and a poorly functioning animal progressing to listlessness and emaciation. Other manifestations of the disease occur as a result of the replacement of sulfur by selenium in sulfur-containing amino acids in body proteins. These amino acids are quite high in keratin and are present in the hooves and hair. The hair becomes rough, coarse, and brittle and is often lost from the mane and switch of the tail, which gives rise to the name "bobtail disease." The coronet swells, and transverse grooves appear on the hooves that are more pronounced than grooves secondary to laminitis.[49] The grooves may crack and the hooves may slough off. More often the hoof remains attached, and the toe grows long with a dorsal concavity because pain in that area leads to less wear. Affected animals may have a stiff-legged gait. In addition, articular erosions may occur, especially in the hock and fetlock joints.[49] Massive soft tissue calcification may occur. The cardiac muscle may contain several hundred times its normal calcium content. There may be decreased circulation to the extremities, making them more susceptible to freezing during cold weather. Although only limited amounts of selenium cross the placenta,[62] excessive selenium ingestion by the mare during pregnancy may result in deformities in the foal at birth.[49]

Selenium toxicity is probably present in animals showing the clinical signs described if greater than the following amounts of selenium are found: 5 ppm in the total ration dry matter; 10 ppb in the drinking water; 0.3 ppm in blood, plasma or serum; 5 to 20 ppm in hair or hoof; 2 to 3 ppm in liver or kidney wet weight. Selenium toxicity must be differentiated from laminitis, freezing of the extremities, ergot toxicity, and fluorosis.

Treatment and prevention of both subacute and chronic selenium toxicity may be achieved with any one of the following: 1) providing salt containing 40 ppm of arsenic, 2) providing drinking water containing 5 ppm of inorganic arsenic, or 3) feeding a ration containing 50 to 100 ppm of arsenilic acid.

Arsenic has been shown to increase biliary excretion of selenium in rats and is reported to be beneficial in the treatment of selenium toxicity in livestock.[10] Arsenic intake should be closely controlled as excesses are toxic. An additional treatment for selenium toxicity in the adult

horse is to administer 4 to 5 g of naphthalene by mouth daily for 5 days, wait 5 days, and then repeat the dose for 5 more days.[10] Initially, Prostigmin administration may be beneficial in clearing the intestinal tract of selenium-containing plants. Affected animals should be removed from selenium-containing feeds and given a low selenium-containing grain and a high-protein ration (20% crude protein). Providing feeds low in selenium, when animals are grazing in pastures containing plants high in selenium, also assists in prevention. Feeding high protein rations may also be protective (refer to Chapter 8 for more information).

Fluorosis

Fluoride requirements are extremely minute, and therefore, deficiencies do not occur. Adding 1 to 2 ppm of fluoride to the drinking water decreases dental caries in humans by an average of 60%, particularly in children. This occurs because fluoride is deposited in the bone and teeth, increasing their crystallinity and hardness and decreasing their solubility, thus impairing osteolysis. However, greater than 2.5 ppm of fluoride in the drinking water will result in mottled enamel during tooth development, but no other effects are observed at levels of less than 8 ppm. Greater than 30 ppm of fluoride in the ration dry matter is toxic during growth, and greater than 50 ppm is toxic during maintenance. At less than 200 ppm, however, toxic effects may not occur in the adult for several years. Ingested fluoride accumulates in the bone and teeth throughout life and is therefore a cumulative poison.

Some of the most common sources of excess fluoride are rock phosphates, phosphatic limestone, or fertilizer grade phosphates that have not been defluoridated. These mineral sources may contain 2 to 5% fluoride prior to defluoridation; each 1% of any one of these phosphate minerals added to the ration will increase the ration's fluoride content by 200 to 500 ppm. Manufacturing plants or mining operations that process minerals containing fluoride (e.g., cryalite, a source of aluminum; fluospar; rock phosphates) and steel processing plants may release large amounts of fluoride into the air, contaminating forage, soil, and water in nearby areas. Contaminated forage is the most common cause of fluorosis in these areas. While forage grown on soils high in fluoride contains high levels of fluoride, cereal grain grown on the same soil is relatively unaffected. Deep wells derived from underground phosphate rock formations may contain excess fluoride.

Fluorosis is characterized almost entirely by signs involving the bone and teeth. It is very insidious and may be confused with any chronic debilitating disease. Teeth generally show the first signs of fluorosis. During the period of calcification, the tooth enamel becomes mottled. Affected teeth are often chalky-white in color with yellowish-brown-to-black mottling that cannot be removed by scraping. In severe cases the teeth become pitted, worn, and eroded to the extent that nerves may be exposed. As a result of these dental changes, eating and drinking cold water may be extremely painful. Feed and water intake decreases, resulting in decreased growth and weight loss. Periosteal hyperostosis, i.e., enlargement, roughening, and thickening of the bone, occurs. Frequently this is first noticeable on the medial surfaces of the proximal one-third of the metatarsal bones. As the condition progresses, the mandible, metacarpal bones, and ribs become involved. These lesions result in spurring and bridging at joints, with subsequent stiffness and lameness. Radiographically, there is thickening and increased density of the bone. Grossly, the bones become chalky-white instead of ivory.

Animals are most commonly affected during growth, although the adult and the fetus may also be affected. Fluoride is transported across the placenta;[107] therefore, excessive intake by the mare during pregnancy may result in mottling of the deciduous teeth of the fetus and a decrease in birth weight.[42,76] However, excess fluoride intake has a minimal effect on the fluoride content of milk,[42] so the nursing animal is not affected.

Diagnosis of fluorosis is based on the clinical signs, finding feed or water fluoride concentrations greater than the values given previously, or finding greater than 1300 ppm fluoride in ribs and caudal vertebrae (normal is less than 1200 ppm). The fluoride present in ribs and caudal vertebrae is 1.5 to 2 times greater than that present in other bones.[42] Urinary fluoride concentrations are sometimes measured but reflect only current, not past, fluoride intake (normal levels in urine are 2 to 6 ppm fluoride). Milk and soft tissue fluoride contents are only minimally affected by dietary fluoride intake.[42]

The effects of fluoride toxicity are not reversible. In addition, no substance will completely prevent the toxic effects of excess fluoride intake; however, aluminum sulfate, aluminum chloride, calcium aluminate, calcium carbonate or limestone, or defluorinated phosphate are beneficial. One of these salts should be added at levels of 2 to 4% in the ration or mixed with equal parts of salt for free-choice consumption. The toxic effects can also be counteracted to some extent with green forage and liberal grain feedings.

References

1. Atinmo T, et al. The effect of dietary protein restriction on serum thyroxine levels of pregnant and growing swine. J Nutr 1978;108(9):1546–1553.
2. Auer JA, Martens RJ, Morris EL. Angular limb deformities in foals. Part I. Congenital factors. Comp Cont Educ Pract Vet 1982;4:S330–S339.
3. Baker HJ, Lindsey JR. Equine goiter due to excess dietary iodine. J Am Vet Med Assoc 1968;153:1618.
4. Beech J, Lindborg S. Potassium concentrations in muscle, plasma and erythrocytes and urinary fractional excretion in normal horses and those with chronic intermittent exercise-associated rhabdomyolysis. Res Vet Sci 1993;55:43–51.
5. Beech J, Fletcher JE, Lizzo F, et al. Effect of phenytoin on the clinical signs and in vitro muscle twitch characteristics in horses with chronic intermittent rhabdomyolysis and myotonia. Am J Vet Res 1988;49:2130–2133.
6. Bergsten G, Holmback R, Lindberg P. Blood selenium in naturally fed horses and the effect of selenium administration. Acta Vet Scand 1970;11:571.
7. Blood DC, Henderson JA, Radostits OM. Veterinary Medicine. 5th ed. Philadelphia: WB Saunders, 1979;891.
8. Bridges CH, Harris ED. Experimentally induced cartilage fractures (osteochondritis dissecans) in foals fed low copper diets. J Am Vet Med Assoc 1988;193:215–221.
9. Brood D. Osteoporosis in a six-year-old pony. Equine Vet J 1975;7:46.
10. Buck WB, Osweiler GD, Van Gelder GA. Clinical and Diagnostic Veterinary Toxicology. Dubuque, IA: Kendall-Hunt, 1976;345.
11. Carlson GP, Mansmann RA. Serum electrolyte and plasma protein alterations in horses used in endurance rides. J Am Vet Med Assoc 1974;165:262.
12. Carlstrom B. Uber die Aetiologie und Pathogenese der Kreuziahme des Pferdes (Haemoglobinaemis paralytica). Scand Arch Physiol 1932;63:164–212.
13. Carroll CL, Huntington PJ. Body condition scoring and weight estimation of horses. Equine Vet J 1988;20:41–45.
14. Chineme CN, Krook L, Pond WG. Bone pathology in hypervitaminosis D, an experimental study in young pigs. Cornell Vet 1976;66:387.
15. Coffman JR. Bone and muscle defects in foals. Mod Vet Pract 1973;54(13):53.
16. Corbellini CN, Krook L, Nathanielsz PW, et al. Osteochondrosis in fetuses of ewes overfed calcium. Calcif Tissue Int 1991;48:37–45.
17. Cymbaluk NF, Schryver HF, Hintz H. Copper metabolism and requirement in mature ponies. J Nutr 1981;111:87.
18. David JB, Cohen ND, Nachreiner R. Equine nutritional secondary hyperparathyroidism. Comp Contin Ed 1997;19:1380–1386.
19. Dill SG, Kallfelz FA, deLahunta A, et al. Serum vitamin E and blood glutathione peroxidase values of horses with degenerative myeloencephalopathy. Am J Vet Res 1989;50:166–168.
20. Divers TJ, Mohammed HO, Cummings JF, et al. Equine motor neurone disease: findings in 28 horses and proposal of a pathophysiological mechanism for the disease. Equine Vet J 1994;26:409–415.
21. Dodd DC, Blakeley AA, Thornbury RS. Muscle degeneration and yellow fat disease in foals. N Z Vet J 1960;78:45–50.
22. Donoghue S, Kronfeld DS, Berkowitz SJ, et al. Vitamin A nutrition of the equine: growth, serum biochemistry and hematology. J Nutr 1981;11:365.
23. Donoghue S, et al. Vitamin A nutrition of the equine: growth, serum biochemistry and hematology. J Nutr 1981;111:365.
24. Drew B, Barber WP, Williams DG. The effect of excess dietary iodine on pregnant mares and foals. Vet Rec 1975;97:93.
25. Driscoll J, Hintz HF, Schryver HF. Goiter in foals caused by excessive iodine. J Am Vet Med Assoc 1978;173:838.
26. El Shorafa WM, Feaster JP, Ott EA, et al. Effect of vitamin D and sunlight on growth and bone development of young ponies. J Anim Sci 1979;48:882.
27. Fallon EH. Proceedings. Cornell Equine Nutrition Conference, Syracuse, NY, 1971;19.
28. Frank N, Hawkins JF, Coutil LL, et al. Primary hyperparathyroidism with osteodystrophia fibrosa of the facial bones in a pony. J Am Vet Med Assoc 1998;212:84–86.
29. Frost HM. Orthopaedic Biomechanics. Springfield, IL: Charles C Thomas Publishers, 1973.
30. Ginther DJ. Occurrence of anestrus, estrus, diestrus, and ovulation over a 12-month period in mares. Am J Vet Res 1974;35:1173.
31. Glade M, Beller D, Bergen J, et al. Dietary protein in excess of requirements inhibits renal calcium and phosphorus reabsorption in young horses. Nutr Rep Int 1985;31:649–659.
32. Glade MJ, Gupta S, Reimers TJ. Hormonal response to high and low planes of nutrition in weanling Thoroughbreds. J Anim Sci 1984;59:658–665.
33. Grondalen T. Osteochondrosis and arthrosis in pigs. III. A comparison of the incidence in young animals of the Norwegian Landrace and Yorkshire breeds. Acta Vet Scand 1973;15:43.
34. Grondalen T, Grondalen J. Osteochondrosis and arthrosis in pigs. IV. Effect of overloading on the distal epiphyseal plate of the ulna. Acta Vet Scand 1974;15:53.
35. Grondalen T, Vangen O. Osteochondrosis and arthrosis in pigs. V. A comparison of the incidence in three different lines of Norwegian Landrace breed. Acta Vet Scand 1974;15:61.
36. Gunson DE, Kowalczyk DF, Shoop CR, et al. Environmental zinc and cadmium pollution associated with generalized osteochondrosis, osteoporosis, and nephrocalcinosis in horses. J Am Vet Med Assoc 1982;180:295–299.
37. Harmon BG. Bioavailability of phosphorus in feed ingredients for swine. Feedstuffs 1977; June 20:16.

38. Harrington DD, Walsh J, White V. Clinical and pathological findings in horses fed zinc deficient diets. In: Proceedings. 3rd Equine Nutrition and Physiology Symposium, 1973;51.

39. Harris P, Snow DH. Role of electrolyte imbalances in the pathophysiology of the equine rhabdomyolysis syndrome. In: Persson SGB, Lindholm A, Jeffcott LB, Eds. Equine Exercise Physiology. 3rd ed. Davis, CA: ICEEP Publications, 1991;435–442.

40. Hedhammar A, et al. Overnutrition and skeletal disease. An experimental study in growing Great Dane dogs. Cornell Vet 1974; 64 (Suppl 5):1.

41. Hennecke DR, Potter GD, Kreider JL. Nutrition and rebreeding. Equine Vet Data 1981; May 15:117–118.

42. Hillman D, Bolenbaugh D, Convey EM. Fluorosis from phosphate mineral supplements in Michigan dairy cattle. Research Report 365, Agriculture Experimental Station. East Lansing, MI: Michigan State University Press, 1978.

43. Hinton MH. The biochemical and clinical aspects of exhaustion in the horse. Vet Annu 1978;18:169.

44. Hintz HF, Schryver HF. Nutrition and bone development in horses. J Am Vet Med Assoc 1976;168:36.

45. Hintz HF, Schryver HF, Lowe JE. Delayed growth and limb conformation in horses. In: Proceedings. Cornell Equine Nutrition Conference, Syracuse, NY, 1976;94.

46. Hodgson DR. Exercise-associated myopathy: is calcium the culprit? (editorial). Equine Vet J 1993;25:1–3.

47. Hunt FB. Genetic defects of bones and joints in domestic animals. Cornell Vet 1968;58:104.

48. Hurtig MB, Green SL, Dobson H, et al. Defective bone and cartilage in foals fed a low-copper diet. Proc Am Assoc Equine Pract 1993;36:637–643.

49. Jones TC, Hunt RD, King NW. Veterinary Pathology. 6th ed. Philadelphia: Lippincott Williams & Wilkins, 1997;729–731.

50. Jordon RM, et al. A note on calcium and phosphorus levels fed ponies during growth and reproduction. In: Proceedings. 3rd Equine Nutrition and Physiology Symposium, 1973;55.

51. Kasstrom H. Nutrition, weight gain and development of hip dysplasia. An experimental investigation in growing dogs with special reference to effect of feeding intensity. Acta Radiol 1975; 334(Suppl):135.

52. Knight DA, Gabel AA, Reed SM, et al. Correlation of dietary mineral to incidence and severity of metabolic bone disease in Ohio and Kentucky. Proc Am Assoc Equine Pract 1985;31: 445–461.

53. Knight DA, Weisbrode SE, Schamall LM, et al. Copper supplementation and cartilage lesions in foals. Proc Am Assoc Equine Pract 1987;33:191–194.

54. Koterba A, Carlson GP. Acid-base and electrolyte alterations in horses with exertional rhabdomyolysis. J Am Vet Med Assoc 1982;180:303–306.

55. Kowalczyk DF, Gunson DE, Shoop CR, et al. The effects of natural exposure to high levels of zinc and cadmium in the immature pony as a function of age. Environ Res 1986;40:285–300.

56. Krook L, Lowe JE. Nutritional secondary hyperparathyroidism in the horse. Vet Pathol 1964;61:44.

57. Krook L, Maylin GA. Fractures in Thoroughbred racehorses. Cornell Vet 1988;78(Suppl 11):5–133.

58. Krook L, Waserman RH. Hypercalcemia and calcinosis in Florida horses: implication of the shrub, *Cestum diunum,* as the causative agent. Cornell Vet 1975;65:26.

59. Lewis LD. Feeding and Care of the Horse. 2nd ed. Philadelphia: Lippincott Williams & Wilkins, 1995.

60. Lilburn MS, Lauterio TJ, Ngiam-Rilling K, Smith JM. Relationships among mineral balances in the diet, early growth manipulation and incidence of tibial dyschondroplasia in different strains of meat type chickens. Poult Sci 1989;68:1263–1273.

61. Mayhew IG, et al. Spinal cord disease in the horse. Cornell Vet 1978;68(Suppl 6):1.

62. Maylin GA, Rubin DS, Lein DH. Selenium and vitamin E in horses. Cornell Vet 1980;70:272.

63. Medows DG. Protein supplements for lactating mares and effects on foal growth. In: Horse Short Course Proceedings, Texas A & M Animal Agricultural Conference, 1979;26.

64. Messer NT. Tibiotarsal effusion associated with chronic zinc intoxication in three horses. J Am Vet Med Assoc 1981;178:294.

65. Muylle E, et al. Hypercalcemia and mineralization of nonosseous tissues in horses due to vitamin D toxicity. Zentralbl Veteriamed 1974;21A:638.

66. Nehrich H, Stewart JA. The effects of prenatal protein restriction on the developing mouse cerebrum. J Nutr 1978;108:368.

67. NRC (National Research Council). Nutrient Requirements of Horses. 5th rev ed. Washington, DC: National Academy Press, 1989.

68. NRC (National Research Council). Nutrient Requirements of Horses. 4th rev ed. Washington, DC: National Academy of Sciences, 1978.

69. Olsson SE. Osteochondrosis, a growing problem to dog breeders. Gaines Progr 1976;Summer:111.

70. Olsson SE, Reiland S. The nature of osteochondrosis in animals. Acta Radiol 1978;(Suppl)358:299–306.

71. Owen JM. Abnormal flexion of the corono-pedal joint of "contracted tendons" in unweaned foals. Equine Vet J 1975;7:40.

72. Owen RR, et al. Dystrophic myodegeneration in adult horses. J Am Vet Med Assoc 1977;171:343.

73. Pearce SG. Copper nutrition in pasture-fed New Zealand Thoroughbreds and its role in developmental orthopaedic disease. PhD Thesis, Massey University, New Zealand, 1997.

74. Pearce SG, Firth EC, Grace ND, et al. The effect of copper supplementation on the evidence of developmental orthopaedic disease in pasture-fed New Zealand Thoroughbreds. Equine Vet J 1998; 30(3):211–218.

75. Petrie L. Hypervitaminosis D and metastatic pulmonary calcification in a cow. Vet Rec 1977;101:480.

76. Phillips PH, Hart EB, Bohstedt G. Chronic toxicosis in dairy cows due to the ingestion of fluorine. Research Bulletin 123, Agriculture Experimental Station. Madison, WI: University of Wisconsin Press, 1934.

77. Pickup J, Wordes AN, Bunyan J. Chronic constipation in dairy cattle associated with a high level of zinc in the water. Vet Rec 1954;66:93.

78. Reddy MK, Etlinger JD, Rabinowitz M, et al. Removal of z-lines and a-actinin from isolated myofibers by a calcium activated protease. J Biol Chem 1975;250:4278–4284.

79. Reed SM. Ataxia and paresis in horses. Part 1. Differential diagnosis. Comp Cont Educ 1981;3:S88.

80. Reiland S. Osteochondrosis in the pig. Acta Radiol 1975; (Suppl)334:1.

81. Reiland S, et al. Osteochondrosis in growing bulls—pathology, frequency and severity on different feedings. Acta Radiol 1978; (Suppl)358:179.

82. Rejno S, Stromberg B. Osteochondrosis in the horse. II. Pathology. Acta Radiol 1978;(Suppl)358:153.

83. Rodney JR. Equine Medicine and Surgery. 2nd ed. Wheaton, IL: American Veterinary Publications, 1972;494.

84. Rodney JR, New Castle DE. Forelimb contracture in the young horse. Equine Med Surg 1977;1:350.

85. Rosenfeld I, Beath OA. In: Geobotony, Biochemistry, Toxicity and Nutrition. San Diego: Academic Press, 1964;141–213.

86. Savage CJ. The influence of nutrition on skeletal growth and induction of osteochondrosis (dyschondroplasia) in horses. PhD Thesis, University of Melbourne, Australia, 1992.

87. Savage CJ, McCarthy RN, Jeffcott LB. Effects of dietary energy and protein on the induction of dyschondroplasia in foals. Equine Vet J 1993;(Suppl)16:74–79.

88. Savage CJ, McCarthy RN, Jeffcott LB. Effects of dietary phosphorus and calcium on induction of dyschondroplasia in foals. Equine Vet J 1993;(Suppl)16:80–83.

89. Savage CJ, McCarthy RN, Jeffcott LB. Histomorphometric assessment of bone biopsies from foals fed diets high in phosphorus and digestible energy. Equine Vet J 1993;(Suppl)16:89–93.

90. Savage CJ, Tidd LC, Ostblom LC, et al. Bone biopsy in the horse. 3. Normal histomorphometrical data according to age and sex. Zentralbl Veterinarmed A 1991;38:793–797.

91. Saville PD, Lieber CS. Increases in skeletal calcium and femur cortex thickness produced by undernutrition. J Nutr 1969;99: 141.

92. Schryver HF, Hintz HF. Recent developments in equine nutrition. Anim Nutr Health 1975;4:6.

93. Schryver HF, Craig PH, Hintz HF. Calcium metabolism in ponies fed varying levels of calcium. J Nutr 1970;100:955–964.

94. Schryver HF, Meakim DW, Lowe JE, et al. Growth and calcium metabolism in horses fed varying levels of protein. Equine Vet J 1987;19:280–287.

95. Schryver HF, Hintz HF, Craig PH. Phosphorus metabolism in ponies fed varying levels of phosphorus. J Nutr 1971;101:1257.

96. Schryver HF, Hintz HF, Lowe JE. Calcium metabolism and sweat losses of exercised horses. Am J Vet Res 1978;39:245.

97. Schryver HF, Hintz HF, Lowe JE. Calcium and phosphorus in nutrition of the horse. Cornell Vet 1974;64:491.

98. Shaver JR, et al. Skeletal manifestations of suspected hypothyroidism in two foals. J Equine Med Surg 1979;3:269.

99. Siassi F, Siassi B. Differential effects of protein-calorie restriction and subsequent repletion on neuronal and non-neuronal components of cerebral cortex in newborn rats. J Nutr 1973;103:1625.

100. Smith JD, Jordan RM, Nelson ML. Tolerance of ponies to high levels of dietary copper. J Anim Sci 1975;41:1645–1649.

101. Sojka JE. Proc Am Coll Vet Intern Med 1996;14:546.

102. Speir SJ, Carlson GP, Harrold D, et al. Genetic study of hyperkalemic periodic paralysis in horses. J Am Vet Med Assoc 1993;202:933–937.

103. Stewart RH, Bertone JJ, Yvorchuk-St Jean K, et al. Possible normokalemic variant of hyperkalemic periodic paralysis in two horses. J Am Vet Med Assoc 1993;203:421–424.

104. Stowe HD. Serum selenium and related parameters of naturally and experimentally fed horses. J Nutr 1967;93:60.

105. Stromberg B, Rejno S. Osteochondrosis in the horse: a clinical and radiologic investigation of osteochondritis dissecans of the knee and hock joints. Acta Radiol 1978;(Suppl)358:139–152.

106. Stromberg B. A review of the salient features of osteochondrosis in the horse. Equine Vet J 1979;11:211.

107. Suttie JW, Miller RF, Phillips PH. Studies of the effects of dietary NaF on dairy cows. I. The physiological effects and the developmental symptoms of fluorosis. J Nutr 1975;63:211.

108. Swartzman JR, Hintz HF, Schryver HF. Inhibition of calcium absorption in ponies fed diets containing oxalic acid. Am J Vet Res 1978;39:1621.

109. Thorp BH, Farquharson C, Kwan APL, et al. Osteochondrosis/dyschondroplasia: a failure of chondrocyte differentiation. Equine Vet J 1993;(Suppl)16:13–18.

110. Tyznich WJ. Nutritional relationships to performance. In: Proceedings California Livestock Symposium, May 1975.

111. Underwood EJ. Trace Elements in Human and Animal Nutrition. 3rd ed. New York: Academic Press, 1971;82.

112. Valberg S, Jonsson L, Lindholm A, Holmgren N. Muscle histopathology and plasma aspartate aminotransferase, creatine kinase and myoglobin changes with exercise in horses with recurrent exertional rhabdomyolysis. Equine Vet J 1993;25:11–16.

113. Valberg SJ, Geyer C, Sorum SA, et al. Familial basis of exertional rhabdomyolysis in Quarter Horse-related breeds. Am J Vet Res 1996;57:286–290.

114. Valberg SJ. Exertional rhabdomyolysis and polysaccharide storage myopathy in Quarter Horses. Proc Am Assoc Equine Pract 1995;41:228–230.

115. Valentine BA, Credille KM, Lavoie J-P, et al. Severe polysaccharide storage myopathy in Belgian and Percheron draught horses. Equine Vet J 1997;29:220–225.

116. Valentine BA, Divers TJ, Lavoie J-P. Severe equine polysaccharide storage myopathy in Draft horses. Clinical signs and response to dietary therapy. Proc Am Assoc Equine Pract 1996;42:294–296.

117. Van Vleet F. Selenium vitamin E deficiency in growing swine postmortem diagnosis and control. In: Proceedings. Mississippi Valley Veterinary Medicine Association Annual Meeting, 1976;1–9.

118. Voss JL. Rupture of the cecum and ventral colon of mares during parturition. J Am Vet Med Assoc 1969;155:745–747.

119. Walthall JC, Mckenzle RA. Osteodystrophia fibrosa in horses at pasture in Queensland. Aust Vet J 1976;52:11.

120. Wendel OW. A study of urinary lactic acid levels in humans. I. Influence on thiamine and pyrithiamine. J Vitaminol 1960;6:16.

121. Wilson TM, et al. Myodegeneration and suspected selenium/vitamin E deficiency in horses. J Am Vet Med Assoc 1976;169:213.

122. Witte ST, Will LA, Olsen CR, et al. Chronic selenosis in horses fed locally produced alfalfa hay. J Am Vet Med Assoc 1993;202:406–409.

123. Yoakam SC, Kirkham WW, Beeson WM. Effect of protein level on growth in young ponies. J Anim Sci 1978;46:483.

6

CHAPTER

Diseases of Bone and Related Structures

GARY M. BAXTER AND A. SIMON TURNER

PHYSIS

Postnatal Development and Growth of the Musculoskeletal System

Longitudinal bone growth results from a series of events occurring at highly specialized regions at one or both ends of the bone. These regions are referred to as the physes (growth plates or, more correctly, the metaphyseal growth plates). The process occurring at the growth plate, termed "endochondral ossification," is characterized by rapidly differentiating and maturing cartilage cells and the replacement of cartilage by bone.

There are two types of growth plates: discoid and spherical. The discoid growth plates are seen at the ends of long bones. Some bones have a physis at each end of the bone, whereas others, such as the third metacarpal/metatarsal bone and the proximal and middle phalanges, have only one. A discoid physis is located between the metaphysis (the flared end of the bone that contains spongy bone) and the epiphysis. An apophysis (which is a type of discoid physis) is an epiphysis that is subject to tensile rather than compressive forces, such as at the olecranon process, calcaneal tuber, and tibial tuberosity. The growth plate of an apophysis contains greater amounts of fibrocartilage than a true discoid physis, which is an adaptation to withstand tensile forces (Fig. 6.1).[101] Spherical physes are located in the small cuboidal bones of the foal's carpus and tarsus. These growth plates develop into bones by centrifugal expansion around a central cartilage core. They begin to ossify in the center and gradually assume the contours of the bone of an adult as bone development reaches the margins of the cartilage model.

Ossification of cartilage at one or both ends of long bones occurs early in life, forming the epiphyses. These develop in a manner similar to ossification of the cartilage models of the small cuboidal bones of the carpus and tarsus. The cellular events consist of vesiculation and chondrocyte death with calcification of matrix, invasion of vessels, and partial resorption and ossification.[101]

Eventually, a subchondral bone plate forms, which is best imagined as a "mini" growth plate. This growth plate contributes to the size of the epiphyses and makes a small contribution to growth in the length of the bone.

Morphology of the Physis

The physis, or growth plate, has a characteristic cellular architecture from birth until the animal matures. The cartilage cells of the growth plate can be divided into a number of zones, which differ in their height and cell number and with respect to their histologic appearance and cellular function. They are arranged more or less in longitudinal columns; cellular division occurs on the epiphyseal side of the cartilage while ossification progresses from the metaphysis to the diaphysis (Figs. 6.2 and 6.3).

Germinal Zone

The germinal (resting) zone, which is the zone nearest the epiphysis, is where cell division is initiated. The chondrocytes undergo mitosis and begin to divide, primarily in a longitudinal direction, although some transverse division occurs. They soon appear as small flattened chondrocytes, providing elongation to the columns of cells. Epiphyseal vessels (arterioles and capillaries) are closely associated with early cellular events and may even provide undifferentiated cells that can add to the pool of chondrocytes that will later divide.

Resting chondrocytes are also elaborated peripherally, forming a cartilaginous ring. This specialized region of the perichondrium is called the "zone of Ranvier." This ring remains in contact with the metaphyseal growth plate. It not only continues to grow on the epiphyseal side but gets resorbed on the diaphyseal side. This is one of the hallmarks of bone growth, i.e., it greatly depends on resorption (disappearance of bone) as well as bone formation. If, for example, bone resorption did not occur and bone grew only in length, then the bone would be disproportionately long and thin.

401

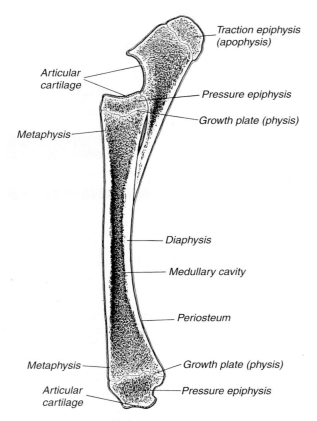

Figure 6.1 Sagittal section of the radius and ulna of a foal.

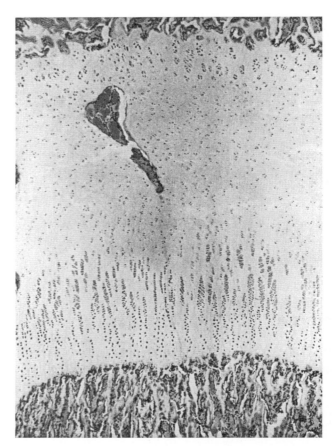

Figure 6.2 High-powered view of the cartilage of the distal radial physis of a horse.

Similarly in the diaphysis, if bone did not become re-sorbed from the inner surface (endosteal side), then continued apposition of bone from the periosteum would produce a bone that was too thick with inadequate marrow cavity.

Proliferative Zone

The proliferative, or growth, zone is where active cell division occurs within the physis. This zone can be quite large, compared with other areas of the growth plate, and can make up more than half of the overall height of the physis. Collagen that is randomly oriented in the region of the resting cells becomes more longitudinally oriented between the columns of proliferating cells.

Zone of Hypertrophy

After the cells are elaborated through cell division, they eventually undergo hypertrophy as a result of increased metabolic activity. At this stage, they no longer have the capability of dividing. The zone of hypertrophy lacks intercellular substance and is a structurally weak region of the growth plate. It is in this zone that physeal fractures occur and where trauma damages the physis (Fig. 6.3).

Zone of Ossification

The zone of ossification, or calcification, is the region in which the matrix between the cells gradually becomes

calcified, beginning with the formation of matrix vesicles. The next histologically distinct zone is the area of vascular penetration. There, blood vessels begin to invade the columns of calcifying cartilage, breaking down delicate transverse septa that have remained between the columns. The blood vessels also provide cellular components (osteoblasts) that will form bone and cells (chondroclasts) that assist in removal of any remaining cartilage. Osteoblasts elaborate the osteoid matrix, the organic part of bone, on the columns of calcifying cartilage (which form a series of projections into the metaphysis). This forms longitudinally orientated bony spicules (inside is a cartilaginous core) in the region called "the primary spongiosa." Eventually, the bone of the primary spongiosa is replaced with secondary spongiosa, which lacks remnants of the cartilage core. As the bone elongates, bone at the diaphyseal end is eroded by osteoclasts at the same rate as new bone is formed on the epiphyseal side of the metaphysis. Thus there is a continuous sequence of events, with cell division (bone formation) at one end and bone destruction (an important process) at the other, contributing to the final shape of the bone (Fig. 6.3).

Vascularity of the Physis

The blood supply to the growth plate originates from the epiphyseal, metaphyseal, and perichondral circula-

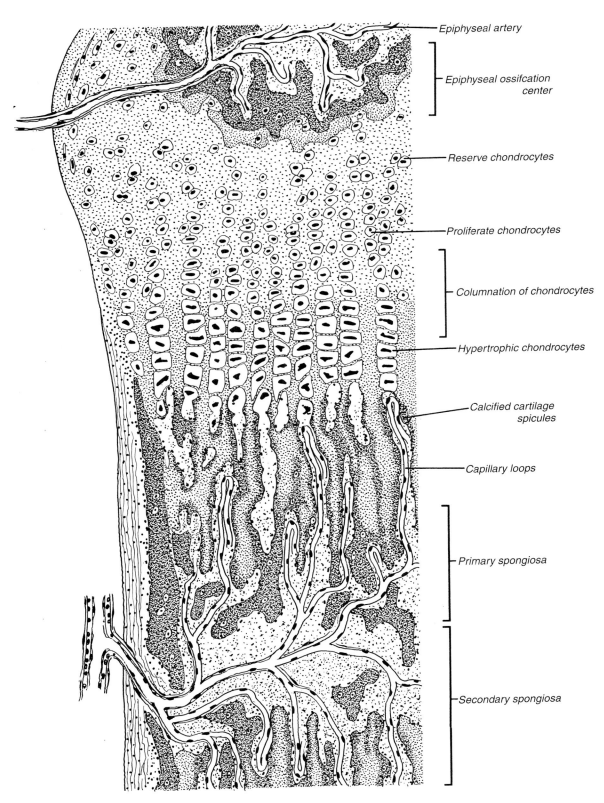

Figure 6.3 Cellular layers of the physis.

tions.[101] Transphyseal vessels (vessels crossing the growth plate) are present in large epiphyses and may serve as a route for spread of infection from the metaphysis to the epiphysis. The metaphyseal circulation forms a series of loops that penetrate the longitudinal septa, enlarging as they return toward the diaphysis, forming a sinusoid. This produces a sluggish pattern of blood flow within the physis, which predisposes the region to bacterial localization and osteomyelitis.[140]

The integrity of the blood vessels within the zone of Ranvier is important for continued appositional growth at the periphery of the epiphyseal growth plate. Disruption of the blood supply of the perichondral region can potentially cause ischemia to the physis, contributing to asynchronous growth and a subsequent angular limb deformity.

Biomechanical Aspects of the Physis of Long Bones

Although the exact mechanism is incompletely understood, tension and compression (within a physiologic range) on the physis are essential for continued orderly bone development and growth. Each growth plate has a biologic range of both tension and compression within which it will respond. Within this range, increasing tension or compression will accelerate physeal growth, whereas decreasing tension or compression will decrease physeal growth.

Beyond the physiologic limits of tension or compression, physeal growth may be significantly decreased or even stopped; the phenomenon is referred to as the Heuter-Volkmann law of physeal growth (Fig. 6.4).[140] This law has an important practical application in the management of foals with angular limb deformities. If it is assumed that a foal with an angular limb deformity of the carpus (e.g., carpus valgus) is exerting an asymmetric load on the distal radial physis, then unrestrained exercise may cause physeal compression that is greater than the physiologic range. This prevents any autocorrection of the angular limb deformity, increasing the likelihood that surgery may be required to alleviate the problem.

Apart from the effects of pressure and tension on the growth plate, the periosteum acts as an anatomic (mechanical) restraint to bone growth by attaching firmly at the zone of Ranvier and being only loosely attached to the diaphysis and metaphysis. Experimental circumferential resection of a portion of the periosteum has been shown to accelerate longitudinal growth of that bone. Houghton and Dekel[58] measured the longitudinal growth of immature rat femurs placed intraperitoneally in diffusion chambers. One femur had circumferential periosteal division and stripping, while the other acted as a control. After 14 days, there was significantly more overgrowth of the periosteally divided femurs than of the control femurs. The bones were under no influence of blood supply in these chambers, discounting the theory that periosteal transection alters bone growth by interfering with metaphyseal vessels and subsequent ischemia. These findings constitute the most logical explanation of why hemicircumferential transection of the periosteum and periosteal elevation increase bone growth in foals with angular limb deformities. After transection of the periosteum, the tension on that side of the bone is relieved, allowing bone growth to continue at an increased rate. When the limb is straight, the periosteum reattaches or regrows and presumably begins to reexert tension on the bone, preventing overcorrection of the deformity.

Cessation of Growth

As growth of the bone ceases, the physis becomes progressively thinner, and finally the epiphysis and metaphysis fuse.[101,102] The cartilaginous growth plate is replaced with trabecular bone, making it incapable of correcting any angular limb deformity. The timing of the physeal closure depends on the specific bone, with some bones closing early in life and others remaining open for several years. Most data on physeal closure are based on radiographic interpretation (loss of a visible physis). Functional physeal closure occurs well before radiographic closure, however, and this difference has important bearing on the timing of surgery used to correct angular limb deformities.

In general, the further distal on the limb the physis is located, the sooner in life it will become functionally inactive. For instance, the distal metacarpal/metatarsal physes close sooner than the distal radial or distal tibial physes, making correction of angular limb deformities of the fetlock and pastern early in life more important than those of the carpus or tarsus. In addition, any injury to the physis, such as excessive pressure, direct trauma, traction, circulatory loss, or shearing forces, can lead to premature cessation of growth or asynchronous growth. This abnormal growth pattern is commonly associated with angular limb deformities, physitis, or bony malformations (e.g., cervical vertebral malformation).[69,154]

Effect of External Trauma on the Physis

When an excessive force is applied to a joint and its nearby physis, an epiphyseal or physeal injury is likely to occur. This is because the cartilaginous growth plate

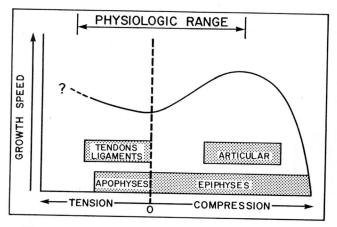

Figure 6.4 Response of the growth plate to compression.

the prognosis and method of treatment may be drastically different in foals than in children because of the dissimilarity in fracture repair between foals and children.[34]

Type 1 Injury

Type 1 injuries are characterized by a complete separation of the physis without any fracture through the bone; the germinal cells of the growth plate remain with the epiphysis (Fig. 6.6). In humans, this type of injury, which is the result of a shearing force, is more common in newborns (from birth injury) and in young children, who have relatively thick growth plates.[117] A similar type of injury occurs in foals and involves the proximal femoral physis (slipped capital femoral epiphysis).

In children, closed reduction is not difficult because the periosteal attachment remains intact around most of the circumference of the physis. The prognosis in children for further growth is excellent, provided the blood supply to the physis is not damaged. The treatment and prognosis for this injury in foals, which almost exclusively involves the proximal femoral physis, are more variable. Closed reduction of a slipped capital femoral epiphysis is impossible, and conservative management usually leads to severe osteoarthritis of the coxofemoral joint.[140] Therefore, open reduction and internal fixation with intramedullary (IM) pins, screws, or the dynamic hip screw (DHS) system is recommended.[63] The prognosis for athletic soundness in these foals is unfavorable, however, and most patients are euthanized without treatment.[63]

Closed reduction for type 1 injuries at other locations in foals is also difficult. Minimally displaced injuries, such as may occur in the proximal humeral physis, may be treated without surgery with good results.

Type 2 Injury

Type 2 injuries are the most common type of physeal injury in children as well as in virtually all domestic animals (Fig. 6.6). The fracture line extends along the physis for a variable distance and then breaks out through a portion of the metaphysis, producing a triangular metaphyseal fragment (Fig. 6.5). Similar to nearly all physeal injuries, the germinal cells remain within the physis. This type of injury usually results from shearing and bending forces. In foals, the distal third metacarpal/metatarsal physis commonly incurs this injury when the mare steps on the foal. The periosteum is torn on the convex side of the angulation but is intact on the concave side. Thus the intact periosteal hinge is always on the side of the metaphyseal fragment.[116] A similar injury also occurs in the proximal tibial physis in slightly older foals.

Closed reduction with casting is usually possible for most metacarpal/metatarsal type 2 physeal injuries; both the intact periosteal hinge and the metaphyseal fragment prevent overreduction. These fractures can also be stabilized with internal fixation using lag screws. In foals, there is no real evidence to indicate to what degree this injury interferes with growth. If the injury involves a physis that has minimal residual growth left (such as the distal physis of the third metacarpal/metatarsal bone or the proximal physis of the proximal phalanx), then the

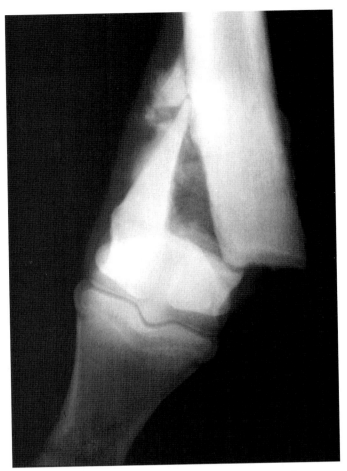

Figure 6.5 Dorsoplantar view of the distal metatarsus of a weanling with a chronic type 2 physeal fracture.

is weaker than the surrounding bone, ligamentous structures, and joint capsule. Physeal and epiphyseal injuries account for approximately 15% of all fractures in children and occur commonly in foals. Injuries that would normally produce a ruptured ligament or joint dislocation in an adult may produce traumatic separation of the physis in a young animal. For example, trauma to the fetlock region usually causes fetlock luxations in adult horses and a distal metacarpal/metatarsal physeal fractures in foals (Fig. 6.5). Joint luxations are rare in young horses.

Classification of Physeal Injuries

The most widely accepted classification of growth plate injuries is based on the Salter-Harris system, which separates the injuries into six types.[117] This system has been applied to domestic animals, including horses, although at times somewhat artificially (Fig. 6.6).[35] The main purpose of the classification system in horses is to permit equine clinicians to communicate effectively when describing such injuries. Pediatricians have used it to correlate the injury with the method of treatment and prognosis with respect to growth disturbance. Some of this information is applicable to foals, but in many cases

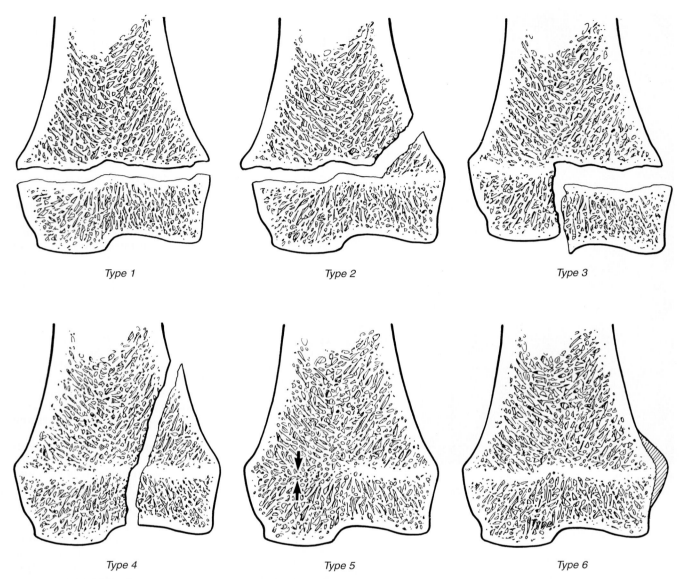

Figure 6.6   Salter-Harris classification of physeal injuries. (Reprinted with permission from Salter RB, Harris WR. Injuries involving the epiphyseal plate. J Bone Joint Surg [Am] 1963;45:587.)

potential for interference with growth is probably negligible. In contrast, type 2 fractures of the proximal tibial physis in young foals, which are best repaired with internal fixation, may result in growth disturbances in the affected limb, because of the increased growth potential remaining in this physis.

Type 3 Injury

Type 3 injuries involve intraarticular fractures that extend from the joint surface to the deep zone of the physeal plate and then along the plate to its periphery (Fig. 6.6).[117] This type of injury is uncommon in children and foals (Fig. 6.7). It is usually caused by an intraarticular shearing force and is usually limited to the distal tibial physis in children. A foal with a type 3 injury requires open reduction and internal fixation to reconstruct the

joint surface to prevent the development of secondary osteoarthritis.

Type 4 Injury

A type 4 injury is a fracture that is intraarticular, extending from the joint surface through the epiphysis, across the entire thickness of the physeal plate, and through a portion of the metaphysis (Fig. 6.6). In children, the most common example of this injury is a fracture of the capitulum of the humerus. This type of fracture does occur in foals, although rarely.

Open reduction and internal fixation with lag screws is necessary not only to restore a normal joint surface but also to obtain perfect apposition of the physeal plate. It has been observed in children that unless the fractured surfaces of the physeal plate are kept perfectly reduced,

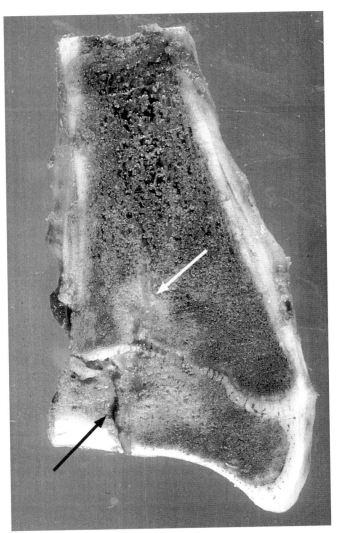

Figure 6.7   Postmortem specimen of the distal tibial of a foal with a type 3 physeal fracture (black arrow) that presumably occurred secondary to infectious physitis. The foal presented with infection of the tarsocrural joint; but radiographs revealed severe lysis within the physis, metaphysis (white arrow), and epiphysis of the distal tibia. The fracture occurred a few days after the start of treatment.

fracture healing occurs across the plate and renders further longitudinal growth impossible. The prognosis for growth after a type 4 injury is poor unless perfect reduction is achieved and maintained.[116]

Type 5 Injury

Type 5 injury is uncommon in foals and children (Fig. 6.6).[117,140] It results from a severe crushing force applied through the epiphysis to one region of the physeal plate. It is seen in the knees and ankles of children and in the distal ulnar physis of dogs. Whether this injury occurs in foals is open to speculation. It may be associated with the distal third metacarpal/metatarsal physes in cases of severe varus deformity of the fetlock or the distal radial physis with severe carpal valgus. Excessive trauma to

one part of the physis may be responsible for the severity of these deformities, although this is difficult to document.

Type 6 Injury

Type 6 injuries are characterized by the development of a periosteal bridge between the metaphysis and epiphysis (Figs. 6.6 and 6.8A). The new bone acts as a restraint to growth on the affected side of the physis and has the same effect as a transphyseal staple or screws and wire. This type of injury may occur as a result of excessive trauma during placement or removal of staples or screws and wire, secondary to local infectious periostitis, or spontaneously from external trauma.

Attempts to alter the growth on the opposite side of the physis usually results in only temporary improvement. Removal of the periosteal bridge, to help restore further growth, and transphyseal bridging on the opposite side of the physis are necessary to correct the problem (Fig. 6.8B). This approach was reported to resolve successfully type 6 lesions of the distal radial physis in three horses.[44]

DEVELOPMENTAL ORTHOPEDIC DISEASES

Developmental orthopedic disease (DOD) complex is a group of abnormalities that occurs in foals and young growing horses.[154] Terms that are often used interchangeably with DOD are osteodystrophy and osteochondrosis, although such terminology is considered erroneous. Most of the diseases included in the DOD complex can be attributed to alterations in bone growth or development (endochondral ossification) at either the metaphyseal or the epiphyseal growth plates. These include physitis, angular limb deformities, osteochondritis dissecans (OCD), subchondral cystic lesions, cuboidal bone collapse or incomplete ossification, juvenile arthritis, cervical vertebral malformation (CVM), and flexural deformities.[69,154]

Clinical signs of these conditions are variable but, because this is an abnormality of developing bone, are usually seen in young horses. Signs include some degree of lameness, alteration in posture or positioning of the limb, crooked legs, joint effusion, limb enlargement, ataxia (CVM only), and possible fractures. In addition, multiple DOD conditions may be present in the same animal.

Although the exact cause for DOD is not known, there are multiple risk factors that appear to predispose young horses to the development of these diseases. Many of the risk factors are of human making (e.g., management and breeding practices), and others have been extrapolated from research work in other species.[37,56,103] For instance, breeding for rapidly growing offspring that, it is hoped, will do better in the show ring and the feeding of rations high in energy and protein appear to predispose the animals to DOD abnormalities, presumably by contributing to rapid bone growth.

Other risk factors are mineral imbalances (e.g., copper deficiency, excess zinc), trauma, and genetic predilection.[118,150] Trace mineral deficiency—copper, in particular—has been incriminated in physitis and angular

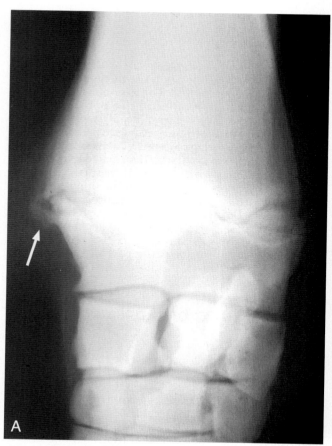

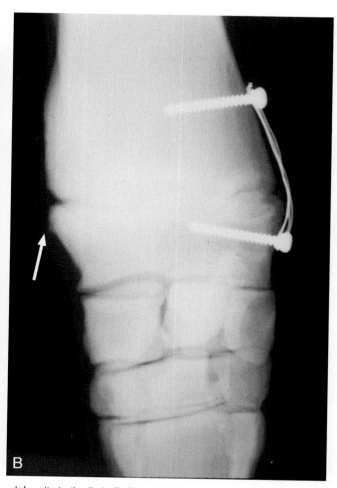

Figure 6.8 Dorsopalmar views of a yearling with a carpal varus deformity. A. An exostosis (arrow) bridged the medial aspect of the distal radial physis and was thought to be causing decreased growth on the medial aspect of the physis, contributing to the deformity in the limb. B. The exostosis was surgically removed (arrow), and transphyseal bridging was performed on the opposite side of the physis to attempt correction of the varus deformity.

deformities in cattle[126] and has been shown to cause clinical signs and joint pathology consistent with osteochondrosis in foals.[65,66] Copper is required for the enzyme lysyl oxidase, which itself is necessary for collagen cross-linking. Therefore, defective collagen cross-linking may impair the strength of bone collagen, producing essentially a "soft bone syndrome," particularly in the metaphyseal regions.[65] Excess zinc or alterations in the calcium to phosphorus ratio in the diet may also lead to clinical problems of DOD, but these are less well defined in horses than is copper deficiency.[118]

Trauma to the metaphyseal or epiphyseal growth plates can contribute to altered growth, subchondral bone damage, and avulsion of defective bone, all of which may also predispose the horse to DOD conditions. Genetics most likely plays a role in the occurrence of these diseases, but its contribution is difficult to determine. In most cases, however, the underlying cause of the DOD condition is multifactorial, usually obscure, and often never determined.[154]

Physitis

Physitis (or, as it is more commonly referred to, epiphysitis) is an important generalized bone disease of young growing horses characterized by enlargement of the growth plates of certain long bones.[150] It usually occurs in young, rapidly growing horses such as foals and weanlings and has a peak incidence between 4 and 8 months of age. Yearlings and even 2-year-old horses may develop the condition, however. The terms "physitis" and "epiphysitis" may be misnomers, since there is no active inflammation within the epiphysis, physis, or metaphysis of affected bones.[21] "Physeal dysplasia" may be a more appropriate term, since the condition is characterized by a disruption of endochondral ossification within the physeal growth cartilage.[19,21] This dysplasia leads to the classic signs of inflammation (heat, pain, and swelling) around the affected physis, however, contributing to use of the common terms physitis and epiphysitis.

Although the exact cause of physitis is unknown, it is most likely multifactorial and may differ from case to case.[19] For instance, in foals with multiple-limb involvement, a nutritional problem affecting the entire animal seems most plausible. In contrast, physitis involving one site is most likely the result of trauma or excessive compression of the affected physis.[111] Foals with severe lameness in one limb may develop physitis and an angular limb deformity in the contralateral limb because of excessive weight bearing. In many cases, however, physitis appears to have a mechanical as well as a nutritional component. Affected animals are frequently heavily muscled and overweight and are being fed excessively for rapid growth. Regions of disturbed ossification within the physis from any of these factors are susceptible to trauma and may predispose the underlying subchondral bone to microfractures. These microfractures could cause clinical signs of inflammation and potentially stimulate bone production and the remodeling that is often seen radiographically in horses with physitis.

Physitis is often referred to as "physeal compression," which further emphasizes the mechanical component of this condition. When compression is applied to a physis, an increased thickening of the physis occurs because of retardation of provisional calcification and increased survival of chondrocytes.[140] This is an autocorrection phenomenon in which the animal compensates for any minor angulation of the limb axis. If the compression is beyond the physiologic limits of the physis, however, complete arrest of endochondral ossification may occur (Fig. 6.4). The result is asynchronous physeal growth and the development of an angular limb deformity in conjunction with physitis.

The clinical appearance of a horse with physitis is characterized by enlargement of the physes primarily of the distal aspects of the radius, tibia, and third metacarpal and third metatarsal bones (Fig. 6.9). The metaphyseal flaring results in an hourglass shape to the bones; the enlargement is often painful to deep palpation, and increased heat can be detected. Physitis of the distal aspect of the cannon bones often involves all four limbs (Fig. 6.10), whereas the distal aspect of the radius and tibia are usually not involved concurrently. Foals with metacarpal/metatarsal physitis are usually younger than foals with physitis in other locations. This may be related to the activity of the physes with respect to bone growth at different ages.

Lameness varies from slight stiffness in gait to overt pain and a reluctance to stand.[19,150] Severely affected animals may have concurrent angular limb (Fig. 6.11) or flexural deformities because of disturbed physeal bone growth and chronic pain, respectively. In addition, phy-

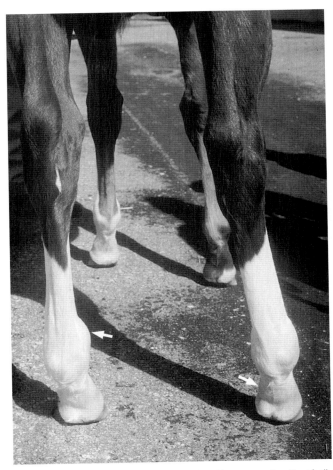

Figure 6.10 A 4-month-old Paint colt with severe physitis of all four distal cannon bones. Note the large swellings of the distal metatarsal physes as well as varus deformities of both rear fetlocks (arrows).

sitis and osteochondrosis affecting the cervical vertebrae may predispose the animal to the vertebral column malformations seen with "wobbler syndrome" in young horses. Severe malformation results in a compressive myelopathy, and a neurologic deficit is appreciated clinically (Fig. 6.12).

The most common radiographic abnormality observed with physitis is paraphyseal bone production, which is often termed "physeal lipping" or "metaphyseal flaring."[19,150] Widening of the physis, asymmetry of the metaphysis, wedging of the epiphysis, metaphyseal sclerosis adjacent to the physis, and an asymmetry of cortical thickness resulting from altered stress on the limb are less commonly observed (Fig. 6.13). Concurrent angular limb deformities or osteochondrosis lesions may also be present.[150]

One of the first steps in treating physitis is to evaluate the feed ration (see Chapter 5). A geographic nutritional deficiency often exists, especially when multiple animals are affected. The ration should be altered accordingly, and many times a reduction in the body weight or the growth rate of the animal is advised. In general, the quantity of protein and energy fed to affected horses should be decreased by feeding less grain and protein

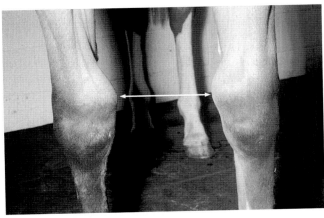

Figure 6.9 Typical swellings on the medial aspects of the distal radial physes (arrow) seen in weanlings or yearlings with physitis. This filly had been receiving an excessive amount of corn as a concentrate in her diet.

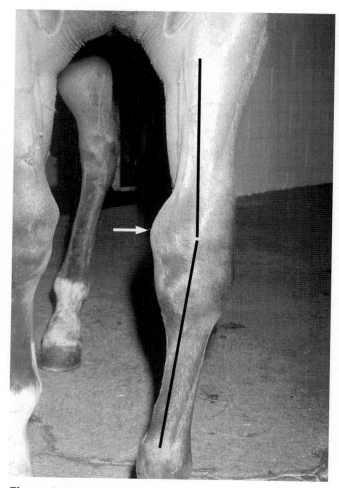

Figure 6.11 Physitis of the medial aspect of the distal radius in a 12-month-old colt, which occurred after being kicked in this area (arrow). A varus deformity of the carpus developed after the trauma (lines).

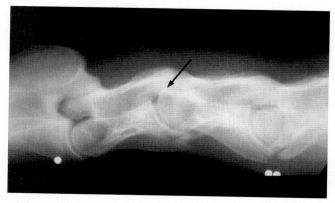

Figure 6.12 Lateral view of the proximal cervical region of a young horse with clinical signs of severe neurologic disease. Note the significant malalignment of the vertebral column (arrow), presumably caused by a developmental abnormality of the bones.

supplements and by either decreasing the quantity of alfalfa hay or replacing it with good-quality grass hay. With nursing foals, the milk production of the mare should be decreased, if possible. In recent years, many feed companies have developed specific balanced rations for growing horses to minimize the development of physitis and other DOD diseases (e.g., Equine Junior, Purina Mills, Inc., St. Louis, MO). We have minimal experience with the success of these rations.

Nonsteroidal anti-inflammatory drugs (NSAIDs) are indicated in most cases to decrease physeal inflammation and to improve the animal's stiff gait. NSAIDs help diminish pain and prevent the development of flexural deformities. These drugs may be required for 2 to 4 weeks at low doses (oral phenylbutazone, every other day, works well). Further trauma to the physis should be prevented by minimizing exercise (confinement) and correcting predisposing causes, such as angular limb deformities. Fortunately, mild cases of physitis are often self-limiting and resolve when skeletal maturity is reached and growth of the affected physis ceases.[140] More severe cases of physitis that have concurrent orthopedic abnormalities may cause residual problems severe enough to limit future athletic soundness.

Angular Limb Deformities

Causes of angular limb deformities in foals include laxity of periarticular supporting tissues, defective or delayed ossification of the tarsal or carpal cuboidal bones, direct trauma to the physis (as from concussion or fracture), traumatic luxation or fracture of the carpal bones, and asynchronous longitudinal growth of the metaphysis and epiphysis. By far the most common reason for angular limb deformities in foals is asynchronous metaphyseal growth. For often-unexplained reasons, one side of the physis grows faster than the other, resulting in a deviation of the normal limb axis.[64]

Trauma in the form of abnormal pressure across the growth plate is believed to be one of the principal underlying causes of asynchronous growth.[64] Trauma may retard calcification of the matured and dying chondrocytes, resulting in thickening of the physeal plate with an increasing number of chondrocytes at the hypertrophied cell layer. If pressure is excessive, chondrocytes may undergo necrosis, and the physis may prematurely close or growth is slowed. Any factor resulting in asymmetric loading across a growth plate can lead to this sequence of events, resulting in an angular limb deformity.[43] Such factors include joint laxity, malpositioning in utero, hypoplasia of the cuboidal bones, poor foot trimming, heavy musculature, excessive activity in foals, or lameness in the opposite limb.[140]

"Valgus" and "varus" are terms used to describe angular limb deformities in foals. These terms, however, have led to confusion not only in the human literature but also in the veterinary field.[60] Valgus and varus indicate a shift outward and inward, respectively, of the distal limb from midline (distal to the site of origin).[60] Typically, the deviation is further characterized by the joint of origin of the angulation. For instance, carpal valgus refers to a deformity in which the carpus is the site of the lesion and the limb distal to this joint (the third meta-

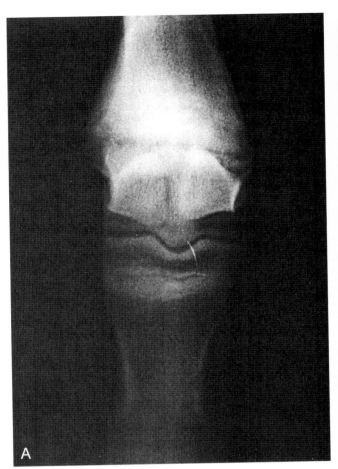 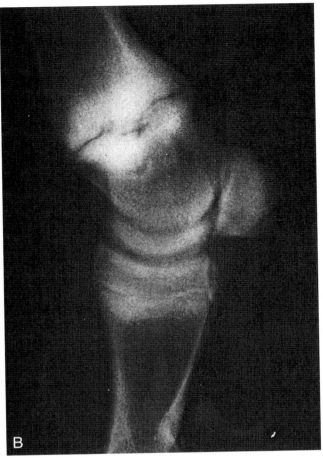

Figure 6.13 Anteroposterior (AP) (A) and lateral (B) views of the fetlock of a foal with severe epiphysitis, showing broadening and asymmetry of the metaphysis and metaphyseal sclerosis. Note the asymmetry of cortical thickness as a result of altered stresses on the limb.

carpal bone and phalanges) is deviated away from the midline of the body (Fig. 6.14). A carpal varus is when the third metacarpal bone and the fetlock are deviated toward midline, distal to the carpus (Fig. 6.11).[35]

Carpal valgus is the most common angular limb deformity seen in foals, followed by fetlock varus, carpal varus, and tarsal valgus.[42,43,64] Tarsal varus is rare, as are deviations of other parts of the limbs.[42,105] Foals with true angular limb deformities caused by asynchronous growth are typically not lame. If lameness is present, physeal trauma, fracture, or collapse of the cuboidal bones should be suspected as the cause of the limb deformity (Fig. 6.15).

Radiographs provide the most conclusive evidence for the location of the angular limb deformity. In the case of asynchronous growth across the distal radial physis, the deviation arises from the distal metaphyseal region rather than within the carpus. This can be verified by drawing lines along the long axes of the bones that bisect, in the case of a deviation of the carpal joint, the radius and the third metacarpal bone.[105,140] The lines bisect at the "pivot point" (Fig. 6.16). The pivot point in asynchronous growth of the distal radius is located within the distal radial physis, and the only radiographic abnormality is limb deviation.

Wedging of the epiphysis on the concave side of the deviation often accompanies limb deviation, but this usually resolves when the limb straightens (Fig. 6.17). Abnormal contour (shape) of the carpal cuboidal bones may also be present with severe carpal valgus, which usually resolves once the limb deviation is corrected. Severe abnormalities or crushing of the carpal or tarsal bones in conjunction with angular limb deformities is, however, a major concern and may contribute to permanent lameness problems even after the deviation is corrected.

An important factor in correcting an angular limb deformity is restriction of exercise. Foals, by their nature, will do everything possible to stay near their dams early in life, and overactivity may cause or perpetuate physeal trauma. Restricting the foal's exercise by confining the mare and foal to a large box stall or a stall and run helps minimize further trauma.[140] This should be continued until the limb has straightened. Foot trimming (or balancing) may also help minimize asymmetric physeal loading. The foot should be trimmed only to balance it, however, not to correct the angular limb deformity (see Chapter 9 for more information). Frequent reevaluations (e.g., every 2 weeks) that include radiographic examination should be performed to monitor the progress of con-

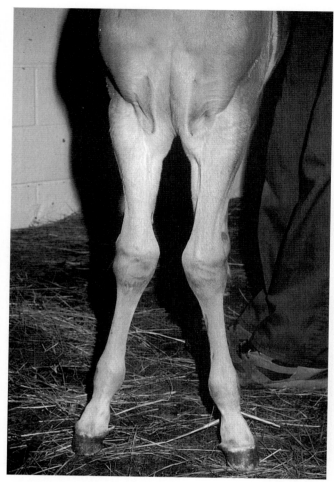

Figure 6.14 Typical clinical appearance of a young foal with bilateral carpal valgus resulting from asynchronous growth of the distal radial physis. The distal aspects of the limbs deviate laterally relative to the carpi.

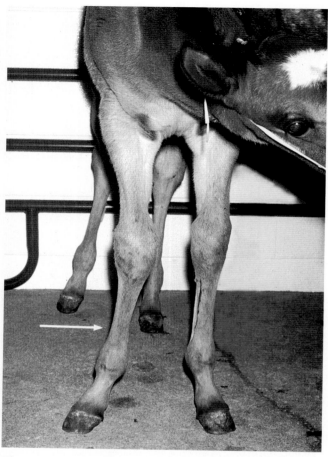

Figure 6.15 A 2-month-old foal with a valgus deformity of the right front carpus (white arrow). The foal was lame at a walk and painful to carpal flexion. Radiographs revealed carpal bone fractures with collapse of the bones, leading to the angular deformity.

servative therapy. Confinement and minor foot trimming can correct a large proportion of foals with angular limb deformities and should always be used as the initial therapy, if possible. Aggressive trimming of the foot may lead to concurrent angular deformities elsewhere in the limb, however, which may worsen the overall condition of the foal.

The growth plate of the distal aspect of metacarpus/metatarsus closes by 2 to 3 months of age, which decreases the time available for conservative therapy. In most cases, angular limb deformities of the fetlock or phalanges should be treated surgically within 30 to 45 days of age or sooner if the defects are worsening. Fretz et al.[42] analyzed a series of foals treated with transphyseal bridging across the distal extremity of the metacarpus or metatarsus. They found that surgery after 60 to 80 days resulted in virtually no improvement of the angular limb deformity but that minor limb deviations of the fetlock may be corrected with surgery after 2 months of age. The distal radial and tibial physes close at a later age; therefore, conservative therapy can be continued longer (60 to 90 days). If the deformity is severe (more

than 15°) or if limb deviation is worsening, however, then surgery should be performed as soon as possible. In most cases of carpal and tarsal deformities, surgery is indicated if the limbs are not straight by 60 days.[64,89] If the limb is nearly straight at this time, the surgeon may wait an additional 30 days, but surgery should not be delayed beyond 3 to 4 months of age. Minor deviations of the carpus and tarsus can be corrected in foals after 6 months of age, because a limited amount of growth potential remains in the physis. This may vary among horses, however, and waiting this long to see if the limb deviation corrects spontaneously is not recommended.

Surgical treatment of foals with angular limb deformities is directed toward accelerating growth on the concave side, slowing growth on the convex side, or a combination of the two. The most commonly used approach is to stimulate growth (endochondral ossification) on the concave side of the deformity[5–7,43] by using hemicircumferential transection of the periosteum (HCTP) and periosteal stripping (PS).[43,59] The mechanism contributing to physeal growth stimulation by PS is thought to be a mechanical release of the periosteal restraint of growth on the side of the physis on which the procedure is per-

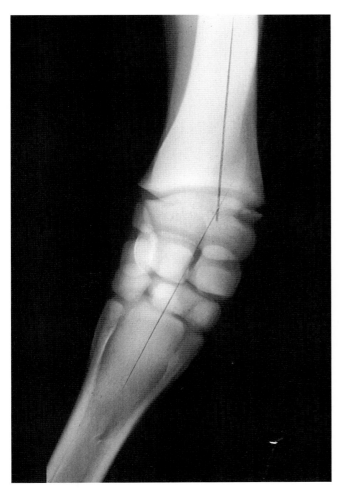

Figure 6.16 Dorsopalmar view of the carpus of a foal with an angular limb deformity. Lines drawn through the centers of the radius and metacarpus demonstrate the location of the growth disturbance within the distal radial physis.

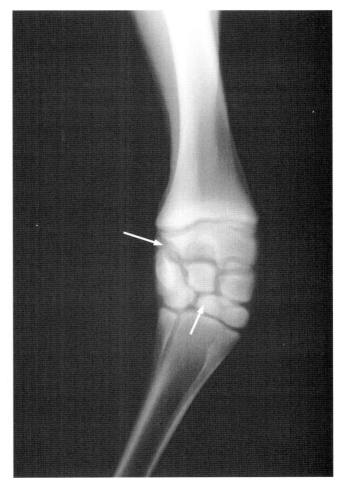

Figure 6.17 Dorsopalmar view of the carpus of a foal with severe carpal valgus. The limb deformity has resulted in wedging of the lateral aspect of the distal radial epiphysis and the lateral aspect of the third carpal bone (arrows).

formed.[58] The advantages of PS are that the procedure is easy to perform, there are minimal complications, and the limb does not overcorrect. PS alone will often not completely correct severe angular limb deformities, however.

Retardation of endochondral ossification on the convex side of the deformity is performed by various transphyseal bridging procedures.[89] The "bridges" are usually in the form of staples or screws and wires spanning the growth plate on one side (Fig. 6.18).[64] After placement of the implants, continued endochondral ossification causes a buildup of internal forces and a gradual decline in growth mainly because of the effects of pressure on the vascularity and subsequent osteogenesis of the physis. Slowed growth on one side of the physis and continued growth on the opposite equalizes the relative length of the medial and lateral aspects of the distal metaphysis, thereby straightening the limb. Once the limb is straight, the implants must be removed or the limb will overcorrect. Once the implants are removed, normal limb growth will continue.

The advantages of the growth retardation procedure are that severe deformities can be corrected quickly and,

some surgeons believe, the procedure is much more effective than HCTP plus PS. The disadvantages of the growth retardation procedure are that it is more difficult to perform, there are more wound healing complications, and if the owners fail to monitor the limb, it can overcorrect. For these reasons, most surgeons use transphyseal bridging for severe deformities that will not correct with HCTP plus PS alone or in older horses in which the growth potential of the physis may be limited. In most situations in which transphyseal bridging is used, it is combined with HCTP plus PS on the same limb (at least we do this). This further speeds resolution of the deformity by promoting growth on one side of the physis while slowing growth on the other side. The details of surgery for growth retardation and stimulation are discussed in Chapter 8.

Incomplete Cuboidal Bone Ossification and Juvenile Spavin

Incomplete ossification of the cuboidal bones of the carpus or tarsus occurs most commonly in premature

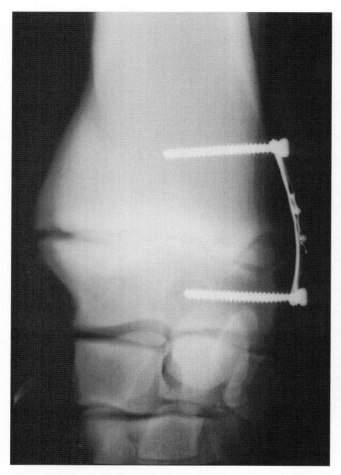

Figure 6.18 Transphyseal bridging (screws and wires) of the lateral aspect of the distal radial physis, used to correct the varus deformity of the carpus of the horse shown in Figure 6.11. Radiographic evidence of physitis (paraphyseal bone formation or lipping) is seen on the medial aspect of the physis.

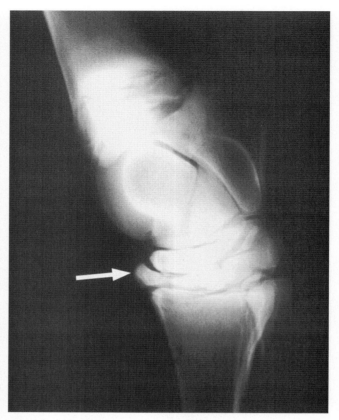

Figure 6.19 Lateral view of the tarsus in a yearling that presented with lameness in the left hindlimb. A valgus deformity of the tarsus was evident clinically, and collapse of the dorsal aspect of the third tarsal bone was evident radiographically (arrow). Collapse of the bone had presumably occurred early in life and was not recognized as a problem until the lameness developed.

foals, twins, or underdeveloped newborn foals. At birth, the cuboidal bones have not ossified sufficiently to withstand the forces of normal weight bearing, predisposing the animal to some degree of carpal or tarsal bone wedging or collapse. Incomplete ossification without collapse is not readily apparent clinically and is best diagnosed with radiography to document abnormal cuboidal bone appearance. Clinical signs associated with cuboidal bone collapse may be evident in the newborn foal as an angular limb deformity of the carpus or tarsus.

Collapse of the tarsal bones is much more common than collapse of the carpal bones. Tarsal collapse is often associated with a sickle or cow-hocked conformation of the tarsus, or the tarsus looks like it has a "curb." The degree of lameness is variable and may not become clinically apparent until later in life. Preventing cuboidal bone collapse in newborn foals with incomplete ossification involves minimizing compressive forces on the bones until they ossify. Confinement, sleeve casts, bandages, or bandages and splints may be used, depending on the severity. In one study, foals with only minor tarsal bone collapse were able to perform as intended, whereas

foals with more severe tarsal bone collapse and fragmentation could not be used for their intended purposes (Fig. 6.19).[31]

In addition, incomplete ossification and mild collapse of the tarsal bones is thought to predispose the horse to juvenile spavin. Horses with juvenile spavin have relatively severe signs of bone spavin at a young age with a history of minimal work (Fig. 6.20). Inherent abnormalities of the central and third tarsal bones are thought to contribute to the development of osteoarthritis in the distal tarsal joints at such an early age.

Osteochondritis Dissecans

Osteochondritis dissecans refers to cartilage or cartilage and bone (osteochondral) fragments or flaps that develop along the articular surfaces of joints in horses. These abnormalities are probably the most common manifestation of the DOD complex in horses. They usually occur along the non-weight-bearing surfaces of the joint and are especially common in the stifle, tarsus, and fetlock joints (Fig. 6.21).[150] Horses with OCD lesions typically are only mildly lame but usually have joint effusion of the affected joint(s). These lesions are often bilateral and may or may not require arthroscopic surgery to

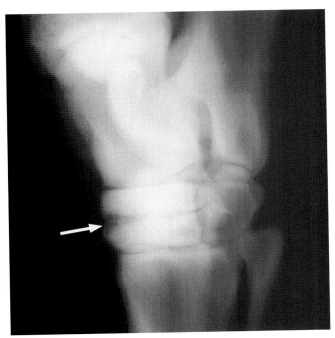

Figure 6.20   Oblique view of the tarsus in a 2-year-old Paint filly with hindlimb lameness. Subchondral bone lysis (arrow) and narrowing of the distal intertarsal joint can be seen.

remove the osteochondral fragment(s). The prognosis for performance of horses with OCD lesions is usually very good (see Chapter 7 for a more detailed discussion).

Subchondral Cystic Lesions

Subchondral cystic lesions (bone cysts or osseous cyst-like lesions) are commonly recognized pathologic entities of bones and joints in horses that may or may not cause lameness. Subchondral cystic lesions may be nonarticular or articular, although most lesions that contribute to lameness involve the weight-bearing area of an articular surface. Nonarticular lesions (which may be classified as subchondral cystic lesions) usually involve the metaphysis and can go undiagnosed because they do not always cause clinical signs and normal bone remodeling may resolve the defect.

The most common age for diagnosis of subchondral cystic lesions or at least the time when clinical signs develop is usually 3 years or younger.[9,61] Horses demonstrate clinical signs related to subchondral cystic lesions over a wide age range, however, and the relationship between when the lesion develops and when the horse begins to show clinical signs is not known.[70] This relationship probably depends on the specific site of the subchondral cystic lesion (most common location is the medial femoral condyle), the age at which the lesion develops, and the occupation of the horse. What causes or initiates the appearance of clinical signs in horses with articular subchondral cystic lesions remains unknown.

Subchondral cystic lesions have been reported to occur at multiple locations in horses.[9,18] The most common sites that contribute to clinical problems involve the stifle (Fig. 6.22), fetlock, pastern, coffin, and elbow joints. Controversy exists over whether these lesions are caused by a defect in endochondral ossification, intraarticular subchondral bone trauma, or a combination of both.[9,18,70] Joint trauma can lead to the development of

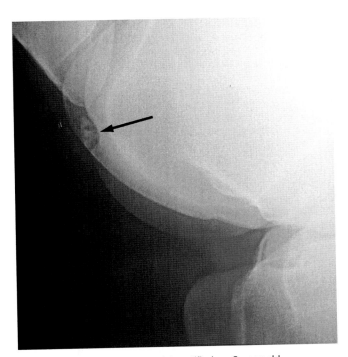

Figure 6.21   Lateral view of the stifle in a 3-year-old Thoroughbred with clinical evidence of femoropatellar joint effusion. Osteochondral fragmentation (arrow) typical of OCD lesions is seen on the lateral trochlear ridge of the femur.

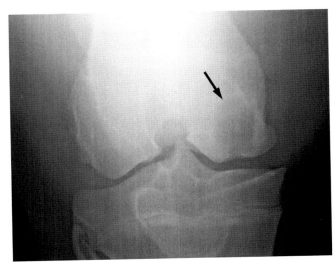

Figure 6.22   Craniocaudal view of the stifle, showing a large subchondral cystic lesion within the medial femoral condyle (arrow) of a yearling Quarter Horse filly. The filly was lame at a walk and had palpable effusion of the medial femorotibial joint.

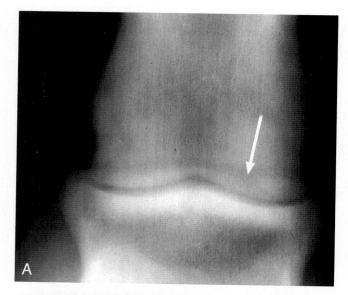

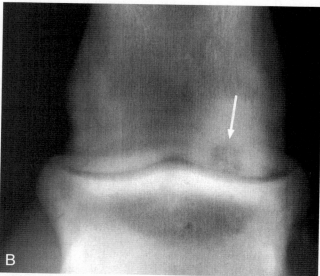

Figure 6.23 Dorsoplantar views of the pastern of a 12-year-old Thoroughbred with a grade 3 (out of 5) hindlimb lameness. A. Minimal abnormalities (arrow) are visible on the initial radiograph. B. A subchondral cystic lesion with surrounding sclerosis (arrow) is evident within the proximal phalanx 6 months later.

subchondral cystic lesions, which has been shown experimentally and has been seen clinically (Fig. 6.23).[9] Many of these lesions, however, are seen in young horses and are bilateral, suggesting a developmental defect.

Subchondral cystic lesions have been described as resulting from an infolding of abnormal cartilage into the underlying bony spongiosa.[9] The infolded cartilage becomes necrotic, and its matrix remains nonmineralized. Thus osteoclasts and blood vessels do not migrate into the defect to enable repair of the defective cartilage and bone. The cystic lining is made up of fibrous tissue with active fibroplasia and capillary proliferation present in the tissue adjacent to the bone.

Treatment of subchondral cystic lesions involves the use of either intraarticular medications (combined with

systemic joint therapies) or surgical debridement of the lesion.[61] Because of the variable prognosis of horses undergoing debridement of the lesion alone, additional treatment of the bone defect is being attempted by some surgeons. Such treatments include packing the entire defect with cancellous bone and packing the depth of the lesion with cancellous bone and then filling the remaining bone defect with fibrin-laden chondrocytes that contain growth factors. The goals of the latter treatment are to promote healing of both the bone and the articular cartilage defects. Nonsurgical treatment is usually recommended initially in most horses because of the variable success of surgical debridement of the lesions, with or without the adjunctive treatments.

LOCAL DISEASES OF BONE

Exercise-Induced Remodeling

Bone is metabolically active under normal physiologic circumstances and in response to many types of injury. Its intricate microstructural and macrostructural organizations, combined with its high rate of metabolic activity, allow it to respond rapidly to many physical and biomechanical demands.[78] Normal daily activity and exercise impose complex forces on the skeletal system that cause different quantities of deformations of bone.

Deformations within a bone are referred to as "strains," and the local force intensities at these sites are the "stresses," defined as a given force per unit area. The direction and magnitude of the stresses and strains depend on the geometry of the bone, the direction and magnitude of the load imposed on the bone, and the material properties of the bone. Equine bone remodels in response to the stresses placed on it according to Wolff's law, which, in brief, states that bone is laid down where it is needed and is resorbed where it is not needed. Two examples of adaptive remodeling in equine bone are 1) the cancellous portions of the proximal sesamoid bones are less porous (stiffer and stronger) in horses trained on dirt tracks than in untrained horses[155] and 2) the shape of the metacarpus changes during training and racing to withstand the added forces applied to the bone.[96,98] These are only a couple of examples of bone's response to exercise, which undoubtedly occurs in every bone during training and performance.

The osteogenic response of bone to remodeling stimuli, such as training and exercise, appears to depend most on the strain magnitude and strain rate. In other words, the greater the load and the more times bone is loaded (repetitions), the greater the remodeling response. Increased magnitude of loading can be achieved by going at higher speeds, training on harder surfaces, or a combination of the two.

Too high loads or excessive repetitions of normal loads are thought to contribute to the development of dorsal metacarpal disease or stress or fatigue fractures in racehorses.[96,97,136] Fatigue fractures indicate that the bone has not remodeled or gained enough strength to withstand the forces (loads) that are being applied to it.[97] In most cases, the exercise regimen should be altered to permit the bone to gain adequate strength to tolerate the higher loads.

If an excessive load is applied to a bone as a single event, the ultimate stresses and strains that the tissue can tolerate are exceeded, and a complete fracture occurs. Single-event trauma is the most likely cause of complete fractures in most horses and foals. Fatigue and stress fractures in bone appear to predispose the horse to complete fractures, however, especially in performance horses, presumably by decreasing the ultimate load that the bone can withstand before fracturing.

Fracture

When a fracture occurs, the bone usually loses structural continuity, and its function is impaired to some degree. The level of altered function and the specific bone that is fractured often determine the type and severity of lameness. For example, a displaced fracture of the olecranon process or a fracture of one of the major load-bearing bones (e.g., radius or tibia) usually produces a severe lameness. Conversely, a so-called osteochondral or "chip" fracture of a carpal bone produces a mild lameness, which may resolve with rest or may predispose the horse to degenerative joint disease, causing a secondary lameness. Most acute fractures cause significant lameness, however, regardless of their size and location. A fracture should always be considered as a possible cause of any non-weight-bearing lameness.

Fractures in horses are usually the result of a single high-energy traumatic event that completely disrupts the bone (breaks the bone into at least two pieces). Incomplete or stress fractures are diagnosed more frequently in performance horses than in other types of horses. Unlike most complete fractures, stress fractures are caused by chronic trauma that weakens the bone, not a single traumatic event that breaks the bone.[136]

Stress fractures of the humerus, tibia (Fig. 6.24), pelvis, and metacarpus/metatarsus have been diagnosed in performance horses (primarily racehorses).[136,137] Initially, these lesions cause some degree of lameness and may contribute to complete fracture of the involved bone with continued use.[137] Diagnosis of incomplete fractures in racehorses can be difficult but is critical to prevent catastrophic bone failure. Scintigraphy can help the clinician locate suspected stress fractures that are not apparent on radiographs.

Treatment of incomplete fractures is much less complicated than treatment of complete fractures and usually involves a period of inactivity combined with a change in training schedule. In contrast, complete fractures of long bones of horses are one of the most difficult injuries to treat successfully, and many horses with severe fractures are still euthanized (Fig. 6.25). The prognosis of repairing complete fractures in horses depends, in part, on the specific bone affected, the temperament of the horse, the age and size of the horse, the specific characteristics of the fracture, and the expertise of the surgeon. Proper stabilization of the fracture for transport to a surgical facility for repair is crucial to achieving a favorable outcome.

Fracture Stabilization and Immobilization

Fractures are a frequently diagnosed problem in horses and often require emergency first aid treatment

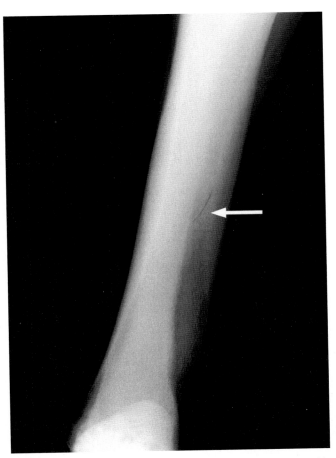

Figure 6.24   Oblique view of the tibia in a young racehorse with a hindlimb lameness that could not be localized with regional nerve blocks. An incomplete spiral fracture of the middle to distal diaphysis of the tibia is evident (arrow).

(Table 6.1). Horses are not readily ambulatory on three limbs and often become anxious when they are unable to place a fractured limb, which potentially can result in further injury. First aid measures should be directed toward minimizing further damage to the fractured limb and maintaining it in a position and condition that will facilitate repair.

The goals of first aid fracture management are to prevent damage to neural and vascular elements of the limb, to prevent skin penetration of the fracture fragments, to minimize further contamination of an existing wound, to relieve the animal's anxiety by stabilizing the fractured limb, and to minimize further damage to the fractured bone ends and surrounding soft tissue.[16,17] Most of these objectives can be accomplished by proper stabilization or splinting of the fracture. Fractures of the upper forelimb and hindlimb in horses are, however, nearly impossible to stabilize with external splints. Luckily, the bones in these locations are surrounded by large muscle groups, which inherently stabilize the fracture ends, making external coaptation less important.

Fracture immobilization serves several purposes. Immobilization in horses is more important to preserve limb vascularity than to prevent hemorrhage at the frac-

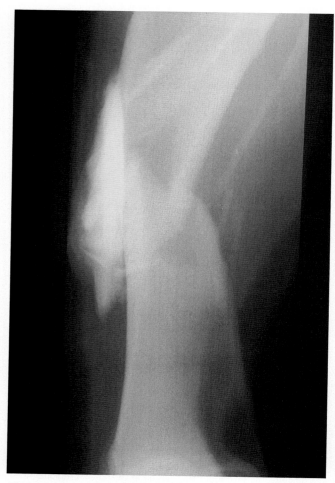

Figure 6.25 Craniocaudal view of the tibia in an adult mare, demonstrating a complete, highly comminuted and severely displaced diaphyseal fracture.

Table 6.1 CONTENTS OF FRACTURE FIRST AID KIT FOR HORSES

Material	Purpose
Cotton, rolled and/or sheet	Padding under splint-cast combination or Robert-Jones bandage
Gauze, sterile and nonsterile	Applying dressing to wounds and Robert-Jones bandage
Razor or portable clippers	Removing hair from around wound
Antibiotic ointment	Topical dressing for open wounds
Support wrap (Vetrap, Elastikon, etc.)	Robert-Jones bandage or bandage under splint-cast combination
White tape	Secure splints or boards to bandage
PVC splints (several lengths)	Splint-cast combination
Fiberglass cast material	Splint-cast combination
Board splints (several lengths) or aluminum rod	Splinting radial and tibial fractures
Drugs (antibiotics, sedatives, NSAIDs)	Tranquilization, pain relief, and treatment of open fractures

PVC, polyvinyl chloride; NSAIDs, nonsteroidal anti-inflammatory drugs.

ture site. Severe hemorrhage infrequently accompanies fractures in horses, but vascular thrombosis from continued stretching and direct trauma often leads to diminished vascularity of the distal limb. Limb immobilization also reduces the animal's anxiety, enabling the horse to regain control of the limb, even though the limb cannot bear weight. Once stabilized, most horses will rest the limb instead of continually trying to place it in a normal stance, which would cause further soft tissue and bone damage. Probably the most important purpose of immobilization is to prevent the development of an open fracture. Loss of intact skin coverage over a fracture is thought to predispose the horse to infection, especially if internal fixation is performed. Equine skin is thin and readily penetrated by sharp bone fragments. In general, fractures of the distal (phalanges) and upper (humerus, ulna, and femur) aspects of the horse's limbs rarely become open, suggesting that proper immobilization of fractures involving the metacarpus/metatarsus, radius, and tibia is most critical to prevent the development of an open fracture during transport. For the purposes of fracture immobilization, the horse's forelimbs and hindlimbs are divided into specific anatomic regions to help guide proper fracture splinting techniques (Fig. 6.26).

PHALANGES AND DISTAL METACARPALS

The phalanges and distal metacarpals are probably the most common sites for fractures to occur in horses, and biomechanically they are dominated by the angle of the fetlock joint.[16,17] Therefore, proper splinting techniques should attempt to counteract the bending force at the fetlock. A cotton bandage combined with a dorsally placed polyvinyl chloride (PVC) splint or a splint-cast combination with the limb maintained in a straight line from the carpus to the hoof appears to provide the optimal immobilization (Fig. 6.27). Minimal padding (light bandage) should be used for the splint-cast combination, whereas a regular cotton bandage should be applied if a dorsal splint alone is used. To facilitate application of the splint and cast material, an assistant should hold the forelimb proximal to the carpus and let the limb hang. The PVC splint is applied to the dorsal aspect of the limb from the carpus to the hoof and secured with white tape. For a splint-cast combination, fiberglass cast material is applied over the entire distal limb to provide further stabilization. Alternatively, a Kimzey splint or Farley compression boot may be used to stabilize fractures in this location. The disadvantages of the commercially available splints are 1) they are expensive to stock for only occasional use and 2) they cannot be easily modified to fit a variety of sizes.

MIDFORELIMB (MIDMETACARPUS TO DISTAL RADIUS)

Fractures in the midforelimb are stabilized best with a Robert-Jones bandage combined with full-limb PVC splints applied caudally and laterally.[16,17] The bandage should be applied in several layers, with each layer of padding (cotton) no more than 1 inch in thickness and compressed with elastic or brown gauze to increase stiffness. The total diameter of the finished bandage should be approximately three times as large as the diameter of the limb at the fracture site. The splints should extend from the elbow to the ground at 90° to each other to

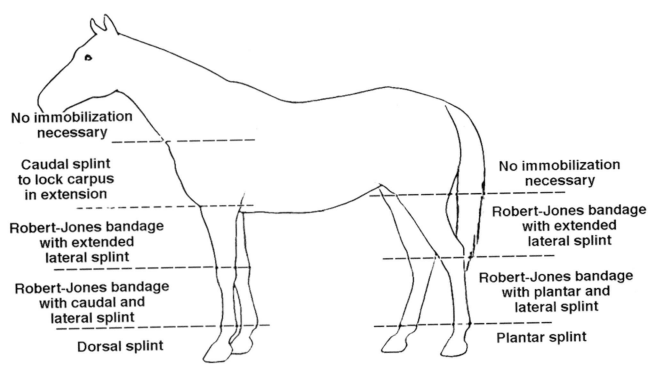

Figure 6.26 Functional division of the horse's limbs, used as a guide for appropriate application of external support to immobilize fractures during transport. (Reprinted with permission from Bramlage LR. First aid and transportation of fracture patients. In: Nixon AL, Ed. Equine Fracture Repair. Philadelphia: WB Saunders, 1996;38.)

help prevent movement of the fracture during transport. The splints should be tightly secured to the bandage with nonelastic white tape. If PVC material is not available, any lightweight, rigid material such as wood, aluminum, or flat steel may be used effectively for splinting. Fractures in this location have the advantage of having portions of the forelimb above and below the fracture site that can facilitate application of splints. Because of the sparse soft tissue coverage of the metacarpal region, however, closed fractures in this location can easily become open if they are not adequately splinted. This is especially true of foals, because their thin skin provides little resistance to bone penetration.

MIDDLE AND PROXIMAL RADIUS

Fractures in the middle and proximal radius cause the upper musculature of the forearm to abduct the distal limb.[16,17] This often results in adduction of the proximal fracture fragment and penetration of skin on the medial side because of lack of soft tissue coverage. Prevention of abduction of the distal limb is the goal when immobilizing fractures in this location. This is best achieved by applying a Robert-Jones bandage similar to that used with midforelimb fractures, but the lateral splint is extended up the lateral aspect of the shoulder, scapula, and chest and taped securely to the proximal forelimb at the level of the axilla. A wide board (15 to 20 cm) or metal rod appears to work better than PVC for this lateral splint. The upper extension of the lateral splint should lie against the shoulder and scapula so that it prevents

abduction of the distal limb during ambulation (Fig. 6.28). A PVC splint that extends from the ground to the elbow should also be placed on the caudal aspect of the limb to provide additional stability for the fracture.

PROXIMAL TO THE ELBOW

The humerus and the ulna are well protected with muscles, which inherently stabilize and protect fractures of these bones. Complete fractures of these bones disable the triceps muscle apparatus, however, making it impossible for the horse to fix the elbow in extension for weight bearing. Restoring the triceps apparatus reduces the anxiety of affected animals and enables them to use the limb for balance during transport. A full-limb cotton bandage with a caudally applied PVC splint keeps the carpus extended and helps restore triceps muscle function. Some horses with ulna fractures will bear considerable weight on the limb after splinting, but walking may be difficult. All fractures in these locations do not require stabilization, however, because the risk of skin penetration is extremely low. Foals may not have the upper forelimb strength to move the limb with a splint in place.

PHALANGES AND DISTAL METATARSALS

Fractures in the distal hindlimb can be managed similarly to those in the forelimb, except that the PVC splint used with the splint-cast combination is best placed on the plantar surface of the limb. Fiberglass cast material is applied over the splint and distal limb in a manner similar to that used with the forelimb. Splints applied to

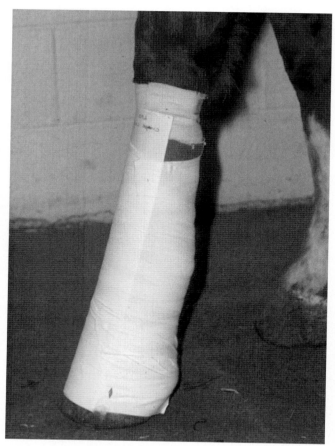

Figure 6.27 A bandage and PVC splint applied to the distal limb of a horse to immobilize a fractured phalanx. The splint was placed dorsally and secured with white nonelastic tape. (Courtesy of Dr. Chris Ray, Amarillo, TX.)

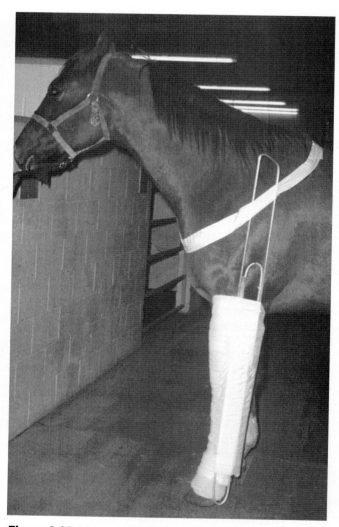

Figure 6.28 A loop of aluminum rod has been shaped to extend from the ground up over the shoulder and scapula to help immobilize a radial fracture. (Courtesy of Dr. Chris Ray, Amarillo, TX.)

the dorsal surface of the hindlimb over a bandage appear to be less useful than in the forelimb because they tend to break more readily. In addition, the Kimzey splint or Farley compression boot may be used to stabilize fractures in this location, as in the forelimb.

MIDDLE AND PROXIMAL METATARSALS

A Robert-Jones bandage, with PVC splints applied laterally and caudally with the calcaneus used as a caudal extension of the metatarsus, provide adequate support for fractures in the middle and proximal metatarsals.[16,17] The Robert-Jones bandage should be less extensive than for the forelimb because it will be difficult to secure the splints to the limb if the bandage on the distal aspect of the metatarsus is too bulky.

TARSUS AND TIBIA

Fractures in the tarsus and tibia are particularly difficult to stabilize adequately because of the reciprocal apparatus and its effect on joint motion in the tarsus and stifle.[16,17] Fractures in this location tend to collapse when the stifle flexes and the tarsus remains in a fixed position. The main principle for stabilization is similar to that of the radius, which primarily involves preventing

abduction of the distal aspect of the limb. There is little muscle coverage on the medial aspect of the tibia, and this is the site prone to become open.

To prevent abduction, a single laterally placed splint that is bent to follow the angulation of the limb and extends proximally above the stifle joint works well. The splint is most effective if it is bent back on itself to mirror the hindlimb contour back to the ground, creating a double splint. The splint is applied over a full-limb Robert-Jones bandage and is best made of lightweight metal, such as aluminum, that can be bent into the proper position, similar to the lateral support of a Schroeder-Thomas splint (Fig. 6.29). An alternative to the metal splint is a wide board (15 to 20 cm) that extends from the ground to the ilium and is applied to the lateral aspect of the bandage.

Fracture Healing

Fracture healing can be considered a series of processes that occur in sequence but are often overlapping. It

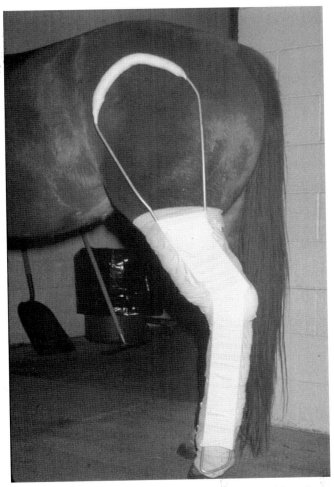

Figure 6.29 An aluminum rod was shaped to extend from the ground up over the stifle and hip of this horse with a tibial fracture. (Courtesy of Dr. Chris Ray, Amarillo, TX.)

can be divided into three distinct phases: inflammatory, reparative, and remodeling.[79] During healing, the bone will unite by one of two patterns: primary or direct healing and secondary or indirect healing. With primary bone healing, the bone ends heal directly by Haversian remodeling in contact and noncontact areas without the formation of a bone callus. Rigid fracture stabilization and correct anatomic reduction of the fracture are required for primary bone healing to occur. With secondary bone healing, fibrous tissue or fibrocartilage is initially formed between the fracture fragments; this is later replaced by new bone. Periosteal and endosteal callus formations unite the bone ends.[79]

PHASES OF THE HEALING PROCESS

The *inflammatory phase* occurs over the first 2 to 3 weeks after injury and is considered critical for the reparative phase of fracture healing that follows. During this phase, the cellular mechanisms necessary for repair and the processes protecting the healing tissue from infection are activated. If the inflammatory response is impaired, tissue healing is compromised. Chemical messengers mediate the inflammatory reaction by causing vasodilation, migration of leukocytes, and chemotaxis of substances necessary for the repair process. In particular, bone morphogenetic proteins play an important role in the initiation of fracture repair.[107]

During the *reparative phase*, the pattern of fracture healing is highly susceptible to mechanical factors, such as interfragmentary motion. With spontaneous fracture healing, periosteal and endosteal callus formation provides interfragmentary stabilization, and bone union occurs by intramembranous and endochondral ossification.[79] This process can take from 2 to 12 months to be completed, depending on the method of fracture fixation that was used, the stability of the fracture, and the size of the fracture gap (fracture displacement).

The *remodeling phase* occurs during and after the reparative phase. Avascular and necrotic regions of bone are replaced by Haversian remodeling.[79] Malalignment of fracture fragments may be corrected during this phase of healing by remodeling of the fracture site and functional adaptation, particularly in young animals. With weight bearing and loading of the fracture, bone is removed from the convex surfaces and laid down on the concave surfaces. This process tends to realign the bone after malunion (Fig. 6.40B). Fracture remodeling cannot correct torsional deformities associated with fracture healing, however. Theoretically, bone can heal completely and regain prefracture strength and function.

Fracture Fixation

In horses, more than in any other domestic animal (except perhaps the racing greyhound) the clinician must carefully define "successful" fracture healing. For centuries, bone has been observed to heal by production of callus, but the result was often angulation, rotation, or limb shortening. With intraarticular fractures, a certain amount of degenerative joint disease often developed. Fixation techniques used to achieve primary bone healing with intraarticular fractures have greatly decreased the morbidity associated with degenerative joint disease in these cases. In addition, improved techniques in internal fixation of long bone fractures have emphasized improving the implants to withstand massive functional forces, thus preventing failure caused by mechanical overload. Such implants must also be strong enough to maintain their integrity until the bone has united, without breaking under fatigue. Despite improvements in fracture fixation equipment, anesthetic protocols, and recovery methods, however, successful repair of some long bone fractures in horses remains difficult.

Stress protection is a phenomenon seen when a bone that has been rigidly immobilized by a plate undergoes certain histologic events, including loss of bone mass without a corresponding reduction in size (quantitative osteopenia).[140] Stress protection results in Haversian remodeling and has generated considerable interest in human and small animal medicine because of the potential for refracture of the bone after removal of the plate. Stress protection is almost an unknown occurrence in the horse, even in foals, because of the great loads imparted on the implants compared with those for humans and other smaller animals.[140] Although the emphasis of research activity in humans and small animals has focused on the development of more flexible implants, the emphasis in horses has been in the reverse direction: to provide stronger implants in an attempt to overcome the massive loading of the implants.

An important consideration in the horse is stress concentration. This is when biomechanical loads are concentrated in a small area of normal or weakened bone, potentially leading to complete bone failure.[140] This primarily occurs in the diaphysis of long bones but may also develop elsewhere in the bone. Examples of stress concentration include drill holes that are not filled with implants during internal fixation and vacant screw holes after implant removal (such as after metacarpal stress fracture repair).[96] In addition, stress concentration occurs at the ends of bone plates, especially if they stop in the middiaphyseal region of a bone, and at intramedullary pinhole sites after removal of external fixators. These are all places where small areas of cortical bone are absent or have been weakened, and they can fail if excessive loading of the bone occurs.

COMPRESSION

The use of various methods of compression in the treatment of fractures in humans and other animals is widely accepted. Under stable conditions, it is recognized that both cancellous and cortical bone heal by primary bone union, without callus formation. Under these circumstances, Schenk and Willenegger[121] showed that healing resulted by proliferation of new osteons growing parallel to the long axis of the bone, first through the necrotic bone ends and then across the fracture. This is termed "primary bone healing" and is the ultimate goal for repairing intraarticular fractures in horses or in any species. Compression across the fracture allows mechanical stability with little or no motion between the fragments, creating more favorable conditions for primary bone healing. Therefore, the function of the implant (plate and/or screws) with internal fixation is to hold the bone fragments under compression with little to no movement until fracture union has occurred.[140]

Compression fixation of fractures is often the goal for fracture repair in horses. Intraarticular fractures when rigidly compressed usually heal rapidly without the development of secondary degenerative joint disease. Long bone fractures repaired with bone plates can heal without exuberant callus that would interfere with nearby soft tissue structures. Compression fixation cannot be achieved in many cases, however, because of the nature of the fracture and the temperament and size of the patient. In general, compression fixation and primary bone healing can be accomplished with most intraarticular fractures in horses but is usually not achieved in long bone fractures. Most long bone fractures will develop some degree of callus formation during the healing process, which in most cases is not a major problem. Specific methods for repair of certain fractures, in particular those amenable to lag screw fixation, are discussed in Chapter 8. Here, we present general principles regarding fracture fixation in horses.

LAG SCREWS

One method for compressing a fracture is to use a lag screw, a basic technique used routinely by carpenters

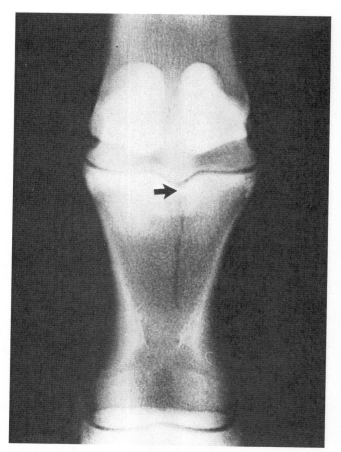

Figure 6.30 This proximal phalangeal fracture is ideal for lag screw fixation, which would minimize the chances of secondary degenerative joint disease of the fetlock joint by accurately reconstructing the intraarticular component of the fracture (arrow).

and engineers. It is particularly suited for intraarticular fractures in horses when accurate anatomic alignment of the joint surface is essential to avoid secondary degenerative joint disease (Fig. 6.30). Lag screws alone are rarely used to repair major long bone fractures in horses or even small foals because they are simply not strong enough. Lag screws are ideally suited for repairing slab fractures of the third carpal bone (Fig. 6.31), condylar fractures of the distal third metacarpal and metatarsal bones, sagittal fractures of the proximal phalanx, and some tarsal bone fractures. In addition, lag screws can be used in conjunction with plates to repair comminuted fractures, by which fracture reconstruction is performed with screws and a so-called neutralization plate is applied or the lag screws are inserted through the plate holes. A variety of sizes of cortical bone screws (3.5, 4.5, or 5.5 mm in diameter) can be used as lag screws. The 5.5-mm screw is used most often in horses because it is stronger and has more holding power than the 4.5-mm screw.

To achieve the lag screw principle, threads must gain purchase in only one bone fragment. For cortical screws, this is achieved by overdrilling the fragment next to the screw head to such a size that the screw threads will not engage that portion of the bone. The hole is termed the

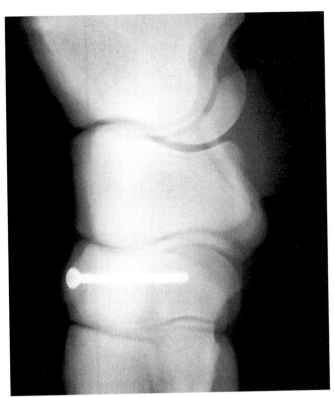

"glide hole" (Fig. 6.32). If the glide hole were not over-drilled, the tightened screw would not be able to close the gap between the fracture fragments, and no compression would be achieved. Therefore, the screw should achieve purchase only in the "far" cortex, or transcortex (i.e., the cortex away from the head).

In some areas, particularly in the metaphysis of bones in foals, the bone may be too soft for cortical screws to gain purchase. Cancellous screws can be used to achieve compression between fragments in these locations. To increase the surface area of contact between the screw and bone, the ratio between the outer diameter and the core in cancellous screws is greater than that found in a cortical screw (Fig. 6.33). A cancellous screw (6.5 mm in diameter) has a smooth shank near the head and a threaded portion near the tip (Fig. 6.34). When employed as a lag screw, the smooth shank must pass through one fragment, and the threaded portion must gain purchase in the other to achieve compression.[140]

Cancellous screws have two lengths of thread at the tip: 16 and 32 mm (Fig. 6.34). The longer threaded cancellous screws should be used whenever possible to achieve maximum holding power. Cancellous screws should be used with caution in dense cortical bone. If a cortical screw has been stripped, however, sometimes the only way to achieve compression is to use a cancellous screw in its place. During the healing process, new bone will form around the smooth shank of the cancellous screw; thus, if screw removal is necessary, the cancellous thread must be able to cut its way through the bone. If the bone around the shank is too dense, the cancellous screw may break at the screw thread junction. Therefore, whenever possible, cortical bone screws should be used in horses, with the exception of young foals with very soft bone.

To exert the maximum amount of interfragmentary compression, a lag screw should be inserted at right an-

Figure 6.31 Lateral view of the carpus in a racehorse after lag screw fixation of a third carpal bone slab fracture. A 3.5-mm cortical screw was used here.

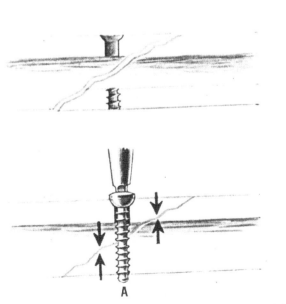

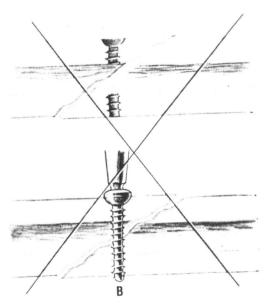

Figure 6.32 A. Correct execution of the lag screw principle. B. Incorrect execution of the lag screw principle. The cortex under the screw head was not overdrilled, and the gap between the bone fragments cannot close. (Reprinted with permission from Mueller ME, et al. Manual of Internal Fixation. 2nd ed. Heidelberg: Springer-Verlag, 1979.)

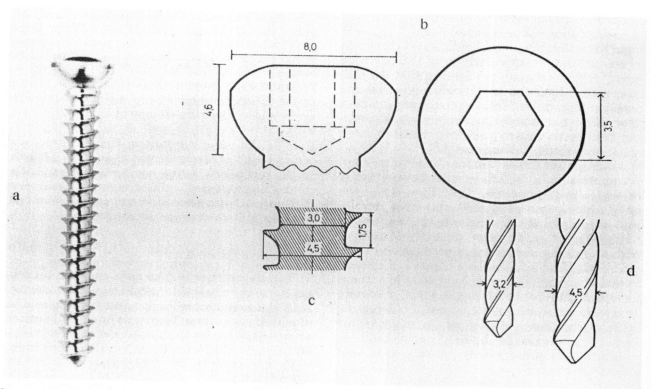

Figure 6.33   Design and dimensions of the ASIF (Association for the Study of Internal Fixation) 4.5-mm cortical screw. (Reprinted with permission from Mueller ME, et al. Manual of Internal Fixation. 2nd ed. Heidelberg: Springer-Verlag, 1979.)

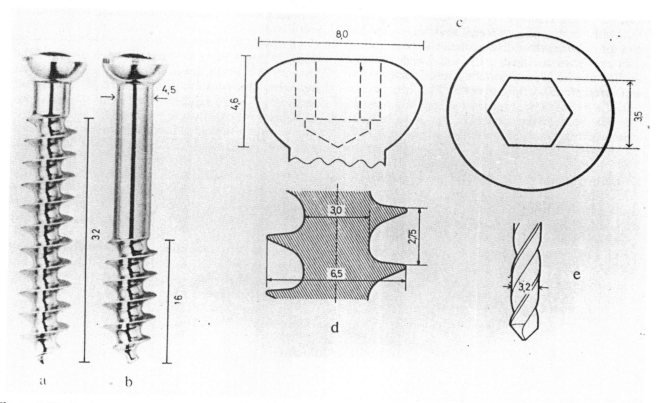

Figure 6.34   Design and dimensions of the ASIF 6.5-mm cancellous bone screw. (Reprinted with permission from Mueller ME, et al. Manual of Internal Fixation. 2nd ed. Heidelberg: Springer-Verlag, 1979.)

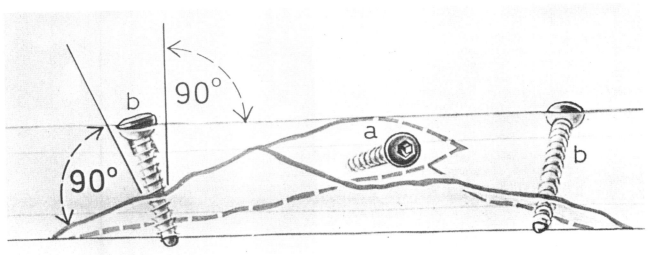

Figure 6.35 Ideal direction of screw placement for achieving maximum interfragmentary compression. (Reprinted with permission from Mueller ME, et al. Manual of Internal Fixation. 2nd ed. Heidelberg: Springer-Verlag, 1979.)

gles to the fracture plane. If the bone is under some axial load, however, the screw should be inserted at right angles to the long axis of the bone. Therefore, the ideal direction for achieving maximum interfragmentary compression and resistance to axial loading is between these two extremes (Fig. 6.35).[140] This is a somewhat hypothetical solution and is not feasible for all equine fractures. For example, in repair of a sagittal fracture of the proximal phalanx, insertion of the screws at right angles to the long axis of the bone usually achieves adequate compression and alignment of the joint surface. In general, two or more lag screws are used, if possible, to prevent rotation of the fragment. This cannot always be achieved, especially for fractures involving the small carpal or tarsal bones.

Pretapped cortical screws are used primarily for lag screw fixation in horses. Self-tapping screws were originally thought to have poorer bone-holding qualities than pretapped screws.[140] When both 5.5- and 6.5-mm screws were inserted into cadaver foal metacarpal/metatarsal bones, the pretapped screws had significantly greater holding power than had the same size self-tapped screws.[157] Similar studies demonstrated, however, that self-tapping screws had the same holding power and pullout strength as pretapped screws.[3,4,120] Use of self-tapping screws may be difficult in dense cortical bone, and the screws may actually break. Self-tapping screws (4.5 mm) inserted into equine third metatarsal bones did not break but could not be inserted continuously.[8] Note that pretapped screws can be placed in the bone with greater precision, thereby producing better holding power.[119,120] In general, most cortical screws inserted into equine bone are pretapped.

Cannulated and bioabsorbable screws are also available for use in horses. Cannulated screws are hollow, enabling screw placement over a guide pin that helps maintain fracture reduction and precise screw positioning during the procedure (Fig. 6.36). They are used commonly in humans but less frequently in veterinary medicine. Cannulated screws are available in a variety of sizes. Concerns about using cannulated screws in horses are

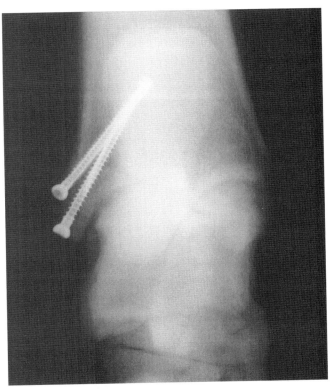

Figure 6.36 Postoperative dorsoplantar view of the tarsus in a horse with a fracture of the medial malleolus of the tibia. The fracture was repaired by using two 4.5-mm cannulated screws.

their questionable strength (because they are hollow) and their expense.[4,8,23] Cannulated 4.5-mm screws had significantly less pullout strength than standard 4.5-mm cortical screws in an in vitro study, suggesting that the interfragmentary compression achieved by these screws may be less than optimal and that screw failure is more likely to occur.[23]

Bioabsorbable screws are made of polylactic acid de-rivatives and, once placed, do not (theoretically) need to be removed. They are used sparingly in horses because of their expense and questionable strength, especially in shear.[38] One in vitro experimental study using equine third carpal slab fractures as a model suggested, how-ever, that bioabsorbable screws have comparable biome-chanical properties to 4.5-mm cortical screws.[93]

OTHER METHODS OF INTERNAL FIXATION

Many fractures in horses, especially those involving long bones, cannot be repaired with lag screws alone. Other methods of repairing long bone fractures include bone plating, tension band wiring (Fig. 6.37), intramed-ullary pinning, intramedullary interlocking nails, and ex-ternal fixators.[4,8] Bone plating provides the most rigid fixation of fractures but cannot be used in all cases be-cause of the specific characteristics of the fracture and the expense. For fractures amenable to bone plating, one or often two plates are used to provide adequate fixation (Fig. 6.38). The plates (usually 4.5 mm thick) are best placed on the tension side of the bone and at right angles to each other, when two plates are used. Either 4.5- or 5.5-mm cortical screws can be used to secure the plates to the bone, and these should be placed as lag screws across the fracture, if possible.

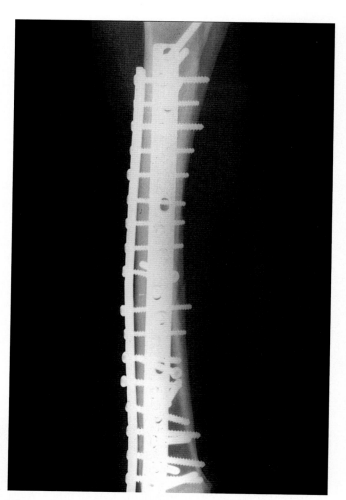

Figure 6.38 Midshaft radial fracture in an adult horse, which was repaired by using two 4.5-mm-diameter broad dynamic compression plates placed at right angles to each other. All screws are 4.5 mm in diameter, although 5.5-mm screws could have been used to provide further stability to the repair.

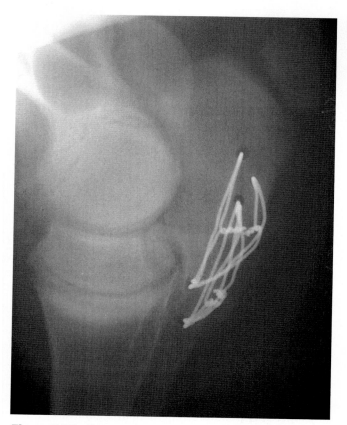

Figure 6.37 Postoperative lateral view of a fractured olecranon in a young foal. The fracture was successfully repaired with tension band wires only.

Special purpose bone plates used occasionally in horses include the dynamic condylar screw (DCS), dy-namic hip screw (DHS), angled blade plate (ABP), and cobra head plate.[4,8] Plate luting refers to placing poly-methylmethacrylate either under the plate or around the screw heads to further increase the strength and stability of the fixation.[100,133] Improved bone-plate contact is achieved; therefore, luting is most beneficial in large horses to increase the overall strength of the implant.[133] Intramedullary interlocking nails are relatively new in equine orthopedics and have primarily been used to re-pair humeral, femoral, and some metatarsal/metacarpal fractures.[8,84] The intramedullary nail is placed within the medullary cavity of the bone and is transfixed to the bone above and below the fracture with bone screws.[84,85] This method of repair is thought to create a more biomechanically sound fixation by placing the implant within the bone rather than applying bone plates to the external surface of the bone. The potential benefit of interlocking nails in equine orthopedics awaits further clinical use.

EXTERNAL METHODS OF FRACTURE FIXATION

External fixators or transfixation pin casts have become more widely used for fracture repair in horses over the past several years.[82,94] They are most useful for stabilizing or preventing collapse of comminuted fractures of the distal limb, where other forms of internal fixation cannot be used. They are also used to treat open fractures when placement of implants would likely result in osteomyelitis.[80,99,109]

The fixator pins (usually 0.25 inch or 6.35 mm in diameter for an average adult horse) can be placed above and below the fracture; but in most cases, pins are placed only above the fracture (Fig. 6.39). Polymethylmethacrylate or stainless-steel side bars can be used as the construct of the fixator to connect the pins if used above and below the fracture, or a fiberglass cast is applied to the limb to support the pins.[80,99,109] For most phalangeal fractures, two to three pins are placed in the distal to middle aspect of the metatarsus/metacarpus, and a half-limb fiberglass cast is applied to the limb to serve as the side bars of the external fixator.[82,83] The transfixation cast permits the horse to ambulate on the limb without further displacement of the fracture during the healing process.

A specially designed external fixator for horses (Nunamaker) that does not use a fiberglass cast may also be used.[99] Catastrophic failure of the bone through one of the external fixator pinholes is the most severe complication of this form of fixation. Other potential problems include infection around the pins, premature pin loosening, chronic pain associated with the pins, and prolonged fracture healing.

Fractures as a Cause of Lameness

Consequences of fracture healing may lead to lameness. This has been termed "fracture disease" in humans and is seen in certain circumstances in horses. A major cause of disability in humans after fracture healing is stiffness of joints from disuse. This is rarely seen in horses and should not be confused with stiffening resulting from ankylosis of joints associated with the development of degenerative joint disease.[140] In fact, joint laxity, especially in young animals with fractures treated with casts, seems to occur more often than joint stiffness in horses.

Most fractures, however, are accompanied by some degree of soft tissue (muscle, tendon, and ligament) damage that may lead to scar tissue formation (Fig. 6.40A). Subsequently, there is obliteration of normal tissue planes, which may impair tendon function, produce stiffening of neighboring joints, and cause flexural deformities in growing animals. A malunion of the fracture may also lead to athletic disability in some horses (Fig. 6.40B). In addition, implant-associated pain from bone plates or screws may cause chronic lameness or poor performance in athletic horses. In some cases, implants used for internal fixation of fractures may need to be removed in performance horses to prevent these problems.

Tendon and muscle flaccidity and atrophy of surrounding muscles are also seen in horses with fractures treated with external immobilization, such as casts. This usually is a temporary problem that is self-correcting with time but may lead to permanent lameness. Other aspects of so-called fracture disease in the nonfractured limb include angular limb deformities caused by excessive axial loading on active growth plates in young horses, stretching of flexor tendons and associated muscles, and support limb laminitis caused by excessive weight bearing. Support limb laminitis with rotation of the distal phalanx is unique to the horse and is a potentially devastating complication of equine fracture repair.

Infection is a serious complication of fractures and can eventually lead to permanent lameness or a nonunion of the fracture. Infection is most likely to occur with open fractures and those repaired with internal fixation.[10] Severe infections may necessitate euthanasia of the animal, whereas milder more chronic infections may necessitate removal of the implants or necrotic bone to resolve the infection. Open, infected fractures that eventually heal are often accompanied by considerably more fibrosis with a greater chance of loss of function of surrounding structures than are closed noninfected fractures. The limb may be permanently thickened as a result of scar tissue and callus formation, which may lead to impaired limb function.[140]

Bone Infections

"Osteitis" and "osteomyelitis" are terms used to describe inflammation of bone involving the periosteum

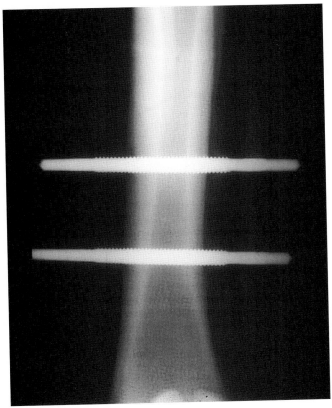

Figure 6.39 Two 6.35-mm-diameter threaded intramedullary pins were placed through the distal metatarsus and incorporated into a fiberglass cast (transfixation pin cast) to prevent collapse of a severely comminuted second phalanx fracture in a mare.

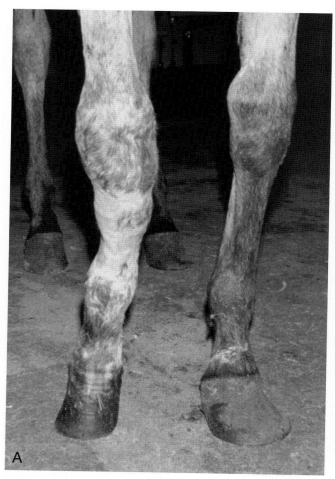

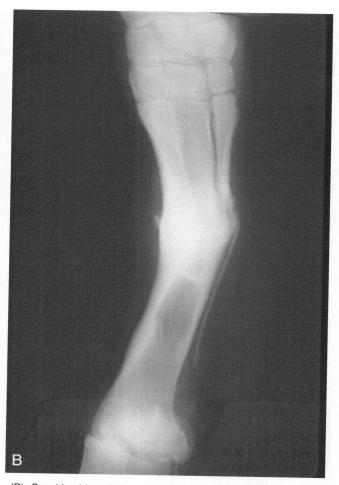

Figure 6.40 Fracture of the third metacarpus several months after treatment with external splinting only. The fracture had healed but was malaligned both clinically (A) and radiographically

(B). Considerable soft tissue swelling and fibrosis were also present in the metacarpal region, which is not uncommon after fracture healing.

and connective tissues of Haversian and Volkmann's canals and the medullary cavity.[71] If the process begins in or involves the periosteum and outer bone cortex, the term "osteitis" or "osteoperiostitis" is used. If the infection involves the medullary cavity, the term "osteomyelitis" is used. The prognoses and treatments for osteitis and osteomyelitis are quite different, and it is important to make a distinction between the two categories of bone infection.[10]

Infectious Osteitis

Osteitis commonly occurs in the extremities of the horse (mostly metacarpal/metatarsal regions) because of the sparse soft tissue coverage in this location. It is usually the result of infection from a nearby septic process or from a break in the skin.[10,15] Osteitis is seen frequently when a horse is kicked but the overlying skin is not broken and may be similar to a bone bruise when no sequestrum develops.

If the skin is broken, exposing the periosteum, the outer layers of cortical bone may eventually die, but the deeper cortical layers of bone survive because of the

blood supply from endosteal vessels. For example, avulsion injuries with bone exposure of the dorsal aspect of the metacarpus/metatarsus frequently develop osteitis and sequestration.[11,15] Bacteria that gain entrance to the bone lodge in the superficial layers of the bone, resulting in a thin layer of dead bone (bone sequestrum) within the wound (Fig. 6.41). Although granulation tissue may advance over the bone sequestrum, the rate of advancement is usually slow. Occasionally, granulation tissue advances under the sequestrum and extrudes it from the wound. The rate of healing of a wound can usually be accelerated by early removal of the sequestrum.

By definition, the two requirements for the formation of a sequestrum are avascularity and infection. Therefore, most surgeons believe that blunt trauma to the bone cortex does not cause sequestration in the absence of infection.[10,11] Sequestration without skin penetration does occur in horses, although it is rare. In cases in which there is no break in the skin, the hematoma may become infected hematogenously, leading to sequestrum formation, fistulation, drainage, and a nonhealing wound. This appears to occur most commonly with injuries to the splint bones, but most cases include skin wounds that lead to secondary bacterial infection.

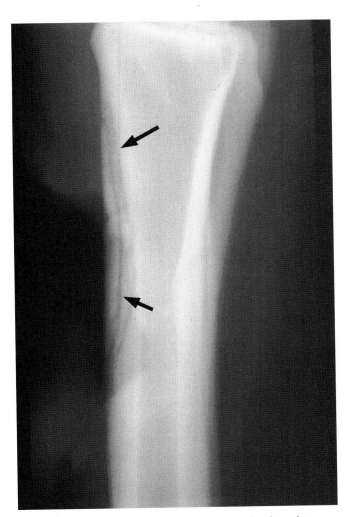

Figure 6.41 Lateral view of the metatarsus, showing a large cortical sequestrum in the dorsoproximal aspect of the metatarsus (arrows). The yearling had severely traumatized the metatarsal region 3 weeks earlier and was lame.

sclerotic margin around the sequestrum—called the involucrum—are usually visible.[10]

Occasionally, an osteitis may resolve spontaneously, especially if there is no infectious component or if the sequestrum is small and extruded from the wound. If bacteria and necrotic bone are present, the wound will be exudative indefinitely until the sequestrum is removed.[140] Wound debridement of unhealthy scar tissue and necrotic bone is usually required for healing to occur. Removal of bone sequestra is best performed with the animal under general anesthesia. Thin cortical sequestra associated with avulsion injuries of the dorsal aspect of the cannon bone can often be removed, however, in the standing, sedated horse. After the surrounding granulation and scar tissue have been excised, the area should be curetted until the bone appears to be healthy. Most wounds are either closed primarily or left to heal by second intention after debridement.

Parenteral antibiotics are of limited value when used alone to treat bone sequestra because of poor penetration of the antibiotics into the necrotic bone. Antibiotics are indicated if there are signs of cellulitis (phlegmon) associated with the lesion and after surgical debridement of the wound. Usually, a wide variety of organisms (secondary pathogens) can be cultured from the wound; occasionally, these bacteria are resistant to antibiotics that are of practical use in the horse. Culturing the sequestrum itself usually gives the most accurate diagnosis of the causative bacteria. The prognosis for horses with osteitis and sequestrum removal is usually excellent.

Osteomyelitis

Osteomyelitis is a more extensive inflammation of the bone than osteitis. It begins within or extends into the medullary cavity. Osteomyelitis in horses can be divided into three categories, based on the origin of the infection: hematogenous, traumatic, and iatrogenic.[10] Osteomyelitis from a hematogenous origin occurs primarily in neonates and only rarely in adults. Traumatic osteomyelitis can occur in any age horse and is usually the result of penetrating wounds or open fractures. Iatrogenic causes of osteomyelitis include surgery, such as internal fixation of fractures, and intraarticular injections of medications.

TYPES

HEMATOGENOUS OSTEOMYELITIS. The localization of hematogenous osteomyelitis in the metaphyseal region can be explained by sluggish metaphyseal blood flow where the blood vessels form terminal sinusoids. This permits bacteria to localize in these areas and establish an infection (Fig. 6.7). The infection in the bone spreads by way of Haversian and Volkmann's cavities, and prostaglandins are considered responsible for bone destruction.[140] Thrombosis of blood vessels also occurs as the infection spreads, producing death of the osteocytes in their lacunae.[10,140] The inflammatory process may increase pressure within the bone, further impairing blood supply. The result is bone necrosis with possible sequestrum formation.

Firth[39] classified hematogenous infections in foals into three categories based on the location of the infection. S-type infections involve the synovial membrane of

Chronic persistent drainage from any wound in the horse suggests the presence of a bone sequestrum or foreign body. Drainage will rarely subside, or at least wound healing will be substantially prolonged, without surgical removal of the sequestrum. This is because the pathogenic organisms reside within the necrotic bone, which is avascular, thereby resisting the animal's immune defenses.

The severity of lameness accompanying osteitis in horses is variable and inconsistent. In addition, the radiographic signs of osteitis depend on the duration that has elapsed between the injury and time of examination. Initially, there may be soft tissue swelling with radiographic evidence of bone resorption. At 7 to 14 days after the injury, periosteal proliferation may be evident. Sequestrum formation may also be visible at that time, as osteoclastic resorption occurs at the periphery of the damaged bone. Radiographic evidence of a sequestrum is usually not visible for a minimum of 2 to 3 weeks after the injury.[15] At that time, the sequestrum and the

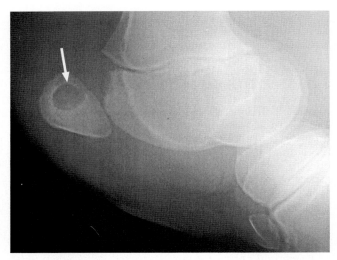

Figure 6.42 Lateral view of the stifle in a foal with lameness and severe effusion of the femoropatellar joint. Lysis within the patella suggests hematogenous osteomyelitis (arrow). The caudal or ventral aspect of the patella directly below the lesion was removed via arthroscopy, and the joint was lavaged.

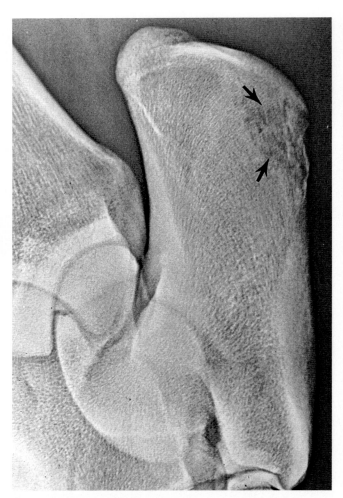

Figure 6.43 Oblique view of the tarsus in a horse with a puncture wound and infection of the calcaneal bursa. Lysis within the proximal aspect of the calcaneus (arrows) suggests concurrent osteitis or osteomyelitis of the bone.

joints, P-type infections involve the physis and usually the metaphysis, and E-type infections involve the epiphysis. These infections are not completely isolated, however, and foals may show multiple types of hematogenous infection at multiple sites (Fig. 6.42). Bone infection caused by *Salmonella* spp., for example, typically involves several bones.[140]

Hematogenous osteomyelitis is frequently secondary to infections elsewhere in the animal's body, such as the umbilicus, gastrointestinal tract, or lungs.[10,39] Foals with a compromised immune system resulting from failure of passive transfer or septicemia appear to be predisposed to hematogenous osteomyelitis. In many of these foals, multiple body systems are involved with signs referable to infection in these regions. Therefore, a complete physical examination is essential. Some foals will recover completely from the initial infection, however, only to develop bone or joint infections several days later when they appear to be very healthy. The most common bacteria that cause hematogenous infections in foals are gram-negative enterics such as *Escherichia coli*.[10,39] Other causative organisms include *Staphylococcus* spp., *Streptococcus* spp., *Rhodococcus* spp., and *Salmonella* spp.

TRAUMATIC OSTEOMYELITIS. An open fracture or a penetrating wound may lead to traumatic osteomyelitis in any age horse (Fig. 6.43). There is usually some degree of trauma to the skin and surrounding soft tissues with these injuries, and the pathogenic organisms may directly enter the medullary cavity through the open wound. Bacteria associated with these types of infections include gram-negative enterics, *Staphylococcus* spp., *Streptococcus* spp., and anaerobes.[10,139] Infection spreads through the bone in a manner similar to that for hematogenous osteomyelitis. Occasionally, there is no overt break in the skin, but the necrotic tissue provides a medium for bacterial proliferation and infection develops from a hematogenous route.

Avascularity is a major factor in the pathogenesis of osteomyelitis; therefore, fractures that leave bone fragments isolated from a blood supply are at risk for developing infection.[10] Treatment of an open fracture without providing absolute stability is usually futile unless the dead, avascular fragments can be removed or reincorporated into the healing fracture so they can be revascularized.[140] Alternatively, some type of external fixator may be used to stabilize the fracture without disrupting the soft tissues around the fracture site.[82,99] In this manner, the potential for osteomyelitis is decreased because no implants are placed near the fracture, and the vascularity to the fracture is not further impaired.

IATROGENIC OSTEOMYELITIS. The cause of osteomyelitis after internal fixation of fractures is usually contamination from an open wound (open fracture). Regardless of the type of internal fixation used, infection after repair of open fractures is much more common than after repair of closed fractures. Contamination of the fracture during the surgical procedure can and does occur, however, particularly if it is prolonged (longer than 3 hours).[10] Usually, the fracture hematoma, avascularity at the fracture site, and the implantation of foreign material (pins, plates, screws, etc.) contribute to the development of osteomyelitis because they provide favorable conditions for bacterial growth. Once bacteria become established where nutrients are available, proliferation occurs within a polysaccharide slime forming a biofilm-enclosed colony. This biofilm or bioslime is formed by bacterial extracapsular exopolysaccharides that bind to surfaces of the implants and help maintain infection by protecting the bacteria from the host defenses. Because of this, osteomyelitis may develop despite prophylactic antibiotic coverage at the time of fracture repair, especially in open fractures. Highly resistant bacteria such as methicillin-resistant *Staphylococcus aureus* and gram-negative enterics often cause these infections.[10]

CLINICAL SIGNS

Hematogenous osteomyelitis may be missed in its early stages and often presents after the lameness has become unresponsive to medical therapy. Frequently, the owner thinks that the lameness was the result of an injury, such as a sprain, or of being stepped on by the mare. There is usually a severe lameness with cellulitis similar to that seen with fractures. Pain is usually elicited by direct pressure and manipulation of the joint(s) adjacent to the infection, and a fever is commonly seen in foals. Clinical signs of traumatic and iatrogenic osteomyelitis are similar and include lameness, soft tissue swelling, retarded wound healing over the implants, drainage, and fistulation. Signs can be present as early as 7 to 10 days after injury or surgery or may be delayed for 3 to 4 weeks.

RADIOGRAPHIC SIGNS

Loss of bone density resulting from a reduction in the calcium salt content of the bone occurs gradually with osteomyelitis. Lytic changes in the bone are not visible until 30 to 50% of the bone mineral has been removed.[104] This is usually evident 10 to 14 days after the onset of infection (Fig. 6.44). In more chronic cases, there are often sclerotic margins around the lytic regions because of new bone formation. Sequestrum formation with a surrounding envelope (called the involucrum) and endosteal and periosteal thickening may also be evident. Occasionally, osteomyelitis may penetrate into an adjacent joint, producing signs of a septic arthritis.

With osteomyelitis after fracture repair, blurring of the cancellous trabeculation and a "moth-eaten" appearance at the fracture site will be seen on radiographs.[140]

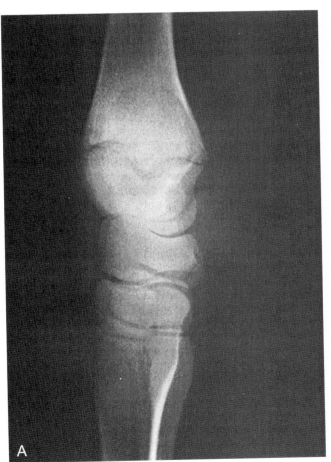
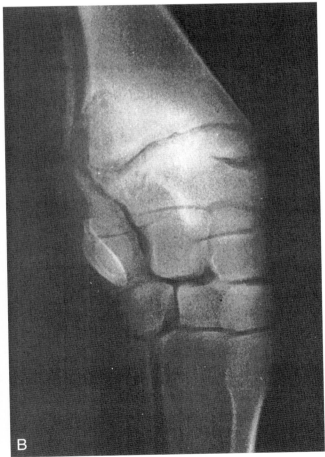

Figure 6.44   Lateral (A) and oblique (B) views of hematogenous osteomyelitis in the distal radius of a foal, showing lytic changes in the bone.

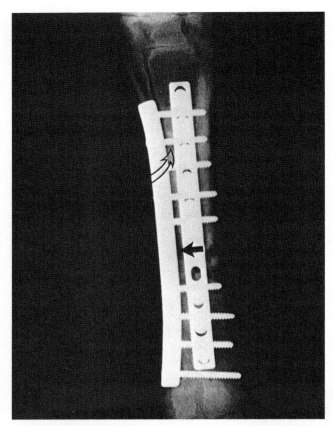

Figure 6.45 Osteomyelitis after internal fixation of a fractured third metacarpal bone. Lysis of the bone is occurring under the plate (solid arrow) and along one of the screw threads (open arrow).

Lysis along the screw threads or under the plate may become evident with time. Usually, a piece of bone that is decalcified and surrounded by a lucent zone is a sign of sequestrum formation. A zone of bone destruction adjacent to the implants typically occurs under the plate and directly along the screw threads (Fig. 6.45). In more chronic cases of osteomyelitis, zones of both bone production and bone destruction are visible radiographically.[10]

TREATMENT

The lameness in many foals with hematogenous osteomyelitis is frequently attributed to trauma but is, in fact, the early stages of infection. Therefore, at the time of initial examination, the infection is often well advanced with obvious radiographic signs, making it difficult to treat medically.[10,114] If, however, acute hematogenous osteomyelitis is suspected in a foal despite there being no radiographic signs, broad-spectrum bacteriocidal antimicrobials should be administered. A blood culture may be taken to determine the causative bacteria, but it is often unrewarding. The duration of antimicrobial use is largely empiric (usually a minimum of 3 weeks) and should be based on the clinical response of the animal. Antimicrobials alone may be unsuccessful, however, because of the ischemic nature of the disease

and poor penetration of the antimicrobial into infected avascular bone. Antimicrobials are best used early in the course of the infection and at high doses. Antimicrobials used most commonly to treat horses and foals with osteomyelitis include penicillin, gentamicin, amikacin, ceftiofur, cefazolin, enrofloxacin, and vancomycin. Prostaglandin synthesis inhibitors (NSAIDs) have been beneficial for treating acute osteomyelitis in humans and animals in conjunction with antimicrobials.[140] They should be used cautiously in foals to avoid possible gastrointestinal ulceration, and concurrent antiulcer medication may be warranted.

If there is no response to medical therapy and/or the osteomyelitis is localized, then surgery in conjunction with medical therapy is recommended. If the lesion can be accessed through a joint, which is often the case with hematogenous infections, then arthroscopy should be used to remove the damaged bone (Fig. 6.42). A sample of the bone should be obtained at surgery and submitted for culture and sensitivity testing. Debridement of infected fractures or open wounds should be performed to remove avascular bone and infected soft tissue and to decrease bacterial numbers.

Cancellous bone grafting is often used with infections of fractures to speed fracture healing. A major priority for treatment of osteomyelitis associated with fractures is to achieve stability of the fracture, however. Stability needs to be maintained not only for fracture healing but also for limiting the spread of infection.[140] Loose implants should be removed and fracture stability should be achieved by other means, such as replating, external fixators, interlocking nails, external immobilization, or a combination of these techniques. If it is impossible to stabilize the fracture with internal fixation, external fixation, or both, euthanasia may be the only alternative, since it is unlikely that the infection will resolve.

Other methods used to treat osteomyelitis include regional perfusion of antimicrobials directly into the medullary cavity of the bone or within the vascular system of the limb.[151–153] The goal is to obtain high tissue concentrations of antibiotics to achieve better bacterial kill. A tourniquet should be placed above and below the site of infusion and maintained for a minimum of 30 minutes to achieve optimal results.[10,151] In addition, antimicrobial-impregnated polymethylmethacrylate (PMMA) may be placed locally into the wound to achieve high antibiotic concentrations in and around the fracture.[57,138] The antimicrobials (amikacin or a cephalosporin) are incorporated into the PMMA during mixing and will elute from the PMMA into the wound for several days to weeks after they are placed. The PMMA is usually molded into bead or cigar shapes and placed adjacent to the implants, fracture, or infection site (Fig 6.46).[57] The use of antibiotic-impregnated PMMA is thought to greatly improve the chances of successful treatment of osteomyelitis in horses, especially that associated with internal fixation.[57]

PROGNOSIS

The prognosis for foals with hematogenous osteomyelitis depends on the individual situation, but if multiple sites are involved, the prognosis is usually poor. If the site of osteomyelitis can be thoroughly debrided, how-

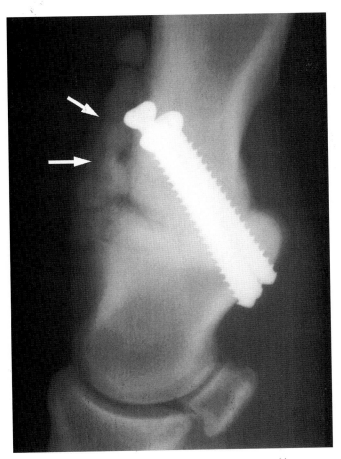

Figure 6.46 Lateral view of the pastern in a horse with a chronic infection of the proximal interphalangeal joint, which had developed from a wound and did not respond to systemic antimicrobials. After debridement of all damaged bone and arthrodesis of the joint, amikacin-impregnated PMMA beads were placed to help treat the infection (arrows). There was no recurrence of the infection after surgery.

ever, the infection can usually be resolved. The prognosis with traumatic osteomyelitis depends on the bone involved and the duration and severity of the infection. Traumatic osteomyelitis is usually less difficult to resolve than iatrogenic infection. Osteomyelitis after internal fixation of a fracture is one of the most difficult diseases to resolve successfully in horses.[10,57] Therefore, the prognosis for these animals is extremely guarded, particularly for adult horses.

Infectious Physitis

Hematogenous infections of the physes are not uncommon in foals and have similar predisposing factors as other bone and joint infections in foals. The physis is often the initial location of hematogenous bacteria and infection, which can subsequently spread to the neighboring epiphysis and joint (Fig. 6.7). Multiple physes can be infected simultaneously, but this is uncommon. Clinical signs, radiographic findings, and treatment are similar to those for other bone infections.

Bone Cysts

True bone cysts that occur in other species (primarily aneurysmal and unicameral) have been reported to occur rarely in horses.[13,68,134] The most common site appears to be the mandible. "Unicameral bone cysts" are solitary intraosseous cysts lined by thin connective tissue membranes.[68] "Aneurysmal bone cysts" are expansile lesions consisting of anastomosing cavernous spaces filled with unclotted blood and lined with fibrous walls of various thicknesses.[77] These cysts usually contain osteoid tissue or osseous components, without elastic laminae or muscle layers.[77] Aneurysmal and unicameral bone cysts are more characteristic of true cystic lesions, since they do not involve an articular surface and are usually solitary, expansile, intraosseous lesions. Most true bone cysts reported in dogs and people occur in the distal or proximal metaphyses of long bones.

The cause of aneurysmal and unicameral bone cysts in any species is uncertain. Unicameral cysts are thought to result from the encapsulation and alteration of a focus of intramedullary hemorrhage, supposedly from trauma. Alternatively, trauma causes a disturbance in endochondral ossification, resulting in a cystic defect within the metaphysis.[22] Aneurysmal bone cysts are generally believed to develop secondary to a preexisting lesion, such as fibrous dysplasia, hematoma from trauma or bleeding disorders, or neoplasia.[134] One case of aneurysmal bone cyst of the distal metaphysis of the metatarsus in a horse was thought to be caused by trauma.[134]

Whether the pathogenesis of aneurysmal and unicameral bone cysts and subchondral cystic lesions are interrelated is controversial. Most of the evidence (including pathogenesis and clinical characteristics) suggests that subchondral cystic lesions, at least in horses, are a distinctly separate clinical entity from aneurysmal or unicameral bone cysts.[9] In addition, aneurysmal and unicameral bone cysts can be difficult to differentiate from some bone tumors in horses (Fig. 6.47).

Treatment of true bone cysts in horses usually involves surgical curettage of the lesion with or without autogenous cancellous bone grafting. Spontaneous resolution of the cyst may also occur, and some bone cysts in people respond to intralesional steroid injections.[77] The prognosis for resolution of bone cysts in horses is usually good, depending on the location of the cyst.

Bone Tumors

Primary bone neoplasia is rare in horses. The most common bone tumors in horses are osteoma, ossifying fibroma, multilobular osteoma or osteochondrosarcoma, and osteosarcoma.[55] Although these tumors may develop at any location, the face and head (mandible, skull, and paranasal sinuses) appear to be the usual sites of occurrence. Osteomas are benign tumors and consist of well-differentiated bone that typically occur within the paranasal sinuses or on the skull. Ossifying fibromas are benign fibro-osseous lesions that usually involve the rostral aspect of the mandible, premaxilla, or paranasal sinuses (Fig. 6.48).[55] Multilobular osteomas or osteochondrosarcomas are rare in horses but usually involve the skull or paranasal sinus (Fig. 6.49). These tumors

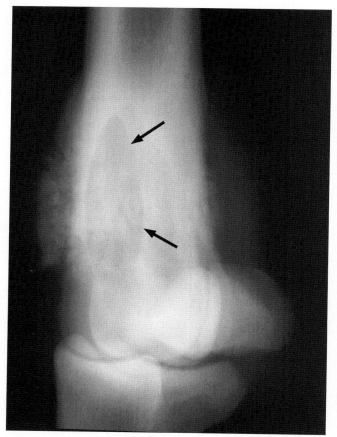

Figure 6.47 Oblique view of the metatarsus of an adult horse with firm swelling of the bone and lameness, revealing a large lytic lesion and extensive periosteal new bone growth indicative of neoplasia (arrows). The lesion was debrided, and a biopsy suggested possible osteosarcoma. Because the lesion showed minimal progression, however, it may have been a true bone cyst and not a tumor.

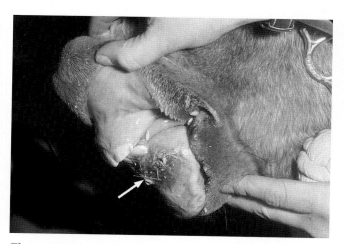

Figure 6.48 Large firm swelling of the rostral aspect of the mandible in a young Quarter Horse filly, consistent with an ossifying fibroma (arrow). A rostral mandibulectomy was performed to completely remove the tumor.

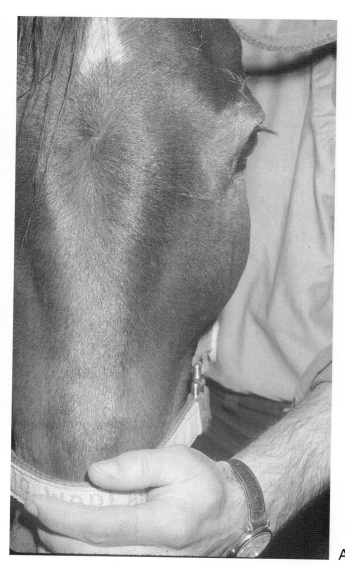

A

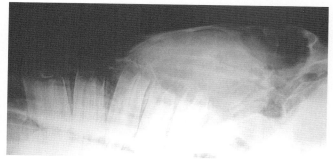

B

Figure 6.49 A. A large external swelling of the paranasal sinus region in a 3-year-old Quarter Horse gelding. B. Lateral view of the same region, showing a large osseous mass within the maxillary sinuses. Biopsy suggested multilobular osteochondroma.

are generally benign but locally aggressive and can be removed surgically. Osteosarcomas are malignant tumors, arising from mesenchyme, in which neoplastic cells produce osteoid or bone.

In horses, the skull, axial skeleton, ribs, and occasionally the limbs are the commonly affected sites. The clinical signs caused by these tumors depend on the location and specific type of neoplasia. The diagnosis of neoplasia is usually made based on its radiographic appearance and is confirmed by histopathology of biopsy or autopsy specimens. Treatment depends on the location of the tumor, involvement of the parent bone, and the specific type of osseous tumor. In general, all tumors except osteosarcomas can potentially be removed successfully with minimal recurrence if complete tumor excision is achieved.[55] Unfortunately, complete tumor excision is not always possible.

Bone Contusions

Bone contusions (bruising, periostitis) from direct or indirect trauma are known to occur in people and contribute to orthopedic pain and lameness. Most joint pain in people is thought to originate from bone and is typically seen as edema of the subchondral bone on MRI (R. Steadman, personal communication, 1998).

With the amount of trauma that horses seem to encounter, bone bruising probably occurs much more often than is currently recognized or diagnosed. Diagnosing bone contusions and bruising in horses is difficult and mostly subjective. This is especially true for bone pain originating in joints. Most bone contusions are diagnosed based on the history, clinical findings, and lack of radiographic abnormalities. With bone contusions, evidence of pain can usually be elicited with direct pressure over the affected site. In addition, bone pain usually causes a more severe lameness than most soft tissue injuries, and pain is often elicited on manipulation of the affected bone or joint.

Radiographs are useful only to document the absence of fractures or other abnormalities within the affected bone or joint. Nuclear scintigraphy is useful for documenting abnormal bone metabolism of the affected site but cannot be used to definitively diagnose a bone bruise. MRI and CT are used in humans for diagnosing bone damage or contusion but are available for use in horses at only a few veterinary institutions.[80,88,132]

Treatment of bone contusions is similar to any type of acute musculoskeletal trauma, and includes inactivity, cold therapy, hydrotherapy, bandaging, and NSAIDs. Suspected bone contusions within joints can also be treated with intraarticular medications. The prognosis of horses with bone contusions is usually good, unless damage to the subchondral bone of a joint contributes to joint pathology and secondary osteoarthritis (Fig. 6.23).

SYSTEMIC DISEASES OF BONE

Osteoporosis

In osteoporosis, the bone mineral density (BMD) of the bone matrix is reduced. The bone becomes porous, light, and fragile and is prone to fracture. Osteoporosis in horses is an uncommon or at least an uncommonly recognized clinical problem. The term "osteopenia" is used if the BMD is reduced but spontaneous fractures do not occur. Clinically, osteopenia is much more commonly recognized in horses than is osteoporosis.

Generalized Osteopenia

The generalized osteoporosis seen in postmenopausal women is not recognized in older horses. Older mares, however, may be more prone to long bone fractures during recovery from general anesthesia. Whether this may be due to declining estrogen levels associated with reproductive senescence is unknown. Osteoporosis is seen occasionally with undernutrition rather than with actual deficiencies in calcium, phosphorus, or vitamin D. In most affected horses, however, osteoporosis is usually associated with a diet low in calcium, high in phosphorus, or low in vitamin D. Osteoporosis is associated with copper deficiency and chronic lead poisoning in lambs, but this has not been seen in foals.[14]

A condition first recognized in Thoroughbred foals may be a manifestation of generalized osteoporosis.[33] The condition is characterized by fractures of the proximal sesamoid bones and typically occurs when foals, trying to keep up with their dams, gallop to exhaustion. Foals seem more prone to the condition if they are confined after birth. During this time of relative inactivity, the bones are not subjected to the stresses required to strengthen them, potentially weakening the skeletal system (Fig. 6.50). Some underlying metabolic problem or deficiency that produces osteoporosis may exist, but at this time it is undefined. Other lameness problems and unexplained fractures in horses may be attributed to generalized osteoporosis, but their pathogenesis and cause are often unexplainable.

Localized Osteopenia

Localized, or disuse, osteopenia is fairly common, especially in horses after rigid external immobilization of their limbs (casting). Disuse osteopenia may also occur in horses with severe or chronic lameness or neuropathies, such as radial nerve paralysis in which weight bearing is reduced. With decreased weight bearing, there is increased resorption of bone and decreased bone formation. One study reported that 6 weeks of cast immobilization of the thoracic limb of a pony caused a significant decrease in weight and specific gravity of the third metacarpal bone.[32] Histologically, the osteopenia in that case was caused by atrophy of osteoblasts with failure of bone apposition.[32,140] Other studies, however, note that external immobilization of the distal limb in horses has only a minor effect on articular cartilage with little clinical significance.[108]

Osteopenia is usually more severe in young animals than in adult horses because of their inherent rapid bone turnover. Bone cortices become thinner and more porotic. Fortunately, it rarely contributes to a clinical problem and is easily reversed when the external immobilization device is removed and the animal commences normal weight bearing. Localized osteopenia is essentially a radiographic diagnosis characterized by lack of

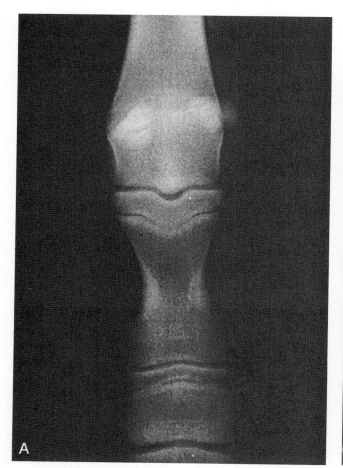 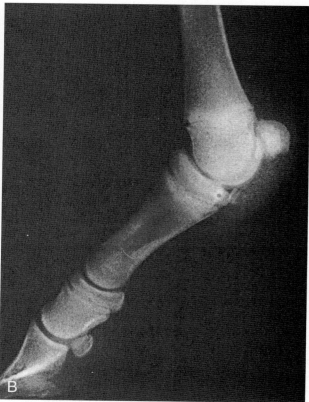

Figure 6.50 AP (A) and lateral (B) views of a fractured proximal sesamoid bone in a Quarter Horse foal. The injury occurred after a period of confinement.

cortical density and a more lucent appearance to the bones (Fig. 6.51).[140] The sesamoids are often the first bones to manifest the problem radiographically. Loss of bone detected radiographically indicates about a 30% BMD loss.

Further experiments have shown that treatment of osteopenia with 25-hydroxycholecalciferol has been beneficial.[32] Fortunately, localized osteopenia after immobilization rarely causes any problems. If the external support is suddenly removed, however, a pathologic fracture may result. To prevent this, the rigidity of the external support should be diminished gradually over time. For example, after cast removal a cotton bandage with a PVC splint incorporated into the bandage should be applied; this will provide less stability than a cast but more support than a bandage alone.[140] After splint removal, successively lighter, less rigid bandages should be applied until no external support of the limb is used. It may take several months before the bone regains normal density and strength after external immobilization. Occasionally, the original BMD is never reached.

Stress protection is another example of localized osteopenia seen in fractured bones that have been repaired with rigid internal fixation devices, such as stainless-steel bone plates.[140] At first, rigid internal fixation enhances healing and permits mobility of neighboring joints. Over

a period of months, however, the bone under the plates becomes porotic, which produces a weakened bone susceptible to fatigue fracture when the plate is removed. Theoretically, plates should be removed as soon as healing has occurred. Plates with a lower modulus of elasticity have been designed to minimize stress protection, especially in people and small animals. In horses, however, osteopenia generally does not occur to the same degree because a much larger animal places a greater force on the healing bone. Therefore, stress protection from internal fixation is of minimal clinical significance in horses. In general, bone plates and other forms of internal fixation are not removed in horses unless they contribute to infection or cause lameness in performance horses.

Osteopetrosis

Osteopetrosis is a rare skeletal disease of horses characterized by an imbalance of bone apposition and resorption. It is an inherited disease of people, rabbits, mice, and cattle and may be an inherited disease in horses.[125] The underlying problem is a failure of bone resorption by osteoclasts. There is complete closure of the medullary canal at the middiaphysis of the bone because the canal has not been remodeled by osteoclasia during de-

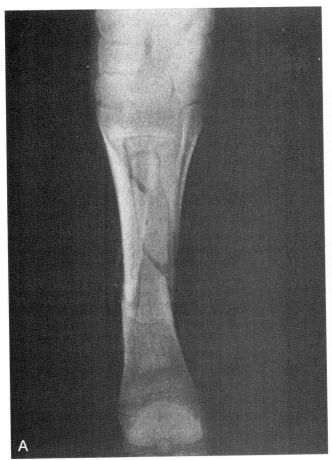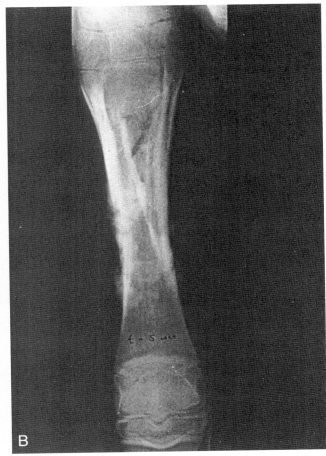

Figure 6.51   A. Radiograph of a fractured third metacarpus in a foal. B. Radiograph 5 weeks later revealing evidence of localized disuse osteoporosis.

velopment from its embryologic state. The disease is also characterized by fractures because of a lack of a normal bone structure. Since there is no evidence of marrow in such bones, an anemia commonly accompanies the condition.

Osteopetrosis has been reported in a Peruvian Paso foal,[125] and it may be an inherited condition in this breed. In the case described by Singer and Whitenack,[125] metaphyseal diameters of long bones were wider than normal, and the cortices were abnormally thick with complete obliteration of the medullary canal. Trabecular bone was soft and could be easily crushed, and the bones were weaker than normal. Large calluses had formed at fracture sites, suggesting that such fractures had occurred in utero. Because of the inherited nature of the disease in other species, owners should be advised against allowing the horse to mate.[125]

Fluorosis

Fluorosis is occasionally seen in horses that ingest small but toxic amounts of fluorine in their diet or drinking water.[124] The source of the fluorine is usually contamination from nearby industries. Plants can become contaminated from industrial fumes, and wells may be-

come contaminated from an industrial effluent (see Chapter 5). In toxic amounts, the fluorine is deposited in bone (for which it has a great affinity). Osteomalacia, osteoporosis, and exostosis formation occur because of excessive mobilization of calcium and phosphorus to compensate for urinary excretion. The exostosis is usually first observed in the third metacarpal/metatarsal bones, commonly as hyperostotic lesions (Fig. 6.52). Periosteal hyperostoses also are seen at tendon and ligament insertion sites.

Clinically, affected horses may be intermittently lame and show signs of generalized unthriftiness. Their gait may be stiff, and they may stand with their feet abnormally placed and, to relieve pain, constantly shift their weight. Their bones are more easily fractured, and if the animal was exposed to fluorine during tooth development, the teeth display classic mottling. Teeth are generally regarded as sensitive indicators of fluorosis.[123] The diagnosis is usually based on clinical and radiographic signs and is confirmed by analysis of fluorine in bone and urine. The diagnosis should be confirmed by examining other animals exposed to a similar environment. The treatment is directed toward prevention as well as general symptomatic treatment of the affected horse (see Chapter 5).

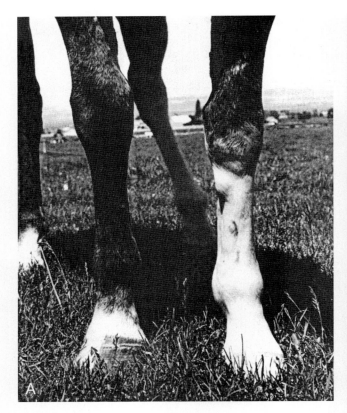

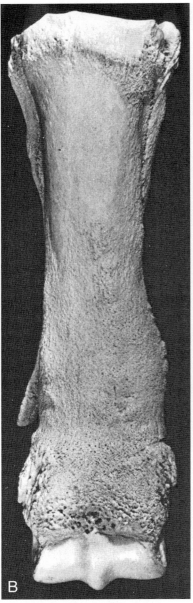

Figure 6.52 A. Enlargement of the metacarpi, caused by fluorosis. B. Fluorosis of the third metacarpal bone with the hyperostotic lesions. (Courtesy of J. L. Shupe, Utah State University, Logan, Utah.)

Hereditary Multiple Exostosis and Solitary Osteochondroma

Hereditary multiple exostosis (multiple cartilaginous exostosis) is an inherited skeletal disorder characterized by numerous abnormal projections from growing bones, resulting in an unusual bone contour.[91,124] The condition affects most of the long bones as well as the ribs, scapula, and pelvis in horses and is used as a model for the condition in humans.[124] The characteristic swellings of hereditary multiple exostosis are usually present at birth, and the lesions are probably initiated during fetal osteogenesis. The swellings are usually bilaterally symmetrical and consist of multiple firm bony enlargements of various shapes and sizes that are firmly attached to bone.[124] Swellings on the limbs do not appear to enlarge

as the animal matures, but others—such as those located on the ribs and scapulae—usually enlarge until maturity is reached (about 4 years of age) (Fig. 6.53). Lameness, if present, is usually the result of impingement of tendons and muscle groups by the bony masses. Some horses may present with a variety of joint and tendon sheath swellings.[73] Grossly, the tumors adopt a variety of shapes, ranging from conical to rounded, pedunculated, multilobulated, and spurlike. Histologically, such tumors appear as osteochondromas and do not appear to undergo malignant transformation.[123] They usually have a small cartilage cap covering underlying spongy cancellous bone. There is no known treatment for this condition.

Solitary osteochondromas occur more commonly in horses than hereditary multiple exostosis and usually develop on the caudomedial aspect of the distal radial metaphysis.[75,131] They are not considered to be an inherited

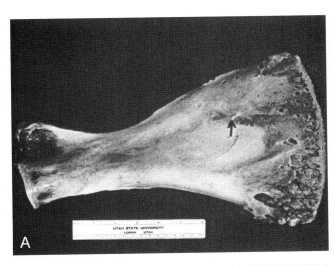

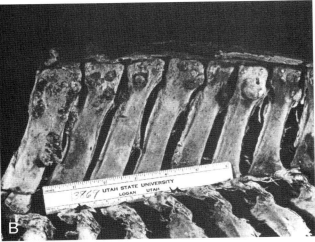

Figure 6.53 Hereditary multiple exostosis involving the scapula (A) and spinous processes of the thoracic vertebra (B). (Courtesy of J. L. Shupe, Utah State University, Logan, Utah.)

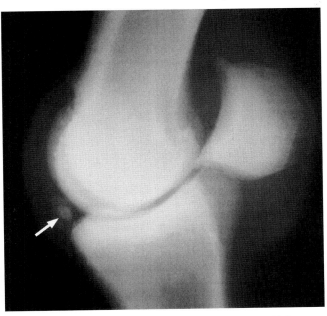

Figure 6.54 Lateral view of the metacarpophalangeal joint, showing osteochondromas (arrow) in a horse 2 years after arthroscopic surgery to remove chip fractures and an enlarged villonodular pad. The osseous densities were not present after surgery but had gradually ossified and enlarged in that time.

condition, as is hereditary multiple exostosis. Horses with osteochondromas on the caudal aspect of the radius usually present with lameness and swelling of the carpal canal. The masses resemble hereditary multiple exostosis, but the lesions are usually not symmetrical.[75,131] Radiographic examination usually reveals an osteocartilaginous exostosis protruding from the caudal aspect of the radius (Fig. 8.284). Large exostoses may cause lameness by interfering with muscle movement, such as the humeral head of the deep digital flexor muscle, or pain from carpal canal effusion.[63,131] Carpal sheath effusion is usually the result of the exostosis and generally does not resolve unless the bone is removed. Surgical approaches for removal of osteochondromas in this region include an incision into the carpal sheath or tenoscopy of the carpal canal.[131]

Solitary osteochondromas may also develop in joints associated with previous trauma or surgery. Small, dislodged pieces of cartilage may become trapped in the synovium, develop a blood supply, and grow to form osseous masses. These do not always cause a clinical problem but will often lead to persistent synovial effu-

sion. The dorsal aspect of the fetlock appears to be particularly susceptible to osteochondroma formation (Fig. 6.54).

Tumoral Calcinosis

Tumoral calcinosis (calcinosis circumscripta) is the formation of calcified, granular, amorphous deposits in the subcutaneous tissues that induce a fibrosing granulomatous reaction.[135] The deposits usually occur in the subcutis near joints and tendon sheaths.[29,46] The condition occurs infrequently in the horse, although it may be more common than is actually recognized.[46] The cause of tumoral calcinosis is unknown.

Affected horses usually present with unsightly swellings that are becoming progressively larger; lameness is uncommon. The swellings are firm and painless, and the skin is usually intact and movable over the swellings. The most common location for tumoral calcinosis lesions is the lateral aspect of the stifle, lateral to the fibula, and beneath the aponeurosis of the biceps femoris and lateral crural fascia. Of 18 cases reported in the literature, lesions occurred over the lateral surface of the tibia close to the femorotibial joint in 16 horses.[46] Radiographically, the lesions are characterized by radio-opaque calcified deposits. On the cut surface of the lesions, there is a honeycomb-like appearance with a calcareous, gritty deposit enclosed in a dense fibrous capsule.

The treatment for calcinosis circumscripta is surgical excision. This should be performed only in cases in which lameness can be directly attributed to the lesion. The lesion may be so firmly attached to the stifle joint capsule that it cannot be dissected free without opening the joint. Therefore, surgical excision of these lesions should be performed cautiously.

Osteodystrophia Fibrosa

Osteodystrophia fibrosa (nutritional secondary hyperparathyroidism) is a generalized bone disease caused primarily by a dietary calcium deficiency in the face of phosphorus excess.[27] It occurs in all equids, although the horse is more susceptible than its relatives.[71] It is most common in horses being fed cereal and cereal by-products, such as bran (diets high in phosphorus and low in calcium), hence the name "bran disease." Adding legume hay, which is high in calcium, to the diet can usually prevent the disease.[27,86] It is also seen in horses grazing on plants high in oxalates, which chelate the calcium and interfere with the absorption of calcium. Horses in Queensland, Australia, developed osteodystrophia fibrosa when grazed on tropical grasses.[140] A subclinical form of the disease may also occur but is difficult to diagnose because the clinical manifestations are subtle.

The underlying pathogenesis in osteodystrophia fibrosa is defective mineralization of bone. The high-phosphorus diet leads to increased absorption of phosphorus and elevation of serum phosphate levels. This tends to lower serum calcium and stimulate the parathyroid gland to increase secretion of parathyroid hormone. Parathyroid hormone increases activation of remodeling, leading to resorption of bone. With bone resorption, there is a compensatory replacement with fibrous tissue.[41] This causes poorly mineralized bone, which is eventually replaced with cellular connective tissue. Horses of both sexes and all ages are susceptible. Lactating mares and foals appear to be at increased risk of developing osteodystrophia fibrosa (see Chapter 5).

The classic form of osteodystrophia fibrosa is called "bighead" because of the predilection of the jaws and flat bones of the skull to respond to parathyroid hormone.[41] The classic clinical signs of the disease include a symmetrical enlargement of the mandible and facial bones (Fig. 6.55A). There is loss of lamina dura around the teeth, resulting from osteoclastic resorption of alveolar margins; the teeth may eventually loosen. This can be identified radiographically and is one of the first signs of the disease. Swelling initially begins just above the facial crest and in the mandible, producing a reduction in intermandibular space (Fig. 6.55B). There may also

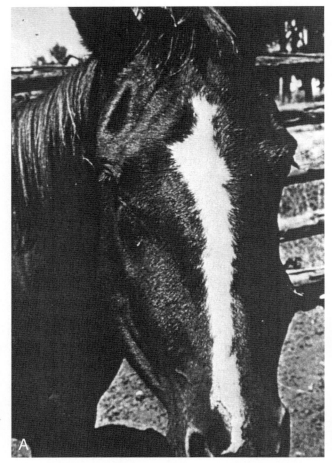
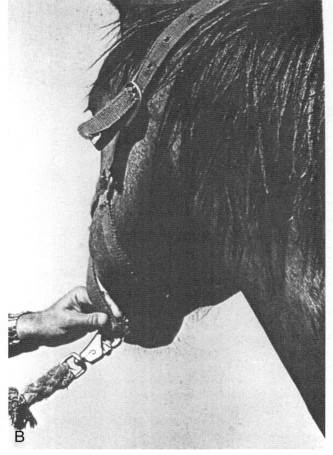

Figure 6.55 A. Symmetrical enlargement of the facial bones that is associated with nutritional secondary hyperparathyroidism. (Courtesy of R. A. McKenzie, Animal Research Institute, Yeerongpilly, Queensland, Australia.) B. Mandibular swelling associated with nutritional secondary hyperparathyroidism.

be enough swelling of the palate, maxillae, and incisor bones to produce dyspnea.

The subclinical form of nutritional secondary hyperparathyroidism may cause a nebulous shifting limb lameness in horses that is difficult to localize with standard perineural anesthesia.[140] The condition may also contribute to unexplained fractures, especially in young horses. In such cases, a dietary history is important for making the diagnosis. Blood calcium and phosphorus levels are usually normal, and the diagnosis is generally based on analysis of the diet and response to treatment with calcium supplementation.

Hypertrophic Osteopathy

Hypertrophic osteopathy (hypertrophic pulmonary osteoarthropathy) is a progressive bilaterally symmetrical proliferation of subperiosteal bone and fibrous connective tissue on the appendicular and axial skeleton and facial bones.[140] It is a relatively rare disease in the horse. The pathogenesis of hypertrophic osteopathy is still unclear. Classically, the disease is associated with a space-occupying pulmonary lesion, such as a neoplasm or chronic suppurative process (e.g., a large abscess, tuberculosis, or a fractured rib with pleural adhesions).[81] The disease rarely occurs in horses with such thoracic lesions but has been associated with a granular cell myoblastoma.[45] The term "hypertrophic osteopathy" is preferred because the disease has also been associated with intraabdominal disorders without pulmonary involvement. Hypertrophic osteopathy was reported in a mare with a dysgerminoma (a neoplasm of ovarian primordial germ cells) that had abdominal metastases but was free of thoracic lesions.[81]

The two most common mechanisms for the development of the disease are classified as neurogenic and humoral. According to the more popular neurogenic theory, an apparent stimulation of the vagus nerve produces an alteration of the vasculature and periosteum of bones by way of an unknown efferent pathway. Support for this theory is based on the fact that in dogs and humans, hypertrophic osteopathy lesions may regress after vagotomy. A humoral mechanism may also exist, since hypertrophic osteopathy has been shown to occur in humans when urinary excretion of estrogen is increased. High levels of circulating estrogen were reported in a mare with hypertrophic osteopathy, although the exact relationship between estrogen levels and hypertrophic osteopathy is purely speculative.[81]

The clinical signs of hypertrophic osteopathy are related to periosteal hyperostoses. There is symmetric enlargement of the long bones of the limb, and all bones in the limb are affected (Fig. 6.56). There is pain and edema of soft tissues, and the horse may have a stiff gait and be reluctant to move. The joint surfaces are rarely involved, although there may be decreased motion in affected joints as well as pain on manipulation. There may be signs referable to pulmonary abnormalities, such as coughing and nasal discharge.

Radiographically, there is a generalized increase in soft tissue swelling and evidence of periostitis. Irregular new bone growth occurs, especially at the proximal and distal ends of the long bones (Fig. 6.57).[140] The differen-

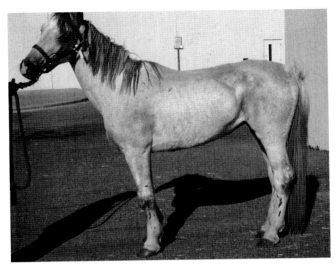

Figure 6.56 All the distal extremities of this horse have swellings associated with hypertrophic osteopathy.

tial diagnosis should include fluorosis, although the gross appearance of the bones, the absence of dental lesions, and blood and urine fluorine levels can usually eliminate fluorosis as the cause. Lateral radiographs of the chest or abdomen may help locate the causative lesion (Fig. 6.58).

CHARACTERISTICS OF EQUINE SKELETAL MUSCLE

Muscle fibers can be classified according to various histochemical (staining) reactions. These staining characteristics are useful in the field of exercise physiology and, when used on muscle biopsies, help diagnose clinical muscle diseases in horses. The contractility of fibers is determined by myosin-adenosine triphosphatase (ATPase) activity, and the muscle fibers can be classified as either slow-twitch (type 1) or fast-twitch (type 2) fibers. Type 2 fibers can be further subdivided into subtypes 2A, 2B, and 2C; type 2C fibers are present only in very young animals.[130] Muscle fibers can also be incubated to determine either succinic dehydrogenase or nicotinamide adenine dinucleotide (NADH) diaphorase activity to assess oxidative capacity (grouped as having high or low activity). The glycogen content of muscle may be determined by the periodic acid Schiff (PAS) reaction, which has revealed that type 1 fibers are lower in glycogen than are type 2 fibers.[130]

Muscle Fiber Types

By using a combination of oxidative capacity and myosin-ATPase activity, three major categories of equine skeletal muscle can be identified,[1,130] including slow-twitch high-oxidative (ST) type 1 fibers, fast-twitch high-oxidative (FTH) type 2A fibers, and fast-twitch low-oxidative (FT) type 2B fibers (Fig. 6.59). Differences between high- and low-oxidative fibers are fairly distinct in the untrained horse, but differentiation becomes more

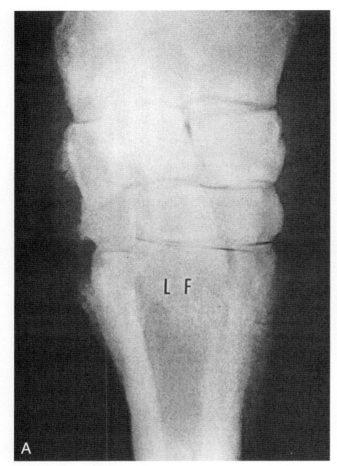

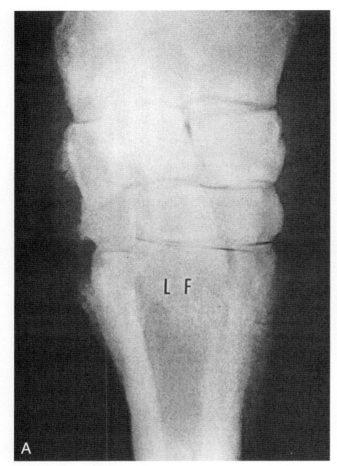

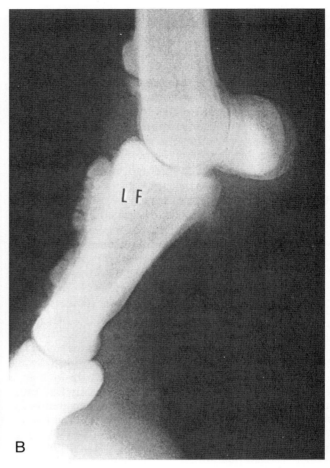

Figure 6.57 Radiographs of the left front (LF) carpal (A) and fetlock (B) joints of a horse with hypertrophic osteopathy, showing irregular new bone growth. (Courtesy of N. Messer, University of Missouri, Columbia, MO.)

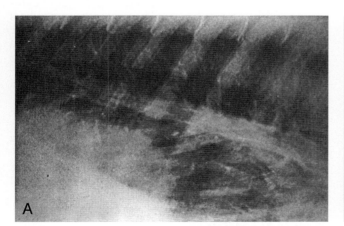

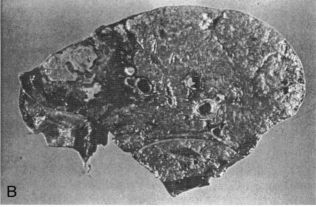

Figure 6.58 A. Radiograph of the thorax of the same horse shown in Figure 6.57, revealing a large pulmonary abscess. B. Necropsy specimen of the lung showing the abscess. (Courtesy of N. Messer, University of Missouri, Columbia, MO.)

difficult as training progresses. In humans, the capacity for muscle performance (i.e., athletic performance) can be related to the individual's muscle fiber profile.[140] Studies have shown that long-distance runners usually have a higher proportion of slow-twitch fibers than the general population, whereas sprinters have a predominance of fast-twitch fibers.[24] In horses, differences in fiber type distribution have been associated with differences in metabolic response to exercise and when muscle fatigue will most likely occur.[129,145]

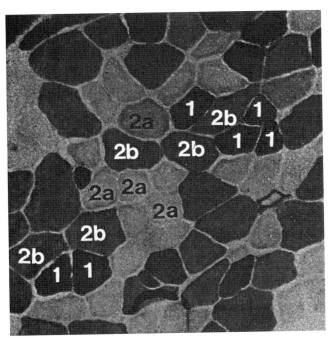

Figure 6.59 Equine skeletal muscle stained for myosin ATPase after preincubation at pH 4. Note the three different muscle fiber types: 1, type 1 (ST) fibers; 2a, type 2A (FTH) fibers; 2b, type 2B (FT) fibers. (Courtesy of D. Hodgson, University of Sydney, Australia.)

Type 1 (ST) fibers are slow-twitch, high-oxidative red fibers that have a lower glycogen storage capacity than type 2 fibers.[130,140] They have poorly developed glycolytic enzyme systems and have a slow speed of contraction. They show little or no fatigue, are good for slow speeds, and are equipped for aerobic metabolism. These are the first fibers formed in myogenesis in the embryo, and they retain their slow-twitch aerobic capacity throughout the animal's life. Snow et al.[127] showed that horses with the highest proportion of these fibers usually have the best performance record in endurance events.

Type 2B (FT) fibers are fast-twitch white fibers that have a well-developed glycolytic pathway but few mitochondria. They fatigue rapidly but are called on for short-term powerful phasic activity. *Type 2A (FTH) fibers* are fast-twitch high-oxidative red fibers that have large glycogen storage capabilities, a well-developed glycolytic pathway, and many mitochondria. These resist fatigue better than type 2B(FT) fibers and are more suited for sustained phasic activity.[130,140]

In humans, the proportion of type 1 to type 2 fibers in muscles is thought to be genetically controlled. This has not been demonstrated in the horse but most likely occurs. In horses, the proportion of fibers in the middle gluteal muscle may be related to the breed and the type of work that the breed has been selected for. It is logical to assume that Quarter Horses and Thoroughbreds, which are involved in sprinting events, have fewer type 1 fibers and more type 2B and type 2A fibers than breeds such as the Arabian, which are used more for endurance events.[128]

Response to Exercise

The proportion of muscle fibers can, to some degree, be altered by training, whereby type 2A and type 2B fibers undergo interconversion.[49] In humans, aerobic training has been associated with increases in oxidative enzyme activities and a marked decrease in type 2B fibers. In horses, however, it appears that the transformation of type 2B to type 2A fibers is rather limited and possibly absent in conventionally trained Thoroughbreds.[130]

Training is thought to increase the cross-sectional area of all three fiber types in horses, similar to what has been observed in human athletes.[140] This view is controversial, however, and other studies have found minimal effects of training on myofiber size.[130] These findings go against the generally accepted opinion that gluteal muscle mass increases with training in horses. The disparity in the results of these studies may be the result of the wide variation in data obtained from muscle biopsies. Muscle biopsies are useful in horses, but samples are too inconsistent to predict performance or the response to training.[110,130] The response of muscle size to training may not be resolved until noninvasive imaging techniques can be used to determine overall muscle mass in horses.

Glycogen depletion within muscle can provide information on muscle fiber composition and possible performance in horses.[140] Glycogen is depleted from type 1 muscle fibers at relatively low intensity levels, since these are the fibers involved in endurance training. As type 1 fibers become depleted, glycogen is lost from the type 2B and type 2A fibers, respectively. Type 2A fibers become depleted of glycogen in some endurance horses presumably because an increase in speed during the ride causes recruitment of these fibers.[127] Proper training, however, prevents a progressive reduction in glycogen content that may affect performance. For instance, training programs involving frequent bouts of prolonged submaximal or high-intensity exercise may lead to a gradual lowering of muscle glycogen content because repletion occurs relatively slowly.[36] Repletion of glycogen occurs in the reverse pattern as depletion, with a preferential repletion of type 2B over type 1 fibers. The practical implication of this is that a period of rest is necessary after strenuous exercise to permit muscle glycogen repletion. Repeated bouts of intensive exercise in Standardbred racehorses has been shown to decrease the glycogen repletion rate in muscle.[67]

Biochemical analysis of muscle biopsies is used to determine the physiologic response of muscle to exercise. Results of several studies indicate that oxidative capacity increases in type 2A fibers with age and training and that the high-oxidative capacity of these fibers is important in racing performance.[112,113] Trained horses have high muscle oxidative capacity, as reflected by high muscle enzyme activities of citrate synthase (CS) and 3-OH-acyl-CoA dehydrogenase. CS is a marker for oxidative capacity, 3-OH-acyl-CoA dehydrogenase is a marker for beta-oxidation of free fatty acids, lactate dehydrogenase (LDH) is a marker for glycolytic capacity, and hexokinase (HK) is a marker for the capacity of glucose phosphorylation. The activities of all of these enzymes can be assayed by using fluorometric techniques.[130] In addition, muscle concentrations of glycogen, lactate, ATP, creatine phosphate, and glucose-6-phosphate (G-6-P) can be measured in muscle tissue. Through biochemical analysis, muscle response to exercise can be determined and findings can be correlated to performance (speed for racehorses). For instance, several studies have indicated that there is a relationship between performance capacity and skeletal muscle ATP content.[112,113] The greatest ATP depletion develops in type 2B fibers, but little depletion occurs in type 1 fibers.

Muscle Degeneration

The response of muscle tissue to injury can vary markedly. From a histologic standpoint, muscle degeneration has been classified into four types:

- *Cloudy swelling.* A mild form of injury that is visible only microscopically. Affected fibers are swollen, finely granular, and opaque, and striations are indistinct. Cloudy swelling may be caused by mild aberrations of cellular metabolism such as would be seen in cases of exertional rhabdomyolysis syndrome.
- *Hyaline (Zenker) degeneration.* A response of the muscle cell to a variety of different conditions, such as white muscle disease and azoturia. Hyaline degeneration affects the cytoplasm but not the sarcolemma.[71] Affected muscle fiber loses its striations and stains homogeneously with eosin. Regeneration occurs by muscle fibers filling the empty portion of the sarcolemma tube.
- *Granular degeneration.* A more severe form of muscle degeneration; the fibers lose both cross striations and longitudinal striations when viewed histologically. The sarcoplasm coagulates into large granules. Many nuclei die, making regeneration difficult; regeneration is possible in cells that have viable nuclei.[71]
- *Fatty degeneration.* An irreversible change in muscle that follows granular degeneration. Histologically, the muscle fiber contains large numbers of fat droplets along with evidence of degeneration.[71]

Muscle Regeneration

Skeletal muscle has the capacity to regenerate as long as other structures, such as the supporting stroma, endomysial tubes, and some viable fragments of muscle fiber, are intact. Jubb and Kennedy[71] classify the regenerative process into three basic types based on the histologic features: budding, proliferation of cellular bands, and recombination of muscle fibers along adjacent surviving sarcoplasm. Which type of muscle regeneration occurs depends on the type and severity of injury and can greatly affect the prognosis.

Regeneration by budding occurs when segments of muscle fiber and sarcolemma are destroyed, such as would occur in a clean incision. The crucial factor is the size of the gap between the free ends of the tube (muscle); large buds forming at the ends of the muscle cells advance across the gap and make contact with similar growths from the other side of the incision. The buds grow just over 1 mm a day, and a certain amount of crossover and interlacing of fibers inevitably occurs. If

the gap is greater than 5 mm or infection or fibroblastic (scar) tissue is present, then bridging may be retarded.[71] Healing of large muscle gaps associated with severe muscle injuries occurs primarily by fibrous tissue and may potentially limit the function of the muscle (e.g., fibrotic myopathy).[2]

If the injury to the muscle cell is milder (e.g., hyaline degeneration when the sarcolemma and endomysium are present), regeneration occurs by proliferation of cellular bands. Macrophages clear away the degenerating substances, nuclei proliferate, and new sarcoplasm appears. Longitudinal and cross striations are restored. Regeneration by fusion of muscle fibers within the same sarcoplasm occurs when there is more severe muscle damage, such as fibers undergoing granular degeneration. Although muscle usually has good regenerative capabilities, in certain conditions muscle may completely lose its ability to regenerate. Such is the case with chronic (of more than 1 year) denervation muscle atrophy resulting from suprascapular nerve injury (sweeney) in horses.[122]

Muscle Atrophy

Muscle atrophy is a diminution in the volume of muscle that is caused by a decrease in individual muscle cell size.[140] Atrophy occurs when muscle is not subjected to sustained periods of tension or activity. It is a potentially reversible phenomenon, since artificial stimulation can reverse the atrophy. Atrophy is seen predominantly in skeletal muscle.

Generalized Muscle Atrophy

Generalized muscle atrophy is associated with poor nutrition, cachexia, malnutrition, and senility. Generalized muscle atrophy is also seen in horses with severe systemic illnesses and is occasionally seen in hospitalized patients that have suffered surgical complications (e.g., peritonitis). In addition to generalized muscle atrophy, there will usually be a loss of fat and a decrease in body weight. Usually, the loss of muscle is symmetric in distribution, but not all muscles are affected to the same degree. Histologically, there will be progressive diminution in size of fibers; individual muscle fibers undergo atrophy at different rates. The diameter of the muscle fibers may be reduced from 40 μm to 15 to 20 μm, as seen in formalin-fixed tissue.[71]

Localized Disuse Muscle Atrophy

Localized muscle atrophy can be categorized into disuse atrophy (associated with immobilization or chronic lameness problems) or neurogenic atrophy (associated with nerve paralysis, e.g., suprascapular nerve injury). Disuse atrophy usually requires a longer duration to become clinically evident, is usually not as severe, and is more likely to be completely reversible than is neurogenic atrophy.[140]

Localized disuse muscle atrophy is commonly seen in horses after cast application, because immobilization produces a hyperextension of the limbs as a result of lack of tone of the flexor muscles and associated tendons. Muscle atrophy after full-limb cast application is usually

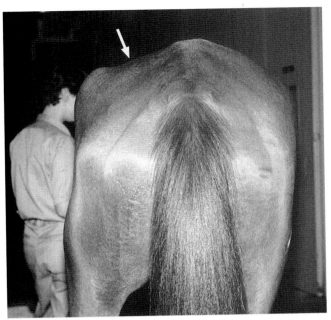

Figure 6.60 Severe disuse atrophy of the left gluteal muscles (arrow), secondary to a chronic pelvic fracture.

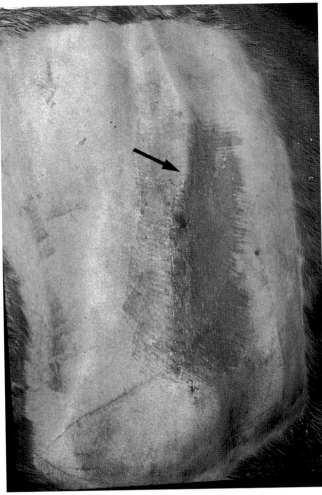

Figure 6.61 Neurogenic atrophy of the supraspinatus muscle over the lateral aspect of the scapula, secondary to damage to the suprascapular nerve. Note the prominent scapular spine (arrow) easily palpable in horses affected with sweeney.

more severe and occurs more rapidly than after half-limb cast application. Localized disuse muscle atrophy is also seen after tendon rupture and fracture of a bone that is required for muscle function, such as the triceps atrophy that occurs with fractures of the olecranon. Pelvic fracture or any severe upper-limb lameness often causes significant disuse atrophy of the gluteal muscles in horses (Fig. 6.60).

If atrophy persists, the muscle will eventually be replaced with fibrous and adipose tissue, regardless of the initiating cause. With severe atrophy, return of muscle volume can be prolonged. Whether localized disuse muscle atrophy can be prevented or reversed with physical therapy, myofascial massage, or muscle stimulation techniques in horses remains unknown and controversial.

Localized Neurogenic Muscle Atrophy

Similar to disuse atrophy, neurogenic atrophy is usually a localized phenomenon and is characteristic of a few well-recognized syndromes in the horse, such as paralysis of the suprascapular nerve (Fig. 6.61) and laryngeal hemiplegia.[122] Damage to the suprascapular nerve is usually caused by pressure from poor-fitting collars in working horses or from trauma from kicks, falls, or scapular fractures in the shoulder region.[122] Regardless of the cause or the specific nerve involved, paralysis of the respective muscles follows denervation and leads to clinical signs of the problem. Other causes of localized neurogenic muscle atrophy include radial nerve damage secondary to humeral fractures, facial muscle atrophy from facial trauma, and multifocal muscle atrophy resulting from equine protozoal myopathy (EPM).[140]

In contrast to generalized and disuse atrophy, neurogenic atrophy usually affects groups of muscle fibers supplied by the damaged nerve. Histologically, clusters of

muscle fibers are seen to degenerate, since each cluster represents a number of terminal nerve endings of a motor unit. Eventually, degeneration with fragmentation occurs subsequent to the atrophy, and fibers lose their ability to proliferate. If muscle regeneration cannot occur, the muscle is ultimately replaced with adipose and fibrous tissue.

Denervated muscle fibers can be reinnervated if the neural sheaths are not injured. Degeneration of a nerve fiber progresses to the nearest node of Ranvier proximal to the site of injury. If the injury is mild, most nerves can regenerate (at about 4 mm a day), and the original continuity to the muscle can be reestablished. If the nerve injury is severe (e.g., transection), however, regrowth of the nerve to the muscle is delayed and may never occur. Also, if concurrent muscle atrophy is severe, even if a functional connection is made, there may be only a limited number of fibers available for reinnervation.[122,140] The result is permanent loss of muscle volume with possible loss of muscle function. This type of neurogenic atrophy is uncommon in horses but may occur after severe lacerations or injuries to the suprascapular nerve.

Calcification and Ossification of Muscle

Calcification occurs when calcium salts are deposited within damaged muscle tissue. The muscle fibers first undergo granular degeneration, at which stage they are apparently highly susceptible to calcification. Calcium deposition occurs in the sarcoplasm of the muscle fiber, although it does not seem to inhibit fiber regeneration if the necessary conditions exist. The most common instance of muscle calcification is seen with degeneration associated with nutritional causes, such as that seen with white muscle disease. In such cases, the fibers are often chalky white in appearance, which can be confirmed histologically.[71]

Ossification is the formation of bone in the connective tissue of muscle that has been chronically traumatized or inflamed.[71] It may also occur as a result of metaplasia or secondary to long bone fractures when there has been displacement of the periosteum. Although uncommon, ossification of muscle is seen primarily in two instances in horses: ossifying myopathy of the semitendinosus muscle[2,140] and ossification of the biceps brachii muscle.[87]

Fibrotic and Ossifying Myopathy

Fibrotic myopathy in horses occurs primarily from repeated tearing or straining of the semitendinosus muscle fibers.[20,76] It may occur after an acute injury if healing is accompanied by extensive fibrosis or adhesion of muscle to surrounding tissues.[2] Fibrotic myopathy may also develop after repeated intramuscular injections or injections of irritating substances into the muscle region. Ossification of the fibrotic tissue occurs uncommonly and is probably related to the chronicity of the problem.[140] Regardless of the cause, the semitendinosus muscle is gradually replaced with fibrous tissue, and irregular jagged plaques of spongy bone may form. Muscle fibers in the region become atrophic. There may also be adhesions to adjacent muscles, including the biceps femoris and semimembranosus.

Because the muscle lacks elasticity, the horse develops a typical goose-stepping gait, characterized by a shortened cranial phase of stride with the limb being pulled back before the foot hits the ground. The gait is most evident at the walk. Palpation of the affected muscle usually reveals firm, nonpainful scar tissue; and radiographs may identify ossification in the affected muscle.[2]

Treatment of horses with advanced fibrosis involves transecting the tendinous attachment of the semitendinosus muscle (semitendinosus tenotomy) on the proximal medial aspect of the tibia.[20] Physical therapy of the limb (walking and pulling the leg forward) is important to help stretch the musculotendinous unit after surgery. The success of this procedure is variable, and recurrence of the condition can develop after an initial improvement in gait.

Alternatively, the muscle itself may be transected (semitendinosus myotomy) at the site of scar formation to achieve a similar elongation of the musculotendinous unit.[76] This technique can be performed with the horse sedated with local anesthesia and standing. This approach has been reported as a successful treatment of horses with fibrotic myopathy.[76] Another option is perform the surgery with the horse anesthetized in lateral recumbency with the affected limb uppermost. Complete surgical removal of the affected scar tissue and muscle is not recommended, because of the numerous postoperative complications and likelihood of refibrosis of the affected area.

Ossification of Biceps Brachii

Fibrosis and ossification of the biceps brachii muscle and tendon are much less common than fibrotic myopathy of the semitendinosus muscle in horses.[87,140] Affected horses usually have a shortened cranial phase of the stride and tend to land on their toes, similar to horses with navicular syndrome. Ultrasound of the tendon is probably the best diagnostic tool for assessing the severity of tendon damage, but radiography can be used to determine the extent of tendon and muscle ossification. Damage to the bicipital bursa may also be diagnosed with ultrasound but is probably most accurately determined by endoscopy (arthroscopy) of the bursa itself. Treatment options are limited. Surgery may not be beneficial for ossification of the biceps brachii, since the tendon and bicipital bursa are often concurrently involved.

Inflammation of Muscle

The term "myositis" is often used as a generic term to describe any painful condition affecting muscle (infectious, traumatic, degenerative, etc.). Strictly speaking, myositis is a reactive inflammation characterized by exudation of lymphocytes and inflammatory cells within the muscle and is most commonly associated with infections or open traumatic injuries. A certain amount of inflammation, however, is seen with true degeneration of muscle that accompanies exercise-related myopathies. Inflammation of skeletal muscle is quite common in horses because of the frequent occurrence of trauma, such as lacerations and wire cuts, and overexertion-related injuries.

Infectious myositis can occur from a variety of causes, including lacerations, penetrating wounds, intramuscular injections, hematogenous spread of infection, and extension of an infective focus into adjacent muscle tissue.[52] The bacteria most likely to cause the infection are *Streptococcus zooepidemicus*, *Streptococcus equi*, *Staphylococci* spp., *Corynebacterium pseudotuberculosis*, and occasionally *Clostridia* spp. *Streptococcus equi* and *Corynebacterium pseudotuberculosis* are common causes of muscle abscessation in horses, which are referred to as strangles and pigeon fever, respectively.

In the horse, bacterial myositis is often accompanied by cellulitis that affects the connective tissue planes as well as the muscle bellies. The cellulitis may respond to treatment, or it may become organized into a true abscess. Initially, the cellulitis may be extremely painful and involve a large surface area, resembling a clostridial myositis. Clostridial myositis rarely develops after traumatic lacerations or blunt injuries in horses, however. Most sites of bacterial myositis are painful to palpation and have some amount of swelling and firmness. Most horses will be lame (and sometimes extremely lame), but this may depend on the severity and site of the infection.[52]

Clostridial myositis most commonly occurs after small penetrating wounds, parturition injuries, castration, and especially intramuscular injections. The species of *Clostridia* involved are commonly found in spore form in soil and feces, and muscles are highly susceptible to bacterial invasion by these organisms (see the sections on tetanus and botulism in this chapter). Under suitable conditions (low oxidative potential and alkaline pH), bacterial spores introduced into the muscle commence vegetative growth. These organisms proliferate, elaborate exotoxins, and cause extensive necrosis of muscle. Death can occur quickly from toxemia, but less severely affected horses will be depressed with systemic signs of toxemia. The affected area is often swollen, and owing to the accumulation of air within the tissues, crepitation may be palpable. The types of wounds often associated with clostridial myositis in horses are usually small and benign, making this condition seem unlikely to occur. Any penetrating wound, however, may result in an anaerobic infection. Fortunately, most wounds in horses are large and open enough so that clostridial myositis is not a major problem.

DIAGNOSIS OF MUSCLE DISORDERS

Physical Examination

Physical examination of the muscles should be included as part of any overall lameness examination of the horse. Examination should include visualization for symmetry and direct digital palpation of the suspected muscle(s) for pain, swelling, heat, and consistency. The symmetry or asymmetry of the muscle is best determined by comparing it—from a distance—with the contralateral side of the animal. The most common sites for disuse muscle atrophy secondary to chronic lameness are the shoulder and scapular region in the forelimb and the gluteal region in the hindlimb. Neurogenic atrophy may develop at any location of nerve injury but primarily occurs over the scapula secondary to suprascapular nerve injury.

In addition, differences in pain, heat, and consistency of the muscle should be compared with the contralateral side if possible. Myalgia or muscle pain may be difficult to determine in horses unless it is severe, especially if the injured muscle is not along the external surface of the body. Detection of occult or subtle muscular injuries in horses by palpation alone is limited, and more advanced diagnostic methods (thermography, nuclear scintigraphy, muscle enzymes, etc.) are not always beneficial either.

A complete lameness examination should be performed to determine if the muscle problem is a primary injury or may be secondary to some other musculoskeletal problem. In our opinion, secondary muscle soreness is much more common than primary muscle injuries as a cause of lameness in horses. Myopathies resulting from overexertion, however, occur in performance horses, similar to the situation in humans, and can cause significant pain and lameness.

Clinical Pathology

When any tissue is damaged, enzymes leak into the circulation and may reflect the degree of tissue damage that has occurred. Serum enzymes most commonly used to evaluate muscle damage or disease are creatine kinase (CK) and aspartate aminotransferase (AST).[51,52] AST is not muscle specific, but large increases tend to be associated with muscle damage. Increases in AST together with increases in the muscle-specific enzyme CK also support the diagnosis of muscle involvement. With acute muscle injury, CK activities peak within 2 to 6 hours and have a half-life of around 2 hours. AST activities peak after about 24 hours and have a half-life of 7 to 8 days. These differences in enzyme activities can be used to evaluate the stage (acute, chronic, recovery) of muscle involvement in horses with rhabdomyolysis.

Enzyme activities are used primarily to help diagnosis of horses with generalized muscle disease, such as exercise-related rhabdomyolysis, since focal muscle injuries often do not cause significant increases in muscle enzymes. Interpretation of muscle enzymes should always be performed in light of the clinical situation, including the animal's daily training routine and stage of fitness. Acute muscle damage causes marked elevations in serum enzymes, whereas slow progressive damage may have levels within normal ranges.

A comparison of muscle enzymes before and after exercise (the so-called exercise test) may also be used to determine the susceptibility of horses to exercise-induced muscular damage. It is recommended samples be taken before and then 2 and 6 hours after exercise to evaluate changes in enzyme activity.[51] A number of variables may affect the results of the exercise test; therefore, the nature of the test and its interpretation are controversial.

In addition, electrolyte abnormalities may either predispose the horse to or be the result of generalized muscle disease. For instance, potassium concentrations in the blood may be increased during clinical episodes of hyperkalemic periodic paralysis (HYPP) in horses but are usually normal between episodes.[25,26] Severe rhabdomyolysis may also cause an increase in blood potassium concentration if severe myonecrosis has occurred. Apparent electrolyte imbalances that may predispose the horse to rhabdomyolysis are, however, best detected by urinary fractional electrolyte excretion tests.[53] These tests must be performed appropriately and interpreted with care.

Thermography

Thermography is a diagnostic tool used to detect surface temperature. It is considered to be more sensitive than digital palpation for detecting temperature differences and, therefore, improving our diagnostic capabilities with soft tissue injuries. Some clinicians believe that using thermography to help diagnose soft tissue injuries is analogous to using nuclear scintigraphy (bone scan) to document bone injuries.[141,142] Note that the results of thermography can be unpredictable; experience using the modality is necessary for accurate interpretation. In addition, surface temperatures can vary markedly because of many uncontrollable factors. Whether thermography can detect deep muscle injuries, such as those of the back and hip in horses, is debatable. Despite these limitations, thermography may be a useful diagnostic tool, complementing digital palpation and helping confirm suspected soft tissue/muscle injuries.[141,142]

Ultrasonography

Ultrasonography is occasionally beneficial for diagnosing muscle injuries in horses. It can be most helpful for documenting suspected muscle tears and ruptures (e.g., with rupture of the gastrocnemius, superficial digital flexor muscle of the hindlimb, semitendinosus, or the peroneus tertius). Disruption of the muscle is not always visible, but there is usually a hematoma/seroma in the vicinity of the muscle damage, suggesting a severe soft tissue injury.

Nuclear Scintigraphy

Nuclear scintigraphy is primarily used to diagnose bone and joint injuries in horses. Certain acute soft tissue (muscle) injuries, however, may be detected on the initial "pool" or "soft tissue phase" of the procedure (see Chapter 4 for details). In one study, abnormal uptake of the radioisotope within skeletal muscle was detected in 10 of 109 racehorses 24 hours after strenuous exercise.[92] These horses had a history of poor performance or subtle lameness problems. From a clinical standpoint, a bone scan is less likely to identify chronic soft tissue injuries than more acute injuries.

Electromyography

Electromyography (EMG) refers to changes in electric potential associated with motor unit twitch. Needle electrodes inserted into the muscle are used to pick up action potentials, which will be absent or abnormal in diseased muscle. This technique is useful for indicating muscle damage and is used primarily for identifying myopathies of neurogenic origin.[122,140] For instance, EMG is used to document suprascapular nerve injuries in suspected cases of sweeney and to diagnose peripheral neuropathies associated with equine protozoal myelitis. Soft tissue swelling and inflammation from the initial traumatic injury, however, may produce erroneous results with the EMG. Therefore, EMG testing is usually delayed until after the initial inflammatory period (1 to 2 weeks).

Biopsy

Microscopic examination of muscle is becoming more widely used to diagnose muscle diseases.[110,130] Muscle biopsies are indicated in horses that have repeated episodes of rhabdomyolysis that do not respond to standard therapies.[146] Definitive diagnosis of polysaccharide storage myopathy (PSSM) requires a muscle biopsy. Two muscle biopsy techniques can be used: open surgical biopsy or percutaneous needle biopsy.[146] In most situations, the open technique is more feasible, since it does

not require a special biopsy punch and produces fewer artifacts.

The open technique is frequently used for biopsy of the semimembranosus muscle because of the ease of approach, lack of a visible scar, and prevalence of abnormal polysaccharide in this muscle. The middle gluteal muscle or other muscles that appear to be actively involved in the disease condition may also be biopsied. The site for biopsy of the semimembranosus muscle is usually 13 cm distal and medial to the tuber ischii.[146] A sample of muscle 3 cm long, 2 cm wide, and 1.5 cm thick is obtained and placed on saline-soaked gauze (Fig. 6.62A). The sample should be handled gently to avoid distortion of the muscle fibers.

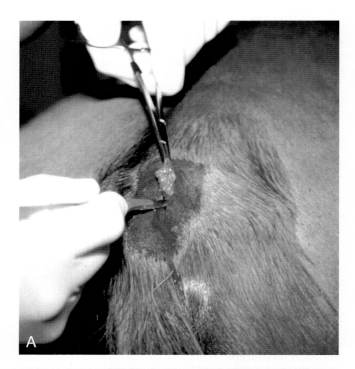

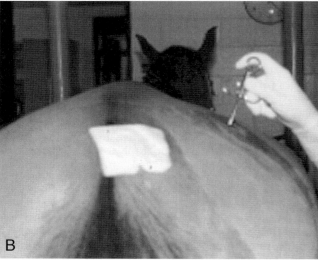

Figure 6.62 Muscle biopsy. A. Open approach. B. Bergstrom needle biopsy. (Courtesy of Dr. Jennifer MacLeay, Colorado State University, Ft. Collins, CO.)

A punch biopsy of the middle gluteal muscle may be obtained with a modified Bergstrom needle 5 mm in diameter (Fig. 6.62B). A trucut biopsy needle cannot be used because it will not provide enough muscle tissue for diagnosis. The punch biopsy is taken at a standardized site 18 cm along a line from the dorsum of the tuber coxae to the base of the tail.[146] The biopsy needle is inserted to a depth of 6 cm in an adult horse and usually obtains a 200- to 400-mg sample of muscle tissue. Samples are placed on saline moistened gauze and shipped overnight (in a waterproof container on ice packs) or can be placed in plastic bags on dry ice for delivery to the laboratory. At the laboratory, histologic and histochemical stains used to evaluate the frozen muscle sections include hematoxylin and eosin (H&E), Gomori's trichrome, reduced nicotinamide adenine dinucleotide phosphate (NADPH), PAS, acid phosphatase, and ATPase activity after preincubation in acidic and alkaline pH.[146] False-negative results may occur owing to small muscle biopsy samples.

Molecular Biologic Techniques

Molecular biology techniques have also been used in horses, primarily to document hereditary muscle disorders such as HYPP.[106] The gene probe for the DNA that codes for the defective sodium channel in this disease can be determined from an ethylenediaminetetraacetic acid (EDTA)-treated blood sample.[106] Suspected carrier horses can also be documented with this test.

PHYSICAL INJURIES TO MUSCLE

Lacerations

Sharp lacerations involving muscle are common in horses and usually result from trauma, such as wire cuts, kicks, lacerations, or running into objects. Although these injuries can be extensive, rarely is there complete loss of limb function, unless an entire group of muscles is transected (e.g., extensor muscles of forelimb) or there is concurrent nerve injury (e.g., sweeney). Initially, there is hemorrhage and edema at the site of injury. Zenker's hyaline degeneration of a certain amount of muscle ensues, depending on the type (crush vs. sharp cut) and severity of the injury.[140] See texts on wound healing for the principles behind the repair of such lacerations (Fig. 6.63). In general, wounds involving muscle tissue of the proximal aspect of a horse's limbs or body heal well, whether they are closed primarily or left to heal by second intention.

Muscle Strains

Muscle strains or small tears, which are often referred to as "pulled muscles," probably occur commonly during exercise in performance horses, as they do in humans.[52] The definitive diagnosis of a pulled muscle can be difficult, especially in more chronic cases. Obvious external swelling is not necessarily present, and pain may be apparent on digital palpation. Abnormalities in the consistency of the muscle, such as increased tension or

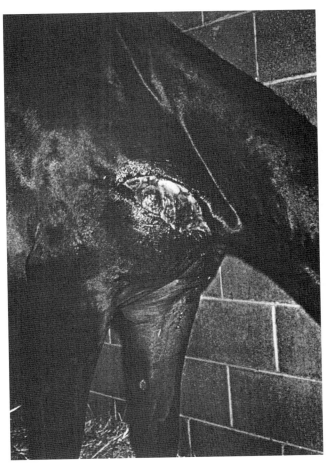

Figure 6.63 Sharp laceration of the shoulder.

"tightness," may be detectable, especially if the longissimus dorsi muscle is involved. Some of the diagnostic procedures discussed earlier may be used to aid diagnosis, but the exact site of muscle damage may never be determined.

As in humans and dogs, localized myositis in horses usually responds to rest and anti-inflammatories, with the possible addition of some form of physiotherapy.[40] Chronic muscle injuries may lead to poor performance or recurrence of the problem, however, when exercise is resumed. Treatments for chronic muscle pain are empirical and may include local injections of corticosteroids, myofascial massage, therapeutic ultrasound, magnetic therapy, cold laser therapy, acupuncture, and chiropractic manipulations.

Myositis of the longissimus dorsi muscles is frequently seen in Standardbreds, hunters, and jumpers.[140] Poor racing performance, poor jumping technique, and twisting over jumps are common complaints. The condition is essentially a localized exertional myopathy involving this muscle group. The resultant muscle spasms lead to a gait alteration in the hindlimbs that resembles bilateral hindlimb lameness. It is most likely an integral part of the sore back syndrome in horses and may be seen secondary to conditions of the stifle or hock.[140]

The clinical signs are usually vague and are frequently mistaken for problems in the limbs. Unfortunately, the condition serves as a catchall for undiagnosed hindlimb lameness in many breeds and uses of horses. Because of the vagueness of the condition, remedies such as chiropractic manipulation, physiotherapy, ultrasound, faradism, and acupuncture have benefited in reputation by successfully treating this condition. Diagnosis is usually based on eliminating other lameness problems and on the response to treatment.

Muscle Rupture or Tearing

Muscle rupture or tearing is a more severe form of a pulled muscle and suggests complete disruption of the muscle fibers. It is not uncommon in performance horses because of violent muscle contraction or repeated overexertion (eventual complete rupture of abnormal muscle).[2,140] Rupture of normal muscle in nonperformance horses may also occur as a result of falls, slips, or struggling to rise and appears to be more common than tendon rupture (e.g., gastrocnemius rupture) (Fig. 6.64).[140]

Muscle rupture is considered the initial injury in many cases of fibrotic myopathy of the semitendinosus muscle. With acute rupture of a muscle, examination usually reveals focal swelling, pain on palpation, and lameness. The ability of the limb to bear weight is generally not altered unless a major supporting muscle is ruptured, such as the gastrocnemius or superficial digital flexor muscle (caudal reciprocal apparatus).

A hematoma usually develops, and occasionally a disruption of the fascia overlying the muscle can be palpated. The hematoma is gradually resorbed, and healing occurs with fibrosis, potentially contributing to future problems, such as fibrotic myopathy. If the hematoma or seroma is large, drainage may be required to permit

healing, because the fluid will separate the tissue planes, leading to delayed healing (Fig. 6.65).

Violent contraction of the muscle may also result in herniation of a muscle belly through the epimysium.[140] Muscle hernias occur when the main body of the muscle bulges through the overlying fascia. We have identified such hernias on the medial and caudal aspects of the thigh associated with severe trauma, such as a fall. These hernias usually have concurrent hematomas and soft tissue swelling, suggesting a severe injury. In such cases, healing of the defects with scar tissue will usually restore limb function. Physical therapy techniques, such as walking and stretching the involved muscles, should be recommended to prevent excessive fibrosis and altered limb function.

SYSTEMIC DISEASES OF MUSCLE

Exertional Rhabdomyolysis Syndrome

Exercise-related or exertional myopathies have been referred to in the literature as paralytic myoglobinuria, exertional rhabdomyolysis, Monday morning disease, myositis, and tying-up syndrome.[115,146] Although the terms encompass a wide range of diseases that are associated with exercise, in all probability they are related and represent different degrees of the same condition. From a pathologic point of view, the term "rhabdomyolysis" is most appropriate; thus the current term is equine or exertional rhabdomyolysis syndrome (ERS).

Horses affected with ERS usually exhibit a stiff gait, muscle cramping, pain, and reluctance to move during or after mild to moderate exercise.[115] Rhabdomyolysis may also occur after endurance rides, transport, or gen-

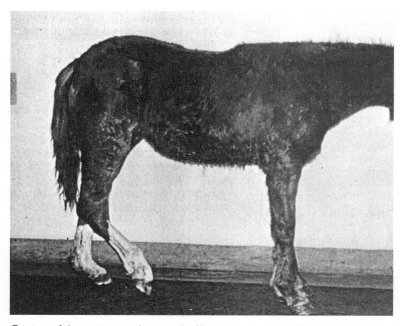

Figure 6.64 Rupture of the gastrocnemius muscle. Note the extended stifle joint with flexion of the hock joint.

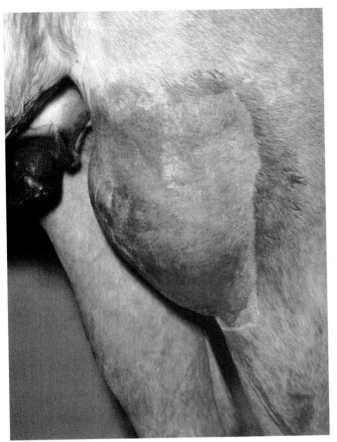

Figure 6.65 Large swelling on the medial aspect of the thigh, secondary to a traumatic fall. The seroma was drained, and the defect was temporarily packed with gauze to facilitate healing.

eral anesthesia. The clinical signs can vary markedly but usually involve the muscles of the back and rear limbs.

Numerous and conflicting causes for the condition have been proposed, including vitamin E and selenium deficiency, electrolyte abnormalities, heat exhaustion in endurance horses, hypothyroidism, and abnormal calcium regulation.[72,115,149] Although the exact cause for ERS is not always determined, there are several risk factors known to precipitate the problem. For instance, horses in training that are rested for 1 to 2 days while maintained on full rations are prone to ERS when they resume exercise. Sudden increases in the duration or intensity of training may precipitate the problem, and horses that are inadequately trained for competition are prone to ERS. This problem is also more common in female horses, especially those that are "high strung"; and certain families or breed lines (such as Quarter Horses) appear to be prone to the condition. The diagnosis is usually based on the typical clinical signs together with increased activity of muscle enzymes (CK and AST) in serum.[115,144]

In humans, many cases of recurrent exertional rhabdomyolysis are caused by errors in skeletal muscle energy metabolism. A similar approach was investigated recently in horses; it used muscle biopsies and examined exercise responses.[143,146] Specific equine exertional my-

opathies that have been identified to date include 1) mitochondrial myopathy resulting from a deficiency in NADH coenzyme Q reductase in an Arabian, 2) a defect in skeletal muscle excitation-contraction coupling resembling malignant hyperthermia in Thoroughbred horses, and 3) a polysaccharide storage myopathy (PSSM) in Quarter Horses involving abnormal glycogen storage.[146,147] More specific causes and multiple causes for ERS most likely exist. Applying the term "tying-up" to all horses with clinical signs of muscle cramping will likely result in failure to recognize specific subsets of ERS.

Treatment of horses with ERS is aimed at reducing the pain, limiting further muscle damage, and restoring fluid and electrolyte balance.[115,148] Affected horses should be moved as little as possible to prevent further muscle damage. Specific treatments include acepromazine to relieve anxiety and improve blood flow to the muscles, NSAIDs, oral or intravenous fluids and electrolytes, intravenous dimethyl sulfoxide (DMSO), dantrolene, and rubeola virus immunomodulator (RVI).

Preventive measures include proper dietary management (adjust ration to level of exercise), vitamin E and selenium, sodium bicarbonate, potassium chloride, phenytoin, acepromazine, dimethylglycine, and RVI injections.[140,148] Standard preventive therapies for most horses with ERS include a period of rest followed by an altered training schedule and the addition of vitamin E, selenium, and electrolytes to the diet (see Chapter 5 for more information).

Hyperkalemic Periodic Paralysis

In the 1980s, a condition characterized by intermittent episodes of muscular weakness and fasciculations was recognized in heavily muscled Quarter Horses, Appaloosas, and Paints.[26,25] Affected horses had a variety of clinical signs, but most would demonstrate muscle weakness and become recumbent and unable to rise.[25] Serum potassium concentrations were increased transiently during episodes. The condition—hyperkalemic periodic paralysis—is now known to be caused by a defect in the skeletal muscle sodium channel that regulates membrane activity; it is an inherited condition.[26,106] The diagnosis can be confirmed using molecular biologic techniques to detect the abnormal DNA that codes for the defective sodium channel in an EDTA blood sample[106] (see Chapter 5 for more information).

Myopathies

Polysaccharide Storage Myopathy

Polysaccharide storage myopathy (PSSM) is a disorder of glycogen storage in Quarter Horse-related breeds, Warmbloods, and draft horses that exhibit signs of exertional rhabdomyolysis.[146,147] The condition often affects horses that are heavily muscled and have a calm demeanor. Clinical signs may be inconsistent, but muscle wastage and an abnormal gait are often present. The condition is diagnosed by identifying abnormal polysaccharide in muscle biopsies taken from horses with typical clinical signs. PSSM can be prevented by replacing grain and sweet feed in the diet with rice bran (a 20% fat supplement) at 0.5 to 3.0 kg a day and by providing regular daily exercise[146] (see Chapter 5 for more information).

Nutritional Myopathy

Nutritional myopathy in foals is usually termed "nutritional muscular dystrophy" or "white muscle disease." It is a well-recognized disease of all domestic animals (calves, pigs, sheep, and foals) and is caused by a dietary deficiency of selenium.[28,90] It is characterized by noninflammatory degeneration of skeletal and cardiac muscle, which can contribute to a variety of clinical signs ranging from recumbency to acute death. Lesions within the affected muscles give them a white appearance on examination, contributing to the name of the disease.

In foals, nutritional myopathy is classically recognized within the first few months of life.[90] Very young foals are more prone to develop the severe form of the disease and may die within a few hours after onset of clinical signs.[90] Older foals may develop a variety of clinical signs, including prolonged recumbency, listlessness, tachypnea, and dysphagia. Nutritional myopathy is rare in adult horses but may affect the muscles of mastication or the limbs, in which case it results in a stiff gait similar to that seen in horses with ERS.

Nutritional myopathy is seen in parts of the world where soil and pastures are low in selenium, such as the eastern and northwestern United States and much of Canada. It has also been reported in Australia, the United Kingdom, the Netherlands, and New Zealand (see Chapter 5 for more information).

Myopathy Associated With Prolonged Recumbency or General Anesthesia

Myopathy associated with extended periods of prolonged recumbency or general anesthesia is seen occasionally in horses. It usually affects focal muscle groups of the dependent limb, but a generalized myopathy can occur. Localized myopathies of the masseter, triceps, and gluteal muscles can be difficult to differentiate clinically from neuropathies involving the facial, radial, and peroneal nerves, respectfully. Horses with generalized myopathy usually exhibit signs of severe pain, have palpable firm muscles, and have difficulty standing. Localized myopathies related to general anesthesia or recumbency are believed to be the result of excessive compression of the muscle groups, which compromises circulation and leads to hypoxia of the tissue.[74] The compression may be related to improper positioning or padding during anesthesia.

The muscles that may be affected in horses in lateral recumbency are the triceps brachii, pectoral, quadriceps femoris, hindlimb extensors, masseter, and flank muscles.[56,156] For horses positioned in dorsal recumbency, the muscles of the longissimus dorsi, gluteal, vastus lateralis, and hindlimb adductor muscles are most frequently affected.[30]

Prolonged anesthesia (more than 2.5 hours), inappropriate positioning, and inadequate padding (particularly in heavily muscled or draft breeds), recent hard exercise, history of muscle cramping, and prolonged hypotension

appear to increase the risk of myopathy after surgery.[47,54] In one clinical study, flexion of the hindlimbs in halothane-anesthetized horses positioned in dorsal recumbency, coupled with a period of hypotension (mean arterial pressure less than 70 mm Hg for more than 45 minutes) was associated with ischemic necrosis of the adductor muscles.[30] In general, mean arterial blood pressure should be maintained above 60 mm Hg to avoid hypoperfusion and hypoxia of dependent muscle groups.[54] Using wick catheters placed in the triceps brachii muscles of laterally recumbent anesthetized horses, pressures between 30 and 50 mm Hg and up to 80 mm Hg have been measured.[74] Interstitial pressures of approximately 20 mm Hg were also measured in the biceps femoris muscle of anesthetized horses.[95]

Blood flow to skeletal muscle is significantly reduced at interstitial pressures over 20 mm Hg, potentially contributing to hypoperfusion of these muscle groups.[95] The high intracompartmental muscle pressures may also alter nerve transmission, which is seen commonly with compartment syndrome in humans and dogs.[40] Therefore, both muscle and nerve abnormalities may exist concurrently, making the distinction clinically difficult.[156]

Clinical signs of localized postanesthetic myopathy depend on the particular muscle affected. Usually, the affected muscles will be firm, painful to palpation, and swollen. The horse may have difficulty supporting weight on the limb or may exhibit pain when weight bearing.[62] With neuropathies, similar clinical signs may be evident, except that no abnormalities of the muscles can be detected. Serum muscle enzyme levels may also be used to help differentiate between a neuropathy and localized myopathy in the postanesthetic patient.[156] Large increases in muscle enzymes may not be evident, however, unless there is severe or generalized muscle damage.

Generalized myopathies usually involve muscles of the nondependent limbs and may be seen regardless of the duration of general anesthesia. Muscles become rigid even before the horse stands from anesthesia. The horse may appear anxious, sweat, and exhibit signs of colic.[54] The animal may not be able to stand, making management of the condition difficult. Myoglobinuria, renal nephrosis, shock, and death are potential sequelae. This syndrome may be the result of the anesthetic agent itself, resembling malignant hypothermia rather than excessive pressure or hypoperfusion of the affected muscles. Luckily, generalized myopathy is rare.

Treatment of localized myopathy or neuropathy in horses is primarily supportive until the muscle or nerve resumes normal function. The time required to restore function is related to the severity of the damage, but most horses are much improved within a few hours to days. Supportive care includes intravenous fluids and vasodilators (acetylpromazine) to promote peripheral blood flow, and anti-inflammatories (phenylbutazone, flunixin meglumine, dimethyl sulfoxide, etc.) to help restore muscle or nerve function.[140,156] Bandaging and splinting of affected limbs may help the horse stand and ambulate more easily, thus relieving much of the animal's anxiety. Horses that can stand on three legs have a good prognosis for recovery from myopathies or neuropathies and generally respond to treatment within 72 hours.[62] Horses that are affected bilaterally and unable to stand have a poor prognosis. In addition, horses with localized myopathy respond much better to treatment than do horses with generalized myopathy.

Tetanus

Tetanus is a highly fatal, infectious disease caused by the toxin of *Clostridium tetani*. The vegetative form of *C. tetani* is a gram-positive bacillus that requires anaerobic conditions for growth and replication. The organism exists primarily in spore form and is commonly found in the intestinal tract and feces of animals and in soils rich in organic material. The most common route of infection is by wound contamination with *C. tetani* spores. When wound conditions favor an anaerobic environment, spore germination, bacterial proliferation, and elaboration of the toxin occur. Wounds most commonly associated with tetanus in horses include puncture wounds, castration sites, metritis after dystocia, retained placenta, and wounds with considerable tissue necrosis.[50] An infected umbilicus is the usual site of *C. tetani* proliferation and toxin formation in neonates.[48]

The clinical signs of tetanus are due to the potent exotoxin tetanospasmin, which is produced locally at the site of *C. tetani* proliferation and acts principally on the central nervous system.[50] In general, the disease causes muscular rigidity, hyperesthesia, and convulsions in horses of all ages.[48,50] The signs reflect spasticity of striated and smooth muscles. Early clinical signs include a stiff gait, reluctance to feed off the ground, and overreactivity to normal external stimuli. More severe clinical signs include spasm of the muscles of mastication (trismus), prolapse of the nictitating membranes, and rigid extension of the neck, back, and limbs ("sawhorse" stance). Once adult animals become recumbent, they generally cannot rise, and attempts to stand cause further clonic muscle spasms and distress. Even slight stimulation usually causes prolonged muscle spasms that may result in self-traumatization. Death usually occurs in 5 to 7 days and is often caused by asphyxia, resulting from spastic paralysis of the respiratory muscles, laryngospasm, or aspiration pneumonia.[50] Average case mortality is approximately 75%.

The current approach to treatment of tetanus is based on the premise that the toxin-ganglioside bond is irreversible and that recovery is caused by the gradual replacement of altered ganglioside by normal metabolic processes.[50] Therefore, recovery is gradual and often takes about 6 weeks. For these reasons, if treatment is undertaken, it is generally symptomatic and supportive with particular emphasis on good nursing care.

Because of the poor success of treating horses with tetanus, prevention is the key. Active immunization against tetanus is reliably achieved with potent commercial aluminum hydroxide-adjuvanted toxoids. The usual recommendations are for a second vaccination 3 to 4 weeks after the first, followed by annual revaccination, with boosters given after lacerations or other tetanus-prone wounds.[50] Annual revaccination for tetanus is recommended, although there is evidence that protective antibody titers may persist for up to 4 years after the first booster vaccination in horses. Equine-origin tetanus antitoxin should be used only to protect unvaccinated

horses after injury or to treat horses with clinical tetanus, because of the risk of acute hepatic necrosis after administration.

Botulism

Botulism is a flaccid neuromuscular paralysis caused by the exotoxin of the gram-positive bacterium *Clostridium botulinum*. The paralysis is the result of interference with acetylcholine release by the exotoxin at the motor endplate.[12] In foals, the disease has been called the shaker foal syndrome, and in adults it is known as forage poisoning.[12] The distribution of *C. botulinum* spores in soils in the United States is variable and is most likely related to the geographic frequency of the disease. The disease generally occurs on an individual case basis, but herd outbreaks can occur. Contaminated feed sources are the usual cause of outbreaks.

There are thought to be three different routes of botulism infection: ingestion of preformed toxin, toxic-infectious, and wound botulism.[12] Ingestion of preformed toxin as with contaminated feed is the most common route of infection and gives rise to the syndrome known as forage poisoning. The toxic-infectious route is thought to occur primarily in foals, and the wound route of infection is uncommon. Infected umbilical remnants in foals and castration sites in adults have been suggested as sources of *C. botulinum* infections.

Clinical signs of botulism reflect flaccid neuromuscular paralysis. The toxin does not affect the central nervous system, so affected animals are bright and alert despite being weak and usually recumbent. Affected animals may also be found dead. The term "shaker foal" was derived from the severe muscle tremors that are frequently seen with this disease. Other signs of neuromuscular paralysis include poor tail, tongue, and eyelid tone or dysphagia.[12] Respiratory difficulties result from paralysis of the intercostal and diaphragmatic musculature, and death is usually the result of respiratory failure.

Treatment consists of polyvalent equine-origin botulism antitoxin to bind circulating toxin and appropriate nursing and nutritional therapy. Before the use of the antitoxin, the mortality rate of horses with botulism was approximately 90%. With the use of botulism antitoxin, the prognosis for survival is greater than 70% in adult horses and even higher in foals.[12] The antitoxin, however, is expensive, should be used early in the course of the disease, and does not guarantee recovery. The recommended dose is 400 mL for adults and 200 mL for foals.

Although treatment of horses with botulism can be effective, prevention of the disease in endemic areas by vaccination programs is recommended and highly successful. Mares should receive a three-dose series of *C. botulinum* toxoid with 1 month between vaccines and the last vaccine in the last month of gestation.[12] Yearly boosters during the last month of gestation should be given thereafter. This regimen provides maximal colostral antibodies to protect susceptible foals. If protection is required in nonbreeding animals, the initial three-series vaccination protocol should be used with yearly boosters in these animals as well.

Myotonia Congenita

Myotonia congenita is a rare skeletal muscle disease in horses that is characterized by prolonged aftercontraction.[140] The disease may be inherited, but the mode of inheritance is unknown, as too few cases have been seen. The biochemical defect involved in myotonia congenita in horses is also unknown. Clinical signs may appear as early as 3 weeks to several months of age. Such animals appear extremely well muscled in the hindquarters. Affected horses, when startled, are stiff and unable to move normally. The first few steps are made with considerable difficulty, often by dragging the hindfeet.

Percussion of affected muscles will result in sustained contraction, with gradual muscle relaxation taking more than 1 minute to occur. The affected muscles feel firm and tense. Muscles of the hindlimbs are usually involved, whereas the head, neck, and forelimbs are unaffected.

Histologically, muscle fibers from such cases show extreme variation in diameter, and many are twice the size of normal equine muscle cells with little inflammatory reaction.[140] There is no known treatment for this condition.

References

1. Aberle ED, et al. Fiber types and size in equine skeletal muscle. Am J Vet Res 1976;37:145.
2. Adams SB. Biology and treatment of specific muscle disorders. In: Auer JA, Ed. Equine Surgery. Philadelphia: WB Saunders, 1992;925–931.
3. Andrea CR, et al. Comparison of pullout strength between ASIF self-tapping and non-self-tapping 4.5 mm. bone screws in adult equine cortical bone. Vet Surg 1998;27:498–499.
4. Auer JA. Surgical equipment and implants for fracture repair. In: Nixon AJ, Ed. Equine Fracture Repair. Philadelphia: WB Saunders, 1996:52–62.
5. Auer JA, Martens RJ. Periosteal transection and periosteal stripping for correction of angular limb deformities in foals. Am J Vet Res 1982;43:1530.
6. Auer JA, Martens RJ, Morris EL. Angular limb deformities in foals. Part I. Congenital factors. Comp Cont Educ Pract Vet 1982;4:330.
7. Auer JA, Martens RJ, Williams EH. Periosteal transection for correction of angular limb deformities in foals. J Am Vet Med Assoc 1982;181:459.
8. Auer JA, Watkins JP. Instrumentation and techniques for equine fracture fixation. Vet Clin North Am Equine Pract 1996;12:283–302.
9. Baxter GM. Subchondral cystic lesions in horses. In: McIlwraith CW, Trotter GW, Eds. Joint Disease in the Horse. Philadelphia: WB Saunders, 1996;384–397.
10. Baxter GM. Treatment of orthopedic infections in horses. Vet Clin North Am Equine Pract 1996;12:303–336.
11. Belknap JK, Baxter GM, Nickels FA. Extensor tendon lacerations in horses: Fifty cases (1982–1988). J Am Vet Med Assoc 1993;203:428–431.
12. Bernard WV. Botulism. In: Robinson NE, Ed. Current Therapy in Equine Medicine. 4th ed. Philadelphia: WB Saunders, 1997;326–328.
13. Blackwell JG, Griffith AD, Crosby WJ. Surgical correction of an alveolar mandibular bone cyst. Equine Pract 1985;7:70–73.
14. Blood DC, Henderson JA, Radostits OM. Veterinary Medicine. Philadelphia: Lea & Febiger, 1979.
15. Booth LC, Feeney DA. Superficial osteitis and sequestrum formation as a result of skin avulsion in the horse. Vet Surg 1982;11:2.
16. Bramlage LR. Current concepts of emergency first aid treatment and transportation of equine fracture patients. Comp Cont Educ Pract Vet 1983;5:S564–S574.
17. Bramlage LR. First aid and transportation of fracture patients. In: Nixon AL, Ed. Equine Fracture Repair. Philadelphia: WB Saunders, 1996;36–42.
18. Bramlage LR. Osteochondrosis related bone cysts. Proc Am Assoc Equine Pract 1993;39:83–84.
19. Bramlage LR. Physitis in foals. Proc Am Assoc Equine Pract 1993;39:57–62.
20. Bramlage LR, Reed SM, Embertson RM. Semitendinosus tenotomy for treatment of fibrotic myopathy in the horse. J Am Vet Med Assoc 1985;186:565.
21. Brown MP, McCallum FJ. Observations on growth plates in limbs of foals. Vet Rec 1976;98:443.
22. Campanacci M, Capanna R, Picci P. Unicameral and aneurysmal bone cysts. Clin Orthop 1986;204:25–36.
23. Colgan SA, et al. A comparison of the Synthes 4.5-mm cannulated screw and the Synthes 4.5-mm standard cortex screw systems in equine bone. Vet Surg 1998;27:540–546.
24. Costill DL, et al. Skeletal muscle enzymes and fiber composition in male and female track athletes. J Appl Physiol 1976;49:149.
25. Cox JH. An episodic weakness in four horses associated with intermittent hyperkalemia and the similarity of the disease to hyperkalemic periodic paralysis in man. Proc Am Assoc Equine Pract 1985;31:383–391.
26. Cox JH, Debowes RM. Episodic weakness caused by hyperkalemic periodic paralysis in horses. Comp Cont Educ Pract Vet 1990;12:83–88.
27. David JB, Cohen ND, Nachreiner R. Equine secondary hyperparathyroidism. Comp Cont Educ Pract Vet 1997;19:1380–1386.
28. Dodd DC. Nutritional myopathy. In: Mansmann RA, McAllister ES, Eds. Equine Medicine and Surgery. 3rd ed. Santa Barbara, CA: American Veterinary Publications, 1982;937.
29. Dodd DC, Raker CW. Tumoral calcinosis (calcinosis circumscripta) in the horse. J Am Vet Med Assoc 1970;157:968.
30. Dodman NH, et al. Postanesthetic hind limb adductor myopathy in five horses. J Am Vet Med Assoc 1988;193:83–86.
31. Dutton DM, et al. Incomplete ossification of the tarsal bones in foals: 22 cases (1988–1996). J Am Vet Med Assoc 1998;213:1590.
32. Eagle MT, Koch DB, Whalen JP. Mineral metabolism and immobilization osteopenia in ponies treated with 25-hydroxycholecalciferol. Cornell Vet 1982;72:372–393.
33. Ellis DR. Fractures of the proximal sesamoid bones in Thoroughbred foals. Equine Vet J 1979;11:48.
34. Embertson RM, Bramlage LR, Gabel AA. Physeal fractures in the horse. II. Management and outcome. Vet Surg 1986;15:230–236.
35. Embertson RM, et al. Physeal fractures in the horse. I. Classification and incidence. Vet Surg 1986;15:223–229.
36. Essen-Gustavsson B, et al. Muscular adaptation of horses during intensive training and detraining. Equine Vet J 1989;21:27.
37. Farnum CE, Wilsman NJ. Ultrastructural histochemical evaluation of growth plate cartilage matrix from healthy and osteochondrotic swine. Am J Vet Res 1986;47:1105–1115.
38. Field JR, Hearn TC, Arighi M. Investigation of bioabsorbable screw usage for long bone fracture repair in the horse: Interfragmentary compression and axial load response in equine cadaver long bone fractures. Vet Clin Orthop Trauma 1995;8:191–205.
39. Firth EC. Specific orthopedic infections. In: Auer JA, Ed. Equine Surgery. Philadelphia: WB Saunders, 1992;932.
40. Fitch RB, Jaffe MH, Montgomery RD. Muscle injuries in dogs. Comp Cont Educ Pract Vet 1997;19:947–958.
41. Frank N. Primary hyperparathyroidism with osteodystrophia fibrosa of the facial bones in a pony. J Am Vet Med Assoc 1998;212:84–86.
42. Fretz PB, Turner AS, Pharr J. Retrospective comparison of two surgical techniques for correction of angular limb deformities in foals. J Am Vet Med Assoc 1978;172:281–286.
43. Gaughan EM. Angular limb deformities in horses. Comp Cont Educ Pract Vet 1998;20:944–946.
44. Gaughan EM. Partial physiolysis with temporary transphyseal bridging for correction of physeal dysplasia and angular limb deformity in two yearling horses. Vet Clin Orthop Trauma 1996;9:101–105.
45. Goodbary RF, Hage TJ. Hypertrophic pulmonary osteoarthropathy in a horse—a case report. J Am Vet Med Assoc 1960;137:602.

46. Goulden BE, O'Callahan MW. Tumoral calcinosis in the horse. N Z Vet J 1980;28:217.
47. Grandy JL, et al. Arterial hypotension and the development of postanesthetic myopathy in halothane-anesthetized horses. Am J Vet Res 1987;48:192–197.
48. Green SL, et al. Tetanus in the horse: A review of 20 cases (1970–1990). J Vet Int Med 1994;8:128.
49. Guy PS, Show DH. The effect of training and detraining in muscle composition in the horse. J Physiol 1977;269:33.
50. Hahn CN, Mayhew IG, MacKay RJ. Diseases of the brainstem cranial nerves (autonomic somatic). In: Colahan PT, Mayhew IG, Merritt AM, Moore JN, Eds. Equine Medicine Surgery. 5th ed. St. Louis: CV Mosby, 1999;935–937.
51. Harris PA. Equine rhabdomyolysis syndrome. In: Robinson NE, Ed. Current Therapy in Equine Medicine. 4th ed. Philadelphia: WB Saunders, 1997;115–121.
52. Harris PA, Dyson SJ. Muscular disorders. In: Robinson NE, Ed. Current Therapy in Equine Medicine. 4th ed. Philadelphia: WB Saunders, 1997;121–124.
53. Harris PA, Gray J. The use of the urinary fractional electrolyte excretion test to assess electrolyte status in the horse. Equine Vet Ed 1992;4:162–166.
54. Hartsfield SM, Matthews NS. Management of physiologic abnormalities during anesthesia in horses. In: Auer JA, Ed. Equine Surgery. Philadelphia: WB Saunders, 1992;215.
55. Hawkins JF. Bone tumors and true cysts. In: White NA, Moore JN, Eds. Current Techniques in Equine Surgery and Lameness. Philadelphia: WB Saunders, 1998;112–115.
56. Hill MA. Causes of degenerative joint disease (osteoarthrosis) and dyschondroplasia (osteochondrosis) in pigs. J Am Vet Med Assoc 1990;197:107–112.
57. Holcombe SJ, et al. Use of antibiotic-impregnated polymethylmethacrylate in horses with open or infected fractures or joints: 19 cases (1987–1995). J Am Vet Med Assoc 1997;211:889–893.
58. Houghton GR, Dekel S. The periosteal control of long bone growth. Acta Orthop Scand 1979;50:635.
59. Houghton GR, Rooker GD. The role of the periosteum in the growth of long bones. J Bone Joint Surg [Br] 1979;61:218.
60. Houston CS, Swischuck LE. Varus and valgus—no wonder they are confused. N Engl J Med 1980;302:471.
61. Howard RD, McIlwraith CW, Trotter GW. Arthroscopic surgery for subchondral cystic lesions of the medial femoral condyle in horses: 41 cases (1988–1991). J Am Vet Med Assoc 1995;206:842–850.
62. Hubbell JAE, et al. Perianesthetic considerations in the horse. Comp Cont Educ Pract Vet 1984;7:S401–412.
63. Hunt DA, et al. Evaluation of an interfragmentary compression system for the repair of equine femoral capital physeal fractures. Vet Surg 1990;18:107–116.
64. Hunt RJ. Angular limb deviations. In: White NA, Moore JN, Eds. Current Techniques in Equine Surgery and Lameness. Philadelphia: WB Saunders, 1998;323–326.
65. Hurtig MB. Defective bone and cartilage in foals fed a low-copper diet. Proc Am Assoc Equine Pract 1990;36:637–643.
66. Hurtig MB, et al. Correlation study of defective cartilage and bone growth in foals fed a low-copper diet. Equine Vet J 1993;16(Suppl):66–73.
67. Hyyppa S, Rasanen LA, Reeta Poso A. Resynthesis of glycogen in skeletal muscle from Standardbred trotters after repeated bouts of exercise. Am J Vet Res 1997;58:162–166.
68. Jackman BR, Baxter GM. Treatment of a mandibular bone cyst by use of a corticocancellous bone graft in a horse. J Am Vet Med Assoc 1992;201:892–894.
69. Jeffcott LB. Osteochondrosis in the horse—searching for the key to pathogenesis. Equine Vet J 1991;23:331–338.
70. Jeffcott LB, Kold SE, Melsen F. Aspects of the pathology of stifle bone cysts in the horse. Equine Vet J 1983;15:304–311.
71. Jubb KV, Kennedy PC. Pathology of Domestic Animals. 2 vols. New York: Academic Press, 1970.
72. Koterba A, Carlson GP. Acid base and electrolyte alterations in horses with exertional rhabdomyolysis. J Am Vet Med Assoc 1982;180:303.
73. Lee HA, Grant BD, Galina AM. Solitary osteochondroma in a horse: A case report. J Equine Med Surg 1979;3:113.
74. Lindsay WA, McDonell W, Bignell W. Equine postanesthetic forelimb lameness: Intracompartmental muscle pressure changes and biochemical patterns. Am J Vet Res 1980;41:1919.
75. Lundvall RL, Jackson LL. Periosteal new bone formation of the radius as a cause of lameness in two horses. J Am Vet Med Assoc 1976;168:612.
76. Magee AA, Vatistas NJ. Standing semitendinosus myotomy for the treatment of fibrotic myopathy in 39 horses (1989–1997). Proc Am Assoc Equine Pract 1998;44:263–264.
77. Malghem J, et al. Spontaneous healing of aneurysmal bone cysts. J Bone Joint Surg [Br] 1989;71:645–650.
78. Markel MD. Bone structure and the response of bone to stress. In: Nixon AJ, Ed. Equine Fracture Repair. Philadelphia: WB Saunders, 1996;3–9.
79. Markel MD. Fracture healing and its noninvasive assessment. In: Nixon AJ, Ed. Equine Fracture Repair. Philadelphia: WB Saunders, 1996;19–29.
80. Martinelli MJ, et al. Magnetic resonance imaging of degenerative joint disease in a horse: A comparison to other diagnostic techniques. Equine Vet J 1996;28:410–415.
81. Mauten DJ, Rendano V. Hypertrophic osteopathy in a mare with a dysgerminoma. J Equine Med Surg 1978;2:445.
82. McClure SR, Honnas CM, Watkins JP. Managing equine fractures with external skeletal fixation. Comp Cont Educ Pract Vet 1995;17:1054–1062.
83. McClure SR, Watkins JP, Ashman RB. An in vitro comparison of the effect of parallel and divergent transfixation pins on the breaking strength of the equine third metacarpal bone. Am J Vet Res 1994;55:1327–1330.
84. McClure SR, Watkins JP, Ashman RB. In vivo evaluation of intramedullary interlocking nail fixation of transverse femoral osteotomies in foals. Vet Surg 1998;27:29–36.
85. McDuffee LA, et al. An in vitro biomechanical investigation of an interlocking nail for fixation of diaphyseal tibial fractures in adult horses. Vet Surg 1994;23:219–230.
86. McKenzie RA, et al. Control of nutritional secondary hyperparathyroidism in grazing horses with calcium plus phosphorus supplementation. Aust Vet J 1981;57:554.
87. Meagher DM, Pool RR, Brown MP. Bilateral ossification of the tendon of the biceps brachii muscle in the horse. J Am Vet Med Assoc 1979;174:272.
88. Mehl ML, et al. The use of MRI in the diagnosis of equine limb disorders. Equine Pract 1998;20:14–17.
89. Mitton LA, Bertone AL. Angular limb deformities in foals. J Am Vet Med Assoc 1994;204:717–720.
90. Moore RM, Kohn CW. Nutritional muscular dystrophy in foals. Comp Cont Educ Pract Vet 1991;13:476–489.
91. Morgan JP, Carlson WD, Adams OR. Hereditary multiple exostosis in the horse. J Am Vet Med Assoc 1962;140:1320.
92. Morris E, et al. Scintigraphic identification of skeletal muscle damage in horses 24 hours after strenuous exercise. Equine Vet J 1991;23:347–352.
93. Murray RC, et al. Biomechanical comparison of the Herbert and AO cortical bone screws for compression of an equine third carpal bone dorsal plane slab osteotomy. Vet Surg 1998;27:49–55.
94. Nemeth F, Back W. The use of the walking cast to repair fractures in horses and ponies. Equine Vet J 1991;23:32–36.
95. Norman WM, Dodman NH, Court MH. Interstitial pH and pressure in the dependent biceps femoris muscle of laterally recumbent anesthetized horses. Vet Surg 1988;17:234–239.
96. Nunamaker DM. Metacarpal stress fractures. In: Nixon AJ, Ed. Equine Fracture Repair. Philadelphia: WB Saunders, 1996;195–199.
97. Nunamaker DM, Butterweck DM, Provost MT. Fatigue fractures in Thoroughbred racehorses: Relationships with age, peak bone strain and training. J Orthop Res 1990;8:604–611.
98. Nunamaker DM, Butterweck DM, Provost MT. Some geometric properties of the metacarpal bone: A comparison between the Thoroughbred and Standardbred racehorse. J Biomech 1989;22:129–134.
99. Nunamaker DM, et al. A new external skeletal fixation device that allows immediate full weight bearing. Vet Surg 1986;15:345–355.

100. Nunamaker DM, et al. Plate luting: A preliminary report of its use in horses. Vet Surg 1986;15:289–293.

101. Ogden JA. The development and growth of the musculoskeletal system. In: Albright JA, Brand RA, Eds. The Scientific Basis of Orthopedics. New York: Appleton-Century-Crofts, 1979.

102. Olsen SE. Morphology and physiology of the growth cartilage under normal and pathologic conditions. In: Sumner-Smith G, Ed. Bone in Clinical Orthopedics. Philadelphia: WB Saunders, 1982;159–196.

103. Olsen SE, Reiland S. The nature of osteochondrosis in animals. Acta Radiol 1987;358(Suppl):299.

104. Owen LN. The pathology of bone infection. In: Sumner-Smith G, Ed. Bone in Clinical Orthopedics. Philadelphia: WB Saunders, 1982;261–272.

105. Pharr JW, Fretz PB. Radiographic findings in foals with angular limb deformities. J Am Vet Med Assoc 1981;179:812.

106. Pickar JG, et al. Altered ionic permeability in skeletal muscle from horses with hyperkalemic periodic paralysis. Am J Physiol 1991; 260:C926–C933.

107. Reddi AH. Initiation of fracture repair process by bone morphogenetic proteins. Clin Orthop 1998;355S:566–572.

108. Richardson DW, Clark CC. Effects of short-term cast immobilization on equine articular cartilage. Am J Vet Res 1993;54: 449–453.

109. Richardson DW, Nunamaker DM, Sigafoos RD. Use of an external skeletal fixation device and bone graft for arthrodesis of the metacarpophalangeal joint in horses. J Am Vet Med Assoc 1986; 191:316–321.

110. Rivero JL. Muscle biopsy as a tool for assessing muscular adaptation to training in horses. Am J Vet Res 1996;57:1412–1416.

111. Rodney JR. Epiphyseal compression in young horses. Cornell Vet 1963;53:567.

112. Roneus N, Essen-Gustavsson B. Skeletal muscle characteristics and metabolic response to exercise in young Standardbreds. Am J Vet Res 1997;58:167–170.

113. Roneus N, et al. Skeletal muscle characteristics in young trained and untrained Standardbred trotters. Equine Vet J 1992;24: 292–294.

114. Rose RJ. Surgical treatment of osteomyelitis in the metacarpal and metatarsal bone in the horse. Vet Rec 1978;102:498.

115. Rossier Y. Management of exertional rhabdomyolysis syndrome. Comp Cont Educ Pract Vet 1994;16:381–386.

116. Salter RB. Birth and pediatric fractures. In: Heppenstall BR, Ed. Fracture Treatment and Healing. Philadelphia: WB Saunders, 1980.

117. Salter RB. Textbook of Disorders and Injuries of the Musculoskeletal System. Baltimore: Lippincott Williams & Wilkins, 1970; 33.

118. Savage CJ. Etiopathogenesis of osteochondrosis. In: White NA, Moore JN, Eds. Current Techniques in Equine Surgery and Lameness. Philadelphia: WB Saunders, 1998;318–322.

119. Schatzker J. Concepts of Fracture Stabilization in Bone in Clinical Orthopedics. Philadelphia: WB Saunders, 1982.

120. Schatzker J, Sanderson R, Murnaghan P. The holding power of orthopedic screws in vivo. Clin Orthop 1975;108:115.

121. Schenk KR, Willenegger H. Zum histologischen bild der sogennanten primarheilung der knockenkompakta nach experimetellen osteomen am hund. Experimentia 1963;19:593.

122. Schneider RK, Bramlage LR. Suprascapular nerve injury in horses. Comp Cont Educ Pract Vet 1990;12:1783–1790.

123. Shupe JL. Fluorosis. In: Colahan PT, et al., Eds. Equine Medicine and Surgery. 4th ed. Goleta, CA: American Veterinary Publications, 1991;1293.

124. Shupe JL, et al. Hereditary multiple exostosis; clinicopathologic features of a comparative study in horses and man. Am J Vet Res 1979;40:751.

125. Singer VL, Whitenack DL. Osteopetrosis in a foal. Equine Pract 1981;3:30.

126. Smart ME, et al. Copper deficiency in calves in north central Manitoba. Can Vet J 1981;21:349.

127. Snow DH, Baxter P, Rose RJ. Muscle fiber composition and glycogen depletion in horses competing in an endurance ride. Vet Rec 1981;108:374.

128. Snow DH, Guy PS. Muscle fiber type composition of a number of limb muscles in different types of horses. Res Vet Sci 1980;28: 137.

129. Snow DH, Harris DC, Gash S. Metabolic response of equine muscle to intermittent maximal exercise. J Appl Physiol 1985;58: 1689–1697.

130. Snow DH, Valberg SJ. Muscle anatomy, physiology, and adaptations to exercise and training. In: Hodgson DR, Rose RJ, Eds. The Athletic Horse. Philadelphia: WB Saunders, 1994;145: 179.

131. Southwood LL, et al. Lateral approach for endoscopic removal of solitary osteochondromas from the distal radial metaphysis in three horses. J Am Vet Med Assoc 1997;210:1166–1168.

132. Spindler KP, et al. Prospective study of osseous, articular, and meniscal lesions in recent anterior cruciate ligament tears by magnetic resonance imaging and arthroscopy. Am J Sports Med 1993; 21:551–557.

133. Staller GS, et al. Contact area and static pressure profile at the plate-bone interface in the nonluted and luted bone plate. Vet Surg 1995;24:299–307.

134. Steiner JV, Rendano VT. Aneurysmal bone cyst in the horse. Cornell Vet 1982;72:57–63.

135. Stone WC, et al. The pathologic mineralization of soft tissue: Calcinosis circumscripta in horses. Comp Cont Educ Pract Vet 1990;12:1643–1648.

136. Stover SM. Stress fractures. In: White NA, Moore JN, Eds. Current Techniques in Equine Surgery and Lameness. 2nd ed. Philadelphia: WB Saunders, 1998;451–459.

137. Stover SM, et al. An association between complete and incomplete stress fractures of the humerus in racehorses. Equine Vet J 1992; 24:260–263.

138. Swalec-Tobias KM, Schneider RK, Besser TE. Use of antimicrobial-impregnated polymethyl methacrylate. J Am Vet Med Assoc 1996;208:841–844.

139. Trotter GW. Osteomyelitis. In: Nixon AJ, Ed. Equine Fracture Repair. Philadelphia: WB Saunders, 1996;359–366.

140. Turner AS. Diseases of bone and related structures. In: Stashak TS, Ed. Adams' Lameness in Horses. 4th ed. Philadelphia: Lea & Febiger, 1987;293–338.

141. Turner TA. Thermography. In: White NA, Moore JN, Eds. Current Techniques in Equine Surgery and Lameness. 2nd ed. Philadelphia: WB Saunders, 1998;606–611.

142. Turner TA, Purohit RC, Fessler JF. Thermography: A review in equine medicine. Comp Cont Educ Pract Vet 1986;11:855–862.

143. Valberg SJ, et al. Familial basis of exertional rhabdomyolysis in Quarter Horse-related breeds. Am J Vet Res 1996;57:286–290.

144. Valberg SJ, et al. Muscle histopathology and plasma aspartate aminotransferase, creatine kinase and myoglobin changes with exercise in horses with recurrent exertional rhabdomyolysis. Equine Vet J 1993;25:11–16.

145. Valberg SJ, et al. Oxidative capacity of skeletal muscle fibers in racehorses: Histochemical versus biochemical analysis. Equine Vet J 1998;20:291–295.

146. Valberg SJ, MacLeay JM, Mickelson JR. Exertional rhabdomyolysis and polysaccharide storage myopathy in horses. Comp Cont Educ Pract Vet 1997;19:1077–1085.

147. Valberg SJ, Townsend D, Mickelson JR. Skeletal muscle glycolytic capacity and phosphofructokinase regulation in horses with polysaccharide storage myopathy. Am J Vet Res 1998;59: 782–785.

148. Valentine BA, et al. Dietary control of exertional rhabdomyolysis in horses. J Am Vet Med Assoc 1998;212:1588–1593.

149. Waldron-Mease E. Hypothyroidism and myopathy in racing Thoroughbreds and Standardbreds. J Equine Med Surg 1979;3: 124.

150. Watkins JP. Osteochondrosis. In: Auer JA, Ed. Equine Surgery. Philadelphia: WB Saunders, 1992:971–984.

151. Whitehair KL. Regional limb perfusion with antibiotics. In: Proceedings. 5th American College of Veterinary Surgeons Symposium, Chicago, 1995;59.

152. Whitehair KL, et al. Regional limb perfusion for antibiotic treatment of experimentally induced septic arthritis. Vet Surg 1992; 21:367.

153. Whitehair KL, et al. Regional perfusion of the equine carpus for antibiotic delivery. Vet Surg 1992;21:279.

154. Williams MA, Pugh DC. Developmental orthopedic disease: Minimizing the incidence of a poorly understood disorder. Comp Cont Educ Pract Vet 1993;15:859–871.

155. Young DR, Nunamaker DM, Markel MD. Quantitative evaluation of the remodeling response of the proximal sesamoid bones to training-related stimuli in Thoroughbreds. Am J Vet Res 1991; 52:1350–1356.

156. Young SS. Post-anesthetic myopathy. Equine Vet Ed 1993;5: 200–203.

157. Yovich JV, et al. Holding power of orthopedic screws: Comparison of self-tapped and pre-tapped screws in foal bone. Vet Surg 1986;15:55–59.

Diseases of Joints, Tendons, Ligaments, and Related Structures

C. Wayne McIlwraith

DISEASES OF JOINTS

Arthritis may be defined simply as inflammation of a joint. It is a nonspecific term and does little to describe the nature of the various specific entities that affect equine joints. The role of inflammation also varies considerably among the different conditions. Such general terms are no longer appropriate in the management of equine joint conditions. Specific diagnoses need to be made to treat the horse effectively and make accurate prognoses.

Knowledge of etiology, pathogenesis, diagnosis, and treatment of each of the different equine joint conditions has advanced considerably since the last edition of this text, and a comprehensive book on equine joint disease has been published recently.[41] To understand joint disease in the horse, a basic knowledge of the anatomy and physiology of joints, as well as their pathobiologic responses, is necessary.

Classification of Joints

Joints are most often classified according to their normal range of motion. Three groups are recognized: 1) synarthroses (immovable joints), 2) amphiarthroses (slightly movable joints), and 3) diarthroses (movable joints). Another classification is based on the specialized forms of connective tissue that are present. These two classifications are interrelated in that the bones of the immovable or slightly movable joints are connected by fibrous or cartilaginous membranes (syndesmoses or synchondroses), whereas the component bony parts of the movable joints, although covered by hyaline cartilage, are completely separated, contained within the joint cavity, and enclosed by a synovial membrane (synovial joints). Synovial joints have two major functions: 1) to enable movement and 2) to transfer load.[73] Synarthroses are generally found in the skull, where bone plates are held firmly to each other by fibrous or cartilaginous elements. Amphiarthroses are characterized by the presence of flattened disks of fibrocartilage connecting the articulating surfaces, as are found between the vertebrae. The entire structure is invested by a fibrous capsule. Diarthroses include most of the joints of the extremities. Since these are the joints that we are essentially concerned with in equine lameness, their anatomy and physiology is described in detail.

General Anatomy

The synovial or diarthrodial joint consists of the articulating surfaces of bone, covered by articular cartilage and secured by a joint capsule and ligaments, and a cavity within these structures containing synovial fluid (Fig. 7.1). The joint capsule is composed of two parts: the fibrous layer, which is located externally and is continuous with the periosteum or perichondrium (and, ultimately, bone), and the synovial membrane, which lines the synovial cavity where articular cartilage is not present.

The fibrous portion of the joint capsule is composed of dense fibrous connective tissue that provides some mechanical stability to the joint. The collateral ligaments are associated with the joint capsule. Intraarticular ligaments normally have a synovial membrane cover. Histologically, the fibrous portion of the joint capsule and the ligaments are principally composed of collagenous fibers. Fourteen genetically distinct collagens have been described. Type I collagen predominates in the fibrous connective tissues of the joint.[73] It is vascular with arteriovenous anastomoses[67] and flow-modifying structures (glomi) reported.[63] The afferent pain fibers of the joint capsule were originally thought to be localized in the fibrous portion, but it was noted that synovial traction was painful.[26] More recently, using immunohistochemistry with substance P as a more sensitive way of identi-

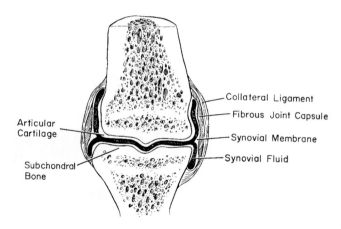

Figure 7.1 Diagram of a typical synovial joint.

Articular Cartilage

Subchondral Bone

Collateral Ligament

Fibrous Joint Capsule

Synovial Membrane

Synovial Fluid

fying the distribution of nociceptor fibers, sensory nerve fibers have been demonstrated in the synovial membrane and subintimal layers as well as collateral ligaments and suspensory ligament and distal sesamoid ligament attachments.[5a,48]

The insertions of the fibrous capsule and articular ligaments into the adjacent bones demonstrate a zonal organization. Parallel bundles of collagen first become invested with the fibrocartilaginous stroma and, as they near the bone, become calcified. The collagenous fibers enter the bone cortex in a manner analogous to that of Sharpey's fibers. This gradual transition of joint capsule and ligaments to mineralized fibrocartilage and then to bone enhances the ability of the insertions to distribute forces evenly and decreases the likelihood of pullout failure.[35]

Stability of the joint is provided by the bony configuration of the joint, the ligamentous and capsular support systems, and the musculotendinous units controlling the joint. In addition, there is a negative hydrostatic pressure within the synovial cavity of normal joints, and this is considered to impart a "suction" and stabilizing effect.[68]

Synovial Membrane Structure and Function

Equine synovial membrane (also called synovium) is normally white to yellowish white, but gross discoloration (pink to brown) may be noted secondary to incidental trauma. It is smooth and glistening in some regions of the joint and is formed into numerous villi in other regions. These villi have specific locations and a diverse morphology.[40] Although villi do proliferate in association with trauma and other insults, they are present in the fetus and, therefore, at birth.[3]

Histologically, the synovial membrane is a modified mesenchymal tissue and consists of two layers. The intima, an incomplete cellular lining layer, lies next to the joint cavity and overlies a deeper layer of connective tissue (fibrous, areolar, or adipose) termed the subsynovial layer, or subintima. Generally, in regions where the synovial membrane is subjected to increased pressure, it is fibrous and flat; where it must move freely and independently of the joint capsule, it is areolar and may be folded. The areolar subintima consists of loose fibrous

connective tissue that continues into the central core of the villi. Numerous blood vessels are present.

The synovial cells of the intima (synoviocytes) form an incomplete layer one to four cells thick, and no basement membrane can be detected (Fig. 7.2).[75] The synoviocytes have been classified at the ultrastructural level into two principal types, designated types A and B.[23] The type A cells resemble macrophages, and the type B cells resemble fibroblasts. Intermediate cells are also observed. A concept has evolved that type A and type B cells are not distinct but merely cells whose differences in morphology reflect the functions they are currently performing.[17]

Numerous blood vessels are present in the subintima and extend to within 5 to 10 microns from the intimal surface.[39] The lymphatic vessels of the synovial membrane lie close to large blood vessels,[9] but their capillaries do not extend as close to the synovial cavity as do the blood capillaries. It appears that each joint has a dual nerve supply consisting of specific articular nerves that reach the joint capsule as independent articular branches of adjacent peripheral nerves and, secondly, articular branches that are nonspecific and arise from related muscle nerves.[11]

The three principal functions of the synovial membrane are phagocytosis, regulation of protein and hyaluronan content of the synovial fluid, and regeneration.[75] The phagocytic ability of type A synoviocytes has been

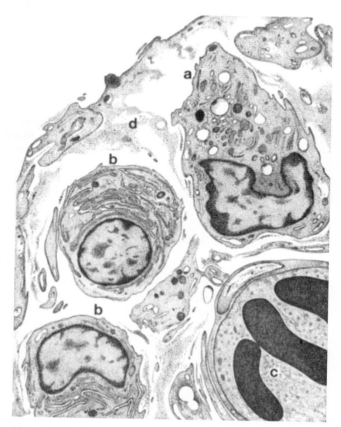

Figure 7.2 Diagram of a portion of synovial membrane demonstrating synoviocytes (types a and b) within the intercellular stroma of the intima, capillary (c), and collagenous matrix of intima (d). Tissue deep to this would be considered subintima.

well demonstrated following the injection of various substances.[7,71] Unwanted materials are engulfed and become contained within phagocytic vacuoles, which in turn fuse with cytoplasmic lysosomes to effect digestion. Excessive phagocytic activity or disruption of lysosomal or cellular membranes releases enzymes into the environment (a typical feature of synovitis).

The synovial membrane acts as an important permeability barrier, which in turn controls synovial fluid composition. Most small molecules cross the synovial membrane by a process of free diffusion that is limited by the intercellular spaces in the synovial membrane rather than by blood vessel fenestrations.[68] It is generally accepted that almost all the protein in synovial fluid is derived from plasma.[8] Only the source of some 2% of protein firmly bound to hyaluronan is unknown, and it has been suggested that it may be derived from type B synoviocytes.[18] In traumatic effusions, the changes in protein content and composition have been associated with both increased vascular permeability[68] and increased protein synthesis by the synoviocytes.[62] Hyaluronan is synthesized by the cells of the synovial membrane.[20a] The function of hyaluronan is discussed below.

The ability of the synovial membrane to reform following synovectomy has been well documented in rabbits,[29,43] and more recently, the process has been described in the horse.[24,72] More recent work in the horse reveals that 120 days after subtotal synovectomy there is evidence of restoration and an intimal layer was present.[72] However, the synovium was devoid of villi and there was subintimal fibrosis.

Another important property of the joint capsule is its ability to allow complete range of motion. The example of a metacarpophalangeal (fetlock) joint, illustrated in Figure 7.3, shows that synovial membrane gathers at the dorsal aspect of the joint in extension and at the palmar aspect in flexion. This property of gathering has been termed redundancy.[68] Inflammation and fibrosis will impede this property and result in joint stiffness. Continued normalcy of the joint capsule is also important because of its role in shock absorption.

Adequate lubrication of synovial membrane is also important for normal joint function and is discussed below.

Articular Cartilage Structure and Function

Grossly, normal articular cartilage appears milky and opaque in the thicker regions but translucent with a slight bluish tinge in the thinner regions. However, the surface is not smooth. Studies using the scanning electron microscope have demonstrated undulations and irregular depressions.[16] The articular cartilage of equine joints is generally of the hyaline type. However, fibrocartilage is also present in synovial joints, as at the junction of articular cartilage, synovial membrane, and periosteum (called the transition zone), and in menisci.[75]

Histologically, adult articular cartilage has been divided into four layers, and the chondrocytes have different appearances within these layers (Fig. 7.4):[3,42]

1. The tangential or superficial layer, containing flattened or ovoid chondrocytes and tangentially oriented collagenous fibrils
2. The intermediate or transitional layer, containing larger chondrocytes that may be single or paired and randomly oriented collagenous fibrils

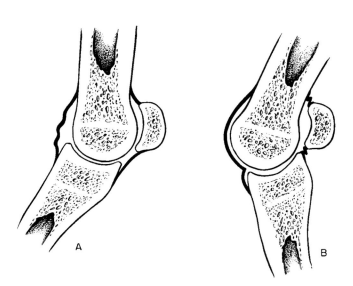

Figure 7.3   Diagram of a metacarpophalangeal joint demonstrating how redundant synovial membrane gathers at the dorsal aspect on extension (A) and at the palmar aspect on flexion (B).

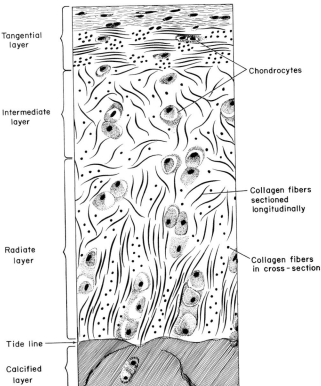

Figure 7.4   Diagram of adult articular cartilage showing the four layers and the arrangement of the chondrocytes and collagenous fibers.

3. The radiate or deeper layer, containing chondrocytes arranged in vertical columns separated by collagenous fibrils that have an overall radial arrangement

4. The calcified cartilage layer, composed of mineralized cartilage and chondrocytes in various stages of degeneration

A basophilic-staining, undulating line of division between the radiate layer and the layer of calcified cartilage is termed the "tide mark" or "tide line."[42] It delineates the elastic, nonmineralized layers of the articular cartilage from the layers of calcified cartilage that has little resilience. The extracellular matrix of the articular cartilage is a complex of collagens, fibrils, amorphous proteoglycans, glycoproteins, and water.[15]

COLLAGENS

Collagen type II comprises 90 to 95% of the collagen in articular cartilage and forms fibrils and fibers intertwined throughout the matrix. Equine type II collagen has been characterized biochemically by cyanogen bromide–cleaved peptide profiles.[75a] Type II collagen is secreted as a procollagen, and the complete sequence of equine type II procollagen messenger RNA has been reported.[58a] The messenger RNA was cloned from a complementary DNA (cDNA) library prepared for messenger RNA isolated from equine articular chondrocytes. The coding sequence is 92.4% homologous with the cDNA of the human sequence, and the propeptide is 95% identical to the human sequence. The authors also showed that chondrocytes harvested from juvenile horses exhibited more synthetic activity in culture with high steady-state levels of messenger RNA for type II procollagen. Type II procollagen is expressed at much lower levels in adult horses than in younger ones. This may have relevance to naturally occurring changes in cartilage in the joints of older horses. These authors also showed that interleukin-1 beta (IL-1β) and tumor necrosis factor alpha (TNF-α) produced a dose-dependent decrease in the steady-state levels of mRNA for type II collagen.

There are also small amounts of types VI, IX, XI, XII, and XIV. The minor collagens help form, and give stability to, the type II fibril network.[47] The collagenous fibrils provide tensile strength to the articular cartilage.[27] In adult articular cartilage, this property chiefly resides in the superficial layers where the collagenous fibers are oriented parallel to the surface of the cartilage. In the intermediate layer of the cartilage the collagenous fibrils are randomly arranged, and they become radially arranged in the radiate layer. The ultrastructural arrangement of the collagenous fibers is more complex than this.[5] Tensile strength is not as critical in these deeper layers in normal cartilage, but if superficial erosion occurs, the collagen of these deeper layers is vulnerable to disruption. It has been shown that in immature cartilage the deeper layers also possess considerable tensile strength, but this is lost with maturation.[61] The tensile properties automatically change with enzymatic degradation of hydroxypyridinolone cross-links, which emphasizes the importance of these cross-links in providing cartilage stiffness, strength, and tension.[64] Collagen fibers are also arranged concentrically around chondrocytes to form a "capsule," and this has been called a chondron. Each chondron contains one or more chondrocytes, is invested by collagenous pericellular capsule, and is surrounded by a proteoglycan-rich territorial matrix.[52] Collagen type VI, fibronectin, and thrombospondin are present in this chondron capsule and help anchor the chondrocyte within the chondron and attach the chondron within the extracellular matrix.[47]

PROTEOGLYCANS

The proteoglycans (previously called mucopolysaccharides) are the other major solid component of the articular cartilage matrix and occupy the spaces between the collagen fibrils. They take several forms and consist of monomers formed by a protein core and glycosaminoglycan (GAG) side chains (Fig. 7.5). Most of the proteoglycans (85%) form large aggregates by noncovalent attachment of the core protein of the proteoglycan to hyaluronan under the stabilization of a link protein (Fig. 7.5). This aggregate is called aggregating proteoglycan, or aggrecan. The major GAGs in adult articular cartilage are chondroitin-6-sulfate and keratan sulfate.[34] Chondroitin-4-sulfate is an important constituent of immature articular cartilage, but its level decreases to a low percentage with cartilage maturity. The GAGs consist of repeating units of disaccharides, whose important feature is their polyanionic nature (carboxyl and sulfate radicals in chondroitin sulfate and sulfate radicals in keratan sulfate) (Fig. 7.6). The charges of the polyanionic GAG side chains both repel each other and attract a hydration shell. These properties in turn provide the articular cartilage with physicochemical stiffness[21] and also affect cartilage permeability.[36,37]

The aggrecan molecules are contained only by the collagen network, and hence the proteoglycans impart compressive stiffness.[28] Enmeshment of the proteoglycans by the collagenous framework and specific interactions be-

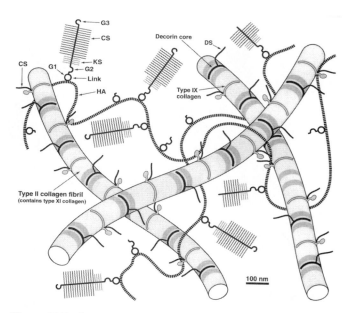

Figure 7.5 Diagrammatic representation of a portion of a proteoglycan aggregate.

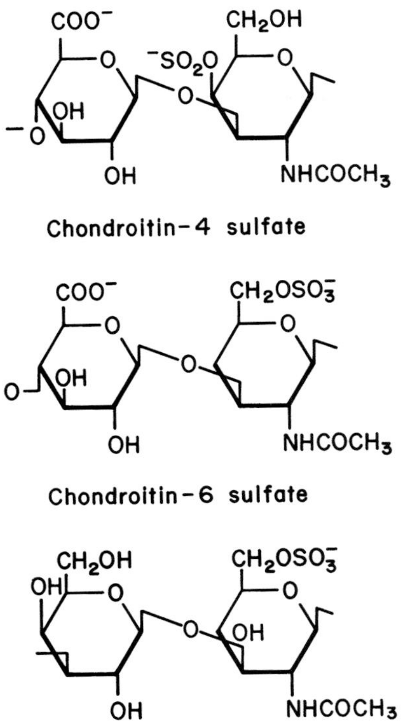

Figure 7.6 Diagram of structures of chondroitin-4-sulfate, chondroitin-6-sulfate, and keratan sulfate.

tween the two components are necessary for the proteoglycans to function.[5] The concentration of collagen is highest in the superficial layer of the articular cartilage and falls sharply with increasing distance from the surface. The proteoglycan content shows a trend in the opposite direction.[38] The average proteoglycan unit in articular cartilage has a molecular mass of 3 million daltons and contains 100 chondroitin sulfate side chains (CS) and 100 keratan sulfate (KS) side chains.[47] Over 100 of these proteoglycan monomers attach to a hyaluronan backbone to form the proteoglycan aggregate aggrecan, which has a molecular mass of over 200 million daltons. The proteoglycan monomer has received much study. There are two globular domains (G1 and G2) at the hyaluronate (HA)-associated end, followed by an extended GAG-containing region (E2), with a third globular domain (G3) at the other end. The N-terminal region of the aggrecan is attached to hyaluronan, and the region that contains most of the GAGs is an extended region lying between G2 and G3.

There are other nonaggregating proteoglycans in articular cartilage including biglycan, decorin, and fibromodulin. Equine decorin from the horse has been characterized biochemically.[51] Investigations of the structure of equine articular cartilage link protein from individuals ranging in age from 1 to 15 years identified three distinct isoforms, and there is alteration with age. Equine decorin was shown to consist of three native fractions with molecular weights comparable with that reported for bovine and human articular cartilage. The gene sequences of

biglycan and decorin from the horse have also been characterized.[58a]

GLYCOPROTEINS

Noncollagenous, nonproteoglycan glycoproteins constitute a small but significant portion of articular cartilage.[73] Link protein is one of these glycoproteins and is one of the few whose function has been defined. There are three fractions of equine link protein (LP1, LP2, and LP3).[13,51] Amino acid sequencing in the horse revealed 96% similarity with human link protein.[13] Other glycoproteins of cartilage include chondronectin (thought to function in adhesion of chondrocytes to type II collagen surfaces); fibronectin (functions to adhere cells to molecules and surfaces); cartilage oligomeric matrix protein (COMP), which has been isolated and characterized from human articular cartilage;[12] thrombospondin; and anchorin C-II, as well as cartilage-derived growth factor.

The articular cartilage is avascular, lacking both blood and lymph vessels. The deep layers of immature cartilage are penetrated extensively by vascular buds from the ossified portion of the epiphysis, and these appear to play an important role in nutrition of the cartilage from the subchondral region.[49] Immature articular cartilage is an articular–epiphyseal complex, with the deeper layers constituting a growth zone. In adults, the articular cartilage is separated from the subchondral vascular spaces by an end plate of bone (the subchondral plate), and nutrition of the articular cartilage occurs by diffusion from the synovial fluid. A lack of recognition of the structural differences between mature and immature articular cartilage has caused confusion between the roles of subchondral and synovial routes of nutrition in the past. Chondrocytes function by anaerobic glycolysis. Under physiologic loads, cartilage can be compressed to 40% of its original height. The depth to which the diffusing nutritional gradient can extend is limited and was calculated by Maroudas (1972) to be a maximal cartilage thickness of 6 mm.[36] Because of this limit, necrosis secondarily occurs when retained thickened cartilage, as develops in some cases of OCD, exceeds diffusion limits.

There are no nerves in articular cartilage, and the bearing surface of the joint depends on nerve endings in the joint capsule, ligaments, muscle, and subchondral bone for appreciation of pain and proprioception.[35]

In summary, articular cartilage is a tissue consisting of aggrecan that is stiff in compression, collagen that is stiff and strong in tension, and a somewhat freely moving fluid carrying mobile ions (interstitial fluid). These components interact to provide the following mechanical and physical characteristics when young and healthy: 1) a permeable matrix that is stiff in compression, 2) a fibrous network capable of withstanding high tensile stresses, 3) a fluid that flows under load or deformation and aids in dissipating high stresses in the tissue, and 4) a high swelling pressure that results in a matrix swollen with water.[45] An important function of aggrecan in cartilage is to retard the rate of stretch and alignment when a tensile load is suddenly applied, and this mechanism may be useful in protecting the cartilage collagen network during physiologic situations.[65]

In an unloaded joint, the opposing articular surfaces are not completely congruent;[16] however, under physiologic loading, because the cartilage is soft, deformation causes increase of contact area (reducing tissue stress levels) and also increases joint conformity (which provides additional stability). The adaptation of the shape of loaded cartilage may also help to form and retain boundary lubrication (see below). As articular cartilage directly under the load is compressed, the surrounding areas are subjected to transverse tensile strains. These forces tend to redistribute fluid away from the compressed area and into the stretched regions. As mentioned above, the major contribution to the osmotic pressure provided by the proteoglycans comes from negatively charged sulfate and carboxyl groups of the GAGs and the associated cations (ionic or Gibbs-Donnan effect).[73] Water is attracted by the high charge density, and this osmotic pressure may contribute up to 50% of the compressive stiffness of the articular cartilage. The swelling pressure is balanced by the tensile stress of the collagen framework.

Mow and colleagues have described the extracellular matrix as a cohesive porous composite. Their biphasic model for articular cartilage considers the tissue as an interacting mixture of two continua: a porous, permeable, elastic solid and an interstitial fluid. Because of swelling pressure, the collagen network of the articular cartilage is under tensile prestress even when unloaded. During compression, the concentration of the organic material and the charge density increase because the interstitial fluid is forced to flow from the matrix. A new equilibrium is reached when the charge density, collagen tension, and applied load are in balance.[44] The deformation of this cartilage in association with fluid exudation is called creep. The compression time curve consists of the creep phase controlled by fluid exudation, and the second phase is related to the collagen proteoglycan matrix component. During prolonged periods of stationary loading, fluid is slowly exuded and redistributed within the cartilage until an equilibrium position is reached, at which stage the increased concentration of the fixed charge density is counterbalanced by the increased osmotic swelling pressure of the proteoglycan. When fluid motion ceases, all the external load is borne by the solid extracellular matrix.

Intermittent pressures created by the interaction of the opposing articular surfaces are needed to pump fluid through the cartilage for nutrition and the removal of metabolic byproducts.[75] Expressed fluid from the articular cartilage resembles synovial fluid except for its low protein content and viscosity.[31] The concentration of fixed charges from GAGs is the prime determinant of cartilage permeability.[37] Simple diffusion would seem sufficient for nutrition of all but the deepest layers of articular cartilage, but joint movement probably facilitates the process.

The structural arrangement of the collagen fibers, proteoglycans, and chondrocytes within articular cartilage produces a complex path for solute movement. The most significant components affecting solute movement are the proteoglycans. As the proteoglycans are interwoven within the collagen fibers, the proteoglycans are constrained from expanding, so the matrix acts like a fine sievelike structural arrangement through which small and large molecules attempt to move. Studies have shown that proteoglycan restricts solute movement within the tissue matrix. The proteoglycans restrict the diffusion of large, uncharged solutes but do not affect the diffusion of small, uncharged solutes. The molecular size and conformation of the solute is also an important factor. Removal of proteoglycans increases the influx of large molecules into the matrix, which suggests that proteoglycan removal may also increase the efflux of large molecules from the tissue matrix.[74] It has been suggested that the marked loss of aggrecan and newly synthesized proteoglycan monomer from the matrix in osteoarthritis (OA) is probably a direct result of the increased mobility of these macromolecules as the tissue matrix components continue to degrade.

It is also well accepted that mechanical forces modulate the metabolic activity of chondrocytes, but the specific mechanisms of mechanical signal transduction in articular cartilage are still unknown.[4,50] One proposal is that chondrocytes may perceive changes in their mechanical environment through cellular deformation.[20] Others have suggested that changes in local interstitial pH may account for the observed biosynthetic response to static compression seen in articular cartilage,[19] but more recently, this has been shown definitely not to be the sole determinant of biosynthesis, and it cannot really account for the long-term response of cartilage tissue to static compression. The GAG content of habitually loaded areas of cartilage is greater than that of habitually unloaded areas.[30] Work in sheep stifle joints has shown that different areas of articular cartilage subjected to differing mechanical stresses contain a phenotypically distinct chondrocyte population.[32] Chondrocyte phenotypes were identified by the relative biosynthesis of aggrecan, biglycan, and decorin.

Articular Cartilage Metabolism and Matrix Turnover

The chondrocytes synthesize all the components of the cartilage matrix. At each stage of growth, development, and maturation the relative rates of matrix synthesis and degradation are adjusted to achieve net growth, remodeling, or equilibrium. A unique interaction exists between chondrocytes and the surrounding matrix. This may be facilitated by a cilium from each chondrocyte that extends into the matrix and acts as a "probe," sensing changes in the matrix composition such as loss of proteoglycan or collagen or increase or decrease in hyaluronan concentration. This information is relayed to the cell. Interaction between the pericellular and territorial matrix and the chondrocyte cell membrane also may include transmission of mechanical signals by changes in matrix tension or compression. Other investigators have provided support for the idea that forces perceived by chondrocytes dictate their shape and then stimulate alterations in cellular biochemistry and matrix metabolism.[22]

Collagen turnover times within articular cartilage have been estimated to be 120 years in the dog and 350 years in adult humans.[73] The slow turnover time of collagen compared with that of proteoglycan is presumably related to the structural features. On the other hand, the protein core of aggrecan is commonly cleaved, particularly the portion between the G1 and G2 domains. Cleavage here leaves a large C-terminal proteoglycan fragment that diffuses out of the tissue. The overall proteoglycan turnover time in adult rabbit and dog articular cartilage is about 300 days.

Dynamic load and the action of cytokines are considered to be involved in matrix turnover. Cytokines of principal interest at the moment are the interleukins and TNF-α. These factors act on chondrocyte receptors and influence the production and activation of metalloproteinases. The activity of matrix metalloproteinase in turn is inhibited by tissue inhibitors of metalloproteinase (TIMP-1 and TIMP-2), and there is a slight excess of TIMP over metalloproteinase concentration in normal articular cartilage.[10] There is further reference to the action of cytokines under "Pathobiology of Joints. . . ."

Not all cytokines cause degradation. There are a number of growth factors, such as insulin-like growth factor 1 (IGF-1) and various members of the transforming growth factor (TGF) superfamily (including bone morphogenic proteins (BMPs)), that are positively involved in articular cartilage synthesis.

Lubrication and Shock Absorption

The synovial joint contains two systems that require lubrication: a soft tissue system involving the sliding of synovial membrane on itself or other tissues and a cartilage-on-cartilage system. Lubrication of the synovial membrane is by boundary lubrication, and hyaluronan is the important component in the synovial fluid that performs this function.[55] The hyaluronan molecules stick to the surface of the synovial membrane and allow the synovial membrane to slide over the opposing surface. This function is important because a major part of the frictional resistance in joint movement is in the synovial membrane and fibrous joint capsule.[35]

Cartilage-on-cartilage lubrication uses two systems: boundary lubrication and hydrostatic lubrication. Boundary lubrication operates at low loads, the necessary component being primarily a glycoprotein lubricating fraction.[53,57] At higher loads, boundary lubrication fails because the lubricant is sheared off the articular cartilage, and the joint is lubricated by hydrostatic or squeeze-film lubrication. In hydrostatic lubrication, the cartilage surfaces are kept apart by a fluid film made of joint fluid and interstitial fluid that weeps from the articular cartilage itself. The squeeze film effect is probably potentiated by the undulation of the cartilage surface and the elasticity of the cartilage, which may lower frictional resistance by elastohydrodynamic effects.[53] Some people have suggested that plugging the cartilage pores by hyaluronate after a squeeze film is present on the surface may facilitate hydrostatic lubrication (called "boosted lubrication"). The concept that cartilage-on-cartilage lubrication is totally independent of hyaluronan has been challenged. When cadaveric joints were used instead of artificial lubricating situations, there was a clear effect of hyaluronan on animal joints with experimentally reduced lubricating ability. It was concluded that lubrication by fluid film was influenced by the viscosity of the lubricant. The viscosity of the synovial fluid was also considered to be important in reducing friction at low loads of articular surfaces, and hyaluronidase digestion of samples caused a significant increase in friction over the control samples.[33,60]

In the past, articular cartilage was considered the shock absorber of the joint. However, force attenuation studies have shown that the bone and periarticular soft tissues are the shock absorbers of the joint, and cartilage provides little shock absorption.[54]

Subchondral Bone

The subchondral plate and epiphyseal bone beneath it form an integral part of the joint structure, providing structural support to the overlying articular cartilage. The subchondral plate consists of cortical bone that varies in thickness depending on the joint. With exercise, remodeling occurs, and the amount of dense cortical bone can increase, at least in the carpus and fetlock, but there is marked variation among horses.[25] The relationship between the mechanical properties and morphometry of the bones of horses has been explored.[78] In the third carpal bone, maximal subchondral bone stiffness occurs 10 mm palmar to the dorsal margin. There is also a significant negative correlation between subchondral stiffness and the porosity of the radial facet of the third carpal bone.

Acquisition of such basic data is important in studying traumatic joint disease in the horse. Early work extrapolated two proposals in humans that OA is associated with an increase in subchondral bone stiffness outside the physiologic range.[56] However, it has been reported that there is no connection between the carpal articular cartilage proteoglycan content of racehorses and the mechanical and morphologic properties of the subchondral bone.[59] Recent work has shown microdamage in the subchondral bone (including microcracks and osteocyte death) to be a relatively early event in exercising horses.[25]

Cytokines and growth factors similar to those present in articular cartilage are present in bone. These include IGF-1, the TGF-β family (which includes BMPs 2 to 7), platelet-derived growth factor, and fibroblast growth factors. These peptides are produced by bone cells and are present in bone matrix. IL-1 and TNF-α are also present in bone. Presumably disease in subchondral bone would expose the articular cartilage to these cytokines. More details on the relationship between articular cartilage and subchondral bone are presented under "Pathobiology of Joints. . . ."

The innervation of the subchondral bone plate has been a subject of controversy. Although examination of histologic preparations by silver staining methods has indicated that the subchondral plate marrow spaces and epiphyseal cortical bone contain nerve fibers of various types, it has been argued that intimate association of these nerve fibers—particularly the small unmyelinated fibers—with penetrating arterioles may indicate that their role is vasomotor.[58,66] (Larger myelinated fibers and nerve endings of various types have been described in diaphyseal bone marrow spaces, periosteum, and periarticular capsular, ligamentous, and synovial structures.) Other doubts have stemmed clinically from the varying pain response from large subchondral defects such as subchondral cystic lesions and the difficulty in effectively eliminating the clinical signs of such entities with intraarticular and regional anesthesia. Other studies have proposed that increased intraosseous pressures are important in the generation of pain and several articular and periarticular diseases.[2]

Recent immunohistochemical techniques identifying substance P (a neuropeptide specifically located in sensory nerves and central nervous system [CNS] elements) have helped study the innervation of the subchondral plate further.[48] Substance P immunoreactive neurofilaments have been identified in the subchondral bone of normal equine metacarpophalangeal joints by use of a specific substance P antiserum. The nerves existed in the small cancellous spaces and diversion canals. Previous immunohistochemical studies of the subchondral plate of diseased human patellae revealed substance P fibers in the periosteum and subchondral plate of patellae affected with degenerative disease.[77] Another interesting finding in the human study was the observation of substance P fibers in erosion channels running through the subchondral plate to the deep surface of the articular cartilage, where nerve terminals were seen. Because erosion channels were not seen in normal patellae, the presence of the substance P fibers in the erosion channels may represent a morphologic change explaining why degenerative patellae become painful.

Embryologic Development and Maturation

A brief review of the embryologic development of joints and their subsequent maturation is relevant to some of the developmental anomalies to be considered below. These events are illustrated diagrammatically in Figure 7.7.

In initial limb bud development there is a concentration of mesenchyme in the center of the limb called the skeletal blastema. A hyaline cartilage model (bone anlagen) develops in the blastema, and a homogeneous interzone composed of undifferentiated mesenchyme appears between the ends of adjacent anlagen (Fig. 7.7A). There is a condensation of two outer layers (fibrous joint capsule and synovial membrane) in the interzone (Fig. 7.7B). The joint capsule and synovial membrane become progressively vascularized. The muscle masses of the fetus then start contracting, and defects appear in the intermediate layer of the interzone (Fig. 7.7C). Expansion of this space forms the synovial cavity (Fig. 7.7D). The outer layers of the interzone form articular cartilage on the ends of the developing bone. Without limb motion, the joint space will not develop, and a mass of cartilage persists across the joint.

Although the main mass of the epiphysis results from chondrification of the blastema, the epiphysis receives a superficial contribution by chondrification of peripheral layers of the joint interzone. Later development also demonstrates the dual nature of the articular cartilage. There is a superficial layer that is destined to serve as articular cartilage and is incapable of ossification, and the deeper layers of the epiphyseal cartilage will become the bony epiphysis. There seems to be a functional difference between articular and epiphyseal chondrocytes of juvenile articular cartilage. The difference is evidenced by the different rates of formation and increase of cytoplasm vesicles and packets.[30]

The process by which cartilage is replaced by bone in the developing epiphysis is identical to that of the metaphyseal growth plate. The cartilage tissue undergoes the developmental sequences of proliferation, maturation, degeneration, and ossification. It is felt that tissue stress histories constitute an important influence during this process.[6] Using finite-element computer models, it has been proposed that the process of endochondral ossification is accelerated by shear stresses (or strain energy) and inhibited or prevented by intermittently applied compressive stresses (hydrostatic pressure). Although these specifics remain theory, mechanical forces are considered to be important but probably more complicated than those proposed so far.

The concept of a direct correlation between the thickness of articular cartilage and magnitude of loading stress placed on articular cartilage is an old one. Simon and co-workers[69,70] proposed that variations in thickness of articular cartilage are closely allied to congruency of opposing articular surfaces of synovial joints. Therefore, in highly congruent joints, thin articular cartilage is sufficient, since the load passing from one bone to the next is distributed over a large area, compared with the

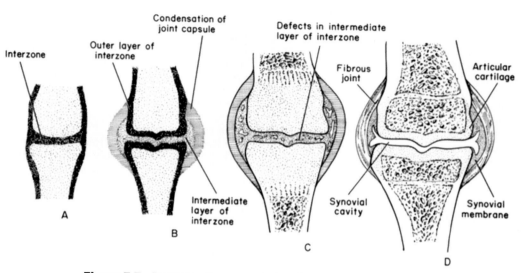

Figure 7.7 Diagrammatic representation of the development of a joint.

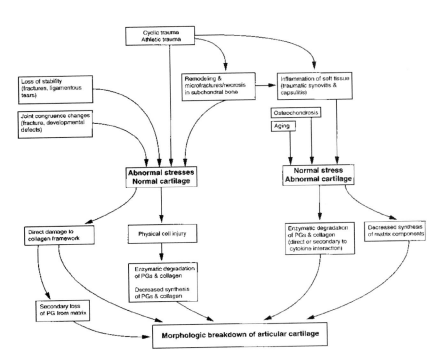

Figure 7.8 Factors involved in articular cartilage degradation in equine osteoarthritis. PG, proteoglycan. (Reprinted with permission from McIlwraith CW, Trotter GW, Eds. Joint Disease in the Horse. Philadelphia: WB Saunders, 1996.)

much larger load that would be experienced if only a focal area of the articulating surfaces was transmitting the load. On the other hand, thicker articular cartilage is found notably in incongruent joints and, because of its increased deformability, is suitably adapted for the distribution of large focal forces to an increased area of the subchondral bone.[69,70,75] Firth and Hartman further studied joint fitting and cartilage thickness in the radio-carpal joint of foals.[14] They found that the thickest cartilage corresponded to the proximal center of the contact area of the opposing articular surface. These areas are all convex to the direction of the ground reaction forces. The situation in the adult, in which convex joint surfaces of the thickest articular cartilage are at the convexity and concave surfaces and the thinnest cartilage at the periphery,[46] appears to be the same as that in the immature equine distal radius. It was felt that the thicker cartilage at these sites may act to protect the cancellous bone of the epiphysis at a time when such immature osseous tissue may not be capable of sustaining the stresses placed upon it. This protective function could be facilitated by the greater ability of thicker (compared with thinner) cartilage to expand laterally when compressed by a given load. It is also known that the restraining effect of the *subchondral* bone on lateral expansion is greater in thinner cartilage.

The epiphyseal cartilage, which is destined to ossify, contains blood vessels within cartilage canals. These canals assist in nutrition of the epiphysis and are directly involved in the osteogenesis of the secondary centers of ossification.[1] They are also partially responsible for interstitial growth of the chondroepiphysis.[76] When epiphyseal cartilage has been converted to bone, the ossifying front ceases to advance, and only the articular cartilage will remain. The ossification of the epiphysis is illustrated in Figure 7.8. Some joint problems are related to errors in these developmental processes.

References

1. Agrawal P, Atre PR, Kulkarni DS. The role of cartilage canals in the ossification of the talus. Acta Anat 1984;119:238–240.
2. Arnoldi C, Linderholm H, Mussbichler H. Venous engorgement and intraosseous hypertension in osteoarthritis of the hip. J Bone Joint Surg [Br] 1972;54:409–421.
3. Barnett CH, Davies DH, MacConaill MA. Synovial Joints: Their Structure and Mechanics. Springfield, IL: Charles C Thomas, 1961.
4. Boustany NN, Gray ML, Black AC, Hunziker EB. Time dependent changes in the response of cartilage to static compression suggest interstitial pH is not the only signaling mechanism. J Orthop Res 1995;13:740–750.
5. Broom ND. Abnormal softening in articular cartilage. Its relationship to the collagen framework. Arthritis Rheum 1982;25:1209.
5a. Caron JP, Neurogenic factors in joint pain and disease pathogenesis. In: McIlwraith CW, Trotter GW, Eds. Joint Disease in the Horse. Philadelphia: WB Saunders, 1996;70–80.
6. Carter DR, Wong M. The role of mechanical loading histories in the development of diarthrodial joints. J Orthop Res 1988;6:804–816.
7. Cochrane W, Davies DV, Palfrey AJ. Absorptive function of the synovial membrane. Ann Rheum Dis 1965;24:2.
8. Curtiss PH. The pathophysiology of joint infections. Clin Orthop 1973;96:129.
9. Davies DV. The lymphatics of the synovial membrane. J Anat 1946;80:21.
10. Dean DD, Martel-Pelletier J, Pelletier JP, et al. Evidence for metalloproteinase and metalloproteinase inhibitor imbalance in human osteoarthritic cartilage. J Clin Invest 1989;84:678–685.
11. Dee R. The innervation of joints. In: Sokoloff L, Ed. The Joints and Synovial Fluid. New York: Academic Press, 1978;177–204.
12. DiCesare PE, Morgelin M, Carlson CS, et al. Cartilage oligomeric matrix protein: Isolation and characterization from human articular cartilage. J Orthop Res 1995;13:422–428.
13. Dudhia J, Platt D. Complete primary sequence of equine cartilage link protein deduced from complementary DNA. Am J Vet Res 1995;56:959–965.
14. Firth EC, Hartman W. An *in vitro* study on joint fitting and cartilage thickness in the radiocarpal joint of foals. Res Vet Sci 1983;34:320–326.

15. Freeman MAR. Adult Articular Cartilage. New York: Grune & Stratton, 1972.

16. Gardner DL, McGillivray DC. Living articular cartilage is not smooth. Ann Rheum Dis 1971;30:3.

17. Ghadially FN. Fine structure of joints. In: Sokoloff L, Ed. The Joints and Synovial Fluid. New York: Academic Press, 1978.

18. Ghadially FN, Roy S. Ultrastructure of Synovial Joints in Health and Disease. New York: Appleton-Century-Crofts, 1969.

19. Gray ML, Pizzanelli AM, Grodzinsky AJ, Lee RC. Mechanical and physicochemical determinants of the chondrocyte biosynthetic response. J Orthop Res 1988;6:777–792.

20. Guilak F, Ratcliffe A, Mow VC. Chondrocyte deformation and local tissue strain in articular cartilage: A confocal microscopy study. J Orthop Res 1995;13:410–421.

20a. Howard RD, McIlwraith CW. Hyaluronan and its use in the treatment of equine joint disease. In: McIlwraith CW, Trotter GW, Eds. Joint Disease in the Horse. Philadelphia: WB Saunders, 1996;257–269.

21. Howell CE, Hart GH, Ittner NR. Vitamin A deficiency in horses. Am J Vet Res 1941;2:60.

22. Hung S-C, Nakamura K, Shiro R, et al. Effects of continuous distraction on cartilage in a moving joint: An investigation on adult rabbits. J Orthop Res 1997;15:381–390.

23. Johansson HE, Rejno S. Light and electron microscopic investigation of equine synovial membrane. A comparison between healthy joints and joints with intra-articular fractures and osteochondrosis dissecans. Acta Vet Scand 1976;17:153.

24. Jones DL, Barber SM, Doige CE. Synovial fluid and clinical changes after arthroscopic partial synovectomy of the equine middle carpal joint. Vet Surg 1993;22:524–530.

25. Kawcak CE, McIlwraith CW, Norrdin RW, et al. Clinical effects of exercise on subchondral bone of carpal and metacarpophalangeal joints in horses. Am J Vet Res 2000;61(10):1252–1258.

26. Kellgren JH, Samuel EP. The sensitivity and innervation of the articular capsule. J Bone Joint Surg [Br] 1950;32:84.

27. Kempson GE, Muir H, Pollard C, Tuke M. The tensile properties of the cartilage on the human femoral head related to collagen and glycosaminoglycans. Biochim Biophys Acta 1973;297:456–472.

28. Kempson GE, Muir H, Swanson SA, Freeman MA. Correlations between stiffness and the chemical constituents of cartilage on the human femoral head. Biochim Biophys Acta 1970;215:70–77.

29. Key JA. The reformation of synovial membrane in the knees of rabbits after synovectomy. J Bone Joint Surg 1925;7:793.

30. Lamar CH, Eller LL, Turek JJ. In vitro characterization of porcine juvenile articular cartilage. Am J Vet Res 1987;48:515–518.

31. Linn FC, Sokoloff L. Movement and composition of interstitial fluid of cartilage. Arthritis Rheum 1965;8:481.

32. Little CB, Ghosh P. Variation in proteoglycan metabolism by articular chondrocytes in different joint regions as determined by post-natal mechanical loading. Osteoarthritis Cartilage 1997;5:49–62.

33. Mabuchi K, Tsukamoto Y, Obara T, Yamaguchi T. The effect of additive hyaluronic acid on animal joints with experimentally reduced lubricating ability. J Biomed Mater Res 1994;28:865–870.

34. Mankin HJ, Lippiello L. The glycosaminoglycans of normal and arthritic cartilage. J Clin Invest 1971;50:1712.

35. Mankin HJ, Radin E. Structure and function of joints. In: McCarty DJ, Ed. Arthritis and Allied Conditions. 9th ed. Philadelphia: Lea & Febiger, 1979;151–166.

36. Maroudas A. Physico-chemical properties of articular cartilage. In: Freeman MAR, Ed. Adult Articular Cartilage. New York: Grune & Stratton, 1972;131–170.

37. Maroudas A. Transport of solutes through cartilage: Permeability to large molecules. J Anat 1976;122:335.

38. Maroudas A, Evans H, Almeida L. Cartilage of the hip joint. Topographical variation of glycosaminoglycan content in normal and fibrillated cartilage. Ann Rheum Dis 1973;32:1.

39. McIlwraith CW. Ultrastructural and histochemical studies of filipin induced equine arthritis. PhD thesis, Purdue University, West Lafayette, IN, 1979.

40. McIlwraith CW, Fessler JF. Arthroscopy in the diagnosis of equine joint disease. J Am Vet Med Assoc 1978;172:263.

41. McIlwraith CW, Trotter GW. Joint Disease in the Horse. Philadelphia: WB Saunders, 1996.

42. Meachim G, Stockwell RA. The matrix. In: Freeman MAR, Ed. Adult Articular Cartilage. New York: Grune & Stratton, 1972; 1–50.

43. Mitchell N, Blackwell P. The electron microscopy of regenerating synovium after subtotal synovectomy in rabbits. J Bone Joint Surg [Am] 1968;50:675.

44. Mow VC, Holmes MH, Lai WM. Fluid transport of mechanical properties of articular cartilage: A review. J Biomech 1984;17:377–394.

45. Myers ER, Mow VC. Biomechanics of cartilage and its response to biomechanical stimuli. In: Hall BK, Ed. Cartilage, vol 1. New York: Academic Press, 1983;313–340.

46. Nickel R, Schummer A, Seiferle E. Lehrbuch der Anatomie der Haustiere, vol 1. Berlin: Paulparey, 1961.

47. Nixon AJ. Articular cartilage surface structure and function. Equine Vet Educ 1991;3:72–75.

48. Nixon AJ, Cummings JF. Substance P immunohistochemical study of the sensory innervation of normal subchondral bone in the equine metacarpophalangeal joint. Am J Vet Res 1994;55:28–34.

49. Ogata K, Whiteside LA, Lesker PA. Subchondral route for nutrition to articular cartilage in the rabbit. J Bone Joint Surg [Am] 1978;60:905.

50. Palmoski MJ, Brandt KD. Effects of static and cyclic compressive loading on articular cartilage plugs in vitro. Arthritis Rheum 1984;27:675–681.

51. Platt D, Bird JLE, Bayliss MT. Aging of equine articular cartilage: Structure and composition of aggrecan and decorin. Equine Vet J 1998;30:43–52.

52. Poole CA, Flint MH, Beaumont BW. Chondrons extracted from canine tibial cartilage: Preliminary report on their isolation and structure. J Orthop Res 1988;6:408–419.

53. Radin EL, Paul IL. A consolidated concept of joint lubrication. J Bone Joint Surg [Am] 1972;54:607.

54. Radin EL, Paul IL. Does cartilage compliance reduce skeletal impact loads? The relative force-attenuating properties of articular cartilage, synovial fluid, periarticular soft tissues, and bone. Arthritis Rheum 1970;13:139.

55. Radin EL, Paul IL, Swann DA, Schottstaedt ES. Lubrication of synovial membrane. Ann Rheum Dis 1971;30:322.

56. Radin EL, Paul IL, Tolkoff MJ. Subchondral bone change in patients with early degenerative arthritis. Arthritis Rheum 1970;13:400.

57. Radin EL, Swann DA, Weisser PA. Separation of a hyaluronate-free lubricating fraction from synovial fluid. Nature 1970;228:377.

58. Reimann I, Christensen S. A histological demonstration of nerves in subchondral bone. Acta Orthop Scand 1977;48:345–352.

58a. Richardson DW, Dodge GR. Cloning of equine type II procollagen and the modulation of its expression in cultured equine articular chondrocytes. Matrix Biol 1997;16:59–64.

59. Richardson DW, Young DR, Clark CC. The relationship of subchondral bone stiffness to overlying cartilage morphology and biochemistry. Trans Orthop Res Soc 1993;18:720.

60. Roberts BJ, Unsworth A, Mian N. The modes of lubrication in human hip joints. Ann Rheum Dis 1982;41:217–224.

61. Roth V, Mow VC. The intrinsic tensile behaviour of the matrix of bovine articular cartilage and its variation with age. J Bone Joint Surg [Am] 62:1102, 1980.

62. Roy S, Ghadially FN, Crane WAJ. Synovial membrane in traumatic effusion. Ultrastructure and autoradiography with tritiated leucine. Ann Rheum Dis 1966;25:259.

63. Scapinelli RB. Studies on the vasculature of the human knee joint. Acta Anat 1968;70:305.

64. Schmidt MB, Schoonbeck JM, Mow VC, et al. The relationship between collagen crosslinking and the tensile properties of articular cartilage. Proc Orthop Res Soc 1987;33:134.

65. Schmidt MB, Mow VC, Chun LE, Eyre DR. Effects of proteoglycan extraction on the tensile behavior of articular cartilage. J Orthop Res 1990;8:353–363.

66. Sherman MS. The nerves of bone. J Bone Joint Surg [Am] 1963;45:522–528.

67. Shively JAC. The morphology of equine synovial membrane. MS Thesis, Purdue University, West Lafayette, IN, 1975.

68. Simkin PA. Synovial physiology. In: McCarty DJ, Ed. Arthritis and Allied Conditions. 9th ed. Philadelphia: Lea & Febiger, 1979; 167–178.

69. Simon WH. Scale effects in animal joints. II. Thickness and elasticity in the deformability of articular cartilage. Arthritis Rheum 1971;14:493–502.

70. Simon WH, Friedenberg S, Richardson S. Joint congruence. A correlation in joint congruence and thickness of articular cartilage in dogs. J Bone Joint Surg [Am] 1973;55:1614–1620.

71. Southwick WO, Bensch KG. Phagocytosis of colloidal gold by cells of the synovial membrane. J Bone Joint Surg [Am] 1971;53:720.

72. Theoret CL, Barber SM, Moyana T, et al. Repair and function of synovium after arthroscopic synovectomy of the dorsal compartment of the equine antebrachiocarpal joint. Vet Surg 1996;25:142–153.

73. Todhunter RJ. Anatomy and physiology of synovial joints. In: McIlwraith CW, Trotter GW, Eds. Joint Disease in the Horse. Philadelphia: WB Saunders, 1996;1–48.

74. Torzilli PA, Arduino JM, Gregory JD, Bansal M. Effect of proteoglycan removal on solute mobility in articular cartilage. J Biomech 1997;30:895–902.

75. Van Sickle DC, Kincaid SA. Comparative arthrology. In: Sokoloff L, Ed. The Joints and Synovial Fluid, vol I. New York: Academic Press, 1978;1–47.

75a. Vachon AM, Kelley FW, McIlwraith CW, Chapman P. Biochemical analysis of normal articular cartilage in horses. Am J Vet Res 1990;51:1905–1911.

76. Wilsman NJ, Van Sickle DC. Cartilage canals, their morphology and destruction. Anat Rec 1972;173:79.

77. Wojtys TM, Beaman DN, Glover RA, Janda D. Innervation of the human knee joint by substance-P fibers. J Arthroscopy 1990;6:254–263.

78. Young DR, Richardson DW, Markel MD, et al. Mechanical and morphometric analysis of the third carpal bone of Thoroughbreds. Am J Vet Res 1991;52:402–409.

PATHOBIOLOGY OF JOINTS AND THEIR REACTION TO INSULT AND INJURY

This section contains some general comments on the reaction of joint tissues to injury and healing responses that occur. Specific pathologic changes as they relate to individual disease entities are considered when those diseases are discussed.

The reaction in the various joint-associated tissues should not be considered in isolation, as evidenced by the example of the carpus of a racehorse. Considerable damage may be inflicted directly to the articular cartilage in regions of concussion, as exemplified by the fractures that occur on the dorsal aspect of the joint. Intraarticular fractures of the carpus cause varying degrees of articular cartilage loss. Ulcerative lesions unassociated with fractures may develop as a consequence of direct concussion. However, cyclic fatigue damage to the collagen network could be an important step in the pathogenesis of a more insidious osteoarthritic entity. Fatigue or damage in the collagen framework could expose chondrocytes to deleterious physical forces, causing injury and metabolic changes. Primary damage to the subchondral bone other than fracture may also occur on the proximal third carpal bone or the distal radial carpal bone and lead to secondary damage to the articular cartilage either from loss of support or secondarily from release of cytokines. Subchondral sclerosis may also lead to further physical damage to the articular cartilage because of decreased shock absorption. Acute synovitis and capsulitis is a common problem in these same joints and may also contribute to the degenerative process by the release of enzymes, inflammatory mediators, and cytokines.[67]

When considering a traumatically injured joint, two basic pathobiologic processes should be considered: 1)

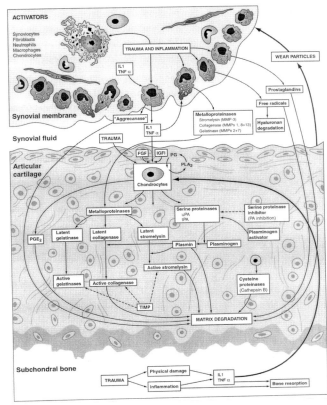

Figure 7.9 Factors involved in enzymatic degradation of articular cartilage matrix. IL-1, interleukin 1; TNFα, tumor necrosis factor alpha; FGF, fibroblast growth factor; PG, prostaglandin; PLA$_2$, phospholipase A$_2$; uPA, urokinase plasminogen activator; tPA, tissue plasminogen activator; PA, plasminogen activator; PGE$_2$, prostaglandin E$_2$; TIMP, tissue inhibitor metalloproteinase. (Modified from Figure 3-7 in McIlwraith CW, Trotter GW, Eds. Joint Disease in the Horse. Philadelphia: WB Saunders, 1996.)

inflammation of the synovial membrane and fibrous joint capsule (synovitis and capsulitis) and 2) physical or biochemical damage to the articular cartilage and bone. Acute synovitis and capsulitis can cause significant clinical compromise and may also contribute to the degenerative process by the release of enzymes, inflammatory mediators, and cytokines.[69] These processes are outlined in Figures 7.8 and 7.9. Aging also causes changes.[87a]

Synovitis and Capsulitis

Treatment of synovitis and capsulitis, particularly the acute form, is indicated to 1) alleviate the immediate compromising effects of inflammation, including pain and reduced function, 2) prevent the development of permanent fibrosis in the joint capsule, which in turn will cause decreased motion and compromised shock absorption capabilities in that joint, and 3) prevent or minimize the development of OA.

Synovitis and capsulitis as primary entities in athletic horses are presumed to be associated with repeated trauma.[66,70] Severe injury to the fibrous joint capsule can also cause instability. Synovial membrane itself is mechanically weak and has no known biomechanical role, but it is recognized that synovial injury may have pathophysiologic consequences in the joint.[27] Some injuries may affect diffusion across the synovial membrane, and others will have a primary effect on the metabolism of the chondrocyte.[27] Mechanically damaged synoviocytes may release degradative enzymes and cytokines that will alter the intraarticular environment and possibly affect articular cartilage. It has also been suggested that high intraarticular pressures in injured joints associated with effusion could suffice to impair the flow of blood through the synovial capillaries. This would not only potentially lower the oxygen tension of the joint, but could potentially lead to reperfusion injury.[56] Flexion of a joint with sufficient synovial effusion could raise the intraarticular pressure to levels of impaired blood flow through the synovial capillaries. Ischemia and reperfusion could lead to the production of oxygen-derived free radicals.[1] In the presence of synovial effusion in the hip, a position of extension and medial rotation causes an increase in intraarticular pressure that may compromise the blood supply to the capital epiphysis of the femur. In inflammatory synovitis in the human knee, the rise in intraarticular pressure with isometric quadriceps contraction related to effusion volume and the inflammatory process prevents reflex muscle inhibition. The latter is normally a locally protective mechanism that minimizes the potential for intermittent ischemia or oxidative injury.[53a]

In addition to direct injury that may occur to the synovial membrane, the reaction of synovial membrane to articular cartilage damage or other mechanical destruction of intraarticular tissues is well recognized. The presence of cartilaginous wear particles increases the cellular production of prostaglandin E_2, cytokines, and the neutral metalloproteinases (collagenase, stromelysin, and gelatinase).[29] Further, the proteoglycans released into synovial fluid cause synovitis.[7]

Synovial membrane inflammation and lysosomal activity in the pathogenesis of equine degenerative joint disease (DJD) was evaluated by the author in an experimental model based on the intraarticular injection of the polyene antibiotic filipin.[70] Filipin is a drug capable of disrupting lysosomes, and this experimental model produced morphologic and biochemical lesions of OA in the articular cartilage. More recent work with cells and tissues of equine joints has shown that synovial cells are a good source of proteolytic enzymes active against both collagen and proteoglycan.[111] Synoviocytes and chondrocytes isolated from healthy joint tissue exhibit no detectable enzyme production, but stimulation of the cells with an extract containing IL-1 produced high levels of stromelysin.[111] Injury or insult to the synovial membrane is important because of the potential to produce a number of effects. The first is direct release of proteinases. Four main classes of proteinases are recognized: metalloproteinases, serine proteinases, cysteine proteinases, and aspartic proteinases. The synthesis of many of them has been shown to be altered by a variety of cytokines and hormones. The various proteinases potentially involved in equine joint disease are considered below.

Proteinases

METALLOPROTEINASES

Metalloproteinases are considered to play a major role in the degradation of the extracellular matrix.[81,90,104] These enzymes are characterized by a re-

quirement for Zn^{2+} in their active site. Calcium is also required for expression of full activity but does not reside in the active site. Neutral proteinase activity was identified by Sapolsky et al. in 1974[103] and identified more specifically as a metalloproteinase (MMP) in 1976.[109] Since that time the enzyme has been shown to be identical to stromelysin or MMP-3.[125] MMPs may be further subdivided into collagenases, gelatinases, and stromelysins. Evidence linking MMPs to matrix degradation includes their presence in increased concentrations in diseased cartilage, topographic relationship to OA lesions, synthesis by articular cells, and activity at physiologic pH.[14] MMPs that have been incriminated in OA include collagenase 1 (MMP-1), collagenase 2 (MMP-8), collagenase 3 (MMP-13), stromelysin 1 (MMP-3), and two gelatinases (MMP-2 and MMP-9). Evidence for varying roles of these MMPs in equine articular cartilage degradation is accumulating and is presented below. The potential for MMPs to degrade collagen and proteoglycans is discussed separately.

Three collagenases have been identified. The one that was recognized first and has been investigated the most is interstitial or tissue collagenase. Interstitial or tissue collagenase (also called MMP-1) is specific for collagen as a substrate and cleaves all three chains of the triple helix at one susceptible point between residues 775 and 776 (glycine and isoleucine, respectively) of the α_1 (I) chain of collagen types I, II, and III.[90,125] Collagenase also cleaves collagen types VII, VIII, and X but does not cleave basement membrane types IV, V, and VI or types IX and XI.[38,125] Interstitial collagenase is produced by a wide variety of cells including macrophages, fibroblasts, synovial cells, osteoblasts, chondrocytes, and endothelial cells.[38,124] There is a second human collagenase, called PMN collagenase (also called MMP-8).[124,125] PMN collagenase is stored in specific granules of polymorphonuclear leukocytes (PMNs) and secreted in response to appropriate stimuli,[124] but recent evidence supports a key role in human OA.[108] Recently, evidence has accumulated in both human and equine studies that the primary collagenase involved in the degradation of type II collagen of articular cartilage may in fact be collagenase 3 (also known as MMP-13).[14,75,108,121] Caron et al.[14] found that MMP-13 is produced by equine chondrocytes and that MMP-13 expression was significantly stimulated by recombinant human (rh)IL-1. The equine MMP-13 cDNA had 93% homology with the human MMP-13 cDNA sequence. MMP-13 is expressed at low levels in stationary equine chondrocyte cultures, and rhIL-1β significantly upregulates this expression. Human MMP-13 was initially cloned from a cDNA library obtained from a human mammary carcinoma.[37] Subsequently, MMP-13 was documented to be a product of human articular chondrocytes.[96] Expression of MMP-13 by chondrocytes in human osteoarthritic cartilage has been demonstrated,[40] and it was shown that MMP-13 turned over type II collagen at least 10 times faster than MMP-1.[74] Experiments with intact type II collagen demonstrated that MMP-13 cleaved type II collagen at the same bond as MMP-1, but this was followed by a secondary cleavage that removed three amino acids from the quarter fragment amino terminus. Other workers have demonstrated higher levels of expression for both MMP-1 and MMP-13 by OA chondrocytes than by normal chondrocytes. In addition, they showed that messenger

RNA for MMP-8 was present in OA cartilage but not in normal cartilage. TNF-α has also been shown to stimulate expression of all three collagenases.[108] Freemont et al.[36] demonstrated gene expression of MMPs 1, 3, and 9 in articular chondrocytes during histologic development of the cartilage lesion of OA using ^{35}S-labeled cDNA probes. In OA, MMP gene expression was greatest in the superficial layer.[36] In contrast, messenger RNAs for MMPs 3 and 9 were expressed deeper in the cartilage: MMP-9 early in the disease, and MMP-3 with a biphasic pattern in early- and late-stage disease. They concluded that the expression of genes for MMPs 3 and 9 is differentially regulated in human articular chondrocytes and, in individual cells, is related to the depth of the chondrocyte below the cartilage surface and the nature and extent of the cartilage lesion.

Consideration of the breakdown of proteoglycan attention has focused on stromelysin (also called proteoglycanase or MMP-3) as well as an undefined enzyme called "aggrecanase." Stromelysin was first purified by Galloway et al. and was termed "proteoglycanase" because it degraded proteoglycan.[39] Stromelysin has a wide variety of substrates including proteoglycans (aggrecan, decorin, fibromodulin, link protein) and types IV, V, VII, IX, and XI collagen (also cleaves type II collagen in nonhelical sites).[90,125,128] Stromelysin is also considered to have a significant role in activating procollagenase to collagenase.[80] A second enzyme closely related to stromelysin and called stromelysin-2 (also MMP-10 and transin-2) has been cloned and characterized. At present its role in inflammatory diseases is unknown.[125] In vitro studies of IL-1–induced cartilage degeneration have revealed evidence of collagen degradation that could be attributable to stromelysin in addition to that attributable to collagenase.[25,82] The molecular cloning and cartilage gene expression of equine stromelysin 1 (MMP-3) has been described recently by Balkman and Nixon (1998).[6]

Initial cleavage of the large aggregating proteoglycan, aggrecan, in situ occurs between the G1 and G2 domains (the E_1 region), which causes release of the GAG-bearing region of proteoglycan, and the G1 domain remains attached to the hyaluronate backbone.[101] Three related metalloproteinases examined (rabbit bone stromelysin and recombinant human stromelysin-1 and stromelysin-2) all cleave cartilage proteoglycans at this location.[34] The specific site of this cleavage is at the asp341–phe342 bond.[33] This may also be the primary site of cleavage during normal proteoglycan turnover in the cartilage matrix. Stromelysin also cleaves link protein in human neonatal cartilage aggrecan at the his16–ile17 bond.[82,83] In addition to cleavage at the asn341–phe342 site (MMP site), cleavage between the G1 and G2 domains also occurs at the glu373–ala374 site, and this has been attributed to an as-yet unidentified enzyme called aggrecanase.[101] Although it was initially felt that neutrophil collagenase (MMP-8) might represent this activity,[35] this has since been proven not to be the case. It has been proposed more recently that aggrecanase is the primary enzyme responsible for breakdown of proteoglycans in cartilage degradation, whereas the principal role of stromelysin is in normal homeostasis and remodeling. Arner et al. also suggested that MMP-8 does not represent cartilage aggrecanase because of the differential breakdown of fragments.[3] In inflammatory synovitis (rheumatoid

arthritis) in humans, high levels of stromelysin in the synovial fluid support the proposal that this enzyme may play a role in the connective tissue degradation observed in this disease.[122a]

This newer information indicates that there are at least two enzyme activities involved in proteoglycan catabolism (the known MMPs and aggrecanase). The sequences or situations in which these act is unknown but could include aggrecanase as the primary degrading enzyme, MMP as the primary enzyme and aggrecanase acting on catabolized molecules, or both enzymes working separately on different molecules.

A 72-kDa gelatin-degrading proteinase (gelatinase) (also called MMP-2, type IV collagenase, and matrilysin) degrades denatured type II collagen and type IV collagen and also has significant activity against fibronectin, elastin, and collagen types V, VII, X, and XI but not against collagens I and VI.[90,125] A second gelatinase (92-kDa) (also called type V collagenase, MMP-9, and invasin) is a major secreted product of stimulated PMN leukocytes and macrophages.[124,125] Equine matrix metalloproteinases 2 and 9 have been characterized in the horse.[16,17] The one-quarter and three-quarter fragments generated by cleavage of fibrin or collagens by collagenases can unwind and are then susceptible to further cleavage by MMP-2 and MMP-9. MMPs 2 and 9 are produced by a variety of equine cell types. These enzymes have been found at elevated levels in synovial fluids from horses with joint disease.[16,17] It is still not clear from current work what role these individual MMPs may play in equine cartilage degradation.

All metalloproteinases are secreted as latent proenzymes that are activated extracellularly. Collagenase is probably normally activated by stromelysin,[80] but collagenase and possibly other metalloproteinases can also be activated by plasmin (produced from plasminogen by the action of tissue or urokinase-type plasminogen activators, kallikrein and cathepsin-B).[26] Stromelysin is activated by plasmin and other proteinases that activate collagenase.[125] Recent evidence suggests that latency is attributable to formation of an intramolecular complex between a single cysteine residue in the propeptide domain and the essential zinc atom in the catalytic domain (these are the only two domains common to all MMPs). Activation is associated with detachment of the cysteine residue from the complex and is referred to as the "cysteine-switch" mechanism of activation.[122]

The metalloproteinases are inhibited by two tissue inhibitors of metalloproteinase, TIMP-1 and TIMP-2.[38,110] They inhibit all known MMPs by forming a 1:1 enzyme–inhibitor complex.[81] TIMP is found in many connective tissues and may be the most important inhibitor found in articular cartilage. A deficiency of TIMP relative to levels of metalloproteinases has been demonstrated in osteoarthritic human cartilage.[23,24] It is currently thought that the balance between MMPs and TIMPs is important for the progression of articular cartilage degradation.

In summary, metalloproteinases are considered to play a major role in articular cartilage degradation. They are secreted as latent proenzymes and activated extracellularly by serine proteinases. Plasmin may activate stromelysin, and stromelysin in turn is an important activator of collagenase. Metalloproteinases are inhibited by TIMPs, and a relative deficiency of the latter may be important in cartilage degradation. With the development of techniques to study equine MMPs, more complete investigations are happening in the horse. Questions that it will be nice have answered include 1) do the aggrecan fragments released into equine synovial fluids reflect cleavage by "aggrecanase" or MMPs; 2) which collagenase plays the major role in type II collagen degradation; 3) when equine articular cartilage is cultured ex vivo with inflammatory cytokines, is there increased degradation of aggrecan type II collagen, and are MMPs involved; and 4) does administration of MMP inhibitors to horses with joint disease lead to clinical improvement and does such improvement correlate with reduced levels of aggrecan and collagen degradation?[44]

SERINE PROTEINASES

Synovitis can also produce plasminogen activators (serine proteinases). Two types of plasminogen activator are recognized. Tissue plasminogen activator (tPA) and urokinase (uPA) both cleave plasminogen to active plasmin. This cascade plays a role in activating metalloproteinase. This system is also regulated by a series of plasminogen activator inhibitors. That IL-1 can stimulate production of tissue plasminogen activator has been established.[119] Other serine proteinases include elastase and cathepsin-G. Neutrophils are the source of elastase and cathepsin-G.

CYSTEINE PROTEINASES

Cathepsins B, H. and L are lysosomal proteinases that belong to the class of cysteine proteinases, of which cathepsin-B and cathepsin-L are best known. Both cathepsin-B and cathepsin-L cleave the internal peptides of collagen. Cathepsin-B also cleaves the hyaluronic acid–binding region from cartilage proteoglycans and degrades the GAG attachment region to small fragments.[77,100] It has been suggested that the proteolytic action of cathepsin-B, at least in human joints, appears to be related to cysteine protease inhibitors.[55] The significance of their role in cartilage degradation is controversial.[66]

ASPARTIC PROTEINASES

Cathepsin D, which is the most prominent lysosomal proteinase acting at acid pH, requires aspartic acid residues as part of the catalytic mechanism. Under inflammatory conditions and during periods of rapid extracellular matrix destruction, it is secreted extracellularly by macrophages in connective tissue cells, mostly as a proenzyme. Under the active metabolic conditions found in inflammatory joint disease, it is possible that CO_2 and lactic acid production could create an environment of sufficiently low pH in the pericellular space to permit the proteolytic activity of cathepsin D. However, there has been no defined work in the horse.

Prostaglandins

Prostaglandins (primarily E group) are produced in inflamed joints and can cause a decrease in the proteoglycan content of the cartilage matrix.[57,99,114] Prostaglandin E_2 (PGE_2) can be released from synovial cells in response to IL-1.[22] The presence of PGE_2 in synovial fluid from inflamed joints has been demonstrated in the

horse,[64,113] and in our laboratory at Colorado State University we use PGE_2 measurements as an index of the level of synovitis. Actions of PGE_2 in joints include vasodilatation, enhancement of pain perception, proteoglycan depletion from cartilage (by both degradation and inhibition of synthesis), bone demineralization, and promotion of plasminogen activator secretion. PGE_2 is released from chondrocytes on stimulation of these cells by IL-1 and TNF-α.

Oxygen-Derived Free Radicals

Oxygen-derived free radicals, including superoxide anion, hydroxyl radicals, and hydrogen peroxide, may be released from injured joint tissues. Studies have demonstrated cleavage of hyaluronic acid by free radicals.[42,43] There is also evidence that superoxide can degrade the α chains of collagen, based on the finding that superoxide treatment inhibits gelatin.[126] Proteoglycans may also be cleaved by free radicals.[22,106] Increased free radical levels in the synovial fluid of horses with equine joint disease have been recently demonstrated.[24a]

Nitric oxide has recently been recognized as an important physiologic mediator. It combines avidly with superoxide anion, and although this was originally thought to provide a protective function, it now seems that this reaction can generate further destructive species including peroxynitrite anion and hydroxyl radicals.[92] The role of nitric oxide in joint disease needs, and is receiving, further attention.

Cytokines and Articular Cartilage Degradation

Much of the destructive proteinase activity described above is released by cytokines. Cytokines are defined as soluble peptides produced by one cell that affect the activity of other cell types. Studies of cytokines in joint tissues suggest that IL-1 and TNF-α modulate the synthesis of metalloproteinases by both chondrocytes[22,106] and synovial cells[21,127] and are important mediators in joint disease. IL-1 and TNF-α may be produced by synovial cells[22] and may therefore be of importance in the deleterious effects of synovitis on articular cartilage. The normal turnover of the extracellular matrix of the articular cartilage is considered to be regulated by chondrocytes under the control and influence of cytokines and mechanical stimuli.[90] Articular cartilage degradation in association with disease represents an exacerbation of these normal processes. Accumulation of knowledge in this regard began with the initial studies by Fell and Jubb[31,32] of cartilage–synovial interactions using in vitro systems. It is widely accepted that cytokines may induce proteoglycan depletion in articular cartilage by either increasing the rate of degradation or decreasing synthesis in association with the release of proteinases and prostaglandins from chondrocytes.[115] Inhibited synthesis seems to be more significant than proteoglycan degradation in studies on the horse, but these experiments have been done in vitro with human recombinant IL-1.[87] Recent recognition of the gene sequence for equine IL-1 by Howard et al.[46,47] at Colorado State University can, one hopes, lead to specific studies with equine tissues as well as equine IL-1. It is felt that IL-1 produces its effects by binding with an IL-1 receptor on the cell. The presence of IL-1 in equine osteoarthritic joints was first reported in 1990 by Morris et al.[76] An equine IL-1–containing extract was produced by May in 1990.[63] To think that IL-1 acts solely on its own in stimulating metalloproteinase release is probably naive. Work is limited in the horse. However, Todhunter showed in an in vitro experiment with canine articular cartilage explants that neither metalloproteinase activity nor proteoglycan degradation were inducible in canine cartilage explants treated with recombinant IL-1α. However, proteoglycan synthesis was significantly decreased by 10 and 100 ng of rhIL-1α/mL. Metalloproteinase activity in the medium accompanied proteoglycan degradation of cartilage treated with lipopolysaccharide and monocyte-conditioned medium. The metalloproteinase released into the medium was identified as prostromelysin by Western blotting.[114a]

In addition to IL-1 being detected with in situ hybridization in osteoarthritic cartilage in humans, it has recently been shown that TNF-α does indeed act on cartilage but only at specific sites where chondrocyte TNF-α receptor expression is high. It is therefore considered that focal loss of cartilage will occur at sites where chondrocyte P55 TNF-R expression is high and sufficient TNF-α is present. It has been suggested that this may explain the focal nature of cartilage loss in some instances of OA.[123] There is evidence that while TNF-α is important in joint swelling, a direct role in tissue destruction is unlikely.[119a] On the other hand, IL-1 is not a dominant cytokine in early joint swelling but has a pivotal role in evasive cartilage damage.

Neuropeptides

It has been pointed out that in addition to its importance in the morbidity (pain sensation) of OA, the nervous system has a potential role in the pathogenesis of the disease.[13] The activation of articular nerves not only provides sensory perception of pain but also results in the release of neurotransmitters that have inflammatory potential. There is evidence that the peripherally released transmitters have deleterious effects on synovial and cartilage cell metabolism, contributing to cartilage matrix depletion. Exposure of monocytes to substance P and other neuropeptides causes the release of the cytokines IL-1, IL-6, and TNF.[58] Elevated synovial fluid concentrations of substance P and other peptides have been observed in humans with joint disease.[62] Substance P levels are also elevated in horses with arthropathies.[12] Substance P is not the only peptide found in nerves; others include the peripheral peptides VIP, MET-enkephalin, and somatostatin.[88]

Fibronectin

The fibronectin content of osteoarthritic cartilage is considerably higher than that of normal cartilage, but the significance of this or the role of fibronectin in the pathologic process has been controversial.[10,73] It has been suggested that the appearance of fibronectin in diseased cartilage matrix may be a feature of the chondrocyte's repair response to the loss of extracellular matrix and that fibronectin may interact with proteoglycan.[73] Further, fibronectin functions as a cellular adherence factor (it is a major cell surface glycoprotein) and is closely associated with the collagen of the extracellular matrix as well as proteoglycans.[73]

Chondrocytes can be a source of some cartilage fibronectin, but plasma or synovial fluid may also be a source.[9] Fibronectin in synovial fluid from osteoarthritic joints is derived from several sources, including synoviocytes, plasma, and increased production by degenerated articular cartilage.[9] There is more recent evidence that fibronectins may contribute to aggrecan degradation in OA and inflammatory joint disease and that the fibronectins mediate their effects through catabolic cytokines.[45]

Mechanical Factors and Subchondral Bone Change in the Pathogenesis of Articular Cartilage Degradation

The role of biomechanical factors has been frequently discussed in relationship to articular cartilage degeneration. It is well recognized that articular cartilage may be subjected to a harsh loading environment.[28] Local intensity of loading is generally defined by mechanical stress (the force/unit area acting on the tissue). The measurement of stress in physiologic situations is not yet possible, and therefore much of the information in vivo is speculative. Some authors suggest that the mechanical factors to which articular cartilage is normally exposed in vivo are insufficient to destroy tissue directly but that when the chemical integrity of the matrix is compromised biochemically, direct mechanical damage becomes possible.[28] However, other authors propose that subfracture impact loads can generate shear stresses that break collagenous cross-links. This substructural damage in turn precedes chondrocyte enzyme production or entry of catabolic enzymes into the matrix.[93] In an experiment on acute transarticular load in the canine patellofemoral joint, it was shown that fractures in the zone of calcified cartilage–bone interface with no visible abnormalities of the articular cartilage. India ink staining revealed superficial damage in the articular cartilage. The authors felt that their experimental model may also simulate the situation with severe ligamentous disruption, in that unrecognized subchondral fractures or fractures in the calcified cartilage may be a common feature of musculoskeletal trauma and a major cause of subsequent osteoarthrosis.[113a] In most situations, mechanical forces are considered more likely to destroy cartilage indirectly through insult to the subchondral bone, synovial membrane, or chondrocytes. Also, while excessive forces may lead to articular cartilage loss, removal of all mechanical stimulation leads to atrophy. Normal cartilage structure and function is maintained by some intermediate level and frequency of loading.[28]

When considering possible pathways for mechanical destruction of articular cartilage, an early concept was that early subchondral bone sclerosis causes a reduction in the joint's shock-absorbing capability and thereby places cartilage at risk of shear-induced tensile failure of cartilage cross-links, particularly under repetitive impulsive loading conditions.[94,95] Recent work in our laboratory has demonstrated that when horses are subjected to athletic exercise on the treadmill, microdamage in the subchondral bone can develop. In looking retrospectively at racehorses, the range of microdamage includes not only microfractures but also primary osteocyte death. It is felt that not only is mechanical support of the articular cartilage lost when subchondral bone microdamage progresses to macrodamage but also potentially cytokine release from the bone can influence the state of the articular cartilage.[54a] We feel that subchondral bone is very important in the development of a number of articular lesions, but it is a lot more complicated than simply being secondary to subchondral stiffness.

Others have challenged the relationship between subchondral stiffness and OA. There is no change in mineral content with impact loading.[107] It has also been suggested that abnormal bony trabeculae cannot fully explain cartilage microfracturing.[107a] Cyclic loading results primarily in deformation of bone.[107] The effect of cyclic loading on cartilage metabolism also needs to be appreciated. Certain regimens will suppress proteoglycan synthesis, whereas others will stimulate it.[85,120] Repetitive cycle loading such as occurs in human runners is not a factor in the pathogenesis of OA.[65] However, there are risk factors in such a group, including prior trauma leading to an internal knee derangement, increased varus angulation of the knees, and long duration of running.[65] It is felt that the fit, physically active individual may be better able to tolerate joint loads as a result of increased muscle tone and possible effects of physical activity on joint nutrition.[59] Forces to joints are dissipated by muscles, soft tissues, ligaments, and bones. Removal of the meniscus or disruption of ligamentous support leads to OA, and this is presumably associated with biomechanical alterations in the joint.[2,30,53,79,89]

The relationship between a single episode of major trauma to a joint and subsequent osteoarthritic change is uncertain. Although a single major impact can cause articular cartilage damage, it has been stated that the histologic features often resemble chondromalacia and thus may be nonprogressive.[19,86] We need to be careful, particularly in the horse, in distinguishing an acute cartilage injury from the development of osteoarthritic lesions.

The concept of OA as an exaggerated process of remodeling of the articular ends of the bone was first suggested by Johnson.[54] He suggested advancement of the tide mark and thickening of the calcified bed in OA, with consequent decrease in the thickness of noncalcified cartilage. Other authors support this concept.[93,109] In addition to the recognized processes of articular cartilage degeneration (chondrocyte necrosis, atrophy, fibrillation, and detachment), cartilage is also altered and lost by advancing endochondral ossification manifested by reduplication of the tide mark and focal vascular resorption and ossification of the calcified layer. These changes in the osteochondral junction in adult life are considered strong evidence of ongoing remodeling.[109] Movement of the zone of calcified cartilage toward the articular surface would cause a decrease in cartilage height, and such a decrease could lead to alterations in the distribution of stresses in both cartilage and subchondral bone.[84,93] Sokoloff proposed three distinct compartments (articular cartilage, osteochondral junction, and adjacent bone and capsular attachments) as an interrelating system that mediates and adapts to mechanical stress.[109] There is evidence that the shape of joints changes throughout life, even in the apparent absence of gross OA.[84] The change in distribution of load to formerly unloaded cartilage

may be an important factor in degeneration of the joint surface.[109] There is also proliferation of osteoarticular tissue in the capsular attachments and subchondral bone marrow. Marginal osteophytosis is a variable, age-related phenomenon in nonosteoarthritic joints. Increased congruency of joints is also considered to affect the nutrition of articular cartilage.

Morphologic and Biochemical Reaction of Articular Cartilage to Insult

As discussed above, trauma can cause an immediate physical defect or initiate a degenerative or degradative process. Degradation of articular cartilage is manifested in a sequence of morphologic changes including chondromalacia or softening, fibrillation (superficial or deep), and erosion (see also the section on osteoarthritis below in this chapter). It has now been well recognized (and the processes reviewed above) that major biochemical changes take place and may indeed precede morphologic defects.[52,115] Some of these processes are outlined in Figures 7.8 and 7.9. The varying degrees in different situations, synovial inflammation (synovitis), release of degradative mediators within the articular cartilage, and/or mechanical and cytokine-related factors from the subchondral bone can contribute to this degradation (see also section on osteoarthritis below).

Formation of Osteophytes and Enthesiophytes

In addition to the central process of articular cartilage breakdown in OA, a second pathologic process characterized by proliferation of new cartilage and bone at the periphery of joints (osteophytosis) occurs. These spurs are usually called osteophytes, but the term "osteochondrophytes" may be more accurate.[78] Osteophyte formation is commonly considered a characteristic component and a secondary consequence of OA, but this concept is to be questioned.[20,61,70]

Using the canine cranial cruciate desmotomy model, Marshall demonstrated that osteophyte formation started early after surgery and could not be related to any major articular cartilage damage or subchondral bone change.[61] He also documented that the first sign of an osteophyte was the appearance of fibrous tissue outside the bone and that this tissue then underwent chondroid metamorphosis and endochondral ossification. Using a filipin-induced equine model, this author demonstrated osteophyte formation unrelated to significant cartilage damage, and formation followed the same sequence of fibrous tissue, then cartilage and bone. This connective tissue response at the junction of the synovial membrane, cartilage perichondrium, and periosteum is characteristic of a marginal osteophyte (there are also central osteophytes in the interior of the joint). Osteophytes need to be distinguished from enthesiophytes, which are bone proliferations at ligament, tendon, or joint capsule insertions into bone. In situations in which osteophytes are consistently associated with structural articular cartilage change and parallel them, it would seem appropriate to consider osteophytes a significant lesion of OA.[78]

Causes proposed for osteophytes include aging,[20] mechanical instability,[61,91] proliferative responses secondary to synovitis,[15,70] and tissue responses to stretching of the synovial membrane at its insertion[4] or forces of any soft tissue attachments in the area of the transition zone.[78] The concept that osteophytes develop as a secondary response to stabilize an osteoarthritic knee or increase available joint surface area is an old one. It is only relatively recently that it was shown marginal osteophytes stabilize the varus–valgus motion of the knee in humans with knee OA.[91] The authors of this study felt that the osteophytes might increase stability by pressing directly against slackened collateral ligaments, thus reducing ligamentous pseudolaxity. They also felt that such osteophytes should not be surgically removed, to prevent even greater instability.

Work with an equine model demonstrates that osteophytes and enthesiophytes can result from chemical synovitis and capsulitis and in the absence of instability (Fig. 7.10).[70] Osteophytes and enthesiophytes are seen in the horse without articular cartilage damage (defined arthroscopically) and also in the absence (in some instances) of clinical significance. Their removal is certainly inappropriate.

Enthesiophytes have been recognized as a consequence of aging in humans.[8] They are also seen in association with instability or without instability in horses. Remodeling and smooth margins to enthesiophytes generally indicate that the enthesiophyte is a sign of previous insult but of doubtful clinical significance.

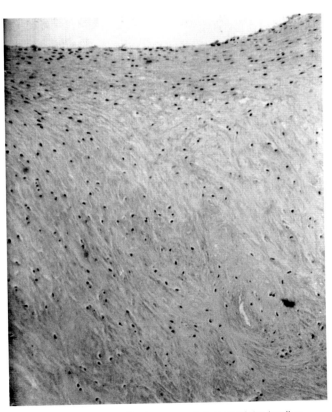

Figure 7.10 Fibrocartilaginous repair typical of the healing achieved with full-thickness articular defect in the horse.

Articular Cartilage Repair

Healing refers to restoration of the structural integrity and function of the tissue after injury or disease, but repair usually has a more restricted meaning.[8] *Repair* refers to the replacement of damaged or lost cells and matrix with new cells and matrix, a process that does not necessarily restore the original structure or function of a tissue. *Regeneration* may be considered a special form of repair in which the cells replace lost or damaged tissue with a tissue identical to the original tissue. It has been suggested that with the exception of bone fractures, most injuries and diseases of the musculoskeletal tissues do not stimulate regeneration of the original tissue.[8] The limited potential of articular cartilage for regeneration and healing has been appreciated for over two centuries. In 1743, Hunter stated "From Hippocrates to the present age, it is universally allowed that ulcerated cartilage is a troublesome thing and that when once destroyed it is not repaired."[49] There is a limited response of cartilage to tissue damage and an inability of natural repair responses from adjacent tissues to produce tissue with the morphologic, biochemical, and biomechanical properties of articular cartilage.

The major limiting factor in the successful rehabilitation of any joint after injury or disease is the failure of osteochondral defects to heal.[69] Three mechanisms have been recognized as possible contributors to articular cartilage repair. *Intrinsic repair* (from within the cartilage) relies on the limited mitotic capability of the chondrocyte and a somewhat ineffective increase in collagen and proteoglycan production. *Extrinsic repair* comes from mesenchymal elements from the subchondral bone participating in the formation of new connective tissue that may undergo some metaplastic change to form cartilage elements. The third phenomenon, known as *"matrix flow,"* may contribute to equine articular cartilage repair by forming lips of cartilage from the perimeter of the lesion that migrate toward the center of the defect.[50,51,112]

The depth of the injury (full or partial thickness), size of defect, location and relation to weight-bearing or non-weight-bearing areas, and the age of the animal influence the repair and remodeling of an injured joint surface.[11,18,72]

With a partial-thickness defect, some repair occurs with increased GAG synthesis and increased collagen synthesis.[72] However, the repair process is never completely effective. In humans, complete repair of chondromalacia of the patella has been reported to occur if matrical depletion and surface breakdown are minimal.[5] However, more recent work with arthroscopic debridement of partial-thickness defects in humans would question any actual regeneration.[105] Also, superficial defects are not necessarily progressive and do not necessarily compromise joint function.

With full-thickness defects, the response from the adjacent articular cartilage varies little from that after superficial lesions and provides only limited repair necessary to replace dead cells and damaged matrix at the margins of the wound. These defects heal by ingrowth of subchondral fibrous tissue that may or may not undergo metaplasia to fibrocartilage (Fig. 7.10).[18,41,51,60,98,118] Subchondral bone defects either heal with bone that grows up into the defect or fill in with fibrocartilaginous ingrowth.[118] Duplication of the tide mark in the calcified cartilage layer is rare, and adherence of the repair tissue to surrounding noninjured cartilage is often incomplete.[41,60]

A number of equine studies demonstrate that the size and location of articular defects have a significant effect on the degree of healing achieved. Convery et al. first reported that large defects were less likely to heal.[18] A more recent study distinguished between large (15 mm^2) and small (5 mm^2) full-thickness lesions in weight-bearing and non-weight-bearing areas of the antebrachiocarpal (radiocarpal), middle carpal (intercarpal), and femoropatellar joints.[51] At 1 month, small defects were filled with poorly organized fibrovascular repair tissue; by 4 months, repair was limited to an increase in the amount of organization of this fibrous tissue, and by 5 months, small radiocarpal and femoropatellar lesions were hardly detectable because of combinations of matrix flow and extrinsic repair mechanisms (see Fig. 7.9). Large lesions showed good initial repair, but at 5 months, perilesional and intralesional subchondral clefts developed.

The repair tissue that forms after full-thickness injury to hyaline cartilage or as a natural repair process in joints with DJD is primarily composed of type I rather than type II collagen, at least at 4 months.[116,117] Identification of type II collagen is the critical biochemical factor distinguishing hyaline cartilage from repair fibrous tissue and fibrocartilage. It is felt that the presence of an abnormal subchondral bone plate and the absence of a tide mark reforming may create a stiffness gradient and that shear stresses of the junction of the repair tissue and underlying bone develop. The propagation of such shear stresses would lead to the degradation of repair fibrocartilage and exposure of the bone. This mechanical failure has been observed experimentally and clinically in the horse.[51,71]

Recently, the author's laboratory analyzed tissue 12 months after creation of full-thickness articular cartilage defects in a weight-bearing area.[48] In a study looking at the long-term effectiveness of sternal cartilage grafting, the repair tissue in the nongrafted defects at 12 months consisted of fibrocartilaginous tissue with fibrous tissue in the surface layers, as was seen in control defects at 4 months (see Fig 7.10). However, on biochemical analysis, the repair tissue of the nongrafted defects had a mean type II collagen percentage of 79%, compared with being nondetectable at 4 months.[117] On the other hand, the GAG content expressed as milligrams of total hexosamine per gram of dried tissue was 20.6 ± 1.85 mg/g, compared with 26.4 ± 3.1 mg/g at 4 months and 41.8 ± 4.3 mg/g DW in normal equine articular cartilage.[48,117]

The fibrocartilaginous repair seen in normal full-thickness defects is therefore biomechanically unsuitable as a replacement bearing surface and has been shown to undergo mechanical failure with use. The lack of durability may be related to faulty biochemical composition of the old matrix and incomplete remodeling of the interface between old and repaired cartilage or to increased stress in the regenerated cartilage because of abnormal remodeling of the subchondral bone plate and calcified cartilage layer. Although recent work implies that it may be possible to reconstitute the normal collagen type in

equine articular cartilage,[48] clearly there is continued deterioration of GAG content, and these are important components in the overall composition of the cartilage matrix.

The presence of a cartilage defect may not represent clinical compromise. In the equine carpus, loss of up to 30% of articular surface of an individual bone may not compromise the successful return of a horse to racing.[71] However, loss of 50% of the articular surface or severe loss of subchondral bone leads to a significantly worse prognosis.

The inadequate healing response may not necessarily apply to immature animals or to non-weight-bearing defects. An example is the young horse after surgery for osteochondritis dissecans (OCD) who shows impressive healing responses or at least functional responses. This may be related to increased chondrocytic capacity for mitosis and matrix synthesis and the presence of intracartilaginous vascularity. Complete restoration of the ultrastructure and surface configuration in a hingelike gliding joint surface such as the femoropatellar joint may be unnecessary for clinical soundness, compared with the more severe loading on an osteochondral defect located on the weight-bearing portion of the medial condyle of the femur or the midcarpal joint. It has been suggested that increasing age may affect the response of cartilage to injury in humans because the ability of the chondrocytes to synthesize and assemble matrix micromolecules could decline with age.[8] Buckwalter cites a study of transplanted chondrocytes, suggesting that older chondrocytes produce a more poorly organized matrix than do younger chondrocytes,[8] and other studies demonstrate that the proteoglycan synthesized by the chondrocytes changes with age.[74,97]

Methods used to attempt manipulation of this healing response have been extensively reviewed elsewhere.[68]

References

1. Allen RE, Blake DR, Nazhat NB, et al. Superoxide radical generation by inflamed human synovium after hypoxia. Lancet 1989; 2:282–283.
2. Allen PR, Denham RA, Swan AV. Late degenerative changes after meniscectomy: Factors affecting the knee after operation. J Bone Joint Surg [Br] 1984;66:667–671.
3. Arner EC, Decicco CP, Cherney R, Tortorella MD. Cleavage of native cartilage aggrecan by neutrophil collagenase (MMP-8) is distinct from endogenous cleavage by aggrecanase. J Biochem 1997;272:9294–9299.
4. Bennett GA, Bauer W. Joint changes resulting from patellar displacement and their relation to degenerative joint disease. J Bone Joint Surg 1937;29:667–682.
5. Bentley G. Articular cartilage changes in chondromalacia patellae. J Bone Joint Surg [Br] 1985;67:769–774.
6. Balkman CE, Nixon AJ. Molecular cloning and cartilage gene expression of equine stromelysin 1 (matrix metalloproteinase 3). Am J Vet Res 1998;59:30–36.
6a. Billinghurst RC, Fretz PB, Gordon JR. Induction of intra-articular tumour necrosis factor in acute inflammatory responses in equine arthritis. Equine Vet J 1995;27:208–216.
7. Boniface RJ, Cain PR, Evans CH. Articular responses to purified cartilage proteoglycans. Arthritis Rheum 1988;31:258–266.
8. Buckwalter JA, Mau DC. Cartilage repair in osteoarthritis. In: Moskowitz RW, Howell DS, Goldberg VM, Mankin HJ, Eds. Osteoarthritis. Diagnosis and Medical/Surgical Management. 2nd ed. Philadelphia: WB Saunders, 1992;71–107.
8a. Bunning RA, Russell RG. The effect of tumor necrosis factor alpha and gamma-interferon on the resorption of human articu-

lar cartilage and on the production of prostaglandin E and of caseinase activity by human articular chondrocytes. Arthritis Rheum 1989;32(6):780–784.

9. Burton-Wurster N, Lust G. Synthesis of fibronectin in normal and osteoarthritic articular cartilage. Biochim Biophys Acta 1984;800:52–58.

10. Burton-Wurster N, Lust G. Deposition of fibronectin in articular cartilage of canine osteoarthritic joints. Am J Vet Res 1985;46: 2542–2545.

11. Calandruccio RA, Gilmer S. Proliferation, regeneration and repair of articular cartilage of immature animals. J Bone Joint Surg [Am] 1962;44:431–455.

12. Caron JP, Bowker RM, Abhold RH, et al. Substance P in the synovial membrane and fluid of the equine metacarpal joint. Equine Vet J 1992;24:364–366.

13. Caron JP, Bowker RM, Toppin DS. Osteoarthritis in the horse: The role of the nervous system. In: Proceedings. 38th Annual Meeting of the American Association of Equine Practitioners, Orlando, FL, 1992;13–20.

14. Caron JP, Tardif G, Martel-Pelletier J, et al. Modulation of matrix metalloproteinase 13 (collagenase 3) gene expression in equine chondrocytes by equine interleukin 1 and corticosteroids. Am J Vet Res 1996;57:1631–1634.

15. Chrisman OD, Fessel JM, Southwick WO. Experimental production of synovitis and marginal articular exostoses in the knee joint of dogs. Yale J Biol Med 1964;37:409–412.

16. Clegg PD, Burke RM, Coughlan AR. Characterization of equine matrix metalloproteinase 2 and 9; and identification of the cellular sources of these enzymes in joints. Equine Vet J 1997;29: 335–342.

17. Clegg PD, Coughlan AR, Riggs CM, Carter SD. Matrix metalloproteinases 2 and 9 in equine synovial fluids. Equine Vet J 1997; 29:343–348.

18. Convery FR, Akeson WH, Keown GH. Repair of large osteochondral defects—An experimental study in horses. Clin Orthop 1972;82:253.

19. Crock HV. Post-traumatic erosions of articular cartilage. J Bone Joint Surg [Br] 1964;46:530–538.

20. Danielsson L, Hernborg S. Clinical and roentgenologic study of knee joints with osteophytes. Clin Orthop 1970;69:302–312.

21. Dayer J-M, Beutler B, Serami A. Cachectin/tumor necrosis factor stimulates collagenase and prostaglandin E_2 production by human synovial cells and dermal fibroblasts. J Exp Med 1985; 162:2163–2168.

22. Dayer J-M, deRochemonteix B, Burrus B, et al. Human recombinant interleukin-1 stimulates collagenase and prostaglandin E_2 production by human synovial cells. J Clin Invest 1986;77: 645–648.

23. Dean DD, Azo W, Martel-Pelletier J, et al. Levels of metalloproteases and the tissue inhibitor of metalloproteases in human osteoarthritic cartilage. J Rheumatol 1987;14:43–44.

24. Dean DD, Martel-Pelletier J, Pelletier JP et al. Evidence for metalloproteinase and metalloproteinase inhibitor imbalance in human osteoarthritic cartilage. J Clin Invest 1989;84:678–685.

24a. Dimock AN, Siciliano PD, McIlwraith CW. Evidence supporting an increased presence of reactive oxygen species in the diseased equine joint. Equine Vet J 2000;32:439–443.

25. Dodge GR, Poole AR. Immunohistochemical detection and immunochemical analysis of type II collagen degradation in human normal, rheumatoid, and osteoarthritic articular cartilage and in explants of bovine articular cartilage cultured with interleukin 1. J Clin Invest 1989;83:647–661.

26. Eckhout Y, Vaes G. Further studies on the activation of procollagenase, the latent precursor of bone collagenase: Effects of lysosomal cathepsin-B, plasmin and kallikrein, and spontaneous activation. Biochem J 1977;166:21–31.

27. Evans CH. Response of synovium to mechanical injury. In: Finerman GAM, Noyes FR, Eds. Biology and Biomechanics of the Traumatized Synovial Joint. Rosemont, IL: American Academy of Orthopedic Surgery, 1992;17–26.

28. Evans CH, Brown TD. Role of physical and mechanical agents in degrading the matrix. In: Woessner JF Jr, Howell DS, Eds. Joint Cartilage Degeneration: Basic and Clinical Aspects. New York: Marcel Dekker, 1993;187–208.

29. Evans CH, Mears DC, Stanitski CL. Ferrographic analysis of wear in human joints: Evaluation by comparison with arthroscopic examination of symptomatic knee joints. J Bone Joint Surg [Br] 1982;64:572–578.

30. Fairbank TJ. Knee joint changes after meniscectomy. J Bone Joint Surg [Br] 1948;30:664–670.

31. Fell HB, Jubb RW. The effect of synovial tissue on breakdown of articular cartilage in organ culture. Arthritis Rheum 1977; 20:1359–1371.

32. Fell HB, Jubb RW. The effect of synovial tissue on the synthesis of proteoglycan by the articular cartilage of young pigs. Arthritis Rheum 1980;23:545–555.

33. Flannery CR, Gordy JT, Lark MW, et al. Identification of a stromelysin cleavage site within the interglobular domain of human aggrecan: Evidence for proteolysis at this site in vivo. In: Proceedings. 38th Annual Meeting of the Orthopaedic Research Society, 1992;84.

34. Fosang AJ, Neame PJ, Hardingham TE, et al. Cleavage of cartilage proteoglycan between G1 and G2 domains by stromelysin [abstract]. J Biochem 1991;266:15579–15582.

35. Fosang AJ, Neame PJ, Last K, et al. The interglobular domain of cartilage aggrecan is cleaved by PUMP, gelatinases and cathepsin B. J Biochem 1992;267:19470–19474.

36. Freemont AJ, Hampson V, Tilman R, et al. Gene expression of matrix metalloproteinases 1, 3 and 9 by chondrocytes in osteoarthritic human knee articular cartilage is zone and grade specific. Ann Rheum Dis 1997;56:542–549.

37. Freije JMP, Diez-Itz AI, Balbin M, et al. Molecular cloning and expression of collagenase-3. A novel human metalloproteinase produced by breast carcinomas. J Biochem 1994;269: 16766–16773.

38. Gadher SJ, Eyere DR, Duance VC, et al. Susceptibility of cartilage collagens type II, III, X and X1 to human synovial collagenase and neutrophil elastase. Eur J Biochem 1988;175:1–7.

39. Galloway WA, Murphy G, Sandy JD, et al. Purification and characterization of a rabbit bone metalloproteinase that degrades proteoglycan and other connective-tissue components. Biochem J 1983;209:741–752.

40. Gilpe G, Magna HA, Reeves LM, et al. Cloning, expression, and type II collagenolytic activity of matrix metalloproteinase-13 from human osteoarthritic cartilage. J Clin Invest 1996;97: 761–768.

41. Grant BD. Repair mechanisms of osteochondral defects in Equidae: A comparative study of untreated in x-irradiated defects. Proc Am Assoc Equine Pract 1975;21:95–114.

42. Greenwald R, Moy W. Inhibition of collagen gelatin by actions of the superoxide radical. Arthritis Rheum 1979;22:251–259.

43. Greenwald R, Moy W. Effect of oxygen-derived free radicals on hyaluronic acid. Arthritis Rheum 1980;23:455–463.

44. Hollander AP. Matrix metalloproteinases as targets for therapy in equine joint diseases. Equine Vet J 1997;29:329–330.

45. Homandberg GA, Davis G, Maniglia C, Shrikhande A. Cartilage chondrolysis by fibronectin fragments causes cleavage of aggrecan at the same site as found in osteoarthritic cartilage. Osteoarthritis Cartilage 1997;5:450–453.

46. Howard RD, McIlwraith CW, Trotter GW, Nyborg J. Cloning of equine interleukin-1 alpha and equine interleukin-1 beta and determination of their full length cDNA sequences. Am J Vet Res 1998;59:704–711.

47. Howard RD, McIlwraith CW, Trotter GW, Nyborg JF. Cloning of equine interleukin-1 alpha and equine interleukin-1 receptor antagonist and determination of their full length cDNA sequence. Am J Vet Res 1998;57:704–711.

48. Howard RD, McIlwraith CW, Trotter GW, et al. Long-term fate and effects of exercise on sternal cartilage autografts used for repair of osteochondral defects in horses. Am J Vet Res 1994; 55:1158–1167.

49. Hunter W. On the structure and diseases of articulating cartilage. Philos Trans R Soc (London) 1743;9:267.

50. Hurtig MB. Experimental use of small osteochondral grafts for resurfacing the equine third carpal bone. Equine Vet J 1988;S6: 23–27.

51. Hurtig MB, Fretz PB, Doige CE, Schnurr DL. Effect of lesion size and location on equine articular cartilage repair. Can J Vet Res 1988;52:137–146.

52. Ikebe T, Harata M, Koga T. Effects of human recombinant tumor necrosis factor alpha and interleukin-1 on the synthesis of glycosaminoglycan and DNA in cultured rat costal chondrocytes. J Immunol 1988;140:827–831.

53. Jackson JP. Degenerative changes in the knee after meniscectomy. Br Med J 1968;2:525–527.

53a. Jawed S, Gaffney K, Blake DR. Intra-articular pressure profile of the knee joint in a spectrum of inflammatory arthropathies. Ann Rheum Dis 1997;56:686–689.

54. Johnson LC. Joint remodeling as the basis for osteoarthritis. J Am Vet Med Assoc 1962;141:1237–1241.

54a. Kawcak CE. Effects of loading on subchondral bone of the equine carpal and metacarpophalangeal joint. PhD dissertation, Colorado State University, Fort Collins, CO, 1998.

55. Killackey JJ, Roughley PJ, Mort JS. Proteinase inhibitors of human articular cartilage. Coll Relat Res 1983;3:419–430.

56. Levick JR. Hypoxia and acidosis in chronic inflammatory arthritis; relation to vascular supply and dynamic effusion pressure. J Rheumatol 1990;17:579–582.

57. Lippiello L, Yamamoto K, Robinson D, Mankin HJ. Involvement of prostaglandin from rheumatoid synovium and inhibition of articular cartilage metabolism. Arthritis Rheum 1978; 21:909.

58. Lotz N, Vaughn JH, Carson DA. Effect of neuropeptides on production on inflammatory cytokines by human monocytes. Science 1988;241:1218–1221.

59. Malemud CJ, Shuckett R. Impact loading and lower-extremity disease. In: Clinical Concepts in Regional Musculoskeletal Illness. New York: Grune & Stratton, 1987;109–135.

60. Mankin HJ. The reactions of articular cartilage to injury in osteoarthritis. I. N Engl J Med 1974;191:1285–1292.

61. Marshall JL. Periarticular osteophytes. Initiation and formation in the knee of the dog. Clin Orthop 1969;62:37–47.

62. Marshall KW, Chiu B, Innaman RD. Substance P and arthritis: Analysis of plasma in synovial fluid levels. Arthritis Rheum 1990;33:87–90.

63. May SA, Hooke RE, Lees P. The characterization of equine interleukin-1. Vet Immunol Immunopathol 1990;24:169–175.

64. May SA, Hooke RE, Peremans KY, et al. Prostaglandin E$_2$ in equine joint disease; personal communication, 1992.

65. McDermott M, Freyne P. Osteoarthritis in runners with knee pain. Br J Sports Med 1983;117:84–87.

66. McIlwraith CW. Current concepts in equine degenerative joint disease. J Am Vet Med Assoc 1982;180:239.

67. McIlwraith CW. General pathobiology of the joint and response to injury. In: McIlwraith CW, Trotter GW, Eds. Joint Disease in the Horse. Philadelphia: WB Saunders, 1996;40–70.

68. McIlwraith CW, Nixon AJ. Joint resurfacing: Attempts at repairing articular cartilage defects. In: McIlwraith CW, Trotter GW, Eds. Joint Disease in the Horse. Philadelphia: WB Saunders, 1996;317–334.

69. McIlwraith CW, Vachon AM. Review of pathogenesis and treatment of degenerative joint disease. Equine Vet J 1988;S6:3–11.

70. McIlwraith CW, Van Sickle DC. Experimentally induced arthritis of the equine carpus: Histologic and histochemical changes in the articular cartilage. Am J Vet Res 1981;42:209–217.

71. McIlwraith CW, Yovich JV, Martin GS. Arthroscopic surgery for the treatment of osteochondral chip fractures in the equine carpus. J Am Vet Med Assoc 1987;191:531–540.

72. Meachim G. The effect of scarification on articular cartilage in the rabbit. J Bone Joint Surg [Br] 1963;45:150–161.

73. Miller DR, Mankin HJ, Shoji H, D'Ambrosia RD. Identification of fibronectin in preparations of osteoarthritic human cartilage. Connect Tissue Res 1984;12:267–275.

74. Mitchell N, Shepherd N. Resurfacing of adult rabbit articular cartilage by multiple perforations through the subchondral bone. J Bone Joint Surg [Am] 1976;58:230.

75. Moldovan F, Pelletier JP, Hambor J, et al. Collagenase-3 (matrix metalloproteinase 13) is preferentially localized in the deep layer of human articular cartilage *in situ*. *In vitro* mimicking effect by transforming growth factor beta. Arthritis Rheum 1997;40: 1653–1661.

76. Morris EA, McDonald BS, Webb AC, Rosenwasser LJ. Identification of interleukin-1 in equine osteoarthritic joint effusion. Am J Vet Res 1990;51:59–64.

77. Morrison RIG, Barrett AJ, Dingle JT. Cathepsin B$_1$ and D action on human articular cartilage proteoglycans. Biochim Biophys Acta 1973;302:411.

78. Moskowitz RW, Goldberg VM. Studies of osteophyte pathogenesis in experimentally induced osteoarthritis. J Rheumatol 1987; 14:311–320.

79. Moskowitz RW, Davis W, Sammarco J, et al. Experimentally induced degenerative joint lesions following partial meniscectomy in the rabbit. Arthritis Rheum 1973;16:397–405.

80. Murphy G, Lockett MI, Stephens PE, et al. Stromelysin is an activator of procollagenase. A study with natural and recombinant enzymes. Biochem J 1987;248:265–268.

81. Nagase H, Woessner Jr JF. Role of endogenous proteinases in the degradation of cartilage matrix. In: Woessner FJ Jr, Howell DS, Eds. Joint Cartilage Degradation: Basic and Clinical Aspects. New York: Marcel Dekker, 1993;159–185.

82. Nguyen Q, Mort JS, Roughley PJ. Preferential mRNA expression of prostromelysin relative to procollagenase and *in situ* localization in human articular cartilage. J Clin Invest 1992;89: 1189–1197.

83. Nguyen Q, Murphy G, Roughley PJ, Mort JS. Degradation of proteoglycan aggregate by a cartilage metalloproteinase. Biochem J 1989;259:61–67.

84. Oegema TR, Thompson RC Jr. Cartilage-bone interface (tide mark). In: Brandt KD, Ed. Cartilage Changes in Osteoarthritis. Ciba-Geigy, 1990;43–52.

85. Palmoski MJ, Brandt KD. Effects of static and cyclic compressive loading on articular cartilage plus *in vitro*. Arthritis Rheum 1984;27:675–681.

86. Peyron JG. Epidemiologic and etiologic approach of osteoarthritis. Semin Arthritis Rheum 1979;8:288–306.

87. Platt D, Bayliss MT. An investigation of the proteoglycan metabolism of mature equine articular cartilage and its regulation by interleukin-1. Equine Vet J 1994;26:297–303.

87a. Platt D, Bird JLE, Bayliss MT. Aging of equine articular cartilage: Structure and composition of aggrecan and decorin. Equine Vet J 1998;30:43–52.

88. Polak JM. More about substance P [editorial]. Equine Vet J 1985;17:1.

89. Pond MJ, Nuki G. Experimentally-induced osteoarthritis in the dog. Ann Rheum Dis 1973;32:387–388.

90. Poole AR. Cartilage in health and disease. In: McCarty DJ, Ed. Arthritis and Allied Conditions. A Textbook of Rheumatology. Philadelphia: Lea & Febiger, 1993;279–333.

91. Pottenger LA, Phillips FM, Draganich LF. The effect of marginal osteophytes on reduction of varus-valgus instability in osteoarthritic knees. Arthritis Rheum 1990;33:853–858.

92. Price JS, Symons JA, Russell RGG. Cytokines: Inflammatory mediators of joint disease. Equine Vet J 1992;24:78–80.

93. Radin EL, Burr DB, Caterson B, et al. Mechanical determinants of osteoarthrosis. Semin Arthritis Rheum 1991;21(Suppl 2): 12–21.

94. Radin EL, Marin RB, Burr DB, et al. Effects of mechanical loading on the tissues of the rabbit knee. J Orthop Res 1984;2: 221–234.

95. Radin EL, Rose RN. The role of subchondral bone in the initiation and progression of cartilage damage. Clin Orthop 1986; 213:34–40.

96. Reboul P, Pelletier JP, Tardif G, et al. The new collagenase, collagenase-3, is expressed and synthesized by human chondrocytes but not by synovial fibroblasts: A role in osteoarthritis. J Clin Invest 1996;97:2011–2119.

97. Repo RB, Mitchell N. Collagen synthesis in mature articular cartilage of the rabbit. J Bone Joint Surg [Br] 1971;53:541–548.

98. Riddle WE. Healing of articular cartilage in the horse. J Am Vet Med Assoc 1970;157:1471.

99. Robinson HJ, Granada JL, Salvati EA. Inflammatory and noninflammatory osteoarthritis of the hip. A study of the prostaglandin E and cathepsin-D levels. Proceedings. 22nd Annual International Meeting of the Orthopaedic Research Society, 1976;27.

100. Roughley PJ, Barrett AJ. The degradation of cartilage proteoglycans by tissue proteinases. Proteoglycan structure and its susceptibility to proteolysis. Biochem J 1977;167:629.

101. Sandy JD, Neame PJ, Boynton RE, Flannery CR. Catabolism of aggrecan in cartilage explants. Identification of a major cleavage site within the interglobular domain. J Biol Chem 1991;266:8683–8685.
102. Deleted in proof.
103. Sapolsky AI, Howell DES, Woessner JF Jr. Neutral proteases and cathepsin-D in human articular cartilage. J Clin Invest 1974;53:1044–1053.
104. Sapolsky AI, Keiser H, Howell DS, Woessner JF Jr. Metalloproteinase of human articular cartilage that digests cartilage proteoglycan at neutral and acid pH. J Clin Invest 1976;58:1031–1041.
105. Schmid A, Schmid F. Ultrastructural studies after arthroscopical cartilage shaving. Arthroscopy 1987;3:137.
106. Schnyder J, Pain T, Dinarello CA. Human monocyte or recombinant interleukin-1s are specific for the secretion of a metalloproteinase from chondrocytes. J Immunol 1987;138:496–503.
107. Seireg A, Kempke W. Behavior of an in vivo bone under cyclic loading. J Biomech 1969;2:455–461.
107a. Serink MT, Nachemson A, Hansson G. The effect of impact loading on rabbit knee joints. Acta Orthop Scand 1977;48:250–262.
108. Shlopov BV, Lie WR, Mainardi CL, et al. Osteoarthritic lesions. Involvement of three different collagenases. Arthritis Rheum 1997;40:2065–2074.
109. Sokoloff L. Osteoarthritis as a remodeling process. J Rheumatol 1987;14(S14):7–10.
110. Slether-Stevenson WG, Krutzsch HC, Liotta LA. Tissue inhibitor of metalloproteinase (TIMP-2). A new member of the metalloproteinase family. J Biol Chem 1989;264:17374–17378.
111. Spiers S, May SA, Bennett D, Edwards GB. Cellular sources of proteolytic enzymes in equine joints. Equine Vet J 1994;26:43–47.
112. Sullins KE, McIlwraith CW, Powers BE, Norrdin RW. The evaluation of periosteal grafts for articular cartilage repair in horses. Abstr Vet Surg 1985;14:66.
113. Tamanini C, Seren C, Pezzoli G, Guidetti M. Concentrazione delle prostaglindine E1-E2 nel liquido sinoviale di cavalli affetti da artropatie. Clin Vet 1980;103:544–549.
113a. Thompson RC, Oegema TR, Lewis JL, Wallace L. Osteoarthropic changes after acute transarticular load. J Bone Joint Surg [Am] 1991;73:990–1001.
114. Tietz CC, Chrisman OD. The effect of salicylate and chloroquine on prostaglandin-induced articular damage in the rabbit knee. Clin Orthop 1975;108:264.
114a. Todhunter RJ, Yeh L-A, Sheldon A, et al. Effects of stromelysin activity on proteoglycan degradation of canine articular cartilage explants. Am J Vet Res 1995;56:1241–1247.
115. Tyler JA, Bird JLE, Gille R, Benton HP. Cytokines, growth factors and cartilage repair in osteoarthritis. In: Russell GG, Dieppe PA, Eds. Current Research and Prospects for Pharmacologic Intervention. IBS Technical Services.
116. Vachon AM, McIlwraith CW, Keeley FW. Biochemical study of repair of induced osteochondral defects of the distal portion of the radial carpal bone in horses by use of periosteal autografts. Am J Vet Res 1991;52:328–332.
117. Vachon AM, McIlwraith CW, Powers BE, et al. Morphologic and biochemical study of sternal cartilage autografts for resurfacing induced osteochondral defects in horses. Am J Vet Res 1992;53:1038–1047.
118. Vachon AM, McIlwraith CW, Trotter GW, et al. Morphologic study of induced osteochondral defects of the distal portion of the radial carpal bone in horses by use of glued periosteal autografts. Am J Vet Res 1991;52:317–327.
119. Vaes G, Eckhout Y. Procollagenase and its activation. In: Burleigh PM, Poole AR, Eds. Dynamics of Connective Tissue Macromolecules. Amsterdam: North Holland, 1975;129–146.
119a. Van den Berg WB, Joosten LAB, van de Loo FAJ. TNF alpha and IL-1 beta are separate targets in chronic arthritis. Clin Exp Rheumatol 1999;17(Suppl 18):5105–5114.
120. van Kempen GPT, Veldhuijzen JP, Kuijer R, et al. Cartilage response to mechanical force in high-dense knee chondrocyte cultures. Arthritis Rheum 1985;28:419–424.
121. Van Wart H. Matrix metalloproteinases in arthritis. In: IBC's Fifth International Congress on Arthritis: Advances in Diagnosis and Treatment. Southboro, MA: International Business Communications, 1995.
122. Van Wart HE, Birkedal-Hansen H. The cysteine-switch: A principle of regulation of metalloproteinase activity with potential applicability to the entire matrix metalloproteinase gene family. Proc Natl Acad Sci USA 1990;87:5578–5582.
122a. Walakovits LA, Moore VL, Bhardwaj N. Detection of stromelysin and collagenase in synovial fluid from patients with rheumatoid arthritis and posttraumatic knee injury. Arthritis Rheum 1992;35:35–42.
123. Webb GR, Westacott CI, Elson CJ. Chondrocyte tumor necrosis factor receptors and focal loss of cartilage in osteoarthritis. Osteoarthritis Cartilage 1997;5:427–437.
124. Werb Z. Proteinases and matrix degradation. In: Kelley WN, Harris ED Jr, Ruddy S, Sledge CB, Eds. Textbook of Rheumatology. 3rd ed. Philadelphia: WB Saunders, 1989;300–321.
125. Werb Z. The biological role of metalloproteinases and their inhibitors. In: Kuettner K, Schleyerbach R, Peyron JG, Hascall VC, Eds. Articular Cartilage and Osteoarthritis. New York: Raven Press, 1992;295–304.
126. Wong S, Halliwell B, Richmond R, Skowroneck W. The role of superoxide and hydroxyl radicals in the degradation of hyaluronic acid induced by metal ions and by ascorbic acid. J Inorg Biochem 1981;14:127–134.
127. Wood DD, Ihrie EJ, Hamerman D. Release of interleukin-1 from human synovial tissue in vitro. Arthritis Rheum 1985;28:853–862.
128. Wu J-J, Lark M, Chun LE, Eyre DR. Sites of stromelysin cleavage in collagens type II, IX, X and XI of cartilage. J Biol Chem 1991;266:5625–5628.

DIAGNOSIS OF JOINT DISEASE

Disease changes in a joint can be detected and evaluated in a number of ways. These include clinical examination to detect pain and gross morphologic change, thermography, radiographic examination, storage phosphorimaging digital (computed) radiography, computed tomography (CT), magnetic resonance imaging (MRI), nuclear imaging, ultrasonography, synovial fluid analysis, and arthroscopy. Prior to evaluating specific joints, a general lameness examination is indicated to localize the problem.

Clinical Examination

There are a number of physical signs of joint disease that may be present singly or in various combinations. These signs include

1. Changes in temperature or color of the overlying skin. Interpretations based on manual palpation are somewhat subjective and variable. Thermography is a more objective means of assessing temperature change, and techniques have been developed.
2. Joint swelling or enlargement, which may be due to a number of events, including synovial fluid effusion, synovial membrane and fibrous capsule thickening (which could be related to edema or fibrosis), swelling of the periarticular tissues, or bony enlargement. The specific nature of this swelling will depend on the stage of the disease (acute or chronic).[15]
3. Tenderness (localized or diffuse). Because of differences between individual animals and their reaction to palpation, care should be exercised in evaluating this parameter when the changes are subtle. Error

is avoided by comparing the reaction with that of the contralateral normal joint.

4. Pain on flexion. Some caution should be exercised here. Normal horses may demonstrate a positive response to a forelimb flexion test, and the response varies directly with the pressure applied to the limb. A positive reaction is a noteworthy sign when there is joint disease. However, one author has proposed caution in relying on a flexion test to diagnose subclinical lameness or predict future problems.[36] The results of a flexion test should always be compared with the response in the contralateral limb. An asymmetric flexion test response is usually meaningful.

5. Crepitation with motion. Again the clinician should be aware of the crepitation that occurs in normal joints, such as that occurring in the fetlock.

6. Limited motion. This may be due to pain, joint effusion, spasm, contracture of periarticular structures, or fibrous or bony ankylosis.

7. Deformities from gross joint destruction or injury-producing subluxation or luxation of the articulating bones.

In some joint conditions, localizing the problem to a particular joint may be difficult. Flexion tests may be useful in these situations to accentuate the lameness. The site of soreness within a particular limb is best defined by the use of nerve blocks and intrasynovial analgesia. More details are available in this text (see Chapter 3), and clinical assessment of joint disease has been recently reviewed.[47]

Radiographic Examination

The radiologic manifestations of joint disease generally reflect the osseous pathologic changes of these conditions. In many instances, radiographic examination will enable a specific diagnosis to be made when the clinical manifestations are nonspecific. Such conditions include intraarticular fractures, OCD, and subchondral cystic lesions. Other conditions such as OA and infective arthritis will have typical radiographic changes later in the course of the disease, but changes are often absent in the early stages. Radiologic signs of OA include a narrow joint space, widened joint space (when there is destruction of the subchondral bone plate), periarticular osteophytes (which do not always indicate articular cartilage damage), and soft tissue swelling.[17,33]

In disease states in which osseous lesions have not yet developed, radiography may still provide some information. Thickening of the subcutaneous and capsular tissues and synovial effusion can be observed radiographically. In the carpal joint, the adipose tissue layer outside the fibrous joint capsule can be used to determine whether the swelling is primarily due to joint effusion or is localized to the soft tissues by looking for displacement of the adipose tissue layer. Similarly, a loss of fat density (relative radiolucency) at the cranial aspect of the femoropatellar joint (present in normal joints because of the patellar fat pad) indicates effusion or inflammation within this joint. The effusion of an early septic arthritis of the coffin joint, for instance, may suffice to cause displacement of the bony ends. However, the radiographic signs of acute traumatic arthritis and septic arthritis may

be indistinguishable, and here the clinician needs to rely on synovial fluid analysis for a differential diagnosis. Periarticular edema can totally obscure a joint effusion. Such details have recently been reviewed elsewhere.[33]

The radiographic manifestations of OCD, subchondral cystic lesions, and DJD have been well described and will be detailed when the conditions are discussed specifically. These diseases are generally diagnosed by use of plain radiographs. However, double-contrast arthrography can be used in some instances to demonstrate the presence of cartilaginous flaps in OCD.[28] Contrast arthrography is used less than before. Its use to diagnose villonodular synovitis has been replaced by ultrasonography. It has limited use for the demonstration of cartilaginous erosion.[44] Contrast arthrography in the shoulder has been described as still useful in cases of osteochondrosis and OCD to allow better evaluation of cartilage attachment in subchondral bone, better evaluation of the length and depth of cartilage lesions, and more accurate definition of the site and shape of osteo-cartilaginous free bodies.[31] Most cases of OCD in which the cartilage was firmly adherent were not candidates for surgical debridement and carried a favorable prognosis. On the other hand, the determination of a free flap by arthrography indicated the need for surgery. Extensive humeral and glenoid cavity lesions were better defined by arthrography, allowing a rational decision between surgical debridement or euthanasia. It was also felt that arthrography defined the size and patency of the communicating canal to a subchondral cystic defect better and separated cases with long, narrow, and poorly patent canals for conservative rather than surgical therapy. For more information on diagnostic radiography see Chapter 4.

Storage Phosphorimaging Digital (Computed) Radiography

Computed radiography is an imaging modality that produces a radiographic image from digital information.[33] Storage phosphorimaging plates made of europium-doped barium fluorohalide are used to record the image, somewhat analogously to a traditional film-screen system. The absorbed energy from the x-ray beam is stored on the plates, and the plates are then placed in a laser reader. The emitted energy released from the plate is detected and digitized, and the digitized information can be viewed on a monitor. The density and latitude can be adjusted to print a hard copy radiograph. The disadvantages of computerized radiography include the high cost and the technical complexity, but one hopes that these disadvantages will be lessened in the future. The advantages are that a single exposure can provide more than one image, and the digital signal can be changed to improve the definition of structure and compensate for over- or underexposure. The image can be edge enhanced to accentuate lesions such as stress fractures. This modality offers an alternative to xeroradiography, which has become almost unavailable.

Imaging

Computed Tomography (CT)

CT can be useful, particularly in conjunction with radiographic studies. CT is excellent for defining unusual fractures (particularly ones that are not visualized on radiographs), stress-induced subchondral bone sclerosis, and other subchondral bone lesions such as cysts or subtle defects. Osteoabsorptiometry has been used experimentally in our laboratory to define the degree of development of subchondral bone sclerosis in exercising horses.[14] For more information see Chapter 4.

Magnetic Resonance Imaging (MRI)

MRI images are sectional images similar to CT images. These images provide very good soft tissue and intraarticular detail and information that presently is only available using arthroscopy. There has been limited ability to do MRI examinations on equine limbs without detaching the legs, but some studies have recently been done in live horses at Washington State University. If appropriate technology (at an appropriate cost) can be developed, it could be a very useful technique for further defining joint disease clinically.

Nuclear Imaging

In nuclear imaging, the image is produced by gamma rays originating from an injected radionuclide. Distribution of the radiopharmaceutical is predictable in normal horses but is increased in areas with higher blood flow and/or increased osteoblastic activity.[33] The distribution pattern is affected by various disease processes, and changes may precede radiographic changes. The technique is therefore useful to localize problems to joints in some situations. Only the bone phase has achieved routine use in the diagnosis of joint disease. Increased uptake by or near joints has been related to OA as well as enthesitis, subchondral bone sclerosis, and septic arthritis. Technetium-99–labeled methylene diphosphonate (MDP) is the most commonly used radionuclide. Indications for scintigraphy include evaluation of horses with multiple causes of lameness, evaluation of a horse with a painful yet radiographically normal joint, and evaluation of joints that cannot be radiographed with the horse standing in a convenient fashion (hip joint and pelvic and back regions). Recent experimental work indicates that nuclear imaging will localize early subchondral microdamage.[14] The author has also found the technique useful for indicating localization of a problem in a carpal joint and convincing the owner of the need for arthroscopic examination. For further details, see Park et al.[33]

The specificity of scintigraphy is low, and a "hot spot" could signify either trauma or osteomyelitis. On the other hand, the sensitivity is high.[54] Image resolution is also a lot lower than that of a radiograph. It also appears that osteoclastic activity contributes little to bony uptake of the radiopharmaceutical, and we have found in research at Colorado State University that lytic processes usually do not show increased uptake of radionuclide (at least in the femoral condyle).[37]

On the other hand, some recent work in humans has shown that scintigraphy will predict radiographic changes in OA of the hand and knee, confirming that subchondral bone activity is a critical factor in the pathogenesis of this disease. Scintigraphy predicted subsequent loss of joint space in patients with established OA of the knee.[6] More recently, a study in the metatarsophalangeal joint of the Standardbred horse confirmed that increased uptake on the plantarolateral aspect of MT-III may precede other stress-related changes and in some horses is associated with a continual stress-related subchondral bone remodeling that results in lameness and later radiographic changes.[41] The author of this study concluded that horses with advanced scintigraphic findings are more likely to have lameness and radiographic evidence of subchondral bone damage.

The value of scintigraphy in diagnosing nondisplaced stress fractures is now well recognized. Some of these fractures could potentially involve joints. See Chapter 4 for more information on nuclear imaging.

Ultrasonography

Diagnostic ultrasonography has been used routinely to evaluate flexor tendons and ligaments. The value of this technique in imaging joints has only been recognized more recently.[5] In addition to imaging collateral and patellar ligaments, it is possible to image other structures within joints. The technique involves careful learning and knowledge of anatomy and has been presented in detail elsewhere.[5] See Chapter 4 for more details.

Synovial Fluid Analysis

Examination of the synovial fluid should be a routine procedure in the evaluation of arthritic conditions, as it can provide valuable information in addition to that gained by clinical and radiologic examination.[21,22,25,47] Conventional analysis will not provide a specific diagnosis; however, it does give an indication of the degree of synovitis and metabolic derangement within the joint. It is more specific in the diagnosis of infective arthritis, as this condition causes the parameters of protein and white cell counts to go beyond a level encountered with other inflammatory conditions (see the section on infective arthritis).

One needs some basic information on synovial fluid to appreciate the changes that occur in joint disease. Synovial fluid is a unique tissue fluid. The distribution of electrolytes and most nonelectrolytes between plasma and joint fluid is in accord with the Gibbs-Donnan equilibrium, which indicates that it is mainly a dialysate of plasma with hyaluronan added.[2] The intercellular space between the synoviocytes in the synovial membrane acts as an important permeability barrier in this filtration process. The source of hyaluronan is the synovial membrane. Studies of the molecular structure of hyaluronan indicate that it is arranged in a random coil with moderate stiffness. Hyaluronan provides synovial fluid with a number of unique properties. It imparts a high viscosity to the fluid. It acts as a boundary lubricant for the synovial membrane. There is evidence that the hyaluronan in the synovial fluid also influences the further composition of the fluid.[32] Data suggest that steric hindrance by hyaluronan may obstruct solute passage through the water surrounding the molecules. In this concept of excluded volume, the size and shape of the molecules presented play an important role. Small molecules are allowed through, whereas large ones, such as fibrinogen, are excluded. With this concept, the quantity and physical state of hyaluronan produced under pathologic conditions may well be the primary determinant of the nature of the remainder of the contents of the synovial fluid. It has also been suggested that the hyaluronate in the perisynovial connective tissue may be of significance in the exclusion of certain plasma proteins from the synovial fluid.[30] However, the exact mechanism by which permeability changes in disease is not yet well defined.

Hyaluronan is depolymerized in untreated inflammatory arthritis,[13] and this has been considered to be the basis of reduced viscosity. However, the situation may be more complex. There are data to show that hyaluronan has a heterogeneous structure and may have three levels of organization. The viscosity of hyaluronan apparently depends on 1) the length of the polysaccharide chain, 2) the conformation of the chain, and 3) interaction between adjacent chains and other molecules.[43] Therefore, the decrease in viscosity may be due to a change in the overall relationship of hyaluronan and other molecules in addition to simple depolymerization.

Normal values for various synovial fluid parameters in the horse and their changes in joint disease have been documented.[34,50] These values are quite variable, and each laboratory should have its own set of normal values. Most of the synovial fluid parameters provide an indication of the relative amount of synovitis and so follow a spectrum of inflammatory activity within the joint. With the exception of infective arthritis, synovial fluid analysis does not usually furnish a specific diagnosis.

Synovial fluid samples are collected using sterile needles and syringes. All sites for arthrocentesis are prepared aseptically. A recent study confirmed that clipping of hair is not a necessary part of the aseptic protocol.[12] In a study that evaluated skin bacterial flora before and after aseptic preparation of clipped and nonclipped arthrocentesis sites (midcarpal joint and distal interphalangeal joint) in horses, the presence of hair did not appear to inhibit the ability of antiseptics to reduce bacterial flora to an acceptable level for arthrocentesis. Sites for arthrocentesis for various joints are given in Chapter 3 and also have been recently detailed in another text.[48] Following aspiration of the fluid into a syringe (Fig. 7.11), the fluid is transferred to both plain and EDTA Vacutainer tubes. Note that excess negative pressure on the syringe when attempting to obtain a fluid sample may cause iatrogenic hemorrhage.

The analysis and interpretation of commonly used parameters are discussed below. Each parameter can provide an assessment of the degree of inflammation present. Defining sharp boundaries for the synovial fluid values in each disease entity is to be discouraged. Cases of OCD and idiopathic synovitis, for instance, produce relatively consistent values; however, the changes in traumatic and infective arthritis may have a wide range.

Appearance

Appearance is evaluated by visual inspection at the time of collection. Normal synovial fluid is pale yellow, clear, and free of flocculent debris (Fig. 7.12). Streaks of blood in the aspirate indicate hemorrhage occurring with needle puncture. Uniformly diffuse hemorrhage represents an acute traumatic situation, whereas dark yellow or pale amber (xanthochromic) samples represent previous hemorrhage and are most often associated with chronic traumatic arthritis. Opacity and flocculent material in the sample indicates synovitis. This change is variable and generally minimal in chronic DJD and OCD but will be more marked in acute synovitis (traumatic or infectious). The intense synovitis associated with infective arthritis results in a serofibrinous to fibrinopurulent sample (see Fig. 7.12). The synovial fluid from infected joints is often bloody due to hemorrhage from the severely pathologic synovial membrane.

Volume

The volume of synovial fluid is increased in most cases of active synovitis. Synovial fluid volume is decreased in some cases of chronic DJD and may manifest as a "dry joint."[35] The presence of a truly dry joint can be correlated with fibrotic synovial membrane. However, failure to obtain synovial fluid on sampling does not automatically mean that a pathologic dry joint exists. Synovial fluid volume is increased in situations of idiopathic synovial effusion such as bog spavin. Volume increases in cases of OCD are variable, but a marked synovial effu-

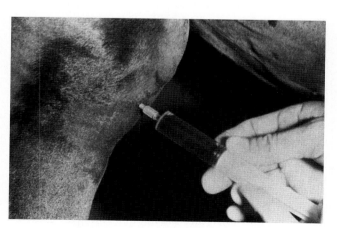

Figure 7.11 Synovial fluid sampling.

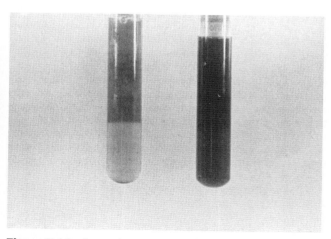

Figure 7.12 Comparison of normal (left) and abnormal (right) synovial fluid samples.

sion is characteristic of the disease in tarsocrural (tibiotarsal) joints. Synovial fluid volume is usually increased in cases of infective arthritis, but this depends on the stage of the disease and the amount of fibrin present in the joint.

Clot Formation

Normal synovial fluid does not clot. This property is attributed to a lack of fibrinogen and other clotting factors (including prothrombin, factor V, factor VII, and tissue thromboplastin).[2] Pathologic synovial fluid clots, and the size of the clot is roughly proportional to the degree of synovitis. This property may be ascertained by observing the clot tube. Fluid should only be collected in a clot tube after sufficient amounts have been collected in the EDTA tube, because the ability to clot is a very nonspecific parameter.

Protein

For convenience, protein concentration is usually measured using a refractometer. The differential protein fractions in synovial fluid may be evaluated using paper electrophoresis following treatment of the sample with hyaluronidase, and this has been performed on normal equine synovial fluid.[34] For routine synovial fluid examination, I do not perform protein electrophoresis.

Synovial fluid protein concentration is approximately 25 to 35% of the plasma protein concentration of the same animal. The normal value for horses has been documented to be 1.81 ± 0.26 g/dL.[50] Generally, normal fluid can be considered to have a protein level of 2 g/dL or less. Synovial fluid has a higher albumin level, lower α_2 and globulin level, and less haptoglobin and various high-molecular-weight proteins than plasma.[34]

Total protein increases with joint inflammation. With increasing inflammation the total synovial protein level approaches that of plasma, and the levels of various protein fractions are comparable to those in serum. The relative amount of albumin decreases, α_2- and γ-globulin levels increase, and fibrinogen is present.

Simple estimation of the total protein concentration is sufficient for routine analysis. One may be reasonably certain that a fluid is not normal when the total protein concentration is above 2.5 g/dL; above 4 g/dL indicates severe inflammation. Noninfective inflammatory conditions generally have concentrations below this level. The protein level may rise above 4 g/dL in infective arthritis. Remember, protein levels should be compared with normal values obtained from the same joint on the contralateral limb if the increase is subtle. Significant differences in protein levels have been demonstrated between different joints in the horse, and significant increases in protein levels have been demonstrated in horses in training.[34]

Viscosity

The viscosity of the synovial fluid is directly related to the hyaluronan content, and it is a measure of the quantity and quality or degree of polymerization of the hyaluronan.[34] Viscosity measurements may be made by measuring the relative viscosity (RV) at a specific temperature, using a viscosimeter in which the viscosity of the synovial fluid sample is compared to that of distilled water.[51] Although the measurement of relative viscosity has been used to monitor the progression of experimental synovitis in ponies,[25] measurement of RV by an individual clinician using the viscosimeter is tedious and is not routinely used to evaluate clinical cases. Because the viscosity of synovial fluid varies with shear rate, some authors have advocated intrinsic viscosity measurement as more meaningful. The author does not measure relative or intrinsic viscosity routinely.

For practical use in the field, a simple estimate of viscosity can be made by watching the fluid drop from the end of the syringe. With normal fluid, the drops usually string out as much as 5 to 7 cm before separating. If the fluid drops from the syringe with the ease of water, viscosity is low. Another test is to place a drop of synovial fluid on the thumb and then touch it with the index finger. Separating the fingers then produces a string 2.5 to 5 cm long before breaking if viscosity is normal (Fig. 7.13). Less stringing occurs with lower viscosity, and fluid from an infected joint will not string. These methods are, of course, subjective and are only useful to detect gross changes. However, because the correlation of viscosity and inflammation is not absolute, these techniques suffice, and precise quantitation is inappropriate. A method of measuring relative viscosity using a white blood cell (WBC) diluting pipette has been developed.[11] The technique is rapid and reproducible with 2% accuracy. It could be of potential value in monitoring horses with clinical cases of arthritis and their response to therapy. I simply do a gross evaluation of viscosity.

A clinician must not place too much significance on viscosity findings. This parameter does not give a complete picture of the rheologic behavior of synovial fluid[39] and should not be considered a direct quantitative or qualitative estimate of the hyaluronan content. I have also noted that some fluid samples from joints with only mild changes had markedly decreased viscosity. A low viscosity indicates that inflammation is present, but the clinician should not interpret too far beyond this.

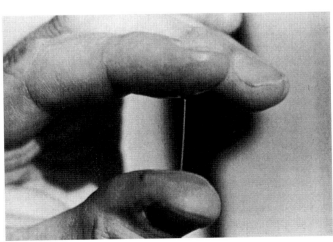

Figure 7.13 Measurement of viscosity of synovial fluid with the fingers.

Mucinous Precipitate Quality

Mucinous precipitate quality (MPQ) is evaluated by adding 0.5 mL of synovial fluid to 2 mL of 2% acetic acid and mixing it rapidly with a glass rod. The precipitate formed (mucin clot) appears to be a salt of anionic hyaluronate and protein made cationic by acidification.[3] When the mucin clot is normal, a tight ropey mass forms in a clear solution, and this conventionally is called a "good" mucin. A softer mass with some shreds in solution constitutes a "fair" mucin, and a "poor" result shows shreds and small soft masses in a turbid solution. Fluids that produce only a few clump flecks of mucin suspended in a cloudy solution are classified "very poor." In general, the more inflamed the joint, the worse the mucin clot. Typically a good-to-fair mucin clot is associated with traumatic and degenerative arthritic conditions, whereas infected joints have very poor mucin tests (due to bacterial enzymes degrading mucin). However, the correlation is a loose one, as poor mucin clots have been observed in the presence of only mild inflammation.[52]

Cytologic Examination

Cells are best preserved when collected in EDTA vials.[42] Total WBC counts may be performed on synovial fluid with hemocytometers. One must use a physiologic saline diluent and not the usual white cell diluent containing acetic acid, for the latter precipitates the hyaluronate–protein complex. Red blood cells may be preferentially lysed by hypotonic saline. Smears for differential cell counts are made in the standard way for peripheral blood smears with minor modifications. If the white cell count is elevated, the smear is made directly from the synovial fluid. Otherwise, the sample should be centrifuged and the sediment resuspended in 0.5 mL of supernatant after which a smear is made. The smears are air dried and stained with Wright's stain or new methylene blue.

Erythrocytes are not considered normal constituents of synovial fluid. Their presence in small numbers is usually attributed to contamination of the sample at the time of arthrocentesis. The erythrocyte count may vary greatly and depends on the amount of contamination during arthrocentesis. Hyperemia in an inflamed synovial membrane will increase the tendency for bleeding. Because of this marked variation, the red cell count does not usually offer useful information.

The white cell count of normal equine synovial fluid has been reported by different workers to be 167 ± 21 and 87 cells/mm^3, respectively.[34,50] Neutrophils, lymphocytes, and large mononuclear cells are observed, but the percentage of neutrophils is generally less than 10%. Quantitative and qualitative changes in the leukocytes can indicate the magnitude of synovial membrane inflammation. Because of the wide range observed in some diseases, one should be cautious about grouping types of effusion and matching them to disease. However, some generalizations are appropriate.

Idiopathic synovitis (bog spavin) and OCD generally have white cell counts below 1000 cells/mm^3. Although these situations have been classified as noninflammatory effusions, histologic examination of the synovial membrane in cases of OCD at least have revealed inflammatory changes.

In traumatic arthritis and OA, the cell count may vary tremendously depending upon the amount of active synovitis present. The cell counts for human patients with DJD are typically low. Synovitis seems to be a more prominent feature of equine DJD. Consequently, counts of 5,000 to 10,000 cells/mm^3 may be encountered. In severe inflammatory effusions the proportion of neutrophils is usually increased.

Cases of infective arthritis have the highest white cell counts. In general, cell counts over 50,000/mm^3 indicate infection, and counts over 100,000 are virtually pathognomonic. Published figures for cases of infective arthritis are $105,775 \pm 25,525$ (59,250 to 178,000).[50] Neutrophils are the predominant cells. One may observe toxic change in the neutrophils, but commonly they appear healthy. Bacteria are not commonly seen on smear examination.

Synovial fluid samples that have cytologic changes typical of infective arthritis will commonly yield negative cultures. Factors involved in this are felt to be the presence of antibiotics, sequestration of the bacteria in the synovial membrane, and the normal bactericidal quality of synovial fluid.[4] Treatment of an infected joint is an emergency, and cytologic examination of synovial fluid is useful for a rapid diagnosis. In instances in which only a drop or two of synovial fluid are available, a simple smear examination will often provide useful information. In some cases there may be an indication for more than a simple bacteriologic examination. Both *Chlamydia* and *Mycoplasma* spp. have been associated with polyarthritic conditions in foals.[18,29]

Gas–liquid chromatography has been useful in providing a specific etiologic diagnosis in septic arthritis. Preliminary work in the horse has identified fatty acid peaks specific for certain bacteria, but this technique has not achieved routine use.[16]

It should be noted that a "gray" zone exists between traumatic arthritis with a high white cell count and infective arthritis with a low white cell count. White cell counts of up to 50,000 have been recorded in cases of traumatic arthritis in humans, but these cases have been differentiated from infectious arthritis by the presence of fat droplets in the synovial fluid.[9] It was theorized that the synovial fluid leukocytosis was secondary to lipid droplet phagocytosis. Lipid globules present intra- and extracellularly in the synovial fluid and in the upper fatty layer following centrifugation of hemorrhagic synovial fluid indicate traumatic arthritis. Although infected joints typically have a high white cell count, there seem to be some situations that are atypical. I have encountered a few cases of seemingly "latent" septic arthritis. Initially the fluid evaluation was more typical of traumatic arthritis, but septic disease became evident a short time later. Fortunately, these cases are rare. At the same time, note that it is quite possible for nonseptic synovitis to develop into septic synovitis. In polyarthritis in foals, the count may sometimes be considerably below 50,000/mm^3.

Enzymes

In general there is a close correlation between the activities of alkaline phosphatase (ALP), aspartate aminotransferase (AAT), and lactic dehydrogenase (LDH) in synovial fluids and the clinical severity of joint disease.[51] The proportionate increase of enzyme activity with the severity of synovitis has been demonstrated experimentally in the equine midcarpal (intercarpal) joint.[25] However, specificity of enzyme levels enabling separation of one diagnostic entity from another has not been demonstrated.

It has been suggested that the increased enzyme activity in the joint fluid may result from one of several mechanisms. These include 1) the release of enzymes from leukocytes, 2) the release of enzymes from necrotic or inflamed synovial tissue, or 3) production and release of increased amounts of enzymes by altered synovial tissue.[55] A positive correlation between the number of leucocytes in the field and the enzyme levels is indirect evidence for the first possibility.

Rejno reported that LDH isoenzyme levels in equine synovial fluid were useful for differentiating whether articular cartilage damage is present or not.[40] He reported that LDH_4 and LDH_5 were present in high amounts in articular cartilage, and an increase in these isoenzymes was the most characteristic feature in synovial joint fluid samples from joints with cartilage damage. However, in a more recent study at Colorado State University we have found the relationship to be less clear. High levels of each isoenzyme were produced with synovial membrane inflammation. Cartilage has a much lower level of all isoenzymes of LDH, and consequently, lesions of the articular cartilage do not make a significant contribution to the overall LDH elevation.[48]

Particle Analysis

The foregoing parameters generally indicate the severity of synovial inflammation in a joint but do not provide an assessment of the severity of cartilage damage. Attempts have been made to assess this by using LDH isoenzymes and also microscopic examination of metachromatically stained sediment after centrifugation.[50] However, the sediment technique has not received common usage.

Synovial Markers

As mentioned above, conventional synovial fluid analysis will not define the degree of articular cartilage damage but merely the degree of synovitis. Previous attempts at techniques such as synovial sediment analysis have not solved the problem. Over the past decade, researchers have developed biochemical and immunologic markers to identify and quantitate breakdown products of the articular cartilage. The principle of markers is that because cartilage degradation involves disruption of the collagen framework as well as loss of proteoglycan, breakdown products of type II collagen and proteoglycan fragments are liberated in increased concentration in the synovial fluid and ultimately the serum.[38] Recently, some of these markers have been looked at with naturally occurring joint disease in the horse.[8] The use of synovial markers has been extensively described in another textbook.[38]

Biochemical tests for identification of proteoglycan fragments and GAGs in synovial fluid include the di-methyl methylene blue (DMMB) assay using conjugation of 19-dimethyl methylene blue to GAGs and comparing the spectrophotometric absorption with that of a chondroitin sulfate standard. The DMMB assay identifies all GAGs present in synovial fluid regardless of origin. Significantly higher levels were found in horses with OCD and traumatic arthritis. However, this test is not very specific.

Immunologic methods appear to provide the most sensitive means of identifying and quantitating types and amounts of articular cartilage components. Polyclonal and, most recently, monoclonal antibodies have been produced against various epitopes on fragments of aggrecan and other molecules that are released from the cartilage. An epitope is an area on the surface of an antigenic molecule against which an immune response is directed. With serum and synovial fluid markers, the epitopes that have been used more frequently are present on fragments of proteoglycans (PGs) liberated from both normal and degenerating articular cartilage. Epitopes have been identified in a number of areas of the PG monomer, including chondroitin sulfate (CS) and keratan sulfate (KS), the hyaluronic acid–binding region (G1), the CS attachment region, the CS-rich region, and the G3 globulin domain and the link protein. Once a monoclonal and polyclonal antibody to a specific epitope has been produced, the amount of epitope can be measured by radioimmunoassay or ELISA test. Antibodies have been produced specific for "native" CS GAG chains as well as those that require predigestion, or "neoepitopes." In our laboratory, we have evaluated CS epitope (846) as well as a KS epitope. The mean value of the CS846 epitope in joints with osteochondral fragmentation was significantly higher than that in control joints. KS fragments in the synovial fluid were not significantly different in the two groups.[8]

Antibodies to the C-propeptide of type II collagen (CP-II) have been developed, and work in our laboratory in the horse found significantly higher C-propeptide levels in joints with fragmentation than in those of controls.[8] More recently, Billinghurst used a specific assay to recognize epitopes in the fragmented and denatured type II collagen molecule, and we are currently evaluating that in our orthopedic research laboratory.[1] Figure 7.14 illustrates the principle behind detecting a marker of degradation.

The use of markers of cartilage degradation and synthesis will be extremely valuable in determining the stage of articular disease, monitoring therapy, or assessing the efficacy of therapeutic agents. Research continues in pursuit of new epitopes and development of more specific antibodies to attempt to identify articular cartilage–specific products to study joint disease and joint metabolism. Metalloproteinase levels, TIMP levels, and cytokine levels are also considered markers in joint disease. Although these are useful in a research situation, they are considered of minimal value in assessing the amount of articular cartilage damage or defining the status of the joint.[49]

Synovial Membrane Biopsy

Changes in the synovial fluid generally reflect the pathologic changes in the synovial membrane. Therefore, histologic examination of the synovial membrane

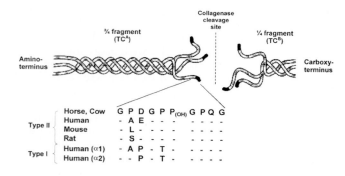

Figure 7.14 Structure of fibrillar type II collagen to show the composition of a collagen fibril with cross-links between the nonhelical telopeptide regions of individual tropocollagen molecules and the helical regions of adjacent molecules. The cleavage site of collagenase is indicated. The cleaved triple helix unwinds to expose "hidden" epitopes on a chains that are not detectable in the native triple helix by antibodies. (Reprinted with permission from McIlwraith CW, Trotter GW, Eds. Joint Disease in the Horse. Philadelphia: WB Saunders, 1996.)

was considered potentially useful in evaluating the status of a diseased joint and aiding differential diagnosis. However, a rather nonspecific reactivity of synovial membrane has been noted.[47] Synovial membrane biopsy specimens have been used to evaluate the development of an experimental synovitis in the equine midcarpal joint.[25] I have also performed synovial biopsies in various types of equine joint disease and found that the specimens provide a means of studying disease progression. On a one-time sampling basis, biopsy specimens do not seem to offer a great deal of information for differential diagnosis. From preliminary work, it appears that the reaction of the synovial membrane in equine joint disease is also nonspecific and the usefulness of synovial membrane biopsy specimens from horses is limited.[23,47]

Arthroscopy

There are limitations in the conventional methods of clinically assessing diseased joints. For example, radiographic examination only demonstrates erosion of the articular cartilage when the erosion is sufficiently advanced that the joint space is narrowed or the subchondral bone shows radiographic change. In addition, although synovial fluid examination may demonstrate the presence of synovitis, the degree of pathologic change in the synovial membrane is difficult to assess.

Examination of the joint with an arthroscope enables evaluation of the nonosseous tissues of the joint, including synovial membrane and associated villi, articular cartilage, intraarticular ligaments, and menisci. Use of the arthroscope in clinical examination and as a research tool has become routine.[20,24] A useful role has been demonstrated for evaluation of both synovial membrane and articular cartilage changes.

The arthroscope was used purely as a diagnostic tool from about 1975 to 1980. Techniques for doing surgery

under arthroscopic visualization started to be developed in 1979 and now virtually all joint surgery is done arthroscopically.[27] The achievements of arthroscopic surgery have tended to overshadow the value of diagnostic arthroscopy. However, diagnostic examination of the entire joint (or as much as possible) is a critical part of any arthroscopic procedure. In most cases, additional damage (not defined by other diagnostic parameters) is encountered, and the prognosis is affected by some of these other changes. In addition, specific diseases are confirmed with diagnostic arthroscopy, including tearing of the medial palmar intercarpal ligament, cruciate ligament tearing, meniscal tearing, degenerative subchondral bone disease, and various degrees of OA.

The characterization of the morphology of the synovial villi is much better with arthroscopy than with arthrotomy. When arthrotomy is performed, villi tend to cling to the synovial membrane and cannot be seen distinctly. In the case of arthroscopy, the villi are suspended in the fluid medium and stand out distinctly (Fig. 7.15). The magnification of the arthroscope also facilitates this definition. In normal joints, villi are located in certain areas, and these must be recognized before one can interpret pathologic changes. Hyperemia and petechiation of the synovial membrane and associated villi may be observed in acute synovitis. Small villi may form in locations where villi were previously absent. New forms of villi may be observed in joints with synovitis. Fusion of villi and formation of fibrinoid strands have also been observed in inflamed joints. With chronicity of the disease process, the villi tend to become thicker and denser. Inflammation of the synovial membrane is commonly present in most joint diseases in the horse. In traumatic and degenerative arthritis, excess villous proliferation may represent an indication for synovectomy. The ability of arthroscopy to monitor changes in the synovial membrane sequentially has been used to study the development of synovitis in the equine midcarpal (intercarpal) joint.[24] Evaluation of synovitis was initially the primary indication for arthroscopic evaluation of

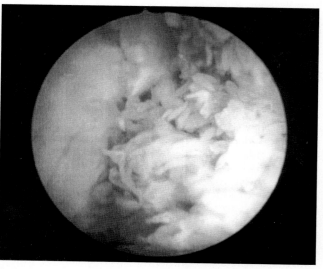

Figure 7.15 Arthroscopic view of chronic synovitis on the right half of the picture, with articular cartilage on the left demonstrating some early changes of osteoarthritis.

soft tissue in the horse. More recently, other specific soft tissue entities have been recognized in equine joints, and their diagnosis is based on arthroscopic evaluation. These include tearing of the medial palmar intercarpal ligament, tearing of the cruciate ligaments, and tearing of the menisci.[20,53] Response to intraarticular analgesia is the usual indication for arthroscopic examination in these cases.

The other clinical diagnostic use of the arthroscope in the horse is the assessment of articular cartilage when radiographic signs are equivocal or nonexistent. Arthroscopic examination allows the recognition of fibrillation, erosion, and wear lines of the articular cartilage (Fig. 7.16). Fibrillation may be more easily recognized by arthroscopy than by gross visualization because of a combination of factors that include transillumination of collagenous fibrils, their suspension in solution, and also the magnification effects.

Carpal chip fragmentation is the most common indication for arthroscopy in the carpus. In most instances, the indication for surgery is based on clinical findings and radiographic conformation. However, arthroscopy further defines the amount of damage to the articular cartilage and bone, and in some instances, fragments that were not demonstrable radiographically are found. Similarly, arthroscopy is used for the treatment of slab fractures and the debridement of subchondral degenerative disease (the latter is defined by skyline radiographs when it is in the third carpal bone but cannot be seen radiographically when on the distal radial carpal bone). As mentioned above, diagnostic arthroscopy is used both to diagnose and to treat tearing of the medial palmar intercarpal ligament. More recently, arthroscopic surgery through the carpal canal is being used to treat osteochondroma of the distal radius. The decision for surgery is usually based on clinical signs, radiology, and/or ultrasonography. The importance of the condition can be confirmed at tenoscopic examination by the presence of an obviously protruding piece of bone and tearing of the deep digital flexor (DDF) tendon–muscle junction. Refer to osteochondroma of the distal radius in Chapter 8 for more information.

Arthroscopic surgery of the dorsal aspect of the fetlock joints is used to treat proximodorsal proximal (first) phalanx chip fragments,[7] villonodular synovitis, and OCD.[20] Arthroscopic examination allows definition of the degree of secondary arthritic change, which has been found to be a negative prognosticator for both proximodorsal first phalanx chip fragments and OCD cases. In the palmar/plantar aspect of the fetlock joint, palmar/plantar P1 fragments are removed, and selected sesamoid fragments are also operated. The degree of change is further defined with arthroscopy.

The most common condition treated in the tarsocrural joint is OCD. Recognition of wear lines on the medial trochlear ridge of the talus is important as it implies a poorer prognosis.[26] Similarly, OCD is the most common condition treated in the femoropatellar joint, but the technique is also used to treat distal patellar fragmentation and patellar fractures. In the femorotibial joint, the first indication used for arthroscopic surgery was subchondral cystic lesions. Now the technique is used for the diagnosis and treatment of cruciate ligament injuries and meniscal tears. Arthroscopy is also used for

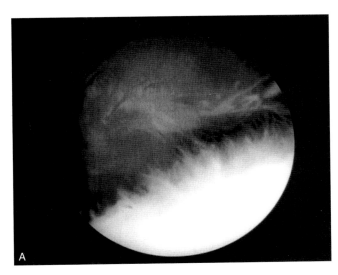

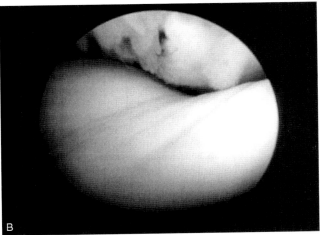

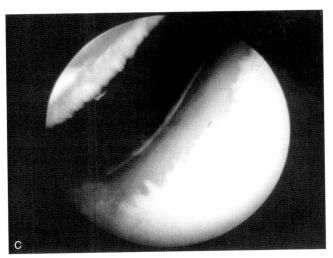

Figure 7.16   Three arthroscopic views of articular cartilage degeneration. A. Fibrillation on the trochlear ridge of the talus. B. Early, mild wear-line formation on the distal metacarpus. C. Full-thickness erosion in the trochlear groove and patella of a femoropatellar joint.

diagnostic and surgical purposes in the pastern, coffin, shoulder, and elbow joints; details are described elsewhere.[20]

References

1. Billinghurst RC, Dahlberg L, Ionescu M, et al. Enhanced cleavage of type II collagen by collagenases in osteoarthritic articular cartilage. J Clin Invest 1997;99:1534–1545.
2. Cohen AS. Synovial fluid. In: Cohen AS, Ed. Laboratory Diagnostic Procedures in the Rheumatic Diseases. Boston: Little Brown & Co, 1967;2–50.
3. Curtiss PH. The pathophysiology of joint infections. Clin Orthop 1973;96:126.
4. DeGara PF. Studies on the bactericidal properties of the synovial fluid. J Clin Invest 1943;22:131.
5. Denoix J-M. Ultrasonographic examination in the diagnosis of joint disease. In: McIlwraith CW, Trotter GW, Eds. Joint Disease in the Horse. Philadelphia: WB Saunders, 1996;165–202.
6. Dieppe P, Cushnaghan J, Young P, Kirwan J. Prediction of the progression of joint space narrowing in osteoarthritis of the knee by bone scintigraphy. Ann Rheum Dis 1993;52:557–563.
7. Foland JW, McIlwraith CW, Trotter GW. Osteochondritis dissecans of the femoropatellar joint: Results of treatment with arthroscopic surgery. Equine Vet J 1992;24:419–423.
8. Frisbie DD, Ray CS, Ionescu M, et al. Measurement of the 846 epitope of chondroitin sulfate and of carboxy propeptides of type II procollagen for diagnosis of osteochondral fragmentation in horses. Am J Vet Res 1999;60:306–309.
9. Graham J, Goldman JA. Fat droplets and synovial fluid leukocytosis in traumatic arthritis. Arthritis Rheum 1978;21:76.
10. Deleted in proof.
11. Hasselbacher P. Measuring synovial fluid viscosity with a white blood cell diluting pipette. A simple, rapid and reproducible method. Arthritis Rheum 1976;19:1358.
12. Hauge BA, Honnas CM, Simpson RB, Peloso JG. Evaluation of skin bacterial flora before and after aseptic preparation of clipped and nonclipped arthrocentesis sites in horses. Vet Surg 1997;26:121–125.
13. Holt PJ, How MJ, Long VJ, Hawkins CF. Mucopolysaccharides in synovial fluid. Effect of aspirin and indomethacin on hyaluronic acid. Ann Rheum Dis 1968;27:264–270.
14. Kawcak CE. Effects of loading on subchondral bone of the equine carpal and metacarpophangeal joint. PhD dissertation, Colorado State University, Fort Collins, CO, 1998.
15. Kawcak CE, McIlwraith CW. Proximodorsal first phalanx osteochondral chip fragments in 320 horses. Equine Vet J 1994;26:392–396.
16. Koch DB. Management of infectious arthritis in the horse. Comp Cont Educ Pract Vet 1979;1:S45.
17. May SA. Radiological aspects of degenerative joint disease. Equine Vet Ed 1996;8:114–120.
18. McChesney AE, Becerra V, England JJ. Chlamydial polyarthritis in a foal. J Am Vet Med Assoc 1974;165:259.
19. Deleted in proof.
20. McIlwraith CW. Diagnostic and Surgical Arthroscopy in the Horse. 2nd ed. Philadelphia: Lea & Febiger, 1990.
21. McIlwraith CW. Synovial fluid analysis in the diagnosis of equine joint disease. Equine Pract 1980;2:44.
22. McIlwraith CW. Tearing of the medial palmar intercarpal ligament of the equine midcarpal joint. Equine Vet J 1992;24:367–371.
23. McIlwraith CW. The use of arthroscopy, synovial fluid analysis and synovial membrane biopsy in the diagnosis of equine joint disease. In: Mansmann RA, McAllister ES, Eds. Equine Medicine and Surgery. Santa Barbara, CA: American Veterinary Publications, 1982;960–974.
24. McIlwraith CW, Fessler JF. Arthroscopy in the diagnosis of equine joint disease. J Am Vet Med Assoc 1978;172:263–268.
25. McIlwraith CW, Fessler JF, Blevins WE, et al. Experimentally induced arthritis of the equine carpus: Clinical determinations. Am J Vet Res 1979;40:11–20.
26. McIlwraith CW, Foerner JJ, Davis M. Osteochondritis dissecans of the tarsocrural joint: Results of treatment with arthroscopic surgery. Equine Vet J 1991;23:155–162.
27. McIlwraith CW, Yovich JV, Martin GS. Arthroscopic surgery for the treatment of osteochondral chip fractures in the equine carpus. J Am Vet Med Assoc 1987;191:531–540.
28. Moore JN, McIlwraith CW. Osteochondrosis of the equine stifle. Vet Rec 1977;100:133.
29. Moorthy ARS, Spradrow PB, Eister MED. Isolation of mycoplasma from an arthritic foal. Br Vet J 1977;133:320.
30. Nettelbladt E, Sundblad L, Jonsson E. Permeability of the synovial membrane to proteins. Acta Rheum Scand 1963;9:28.
31. Nixon AJ, Spencer CP. Arthrography of the equine shoulder joint. Equine Vet J 1990;22:107–113.
32. O'Farrell T, Costello BG, Osteochondritis dissecans of the talus: The late results of surgical treatment. J Bone Joint Surg [Br] 1980;62:131.
33. Park RD, Steyn PF, Wrigley RH. Imaging techniques in the diagnosis of equine joint disease. In: McIlwraith CW, Trotter GW, Eds. Joint Disease in the Horse. Philadelphia: WB Saunders, 1996;145–164.
34. Persson L. On the synovia in horses. Acta Vet Scand 1971;35 (S1):1.
35. Raker CW, Baker RH, Wheat JD. Pathophysiology of equine degenerative joint disease and lameness. Proceedings. 12th Annual Meeting of the American Association of Equine Practitioners, Los Angeles, CA, 1966;229–241.
36. Ramey DW. Prospective evaluation of forelimb flexion tests in practice: Clinical response, radiographic correlations and predictive value for future lameness. Proc Am Assoc Equine Pract 1997;43:116–120.
37. Ray CS, Baxter GB, McIlwraith CW, et al. Development of subchondral cystic lesions after articular cartilage and subchondral bone damage in young horses. Equine Vet J 1996;28:225–232.
38. Ray CS, Poole AR, McIlwraith CW. Use of synovial fluid and serum markers in articular disease. In: McIlwraith CW, Trotter GW, Eds. Joint Disease in the Horse. Philadelphia: WB Saunders, 1996;203–216.
39. Rejno S. Viscosity of equine synovial fluid. Acta Radiol Scand 1976;17:169.
40. Rejno S. LDH and LDH isoenzymes of synovial fluid in the horse. Acta Vet Scand 1976;17:178.
41. Ross MW. Scintigraphic and clinical findings in the Standardbred metatarsophalangeal joint: 114 cases (1993–1995). Equine Vet J 1998;30:131–138.
42. Sevelius F, Tufvesson PG. Treatment for fractures of the sesamoid bone in horses. J Am Vet Med Assoc 1963;142:981.
43. Swann DA. Macromolecules of synovial fluid. In: Sokoloff L, Ed. The Joints and Synovial Fluid. New York: Academic Press, 1978.
44. Swanstrom OG. Arthrography of the equine fetlock. MS Thesis, Purdue University, West Lafayette, IN, 1969.
45. Deleted in proof.
46. Deleted in proof.
47. Trotter GW, McIlwraith CW. Clinical features and diagnosis of equine joint disease. In: McIlwraith CW, Trotter GW, Eds. Joint Disease in the Horse. Philadelphia: WB Saunders, 1996;120–145.
48. Trotter GW, McIlwraith CW, Wagner AM. Unpublished data, 1980.
49. Vaatainen U, Lohmander LS, Thonar E, et al. Markers of cartilage and synovial metabolism in joint fluid and serum of patients with chondromalacia of the patella. Osteoarthritis Cartilage 1998;6:115–124.
50. Van Pelt RW. Interpretation of synovial fluid findings in the horse. J Am Vet Med Assoc 1974;165:91.
51. Van Pelt RW. Properties of equine synovial fluid. J Am Vet Med Assoc 1962;141:1051.
52. Wagner AF, McIlwraith CW, Martin GS. Effect of intra-articular injection of orgotein and saline on equine synovial fluid parameters. Am J Vet Res 1982;43:594.
53. Walmsley JP. Vertical tears of the cranial horn of the meniscus and its cranial ligament in the equine femorotibial joint: 7 cases and their treatment by arthroscopic surgery. Equine Vet J 1995;27:20–25.
54. Weaver MP. Twenty years of equine scintigraphy—coming of age? Equine Vet J 1995;27:163–165.
55. West M, Poske RM, Black AB, et al. Enzyme activity in synovial fluid. J Lab Clin Med 1963;62:175–183.

SPECIFIC DISEASES OF JOINTS: IDIOPATHIC SYNOVITIS (BOG SPAVIN AND ARTICULAR WINDPUFFS)

Effective management of joint diseases in the horse necessitates the classification and definition of the various disorders. In some instances, however, a joint condition may progress from one classification to another, and the treatment and prognosis must change accordingly. For example, a case of traumatic arthritis or infective arthritis may progress to OA.

The term "idiopathic synovitis" refers to a chronic synovial effusion of a joint of uncertain pathogenesis and unassociated with lameness, tenderness, heat, or radiographic changes. The disease is typified by bog spavin of the tarsocrural (tibiotarsal) joint. Another example is windpuffs of the fetlock.

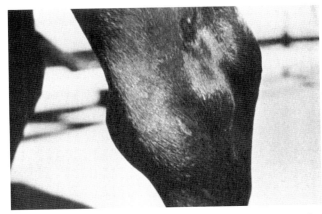

Figure 7.17   Idiopathic synovitis of the tarsocrural (tibiotarsal) joint (bog spavin).

PATHOGENESIS

Bog spavin (tarsal hydrarthrosis) has been classified as a noninflammatory effusion.[2] However, it is probably more accurate to classify bog spavin as a chronic low-grade synovitis, because inflammatory changes can be seen on histologic examination of the synovial membrane. There are minor changes in synovial fluid samples that indicate a low-grade synovitis. The gross appearance of the fluid ranges from pale yellow and clear in 50% of cases to pale yellow with some opacity in others. The relative viscosity is decreased and the MPQ ranges from normal in 50% of cases to very poor. The protein level is within normal range, and white cell counts have been reported to range from 25 to 1131, compared to 67 to 356 cells/mm[3] for controls.[4] ALP, LDH, and AAT levels in synovial effusions exceed the activity levels in normal equine tarsal synovial fluid.[2] These synovial fluid parameters return toward normal after treatment with anti-inflammatory agents.[2,4]

Bog spavin is more often seen in horses with faulty tarsal conformation (straight hocks, sickle hocked, or cow hocked), which suggests that abnormal biomechanical stresses on the soft tissues of the joint are possibly a factor.[2] In addition, strain and minor trauma, regardless of tarsal joint conformation, have been considered causes of the disease.[3] Other stresses such as lameness in another limb, heavy training, or poor shoeing could also be involved in some instances. Although nutritional abnormalities, including disorders of calcium, phosphorus, vitamin A, and vitamin D intake, have been suggested as causing the problem, there is no scientific evidence for this. The only instance in which a nutritional basis for the condition has been demonstrated is when OCD is the basis for clinical signs. OCD of the tarsocrural (tibiotarsal) joint typically presents as bog spavin, and lameness is often not obvious. Radiographs are absolutely necessary for definitive diagnosis of idiopathic synovitis of this joint.

Once synovial distension of a joint occurs, the condition may be self-perpetuating because of the resultant increase in the intercellular spaces between the synoviocytes and the dilution of hyaluronic acid by the effusion (this could decrease the permeability control of the hyaluronate layer over the synovial membrane).

Windpuffs are often associated with straight fetlocks. Young horses under a heavy training schedule will some-

times develop windpuffs of the fetlock joint. More often, however, the presence of synovial effusion in a young horse's fetlock signals OCD (defined by radiographs), as tarsocrural effusion signals OCD in that joint. Other horses under heavy work can be similarly affected and a blemish can remain throughout life.

CLINICAL SIGNS

Bog spavin manifests as a distended tarsocrural (tibiotarsal) joint with three characteristic fluctuant swellings, the largest of which is at the dorsomedial aspect of the joint (Fig. 7.17). With moderate-to-severe distension, the medioplantar and lateroplantar pouches are also distended. These are located on either side of the plantar aspect of the joint, at the level of the tarsocrural articulation joints, and are more distal than the swellings of thorough-pin. The three areas of distension are where the joint capsule is not covered by ligaments, tendons, or retinacula. Bog spavin may also involve distension of the proximal intertarsal synovial joint because of its communication with the tarsocrural joint sac on the dorsal aspect of the tarsus. However, any distension in this joint is overshadowed by the distension in the tarsocrural joint. When pressure is exerted on any one of the swellings in the tarsocrural joint, the other enlargements increase in size, and increased tension on the joint capsule may be palpated. If the joint distension is severe, a mechanical alteration in the gait (decreased hock flexion and decreased cranial phase of stride) may be noted during exercise. Synovial fluid changes are discussed above.

Articular windpuffs manifest as distension of the palmar (or plantar) recess of the metacarpophalangeal or metatarsophalangeal joint (Fig. 7.18). Again no lameness, heat, or pain should be present. The swelling in longstanding cases may harden as a result of fibrosis in the region.

DIAGNOSIS

Diagnosis of bog spavin is based on the typical clinical appearance. The problem should not be confused with thorough-pin (see page 630), which occurs caudally and above the point of the hock. The clinician should attempt to identify any etiologic factors associated with bog

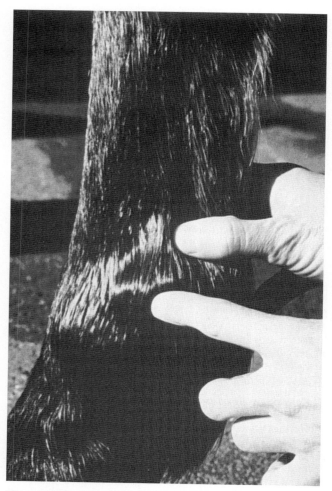

Figure 7.18 Idiopathic synovitis in the metacarpophalangeal joint (windpuffs).

spavin. OCD (or chip fragmentation) should be ruled out by radiographic examination, and the condition distinguished from traumatic synovitis. Similarly, any evidence of lameness or sensitivity of the fetlock associated with palmar recess distension disqualifies the condition as one of simple windpuffs, and OCD needs to be ruled out in this joint.

TREATMENT

In many instances, the best treatment for idiopathic synovitis, after recognition and elimination of any primary problems, is to do nothing. A number of weanlings and yearlings will have bog spavin in one or both hocks, and the problem disappears as they get older. Bog spavins associated with conformation defects cannot be eliminated, and the results of any attempt at treatment will only be temporary. The owners should be made aware of this before treatment is instituted and also warned that other problems may develop in association with the conformational defect. Although no specific nutritional abnormalities have been identified, the nutritional status of an individual should be ascertained to be normal when a case of bog spavin is encountered.

In a persistent case of bog spavin for which treatment of the blemish is desired, there are a number of alternatives. Drainage of the joint is rational, based on the idea that increased distension of the synovial membrane can potentially increase synovial effusion. However, drainage alone is not usually satisfactory and will result in a return of the condition. The use of joint lavage as well as drainage could be considered (see the traumatic arthritis section in this chapter). The use of drainage followed by the injection of corticosteroids has been described.[4] Varying amounts of 6α-methylprednisolone (Depo-Medrol) are used, depending on the extent of the initial effusion. A second and occasionally third injection are given if excessive synovial effusion reforms. Other clinicians have had less consistent results with the use of corticosteroids. The use of bandaging following injection may give more consistent results.

A progesterone derivative 6α-methyl-17α-hydroxy-progesterone acetate (6-MAP) (Depo-Provera) administered intraarticularly has also been used successfully in the treatment of bog spavin.[2] In addition to being a potent progesterone agent, 6-MAP has the 6α-methyl group that confers significant anti-inflammatory activity on the drug. A good percentage of the cases responded to one injection (150 to 200 mg); 30% received a second injection when synovial effusion re-formed.[2] A return of synovial fluid parameters toward normalcy was again observed with this treatment.

Another treatment used for bog spavin has been drainage followed by intraarticular injection of orgotein (Palosein). Orgotein is a copper-zinc protein with potent anti-inflammatory properties attributable to its superoxide dismutase activity.[1] Superoxide radical (O_2^-) is released by activated inflammatory cells and can induce marked local tissue damage. Orgotein has marked ability to reduce synovial inflammation.[1] It seems quite effective in reducing synovial effusion in some cases of bog spavin. A 5-mg dose is used in the tarsocrural joint. Intraarticular atropine (9 mg) has also been used with success.

With articular windpuffs, treatment is generally limited to the use of pressure wraps and osmotic agents in performing horses. The blemish is less obvious, and unless problems with lameness or pain develop, there is little indication for any specific intraarticular treatment.

PROGNOSIS

The prognosis for complete elimination of effusion in idiopathic synovitis is always guarded, because none of the treatments can be considered 100% successful.

References

1. Beckmann R, Flohe L. The pathogenic role of superoxide radicals in inflammation: Efficacy of exogenous superoxide dismutase. Bull Eur Physiopathol Respir 1981;17(Suppl):275–286.
2. Van Pelt RW. Intra-articular injection of 6-methyl, 17-hydroxyprogesterone acetate in tarsal hydrarthrosis (bog spavin) in the horse. J Am Vet Med Assoc 1967;151:1159.
3. Van Pelt RW, Riley WF. Tarsal hydrarthrosis in the horse: Response to intra-articular injection of synthetic steroids. Can Vet J 1969;10:130.
4. Van Pelt RW, Riley WF. Therapeutic management of tarsal hydrarthrosis (bog spavin) in the horse by intra-articular injection of prednisolone. J Am Vet Med Assoc 1967;151:328.

SPECIFIC DISEASES OF JOINTS: TRAUMATIC ARTHRITIS

In its broadest sense, the term "traumatic arthritis" includes a diverse collection of pathologic and clinical states that develop after single or repetitive episodes of trauma and may include one or all of the following: 1) synovitis (inflammation of the synovial membrane), 2) capsulitis (inflammation of the fibrous joint capsule), 3) sprain (injury of specific ligaments associated with the joint), 4) intraarticular fractures, and 5) meniscal tears (femorotibial joints).

Any of the above situations can potentially progress to OA. To facilitate discussion of pathogenesis, diagnosis, and treatment, it is convenient to divide articular trauma into three entities:

Type 1. Traumatic synovitis and capsulitis without disturbance of articular cartilage or disruption of major supporting structures. This includes acute synovitis and most sprains.
Type 2. Disruptive trauma with damage to the articular cartilage or complete rupture of major supporting structures. This includes severe sprains (A), meniscal tears (B), and intraarticular fractures (C).
Type 3. Posttraumatic OA. This includes disruptive trauma in which major residual damage is present. Patients may have deformity, limited motion, or instability of joints.

There is considerable overlap in that cases of osteochondral fragmentation in the carpus or fetlock typically present as synovitis/capsulitis. The pathobiology associated with injury to each of the tissues of the joint is detailed above in this chapter. There is obvious overlap between the entities of articular trauma, and this needs to be recognized. However, each entity is discussed separately because the specific treatments for each condition are most conveniently dealt with in this fashion. Note that failure to obtain a good response to treatment of traumatic synovitis and capsulitis commonly implies other damage within the joint. If one takes a problem-based approach and treats specifically for each problem present in the joint, the best results will be attained.

Traumatic Synovitis and Capsulitis (Type 1 Traumatic Arthritis)

In this section we consider synovitis and capsulitis in general terms, but specific reference is made to the joints most often affected with this condition. Sprains, luxations, and intraarticular fractures are considered separately.

Some confusion exists regarding the terms "carpitis" and "osselets." Carpitis is an acute or chronic inflammation of the carpal joint that may involve the fibrous joint capsule, synovial membrane, associated ligaments, and bones of the carpus. It can also progress to OA. For our purpose, however, we will consider the problem one of synovitis and capsulitis with minimal loss of integrity to the associated ligaments (type 1 traumatic arthritis). Osselets has been defined as traumatic arthritis of the metacarpophalangeal joint.[1] It is more appropriate to restrict the term osselets to describe the thickening associated with synovitis and capsulitis of the fetlock. Ossification can develop as a chronic change. Osselets are essentially a chronic capsulitis associated with trauma. The term is used a lot less these days, and veterinarians generally refer to synovitis and capsulitis by such specific names.

PATHOGENESIS

Traumatic synovitis and capsulitis may result from single or multiple episodes of trauma to a joint. The most common clinical situations are in the carpal or fetlock joints of the young racehorse, but the problem also occurs frequently in the distal interphalangeal (coffin) and distal tarsal joints. Continued repeated trauma to the joint ("use-trauma"), rather than an isolated traumatic episode, is the central etiologic concept in synovitis and capsulitis. Racing places repeated stress on both the hard and soft tissues of the joint. Inadequate conditioning may lead to early fatigue and overextension of the carpus. Conformational defects cause abnormal stresses on the joint. This results in weight being placed on the dorsal edges of the carpal bones for instance, and this can cause direct damage to the articular cartilage or result in intraarticular fractures. Redundant synovial membrane and its associated villi are also traumatized, resulting in synovitis. Capsulitis may develop secondary to synovial membrane inflammation, but the primary damage to the fibrous capsule occurs directly at its attachment to the bone. Tears in the fibrous joint capsule result in inflammation and subsequent bone formation (which gives rise to enthesiophytes). The joint distension associated with synovial effusion could also increase the chance of capsular tearing.

Similar events result in damage to the fetlock joint. Synovitis occurs, resulting in synovial effusion and joint capsule distension. Capsulitis also occurs. The capsulitis is centrally located over the dorsal aspect of the fetlock and is a more severe clinical component in this joint than it is in the carpal joint. In the acute stage of the inflammatory process, the term "green osselets" is used for this capsular inflammation. The sequence of events by which lesions develop in the fetlock is uncertain. It is likely that synovial effusion in association with synovitis occurs initially, resulting in a minor problem. If the problem is unrecognized in the face of continued training, thickening of the fibrous joint capsule develops and degenerative changes progress.[5] Direct damage to the fibrous joint capsule with concussion or pulling on the fibrous attachment of joint capsule to bone is considered of major importance in the pathogenesis of osselets. The tearing at the attachments of joint capsule to bone does not remain as a soft tissue lesion. New bone growth appears at the dorsal aspect of the distal extremity of the third metacarpal bone and the proximal extremity of the proximal phalanx, secondary to the tearing of the periosteum, and cartilage degeneration can also result. In addition, or separately, the attachment of the lateral digital extensor may be pulled sufficiently to produce periostitis in that area.

CLINICAL SIGNS

In acute carpitis, lameness is evident and there is shortening of the cranial phase of the stride due to decreased flexion of the carpus. The horse typically travels

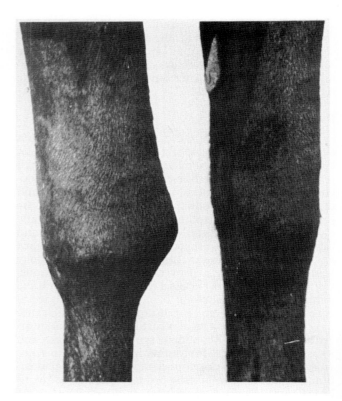

Figure 7.19 Acute, severe carpitis. Limb is held in a partially flexed position to maximize joint volume and minimize joint pressure.

at the trot, with the legs placed more widely apart. Swelling is present because of joint distension. There will be a variable amount of swelling in the joint capsule itself and other periarticular tissues. There is a tendency for the horse to hold the carpus slightly flexed in the standing position in severe cases (Fig. 7.19). This maximizes intracapsular volume and reduces intracapsular pressure.[8] Digital pressure on the joint may provoke pain. Carpal flexion may be used to define stiffness in the joint and the degree of pain.

In chronic carpitis, lameness may not be evident until the horse is used at a fast gait. Carpal flexion may be used to accentuate lameness. A hard thickening will be palpated at the dorsal aspect of the joint. The relative amounts of fibrous or bony tissue in this swelling needs to be ascertained by radiographic examination. Radiographs may also reveal enthesiophytosis on the dorsal aspect of the carpal bones as a result of previous tearing of the fibrous joint capsule attachments to the bone. These enthesiophytes are not necessarily a sign of OA and will generally cause no clinical problem unless there is continued capsular tearing or disease.

With synovitis/capsulitis in the metacarpophalangeal joint, the horse moves with a choppy gait if bilaterally affected. If only one limb is involved, the horse has an obvious lameness of that limb. Synovitis is evidenced by synovial fluid distension of the palmar recess. Pain and heat may be present. The capsular inflammation of osselets is manifested as swelling on the dorsal aspect of the joint. This swelling may extend at least half way around

the joint. In the acute phase, pressure over the involved region will cause the animal to flinch. In a later stage, hard thickening may be present. The sensitivity to palpation and flexion will be variable. Radiographs should be taken to determine if new bone growth is present and to evaluate its relationship to the articular surfaces. Early cases have no radiographic changes, but enthesiophytes may be subsequently observed on the dorsal surface of the proximal aspect of the proximal phalanx and may also occur on the dorsal aspect of the distal extremity of the third metacarpal bone. In addition, ossification may develop in the joint capsule itself. In chronic inflammatory conditions of the fetlock, remodeling changes in the distal extremity of the third metacarpal bone may also be apparent in radiographs[3] (Fig. 7.20).

Synovitis and capsulitis of the tarsocrural joint manifest as synovial effusion accompanied by varying degrees of lameness, heat, and periarticular swelling. Radiographs are made to eliminate more serious problems. Synovitis in the tarsocrural joint may be particularly reactive, with chronic proliferation of synovial villi pre-

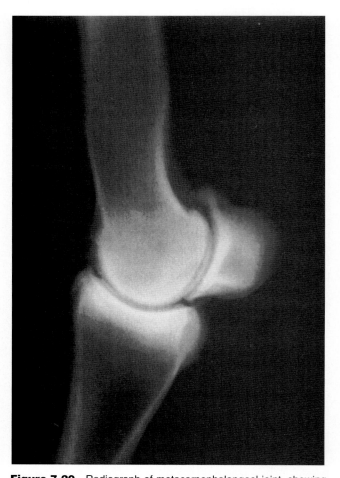

Figure 7.20 Radiograph of metacarpophalangeal joint, showing loss of bone cortex on the distal palmar aspect of the third metacarpal bone, presumably caused by a combination of pressure from inflammatory change and fibrosis of the palmar recess. There is also osteophytosis on both the apical and basilar regions of the sesamoid bone and an osteophyte on the proximodorsal aspect of the first phalanx.

cluding a successful outcome with medical treatment. Traumatic arthritis of the femoropatellar joint usually manifests with obvious synovial effusion, and the problem can usually be localized reasonably easily. However, when there is traumatic synovitis/capsulitis of the femorotibial joint, the tight encapsulation of these small, separate compartments means that joint distension is not a common feature. There may be some effusion in the femoropatellar joint due to pressure going through the communication between the medial femorotibial joint and the femoropatellar joint. In severe traumatic injuries, such as meniscal tears, synovial effusion of the femorotibial joint itself can be detected. In many instances in the femorotibial joint, intraarticular analgesia is often used to achieve a specific diagnosis. Intrasynovial analgesia is not needed routinely for problems in the carpus and fetlock, but when a problem in one of these joints has failed to respond to medical treatment and clear indication is needed for diagnostic arthroscopy, intraarticular analgesia is used. Synovitis/capsulitis of the distal interphalangeal (coffin joint) is a common problem. These horses have a short choppy gait. Usually some effusion may be detected above the coronet. Placement of a needle in the joint reveals greatly increased fluid pressure and confirms the diagnosis.

DIAGNOSIS AND DIFFERENTIAL DIAGNOSIS

Radiographs are commonly made to eliminate the possibility of osteochondral damage. This is not always routine in sports medicine practices if the clinician feels comfortable that the problem is primarily localized in soft tissues. On the other hand, if there is failure to respond to therapy or the synovial fluid tap at the time of treatment reveals changes suggesting more structural damage (and obviously if the lameness is sufficiently severe), radiographs must be taken. Synovial fluid analysis (even gross inspection) is always useful. Color and viscosity can be evaluated while one is aspirating fluid or injecting the joint. With severe lameness associated with synovial effusion, synovial fluid analysis should always be performed to rule out infective arthritis. As implied above, diagnostic arthroscopy may be the only way to truly define the internal state of the joint and the degree of disease.

TREATMENT

There are a number of treatments for acute synovitis with or without accompanying capsulitis.[9] The aim of these treatments is to return the joint to normal as quickly as possible. In addition to bringing relief to the patient and allowing it to return to normal work, suppression of synovitis and capsulitis is important to prevent the products of inflammation from compromising the articular cartilage and leading to OA. These processes are discussed above in the pathobiology section. In addition to the potential deleterious effects of synovitis on articular cartilage, it is important to provide pain relief and minimize the potential microinstability associated with excessive synovial effusion. It has also been shown experimentally in the rabbit that joint inflammation weakens intraarticular ligaments in addition to affecting the cartilage.

REST AND IMMOBILIZATION. The usefulness of rest in patients with acute inflammation and capsular injury is obvious. The realities of racing or other athletic activities often prevent proper application of this modality, which would allow a complete recovery in many cases. Bandage support may also assist healing of an acutely damaged joint. A pressure bandage stimulates mechanoreceptors, and this in turn can decrease pain sensation. Immobilization is important when there is any destabilizing injury but is not ideal if the problem is limited to synovitis/capsulitis. Prolonged immobilization may lead to muscle atrophy and adhesion formation within the joint as well as articular cartilage atrophy. Casting is only appropriate in cases of destabilizing injury. Passive flexion of limbs may help retain mobility and some hand walking is recommended in most instances. The author uses passive flexion of the fetlock routinely after surgery to maintain capsular range of motion and minimize adhesions and fibrosis, and if it is considered appropriate (if the patient is willing), for primary capsular injury as well. Hand walking should always be continued, even if training is stopped. If there is no destabilizing injury, hand walking will maintain motion of the joint capsule as well as prevent atrophic change in the articular cartilage.

PHYSICAL THERAPY. Hydrotherapy may be useful immediately after a traumatic joint injury. Although the use of cold or hot water seems to be debated regularly, it is reasonable to assume that cold hydrotherapy is indicated in the acute stage of joint injury to retard the inflammatory processes of exudation and diapedesis and reduce edema.[6] The application of ice is extremely beneficial as a primary treatment for most acute joint injuries. After 48 hours, hot hydrotherapy may be indicated to relieve pain and reduce tension in inflamed tissues. The vasodilatory effect can aid in fluid resorption as well as providing phagocytic cells.[1]

Swimming has also been used in the convalescent period with joint injury to maintain the horse's condition while relieving joint trauma. It is the closest one can approximate non-weight-bearing motion as practiced in human sports medicine. It is also possible that the massaging effect of the water on the limbs may help prevent fibrosis of the joint capsule. However, swimming does not maintain joint tone, and quick return of the horse to fast work is potentially dangerous.

There has been considerable use made in recent years of modalities such as electromagnetic therapy, electrostimulation, and low-level laser for various musculoskeletal conditions including traumatic joint disease. There have been no controlled studies documenting their value, but anecdotally, people who use these various modalities consider that symptomatic relief is achieved.

Any process that causes chronic fibrosis in the capsular tissues is contraindicated because it decreases joint motion and decreases the shock-absorbing capabilities of the joint capsule. Diathermy and ultrasound have been used to produce deep heat in the tissues and to enhance vascularity and healing.[6] Repeated applications of ultrasound will cause bone resorption (osteoporosis). However, these techniques have not attained a prominent place in the treatment of joint conditions. Liniments are also commonly used.[1] The massaging effect of their application is probably as useful as their ability to produce heat.

DIMETHYL SULFOXIDE (DMSO [DOMOSO]). The polar chemical solvent DMSO has been used alone in the horse or mixed with corticosteroids to reduce soft tissue swelling and inflammation resulting from acute trauma.[7] Its main value in this regard is considered to be the reduction of edema.[13] More recently, DMSO has been shown to possess superoxide dismutase activity, whereby it can inactivate superoxide radicals. The drug also enhances penetration of various agents through the skin, and a threefold increase in the penetration of percutaneous steroid when mixed with DMSO has been reported.[13] Also, when cortisone was dissolved in DMSO, the dilution of cortisone necessary to stabilize lysosomes was reduced from 1/10 to 1/1000. Work has also shown increased blood flow through experimental flaps and the presence of vascular dilation with DMSO application. This may also help with the resolution of soft tissue inflammation. The drug is bacteriostatic and produces collagen dissolution, which may help in restoring pliability to fibrosed tissue.[13]

Such properties provide some rationale for its use in joint inflammation, and the development of adjuvant polyarthritis in the rat is significantly inhibited by the local use of DMSO. The drug has a definite antiarthritic effect that seems independent of its ability to promote the absorption of corticosteroids.[4] The local antiarthritic effect of hydrocortisone was increased 10-fold when DMSO was used as a carrier.[4] DMSO has been used in the treatment of synovitis in horses.[12] It is important to use the medical grade DMSO (liquid or gel), and gloves should be worn during its application.[11]

JOINT LAVAGE. The technique of joint lavage was initially proposed to remove cartilaginous debris that caused synovitis.[10] Production of synovitis with articular cartilage fragments and purified chondroitin sulfate has been demonstrated experimentally.[2] In addition, synovitis of inflamed synovial membrane acts as a source of deleterious mediators (discussed under "Pathobiology of Joints . . . "), and this constitutes an additional reason for the use of joint lavage.

Lavage may be done with the patient standing or under general anesthesia. Obviously, one can do more extensive lavage under general anesthesia. Clipping and aseptic preparation of the joint are performed, after which two 12- to 14-gauge needles are inserted in the joint. The use of a fluid pump saves time for lavage. The clinical results from joint lavage are particularly gratifying in a patient with severe lameness associated with acute synovitis. After completion of lavage, therapeutic agents such as hyaluronan may be administered. Joint lavage is used most commonly in association with arthroscopic surgery and is considered responsible for a significant part of the benefit achieved from surgery. It can, however, also be done with the patient standing; although the volume put in the joint is lower than that under general anesthesia, it still seems quite effective; there are no known data on minimum volume or flow requirements.

References

1. Adams OR. Lameness in Horses. 3rd ed. Philadelphia: Lea & Febiger, 1974.
2. Chrisman OD, Fessel JM, Southwick WO. Experimental production of synovitis and marginal articular exostoses in the knee joints of dogs. Yale J Biol Med 1965;37:409.
3. Ferraro GL. Selected injuries of the fetlock. Proceedings. 24th Annual Meeting of the American Association of Equine Practitioners, St. Louis, MO, 1978;315–317.
4. Gorog P, Kovacs IB. Antiarthritic and antithrombotic effects of topically applied dimethyl sulfoxide. Ann NY Acad Sci 1975;243:91.
5. Haynes PF. Disease of the metacarpophalangeal joint and metacarpus. Vet Clin North Am [Large Anim Pract] 1980;2:33.
6. Hickman J. Veterinary Orthopaedics. Philadelphia: JB Lippincott, 1964.
7. Koller LD. Clinical application of DMSO by veterinarians in Oregon and Washington. VM/SAC 1976;71:591.
8. Mankin HJ, Radin E. Structure and function of joints. In: McCarty DJ, Ed. Arthritis and Allied Conditions. 9th ed. Philadelphia: Lea & Febiger, 1979;151–166.
9. Milne EJ. Medical treatment of equine osteoarthritis and tenosynovitis. J Am Vet Med Assoc 1962;141:1269.
10. Norrie RD. The treatment of joint disease by saline lavage. Proceedings. 21st Annual Meeting of the American Association of Equine Practitioners, Boston, MA, 1975;91–94.
11. Rubin LF. Toxicity of dimethyl sulfoxide, alone and in combination. Ann NY Acad Sci 1975;8.
12. Tiegland MB, Metcalf JW, Levesque F. Observations on the therapeutics of DMSO. Proceedings. 11th Annual Meeting of the American Association of Equine Practitioners, Miami Beach, FL, 1965;371–375.
13. Wood DC, Wood J. Pharmacologic and biochemical considerations of dimethyl sulfoxide. Ann NY Acad Sci 1975;243:7.

MEDICATIONS FOR JOINT DISEASE: NONSTEROIDAL ANTI-INFLAMMATORY DRUGS

The most common nonsteroidal anti-inflammatory drug (NSAID) is phenylbutazone. NSAIDs are substances other than steroids that suppress one or more components of the inflammatory response.[7a,17] Such a broad definition includes both phenylbutazone-type drugs and the new intraarticular preparations such as HA, polysulfated GAG (PSGAG), and pentosan sulfate. The term NSAID tends to be used more restrictively to describe anti-inflammatory agents that inhibit some component of the enzyme system that converts arachidonic acid into prostaglandins and thromboxanes (Fig. 7.21).[22] Various NSAIDs are available for, and used in, the treatment of joint disease in the horse.[13]

As defined above, all NSAIDs inhibit cyclooxygenase activity to some degree.[31] With phenylbutazone, this effect is marked and is one of the most important aspects of its therapeutic potential. However, other agents such as carprofen are relatively weak cyclooxygenase inhibitors, leading to the conclusion that in addition to these agents' effects on prostaglandins, other mechanisms may contribute to their overall anti-inflammatory activity. Drugs such as ketoprofen inhibit 5-lipoxygenase in vitro in addition to cyclooxygenase, but this property has not been demonstrated in vivo.[7] Meclofenamate also inhibits human PMN chemotaxis as well as degranulation and generation of superoxide free radicals. However, the significance of such findings to clinical anti-inflammatory therapy remains unclear. Although it is clear that in low doses aspirin and most of the newer NSAIDs inhibit the biosynthesis of prostaglandins from arachidonic acid (and stable prostaglandins have been shown to mediate fever, hyperalgesia, vasodilation (edema), and several

genase. This has a profound effect on platelet function. Aspirin is commonly administered at about 25 to 35 mg/kg orally. Aspirin has had limited clinical use in the horse.[17] However, its unique effect on platelets at low dose rates would suggest a rationale for its use in conditions such as navicular syndrome, chronic laminitis, and thromboembolic colic in which vasoactive agents are advocated and have been found of some value. Daily dosing or even administration of aspirin every 2 days should reduce clotting and thrombus formation in horses.

Meclofenamic Acid (Arquel)

Meclofenamic acid is used in the oral granule form at a dosage of 2.2 mg/kg/day. Compared with other NSAIDs it has an onset of action that is slow, requiring 36 to 48 hours for full effect.[6] Clinical experience suggests that it is particularly useful in the treatment of chronic musculoskeletal problems.[30] In clinical trials with 304 horses, it benefited 78% of the horses with navicular syndrome, 76% of those with laminitis, and 61% of those with OA.[6] In a double-blind study comparing 7-day treatments of phenylbutazone (4.4 mg/kg) and meclofenamic acid (2.2 mg/kg), meclofenamic acid produced a favorable clinical response in 60% of the animals suffering from navicular syndrome or OA, whereas phenylbutazone only benefited 36% of such patients.[17] However, the drug has not achieved routine use because of the differential costs.

Excessive doses of meclofenamic acid produce signs of toxicity similar to those of phenylbutazone (the dose 13 to 18 mg/kg). Signs include anorexia, depression, weight loss, edema, diarrhea, oral ulceration, and reduced hematocrit.[17]

Flunixin (Banamine, Finadyne)

Flunixin is used clinically in the horse at a dose of 1.1 mg/kg. Whether it is given orally or parenterally, the onset of action occurs after about 2 hours and persists for as long as 30 hours.[22] The maximal effect is obtained between 2 and 16 hours. Because the drug has a short plasma half-life, it is assumed that there is accumulation of the drug at inflammatory foci (the measured range is 1.6 to 2.5 hours for $t_{1/2}$). Flunixin is rapidly absorbed after oral intramuscular administration, with plasma levels occurring within 30 hours. Like all NSAIDs except salicylate, it is more than 90% protein bound. In experimental systems for studying inflammation, a single intravenous dose of 1.1 mg/kg of flunixin suppressed PGE_2 production in inflammatory exudates for 12 to 24 hours. This dose also inhibited the ex vivo production of thromboxane ETXB2 by equine platelets. Flunixin has been used most frequently for the treatment of colic, but it is useful in the treatment of lameness in horses. However, for economic reasons phenylbutazone is preferred when the latter drug is efficacious.

No adverse clinical or biochemical signs have been recorded in horses given three times the recommended dose of flunixin for 10 days or five times the recommended dose for 5 days. However, toxicity has been reported in ponies and foals.

Naproxen (Equiproxen, Naprosyn)

Naproxen is given orally at a dose of 10 mg/kg. It is used much less than phenylbutazone for musculoskeletal conditions. It was originally marketed primarily for muscular conditions, but experience in humans shows it to be very valuable in joint conditions. Naproxen has relatively close anti-inflammatory and analgesic doses and would therefore be expected to have a greater anti-inflammatory effect than drugs such as phenylbutazone and aspirin. Naproxen does indeed seem to be more effective than phenylbutazone in an experimental model of equine myositis. In horses with clinical cases of azoturia, naproxen produced a favorable response in 90%, with an average time for remission of 5 days[22] Naproxen also seems to have a wide safety margin, with no sign of toxicity in horses given the drug at three times the recommended dose for 42 days.

Carprofen (Zenecarp, Rimadyl)

Carprofen is a relatively recent addition to the NSAID armamentarium. It has a longer $t_{1/2}$ than the other NSAIDs. It is used in the horse at a dose of 0.7 mg/kg administered intravenously and can be given once daily. Carprofen has been tested in the horse for its anti-inflammatory and analgesic activity. A single dose of 0.7 mg/kg reduced the concentration of PGE_2 and inflammatory exudate for up to 8 hours and the ex vivo generation of TXB2 in blood for up to 15 hours.[19] The reduction in eicosanoid production by carprofen was modest compared with the reductions produced by therapeutic doses of phenylbutazone and flunixin.[16] However, carprofen demonstrated an anti-inflammatory effect at 12, 24, 36, and 48 hours by way of reduced volume of a swollen area experimentally created in the necks of ponies.[19] Subsequent studies have demonstrated greater inhibition of PGE_2 and inflammatory exudate by carprofen at 4 mg/kg administered intravenously, and this dose also causes moderate but significant inhibition of LTB4, which indicates inhibition of 5-lipoxygenase at the high dose rate. Carprofen is better tolerated at the dose of 0.7 mg/kg given by the oral or intravenous route. Intramuscular administration resulted in an increase in CPK levels, suggesting muscle damage.[23] In a randomized, controlled study of OA in dogs, carprofen was of significant benefit.[33]

Ketoprofen (Ketofen)

Ketoprofen (Ketofen) was originally marketed as a dual inhibitor of cyclooxygenase and 5-lipoxygenase.[2] Such activity would broaden the anti-inflammatory potential of the compound, in theory making it superior to other NSAIDs. However, such claims are based on early in vitro data[7] and have been challenged with results from experimental models in rats. Ketoprofen had no effect on LTB-4 concentration in such models at doses that produced virtually 100% inhibition of PGE_2 and TXB-2 production.[28] In two studies involving ketoprofen and exudate eicosanoid concentrations in the horse, the drug significantly reduced PGE_2 but not LTB-4 levels. The dose rate used was 2.2 mg/kg once or twice daily (two doses). In another study, synovitis was induced in the midcarpal joints of 12 horses by injection of carra-geenan. Although intravenous administration of keto-profen significantly reduced PGE$_2$ concentrations in sy-novial fluid at 6 and 9 hours after administration, the LTB-4 levels were unaffected. Joint effusion was reduced at 3 hours, and lameness was reduced at 3 and 6 hours after ketoprofen treatment.[25] At clinical doses of 2.2 mg/kg/day, the drug should not be considered superior to other NSAIDs on the basis of claims about its ability to inhibit 5-lipoxygenase.

In a recent study with experimentally induced synovi-tis in horses (sterile carrageenan), the analgesic and anti-inflammatory effects of ketoprofen (2.2 and 3.6 mg/kg) and phenylbutazone (4.4 mg/kg) were compared. All NSAID-treated horses had PGE$_2$, compared with saline-treated horses. The effect lasted longer with phenylbuta-zone-treated horses than with ketoprofen-treated horses.[26] There were no treatment effects on leukotriene B4 (which supposedly happened if ketoprofen was in-deed inhibiting the lipoxygenase pathway). Only phenyl-butazone treatment reduced lameness, joint temperature, and synovial fluid volume. The conclusion was that phenylbutazone was more effective than ketoprofen in reducing lameness, joint temperature, synovial fluid vol-ume, and synovial fluid PGE$_2$. The results do not support lipoxygenase inhibition by either NSAID.

References

1. Abramson SB, Weissmann G. The mechanisms of action of nonste-roidal anti-inflammatory drugs. Arthritis Rheum 1989;32:1–9.
2. Betley M, Sutherland SF, Gregoricka MJ, Pollett RA. The analgesic effect of ketoprofen for use in treating equine colic as compared to flunixin meglumine. Equine Pract 1991;13:11–16.
3. Brandt KD. Nonsteroidal anti-inflammatory drugs and articular cartilage. J Rheumatol 1987(S14);14:132–133.
4. Brandt KD, Slowman-Kovacs S. Nonsteroidal anti-inflammatory drugs in treatment of osteoarthritis. Clin Orthop 1986;213:84–91.
5. Collins LG, Tyler DE. Phenylbutazone toxicosis in the horse: A clinical study. J Am Vet Med Assoc 1984;184:699–703.
6. Cotter GH, Riley WF, Beck CC, et al. Arquel (Cl-1583). A new nonsteroidal anti-inflammatory drug for horses. Proc Am Assoc Equine Pract 1973;19:81–90.
7. Dawson W, Boot JR, Harvey J, Walker JR. The pharmacology of benoxaprofen with particular reference to effects on lipoxygenase product formation. Eur J Rheumatol Inflamm 1982;5:61–68.
7a. Ferreira SH. Prostaglandins, aspirin-like drugs and analgesia. Nature 1972;240:200–203.
8. Higgins AJ, Lees P. Phenylbutazone inhibition of prostaglandin E$_2$ production in equine acute inflammatory exudate. Vet Rec 1983; 113:622–623.
9. Higgs GA, Eakins KE, Mugridge KG, et al. The effects of non-steroid anti-inflammatory drugs on leukocyte migration in carra-geenan-induced inflammation. Eur J Pharmacol 1980;66:81–86.
10. Huskisson EC, Woolf DL, Balme HW, et al. Four new anti-inflam-matory drugs: Responses and variations. Br Med J 1976;1: 1048–1049.
11. Insel PA: Analgesic-antipyretics and anti-inflammatory drugs: Drugs employed in the treatment of rheumatoid arthritis in gout. In: Gilman AG, Rall TW, Nies AS, Taylor P, Eds. The Pharmaco-logical Basis of Therapeutics. 8th ed. New York: Pergamon Press, 1990;638–681.
12. Jolly WT, Whittem T, Jolly AC, Firth EC. The dose-related effects of phenylbutazone and a methylprednisolone acetate formulation (Depo-Medrol®) on cultured explants of equine carpal articular cartilage. J Vet Pharmacol Ther 1995;18:429–437.
13. Kallings P. Nonsteroidal anti-inflammatory drugs. Vet Clin North Am Equine Pract 1993;9:523–541.
14. Landoni MF, Foote R, Frean S, Lees P. Effects of flunixin: Tolfena-mic acid, R(−) and S(+) ketoprofen on the response of equine

15. synoviocytes to lipopolysaccharide stimulation. Equine Vet J 1996; 28:468–475.
15. Lee SH, Soyoola E, Chanmugam P, et al. Selective expression of mitogen-inducible cyclooxygenase in macrophages stimulated with lipopolysaccharide. J Biol Chem 1992;267:25934–25938.
16. Lees P, Ewins CP, Taylor JBO, Sedgwick AD. Serum thromboxane in the horse and its inhibition by aspirin: Phenylbutazone and fluni-xin. Br Vet J 1987;143:462–476.
17. Lees P, Higgins AJ. Clinical pharmacology in therapeutic uses of non-steroidal anti-inflammatory drugs in the horse. Equine Vet J 1985;17:83–96.
18. Lees P, Taylor KBO, Higgins AJ, Sharma SC. Phenylbutazone and oxyphenbutazone distribution into tissue fluids in the horse. J Vet Pharmacol Ther 1986;9:204–212.
19. Lees P, McKellar Q, May SA, Ludwig B. Pharmacodynamics and pharmacokinetics of carprofen in the horse. Equine Vet J 1994; 26:203–208.
20. Deleted in proof.
21. MacKay RJ, French TW, Nguyen HT, Mayhew IG. Effects of large doses of phenylbutazone administration in horses. Am J Vet Res 1983;44:774–780.
22. May SA, Lees P. Nonsteroidal anti-inflammatory drugs. In: McIl-wraith CW, Trotter GW, Eds. Joint Disease in the Horse. Philadel-phia: WB Saunders, 1996;223–237.
23. McKellar QA, Bogan JA, Fellenberg RL, et al. Pharmacokinetic, biochemical and tolerance studies on carprofen in the horse. Equine Vet J 1991;23:280–284.
24. Mead EEA, Smith WL, Dewitt DL. Differential inhibition of pros-taglandin endoperoxide synthase (cyclo-oxygenase) isozymes by aspirin and other non-steroidal anti-inflammatory drugs. J Biol Chem 1993;268:6610–6614.
25. Owens JG, Kamerling SG, Keowen ML. Anti-inflammatory effects and pharmacokinetics of ketoprofen in a model of equine synovitis. Proceedings of the 6th International Congress European Associa-tion of Veterinary Pharmacology and Toxicology, Oxford, Black-well, 1994;170–171.
26. Owens JG, Kamerling SG, Stanton SR, et al. Effects of pretreatment with ketoprofen and phenylbutazone on experimentally induced synovitis in dogs. Am J Vet Res 1996;57:866–874.
27. Palmoski MJ, Brandt KD. Benoxaprofen stimulates proteoglycan synthesis in normal canine knee cartilage in vitro. Arthritis Rheum 1983;26:771–774.
28. Salman JA, Tilling LC, Moncada S. Benoxaprofen does not inhibit formation of leukotriene B4 in a model of acute inflammation. Biochem Pharmacol 1984;33:2928–2930.
29. Slowmans-Kovacs SD, Albrecht ME, Brandt KD. Effects of salicy-late on chondrocytes from osteoarthritic and contralateral knees of dogs with unilateral anterior cruciate ligament transection. Ar-thritis Rheum 1989;32:486–490.
30. Snow DH, Baxter P, Whiting B. The pharmacokinetics of meclofen-amic acid in the horse. J Vet Pharmacol Ther 1981;4:147–156.
31. Vane JR. Inhibition of prostaglandin synthesis as a mechanism of action for aspirin-like drugs. Nature 1971;231:232–235.
32. Vane JR, Botting RM. New insights into the mode of action of anti-inflammatory drugs. Inflamm Res 1995;44:1–10.
33. Vasseur PB, Johnson AL, Budsberg SC, et al. Randomized, con-trolled trial of the efficacy of carprofen, a nonsteroidal anti-inflam-matory drug, in the treatment of osteoarthritis in dogs. J Am Vet Med Assoc 1995;206:807–811.
34. Xie W, Robertson DL, Simmons DL. Mitogen-inducible prosta-glandin G/H synthase: A new target for non-steroidal anti-inflam-matory drugs. Drug Dev Res 1992;25:249–265.

MEDICATIONS FOR JOINT DISEASE: INTRAARTICULAR CORTICOSTEROIDS

Although it has been implied by some that intraarticu-lar corticosteroids have been replaced by HA and PSGAG, many clinicians have returned to, or persisted in the use of, corticosteroids.[29] The untoward effects of intraarticular corticosteroids in horses have been repeat-edly cited in the veterinary literature and more recently in the lay press. The first report of intraarticular corticosteroid use was in 1955.[59] More recently, various investigators have attempted critical evaluations of the effects of corticosteroids in equine joints,[5,9–11,20,39,46,48] and these results are helping to delineate a more definitive role for these agents in the management of joint disease.

Historical Perspectives

Wheat first reported the use of hydrocortisone to treat clinical muscular conditions in 94 horses and cattle.[59] This report was followed by a series of investigations by Van Pelt and co-workers evaluating a number of corticosteroid preparations as treatments for a variety of clinical conditions.[11,51–56] A few clinical trials have been reported since.[18,19,30,44,57] Mostly favorable results have been reported, but all studies were poorly controlled.

The first paper indicting corticosteroids as harmful in the horse was written by O'Connor in 1968.[34] The report was based on some papers in the human literature. The statement "An endless destructive cycle is set into motion, which if continued will produce a steroid arthropathy which can render the horse useless" was cited, and the reference was an abstract written by an anonymous author.[1] Six other human-based references (four textbook chapters and two journal papers) were quoted in this paper, and one of them alluded to corticosteroids producing Charcot-like arthropathy. Charcot's arthropathy is a neurogenic disease that results in the loss of sensation, loss of proprioceptive control, instability, and arthritis (most often seen as a sequel to syphilis). There has never been any scientific demonstration of a comparable response associated with corticosteroid use in horses.

A noted veterinary pharmacologist made some rather alarming statements in discussing corticosteroids in his textbook.[45] Examples include "A patient on corticosteroids can walk all the way to the autopsy room" and "A horse can wear a joint surface right down to the bone running on a glucocorticoid-injected joint." Photographs of a normal fetlock from an immature horse and a severely degenerative fetlock (that had been injected with corticosteroids) were also included. However, no substantiation was made for corticosteroids causing such gross damage. Instances of DJD caused by corticosteroids were persistently presented without proof of such pathogenesis.[45]

More recently, the beneficial versus deleterious effects of corticosteroids have been revisited in humans[14,15,32,43,58] and in horses.[29] Recent studies have looked at the morphologic and biochemical changes in equine articular cartilage under the influence of corticosteroids, with or without the added effect of exercise,[3,5,9,39,48] as well as articular cartilage matrix metabolism and synovial membrane hyaluronan production under the influence of corticosteroids.[3,36,46,50] Much new information has been gained, and it is clear that many previous generalizations are wrong and that there are many differences with regard to the type and dose of corticosteroid used, as well as the reaction of individual tissues.

Effect of Corticosteroids

Corticosteroid effects have been reviewed recently.[47] They are exerted through interaction with steroid-specific receptors in the cytoplasm of steroid-responsive tissues.[21,33,43] The corticosteroid binds to the receptor, resulting in a change in the allosteric nature of the receptor–steroid complex. This then allows the complex to bind reversibly to specific sites on the nuclear chromatin of glucocorticoid-responsive genes. Different corticosteroids interact differently with these receptors.[21] Due to this interaction, transcription of genes is modulated in messenger RNA coding for proteins, and this produces the hormonal effect.[21,43]

Corticosteroids are potent anti-inflammatory agents and inhibit inflammatory processes at virtually all levels. Traditionally, the primary anti-inflammatory effect of corticosteroids has been related to stabilization of lysosomal membranes, with a concomitant decrease in the release of lysosomal enzymes. However, the anti-inflammatory effects are considerably more complex than this.[2] Glucocorticoid receptors have been demonstrated in neutrophils, lymphocytes, and eosinophils, and it is possible that all glucocorticoid anti-inflammatory effects are exerted through receptor-mediated mechanisms.[2] A major effect of corticosteroids is their inhibition of movement of inflammatory cells (including neutrophils and monocyte–macrophages) into a site of inflammation.[2,21,33,43] Corticosteroids also affect neutrophil function but to a lesser extent than movement, and the effect on neutrophil function seems to be dose dependent.[2,21,33,43] It has been suggested that at physiologic (lower) doses of corticosteroids, the effects on neutrophilic phagocytosis, lysosomal membrane stabilization, and inhibition of lysosomal enzyme release and neutrophilic chemotaxis may be less significant to how corticosteroids elicit their effect than previously believed.[2] There is also some evidence that the inhibitory effects of corticosteroids on prostaglandin production by leukocytes is more profound on monocytes–macrophages than it is on neutrophils.[22,23] A poor correlation has been reported between neutrophil numbers and PGE_2 concentrations in synovial fluid after corticosteroid treatment of chronic inflammatory joint disease in humans, suggesting either alternative sources of prostaglandin (macrophage) or differential effects of corticosteroids on cellular function.[4]

Corticosteroids affect the humoral aspects of inflammation, predominantly by inhibition of prostaglandin production.[2,4,37,49] Much evidence supports inhibition of the generation of proinflammatory metabolites (prostaglandins) from arachidonic acid as the primary mechanism of anti-inflammatory action of corticosteroids (Fig. 7.22).[4,37,49] This action is considered to be largely due to the inhibition of phospholipase A_2 by the steroid-inducible group of proteins called lipocortins.[6,7,37,49,60] NSAIDs exert their effect at an adjacent location along the pathway of eicosanoid production, with corticosteroids being effective at inhibiting both the cyclooxygenase and lipoxygenase pathways and NSAIDs mainly acting by inhibiting the cyclooxygenase pathway, thereby limiting production of prostacyclin and thromboxane. It has been suggested recently that in addition to inhibition of the proinflammatory prostaglandin pathways, corticosteroids may have other anti-inflammatory effects at different levels, and the finding that some prostaglandins also exhibit anti-inflammatory effects complicates the complete definition of the anti-inflammatory mode of action of corticosteroids.

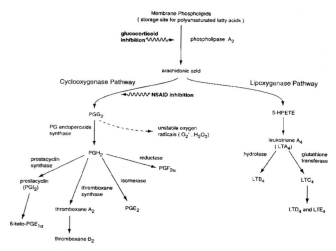

Figure 7.22 Schematic representation of the cyclo-oxygenase and lipo-oxygenase pathways of arachidonic acid metabolism demonstrating where corticosteroids exert their influence. (Reprinted with permission from McIlwraith CW, Trotter GW, Eds. Joint Disease in the Horse. Philadelphia: WB Saunders, 1996, Fig 14-3.)

The eicosanoids are important in both induction and maintenance of inflammation, and once produced, they can interact with various cytokines. This further complicates accurate definition of modes of action. Many of the effects of IL-1 are associated with stimulation of prostaglandin production and inflammation, and TNF is known to induce production of PGE$_2$ in macrophages.[60] PGE$_2$ has been shown to suppress TNF activity, and phospholipase A$_2$ synthesis is enhanced by IL-1, TNF, and lipopolysaccharide.

Data on specific activity of proteinases under the influence of corticosteroids varies. In one study in humans, messenger RNA expression for collagenase and TIMP as well as histologic inflammation scores were decreased after triamcinolone administration in arthritic joints.[8] However, corticosteroids did not suppress stromelysin activity by activated equine synovial cells in vitro.[27] In another study in humans, the presence of hydrocortisone caused decreased PGE$_2$ concentrations, increased TIMP concentrations, and decreased collagenase concentrations in normal, osteoarthritic, and rheumatoid synovial membranes.[28]

Low doses of corticosteroids have also been associated with inhibition of plasminogen activator activity in human synovial fibroblasts.[16] Although HA synthesis has been observed to be decreased by corticosteroids in cultures of human skin fibroblasts as well as canine synovial membrane,[24,42] synovial fluid concentrations of HA were increased after intraarticular corticosteroid injection in horses.[50]

A number of early reports described deleterious effects of corticosteroids on normal articular cartilage.[17,24,25,38,40,41] Cortisone acetate administration in mice resulted in a decrease in chondrocyte size and impaired organelle development in association with both single and repeated systemic corticosteroid injections.[40] A study of intraarticular corticosteroids (once weekly for 2 to 12 weeks) in rabbits noted progressive loss of endoplasmic reticulum, mitochondria, and Golgi apparatus.[41] The same author also noted progressive loss of proteoglycans as well as an overall decrease in protein, collagen, and proteoglycan synthesis, and gross evidence of cartilage thinning, fibrillation, and fissuring. In many of these studies, corticosteroids were administered daily for periods of up to 12 weeks or very high dosages were used.

Equine Studies

Methylprednisolone Acetate (Depo-Medrol)

A number of studies have evaluated the effect of methylprednisolone acetate (MPA) injected into normal equine joints. The first was done by Marcoux in 1977.[26] Methylprednisolone (80 mg) was injected into equine carpal joints, and the response was compared with the response to repeated injections of blood (simulating hemarthrosis). Marcoux injected 80 mg of MPA per joint in all four carpal joints of six horses for a total of five injections. The four joints of each horse were injected with either 80 mg of MPA, MPA plus blood, blood alone, or the vehicle associated with corticosteroid; two joints of each horse therefore received MPA. The author concluded that repeated injections did not have any direct toxic effects on the articular cartilage and that injection of the vehicle did not alter the articular structures. However, evaluation methods were not well described. Levels of MPA were still elevated in the joint 47 days after a single injection. White deposits were also noted in the synovial membrane of all MPA-injected joints.

In a second study, eight mature horses with no prior signs of joint disease or history of intraarticular therapy were treated with eight weekly intraarticular injections of MPA.[5] Treatments were given at a dose of 120 mg/joint into the antebrachiocarpal (radiocarpal) and middle carpal (intercarpal) joints, with the left joints used as untreated controls. There were no gross differences, but chondrocyte necrosis and hypocellularity were observed, and the rates of proteoglycan and collagen synthesis were reduced in MPA-injected joints. After eight weekly injections, the proteoglycan content of the articular cartilage was reduced to 56.52% of the control values, and the proteoglycan content decreased further at 4- and 8-week recovery periods to 40.77 and 35.17% of the control values, respectively. The rate of proteoglycan synthesis as measured by ^{35}SO$_4$ uptake was reduced to 17.04% of the control values after the last injection. Four and 8 weeks later, the rates of synthesis increased to 55.31 and 71.28% of the control values, respectively, indicating a positive response. The authors asked whether cartilage that had lost 50% of its proteoglycan would be vulnerable to breakdown with exercise. The doses used in this study are high, and with both joints injected, they become particularly high.

In a third study, we injected 100 mg MPA three times at 2-weekly intervals into the middle carpal joints of four normal horses, and tissues were collected 2 weeks after the last injection.[48] Horses remained clinically normal during the study, and no significant radiographic changes were observed. However, safranin O matrix staining intensity and uronic acid content were significantly lower in the treated joints. Articular cartilage fibrillation was not evident in any joints. The latter two studies did show, however, that some regressive changes occurred to normal equine articular cartilage when 6α-MPA was used.

MPA has also been evaluated using equine osteochondral fracture models.[9,11,31] Synovitis is a common feature of all of these. Meagher created large osteochondral fractures of the distal aspect of the radial carpal bone bilaterally in five horses, using arthrotomy; another horse was used as a nonoperated control. Fragments were 1 cm wide and 2.5 cm long, which is more like a slab fracture. Three weeks later these horses were galloped for 4.5 to 5 miles by chasing them around a pasture in a pickup truck. One middle carpal joint received 120 mg of MPA; the other one was an untreated control. The first injection was given 3 weeks after surgery, and injections were repeated every 2 weeks for four injections. Horses were galloped from the 22nd day until the 78th day. Changes occurred, including cartilage erosion and periarticular proliferation in the nontreated joints (probably related to instability or arthrotomy), with change being more severe in the joints injected with MPA. This study was considered to confirm previous statements that adequate rest is required after injection of intraarticular corticosteroids.

Most recently, we have reevaluated the effects of intraarticularly administered MPA in exercised horses with our arthroscopic carpal osteochondral fragmentation model. Eighteen horses were randomly assigned to one of three groups (six horses in each group). An osteochondral chip fragment was created in one randomly chosen middle carpal joint of each horse. Both middle carpal joints in the placebo-control group (CNT) horses were injected intraarticularly (IA) with a polyionic fluid. The MPA-control group horses (MPA CNT) were injected with 100 mg of MPA IA in the middle carpal joint without an osteochondral fragment, and the opposite middle carpal joint was injected with a similar volume of polyionic fluid. The MPA-treated group horses (MPA TX) were treated with 100 mg of MPA IA in the joint that contained the osteochondral fragment, and the opposite middle carpal joint was injected with a single volume of polyionic fluid. All horses were treated IA on days 14 and 28 after surgery and exercised on a high-speed treadmill for 6 weeks, starting on day 15 after surgery.

In this experiment there was no significant clinical improvement in the degree of lameness associated with MPA administration. The lack of significant reduction of joint pain (manifested by lameness) was in contrast to our previous work with triamcinolone acetonide (TA) and also with anecdotal reports of decreased lameness associated with the clinical use of MPA. Joints that contained an osteochondral fragment and were treated with MPA had lower prostaglandin E_2 concentrations in the synovial fluid and lower scores for intimal hyperplasia and vascularity (there was no effect on cellular infiltration) in synovial membrane than placebo-treated joints. However, other parameters observed postmortem and evaluated in the articular cartilage (histologic and histochemical evaluation of articular cartilage GAG content and rate of GAG synthesis) suggested possible deleterious effects of intraarticular MPA administration compared with controls.

There was lower synovial fluid volume in 10 of 12 MPA-treated joints, independent of fragmentation. These findings are compatible with anecdotal clinical reports of "red, dry joints" in association with MPA administration and are in contrast to results with intraarticular administration of TA in which similar color or volume changes were not seen. There was also a higher color score attributable to MPA plus fragmentation. Synovial fluid protein concentration was higher in fragmented joints, but on day 72 after surgery, all joints from horses receiving MPA treatment had significantly more total protein in the synovial fluid than nonfragmented joints in the control group horses. Fragmented joints from MPA-control group horses had higher total protein concentrations in the synovial fluid than did fragmented joints or control group horses, suggesting that MPA administration in a nonfragmented joint increased protein concentration, compared with saline administration, and this also is in contrast to the decreased protein levels in synovial fluid after TA administration.

Significantly higher GAG concentration was seen in the synovial fluid from joints injected directly with MPA, and this was considered to be a direct result of MPA administration. GAG synthesis in the articular cartilage decreased under the influence of MPA, so it was felt that increased fluid GAG levels were most likely resulting from increased degradation of GAG in the articular cartilage. Increased HA levels were also associated with MPA administration, which has also been reported after administration of other corticosteroids.[12] In addition, all joints receiving MPA treatment had significantly poorer modified Mankin scores on histologic evaluation, illustrating the deleterious effect of intraarticular administration of MPA on articular cartilage. This is again in contrast to the lack of deleterious effects with betamethasone[9] and the improvement in Mankin scores associated with TA administration.[10] Although a significant loss of safranin O–fast green (SOFG) staining is observed in nonfragmented joints treated with MPA, compared with the contralateral joints, no differences between joints were observed in the MPA-treated or control groups, and there was poor correlation between SOFG staining and biochemical analysis of the GAG content of the articular cartilage. Recent studies question the accuracy of SOFG staining in assessing the GAG content of the articular cartilage,[12] and we feel that the results of SOFG staining need to be interpreted with caution.

Biochemical analysis of the total articular cartilage GAG content did not reveal a detrimental effect with MPA treatment. However, cartilage from joints opposite those receiving MPA had significantly higher GAG content than either contralateral joints or joints from the control group horses. This suggests that there may be a beneficial remote effect on GAG content of cartilage associated with MPA administration. Similar remote effects were seen with TA. Although total articular cartilage GAG content was not adversely affected by MPA administration, GAG synthesis on day 72 after surgery was lower in MPA-treated joints than in joints from control horses, suggesting a direct negative effect on articular cartilage GAG synthesis associated with MPA treatment. This is in contrast to previous data following TA administration, which showed no negative effects on the rate of GAG synthesis, but is consistent with previous in vitro and in vivo studies.

In conclusion, there was no significant clinical improvement in lameness associated with MPA, although there was a decrease in PGE$_2$ levels in the synovial fluid and lower synovial membrane vascularity and intimal hyperplasia scores. On the other hand, there were deleterious effects on articular cartilage with direct administration of MPA, with possible deleterious effects associated with MPA in the contralateral joint. These findings are in contrast to the positive effects seen when TA was assessed using the same model but are consistent with previous studies in which MPA was administered intraarticularly in normal and abnormal joints. Our studies further confirm the potential detrimental effects of MPA in articular cartilage in horses. More recently, the effect of intraarticular MPA on the biomechanical properties of articular cartilage has been evaluated.[32a] Eight 2-year-old horses had MPA or 2.5 mL of pH-adjusted polyethylene glycol, sodium chloride, and Myristyl-γ-picolinium chloride. They were injected at 14-day intervals for a total of four treatments per horse (100 mg MPA each time). Horses underwent a standard treadmill exercise protocol until euthanasia at day 70. There were significant differences demonstrated between intrinsic material properties and thickness of the cartilage between MPA-treated and diluent-treated joints. Diluent-treated cartilage had a 97% increase in compressive stiffness modulus, was 121% more permeable, and had an 88% increase in shear modulus compared with MPA-treated articular cartilage. Diluent-treated cartilage was also 24% thicker than MPA-treated cartilage. These findings indicate that repetitive intraarticular administration of MPA to exercising horses alters the mechanical integrity of articular cartilage, which could lead to early cartilage degeneration.

In another study, the effect of MPA was tested in joints that also had lipopolysaccharide-induced synovitis. Intraarticular MPA alone was associated with decreased proteoglycan synthesis and increased protein and collagen synthesis in the articular cartilage. Total protein synthesis by synovial membrane was also increased by MPA alone. In contrast, no differences in protein or proteoglycan synthesis were observed in explants from the joints with synovitis, with or without intraarticular MPA. The results suggested that the effect of intraarticular MPA on joint metabolism differed in inflamed and normal joints. The authors also suggested caution in interpretation of in vitro culture results when investigating the effect of intraarticular corticosteroids on chondrocyte function.[46a] Caron et al. showed that MPA inhibited the stimulation of MMP-13 expression by rhIL-1α.[4a]

We have recently done an in vitro study with cartilage explants to try to determine a minimally effective dose for MPA. A traditional dose in a carpal joint, for instance, has been 100 mg. Our hypothesis was that we could perhaps inject considerably less MPA and still have the same effect. Clinical reports from equine veterinarians confirm that they indeed do get clinical responses with lower doses. However, in our in vitro study using human recombinant IL-1 with equine cartilage explants, we needed a dose equivalent to 100 mg to achieve effective suppression of IL-1–mediated degradation in the cartilage. We plan to do this work again with our newly acquired equine IL-1.

In the meantime, we need to be cautious with the use of MPA. We should try to use as low a dose as possible and be well aware of the deleterious side effects. Personally, I prefer using betamethasone or TA (described below).

Betamethasone

Using an osteochondral fragment–exercise model that we developed, we evaluated betamethasone esters. Osteochondral fragments were created arthroscopically on the distal aspect of both antebrachiocarpal bones in 12 horses to evaluate the effects of intraarticular betamethasone with and without exercise.[9,11] One middle carpal joint of each horse was injected with 2.5 mL of betamethasone 14 days after surgery, and the procedure was repeated at 35 days. The opposite joint was injected with 2.5 mL of saline as a control. Six of the horses were maintained in box stalls throughout the study as nonexercised controls, and six were exercised 5 days per week on a high-speed treadmill with a regimen of 2 minutes trot, 2 minutes gallop, 2 minutes trot. Three weeks after the second injection, horses were clinically examined for lameness and synovial effusion, radiographs were taken, and the horses were euthanized.

Mild lameness was seen in all horses in the exercised group at the end of the study. Four of these were lame in the saline-injected limb, one in the corticosteroid-treated limb, and one had bilateral lameness. Of the five nonexercised horses evaluated for lameness (one horse was removed from the study), two were lame in the saline-injected joint, two in the steroid-treated limb, and one was sound. No differences between the steroid-treated limbs and the control limbs in either exercise group were noted on radiographs or on palpation. Firm reattachment of the osteochondral fragment was seen in all but three joints. Gross articular cartilage damage subjectively seemed worse in the exercised horses, but steroid- and saline-treated joints of the same horse did not differ. The results of histologic examination showed no consistent detrimental effects of betamethasone, with or without exercise. Histochemical staining showed a decrease in GAGs in the steroid-treated limbs of rested horses, although the decrease was not significant at $P < .05$. The exercised horses had similar levels of GAGs in treated and control joints. Chemical assays showed no significant difference in water content or uronic acid concentration (a measure of GAG content) of the treated and control joints. The use of betamethasone in this carpal chip model showed no consistent detrimental effects in either rested or exercised horses. This was our first evaluation of an intraarticular corticosteroid using our arthroscopic fragmentation–exercise model. At that stage our laboratory was not doing good biochemical analyses of GAG content or GAG synthetic rate. In subsequent experiments, we have modified our fragmentation (to increase the severity of synovitis and decrease the tendency for healing of the fragment) and also are evaluating the articular cartilage by more sophisticated means.

This paper also addressed the question of whether exercise after corticosteroid injection causes significant deleterious effects on articular cartilage, at least in the short term. It showed that exercise did not harm articular cartilage exposed to betamethasone. It implied that there may be considerable differences in metabolic responses of articular cartilage to the various corticosteroids used routinely and also pointed out that no evaluation of therapeutic dose (in the way of dose titration studies) has ever been done with any of the intraarticular corticosteroids used in the horse.[29]

Triamcinolone Acetonide

Our work with TA suggests that it may indeed be chondroprotective in the horse.[11] In this study 18 horses were trained on a high-speed treadmill and then had an osteochondral fragment created at the distal aspect of the radial carpal bone of one randomly chosen midcarpal joint. Six horses were treated with intraarticular injection of polyionic fluid in both middle carpal joints (CNT), six horses were treated with 12 mg TA intraarticularly in the middle carpal joint without an osteochondral fragment (the opposite midcarpal joint was treated intraarticularly with a similar volume of polyionic fluid [TA CNT]), six horses were treated with 12 mg TA in the joint that contained the osteochondral fragment (the opposite middle carpal joint was treated intraarticularly with a similar volume of polyionic fluid) (TA TX). TA and placebo treatments were repeated on days 13 and 27 after surgery, and treadmill exercise proceeded 5 days per week, beginning on day 14 and ending on day 72. Clinical examinations were performed at the beginning and end of the study. Synovial fluid samples were obtained from the joints on days 0, 14, 21, 28, 35, and 72 and analyzed for total protein, nucleated cell counts, HA levels, GAG, and PGE_2. Euthanasia was done on day 72, and synovial membrane samples were taken and assessed histologically. Articular cartilage samples were aseptically collected to determine GAG content of the cartilage as well as GAG synthetic rate. A split plot with repeated measures design was used as the statistical model, and a multivariant analysis of variance was performed to determine statistical significance of both main and interaction effects of independent variables.

Horses that were treated intraarticularly with TA in a joint containing a fragment (TA TX) were less lame than horses in the CNT and TA CNT groups. Horses treated with TA in either joint had lower protein and higher HA and GAG concentrations in synovial fluid. Synovial membrane from CNT and TA CNT horses had less inflammatory cell infiltration, intimal hyperplasia, and subintimal fibrosis. Articular cartilage morphologic parameters evaluated with a standardized scoring system were significantly better from TA CNT and TA TX groups, irrespective of which joint received TA. There was less staining with SOFG in the TA CNT group than in either the TA TX group or the CNT group, although the GAG synthetic rate was higher in the TA CNT group than in the other two groups.

In conclusion, the results from this study supported favorable effects of TA on the severity of clinically detectable lameness and on synovial fluid, synovial membrane, and articular cartilage morphologic parameters, both with direct intraarticular administration and remote site administration, compared with effects of placebo treatments. The beneficial effects were recorded in both synovial membrane morphologic and biochemical articular cartilage parameters. Increased HA concentrations were observed in TA-treated joints, which also suggests a favorable corticosteroid effect on synoviocyte metabolism. This research supports a chondroprotective effect of corticosteroids in a controlled model of OA and is in marked contrast to the detrimental effects of corticosteroids seen in in vivo osteochondral fragment models in which MPA was used.

The same study assessed the effect of TA on dynamics of bone remodeling and fragility.[20] Third carpal bones from joints with fragments showed significantly more vascularity, single-labeled surface, and total labeled surface of mineralizing surface in subchondral and subjacent trabecular bone. Trends were also seen toward high vascular canal volume and osteochondral junction remodeling sites in third carpal bones from fragmented joints. No significant differences were seen in microdamage density or size of fragmented and nonfragmented joints. No significant influence of TA treatment was seen on any parameter measured. The results from this study show that osteochondral fragmentation induces significant changes in remodeling of opposing bone and that administration of corticosteroids into joints with fragmentation does not significantly alter bone remodeling or fragility. This information is particularly useful in view of the extrapolation from human clinical work that has suggested that intraarticular corticosteroids in horses may cause osteoporosis in the adjacent bone.

In summary, the critical evaluation of intraarticular TA administration in this study revealed no substantial detrimental effects and some chondroprotective effects on joint tissues.

Clinical Impressions

There have also been some clinical reports questioning the extent of the deleterious effects of corticosteroids. McKay and Milne looked at Thoroughbreds that received intraarticular corticosteroids on the racetrack.[30] No conclusive evidence of corticosteroid arthropathy in racehorses was seen when there was no prior radiographic evidence of osseous changes in the joint. In a review of case records by Owen in which the intraarticular injection of a corticosteroid had been considered to result in arthropathy, all subjects had evidence of prior osseous changes in the joint, including three cases of carpal chip fractures, two of osselets, one of a proximal first phalanx chip fracture, and one of a fractured tuber scapulae in the shoulder.[35] This author pointed out that the term "Charcot's arthropathy" in humans was sometimes used incorrectly to describe corticosteroid-induced arthropathy. Unfortunately, the lay public has been told that corticosteroids purely inhibit pain and therefore permit horses to continue to run and to degenerate their joints. It would seem that the beneficial effects of corticosteroids go far beyond being painkillers. Some of the beneficial effects in clinical practice have been outlined by Genovese.[13]

References

1. Anon. Abstracts of medical literature. JAMA 1958;173:2302.
2. Axelrod L. Glucocorticoids. In: Harris ED, Kelley WN, Ruddy S, Sledge CB, Eds. Textbook of Rheumatology. 4th ed. Philadelphia: WB Saunders, 1993;779.
3. Bertone AL, Carter BG, Weisbrode SE, et al. Influence of steroid suppression on more and less weightbearing osteochondral defects in equine tarsocrural joints. Proc Vet Orthop Soc 1993;20:8.
4. Bombardieri S, Cattani P, Ciabattoni G, et al. The synovial prostaglandin system in chronic inflammatory arthritis: Differential effects of steroidal and nonsteroidal anti-inflammatory drugs. Br J Pharmacol 1981;73:893–901.
4a. Caron JP, Tardiff G, Martel-Pelletier J, et al. Modulation of matrix metalloproteinase 13/collagenase 3 gene expression in equine chondrocytes by interleukin 1 and corticosteroids. Am J Vet Res 1996;57:1631–1634.
5. Chunekamrai S, Krook L, Lust G, et al. Changes in articular cartilage after intra-articular injections of methylprednisolone acetate in horses. Am J Vet Res 1989;50:1733–1741.
6. Clements PJ, Paulus HE. Nonsteroidal anti-inflammatory drugs (NSAIDs). In: Kelley WN, Harris ED, Ruddy S, Sledge CB, Eds. Textbook of Rheumatology. 4th ed. Philadelphia: WB Saunders, 1993;700.
7. DiRosa M. Role in inflammation of glucocorticoid-induced phospholipase inhibitory proteins. Prog Biochem Pharmacol 1985;20:55–62.
8. Firestein GS, Paine MM, Littman BH. Gene expression (collagenase, tissue inhibitor of metalloproteinases, complement, and HLA-DR) in rheumatoid arthritis and osteoarthritis synovium. Arthritis Rheum 1991;34:1094–1105.
9. Foland JW, McIlwraith CW, Trotter GW, et al. Effect of betamethasone and exercise on equine carpal joints with osteochondral fragments. Vet Surg 1994;23(5):369–376.
10. Frisbie DD, Kawcak CE, Baxter GM, et al. The effects of 6-alpha-methylprednisolone acetate on an equine osteochondral fragment exercise model. Am J Vet Res 1998;59(12):1619–1628.
11. Frisbie D, Kawcak CS, McIlwraith CW, et al. Unpublished data, 1995.
12. Frisbie DD, Kawcak CE, Trotter GW, et al. Effects of triamcinolone acetonide on an *in vivo* osteochondral fragment exercise model. Equine Vet J 1997;29:349–359.
13. Genovese RL. The use of corticosteroids in racetrack practice. In: Proceedings. Symposium on Effective Use of Corticosteroids in Veterinary Practice. Princeton, NJ: ER Squibb, 1983;56–65.
14. Gray RG, Gottlieb NL. Intra-articular corticosteroids: An updated assessment. Clin Orthop 1983;177:235–263.
15. Gray RG, Tenenbaum J, Gottlieb NL. Local corticosteroid injection treatment in rheumatic disorders. Semin Arthritis Rheum 1981;10:231–254.
16. Hamilton JA, Bootes A, Phillips PE, et al. Human synovial fibroblast plasminogen activator. Modulation of enzyme activity by anti-inflammatory steroids. Arthritis Rheum 1981;24:1296–1303.
17. Higuchi M, Masuda T, Susuda K, et al. Ultrastructure of the articular cartilage after systemic administration of hydrocortisone in the rabbit: An electron microscope study. Clin Orthop 1980;152:296–302.
18. Houdeshell JW. Field trials of a new long acting corticosteroid in the treatment of equine arthropathies. VM/SAC 1969;64:782–784.
19. Houdeshell JW. The effect of a corticosteroid combination on blood and synovial fluid in horses. VM/SAC 1970;65:963–966.
20. Kawcak CE, Norrdin RW, Frisbie DD, et al. Effects of osteochondral fragmentation and intra-articular triamcinolone acetonide treatment on subchondral bone in the equine carpus. Equine Vet J 1998;30:66–71.
21. LaPointe MC, Baxter JD. Molecular biology of glucocorticoid hormone action. In: Schleimer RP, Claman HN, Oronsky AL, Eds. Anti-inflammatory Steroid Action: Basic and Clinical Aspects. San Diego: Academic Press, 1989;3.
22. Lees P, Higgins AJ. Influence of betamethasone on the composition of inflammatory exudate in the horse: A preliminary report. Equine Vet J 1984;16:539–541.
23. Lees P, Higgins AJ, Sedgwick AD, et al. Actions of betamethasone in models of acute nonimmune inflammation. Br Vet J 1987;143:143–158.
24. Mankin HJ, Conger KA. The effect of cortisol on articular cartilage of rabbits. I. Effect of a single dose of cortisol on glycine-C14 incorporation. Lab Invest 1966;15:794–800.
25. Mankin HJ, Conger KA. The acute effects of intra-articular hydrocortisone on articular cartilage in rabbits. J Bone Joint Surg [Am] 1966;48:1383–1388.
26. Marcoux M. The effects of methylprednisolone and blood on equine articular structures. Proc Am Assoc Equine Pract 1977;23:333–341.
27. May SA, Hooke RE, Lees P. The effect of drugs used in the treatment of osteoarthrosis on stromelysin (proteoglycanase) of equine synovial cell origin. Equine Vet J 1988;S6:28–32.
28. McGuire MB, Murphy G, Reynolds JJ, et al. Production of collagenase and inhibitor hydrocortisone and indomethacin. Clin Sci 1981;61:703–710.
29. McIlwraith CW. The usefulness and side effects of intra-articular corticosteroids—What do we know? Proceedings. 38th Annual Meeting of the American Association of Equine Practitioners, Orlando, FL, 1992;21–30.
30. McKay AG, Milne FJ. Observations of the intra-articular use of corticosteroids in the racing Thoroughbred. J Am Vet Med Assoc 1976;168:1039–1041.
31. Meagher DM. The effects of intra-articular corticosteroids and continued training on carpal chip fractures of horses. Proc Am Assoc Equine Pract 1970;16:405–412.
32. Munck A, Guyre PM. Anti-inflammatory steroid action: Basic and clinical aspects. San Diego: Academic Press, 1989;30–47.
32a. Murray RC, deBowes RM, Gaughan EM, et al. The effects of intra-articular methylprednisolone and exercise on the mechanical properties of articular cartilage in the horse. Osteoarthritis Cartilage 1998;6:106–114.
33. Nelson A, Conn D. Glucocorticoids in rheumatic disease. Mayo Clin Proc 1980;55:758–769.
34. O'Conner JT. The untoward effects of the corticosteroids in equine practice. J Am Vet Med Assoc 1968;153:1614–1617.
35. Owen R, Ap R. Intra-articular corticosteroid therapy in horses. J Am Vet Med Assoc 1980;177:710–713.
36. Roneus B, Lindblad A, Lindholm A, et al. Effects of intra-articular corticosteroid and sodium hyaluronate injections on synovial fluid production and synovial fluid content of sodium hyaluronate and proteoglycans in normal equine joints. Zentralbl Veterinarmed A 1993;40:10–16.
37. Russo-Marie F, Duval D. Prostaglandin Synthetase Inhibitors: New Clinical Applications. New York: Alan R. Liss, 1980;13–29.
38. Shaw NE, Lacey E. The influence of corticosteroids on normal and papain-treated articular cartilage in the rabbit. J Bone Joint Surg [Br] 1973;55:197–205.
39. Shoemaker RS, Bertone AL, Martin GS, et al. Effects of intra-articular administration of methylprednisolone acetate on normal articular cartilage and on healing of experimentally induced osteochondral defects in horses. Am J Vet Res 1992;53:1446–1453.
40. Silberberg M, Silberberg R, Hasler M. Fine structure of articular cartilage in mice receiving cortisone acetate. Arch Pathol 1966;82:569–582.
41. Silberman M, Lewinson D, Toister Z. Early cartilage response to systemic glucocorticoid administration: An ultrastructural study. Metab Bone Dis Relat Res 1980;2:267–279.
42. Smith TJ. Glucocorticoid regulation of glycosaminoglycan synthesis in cultured human skin fibroblasts: Evidence for a receptor-mediated mechanism involving effects on specific de novo protein synthesis. Metabolism 1988;37:179–184.
43. Sternberg EM, Wilder RL. Corticosteroids. In: McCarty DJ, Koopman WJ, Eds. Arthritis and Allied Conditions. 12th ed. Philadelphia: Lea & Febiger, 1993;665.
44. Swanstrom OG, Dawson HA. Intra-articular Betasone and Depo-Medrol: A comparative study. Proc Am Assoc Equine Pract 1974;20:249–254.
45. Tobin T. Steroidal-anti-inflammatory agents: The corticosteroids and ACTH. In: Tobin T, Ed. Drugs and the Performance Horse. Springfield, IL: Charles C Thomas, 1981;132–148.

46. Todhunter RJ, Fubini SL, Lust G. *In vitro* dose-response study on effect of methylprednisolone acetate (Depo-Medrol) on proteoglycan metabolism in equine articular cartilage. Vet Surg 1993; 22:402.

46a. Todhunter RJ, Fubini SL, Veriner-Singer M, et al. Acute synovitis and intra-articular methylprednisolone acetate in ponies. Osteoarthritis Cartilage 1998;6:94–105.

47. Trotter GW. Intra-articular corticosteroids. In: McIlwraith CW, Trotter GW, Eds. Joint Disease in the Horse. Philadelphia: WB Saunders, 1996;237–256.

48. Trotter GW, McIlwraith CW, Yovich JV, et al. Effects of intra-articular administration of methylprednisolone acetate on normal equine articular cartilage. Am J Vet Res 1991;52:83–87.

49. Tsurufuji S, Ohuchi K. *In vivo* models of inflammation: A review with special reference to the mechanisms of action of glucocorticoids. In: Schleimer RP, Claman HN, Oronsky AL, Eds. Anti-inflammatory Steroid Action: Basic and Clinical Aspects. San Diego: Academic Press, 1989;259.

50. Tulamo R-M. Comparison of high-performance liquid chromatography with a radiometric assay for determination of the effect of intra-articular administration of corticosteroid and saline solution on synovial hyaluronate concentration in horses.

51. Van Pelt RW. Clinical and synovial fluid response to intra-articular synovial injection of 6α-methylprednisolone acetate into horses and cattle. J Am Vet Med Assoc 1963;143:738–748.

52. Van Pelt RW. Intra-articular injection of 6α-methyl, 17 α-hydroxyprogesterone acetate in tarsal hydrarthrosis (bog spavin) in the horse. J Am Vet Med Assoc 1967;151:1159–1171.

53. Van Pelt RW, Riley WF. Tarsal hydrarthrosis in the horse: Response to intra-articular injection of synthetic steroids. Can Vet J 1969;10:130–135.

54. Van Pelt RW, Tillotson PJ, Gertsen KE. Intra-articular injection of betamethasone in arthritis in horses. J Am Vet Med Assoc 1970;156:1589–1599.

55. Van Pelt RW, Tillotson PJ, Gertsen KE, et al. Effects of intra-articular injection of flumethasone suspension in joint diseases of horses. J Am Vet Med Assoc 1971;159:739–753.

56. Van Pelt RW, Tillotson PJ, Gertsen KE, et al. Effects of intra-articular flumethasone suspension on synovial effusion enzyme activity of arthritic horses. J Am Vet Med Assoc 1972;160:186–190.

57. Vernimb GD, Van Hoose LM, Hennessey PW. Onset and duration of corticosteroid effect after injection of Betasone for treating equine arthropathies. Vet Med Small Anim Clin 1977;72:241–244.

58. Weiss MM. Corticosteroids in rheumatoid arthritis. Semin Arthritis Rheum 1989;19:9–21.

59. Wheat JD. The use of hydrocortisone in the treatment of joint and tendon disorders in large animals. J Am Vet Med Assoc 1955;127:64–67.

60. Zurier RB. Prostaglandins, leukotrienes, and related compounds. In: Kelley WN, Harris Ed, Ruddy S, Sledge CB, Eds. Textbook of Rheumatology. 4th ed. Philadelphia: WB Saunders, 1993; 201.

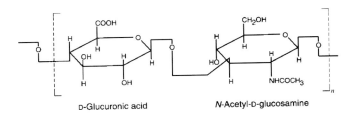

Figure 7.23 Molecular structure of the hyaluronic acid disaccharide. (Reprinted with permission from McIlwraith CW, Trotter GW, Eds. Joint Disease in the Horse. Philadelphia: WB Saunders, 1996, Fig 15-1.)

MEDICATIONS FOR JOINT DISEASE: SODIUM HYALURONATE (HYALURONAN)

Hyaluronic acid (hyaluronan) is a linear polydisaccharide and polyionic nonsulfated GAG. The disaccharide units are linked by 1–4 glycosidic bonds to form a long, unbranched chain consisting of 10,000 to 12,000 disaccharide units[9,11] forming particles of widely varying size (Fig. 7.23). Under physiologic conditions, hyaluronic acid is anionic and associated with monovalent cations. It has been suggested that when the cation of a polysaccharide is undetermined, the compound is properly referred to as hyaluronan (HA).[11] Estimates of molecular mass vary and depend on the source of the compound, the method of isolation, and the method used for determination. Studies in humans and animals have determined the molecular mass of synovial fluid HA to be 2 to 6 million daltons.[12] Concentration of synovial fluid HA varies between species and between joints of an individual, with the smaller joints generally exhibiting a higher concentration.[6,51] The various methods used in the determination of equine synovial fluid HA concentration have resulted in a range of normal values. Values for normal equine synovial fluid have fallen into the range of 0.33 to 1.5 mg/mL, depending on the investigator and the technique used. The wide range of reported values indicates that comparison of absolute values between studies is impossible.

Synthesis and Function of Endogenous Hyaluronate

HA is an integral component of both synovial fluid and articular cartilage in normal synovial joints. Synovial fluid HA is synthesized by the synoviocyte of the synovial membrane. HA that is incorporated in the extracellular matrix of articular cartilage is synthesized locally by the chondrocyte. HA is removed from the joint via the lymphatic system. Once in the peripheral circulation, HA is rapidly taken up, primarily by the liver, and degraded by endothelial cells of the hepatic sinusoids.[11,18] It has been shown recently that in addition to the liver, the articular tissues are capable of local degradation of HA; however, no degradation is apparent within the joint cavity.[43]

HA confers viscoelasticity to synovial fluid, and this viscoelasticity is proportional to, and dependent upon, the concentration and degree of polymerization of HA in the fluid.[29,34] HA is responsible for boundary lubrication of the synovial membrane and was recently shown to be a significant factor in the lubrication of articular cartilage.[57,66] HA may also influence the composition of synovial fluid through steric hindrance of active plasma components and leukocytes from the joint cavity.[47] Solutions containing HA have the ability to exclude solutes and particles from the solution in proportion to the size of the particle, concentration, and molecular weight of the HA in solution.[17,47] Solutions containing HA may also modulate the chemotactic response within the extracellular fluid of connective tissues through reduction of cell migration[20] and reduced rates of perfusion and flow of solutes.[48]

A molecule of HA is the nucleus of the proteoglycan aggregates (aggrecan) in the extracellular matrix of articular cartilage. It is believed that the compressive stiffness in articular cartilage depends on the integrity of the matrical proteoglycans.[23]

Possible Mechanism of Action of Exogenous Sodium Hyaluronate

Beneficial effects after intraarticular administration of HA have been reported in a number of equine studies[16,24,38,53,58–61,67,72] as well as studies in other animals. The mechanism by which beneficial effects have been achieved remains controversial. The therapeutic effect(s) of exogenously administered HA may result from supplementation of the actions of depleted or depolymerized endogenous HA or, alternatively, result from other properties that have been ascribed to HA on the basis of experimental work, including modulation of increased synthesis of endogenous HA. The mechanisms by which HA has been hypothesized to benefit diseased joints are varied and highly speculative.

Alterations in synovial fluid HA concentration and molecular weight in various pathologic states have been described but the results are somewhat conflicting. Generally there is a reduction in synovial HA concentration and molecular weight with equine joint disease. The concentration has been reported to be lower in horses with traumatic arthritis.[35] On the other hand, in another study, synovial fluid from equine joints with acute traumatic synovitis did not differ significantly in HA concentration from fluid from normal joints.[62] In a third study, there was no significant difference in the concentration of synovial fluid HA between normal equine joints and those with acute or chronic arthritis; however, joints with septic arthritis and those with radiographic evidence of OA had lower concentrations than controls.[71] The molecular weight of synovial fluid HA from nonclinical equine joints and that from joints with acute or chronic arthritis did not differ significantly.

The mechanisms by which HA has been hypothesized to benefit diseased joints have been varied and highly speculative. It has not been determined what concentration or degree of polymerization of HA is necessary for effective intraarticular soft tissue lubrication. In one study using a synovial membrane assay to evaluate the ability of various solutions containing HA to lubricate soft tissues, synovial fluid from human rheumatoid arthritis patients had lubricating properties similar to those of normal bovine synovial fluid.[66] The half-life of exogenous intraarticular HA injected into normal equine joints has been estimated to be 96 hours.[36] The half-life of exogenously administered HA is lower in diseased joints. In a sheep experimental model the half-life was reduced from 20.8 hours in normal joints to 11.5 hours in arthritic joints.[21] However, although most exogenously administered HA is rapidly cleared from the joint, a proportion remains associated with synovial tissues.[44] It has been suggested that some of the exogenous HA and its breakdown products localize in the intercellular space surrounding the synoviocytes, influencing the metabolic activity of these cells.[26] The mechanism by which exogenous HA produces clinical benefit beyond its presence in the joint is of great interest.

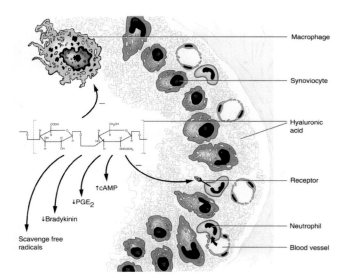

Figure 7.24 Potential anti-inflammatory effects of hyaluronan. These include steric inclusion of plasma components and white blood cells from the synovial fluid, inhibition of macrophage chemotaxis and phagocytosis, inhibition of neutrophil function through interaction with a cell surface membrane receptor, scavenging of free radicals, reduction of the levels of bradykinin and prostaglandin (PG)E2, and an increase in cAMP levels. (Reprinted with permission from McIlwraith CW, Trotter GW, Eds. Joint Disease in the Horse. Philadelphia: WB Saunders, 1996, Fig 15-4.)

Other effects of exogenous HA have been identified experimentally. Anti-inflammatory effects have been demonstrated in a number of in vitro studies and include an inhibition of chemotaxis of granulocytes and macrophages and migration of lymphocytes, as well as reduction of phagocytosis by granulocytes and macrophages (Fig. 7.24).[8,13,14,19,26,32,33,49,55,70] It has been suggested that the anti-inflammatory effect of HA is the result of reduced interaction of enzymes, antigens, or cytokines with target cells through steric hindrance.[18,20,48,55] Recent evidence suggests that reduced chemotaxis and phagocytosis of activated neutrophils are mediated through the interaction of HA with the CD44 cell receptors of neutrophils.[68] HA inhibited neutrophil-mediated degradation in a concentration- and molecular weight–dependent fashion, and it has been shown to be effective in reducing the production of PGE_2 by IL-1–stimulated rabbit chondrocytes.[4,68] In a controlled clinical trial in human arthritic patients, HA treatment reduced synovial fluid levels of PGE_2 and elevated levels of cyclic AMP.[56] These studies suggest that the anti-inflammatory properties of HA may be attributable in part to its ability to reduce production of soluble inflammatory mediators and to augment signal transduction pathways. The proliferation of rabbit synovial cells in culture was inhibited by the addition of HA to the culture medium. This effect depended markedly on the molecular weight and concentration of HA. At the molecular weight and concentration of HA present in normal synovial fluid, proliferation was inhibited. At lower molecular weights or concentrations, as found in rheumatoid synovial fluid, HA was significantly less inhibitory.

Thus, changes in synovial fluid HA associated with arthropathies may contribute to a favorable environment for rheumatoid pannus expansion.[31]

Recently, a commercial preparation of 800-kDa HA (Artz, Seikagaku Inc.) was tested in an in vitro cartilage chondrolytic system. The HA was effective in blocking the ability of a fibronectin fragment to cause cartilage degradation and release of half of the total cartilage PG from cartilage, and this was associated with a decreased concentration of fibronectin fragment on the superficial cartilage surface and decreased penetration into the cultured cartilage tissue. The blocking activity appeared to be associated with the ability of HA to block penetration of the fibronectin fragment rather than with direct effects on cartilage tissue.[37] In a study evaluating the value of HA in a canine stifle immobilization model, it was found that the immunolocalization of TNF-α was absent or greatly reduced in articular cartilage of the injected stifle along with increased retention of proteoglycan histochemical staining. Immunoreactivity of TNF receptors was similar to that of TNF-α. In this study the pattern of distribution of stromelysin in regions where proteoglycans were degraded supported the role of stromelysin in the destruction of proteoglycans in atrophic articular cartilage.[41a]

Effect of Molecular Weight

It has been stated repeatedly that injection of HA into a pathologic joint results in increased synthesis of high-molecular-weight endogenous HA by synoviocytes.[38,59,61,69] Many of these authors reached this conclusion on the basis of a hypothesis by Asheim and Lindblad in 1976[5] and opinions expressed by Balazs.[15] A direct effect on HA synthesis was not clearly demonstrated, however. A later in vitro study demonstrated that HA at a molecular weight above 5×10^2 kDa stimulated the synthesis of hyaluronate in a concentration-dependent manner. However, HA preparations with a molecular weight below 5×10^2 kDa had little or no effect except at high concentrations, when HA synthesis was depressed.[65] In a more recent study on the influence of exogenous HA on the synthesis of HA and collagenase by equine synoviocytes (monolayer culture), it was found that exogenous HA influenced neither the rate of synthesis nor the hydrodynamic size of the newly produced HA by control or principal cell cultures. The authors concluded that the principal mechanism of action of HA did not appear to be stimulation of HA synthesis or augmented molecular weight or marked inhibition of collagenase synthesis.[45a] Exposure of synoviocytes from normal and diseased joints to a number of commercial HA preparations failed to influence endogenous HA biosynthetic activity significantly and, at higher concentrations, stimulated collagenase synthesis significantly. This study provided some objective evidence that HA in the extracellular environment may modulate the synthesis of HA by synoviocytes. Whether these in vitro effects occur in vivo has not been clearly demonstrated. It is also possible that normalization of synovial fluid HA concentration and molecular weight may occur secondarily as a result of other benefits derived from the exogenous HA therapy rather than through direct pharmacologic effects.

Direct Effects on Cartilage Healing

It is doubtful that exogenous HA has any direct effect on articular cartilage. There is decreased proteoglycan aggregation in articular cartilage with OA (and proteoglycan aggregation is mediated by a link protein to an HA backbone), and various investigators have demonstrated in vitro that addition of HA to a medium of disaggregated proteoglycan subunits results in aggregation.[14a] In view of these findings, some authors have theorized that one of the benefits of intraarticular HA lies in its ability to increase proteoglycan aggregation in articular cartilage. However, there are no convincing data to support proteoglycan-aggregating effects of exogenous HA in hyaline cartilage in vivo. If one considers the molecular size of pharmaceutical HA, it would seem unlikely that exogenous HA would gain access to the cell membrane of the chondrocyte. Exogenously administered HA has been shown to interact with proteoglycans and the chondrocyte cell surface via the HA binding domain of the proteoglycan molecule.

There have been no demonstrated direct effects on intact articular cartilage. However, in vitro studies have demonstrated that high concentrations of HA suppress IL-1α– and TNF-α–induced release of $^{35}SO_4$ proteoglycans from chondrocytes in culture.[42,64] The influence of intraarticularly injected high-molecular-weight HA on the healing of superficial and deep lesions of the articular cartilage in an experimental animal model has been investigated.[73] The HA injections appeared to have no effect, either positive or negative, on the healing of intracartilaginous and osteochondral joint lesions. However, the positive effects of high-molecular-weight HA on experimentally induced cartilage degeneration have been recognized. In one study using a partial meniscectomy of OA in the rabbit knee, high-molecular-weight HA injected intraarticularly twice a week, starting immediately after surgery, inhibited cartilage degeneration in both the femoral condyle and the tibial plateau. High-molecular-weight HA offered better protection than a lower-molecular-weight product and, therefore, showed that at least in the rabbit model, intraarticular high-molecular-weight HA was more effective than lower-molecular-weight HA in inhibiting cartilage degeneration and early OA.[41]

Clinical Use of Hyaluronan

The first report of the clinical use of HA for intraarticular treatment of equine joint disease was published in 1970[61], in which traumatic degenerative equine arthritis was treated with MPA or an HA/MPA combination in 20 racing Thoroughbreds and Standardbreds. The investigators concluded that the combination of HA and MPA resulted in better and more lasting improvement than the corticosteroid alone. In 1976, Asheim and Lindblad provided the first report of treatment of equine traumatic arthritis with intraarticular HA alone, in 54 joints of 45 racehorses previously treated unsuccessfully by conventional means. Through a 1-year observation period, 38 of 45 horses were free of lameness, and 32 returned to the racetrack after treatment.[5] Since these early reports, numerous clinical and experimental studies have been conducted to evaluate the efficacy of HA in the treatment of equine joint disease.[14,19,21,24,30,36,38,44,50,53,59,67,72] Clinical reports have generally supported the use of HA, but in many of them, the evaluations are subjective and the definitions of criteria for successful treatment are absent. The duration of posttreatment observation periods vary, and some studies were of short duration. Most studies include response to intraarticular anesthesia as a criterion for case selection, which helps in localizing the problem but provides little information about the specific diagnosis. A number of studies state or imply that the condition treated was OA, but the criteria for OA were not presented. It would seem that many of the cases were synovitis and/or capsulitis rather than OA.

Attempts have been made to assess the clinical response to HA therapy in the horse more objectively.[30,43] In a model using bilateral osteochondral fractures created by arthrotomy, the authors concluded that HA had a protective effect on the articular cartilage and resulted in reduced lameness. However, the conclusion that HA treatment was responsible for the return to normal weight-bearing is suspect, since both treated and non-treated limbs returned to presurgical weight-bearing values. The effectiveness of intraarticular hylan, a derivative of HA modified by cross-linking, was evaluated in a double-blind study that used gait analysis.[50] In this study, treatment with hylan did not significantly alter any of those variables, compared with baseline or control values, and the conclusion was that at least in this model of acute synovitis (amphotericin), there was no beneficial effect.

A chondroprotective effect for HA was reported based on a study involving experimentally induced arthritis in dogs.[1,63] However, treatment with HA has been reported to result in exacerbation of histologic, biochemical, and gross morphologic changes associated with OA experimentally induced in sheep by medial meniscectomy.[27,28] Treatment with HA improved weight-bearing and resulted in a lower gross pathologic score for OA but a higher score for osteophytosis and a higher histologic score for OA as well as reduced proteoglycan content. One of the arguments espoused by proponents of the use of HA has been its actions of physiologic therapeutic modality in the treatment of joint disease, allowing rapid return to athletic function without the risk of deleterious effects that have been associated with some other treatments. This notion of safety has been challenged, and the sheep meniscectomy study demonstrates that rapid return to function may not be an appropriate goal in every case.

Controversy exists concerning the relationship between molecular weight of exogenous HA and the clinical efficacy of treatment in equine joint disease. Certain advantages have been claimed in promotional material for products of higher molecular weight.[46] Although many of the in vitro effects of HA have been shown to be enhanced with higher-molecular-weight HA (including inhibition of fibroblast proliferation, inhibition of phagocytosis, enhanced synthesis of HA by cultured synoviocytes, and inhibition of PGE_2 production by IL-1–stimulated chondrocytes),[12,13,20,32,49,65] the correlation between molecular weight and clinical effect is less clear. In a comparative study of five sodium hyaluronate products in the treatment of traumatic arthritis in horses,

horses treated with HA of molecular weight above 2×10^3 kDa stayed sound significantly longer than those treated with HA below 2×10^3 kDa.[54] In another blinded study, the clinical effects of sodium hyaluronates with molecular weights of 0.13×10^3 and 2.88×10^3 kDa were compared in the treatment of 69 racing Thoroughbreds with carpitis. There were no clinically significant differences in the response to the two drugs, questioning whether the molecular weight of administered HA had any effect on therapeutic response.[7] The posttreatment observation period in this study was 2 weeks; therefore, the duration of effect was not evaluated.

Recently, a randomized, double-blind, and placebo-controlled clinical study was carried out in Standardbred trotters. Seventy-seven trotters with moderate-to-severe lameness were grouped according to number of affected joints and, within each group, were randomized for treatment with PSGAG, HA, or placebo for 3 weeks. The horses were inspected weekly, with final examination 2 to 4 weeks after the end of treatment. The mean and initial lameness scores were significantly reduced during treatment and at the last examination in all three groups ($P < .01$).[25] Additionally, the prevalence of sound horses increased significantly from 1 to 3 weeks of treatment and to the last examination in all three groups ($P < .03$). Comparison of the two treatment groups with regard to the development of the lameness curve and time until soundness indicated a small, nonsignificant difference in favor of HA. No significant difference was detected between the two treatment groups in prevalence or cumulative incidence of soundness. The study found the two drugs to be better than placebo in reduction of lameness score during the treatment period ($P = .03$) and the total study period ($P < .01$), time until soundness ($P = .04$), and prevalence of sound horses at the last examination ($P < .01$). All three treatments affected traumatic arthritis in horses, but HA and PSGAG gave better results than placebo.

Viscosupplementation

It has been known for many years that synovial fluid from osteoarthritic joints has lower elasticity and viscosity than that from normal joints and that the decrease in rheologic properties of synovial fluid results from reduction in molecular size and concentration of HA in the synovial fluid.[3,12] This phenomenon led Balazs to introduce viscosupplementation therapy, which is the injection of HA or its derivative in an attempt to return the elasticity and viscosity of the synovial fluid to normal or higher levels.[10,52] Viscosupplementation with HA has been used as a specific therapeutic technique in OA, especially in Italy and Japan. However, 6 to 10 injections are often required to achieve efficacy. Suggested reasons for this have included that the elastoviscous properties of current HA preparations are inadequate to restore the elasticity and viscosity of the synovial fluid in the arthritic knee sufficiently or that the injected HA is eliminated from the joint too quickly to be effective.[3]

Because of this limitation in viscosupplementation with conventional HA preparations, hylans (chemically cross-linked hyaluronans) were developed to improve the efficacy of viscosupplementation therapy of OA. Cross-linked HA improves its utility for viscosupplementation in several ways: 1) the rheologic properties are increased; 2) it has a longer retention time in the synovial space; and 3) because of the cross-links, it becomes more resistant to free radical production. One particular combination of hylan, G-F20 (Synvisc) has been developed specifically as a device for viscosupplementation therapy in OA of the knee. In a Canadian multicenter trial of human OA, patients treated with Synvisc had a response equaling that to NSAIDs (without the consequent side effects).[3] The results of four clinical trials in Germany also validated the efficacy and safety of Synvisc.[2] In another, more recent study in Canada, 1537 injections were performed in 336 patients involving 458 knees.[45] The overall response and the change of activity level were judged better or much better for 77 and 76% of the treated knees after the first course of treatment (three weekly injections) and 87 and 84% after a second course. The mean time elapsing between the first and second course (8.2 ± 0.5 months) is an evaluation of the duration of benefits. Local adverse events were observed in 28 patients (32 knees), with an overall rate of 2.7% adverse events per injection. The adverse events were characterized by pain and/or transient swelling in the injected joint, mostly mild or moderate in intensity. The conclusion was that Synvisc provided good clinical benefit and an acceptable safety profile in current clinical practice. The occurrence of adverse events after an intraarticular injection is infrequent and unpredictable. Hylan G-F20 is a cross-linked HA preparation with an average molecular weight over 6 million. Purified human umbilical hyaluronate and a commercial preparation of HA (Healon) intended for intraarticular viscosupplementation did not demonstrate the same boundary-lubricating ability as bovine synovial fluid or purified lubricin. The data did show that HA possesses some boundary-lubricating ability in excess of that produced by physiologic saline alone but could not replicate the boundary lubrication provided by synovial mucin. This study also supported earlier observations of an interaction between lubricin and HA, however.[39]

As mentioned above, a double-blind study with amphotericin-induced synovitis was done in the middle carpal joint of horses. The response to treatment with hylan was compared with that in untreated horses using 3-D motion analysis, synovial fluid analysis, and synovial histologic examination. Treatment with hylan did not significantly alter any of these variables, compared with baseline control values. When one considers where hylan has been used in humans compared with an acute synovitis model in the horse, it may be that viscosupplementation is more appropriate for OA.

Intravenous Hyaluronan

A formulation of HA for intravenous administration has been developed for use in horses and has been licensed for several years. It is given as a 40-mg (4-mL) intravenous injection and goes under the trade name of Legend in the United States and Hyonate everywhere else. Anecdotal information from personal communication with veterinarians and from personal experience suggests efficacy. However, data from a controlled study have only recently become available. A controlled investigation of intravenously administered HA was done

using an osteochondral fragmentation model of equine arthritis.[40] Osteochondral fragments were created unilaterally on the distal aspect of the radial carpal bone of 12 horses, and the horses were subjected to a controlled program of exercise using a high-speed treadmill. Six horses were treated with 40 mg of sodium hyaluronate intravenously on days 13, 20, and 27 after osteochondral fragmentation, and six control horses were similarly treated with physiologic saline. Horses treated with HA intravenously had lower lameness scores (i.e., were less lame), significantly better synovial membrane histologic scores (cellular infiltration and vascularity), and significantly lower concentrations of total protein and PGE_2 in synovial fluid 72 days after surgery than placebo-treated horses. Treatment with IV-administered HA had no significant effects on GAG synthetic rate or morphologic scores in articular cartilage (i.e., no deleterious effects occurred with HA treatment), and synovial fluid HA levels did not change.

The mechanism by which intravenously administered HA achieves therapeutic levels intraarticularly is uncertain. Assuming that the plasma clearance of HA in the horse is similar to that in rabbits,[34] it must be assumed that the beneficial effects seen in the experimental study are associated with localization of HA (or part of the molecule) at the synovial membrane level. The synovial membrane of the horse is highly vascularized, and perhaps intravenous administration provides the synoviocyte with more exposure to exogenous HA than intraarticular administration. A possible mechanism of action is illustrated in Figure 7.24. HA receptors are not confined to connective tissue cells. There are three main groups of HA cell receptors identified to date: CD 44, RHAMM, and ICAM-1. Some have yet to be classified, and the first and third of these were already known as cell adhesion molecules with other recognized ligands before their HA binding was discovered.[22] CD44 is a multipurpose receptor that is widely distributed in the body, and recent studies in our laboratory have shown expression of this receptor on equine synoviocytes, neutrophils, and lymphocytes. Although there is low expression of CD44 receptors on chondrocytes in normal cartilage, we have shown increased expression in osteoarthritic equine chondrocytes.

Intravenous HA has achieved widespread use clinically in the United States. It has been used as a direct therapeutic agent as well as on a prophylactic basis. A prospective blinded study was done in 1996 to evaluate the effects of regular injections of intravenous HA at 2-weekly intervals.[31a] Seventy horses were treated from May 1 to December 1, and 70 horses received placebo (racing Quarter Horses). Positive trends were noted, but the hypothesis that prophylactic use of HA would cut down the amount of other medication was not proven.

References

1. Abatangelo G, Botti P, Delbue M, et al. Intra-articular sodium hyaluronate injections in the Pond-Nuki experimental model of osteoarthritis in dogs. I. Biochemical results. Clin Orthop 1989; 241:278–285.
2. Adams ME. An analysis of clinical studies of the use of crosslinked hyaluronan, hylan, in the treatment of osteoarthritis. J Rheumatol Suppl 1993;39:16–18.
3. Adams ME, Atkinson MH, Lussier AJ, et al. The role of viscosupplementation with hylan G-F20 (Synvisc®) in the treatment of

osteoarthritis of the knee: A Canadian multicenter trial comparing hylan G-F20 alone, hylan G-F20 with nonsteroidal anti-inflammatory drugs (NSAIDs) and NSAIDs alone. Osteoarthritis Cartilage 1995;3:213–226.

4. Akatsuka M, Yamamoto Y, Tobetto K, et al. *In vitro* effects of hyaluronan on prostaglandin E_2 induction by interleukin-1 in rabbit articular chondrocytes. Agents Actions 1993;38:122–125.

5. Asheim A, Lindblad G. Intra-articular treatment of arthritis in racehorses with sodium hyaluronate. Acta Vet Scand 1976;17: 379–394.

6. Auer JA, Fackelman GE, Gingerich DA, Fetter AW. Effect of hyaluronic acid in naturally occurring and experimental osteoarthritis. Am J Vet Res 1980;41:568–574.

7. Aviad AD, Arthur RM, Brencick VA, et al. Sinacid vs Hylartin-V in equine joint disease. Equine Vet Sci 1988;8:112–116.

8. Balazs EA, Darzynkiewiez Z. The effect of hyaluronic acid on fibroblasts, mononuclear phagocytes and lymphocytes. In: Kulonen E, Pikkarainen JPKK, Eds. Biology of Fibroblasts. London: Academic Press, 1973;237.

9. Balazs EA, Denlinger JL. The role of hyaluronic acid in arthritis and its therapeutic use. In: Peyron JG, Ed. Osteoarthritis in current clinical and fundamental problems. Paris: Ciba Geigy, 1984; 165–174.

10. Belazs EA, Denlinger JL. Viscosupplementation: A new concept in the treatment of osteoarthritis. J Rheumatol 1993(S39);20:3–9.

11. Balazs EA, Laurent TC. Nomenclature of hyaluronic acid. Biochem J 1986;235:903.

12. Balazs EA, Watson D, Duff IF, Roseman S. Hyaluronic acid in synovial fluid. I. Molecular parameters of hyaluronic acid in normal and arthritic human synovial fluid. Arthritis Rheum 1967; 10:357–376.

13. Brandt KD. Modification of chemotaxis by synovial fluid hyaluronate [abstract]. Arthritis Rheum 1970;13:308.

14. Brandt KD. The effect of synovial fluid hyaluronate on the ingestion of monosodium urate crystals by leukocytes. Clin Chem Acta 1974;55:307–315.

14a. Brandt KD, Palmoski MJ, Perricone E. Aggregation of cartilage proteoglycans. II. Evidence for the presence of a hyaluronate-binding region on proteoglycans from osteoarthritic cartilage. Arthritis Rheum 1976;19:1308.

15. Burkhardt D, Ghosh P. Laboratory evaluation of anti-arthritic drugs as potential chondroprotective agents. Semin Arthritis Rheum 1987;17:3–34.

16. Cannon JH. Clinical evaluation of intra-articular sodium hyaluronate in the Thoroughbred horse. Equine Vet Sci 1985;5:147–148.

17. Comper WD, Laurent TC. Physiological function of connective tissue polysaccharides. Physiol Rev 1978;58:255–315.

18. Eriksson S, Fraser JRE, Laurent TC, et al. Endothelial cells are a site of uptake and degradation of hyaluronic acid in the liver. Exp Cell Res 1983;144:223–228.

19. Forrester JB, Balazs EA. Inhibition of phagocytosis by high molecular weight hyaluronate. Immunology 1980;40:435–446.

20. Forrester JV, Wilkinson PC. Inhibition of leukocyte locomotion by hyaluronic acid. J Cell Sci 1981;48:315–330.

21. Fraser JR, Kimpton WG, Pierscionek BK, Cahill RNP. The kinetics in normal and acutely inflamed synovial joints: Observations with experimental arthritis in sheep. Semin Arthritis Rheum 1993;22:9–17.

22. Fraser JRE, Laurent TC. Hyaluronan. In: Comper WD, Ed. Extracellular Matrix, vol 2, Molecular Components and Interactions. The Netherlands: Harwood Academic Publishers, 1996; 141–199.

23. Freeman MAR, Kempson GE. Load carriage. In: Freeman MAR, Ed. Adult Articular Cartilage. New York: Grune & Stratton, 1972;228–246.

24. Galley RH. The use of hyaluronic acid in the racehorse. Proc Am Assoc Equine Pract 1986;32:657–661.

25. Gaustad G, Larsen S. Comparison of polysulfated glycosaminoglycan and sodium hyaluronate with placebo in treatment of traumatic arthritis in horses. Equine Vet J 1995;27:356–362.

26. Ghosh P. Osteoarthritis and hyaluronan—palliative or disease-modifying treatment? Semin Arthritis Rheum 1993;22:1–3.

27. Ghosh P, Read R, Armstrong S, et al. The effects of intra-articular administration of hyaluronan in a model of early osteoarthritis

in sheep. I. Gait analysis and radiological and morphological studies. Semin Arthritis Rheum 1993;22:18–30.

28. Ghosh P, Read R, Numata Y, et al. The effects of intra-articular administration of hyaluronan in a model of early osteoarthritis in sheep. II. Cartilage composition and proteoglycan metabolism. Semin Arthritis Rheum 1993;22:31–42.

29. Gibbs DA, Merrill EW, Smith KA. Rheology of hyaluronic acid. Biopolymers 1968;6:777–791.

30. Gingerich DA, Auer JA, Fackelman GE. Force plate studies on the effect of exogenous hyaluronic acid on joint function in equine arthritis. J Vet Pharmacol Ther 1979;2:291–298.

31. Goldberg RL, Toole BP. Hyaluronate inhibition of cell proliferation. Arthritis Rheum 1987;30:769–778.

31a. McIlwraith CW, Goodman NL, Frisbie DD. Prospective study in the prophylactic value of intravenous hyaluronan in two year old racing Quarter Horses. Proceedings. 44th Annual Meeting of the American Association of Equine Practitioners, Baltimore, MD, 1998;269–271.

32. Grecomoro G, Martorana U, DiMarco C. Intra-articular treatment with sodium hyaluronate in gonarthrosis: A controlled clinical trial versus placebo. Pharmatherapeutica 1987;5:137–141.

33. Hakansson L, Hallgren R, Benge P. Effect of hyaluronic acid on phagocytosis of opsonized latex particles. Scand J Immunol 1980; 11:649–653.

34. Hamerman D, Rojkind M, Sandson J. Protein bound to hyaluronate: Chemical and immunological studies. FASEB J 1966;25: 1040–1045.

35. Hilbert BJ, Rowley G, Antonas KN. Hyaluronic acid concentration in synovial fluid from normal and arthritic joints of horses. Aust Vet J 1984;61:22–24.

36. Hilbert BJ, Rowley G, Antonas KN, et al. Changes in the synovia after the intra-articular injection of sodium hyaluronate into normal horse joints and after arthrotomy and experimental cartilage damage. Aust Vet J 1985;62:182–184.

37. Homandberg GA, Hui F, Wen C, et al. Hyaluronic acid suppresses fibronectin fragment mediated cartilage chondrolysis: I. *In vitro*. Osteoarthritis Cartilage 1997;5:309–319.

38. Irwin DHG. Sodium hyaluronate in equine traumatic arthritis. J South Afr Vet Assoc 1980;50:231–233.

39. Jay GD, Haberstroh K, Cha C-J. Comparison of the boundary-lubricating ability of bovine synovial fluid, Lubricen and Healon. J Biomed Mater Res 1998;40:414–418.

40. Kawcak CE, Frisbie DD, Trotter GW, et al. Effects of intravenous administration of sodium hyaluronate on carpal joints in exercising horses after arthroscopic surgery and osteochondral fragmentation. Am J Vet Res 1997;58:1132–1140.

41. Kikuchi T, Yamada H, Shimmei M. Effect of high molecular weight hyaluronan on cartilage degeneration in a rabbit model of osteoarthritis. Osteoarthritis Cartilage 1996;4:99–110.

41a. Kincaid SA, Kurkendall JA, Beard AR, Kammerman JR. Influence of hyaluronate on regulators and products of articular chondrocyte metabolism. In: Hyaluronic Acid Workshop. Kansas City, MO: Bayer, 1995;54–63.

42. Larsen NE, Lombard KM, Parent E, Balazs EA. Effect of hylan on cartilage and chondrocyte cultures. J Orthop Res 1992;10: 23–32.

43. Laurent UB, Fraser JR, Laurent-Engstrom A, et al. Catabolism of hyaluronan in the knee joint of the rabbit. Matrix 1992;12: 130–136.

44. Laurent UBG, Fraser JRE, Engstrom-Laurent A, et al. Catabolism of hyaluronan in the knee joint of the rabbit. Matrix 1992;12: 130–136.

45. Lussier A, Cibidino AA, McFarlane CA, et al. Viscosupplementation with hylan for the treatment of osteoarthritis: Findings from clinical practice in Canada. J Rheumatol 1996;23:1579–1585.

45a. Lynch TM, Caron JP, Arnoczky SP, et al. Influence of exogenous hyaluronan on synthesis of hyaluronan and collagenase by equine synoviocytes. Am J Vet Res 1998;59:888–892.

46. McIlwraith CW. Intra-articular medication for traumatic joint problems: Do we understand the choices? Comp Cont Educ Pract Vet 1989;11:1287–1311.

47. Ogston AG, Phelps CF. The partition of solutes between buffer solutions and solutions containing hyaluronic acid. Biochem J 1960;78:827–833.

48. Ogston AG, Sherman TF. Effects of hyaluronic acid upon diffusion of solutes and flow of solvent. J Physiol 1961;156:67–74.
49. Partsch G, Schwarzer C, Neumuller J, et al. Modulation of the migration and chemotaxis of PMN cells for hyaluronic acid. Z Rheumatol 1989;48:123–128.
50. Peloso JG, Stick JA, Caron JP, et al. Effects of hylan on amphotericin-induced carpal lameness in equids. Am J Vet Res 1993;54:1527–1534.
51. Persson L. On the synovial in horses: A clinical and experimental study. Acta Vet Scand 1971;35:29–43.
52. Peyron JG. A new approach to the treatment of osteoarthritis: Viscosupplementation. Osteoarthritis Cartilage 1993;1:85–87.
53. Phillips MW. Intra-articular sodium hyaluronate in the horse: A clinical trial. Proc Am Assoc Equine Pract 1980;26:389–394.
54. Phillips MW. Clinical trial comparison of intra-articular sodium hyaluronate products in the horse. Equine Vet Sci 1989;9:39–40.
55. Pisko EJ, Turner RA, Soderstrom LP, et al. Inhibition of neutrophil phagocytosis and enzyme release by hyaluronic acid. Clin Exp Rheumatol 1983;1:41–44.
56. Punzi L, Schiavon F, Cavasin F, et al. The influence of intra-articular hyaluronic acid on PGE_2 and cAMP of synovial fluid. Clin Exp Rheumatol 1989;7:247–250.
57. Radin EL, Paul IL. A consolidated concept of joint lubrication. J Bone Joint Surg [Am] 1972;54:607–616.
58. Roneus B, Lindblad A, Lindholm A, Jones B. Effects of intra-articular corticosteroid and sodium hyaluronate injections on synovial fluid production and synovial fluid content of sodium hyaluronate and proteoglycans in normal equine joints. Zentralbl Veterinarmed A 1993;40:10–16.
59. Rose RJ. Intra-articular use of sodium hyaluronate for the treatment of osteoarthrosis in the horse. NZ Vet J 1979;27:528.
60. Ruth DT, Swites BJ. Comparison of the effectiveness of intra-articular hyaluronic acid and conventional therapy for the treatment of naturally occurring arthritic conditions in horses. Equine Pract 1985;7:25–29.
61. Rydell NV, Butler J, Balazs EA. Hyaluronic acid in synovial fluid. VI. Effect of intra-articular injection of hyaluronic acid on the clinical symptoms of arthritis in track horses. Acta Vet Scand 1970;11:139–155.
62. Saari H, Konttinen YT, Tulamo RM, et al. Concentration and degree of polymerization of hyaluronate in equine synovial fluid. Am J Vet Res 1989;50:2060–2063.
63. Schiavinato A, Lini E, Guidolin D, et al. Intra-articular sodium hyaluronate injections in the Pond-Nuki experimental model of osteoarthritis in dogs. II. Morphological findings. Clin Orthop 1989;241:286–299.
64. Shimazu A, Jikko A, Iwamato M, et al. Effects of hyaluronic acid on the release of proteoglycans from the cell matrix in rabbit chondrocyte cultures in the presence and absence of cytokines. Arthritis Rheum 1993;36:247–253.
65. Smith MM, Ghosh P. The synthesis of hyaluronic acid by human synovial fibroblasts is influenced by the extracellular environment. Rheumatol Int 1987;7:113–122.
66. Swann DA, Radin EL, Nazimiec M, et al. Role of hyaluronic acid in joint lubrication. Ann Rheum Dis 1974;33:318–326.
67. Swanstrom OG. Hyaluronate (hyaluronic acid) and its use. Proc Am Assoc Equine Pract 1978;24:345–348.
68. Tamoto K, Tada M, Shimada S, et al. Effects of high molecular weight hyaluronates on the functions of guinea pig polymorphonuclear leukocytes. Semin Arthritis Rheum 1993;22:4–8.
69. Tobetto K, Nakai K, Akatsuka M, et al. Inhibitory effects of hyaluronan on neutrophil-mediated cartilage degradation. Connect Tissue Res 1994;29:181–190.
70. Treadway WJ, Sederstrom LP, Turner RA, et al. The role of hyaluronic acid flux on modulation of neutrophil function. Arthritis Rheum Suppl 1981;24:94.
71. Tulamo RM, Heiskanen T, Salonen M. Concentration and molecular weight distribution of hyaluronate in synovial fluid from clinically normal horses and horses with diseased joints. Am J Vet Res 1994;55:710–715.
72. Vernon GT. Clinical successes and failures using a new hyaluronic acid—Synacid. Proc Am Assoc Equine Pract 1983;29:397–402.
73. Wygren A, Falk J, Wik O. The healing of cartilage injuries under the influence of joint immobilization and repeated hyaluronic acid injections. An experimental study. Acta Orthop Scand 1978;49:121–133.

MEDICATIONS FOR JOINT DISEASE: POLYSULFATED POLYSACCHARIDES

Polysulfated Glycosaminoglycan

Polysulfated GAG (PSGAG) belongs to a group of polysulfated polysaccharides and includes, in addition to Adequan, pentosan polysulfate (Cartrophen), and GAG (peptide complex [Rumalon]). This group has often been referred to as having chondroprotective properties (discussed above), and because of this, PSGAG has been traditionally used when cartilage damage is considered to be present rather than in the treatment of acute synovitis.[44] Using the new alternative terminology for chondroprotective drugs, PSGAG would now be referred to as a disease-modifying OA drug (DMOAD). Therapy with such drugs is meant to prevent, retard, or reverse the morphologic cartilaginous lesions of OA, with the major criterion for inclusion being prevention of cartilage destruction. Based on some work in the horse, this classification would seem to be valid.

Adequan is the commercially available PSGAG formulation in veterinary medicine, and Arteparon is the previously used human product. The chemical structure of the two products is identical, and only the concentration of the active ingredient varies.[60] The principal GAG present in PSGAG is chondroitin sulfate (Fig. 7.25). PSGAG is made from an extract of bovine lung and trachea modified by sulfate esterification.

Mechanism of Action

There have been numerous in vitro and in vivo studies of PSGAG.[2,7,60] PSGAG is a heparinoid. There have been varying opinions about binding of PSGAG in cartilage, but affinity for proteoglycans, collagen, and noncollagenous protein has been proposed.[2,6] PSGAG has been shown to inhibit the effects of various enzymes associated with cartilage degradation, including neutral metalloproteinases (both collagenase and stromelysin)[2,3,34,43] and serine proteinases,[39,57] as well as lysosomal elastase,[8,10] cathepsin B,[21] and cathepsin G,[8] and may also

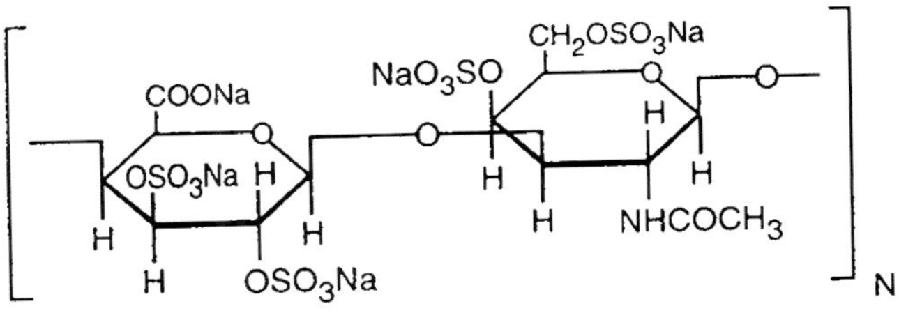

Figure 7.25 Structural formula of polysulfated glycosaminoglycan (PSGAG). This structure shows all hydroxyl groups, sulfated or esterified, but chemical analysis indicates sulfate substitution of 3 to 4 esters per disaccharide. (Reprinted with permission from McIlwraith CW, Trotter GW, Eds. Joint Disease in the Horse. Philadelphia: WB Saunders, 1996;270, Fig 16-1.)

influence synoviocyte metabolism.[38] PSGAG has also been shown to have a direct inhibitory effect on PGE_2 synthesis.[22] Some other work in which PSGAG reduced proteoglycan breakdown associated with conditioned synovial membrane suggests an anti–IL-1 effect.[26,37] In addition to antidegradative effects, PSGAG stimulates the synthesis of sodium hyaluronate both in vitro,[48,53] in vivo,[47,64] and in the horse.[14] However, increased HA content in synovial fluid has been seen in association with other intraarticular medications by our research group, and the significance is to be questioned. In addition, enhanced GAG synthesis has been demonstrated in vitro in association with PSGAG. In radioactive labeling studies,[1,32,63,65] it was demonstrated that both glucosamine (proteoglycan) and proline (collagen) had increased labeling after treatment of human osteoarthritic cartilage with PSGAG (this effect was less marked with normal human articular cartilage).[1]

In Vitro Equine Studies

In a study on equine synoviocytes stimulated to produce stromelysin (measured by the caseinase degradation assay), PSGAG was the only drug tested that inhibited stromelysin (others tested were phenylbutazone, flunixin, betamethasone, and sodium hyaluronate).[43]

There have been three in vitro studies on the effects of PSGAG on equine cartilage, and the results are somewhat contradictory. Initially it was reported that PSGAG caused increased collagen and GAG synthesis in both articular cartilage explants and cell cultures from normal and osteoarthritic equine articular cartilage.[27] The same author also reported that collagen and GAG degradation was inhibited by PSGAG in cell culture studies and also that osteoarthritic tissues were more sensitive to PSGAG than normal tissues. However, another investigator using smaller doses of PSGAG (50 and 200 μg/mL vs. 25 to 50 mg/mL) and normal equine articular cartilage explants found dose-dependent inhibition of proteoglycan synthesis, little effect on proteoglycan degradation, and no effect on proteoglycan monomer size.[15] In a following study using osteoarthritic equine articular cartilage explants and small (0.025 mg/mL) and large (25 mg/mL) doses of PSGAG, the same investigator found a decrease in proteoglycan synthesis, little effect on proteoglycan degradation, no change in the size of the proteoglycan monomer, and no change in the aggregability of the monomer.[16] Three nonequine in vitro studies and one equine study have shown decreased degradative effects of certain enzymes on articular cartilage in the presence of PSGAG.[3,34,35,43] However, the precise mechanisms of action of PSGAG are uncertain, and the interaction of PSGAG with cytokines involved in joint disease has not been well investigated.

In Vivo Studies

The earliest animal studies were not done in horses. Using a canine lateral meniscectomy model, Ueno demonstrated dramatic morphologic differences between articular cartilage from control and PSGAG-treated joints. PSGAG was given intramuscularly at 25 mg/kg for 13 treatments.[62] Later work with a canine meniscectomy model also showed a protective effect when PSGAG was administered subcutaneously.[32] These authors suggested that PSGAG likely acts by inhibiting matrix-degrading enzymes. Favorable effects (lower active neutral metalloproteinase activity, increased chondrocyte counts, and maintenance proteoglycan content) have also been reported using intraarticularly administered PSGAG in a meniscectomy model of OA in rabbits.[34,35] PSGAG has also been tested on the canine anterior cruciate ligament transection model and is reported to have both prophylactic and therapeutic effects.[4,5] PSGAG has been tested using the rat air pouch model of inflammation, and both improved proteoglycan content extractability and aggregation and reduction of leukocyte infiltration into the pouch were noted.[23] It was felt that reduced leukocyte infiltration would reduce cartilage exposure to leukocyte-derived proteinases and other mediators of cartilage damage. PSGAG was also tested in clinical cases of OA in boars (intramuscularly at 5.2 mg/kg for six treatments, and saline was put into control joints). Lameness was significantly decreased, and there was increased HA in the synovial fluid.[13] The drug has also been used in the treatment of canine hip dysplasia.[21]

The first equine investigation involved 250-mg injections of PSGAG intraarticularly twice weekly for 3 weeks and then once weekly for the next 3 weeks in clinical equine patients with joint swelling and lameness.[56] A significant improvement in synovial fluid protein concentration and synovial fluid viscosity was reported as well as an overall impression of improved clinical signs (lameness, swelling and effusion, and flexion). Intraarticular PSGAG was then tested using a Freund's adjuvant–induced model in the carpus of 30 horses. This study concluded that the clinical signs of arthritis were reduced in treated animals.[31] The latter investigators, in a clinical trial in 109 horses, also felt that PSGAG improved clinical signs more frequently than in untreated horses.

PSGAG was then tested in our laboratory on chemically induced and physically induced lesions in the horse.[61,67] Treatment with intraarticular injections of 250 mg of PSGAG once weekly for 5 weeks in carpal joints injected with sodium monoiodoacetate revealed less articular cartilage fibrillation and erosion, less chondrocyte death, and markedly improved safranin O staining. PSGAG, however, did not have any effect on physically induced lesions (partial and full thickness). Our conclusions from this study were that PSGAG could markedly decrease the development of OA but was of no benefit in healing cartilage lesions already present at the initiation of treatment. A second study using intramuscular PSGAG (500 mg every 4 days for seven treatments) showed relatively insignificant effects with treatment. The effects were limited to slightly improved safranin O staining in sodium monoiodoacetate joints when PSGAG was used.

More recent studies have evaluated the effects of PSGAG, with or without exercise, on the repair of articular cartilage defects and on the development of OA in the carpus of ponies.[58,59] The authors concluded that PSGAG was beneficial in ameliorating the clinical, radiographic, and scintigraphic signs of joint disease. In another study, the effects of both HA and PSGAG were evaluated in the repair of equine articular cartilage defects in ponies.[11] Neither drug showed any beneficial effects. However, the project was terminated 11 weeks after defect induction.

Potential Complications of Intraarticular Use

Intraarticular infection after intraarticular injection is always a potential risk. However, research has demonstrated that PSGAG may have greater potential in this regard. Potentiation of a subinfective dose of *Staphylococcus aureus* in the middle carpal joint of horses has been demonstrated in our laboratory.[29,30] Using a subinfective dose, infection occurred in eight of eight PSGAG-injected joints, whereas it occurred in only three horses that received intraarticular HA and four that received intraarticular MPA. This infection could be prevented by 125 mg of amikacin but was not abolished by prior filtration of Adequan. In another study, PSGAG was shown to inhibit equine complement activity.[50] The classical and ultimate complement pathways have bactericidal activity, and both were shown to be inhibited by PSGAG in vitro. This inhibition could be a factor in the ability of bacteria to induce septic arthritis.

Because PSGAG is classified as a heparinoid, some effect on the hemostatic mechanisms is expected.[12,20,28] Local hematomas were sometimes described as transient complications in early clinical trials in humans, and heparin-associated thrombocytopenia is known to occur with heparin use in people.[28] However, in earlier reports, the drug was used extensively in people, with a low complication rate. It has been suggested that the risk of hemarthrosis in humans is high.[12] It is therefore interesting that hemarthrosis has not been seen in the horse, despite extensive use. In addition, one of the author's primary uses of Adequan is following arthroscopic surgery in which there is considerable articular cartilage loss and subchondral bone exposure. These joints typically have persistent effusion that could be classified as hemarthrosis, and the use of intraarticular PSGAG seems to treat this condition quite effectively.

Intramuscular Use of PSGAG

Most Adequan is used intramuscularly. As discussed above, the positive effects seen with intraarticular PSGAG in the monoiodoacetate model could not be emulated by the intramuscular route. However, defects in this monoiodoacetate model have since been recognized. There is minimal objective data supporting effectiveness of intramuscular Adequan, but the drug is widely used, and anecdotal reports support its value. The issue of absorption after intramuscular injection was addressed by Burba et al.[14] In this study, PSGAG was labeled with tritium, and scintillation was done on synovial fluid and joint tissues. It was felt that levels of drug consistent with those seen in other nonequine studies were obtained, and it was concluded that therapy every 4 days was effective in maintaining antiinflammatory levels in the joint.

Clinical Use of PSGAG

I primarily use Adequan following surgery when there is significant loss of articular cartilage (grade III or grade IV damage). Typically, these horses have persistent bloody synovial effusion. The use of intraarticular Adequan has marked beneficial effects in these instances. I like to give one injection intraarticularly (I use 0.5 mL amikacin concurrently) and then follow up with intramuscular therapy at weekly intervals at a dose of 500 mg. The drug is also used to considerable extent on a prophylactic basis. Caron et al.[15a] did a survey of 1522 equine practitioner members of AAEP seeking information on Adequan use. Of practitioners responding, 90.5% reported use of PSGAG. Use of PSGAG was significantly more common by practitioners involved predominantly with racehorses or show horses. Standardbred racehorse practitioners had a significantly higher level of intraarticular use of Adequan. Overall, PSGAG was reported to be perceived as moderately effective for all four categories of joint disease: idiopathic synovitis, acute synovitis (with lameness), subacute OA (mild radiographic changes), and chronic OA (moderate-to-severe radiographic changes). PSGAG was considered more effective than HA for the treatment of subacute OA and less effective for idiopathic joint effusion and acute synovitis.

Pentosan Polysulfate

The use of this drug in the treatment of equine joint disease has been extensively reviewed recently.[40] Although pentosan polysulfate (PPS) as the sodium salt (NAPPS) has been used in Europe for over 30 years as an antithrombotic–antilipidemic agent, its potential as a disease-modifying antiarthritic agent has only been realized in recent years. Also, a new calcium derivative of PPS (CAPPS) has recently been developed that is absorbed more effectively after oral administration than NAPPS, and this offers hope for wider use of this drug. PPS could also be considered a disease-modifying OA drug. Little and Ghosh pointed out that PPS, unlike NSAIDs, does not possess analgesic activity.[40] Therefore, to provide symptomatic relief and efficacy, a drug such as PPS must be capable of correcting the pathobiologic imbalances that are present within the OA joint, and these authors feel that PPS fulfills these requirements.

PPS is not derived from animal or bacterial sources, but rather, the "backbone" of PPS is isolated from beechwood hemicellulose, which consists of repeating units of (1–4)-linked β-D-xylanopyranoses.[17] An anabolic effect on chondrocytes has been demonstrated in a focal model of OA induced by unilateral meniscectomy in sheep.[41] Studies on chondrocytes in agarose culture showed that PPS stimulated proteoglycan synthesis.[51] Also, in an experimental model of joint disease in rabbits, oral administration of CAPPS (10 mg/kg every 7 days) maintained the normal articular cartilage ratio of aggrecan to dermatan sulfate (interpreted by the authors as chondrocyte phenotype).[54] PPS also stimulates HA synthesis by cultured synoviocytes obtained from both rheumatoid and osteoarthritic joints.[36] These in vitro effects of PPS on HA synthesis were confirmed in a rat air pouch model of inflammation and in another study.[23,24]

A number of in vitro and in vivo studies have shown that PPS will inhibit various processes that induce degeneration of the articular cartilage matrix. For example, PPS has been shown to inhibit MMP3.[46] There is a suggestion that PPS may modulate receptor-mediated binding of cytokines.[40] In an ovine model of OA (medial meniscectomy), weekly intraarticular injections of PPS for 4 weeks improved joint function and reduced mean radiographic scores and Mankin histologic scores of articular cartilage damage in the femoral condyle.[25]

There are no published studies describing the application of PPS for equine joint disease, but the drug has been used in Australia. Anecdotally, treatment is considered to improve the clinical parameters of synovial effusion and lameness in most horses, when used clinically. Marked alleviation of lameness after racing was the most noted change with this drug.[40] It is also felt that the vascular effects of the drug could aid or decrease the rate of subchondral bone necrosis and sclerosis.

An interesting study involved simultaneous administration of NAPPS and IGF-1 early in the pathogenesis of iatrogenic canine OA. The combination of drugs significantly reduced the severity of lesions, whereas IGF-1 alone had little effect.[52] The presence of PPS appeared to decrease the amount of total and active metalloproteinase in the cartilage. The authors suggested that the PPS reduced the enzymatic breakdown of IGF-1, binding protein, or receptor, thus allowing IGF-1 to exert its influence.

Oral Glycosaminoglycans

Oral GAG products available for horses include a purified chondroitin sulfate product from bovine trachea (Flex-Free) and a complex of GAGs and other nutrients from the sea mussel *Perna canaliculus* (Syno-Flex). More recently, a combination of glucosamine hydrochloride, chondroitin sulfate, manganese, and vitamin C has been marketed as a "nutraceutical" (Cosequin). There have been some positive anecdotal reports for such supplements.[9,19,42,45,49] Cosequin has been evaluated using the Freund's adjuvant model of inflammatory joint disease in horses.[66] The oral supplement was used at the recommended dose beginning 10 days prior to arthritis induction and continuing for a further 26 days. No benefit was demonstrated based on clinical parameters (lameness, stride length, carpal circumference, carpal flexion) and synovial fluid analysis (protein). However, it is questionable whether the Freund's adjuvant model simulates any clinical equine joint entity, and one must question the value of studies using this model.

Oral administration of glucosamine sulfate has been associated with decreased pain and improved range of motion compared with placebo in a controlled clinical trial in humans.[49] In another controlled study, glucosamine sulfate was as effective as ibuprofen in relieving symptoms of OA in people.[45] In vitro studies using glucosamine sulfate have demonstrated increased GAG and proteoglycan synthesis, and in vivo studies have demonstrated anti-inflammatory activity through inhibition of lysosomal enzyme activity and free radical production.

There is conflicting evidence regarding the enteral absorption of orally administered GAGs.[9,18,19,42] The initial focus with oral GAGs was on chondroitin sulfate, and there has been some supportive evidence presented

for absorption of active molecules.[19,21] In interpretation of such studies, however, one has to be careful whether radiolabeled macromolecular sulfate or chondroitin sulfate or labeled but inactive monomer or other degradation products are being absorbed. It is not valid to extrapolate from antienzymic data (involving intact chondroitin sulfate molecules) and the detection of tritium label in tissues. Some earlier studies that failed to show absorption have been since criticized for the lack of specificity of the methods used. However, favorable absorption of chondroitin sulfate and dermatan sulfate from the gastrointestinal tract with reduced N-acetylglucosaminodase and granulocyte elastase activity as well as increased HA concentration in treated patients has been reported.[19] For instance, in another study, when chondroitin sulfate was administered to healthy human volunteers and serum concentrations of GAGs determined using the DMMB assay, it was reported that neither intact nor depolymerized chondroitin sulfate was effectively absorbed.[9] This paper was criticized for low dosage and the low sensitivity of the DMMB assay used.[42]

As mentioned in the section above, absorption of CAPPS after oral administration in rats has been reported as effective and high enough to maintain cartilage proteoglycan concentration and biosynthesis.[54] There was also some evidence for oral bioavailability of glucosamine sulfate and tropism for articular cartilage after oral administration.[45] The pharmacokinetics, organ distribution, metabolism, and excretion of glucosamine were studied in the dog using uniformly labeled [^{14}C]-glucosamine sulfate intravenously or orally in single doses. In humans, unlabeled glucosamine sulfate was given intravenously and orally, and glucosamine was measured in plasma and urine with a glucosamine-specific ion-exchange chromatographic method. The result showed that the bioavailability, pharmacokinetics, and excretion pattern of glucosamine were consistent with those found in the dog with radiolabeled glucosamine and with those reported in a previous study in the rat.[52a] In the dog study, radiolabeled glucosamine was given intravenously and orally, and the distribution of radioactivity was the same in both cases.

In one human study, cartilage biopsies were taken before and after 4 weeks of glucosamine sulfate oral supplementation in a few treated subjects as well as assessing the overall results clinically. Joint pain analgesic use was reduced and joint function improved with glucosamine sulfate administration. Electron microscopy showed a typical picture of established OA. Those given glucosamine sulfate were considered to show "a picture more similar to healthy cartilage."[49a] Exogenous glucosamine increases matrix production and seems likely to alter the natural history of OA. Glucosamine also has a mild anti-inflammatory activity, probably via a free radical scavenging effect.[49b] Numerous in vitro studies have demonstrated that glucosamine stimulates the synthesis of proteoglycan and collagen by chondrocytes.[36a]

An additional mechanism by which chondroitin sulfate may benefit joint tissues is the prevention of fibrin thrombi in synovial or subchondral microvasculature. The antisynovitis effect may be significant. It is interesting that in a study with extract of *Perna canaliculus* in humans, at the end of 6 months, 19 of the 28 rheumatoid patients (67.9%) and 15 of the 38 osteoarthritic patients (39.5%) felt they had benefited from the treatment.[26a] However, other studies have questioned both the GAG content and the therapeutic value of this extract.

There is better evidence for glucosamine absorption than for chondroitin sulfate absorption. Glucosamine is an amino monosaccharide that is a basic constituent of the disaccharide units of GAGs of articular cartilage.[51] Glucosamine is the hexosamine present in keratan sulfate and is the precursor of D-galactosamine (the hexosamine in chondroitin sulfate).[60] Exogenous glucosamine has been suggested as the preferred substrate for GAG synthesis because a higher energy expenditure is required with endogenous glucose.[51] There is good evidence for effective absorption of glucosamine sulfate (up to 87%) after oral administration in humans. In vitro studies have also documented enhanced chondrocyte synthesis of GAGs and collagen by glucosamine. Although research mainly documents the effects of glucosamine as the sulfate salt, the veterinary product contains glucosamine hydrochloride.

New oral GAG/glucosamine products continue to be developed. There is quite an explosive market in both humans and horses, despite very little scientific validation. A controlled study is needed to address the effectiveness of these oral GAG-type products and to evaluate their efficacy relative to other systemically administered products such as Adequan.

A clinical trial was conducted in 25 horses over a 6-week period. In this study, Cosequin was associated with decreased lameness, improved lameness, and improved lameness scores, but there were no controls.[33]

References

1. Adam M, Krabcova M, Musilova J, et al. Contribution to the mode of action of glycosaminoglycan-polysulfate (GAGPS) upon human osteoarthritic cartilage. Arzneimittelforschung 1980;30:1730–1732.
2. Altman RD, Dean DD, Muniz O, et al. Therapeutic treatment of osteoarthritis with glycosaminoglycan polysulfuric acid ester. Arthritis Rheum 1989;32:1300–1307.
3. Altman RD, Dean DD, Muniz O, et al. Prophylactic treatment of canine osteoarthritis with glycosaminoglycan polysulfuric acid ester [abstract]. Arthritis Rheum 1989;32:759–766.
4. Deleted in proof.
5. Altman RD, Kapila P, Dean DD, et al. Future therapeutic trends in osteoarthritis. Scand J Rheumatol 1989;S77:37–42.
6. Andrews JL, Sutherland J, Ghosh P. Distribution and binding of glycosaminoglycan polysulfate to intervertebral disc, knee joint cartilage and meniscus. Arzneimittelforschung 1985;35:144–148.
7. Annefeld M. The effect of chondroprotective substances (GAGPS) on articular cartilage of the rat. Therapiewoche 1984;34:3476–3481.
8. Baici A, Fehr K. Inhibition of human lysosomal elastase by Arteparon. In: Dettmer N, Greiling H, Eds. International Drug Symposium, Arteparon. IXth European Congress of Rheumatology, Wiesbaden. Basle: Eular Publishers, 1982;19.
9. Baici A, Horler D, Moser B, et al. Analysis of glycosaminoglycans in human serum after oral administration of chondroitin sulfate. Rheumatol Int 1992;12:81–88.
10. Baici A, Salgam P, Fehr K, et al. Inhibition of human elastase from polymorphonuclear leukocytes by a glycosaminoglycan polysulfate (Arteparon). Biochem Pharmacol 1980;29:1723–1727.
11. Barr ARS, Duance VC, Wotton SF, et al. Influence of intra-articular sodium hyaluronate and polysulphated glycosaminoglycans on the biochemical composition of equine articular surface repair tissue. Equine Vet J 1994;26:40–42.
12. Bauer F, Schulz P, Reber G, et al. Anticoagulant properties of three mucopolysaccharides used in rheumatology. Thromb Haemost 1983;50:652–655.
13. Brennan JJ, Aherne F, Nakano T. Effects of glycosaminoglycan polysulfate treatment on soundness, hyaluronic acid content of synovial fluid and proteoglycan aggregate in articular cartilage of lame boars. Can J Vet Res 1987;51:394–398.
14. Burba DJ, Collier M. In vivo kinetic study on uptake and distribution of intramuscular tritium-labeled polysulfated glycosaminoglycan in equine synovial fluid and articular cartilage [abstract]. Proc Am Assoc Equine Pract 1991;37:241–242.
15. Caron JP, Eberhart SW, Nachreiner R. Influence of polysulfated glycosaminoglycan on equine articular cartilage in explant culture. Am J Vet Res 1991;52:1622–1625.
15a. Caron JP, Kaneene JB, Miller R. Results of a survey of equine practitioners on the use and perceived efficacy of polysulfated glycosaminoglycan. Am J Vet Res 1996;209:1564–1568.
16. Caron JP, Toppin DS, Block JA. Effect of polysulfated glycosaminoglycan on osteoarthritic equine articular cartilage in explant culture. Am J Vet Res 1993;54:1116–1121.
17. Collier S, Ghosh P. Evaluation of the effect of antiarthritic drugs on the secretion of proteoglycans by lapine chondrocytes using a novel assay procedure. Ann Rheum Dis 1989;48:372–381.
18. Conte A, Volpi N, Palmiera L, et al. Biochemical and pharmacokinetic aspects of oral treatment with chondroitin sulfate. Arzneimittelforschung 1995;45:918–925.
19. Conte A, DeBernardi M, Palmieri L, et al. Metabolic fate of exogenous chondroitin sulfate in man. Arzneimittelforschung 1991;41:768–772.
20. DeHaan JJ, Beale BS, Clemmons RM, et al. The effects of polysulfated glycosaminoglycan (Adequan®) on activated partial thromboplastin time, prothrombin time, complete blood count, biochemical profile and urinalysis in cats. Vet Compar Orthop Traumatol 1994;7:77–81.
21. DeHaan JJ, Goring R, Beale BS. Evaluation of polysulfated glycosaminoglycan for the treatment of hip dysplasia in dogs. Vet Surg 1994;23:177–181.
22. Dietmar EGG. Effects of glycosaminoglycan-polysulfate and two nonsteroidal anti-inflammatory drugs on prostaglandin E_2 synthesis in Chinese hamster ovary cell cultures. Pharmacol Res Commun 1983;15:709–717.
23. Francis DJ, Forrest MJ, Brooks PM, et al. Retardation of articular cartilage degradation by glycosaminoglycan polysulfate, pentosan polysulfate, and DH-40J in the rat air pouch model. Arthritis Rheum 1989;32:608–616.
24. Francis DJ, Hutadilok N, Kongtawelert P, et al. Pentosan polysulfate and glycosaminoglycan polysulfate stimulates synthesis of hyaluronan in vivo. Rheumatol Int 1993;13:61–64.
25. Ghosh P, Armstrong S, Read R, et al. Animal models of early osteoarthritis: Their use for the evaluation of potential chondroprotective agents. In: Van den Berg WB, van der Kraan PM, van Lent PLEM, Eds. Joint Destruction in Arthritis and Osteoarthritis. Austin, TX: Birkhauser, 1993;195.
26. Ghosh P, Smith M, Wells C. Second-line agents in osteoarthritis. In: Dixon JS, Furst DE, Eds. Second-line Agents in the Treatment of Rheumatic Diseases. New York: Marcel Dekker, 1992;363.
26a. Gibson RG, Gibson SLM, Conway V, Chappell D. Perna canaliculus in the treatment of arthritis. Practitioner 1980;224:955–960.
27. Glade MJ. Polysulfated glycosaminoglycan accelerates net synthesis of collagen and glycosaminoglycans by arthritic equine cartilage tissues and chondrocytes. Am J Vet Res 1990;51:779–785.
28. Greinacher A, Michels I, Schafer M, et al. Heparin-associated thrombocytopenia in a patient treated with polysulfated chondroitin sulphate: Evidence of immunological cross-reactivity between heparin and polysulphated glycosaminoglycan. Br J Haematol 1992;81:252–254.
29. Gustafson SB, McIlwraith CW, Jones RL. Comparison of the effect of polysulfated glycosaminoglycan, corticosteroids, and sodium hyaluronate in the potentiation of a subinfective dose of Staphylococcus aureus in the midcarpal joint of horses. Am J Vet Res 1989;50:2014–2017.
30. Gustafson SB, McIlwraith CW, Jones RL. Further investigations into the potentiation of infection by intra-articular injection of

polysulfated glycosaminoglycan and the effect of filtration and intra-articular injection of amikacin. Am J Vet Res 1989;50: 2018–2022.

31. Hamm D, Goldman L, Jones EW. Polysulfated glycosaminoglycan: A new intra-articular treatment for equine lameness. Vet Med 1984;6:811–816.

32. Hannan N, Ghosh P, Bellenger C, et al. Systemic administration of glycosaminoglycan polysulphate (Arteparon) provides partial protection of articular cartilage from damage produced by meniscectomy in the canine. J Orthop Res 1987;5:47–59.

33. Hanson R. Oral glycosaminoglycans in treatment of degenerative joint disease in horses. Equine Pract 1996;18:18–22.

34. Howell DS, Carreno M, Pelletier J-P, et al. Articular cartilage breakdown in a lapine model of osteoarthritis. Clin Orthop 1986; 213:69–76.

35. Howell DS, Muniz O, Carreno MR. Effect of glycosaminoglycan polysulfate ester on proteoglycan-degrading enzyme activity in an animal model of osteoarthritis. Adv Inflamm Res 1986;11: 197–206.

36. Hutadilok N, Smith M, Cullis-Hill D, et al. Pentosan polysulfate stimulates hyaluronate and DNA synthesis in synovial fibroblasts and partially reduces the suppressive effect of hydrocortisone on fibroblast metabolism. Curr Ther Res 1988;44:845–860.

36a. Jimenez SA. The effect of glucosamine on human chondrocyte gene expression. The 9th EULAR Symposium, Madrid, Spain, 1996;8–10.

37. Jones IL, Sandstrom T. Enhanced breakdown of bovine articular cartilage proteoglycans by conditioned synovial medium *in vitro*. Arzneimittelforschung 1985;35:141–144.

38. Kleesiek K, Greiling H. Effect of anti-inflammatory agents on the glycosaminoglycan metabolism in cultured human synovial cells. Rheumatol Int 1982;2:167–174.

39. Kruze D, Fehr K, Menninger H, et al. Effect of antirheumatic drugs on neutral protease from human leukocyte granules. Z Rheumatol 1976;35:337–346.

40. Little C, Ghosh P. Potential use of pentosan polysulfate for the treatment of equine joint disease. In: McIlwraith CW, Trotter GW, Eds. Joint Disease in the Horse. Philadelphia: WB Saunders, 1996;281–292.

41. Little C, Ghosh P, Bellinger C. Meniscectomy increases aggrecan, decoran (PGS2) and biglycan (PG–S1) metabolism in cartilage. Proceedings. 39th Annual Meeting of the Orthopaedic Research Society, San Francisco, 1993;18:707.

42. Lualdi P. Bioavailability of oral chondroitin sulfate [letter]. Rheumatol Int 1993;13:39–43.

43. May SA, Hooke RE, Lees P. The effect of drugs used in the treatment of osteoarthrosis on stromelysin (proteoglycanase) of equine synovial cell origin. Equine Vet J 1988;S6:28–32.

44. McIlwraith CW. Intra-articular medication for traumatic joint problems: Do we understand the choices? Comp Cont Educ Pract Vet 1989;11:1287–1311.

45. Muller-Fassbender H, Bach G, Haase W, et al. Glucosamine sulfate compared to ibuprofen in osteoarthritis of the knee. Osteoarthritis Cartilage 1994;2:61–69.

46. Nethery A, Giles I, Jenkins K, et al. The chondroprotective drugs, Arteparon and sodium pentosan polysulfate, increase collagenase activity and inhibit stromelysin activity *in vitro*. Biochem Pharmacol 1992;44:1549–1553.

47. Nishikawa H, Mori I, Umemoto J. Influences of sulfated glycosaminoglycans on biosynthesis of hyaluronic acid in rabbit knee synovial membrane. Arch Biochem Biophys 1985;240:146–153.

48. Nishikawa H, Mori I, Umemoto J. Glycosaminoglycan polysulfate-induced stimulation of hyaluronic acid synthesis in rabbit knee synovial membrane: Involvement of binding protein and calcium ion. Arch Biochem Biophys 1988;266:201–209.

49. Noack W, Fischer M, Forster K, et al. Glucosamine sulfate in osteoarthritis of the knee. Osteoarthritis Cartilage 1994;2:51–59.

49a. Pujalte JM, Llavore E, Ylescupidez FR. Double-blind clinical evaluation of oral glucosamine sulfate in the basic treatment of osteoarthrosis. Curr Med Res Opin 1980;7:110–114.

49b. Raiss R. Einfluss von D. Glucosaminsulfat auf experimentell geschaedigten Gelenkknorpel. Fortschr Med 1985;103:658–668.

50. Rashmir-Raven AM, Coyne CP, Fenwick BW, et al. Inhibition of equine complement activity by polysulfated glycosaminoglycans. Am J Vet Res 1992;53:87–90.

51. Reichelt L, Forster K, Fischer M, et al. Efficacy and safety of intramuscular glucosamine sulfate in osteoarthritis of the knee. Arzneimittelforschung 1994;44:75–80.

52. Rogachefsky RA, Dean DD, Howell DS, Altman RD. Treatment of canine osteoarthritis with insulin-like growth factor (IGF-1) and sodium pentosan polysulfate. Osteoarthritis Cartilage 1993; 1:105–114.

52a. Setnikar I, Giacchetti C, Zanolo G. Pharmacokinetics of glucosamine in the dog and in man. Arzneimittelforschung 1986;36: 729–735.

53. Smith MM, Ghosh P. The effects of some polysulfated polysaccharides on hyaluronate synthesis by human synovial fibroblasts. Recent advances in connective tissue research. Agents Actions 1987;518:55–62.

54. Smith MM, Ghosh P, Numata Y, et al. The effects of orally administered calcium pentosan polysulfate on inflammation and cartilage degradation produced in rabbit joints by intra-articular injection of a hyaluronate-polylysine complex. Arthritis Rheum 1993; 37:125–136.

55. Stancikova M, Trnavsky K, Keiloca H. The effect of antirheumatic drugs on collagenolytic activity of cathepsin B_1. Biochem Pharmacol 1977;26:2121–2124.

56. Tew WP. Demonstration by synovial fluid analysis of the efficacy in horses of an investigational drug (L-1016). J Equine Vet Sci 1982;March/April:42–50.

57. Theiler R, Thosh P, Brooks P. Clinical, biochemical and imaging methods of assessing osteoarthritis and clinical trials with agents claiming "chondromodulating" activity. Osteoarthritis Cartilage 1994;2:1–23.

58. Todhunter RJ, Minor RR, Wootton J, et al. Effects of exercise and polysulfated glycosaminoglycan on repair of articular cartilage defects in the equine carpus. J Orthop Res 1993;11:782–795.

59. Todhunter RJ, Freeman KP, Yeager AE. Effects of exercise and polysulfated glycosaminoglycan on the development of osteoarthritis in equine carpal joints with osteochondral defects. Vet Surg 1993;22:330–342.

60. Trotter GW. Polysulfated glycosaminoglycan (Adequan®). In: McIlwraith CW, Trotter GW, Eds. Joint Disease in the Horse. Philadelphia: WB Saunders, 1996;270–280.

61. Trotter GW, Yovich J, McIlwraith CW, et al. Effects of intramuscular polysulfated glycosaminoglycan on chemical and physical defects in equine articular cartilage. Can J Vet Res 1989;43: 224–230.

62. Ueno R. Results of the treatment of experimental arthrosis of the knee joint with a mucopolysaccharide polysulfuric acid ester. Z Orthop 1973;111:886–892.

63. Vacha J, Pesakova V, Krajickova J, et al. Effect of glycosaminoglycan polysulfate on the metabolism of cartilage ribonucleic acid. Arzneimittelforschung 1984;34:607–609.

64. Verbruggen G, Veys EM. Influence of an oversulphated heparinoid upon hyaluronate metabolism of the human synovial cell *in vivo*. J Rheumatol 1979;6:554–561.

65. Verbruggen G, Veys EM. Influence of sulfated glycosaminoglycan upon proteoglycan metabolism of the synovial lining cells. Acta Rheum Belg 1977;1:75–92.

66. White GW, Jones EW, Hamm J, et al. The efficacy of orally administered sulfated glycosaminoglycan in chemically-induced equine synovitis and degenerative joint disease. J Equine Vet Sci 1994;14:350–353.

67. Yovich J, Trotter GW, McIlwraith CW, et al. Effects of polysulfated glycosaminoglycan on chemical and physical defects in equine articular cartilage. Am J Vet Res 1987;48:1407–1414.

NEW HORIZONS

Work is continuing to find more effective agents not only for the treatment of traumatic synovitis and capsulitis but also to help articular cartilage repair, or at least improve, cartilage metabolism in OA. One such regimen, the addition of growth factors IGF-1 and NAPPS in the treatment of canine anterior cruciate ligament–deficient OA, has been described recently.[2]

The development of metalloproteinase inhibitors offers the potential to specifically inhibit one of the important groups of enzymes capable of degrading both collagen and proteoglycans in the articular cartilage. It has been demonstrated that metalloproteinase inhibitors will also inhibit the secretion of cytokines and cytokine receptors in human monocytic cells.[1]

The other area of great potential development is specific inhibition of cytokines by the use of IL-1 receptor antagonist or anti-TNF antibodies or the addition of anabolic growth factors.[2] Gene therapy with IL-1 receptor antagonist has recently been demonstrated in our laboratory to significantly decrease both the development of experimentally induced OA in the horse and lameness.[3]

References

1. Gallea-Robache S, Morand V, Millet S, et al. A metalloproteinase inhibitor blocks the shedding of soluble cytokine receptors and processing of transmembrane cytokine precursors in human monocytic cells. Cytokine 1997;9:340–346.
2. Rogachefsky RA, Dean DD, Howell DS, Altman RD. Treatment of canine osteoarthritis with insulin-like growth factor-1 (IGF-1) and sodium pentosan polysulfate. Osteoarthritis Cartilage 1993;1:105–114.
3. Frisbie DD, Ghivizzani S, Robbins PD, et al. Evaluation of equine interleukin-1 receptor antagonist developed using gene transfer for the treatment of joint disease [abstract]. Vet Surg 1999;393.

SYNOVECTOMY

The surgical excision of synovial membrane from joints has appeared for over a century in the medical literature. Synovectomy is still done today with successful results and, after development of arthroscopic techniques and instrumentation, has greatly decreased the morbidity of the procedure. Now that the significance of traumatic synovitis in the horse is realized, there is a rationale for synovectomy. In addition, it is indicated for localized chronic proliferation such as villonodular synovitis. The primary indication for synovectomy in human orthopedics is rheumatoid arthritis resistant to 6 to 12 months of medical management. The primary indication in horses is traumatic synovitis and includes chronic proliferative synovitis, villonodular synovitis, as well as hemarthrosis. The technique is also useful in infective arthritis. Radiation synovectomy has been used as an alternative to surgical synovectomy but has not found general acceptance in human orthopedics in the United States because of the risks, which include leakage of the isotope external to the joint capsule, carcinogenesis, chondronecrosis, and radioactive exposure of medical personnel.[3] In a recent report on the use of radiation synovectomy with rhenium-186 in rheumatoid arthritis, the best clinical results and slowest progression in radiologic destruction were achieved with a combined injection of rhenium-186 and triamcinolone hexacetonide.[1]

Arthroscopic synovectomy appears to be appropriate for several primary synovial diseases. As stated in a human textbook, the major drawbacks to arthroscopic synovectomy include the need for the surgeon to be skilled in advanced arthroscopic technique and the need for specialized instrumentation. In the case of the equine surgeon, the additional requirement over what might be commonly available is motorized resection equipment. With the use of arthroscopic synovectomy, the ability

to maintain high fluid flows with a motorized pump is critical.[2] However, recent work with subtotal synovectomy in the carpus demonstrated that although there was evidence of restoration and an intimal layer was present, the synovium was devoid of villi and there was subintimal fibrosis.[4]

References

1. Gobel D, Gratz S, von Rothkirch T, et al. Radiosynoviorthesis with rhenium-186 in rheumatoid arthritis: A prospective study of three treatment regimens. Rheumatol Int 1997;17:105–108.
2. McIlwraith CW. Diagnostic and Surgical Arthroscopy in the Horse. 2nd ed. Philadelphia: Lea & Febiger, 1989;227.
3. Rosenberg TD, Jaureguito JW, Kolowich PA, Tearse DS. Synovectomy of the knee. In: McGinty JB, Caspari RB, Jackson RW, Poehling GG, Eds. Operative Arthroscopy. 2nd ed. Philadelphia: Lippincott-Raven, 1996;459–467.
4. Theoret CL, Barber SM, Moyana T, et al. Repair and function of synovium after arthroscopic synovectomy of the dorsal compartment of the equine antebrachiocarpal joint. Vet Surg 1996;25:142–153.

SPECIFIC DISEASES OF JOINTS: CHRONIC PROLIFERATIVE SYNOVITIS (VILLONODULAR SYNOVITIS)

Chronic proliferative synovitis was originally called villonodular synovitis based on its apparent resemblance to the nodular form of pigmented villous synovitis in humans.[5] Histologically, however, there is a lack of pigmentation of the intracapsular mass by hemosiderin. Characteristic histologic features in the horse are dense fibrous connective tissue with nodules containing fibroblastic and vascular proliferation often surrounding regions of collagen necrosis. Few inflammatory cells have been found within the lesions, and a covering layer of synoviocytes is often absent.[7] The mass arises from a fold, or plica, of tissue that normally projects distad from the dorsoproximal attachment of the joint capsule in the metacarpophalangeal joint. To distinguish it from villonodular synovitis in humans, it is probably more appropriate to call the disease a chronic proliferative synovitis.[6]

PATHOGENESIS

The pathogenesis appears to be a traumatic one. Histologic characteristics support a traumatic pathogenesis rather than a response to joint inflammation. The histologic findings also suggest that synovial pad lesions are not acute and probably result from chronic repetitive trauma with attempted healing. There is secondary erosion, fragmentation of cartilage and bone beneath the mass, and it is presumed that this erosion of cortical bone under the lesion is due to local pressure of the mass on the bone or possibly trauma to the underlying cortical bone.[7]

CLINICAL SIGNS AND DIAGNOSIS

The typical presenting signs are lameness and joint effusion (associated with one or both metacarpophalangeal joints). The disease is typical of the racing Thoroughbred and racing Quarter Horse. Soft tissue thickening in the proximodorsal aspect of the joint may be palpated. Bone remodeling and concavity on the distodorsal aspect of the metacarpus above the condyles is

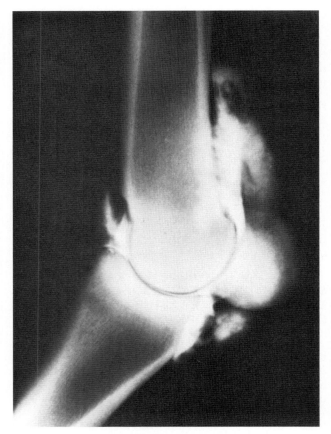

Figure 7.26 Contrast arthrogram of metacarpophalangeal joint with villonodular synovitis showing filling defect created by proliferative lesion.

common (seen in 93% of joints in the study by White[7]). Fragmentation of the proximodorsal proximal (first) phalanx may also be seen on radiographs. In the occasional case, there is ossification within the villonodular mass, which shows up as a rounded density associated with the distal dorsal aspect of the metacarpus (Fig. 7.26). Although this condition is classically described as being diagnosed with contrast radiography, this is rarely practiced because diagnostic ultrasound is a consistently useful (and noninvasive) technique. In one series of cases, 54 joints (71%) were examined by ultrasound. The mean ± SD thickness of the synovial pads was 11.3 ± 2.8 mm (range, 7 to 14 mm) in the sagittal ridge. The medial synovial pad was usually 2.5 ± 0.5 mm thicker than the lateral synovial pad. The edges of the synovial pads were more rounded than normal synovial pads, and hypoechoic areas were often evident. The medial synovial pad was abnormal in 30 joints, both medial and lateral pads were enlarged in 19 joints, and the lateral pad only was abnormal in 5 joints.

TREATMENT

Medical treatment (intraarticular HA) has been described in eight horses. Three of these horses returned to racing, but only one at a similar or better level than before injury. Five horses were retired for breeding purposes because of continued fetlock joint problems.

Arthroscopic surgery is the recommended definitive treatment.[4] The technique typically involves a lateral arthroscopic approach and a medial instrument approach in the dorsal pouch of the affected fetlock. The surgery is often combined with removal of proximodorsal first phalanx chip fragments. If the lateral pad is enlarged, swapping the arthroscope and instrument to the medial and lateral portals, respectively, may be necessary. Generally the enlarged pads are severed at the base and removed with Ferris-Smith rongeurs. Motorized equipment can be useful as well.

In one report of arthroscopic surgery, 68 joints in 55 horses were treated. Osteochondral fragmentation or fibrillated cartilage of the third metacarpus beneath the enlarged pads was identified in 60 joints (88%) and wear lines were seen in the metacarpal condyles in 27 joints (40%). Forty-four percent of joints had bone chips removed from the proximal first phalanx.

PROGNOSIS

Follow-up of 50 of the 55 horses at arthroscopic surgery showed that 43 (68%) horses returned to the same or higher level of race performance after surgery, 9 (18%) returned to a lower level, and 7 (14%) were unable to race. The presence of proximal first phalanx fragments, metacarpal lesions, synovial pad thickness, or bilateral or unilateral joint involvement had no association with outcome. Horses that returned to racing at or above their presurgery race level were significantly ($P = .05$) younger than horses that returned at a lower level of performance or did not race.[7] Many of the horses in this study were back in work 6 to 8 weeks after arthroscopic surgery. Studies smaller but earlier than the one cited above reported 8 of 12 horses returning to race training after treatment by arthrotomy[2] and 12 of 13 racing again after arthroscopic surgery.[3]

References

1. Dabareiner RM, White NA, Sullins KE. Metacarpophalangeal joint synovial pad fibrotic proliferation in 63 horses. Vet Surg 1996;25:199–206.
2. Jann HW, Fackelman GE, Koblik PD, et al. Electrosurgical arthrotomy and excision of soft tissue masses in the metacarpophalangeal joint of the horse. Vet Surg 1986;6:429–434.
3. Kannegieter NJ. Chronic proliferative synovitis of equine metacarpophalangeal joint. Vet Rec 1990;127:8–10.
4. McIlwraith CW. Diagnostic and Surgical Arthroscopy in the Horse. 2nd ed. Philadelphia: Lea & Febiger, 1990;100–102.
5. Nickels FA, Grant BD, Lincoln SD. Villonodular synovitis of the equine metacarpophalangeal joint. J Am Vet Med Assoc 1976;168:1043.
6. Van Veenendaal JC, Moffatt RE. Soft tissue masses in the fetlock joint of horses. Aust Vet J 56:533, 1980.
7. White NA. Synovial pad proliferation in the metacarpophalangeal joint. In: White NA, Moore JN, Eds. Current Practice of Equine Surgery. Philadelphia: JB Lippincott, 1990;555–558.

SPECIFIC DISEASES OF JOINTS: SPRAINS AND LUXATIONS, MENISCAL TEARS, AND OSTEOCHONDRAL FRAGMENTATION

Sprains and Luxations (Type 2A Traumatic Arthritis)

Sprain

A sprain may be defined as the stretching or tearing of a supporting ligament of a joint by forced movement beyond its normal range.[41] In its simplest form there is minimal disruption of fibers, swelling, pain, and dysfunction. Severe sprains may cause total rupture of ligaments, marked swelling, hemorrhage, and joint instability, which may be permanent if untreated. As a normal force is applied, the ligament becomes tense and then gives way at one of its attachments or at some point in its substance. If the attachment pulls loose with a fragment of bone, it is called a "sprain fracture" or an "avulsion fracture." Sprains may be classified, and their treatment will vary.

A mild sprain is one in which a few fibers of the ligament have been stretched or torn with some hemorrhage into the ligament, but integrity is not lost. This type of problem will present clinically as capsulitis unless an intraarticular ligament is involved, in which case synovitis will be present. Rest and a support bandage are the appropriate treatment for this problem.

A moderate sprain is one in which some portion of the ligament is torn and some functional loss is sustained. The amount of damage may vary from a tear of a relatively small portion of the ligament to almost complete avulsion, but wide retraction of the torn ligament ends is not a feature. Union can therefore proceed in an orderly manner as a result of healing with fibrosis. The use of a cast is indicated in the appropriate joint to support this healing. Clinically, there may be some laxity in the joint but not complete loss of integrity to the ligament, and surgical intervention is not generally indicated.

In severe sprain there is complete loss of function of the ligament, and separation of the ends occurs. The loss of integrity of the ligament may result in luxation of the joint. Some form of surgical intervention is generally indicated with a severe sprain, but this depends on the ligament and the joint. The different types of luxations associated with ligamentous rupture are discussed in the next section.

Various forms of ligament sprain and luxation may occur within the stifle joint. Upward fixation of the patella involves displacement of the patella, but there is no loss of integrity to any ligaments with this problem, and the fixation is usually temporary. Standardbred racehorses develop problems in the stifle resulting in soreness that can be associated with ligamentous abnormalities. The condition of loose patella has been associated with laxity of the patellar ligaments.[28] The patella is looser than normal, resulting in a secondary gonitis, and this results in soreness in the stifle and secondary back soreness. The condition is commonly treated by injecting an internal blistering agent (Hypodermin) in the area of attachment of the patellar ligaments, and the resulting cicatrization may resolve the problem.[8] Repeat injections are sometimes necessary. There is no primary problem of the patellar ligaments; the problem is one of lack of conditioning in the quadriceps femoris musculature with subsequent loosening in the patella (it is typical of young horses early in training). Proper conditioning is a better method of treatment. Stifle soreness also occurs with jarring, which results when heavy caulks and other adhering agents are used on the shoes. These shoes are commonly applied to Standardbreds that are raced during the winter. It seems that the jarring results in a degree of sprain to the ligaments of the stifle. It should not be considered a luxation.

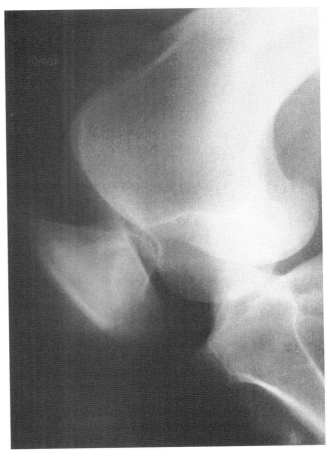

Figure 7.27 Distal luxation of the patella. (Reprinted with permission from McIlwraith CW, Warren RC. Distal luxation of the patella in a horse. J Am Vet Med Assoc 1982;181:67–69.)

Congenital lateral and medial luxations of the patella occur, but acquired traumatic luxations in this direction have not been reported (lateral luxation may recur in severe cases of OCD with severe loss of the lateral trochlear ridge of the femur). I have observed luxation of the patella distad[34] (Fig. 7.27), with the stifle consequently locked in flexion. The luxation was reduced under anesthesia, and there was apparently no loss of ligamentous integrity. Various degrees of sprain of collateral or cruciate ligaments are recognized in the horse. Mild sprains (desmitis) have been recognized in the collateral ligaments using ultrasonography. Severe sprains cause instability, and rupture of collateral ligaments can be evident on a stressed radiograph (Fig. 7.28). Similarly, rupture of cruciate ligaments can be recognized on stressed radiographs, and when this severe an injury is present, the prognosis is poor. However, with experience in arthroscopic surgery of the femorotibial joints, mild-and-moderate sprains have also been recognized (Fig. 7.29) and are amenable to arthroscopic treatment.

TEARING OF MEDIAL PALMAR INTERCARPAL LIGAMENT

A specific entity diagnosed by arthroscopy occurring in the medial palmar intercarpal ligament in the equine middle carpal joint was first described in 1990 by

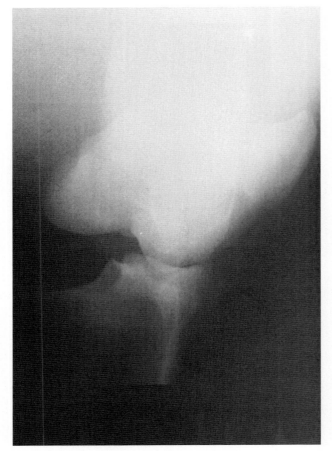

Figure 7.28 Radiograph of stifle with combined rupture of the medial collateral and cruciate ligaments.

McIlwraith[30] in 24 cases, and 45 cases were reported in 1992.[32] Damage to intracarpal ligaments in three joints was also mentioned in a study of 150 carpal joints by Kannegieter and Burbridge in 1990,[23] and two cases of medial intercarpal ligament damage and three of lateral ligament damage were reported by Kannegieter in 1990.[22] Further reports have been written by Phillips and Wright in 1994, Whitton et al. in 1997,[49] and Davankar et al. in 1996.

The medial palmar intercarpal ligament consists of two portions. Both portions attach proximally on the radial carpal bone. The medial portion tends to attach on the second carpal bone, and the lateral portion on the third carpal bone (Fig. 7.30). In the series of McIlwraith, the condition was recognized in 45 middle carpal joints in 42 horses (37 racehorses, 5 nonracehorses). Of the 37 racehorses, there were 20 Quarter Horses, 14 Thoroughbreds, and 3 Standardbreds. Patients were referred for arthroscopic surgery for removal of osteochondral chip fragments that were diagnosed radiographically or for diagnostic arthroscopy of a persistent carpal problem. The problem was unilateral in 39 horses and bilateral in 3. The presenting clinical signs were lameness and/or persistent synovial effusion. In one instance, the presenting complaint was hemarthrosis. Osteochondral chip fragments were present in the joint affected with tearing in 23 horses. In 6 horses in which

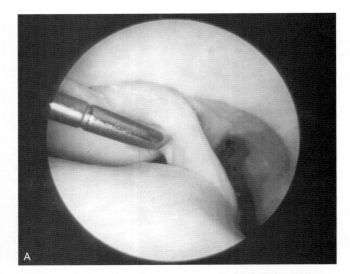
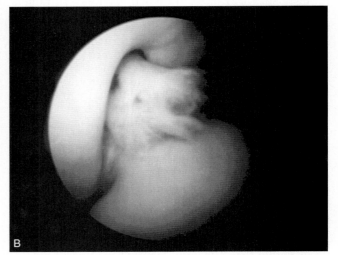
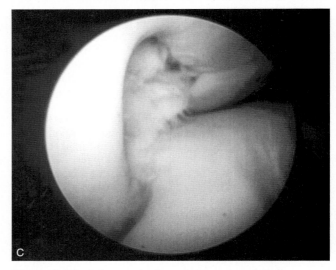

Figure 7.29 Arthroscopic views. A. Normal medial palmar intercarpal ligament with a probe delineating the medial and lateral portions. B. Tearing of the lateral portion of a medial palmar intercarpal ligament. C. The same ligament after debridement of frayed fibers.

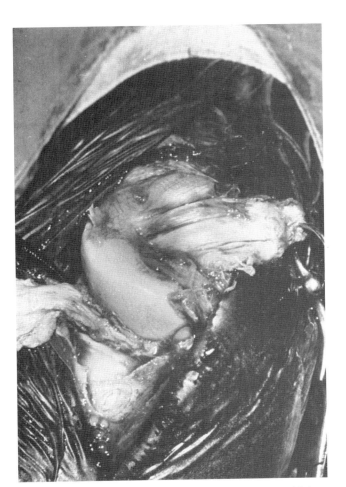

Figure 7.30   Traumatic luxation of metacarpophalangeal joint. Ruptured collateral ligament is held in towel forceps.

the osteochondral fragments were present in other joints, synovial effusion was greatest in the middle carpal joint, with ligamentous tearing. In most of the 22 middle carpal joints where carpal chip fragmentation and ligamentous tearing were present concomitantly, the clinical compromise was more severe than normally seen with that degree of osteochondral fragmentation. A ligament was designated as torn when a defect was present in the ligament (Fig. 7.29). This usually took the form of frayed fibers suspended in the irrigating solution, presenting a transverse type of defect in the dorsal aspect of the lateral portion of the ligament. However, longitudinal tearing was present in one case, and tearing was noted in the palmar aspect of the ligament in two others. Shredded fibers were trimmed in most instances, which allowed better definition of the amount of ligament considered torn. The degree of damage ranged from 10 to 100% of the total width. The degree of tearing was estimated to be 70 to 90% in six joints, 50% in 11, 30% in 7, 20 to 25% in 7, and 10 to 15% in 9. A total loss of integrity was diagnosed in 2 joints. Long-term follow-up was obtained for 31 horses; 17 had successful and 14 had unsuccessful results. Of the horses with successful results, 13 were estimated to have 30% or less damage to the total ligamentous width, and 3 with 50% damage to the liga-

ment raced successfully after treatment with intraarticular corticosteroids. One horse with more than 30% damage was considered to be successful without the use of intraarticular corticosteroids. Of the 14 horses with unsuccessful results, all but 2 had 50% or more estimated damage to the medial palmar intercarpal ligament. Of the two exceptions, one had 30% damage but also had a sagittal fracture of the third carpal bone, and the second horse's lack of success was considered to be unrelated to the carpus.

Studies of the anatomy of the palmar intercarpal ligaments have concluded that the medial palmar intercarpal ligament resists dorsomedial displacement of the radial carpal bone where the lateral palmar intercarpal ligament resists dorsolateral displacement of the ulna and intermediate carpal bones.[49] A biomechanical study of cadaver carpal joints found that the palmar intercarpal ligaments contribute 22.7 ± 2.2% of dorsal displacement.[50] It was felt that despite their small size, they play an important role in the restraint of dorsal displacement of the proximal row of carpal bones.

Luxations

Luxation or dislocation of the joint may be complete or partial (subluxation). Most luxations involve loss of integrity of one or more joint ligaments (severe sprain) as well as damage to other joint structures such as the fibrous joint capsule and surrounding tendons (Fig. 7.30). Complete luxations are probably the most common in the pastern, fetlock, and hock joints. Luxation of the pastern may occur with associated fractures of the middle phalanx (Fig. 7.31) or be unassociated with an avulsion fracture (Fig. 7.32). In both instances some form of healing may be achieved by long-term casting, but OA is generally anticipated. Exceptions have been noted.[3] Surgical arthrodesis is often indicated as the treatment for this condition. Subluxation of the fetlock may occur in association with rupture of one of the collateral ligaments. Because of the necessary function in this joint, one attempts to maintain integrity of the ligaments and avoid ankylosis. Casting may be used as a method of treatment. I have used screw and wire bridging to provide initial replacement of a ruptured collateral ligament. The use of carbon fiber implants has been reported in two cases.[10] OA may be anticipated following subluxation of the fetlock, but surgical arthrodesis is used as a last resort. A case of shoulder luxation was reported in a 3-year-old Thoroughbred filly.[29] The injury had occurred on a wet pasture 2 weeks prior to presentation. There was no weight-bearing lameness, and the humeral head was displaced lateral to the scapula. Under general anesthesia the luxation was reduced, and the filly was allowed to recover in a swimming pool recovery system. Eight months after surgery, the filly had returned to light work without evidence of lameness, and muscle atrophy evident at the time of admission had resolved. In the case of shoulder luxation, there is no ligamentous injury involved, but there is disruption of fibrous joint capsule and musculature. Subluxation of the shoulder joint has also been seen (see Chapter 8, shoulder luxation/subluxation). Displacement of the carpal bones (carpal luxation) is usually associated with comminuted fractures.

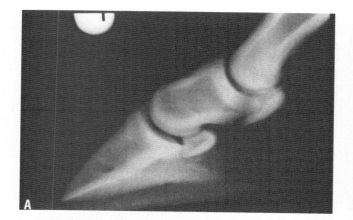
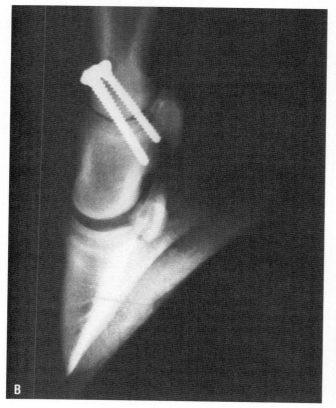

Figure 7.31 Radiographs of luxation of pastern joint associated with an avulsion fracture of the palmar aspect of the proximal end of the middle phalanx. A. Prior to repair. B. After surgical arthrodesis.

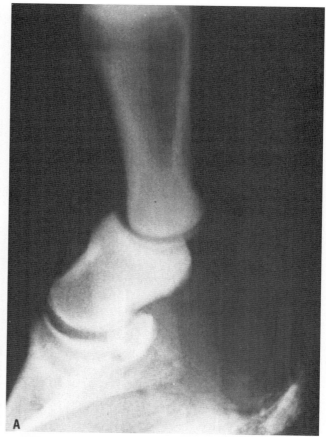
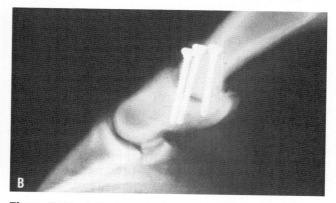

Figure 7.32 A. Radiograph of luxated pastern unassociated with fracture. B. Radiograph of pastern after surgical arthrodesis.

Luxations of the various tarsal joints are not uncommon. A severe form of luxation occurs in the tarsocrural (tibiotarsal) joint, and in this instance, the tibia is generally displaced distocraniad. Reduction of this dislocation is very difficult and is often not achieved. Luxations of the intertarsal joints (Fig. 7.33) or tarsometatarsal joint, while still severe injuries, do not usually present the same problem with reduction. Long-term continued function of these joints is not required, and surgery and treatment are generally aimed at eventually producing an ankylosis. Results have been inconsistent with casting alone, and surgical arthrodesis is recommended. An incision

through the skin and subcutaneous tissue usually allows opening of the luxated joint. The articular cartilage is removed, and some form of internal fixation across the joint may be attempted. Following surgical arthrodesis of the hock or pastern, the limbs are retained in a cast for 6 weeks.

Coxofemoral luxation is rare in the horse, largely because of the ligamentous support to the hip joint. The acetabulum is surrounded by the fibrocartilaginous acetabular lip, and in addition to the ligament of the head of the femur (round ligament), an accessory femoral ligament passes from the symphysial (prepubic) tendon

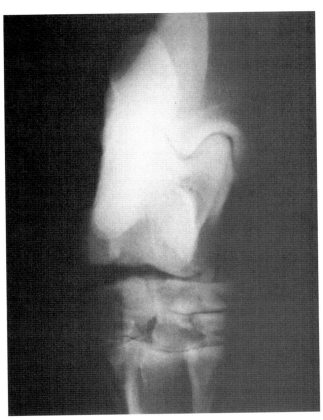

Figure 7.33   Luxation of proximal intertarsal joint.

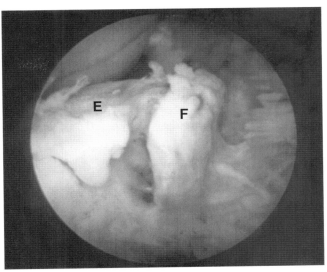

Figure 7.34   Arthroscopic view of chip fragment on distal radial carpal bone (F) accompanied by significant articular cartilage fragmentation and erosion (E).

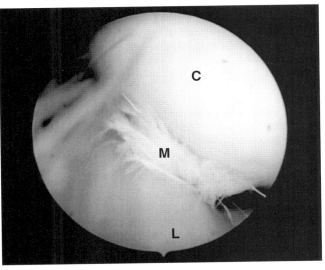

Figure 7.35   Arthroscopic view of tear in the axial portion of the medial meniscus in a left femorotibial joint. C, medial condyle of femur; L, cranial ligament of medial meniscus; M, torn portion of meniscus.

through the acetabular notch (bound by the transverse acetabular ligament) to the femoral head. Upward fixation of the patella commonly accompanies coxofemoral luxation.[5] It is suggested that the patella is retained in upward fixation when dislocation of the hip occurs because as the latter produces rotation of the limb, the rectus femoris muscle loses its normal leverage and is unable to release the patella.[43] Reduction of a coxofemoral luxation is generally unsuccessful with the use of traction and manipulation. A successful case in a 3-week-old foal has been reported, but the follow-up was only 6 weeks.[39] Femoral head removal has been used as a treatment in ponies. In another report, a brood mare with a luxated hip was left with the hip luxated and was able to function satisfactorily after medial patellar desmotomy for relief of the associated upward fixation of the patella.[5] Rupture of the ligament of the head of the femur without luxation of the joint may also occur. Although the joint is in position, the prognosis is unfavorable, since an increase in the range of motion of the femoral head can be anticipated to cause severe DJD before ligamentous regeneration can occur.[1]

Meniscal Tears (Type 2B Traumatic Arthritis)

Meniscal injuries are restricted to the femorotibial joints. These injuries have been recognized increasingly with diagnostic arthroscopy of the femorotibial

joints.[30,48a] A limited amount of the menisci is visible in the femorotibial joints when the cruciate ligaments are intact. However, the visible portion is a common location for meniscal tears, which typically occur on the most axial portion in a sagittal direction (Fig. 7.34). Treatment with arthroscopic resection of the torn portion has had successful results. Associated damage can also occur in the cranial ligaments of the medial or lateral meniscus. Horses typically present with obvious lameness, and in some instances, femorotibial effusion can be detected (Fig. 7.35). The condition is confirmed by diagnostic arthroscopy.

An open surgical procedure has been reported for removal of the medial meniscus in the horse.[48] However, with the ability to treat meniscal injuries arthroscopically and the recognition of the morbidity associated with entire menisci in humans, the author does not consider there is ever an indication for open meniscectomy in the horse.[43]

Intraarticular Fractures (Type 2C Traumatic Arthritis)

Intraarticular fractures represent an arthritic entity, and their review is appropriate. They are particularly important in that they can potentially lead to OA. If they are not treated in an appropriate and timely fashion, OA is inevitable.

Osteochondral Fragmentation

PATHOBIOLOGIC PRINCIPLES

The development of fragmentation in equine joints has two main sources: traumatic injury and OCD. Treatment of the latter condition is presented elsewhere in this chapter. The most common instances of traumatically induced osteochondral chip fragmentation are in the carpal and fetlock joints.

Although chip fractures have been frequently considered acute injuries and recognized with acute clinical signs, it has been suggested relatively recently that they are a secondary complication affecting joint margins previously altered by OA.[42] It has been proposed that chip fractures of the joint margins in the carpus, at least, arise from two different pathogenetic processes: 1) fragmentation of the original tissue of the joint margin (this lesion starts as progressive subchondral bone sclerosis induced by repetitive trauma of training and racing, with eventual damage to articular cartilage because of the noncompliant subchondral bone; eventually the sclerotic bone undergoes ischemic necrosis and subsequent fragmentation) or 2) within the base of periarticular osteophytes forming in OA. Experience with arthroscopic surgery of carpal fragmentation supports both these roles in various instances. On the other hand, "fresh" fracture lines through an articular surface that otherwise appears grossly normal forces the conclusion that if the above proposals are true, then such change can only be at the microscopic level in some instances.

Fragmentation of the osteochondral articular surfaces causes direct physical effects due to loss of a smooth congruent articular surface as well as release of cartilage and bone debris, which may lead to synovitis. Sufficiently severe compromise of the articular surface leads to instability, as does tearing of fibrous joint capsule and ligaments. Synovial membrane in turn has the potential to respond directly to mechanical trauma and/or indirectly to injury elsewhere in the joint.[42] Damage to articular cartilage releases wear particles and, possibly, other soluble breakdown products. These materials in turn can activate the synovial membrane, resulting in increased production of proteinases, prostaglandins, cytokines, and other biochemical mediators.[11] These pathobiologic processes are discussed above in this chapter.

The chronic effects that result in the loss of motion after joint surgery also need to be recognized. Arthro-fibrosis is recognized as an important problem in humans, although the etiology is still unknown. The use of skilled arthroscopic techniques is critical in the minimization of arthrofibrosis.[12] However, arthrofibrosis may still be a complication despite proper surgical technique and rehabilitation. Orthopedic surgeons use such methods as elevation, compression, heat, cold, immobilization, mobilization, and anti-inflammatory medications to try to minimize swelling and stiffness in humans.[21,36]

Direct compromise to the articular surface is discussed above. Additional factors that need to be considered include the possibility of chondrocytes within articular cartilage being damaged or undergoing necrosis subsequent to impact loads that do not cause gross morphologic damage[44] as well as the presence of a step in the articular surface contributing to posttraumatic OA.[26] Mechanical injuries of the articular cartilage have been divided into three types: 1) disruption or alteration of the macromolecular framework, loss of matrix components, or cell injury without visible disruption; 2) disruption of articular cartilage alone (chondral fractures); and 3) mechanical disruption of articular cartilage and subchondral bone (osteochondral fractures). Each of these types of articular cartilage damage represents a different problem for repair and stimulates a different response.[6a] While damage to the cartilage matrix without tissue disruption has not been studied extensively, experimental evidence shows that loss of proteoglycans or alteration of their organization (decreased proteoglycan aggregation) occurs before other signs of significant matrix injury. The loss of proteoglycans (by increased degradation or decreased synthesis) will cause loss of cartilage stiffness and may cause greater loading of the collagen framework, which in turn increases the vulnerability of subchondral bone to damage by impact loading. However, whether cartilage "softening" progresses to matrix disruption is not known. With regard to chondral fractures, compression and shear forces can rupture the cartilage matrix, producing fissures, flaps, or fractures. Osteochondral fractures result from similar forces. In humans, chondral fractures generally occur in skeletally mature people, while osteochondral fractures typically occur in skeletally immature people or young adults.[35] Such distinction has not been recognized in the horse.

OSTEOCHONDRAL FRAGMENTATION OF THE CARPUS

Osteochondral chip fractures of the equine carpus are common in racehorses. Patients present with synovial effusion and various degrees of lameness. In cases of osteochondral fragmentation with minimal associated damage, the main clinical sign is that the horses jog with a wide-based stance. The presence of fragmentation is confirmed with radiographs. Deficiencies have been noted in the radiographic demonstration of some fragments and in the amount of associated articular damage.[35]

Arthroscopic surgery for the removal of these osteochondral fragments is indicated for the immediate relief of clinical signs as well as to prevent further development of OA. Carpal chip fragments are considered to cause pain because of their tugging on synovial membrane attachments, to induce synovitis, and to cause damage to the opposing articular surface (kissing lesions). All these factors may contribute to the cycle of OA, and this cycle is self-perpetuating after removal of the chip fragments if surgical intervention is not timely. Other factors enter into case selection for surgery, particularly the athletic ability of the horse and economics.

All osteochondral chip fragments in the carpus are operated using arthroscopic technique, which has been extensively described elsewhere.[30,35] Arthroscopic surgery for the removal of any osteochondral fragment from either carpal joint involves triangulation technique using two portals that remain consistent for all locations of fractures in these joints. The position of the arthroscope and instrument relative to the appropriate lesion is illustrated in Figure 7.36, using the distal radial carpal bone as an example. The arthroscope is placed through the lateral portal with the lens angle proximad, and the instruments are brought through the medial portal.[30] A diagnostic examination is always performed first.

Carpal chip fragments can be divided into four categories, and the techniques used for their removal vary accordingly. If the chip is fresh and mobile on palpation, grasping forceps are immediately inserted, the chip is grasped, the forceps are rotated to free the chip of soft tissue attachments (if they are significant), and the chip is removed. Ferris-Smith intervertebral disk rongeurs are the most commonly used forceps for removal of fragments. In the second category of chip fragments, synovial membrane and fibrous capsule attachments of the fracture line are stronger, and the chip cannot be displaced with initial probing. In this case, an elevator is used to separate the chip from the parent bone. Ideally the fragment should not be completely separated, as it then becomes a loose body and is more difficult to remove. A third category (uncommon) is a longstanding fragment

when bony reattachment is developing. An osteotome may be used to free the fragment from the bone. A fourth category of chip fragment involves extensive bony reattachment and a proliferative response as well. These cases are amenable to the osteotome, but use of a motorized arthrobur is often appropriate. These patients are generally poor candidates for arthroscopic surgery and should not represent a major portion of any surgeon's caseload. It is common to find more damage than anticipated at arthroscopy (see Fig 7.34).

Once the chip is removed, the defect is debrided, and underlying cartilage or flakes of cartilage at the base of the lesion are removed by using a bone curet and forceps. Soft defective tissue in the base of the defect is commonly recognized and is also curetted. Debridement of articular defects is based on our current knowledge of an articular cartilage lesion (see next section). After debridement the joint is flushed using the egress cannula.

The horse is re-covered in a sterile padded bandage. Phenylbutazone is administered postoperatively. Perioperative antibiotics are not usually administered unless there are recent concerns of intraarticular contamination or respiratory infections. It has been shown that 100 *S. aureus* organisms are required to achieve infection in an equine joint.[19] If there has been intervention (joint injection or intrasynovial anesthesia) in a joint within the previous 2 to 3 weeks, the use of prophylactic antibiotics could be appropriate. The skin sutures are removed 10 to 14 days after surgery, and a program of hand walking begun at this time. Complications from surgery are few.

Compared with the benefits from arthrotomy, we consider the benefits from arthroscopic surgery to include increased diagnostic accuracy (and, therefore, more definitive treatment of the condition), less tissue damage and better cosmetic appearance of the joints, more complete irrigation of the joint and elimination of debris, less postoperative pain, the ability to operate multiple joints concurrently, and improved performance after surgery.[35] Postsurgical information has been reported for 445 racehorses.[35] After surgery, 303 (68.1%) raced at a level equal to or better than preinjury levels, 49 (11.0%) had decreased performance or still had problems referable to the carpus, 23 (5.2%) were retired without returning to training, 28 (6.3%) sustained another chip fracture, 37 (7.2%) developed other problems, and 10 (2.2%) sustained collapsing slab fractures while racing. Earlier reports with arthrotomy considered return to competition or starting in one race to be a success.[27,52] Using such criteria for success would mean 88.6% of Thoroughbreds and 88.8% of Quarter Horses were successful in our study.[35] However, we believe that the same level or higher is a more reliable criterion and at least eliminates the variable of the horse's ability.[33]

When horses were separated into four categories of articular damage, the performance of the two most severely affected groups was significantly inferior. Some 133 of 187 horses with grade 1 damage (71.1%), 108 of 144 horses with grade 2 damage (75%), 41 of 77 horses with grade 3 damage (53.2%), and 20 of 37 horses with grade 4 damage (54%) returned to racing equal to or better than before injury. The success rate in horses with grade 1 and grade 2 lesions was significantly higher than in those with grade 3 and grade 4 lesions ($P < .01$).[35]

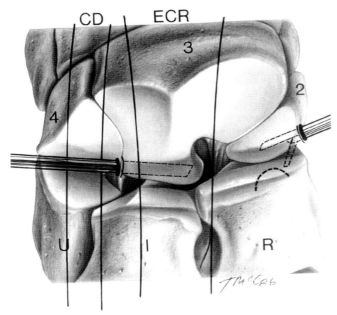

Figure 7.36 Diagram of technique for the removal of carpal chip fragment. (Reprinted with permission from McIlwraith CW. Fractures of the carpus. In: Nixon AJ. Equine Fracture Repair. Philadelphia: WB Saunders, 1996;211.)

OSTEOCHONDRAL FRAGMENTATION IN THE FETLOCK JOINT

This section includes osteochondral chip fragments of the dorsal and palmar/plantar aspects of the first phalanx and osteochondral fractures of the proximal sesamoid bones.

PROXIMODORSAL OSTEOCHONDRAL FRACTURES OF THE PROXIMAL (FIRST) PHALANX. These fracture fragments are common in racehorses. All but 1 of 63 horses in a 1986 retrospective study reporting on arthroscopic surgery for the removal of these fragments were racehorses.[53] However, more recently, cases of rounded fragments of long-term duration have been recognized in nonracehorses and may represent a different entity.[24]

The typical signalment in a racehorse is the presence of synovial effusion in the fetlock joint, varying degrees of lameness, some dorsal soft tissue swelling, and pain upon flexion of the joint. The injury occurs typically during strenuous exercise. The clinical signs are most prominent during the first few days after injury. Lameness is mild to moderate. Fragments may occur on one medial or lateral eminence (most commonly in the former).[30] Clinical signs may decrease with rest and become apparent again with exercise. In most instances, the fragment is considered to be the result of trauma (compression of the dorsoproximal portion of the proximal phalanx against the distal part of the third metacarpal bone when extreme extension of the fetlock joint occurs during racing or fast training).[9,20] It has also been suggested that these fragments are a secondary complication affecting joint margins altered by DJD and that the fractures can arise by fragmentation of the original tissue of the joint margin or within the bony base of a periarticular lip that forms in DJD.[42] Recognition of fragments that are rounded and chronic in young horses as incidental findings suggest developmental pathogenesis in some instances. However, developmental pathogenesis is not considered to be the usual situation in the racehorse, as has been implied by some authors.[25]

The treatment of choice when the fragment is causing clinical signs is surgical removal using arthroscopic surgery, even when the fragment is small (Fig. 7.37).[24,30,53] However, many of these chip fractures are treated conservatively, and satisfactory repair and athletic activity can result if the joint is kept at rest for 3 to 6 months.[2] Because of the occurrence of calcification over the dorsal aspect of the equine metacarpophalangeal joint after removal of chip fragments using arthrotomy, conservative treatment was recommended in the past.[2] It was felt at that time that removal of most of the chip fragments was not necessary to restore a horse to a functional state, in that the complication of calcification of the capsule and associated lameness could be avoided. Surgical morbidity has been decreased or eliminated with the use of arthroscopic surgery. Although it has been proposed that most fractures will heal with time, and this is possibly true, no follow-up study on racing performance after conservative treatment has been reported. In an initial study on the use of arthroscopic surgery for the treatment of these fractures, the training period during which fragmentation occurred was known for 50 of 63 horses. Of these 50 horses, the interval between injury and ar-

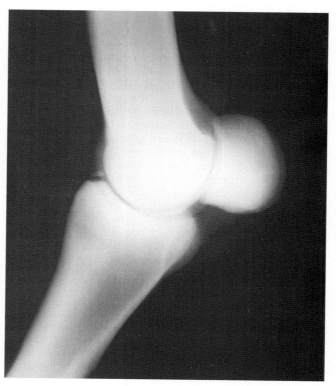

Figure 7.37 A small chip fragment off the proximodorsal aspect of first phalanx.

throscopic surgery was less than 5 weeks for 13, 2 to 4 months for 23, and more than 6 months for 14 horses.[53] Most of these latter instances involved horses that had not responded well to conservative treatment and training had been continued.

Osteochondral chip fragments are removed using arthroscopic technique in the dorsal pouch of the metacarpophalangeal (metatarsophalangeal) joint.[30] The arthroscopic portal is located in the proximolateral aspect of the distended dorsal joint pouch.[24] If the fragment is located on a proximolateral eminence, it is removed first using a lateral arthroscopic portal. Proximomedial fragments are removed using a medial portal. These techniques are described in more detail in another text.[30] The usual sequence of instrument use is egress cannula insertion to clear the visual field, an elevator to break the fragment, fragment removal with Ferris-Smith rongeurs, and debridement of the fracture bed. The presence of any associated articular cartilage erosion and wear lines on the distal metacarpus or metatarsus is noted during surgery. After debridement of the defect, the joint is flushed with fluid, using a 4.5-mm egress cannula, and the skin portals are closed. The horse is re-covered, with the leg in a sterile bandage.

The results of arthroscopic surgery for the treatment of these chip fractures were initially reported for 74 fetlock joints of 63 horses (35 Thoroughbreds and 28 Quarter Horses) during a 2-year period.[53] In a more recent and extensive study, results have been recorded for 320 horses with 446 osteochondral fragments removed from 417 fetlock joints.[18,24] Some 295 of the horses were racehorses, including 181 Thoroughbreds, 111 Quarter

Horses, 2 Standardbreds, and 1 racing Arabian. There were 25 nonracehorses. A single metacarpophalangeal joint was operated in 209 horses, while both metacarpophalangeal joints were operated in 94. Fragmentation of the proximodorsal first phalanx was the only lesion in the fetlocks of 93 horses. Some 134 horses had other lesions in the fetlock along with fragmentation. These included 64 with wear lines, 11 with articular cartilage erosion, 13 with chronic proliferative synovitis, 3 with OCD, and 43 with a combination of the above lesions. Carpal arthroscopy for removal of osteochondral chips was performed additionally in 93 of these horses. Follow-up was available for 260 horses. Of these, 191 (73.5%) returned to their intended use. This included 141 (54.2%) that returned to the same level of performance, 50 (19.2%) horses that returned to performance but at a lower level, 18 hoses (6.9%) that developed another fragment, and 51 (19.6%) horses that did not return to their intended use. Of the 244 racehorses with follow-up, 179 (73.4%) returned to racing, and 129 (52.9%) of these raced at the same or higher level; 18 (7.4%) of the racehorses developed another fragment, and 47 (19.2%) were in the failure category. Horses that sustained chip fragmentation alone without other intra-articular changes in the fetlock joints had a higher return to use than those with other (including articular cartilage erosions or wear lines) lesions (86 vs. 75%). This difference was significant.[24]

PROXIMAL PALMAR/PLANTAR (FIRST) PHALANX FRAGMENTATION. Bony fragments associated with the palmar or plantar aspect of the metacarpophalangeal and metatarsophalangeal joints were first described in 1972 by Birkeland.[6] Opinions differ as to the pathogenesis of these fragments, but several authors propose that they result from fracture.[6,40] Lameness caused by the bony fragments is usually evident only at the horse's maximal performance.[4,13,32a] A history of swelling of the fetlock joint and lameness that increases after fast work is common.[40] The lameness is usually mild, and flexion of the fetlock joint will increase the lameness. It was noted in one study that intraarticular injection of local anesthetic abolished lameness in only 12 of the 43 horses investigated, whereas high volar or plantar nerve block successfully abolished lameness in all cases.[40] Not all fragments at this location give rise to lameness.[17,18] Fragments were also observed in the palmar/plantar part of the metacar-

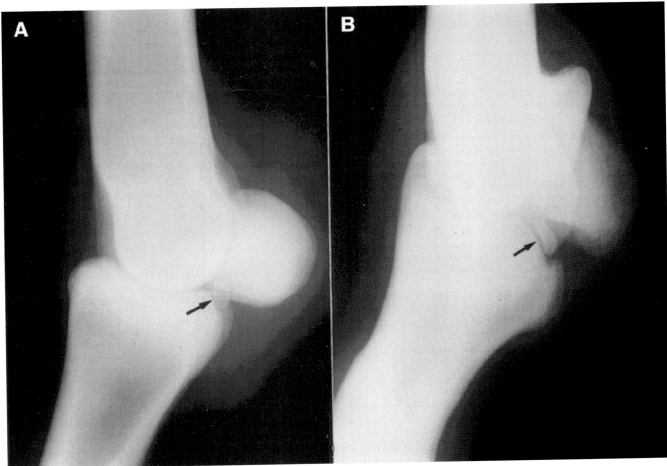

Figure 7.38   Lateral (A) and 30: downwardly angled oblique (B) views of a fragment (arrows) from the proximal plantar aspect of the first phalanx. (Reprinted with permission from McIlwraith CW. Diagnostic and Surgical Arthroscopy in the Horse. 2nd ed. Philadelphia: Lea & Febiger, 1990;106.)

pophalangeal and metatarsophalangeal joint in 89 (11.8%) of 753 yearling Standardbred trotters.[18]

Two types of fragments have been described: 1) type I osteochondral fragments of the palmar/plantar aspect[13] (also called bony fragments of the palmar/plantar part of the metacarpophalangeal and metatarsophalangeal joint)[45] and 2) type II osteochondral fragments of the palmar/plantar aspect of the fetlock joint[13] (also called ununited proximoplantar tuberosity of the proximal phalanx).[17] Lameness is usually slight with type 1 fragments and may be performance limiting only at the upper levels of competition or performance. Fragments are best demonstrated on dorsoproximal lateral–palmaro (plantaro)distal medial or dorsoproximal medial–palmaro(plantaro)distal lateral oblique views (Fig. 7.38).[18,45] Lameness may develop in association with type II fragments but is uncommon.

The patient that has a demonstrable lameness referable to the fetlock in addition to a radiographically demonstrable lesion is a definite surgical candidate. In these cases, arthroscopic surgery is an effective means of treatment.[15] "Prophylactic" removal is also practiced in young horses. The horse is operated in lateral or dorsal recumbency, depending on the preference of the surgeon. The arthroscope is placed in the plantar or palmar joint pouch after distending the joint with sterile polyionic fluid. The arthroscope is positioned to visualize the distal

part of the joint. An assistant facilitates this step by flexing the joint. After the correct position is ascertained with a needle, an instrument portal is made distal to the arthroscopic portal so that an instrument moves along the base of the sesamoid. The fragment can sometimes be visualized, but in other situations a probe is used to ensure its location. It can be found between the base of the sesamoid and the first phalanx under the central area of the sesamoid bone. The fragment is separated from the soft tissue with a knife and removed by using Ferris-Smith cup rongeurs. Debridement of the proximal first phalanx is not usually necessary.

Surgery is rarely indicated with type II osteochondral fragments (or ununited proximoplantar tuberosity of the proximal phalanx) (Fig. 7.39). This lesion was seen in 18 (2.4%) of 753 Standardbred yearlings radiographed.[18] All fragments were in the pelvic limb. The condition was seen laterally in 16 horses, while one horse had a medial and lateral tuberosity affected, and another had only one medial tuberosity affected. Lameness was not observed in any horse prior to first examination. On follow-up examination, 12 lesions in 11 horses had united to the proximal phalanx after 6 to 12 months. One horse was unchanged after 7 months, and the remaining 4 horses had a radiographic worsening of the condition, with the ununited proximoplantar tuberosity being more dislocated. Three of these 4 horses also had

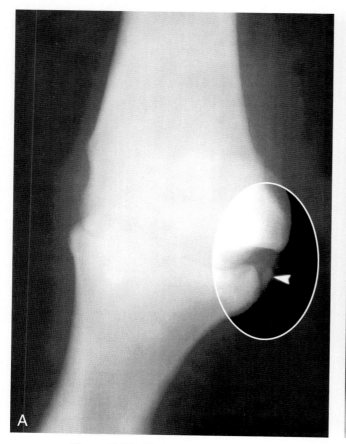 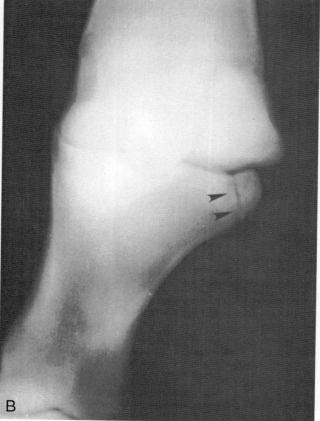

Figure 7.39 Two examples of type II osteochondral fragments (or ununited proximoplantar tuberosity of the proximal phalanx).

calcification of the distal sesamoid ligament and periosteal proliferation. Two of the horses with the most severe radiographic changes developed lameness and subsequently underwent surgery to remove the fragment. Removal of type II fragments, if considered necessary, is achieved using an arthrotomy technique distal to the sesamoid bone.[7,13] A vertical 4-cm skin incision is made on the abaxial surface of the fetlock joint at the level of the proximal first phalanx, which is palpable, and dorsal to the palmar digital artery, vein, and nerve, which are retracted caudally. The incision is continued through the distal part of the anular ligament of the fetlock and joint capsule immediately distad to the collateral sesamoid ligament and proximal to the proximal surface of the first phalanx. A retractor is used, and with the fetlock flexed, exposure of the fracture site is possible. The fracture fragment is dissected free and removed. Lag screw of a large fracture has also been done.

In the case of type I fragments operated with arthroscopic surgery, hand walking is started at 2 weeks and gradually increased over the next 6 weeks. A period of 2 to 3 months rest before training is resumed is recommended. The convalescent time for fractures removed using arthrotomy is 6 months.

Successful results with type I osteochondral fragments have been obtained with arthroscopic surgery.[32a] Recently, a series of type I fragments have been reported.[14] In an earlier series of 19 horses, 10 were treated with arthrotomy and all returned to full use, whereas of 7 treated intraarticularly with corticosteroids, only 1 was able to return to full use.[4] In another study of palmar/plantar process fractures in 15 horses, all horses that were operated on were sound within 6 months after surgery, and 14 returned to an equal or better level of performance.[7] Because of lack of definition of the location of fragments and low numbers, prognostic figures are not really available with type II fragments.

OSTEOCHONDRAL CHIP FRACTURES OF PROXIMAL SESAMOID BONES. Osteochondral chip fragments amenable to removal occur at the apical, abaxial, and basilar margins of the proximal sesamoid bones (Fig. 7.40). Arthroscopic techniques for the removal of these fragments have been developed. Previous dogma has proposed limitations for fragment removal based on the size of the fragment and the degree of attachment to the suspensory and distal sesamoid ligaments. However, current follow-up on the author's cases that have been treated arthroscopically suggest that limitations should be strictly defined. As a generalization, however, the idea that the prognosis will worsen with greater involvement of both bone and soft tissue attachments is still considered reasonably valid. The diagnosis is made radiographically, and special views are used to clearly delineate the articular involvement of abaxial fragments. Arthroscopic surgery for removal of sesamoid fragments is performed with the horse in either lateral or dorsal recumbency. The arthroscope is placed in the most proximal portion of the palmar or plantar pouch of the fetlock joint. With partial flexion of the joint, a needle is used to ascertain the ideal placement of the instrument portal. Sharp dissection is used to separate apical and abaxial fragments from the suspensory ligament as well as the intersesamoid ligament in the case of apical fragments. A curved blade is used

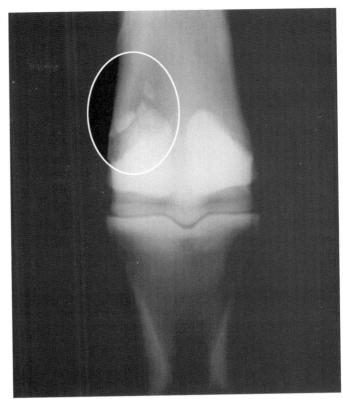

Figure 7.40   Comminuted fragmentation of the apical and abaxial areas of the sesamoid bone. The horse was able to return to athletic activity after arthroscopic surgery.

to continue dissection, and the fragments are removed after separation. Soft tissue attachments are trimmed. Fragmentation involving the apex and abaxial portions of the sesamoid bone involving more than one-third of the articular surface is not considered an ideal candidate for removal. A series of cases of abaxial sesamoid fractures has been reported recently.[46a]

Basilar sesamoid fragments are candidates for arthroscopic removal if no other pathologic changes are present in the fetlock joint (Figs. 7.41 and 7.42). A reasonable number of fragments are small enough that their removal does not compromise distal sesamoid ligament attachments. The exact size limitations are still being defined. The horses are operated in the flexed position with the instrument coming across the base of the sesamoid. Sharp dissection is used to sever the fragment from capsular and distal sesamoid ligament attachments. The defects are then debrided (bone and soft tissue), and the joints flushed.

OSTEOCHONDRAL FRAGMENTATION OF THE TARSUS

Intraarticular chip fragments in the tarsocrural joint are relatively uncommon but do occur. Small fragments from the proximal aspect of the medial trochlear ridge have been encountered after traumatic injury.[30] In these cases, the fragments may be removed arthroscopically, and both the arthroscopic and the instrument portal are through the medial plantar pouch. The fragment(s) are removed, and the defects in the medial trochlear ridge

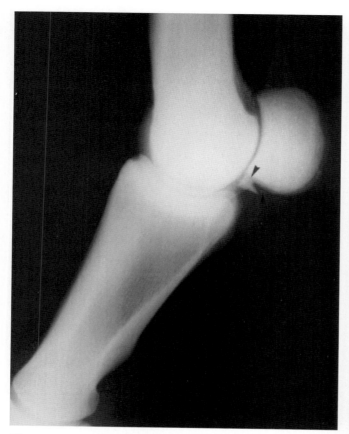

Figure 7.41 A small basilar chip fragment of the sesamoid bone that was removed with arthroscopic surgery. The horse returned to racing.

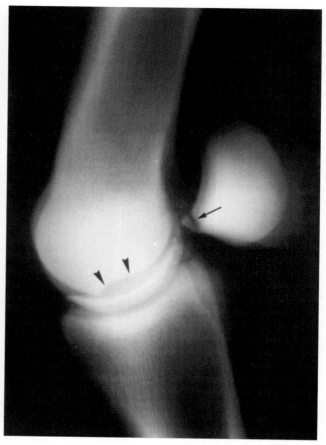

Figure 7.42 Fragment from the base of a sesamoid bone (long arrow) in a fetlock joint that also exhibits palmar metacarpal disease (short arrows). In such a case, surgery is contraindicated, and the pathogenesis of the fragment is pathologic.

debrided. Osteochondral fragments also occur in the dorsal pouch of the proximal intertarsal joint, and their successful treatment with arthroscopic surgery has been described.[47]

The most common fractures associated with the tarsocrural joints are lateral malleolar fractures. Only a small portion of the lateral malleolus is intraarticular, and most of these fragments are enclosed within joint capsule and collateral ligament (Fig. 7.43). Unless the fragment is very small and intraarticular, arthroscopic surgery is not the appropriate treatment. The clinical and radiologic features as well as the surgical technique and results for removal of these fragments have been reported in 16 horses.[51] Fourteen fractures were unilateral and two were bilateral. The history included a known traumatic incident in 14 of the 16 horses. All animals had tarsocrural joint effusion, and 10 had palpable thickening of the lateral collateral ligament. A fracture was identified in all dorsoplantar and 14 of 18 dorsomedial–plantarolateral oblique radiographic projections. Nine fractures were simple and 9 were comminuted. All were removed via a tarsocrural arthrotomy (dorsolateral in 14, plantarolateral in 3, and dorsolateral and plantarolateral in 1). Horses were returned to work 6 months after surgery. Fifteen horses were free of lameness after 17 to 62 months, with 13 animals performing at a level similar to their preinjury standard.

OSTEOCHONDRAL FRAGMENTATION OF THE FEMOROPATELLAR JOINT

Osteochondral fragmentation of the distal aspect of the patella has been described by the author and is associated with medial patellar desmotomy.[31] Based on an experimental study, it is felt that the medial patellar desmotomy creates a period (probably temporary) of instability, which leads to traumatically induced fragmentation of the distal aspect of the patella.[16] It is not necessarily a single traumatic event, however.

Horses present with fibrous thickening associated with the patellar desmotomy and synovial effusion in most instances. Radiographic changes include bony fragmentation, spurring (with or without an associated subchondral defect), subchondral roughening, and subchondral lysis of the distal aspect of the patella. Horses may be treated with arthroscopic surgery. The lesions at arthroscopy vary from flaking, fissuring, undermining, or fragmentation of the articular cartilage to fragmentation or lysis of the bone at the distal aspect of the patella. Of 12 horses reported initially, 8 became sound at their intended use, 1 was sold in training without problems, 1 was in training without problems, 1 never improved, and 1 was in convalescence.[31]

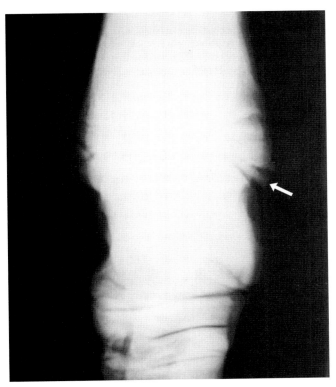

Figure 7.43 Dorsoplantar radiograph demonstrating a fracture of the lateral malleolus of the tibia.

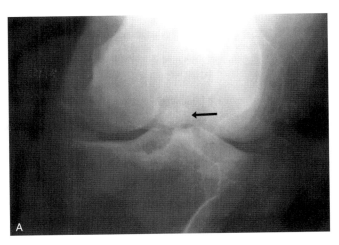

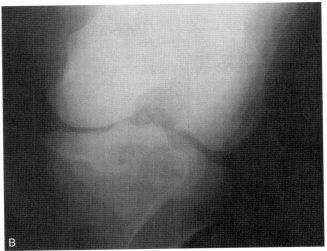

Figure 7.44 Cranial caudal radiograph of a jumper with a fracture of the intercondylar eminence of the tibia before (A) and after (B) arthroscopic removal.

Fracture fragments also occur from the lateral and medial aspects of the patella.[30] These are associated with an acute traumatic event (direct trauma on the patella is the usual situation). There is severe lameness referable to the stifle, as well as swelling, including femoropatellar effusion. Conventional radiographs may show sufficient changes, but a skyline radiograph of the femoropatellar joint is usually necessary to define the fracture. These cases have been treated with arthroscopic removal of the fragments using the same arthroscopic portal as that used for operating OCD. A medial or lateral portal, as appropriate, is used. It is important to have correct direction, as the fragmentation often extends from dorsal to proximal limits of the patella.

OSTEOCHONDRAL FRAGMENTATION OF THE FEMOROTIBIAL JOINT

Traumatic injuries in the femorotibial joints have become more recognized in recent years with the development of femorotibial arthroscopic techniques. The most common injuries are ones involving the cruciate ligaments and menisci. However, traumatic injury to articular cartilage and/or bone may also occur in the joint. Fractures of the intercondylar eminence of the tibia occur and can range from being small to quite large (Fig. 7.44). These were previously diagnosed as avulsions of the cruciate ligament and considered to represent a loss of cruciate integrity. However, a large part of the eminence does not provide attachment to the cruciate ligament, and arthroscopic removal of these fragments is appropriate and can yield a good prognosis.

DEBRIDEMENT OF ARTICULAR SURFACE DEFECTS

The limitations of articular cartilage repair have long been recognized and are discussed above (page 475). Fibrocartilage is biochemically and biomechanically defective, is unsuitable as a replacement bearing surface, and has been shown to undergo mechanical failure with use. This lack of durability may be related to faulty biochemical composition of the matrix or incomplete remodeling of the interface between old and repair cartilage, as well as abnormal stresses and degeneration associated with abnormal remodeling of the subchondral bone plate and calcified cartilage layer.

Loss of articular cartilage occurs in association with acute traumatic injury and also from OA. A cartilage defect may not represent clinical compromise, at least in some acute situations. Loss of up to 30% of the visible articular surface of a carpal bone, for instance, does not compromise the successful return of the horse to racing.[35] On the other hand, a 50% loss of the articular surface or a severe loss of subchondral bone carries a significantly poorer prognosis.

The repair of articular cartilage necessitates considering two situations: 1) superficial defects that do not penetrate the full thickness of the articular cartilage and 2) full-thickness defects. Superficial defects in equine articular cartilage do not heal, whereas full-thickness defects heal through formation of granulation tissue and its subsequent metaplasia resulting in a mixture of fibrous tissue and fibrocartilage (see Chapter 3). However, partial-thickness defects, while not healing, are not necessarily progressive, and the author's approach to debridement of such defects is conservative. The use of partial-thickness chondrectomy down to relatively healthy chondral tissue (shaving) has been used in humans to smooth the fragmented cartilage area, and this may decrease further tissue exfoliation, producing (in conjunction with joint lavage) early remission of synovitis. However, controlled work is necessary to evaluate the usefulness of such debridement. In one study, articular cartilage was shaved on the underside of the rabbit patella with no evidence of repair and no evidence of degenerative changes in either the superficially or deeply shaved areas.[38] Results of ultrastructural studies after arthroscopic cartilage shaving suggest that shaving does not help.[46] The results of a study in humans that involved follow-up arthroscopy for chondromalacia of the knee, with or without cartilaginous shaving, led to the conclusion that only loosely hanging articular cartilage material should be shaved and softened or nonloose fissured articular cartilage should be spared.[15]

With full-thickness lesions, inadequate healing has been well substantiated, and as yet, no surgical procedure has been shown to change this situation significantly. A relatively conservative approach with debridement of deeper defects thus is used. Any rough edges of the defect are smoothed, and adjacent undermined or fragmented cartilage is removed, usually using a forceps or bone curet. This protocol is based on the belief that any type of loose articular cartilage or bone is irritating, and its prospects of healing onto bone virtually nil. Full-thickness defects are debrided to the level of subchondral bone, and any soft defective bone is removed.

The author also feels that deeper extensive debridement using motorized equipment is unnecessary and can cause problems in the carpus and fetlock. If the debridement extends beyond the level of attachment of the joint capsule, increased capsulitis and enthesitis postoperatively is a possibility.

Relating some of these ideas to follow-up management, the material that fills the defects left by fresh localized chip fragments is not of major concern. The area of the defect is not critical to the horse's joint function, and if other sources of irritation have been removed, athletic function should be limited only by soft tissue handling, and an early return to training can be achieved. When the lesions are more severe, the importance of an intact subchondral bone support becomes more relevant. However, as mentioned above, methods of modulation for optimal healing have yet to be developed.

The potential usefulness of debridement in cases of extensive OA is commonly questioned. Debridement has been shown to be a useful technique in OA in humans, but its primary usefulness has been for partial meniscectomy, limited debridement of loose articular cartilage, and removal of loose bodies in joints that also happen to have degenerative changes.[37] It is felt the same principles apply in the equine situation. When OA is present prior to surgery, the prognosis is always guarded, because removal of fragmentation does not result in athletic soundness in most cases. Early arthroscopic treatment of osteochondral fragmentation is critical to minimizing the development of OA.

References

1. Adams OR. Lameness in Horses. 3rd ed. Philadelphia: Lea & Febiger, 1974.
2. Baker CW. Calcification of the equine metacarpophalangeal joint following removal of chip fractures. Arch Am Coll Vet Surg 1975; 4:66.
3. Barber SM. Interphalangeal joint subluxation in horses. J Am Vet Med Assoc 1982;181:1468.
4. Barclay WP, Foerner JJ, Philips TN. Lameness attributable to osteochondral fragmentation of the plantar aspect of the proximal phalanx in horses: 19 cases (1981–1985). J Am Vet Med Assoc 1987;191:855–857.
5. Bennett D, Campbell JR, Rawlinson JR. Coxofemoral luxation complicated by upward fixation of the patella in the pony. Equine Vet J 1977;9:192.
6. Birkeland R. Chip fractures of the first phalanx in the metatarsophalangeal joint of the horse. Acta Radiol Suppl 1972;29:73–77.
6a. Buckwalter JA. Mechanical injuries of articular cartilage. In: Finerman GAM, Noyes FR, Eds. Biology and Biomechanics of the Traumatized Synovial Joint: The Knee as a Model. Rosemont, IL. American Academy of Orthopaedic Surgeons, 1992;83–96.
7. Bukowiezki CF, Bramlage LR, Gabel AA. Palmar/plantar process fractures of the proximal phalanx in 15 horses. Vet Surg 1986; 15:383–388.
8. Churchill EA. Lameness in the Standardbred. In: Harrison JC, Ed. Care and Training of the Trotter and Pacer. Columbus, Ohio: US Trotting Association, 1968;795–873.
9. Copelan R, Bramlage LR. Surgery of the fetlock joint. Vet Clin North Am 1983;2:221–231.
10. Edwards GB, Vaughan LC. Use of carbon fibre implants in the treatment of fetlock joint dislocation in two horses. Vet Rec 1984; 114;87–88.
11. Evans CH, Mears DC, Cosgrove JL. Release of neutral proteinases from mononuclear phagocytes and synovial cells in response to cartilaginous wear particles in vitro. Biochim Biophys Acta 1981;677:287–294.
12. Finerman GAM, Noyes FR, Eds. Biology and Biomechanics of the Traumatized Synovial Joint: The Knee as a Model. Rosemont, IL. American Academy of Orthopaedic Surgeons, 1992.
13. Foerner JJ, Barclay WP, Philips TN, MacHarg MA. Osteochondral fragments of the palmar/plantar aspect of the fetlock joint. Proceedings. 33rd Annual Meeting of the American Association of Equine Practitioners, New Orleans, LA, 1987;739–744.
14. Fortier LA, Foerner JJ, Nixon AJ. Arthroscopic removal of axial osteochondral fragments of the plantar/palmar proximal aspect of the proximal phalanx in horses: 119 cases (1988–1992). J Am Vet Med Assoc 1995;206:71–74.
15. Friedman MJ, et al. Chondromalacia of the knee: The comparison between those treated with and without intra-articular shaving. Arthroscopy 1987;3:131.
16. Gibson KT, McIlwraith CW, Park RD, et al. Production of patellar lesions by medial patellar desmotomy in normal horses. Vet Surg 1989;18:466–471.
17. Grondahl AM. The incidence of bony fragments in osteochondrosis in the metacarpo- and metatarsophalangeal joints of Standardbred trotters. A radiographic study. J Equine Vet Sci 1992;12: 81–85.
18. Grondahl AM. Incidence and development of ununited proximoplantar tuberosity of the proximal phalanx in Standardbred trotters. Vet Radiol Ultrasound 1992;33:18–21.
19. Gustafson SB, McIlwraith CW, Jones RL. Comparison of the effects of polysulfated glycosaminoglycans, corticosteroids and sodium hyaluronate in the potentiation of a subinfective dose of

Staphylococcus aureus in the midcarpal joint of horses. Am J Vet Res 1989;50:2014–2017.

20. Haynes PF. Diseases of the metatarsophalangeal joint and metacarpus. Vet Clin North Am [Large Anim Pract] 1980;2:33–85.

21. Johnston-Jones K, Gebhard JS, Kabo JM, Meals RA. The effect of terfenadine on joint stiffness and bone healing after periarticular fracture. In: Proceedings. 38th Annual Meeting of the Orthopaedic Research Society, 1992;266.

22. Kannegieter NJ. Inter-carpal ligament damage as a cause of lameness in the horse. In: Proceedings. 12th Bain-Fallon Lectures, Austrian Equine Veterinary Association, 1992;175–176.

23. Kannegieter NJ, Burbidge HM. Correlation between radiographic and arthroscopic findings in equine carpus. Aust Vet J 1990;67:132–133.

24. Kawcak CE, McIlwraith CW. Proximodorsal first phalanx osteochondral chip fragments in 336 horses. Equine Vet J 1994;26:392–396.

25. Krook L, Maylin GA. Fractures in Thoroughbred racehorses. Cornell Vet 1988;78:5–74.

26. Lefkoe TP, Trafton PG, Dennehy DT, et al. A new model of articular step-off for the study of post-traumatic arthritis. In: Proceedings. 38th Annual Meeting of the Orthopaedic Research Society, 1992;207.

27. Lindsay WA, Horney FD. Equine carpal surgery: Review of 89 cases and evaluation of return to function. J Am Vet Med Assoc 1981;179:682–685.

28. Mackay-Smith MP, Raker CW. Mechanical defects of the equine stifle—Diagnosis and treatment. Proceedings. Annual Meeting of the American Veterinary Medical Association, 1963;142:82–85.

29. Madison JB, Young D, Richardson D. Repair of shoulder luxation in a horse. J Am Vet Med Assoc 1991;198:455–457.

30. McIlwraith CW. Diagnostic and Surgical Arthroscopy in the Horse. 2nd ed. Philadelphia: Lea & Febiger, 1990.

31. McIlwraith CW. Osteochondral fragmentation of the distal aspect of the patella in horses. Equine Vet J 1990;22:157–163.

32. McIlwraith CW. Tearing of the medial palmar intercarpal ligament in the equine midcarpal joint. Equine Vet J 1992;24:367–371.

32a. McIlwraith CW, Foerner JJ. Removal of osteochondral fragments from the proximal palmar or plantar aspect of the first phalanx. In: McIlwraith CW, Ed. Diagnostic and Surgical Arthroscopy. 2nd ed. Philadelphia: Lea & Febiger, 1989.

33. McIlwraith CW, Turner AS. Assessing success of surgery. Equine Vet J 1986;18:165–166.

34. McIlwraith CW, Warren RC. Distal luxation of the patella in a horse. J Am Vet Med Assoc 1982;181:67.

35. McIlwraith CW, Yovich JV, Martin GS. Arthroscopic surgery for the treatment of osteochondral chip fractures in the equine carpus. J Am Vet Med Assoc 1987;191:531–540.

36. Meals RA. Post-traumatic limb swelling and joint stiffness are not causally related experimental observations in rabbits. Clin Orthop 1993;287:292–303.

37. Merchan ECR, Galindo E. Arthroscope-guided surgery versus nonoperative treatment for limited degenerative osteoarthritis of the femorotibial joint in patients over 50 years of age: A prospective comparative study. Arthroscopy 1993;9:663–667.

38. Mitchell N, Shepherd N. Effects of patellar shaving in the rabbit. J Orthop Res 1987;5:388–392.

39. Nyack B, Willard MJ, Stott J, Padmore CL. Nonsurgical repair of coxofemoral luxation in a Quarter Horse filly. Equine Pract 1982;4:11.

40. Pettersson H, Ryden G. Avulsion fractures of the caudoproximal extremity of the first phalanx. Equine Vet J 1982;14:333–335.

41. Pinals RS. Traumatic arthritis and allied conditions. In: Arthritis and Allied Conditions. 9th ed. Philadelphia: Lea & Febiger, 1979.

42. Pool RR, Meagher DM. Pathologic findings and pathogenesis of racetrack injuries. Vet Clin North Am: Equine Pract 1990;6:1–30.

43. Raker CW. Clinical observations of bone and joint disease in horses. Cornell Vet 1968;58:15.

44. Repo RU, Finlay JV. Survival of articular cartilage after controlled impact. J Bone Joint Surg [Am] 1977;59:1068–1076.

45. Sandgren B. Bony fragments in the tarsocrural and metacarpo- or metatarsophalangeal joints in the Standardbred horse—a radiographic survey. Equine Vet J 1988;(Suppl 6):66–70.

46. Schmid A, Schmid F. Ultrastructural changes after arthroscopic or cartilage-shaving. Arthroscopy 1987;3:1–7.

46a. Southwood L, Trotter GW, McIlwraith CW. Arthroscopic removal of abaxial fracture fragments of the proximal sesamoid bone in horses: 47 cases (1989–1997). J Am Vet Med Assoc 1998;213:1016–1021.

47. Stephens PR, Richardson DW, Ross MW, Ford TS. Osteochondral fragments within the dorsal pouch or dorsal joint capsule of the proximal intertarsal joint of the horse. Vet Surg 1989;18:151–157.

48. Valdez H, Adams OR. Surgical approach for medical meniscectomy in the horse. J Am Vet Med Assoc 1978;173;766.

48a. Walmsley JP. Vertical tears of the cranial rim of the meniscus and its cranial ligament in the equine femorotibial joint: 7 cases and their treatment by arthroscopic surgery. Equine Vet J 1995;27:20–25.

49. Whitton RC, McCarthy PH, Rose RJ. The intercarpal ligaments of the equine midcarpal joint. Part I: The anatomy of the palmar and dorsomedial intercarpal ligaments of the midcarpal joint. Vet Surg 1997;26:359–366.

50. Whitton RC, Rose RJ. The intercarpal ligaments of the equine midcarpal joint. Part II: The role of palmar intercarpal ligaments in the restraint of dorsal displacement of the proximal row of carpal bones. Vet Surg 1997;26:367–373.

51. Wright IM. Fractures of the lateral malleolus of tibia in 16 horses. Equine Vet J 1992;24:424–429.

52. Wyburn RS, Goulden DE. Fractures of the equine carpus: Report on 57 cases. NZ Vet J 1987;22:133–143.

53. Yovich JV, McIlwraith CW. Arthroscopic surgery for osteochondral fractures of the proximal phalanx in the metacarpophalangeal and metatarsophalangeal (fetlock) joints in horses. J Am Vet Med Assoc 1986;188:273–279.

SPECIFIC DISEASES OF JOINTS: OSTEOARTHRITIS (DEGENERATIVE JOINT DISEASE)

OA may be considered as a group of disorders characterized by a common end stage: progressive deterioration of the articular cartilage accompanied by changes in the bone and soft tissues of the joint. The deterioration of the articular cartilage is characterized by local splitting and fragmentation (fibrillation) of articular cartilage. Synovitis and joint effusion are often associated with the disease. Clinically, the disease is characterized by pain and dysfunction of the affected joint. Human OA has been classified conventionally into primary and secondary varieties.[23] The term "primary" is used when the causes are unidentified and is typified by the insidiously developing disease of old people. The term "secondary" is used when an etiologic factor can be demonstrated. The "term degenerative joint disease" has been used as a synonym for primary OA. However, as more etiologic factors become identified, the distinction between primary and secondary lessens, and osteoarthritis is now used synonymously with all forms of OA.[35] With the exception of idiopathic synovitis, all the other joint conditions described in this chapter could potentially lead to OA if they are severe enough or treated inappropriately.

There have been various interpretations of OA in the horse.[41] The morphologic changes have been well defined in these accounts, but OA is not a simple morphologic event. Biochemical and molecular events have been recognized in recent years. These events are reviewed above in the pathobiology section.

Clinical Entities

To facilitate discussion of pathogenesis, diagnosis, and treatment, it is appropriate to divide OA in the horse

Table 7.1 DEGENERATIVE JOINT DISEASE ENTITIES
IN THE HORSE

Type
1. Acute—associated with synovitis and high-motion joints
2. Insidious—associated with low-motion joints
3. Incidental or "nonprogressive" articular cartilage erosion
4. Secondary to other identified problems
(a) Intraarticular fractures
(b) Dislocations/ligamentous rupture
(c) Wounds
(d) Septic arthritis
(e) Osteochondrosis
5. Chondromalacia

into four entities and a fifth condition of uncertain status (Table 7.1). The first type typically affects athletes. It is commonly associated with racing and affects the highly mobile joints such as the carpal and metacarpophalangeal joints.[33,39] Acute inflammatory changes (synovitis and capsulitis) accompany, and usually precede, the degenerative process. The second type may be insidious and involves the high load–low motion joints such as the interphalangeal (ringbone) and intertarsal (bone spavin) joints. This type was initially classified as a disease that predominates in mature and aged horses,[39] but it is also a major problem in young competitive horses. The third type includes a series of changes in the articular cartilage that may be recognized during routine necropsies[9,36,56,71,76] but are of questionable clinical significance.[56,76] Sippel noted that the extent of various joint changes in equine joints at routine necropsy did not correlate with the amount of lameness but was more associated with age.[76] This entity may be comparable to the degeneration observed with age in human joints (also called primary OA).[78] The fourth type of DJD includes cases that develop secondary to some other primary joint problems such as intraarticular fractures, unresolved osteochondrosis,[80] tarsal bone collapse,[52,75] flattening and erosion of the distal palmar aspect of the third metacarpal bone,[21,58] and infective arthritis. The fifth type of OA is reserved for chondromalacia of the patella, which is characterized by cartilage fibrillation on the articular surface of the patella.

Pathologic Changes

Destruction of the articular cartilage is the essential pathologic component in a series of events, some degenerative and some regenerative, which ultimately affect all the tissues and structures of the joint. As implied above, the intensity and clinical significance of these changes will vary, and there will be a variety of characteristic manifestations depending on the joint affected. However, destruction of articular cartilage is the sine qua non for OA, and its characteristics are reviewed here before specific changes are considered.

On gross observation the articular cartilage first loses its normal luster and consistency, becoming yellow and

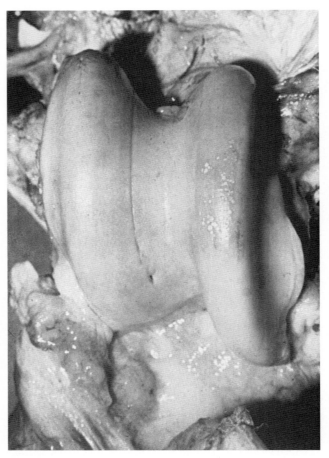

Figure 7.45 Early osteoarthritis with discoloration and blister formation in the articular cartilage.

soft (Fig. 7.45). Blister formation is a common early change (Fig. 7.45),[36] and this leads to pitting and superficial fraying of the cartilage. Progressive loss of cartilage is then manifested in a number of ways and has been assigned a variety of terms. Thinning of the cartilage involves an even decrease in its thickness and may be physiologic, as in the "butterfly area" of articulation between the third metacarpal or third metatarsal bones and the proximal sesamoid bones. "Wearing" is another term that may be considered synonymous with superficial erosions;[56] it is manifested as partial-thickness loss of cartilage (see Fig. 7.54). "Ulcerations" are localized defects in cartilage that probably follow blister formation. "Erosion" represents full-thickness loss of cartilage.[56,76] It may be localized or widespread (see Fig. 7.54). When the subchondral bone becomes exposed, the term "eburnation" is used to describe the polished sclerotic appearance that develops.[78,79] With continued wear, "grooving" may develop within the eburnated subchondral bone (Fig. 7.46). Other changes are illustrated in Figure 7.47. Grooves or "wear lines" are a frequent finding of articular cartilage of equine ginglymal joints and appear as lines running in the direction of joint motion.[36,56,71,76] They vary in width up to 3 mm and may be superficial or deep (Fig. 7.48).

The essential histologic lesion is progressive disruption of the articular cartilage along the planes of the col-

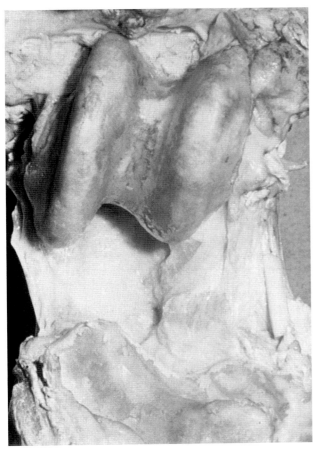

Figure 7.46   Osteoarthritis with partial-thickness and full-thickness erosion of articular cartilage.

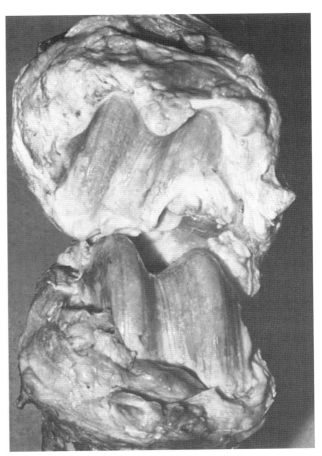

Figure 7.47   Degenerative joint disease with grooving in eburnated subchondral bone.

lagenous fibrils of the matrix. When the disruption is confined to the tangential layer of the matrix, the process has been referred to as "flaking"[77] or "early fibrillation"[79] (Fig. 7.49). When the process extends to the radiate layer it is described as "fibrillation" (Fig. 7.50).[15,77] Early fibrillation is manifested as discoloration or thinning at the gross pathologic level. Fibrillation into the intermediate layer may be represented by superficial erosion. Blisters are considered to represent a sequence of focal edema and localized fibrillation.[36] As fibrillation extends through the radiate layer, vertical clefts are formed, and full-thickness fragmentation and loss of articular cartilage can occur (Fig. 7.51). This degree of change is represented grossly by full-thickness erosion. Wear lines are represented histologically by varying layers of fibrillation, with deep ones appearing similar to deep erosions.[56] Fibrillation is purely a morphologic endpoint and can result from many different normal and abnormal factors.[25]

There is a variable amount of necrosis among the chondrocytes of fibrillated cartilage.[50] Multicellular clusters, or chondrons, develop from other viable chondrocytes and are considered a reactive response (see Fig. 7.59). In addition to the above morphologic changes, histochemical staining indicates depletion of proteoglycans from the articular cartilage, and the water content of the cartilage increases.[45]

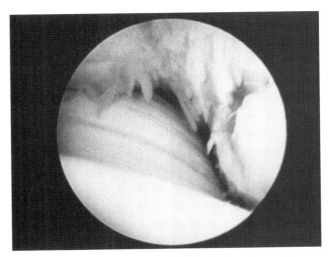

Figure 7.48   Wear lines of the distal articular surface of the third metacarpal bone as visualized at arthroscopy.

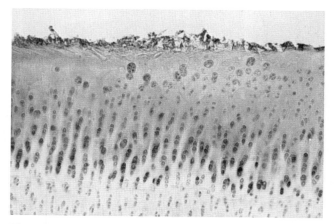

Figure 7.49 Early morphologic change in articular cartilage with osteoarthritis. There is disruption of the tangential layer and chondron formation in the intermediate layer.

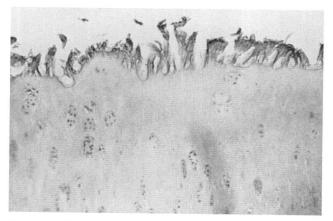

Figure 7.50 More advanced morphologic change in articular cartilage with osteoarthritis. Fibrillation of the matrix has extended into the intermediate layer. There is overall loss of chondrocytes and some chondron formation.

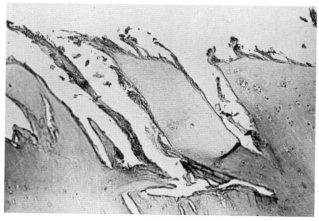

Figure 7.51 Full-thickness fibrillation with severe osteoarthritis. Fibrillated pieces of cartilage are being shed from the bone.

Lesions that accompany articular cartilage changes include marginal ripping or osteophytosis and subchondral bone sclerosis.[36,68,76] The latter is the result of reactive new bone formation in the subchondral end plates. Subchondral cyst formation has been reported as a secondary change in equine OA[58] but is not observed as commonly as it is in humans. (One needs to distinguish secondary subchondral cysts from the cystic bony lesions of osteochondrosis.) Inflammatory changes (acute and chronic) in the synovial membrane and fibrous joint capsule also occur, resulting in villous hypertrophy of the synovial membrane and fibrosis of the joint capsule.[40,70]

In the highly mobile joints of the racehorse (type 1 OA), changes are first seen near the joint margins.[70] There is a sequence of cartilage discoloration, fraying, erosion, and ulceration in discrete areas. Wear lines are common, secondary to chronic osteochondral fragmentation in the carpus and fetlock. Synovitis is prominent in early OA of these joints. In addition to marginal osteophyte formation, fibro-osseous proliferation occurs over the central dorsal surface of the carpal bones and the distal end of the radius. These changes are associated with concurrent traumatic damage to the attachments of the joint capsule and ligaments.[70]

DJD of the interphalangeal (ringbone) and distal intertarsal and tarsometatarsal joints (bone spavin) (type 2 OA) is characterized by periosteal proliferation, with a tendency toward bony ankylosis in advanced cases. In some cases, the periarticular proliferative changes may be present in the absence of intraarticular OA.[30] When OA of the proximal interphalangeal joint develops, the typical pathologic changes are severe and include widespread erosion, subchondral bone sclerosis and eburnation (in most cases), and marginal osteophytes as well as periosteal exostoses. An exceptional characteristic that may be found in bone spavin and in a few instances of ringbone is lysis of subchondral bone, as opposed to the subchondral sclerosis typically seen in other joints.[53]

The various changes in the articular cartilage found in the third (nonclinical) group include blisters, wear lines, ulcerations, and superficial erosions.[36,76] Wide areas of erosion or eburnation are not observed. Another nonclinical cartilage defect routinely observed at specific sites in various joints is the synovial fossa.[71,76] Synovial fossae, or fossae nudatae, are sharply defined depressions of the articular cartilage. In the floor of the fossa the cartilage is reduced to a thin sheet of very irregular thickness separated from the articular surface by a loose pannus. The locations of synovial fossae have been well described by Sippel.[76] Synovial fossae develop postnatally,[74] are seen in all horses over 3 years old, and are unassociated with lameness.[76] It seems that in the later development of the fossae, the cartilage in the floor of the fossa may be completely removed and replaced by pannus, which is vascularized by the spread of vessels either from the neighboring synovial tissue or from the underlying marrow.[29] However, this does not clarify the origin or development of the fossae. They have been considered to be due to lack of proper contact, but the fossae do not consistently form in areas of no contact. Regular sites for synovial fossae in the horse include 1) the distal end of the humerus, 2) the proximal extremities of the radius and ulna (see Fig. 7.62), 3) the intermediate ridge of the distal end of the tibia, and 4) the intertrochlear groove of the tibiotarsal bone. Less common sites for synovial fossae in the horse include the distal ends of the third metacarpal and metatarsal bones, appositional surfaces of the proximal and middle phalanges, and the medial trochlear ridge of the talus.[76] The main importance of synovial fossae is recognition of their existence so they are not confused with cartilaginous erosions of OA.

CORRELATION BETWEEN PATHOLOGIC CHANGES AND CLINICAL SIGNS

It was noted above that some articular cartilage lesions may be of questionable clinical significance. Most of the lesions in Sippel's series were clinically insignificant, and this study helped define a baseline of normal, age-related changes as well as identify the sites for synovial fossae.[76]

It has been recognized in humans that fibrillation in articular cartilage can develop in the absence of clinical signs of OA.[23] Two types of alterations in articular cartilage have been described in the human hip.[8] The first, "nonprogressive," is limited to cartilage alteration and is related to age. The second type, a "progressive" lesion, is that of OA. Whether the aging "nonprogressive" lesion has the potential to progress to clinical disease is not clear. Such a classification system may be appropriate to the horse to distinguish the nonclinical lesions (observed incidentally at necropsy) from the clinically significant ones.

Even in clinically affected joints, the relationship between the amount of lameness and the cartilage degeneration is not easily established. Clinical problems in the fetlock have been considered to correlate with the articular cartilage lesions.[58,71] However, in another careful study in the fetlock, there was a good correlation between lameness and the pathologic changes in the synovial membrane and fibrous joint capsule.[56] Degenerative cartilage lesions were not well correlated with evidence of pain, and wear lines were seen in most cases. Degenerative cartilage lesions were not considered to be painful if they did not involve subchondral bone.

In summary, although articular cartilage lesions are the indispensable criteria of OA, they may not be the centrally important cause of clinical disease. The clinical significance of lesions that extend into subchondral bone is not disputed; however, the clinical significance of more superficial lesions associated with age and wear and tear requires better definition. Also, cartilage breakdown products have been shown to cause synovitis when injected into joints.[10] The amount that articular cartilage damage contributes to synovitis in equine OA is not known.

USE TRAUMA AS AN ETIOLOGIC CONCEPT

In more recent times, "use trauma" has become the central etiologic concept for OA.[39,70,71] The various forms of traumatic arthritis described above can all potentially lead to DJD. Although trauma is considered to be the important factor in initiating OA,[70] the pathways by which trauma leads to disease need careful examination, particularly in OA of the high-motion joints.

Considerable damage may be inflicted directly to the cartilage in regions of concussion, as exemplified by fractures of the carpus. It has been postulated that ulcerative lesions may develop as a consequence of direct concussion when the joint moves beyond its closed-packed position into overextension.[71] The closed-packed position is achieved when the joints move into perfect congruity at the time of maximal loading.[3,84] It has also been suggested that abnormal movement may also cause synovial fluid turbulence and joint lubrication defects, with resulting frictional wear.[71] This idea was based on hydrodynamic lubrication concepts that are now considered untenable.[64] These principles are outlined above. In a recent study with a synthetic-bearing test system, no deficiency in the boundary-lubricating ability of synovial fluid from horses with OA could be found.[18]

In humans, wear and tear on the articular cartilage has also been related to the changing geometry of diarthrodial joints with age.[7] It has been reported that there is greater congruity of the articulating surfaces in older people and the distribution of load and the magnitude of local stress consequently change. Age-related degenerative changes occur in the unloaded, rather than the loaded, part of the joint. The significance of this age-related change in congruity may be that with the redistribution of load on formerly unloaded cartilage, areas of the joint that have become deficient in proteoglycans because of extended lack of use come to bear considerable stress, and they are poorly suited to these loads and break down with physical stress. Whereas this aspect cannot be directly extrapolated to OA in the young racehorse, it may be relevant. The change from non-weight-bearing to weight-bearing may be relevant to varying training programs and change in work. Training is probably necessary to have the cartilage in the best state to resist wear. It has been shown that with loading on previously unloaded cartilage, it is possible to modulate the GAG content of the cartilage.[37]

Direct damage to the cartilage is not the only route by which trauma contributes to OA, and cartilage degeneration is not necessarily the primary lesion. There is evidence in humans to suggest that trauma causes microfractures of the subchondral bone, which subsequently stiffens. This results in decreased shock absorption and subsequent cartilage degeneration.[65–67] In many cases of OA of the high-motion joints of young racehorses, the initial changes in the joint are characterized by acute synovitis and capsulitis (type 1 traumatic arthritis). To appreciate the importance of this synovitis/capsulitis in the pathogenesis of OA, it is appropriate to review the pathobiologic events associated with synovitis (presented above).

The pathogenesis of the other OA entities in the horse can be discussed more briefly. The more insidious entities of the interphalangeal, intertarsal, and tarsometatarsal joints (type 2 DJD) have some unique characteristics. Use trauma is the obvious etiologic factor. Standardbreds, Quarter Horses, and jumping horses all have particular demands placed on their hock joints, and any of the insults can be exacerbated by conformational defects, shoeing that does not allow normal sliding of the hoof, and other factors. Similarly, ringbone is seen commonly in horses when a lot of jarring motion is placed on their hindlimbs, such as in a working Quarter Horse. Rupture of collateral ligaments with luxation or subluxation (type 2A traumatic arthritis) acts as a particularly severe traumatic insult and often results in DJD. The marked periosteal bone production that characterizes these diseases is presumably associated with stretching and tearing of the joint capsule and ligamentous attachments. The observation of nonarticular bony proliferation in the pastern (denoted "false ringbone"[31]) tempts speculation that periarticular changes are the precursor of intraarticular degeneration ("true ringbone"), but the relationship has not been defined. A relationship between ringbone and conformation has been established in the Norwegian Dole.[28] Ringbone is similar to the entity of Heberden's node in humans, and both genetic and environmental factors have been incriminated with this disease entity.[77] Why bone spavin and ringbone are sometimes associated with subchondral lysis and sometimes with subchondral sclerosis is unknown. An entity of pastern DJD associated with osteochondrosis in weanling-age horses has been recognized.[82]

The series of changes that are poorly correlated with clinical problems (group 3) may reflect intrinsic degeneration associated with age. It is equally logical, however, to superimpose the trauma of continued use on this intrinsic degeneration when considering the pathogenesis of these lesions.

The fourth group of equine DJD consists of problems in which a primary cause other than use-trauma has been identified. However, the pathogenesis in some of these primary diseases such as OCD,[80] tarsal bone collapse,[52,75] and erosion of the distal palmar aspect of the metacarpus[21,58] is still uncertain. Osteochondrosis in some joints is often sufficiently severe to cause DJD, while in others it rarely does so. Such variation is discussed in the osteochondrosis section in this chapter. DJD can follow infectious arthritis when the septic process has been treated successfully but not before cartilage degeneration has occurred. The pathogenesis of articular cartilage destruction in infectious arthritis is discussed in the infectious arthritis section in this chapter.

The concepts of marginal osteophyte formation also need clarification. Bony proliferations generally have one or two patterns of growth in DJD. The bony proliferations that develop within joint capsule and ligamentous attachments to the periosteum are considered to be associated with tearing and stretching of the attachments. The origin of the osteophytes that arise at the marginal transition zone (junction of articular cartilage, synovial membrane, and periosteum) is more controversial. They have been described as a response to limit, and they control the initial pathologic lesion (erosion of cartilage) by extending the surface area of the articular cartilage and thereby reducing concussion and limiting motion of the joint.[31,36] However, osteophytes can develop at the transition zone before any morphologic cartilage damage is observed.[43,48] It has been proposed that the formation of these osteophytes is initiated at the transition zone by the release of GAGs from the cartilage matrix.[11] A number of irritants cause such changes,[77] and there is a poor correlation between the degree of articular cartilage change and osteophyte production.[47,77] There is experimental evidence that synovitis can produce osteophytes in equine joints.[43] It seems likely that osteophytes are produced by multipotential cells in response to a number of substances that are released in inflamed and/or degenerate joints. It has been suggested that direct trauma[69]

and instability[48] may also be involved in the pathogenesis of marginal osteophytes.

DIAGNOSIS

The clinical signs vary with the type and degree of OA as well as with the amount of acute inflammation. In high-motion joints with acute synovitis, there will be lameness, heat, swelling of the joint (synovial effusion, joint capsule, and periarticular components), and pain on flexion. In more chronic cases, joint enlargement is associated with fibrous tissue deposition (some bony enlargement may also be present), but some acute inflammatory signs may persist. There is decreased motion. Localization of the problem may be confirmed by local nerve blocks or intrasynovial analgesia. Obviously, the above-mentioned signs are similar to those of traumatic synovitis and capsulitis described above, and identification of the disease as OA is based on radiographs and/or arthroscopy. (Heat or joint effusion are not usually observed in cases with flattening of the distopalmar aspect of the third metacarpal bone.[11])

In the low-motion joints, the most prominent signs are joint enlargement and exacerbation of the lameness

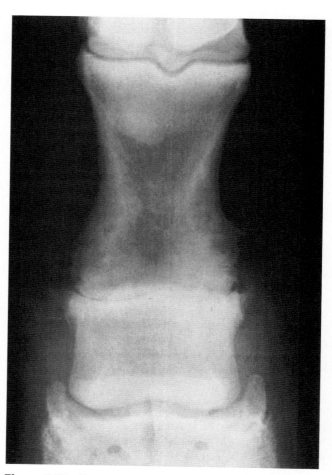

Figure 7.52 Dorsopalmar radiograph of pastern joint with osteoarthritis showing decreased joint space, subchondral sclerosis, and marginal osteophytosis. This case was treated by surgical arthrodesis.

with flexion. The radiographic diagnosis of OA is well documented.[30,53,57,59] The characteristic radiographic features of OA include narrowing or loss of joint space, subchondral bone sclerosis, marginal osteophyte formation, and periosteal bone proliferation (Figs. 7.52 and 7.53). Alternatively, ankylosis may develop (Fig. 7.54). Subchondral lysis is often observed in DJD of the distal intertarsal (centrodistal) joint (Fig. 7.55). The special radiographic features of chronic synovitis in the fetlock (concavity of the cranial aspect of the sagittal ridge of the third metacarpal bone and indentation of the caudal aspect of the third metacarpal bone in association with chronic effusion[30]) are described above. These may be observed in cases of OA of the fetlock in association with additional radiographic changes.[57]

The clinical signs in the fourth OA group are generally characteristic of the specific primary problem. The clinical features of osteochondrosis and infective arthritis are described elsewhere. Degenerative changes resulting from these conditions are typically recognized with radiographic examination, arthroscopy, or arthrotomy. Degenerative changes associated with intraarticular fractures are also recognized radiographically and can be further defined with arthroscopy.

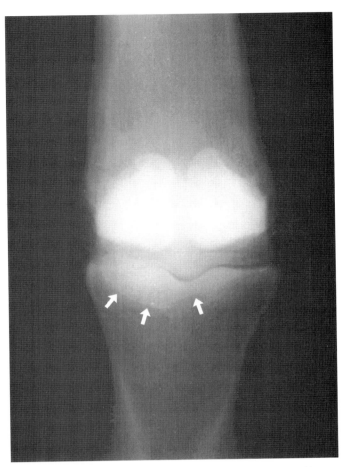

Figure 7.54 Osteoarthritis of the fetlock joint demonstrated by collapse of the medial joint space, shifting in the sagittal ridge-sagittal groove positioning, and subchondral sclerosis. This horse was treated with fetlock arthrodesis.

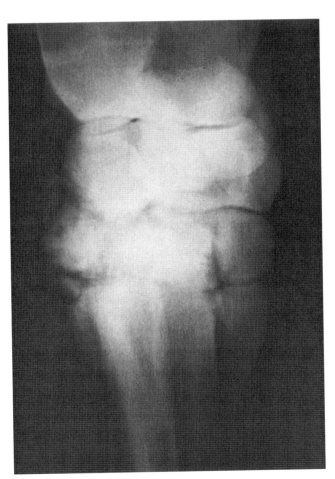

Figure 7.53 Severe osteoarthritis of the midcarpal and carpometacarpal joints consequent to a slab fracture. There is loss of joint space and considerable periosteal bone proliferation.

There is considerable disparity between radiographic and pathologic changes.[55,57] Marked cartilage degeneration can be present with equivocal radiographic signs. Contrast arthrography provides limited additional information.[57] The use of arthroscopy in diagnosing cartilage degradation in the absence of radiographic signs is discussed above. As mentioned, conventional synovial fluid analysis has not been very useful in characterizing the degree of cartilage degeneration, but newly developed markers are useful.

TREATMENT

OA is the result of a number of different pathologic processes and the choice of treatment and its effectiveness will depend on the stage of the disease and the degree of active inflammation present. Specific treatments toward the resolution of cartilage degeneration and proliferative bony change are limited, but attention to any soft tissue inflammation may be of considerable benefit to the patient. The rationale for the various treatment techniques, whether traditional or new, should be examined with reference to current information and pathogenesis of OA in the horse.[13]

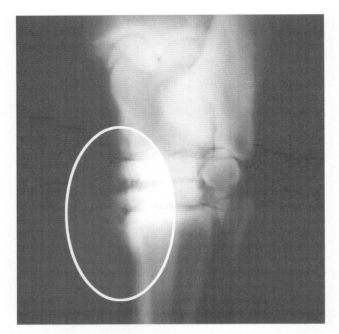

Figure 7.55 Oblique radiograph of tarsus with osteoarthritis of the distal intertarsal and tarsometatarsal joint. Note the periosteal proliferation and subchondral lysis.

The principles of treatment of clinical DJD can be divided into three areas. The first is prevention or treatment of any primary cause. Use-trauma can seldom be eliminated, but in cases of intraarticular fractures, infective arthritis, or osteochondrosis, for example, proper treatment of the primary problem is appropriate. The second principle is treatment of active soft tissue disease contributing to articular cartilage degeneration. This includes the use of rest, physical therapy, anti-inflammatory drugs, joint lavage, sodium hyaluronan, PSGAG, and synovectomy. The third principle is treatment (if possible) of the cartilage degeneration of fulminant DJD. This may include articular cartilage curettage, osteophyte removal, subchondral drilling, micropicking, and surgical arthrodesis, as well as some recently developed medications that are considered to promote cartilaginous healing. There is good evidence to suggest that the chondrocytes in OA articular cartilage are metabolically hyperactive,[46] but at a certain point in the osteoarthritic process, reparative cellular activity and proteoglycan synthesis appear to fail, leading to progressive cartilage destruction.[54] Not only do cytokines such as IL-1 and TNF-α play a central role by inducing expression of cartilage-degrading enzymes such as matrix metalloproteinases and depressing the synthesis of major matrix components, but it is felt that other changes may take place in the normal mechanisms of growth factor stimulation. For instance, in rabbit experimental OA there is a decrease of cartilage TGF-β receptor expression. TGF-β receptor II is absolutely required to bind TGF-β and form a heteromeric complex with TGF-βr1. It is felt that this may cause reduced sensitivity of the articular chondrocytes to TGF-β during development of the osteoarthritic process. This would mean that the repair potential is no longer capable of balancing the erosive process,

thus an irreversible degradation takes place. Elucidation of these mechanisms and appropriate growth factor augmentation and other biologic manipulations may help heal articular cartilage in the future.[6]

Specific treatment methods are discussed below.

REST AND PHYSICAL THERAPY. The use of rest in the treatment of synovitis/capsulitis is discussed under "Specific Diseases of Joints: Traumatic Arthritis." Discontinuation of hard work is important in the management of many cases of OA.[51,70] During this rest period, daily walking and passive joint manipulation are appropriate. The use of rest is primarily aimed at restoration of soft tissue function. How much positive effect rest has on the resolution of cartilage erosion or bony proliferation is uncertain. However, there is some evidence that appropriate exercise can modulate the quantity and quality of the cartilage GAGs.[37] In a study in rabbits in which full-thickness articular cartilage defects were created, the metaplasia of the healing tissue from undifferentiated mesenchymal tissue to hyaline articular cartilage was much more rapid and complete when the joints were subjected to continuous passive motion than with either immobilization or intermittent active motion. Whereas such a treatment modality is impractical in the horse, the work demonstrates that the healing response in articular cartilage can be modulated to some degree. Ultrasound has been used.[38]

DIMETHYL SULFOXIDE. The use of DMSO in traumatic arthritis is discussed above. The use of DMSO may help resolve acute inflammation as well as chronic fibrosis.[83] It has also been suggested that DMSO plays a role in OA because of its local analgesic properties rather than any specific anti-inflammatory effect.[5] Whatever the situation, advantages in pain relief have been demonstrated in human OA.

JOINT LAVAGE. The rationale for joint lavage has already been discussed with traumatic arthritis. This technique may be useful in DJD if active synovitis is still present. As noted above, cartilage breakdown products can promote or induce synovitis.[10] An additional rationale is that lavage may rid the joint of deleterious factors such as MMPs, PGE$_2$, cytokines, and free radicals.

CONVENTIONAL MEDICATIONS. NSAIDs, corticosteroids, HA, and PSGAGs have all been used in the treatment of arthritis. It is generally accepted that they provide symptomatic relief to synovitis and do little to help articular cartilage. Drugs that are currently used in the treatment of OA can be divided into two classes: those that act symptomatically and those that have the potential to alter the course of the disease. The ones that fall into the second category have been classified as DMOADs.[19] To be accepted as a DMOAD, it needs to be demonstrated that the drug will prevent articular cartilage destruction while providing efficacy in vivo.[81] Classically, corticosteroids have been criticized because of their supposed deleterious effects. However, recent work in our laboratory has demonstrated enhancement of GAG content and GAG synthetic rate in the articular cartilage of joints containing chip fractures, experiencing synovitis, and being injected with TA. The GAG content and GAG synthetic rate were higher in the joints treated with corticosteroid than in others. There have been numerous in vitro and in vivo studies with these medications (discussed above). At the present time, often the only treatments available are indeed such conventional medications.

NEW TREATMENT HORIZONS. Recognition of the role of cytokines and metalloproteinases in the degradation of articular cartilage is leading to investigation of newer types of drugs.[62] Inhibitors of metalloproteinases are being evaluated in our laboratory as well as elsewhere. In addition, our sequencing of the equine gene IL-1 receptor antagonist offers the potential to either manufacture the protein for use as a therapeutic agent to specifically inhibit IL-1 or, alternatively, investigate the use of gene therapy. In the latter technique, the gene is transfected into synoviocytes by use of a viral vector. The challenge at the present time is to get good expression of protein from the synoviocyte transfected with the IL-1RA gene. We are currently undertaking work in this direction.

SYNOVECTOMY. The potential benefits of lowering the level of mediators that are potentially deleterious to the articular cartilage are described under "Specific Diseases of Joints: Traumatic Arthritis." In chronic OA, synovectomy to remove fibrotic nonproductive synovial membrane may also be of benefit in certain instances.

COUNTERIRRITATION. The use of counterirritation in the form of rubefacients (braces and paints), vesicants (blisters), and thermocautery (firing) has been historically popular in the treatment of joint and tendon conditions. The rationale behind these methods is the creation of hyperemia within the diseased tissue, but experimental work questions this principle.[51] Most people now agree that the primary usefulness of the more severe forms of counterirritation is the enforced rest they cause. The various counterirritants can be classified as follows:[4]

SURGICAL CURETTAGE OF CARTILAGE AND BONE. It has been suggested that superficial defects in equine articular cartilage do not heal and that full-thickness defects heal through metaplasia of granulation tissue that arises at the articular margin or in the subchondral marrow spaces below.[70a] A number of surgeons routinely curette partial-thickness defects to get "healing." However, the importance of small partial-thickness defects has been questioned,[77] and the new replacement tissue after full-thickness curettage is of uncertain quality and commonly defective.[17,26,32] Although it has generally been accepted that there is a process of metaplasia from granulation tissue to fibrocartilage to hyaline cartilage, more recent work demonstrates the presence of hyaline cartilage at a relatively early stage and deterioration of the new cartilage into fibrotic material later. For these reasons, articular curettage should only be performed in selected cases. It has also been suggested that 12 months of rest is no advantage over 4 months of rest following osteochondral curettage.[26]

In addition to curettage of pannus-type tissue, it would seem that penetration or removal of sclerotic subchondral bone may be necessary to achieve formation of new tissue in the defect.[22] With osteoarthritic cartilage defects the subchondral plate is often sclerotic and ischemic. It has been felt, therefore, that complete removal of the subchondral plate (spongialization) or its penetration with holes (forage) provides an increased opportunity for tissue to fill the cartilage defect.[22] However, experience has shown that these techniques can compromise the subchondral bone and that the use of subchondral micropicking has rationale.[24a] Arthroscopic debridement is practiced by some orthopedists in human OA. Its benefits are controversial, but the associated lavage is considered by most to provide pain relief at least.

Debridement of articular cartilage defects has been reviewed extensively in recent publications.[42]

REMOVAL OF OSTEOPHYTES. Although some authors generally recommend removing osteophytes, remember that these hypertrophic changes are a reactive response that may not be related to any clinical problem and may not represent severe DJD.[53] In my opinion, osteophytes should be removed if they are large and positioned so that they will potentially fracture or interfere with function (prophylactic removal). Removal of nonarticular exostoses typical of periosteal proliferation is not indicated.

PROMOTION OF CARTILAGE HEALING. Various techniques have been used to augment articular cartilage healing including subchondral drilling, subchondral microfracturing, periosteal grafting, sternal cartilage grafting, and grafting of cultured chondrocytes. The use of these techniques in the horse has been reviewed recently elsewhere.[42a] Augmentation with growth factors as a potential means of healing articular cartilage is also being evaluated as a treatment for both localized lesions and more generalized OA.[42,60,72] A number of basic questions need to be answered before such methods become practical, including when certain growth factors are needed, for how long, and in what concentrations. Although it is yet to be demonstrated that there is any benefit to the articular cartilage defects per se, it is accepted that the associated lavage and recognition of meniscal tears and synovial hyperplasia and their treatment will be beneficial.[34,50a]

SURGICAL ARTHRODESIS. For many cases of end-stage OA, the only methods available for pain relief are total joint replacement or arthrodesis. Joint replacement has been described in horses[27] but is not practiced. In low-motion joints, surgical arthrodesis is a useful treatment for OA. Results are particularly satisfying in the pastern[49,73] and distal tarsal joints. Primary arthrodesis of the intertarsal and tarsometatarsal joints can be rewarding in cases of luxation if curettage of the articular cartilage, internal fixation, and external support are all combined in the treatment method. Arthrodesis of the scapulohumeral joint (for an arthritic problem) has been reported in a miniature horse.[2] Fetlock arthrodesis is also used to treat nonresponsive OA of the fetlock joint (Fig. 7.55).

References

1. Adams OR. Lameness in Horses. 3rd ed. Philadelphia: Lea & Febiger, 1974.

2. Arighi M, Miller CR, Pennock PW. Arthrodesis of the scapulo-humeral joint in a miniature horse. J Am Vet Med Assoc 1987; 191:713–714.
3. Auer JA. Diseases of the carpus. Vet Clin North Am [Large Anim Pract] 12:81, 1980.
4. Auer JA, Fackelman GE. Treatment of degenerative joint disease of the horse: A review and commentary. Vet Surg 1981;10:80.
5. Baum J. The present and potential role of dimethyl sulfoxide in connective tissue disorders. Ann NY Acad Sci 1975;243:391.
6. Boumediene K, Conrozier T, Mathieu P, et al. Decrease of cartilage transforming growth factor-beta receptor II expression in the rabbit—Potential role in cartilage breakdown. Osteoarthritis Cartilage 1998;6:146–149.
7. Bullough PG. The geometry of diarthrodial joints, its physiologic maintenance and the possible significance of age-related changes in geometry-to-load distribution and its development of osteoarthritis. Clin Orthop 1981;156:61.
8. Byers PD, Contepomi CA, Farkas TA. A postmortem study of the hip joint. Ann Rheum Dis 1970;29:15.
9. Callender GR, Kelser RA. Degenerative arthritis. A comparison of the pathological changes in man and equines. Am J Pathol 1938;14:253.
10. Chrisman OD. Biochemical aspects of degenerative joint disease. Clin Orthop 1969;64:77.
11. Chrisman OD, Fessel JM, Southwick WO. Experimental production of synovitis and marginal articular exostoses in the knee joints of dogs. Yale J Biol Med 1965;37:409.
12. Deleted in proof.
13. Clegg PD, Carter SD, Riggs CM. Osteoarthritis—What hope for effective therapy? Equine Vet J 1997;29:331–332.
14. Deleted in proof.
15. Collins DH. The Pathology of Articular and Spinal Diseases. London: Edward Arnold, 1949.
16. Coventry MB, Scanlon PW. The use of radiation to discourage ectopic bone. J Bone Joint Surg [Am] 1981;63:201.
17. Convery FR, Akeson WH., Keown GH. The repair of large osteochondral defects—An experimental study in horses. Clin Orthop 1972;82:253.
18. Davis WH. Boundary lubricating ability in synovial fluid in degenerative joint disease. Ph.D. Thesis, State University of New York, Stony Brook, 1977.
19. Dieppe P. Toward effective therapy for osteoarthritis. Rheum Eur 1995;24:118–120.
20. Deleted in proof.
21. Ferraro GL. Selected injuries of the fetlock. In: Proceedings. 24th Annual Meeting American Association of Equine Practitioners, St. Louis, MO, 1978;315–317.
22. Ficat RP, Ficat C, Gedeon P, Toussaint JB. Spongialization: A new treatment for diseased patellae. Clin Orthop 1979;144:74–83.
23. Freeman MAR. Adult Articular Cartilage. New York: Grune & Stratton, 1972.
24. Frisbie DD, Kawcak CE, Trotter GW, et al. The effects of triamcinolone acetonide on an in vivo equine osteochondral fragment exercise model. Equine Vet J 1997;29:349–359.
24a. Frisbie DD, Trotter GW, Powers BE, et al. Arthroscopic subchondral bone plate microfracture technique augments healing of large osteochondral defects in the radial carpal bone and medial femoral condyle of horses. Vet Surg 1999;28:242–255.
25. Gardiner DL. General pathology of the peripheral joints. In: Sokoloff L, Ed. The Joints and Synovial Fluid 11. New York: Academic Press, 1980;315–425.
26. Grant BD. Repair mechanisms of osteochondral defects in Equidae: A comparative study of untreated and x-irradiated defects. In: Proceedings. 21st Annual Meeting of the American Association of Equine Practitioners, Boston, MA, 1976;95–114.
27. Grossman BS, Grant BD, Sande RD, et al. A prosthetic implant for the equine carpal joint: Surgical technique and results. Vet Surg 1980;9:93.
28. Haakenstad LH. Chronic bone and joint diseases in relation to conformation in the horse. Equine Vet J 1969;1:248.
29. Haines RW. Destruction of hyaline cartilage in the sigmoid notch of the human ulna. J Anat 1976;122:331.
30. Haynes PF. Disease of the metacarpophalangeal joint and metacarpus. Vet Clin North Am [Large Anim Pract] 1980;2:33.

31. Hickman J. Veterinary Orthopaedics. Philadelphia: JB Lippincott, 1964.
32. Howell DS, Sapolsky AI, Pita JC, Woessner JF. The pathogenesis of osteoarthritis. Semin Arthritis Rheum 1976;4:365–383.
33. Hunt MDN. Traumatic arthritis in young Thoroughbreds. Proc R Soc Lond 1965;58:370.
34. Jackson RW. Arthroscopic treatment of degenerative arthritis. In: McGinty JB, Caspari RB, Jackson RW, Poehling GG, Eds. Operative Arthroscopy. 2nd ed. Philadelphia: Lippincott-Raven, 1996;405–409.
35. Jappe HL. Metabolic, Degenerative and Inflammatory Diseases of Bones and Joints. Philadelphia: Lea & Febiger, 1972.
36. Kelser RA, Callender GR. Equine degenerative arthritis. Vet Med 1938;38:307.
37. Kincaid SA, Van Sickle DC. Regional histochemical and thickness variations of adult articular cartilage. J Am Vet Med Assoc 1981; 42:428.
38. Lang DC. Ultrasonic treatment of musculoskeletal conditions in the horse, dog and cat. Vet Rec 1980;106:427–431.
39. Mackay-Smith MP. Pathogenesis and pathology of equine osteoarthritis. J Am Vet Med Assoc 1962;141:1246.
40. McIlwraith CW. Current concepts in equine degenerative joint disease. J Am Vet Med Assoc 1982;180:239.
41. McIlwraith CW. General pathobiology of the joint and response to injury. In: McIlwraith CW, Trotter GW, Eds. Joint Disease in the Horse. Philadelphia: WB Saunders, 1996;40–70.
42. McIlwraith CW, Nixon AJ. Joint resurfacing: Attempts at repairing articular cartilage defects. In: McIlwraith CW, Trotter GW, Eds. Joint Disease in the Horse. Philadelphia: WB Saunders, 1996; 317–334.
43. McIlwraith CW, Van Sickle DC. Experimentally induced arthritis of the equine carpus: Histologic and histochemical changes in the articular cartilage. Am J Vet Res 1981;42:207.
44. Deleted in proof.
45. Mankin HJ. The reaction of articular cartilage to injury and osteoarthritis. N Engl J Med 1974;291:1335.
46. Mankin HJ, Johnson ME, Lippiello L. Biochemical and metabolic abnormalities in articular cartilage from osteoarthritic human hips. Distribution and metabolism of amino sugar-containing macromolecules. J Bone Joint Surg [Am] 1981;63:131.
47. Marshall JL. Discussion following Dr. Morgan's paper. Cornell Vet 1968;58(Suppl):46.
48. Marshall JL. Periarticular osteophytes. Irritation and formation in the knee of the dog. Clin Orthop 1969;62:37.
49. Martin GS, McIlwraith CW, Turner AS, et al. Long-term results and complications of proximal interphalangeal arthrodesis in the horse. J Am Vet Med Assoc 1984;184:1136–1140.
50. Meachim G, Collins DH. Cell counts of normal and osteoarthritic articular cartilage in relation to the uptake of sulfate [$^{35}SO_4$] in vitro. Ann Rheum Dis 1962;21:45.
50a. Merchan ECR, Galindo E. Arthroscope-guided surgery versus nonoperative treatment for limited degenerative osteoarthritis of the femorotibial joint in patients over 50 years of age: A prospective comparative study. J Arthrosc Rel Surg 1993;9:663–667.
51. Milne EJ. Medical treatment of equine osteoarthritis and tenosynovitis. J Am Vet Med Assoc 1962;141:1269.
52. Morgan JP. Necrosis of the third tarsal bone in the horse. J Am Vet Med Assoc 1967;151:1334.
53. Morgan JP. Radiographic diagnosis of bone and joint diseases in the horse. Cornell Vet. Suppl 1 1968;58:28.
54. Moskowitz RW, Goldberg VM, Malemud C. Metabolic responses of cartilage in experimentally induced osteoarthritis. Ann Rheum Dis 1981;40:584.
55. Nilsson G. Lameness and pathologic changes in the distal joints and the phalanges of the Standardbred horse. A correlative study. Acta Vet Scand Suppl 1 1973;44:83.
56. Nilsson G, Olsson SE. Radiologic and pathoanatomic changes in the distal joints and the phalanges of the Standardbred horse. Acta Vet. Scand Suppl 1 1973;44:1.
57. O'Brien TR. Disease of the Thoroughbred fetlock joint: A comparison of radiographic signs with gross pathologic lesions. Pro-

ceedings. 23rd Annual Meeting of the American Association of Equine Practitioners, Vancouver, Canada, 1977;367–380.

58. O'Brien TR, Hornoff WJ, Meagher DM. Radiographic detection and characterization of palmar lesions in the equine fetlock joint. J Am Vet Med Assoc 1981;178:231.

59. O'Brien TR, Morgan JP, Park RD, Lebel JL. Radiography in equine carpal lameness. Cornell Vet 1971;61:646–660.

60. Osborn KD, Trippel SV, Mankin HJ. Growth factor stimulation of adult articular cartilage. J Orthop Res 1989;7:35–42.

61. Deleted in proof.

62. Pelletier JP, McCollum R, Tardif G, et al. Tenidap, a new anti-rheumatic drug, reduces IL-1R expression and IL-1-induced expression of metalloproteinases in cartilage human chondro-cytes. Osteoarthritis Cartilage 1993;1:39.

63. Deleted in proof.

64. Radin EL, Paul IL. A consolidated concept of joint lubrication. J Bone Joint Surg [Am] 1972;54:607.

65. Radin EL, Paul IL. Does cartilage compliance reduce skeletal impact loads? The relative force-attenuating properties of articular cartilage, synovial fluid, periarticular soft tissues, and bone. Arthritis Rheum 1970;13:139.

66. Radin EL, Paul IL, Rose RM. Role of mechanical factors in pathogenesis of primary osteoarthritis. Lancet 1972;519.

67. Radin EL, Paul IL, Tolkoff MJ. Subchondral bone change in patients with early degenerative arthritis. Arthritis Rheum 1970;13:400.

68. Raker CW. Orthopedic surgery: Errors in surgical evaluation and management. Proceedings. 19th Annual Meeting of the American Association of Equine Practitioners, Atlanta, GA, 1973;205–212.

69. Raker CW. Clinical observations of bone and joint disease in horses. Cornell Vet 1968;58:15.

70. Raker CW, Baker RH, Wheat JD. Pathophysiology of equine degenerative joint disease and lameness. Proceedings. 12th Annual Meeting of the American Association of Equine Practitioners, Los Angeles, CA, 1966;229–241.

70a. Riddle WE. Healing of articular cartilage in the horse. J Am Vet Med Assoc 1970;157:1471.

71. Rodney JR. Biomechanics of Lameness in Horses. Baltimore: Williams & Wilkins, 1969.

72. Rogachefsky RA, Dean DD, Howell DS, Altman RD. Treatment of canine osteoarthritis with insulin-like growth factor-1 (IGF-1) and sodium pentosan polysulfate. Osteoarthritis Cartilage 1993;1:105–114.

73. Schneider JE, Carnine BL, Guffy MM. Arthrodesis of the proximal interphalangeal joint in the horse: A surgical treatment for high ringbone. J Am Vet Med Assoc 1978;173:1364.

74. Schultz K. Untersuchungen uber die sogennanter synovial gruben, fossae nudatae, beim pferd. Arch Wiss Prakt Tierheilkd 1915;41:245.

75. Shaver JR, et al. Skeletal manifestations of suspected hypothyroidism in two foals. J Equine Med Surg 1979;3:269.

76. Sippel WL. Equine degenerative arthritis. M.S. Thesis, Cornell University, Ithaca, NY, 1942.

77. Sokoloff L. Pathology and pathogenesis of osteoarthritis. In: McCarty DJ, Ed. Arthritis and Allied Conditions. 9th ed. Philadelphia: Lea & Febiger, 1979;1135–1153.

78. Sokoloff L. The Biology of Degenerative Joint Disease. Chicago: University of Chicago Press, 1969.

79. Sokoloff L. The general pathology of osteoarthritis. American Academy of Orthopaedic Surgeons Symposium on Osteoarthritis. St. Louis: CV Mosby, 1976;23–33.

80. Stromberg B, Reino S. Osteochondrosis in the horse. I. A clinical and radiologic investigation of osteochondritis dissecans of the knee and hock joints. Acta Radiol Suppl 1 1978;358:140.

81. Theiler R, Ghosh P, Brooks P. Clinical, biochemical and imaging methods of assessing osteoarthritis and clinical trials of agents claiming "chondromodulating" activity. Osteoarthritis Cartilage 1994;2:1–23.

82. Trotter GW, McIlwraith CW, Norrdin RW, Turner AS. Degenerative joint disease with osteochondrosis of the proximal interphalangeal joint in young horses. J Am Vet Med Assoc 1982;180:1312–1318.

83. Wood DC, Wood J. Pharmacologic and biochemical considerations of dimethyl sulfoxide. Ann NY Acad Sci 1975;243:7.

84. Wyburn RS, Goulden BE. Fractures of the equine carpus: A report on 57 cases. NZ Vet J 1974;22:133.

SPECIFIC DISEASES OF JOINTS: DEVELOPMENTAL ORTHOPEDIC DISEASE AND ITS MANIFESTATION IN JOINT DISEASE

Developmental Orthopedic Disease

The term "developmental orthopedic disease" (DOD) was coined in 1986 to encompass all orthopedic problems seen in the growing foal.[61] It is a term that encompasses all general growth disturbances of horses and is therefore nonspecific. It has yet to be determined how closely related the various forms of DOD may be, and the term should not be used as a synonym for "osteochondrosis." It is felt inappropriate that subchondral cystic lesions, physitis, angular limb deformities, and cervical vertebral malformations all be presumed to be manifestations of osteochondrosis. In addition to problems associated with the articular–epiphyseal cartilage complex and metaphyseal growth plate or physis, flexural deformities are a significant problem of growing foals and need to be included within the spectrum of DOD. The spectrum of conditions currently classified as DOD was earlier designated "metabolic bone disease."[11,19] However, this term is considered misleading because it refers specifically to bone, whereas many of these problems are seen essentially as joint and growth plate conditions. Severe forms of DOD are seen in which histomorphometry reveals little or no observations in bone metabolism.[102] Use of the term "metabolic bone disease" has been defended,[18] but "developmental orthopedic disease" has become the generally accepted term.

When the term "developmental orthopedic disease" was first coined, it was categorized as including the following:[61]

- Osteochondrosis—Osteochondrosis is a defect in endochondral ossification that can result in a number of different manifestations, depending on the site of the endochondral ossification defect. These manifestations include OCD of cartilaginous origin (to distinguish it from human OCD, which originates in the bone). They also include *some* subchondral cystic lesions—not all subchondral cystic lesions or osseous cystlike lesions are necessarily manifestations of osteochondrosis.[38,58,63,93] There is evidence that traumatic factors or primary defects on the articular cartilage may be an originating cause in some cases. Another manifestation is *some* physitis. Defects in endochondral ossification in the metaphyseal side of the physis are associated with some clinical problems in this area. However, these are not the only form of problems in the physis. Some cervical vertebral malformations are also included. The exact role of osteochondrosis in the pathogenesis of cervical vertebral malformations is still uncertain.[53] Finally, some angular limb deformities are associated with retained cartilage associated with the physis. There is considerable controversy over what syndromes fall within the osteochondroses.[87] This is discussed further under osteochondrosis. Based on pathologic studies, for instance, Pool feels that there is no evidence that osteochondrosis plays a role in the pathogenesis of cervical vertebral stenosis.

- Acquired angular limb deformities
- Physitis
- Subchondral cystic lesions[82,94,116]
- Flexural deformities—these may be secondary to osteochondrosis or physitis
- Cuboidal bone malformation

It would be appropriate to add a seventh entity to the spectrum of DOD—juvenile arthritis[19] or juvenile DJD and bony fragments of the palmar/plantar surface of the first phalanx of Standardbred horses.[2,16,29,70,71,99,118] Currently these are considered to be traumatic lesions.

The above entities are considered DODs.[74] Individual instances may or may not be associated with osteochondrosis. The panel also distinguished palmar metacarpal disease (previously called OCD of the distal metacarpus[40,73] as a traumatic entity and stated that it did not fit within DOD.[89] However, some authors describe the condition as traumatic osteochondrosis of the palmar/plantar surface of the condyle of the cannon bone, which continues to confuse the issue somewhat. Pool has emphasized that the following DODs are not manifestations of osteochondrosis: 1) palmar metacarpal disease, 2) first

phalanx fragments, 3) juvenile arthrosis of the pastern, and 4) cervical vertebral malformations.[86] He also suggests a need to differentiate between primary (idiopathic) developmental lesions and secondary (acquired) lesions of equine osteochondrosis (discussed in more detail below). Because this chapter is focused on joint disease, we restrict our discussion to the entities that involve joints.

Osteochondrosis

Osteochondrosis (dyschondroplasia) was initially defined as a disturbance of cellular differentiation in the growing cartilage.[75] Osteochondrosis is considered to result from a failure of endochondral ossification and thus may affect either the articular–epiphyseal cartilage complex or the metaphyseal growth plate. The loss of normal differentiation into cartilage cells was considered to mean that the transitional calcification of the matrix does not take place, and vessels from the marrow cavity and blood vessels do not penetrate the cartilage.[113] As a consequence, endochondral ossification ceases, and cartilage is retained. This failure of endochondral ossification leads to necrosis in the basal layers of the thickened retained cartilage. It was initially proposed that subsequent physical stresses give rise to fissures in this

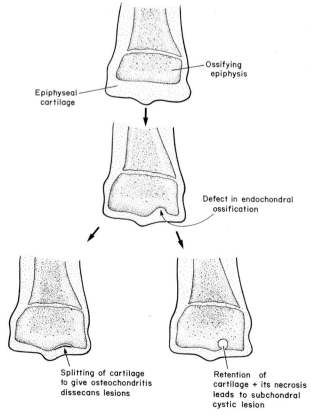

A

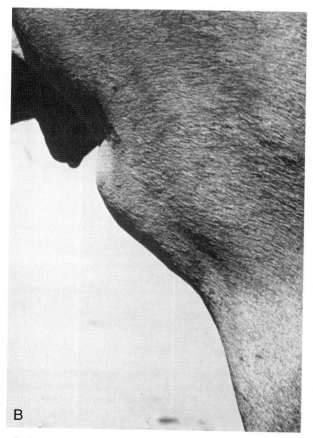

B

Figure 7.56   A. Diagram of pathogenesis of osteochondritis dissecans and subchondral cystic lesions in relation to the generalized condition of osteochondrosis. B. Femoropatellar

effusion in association with osteochondritis dissecans of the lateral trochlear ridge of the femur. *(continued)*

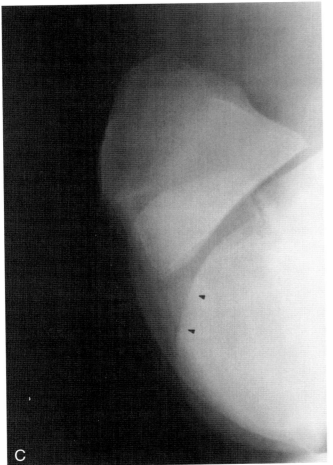

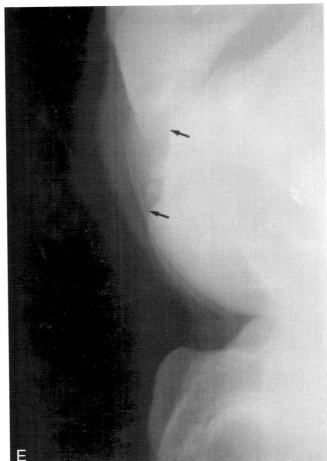

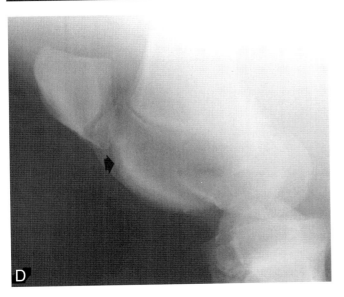

Figure 7.56 (continued) C–E. Lateral to medial radiographs showing OCD lesions of the lateral trochlear ridge of the femur with increasing severity: flattening with some lucency appearing in the lateral trochlear ridge (C), a grade 1 defect (D), and a grade 2 defect (E).

damaged cartilage and that progressive breakdown of the cartilage can then lead to the syndromes designated as OCD or periarticular subchondral bone cysts (Fig. 7.56).

The initial proposals that these entities are part of the generalized condition of osteochondrosis resulted from studies in other species and extrapolation to the condition in the horse.[91,92,95–97,113] As a result of these various studies, Olsson suggested that dyschondroplasia was a better alternative to osteochondrosis because the initial lesion occurred in growing cartilage.[75] However, based on different instances of clinical disease, I feel that the assertion that all osteochondrosis entities in the horse are in fact associated with a primary dyschondroplasia should be questioned. While typical lesions of thickening in the articular cartilage, as well as thickening and separation, have been seen in clinical cases as well as experimentally produced disease,[19,101,103,104] cases have been seen at surgery where dissection between cartilage and bone had occurred without a defect in the normal subchondral bone contour and without thickening of cartilage. Cases have also been encountered in which radiographic lucency developed in the bone after endochondral ossification had apparently ceased.[65] It would seem that "osteochondrosis" is as specific a term as we want to use at the moment, as it covers all conditions involving the articular–epiphyseal cartilage complex and epiphyseal bone, as well as metaphyseal growth plate and metaphyseal bone. Until we define the pathogenesis better and indeed prove that currently described "models" of osteochondrosis are representative of, or identical to, the clinical syndrome, the use of any more specific terms is inappropriate.

Stromberg described the second stage of osteochondrosis as involving necrosis of the basal layers of the thickened retained cartilage with subsequent pressure and strain within the joint giving rise to fissures in this damaged cartilage. The fissures may extend from the deep necrotic layer to the surface of the cartilage, and such dissecting lesions cause clinical signs of synovitis and pain and should be called "osteochondritis dissecans." The terms "osteochondrosis," "osteochondritis dissecans," and "osteochondrosis dissecans" have been used regularly as synonyms, and their meaning is still somewhat controversial. Previously, "osteochondrosis" referred to the disease, "osteochondritis" was defined as the inflammatory response to the disease, and "osteochondritis dissecans," the condition when a flap can be demonstrated,[90] and this is a simple, but fairly appropriate, representation.

Pool proposed that it might be useful to distinguish foals with idiopathic (constitutional defects in the cartilage model) and acquired (defect in endochondral ossification with a known cause) osteochondrosis. Examples of the latter would be a traumatic osteochondrosis or zinc-induced osteochondrosis.[87] Hurtig and Pool implied that a useful classification scheme of equine osteochondrosis was still needed.[45] They pointed out that the human classification scheme had introduced a confusing array of distantly related conditions. They felt that lesions without clear evidence of defective bone formation should not be included in osteochondrosis. These include cervical vertebral malformation, proximal palmar/plantar osteochondral fragments, physeal dysplasia, subchondral bone cysts, flexural limb deformities, and angular limb deformities. They should, however, remain under the larger syndrome of DOD. Pool and Hurtig proposed that lesions disrupting the articular surface through defective bone and cartilage formation could be categorized as follows:

1. The *typical pattern* of osteochondrosis is manifested by one or two lesions in a characteristic location and may be bilaterally symmetric (although one joint may be clinically silent). This would be consistent with an event or trauma during a specific period of time during the "window of susceptibility."[45] Typical sites include OCD of the lateral trochlear ridge of the femur, cystic lesions of the medial femoral condyle, and OCD of the medial trochlear ridge of the femur, distal intermediate ridge, lateral trochlear ridge, medial malleolus, OCD of the tarsocrural joint, and OCD of the distal dorsal metacarpus.

2. *Atypical pattern* refers to horses with multiple articular, and sometimes physeal, lesions in characteristic sites and other random locations in the skeleton. Such horses have widespread articular disruption reminiscent of experimental models and have usually suffered nutritional or toxic insults.

3. A *mixed pattern* includes more joint lesions in different locations than the typical pattern.[66]

Personally, the author continues to classify lesions according to their specific morphology and clinical significance.

Pathogenesis of Osteochondrosis

It is probably useful to consider osteochondrosis involving a susceptibility of the joint surface to injury during development.[5,45] It has been conventional to use the term "osteochondrosis" to describe the process of abnormal bone and cartilage formation and to use the term "osteochondritis dissecans" to describe the subsequent lesions that penetrate the joint surface creating inflammation and effusion.[45,64] Although dyschondroplasia may be a more descriptive term because it emphasizes a primary defect in cartilage formation rather than bone, it can be confused with other generalized metabolic conditions, and it has yet to be proven that the clinical entities we see start in cartilage per se. On the other hand, certain etiologic factors have been recognized that contribute to the development of the clinical manifestations of OCD (and subchondral cystic lesions) that we see. Equine OCD is a localized defect in a bone and cartilage at the joint surface that develops during a short period in the horse's life.[45] These factors have been varied, but that there is a multifactorial etiology has generally been accepted.

Historically, OCD was initially considered to be due to a vascular or ischemic necrosis of the subchondral bone.[1,108] The problem has also been described as an osteochondral fracture.[72] Rooney recognized the problem as a defect in endochondral ossification of epiphyseal cartilage.[98] He considered that ischemic necrosis at or near the chondro-osseous junction stopped invasion of the growing cartilage by capillaries and thus stopped the process of endochondral ossification. Some histologic studies of various lesions in the horse have revealed little evidence of primary bone or cartilage necrosis, and subchondral avascularity was not seen.[67,97] On the other hand, recent work in the pig suggests that the viability of epiphyseal cartilage and the articular–epiphyseal cartilage complex depends highly on inadequate blood supply from cartilage canal vessels and strongly implicates a defect in blood supply in the pathogenesis of osteochondrosis.[9] Based on pathologic observations of early lesions of osteochondrosis in young horses, it has been proposed that subchondral blood vessels in the epiphyseal physis give rise to arcades of thin capillary-size vessels that extend radially from the subchondral bone into the cartilage and that these vessels are disrupted and chondrocytes in the epiphyseal physis that they supply undergo necrosis. With cessation of endochondral ossification in this area, the bony base of the trochlear ridges fails to grow outwardly to replace the cartilage and form a normal ridge. When the lesion develops in a very young horse, a much larger defect often occurs because a large amount of the bony base of the ridge was never formed. On the other hand, when the onset of the lesions occurs prior to skeletal maturity, the lesion on the trochlear ridge may go unnoticed because ridge development is nearly complete.[88] Pool feels that shear forces are likely to be the cause of the disruption of these radially oriented capillaries.

In many clinical instances in the horse, changes consistent with various stages of the proposed pathogenic pathway have been identified. On the other hand, exceptions are noted to the central concept of either thickening of articular cartilage or a defect in the subchondral bone.[64]

The concept of dyschondroplasia has its proponents, and one laboratory in particular is focusing on assessing various abnormalities in the growth cartilage of normal foals as well as those with osteochondrosis.[49] Differences in the normal growth cartilage of foals and those with lesions of osteochondrosis (dyschondroplasia) have included collagen localization, degradative enzymes, and growth factor expression. These authors have also classified dyschondroplastic lesions into two groups on the basis of histologic findings. Dyschondroplasia is a widely recognized disorder of young, rapidly growing poultry.[59a] Avian tibial dyschondroplasia is characterized by an avascular mass of cartilage containing partly hypertrophied (transitional) chondrocytes. In situ biochemistry and immunocytochemistry of chondrocytes indicate that the accumulation of cartilage is not caused by increased chondrocyte proliferation or decreased osteoclast/chondroblast activity. Neither is anaerobic glycolysis increased in the transitional chondrocytes, showing that oxygen supply to these cells is not limiting. Initial studies have confirmed that the disease results from a failure of chondrocytes to differentiate fully, which is supported by an investigation in which genetic selection for tibial dyschondroplasia resulted in accumulations of transitional chondrocytes. Transitional chondrocytes contain high concentrations of TGF-β and the product of the proto-oncogene c-myc, but in tibial dyschondroplasia these cells are deficient in TGF-β and c-myc. Concentrations of ALP and type X collagen messenger RNA are increased, but a lower concentration of type X collagen within the matrix indicates a defect in its secretion or incorporation.[115]

Endochondral ossification involves chondrocyte proliferation, maturation, and replacement of mineralized cartilage with bone and is controlled by a complex interaction of systemic factors including growth hormone, IGF-1, and thyroid hormones, as well as a number of local growth factors such as TGF-β, IGF-1 and -2, and basic fibroblast growth factor (FGF).[33] TGF-β has also been shown to have an important role in growth cartilage metabolism, particularly in the control of chondrocyte differentiation and hypertrophy, and the TGF-β1 isoform has been particularly implicated in the process in mammals. A study assessed the distribution pattern of

TGF-β1 messenger RNA and protein in normal prenatal and postnatal growth cartilage as well as cartilage from lesions of dyschondroplasia in the horse. TGF-β1, mRNA expression, and immunoreactivity were detected in the proliferative and upper hypertrophic zones in both prenatal and postnatal normal articular/epiphyseal cartilage. However, mRNA for TGF-β1 was only detected in the mid and lower hypertrophic zones. In focal lesions of dyschondroplasia, mRNA expression and immunoreactivity were lower than in normal cartilage, but strong mRNA expression was observed in the chondrocyte clusters immediately surrounding a lesion of dyschondroplasia. The authors felt that TGF-β1 could be involved in the pathogenesis of dyschondroplasia.[33] The same laboratory has also assessed the presence and activity of cathepsin B and cathepsin D, collagenase, TIMP, and types II and VI collagen in specimens of cartilage or the media of explant or chondrocyte cultures.[33]

In identifying etiologic factors associated with osteochondrosis, there are clinical and pathologic reports[15,20,62,64,65] and experimental studies in the horse.[15,19,20,41–44,54–56,62,79–81,102–106] One problem with the latter is determining how much the experimentally produced lesions have in common with the lesions we see clinically. Major factors that seem to predispose the growing animal to osteochondrosis include rapid growth, genetic predisposition, nutritional excesses or imbalances, and superimposed trauma to the cartilage. In pigs it has been demonstrated that high growth rate is the main reason for the high incidence of osteochondrosis, and the high growth rate is the result of both genetic selection and caloric intake.[95,96]

Genetic Predisposition

A radiographic survey by Hoppe and Phillipson[39] in Standardbred trotters and Swedish Warmbloods showed that one stallion of each breed had a significantly higher frequency of OCD among his progeny than the other stallions ($P < .001$). The various OCD frequencies in the progeny groups of the "normal" young horses also indicated an inherited predisposition for OCD, but there were not enough data for detailed analysis.[39a] In another study, Shougaard et al. showed radiographic evidence of a significantly higher proportion of osteochondrosis in the progeny of one of eight stallions, even though the stallion itself did not show radiographic signs of osteochondrosis.[109] Since that time, there have been two more studies on the heritability of osteochondrosis in the tibiotarsal joint in Standardbred trotters.[29,30,84,85] Both of these studies also examined the heritability of bony fragments from the palmar/plantar aspect of the first phalanx.

The study of Grondahl and Dolvik[29] involved radiography of the tarsocrural and metacarpophalangeal and metatarsophalangeal joints in 753 Standardbred trotters (6 to 21 months old) that were born in 1998.[29] The survey population was drawn at random from all parts of Norway and represented approximately 60% of Standardbred trotters born that year. Osteochondrosis in the tarsocrural joint was diagnosed in 108 (14.3%) horses, and the prevalence of disease in progeny groups of more than 10 horses ranged from 0 to 69%. Bony fragments in the palmar/plantar portion of the metacarpophalangeal and metatarsophalangeal joints were diagnosed in 89

(11.8%) horses, and the prevalence of disease in progeny groups of more than 10 ranged from 0 to 41%. Heritability analysis was restricted to 644 horses comprising groups of five or more progeny from 39 stallions. The heritability of osteochondrosis in the tibiotarsal joint and bony fragments in the palmar/plantar portion of the metacarpophalangeal and metatarsophalangeal joints was estimated to be 0.52 and 0.21, respectively, using a nonlinear model. The authors recognized that they were unable to interpret various environmental effects and control for them. The authors noted that in their study, the heritability of OCD in the tibiotarsal joint (0.52) was higher than that reported by Shougaard et al.[109] (0.26 ± 0.14). Shougarrd et al. investigated the degree of heritability by means of the chi square value for binomial data on the basis of nine progeny groups and a morbidity of 12%. In the Norwegian study, the high heritability was to some degree caused by the high morbidity in one progeny group (69%) and could therefore represent an overestimate. A lack of correlation between the heritability of tibiotarsal lesions and fetlock lesions was considered to indicate that few common genes code for these two lesions.

The study by Philipsson et al.[84] used 793 progeny of 24 Swedish Standardbred trotter stallions, based on radiographs of the tarsocrural joint for OCD and the fetlock joints for palmar/plantar osteochondral fragments. These horses were a random sample of about 35 progeny of each of 24 stallions. Twenty of these stallions were randomly drawn from the Swedish trotter population, most of which had an American origin, whereas four stallions were chosen because of their own defects. Because all stallions had been radiographed when they were selected for breeding, it was also possible to apply a third method of detecting any hereditary role in osteochondrosis. This was done by comparing the incidence of OCD in the progeny of affected and nonaffected stallions. The occurrence of OCD was nearly three times as high among the progeny of stallions affected with OCD in the hock as among those of the nonaffected stallions. The difference was much smaller with the occurrence of plantar osteochondral fragments in the fetlock. The results in all progeny groups showed differences in the incidence in hock OCD in different progeny stallions from 0 to more than 40%, which strongly indicates that hereditary factors contribute to the development of OCD in the tarsocrural joint. The heritability estimates were 0.27 for tarsocrural OCD and 0.17 for proximal palmar/plantar lesions. These authors felt that the high estimate of heritability by Grondahl and Dolvik[30] was probably due to the very high incidence in one particular progeny group (9 of 13). The authors commented that although heritability coefficients indicate that selection against both OCD in the hock and palmar/plantar fragments in the fetlock could be effective for horses, the selection would need to be based on progeny testing because stallions that are free of the diseases can produce progeny with a relatively high incidence of lesions. Another issue of importance is evaluation of the consequences of these disease processes on future longevity and performance. Even though the defects have proven to be partly under genetic control, breeding policies must also consider the importance of the defects on future soundness and the ability to perform.

In a recent review on genetic implications, Philippson said that the studies indicate that inheritance is not a function of a single pair of genes but rather is polygenetic. When evaluating the relative contribution of genetic and environmental factors, the most common approach when polygenetic effects are assumed is to estimate the heritability of a trait. Heritability estimates the proportion of the total variation in the abnormal trait that can be associated with the additively inherited genes (i.e., such genetic effects that are transmitted from one generation to the next).[83] Philippson felt that a prerequisite for any selection scheme is that the heritable trait in question is of importance, economically or ethically, for the purpose of use of the animals. He used the example of Standardbred trotters used for breeding. Stallions are usually selected from animals superior in racing ability. If these horses are raced without having been treated surgically, such a selection scheme favors horses free from significant defects. On the other hand, he felt that riding horse populations were different, because stallions might be selected without a competition career and after a short performance test (not always the case). Under these conditions, it may well be justified to exclude from breeding those stallions that are found to have osteochondrosis, but it still requires knowledge that the type of osteochondrosis selected against has a negative effect on the use of the horse. The author felt that the level of heritability in osteochondrosis of 0.25 to 0.35 is of the same magnitude as important traits in cattle, such as milk yield and growth rate. Remember, however, that all of these studies have looked at OCD in the hock only (excluding palmar/plantar fragments as an entity of OCD).

Wagner performed a study in which 12 wobbler mares were bred to two affected stallions.[117] Although the resulting offspring did not show signs of ataxia, seven developed contracted tendons, four had lesions of "osteochondrosis" in the cervical spine, and five had physeal abnormalities. However, there was no control group and the "normal" incidence of DOD problems varies from place to place.[117] Hereditary aspects have been suggested with human OCD.[112]

Growth and Body Size

A high growth rate was first recognized to be associated with a high incidence of osteochondrosis in dogs and pigs.[32,95] Stromberg reported a predominance of osteochondrosis in large-framed and rapidly growing horses, and many others have noted this anecdotally.[113] However, only recently have there been any studies with data. Green reviewed reports with many different breeds, geographic locations, and diets and noted an essentially similar pattern of growth in all animals.[28] Jeffcott noted that the most intense phase of growth occurs in the first 3 months of life and said that this was when lesions of osteochondrosis are most likely to occur.[47] That is not when we recognize the highest incidence of lesions clinically, but we cannot dispute that the statement is incorrect with regard to actual development of a lesion. It has also been reported that the growth rate appears higher in the hindlimb than in the forelimb in foals,[27] and osteochondrosis is indeed recognized very frequently in hindlimb sites. A study by Staun et al.[111] was cited by Jeffcott[47] in which no evidence of signs of osteochondrosis were found in a study of compensatory growth. Stallion size is not related to the incidence of osteochondrosis in the offspring,[39] which is not surprising since the dam has a greater influence on progeny size. Growth rate is also, obviously, associated with a number of factors.[36,37]

In more recent work, the incidence of OCD lesions occurring in either the fetlock, hock, shoulder, or stifle on a commercial Thoroughbred farm were studied over a 4-year period. DOD was defined as osteochondrotic lesions occurring in either the fetlock, hock, shoulder, or stifle. Lesions were initially diagnosed radiographically after a foal displayed either lameness or joint effusion, meaning that it was a true clinical incidence study rather than a radiographic study. Other manifestations of OCD such as physitis, flexural deformities, and angular limb deformities were not included in the study since they are more difficult to quantify. No foals were diagnosed as wobblers during this 4-year period. OCD was diagnosed in 10% of the 271 foals monitored. Fetlock OCDs tended to occur before 180 days of age, while hock, shoulder, and stifle OCDs occurred around 300 to 350 days of age. Foals that developed hock and stifle OCDs as yearlings tended to be large foals at birth that grew rapidly from 3 to 8 months. Foals that developed hock OCDs averaged 5 kg heavier than the Kentucky average at 25 days of age. By 240 days, these foals were 14 kg heavier than the population average. Foals that developed stifle or shoulder lesions averaged 5.5 kg heavier than the Kentucky average at 25 days of age and 17 kg heavier at 120 days of age. By 300 days of age, these foals were 12 kg heavier than the Kentucky average. Foals that developed fetlock OCDs before 6 months of age were born early in the year (January, February, or March). Their weight tended to be average. When foals were diagnosed with fetlock lesions at a later date, they tended to be of normal size during the first 110 days but grew heavier than the Kentucky average after weaning. The authors felt that the types of lesions seen could have been the result of excessive biomechanical forces exerted on otherwise normal cartilage. Early fetlock OCDs could have resulted from inadequate subchondral bone formation due to restricted activity in foals born early in the year and housed indoors at night. Hock and stifle lesions may have occurred in heavy foals that grew rapidly after weaning.[77]

In a radiographic survey in Sweden, 77 Standardbred foals (35 colts, 42 fillies) were examined six times, from birth to the age of 16 months. In addition to the radiographic examination of the tarsocrural and fetlock joint areas, the horses were measured for height at the withers and at the croup, circumference of the girth and carpus, and length of cannon, and their conformation was assessed according to a standardized protocol. Examinations included clinical examination and palpation of the extremities, with all examinations being done by the same person. The foals were weighed each month. The metric observations were precorrected according to a model including the effects of sex, year of birth, and the regression on individual recording age. Eight foals (4 colts, 4 fillies) that developed radiographic signs of tibiotarsal OCD had a higher body weight at birth (54 vs. 51 kg) and continued to be heavier and have a significantly higher average daily weight gain than did unaf-

fected foals (at 12 months, weight, 337.8 vs. 316.8 kg; growth rate, 0.8 vs. 0.74 kg/day). They also had a larger frame than did horses without tarsocrural OCD, including a greater height at the withers and at the croup and a markedly larger circumference of the carpus and the cannon. Enlargement of the distal physeal region of the metacarpus was more common and more pronounced between 3 and 8 months of age in horses with tarsocrural joint OCD. However, 11 foals with palmar/plantar fragments or ununited palmar/plantar eminences were slightly lighter, and the average daily weight gain as well as different body measurements was similar in affected and unaffected horses. There was no relationship between the radiologic findings of these palmar/plantar fragments and the degree of synovial effusion or other clinical signs in the area. The authors felt that the early radiologic signs of OCD and the observed difference in body size at birth indicated that the pregnancy period and the first month in the foal's life were of major importance for the development of OCD. They also felt that the differences in body weight, body measurements, and clinical signs among horses affected by tarsocrural OCD and fetlock palmar/plantar fragments indicate that the pathogenesis of these lesions differ.[100]

Mechanical Stress and Trauma

It has long been recognized clinically that mechanical stresses precipitate the onset of clinical signs, presumably by avulsing an OCD flap or fragment.[62] The role of trauma as a primary initiator of a lesion is more controversial. Pool has pointed out that there are no unique histologic features that consistently distinguish the lesion of osteochondrosis from that of trauma to a developing osteochondral junction and that the radial vessels supplying the chondrocytes in the epiphyseal physis may be sheared and cause a primary osteochondrosis lesion.[88] He feels that biomechanical forces are an important factor that is superimposed upon an idiopathic lesion to produce defective cartilage. Reflection back to the classic paper by Konig in 1887 is appropriate in considering the potential role of trauma in the pathogenesis. He claimed that loose bodies in the knee joints of young people had three causes: 1) very severe trauma, 2) lesser trauma causing contusion and necrosis, and 3) minimal trauma acting on an underlying lesion—for which he suggested the name "osteochondritis dissecans" (of which he is considered the originator).[3] More recently, Pool and Hurtig have proposed that studies in horses and other animals make it likely that the typical locations of OCD are sites of high mechanical load and areas where developing cartilage is thick and has a tenuous blood supply.[60a,78,78a] They feel that traumatic and vascular insult should be considered. In the case of intermediate ridge OCD in the hock, they have felt that toed-out upright conformation could be a contributory factor, with the intermediate ridge being forced against the axial wall of the trochlear of the talus by rotation of the distal limb.[87] They also point out that the foals are also heavier at birth.[10] Plantar fragments in hind fetlocks are considered to be traumatic in origin.[13]

Defects in Vascularization

OCD was initially attributed to vascular or ischemic necrosis of the subchondral bone.[1,108] Some histologic studies of various lesions in the horse have revealed little evidence of primary bone or cartilage necrosis, and subchondral avascularity was not recognized.[67,97] Recent work in the pig suggests that the viability of epiphyseal cartilage and the articular–epiphyseal cartilage complex depends highly on an adequate blood supply from cartilage canal vessels and strongly implicates a defect in blood supply in the pathogenesis of osteochondrosis.[9] As discussed above, based on pathologic observations of early lesions of osteochondrosis in young horses, Pool feels that subchondral blood vessels in the epiphyseal physis give rise to arcades of thin capillary-sized vessels that extend radially from the subchondral bone into the cartilage and that these vessels are disrupted by shear forces, and chondrocytes in the epiphyseal physis that they supply undergo necrosis.[88] When the lesion develops in a very young horse, a much larger defect occurs because a large amount of the bony bases of the articular surface were never formed. On the other hand, when the onset of the lesions occurs prior to skeletal maturity, the lesion on the trochlear ridge may go unnoticed because articular development is nearly complete.[88] Hurtig and Pool feel that the idea of direct mechanical shearing of cartilage canals is more likely to account for distribution of lesions in equine osteochondrosis than simple ischemic necrosis of epiphyseal bone.[45] They feel that the idea is consistent with some sites in the horse where biomechanical forces are high and the cartilage is normally quite thick, making it more prone to shearing forces. The lateral trochlear ridge of the femur is one such site, where running at speed can create direct compression of the lateral ridge[60a] and where the lateral ridge may resist the tendency for the patella to luxate laterally.[35] They also feel that stress concentration would increase as the limb is adducted in foals that have a toed-out conformation. Cartilage could be deformed in association with occluded vascular canals, leading to chondronecrosis.

Nutrition

Overnutrition as a predisposing cause of osteochondrosis has been extrapolated from work in dogs[32] and pigs.[95,96] Lesions considered consistent with osteochondroses have been induced in horses by feeding 130% National Research Council (NRC) requirements for carbohydrate and protein.[22] Samples were taken from the distolateral radial growth plate cartilage serially harvested from weanling Thoroughbreds after 0, 3, 6, and 9 months on these diets. The higher plane of nutrition is associated with lower cartilage hexosamine and hydroxyproline contents and higher DNA content. Similar observations were made in the articular cartilage collected from the radiohumeral joint at 9 months. The authors also noted that the changes in body weight were 15.5% greater in the horses fed the higher ration. There was no difference in the growth rates of the withers, heart girths, or cannon bones. The high plane of energy and protein did not significantly accelerate any measure of longitudinal growth.

Another series of controlled experiments showed that high-energy diets of 129% NRC requirements consistently produced lesions of osteochondrosis in weanling foals, compared with a control diet based on 100% NRC requirements.[102–104] Thirty mixed-bred foals aged 2.5

to 6.5 months with no clinical or radiographic signs of osteochondrosis were fed one of four diets for 16 to 18 weeks. Twelve horses were fed a control diet with 100% NRC recommendations for digestible energy and crude protein, 6 were fed a diet with 126% of NRC levels for crude protein (CP), and 12 foals were fed a diet with 129% of NRC levels of digestible energy (DE). The diets were composed of three different formulations of rice-based pellets with added maize oil for the high-DE diet and oat and chafe. Average daily gain in humeral length and wither height was slightly, but not significantly, different in the foals on the high-DE diet from that of foals fed the control or high-CP diet. Clinical and radiographic signs of osteochondrosis were seen in 6 of 12 foals fed the high-DE diet. None of the foals fed the high-CP or control diets showed any clinical or radiographic signs of osteochondrosis. The number and severity of lesions found postmortem was much greater in the high-DE group than in the control and high-CP groups. Multiple lesions of osteochondrosis were detected in 11 foals fed the high-DE diet, in 1 foal fed the high-CP diet, and in 1 foal fed the control diet. Histologic lesions were confirmed in 18 foals: all 12 of the high-DE foals, 4 of the high-CP foals, and 2 of the 12 control foals. The number of histologic lesions was significantly greater in the high-DE foals than the control group ($P < .0001$). The incidence of lesions in the foals fed high CP did not differ significantly from that in the control foals ($P = .11$).[105]

Glade et al. found that high-energy/protein diets fed young horses resulted in earlier glucose and insulin peaks and proposed that the intense early insulin secretion and clearance stimulated conversion of thyroxin (T_4) to triiodothyronine (T_3).[23] Higher T_3 concentrations inhibit thyroid-stimulating hormone via negative feedback, so T_4 secretion decreases, and a periodic postprandial transient hypothyrotoxemia may be induced. Because final stages of chondrocytic differentiation in collagen and proteoglycan synthesis appear to depend on thyroid hormones, there is the potential for a problem here. It was reported in one study that foals aged 6 to 8 months receiving diets containing 130% of the recommended dietary intake of protein exhibited significant lower calcium and phosphorus levels due to a calciuric effect of the high-protein diet.[21] However, Schryver et al. studied the effect of dietary protein concentration on foals between 4 and 13 months of age and were unable to confirm the findings of Glade et al. and suggested that metabolic adaptation to the high-protein diet could occur.[110] Another author pointed out other different factors between the two experiments that made comparisons impossible.[17] As noted above, in the study by Savage et al.,[105–107] elevated crude protein levels in the ration did not influence the incidence of osteochondrosis. It was also noted that foals receiving diets with 9% protein were subject to reduced growth in cannon bone diameter without effect on height growth. This was interpreted to demonstrate inhibition of bone remodeling by a low-protein diet, which may contribute to the incidence of angular and other deformities.[59]

Mineral Imbalances

Various mineral imbalances have been implicated in the pathogenesis, including high calcium, high phosphorus, low copper, and high zinc levels. While high calcium levels and hypercalcitoninism have been implicated in the pathogenesis of osteochondrosis,[59] work in the pig does not support any influence of high calcium levels,[76,95] and experimental work in the horse with three times the NRC level of calcium in the diet failed to produce lesions of osteochondrosis.[104] The incidence of clinical physitis and flexural deformities was not related to marginally deficient phosphorus intake in a study of the effect of dietary energy and phosphorus content on blood chemistry and development of growing foals.[11] In this study, excessive dietary phosphorus also appeared to increase significantly the incidence of osteochondrosis in unexercised foals, while excessive levels of dietary calcium did not have this effect unless they were combined with excessive (129% NRC level for DE) digestible energy. It was presumed that the latter result was caused by the effect of high DE rather than by calcium. In the high-phosphorus group, the foals showed no clinical signs of nutritional secondary hyperparathyroidism despite getting significantly more osteochondrosis lesions. It was suggested that dietary intake of excess phosphorus could depress calcium absorption or retention and induce a relative calcium deficiency, but no signs of this were evident after 17 weeks on the diet. The average daily gain was nonsignificantly depressed in foals fed excess phosphorus, which appeared to be due to a palatability problem causing decreased intake.

Low copper levels have been implicated as a cause of osteochondrosis. In experimental studies, a marked copper deficiency (1.7 ppm) produced both flexural deformities and osteochondrosis-like lesions.[6] The authors also noticed a softening of articular cartilage and suggested that low copper stasis may lead to reduced cross-linking of collagen by lysyl oxidase, predisposing to physeal and articular fractures. In another study of eight Thoroughbred foals in which osteochondrosis developed before weaning, seven had serum copper and ceruloplasmin concentrations below normal.[7] Three of these foals on one farm had serum zinc contents high enough to suggest zinc toxicosis, but no evidence for environmental exposure to excess zinc was found.

An epidemiologic study of developmental orthopedic disease in young horses by Knight et al.[53] suggested a relationship between copper and zinc concentrations in the diet and clinical signs of DOD. Joint lesions had been reported in growing foals fed low-copper diets (8 ppm) in 1949 by Kupps and Howell, but these observations were ignored in developing NRC levels for copper at that time. Dose response studies have been done in relationship to copper by Knight et al.[56] and Hurtig et al.[43] In the study by Knight et al., foals were killed at 90 days, after the mares were subjected to rations containing 32 or 13 ppm copper and foals received 55 or 15 ppm of copper, respectively. In foals killed at 90 days, there were over twice (9 vs. 4) as many lesions of osteochondrosis and more than four times (9 vs. 2) as many articular lesions of osteophyte formation or thinning in copper-control foals than in copper-supplemented foals. However, these differences were predominantly due to a higher number of lesions in one copper-control foal. The differences at 90 days were not significant, but there was a significant reduction in prevalence of lesions in copper-supplemented foals killed at 120 days of age. Typical

lesions were subchondral thickening of the articular–epiphyseal complex, with separation from the subchondral bone.

Hurtig et al. conducted a blind randomized study in Quarter Horse foals with high (25 ppm) and low (7 ppm) copper diets.[41] Foals in the low-copper group had declining liver copper values and developed OCD lesions, physitis, and limb deformities over a 6-month period. Erosion and separation of cartilage from the subchondral bone in the dorsal facets of the cervical spine were the most consistent postmortem lesions (it was not possible to diagnose these lesions clinically). Foals fed the high-copper diet had no significant musculoskeletal lesions. Scintigraphy failed to detect occult or known lesions in the limbs and cervical spines. X-rays were mediocre at detecting lesions. Microscopic examination of growth plates and metaphyseal bone from affected foals showed that fractures disrupted or displaced the normal growth plate architecture and interfered with orderly bone growth, similar to copper deficiency in cattle. Bone morphometry indicated less subchondral bone volume in the distal cannon bone, and there were fewer newly formed trabeculae in the primary spongiosa and metaphysis in the distal tibia in copper-deficient foals. Biochemical studies were limited to four control and six low-copper foals. Of the six low-copper foals, four were severely affected with multiple lesions. The biochemical assays showed significantly reduced collagen pyridinoline cross-linkages in articular cartilage, growth plate cartilage, and bone in the OCD-affected foals. Articular cartilage proteoglycanase and gelatinase had elevated levels in the low-copper group and were present in an active form. All metalloproteinase activities were low in growth plate cartilage (presumed to be due to the presence of TIMP). In further examination of the growth plate of these foals, it was felt that the concept of cartilage thickening was a myth, at least in the growth plate, and that the defect was in the transition between calcified cartilage and primary spongiosa.[42] They interpreted the lesion as one of reduced structural strength rather than arrested or abnormal endochondral ossification. Further studies have led to the proposal that cartilage defects and microfractures of metaphyseal and subchondral bone may be due to biomechanically inferior connective tissues rather than failure of chondrocyte differentiation and provisional calcification. This defect in connective tissues could be associated with defective collagen cross-linking and altered matrix remodeling (elevated levels of stromelysin and gelatinase were found in the OCD-affected foals in the low-copper group).[44]

In some recent work from New Zealand, the effect of copper status on evidence of bone and cartilage lesions was investigated in 21 Thoroughbred foals. It was found that mare copper supplementation significantly decreased the radiographic indices for physitis in the distal third metatarsal bone of the foals at 150 days and the prevalence of articular cartilage lesions. Articular cartilage lesions were minor in all foals, with no evidence of clinical OCD in vivo, with the exception of minor radiographic changes assessed postmortem. Copper supplementation of the foal had no effect on any of the bone and cartilage parameters. Copper supplementation of the mares did not abolish DOD in the growing foals, emphasizing the probable multifactorial nature of this condition. Although the copper intake of control foals in the present study was within the range considered by Hurtig and Pool to be mildly deficient, there was no histomorphometric evidence of tissue fragility in the primary spongiosa of the distal radius of these foals, compared with supplemental foals.[45] The articular cartilage lesions were similar to those found in the studies of Knight et al. (1990) and Hurtig et al. (1993).[43,56] The authors felt that the low incidence and severity of lesions in their foals differed from the findings of Knight and Hurtig because it is possible that in the American studies a greater dietary copper requirement exists compared with that of the pasture-fed foals in New Zealand. Pearce et al.[81] did not find articular lesions in the cervical vertebrae. In their study, copper supplementation of the mare and not the foal decreased articular cartilage lesions and the radiographic indices of physitis in foals at 150 days. On the other hand, there was no relationship between neonatal liver copper stores and either radiographic physitis scores or articular cartilage lesions. It was suggested that copper supplementation of mares could provide a convenient treatment regimen on farms experiencing an increased incidence of DOD.[80] In associated papers, the same group found that increasing the copper intake of the mare was effective in enhancing the copper status of the foals (liver copper).[79] They also found that although copper supplementation of the foals is reflected in liver copper concentrations, it is poorly reflected in bone, other soft tissue copper concentrations, and circulating copper status indices.[81] Mare treatment also did not affect plasma copper concentration, red blood cell copper concentration, plasma ceruloplasmin activity, or copper concentration in bone and organs other than the liver.[81]

Cymbaluk and Smart[12] have cautioned that equine veterinarians and owners are currently overemphasizing copper intake to the exclusion of adequate energy and protein macromineral intake. Although there is evidence that copper may control some aspects of osteochondrosis, we need to pay attention to general sound nutritional management and not presume that copper supplementation alone will cure this multifactorial problem.[12,50] Because zinc appears to be the main copper antagonist for horses, dietary copper supplementation must always consider zinc intake. Zinc to copper ratios of 4:1 or 5:1 for all breeds of horses have been recommended.

Excessive zinc intake has been related directly to equine osteochondrosis.[68] The effects of environmental exposure to zinc and cadmium were studied in pregnant pony mares following observations of lameness, swollen joints, and unthriftiness, particularly in foals.[31] Two foals born and raised near a zinc smelter were lame and had joint swellings that were attributable to severe generalized osteochondrosis. Lesions resembling osteochondrosis were found in the limbs and cervical vertebrae, and on the basis of increased tissue levels of zinc and cadmium, the authors concluded that increased exposure to zinc and possibly cadmium resulted in the development of osteochondrosis. On the other hand, some experimental work insinuated that certain levels of zinc (supplementation) are appropriate when copper levels are also adequate.[57] Because of the multifactorial nature of the disease, correction of nutritional imbalances does not eliminate this disease.[46]

Endocrine Factors

Endocrinologic causes have been implicated in the pathogenesis. It has been postulated by Glade that the production of osteochondrosis lesions in association with overfeeding is mediated by the endocrine system.[36] It was initially suggested, in dogs, that lesions of osteochondrosis might be an endocrine disorder in 1970.[60] There is evidence for hormonal imbalances being significant in dogs; histologic changes similar to those seen with osteochondrosis were produced by administration of somatotropin–thyrotropin and thyrotropin–corticotropin combinations.[78a] There is also some evidence for hormonal factors in pigs.[69] Glade has proposed that feeding initiates increased concentrations of insulin and T4. High concentrations of insulin could inhibit growth hormone, although the exact mechanism is not known.[20] High-energy and high-protein diets were associated with earlier peaking of insulin levels postprandially, and there were thought to be stimulatory effects on clearance of T4 and coincident increases of T3.[23] Glade and Belling suggested that the episodic transient hypothyroidemia produced by high-soluble-carbohydrate diets could cause osteochondrosis.[36]

Long-term administration of dexamethasone has been associated with the production of osteochondrosis-like lesions.[24–26] It was considered that glucocorticoids induced parathyroid hormone resistance at the level of the osteocyte, causing inhibition of osteocytic osteolysis. Glucocorticoids also induced decreased GAG levels, and this decrease in turn inhibits capillary penetration of the cartilage. The failure of endochondral ossification could also be mediated through induced defects in vitamin D metabolism. In addition to $1,25\text{-}OH_2(D3)$ promoting the availability of both calcium and phosphate, it has been shown that the other active vitamin D metabolite ($24,25\text{-}OH_2D3$) promotes the synthesis of proteoglycan by chondrocytes and is necessary for the normal differentiation of epiphyseal cartilage.[51] These are not necessarily the same as what we see clinically. It has also been pointed out that corticosteroids are potent inhibitors of lysyl oxidase, and a deficiency of lysyl oxidase can produce histologic lesions similar to those seen in clinical cases of osteochondrosis.

Site Vulnerability

Because the lesions of equine osteochondrosis occur at specific anatomic sites, this obviously suggests site vulnerability. This predilection could be related to delay of endochondral ossification or trauma due to excessive stress at that region. In osteochondrosis of the cervical articular process in the horse, those regions of the intervertebral joint that are under constant load because of flexion ossify last, and the lesions regularly develop in those areas.[98] In nearly all instances, the sites of occurrence of OCD in the horse are very close to the limits of articulation. Differences in GAG content have been demonstrated between articular and nonarticular margins in canine shoulders,[52] and also, GAG contents can be modulated by changing a nonarticular into an articular surface by making the dog step up onto a raised surface. As noted above, in the equine tarsocrural joint at least, the thickest cartilage in the distal tibia (caudal part of the intermediate ridge) and distal femur (medial trochlear ridge) do not correspond with the most common sites of osteochondrosis in these bones (cranial part of the intermediate ridge and lateral trochlear ridge, respectively).[14]

Some strong arguments have been made for involvement of mechanical factors in the pathogenesis of natural cases of equine osteochondrosis.[45] For example, 1) many horses are affected in only one site and one joint,[64] 2) lesions of OCD have been reported in sites where ossification has ceased, indicating that defective endochondral ossification was an unlikely cause,[64,65] and 3) retained cartilage is not commonly found in the growth plates of foals. There is limited radiographic and histologic evidence of retained cartilage in equine OCD lesions. Fragments of distal intermediate ridge OCD of the tibia, for example, appear to be separated from the parent bone very early in life and have undergone revascularization of even some appositional growth. Retained cartilage is rarely found. It has been proposed that when islands of cartilage are found it is uncertain whether these are residues of traumatically induced callus or displaced hypertrophic cartilage. Further, 4) it is common in routine cases to find fragments of normal-thickness cartilage separated from apparently normal subchondral bone, which is inconsistent with the proposal for fissures developing from thickened articular cartilage.[64]

Lesions are frequently bilateral in the femoropatellar and tarsocrural joint and quadrilateral in the fetlock joint, while infrequently involving different joints in the same animal. Does this suggest a "window of vulnerability" in the endochondral ossification of that specific joint when an environmental insult may have occurred?[88] If the causative factor was present intermittently or for a transient period during the foal's growth period, this could explain the development of the disease in only one pair of joints. It is not possible from these data to ascertain different periods of onset of the disease process in different joints.

Exercise (or Lack Thereof)

Adequate exercise in foals would logically be important to maintain cartilage and bone quality. There are some data suggesting a "protective" effect of exercise.[8] In this study done on early weaned Warmblood foals, there was a dramatically lower incidence of osteochondrosis in foals subjected to forced exercise and a high-energy diet than in foals fed the same diet but with limited exercise.

Osteochondritis Dissecans

There is general agreement that osteochondritis dissecans involves a dissecting lesion with formation of a chondral or osteochondral flap(s). Flaps may become detached and form joint mice. Blood vessels from the periphery of the joint frequently remain in communication with cartilage flaps or detached flakes, leading to calcification or ossification of the avulsed cartilage. Release of necrotic debris into the joint along the fissures is considered to cause synovitis and pain.[114] The latter conclusion needs to be questioned, based on the cases seen with intact cartilage separated from the bone, manifesting with lameness and synovial effusion.[65]

As alluded to above, lesions have been found at arthroscopy in some instances that consisted of cartilage separated from bone, and the cartilage did not appear to be thickened. Many histologic studies of porcine osteochondrosis have revealed areas of necrosis in the articular–epiphyseal cartilage complex without concurrent or prior thickening of the cartilage.[34,35] In earlier histologic studies of equine material,[56,97] some subchondral bone involvement has also been demonstrated. However, it must be questioned whether persistence of hypertrophied cartilage is a necessary event prior to development of an OCD lesion,[64] based on instances seen at arthroscopic examination or in follow-up histologic examination in which dissection or separation occurs close to the cartilage–bone interface rather than in the underlying cancellous bone between normal cartilage and a normal bone–cartilage junction, as it commonly does in humans.[88]

As mentioned above, one entity in the horse on the palmar aspect of the distal third metacarpal bone has its origin within the bone and was initially described as OCD.[40,73] It has since been recognized that this name implies that this lesion is a developmental joint disease, which it is not.[89] It is still classified as traumatic osteochondrosis by some. The diagnosis and treatment of the important entities of OCD in the horse are discussed below.

References

1. Adams OR. Lameness in Horses. 3rd ed. Philadelphia: Lea & Febiger, 1974.
2. Alvarado AF, Marcoux M, Berton L. The incidence of osteochondrosis on a Standardbred breeding farm in Quebec. Proceedings. Annual Meeting of the American Association of Equine Practitioners, Boston, MA, 1989;35:293–307.
3. Barrie HJ. Osteochondritis dissecans. 1887–1987. A centennial look at Konig's memorable phrase. J Bone Joint Surg [Br] 1987; 69:693–695.
4. Bramlage LR. Clinical manifestations of disturbed bone formation in the horse. Proceedings. 33rd Annual Convention of the American Association of Equine Practitioners, 1987;135–138.
5. Bramlage LR. Investigation of farm-wide incidence of bone formation problems in the horse. Proceedings. 39th Annual Convention of the American Association of Equine Practitioners, San Antonio, TX, 1993;45–48.
6. Bridges CH, Harris ED. Experimentally induced cartilaginous fractures (osteochondritis dissecans) in foals fed low-copper diets. J Am Vet Med Assoc 1988;193:215–221.
7. Bridges CH, Womack JE, Harris ED, Scrutchfield WL. Considerations of copper metabolism in osteochondrosis of suckling foals. J Am Vet Med Assoc 1984;185:173–178.
8. Bruin G, Creemers JJHM, Smolders EEA. Effect of exercise on osteochondrosis in the horse [abstract]. Proceedings. Equine Osteochondrosis in the 90's, Cambridge University, 1992;41–43.
9. Carlson CS, Meuten DJ, Richardson DC. Ischemic necrosis of cartilage in spontaneous and experimental lesions of osteochondrosis. J Orthop Res 1991;9:317–329.
10. Carlsten J, Sandgren B, Dalin G. Development of osteochondrosis in the tarsocrural joint and osteochondral fragments in the fetlock joints of Standardbred trotters. I. A radiological survey. Equine Vet J 1993;(S16):42–47.
11. Cymbaluk NF, Christison GI. Effects of dietary energy and phosphorus content on blood chemistry and development of growing horses. J Anim Sci 1989;67:951–958.
12. Cymbaluk NF, Smart ME. A review of possible metabolic relationships of copper to equine bone disease. Equine Vet J 1993; S16:19–26.
13. Dalin G, Sandgren B, Carlsten J. Plantar osteochondral fragments in the metatarsophalangeal joints in Standardbred trotters; result of osteochondrosis or trauma? Equine Vet J 1993;S16:62–65.

14. Firth EC, Greydanus Y. Cartilage thickness measurement of foals. Res Vet Sci 1984;42:35–46.

15. Fisher AT, Barclay WP. Osteochondrosis dissecans in the horse. Comp Cont Educ Pract Vet 1984;6:123–131.

16. Foerner JJ, Barclay WP, Phillips TN, MacHarg MA. Osteochondral fragments of the palmar/plantar aspect of the fetlock joint. Proceedings. 33rd Annual Convention of the American Association of Equine Practitioners, New Orleans, LA, 1987;32:739–744.

17. Frape DL. Calcium balance and dietary protein content. Equine Vet J 1987;19:265–270.

18. Gabel AA. Metabolic bone disease: Problems in terminology. Equine Vet J 1988;20:4–6.

19. Gabel AA, Knight DA, Reed SM, et al. Comparison of incidence and severity of developmental orthopedic disease on 17 farms before and after adjustment of ration. Proceedings. 33rd Annual Convention of the American Association of Equine Practitioners, New Orleans, LA, 1987;163–170.

20. Glade MJ. Control of cartilage growth in osteochondrosis: A review. J Equine Vet Sci 1986;6:175–187.

21. Glade MJ, Beller D, Bergman J, et al. Dietary protein in excess of requirements inhibits renal calcium and phosphorus reabsorption in young horses. Nutr Rep Int 31:649–659.

22. Glade MJ, Belling TH. A dietary etiology for osteochondrotic cartilage. J Equine Vet Sci 1986;6:151–155.

23. Glade MJ, Gupta S, Reimers TJ. Hormonal responses to high and low planes of nutrition in weanling Thoroughbreds. J Anim Sci 1984;59:658–665.

24. Glade MJ, Krook L. Glucocorticoid-induced inhibition of osteolysis and the development of osteopetrosis, osteonecrosis and osteoporosis. Cornell Vet 1982;72:76–91.

25. Glade MJ, Krook L, Schryver HF, Hintz HF. Morphologic and biochemical changes in cartilage of foals treated with dexamethasone. Cornell Vet 1983;73:170–192.

26. Glade MJ, Lowe JE, Hintz HF, et al. Growth suppression and osteochondritis dissecans in weanlings treated with dexamethasone. Proceedings. 25th Annual Convention of the American Association of Equine Practitioners, Miami Beach, FL, 1979;24:361–366.

27. Goyal HO, MacCallum FJ, Brown MP, Delack JB. Growth rates of the extremities of limb bones in young horses. Can Vet J 1981;22:31–33.

28. Green DA. A study of growth rate in Thoroughbred foals. Br Vet J 1969;125:539–546.

29. Grondahl AM, Dolvik NI. Heritability of osteochondrosis in the tibiotarsal joint and of bony fragments in the fetlocks of Standardbred trotters. Proceedings. Equine Osteochondrosis in the 90's, Cambridge University, 1992;14–15.

30. Grondahl AM, Dolvik NI. Heritability estimations of osteochondrosis in the tibiotarsal joint and of bony fragments in the palmar/plantar portion of the metacarpophalangeal and metatarsophalangeal joints of horses. J Am Vet Med Assoc 1993;203:101–104.

31. Gunson DE, Kowalczyk DF, Shoop CR, Ramberg CF. Environmental zinc and cadmium pollution associated with generalized osteochondrosis, osteoporosis and nephrocalcinosis in horses. J Am Vet Med Assoc 1982;180:295–299.

32. Hedhammar A, Wu F, Krook L, et al. Overnutrition and skeletal disease. An experimental study in growing Great Dane dogs. Cornell Vet 1972;(Suppl)5:1.

33. Henson FMD, Schofield PN, Jeffcott LB. Expression of transforming growth factor-â1 in normal and dyschondroplastic articular growth cartilage of the young horse. Equine Vet J 1997;29:434–439.

34. Hill MA, Kincaid SA, Visco DM. Use of histochemical techniques in the characterisation of osteochondrosis affecting pigs. Vet Rec 1990;127:29–37.

35. Hill MA, Ruth GR, Hilley HD, Hansgen DC. Dyschondroplasias, including osteochondroses, in boars between 25 and 169 days of age: Histologic changes. Am J Vet Res 1984;45:903–916.

36. Hintz HF. Factors which influence developmental orthopedic disease. Proceedings. 33rd Annual Convention of the American Association of Equine Practitioners, New Orleans, LA, 1987;159–162.

37. Hintz HF, Hintz RL, Van Vleck LD. Growth rate of Thoroughbreds, effect of age of dam, year and month of birth and sex of foal. J Anim Sci 1979;48:480–487.

38. Hogan PM, McIlwraith CW, Honnas CM, et al. Surgical treatment of subchondral cystic lesions of the third metacarpal bone: Results in 15 horses (1986–1994). Equine Vet J 1997;29:477–482.

39. Hoppe F, Phillipsson J. A genetic study of osteochondrosis in Swedish horses. Equine Pract 1985;7:7–15.

39a. Hoppe F. Osteochondrosis in Swedish horses. A radiological and epidemiological study with special reference to frequency and heredity. PhD dissertation, Swedish College of Agricultural Sciences, Uppsala, Sweden, 1984.

40. Hornoff WJ, O'Brien TR, Pool RR. Osteochondritis dissecans of the distal metacarpus in the adult racing Thoroughbred horse. Vet Radiol 1981;22:98.

41. Hurtig MB, Green SL, Dobson H, Burton J. Defective bone and cartilage in foals fed a low copper diet. Proceedings. 35th Annual Convention of the American Association of Equine Practitioners, Lexington, KY, 1990;637–643.

42. Hurtig MB, Green SL, Dobson H, Burten J. Correlation of the clinical signs, diagnostic imaging and gross pathology of defective cartilage and bone growth in copper-deficient foals [abstract]. Proceedings. Equine Osteochondrosis in the 90's, Cambridge University, 1992;27–28.

43. Hurtig M, Green SL, Dobson H, et al. Correlative study of defective cartilage and bone growth in foals fed a low-copper diet. Equine Vet J 1993;S16:66–73.

44. Hurtig MB, Mikuna-Takagaki Y, Choi J. Biochemical evidence for defective cartilage and bone growth in copper deficient foals [abstract]. Proceedings. Equine Osteochondrosis in the 90's, Cambridge University, 1992;28–30.

45. Hurtig MB, Pool RR. Pathogenesis of equine osteochondrosis. In: McIlwraith CW, Trotter GW, Eds. Joint Disease in the Horse. Philadelphia: WB Saunders, 1996;335–357.

46. Jackson SJ, Pagan JD. Developmental orthopedic disease. Multiple causes—No sure cures. J Equine Vet Sci 1993;13:9–10.

47. Jeffcott LB. Osteochondrosis in the horse—Searching for the key to pathogenesis. Equine Vet J 1991;23:331–338.

48. Jeffcott LB. Problems and pointers in equine osteochondrosis. Equine Vet J 1993;S16:1–3.

49. Jeffcott LB. Studies on endochondral ossification in the horse and their application to osteochondrosis. Report to horserace betting levy board. Personal communication, 1997.

50. Jeffcott LB, Davies ME. Copper status and skeletal development in horses: Still a long way to go. Equine Vet J 1998;30:183–185.

51. Kanis JA. Vitamin D metabolism and its clinical application. J Bone Joint Surg [Br] 1982;64:542.

52. Kincaid SA, Van Sickle DC. Regional histochemical and thickness variations of adult articular cartilage. J Am Vet Med Assoc 1981;42:428.

53. Knight DA, Gabel AA, Reed SM, et al. Correlation of dietary minerals to incidence and severity of metabolic bone disease in Ohio and Kentucky. Proceedings. 31st Annual Meeting of the American Association of Equine Practitioners, Toronto, Canada, 1985;445–561.

54. Knight DA, Schmall LM, Reed SM, et al. The influence of dietary copper and growth rate on cartilage defects in foals [abstract]. Proceedings. Equine Osteochondrosis in the 90's, Cambridge University, 1992;22–23.

55. Knight DA, Schmall LM, Reed SM, et al. Effects of dietary copper on trace element concentrations of mare's milk and the serum and tissues of their foals [abstract]. Proceedings. Equine Osteochondrosis in the 90's, Cambridge University, 1992;23–24.

56. Knight DA, Weisbrode SE, Schmall LM, et al. The effects of copper supplementation on the prevalence of cartilage lesions in foals. Equine Vet J 1990;22:426–432.

57. Knight DA, Weisbrode SE, Schmall LM, et al. Effect of varying copper:zinc ratios on the frequency of cartilage lesions in foals [abstract]. Proceedings. Osteochondrosis in the '90s. University of Cambridge 1992;25–26.

58. Kold SE, Hickman J, Melsen F. An experimental study of the healing process of equine chondral and osteochondral defects. Equine Vet J 1986;18:18–24.

59. Krook L, Maylin GA. Fractures of Thoroughbred racehorses. Cornell Vet 1988;78:5–133.

59a. Leach RM, Nesheim MC. Nutritional, genetic and morphological studies of an abnormal cartilage formation in young chicks. J Nutr 1965;86:236–244.

60. Lundgren G, Reiland S. Osteochondrosis in adolescent animals: An endocrine disorder? Calcif Tissue Res 1970;S4:150–151.

60a. Maquet P. Biomechanique du genou et gonarthrose. Rev Med Liege 1969;24:170.

61. McIlwraith CW, Ed. Developmental Orthopedic Disease Symposium. Amarillo, TX: American Quarter Horse Association, 1984; 1–77.

62. McIlwraith CW. Osteochondrosis. In: Stashak TS, ed. Adams' Lameness in Horses. 4th ed. Philadelphia: Lea & Febiger, 1987; 396–410.

63. McIlwraith CW. Subchondral cystic lesions in the horse—The indications, methods and results of surgery. Equine Vet Educ 1990;2:75–80.

64. McIlwraith CW. Inferences from referred clinical cases of osteochondrosis dissecans. Equine Vet J 1993;S16:27–30.

65. McIntosh SC, McIlwraith CW. Natural history of femoropatellar osteochondrosis in three crops of Thoroughbreds. Equine Vet J 1993;S16:54–61.

66. McLaughlin BG, Doige CE, Fretz PB, Pharr JW. Carpal bone lesions associated with angular limb deformities in foals. J Am Vet Med Assoc 1981;178:224–230.

67. Meagher DM, Pool RR, O'Brien TR. Osteochondritis of the shoulder joint in the horse. Proceedings. 19th Annual Meeting of the American Association of Equine Practitioners, Atlanta, GA, 1973;247–256.

68. Messer NT. Tibiotarsal effusion associated with chronic zinc intoxication in three horses. J Am Vet Med Assoc 1981;178:294.

69. Nakano T, Aherne FX, Thompson JR. Effects of feed restriction, sex and diethylstilbestrol on the occurrence of joint lesions with some histological and biochemical studies of the articular cartilage of growing-finishing swine. Can J Anim Sci 1979;59:491.

70. Nilsson G, Olsson SE. Radiographic and patho-anatomic changes in the distal joints and phalanges of the Standardbred horse. Acta Vet Scand 1973;44:1–57.

71. Nixon AJ. Osteochondrosis and osteochondritis dissecans of the equine fetlock. Comp Cont Educ Pract Vet 1990;12:1463–1465.

72. O'Brien TR. Radiology of the equine stifle. Proceedings. 19th Annual Meeting of the American Association of Equine Practitioners, Atlanta, GA, 1973;271–287.

73. O'Brien TR, Hornoff WJ, Meagher DM. Radiographic detection and characterization of palmar lesions in the equine fetlock joint. J Am Vet Med Assoc 1981;178:231.

74. O'Donohue DD, Smith EH, Strickland KL. The incidence of abnormal limb development in the Irish Thoroughbred from birth to 18 months. Equine Vet J 1992;24:305–309.

75. Olsson SE. Introduction. Acta Radiol Suppl 1978;358:9–14.

76. Olsson SE, Reiland S. The nature of osteochondrosis in animals. Summary and conclusions with comparative aspects on osteochondritis dissecans in man. Acta Radiol Suppl 1978;S358: 299–306.

77. Pagan JD, Jackson SG. The incidence of developmental orthopaedic disease on a Kentucky Thoroughbred farm. World Equine Vet Rev 1996;20–26.

78. Paatsama S, Rokkanen P, Jussila J. Etiological factors in osteochondritis dissecans. Acta Orthop Scand 1975;46:906–918.

78a. Paatsama S, Rokkanen P, Jussila J, Sittnikow K. Somatotropin, thyrotropin and corticotropin hormone-induced changes in the cartilages and bones of the shoulder and knee joints in young dogs. J Small Anim Pract 1971;12:595–601.

79. Pearce SG, Firth EC, Grace ND, Fennessy PF. Effect of copper supplementation on the evidence of developmental orthopaedic disease in pasture-fed New Zealand Thoroughbreds. Equine Vet J 1998;30:211–218.

80. Pearce SG, Grace ND, Firth EC, et al. Effect of copper supplementation on the copper status of pasture-fed young Thoroughbreds. Equine Vet J 1998;30:204–210.

81. Pearce SG, Grace ND, Wichtel JJ, et al. Effect of copper supplementation on copper status of pregnant mares and foals. Equine Vet J 1998;30:200–203.

82. Petersson H, Sevelius F. Subchondral bone cysts in the horse: A clinical study. Equine Vet J 1986;1:75.

83. Philipsson J. Pathogenesis of osteochondrosis—Genetic implications. In: McIlwraith CW, Trotter GW, Eds. Joint Disease in the Horse. Philadelphia: WB Saunders, 1996;359–362.

84. Philipsson J, Andreasson E, Sandgren B, et al. Osteochondrosis in the tarsocrural joint and osteochondral fragments in the fetlock joints in Swedish Standardbred trotters—II. Heritability estimations. Proceedings. Equine Osteochondrosis in the 90's, Cambridge University, 1992;17–18.

85. Philipsson J, Andreasson E, Sandgren B, et al. Osteochondrosis in the tarsocrural joint and osteochondral fragments in the fetlock joints in Standardbred trotters. II. Heritability. Equine Vet J 1993; S16:38–41.

86. Pool R. Difficulties in definition of equine osteochondrosis—Differentiating developmental and acquired lesions. Proceedings. Osteochondrosis in the 90s, Cambridge University, 1992;10.

87. Pool RR. Difficulties in definition of equine osteochondrosis; differentiation of developmental and acquired lesions. Equine Vet J 1993;S16:5–12.

88. Pool RR. Pathologic manifestations of osteochondrosis. In: McIlwraith CW, Ed. Proceedings. Developmental Orthopedic Disease Symposium. Amarillo, TX: American Quarter Horse Association, 1986;3–7.

89. Pool RR, Meagher DM. Pathologic findings and pathogenesis of racetrack injuries. Vet Clin North Am [Equine Pract] 1990;6: 1–30.

90. Poulos P. Radiologic manifestations of developmental problems. In: McIlwraith CW, Ed. Proceedings. Developmental Orthopedic Disease Symposium. Amarillo, TX: American Quarter Horse Association, 1994;1–2.

91. Poulos PW Jr. Tibial dyschondroplasia (osteochondrosis) in the turkey. Acta Radiol Suppl 1978;358:197–227.

92. Poulos PW Jr, Reiland S, Elwinger K, Olsson S. Skeletal lesions in the broiler, with special reference to dyschondroplasia (osteochondrosis). Acta Radiol Suppl 1978;358:229–275.

93. Ray CS, Baxter GM, McIlwraith CW, et al. Development of subchondral cystic lesions following subchondral bone trauma in horses. Equine Vet J 1997.

94. Reid CF. Radiographic diagnosis and appearance of periarticular cyst-like lesions primarily reported as periarticular "bone cysts." Proceedings. 16th Annual Convention of the American Association of Equine Practitioners, Montreal, Canada, 1970;185–187.

95. Reiland S. Morphology of osteochondrosis and sequelae in the pig. Acta Radiol Suppl 1978;358:45–90.

96. Reiland S, Ordell N, Lundeheim N, Olsson SE. Heredity of osteochondrosis, body constitution and leg weakness in pigs. Acta Radiol Suppl 1978;358:123–137.

97. Rejno S, Stromberg B. Osteochondrosis in the horse. II. Pathology. Acta Radiol Suppl 1978;358:153–178.

98. Rooney JR. Osteochondrosis in the horse. Mod Vet Pract 1975; 56:41–43, 113–116.

99. Sandgren B. Bony fragments in the tarsocrural and metacarpophalangeal or metatarsophalangeal joints in the Standardbred horse—A radiographic survey. Equine Vet J 1988;S6:67–70.

100. Sandgren B, Dalin G, Carlsten J. Osteochondrosis in the tarsocrural joint and osteochondral fragments in the fetlock joints of Standardbred trotters. II. Body measurements and clinical findings. Equine Vet J S16:48–53.

101. Savage CJ. The influence of nutrition on skeletal growth and induction of osteochondrosis (dyschondroplasia) in horses. PhD thesis, University of Melbourne, Australia, 1993.

102. Savage CJ, McCarthy RN, Jeffcott LB. Developmental orthopedic disease versus metabolic bone disease—A histomorphometrical study [abstract]. Proceedings. Equine Osteochondrosis in the 90's, Cambridge University, 1992;45–46.

103. Savage CJ, McCarthy RN, Jeffcott LB. Induction of dyschondroplasia in foals. I. Effects of dietary energy and protein [abstract]. Proceedings. Equine Osteochondrosis in the 90's, Cambridge University, 1992;38–29.

104. Savage CJ, McCarthy RN, Jeffcott LB. Induction of dyschondroplasia in foals. II. Effects of dietary phosphorus and calcium. Proceedings. Equine Osteochondrosis in the 90's, Cambridge University, 1992;40–41.

105. Savage CJ, McCarthy RN, Jeffcott LB. Effects of dietary energy and protein on induction of dyschondroplasia in foals. Equine Vet J 1993;S16:74–79.

106. Savage CJ, McCarthy RN, Jeffcott LB. Effects of dietary phosphorus and calcium on induction of dyschondroplasia in foals. Equine Vet J 1993;S16:80–83.

107. Savage CJ, McCarthy RN, Jeffcott LB. Histomorphometric assessment of bone biopsies from foals fed diets high in phosphorus and digestible energy. Equine Vet J 1993;S16:89–93.

108. Schebitz H. Degenerative arthritis of the shoulder joint following aseptic necrosis of the humeral head in foals. In: Proceedings. 11th Annual Meeting of the American Association of Equine Practitioners, Miami Beach, FL, 1965;359–370.

109. Schougaard H, Falk-Ronne J, Phillipson J. A radiographic survey of tibiotarsal osteochondrosis in a selected population of trotting horses in Denmark and its possible genetic significance. Equine Vet J 1990;22:288–289.

110. Schryver HF, Meakin DW, Lowe JE, Williams LV, Soderholm LV, Hintz HF. Growth and calcium metabolism in horses fed various levels of protein. Equine Vet J 1987;19:280–287.

111. Staun HF, Linneman F, Eriksen L, Neilson K, et al. (As cited by Jeffcott) Influence of feeding intensity on the development of the young growing horse until 18 months of age. Beret Statens Husdybrugsfors 1987;630:1–79.

112. Stougaard J. The hereditary factor in osteochondritis dissecans. J Bone Joint Surg [Br] 1961;43:256–258.

113. Stromberg J. A review of the salient features of osteochondrosis in the horse. Equine Vet J 1979;11:211–214.

114. Stromberg B, Rejno S. Osteochondrosis in the horse. I. A clinical and radiologic investigation of osteochondrosis dissecans of the knee and hock. Acta Radiol Suppl 1978;358:139–152.

115. Thorp BH, Farquharson C, Kwan APL, Loveridge N. Osteochondrosis/dyschondroplasia: A failure of chondrocyte differentiation. Equine Vet J 1993;S16:13–18.

116. Verschooten F, deMoor A. Subchondral cystic and related lesions affecting the equine pedal bone and stifle. Equine Vet J 1982;14:47–54.

117. Wagner PC, Grant BD, Watrous BJ, et al. A study of the heritability of cervical vertebral malformations in horses. Proceedings. 31st Annual Convention of the American Association of Equine Practitioners, Toronto, Canada, 1985;31:43–50.

118. Watrous BJ, Hultgren BD, Wagner PC. Osteochondrosis in juvenile spavin in equids. Am J Vet Res 1991;52:607–612.

SPECIFIC DISEASES OF JOINTS: OSTEOCHONDRITIS DISSECANS

OCD is a frequent cause of lameness in young athletic horses and is the most frequent condition of the complex requiring surgical intervention. As discussed above, the terms "osteochondrosis," "osteochondritis dissecans," and "osteochondrosis dissecans" have been used regularly as synonyms, and their meaning is still somewhat controversial. The terms have been distinguished as follows: "osteochondrosis" refers to the disease, "osteochondritis" to the inflammatory response to the disease, and "osteochondritis dissecans" to the condition when a flap can be demonstrated.[54] This section addresses the clinical aspects of OCD, including clinical signs, diagnosis, treatment options, and prognosis. Although arthroscopic surgery is the most commonly recommended treatment to achieve athletic activity and prevent DJD, certain situations have been recognized in which conservative treatment is successful.

Three categories of OCD lesions are recognized: 1) those showing clinical and radiographic signs, 2) those showing clinical signs without radiographic (but arthroscopic) signs, and 3) those showing radiographic signs but no clinical signs. Data from the first two categories of disease have been tabulated for the most commonly selected joints from the author's surgical case reports.[37] The relative incidence of clinical signs versus radio-graphic lesions has also been documented in the femoropatellar joint by McIntosh and McIlwraith.[42] Similar data for other joints are needed. The clinical aspects of OCD are presented for the individual joints where OCD is most common.

Osteochondritis Dissecans of the Femoropatellar Joint

OCD was first described in the femoropatellar joint of the horse by Nilsson in 1947.[45] The lesion described by Nilsson was believed to be similar to lesions currently referred to as OCD. Similar lesions were later described as osteochondral fractures in 1973.[50] Since that time there have been a number of reports concerning pathologic and surgical aspects of the condition.[20,36,40,44,51,55,65–68]

In a recent study, 50% of the horses operated for femoropatellar OCD were Thoroughbreds.[20] There were 53 females in the group and 108 males (82 intact and 26 gelded). Approximately 60% of the horses were 1 year of age or less at presentation, and the younger animals tended to have more severe lesions.[20]

CLINICAL SIGNS

Clinical signs may develop at any age. More mature animals frequently present with a sudden onset of clinical signs thought to be associated with the displacement of osteochondral fragments. Less frequently, clinically silent lesions may be identified in mature horses, and a sudden onset of clinical signs may also occasionally be seen in cases in which fragmentation has not yet developed. In one study on one farm, the average age of identification of femoropatellar OCD problems was 12.6 months, 9 months, and 6 months, in three consecutive years.[42]

Horses with OCD of the femoropatellar joint usually present with varying degrees of distension of the femoropatellar joint and varying degrees of lameness, depending on the severity of the lesions. Distension of the femoropatellar joint is the more consistent presenting sign (Fig. 7.56). However, the clinicopathologic changes in the synovial fluid are usually minor. Lameness varies from nondiscernable to severe. Other common abnormalities of gait include reduced cranial phase to the stride and lowered foot arc. Young animals with severe lesions may have difficulty rising. Concurrent flexural deformities have also been reported.[40,44] Lateral luxation of the patella in association with OCD of the lateral trochlear ridge of the femur has been seen.[36] Unilaterally affected animals are often asymmetrically muscled, whereas bilateral cases frequently exhibit poor hindlimb muscle development.[67] The disease is commonly bilateral. In one recent series, 91 horses were bilaterally affected (57%), and 70 horses had unilateral disease (43%).[20]

DIAGNOSIS

Lateral-to-medial radiographs provide the most useful information with regard to the location and nature of the lesions (Fig. 7.56). Caudolateral-to-craniomedial oblique projections may provide additional information with regard to the depth of the lesion on the lateral trochlear ridge of the femur. The most common defect seen radiographically is an irregularity or flattening in the subchondral bone of the lateral trochlear ridge of the femur that may be localized or generalized (Fig. 7.56). Lesions manifesting as defects on radiographs usually manifest with an OCD flap or elevated cartilage. Partially mineralized flaps or islands of mineralized tissue in other defects may be observed. Mineralized free bodies or joint mice that have detached from the primary defect may be present loose within the joint or attached to synovial membrane. Irregular subchondral defects without joint mice tend to be seen in younger horses. Similar lesions may be seen on the medial trochlear ridge but are usually limited to irregularities of contour and are not as extensive. In a number of instances, a separation of cartilage from the medial trochlear ridge without any defect in the subchondral bone (and therefore no radiographic signs) is seen at surgery. Primary OCD of the patella is relatively rare but is seen in some instances. In severe cases of OCD of the trochlear ridges, remodeling of the patellar contour may be visible. Localized defects of the patellar contour visualized on radiographs may represent primary osteochondrosis or secondary change. Care must be taken to avoid diagnosing the radiographic changes of endochondral ossification on the trochlear ridges of young foals as OCD lesions (Fig. 7.57).[1]

In one series of cases, 32 horses had loose bodies in at least one joint.[20] Grades determined from surgery reports were equal to the radiographic grades in 111 cases, but 46 horses had lesions at surgery that were worse than those seen radiographically. In a related study, the radiographs of 72 femoropatellar and femorotibial joints from 50 horses that had arthroscopic surgery were evaluated.[64] Ninety-four arthroscopically evaluated areas were graded according to a predetermined system (based on surgery reports). Radiographic grade was then compared with arthroscopic findings in the same location, and statistical analysis was performed to determine the association between radiographic subchondral bone changes and arthroscopic findings. Radiographically normal areas in the femoropatellar joint were arthroscopically positive for cartilaginous changes in 40% of the femoropatellar joints. Areas of mild subchondral bone flattening (grade I) in the lateral trochlear ridge of the femur were arthroscopically positive for cartilage changes 78% of the time. Some 96% of moderate-to-severe subchondral bone changes (grades II to V) were arthroscopically positive for cartilage damage. This research demonstrated that 1) a significant number of radiographically normal joints have cartilage changes, 2) areas of mild subchondral bone flattening have cartilage changes present in most cases, and 3) areas of moderate-to-severe subchondral bone change have arthroscopically detectable cartilage changes.

Lesions of OCD in other than in the femoropatellar joint may occur at the same time but in low incidence. In the previously mentioned series of 161 horses, 10 horses underwent surgery for other OCD lesions at the time of the femoropatellar arthroscopy.[20] Five had OCD of both metatarsophalangeal joints, 4 had OCD of the tarsocrural joint, and 1 had OCD of the scapulohumeral joint. Two other horses had subchondral cystic lesions of the medial femoral condyle.

TREATMENT

Conflicting reports have been published concerning the management of OCD of the equine femoropatellar joint. In 1977, Wyburn reported that satisfactory results were achieved with conservative therapy if osteochondral fragments were not seen radiographically but that surgery was indicated if free bodies were noted.[68] However, two later reports showed that fragments were often found at surgery that could not be detected radiographically.[40,51] Another group of authors also felt that 54% of stifle cases (OCD of femoropatellar joint and subchondral cystic lesions of the femorotibial joint were not distinguished) were improved after conservative therapy,[57] but examination of the results show them to be inferior to those reported with surgery.[20] Stromberg and Rejno reported radiographic evidence that young horses that had large subchondral defects and were not treated surgically developed DJD.[65] Steenhaut et al. also considered the outcome without surgical treatment to be poor.[63] Favorable results after surgical treatment by using arthrotomy have been reported.[51,65,66] The advantages of using arthroscopic surgery to treat femoropatellar OCD are now well recognized, and the results of surgery with this technique have been published.[20,33,40]

More recent work indicates that conservative treatment can be appropriate in some instances. A recent study demonstrated considerable success in Thoroughbreds (based on subsequent racing performance) with conservative treatment.[42] In this study a careful assessment of foals led to the detection of lesions at an early age, and it was concluded that with confinement, early radiographic lesions of OCD (subchondral bone contour irregularity and subchondral lysis) were potentially reversible. On a farm with a high incidence of femoropatellar OCD, three crops of foals were evaluated. Of 11 cases not operated on in 1989 (some other cases were operated on), 6 raced, 3 had no follow-up, 1 became a jumper, and 1 was operated on later. In 1990, 9 foals with clinical and radiographic lesions of OCD were treated conservatively; 2 had raced, 2 were still unraced at the time of the report, 3 had lameness, and 2 were used for nonracing careers. In 1991 there were 10 cases diagnosed (5 had no radiographic lesions initially but subsequently developed them, and 1 never had a radiographic lesion but had persistent synovial effusion). Four horses were sold as yearlings, reportedly without synovial effusion or lameness, 1 died of unrelated causes, 10 are currently racing or training, and 1 subsequently developed OCD of the metatarsophalangeal joints. A trend in these data indicated that lesser lesions healed with conservative treatment, and more severe ones persisted in having clinical signs. There were two exceptions (successful results when the lesion was large) to this rule.

A case can be made for arthroscopy in all cases, since unsuspected intraarticular pathologic changes are often found, and early management of these problems could be instituted. It has been stated that once a radiographic diagnosis of OCD has been made in humans, arthroscopic staging of the disease and treatment is the next logical step and that conservative treatment by casting, immobilization, and limitations of activities (particularly in children) should be tried initially before resorting to surgery.[18] It is still difficult to predict when a lesion will

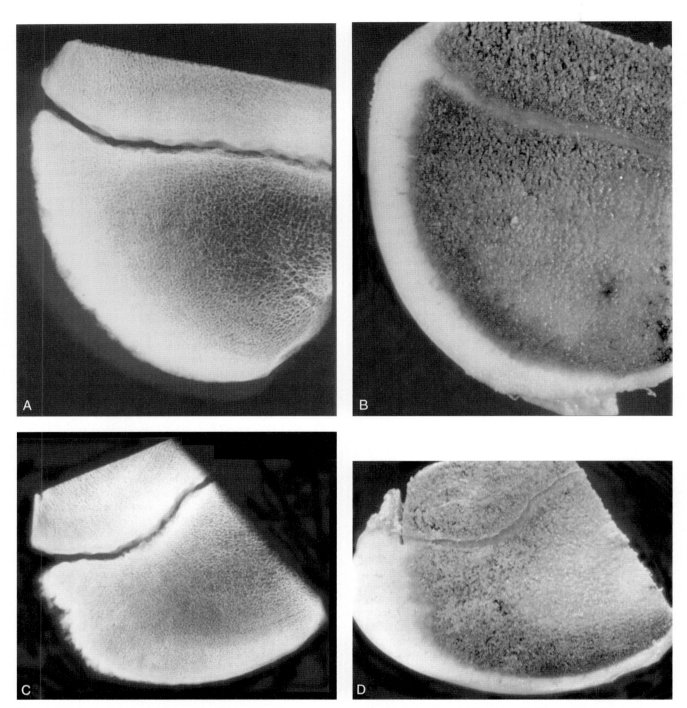

Figure 7.57 Radiographs (A and C) and sagittal sections at postmortem (B and D) of the normal endochondral ossification pattern in a 6-week-old foal. A and B. Lateral trochlear ridge of the femur. C and D. Medial trochlear ridge of the femur. (Reprinted with permission from McIlwraith CW, Trotter GW, Eds. Joint Disease in the Horse. Philadelphia: WB Saunders, 1996, Fig 22-7.)

heal and when a lesion will persist, particularly if arthroscopy is not done.[18] If conservative treatment is to be attempted, restriction of exercise with confinement is the critical factor. Restricted activity is the basis for the conservative management of human juvenile OCD but is not consistently successful.[2]

The treatment of femoropatellar OCD by using arthroscopic surgery has been extensively described elsewhere.[20,33,35,40] The lesion in the joint is evaluated thoroughly, as not all lesions are detected radiographically, and each lesion is assessed using a probe. Elevators are used to separate OCD flaps. The flaps are generally removed by use of rongeurs, and the underlying lesions are debrided by use of curets, motorized equipment, or both. Loose bodies are also removed. Debridement of all pathologic tissue is necessary.

The results of arthroscopic surgery for the treatment of OCD of the femoropatellar joint have been reported in 252 femoropatellar joints in 161 horses.[20] Follow-up information was obtained on 134 horses, including 79 racehorses and 55 nonracehorses. Eighty-six (64%) of these 134 horses returned to their intended use, 9 (7%) were in training, 21 (16%) were unsuccessful, and 18 (13%) were unsuccessful because of other defined reasons. Of the 18 horses that were unsuccessful because of other reasons, 14 developed unassociated lameness (10 forelimb and 4 hindlimb), 1 died of colic, 1 became a wobbler, 1 developed a fatal case of enteritis, and 1 died under anesthesia during surgery for an unrelated problem in another clinic. The time from surgery until horses started training was dictated in many cases by the age of the horse. Horses that had already performed or trained before surgery returned to training 4 to 6 months after surgery. Sufficient follow-up was available for 11 of the 12 horses that had surgery for OCD in other joints at the time of femoropatellar surgery. Six of these horses (55%) were successful, 3 (27%) were unsuccessful, and 2 (18%) were unsuccessful for other reasons.[20]

There was a significant effect of lesion size on prognosis. Horses with grade 1 lesions (<2 cm in length) had a significantly higher success rate (78%) than horses with grade 2 (2 to 4 cm) or grade 3 (>4 cm) lesions (63% and 54% success rates, respectively).[20] Significantly higher success was also noted for horses operated on at 3 years than for the remainder of the study population. A significantly lower success rate was noted for yearlings than for the remainder of the population. It was felt that the lowest success rate in horses operated on as yearlings probably reflects the fact that more severe lesions occurred in the yearling horses (16% grade 1, 13% grade 2, 46% grade 3) and less severe lesions occurred in the 3-year-old group (52% grade 1, 38% grade 2, 10% grade 3). There was no significant difference in outcome as related to sex of the animal involved, racehorse versus nonracehorse, lesion location, unilateral versus bilateral involvement, presence or absence of patellar or trochlear groove lesions, or presence or absence of loose bodies.

Although the results of this study may at first seem somewhat discouraging in that only 64% of the horses returned to, or achieved, the intended level of performance, note that many of these horses were operated on at relatively young ages and consequently had not yet proven themselves as athletes (over 50% were 1 year of age or younger). A study on racing performance in Thoroughbreds indicated that approximately 60% of all named foals should start a race.[17] The inclusion of only named foals (registered with the Jockey Club) would exclude those that showed no potential or developed other problems at a young age and were consequently not registered. Many of the horses had surgery before they were named, and this led us to believe that a 64% success rate is comparable with successful performance in the normal population of racing Thoroughbreds.[20]

Although a permanent clinical cure can often be associated with surgery, limited data show that the healing tissue differs from normal osteochondral tissue.[35] On the basis of long-term follow-up radiographs of horses operated on by the author that are sound, irregular subchondral contours frequently persist, which suggests that subchondral bone remodeling does not take place in the femoral trochlear ridges. In humans, OCD may affect the trochlear ridges but more commonly affects the femoral condyles.[61] Surgical treatments include the removal of flaps, drilling through the lesion into bone, and fixation of the flap.[2,18,61]

Osteochondritis Dissecans of the Femorotibial Joints

Subchondral cystic lesions are the most common entity of DOD involving the femoral condyles. However, cases of OCD of the femoral condyles have been encountered. Lesions of OCD may accompany subchondral cystic lesions or occur on their own (most commonly in Thoroughbreds). The lesions manifest radiographically as an irregular defect in the subchondral bone, best seen on a flexed lateral view. They appear arthroscopically as typical OCD lesions and have responded to surgical treatment. A series of lesions of the femoral condyle, some of which may be lesions of osteochondrosis, has also been reported recently.[25] Because these cases have been recognized infrequently, figures for prognosis do not exist.

Osteochondritis Dissecans of the Tibiotarsal (Tarsocrural) Joint

OCD of the tarsocrural joint was first described as an entity in the horse in 1972.[16] Before this, however, seven cases of a condition that appears identical to OCD were described by Birkeland and Haakenstad as intracapsular bony fragments of the distal tibia.[10] These authors later described the lesions as OCD.[11] There have been a number of recent reports documenting the incidence, clinical signs, and results of treatment of OCD of the tarsocrural joint.[3,5,13,22,27,28,32,39,58,65]

OCD of the tarsocrural joint is seen most frequently in Standardbred horses.[3,10,11,13,16,22,27,28,39,58,65] In the largest series of clinical cases published to date, 154 of 225 horses were intended for racing (106 Standardbreds, 30 Thoroughbreds, and 18 Quarter Horses), and the remaining 71 included 20 Arabians, 18 Quarter Horses, 13 Warmbloods, 4 American Saddlebreds, 4 Appaloosas, 4 Thoroughbreds, 3 Draft Horses (1 Clydesdale, 1 Percheron, 1 Shire), 2 Paint horses, 1 Morgan, 1 National Show Horse, and 1 Lipizzaner.[39]

CLINICAL SIGNS AND DIAGNOSIS

The presenting clinical signs were synovial effusion of the tarsocrural (tibiotarsal) joint and lameness. Synovial effusion of the joint is the most common reason for cases being presented, particularly in animals being presented prior to being put into training. Of 303 joints with tarsocrural OCD in which the presence or absence of synovial effusion was recorded, synovial effusion was the presenting clinical sign in 261 joints (86.1%).[39] Obvious lameness is often not observed. Older horses (>2 years) or racehorses may be presented for lameness. The degree of

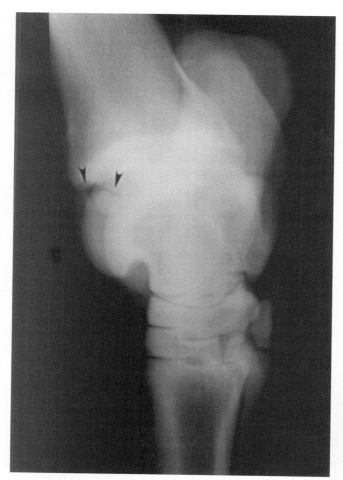

Figure 7.58 Dorsomedial-plantarolateral oblique radiograph showing an OCD fragment(s) of the distal intermediate ridge of the tibia.

lameness was not recorded consistently but was usually designated as mild. The exception was when severe lesions were present on the lateral trochlear ridge of the talus (lesions involving the entire visible portion of the lateral trochlear ridge of the talus when viewed arthroscopically in the flexed position). Racehorses presented most often at 2 years of age, having trained or raced, whereas nonracehorses presented most often as yearlings prior to training.[39] The age range was from yearling or less, up to 14 years. Lesions of OCD of the distal articular surface of the tibia have been reported postmortem in a 3-day-old foal euthanized for neonatal maladjustment syndrome.[55]

The radiographic manifestations depend on the location of the lesions. Based on a series of 318 joints reported, lesions were seen most frequently in the intermediate ridge of the distal tibia, followed by the lateral trochlear ridge of the talus and medial malleolus, respectively. Lesions were also seen in multiple sites in 22 joints, and loose bodies were present in 8 joints. Five of these had separated from intermediate ridge lesions, and 3 had separated from lateral trochlear ridge lesions.[39] The lesions on the distal intermediate ridge of the tibia commonly consist of separation of a bony fragment from

the dorsal aspect of the intermediate ridge and are best demonstrated on the dorsomedial–plantarolateral oblique radiograph (Fig. 7.58). OCD lesions of the intermediate ridge of the tibia have been rated on a scale of 0 to 5, according to the defects and the presence and size of the fragments within them.[27] Most of the author's surgical cases are either grade 4 or grade 5 (some grade 3) using this classification, and Hoppe grade 1 and 2 lesions (defect but no fragment) are rare, at least in cases with clinical signs. Intermediate ridge lesions were classified into three sizes in a separate study to evaluate the possibility of the size of the fragment affecting prognosis. Fragment size did not influence prognosis, and the usefulness of such a grading system is questionable.[39] Lesions on the lateral trochlear ridge are best demonstrated with dorsomedial–plantarolateral oblique radiographs (Fig. 7.59), but loose bodies may be elsewhere. Radiographs may not accurately depict the amount of articular cartilage dissection extending beyond the subchondral bone defect in some lateral trochlear ridge lesions.[39] Lesions of the medial malleolus of the tibia may be demonstrated with a dorsoplantar or dorsolateral–plantaromedial oblique radiograph (Fig. 7.60). These lesions are depicted relatively accurately by radiographs. Lesions of

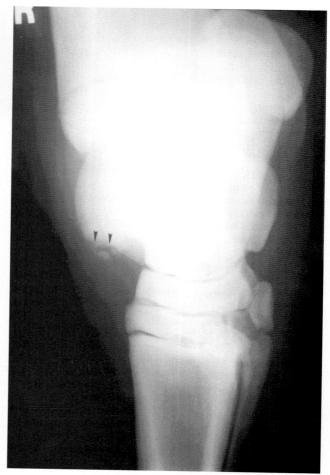

Figure 7.59 Dorsomedial-plantarolateral oblique radiograph demonstrating an OCD lesion at the distal aspect of the lateral trochlear ridge of the talus.

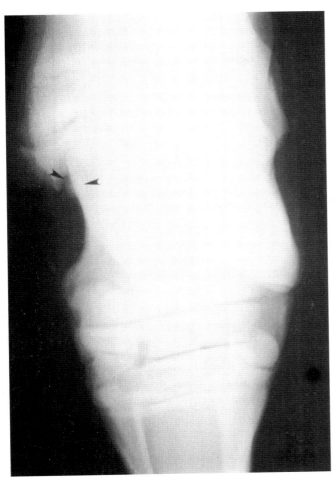

Figure 7.60   Dorsoplantar radiograph demonstrating OCD of the medial malleolus of the tibia.

the trochlear ridge of the talus may be demonstrated with dorsolateral–plantaromedial oblique or lateral–medial radiographs.

A longitudinal study of 77 Standardbred foals that were examined and radiographed six times from birth to the age of 16 months provides information on the timing of the development of radiographic lesions. Eight horses (10.4%) showed lesions of OCD in the tarso-crural joints at the age of 12 months (considered to have permanent OCD). These 8 horses all showed abnormal ossification and/or OCD before 3 months of age, and in 4 of these, the lesions were present before 1 month of age. The authors also recognized abnormal endochon-dral ossification of the subchondral bone at the sites of predilection for hock OCD that reverted to normal in 11 other horses. All of these were radiographically nor-mal after the examination at 7 or 8 months, and there were no other lesions at examination at 16 months.[13] In another study in Norway, radiographs were taken of the tarsocrural joints in 753 Norwegian Standardbred trot-ters, all yearlings. OCD lesions of the intermediate ridge of the distal tibia and/or the lateral trochlear ridge of the talus were diagnosed in 108 (14.3%) horses. The lesional changes were bilateral in 49 (45.4%) affected horses. Radiographs were repeated in 79 horses after 6 to 18

months and revealed OCD in only one additional joint. No clinical evaluation was reported in this latter study.

Lesions may be identified during arthroscopy that were not apparent on radiographs. In one study, OCD lesions were present at arthroscopy in 13 joints without being identified by radiographic examination. In 4 of these cases, there was synovial effusion without radio-graphic change in the joint contralateral to the one with the radiographic lesion (3 on distal intermediate ridge and 1 on medial malleolus).[39] In 9 other cases, the lesions (4 medial malleolus, 3 lateral trochlear ridge, and 2 me-dial trochlear ridge) were found during arthroscopy of a joint with other radiographically apparent lesions. Loose bodies were detected by different radiographic views, de-pending on their location. OCD can frequently be diag-nosed on radiographs when no clinical signs are pres-ent.[3,13,28,58] Distinguishing these cases from ones with clinical signs is important when assessing the need for surgery or the results of conservative treatment.[3,5,13,28,32]

Radiographic changes observable in the tarsus that are not lesions of OCD include spurs or fragments (dew-drop lesions) of the distal end of the medial trochlear ridge of the talus, an irregularly shaped depression (syno-vial fossa) in the central region of the intertrochlear groove of the talus, and some flattening of the medial trochlear ridge centrally, which may be seen particularly in heavy horses.[60] Separated OCD fragments can occa-sionally lodge in the proximal intertarsal joint.

TREATMENT

The need for surgery on individual cases of OCD of the tarsocrural joint is still questioned by some, but the literature supports a surgical approach.[10,16,39,65] Hoppe concluded that horses affected with OCD seemed to have a poorer performance capacity than normal horses, but their performance was improved by surgical treatment.[28] Some of the discrepancy in opinions is based on radio-graphic surveys that lack any clinical data.[3,22]

When clinical signs are present, surgical treatment is preferred, particularly if an athletic career is planned.[39] Arthroscopic surgery is used, and follow-up results sup-port its value.[5,39] Some horses have had full athletic ca-reers despite lesions being present radiographically, and it is presumed that lack of clinical signs is associated with some form of stability between the lesion and parent bone. In contrast, horses often develop problems when in training, and lameness is a factor in many of these cases. Resolution of synovial effusion is also of particular importance to nonracehorse owners. Case selection is important, however. Radiographic changes in the distal tarsal joints (such changes are seen quite often) should be noted when discussing prognosis. As mentioned above, dewdrop lesions or the presence of calcified fragments at the distal end of the medial trochlear ridge of the talus are not indications for surgery, as they are usually extra-articular. If a free OCD fragment is present in the proxi-mal intertarsal joint, then removal is indicated. Lateral malleolus fragments are usually of traumatic origin and are rarely a manifestation of OCD. Arthroscopic surgery techniques have been described elsewhere.[18,39]

PROGNOSIS

In a study in which postsurgical follow-up was ob-tained for 183 horses, 140 (76.5%) raced successfully or performed their intended use after surgery.[39] Of the remaining 43, 11 were considered to still have a tarso-crural joint problem, 19 developed other problems precluding successful performance, 8 were considered poor racehorses without any lameness problems identified, 3 were killed because of septic arthritis, and 2 died from other causes. There was no effect of age, sex, or limb involvement on the outcome. The success rate relative to location of the lesion was 139 of 177 (78.5%) for the distal intermediate ridge of the tibia, 24 of 31 (72.7%) for the lateral trochlear ridge of the talus, 7 of 9 (77.8%) for the medial malleolus of the tibia, 3 of 3 for the medial trochlear ridge of the talus (100%), and 17 of 22 (77.3%) pooled for multiple lesions (no significant differences). The success rate relative to the three size groups for intermediate ridge lesions was 27 of 33 (81.8%) for lesions 1 to 9 mm in width, 86 of 116 (74.1%) for lesions 10 to 19 mm in width, and 41 of 47 (87.2%) for lesions 20 mm or more in width.[39]

When success rate was considered relative to the findings of additional lesions at arthroscopy, 16 of 19 (84.1%) with articular cartilage fibrillation, 5 of 10 (50%) (did not affect prognosis) with articular cartilage degeneration or erosion, 3 of 5 (60%) with loose fragments, 0 of 2 with proliferative synovitis, and 0 of 1 with joint capsule mineralization were successful. There was a significantly poorer outcome in racehorses with articular cartilage degeneration or erosion ($P < .05$).

Follow-up data on the degree of synovial effusion resolution was obtained for 217 joints that had effusion preoperatively. The synovial effusion resolved in 117 of 131 racehorse joints (89.3%) and 64 of 86 nonracehorse joints (74.4%). Of the 22 nonracehorse joints without resolution, the owner calculated that 75% resolution occurred in 12, and 50% resolution had occurred in another four. The resolution of synovial effusion was also documented relative to location of lesion. The outcome for synovial fluid resolution was significantly poorer ($P < .05$) for lesions of the lateral trochlear ridge of the talus or medial malleolus of the tibia than for lesions of the distal intermediate ridge of the tibia.[39]

There was no relationship between postoperative performance and resolution of effusion. In 165 horses in which effusion was resolved, 141 raced or performed successfully (85.4%). Of the 30 horses in which effusion was not resolved, 25 raced or performed successfully (83.3%). Five horses that had OCD in the tarsocrural joint also had proximal plantar lesions of the first phalanx (4 had successful results and 1 was lost to follow-up). Two horses had concurrent lesions of the lateral trochlear ridge of the femur (1 was successful and 1 was lost to follow-up).

Recently, the results of 64 Thoroughbreds and 45 Standardbred horses treated for OCD of the tarsocrural joint with arthroscopic surgery prior to 2 years of age were reported and were compared with those of other foals from the dams of the surgically treated horses (siblings).[5] For the Standardbreds, 22% of those that had surgery raced as 2-year-olds and 43% raced as 3-year-olds, compared with 42 and 50% of the siblings that raced as 2-year-olds and 3-year-olds, respectively. For the Thoroughbreds, 43% of those that had surgery raced as 2-year-olds and 78% raced as 3-year-olds, compared with 48 and 72% of the siblings that raced as 2-year-

olds and 3-year-olds, respectively. The median number of starts for surgically treated horses was lower than the median number of starts for siblings for all groups except 3-year-old Thoroughbreds. Median earnings were lower for affected horses than for siblings for both breeds and both age groups. There was a tendency for horses with multiple lesions to be less likely to start a race than horses with only a single lesion; however, the difference was significant only for 2-year-old Standardbreds. Affected Standardbreds and Thoroughbreds were less likely to race as 2-year-olds than were their siblings.[3] The authors noted that while the percentage of horses that raced was lower than that previously reported,[5,39] it was inappropriate to compare this study with previous studies because selection criteria and control groups were different and racing performance was not analyzed by year in previous studies. The authors stated that they currently recommended removal of any osteochondral fragment associated with joint effusion but warned owners that affected foals may already have or may develop other orthopedic conditions that could limit their performance. In another study, horses treated for osteochondrosis of the cranial intermediate ridge of the tibia performed as well as matched controls.[32]

Osteochondritis Dissecans of the Metacarpophalangeal and Metatarsophalangeal Joints

There is some divergence of opinion as to what is considered OCD within the fetlock and also those entities that might be considered appropriate to include within DOD.[4,19,23,38,41,70] The following conditions should be addressed:

1. *OCD of the dorsal aspect of the distal metacarpus and metatarsus.* It is undisputed that this is a manifestation of OCD.[36,41,70] The condition was initially described as OCD of the sagittal ridge of the third metacarpal and metatarsal bones,[41] but the term was modified after recognition that the disease process commonly extends onto the condyles of the metacarpus and metatarsus.[70] In one radiographic study, OCD changes in the dorsal aspect of the sagittal ridge of the third metacarpus or metatarsus were seen in 118 of 753 yearling Standardbred trotters with 61 forelimbs and 147 hindlimbs affected.[23] In a second study, in which cases were evaluated and treated on the basis of clinical signs, the problem was assessed in 65 horses.[70] These lesions usually involve the proximal aspect of the distal dorsal metacarpus or metatarsus. In some instances the most distal aspect of the metacarpus or metatarsus is involved. When this is the case, the lesion is within the metacarpophalangeal or metatarsophalangeal articulation.[36]

2. *Proximal palmar/plantar first phalanx fragments.* Bony fragments associated with the palmar or plantar part of the metacarpophalangeal and metatarsophalangeal joints were first described in 1972 by Birkeland.[9] Opinions differ as to whether these fragments are the results of fractures[9,12,52] or osteochon-

drosis.[19,46,56] Because follow-up radiographic examination showed that such fragments seldom develop in horses beyond 1 year of age, this condition is considered a manifestation of DOD.[13,23] More recent studies suggest that although these fragments do indeed show up in young horses, they are the results of a traumatic avulsion associated with the short distal sesamoid ligament.[14] Lameness caused by the bony fragments has been reported to be evident only at the horse's maximal performance,[4,19,35] and some fragments at this site do not cause lameness.[4,26,58] In one radiographic study, these fragments were observed in the palmar–plantar aspect of the metacarpophalangeal and metatarsophalangeal joints in 89 (11.8%) of 753 yearling trotters.[23] Fragments were recorded in 7 forelimbs and 86 hindlimbs, and bilateral occurrence was observed in the hindlimbs of 11 horses. Eleven of 77 foals developed palmar–plantar fragments in another study.[13]

3. *Proximodorsal first phalanx fragments.* These fragments, at least in racehorses, have long been considered to be traumatic in origin and to cause lameness.[36,69] One group of authors has proposed that these fractures in Thoroughbred racehorses are manifestations of osteochondrosis,[31] but this is not generally accepted, at least in Thoroughbreds. However, dorsal bony fragments in the metacarpophalangeal and metatarsophalangeal joints were diagnosed in 36 (4.8%) of 753 yearling Standardbred trotters in a radiographic survey;[23] 11 horses had two affected joints, and 1 horse had three affected joints. The condition was seen in 35 forelimbs and 14 hindlimbs. The author also considered these to be manifestations of DOD.[23] Similar fragments may be found in Warmblood horses as well, and some of these fragments could be osteochondrosis related. Most clinical conditions, however, are considered to be traumatic in origin and are not discussed further here.

The fourth condition that has been labeled OCD is the condition that was initially described as OCD of the palmar metacarpus.[29] This condition is now generally accepted to be a traumatic entity and not a syndrome of osteochondrosis.[53] It also is not considered further here.

Osteochondritis Dissecans of the Dorsal Aspect of the Distal Metacarpus and Metatarsus

INCIDENCE, CLINICAL SIGNS, AND DIAGNOSIS

Figures on incidence of this condition are given in the section above. Synovial effusion is usually the first indication of a problem (Fig. 7.60). The degree of associated lameness will vary, but flexion of the fetlock will usually provoke lameness.[41,70] Confirmation of OCD is made by radiography. If OCD is diagnosed in one fetlock, the other three are radiographed, because clinically silent lesions are commonly found. Although there may be no synovial effusion in these latter joints and lameness is inapparent, a positive response is often induced with flexion.

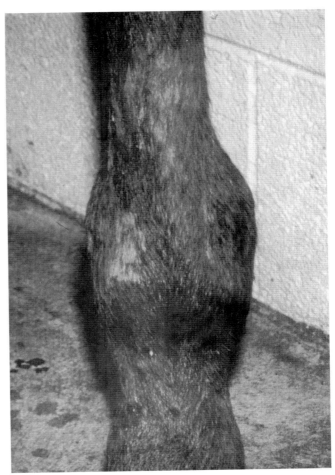

Figure 7.61 Synovial effusion in a left hind fetlock that has OCD of the distal dorsal aspect of the metacarpus.

For purposes of treatment decision and prognosis, the lesions have been divided into three types: type I includes those with a defect or flattening as the only visible radiographic lesion (Fig. 7.61), type II includes those in which a defect or flattening with fragmentation is associated with the defect (Fig. 7.62), and type III includes those that have a defect or flattening, with or without fragmentation, plus one or more loose bodies (Fig. 7.63). Oblique radiographs should be taken as well as dorsopalmar (plantar) and lateral radiographs to discern involvement of the medial or lateral condyles of the distal metacarpus or metatarsus.[41]

TREATMENT

When this condition was first reported, there were eight cases in the series.[70] Two cases of type II OCD were euthanized, four cases of type I OCD were treated conservatively, one case of type II OCD was treated conservatively, and one case of type II OCD was operated arthroscopically. Based on these small numbers, a working hypothesis was made that if the defects were without fragmentation (type I lesion), conservative treatment would generally be successful. In contrast, it was hypothesized that defects with fragmentation needed surgery.

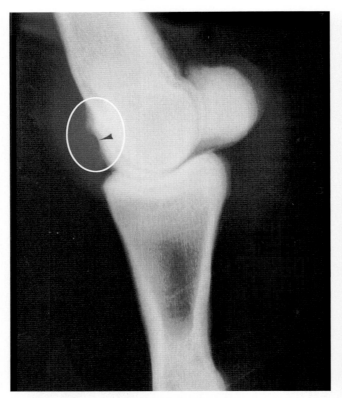

Figure 7.62 Type I OCD of distal dorsal metatarsus. It is anticipated that this lesion would have healed with conservative treatment.

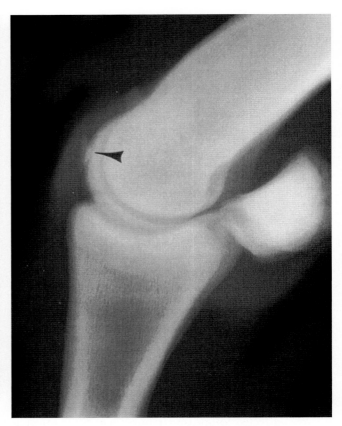

Figure 7.63 Type II OCD of distal dorsal metacarpus with obvious fragment contained within defect.

This hypothesis became our current recommendations for treatment on the basis of follow-up data.[41]

Of 15 horses with type I lesions that were treated conservatively, 12 resolved clinically, and 8 of these showed remodeling of the lesions with improvement on radiographic examination.[41] In 3 horses, the clinical signs persisted. In 2 of these, the radiographs showed no change, and the horses eventually underwent surgery. In the other case, the clinical and radiographic signs progressed, but the horse was not operated on. In 8 cases of type II lesions for which owners requested conservative management, 2 eventually underwent surgery because of the persistence of clinical signs. Clinical signs persisted in 5 other horses, but surgery was not performed. The clinical signs improved in only 1 horse. In most of these cases in which clinical signs persisted, the fragmentation also progressed radiographically or, at least, did not resolve (Fig. 7.20). This study also showed that clinical signs of effusion may appear before definitive radiographic changes. Some type I lesions progressed. Such cases do not develop osseous fragmentation, but the lesions progressed to larger defects, particularly on the condyles (seen on oblique view radiographs). A few cases of type II lesions improved radiographically. These were generally cases with small fragments, and the fragment fused in place, resulting in a bony protuberance at this location.[41] In the above group of conservatively managed horses, most horses were foals from 1988. At that time, the horses on the farm were followed radiographically without any particular management change. In 1989, creep feed was discontinued for foals in which any swelling developed, and this was successful in reducing problems. During 1990, the energy intake was routinely restricted, with an apparent decrease in problems.[41]

Surgery is usually recommended for type II or type III lesions. Most of the cases in a series of 42 horses operated on with arthroscopic surgery and previously reported were type II or type III lesions. Some type I lesions were operated on if they had not responded to conservative management. In other instances, type I lesions were operated on in individual joints if a type II or type III lesion was present in another fetlock joint in the same horse. This was before our retrospective data with conservative cases revealed that type I lesions did not usually require surgical treatment. The technique for arthroscopic surgery for the treatment of this condition has been described elsewhere.[35] The series of 42 horses previously reported included 20 Thoroughbreds, 8 Quarter Horses, 7 Arabians, 4 Warmbloods, 1 Standardbred, 1 Percheron, and 1 Appaloosa. There were 18 fillies, 15 colts, and 9 geldings. The forelimbs were involved in 10 horses, the hindlimbs were involved in 15, and both the forelimbs and hindlimbs were involved in 17 horses. One fetlock was operated on in 10 horses, two fetlocks in 17, three fetlocks in 1, and four fetlocks in 14 horses. In 48 joints, the proximal 2 cm of the sagittal ridge were involved, whereas in 11 joints the lesions extended distad for more than 2 cm. In 14 joints, the lesions involved the lateral or medial condyles of the metacarpus or metatarsus, with or without lesions of the sagittal ridge.[41]

PROGNOSIS

Of the 42 horses operated on, follow-up was obtained in 28. Eight cases were convalescing, and in 6 cases follow-up was unavailable. Surgery was successful in 16 cases (57.1%), and 12 cases were unsuccessful (42.8%). Of the 12 unsuccessful cases, 7 horses were considered to still have a problem in the fetlock (25%), 3 cases were unsuccessful because of other reasons, 1 case was unsuccessful for unidentified reasons but was considered to be normal in the fetlock joint, and 1 horse died. The success rate was found to be related to certain other factors. There was a trend for the success rate to be higher for surgery in hindlimbs than in forelimbs ($P = .09$). The lack of statistical significance in some instances is probably related to low overall numbers. In the forelimbs, only 2 cases were successful, whereas 6 were unsuccessful. In the hindlimbs, 7 cases were successful, and 3 were unsuccessful. When both fore- and hindlimbs were involved, there were 7 successes and 3 failures. Type III lesions had 4 successes and 4 failures; type II lesions had 10 successes and 4 failures. The difference, however, was not statistically significant ($P = .25$). There was no statistical difference between proximal or distal lesions. In contrast, there were statistical differences in the success rate depending on whether there was articular cartilage erosion or wear lines on the articular surfaces. Only 3 of 12 cases with erosions or wear lines were successful, whereas 13 of 16 with no erosions were successful ($P = .0029$). There was also a significantly inferior result when a defect was visible on the condyle on oblique radiographs. When a defect was visible, 6 of 13 were successful; if a defect was not visible, 10 of 15 were successful ($P = .0274$). Osteophytes were also negative prognostic indicators. Three of 9 with osteophytes present on the first phalanx were successful, whereas 13 of 19 with no osteophytes were successful ($P = .1792$).

It was concluded that surgical management of type II and type III lesions will allow athletic activity in most cases, but clinical signs will persist in 25%. Whether surgery will be successful or not is affected by the extent of the lesions as evident arthroscopically (and in some instances radiographically) as well as the presence of osteophytes and of erosion and wear lines.

Proximal Palmar–Plantar First Phalanx Fragments

INCIDENCE, CLINICAL SIGNS, AND DIAGNOSIS

Two types of fragments have been described: 1) type I osteochondral fragments of the palmar–plantar aspect of the first phalanx,[4,19] also called bony fragments of the palmar–plantar part of the metacarpophalangeal and metatarsophalangeal joints,[23] and 2) type II osteochondral fragments of the palmar–plantar aspect of the fetlock joint,[19] also called ununited proximoplantar tuberosity,[24] or united plantar eminence[13] of the proximal phalanx. As discussed above, these fragments have been found frequently on radiographs of yearling trotters.[23]

Type I fragments usually occur in the hind fetlock joints, and the consistent complaint is that the horse has a hindlimb problem that occurred at the upper level of the horse's performance ability and prevented it from competing successfully. Metatarsophalangeal joint distension is uncommon.[4,19] There may be a response to flexion tests, and intraarticular anesthesia will usually eliminate the existing lameness or response to flexion. Fragments are best demonstrated on lateromedial oblique and dorsal 20° proximal 75° lateral–plantarodistomedial views. Dorsoplantar radiographs may also demonstrate the fragments. In one series of clinical cases, the fragments were most commonly seen medially.

Lameness may develop in association with type II fragments but is uncommon. These fragments are easily recognized on conventional oblique radiographs (see page 527).[24]

In a longitudinal study of 77 Standardbred foals examined and radiographed six times from birth to the age of 16 months, 11 foals (14.3%) showed either palmar/plantar fragments (or bony defects greater than 5 mm at the site of attachment of the short sesamoid ligaments to the proximal phalanx) or ununited palmar/plantar eminences of the proximal phalanx. At four or more examinations from birth to 16 months, some were considered to have permanent lesions. All 11 foals had the lesions identified before the age of 5 months, and 6 before the age of 3 months. In 7 horses, early radiographic changes reverted to a normal appearance before the age of 8 months.[13] The extraarticular osteochondral fragments or ununited proximal plantar eminences cannot be considered permanent until after the age of 1 to 2 years, because these fragments may unite to the proximal eminence of the proximal phalanx after 2 years of age, but in such cases early signs of unification are seen after 12 months of age.

TREATMENT

If type I osteochondral fragments are incidental findings at radiography, treatment is not usually indicated. To be considered a surgical candidate, the patient must have demonstrable lameness referable to the fetlock in addition to a radiographically demonstrable lesion. In these cases, arthroscopic surgery is an effective method of treatment.[19,35] In one series of 19 horses, 10 were treated with arthrotomy, and all returned to full use. Seven horses were treated intraarticularly with corticosteroids and only 1 horse was able to return to full use.[19] Successful results have been obtained more recently with arthroscopic surgery.[19,21,35] In 55 of 87 (63%) racehorses and in 100% of 9 nonracehorses, performance returned to preoperative levels after surgery. Standardbred racehorses constituted 109 of the 119 (92%) horses. At surgery, evidence of full-thickness cartilage fibrillation was noticed in nine metatarsophalangeal joints but was not found in any metacarpophalangeal joints. Synovial proliferation in the area of, and immediately adjacent to, the fragment was recorded in an additional four metatarsophalangeal joints. A significant ($P < .0001$) association between abnormal surgical findings and unsuccessful outcome was found with 10 of 32 (31%) unsuccessful horses with evidence of articular cartilage loss or synovial proliferation. Only 1 of 55 (2%) successful horses had synovial proliferation evident at surgery, and none had evidence of articular cartilage damage.[49] All osteochondral fragments removed in this study were type I fragments.

With type II osteochondral fragments (or ununited proximoplantar tuberosity of the proximal phalanx), surgery is rarely indicated. Ununited proximoplantar tuberosity (UPT) was seen in 18 (2.4%) of 753 Standardbred yearlings radiographically in one report.[24] All fragments were in the pelvic limb. The condition was seen laterally in 16 horses, while one horse had a medial and lateral tuberosity affected, and another only one medial tuberosity. Lameness was not observed in any horse prior to first examination. On follow-up examination, 12 UPTs in 11 horses had united to the proximal phalanx after 6 to 12 months. One horse was unchanged at 7 months, and the remaining 4 had radiographic worsening of the condition, with the UPT being more dislocated. Three of these 4 horses also had calcification of the distal sesamoid ligaments and periosteal proliferation. Two of the horses with the most severe radiographic changes developed lameness and subsequently underwent surgery to remove the fragment. This gives an incidence of clinically significant disease for UPT in 2 of 16 horses diagnosed and followed (12.5%). In 11 of 18 horses, type I osteochondral fragments of the plantar part of the metacarpophalangeal joint were seen together with UPT in the same pelvic limb. Occurrence of the latter condition may be an indication for surgery. A common etiologic factor could explain the incidence of simultaneous occurrence of these two conditions. It has been proposed that clinical signs in conjunction with a UPT may be caused by tension on the distal sesamoid ligaments with training. Wear and tear of the attachment of these ligaments could possibly stimulate dislocation of the fragment, ligamentous calcification, or periosteal proliferation, and the author therefore recommended restricting training of horses with radiographic evidence of the disease.[24] The author also recommended that owners of these horses have them radiographed regularly (every 4 months) and consider surgery if radiographic or clinical evidence indicates progression of the condition.[24] Such cases are unusual.

Osteochondritis Dissecans of the Scapulohumeral Joint

OCD of the shoulder is the most severely debilitating form of OCD seen in the horse. It is, however, less common than the entities discussed above. Primary lesions of OCD occur on the glenoid as well as the humeral head, and the disease often affects a major part of the joint surfaces. Severe, diffuse OCD lesions as well as single or multiple cystic lesions may occur in the glenoid. Secondary DJD was recorded in 35 of 54 cases.[49] OCD of the shoulder is less common than that of the femoropatellar, tarsocrural, or fetlock joints. A series of 54 cases has been reported.[49] In a series of 58 joints in 48 horses operated by the author, there were 19 Quarter Horses, 14 Thoroughbreds, 6 Crossbreds, 3 Arabians, 3 Warmbloods, 2 Morgans, and 1 American Paint horse. The problem was unilateral in 38 horses and bilateral in 10 (Howard RD, McIlwraith CW, unpublished data). The humeral head was involved in 12 cases, the glenoid in 11,

and both the humeral head and glenoid were involved in the 26 other joints that had arthroscopic surgery.

CLINICAL SIGNS AND DIAGNOSIS

Most cases of OCD of the shoulder present as yearlings or younger (it has been reported at 3 months) and manifest with a history of intermittent forelimb lameness of insidious onset. The forelimb lameness often exhibits a swinging component, with reduced limb protraction common. It is also common to see muscle atrophy over the shoulder, and pain may be demonstrated using direct pressure over the joint or by pulling the leg upward and craniad, caudad, or into an adducted position. Stumbling may result from inadequate foot clearance and the shortened anterior phase of stride. A small foot with a long heel and club-footed appearance often develops on the affected limb because of the altered gait. Synovial effusion cannot usually be detected because of the muscles and tendons overlying the scapulohumeral joint. The presentation of a horse 1 year old or younger for forelimb lameness, with chronicity evidenced by a smaller foot and with muscle atrophy over the shoulder, is considered by us to be sufficient reason to take standing radiographs of the shoulder.

The problem may be localized to the shoulder using intraarticular analgesia. This diagnostic aid is important, as the condition can often only be diagnosed definitively by taking radiographs under general anesthesia. A 3-inch, 18-gauge spinal needle is used for intraarticular analgesia of the shoulder. The needle is inserted cranial to the infraspinatus tendon at the level of the greater tuberosity of the humerus. The needle is inserted slightly caudad and ventrad (see Chapter 3 for more information). Mepivacaine or lidocaine (20 mL) is injected. A 100% response to the block is not necessary to consider the test result positive. It is relatively common for an OCD lesion in the shoulder to show intact cartilage at the surface and a dissection plane with subchondral cavitation beneath when evaluated arthroscopically. A dramatic response to local analgesia cannot be expected in such cases.

When OCD involves the humeral head, the most common radiographic change is flattening or indentation of the caudal aspect of the humeral head (Fig. 7.64). Lesions in the glenoid manifest as either diffuse areas of subchondral lucency or as cystic lesions (usually multiple). Subchondral bone irregularities are a significant sign in either the humeral head or the glenoid. Lesions may occur in both locations in the same joint. Osteophyte formation (caudal humeral head) is reasonably common, and subchondral sclerosis may also be seen. Cystic lesions in the glenoid have been seen as solitary lesions. Free bony fragments are rare.

TREATMENT

Conservative nonsurgical treatment of osteochondrosis of the shoulder has not been successful for athletic performance.[43,49,57] Animals have been treated successfully with arthrotomy.[15,34,48,59] Extensive soft tissue dissection is necessary, however, and the craniomedial aspect of the joint may not be visualized.[59] The development of arthroscopic surgery techniques has provided advantages over arthrotomy in both avoiding these complications and providing additional benefits, partic-

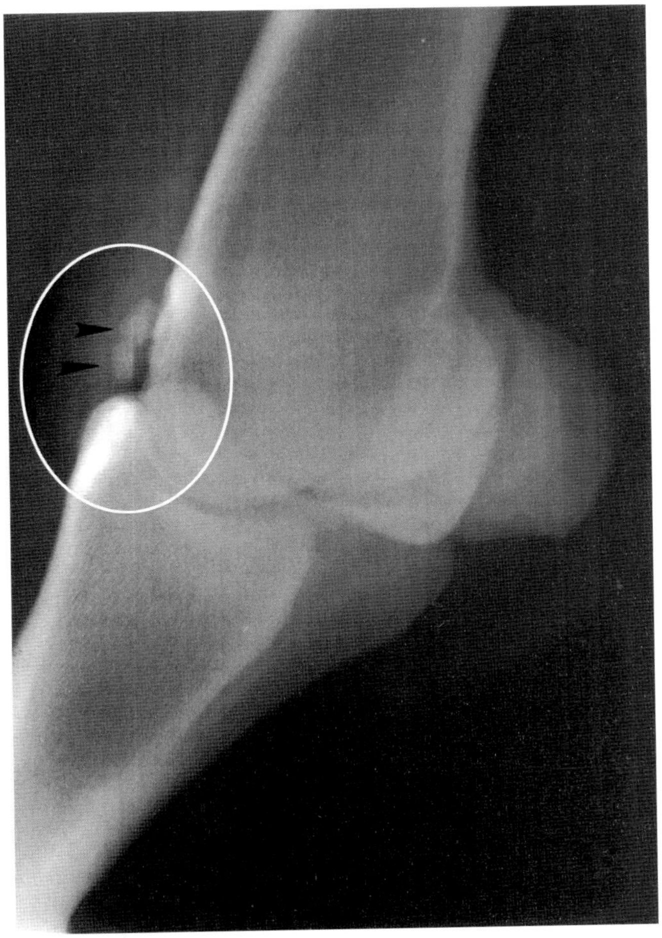

Figure 7.64   Type III OCD with two loose fragments visible on this oblique radiograph of the fetlock.

ularly improved visualization of the whole joint and a lack of surgical morbidity[6-8,35,47]; however, the arthroscopic technique is not easy, and it becomes extremely difficult in an adult horse.

Because of the generalized pathologic changes present in many instances, surgical cases should be selected carefully. However, surgery will benefit some horses, even when secondary degenerative changes are present.[7] Although the ability of the young equine joint to heal after curettage of major defects is impressive, we still lack sufficient numbers to give realistic percentages. With very severe cases, a poor prognosis is offered, and surgery is not recommended.

At arthroscopic surgery the lesions are usually more extensive than could be surmised from the radiographs.[7] In most instances, the cartilaginous changes extend beyond the limits of the subchondral bone abnormalities observed on radiographs, particularly in the glenoid. In some horses in which a lesion is limited radiographically to the glenoid or the humeral head, additional lesions are found arthroscopically on the opposing articular surface. The most common arthroscopic abnormalities of the humeral head are cartilage discoloration with undermining or erosion down to subchondral bone on the caudal aspect of the articular surface. In some instances, a lesion

is not visible initially, and probing is required to ascertain the area of undermined cartilage. The most common arthroscopic abnormality in the glenoid is cracked and undermined articular cartilage with fissure formation and fibrillation. An additional common finding is defective, friable subchondral bone, and these lesions may extend quite deeply (however, young horses have subchondral bone of a softer consistency, and it is sometimes difficult to differentiate pathologic from nonpathologic bone). Problems with arthroscopic surgery in the shoulder include difficulty with arthroscopic placement, difficulty establishing triangulation with the instrument portal, extravasation of fluids, difficulty in reaching potential lesions, and damage to instruments.[7,47]

PROGNOSIS

The results of arthroscopic surgery for OCD and subchondral cystic lesions of the shoulder were initially described for 13 shoulders in 11 horses.[7] The lameness decreased in all 11 horses after surgery, with 9 of the 11 horses reported as becoming sound, and 2 remaining lame. On long-term follow-up, 5 horses were athletically sound and were being shown, ridden, or raced after 5 to 20 months. A sixth horse was sound when beginning race training. A seventh horse was pasture sound and was to begin race training in several months at the time of the report. An eighth horse showed well in halter for 12 months, but shoulder lameness returned; this horse was donated and necropsy was performed. The ninth, tenth, and eleventh horse remained lame. Complications included the development of subchondral cystlike lesions and signs of DJD. Follow-up radiographic assessment of 6 of the 9 sound horses revealed improvement in the contour of the humeral head and joint space and more even density of the humeral epiphysis and glenoid of the scapula in 6 horses. One of these horses showed marked improvement in subchondral bone density and the surface contour of the glenoid cavity. In 2 of the remaining 5 horses, the caudal border of the glenoid cavity had remodeled to appear more like the contralateral joint. In the fourth of the 6 sound horses, radiographs obtained 1 year later showed a subchondral cystic lesion in the bone adjacent to the scapula that had definitely not been present previously, but the horse was still sound and remained so. The contour of the glenoid articular surface on its caudal border was smoother postoperatively, the subchondral osteosclerosis was reduced in thickness, and the horse was athletically sound. In the fifth horse in this group, an osteophyte on the humerus had enlarged, but definite improvement was noted in the joint contour of both the humeral head and glenoid cavity. Radiographs obtained from 1 of the 2 horses that improved but was still lame showed no improvement in the glenoid lesion. In the horse that deteriorated clinically in which euthanasia was chosen, the humeral epiphysis was severely deformed, with a defect in the articular surface contour, a subchondral cystic lesion, and a small intraarticular fracture of the cranial margin of the glenoid cavity.

A larger, long-term follow-up study has recently been completed. Of 48 horses operated on by the author, complete follow-up was obtained in 35. Sixteen had successful outcomes (45.7%) and 19 had unsuccessful outcomes (54.3%). Five additional horses were in various stages of convalescence or training, and 8 horses were lost to follow-up (Howard RD, McIlwraith CW, unpublished data).

An alternative arthroscopic technique has been reported in 8 normal horses and 2 cases of osteochondrosis.[47]

References

1. Adams WH, Thilsted JP. Radiographic appearance of the equine stifle from birth to six months. Vet Radiol 1985;26:126–132.
2. Aglietti P, Buzzi R, Bassi PB, Fioriti M. Arthroscopic drilling in juvenile osteochondritis dissecans of the medial femoral condyle. Arthroscopy. J Arthritis Relat Surg 1994;10:286–291.
3. Alvarado AF, Marcoux M, Breton L. The incidence of osteochondrosis on a Standardbred breeding farm in Quebec. Proceedings. 35th Annual Convention of the American Association of Equine Practitioners, Lexington, KY, 1990;293–307.
4. Barclay WP, Foerner JJ, Phillips TN. Lameness attributable to osteochondral fragmentation of the plantar aspect of the proximal phalanx in horses: 19 cases (1981–1985). J Am Vet Med Assoc 1987;191:855–857.
5. Beard WL, Bramlage LR, Schneider RK, Embertson RM. Postoperative racing performance in Standardbreds and Thoroughbreds with osteochondrosis of the tarsocrural joint: 109 cases (1984–1990). J Am Vet Med Assoc 1994;204:1655–1659.
6. Bertone AL, McIlwraith CW. Arthroscopic approaches in intra-articular anatomy of the equine shoulder joint. Vet Surg 1987;116:317–322.
7. Bertone AL, McIlwraith CW, Powers BE, et al. Arthroscopic surgery for the treatment of osteochondrosis in the equine shoulder joint. Vet Surg 1987;16:303–311.
8. Bertone AL, McIlwraith CW. Osteochondrosis of the equine shoulder. Treatment with arthroscopic surgery. Proceedings. 33rd Annual Convention of the American Association of Equine Practitioners, New Orleans, LA, 1987;683–686.
9. Birkeland R. Chip fractures of the first phalanx in the metatarsophalangeal joint of a horse. Acta Radiol 1972;29(Suppl):73–77.
10. Birkeland R, Haakenstad LH. Intracapsular bony fragments of the distal tibia of the horse. J Am Vet Med Assoc 1968;152:1526–1529.
11. Birkeland R, Haakenstad LH. Osteochondritis dissecans. Ii heseledtet hos hust. Kirurgiskog konservativ behandling. Proceedings. 12th Nordic Veterinary Congress, Reykjavik, Iceland, 1974;34.
12. Bukowiecki CF, Bramlage LR, Gabel AA. Palmar/plantar process fractures of the proximal phalanx in 15 horses. Vet Surg 1986;15:383–388.
13. Carlsten J, Sundgren B, Dalin G. Development of osteochondrosis in the tarsocrural joint and osteochondral fragments in the fetlock joints of Standardbred trotters. I. A radiological study. Equine Vet J 1993;(Suppl)16:42–47.
14. Dalin G, Sandgren B, Carlsten J. Plantar osteochondral fragmentation in the fetlock joints of Standardbreds: Results of osteochondrosis or trauma? Equine Vet J Suppl 1993;16:62–65.
15. DeBowes RM, Wagner PC, Grant BD. Surgical approach to the equine scapulohumeral joint through a longitudinal infraspinatus tenotomy. Vet Surg 1982;11:125–128.
16. DeMoor A, Verschooten F, Desmet P, et al. Osteochondritis dissecans of the tibiotarsal joint of the horse. Equine Vet J 1972;4:139–143.
17. Dink D. Advantages of a February foal. Thoroughbred Times 1990;18:28–32.
18. Ewing JW, Voto SJ. Arthroscopic surgical management of osteochondritis dissecans of the knee. J Arthrosc Rel Surg 1988;4:37–44.
19. Foerner JJ, Barclay WP, Phillips TN, et al. Osteochondral fragments of the palmar/plantar aspect of the fetlock joints. Proceedings. 33rd Annual Convention of the American Association of Equine Practitioners, New Orleans, LA, 1987;739–744.
20. Foland JW, McIlwraith CW, Trotter GW. Osteochondritis dissecans of the femoropatellar joint: Results of treatment with arthroscopic surgery. Equine Vet J 1992;24.419–423.
21. Fortier LA, Foerner JJ, Nixon AJ. Arthroscopic removal of axial osteochondral fragments of the plantar/palmar proximal aspect of the proximal phalanx in horses: 119 cases (1988–1992). J Am Vet Med Assoc 1995;206:71–74.
22. Grondahl AM. The incidence of osteochondrosis in the tibiotarsal joint of Norwegian Standardbred trotters. A radiographic study. J Equine Vet Sci 1991;11:272–274.
23. Grondahl AM. The incidence of bony fragments in osteochondrosis in the metacarpo- and metatarsophalangeal joints of Standardbred trotters. A radiographic study. J Equine Vet Sci 1992;12:81–85.
24. Grondahl AM. Incidence and development of ununited proximoplantar tuberosity of the proximal phalanx in Standardbred trotters. Vet Radiol Ultrasound 1992;33:18–21.
25. Hance SR, Schneider RK, Embertson RM, et al. Lesions of the caudal aspect of the femoral condyles in foals: 20 cases (1980–1990). J Am Vet Med Assoc 1993;202:637–646.
26. Hardy J, Marcoux M, Breton L. Prevalence et des fragments articulaires retroubes au boulet chez le chevel Standardbred. Med Vet Quebec 1987;17:57–61.
27. Hoppe F. Radiological investigations of osteochondrosis dissecans in Standardbred Trotters and Swedish Warmblood horses. Equine Vet J 1984;16:425–429.
28. Hoppe F. Osteochondrosis in Swedish horses. A radiological and epidemiological study with special reference to frequency and heredity. PhD dissertation, Swedish College of Agricultural Sciences, Uppsala, Sweden, 1984.
29. Hornof WH, O'Brien TR, Pool RR. Osteochondritis dissecans of the distal metacarpus in the adult racing Thoroughbred horse. Vet Radiol 1981;22:98–106.
30. Deleted in proof.
31. Krook L, Maylin GA. Fractures in Thoroughbred racehorses. Cornell Vet 1988;78:5–47.
32. Laws EG, Richardson DW, Ross MW, et al. Racing performance in Standardbreds following conservative and surgical treatment for tarsocrural osteochondrosis. Equine Vet J 1993;25:199–202.
33. Martin GS, McIlwraith CW. Arthroscopic anatomy of the equine femoropatellar joint and approaches for the treatment of osteochondritis dissecans. Vet Surg 1985;14:99–104.
34. Mason A, McLean AA. Osteochondrosis dissecans of the head of the humerus in two foals. Equine Vet J 1977;9:189–191.
35. McIlwraith CW. Diagnostic and Surgical Arthroscopy in the Horse. 2nd ed. Philadelphia: Lea & Febiger, 1990;113–159.
36. McIlwraith CW. Diseases of joints, tendons, ligaments and related structures. In: Stashak TS, Ed. Adams' Lameness in Horses. 4th ed. Philadelphia: Lea & Febiger, 1987; 339–447.
37. McIlwraith CW. Inferences from referred clinical cases of osteochondritis dissecans. Equine Vet J 1993;16:27–30.
38. McIlwraith CW. What is developmental orthopedic disease, osteochondrosis, osteochondritis, metabolic bone disease? Proceedings. 39th Annual Convention of the American Association of Equine Practitioners, San Antonio, TX, 1993;35–44.
39. McIlwraith CW, Foerner JJ, Davies M. Osteochondritis dissecans of the tarsocrural joint: Results of treatment with arthroscopic surgery. Equine Vet J 1991;23:155–162.
40. McIlwraith CW, Martin GS. Arthroscopic surgery for the treatment of osteochondritis dissecans of the equine femoropatellar joint. Vet Surg 1985;14:105–116.
41. McIlwraith CW, Vorhees M. Management of osteochondritis dissecans of the dorsal aspect of the distal metacarpus and metatarsus. Proceedings. 35th Annual Convention of the American Association of Equine Practitioners, Lexington, KY, 1990;547–550.
42. McIntosh SC, McIlwraith CW. Natural history of femoropatellar osteochondrosis in three crops of Thoroughbreds. Equine Vet J 1993;16:54–61.
43. Meagher DM, Poole RR, O'Brien TR. Osteochondritis dissecans of the shoulder joint in the horse. Proceedings. 19th Annual Convention of the American Association of Equine Practitioners, Atlanta, GA, 1973;19:247–256.
44. Moore JN, McIlwraith CW. Osteochondrosis of the equine stifle. Vet Rec 1977;100:133–136.
45. Nilsson F. Hastens goniter. Sven Vet Tidskr 1947;52:1–14.
46. Nixon AJ. Osteochondrosis and osteochondritis dissecans of the equine fetlock. Comp Cont Educ Pract Vet 1990;12:1463–1475.
47. Nixon AJ. Diagnostic and surgical arthroscopy of the equine shoulder joint. Vet Surg 1987;16:44–52.

48. Nixon AJ, Stashak TS, McIlwraith CW, et al. A muscle-separating approach to the equine shoulder for the treatment of osteochondritis dissecans. Vet Surg 1984;13:247–256.

49. Nyack B, Morgan MB, Poole RR, et al. Osteochondrosis of the shoulder joint of the horse. Cornell Vet 1981;71:149–163.

50. O'Brien TR. Radiology of the equine stifle. Proceedings. 19th Annual Convention of the American Association of Equine Practitioners, Atlanta, GA, 1973;19:271–287.

51. Pascoe JR, Pool RR, Wheat JD, et al. Osteochondral defects of the lateral trochlear ridge of the distal femur of the horse. Clinical, radiographic and pathologic examination and results of surgical treatment. Vet Surg 1984;13:99–110.

52. Pettersson H, Ryden G. Avulsion fractures of the caudoproximal extremity of the first phalanx. Equine Vet J 1982;14:333–335.

53. Pool RR, Meagher DM. Pathologic findings and pathogenesis of racetrack injuries. Vet Clin North Am 1990;6:1–30.

54. Poulos P. Radiologic manifestations of developmental problems. In: McIlwraith CW, ed. AQHA Developmental Orthopedic Disease Symposium. Amarillo, TX: American Quarter Horse Association, 1986;1–2.

55. Rejno S, Stromberg B. Osteochondrosis in the horse. II. Pathology. Acta Radiol Suppl 1978;358:153–178.

56. Roneus B, Carlsten J. Bone fragments in fetlock and hock joints in young Standardbred trotters. Sven Vet Tidskr 1989;41:417–422.

57. Rose JA, Sandee RD, Rose EM. Results of conservative management of osteochondrosis in the horse. Proceedings. 31st Annual Convention of the American Association of Equine Practitioners, Toronto, Canada, 1985;617–626.

58. Sandgren B. Bony fragments in the tarsocrural and metacarpo- and metatarsophalangeal joints in the Standardbred horse—A radiographic study. Equine Vet J 1988;6(Suppl):66–70.

59. Schmidt GR, Dueland R, Vaughan JT. Osteochondrosis dissecans of the equine shoulder joint. Vet Clin North Am (Small Anim Pract) 1975;70:542–547.

60. Shelley J, Dyson S. Interpreting radiographs. V. Radiology of the equine hock. Equine Vet J 1984;16:488–495.

61. Smith JB. Osteochondritis dissecans of the trochlea of the femur. Arthroscopy 1990;6:11–17.

62. Spurlock GH, Gabel AA. Apical fractures of the proximal sesamoid bones in Standardbred horses. J Am Vet Med Assoc 1983;183:76–79.

63. Steenhaut M, Verschooten F, deMoor A. Osteochondritis dissecans of the stifle joint in the horse. Vlaams Dierg Tigdchrift 1982;5:173–191.

64. Steinheimer DN, McIlwraith CW, Park RD, Steyn PF. Comparison of radiographic subchondral bone changes with arthroscopic findings in the equine femoropatellar and femorotibial joints: A retrospective study of 72 joints (50 horses). Vet Radiol 1995;36:478–484.

65. Stromberg C, Rejno S. Osteochondrosis in the horse. I. A clinical and radiological investigation of osteochondritis dissecans of the knee and hock joint. Acta Radiol 1978;358(Suppl);139–152.

66. Trotter GW, McIlwraith CW, Norrdin RW. Comparison of two surgical approaches to the equine femoropatellar joint for the treatment of osteochondritis dissecans. Vet Surg 1983;12:33–40.

67. Wright IM, Pickles AC. Osteochondritis dissecans (OCD) of the femoropatellar joint. Equine Vet Educ 1991;3:86–93.

68. Wyburn RS. A degenerative joint disease in the horse. NZ Vet J 1977;25:321–322, 335.

69. Yovich JV, McIlwraith CW. Arthroscopic surgery for osteochondral fractures of the proximal phalanx of the metacarpophalangeal and metatarsophalangeal (fetlock) joints in horses. J Am Vet Med Assoc 1986;188:273–279.

70. Yovich JV, McIlwraith CW, Stashak TS. Osteochondritis dissecans of the sagittal ridge of the third metacarpal and metatarsal bones in horses. J Am Vet Med Assoc 1985;186:1186–1191.

SPECIFIC DISEASES OF JOINTS: SUBCHONDRAL BONE CYSTS

Subchondral bone cysts and, in particular, their pathogenesis and treatment, still incite considerable controversy. We have not even been able to agree on terminology. Although the lesions were initially described as subchondral bone cysts, other authors describe them as subchondral cystic lesions or osseous cystlike lesions to avoid the implication that they are true cysts. Examined pathologically, this author feels that they do conform to most people's definition of a cyst in that they have a lining.

Their etiology is also multifactorial.[18] They occur in a number of locations. Subchondral bone cysts were first reported as a clinical entity in 1968.[22] In that report there were 12 cases in the phalanges and one in the radial carpal bone. A series was reported in 1982 in the stifle and distal phalanx.[30] A third series of 69 cases with 64 horses was reported in 1970 under a modified name, osseous cystlike lesions.[24] In that series there were 15 instances of cysts in the carpal bones, 10 in the third metacarpal bone, 3 in the radius, 5 in the proximal sesamoid, 6 in the proximal phalanx, 4 in the middle phalanx, 5 in the distal phalanx, 6 in the navicular bone, 12 in the femur, 2 in the tibia, and 3 in the tarsal bones. Since that time, the most common site of clinical cases reported has been the medial condyle of the femur.[7,8,10,12,16,17,27,33]

ETIOLOGY AND PATHOGENESIS

A number of authors[15,28] have proposed that subchondral cystic lesions are manifestations of osteochondrosis, and the author feels that with young horses and particularly in bilateral cases, this is the likely cause. On the other hand, there has been progressive recognition that subchondral bone cysts occur in older horses, and some have been identified with an initial articular defect.[14,34] In an early study by Kold, Hickman, and Melson, a subchondral bone cyst was produced experimentally in a pony by creating a linear cartilaginous defect in a central weight-bearing area of the medial femoral condyle.[11] More recent work in our laboratory did not duplicate this finding but yielded interesting data.[23] A full-thickness linear defect was created in the articular cartilage of the medial femoral condyle in six femorotibial joints in a group of exercised horses, and in all cases, no subchondral bone cysts formed. However, in the same study, concurrent elliptical cartilaginous and subchondral bone defects (5 mm diameter and 3 mm deep) in the medial femoral condyle resulted in the development of cystic lesions in five of six horses. This experimental finding, as well as the anecdotal clinical evidence, lends support to the theory that direct mechanical trauma to the subchondral bone plays a role in the development of subchondral bone cysts.

Some recent work from a collaborative study between our laboratory and a laboratory in Zurich has demonstrated that the fibrous tissue contents of subchondral bone cysts in horses produce PGE_2 as well as the matrix metalloproteinases, collagenase, gelatinase, and stromelysin. Further evidence that these mediators may play an important role in the pathologic bone resorption associated with subchondral bone cysts is provided by the observation that conditioned media of explant cultures of fibrous tissue of subchondral bone cysts and cyst fluid was capable of recruiting osteoclasts and increasing their activity in a bone resorption assay.[31] Such active bone resorption may play a role in the pathogenesis of subchondral bone cysts and also may be significant in the continued enlargement of cystic lesions well after the cessation of endochondral ossification.

As an "intermediate" hypothesis, it has been thought that compressive forces encountered in normal weight-bearing may encourage the formation of subchondral bone cysts by contributing to the deformation of thickened cartilage previously compromised by a disturbance in the endochondral ossification process.[3,11] Associated with this is the observation that subchondral bone cysts tend to occur at the location in a joint that is subjected to maximal weight-bearing during the support phase of the stride.[14,21] Bramlage has also suggested on the basis of the medial femoral condyle being a high-risk site for infarction and blood supply intervention that this may be a means by which disturbed ossification occurs and could explain the incidence of cysts in the medial femoral condyle.[3]

SITES OF OCCURRENCE AND DIAGNOSIS

FEMOROTIBIAL JOINT. Subchondral cystic lesions of the medial condyle of the femur are the most common entity described. They are most common in young horses but have been diagnosed in horses up to 12 years of age. The typical history is lameness (often intermittent), appear-

ing when a young horse undergoes training or is subjected to increased athletic activity, when other causes of hindlimb lameness are eliminated. There may be few visual signs in the femorotibial area. Synovial effusion of the femorotibial joint is very difficult to detect because of the anatomy. However, over 50% of cases manifest with some femoropatellar effusion.[7] This is presumably associated with increased pressure of fluid in the femorotibial joint opening the flaplike communication between the medial femorotibial and femoropatellar joints. The lesion is defined with radiographs, and its clinical significance may be confirmed with a medial femorotibial intraarticular block (Fig. 7.65). Although increased scintigraphic uptake associated with subchondral cystic lesions on preoperative scintigrams has been reported,[26] it is not a consistent diagnostic feature. Two studies have reported lack of increased radionuclide uptake in the presence of cyst enlargement.[23,26]

CARPUS. Lesions occur in both distal radius and carpal bones (Figs. 7.66 and 7.67). These lesions are seen regularly, but they may be clinically insignificant.[4,5] Clinical evidence needs to be proven by local analgesia[4] and response to intraarticular analgesia is not consistent. A specific subcarpal injection and/or local infiltration of analgesic solution is often necessary. An alternative is the use

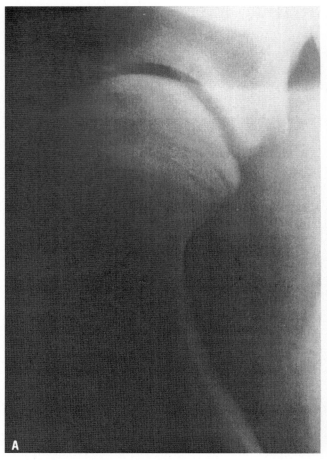
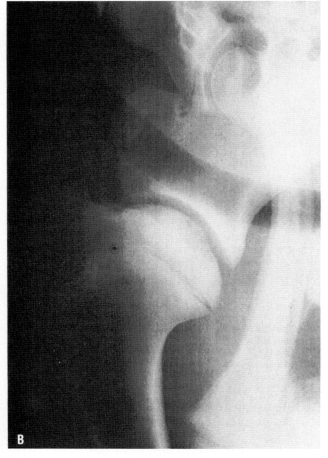

Figure 7.65 Radiograph of osteochondritis dissecans of the shoulder. A. Flattening of caudal aspect of the humeral head and irregularities in the glenoid. B. More concave defect in humeral head.

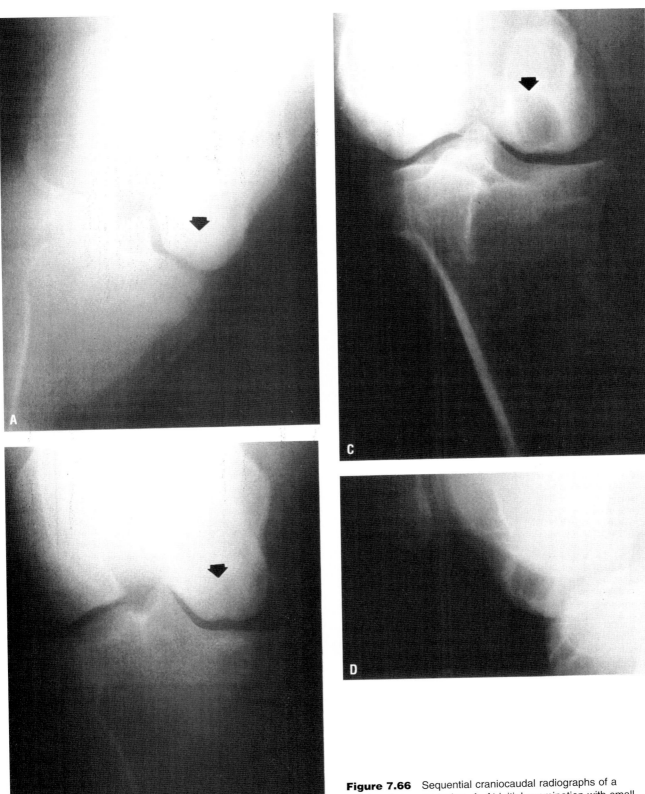

Figure 7.66 Sequential craniocaudal radiographs of a subchondral cystic lesion. A. At initial examination with small defect (arrow). B. Five months later an increased area of lucency (arrow) is present. C. After a further 11 months the lesion is more lucent and increased in area. D. Lateral radiographs of lesion taken at the same time as C.

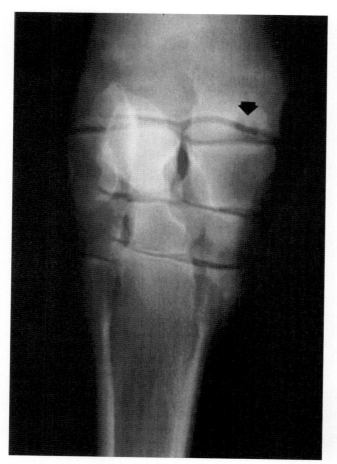

Figure 7.67 Radiograph of subchondral cystic lesion of distal (arrow) radius.

of an ulnar, median, and musculocutaneous nerve block combination to at least localize to the region.

FETLOCK JOINT. Subchondral cystic lesions may occur in the distal metacarpus (metatarsus) or the proximal first phalanx. Subchondral cystic lesions of the third metacarpal bone are the most common and typically involve forelimbs. In a series of 15 cases recently described,[6] cystic lesions most commonly involved the medial condyle of the third metacarpus. They can also occur in the lateral condyle and in the sagittal ridge. Most (10 of 15) of the horses in this study were age 2 years or less at the onset of clinical signs, but 5 horses were more than 6 years of age and had been performing successfully in their respective careers for a number of years without lameness (additional evidence of a nondevelopmental process). Because synovitis is not a consistent feature, localization of lameness to the fetlock may not be obvious. Regional anesthesia can be useful. Radiographs confirm the diagnosis, with dorsopalmar and standing lateromedial views being routine, and for several horses, an elevated 45° dorsopalmar view providing more detail (Fig. 7.68).[6] Fourteen of 15 horses had a history of moderate lameness attributable to the metacarpophalangeal joint, and the lesion was an incidental finding in 1 horse. The duration of lameness ranged from 4 weeks to 8

months, it was either acute in onset or occurred intermittently, and it was associated with exercise. Fetlock flexion significantly exacerbated the lameness in all cases. Synovial effusion was absent in 8 (53%) cases. Although it has been considered that lameness from subchondral cystic lesions can be attributed to acute synovitis occurring from shedding of inflammatory debris from the cystic lesion into the joint,[3] the lack of synovial effusion and the presence of lameness in cases in the fetlock suggests that other mechanisms are involved. The recent demonstration of nociceptive nerve fibers in the subchondral bone plate of the distal metacarpus[21] provides an alternative explanation for the pain. It has also been suggested that there may be an increase in intraosseous pressure within the bone surrounding the cystic cavity and that this is also the reason for the deposition of woven bone (sclerosis) around the periphery of cystic lesions.[3]

PASTERN JOINT. Two separate entities should be considered in the discussion of subchondral cystic lesions of this joint.[19] In both instances, the cystic lesions usually occur on the distal aspects of the first phalanx. The first entity is a single (or multiple with minimally associated OA) lesion. Such lesions occur in young mature horses, and the cases described by Pettersson and Sevelius[22] seem

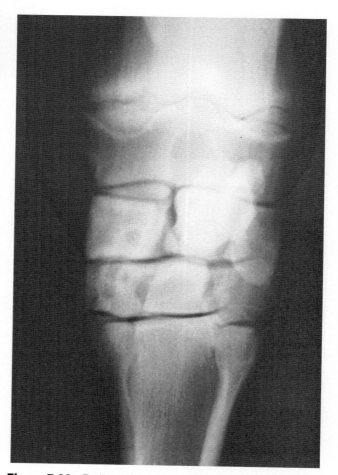

Figure 7.68 Radiograph of subchondral cystic lesions in radial second and third carpal bones.

to fall within this category. The second entity is multiple cystic lesions of the distal first phalanx in association with severe OA that typically occurs in very young animals.[29] These are most commonly observed in Quarter Horses. The severe loss of articular cartilage associated with this entity is particularly unusual compared with other locations where subchondral bone cysts occur.

In each case, diagnosis is often made by recognition of lameness and evidence of swelling in the pastern region. Obvious clinical ringbone is evident when there are multiple cysts with OA. The diagnosis is usually made definitively with radiographs (dorsopalmar and lateral-to-medial views) (Figs. 7.69 and 7.70). In cases with single cysts, localization of the lameness to the pastern by intraarticular or regional infiltration of analgesic solution is appropriate. Subchondral cystic lesions of the proximal aspect of the middle phalanx are sometimes seen as incidental findings on prepurchase radiographs (Fig. 7.71). It is important to ensure that the lesion is indeed the cause of clinical lameness.

COFFIN JOINT. Subchondral cystic lesions of the distal (third) phalanx were reported in the initial series by Pettersson and Sevelius[22] and received closer attention by Verschooten and DeMoor.[30] The problem can be localized clinically with intraarticular anesthesia or distal palmar anesthesia. Communication of the cystic lesion with the joint may be established by observation of plain radiographs or xeroradiographs; alternatively, an arthrogram may be used. Cystic lesions may occur on either the distal aspect of the middle (second) phalanx (less commonly) or the proximal aspect of the distal phalanx (most common).

SHOULDER. Cystic lesions of the glenoid are commonly associated with OCD of the humeral head in young horses. In most instances, they are considered to be a manifestation of osteochondrosis.[2] Cystic lesions can occur as a primary entity on the glenoid alone as well. The presenting clinical sign is forelimb lameness in a horse, usually under 1 year of age. There is commonly some shoulder muscle atrophy as well as a smaller foot on the affected side. The disease is confirmed by radiographs, and confirmation that the radiographic lesions are clinically important can be achieved by a response (partially sufficient) to intraarticular infiltration of local anesthetic solution.

ELBOW. Subchondral cystic lesions occur in the elbow. They most commonly involve the proximomedial aspect of the radius but have been seen occasionally in the distal medial aspect of the humerus.[1] They present as forelimb

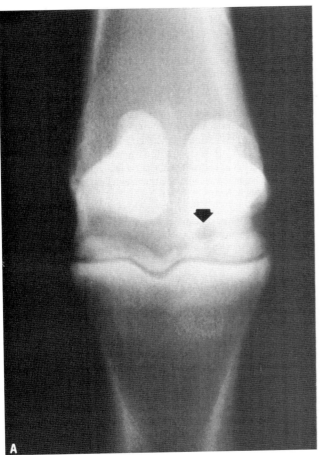 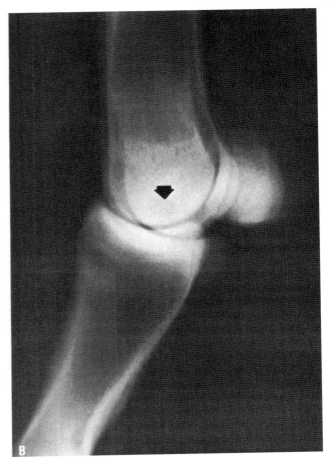

Figure 7.69   Dorsopalmar (A) and lateral (B) views of subchondral cystic lesion (arrows) in the distal extremity of the third metacarpal bone.

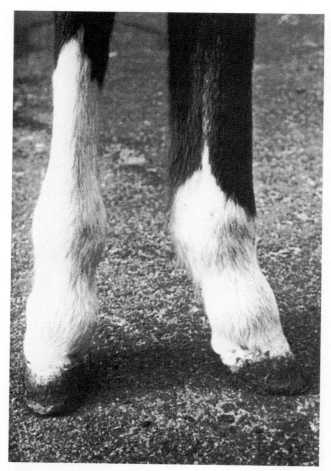

Figure 7.70 Clinical presentation of subchondral cystic lesions of the distal aspect of the proximal phalanx.

lameness, and diagnosis is confirmed by radiographs and (most commonly) elimination of other sites of lameness.

TREATMENT

FEMOROTIBIAL JOINT. The ideal treatment is the subject of debate. Success with conservative treatment (rest and anti-inflammatory agents) has been reported;[8,27] however, older horses had a worse prognosis.[27] In the author's experience, some horses progress to athletic activity (including racing) without surgery, but most have persistent problems. Surgery is recommended, therefore, when athletic soundness is required. The client should be advised that although some horses may recover spontaneously, the prognosis for athletic activity increases from about 20 to 75% after surgery. In terms of evaluating "success," we have found that with conservative treatment, some horses can go on to alternative and less-demanding careers. For instance, we have horses that are bred to race but end up being riding horses with conservative therapy. Success can only be considered truly achieved when the horse has returned to the complete activity that it was undertaking before or for which it is bred and at the same level.

Historically, there have been a number of surgical treatments. From 1975 to 1978, I attempted surgical treatment using an extraarticular approach and packing the defect with cancellous bone graft. None of the initial six cases I treated in this fashion achieved athletic soundness. This was attributed to inadequate curettage at the edge of the cyst and lack of penetration of the sclerotic bone. A similar periarticular approach was described as successful by White and Pradas in 1988.[32] From 1979 to 1989, I used an intraarticular approach with arthrotomy into the medial femorotibial joint between the middle and medial patellar ligaments with the joint flexed.[16] Of 42 horses that did not have evidence of OA prior to surgery, all improved, and 35 were not lame when returned to athletic activity.[33] Of four with osteoarthritic signs prior to surgery, two remained lame and two improved. Surgery is currently recommended for cases that have not responded to at least 3 months of rest. However, a longer delay is not necessarily detrimental; several horses were lame for a year or more before becoming sound after surgery.

Surgery by arthrotomy using cancellous bone graft placed in the curetted cavity has also been reported to provide good results.[9] However, we have found that leaving the cavity empty removed the need for bone graft harvesting and produced similar results.[13] In the arthrotomy study that we did, radiographic changes observed in 14 horses (22 operated lesions) after surgery varied from reduction of the sclerotic bone margin with retention of a lytic cystlike area to partial healing.[33] Nearly complete filling was observed in two lesions. There appeared to be no relationship between the degree of radiographic density postoperatively and eventual soundness.

Since 1989 I have used arthroscopic surgery as described by Lewis[12] to treat these lesions. Excellent visualization of the cystic lesion can be obtained. In a follow-up study using censored analysis we found that our success rate was 70%.[7] In eight horses in this study the cystic lesion increased in size, and this increase in size postsurgery was correlated with the use of subchondral bone drilling. We have since ceased using subchondral bone drilling and have added intralesional injection of 40 mg of MPA (Depo-Medrol) to the regimen. The latter technique was based on some data from the treatment of unicameral bone cysts in humans. I now feel that the use of adjunctive MPA is probably supported by our recent findings of inflammatory mediators in the lining of the cysts. Since we started using corticosteroids at the time of surgery, we have had no cases in which the cyst has increased in size postoperatively.

Concave defects and flattened defects of the femoral condyle have been encountered, and we have treated these in various fashions. Currently we only treat them arthroscopically if they are symptomatic.

CARPUS. I currently recommend surgery for cystic lesions in the carpus if there has been no response to 6 months of conservative treatment and the clinical problem responds to local analgesia. Four cases of distal radial cysts have been reported as responding successfully to conservative management.[25]

FETLOCK JOINT. I have had very poor results with conservative management of cystic lesions of the distal metacarpus and consequently recommend arthroscopic surgery.[17,20] Arthroscopic surgery is somewhat difficult

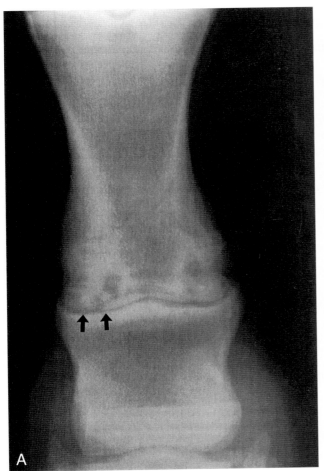

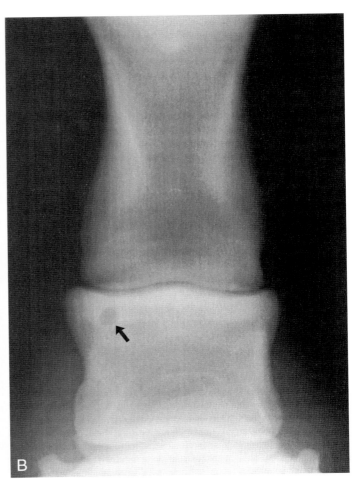

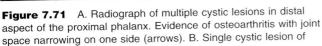

Figure 7.71 A. Radiograph of multiple cystic lesions in distal aspect of the proximal phalanx. Evidence of osteoarthritis with joint space narrowing on one side (arrows). B. Single cystic lesion of proximal aspect of middle phalanx noted as an incidental finding on prepurchase examination.

because of the need for maximum flexion to expose the communication of the cystic lesion with the articular surface of the distal metacarpus or metatarsus. However, it can be done, and this is the routine treatment for our cases now. Recently, the results of surgical treatment in 15 horses have been described.[6] Cystic lesions were curetted arthroscopically in 12 horses and through a dorsal pouch arthrotomy in 3 horses. Concurrent osteostixis of the cystic cavity was performed in 7 horses. Twelve of 15 horses (80%) were sound for intended use after surgical treatment, 2 horses did not regain soundness, and follow-up information was unavailable for 1 horse. Mild periarticular osteophyte formation and enthesiophyte formation of the dorsal joint capsule attachments were present in 5 of 9 horses. Bony ingrowth of the cystic lesion was detectable in 8 horses, and enlargement of the cystic cavity was observed in 1 horse (this horse had also had subchondral bone drilling). Based on this study, it would appear that the surgical treatment of subchondral bone cysts of the distal metacarpus can result in a favorable outcome for athletic use.

PASTERN JOINT. Subchondral cystic lesions in the distal aspect of the first phalanx that are single (or multiple with minimally associated OA) may respond well to conservative treatment and be functionally sound. Ample time is therefore given before treatment is instituted. These lesions tend to occur in young mature horses. In the second entity where there are multiple cystic lesions of the distal first phalanx in association with severe OA in very young animals,[29] the prognosis is poor, and the only treatment is surgical arthrodesis. This has been done successfully.[29]

COFFIN JOINT. There is general agreement that the prognosis with conservative treatment is guarded to poor. The author has not seen a horse achieve athletic soundness following conservative management. However, this statement is made with reference to cystic lesions associated with the coffin joint rather than cystic lesions in the more distal aspect of the distal (third) phalanx, which do not communicate with the joint and represent a different entity in terms of pathogenesis and treatment. The author has used two different approaches with subchondral cystic lesions. In the case illustrated arthroscopically, communication of the cystic lesion with the joint was in the area of the extensor process. We approached the case arthroscopically and debrided the cyst with a burr. On the other hand, other cases require curettage through a created defect in the hoof wall. I still give a guarded prognosis in these cases because insufficient numbers are available and we have experienced some unsuccessful results.

SHOULDER. Cystic lesions in the shoulder do not respond to conservative treatment. The only option for successful treatment is arthroscopic surgery and debridement of the cystic lesion. The prognosis in these instances depends on the amount of cartilage collapse and undermining osteochondrosis.

ELBOW. Although we previously reported that surgical intervention of these cases is preferred to conservative management, more case experience and longer follow-up cause questioning of these initial conclusions.[1] The surgical approach goes through the proximomedial aspect of the radius with enucleation of the cyst. The procedure is somewhat cumbersome because it requires radiologic monitoring. In one case, a comminuted proximal radius fracture was sustained during anesthetic recovery from curetting such a case. At the present time the author prefers at least 3 months of conservative treatment before contemplating surgery.

SUMMARY

Controversy still exists with regard to subchondral bone cysts in the horse, but in the last 10 years we have gathered much useful information on both pathogenesis and treatment. Osteochondrosis is clearly not the only means of acquiring a subchondral bone cyst. We also have good data on the response to surgical treatment of the femorotibial and fetlock joints. We have less extensive data on the treatment in the carpal, pastern, coffin, and elbow joints. Whether cancellous bone graft augments healing is still controversial. At the moment the author feels that the most important principles are enucleation of the cyst and suppression of any ongoing inflammatory reaction that can cause progressive lysis after surgical curettage.

References

1. Bertone AL, McIlwraith CW, Powers BE, Stashak TS. Subchondral osseous cystic lesions of the elbow of horses: Conservative vs surgical management. J Am Vet Med Assoc 1986;189:540–546.
2. Bertone AL, McIlwraith CW, Powers BE. Arthroscopic surgery for the treatment of osteochondritis dissecans in the equine shoulder joint. Vet Surg 1986;16:303–311.
3. Bramlage LR. Osteochondrosis related bone cysts. Proceedings. 39th Annual Meeting of the American Association of Equine Practitioners, San Antonio, TX, 1993;83–85.
4. Ellis DR. Some observations on bone cysts in the carpal bones of young horses. Equine Vet J 1985;17:63–65.
5. Grant BD. The carpus. In: Mansmann RA, McAllister ES, Eds. Equine Medicine and Surgery. Vol. 2. 3rd ed. Santa Barbara, CA: American Veterinary Publications, 1982;1125.
6. Hogan PC, McIlwraith CW, Hollis CM, et al. Surgical treatment of subchondral cystic lesions of the third metacarpal bone: Results in 15 horses (1986–1994). Equine Vet J 1997;29:477–482.
7. Howard RD, McIlwraith CW, Trotter GW. Arthroscopic surgery for subchondral cystic lesions of the medial femoral condyle in horses. 41 cases (1988–1991). J Am Vet Med Assoc 1995;206:842–850.
8. Jeffcott LB, Kold SE. Clinical and radiological aspects of stifle bone cysts in the horse. Equine Vet J 1982;14:40–46.
9. Kold SE, Hickman J. Use of an autogenous cancellous bone graft in the treatment of subchondral bone cysts in the medial femoral condyle of the horse. Equine Vet J 1983;15:312–316.
10. Kold SE, Hickman J. Results of treatment of subchondral bone cysts in the medial condyle of the equine femur with an autogenous cancellous bone graft. Equine Vet J 1984;16:414–418.
11. Kold SE, Hickman J, Melsen F. An experimental study of the healing process of equine chondral and osteochondral defects. Equine Vet J 1986;18:18–24.
12. Lewis RD. A retrospective study of diagnostic and surgical arthroscopy of the equine femorotibial joint. Proc Am Assoc Equine Pract 1987;23:887–893.
13. McIlwraith CW. Diseases of joints, tendons, ligaments and related structures. In: Stashak TS, Ed. Adams' Lameness in Horses. 4th ed. Philadelphia: Lea & Febiger, 1987;396–418.
14. McIlwraith CW. Influences from referred clinical cases of osteochondritis dissecans. Equine Vet J 1993;S16:27–30.
15. McIlwraith CW. Osteochondrosis. In: Stashak TS, Ed. Adams' Lameness in Horses. 4th ed. Philadelphia: Lea & Febiger, 1987;396–410.
16. McIlwraith CW. Subchondral cystic lesions. Vet Clin North Am (Large Anim Pract) 1983;5:350–355.
17. McIlwraith CW. Subchondral cystic lesions in the horse—the indications, methods and results of surgery. Equine Vet Educ 1990;2:75–80.
18. McIlwraith CW. What is developmental orthopedic disease, osteochondrosis, osteochondritis, metabolic bone disease? Proceedings. American Association of Equine Practitioners, San Antonio, TX, 1993;35–44.
19. McIlwraith CW, Goodman NL. Conditions of the interphalangeal joints. Vet Clin North Am (Equine Pract) 1989;5:161–178.
20. Nixon AJ. Osteochondrosis and osteochondritis dissecans of the equine fetlock. Comp Cont Educ Pract Vet 1990;12:1463–1475.
21. Nixon AJ, Cummings JF. Substance P immunohistochemical study of the sensory innervation of normal subchondral bone in the equine metacarpophalangeal joint. Am J Vet Res 1994;55:28–34.
22. Pettersson H, Sevelius F. Subchondral bone cysts in the horse: A clinical study. Equine Vet J 1968;1:75–80.
23. Ray CS, Baxter GM, McIlwraith CW, et al. Development of subchondral cystic lesions following subchondral bone trauma in horses. Equine Vet J 1996;28:225–232.
24. Reid CF. Radiographic diagnosis and appearance of osseous cyst-like lesions in horses previously reported as periarticular subchondral bone cysts. Proceedings. American Association of Equine Practitioners, 1970;16:185–187.
25. Specht TE, Nixon AJ, Colahan PT, Moor BG. Subchondral cyst-like lesions in the distal portion of the radius of four horses. J Am Vet Med Assoc 1988;193:949–952.
26. Squire KRE, Fessler JF, Cantwell HD, Widmer WR. Enlarging bilateral femoral condylar bone cysts without scintigraphic uptake in a yearling foal. Vet Radiol Ultrasound 1992;33:109–113.
27. Stewart B, Reid CF. Osseous cyst-like lesions of the medial femoral condyle in the horse. J Am Vet Med Assoc 1982;180:254–258.
28. Stromberg J. A review of the salient features of osteochondrosis in the horse. Equine Vet J 1979;11:211–214.
29. Trotter GW, McIlwraith CW, Norrdin RW, Turner AS. Degenerative joint disease with osteochondrosis of the proximal interphalangeal joint in young horses. J Am Vet Med Assoc 1982;180:1312–1318.
30. Verschooten F, DeMoor A. Subchondral cystic and related lesions affecting the equine pedal bone and stifle. Equine Vet J 1982;14:47–54.
31. von Rechenberg B, Guenther H, McIlwraith CW, et al. Fibrous tissue of subchondral cystic lesions in horses produces local mediators and neutral metalloproteinases and causes bone resorption in vitro. Vet Surg 2000;29(5):420–429.
32. White KK, Prades M. Grid-assisted periarticular approach to subchondral cysts [abstract]. J Am Vet Med Assoc 1988;192:1762.
33. White KK, McIlwraith CW, Allen D. Curettage of subchondral bone cysts in medial femoral condyles of the horse. Equine Vet J Suppl. 1988;6:120–124.
34. Yovich JV, Stashak TS. Subchondral osseous cyst formation after an intra-articular fracture in a filly. Equine Vet J 1989;21:72–74.

SPECIFIC DISEASES OF JOINTS: INFECTIVE (SEPTIC) ARTHRITIS

The term "infective" arthritis is being used here and is considered the most appropriate.[43] However, "septic" or "infectious" arthritis has achieved common usage by others as well as the author. It has been recently pointed out that infectious is frequently defined as "capable of being spread from one host to another with or without direct contact," and thus equine influenza virus or equine herpesvirus could be regarded as an infectious organism. (May S, personal communication, 1994). "Infective" by usage is more restricted in its definition, and *Churchill's Medical Dictionary* defines it as "capable of causing infection." It is therefore felt that in the case of infective arthritis, bacteria could not be regarded as infectious as it is in the case of respiratory virus, although the bacteria could be regarded as infective because they are capable of causing infection.

Infective arthritis is the most severe problem encountered in the equine joint. It can result in rapid destruction of the articular cartilage, and when septic osteomyelitis is also present, there may be irreversible loss of articular surface at the time of presentation.[53]

Three syndromes of infective arthritis can be identified in the horse: 1) hematogenous, 2) local penetration or traumatic, and 3) iatrogenic (usually associated with intraarticular injection). Hematogenous infective arthritis is most commonly observed in young foals. In past literature the classic organisms causing infective arthritis in foals have been cited as *Actinobacillus* spp., *Streptococcus* spp., and *Salmonella* spp.[56] More recently, *Escherichia coli* and other *Enterobacteriaceae* have emerged as the most common isolates.[11,34] Septic arthritis in foals has been divided into type S (septic arthritis), type E (septic arthritis and osteomyelitis of the epiphysis), type P (septic arthritis and osteomyelitis of the physeal area), and type T (involving central tarsal bone flaps).[19] Osteomyelitis is a common and classical accompaniment to infection of the joint in the foal.[19] The clinical findings in 78 foals affected with septic polyarthritis were presented by Firth and correlated with radiologic and pathologic findings. More than two-thirds of the foals that were necropsied had septic polyosteomyelitis in addition to septic polyarthritis.[19] It is considered that hematogenous seeding of the synovial membrane can be due to either direct lodgment of organisms within the synovial vessels or spread from an adjacent focus of osteomyelitis by means of vascular continuity between the bone and the synovial membrane.[59,64]

Umbilical infection is the classically described origin of the problem, but this should not be considered an exclusive route of infection. The disease may be associated with pneumonia, enteritis, or any other form of systemic infection. Although an affected foal usually has concurrent septicemia, systemic involvement may not be clinically apparent. Frequently a traumatic cause (stepped on or kicked by the mare) is assumed in affected foals.[38] The potentiation of hematogenous infection by local trauma has been reported elsewhere.[59] Hematogenously induced septic arthritis has been reported in older people, and concurrent medical illnesses are observed in most patients.[76] Most patients also show evidence of joint damage prior to the development of septic arthritis.

These authors also cited hematogenous spread in 33 to 86% of patients and evidence of direct injury to the joint in 14 to 71% of patients when they reviewed other studies.[76] Osteomyelitis and infective arthritis have been recognized as a complication of *Rhodococcus equi* infection in foals.[51] In a study of 18 cases of *R. equi* infection, 9 foals (50%) had cutaneous or musculoskeletal abnormalities in addition to the typical clinical signs of respiratory disease in the development of pulmonary abscessation. In two instances there was osteomyelitis of the physis.[51] Intrauterine infection can occur.[38] In many instances, osteomyelitis of the adjacent epiphysis or metaphysis is the primary localizing focus. Other influences may increase the incidence of infective arthritis in foals; a good example is complete or partial failure of passive transfer of immunoglobulins. It has been suggested that decreased acidity in the stomach of the newborn may allow escape of organisms usually destroyed into the lower gastrointestinal tract, and systemic invasion may then occur. In addition, both mycoplasma and chlamydial infections have also been associated with polyarthritis in foals.[40,46]

Bacteria in the bloodstream gain access more readily to synovial fluid than to spinal fluid, aqueous humor, or urine.[15] It has been suggested that the configuration of the capillary tufts in the synovial membrane favor entrapment of organisms.[47] These factors may promote the establishment of infection within the synovial membrane of the foal.

Direct trauma is a common cause of infective arthritis in older animals. Direct penetration of the joint is the usual event but is not essential. Tissue destruction and cellulitis in the region of the joint can lead to an open joint and infective arthritis. The elbow is a good example, where absence of muscular tissue on the lateral aspect of the joint leaves it poorly protected.[17] Various factors may dictate the establishment of infection after such a penetrating wound. Penetrating wounds with subsequent infective arthritis are associated with retained foreign material in people.[58] In a retrospective study of open joint injuries at Colorado State University, 16 horses were euthanized on the day of admission; of the horses treated, 53% that were examined within the first 24 hours developed septic arthritis, and the overall survival was 65%. Ninety-two percent of horses examined within 2 to 7 days of injury developed septic arthritis, with 38.5% surviving. All horses evaluated a week or more after joint injury had septic arthritis, and 50% survived. Horses examined more than 24 hours after injury had a significantly higher chance of developing septic arthritis and thus were significantly less likely to survive the injury.[22] However, the one significant risk factor for establishment of infective arthritis was failure to initiate antibiotic therapy within 24 hours of the penetrating injury. Common organisms involved in septic arthritis due to trauma or a penetrating injury include *Streptococcus* spp., *Staphylococcus* spp., *E. coli*, and anaerobes. With iatrogenic septic arthritis, intraarticular injection or surgical procedures are the inciting cause. *Staphylococcus* spp. are the most likely organisms. In one study in 15 Standardbreds, 86% of the isolates were staphylococci.[33] In a study of 43 children with 45 hip joint infections, concomitant osteomyelitis in the proximal femur produced a worse prognosis than if the infection was confined to the synovium of the hip. In addition, patients whose hips were infected with *Staphylococcus aureus* were more likely to have a poor prognosis than those whose hips were infected with another organism. Almost all children who were treated within 4 days of symptoms had a satisfactory outcome.[2]

EPIDEMIOLOGY

Predisposing conditions have been identified for infective arthritis. Hypogammaglobulinemia, from either genetic defects or failure of passive transfer, is associated with a higher risk of infection with both common and uncommon pathogens in the young.[3] Approximately one-third of children with osteomyelitis or infective arthritis have deficiencies in IgA and IgG. Patients with rheumatoid arthritis have a significantly increased risk of secondary joint infection, and rheumatoid arthritis is associated with approximately 50% of human cases of infective arthritis.[24] Rheumatoid and other immunologic arthritides are rare in the horse, and this association has not been reported. Systemic sepsis is a risk factor for bone or joint infection. Foals with higher sepsis scores have more joint infections.[19] Trauma also predisposes to infection.

The incidence of infection varies for each joint. In one study in horses, the tarsocrural joint was the most commonly affected (34%), followed by the fetlock (20%), carpus (18%), and stifle (9%).[61]

Isolates in the various syndromes of infective arthritis are discussed above. In a study of 233 horses with musculoskeletal infection (including septic arthritis/tenosynovitis or osteomyelitis that developed after fracture repair), *Enterobacteriaceae* (28.8%) were the most common bacterial group isolated, followed by non-beta-hemolytic streptococci (13%), coagulase-positive staphylococci (11%), beta-hemolytic streptococci (9.4%), and coagulase-negative staphylococci (7.3%). The remainder of the organisms were other gram-negatives (15.8%), other gram-positives (2.3%), and miscellaneous (2.6%).[45] With iatrogenic infection, *Staphylococcus* spp. were isolated in 69 and 86% in two studies, respectively.[33,61] Gram-negative organisms were isolated from 92.5% of joint cultures from foals, and *E. coli* was isolated from 27% of foals.[61] Anaerobes were isolated in 10.3% of all equine cases and 26.3% of infections caused by wounds. Figures vary in the percentage of cases having no bacterial growth, but in four studies, the no-growth percentages were 7,[33] 27,[61] 31,[77] and 45%.[37]

PATHOBIOLOGY

Bacterial colonization of the synovial membrane causes an inflammatory reaction and will vary in intensity. However, in general, it represents the most severe form of synovitis we see in the horse. Inflammation may range from mild changes with cellular infiltration to necrosis of the synovial membrane and formation of extensive fibrinopurulent exudation. Thrombosis of the synovial membrane and necrosis and pannus formation results in markedly disturbed function in the joint. Of equal or more significance is the release of various mediators potentially destructive to the articular cartilage. Organisms vary in their aggressiveness and colonization of the synovial membrane. With *S. aureus,* an accessory

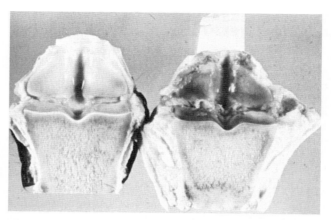

Figure 7.72 Severe loss of articular cartilage in right fetlock joint in a case of infective arthritis that did not respond to treatment.

gene regulator (collagen adhesion gene) influences virulence.[1,54] Organisms with an inactivated copy of the chromosomal collagen adhesion gene produced a 27% infection rate, and those with a functional chromosomal collagen adhesion gene produced a 70% joint infection rate in a murine model of arthritis.[54] On the surface of *S. aureus,* collagen receptors that mediate bacterial adherence to cartilage can be blocked with receptor-specific antibodies.[71]

Articular cartilage degradation can occur rather quickly in many models of joint infection (Fig. 7.72). However, grossly visible articular cartilage degradation is not apparent in most equine infective arthritis models or clinical cases of equine infective arthritis at the time of initial assessment.[61] Collagen loss is a prerequisite for visible cartilage destruction.[16,27] Loss of GAGs and proteoglycans from the matrix precedes this loss of collagen. Within 48 hours of infection, 40% of the GAGs can be lost from the articular cartilage, and by 3 weeks, 50% of the collagen.[67] The staphylococcal proteoglycan-releasing factor has been found in the bacterial growth medium of cartilage cultures.[67] The authors felt that staphylococci or a staphylococcal filtrate could induce rapid proteoglycan loss from viable articular cartilage in a manner analogous to that seen with bacterial life or polysaccharide catabolin and other mediators of cartilage degradation. In an in vitro study evaluating the effect of synovial membrane infection on equine synoviocytes and chondrocytes, IL-1β and IL-6 were significantly increased in synovium explants incubated with *S. aureus* or infected–filtered media (collected from the infected group and filtered). In addition, proteoglycan synthesis and total GAG and chondroitin sulfate concentrations were significantly lower in cartilage from the infected–filtered group. The study emphasized the role of synovium in the pathogenesis of septic arthritis. The concentration of HA was also lower with synovial infection and in normal synoviocytes exposed to conditioned medium and in conditioned synoviocytes released in inflammatory mediators that contributed to articular cartilage degeneration.[25] Factors capable of causing degradation include neutral metalloproteinases, PGE$_2$, free radicals, and cytokines (particularly IL-1). These mediators are discussed above, but joint sepsis induces the highest level of such mediators. In addition to direct enzymatic destruction, it has been suggested that this collagen loss is associated with mechanical wear on vulnerable collagen, and the increased wear that is observed in contact areas of the joint supports this idea.

Other factors such as joint effusion, intraarticular fibrin, and altered cartilage biomechanics contribute to the pathobiology of the infective arthritic process. In a study with children with hip pain, positional severe increases in intraarticular pressure were correlated with pain and the volume of synovial fluid aspirated.[28] Using nuclear scintigraphy, edema of the physis evident in joints with high intraarticular pressure was relieved with joint fluid aspiration.[28] More recently, it was shown that increased intraarticular pressure induced by the intraarticular injection of synovial fluids in horses significantly reduced blood flow to the synovial membrane and fibrous layer of the joint capsule.[26] Such ischemia to articular soft tissues and subchondral bone can further damage the joint.

CLINICAL SIGNS AND DIAGNOSIS

The clinical signs of infective arthritis include severe lameness, swelling, effusion plus thickening and edema, and pain on manipulation (Fig. 7.73). Although there

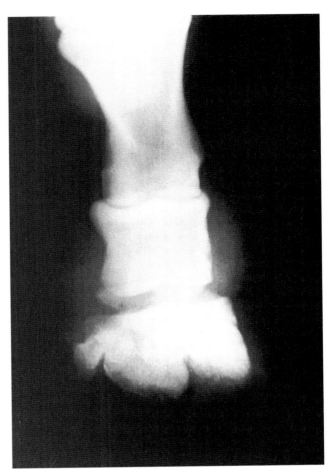

Figure 7.74 Increased joint space in distal interphalangeal joint associated with early infective arthritis.

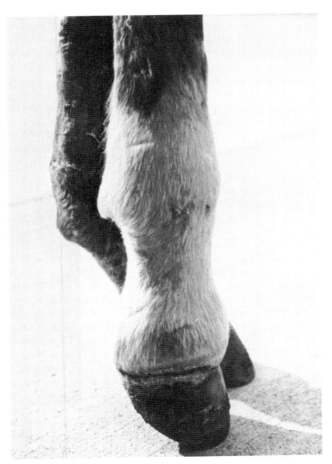

Figure 7.73 Non-weight-bearing lameness and swelling over the coronary band in a case of infective arthritis of the coffin joint.

may be obvious and severe periarticular swelling in some traumatic entities, edema is more typical of sepsis.

Radiographically, osteomyelitis is often identified in foals. For this reason, radiographs should be routinely made. Osteomyelitis has been reported in 50 to 80% of foal cases.[18,19,38] Osteomyelitis is uncommon in adult horses, but fractures associated with trauma may occur, and removal of these fragments may be required to eliminate infection. Joint space narrowing due to loss of cartilage will only be apparent in long-term cases (with the exception of a severe osteoarthritic joint in which infection develops). In retrospective examination of adult horses treated for joint infection, few developed OA. However, in some joints, a sequence is seen of increased joint space early (Fig. 7.74) followed by decreased joint space with development of subchondral lysis and periarticular proliferation (Fig. 7.75).

Synovial fluid analysis is a significant diagnostic aid, often allowing a definitive diagnosis (Fig. 7.76). Changes include gross appearance (cloudy, purulent, sometimes hemorrhagic) (Fig. 7.77), decreased viscosity, and increased white cell count to above 30,000/mm³ (usually 100,000/mm³) with more than 95% neutrophils. The protein generally increases to above 4 g/dL, and the pH is decreased. The sequential clinical and synovial fluid

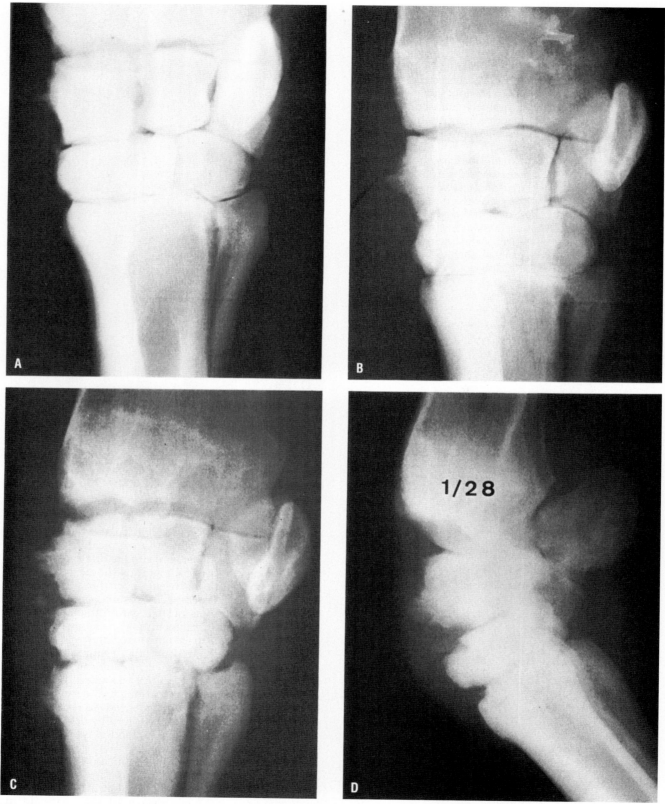

Figure 7.75 Radiographs of carpal joint with septic arthritis, showing a sequence of changes. A. Early periosteal proliferation. B. Loss of midcarpal (intercarpal) joint space with articular cartilage lysis. C and D. Extensive periosteal reaction and irregular widening of joint space in association with subchondral lysis.

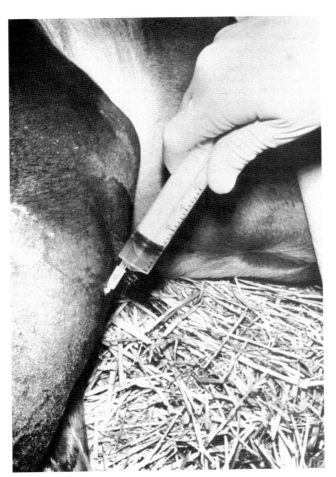

Figure 7.76   Aspiration of turbid synovial fluid in a case of infective arthritis.

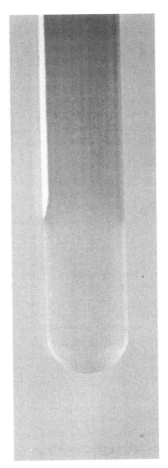

Figure 7.77   Cloudy turbid synovial fluid typical of infective arthritis.

changes associated with acute infective arthritis in the horse were outlined by Tulamo et al.[74] In this study, high, persistent neutrophilia (90% +) was the hallmark sign. Generally, counts of 100,000 cells were seen 12 to 24 hours after induction of septic arthritis. The total protein also rises rapidly, and a drop in pH is a good indicator. In this study, corticosteroids delayed the onset of clinical signs in some horses for up to 3 days (although synovial fluid signs were seen earlier). Another study found that clinical signs may not reach a maximum until 10 days after injection.[23]

Culture of the organism is an important part of the management of septic arthritis. Synovial fluid culture is routine. Synovial membrane biopsies are not done routinely. In a retrospective report of 64 cases of horses with suspected infectious arthritis, positive cultures were obtained from 55% of the joints. Culturing of synovial fluid yielded bacterial growth more often than culturing of synovial membrane, and histologic evaluation (hematoxylin and eosin [H & E] and Gram stain) of synovial membrane biopsy specimens provided little information to help distinguish infected from culture-negative joints.[37] In an experimental study in dogs in which joints were inoculated with *Staphylococcus intermedius*, incubating synovial fluid for 24 hours in blood culture me-

dium was significantly more reliable than synovial membrane biopsy or synovial fluid on aerobic culturette.[44] In the author's hospital, it is considered critical to use a nutrient broth such as brain–heart infusion broth or a blood culture medium. Cultures are in a relatively anaerobic atmosphere (5% CO_2), and we also make use of sodium polyanetholesulfonate (SPS) to prevent coagulation and inhibit aminoglycoside and trimethoprim antibiotics, as well as complement and lysozyme activity. This enhances our success rate of culture, which is approximately 70%. Both anaerobic and aerobic culture methods should be used. Although it has been suggested that the use of synovial membrane biopsy can improve the rate of positive culture, a critical study of this did not reveal such a change.[37] The use of gas liquid chromatography is of potential benefit in obtaining an etiologic diagnosis but has not achieved routine use.

Because the treatment of infective arthritis is an emergency and needs to be started before the results of bacterial culture are available, the clinical signs and synovial fluid analysis report are relied on heavily. Variations from the usual situation will occur. In foals with polyarthritis, the parameters are sometimes less spectacular. In one series the WBC count ranged from 4,122 to 178,000.[75]

Some joint problems associated with streptococcal or corynebacterial infections may be immune-mediated synovitis problems rather than infections.[31] This means that a foal that presents with pneumonia and polyarthritis with less spectacular WBC counts than with a typical septic joint may have an immune-mediated problem. Low-grade infections in joints are a problem for diagnosis. Focal infection of synovial membrane may manifest with very low grade clinical signs, but it is still important because the condition can smolder and eventually cause severe degenerative changes. There also can be a noninfective reactive synovitis in a joint adjacent to an area of infection such as cellulitis. In these instances, diagnosis can be confusing, and joint aspiration runs the risk of introducing infection.

DNA hybridization combined with polymerase chain reaction (PCR) has been considered a hopeful new field for sensitive and early microbial identification.[62] In a recent experimental equine study, PCR was able to detect bacteria in equine synovial fluid within 24 hours of inoculation.[14] MRI is frequently considered the best imaging modality to diagnose and anatomically pinpoint most soft tissue infections, including septic arthritis. Radionuclide imaging is another option. The use of indium-111 WBC imaging in 39 patients for the evaluation of musculoskeletal sepsis (55 images) resulted in 40 negative and 50 positive indium-111 WBC images. These were correlated with operative culture and tissue pathology, aspiration culture, and clinical findings. Thirty-eight of the images were performed to evaluate possible total joint sepsis (8 positive and 30 negative images), and 17 to evaluate non–arthroplasty-related musculoskeletal sepsis (7 positive and 10 negative images). Overall, there were 13 true-positive, 39 true-negative, 2 false-positive, and 1 false-negative image. It was concluded that indium-111 WBC imaging is a sensitive and specific means of evaluating musculoskeletal sepsis, especially following total joint replacement.[50]

TREATMENT

Treatment of infective arthritis is designed to 1) eliminate the causative organism(s) and 2) remove the harmful products of synovial inflammation and fibrin that can damage the articular cartilage.[41] In types E and P septic arthritis in foals, attention must also be paid to treating osteomyelitis.

Potent, broad-spectrum antibiotic regimens should be used before culture results are available. Systemic antibiotic therapy is always practiced. Penicillin/gentamicin in combination, cephalosporins, amikacin, and trimethoprim–sulfa combinations are the most commonly used. New data provide evidence indicating that allowing antimicrobial concentrations to decrease below the minimal

inhibitory concentration (MIC) will cause the bacterial population to become more susceptible to the antimicrobial drug, and the traditional approach of maintaining antimicrobial drug concentrations above the bacteria's MIC for the duration of the interval has been questioned.[12] This has led to less frequent administration of drugs such as gentamicin.

Selection of antibiotics in the initial stage should be based on the clinician's knowledge of the most likely pathogen in his or her clinical practice and the likely sensitivity. Synovial fluid culture at the time of initial presentation, however, is still an important part of the treatment. When culture and sensitivity results are known, the antibiotic regimen often changes. Continued culturing of a sensitive organism after 3 weeks of systemic antibiotic administration has been noted in horses, and systemic administration of antibiotics should be continued for an appropriate time.[8] It was also noted in a study with trimethoprim (5 mg/kg)/sulfadiazine (25 mg/kg) combination that twice-daily administration was necessary to maintain an adequate MIC in an experimentally induced septic arthritis model using *S. aureus*.[5] The author examined the antibiotic sensitivity of equine isolates at Colorado State University over a period of 2 years (Table 7.2).[42]

Based on retrospective examination of these isolates at Colorado State University, it was concluded that sodium ampicillin, for instance, is not a good drug for use in equine septic arthritis cases. Different bacterial isolates and susceptibility patterns will be recognized in other institutions. As mentioned above, a study at Florida in neonates revealed that the predominant organisms now are gram negatives (*Klebsiella* spp., *E. coli*, *Salmonella* spp.), and amikacin–penicillin is the preferred initial treatment for such organisms.

In another major study in which bacterial culture and susceptibility results were analyzed from 233 horses with septic arthritis/tenosynovitis or osteomyelitis that developed after fracture repair, 424 bacterial types were isolated; 386 were aerobic or facultative, and 38 were anaerobic. *Enterobacteriaceae* (28.8%) were most commonly isolated, followed by non–beta-hemolytic streptococci (13%), coagulase-positive staphylococci (11.8%), beta-hemolytic streptococci (9.4%), and coagulase-negative staphylococci (7.3%). The remainder of the organisms were other gram-negative (15.8%), other gram-positive (2.3%), and miscellaneous (2.6%) bacteria.

Penicillin and ampicillin were highly effective against beta-hemolytic streptococci but were ineffective against other bacteria. Ampicillin was no more effective than penicillin against most bacteria. Amikacin was the most effective antibiotic against the wide range of bacteria iso-

Table 7.2 PERCENTAGE OF ISOLATES SUSCEPTIBLE TO AN ANTIDOTE[42]

	Penicillin	Ampicillin	Cephalothin	Gentamicin	TMS
Streptococcus spp.	99	99	100	72	97
Salmonella spp.	0	83	100	100	100
Actinobacillus spp.	87	87	100	100	100
Escherichia coli	0	64	94	100	83
Staphylococcus spp.	27	27	100	100	100

lated in the study (highly effective against coagulase-positive staphylococci, *Enterobacteriaceae*, and *Pseudomonas* spp. and also effective against coagulase-negative staphylococci and *Actinobacillus* spp.). Gentamicin was not highly effective against any bacterial group but was effective against coagulase-positive and -negative staphylococci and *Pseudomonas, Salmonella*, and *Actinobacillus* spp. Cephalothin was highly effective against beta-hemolytic streptococci, coagulase-positive staphylococci, and *Actinobacillus* spp., as well as coagulase-negative staphylococci. It is therefore highly useful in iatrogenic infections. Trimethoprim–sulfonamides were highly effective against *Actinobacillus* spp. and were effective against coagulase-positive staphylococci, beta-hemolytic streptococci, non-beta-hemolytic streptococci, and *Rhodococcus equi*.

The authors pointed out that because of the narrow spectrum of activity of trimethoprim–sulfonamides against the common pathogenic organisms, these drugs should be used only after culture and susceptibility results are known. This is most commonly done in clinical practice. If we have a sensitive organism, the animal is discharged on oral trimethoprim–sulfonamides. Chloramphenicol was effective against a wide range of organisms, but human health hazard precludes its general recommendation. These authors felt that the combination of a cephalosporin and amikacin provided the best coverage against the bacteria isolated in this study. These factors need to be weighed against the risk of antibiotic pressure causing major resistance, and as emphasized above, these sensitivity patterns do not necessarily reflect sensitivity patterns in other places where there has been less antibiotic pressure.

In a study of the effect of induced synovial inflammation on pharmacokinetics and synovial concentrations of sodium ampicillin and kanamycin sulfate after systemic administration in ponies, it was found that antibiotics entered the synovial fluid of the inflamed joints more quickly and attained higher concentrations than in fluid of uninflamed joints.[20]

Antimicrobial concentrations that exceed the in vitro MIC for an isolate do not ensure antimicrobial effectiveness, because the higher bacterial concentrations that often are present in vivo can markedly decrease antibacterial effectiveness (the inoculum effect), and protein binding may lower the concentration of active drug. Recognition of the inoculum effect provides some rationale for the use of intraarticular antibiotics. It was demonstrated relatively recently that a single IA injection of gentamicin is more effective in sterilizing a joint than systemic gentamicin. Joints were experimentally inoculated with *E. coli* and (with clinical signs present at 24 hours) subjected to the following treatment regimens:

1. A single IA injection of 150 mg of gentamicin
2. Systemic administration of 2.2 mg/kg IV four times
3. IA, buffered (150 mg) Gentocin, (3 mg) sodium bicarbonate

In these three groups, the percentage of positive isolates 24 hours after the commencement of treatment was 0%, 80%, and 66%, respectively.[35] Results of a related study showed that the mean apparent half-life of gentamicin in the synovial fluid after IA administration (259 minutes) was 2.8 times longer than that in the plasma after IV administration (92 minutes). Also, the mean synovial fluid concentration of gentamicin remained well above the minimal concentration of gentamicin for many common equine bacterial pathogens for 24 hours after IA administration of gentamicin in any combination. The peak mean synovial fluid concentration after IA administration of unbuffered gentamicin was significantly higher than that after IV administration and significantly lower than that after simultaneous IV and IA administration (1.828, 2.53, and 5.720 µg/mL, respectively).[36] Other work has shown that previous concerns about the acidity of aminoglycosides causing chemical synovitis are unwarranted, particularly considering the value of IA administration.[69] The use of intraarticular antibiotics as a supplement to systemic antibiotics is considered appropriate.

The penetration of antibiotics into equine bone (normal or pathologic) is still poorly understood.[49] Bone necrosis is the crux of the therapeutic problem in the treatment of osteomyelitis, and debridement is necessary. The use of regional antibiotic perfusion has also been explored recently. The antibiotic is delivered under pressure into an infected area via the venous system, and the technique would seem applicable to osteomyelitis and/or infective arthritis.[80] The antibiotic reaches chronically infected tissue by diffusion from the surrounding vascular tissue. Successful use has been documented with both clinical and experimentally induced septic arthritis.[80] Guidelines for the number of perfusions and numbers with results have yet to be established.

In addition to antibiotic therapy, some method of drainage of an infected joint is important for a number of reasons. The presence of a purulent effusion retards the action of many antibiotics by decreasing the metabolic rate of the bacteria.[48] In addition, pH values drop in septic effusions, and the activity of aminoglycosides is reduced significantly with a decrease in pH. The major indication for joint drainage is removal of substances deleterious to the articular cartilage. There are various opinions on the best methods of treatment and the relative urgency of using them in both humans and horses. There is certainly general agreement that the earlier the problem is treated, the better the results. Some authors are quite conservative, and one proposed that aspiration was therapeutic and arthrotomy was often unnecessary in treating acute septic arthritis in children. As early as 1956, papers advocated more aggressive treatment by routine arthrotomy.[82] In a paper published in 1983 on septic arthritis of the wrist in 28 patients (29 wrists) who were treated with early surgical drainage, parenteral antibiotics, and early motion after surgical decompression (*S. aureus* was the most commonly cultured organism), the authors noted that of the 10 wrists with a good or excellent result, all had had the arthrotomy within 10 hours after diagnosis and of the 13 with a fair or poor result, surgery had been delayed for 16 hours or longer. The authors also maintained that the long-term results deteriorated in direct proportion to increasing time until treatment and the number of procedures performed.[57] At this time the author started using arthrotomy in equine septic cases. Another author discussing pyarthrosis of the knee recognized that several different methods of treatment could be used. However, based on a retrospective study of septic arthritis of the knee in which multiple needle arthrocentesis was contrasted with formal arthrotomy drainage, the patients with a history of septic arthritis longer than 3 days and those with *S. aureus* or enteric gram-negative organisms on culture benefited from open drainage procedures in lieu of repeated aspiration.[32] Other authors have reported good results with a closed irrigation–suction system. However, if such a system is used, there must be a flow-reversal system using a double tube that prevents obstruction of the tube. In this series of 154 patients with acute and chronic bone and joint infections treated with closed irrigation, in 172 closed irrigation–suction procedures 86% of the patients were treated successfully.[30]

More recently, an arthroscopic management protocol was recommended and reported to be successful. In 1986, 30 cases of septic arthritis of the knee treated by arthroscopic decompression and lavage coupled with parenteral and oral antibiotics were reported. Twenty-two cases were considered to have a hematogenous origin and eight were caused by penetrating trauma. Excellent results were obtained in 28 (93.3%) of 30 patients, and good results were obtained in 2 (6.7%) of 30 patients. Twenty-eight of these patients had the onset of symptoms within 72 hours prior to arthroscopy. There were no poor results or recurrences, and no cases of osteomyelitis occurred. The average hospital stay was 3.5 days, and it was felt that this method of treatment markedly reduced the morbidity and hospital stay of patients with a septic knee.[65] Arthroscopic cleaning and debridement were "performed as indicated." There was little detail on this. Another multicenter study involving 46 cases of septic arthritis of the knee treated by arthroscopic drainage was reported in 1989. There were 11 cases of hematogenous arthritis, 15 secondary to puncture and infiltration, and 20 postoperative cases. There was a 63% positive culture rate. After thorough articular lavage (average, 7 L) and prolonged antibiotic therapy (average, 2 months), there were 36 bacteriologic cures (78.3%), 5 failures (10.9%) due to persistent articular sepsis, and 5 recurrences of the infection (2.9%) after an initial remission. There were 5 secondary flareups, and 4 of these recovered after repeat arthroscopy and 1 after synoviocentesis.[72] A third study was published in 1990.[52] These authors described the joint being thoroughly irrigated with saline solution to eliminate as much debris as possible; after this, the arthroscope was used to perform a complete joint assessment. When fibrinous debris, necrotic synovium, loose cartilage fragments, or loculated pockets of adhesions were present, the high-speed motorized shaver was used to debride the involved compartments. No synovectomy was performed. Synovial plica present superiorly, medially, or inferiorly were cut and excised because they can hide pockets of infection. Drainage catheters were inserted at the end of the joint through inferomedial and inferolateral portals. One of the plastic drains was connected to a continuous irrigation saline solution and the other to a suction apparatus. Five to 6 L of normal saline were used daily. No antibiotics were used in the solution. Most patients were seen 2 to 5 days after the onset of symptoms. After the initial culture and sensitivity results were obtained and broad-spectrum antibiotics were administered, all patients were taken to the operating room on an emergency basis. At an average follow-up evaluation of 36 months (range, 14 to 48 months), the results

were excellent to good, without evidence of recurrence. The authors suggested that when more reported series are available, arthroscopic techniques will be universally accepted as the most reasonable alternative to repeated needle aspirations or arthrotomy in the management of septic arthritis in accessible joints. They felt that there was enough evidence, both clinical and experimental, and suggested that a successful outcome depends primarily on rapid and aggressive institution of the change in methods of management. The initial use of antibiotics, particularly in children not treated by primary decompression, has been advocated by others.[63] However, there needs to be obvious response within 36 hours, and if little or no improvement occurs, surgical decompression is indicated.

Although not reflected in the arthroscopic papers, synovectomy was recommended as a treatment in earlier times.[73] However, the authors found that synovectomy was useful in the knee but not in the hip. Methods of joint drainage used in the horse include through-and-through lavage, arthrotomy, arthroscopic surgery, and drain implantation.

In an attempt to compare the use of antibiotics alone with the use of lavage and arthrotomy in the horse, we performed a controlled study with an experimentally induced equine septic arthritis model using *S. aureus*.[8] Using a randomized block design, 12 joints were treated by through-and-through lavage on days 1 and 3 or days 1, 3, and 6. In a fourth group, an arthrotomy was performed on day 1, and subsequent lavage was performed via an indwelling drain every 12 hours for 4 days. All groups were treated with systemic antibiotics (the control group with systemic antibiotics alone). Joint drainage by either lavage or arthrotomy did not affect the bacterial isolation rate. Articular cartilage specimens from joints treated with antibiotics alone had less safranin O staining in the articular cartilage than those from other treatment groups. Arthrotomy with lavage resulted in less synovitis and less fibrin formation than treatment by through-and-through lavage performed one to three times. There was no significant difference between the one, two, or three times lavage-treatment groups. Delayed healing, fibrosis, and excessive granulation tissue complicated healing of all arthrotomy incisions, but this was the only effective way of eliminating fibrin from the joint, at least in this experiment.[8] For humane reasons, we never had a control group without antibiotics. Work in rabbits demonstrates that there is extremely rapid loss of GAG and collagen and that early antibiotic (prophylactic) treatment prevents the loss of GAGs and collagen. There was felt to be less protection against loss of GAG however.[68]

In related work with our equine model, we demonstrated that there was no significant difference between using lavage with a balanced electrolyte solution and lavage with 0.1% povidone iodine.[7] In another study, three concentrations of povidone iodine (0.1, 0.2, and 0.5% weight/volume) and one concentration of chlorhexidine (0.5% weight/volume) were tested.[9] The control was again balanced electrolyte solution. The 0.5% povidone iodine and 0.5% chlorhexidine solutions produced severe lameness, soreness to joint palpation, and limb enlargement. Histologic evaluation confirmed the presence of moderate-to-severe neutrophilic synovitis in these treatment groups. We therefore felt that it was inappropriate to use 0.5% povidone iodine or 0.5% chlorhexidine.[8] More recently, the use of 0.05% chlorhexidine lavage was reported in the tarsocrural joint.[81] Even with this low concentration, there was synovial ulceration, inflammation, and abundant fibrin accumulation, and the authors did not recommend using this as a lavage solution.[81]

It was suggested more recently that delayed closure (tertiary closure) of the arthrotomy incision obviates complications.[62] In this report, 26 horses were treated by open drainage with small (3 cm) arthrotomy. All horses had lavage, and 24 left the hospital (infection was eliminated in 25). The arthrotomy healed by granulation in 16 cases and was sutured in 9. Twenty-three horses were treated also with intraarticular antibiotics. Partial synovectomy may also be performed through an arthrotomy. One author talks of using a Sims uterine curet to remove synovial membrane.

As expected, arthroscopic surgery has been used more recently to treat infective arthritis in the horse as in humans.[10] Removal of fibrin as well as synovectomy can be performed. In an effort to clarify the relative success of arthroscopy and partial synovectomy versus arthrotomy, an experimental study was done using the *S. aureus* model with evaluation at 14 days.[4] It was shown that arthrotomy eliminated joint infection earlier, with less lameness and decreased joint circumference. On the other hand, there was more joint contamination (ascending infection) with arthrotomy. The synovectomy in this study was done with rongeurs, and a more effective means of synovectomy using motorized arthroscopic equipment could be expected to make a difference here.[4] The use of arthroscopic technique certainly has advantages in that it allows superior evaluation of the joint and avoids the morbidity of arthrotomy. I feel it is possible to remove fibrin in a manner comparable to arthrotomy, and I now do arthroscopy on all infected joints but still often leave a small arthrotomy hole and implant a drain for flushing.

The use of closed suction drainage in 13 cases of tarsocrural septic arthritis has also been reported. Eleven of the 13 clinical cases also had arthroscopic lavage and debridement.[60] A flat, fenestrated (Jackson-Pratt) drain was used. The drains were removed on the basis of synovial fluid characteristics at 5 to 26 days. Although ingress lavage was also done in some cases, the authors do not recommend it because *Pseudomonas* superinfection developed in one horse in association with the use of an ingress catheter. The authors noted that although arthroscopy was not necessary, it facilitated fibrin removal, lavage, and partial synovectomy.[60] The installation of continuous tube irrigation in the septic knee at the time of arthroscopy has also been described for the treatment of septic arthritis in humans.[21] Four irrigation catheters are placed through stab wounds, and the portals are each closed with a single stitch to prevent leakage of the system. An average of 4 L of normal saline and antibiotic solution is used to lavage the joint. The authors recommended large-bore catheters (6.2 mm) to ensure a patient-durable system. The implantation of four tubes in the joint allows preservation of the irrigation circuit if some of the drains become obstructed and require withdrawal prior to planned discontinuation of the system during the week after surgery. Each joint is perfused after surgery with an average of 60 mL of antibiotic solution per hour. Inflow and outflow of the closed-circuit system are carefully monitored.

New systems are being developed to maintain intraarticular concentrations of antibiotics. Alternatives have been developed to obviate the need for daily intraarticular injections of antibiotics. Polymethyl methacrylate beads impregnated with antimicrobials have been used for many years in orthopedic surgery. However, the beads are nonabsorbable and removal is necessary to avoid the risk of damage to the joint. Different bioabsorbable polymers have become available. A study was recently described in horses that used two biodegradable drug-delivery systems for elution of gentamicin and elimination of synovial membrane infection. The antibiotic-impregnated biodegradable drug-delivery system released more than 500 μg/mL of active gentamicin for 10 days. Both antibiotic-impregnated biodegradable delivery systems eliminated infection within 24 hours. Although this was an in vitro system, the authors also concluded that there were no adverse effects on synovial viability or synovial HA production.[13] Regional perfusion with antibiotics has also been used.[78,79]

ADJUNCTIVE MEDICAL TREATMENT

Adjunctive treatment should include the use of NSAIDs (usually phenylbutazone). In an experimental study of staphylococcal septic arthritis in a rabbit model 3 weeks after infection, the combined treatment with anti-inflammatory drug naproxen sodium and antibiotics reduced the loss of GAG and collagen from the cartilage of the infected knee by 15 and 30%, respectively, compared with antibiotic treatment alone. Continuing treatment with naproxen sodium for 7 weeks reduced the loss of collagen by 50% compared with antibiotic treatment alone. A longer period of treatment with naproxen sodium showed little further effect on the loss of GAG than was observed after 3 weeks. Treatment with this drug and antibiotics reduced swelling of the knee and levels of PGE$_2$ in the synovial fluid and supports the hypothesis that decreasing postinfectious inflammation by adding a NSAID to the standard antibiotic regimen reduces cartilage damage from staphylococcal septic arthritis.[66] Recent studies have shown a beneficial effect of postoperative intraarticular use of sodium hyaluronate (Sullins KE, unpublished data, 1991). Sequential synovial fluid analyses should be done to monitor progression of treatment.

Other general postoperative care consists of close physical monitoring, continued systemic antibiotic administration, repeated synovial cultures, and aseptic cleaning and bandaging of incisions and arthrocentesis portals. During the early phases of inflammation, joint rest is indicated to minimize joint injury and decrease pain. In the horse, this usually means intermittent active motion such as that afforded by stall rest. Passive range-of-motion exercise may be initiated in the early stage and might help regain soft tissue flexibility that is lost through immobilization and fibrosis of the joint capsule and also minimize synovial adhesions. Corticosteroids are a potent anti-inflammatory agent and there is some experimental work to justify their use.[83] The effect of adding intraarticular corticosteroids to systemic antibiotics in experimental septic arthritis was examined in rabbits infected with *Staphylococcus epidermidis*. At 15 days, the group treated with systemic antibiotics and intraarticular corticosteroids had significantly lower scores in joint sections than the group treated with antibiotics alone, because of less damage expressed in clustering of chondrocytes, pannus formation, proteoglycan depletion, and synovitis.[83] The authors concluded that the addition of local corticosteroids to systemic antibiotics in septic arthritis seems to be harmless and improves joint histologic–histochemical parameters in the experimental setting.[83] This author considers this a rather dangerous practice on the basis of earlier experimental work of ours in an experimental model of septic arthritis induced by *S. aureus* in the horse, which showed that despite clinical resolution after 3 weeks, many joints still cultured positive for the organism. The study in rabbits only went to 15 days.[83]

Other substances and procedures are of potential benefit postoperatively, including PSGAGs and DMSO. In the author's practice, a 20% solution of DMSO is usually flushed through the joint at the completion of lavage. DMSO may both reduce inflammation (it is a free radical scavenger) and provide antibacterial activity. With all these medications, care must be taken to ensure that no drugs that may potentiate infection are used intraarticularly. Recognition that clinically "cured" joints can still have organisms cultured from them is important.

Physical therapy may also be useful, as well as modalities such as electromagnetic therapy.

In some cases where the above-described treatments have not been successful, a functional result can still be obtained with ankylosis of the joint. Spontaneous ankylosis will occur in some cases, particularly in the distal interphalangeal (coffin) joint (Fig. 7.76). In a report of septic arthritis of the distal interphalangeal joint in 12 horses, ankylosis of the affected joint developed in 5 horses, 4 of which were pasture sound. This corresponds to my experiences.[29] We have also performed elective arthrodesis of coffin joints in horses that did not respond to other treatment modalities.

Prognosis

The prognosis for any case of septic arthritis in the horse is guarded because lack of response to treatment can occur in all types of cases. Young animals have a better capacity for joint healing after infection is controlled than older animals. Various papers have reported the success rate of treatment for infective arthritis. Schneider et al. reported that infection was eliminated in 25 of 26 horses, and 24 survived and were released from the hospital.[61] Of 13 horses treated with closed-suction drainage by Ross et al., 10 horses returned to their previous level of competition or were sound. One horse raced but had lameness of the affected tarsocrural joint and dropped in racing class, 1 horse was euthanized because of laminitis in the supporting limb, and 1 horse was lame but useful as a breeding animal.[60] In a report of monoarticular infective arthritis in 34 cases from Ghent, Belgium, 9 horses were reported to recover completely, 2 returned to stud and were not visibly lame but were not worked, 3 horses improved but when worked hard suffered from residual lameness, 6 horses remained lame as a result of OA, 13 horses were euthanized, and 1 horse

was lost to follow-up.[55] In a series of 15 Standardbred racehorses that were infected after intraarticular injection, 12 of 15 were treated. All received parenteral antibiotic therapy, and all but one had its joint lavaged either with nonsurgical through-and-through techniques only (3), surgically with arthrotomy (1), or arthroscopy (7). Eleven of 12 horses returned to racing. Outcome was judged as satisfactory (3 of 12), if the horse had returned to racing levels similar to or better than before treatment, or unsatisfactory (9 of 12), if a horse had poorer performance or could not return to racing. The 3 horses with satisfactory follow-up had been treated with arthroscopy and postsurgical closed-suction drainage. The results of bacterial cultures suggested that the antimicrobial agent used initially should be effective against penicillin-resistant staphylococci.[33] Such a low return to satisfactory athletic performance after iatrogenic septic arthritis has important treatment and legal consequences.

In some instances of septic arthritis, despite all efforts with antibiotics and drainage techniques, one may see temporary success, but an insidious degradation continues. Some possible causes of continued destruction in cartilage are 1) the inability of the injured chondrocyte to replace the depleted matrix, 2) the continued inflammatory process secondary to tissue-fixed bacterial products, and 3) an immunologic disease of articular cartilage initiated by the septic process. However, ankylosis may allow a tolerable level of soundness (Fig. 7.78).

In summary, very early in the disease of septic arthritis, systemic antibiotic treatment and synovial aspiration may be adequate therapy. However, if clinical improve-

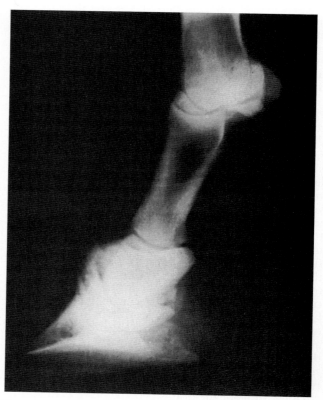

Figure 7.78 Bony ankylosis developing in a coffin joint after infective arthritis.

ment is not evident within 24 to 48 hours, drainage techniques must be instituted. It is common in the field to start with synovial distension–irrigation and/or joint lavage, but more and more we have recognized that we need to go rapidly to arthroscopic surgery.

References

1. Abdelnour A, Arvidson S, Bremell T, et al. The accessory gene regulator (ARG) controls *Staphylococcus aureus* virulence in a murine arthritis model. Infect Immun 1993;61:3879–3885.
2. Bennett OM, Namnyak SS. Acute septic arthritis of the hip joint in infancy and childhood. Clin Orthop 1992;281:123–132.
3. Bertone AL, Caprile KA, Davis DM, et al. Serum and synovial fluid concentrations of gentamicin administered chronically to horses with experimentally-induced infectious arthritis [abstract]. Vet Surg 1990;19:57.
4. Bertone AL, Davis DM, Cox HU, et al. Arthrotomy versus arthroscopy and partial synovectomy for treatment of experimentally induced infectious arthritis in horses. Am J Vet Res 1992;53:585–591.
5. Bertone AL, Jones RL, McIlwraith CW. Serum and synovial fluid steady-state concentrations of trimethoprim and sulfadiazine in horses with experimentally induced infectious arthritis. Am J Vet Res 1988;49:1681–1687.
6. Bertone AL, McIlwraith CW. A review of current concepts in the therapy of infectious arthritis in the horse. Proceedings. American Association of Equine Practitioners, New Orleans, LA, 1987;32:323–339.
7. Bertone AL, McIlwraith CW, Jones RL. Povidone iodine lavage treatment of experimentally induced equine infectious arthritis. Am J Vet Res 1987;48:712–715.
8. Bertone AL, McIlwraith CW, Jones RL, et al. Comparison of various treatments for experimentally induced equine infectious arthritis. Am J Vet Res 1987;48:519–529.
9. Bertone AL, McIlwraith CW, Powers BE, et al. Effect of four antimicrobial lavage solutions on the tarsocrural joints of horses. Vet Surg 1986;15:305–315.
10. Blitzer CM. Arthroscopic management of septic arthritis of the hip. Arthroscopy 1993;9:414–416.
11. Brewer B, Koterba A. Bacterial isolates and susceptibility patterns in a neonatal intensive care unit. Comp Cont Educ Pract Vet 1990;12:1773–1781.
12. Brown AS. Minimum inhibitory concentrations and postantimicrobial effects as factors in dosage of antimicrobial drugs. J Am Vet Med Assoc 1987;199:871–872.
13. Cook VL, Bertone AL, Kowalski JJ. Biodegradable drug delivery systems for gentamicin release and treatment of synovial membrane infection. Vet Surg 1999;28:233–241.
14. Crabil MR, Cohen ND, Martin LJ, et al. Detection of bacteria in equine synovial fluid by use of polymerase chain reaction. Vet Surg 1996;25:195–198.
15. Curtis PH. Changes produced in the synovial membrane and synovial fluid by disease. J Bone Joint Surg [Am] 1964;46:873.
16. Curtis PH, Cline L. Destruction of articular cartilage in septic arthritis. II. *In vivo* studies. J Bone Joint Surg [Am] 1965;47:1595.
17. Edwards GB, Vaughan LC. Infective arthritis of the elbow joint in horses. Vet Rec 1977;103:227.
18. Firth EC. Current concepts in infectious polyarthritis in foals. Equine Vet J 1983;15:5–9.
19. Firth EC, Dik KJ, Goedegebuure SA, et al. Polyarthritis and bone infections in foals. Zentralbl Veterinarmed [B] 1980;27:102–124.
20. Firth EC, Klein WR, Nouws JFM, Wensing TL. Effect of induced synovial inflammation on pharmacokinetics and synovial concentration of sodium ampicillin and kanamycin sulfate after systemic administration in ponies. J Vet Pharmacol Ther 1988;11:56–62.
21. Gainor BJ. Installation of continuous tube irrigation in the septic knee at arthroscopy. A technique. Clin Orthop 1984;183:96–98.
22. Gibson KT, McIlwraith CW, Turner AS, et al. Open joint injuries in horses: 58 cases (1980–1986). J Am Vet Med Assoc 1989;194:398–404.
23. Gustafson SB, McIlwraith CW, Jones RL. Comparison of the effect of polysulfated glycosaminoglycans, corticosteroids and sodium hyaluronate in the potentiation of a subinfective dose of *Staphylococcus aureus* in the midcarpal joint of horses. Am J Vet Res 1989;50:2014–2017.
24. Hammerman D. Cartilage in the rheumatoid joint. Clin Orthop 1969;64:91.
25. Hardy J, Bertone AL, Malemud CJ. Effect of synovial membrane: Infection in vitro on equine synoviocytes and chondrocytes. Am J Vet Res 1998;59:293–299.
26. Hardy J, Bertone AL, Muir WW. Joint pressure influences synovial tissue blood flow as determined by colored microspheres. J Appl Physiol 1996;80(4):1225–1232.
27. Harris ED Jr, Cohen GL, Krane SM. Synovial collagenase: Its presence in culture from joint disease of diverse etiology. Arthritis Rheum 1969;12:92.
28. Hasegawa Y, Ito H. Intracapsular pressure in hip synovitis in children. Acta Orthop Scand 1991;62:333–336.
29. Honnas CM, Welch RD, Ford TS, et al. Septic arthritis of the distal interphalangeal joint in 12 horses. Vet Surg 1992;21:261–268.
30. Kawashima M, Torisu T, Kamo Y, et al. The treatment of pyogenic bone and joint infections by closed irrigation suction. Clin Orthop 1980;148:240–244.
31. Koch DV. Management of infectious arthritis in the horse. Comp Cont Educ Pract Vet 1979;1(S45).
32. Lane JG, Falahee MH, Wojtys EM, et al. Pyarthrosis of the knee. Treatment considerations. Clin Orthop 1990;252:198–204.
33. LaPointe JM, Laverty S, Lavoie JP. Septic arthritis in 15 Standardbred racehorses after intra-articular injection. Equine Vet J 1992;24:430–434.
34. Leitch M. Musculoskeletal disorders in neonatal foals. Vet Clin North Am (Equine Pract) 1985;1:189–207.
35. Lloyd KCC, Stover SM, Pascoe JR, Adams P. Synovial fluid pH, cytologic characteristics, and gentamicin concentration after intra-articular administration of drug in an experimental model of infectious arthritis in horses. J Am Vet Med Assoc 1990;51:1363–1369.
36. Lloyd KCC, Stover SM, Pascoe JR, et al. Plasma and synovial fluid concentrations of gentamicin after intra-articular administration of buffered and unbuffered gentamicin. Am J Vet Res 1988;49:644–662.
37. Madison JB, Sommer M, Spencer PA. Relations among synovial membrane histopathologic findings, synovial fluid cytologic findings, and bacterial culture results in horses with suspected infectious arthritis: 64 cases (1979–1987). J Am Vet Med Assoc 1991;198:1655–1661.
38. Martens RJ, Auer JA, Carter GK. Equine pediatrics: Septic arthritis and osteomyelitis. J Am Vet Med Assoc 1986;188:582–585.
39. Deleted in proof.
40. McChesney AE, Becerra V, England JJ. Chlamydial polyarthritis in a foal. J Am Vet Med Assoc 1974;165:259.
41. McIlwraith CW. Treatment of infectious arthritis. Vet Clin North Am (Large Anim Pract) 1983;5:363–379.
42. McIlwraith CW. Antibiotic use in musculoskeletal disease. Proceedings. 32nd Annual Meeting of the American Association of Equine Practitioners, Nashville, TN, 1986;241–249.
43. McIlwraith CW, Trotter GW. Joint Disease in the Horse. Philadelphia: WB Saunders, 1996.
44. Montgomery RD, Long IR, Milton JL, et al. Comparison of aerobic culturette, synovial membrane biopsy and blood culture medium in detection of canine bacterial arthritis. Vet Surg 1989;18:300–303.
45. Moore RM, Schneider RK, Kowalski J, et al. Antimicrobial susceptibility of bacterial isolates from 233 horses with musculoskeletal infection during 1979–1989. Equine Vet J 1992;24:450–456.
46. Moorthy ARS, Spradrow PB, Eister MED. Isolation of *Mycoplasma* from an arthritic foal. Br Vet J 1977;133:320.
47. Nade S. Acute septic arthritis in infancy and childhood. J Bone Joint Surg [Br] 1983;65:234.
48. Neal D, et al. Lavage of septic joints in rabbits: Effects of chondrolysis. J Bone Joint Surg [Am] 1976;58:393.
49. Nelson CL, Hickman SG, Skinner RA, et al. Comparison of gentamicin dosing regimens in the treatment of experimental osteomyelitis. Trans Annu Meet Orthop Res Soc 1994;40:20.
50. Ouzounian TJ, Thompson L, Grogan TJ. Evaluation of musculoskeletal sepsis with indium-111 white blood cell imaging. Clin Orthop 1987;221:304–311.
51. Paradis MR. Cutaneous and musculoskeletal manifestations of *Rhodococcus equi* infection in foals. Equine Vet Educ 1997;9:266–270.
52. Parisien JS, Shaffer B. Arthroscopic management of pyarthrosis. Clin Orthop 1992;275:243–247.

53. Pascoe JR. For want of a joint the horse was lost [editorial]. Equine Vet J 1992;24:412–414.
54. Patti J, Bremell T, Krajewska-Bietrasik D, et al. The *Staphylococcus aureus* collagen adhesion is a virulence determinant in experimental septic arthritis. Infect Immun 1994;62:152–161.
55. Peremans K, Verschooten F, DeMoor A, et al. Monoarticular infectious arthritis in the horse: 34 cases. J Equine Vet Sci 1991;11:27–31.
56. Platt H. Joint ill and other bacterial infections on Thoroughbred studs. Equine Vet J 1977;9:141.
57. Rashkoff ES, Burkhalter WE, Mann RJ. Septic arthritis of the wrist. J Bone Joint Surg [Am] 1983;65:824–828.
58. Reginato AJ, Ferreiro JL, O'Connor CR, et al. Clinical and pathologic studies of 26 patients with penetrating foreign body injury to the joints, bursae and tendon sheaths. Arthritis Rheum 1990;33:1753–1762.
59. Resnick D, Niwayama G. Osteomyelitis, septic arthritis and soft tissue infections: The mechanisms and situations. In: Resnick D, Niwayama G, Eds. Diagnosis of Bone and Joint Disorders. Philadelphia: WB Saunders, 1981:2042–2129.
60. Ross MW, Orsini JA, Richardson DW, Martin RB. Closed suction drainage in the treatment of infectious arthritis of the equine tarsocrural joint. Vet Surg 1991;20:21–29.
61. Schneider RK, Bramlage LR, Meckleburg LM, et al. Open drainage, intra-articular and systemic antibiotics in the treatment of septic arthritis/tenosynovitis in horses. Equine Vet J 1992;24:443–449.
62. Schurman DJ, Smith RL. Joint infection. Acta Orthop Scand 1998(S281):14–16.
63. Scoles PV, Aronoff SC. Antimicrobial therapy of childhood skeletal infections. J Bone Joint Surg [Am] 1984;66:1486–1492.
64. Shaw BA, Kasser JR. Acute septic arthritis in infancy and childhood. Clin Orthop 1990;257:212–225.
65. Smith MJ. Arthroscopic treatment of the septic knee. Arthroscopy 1986;2:30–34.
66. Smith RL, Kajiyama G, Schurman DJ. Staphylococcal septic arthritis: Antibiotic and nonsteroidal anti-inflammatory drug treatment in a rabbit model. J Orthop Res 1997;15:919–926.
67. Smith RL, Schurman DJ. Bacterial arthritis. A staphylococcal proteoglycan-releasing factor. Arthritis Rheum 1986;29:1278–1386.
68. Smith RL, Schurman DJ, Kajiyama G, et al. The effect of antibiotics on the destruction of cartilage in experimental infectious arthritis. J Bone Joint Surg [Am] 1987;60:1063–1068.
69. Stover SM, Pool RR. Effect of intra-articular gentamicin sulfate on normal equine synovial membrane. Am J Vet Res 1985;46:2485–2491.
70. Deleted in proof.
71. Switalski LM, Patti JM, Butcher W, et al. A collagen receptor on *Staphylococcus aureus* strains isolated from patients with septic arthritis mediates adhesions to cartilage. Mol Microbiol 1993;7:99–107.
72. Thieng JA. Arthroscopic drainage in septic arthritides of the knee: A multicenter study. Arthroscopy 1989;5:65–69.
73. Torholm C, Hedstrom S-A, Sunden G, et al. Synovectomy in bacterial arthritis. Acta Orthop Scand 1985;54:748–753.
74. Tulamo R-M, Bramlage LR, Gabel AA. The influence of corticosteroids on sequential clinical and synovial fluid parameters in joints with acute infectious arthritis in the horse. Equine Vet J 1989;21:332–337.
75. VanPelt RW, Riley WF. Clinicopathologic findings and therapy in septic arthritis in foals. J Am Vet Med Assoc 1969;155:1467.
76. Vincent EM, Amirault JD. Septic arthritis in the elderly. Clin Orthop 1990;251:241–245.
77. Welsh RD, Watkins JP, DeBowes RM, et al. Effects of intra-articular administration of dimethyl sulfoxide on chemically induced synovitis in immature horses. Am J Vet Res 1991;52:934–939.
78. Whitehair KJ, Adams SB, Parker JE, et al. Regional limb perfusion with antibiotics in three horses. Vet Surg 1992;21:286–292.
79. Whitehair KJ, Blevins WE, Fessler JF, et al. Regional limb perfusion of the equine carpus for antibiotic delivery. Vet Surg 1992;21:279–285.
80. Whitehair KJ, Bowersock TL, Blevins WE, et al. Regional limb perfusion for antibiotic treatment of experimentally induced septic arthritis. Vet Surg 1992;21:367–373.
81. Wilson DG, Cooley AJ, MacWilliams PS, et al. Effects of 0.05% chlorhexidine lavage on the tarsocrural joints of horses. Vet Surg 1994;23:442–447.
82. Wilson NIL, DiPaola M. Acute septic arthritis in infancy and childhood. 10 years experience. J Bone Joint Surg [Br] 1986;68:584–587.
83. Wysenbeck AJ, Volchek J, Amit M, et al. Treatment of staphylococcal septic arthritis in rabbits by systemic antibiotics and intra-articular corticosteroids. Ann Rheum Dis 1998;57:687–690.

OTHER SPECIFIC DISEASES OF JOINTS

Synovial Hernia, Ganglion, and Synovial Fistula

A synovial hernia is a cystic structure arising from the herniation of synovial membrane through a defect in the fibrous joint capsule or the fibrous sheath of a tendon. A ganglion is a cystic swelling containing mucinous material but without a distinctive lining that occurs in close association to a joint or tendon sheath.[26] Contrary to previous equine reports,[1,34] these two conditions should not be considered synonymous. That ganglia arise as outpouchings of the joint capsule or tendon sheath is not generally accepted. Although there is usually an attachment between a ganglion and the joint capsule, pathologic studies give the impression that the ganglion does not initially connect with the joint and that any communication with the joint occurs secondary to degeneration of the capsule, which then ruptures. Ultrastructural studies have failed to show evidence of synovial membrane lining within a ganglion,[29] and careful dissection has failed to show consistent communication with the synovial space.[23] Studies suggest that the ganglion arises from multifunctional mesenchymal cells. Despite the differences in the pathogenesis of the two conditions, they may be hard to distinguish clinically because, after formation, ganglia can communicate with the joint capsule. Differential diagnosis necessitates histologic examination of the structures for the presence of synovial membrane. In one report in the equine literature, the structure was described as both ganglion and synovial hernia, but histopathology was not performed.[34]

Intersynovial fistulas occur with communication between one synovial cavity and another, associated with breakdown of soft tissue between adjacent synovial membranes. They typically arise between a joint and a tendon sheath.[14,21] They are considered to have a traumatic origin, being observed in association with carpitis and other inflammatory conditions. They have been reported between the common digital extensor tendon sheath and the midcarpal (intercarpal) joint, common digital extensor sheath and antebrachiocarpal (radiocarpal) joint,[14] and extensor carpi radialis tendon sheath and midcarpal joint.[21] They have also been reported under the long digital extensor tendon in the region of the pastern,[1] and they may occur in association with the proximal (pastern) or distal (coffin) interphalangeal joint. Trauma is considered to be the pathogenesis, but this is not identified in all cases.[21] The conditions are relatively uncommon.

DIAGNOSIS

A synovial hernia or ganglion presents as a subcutaneous, fluid-filled swelling (Fig. 7.79). Pressure of the swell-

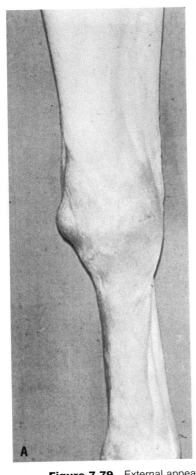

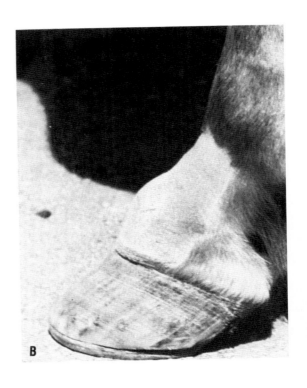

Figure 7.79   External appearance of synovial hernia. A. Midcarpal joint. B. Distal interphalangeal joint.

ing may cause movement of fluid into the associated joint or tendon sheath. The condition is confirmed by contrast radiology (Fig. 7.80). Ganglia may be multilocular, whereas synovial hernias tend to show up as single cavities.

An intersynovial fistula between tendon sheath and joint typically presents with a distended sheath and appears similar to tenosynovitis. Synovial fluid can usually be massaged between the tendon sheath and the joint. Again, contrast radiology confirms the diagnosis. A synovial hernia is usually a cosmetic problem, but a fistula may cause lameness. It is not clear whether the lameness is associated with tenosynovitis per se or the fistula.

TREATMENT

Surgery is the treatment of choice for all of these conditions (Fig. 7.81). In some instances, however, particularly synovial hernia, the indication is for cosmetic reasons, and treatment may not be considered worthwhile. Although a number of treatments have been used for ganglions in humans, surgical excision provides the lowest rate of recurrence.[26] The surgical treatment of a synovial hernia involves complete excision and suturing of the defect in the fibrous joint capsule. The dissection of a hernia is straightforward, but a ganglion may have diffuse tissue and multiple tracts present and be more

difficult. Failure to remove all of the lesion invites recurrence.[34]

The treatment of an intersynovial fistula involves exposure of the fistula, removal of redundant synovial membrane, and closure of the fibrous investment of the joint and tendon sheath.

Immune-Mediated Joint Disease

There is little documentation of immune-mediated joint disease in the horse. Rheumatoid arthritis is undocumented in the horse, and the presence of a polyarthritis approximating the clinical criteria of rheumatoid arthritis as described in humans and the dog has generally not been recognized.

I was involved in the diagnosis of what appeared to be the first reported case of arthritis associated with systemic lupus erythematosus (SLE) in a horse in 1980.[17] The horse was an 11-year-old Quarter Horse gelding that had been bought recently at a sale. It was noticed to have synovial effusion in all four fetlock joints, and there was mild pain on flexion in each joint. The right carpus was similarly affected. Radiographs indicated no changes. The synovial fluid analyses were mildly inflammatory, with neutrophils being the predominant white cells. Diagnosis was made on the basis of both a positive

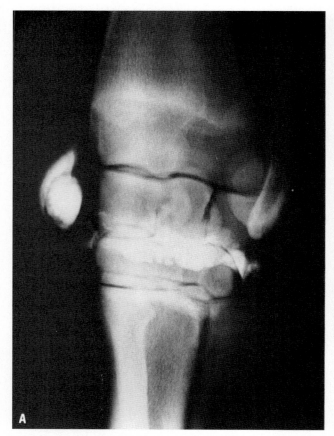

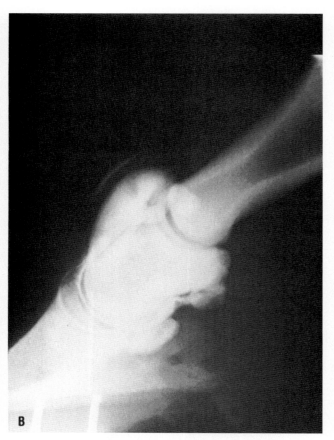

Figure 7.80 Contrast arthrograms of synovial hernias depicted in Figure 7.75. Contrast material can be noted within the hernias as well as within the joints. A. Midcarpal joint. B. Distal interphalangeal joint.

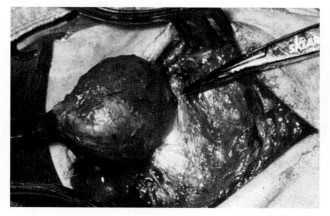

Figure 7.81 Synovial hernia of midcarpal joint exposed at surgery. Forceps indicate the defect in the fibrous joint capsule through which synovial membrane is herniated.

antinuclear antibody (ANA) titer between 1:160 and 1:320 and an anti–double-strand DNA titer as determined by the *Crithidia* assay of 1:40. Based on analyses of control samples, these were sufficiently high dilutions for the diagnosis of SLE. Tests for rheumatoid factor were negative. The horse was treated with a schedule of decreasing doses of prednisolone. SLE is a multisystem immune-mediated disease that may theoretically cause pathologic manifestations in any organ of the body.[5] In cases seen in the dog and human, joint problems are the most common presenting sign.[4,11] Shifting limb lameness is the most common complaint in the dog. Arthrocentesis is consistent with a noninfectious inflammatory arthritis and often shows a markedly increased number of neutrophils. Most SLE patients have high titers of ANA antibodies, and such titers are found only rarely in other conditions.[33] Since then, two cases of sterile polyarthritis have been reported in the horse in which an LE cell preparation was positive and the horses had ANA titers.[1a,36a]

Most canine patients with SLE present as with polyarthritis, but the disease may be mono- or polyarticular in manifestation. As a general recommendation, it would seem that an equine patient presenting with nonseptic inflammatory polyarthritis should be tested for ANA and rheumatoid factor. If the disease is diagnosed, prednisolone should be the first line of treatment, as it is most useful in a large number of cases in other species. Early diagnosis improves the prognosis.

As mentioned in the infectious arthritis section, there is another clinical situation in the horse which could be described as an immune-mediated arthritis. Polyarthritides and polytenosynovitis with an effusion that was often transient have been observed in foals following either *Streptococcus* upper respiratory infection or *Rho-*

dococcus lung infection.[18] Lameness was usually minimal. Synovial analysis revealed WBC counts up to 10,000/mm³, a high mononuclear cell component, and protein elevations to 3.4 to 4 mg/dL. Cultures were routinely negative, and organisms were not observed on histopathology of the synovial membrane. It was postulated that the arthropathy in these foals might be immune-mediated and that either antibody is attacking the synovial membrane or antigen-antibody complexes are being deposited on the synovial membrane and binding complement. The result of this is a transient synovitis. Research is continuing on these horses. The possibility of some arthritic problems in foals associated with an allergic response to the presence of an abscess remote from the joint and not involved with infection directly had been suggested previously.[7] A good example of a similar situation is rheumatic fever in humans, a disease primarily of children, which is usually preceded by streptococcal pharyngitis.[36] Clinical symptoms referable to the heart, joints, or CNS may develop from what is thought to be an autoimmune reaction triggered by the streptococcal infection. Four cases of immune-mediated polysynovitis in four foals were reported in 1988. A syndrome of nonerosive sterile arthritis was seen, characterized by inflammation of many joints (four to nine) and stiffness. The presence of immunoglobulin (fluorescein-labeled antiequine IgG staining) was verified in the synovial membrane in three of four foals (anti-IgG staining was not attempted in one case). All of the foals had a primary disease focus in the thorax (three of four *R. equi* pneumonia). The one surviving foal was responsive to prednisone treatment.[21a]

Nonerosive, noninfectious arthritis is also recognized as an important manifestation of a number of chronic systemic diseases in the dog and human.[27] In a series of 63 cases of noninfectious, nonerosive arthritis in the dog, 29 had SLE, 15 had arthritis associated with some chronic infectious process (these are usually monoarticular or pauciarticular), and 19 had a similar type of arthritis but without serologic evidence of SLE or any chronic infectious disease process. An immune basis is suspected in arthritis associated with chronic disease and may be associated with circulating immune complexes produced secondary to the infectious process.[27]

Based on the discussion above, one should keep an open mind regarding immune-related joint problems in the horse. A precedent is obviously created for the existence of the disease, and more careful examination of patients is necessary to determine the incidence properly.

Congenital Joint Anomalies

Congenital deformities in joints are not commonly encountered in the horse, but various entities have been recognized and are seen occasionally.

Arthrogryposis

Arthrogryposis has been defined as a deformity of the limbs characterized by curvature of the limbs, multiple articular rigidities, and muscle dysplasia.[16] It is probably an entity only in superficial terms, being pathologically and pathogenetically diverse. However, some muscular dysfunction must be present to fulfill the criteria of the disease. In some instances, the primary defect may be in the skeletal muscle, but in many and perhaps most cases, the primary defect is in the spinal column or cord, and the lesions in the muscle are secondary to innervation dysfunction. It is considered probable that unbalanced leverage on the bones of the limb causes the arthrogryposis, and the sustained inequalities in tension and immobility eventually result in modification of the joint capsule and the articular surfaces so that fixation persists even after the muscles are severed. In the veterinary literature it has been classified as a disease of muscle rather than joints.[16]

A number of veterinary reports give little attention to the status of the muscles, and it is difficult to decide in some instances if true arthrogryposis is the problem. In addition, the term has been used by some to include any syndrome or developmental disorder in which there is contracture or stiffness of joints. Because of this, we need to recognize arthrogryposis-like conditions in addition to the true disease. In humans, the classical condition of arthrogryposis multiplex congenita is a very specific clinical disorder.[37] It appears to be an environmental disease of early pregnancy associated with one of a variety of unfavorable intrauterine factors, including structural uterine deformity, vascular abnormality, hormonal imbalance, increased pressure, and possible intrauterine infection. It is considered that an unknown environmental agent has probably been present to a significant degree only in recent decades.[37]

Arthrogryposis has been well documented in calves and has been associated with heredity, lupine ingestion, manganese deficiency, and viral infection.[11,25] Other conditions such as cleft palate, scoliosis, and kyphosis frequently accompany the condition.

In a review of congenital defects of foals, arthrogryposis was not listed.[12] However, there are some reports of conditions that appear to be valid to classify as arthrogryposis-like, even though details on muscular or neural change were not mentioned.[13] Flexion deformities of the proximal (pastern) and distal (coffin) interphalangeal joints with ankylosis have been described as a congenital defect in 8 of 26 foals sired by the same Anglo–Arabian stallion.[28] There was rigid fixation of the two interphalangeal joints in one or both forelimbs. The foals could not stand and were destroyed. Another report describes ankylosis of joints in foals born from mares that had eaten hybrid Sudan grass pasture. Pathologic details were lacking in this case also.

Contracted foals, a syndrome seen in aborted fetuses as well as foals and yearlings, is characterized by bilateral flexion deformities in the limbs, asymmetric formation of the cranium, torticollis, and scoliosis.[31,32] Hypoplasia and malformation of the joint articulations are also present. Other congenital flexion deformities (contracted tendons) observed in foals generally do not have joint anomalies, although there has been one report of hypoplasia of the distal limb in a case of a unilateral flexion deformity.[24]

Abnormal articulations have been associated with flexion deformities of the carpus (dorsal deviation of carpal joints).[1] Generally the joint is stiff but not deformed.

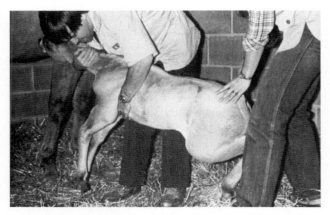

Figure 7.82 Foal with bilateral congenital lateral luxation of the patella. The foal was unable to stand.

This condition could be considered arthrogryposis-like but should not really be classified as arthrogryposis.

Lateral Luxation of the Patella

This condition is usually congenital and may or may not be associated with hypoplasia of the lateral trochlear ridge of the femur. The term "patella ectopia" has been used when there is no hypoplasia of the trochlea. Foals present with a typical squatting stance with hip, stifles, and hocks in extreme flexion (Fig. 7.82). The patella is positioned laterally. The condition can be confirmed radiographically. If hypoplasia of the trochlear ridge is present, the prognosis is poor. Surgical treatment may be attempted in unilateral cases and involves retinacular release on the lateral side and an imbrication procedure on the medial aspect of the joint.[20] It is not recommended for bilateral cases.

Absence (Agenesis) of the Patella

Absence of the patella has been reported in one case.[19]

Upward Fixation of the Patella

Upward fixation of the patella is mentioned here because it is considered to have an hereditary predisposition brought about by long, straight-limbed conformation.[1] However, other factors are also implicated in the condition, and it may be seen secondarily to coxofemoral luxation. These are discussed more fully in Chapter 8.

Hip Dysplasia

Hip dysplasia has been reported as a well-defined syndrome in the Norwegian Dole.[10] There have also been single case reports in a Shetland pony colt,[22] a Standardbred colt,[15] and an Andalusian–Arabian crossbred filly.[35] The Shetland pony colt presented with flattening of the acetabulum in the femoral head, a lack of femoral neck angulation, and secondary osteoarthritic change. These osteoarthritic lesions progressed in follow-up radiographs. The disease in the crossbred filly was typified by joint laxity and secondary DJD.[35] In the normal horse population this disease appears to be rare.

Bipartite Sesamoid Bones and Tripartite Navicular Bones

A condition typified by what appeared to be congenital "fractures" occurring bilaterally in the proximal sesamoid bones in foals and accompanied by any detectable heat, pain, swelling, or history of lameness has been mentioned by Adams.[1] He recognized this disease as a congenital imperfection of the bone and termed it "bipartite sesamoids." Another author has suggested that the lesions observed by Adams were probably traumatic fractures without reaction,[6] but there was no supportive evidence for the statement. We as well as others[2] have observed tripartite navicular bones occurring bilaterally, and the bilateral nature of this lesion makes it difficult to accept it as acquired.

Tumors

Tumors associated with joints in the horse are very uncommon. Chondrosarcoma of a metatarsophalangeal joint has been reported.[30] The case occurred in a 4-year-old Arabian mare that presented slightly lame, with a swollen joint. There was bone resorption in both the distal end of the third metatarsal bone and the proximal end of the proximal phalanx, without bony proliferation. Pathologically, the mass invaded bone, and smaller masses were distributed along the synovial membrane of the joint itself. The origin of the tumor was uncertain, but such tumors can arise in soft tissues as well as cartilage or bone. The articular cartilage was normal. The tumor was slow growing, and there were no metastases.

Metastatic melanoma involving the elbow and shoulder joint has been reported in a horse.[9] The horse was generally affected with the melanoma but did present clinically as a lameness problem.

I have encountered a case of fibroma associated with the femoropatellar joint. The horse exhibited a hard swelling proximal to the patella within the quadriceps femoris muscle that was progressing in size. Surgical removal of the fibroma involved entering the femoropatellar joint space and resectioning the distal end of the tumor from the joint capsule (Fig. 7.83). A hematoma of the synovial membrane within the fetlock joint has

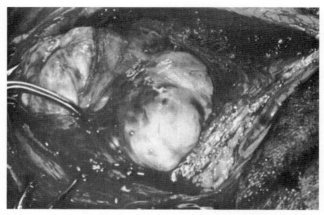

Figure 7.83 Surgical exposure of a fibroma associated with the femoropatellar joint capsule.

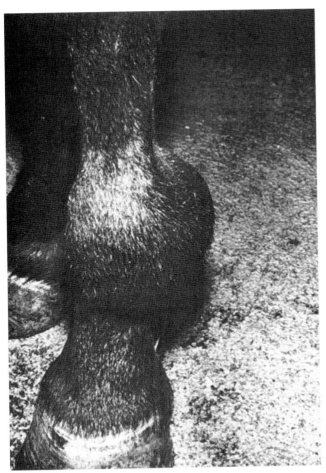

Figure 7.84 Swelling of fetlock associated with a hematoma of the synovial membrane.

also been encountered. Both lameness and local swelling were present. The lesion appeared as a spherical mass within the metacarpophalangeal joint, and treatment involved removal of synovial membrane involving the tumor (Fig. 7.84).

Another condition that could be considered a joint-associated tumor is tumoral calcinosis (calcinosis circumscripta). This condition commonly occurs in association with the femorotibial joint, but it is occasionally reported elsewhere. The condition is characterized by formation of one or more hard, circumscribed, subcutaneous swellings and is typically found over the lateral surface of the crus (gaskin), close to the femorotibial joint.[3,8] Lameness is not usually present. Caudal–cranial radiographs demonstrate the lesion as a distinctly encapsulated mass of soft tissue density irregularly infiltrated with small, highly radiopaque amorphous granules. The lesion tends to lie beneath the aponeurosis of the biceps femoris or the lateral fascia of the leg.[3] In some cases, the swellings are well demarcated and easily dissected from the surrounding structures. In others, however, the lesions involve the joint capsule of the femorotibial articulation so that entry into the joint is required for complete removal of the mass. This surgery has resulted in some deleterious outcomes.[3] If the condition is not caus-

ing a real clinical problem, conservative treatment should be considered. The etiology of the condition is not known.

References

1. Adams OR. Lameness in Horses. 3rd ed. Philadelphia: Lea & Febiger, 1974.
1a. Byars TD, Tyler DE, Whitlock RH, et al. Nonerosive polysynovitis in a horse. Equine Vet J 1984;16:141–143.
2. Chrisman OD. Biochemical aspects of degenerative joint disease. Clin Orthop 1969;64:77.
3. Dodd DC, Raker CW. Tumoral calcinosis circumscripta in the horse. J Am Vet Med Assoc 1970;157:968.
4. Drazner FH. Systemic lupus erythematosus in the dog. Comp Cont Educ Pract Vet 1980;2:243.
5. Dubois EL. Lupus Erythematosus. 2nd ed. Los Angeles: University of Southern California Press, 1976;90–108.
6. Ellis DR. Fractures of the proximal sesamoid bones in thoroughbred foals. Equine Vet J 1979;11:48.
7. Evans LH. Surgical treatment for the polyarthritis-septicemia complex in young foals. Am Coll Vet Surg Arch 1977;6:44.
8. Goulden BE, O'Callighan MW. Tumoral calcinosis in the horse. NZ Vet J 1980;28:217.
9. Grant B, Lincoln S. Melanosarcoma as a cause of lameness in a horse (a case report). Vet Med Sm Anim Clin 1972;67:995.
10. Haakenstad LH. Chronic bone and joint diseases in relation to conformation in the horse. Equine Vet J 1969;1:248.
11. Hartley WJ, De Saram WG, Della-Porta AJ, et al. Pathology of congenital bovine epizootic arthrogryposis and hydranencephaly and its relationship to Akabane virus. Aust Vet J 1977;53: 319–325.
12. Huston R, Saperstein G, Leipold HW. Congenital defects in foals. J Equine Med Surg 1977;1:146.
13. James LF. Plant-induced congenital malformations in animals. World Rev Nutr Diet 1977;26:208.
14. Johnson JE, Ryan GD. Intersynovial fistula in the carpus of a horse. Cornell Vet 1975;65:84.
15. Jogi P, Norberg I. Malformation of the H-joint in a Standardbred horse. Vet Rec 1962;74:421.
16. Jubb KVF, Kennedy PC. Pathology of Domestic Animals, vol. 2. New York: Academic Press, 1963.
17. Eales FL, McIlwraith CW, Schultz RD. Unpublished data, 1980.
18. Koch DB. Management of infectious arthritis in the horse. Comp Cont Educ Pract Vet 1979;1:S45.
19. Kostyra J. Congenital absence of patella in a foal. Med Vet 1963; 19:95.
20. Leitch M, Kotlikopp M. Surgical repair of congenital lateral luxation of the patella in the foal and calf. Vet Surg 1980;9:1.
21. Llewellyn HR. A case of carpal intersynovial fistula in a horse. Equine Vet J 1979;11:90.
21a. Madison JB, Scarratt WK. Immune-mediated polysynovitis in four foals. J Am Vet Med Assoc 1988;192:1581–1584.
22. Manning JP. Equine hip dysplasia-osteoarthritis. Mod Vet Pract 1963;44:44.
23. McEvedy BV. Simple ganglia. Br J Surg 1962;49:585.
24. Mitchell PJ, Parkes RD. Congenital hypoplasia in a foal [letter]. Vet Rec 1974;95:176.
25. Nawrot PS, Howell WE, Leipold HW. Arthrogryposis: An inherited defect in newborn calves. Aust Vet J 1980;56:359.
26. Nelson CL, Sawmiller S, Phalen GS. Ganglions of the wrist and hand. J Bone Joint Surg [Am] 1972;54:1459.
27. Pederson NC, Weisner K, Castles JJ, et al. Noninfectious canine arthritis: The inflammatory, nonerosive arthritides. J Am Vet Med Assoc 1976;169:304.
28. Prawochenski R. A new lethal factor in the horse. J Hered 1936; 27:410.
29. Psaila JV, Mansel RE. The surface ultrastructure of ganglia. J Bone Joint Surg [Br] 1978;60:228.
30. Riddle WE Jr, Wheat JD. Chondrosarcoma in a horse. J Am Vet Med Assoc 1971;158:1674.
31. Rooney JR. Congenital equine scoliosis and lordosis. Clin Orthop 1969;62:25.
32. Rooney JR. Contracted foals. Cornell Vet 1966;56:172.

33. Schultz RD. Basic veterinary immunology: An overview. Vet Clin North Am 1978;8:555.
34. Schumacher J, Auer J. A case report of a carpal ganglion in a horse. J Equine Med Surg 1979;3:391.
35. Spiers VC, Wrigley R. A case of bilateral hip dysplasia in a foal. Equine Vet J 1979;11:202.
36. Taranta A. Rheumatic fever, clinical aspects. In: McCarty DJ, Ed. Arthritis and Allied Conditions. Philadelphia: Lea & Febiger, 1972;764–820.
36a. Urins A, Feldman BF. Lupus erythematosus-like syndrome in a horse. Equine Pract 1983;5:18–25.
37. Wynne-Davies R, Williams PF, O'Connor JCB. The 1960's epidemic of arthrogryposis multiplex congenita. J Bone Joint Surg [Br] 1981;63:76.

DISEASES AND PROBLEMS OF TENDONS, LIGAMENTS, AND TENDON SHEATHS

The areas covered in this section include the anatomy and physiology of tendons and ligaments, developmental and traumatic problems of tendons and ligaments, and conditions of tendon sheaths. In the section on developmental problems of tendons and ligaments, we discuss limb deformities that have been classically attributed to, and called, tendon defects (e.g., contracted tendons). As explained, the pathogenesis is not necessarily a primary problem of the tendon, but for reasons of both convenience and convention, they are discussed in this section.

Anatomy and Physiology

Tendon Structure

A tendon is a dense band of fibrous connective tissue that acts as an intermediary in the attachment of muscle to bone. Ligaments are similar bands of dense connective tissue that connect bones. Tendons are composed of dense, regular connective tissue and have a specific arrangement that reflects the mechanical requirements of this tissue.[25] Mammalian tendons consist of longitudinally arranged units termed fascicles (100 to 300 μg in diameter), which in turn are composed of collagen fibrils (type I collagen) within a matrix of proteoglycans, glycoproteins, elastic fibers, ions, and water. Fibroblasts (tenoblasts) are arranged in long parallel rows in the spaces between the collagenous bundles. The basic unit of tendon structure, the primary tendon bundle, may be defined as coherent bundles of collagenous fibrils lying between rows of fibroblasts and encircled by their anastomosing processes.[48] These primary bundles group into secondary bundles or fascicles, and these in turn are aggregated into larger tertiary tendon bundles. The collagenous fibrils within a primary bundle are arranged in a parallel manner but follow a helical course along the length of the tendon.[50]

Collagen fibrils are the fundamental units of tensile strength in the tendon and are cylindrical structures composed of mainly type I collagen molecules in a specific axial and lateral arrangement.[155] The fibrils follow a planar zigzag waveform along the longitudinal axis of the tendon, which is termed the "crimp."[39] Crimp is a feather of the fibril bundles rather than isolated fibrils. It is quantified by the crimp angle and crimp length, measured at the level of the fascicle by use of polarizing optics.[39] Collagen fibers are submicroscopic units be-

lieved to be at least several millimeters long. It has been stated that the strength of the collagen fibril is determined by intermolecular cross-links between the collagen molecules within the fibril.[10] They also may be classified as "large" or "small" diameter in equine digital flexor tendons.[150,151] A diameter–area distribution has been derived from the diameter–frequency distribution for a collagen fibril population.[151] The *mass-average diameter* (MAD) is effectively the mean of this distribution and is correlated positively with overall tendon strength.[149,152]

Knowledge of the biochemistry of tendon, in the horse at least, has lagged behind biochemical knowledge of articular cartilage. It is known that tendons are composed predominantly of extracellular matrix in which the major structural protein is type I collagen fibrils. However, a number of noncollagenous proteins have attracted interest recently because of their interactions with the fibrillar collagen network, other matrix components, and tenocytes.[184] Proteoglycans, including aggrecan, decorin, biglycan, and fibromodulin, have been investigated in tendon.[214,214a] Noncollagenous extracellular matrix is not homogeneous along the tendon, which is presumed to reflect the different biomechanical environments experienced in different regions of the tendon. Aggrecan is characteristic of the pressure-resisting matrix of articular cartilage predominating in the compressed region of tendons where they pass over bony prominences. On the other hand, the small proteoglycans (especially decorin) are the major proteoglycans of a tensional tendon. The proteoglycans constitute only a small proportion of the noncollagenous proteins in tendons and ligaments, and most of the other noncollagenous proteins are still unknown.[184] One noncollagenous glycoprotein, cartilage oligomeric matrix protein (COMP), has been shown to be a constituent of tendon extracellular matrix.[39a,184] Recent work by Smith et al. suggests that COMP is synthesized in response to load and is necessary for tendon to resist, load.

It is generally accepted that ligaments, tendons, and fascia are similar histologically, and they are commonly grouped into a family of "dense, regularly arranged connective tissue." However, some work in the rabbit has demonstrated some differences between tendon and ligament.[4a] The findings suggest that ligaments are more metabolically active than tendons, with plumper cellular nuclei, higher DNA content, more reducible cross-links, and more type III collagen than tendons. Both tendons and ligaments contain the reducible collagen cross-links dihydroxylysinonorleucine (DHLNL), hydroxylysinonorleucine (HLNL) and histidinohydroxymerodesmosine (HHMD). Ligamentous tissues contain higher concentrations of DHLNL than of HLNL. Tendon fibroblasts do not contribute clinically to tendon strength, but their viability is of paramount importance to the maintenance of this strength. The tendon, a dynamic structure, renews its collagen. As fibrils are broken down, the fibroblasts replace them.

Structures Associated With Tendons

Consisting of trabeculae of loose connective tissue, the endotendon lies between the tendon bundles and carries vessels, nerves, and lymphatics. The endotendon is

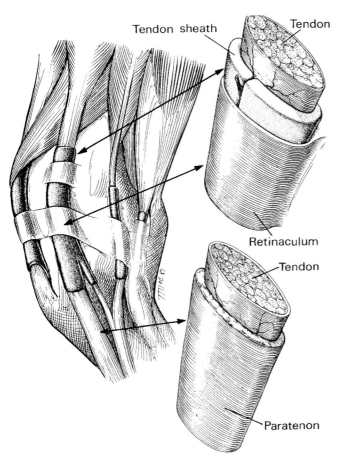

Figure 7.85 Diagram of tendons and their relationship to paratendon (paratenon) and tendon sheaths.

an extension of the epitendon (or peritendon), a delicate layer of loose connective tissue that closely invests the tendon surface (Fig. 7.85). Outside the epitendon the tendon is either enclosed by a sheath of the loose vascular connective tissue of the paratendon or, where a change of direction or increased friction occurs, a tendon sheath (Fig. 7.85). The paratendon is elastic and pliable, with long fibers that allow the tendon to move back and forth.[74,125]

The tendon sheath is comparable to the joint capsule, with an outer fibrous sheath and an inner synovial membrane. The synovial lining is folded around the tendon so that parietal and visceral layers can be distinguished, and the two layers are continuous along a fold called the "mesotenon" or "mesotendon." The presence of a mesotendon is apparently not always consistent.[222] Using the digital flexor tendons as an example of the relative position of these structures, as the tendons pass through the carpal canal, they are enveloped in a tendon sheath with a mesotendon present. Distal to the carpal canal in the midmetacarpus, the tendon is surrounded by paratendon. The tendon then enters the digital synovial sheath where there is reportedly no mesotendon, but the DDF tendon has a distal vinculum (band) at the level of the pastern joint.[190]

Anular ligaments, or retinacula, are strong fibrous bands that act to maintain the tendon in its correct posi-

tion when it passes over surfaces that could cause it to change position or "bow-string" (Fig. 7.85).[175]

Blood Supply to Tendons

A tendon may receive blood from four sources: the muscle or bone to which the tendon is attached, a mesotendon or vinculum within a synovial sheath, and the paratendon, if no sheath exists. The muscle and bone only supply the proximal and distal 25% of the tendon with blood, and the paratendon can be assumed to play an important role.[222] Observations made in the equine forelimb indicate that proximally and distally, the superficial digital flexor (SDF) tendons and DDF tendons receive vessels from their muscles and periosteal insertions, respectively. Within the carpal sheath, the primary branches of the median artery supply the surfaces of these tendons via the mesotendon, and other branches run parallel to the flexor tendons into the metacarpus.[222] Between the carpal and digital sheaths the tendons are surrounded by the paratendon, from which vessels enter the tendon. In the digital sheath, the SDF tendon receives blood caudally from vessels passing through the anular ligament of the fetlock and dorsally from vessels arising from the common digital artery that travel on the surface of the tendon and the digital sheath. Similarly, vessels from the digital artery supply the superficial flexor tendon distal to the fetlock, but there is no anastomosis between these two groups of vessels.[182] The deep flexor tendon is supplied proximally within the digital sheath by branches from the medial palmar artery (common palmar digital a. III) and is supplied distally by a vinculum. Regions of decreased vascularity have been found in the flexor tendons and related to a predisposition to degenerative change.[53]

Mechanical Properties of Tendons

Tendons possess great tensile strength and have low extensibility. In mechanical terms, the tendon serves primarily as a force transmitter. Other mechanical functions more recently attributed to tendons include that of a dynamic amplifier during rapid muscle contraction, an elastic energy store, and a force attenuator during rapid and unexpected movement.[50]

In uniaxial tension, the tendon initially appears highly compliant, but on further extension, there is a stiffer region of response (Fig. 7.86). This transition is considered to correspond to the disappearance of the waveform on the surface of the tendon and occurs at approximately 3% extension. Within this elastic range the waveform reappears on removal of the force. Unwinding of the helices is also considered to occur in this zone. Beyond this initial elastic phase, the mechanical characteristics of the tendon change and possess viscoelastic properties, and apparently irreversible structural changes take place.[169,195,222] Under constant load the tendon extends progressively with time (creep) (Fig. 7.86). It is considered that these viscoelastic changes do not occur in the primary tendon bundles but in the adjacent ground substance, and they are not a property of the collagen itself.[193]

In the typical nonlinear stress–strain curve the tendon demonstrates when mechanically tested in vitro,[32] the

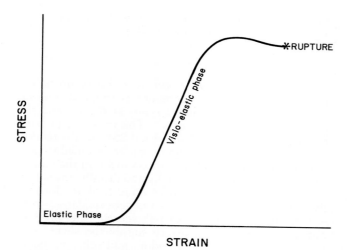

Figure 7.86 Diagram of stress-strain characteristics of a tendon. An initially lax response (elastic phase) precedes a stiff, nearly linear region (viscoelastic phase). Rupture occurs at about 8% elongation. (Reprinted with permission from Evans JH, Barbenel JC. Structured and mechanical properties of tendon related to function. Equine Vet J 1975;7:5.)

initial compliant region is termed the "toe." This region is considered to correspond to opening out of the crimp, and when the "toe limit strain" is reached, the straightened fibrils are stretched and the tendon begins to behave in a linear, elastic fashion. A collagen fibril bundle with a low crimp angle will reach its elastic limit at the end of the linear region at a lower level of strain than a bundle with a larger crimp angle.[229]

The magnitude of normal "physiologic forces" on equine tendons and its relation to the previous findings and rupture strength are still poorly defined. To understand the significance of the dynamic characteristics of a tendon, one must know whether the tendon is behaving in an elastic or viscoelastic manner. This working range needs to be defined. It has been suggested that because the second phase of the stress–strain curve for a tendon (Fig. 7.86) causes residual damage, normal physiologic activity never exceeds the elastic limit.[222] However, other authors believe that many forces fall within the transition area. Between the 3 and 5% strain level, the normal linear stress–strain relationship is maintained, but at the 5 to 6% level, more rapid extension ensues, which finally leads to total separation of the tendon.[222] Another point related to the significance of this work is whether overextension resulting in obliteration of the normal wave pattern causes a clinical lesion or whether such extensions return to normal and in what period of time. It is known that in the linear stress (5 to 6%) zone the normal wave pattern does not return after release of the tensile force. Histologic sections taken from tendons with acute and chronic lesions indicate loss of the wave pattern referred to above. Hall effect strain gauges have measured strains of 10 to 15% in the superficial flexor tendon of galloping Thoroughbreds.[189] An in vitro study in the horse has indicated an elastic strain limit of approximately 10%.[232] This implies that to fulfill an energy storing role, the SDF tendon has a very low safety margin during the weight-bearing phase of the gallop.[152]

Recently, the histologic variations of the equine SDF tendon were assessed by site and horse's age and activity, and these data correlated with previously reported segmental mechanical results.[37] Seven segments of each SDF tendon were delineated and examined histologically. Each segment was examined and graded for fiber undulation, cellularity, number and size of interfascicular connective spaces (ICS), presence or absence of focal and diffuse chondroid metaplasia, and differentiation of the dorsal and palmar borders of the tendon. Fiber undulation and cellularity decreased significantly with age. The proximal and middle metacarpal segment fibers were significantly less undulated and their interfascicular connective spaces were smaller than those of the other segments, especially in older horses. Focal chondroid metaplasia developed from 5 years onward, mainly in the sesamoidean segments. Diffuse chondroid metaplasia was characteristic of the digital region in horses more than 6 years of age. The dorsal border of the metacarpal–digital region tended to differentiate into fibrocartilage in association with age. The posterior border was generally differentiated as nonfascicular dense connective tissue. There was a decrease in the number and size of the interfascicular connective spaces with activity. The authors were able to correlate the lesser undulation of the proximal and middle metacarpal segment fibers with their mechanical behavior (stress–strain curve) and relative weakness within the SDF tendon. Focal chondroid metaplasia and fibrocartilage on the dorsal border are normal features related to the compression stresses undergone by the sesamoidean region of the tendon.

Response of Equine Flexor Tendons and Suspensory Ligament to Exercise

In general, skeletal tissues are presumed to have the ability to undertake functional adaptation. With increasing mechanical demand, a tissue response of increased mass or change in architecture is anticipated. In muscle, hypertrophy occurs with enhanced exercise, and bone also responds to function by increasing its mass in architecture for exercise regimens that are osteogenic. Functional adaptation of tendons and ligaments, however, is poorly understood, and as mentioned above, the functional loading magnitude in the SDF tendon is close to failure level for that structure. Several recent studies have suggested that galloping exercise causes microtrauma to the core region of the SDF tendon.[22,153,154,229] It has been hypothesized that accumulation of microtrauma weakens the tendon, eventually resulting in partial or complete rupture.

A study comparing young Thoroughbreds that had a specific 18-month exercise program (treadmill) with a control group that had walking exercise only found that the crimp angle and length in the central region of the SDF tendon was significantly lower in exercised horses than in control horses. The crimp angle was also significantly lower in the central region than in the peripheral region of the tendon in four of the five exercised horses, as was the crimp length in three of the four horses.[155] The crimp angle in the peripheral region was significantly larger in exercised horses than in the controls, which may indicate functional adaptation due to differing mechanical environment between the two tendon regions. The results of this study supported previous evidence that galloping exercise modifies normal age-related changes in crimp morphology in the core of the SDF tendon. The authors concluded that such changes indicate microtrauma and would be detrimental for tendon strength. As this is an area of problems with clinical tendinitis, the authors felt that training regimens that do not adversely affect central region crimp morphology would help to prevent tendinitis. In untrained horses, a crimp angle that is significantly lower in the tendon core than in the periphery has been observed only in animals age 10 years or more.[151] Lower crimp angles in the tendon core of exercised younger horses are suggested to represent acceleration of collagen fibril fatigue induced by the rapid high-strain cycles during galloping.

Patterson-Kane and co-workers have also looked at the MAD. The MAD for core regions of Thoroughbred superficial digital flexor (SDF) tendon was reduced significantly in response to a specific 18-month training program.[153] This was considered to be attributable to breakdown of larger-diameter fibrils, resulting in weakening of the tendon structure in this region. On the other hand, the MAD from the central region of the suspensory ligament in trained horses did not differ significantly from that of control horses. Similarly, in the DDF tendon there was no difference in central or peripheral regions between trained and control group horses. It was felt in this study[152] that the suspensory ligament and DDF tendon did not undergo significant changes in the ultrastructure of the tensile units in response to training, whereas the SDFT had evidence of microtrauma, which may indicate preferential loading of the SDFT at a gallop.

Postmortem examination of apparently normal equine flexor tendons has revealed an abnormal macroscopic appearance in the central core, characterized by a reddish discoloration.[22] Physical damage to the collagen fibers in this area has been demonstrated (tendinitis usually occurs in the central core of the mid metacarpal region also). Biochemical analysis of the extracellular matrix in these "degenerative" areas demonstrates an increase in total sulfated GAG content, an increase in the proportion of type III collagen, and a decrease in collagen-linked fluorescence in the central core of "degenerated" tendons relative to tissue from the peripheral region of the same tendon and also central regions of "normal" tendon.[21] Dry matter content and total collagen content were not significantly different between tendon zones or normal and "degenerated" tendons. The authors felt that these changes suggest a change in cell metabolism and matrix turnover in the central core of the tendon that could represent an early healing response by the cells that is initiated as a result of microdamage to the matrix. There were, however, differences from other scar tissue and ligament; for example, the levels of hydroxylysyl pyridinolone were unchanged in both peripheral and central zone tissue of degenerate tendon, while in ligament there are lower levels of this mature cross-link after injury. Immature reducible cross-link was present at only low levels, suggesting that increased collagen turnover is occurring over a longer time course than that expected during gross tendon injury. Previously, the first author also found no difference in matrix composition between central and peripheral zones of su-

perficial digital flexor tendon in young, unexercised horses. Stimulus for this increased collagen turnover, type III collagen deposition, and GAG synthesis is unclear but could be associated with change in biochemical environment such as oxygen tension or hypothermia as a result of repetitive loading cycles. It is anticipated that this observed macroscopic change in the tendon could result in a loss of mechanical integrity of the core of the tendon.[23]

Response to Injury and Tendon Healing

Both extrinsic and intrinsic components can be involved in tendon healing. When the tendon was considered an inert, almost avascular structure with little potential for repair, healing was thought to take place solely by ingrowth of fibroblasts and capillaries from the peritendinous tissues. While this extrinsic healing is an important and major component (or possibly an exclusive component with severe disruption of an equine tendon), intrinsic repair does exist, and the potential for intrinsic repair of tendons has been recognized.[119] It would seem that endotendon cells can function as active fibroblasts. Maximization of the intrinsic healing and minimization of extrinsic healing will potentially lead to fewer problems with peritendinous adhesions.

As with wound healing elsewhere in the body, tendon healing begins with an inflammatory reaction. There is outpouring of fibrin and inflammatory cells proportional to the size of the wound and the amount of trauma.[103] Fibroplasia is influenced by the inflammatory reaction. If there is traumatized, ischemic tissue with foreign material, a greater inflammatory reaction occurs, which is a significant stimulus for formation of excessive granulation tissue and collagen deposition.[103]

The contribution of capillaries from the paratendon is important in tendon healing.[13] They contribute oxygen for cellular survival and hydroxylation of proline during synthesis of collagen, deliver inflammatory cells for removal of debris and suture, and supply the amino acids essential for protein synthesis. However, the tendon can and does contribute significantly to its own healing. This was demonstrated by isolating segments of severed tendons from their blood supply, repairing them, and placing them in intact tendon sheaths bathed only by synovial fluid.[103] The cells of tendons treated in this manner survive, except for those in the center. The epitendon, as well as the endotendon, becomes hyperplastic. The fibroblasts can then effect primary repair. Unfortunately, most tendon injuries in the horse involve loss of tendinous tissue as well as contamination, and primary intrinsic repair is overshadowed by an extensive response from the peritendinous tissues. This response causes peritendinous fibroplasia and adhesions in addition to tendon healing and precludes restoration of normal gliding function.

While limited passive motion aids in longitudinal orientation of collagenous fibrils and bundle formation in tendon repair, more severe active motion inhibits early repair of the tendon.[103,174] This situation constitutes the major dilemma in the management of equine tendon injuries. Work in dogs showing that early controlled passive motion stimulated an intrinsic healing response in a clinically relevant tendon-repair model supports the idea of early controlled motion.[66] The gliding surface was restored at an early stage, and the tendon healed more rapidly than in immobilized repairs.

Developmental Problems in Tendons and Ligaments

Flaccidity or Weakness of Flexor Tendons in Foals

In its mildest form, flaccidity or weakness of flexor tendons is a common condition in newborn foals, generally affecting only the hindlimbs, but sometimes all four limbs. It usually corrects itself spontaneously and can almost be considered a physiologic variant rather than a disease. However, the problem has been associated with systemic illness or lack of exercise. The affected foals walk on the palmar (plantar) part of the hoof and do not bear weight on the toe (Fig. 7.87). They essentially rock back on the bulbs of the heel.

In foals that do not correct themselves within 1 to 2 weeks, the treatment involves corrective trimming and exercise. The heels are trimmed to eliminate the "rocker" effect and to provide a flat weight-bearing surface[138] (Fig. 7.88). The toes should not be trimmed. The use of protective bandages or casts will exacerbate the tendon weakness. In more severely affected foals, a small exten-

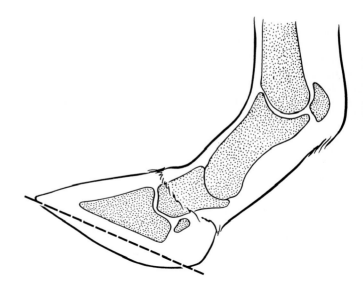

Figure 7.88 Diagram of trimming for flaccid tendons.

sion shoe with a 1.5-inch heel extension should be attached to the foot. The use of plywood or polyvinyl chloride (PVC) pipe attached with wiring or acrylic cement has been described.[58] A small metal plate or a door hinge applied with adhesive tape can also work. When the rounded portion of the hinge is at the back, a raised-heel effect is also obtained. Wooden tongue depressors applied with adhesive tape can be used in neonatal foals. Application of extension shoes are more problematic in the front limbs but are rarely needed here.

Digital Hyperextension in Foals

Digital hyperextension is apparent at birth or shortly after and is characterized by extreme extension (dorsiflexion) of the interphalangeal joints.[55] It is a rare condition. It appears as an extreme form of the flaccid tendon problem but must be considered a separate entity. The etiology is unknown. Electromyographic examinations have not demonstrated any pathologic changes in the musculature of the flexor group.[55] Severely affected animals bear weight on the palmar or plantar surface of the phalanges and sesamoid bones (Fig. 7.89).

Conservative methods of treatment such as the use of elongated shoe branches or support bandages are not usually successful. A surgical procedure for shortening of the superficial and DDF tendons has been described,[55] but results of this surgery are variable.

As discussed, less severe forms of digital hyperextension in foals usually resolve spontaneously, although the bulbs of the heels may need protection to prevent pressure ulcers developing. In general, farrier treatment consists of trimming the heel to allow a longer base of support and reduce rocking back in the heels, and in severe cases, caudal extensions that could be applied potentially by taping, gluing, or nailing have been described. Taping is unsatisfactory and difficult to achieve without constricting the hoof capsule.[38] Nailed-on shoes require very skillful forgery ability and risk damage to the sensitive structures of the hoof. Glue-on shoes (Dalic) can be effec-

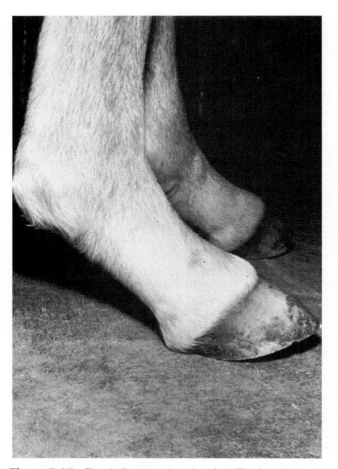

Figure 7.87 Flaccid flexor tendons in a foal. The feet have been trimmed. The problem resolved in a short time.

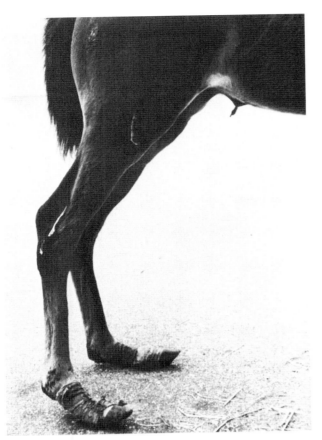

Figure 7.89   Severe digital hyperextension.

tive in some cases. A new technique using hoof repair composite and aluminum plates to make caudal extensions has been described and is also an option in cases of severe flexor tendon laxity (digital hyperextension).

Contracted Tendons or Flexural Deformities

The term "contracted tendons" has been used traditionally to represent various flexural deformities in the limbs.[170] However, the potential for contraction of dense tendinous tissue is obviously limited. The primary defect is not usually in the tendon itself. In many instances the effective functional length of the musculotendinous unit is less than necessary for normal limb alignment to be maintained, but this should not imply a primary defect in the tendon itself. The term "contracted tendons" has become common usage, and it describes the condition effectively. However, the reader is urged to be aware of other possible pathogenetic mechanisms and to recognize that these are not completely understood.

Flexural deformities are considered congenital (apparent at the time of birth) or acquired (developing during the growth period). Various etiologic factors have been incriminated in each group.

Congenital Flexural Deformities

PATHOGENESIS

Congenital flexural deformities have been attributed to uterine malpositioning.[49,71,98] Although this is plausi-

ble and may occur in some instances, it is unlikely to be very common, as the fetus commonly changes position. More complex influences that have been implicated include genetic factors and teratogenic insults during the embryonic stage of pregnancy.

There was one report of eight foals with severe fetlock flexion considered to result from a recent dominant gene mutation in the sire[93] and another report of three cases of congenital flexor contracture in foals from mares on a farm where an influenza outbreak occurred while the mares were pregnant.[57] Congenital limb deformities have also been found in association with ingestion of locoweed by pregnant mares.[128] Although such evidence is often circumstantial, it does point out the need for continuing investigation into the role of toxic and infectious agents in congenital deformities. Another reported contracted foal syndrome involved torticollis, scoliosis, and hypoplasia of the vertebral articular facets and distal extremities of the third metacarpal and metatarsal bones, with flexion contracture of the fetlock, carpal, and tarsal joints.[171] The etiologic basis of this syndrome is unknown, but it was hypothesized that the pathogenesis of the flexural deformities originated from joint instability associated with the bony malformations that resulted in compensatory muscle contracture.[171] Similar pathologic manifestations have also been reported in two Clydesdale foals. However, one of these foals had a severe extension deformity rather than a flexion deformity.[26] Defects in cross-linking of elastin and collagen due to lathyrism will cause flexural deformities in other species.[102] Such biochemical lesions could feasibly be involved in some cases of congenital flexural deformities in foals.

Congenital flexural deformities have also been associated with equine goiter.[12] In another report, rupture of the common digital extensor tendons, forelimb contracture, and mandibular prognathism were common findings in association with severe hyperplastic goiter.[130]

Arthrogryposis may also produce flexural deformity. This condition has been well documented in calves but is less well defined in horses. A condition appearing clinically similar to arthrogryposis occurring as a result of the mare ingesting hybrid Sudan grass pasture has been reported.[161]

CLINICAL MANIFESTATIONS

Congenital flexural deformities may affect one or more limbs. The common manifestations are fetlock and carpal flexural deformities. Congenital flexural deformities of the pastern, tarsus, and distal interphalangeal joint are rare but have been reported.[200,217] With fetlock flexural deformities, the foals may be able to stand but knuckle over at the fetlock (Fig. 7.90). In severe instances, the foals will walk on the dorsal surface of the fetlock. Generally, both SDF and DDF muscle–tendon units are shortened in these cases. Some authors suggest that the suspensory ligament (interosseus medius muscle) is the primary structure involved.[34,35] Involvement of the DDF tendon alone may manifest as a flexural deformity of the distal interphalangeal joint. Congenital flexure deformities of the carpus are common (Figs. 7.91 to 7.93). Individual tendon involvement is difficult to define in these cases, and frequently, contracture of the carpal fascia

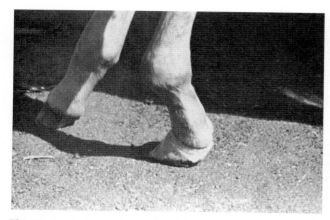

Figure 7.90 Congenital flexion deformity of metacarpophalangeal joint. A toe extension has been placed on the hoof but is not helping the condition.

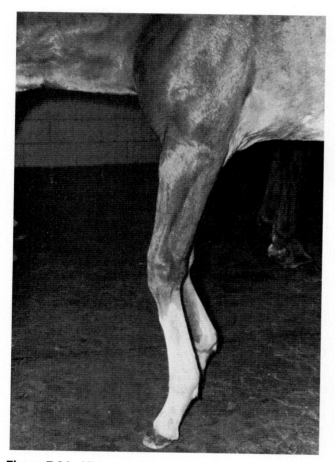

Figure 7.91 Mild congenital carpal flexure deformity. This case recovered spontaneously.

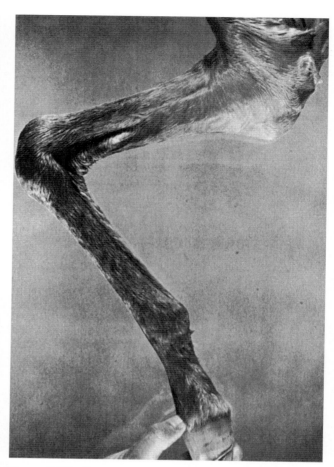

Figure 7.92 Severe congenital carpal flexure deformity with limb in maximal extension possible.

TREATMENT

Some foals with congenital flexural deformities (particularly associated with the carpus) improve spontaneously, and these rarely require treatment. They include mild carpal and fetlock flexural deformities. Most fetlock flexural deformities usually respond well to splinting. Splints can be made from 4-inch diameter thick-walled pipe tubing and may also be bent with heat to whatever conformation is desired. With a severe fetlock deformity, a straight splint is used, and as relaxation is achieved, a bent splint is applied to force the fetlock back into normal position (Figs 7.94 and 7.95). During weight bearing, tensional forces are now constantly applied to the flexor units, which will induce flexor relaxation. All splinting devices require strategic placement of padding, constant evaluation, and changing of the splints to prevent skin necrosis. Severe problems can result from faulty use of splints and bandages (Fig. 7.96). With the use of these PVC splints at the appropriate angle, the risk of skin problems is markedly reduced. Distal interphalangeal joint deformities can respond to the application of toe extensions that protect, and prevent excessive wear of, the toe and also induce the inverse myotatic reflex. Because the hoof wall of foals is thin and soft, nailing or wiring shoes to the foot is difficult, and gluing on is appropriate. A cheap alternative to glue-on shoes is the

and palmar ligament seems to be the primary component. With carpal contractures, for instance, complete removal of the palmar joint structures and severing of the flexor tendons was required to straighten the joint.[171] Rotational deformities may also accompany flexure deformities.

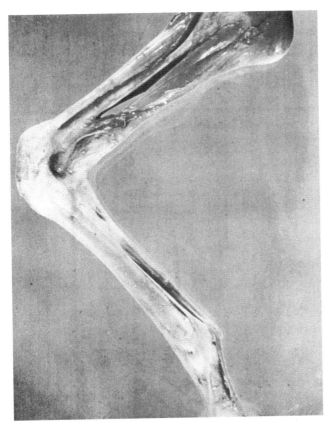

Figure 7.93   Same forelimb as in Figure 7.92 after being skinned. After all tendons were severed, extension of carpus was still not possible.

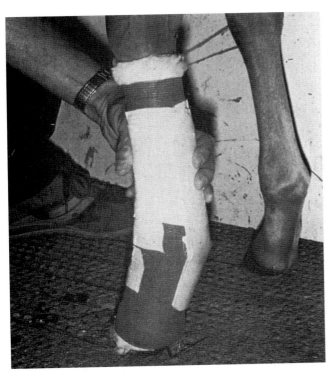

Figure 7.94   Splinting of a congenital fetlock flexion deformity. Limb is bandaged and prebent PVC splint is in position.

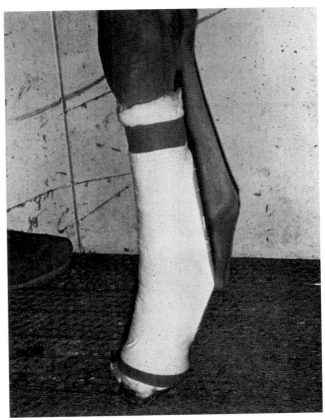

Figure 7.95   Splint held in place with adhesive tape.

use of a toe extension device made with PVC. The basic principle of splinting or toe extension treatment is forced extension of the limb to induce the inverse myotatic reflex and consequent relaxation of the flexor muscles. Various splints and devices have been recommended,[1,9] but the most effective material in my opinion is PVC tubing.

The use of oxytetracycline to treat congenital flexural deformities is now routine. The practice was first described in 1985 by Lokai,[112] and a paper on case selection from the same author was published in 1992.[113] The author described the use of oxytetracycline on a preliminary basis in the previous edition of this text. In describing case selection of 123 foals, Lokai said that all foals were less than 14 days of age. "Contracted" foals were not included; only foals that could place some part of the foot on the ground were included, and the only previous treatment in any of the foals was splinting of the limb for 24 hours (8 of 123). All foals were treated with 3 g of oxytetracycline intravenously (undiluted) using various brand names and concentrations. Every other foal was not treated for 3 days after foaling to give equal time for natural correction before treatment was instituted (delayed treatment). Foals not showing 80% correction within 48 hours (21 foals) of first treatment were reinjected with a second 3-g IV dose. No external splinting was used with any IV treatment. Of 123 cases, there was a 94% overall success rate (normal function restored within 72 hours after injection). The 3-g doses of undiluted oxytetracycline were used in the 50 mg/mL

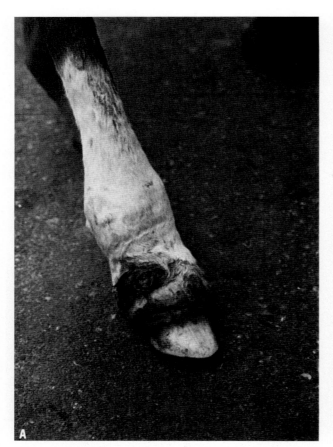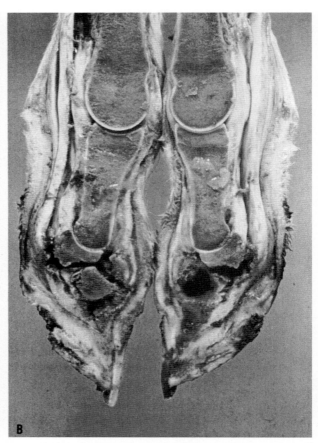

Figure 7.96   A and B. Gangrene of distal limb associated with poor splinting technique and failure to remove splint when lameness developed.

concentration and 100 mg/mL concentration. There are potential side effects.[236] No diarrhea was seen, and in delayed-treatment cases, the same response was evident after IV therapy. Of the 123 foals, 96 had one forelimb involved, 10 had both forelimbs involved, 8 had both hindlimbs involved, and 9 had both forelimb and rear limb involved. Success rate in the forelimb was 104 of 106 (98%); in the rear limb, 6 of 8 (75%); and in both forelimb and rear limb, 6 of 9 (66%).

Although the mechanism of action of oxytetracycline in the treatment has not been investigated extensively, it has been hypothesized that chelation of calcium in skeletal muscle will occur and chelation of calcium in skeletal muscle has been documented.[113] Oxytetracycline has been shown to be a neuromuscular blocking agent.[158] It has been suggested that if a neuromuscular blockade is responsible for the flexor tendon relaxation obtained after oxytetracycline treatment, then maximal clinical effect would be expected when the plasma concentration of oxytetracycline was at its highest, and one would also expect that muscle groups other than flexor muscles would be affected as well. The mechanism of treatment is still uncertain. Controlled studies showed no significant changes in blood chemistry values after administration of oxytetracycline other than those typically observed in newborn foals. A significant decrease in mean metacarpophalangeal joint angles was observed in foals 24 hours

after treatment with oxytetracycline, compared with those of foals treated with saline or oxytetracycline vehicle. The mean metacarpophalangeal joint angle returned to pretreatment value by 96 hours.[118] It was concluded that oxytetracycline appeared to be an effective method for obtaining a short-term moderate decrease in metacarpophalangeal joint angle in newborn foals. Another study looked at metacarpophalangeal joint angulation during locomotion in normal foals before and after treatment with a high dose of oxytetracycline and found that maximum metacarpophalangeal joint angle, which occurred during the stance phase of the stride, and range of joint motion were significantly higher in foals in the treatment group than in foals in the control group.[101] The dose and schedule of oxytetracycline used in this study (two doses of 3 g IV at 4 and 5 days of age) has been shown to be safe in foals with normal renal function.[231]

If the above conservative methods for treating congenital flexure deformities are not successful, casts may be used to provide extension, but their indications are limited to severe contractures that cannot be extended completely. In this instance, casting may weaken the muscles enough to allow sufficient extension after the cast is removed. The prognosis is generally poor in cases that require cast application. Cast management in foals has risks, and use of a combined plaster/fiberglass cast is recommended. A thin layer of plaster is applied initially, and the cast is completed using one of the light-weight commercial casting materials. Corrective shoes may be useful in some instances.[35]

When corrective shoes with toe extensions are used, the clinician should ensure that any toe abscesses are recognized. These can occur due to entry of infection at the white line of the toe in association with excessive wear or pressure.

The final alternative in treatment of congenital tendon contractures is surgery. Flexor tenotomies[1,124] and carpal (inferior) check desmotomies have been used successfully (the methods are described in the acquired flexure deformities section) but are not commonly indicated. A case of congenital flexure of the right hock associated with an abnormally short peroneus tertius muscle has been recently described.[200] The problem was successfully treated by resection of a portion of the peroneus tertius.[200] In cases not amenable to conservative treatment, the use of surgery is unrewarding. Transection of the palmar carpal ligament in the palmar carpal joint capsule has been used in the treatment of carpal flexural deformities.[217] It is presumed that the clinical compromise would be significant if an athletic career is envisaged. The same authors also reported on the treatment of a congenital pastern flexural deformity using surgical realignment and arthrodesis of the joint with lag screws.

Acquired Flexural Deformities

PATHOGENESIS

Acquired flexure deformities can be unilateral or bilateral and usually occur as flexural deformities of the distal interphalangeal or metacarpophalangeal joint. The pathogenesis of acquired flexural deformities is frequently related to pain. Any pain in the limb may, potentially, initiate a flexion withdrawal reflex that results in flexor muscle contraction and an altered position of the joint. Pain can arise from physitis, OCD, septic arthritis, soft tissue wounds, or hoof infections, with or without involvement of the distal phalanx. Physitis is commonly observed in animals with flexural deformities. Flexural deformities have also been associated with OCD in the shoulder and stifle joints.

Poor nutritional management often has been incriminated as a cause of flexural deformities in young growing foals. Both overfeeding and imbalanced rations have been implicated.[128,147] Physitis, OCD, and flexural deformities have all been related to intake of excess energy during growth. However, the relationship is not consistent, and evidence that excess energy intake causes flexural deformities in the horse is anecdotal. Associations can be made clinically between increased caloric intake and fetlocks becoming more upright.

In addition to trauma and lack of exercise, another environmental factor that has been suggested is stance. One author has pointed out that young horses place one foot forward and one back when eating from the ground and that the club foot is consistently on the one that is placed back.[18] A genetic predisposition in terms of potential for rapid growth may also be involved. In Denmark, the condition has been noted to occur in foals that are born late in the winter season and are kept inside in stall boxes without the possibility of exercising on the

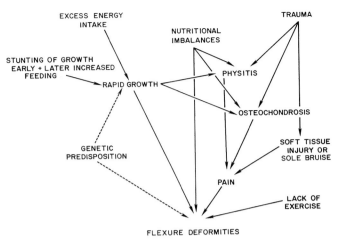

Figure 7.97 Suggested pathogenetic pathways for acquired flexure deformities.

hard surface and stretching the stay apparatus.[186] Suggested pathogenetic pathways for acquired flexural deformities are illustrated in Figure 7.97.

The mechanism by which suggested etiologic factors produce flexural deformities is still uncertain. One author has suggested that rapid bone growth without exercise results in a failure of tendons and ligaments to develop at the same rate as bone lengthening.[147] Flexor muscles are stronger than extensor muscles, and the foal consequently develops a flexural deformity. Another author has related the mechanism of flexural deformity development to discrepancy between bone growth and the capacity for lengthening the check ligaments.[52] These theories are not entirely compatible with our knowledge of bone growth of the distal limbs. Bone growth from the midmetacarpus/metatarsus distad is very limited beyond 2 months of age, and many cases develop after this period.

True tendon contracture of a flexor tendon can occur occasionally following some cases of severe traumatic injury to the tendon and is associated with contraction of fibrous tissue in the reparative process.

CLINICAL MANIFESTATIONS

Clinically, there are two distinct entities. Flexural deformity of the distal interphalangeal (DIP) joint, or so-called DDF contracture, results in a raised heel and a "club foot" (Fig. 7.98). For purposes of prognosis and therapy evaluation, this deformity has been subdivided into stages 1 and 2.[127] Stage 1 contracture is when the dorsal surface of the hoof does not pass beyond vertical (Fig. 7.99). When the dorsal surface of the hoof passes beyond vertical, the situation is classified as stage 2 (Fig. 7.100). The primary abnormality with flexural deformity of the DIP joint appears to be a relative shortening of the DDF musculotendinous unit. However, once the problem has progressed to a stage 2 contracture, pathologic changes develop in the joint capsule and other tissues of the coffin joint, resulting in an irreversible state of fibrous ankylosis if not treated promptly. Radiographic changes in the distal phalanx have been correlated with

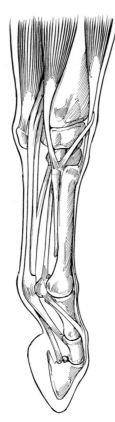

Figure 7.98 Diagram of flexure deformity of distal interphalangeal (coffin) joint.

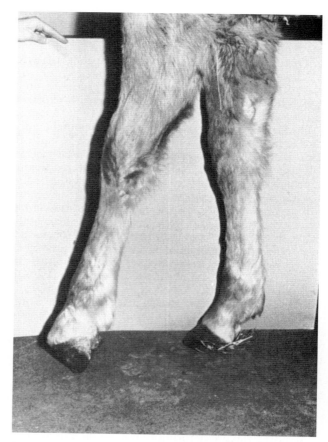

Figure 7.100 Stage 2 acquired flexure deformity of distal interphalangeal joint.

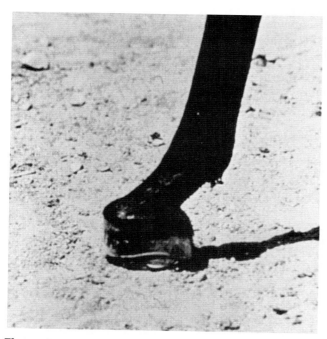

Figure 7.99 Acquired flexure deformity of distal interphalangeal joint (stage 1). The elongated heel gives the typical "club-foot" appearance.

clinical severity in nine foals with flexural deformity of the DIP. Varying degrees of osteolysis in the distal part of the distal phalanx were observed,[5] and the foals with the most pronounced clinical signs also displayed the most prominent radiologic changes.

Flexural deformities of the DIP joint may occur rapidly over 3 to 5 days, so that the heel of the hoof rises off the ground, causing the foal to walk on the toe. In more slowly developing cases, the heel maintains contact with the ground and grows excessively long. Hooves of this deformity have been termed club feet or boxy feet. The coronary band may also appear prominent in horses with club feet.[3] Deformity of the dorsal hoof wall with dishing and distraction of the sensitive and insensitive laminae may occur in longstanding disease, and this in turn may lead to seedy toe and toe abscesses. Because osteitis and remodeling of the distal phalanx can also occur, radiographs of the foot should be taken as part of the evaluation.

The other clinical entity, flexural deformity of the fetlock joint, has been classically referred to as contracture of the superficial digital flexor (SDF) tendon. It is characterized by knuckling at the fetlock with the hoof itself remaining in normal alignment (Figs 7.101 and 7.102). These cases should be called fetlock flexural deformities or metacarpophalangeal flexure deformities (the clinical problems are usually in the forelimbs), as the term SDF contracture is a gross oversimplification. The angle of

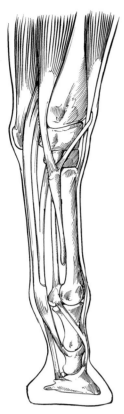

Figure 7.101   Diagram of flexure deformity of metacarpophalangeal joint. Note that the deep digital flexor tendon has to pass through a shorter distance when the fetlock is in this position.

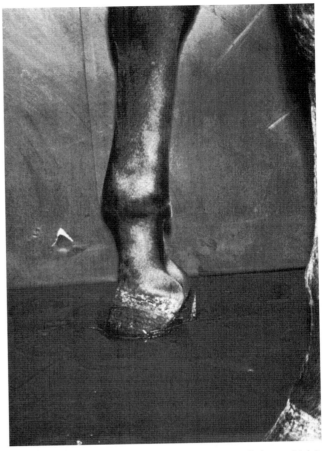

Figure 7.102   Flexure deformity of metacarpophalangeal joint.

the affected joint increases from a normal angle of 135° (measured from the dorsal surface of the limb) to 180° and more. DDF involvement is commonly present in these cases as well, and it would be more appropriate to describe the condition as combined superficial and DDF contracture. In longstanding cases, the suspensory ligament becomes involved secondarily, and osteoarthritic changes occur in the fetlock joint.

Flexural deformities of the DIP joint have been described typically as occurring in foals and weanlings, and flexural deformities at the metacarpophalangeal joints have been considered more typical of 1- to 2-year-old animals.[147] Such a distribution was thought to be related to the suspensory ligament (interosseus medius muscle) losing muscle fiber content and thus elasticity during the first year of life.[172] In foals, the extensor branch of the suspensory ligament stretches and the distal interphalangeal joint flexes under the influence of DDF contracture. After 1 year of age, the extensor branch of the suspensory ligament cannot stretch, and the extensor tendon can only stretch proximal to its junction with the extensor branches of the suspensory ligament. In these cases, fetlock knuckling will occur. Some of these assumptions are controversial, and the sequence of events requires investigation. The relationship between age and the type of flexure deformity is not absolute. Fetlock knuckling does tend to occur in older animals, but flexure deformi-

ties of the DIP joint are also observed in animals over 12 months of age.[127]

In all cases of flexural deformities, careful palpation of the limbs in both the standing and flexed positions to determine which structures are involved is necessary (Fig. 7.103). With flexural deformities of the distal interphalangeal joint, the structures involved are easily ascertained. However, with fetlock flexural deformities, it is important to ascertain which tendon seems to be primarily affected. This decision is very important when selecting treatment.

TREATMENT

Conservative methods of treatment including dietary changes, exercise, and hoof trimming should be used and are appropriate if affected animals are presented early. It is important to check that the patient is on a balanced nutritional regimen. Energy intake should be reduced in rapidly growing foals. Recognition of cases in foals obviously underfed emphasizes that this is not simply an overnutrition disease. The animal should be exercised and anti-inflammatory agents used judiciously if pain is considered to be a cause of the problem.

NONSURGICAL TREATMENT. Animals with flexural deformities of the DIP joint should have the heels trimmed

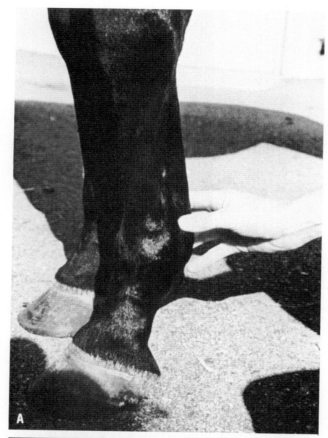

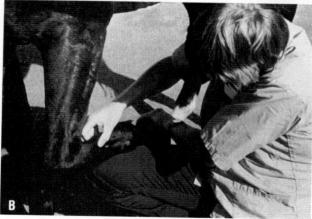

Figure 7.103 Palpation of tendons. A. Standing. B. With the carpus flexed and fetlock extended.

short so that tension is placed on the flexor tendons to induce the inverse myotatic reflex. Hoof trimming works for mild cases. It is important to combine heel trimming with acrylic on the toe when the toe of the hoof is worn, bruised, or deformed. For fetlock flexure deformities, it was generally recommended in the past to raise the heels by corrective shoeing. It was thought that raising the heel creates a relative relaxation of tension in the deep flexor tendon, which in turn leads to selective overloading of the remaining support structures and dropping of the fetlock.[52] Research has indicated that although mean tendon strain in the DDF tendon changes with hoof angle, there is no significant difference in strain in either the SDF tendon or suspensory ligament with changing hoof angle.[111] This finding, coupled with the realization that the DDF tendon is involved in some instances of fetlock flexure deformities, makes rationalization of raising the heel and increasing the hoof angle difficult. However, clinical cases commonly respond to this regimen. A more recent study has confirmed that the use of wedges on the heels produces DDF strain but has very little effect on reducing SDF strain. However, this study did find a dramatic increase in strain on the extensor branch of the suspensory ligament with placement of wedges that raised the hoof beyond 61°.[199] Therefore the author still recommends raising the heels for flexural deformities of the metacarpophalangeal joint.

SURGICAL TREATMENT. Surgical intervention is indicated in cases unresponsive to conservative methods of therapy. Immediate surgical intervention is also indicated on initial presentation of cases when rapid correction of the flexure deformity is necessary to prevent development of permanent degenerative joint changes.

Stage 1 DDF contracture (DIP joint flexure deformity) should be treated by carpal (inferior) check ligament desmotomy (Fig. 7.104). This treatment for flexural deformity of the DIP joint was originally described by Lysholt and Sonnichsen.[115] The value of this technique has been documented in both the European literature[96,108,185,186] and in the United States, initially by McIlwraith and Fessler, with long-term results reported by Wagner et al. in 1985.[127] Normal limb alignment is usually obtained immediately following surgery, but in some cases, flexor relaxation progresses for 7 to 10 days postoperatively as the digital flexor muscles relax in response to increased tensile forces imposed on them after sectioning of the carpal check ligament. Some cases in which the dorsal surface of the hoof is beyond vertical (mild stage 2) may respond to inferior check ligament desmotomy, particularly if a toe extension is applied postoperatively to increase the tensile forces on the deep flexor tendon, but a consistent result cannot be anticipated in all severe cases. Compared with tenotomy of the DDF tendon, inferior check ligament desmotomy causes less postoperative pain and has a superior postoperative appearance, and the long-term functional capability of the operated limb is much improved.[24] It is a safe, effective method of correcting the problem before secondary changes develop. In a long-term follow-up study in 40 horses with flexural deformity of the DIP joint, the condition had been diagnosed and treated in 26 horses before they were 1 year old and 14 horses more than 1 year of age.[215] The former group was classified as acute and the latter one as chronic. Nine months to 4 years after surgery, 35 of 40 horses (24 from the acute group and 11 from the chronic group) were not lame and were being used as athletes. Thirty-three horses were being used for what the owner had intended before the development of the flexural deformity, and 7 were not. Of these 7 horses, 6 had complications related to the deformity and 1 had complications resulting from surgery. The authors pointed out that if surgery and corrective shoeing is undertaken as soon as it is apparent that nonsurgical treatment is not proving successful, the chances for complete success and less scarring are increased. However, surgery and corrective

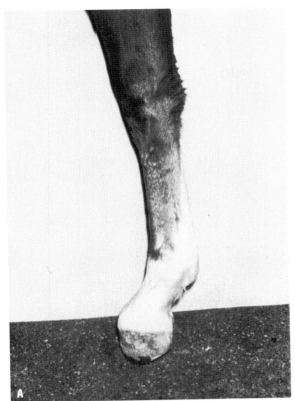
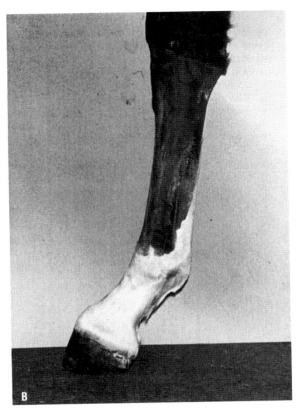

Figure 7.104   Stage 1 flexure of deformity of distal interphalangeal joint before (A) and after (B) carpal (inferior) check desmotomy.

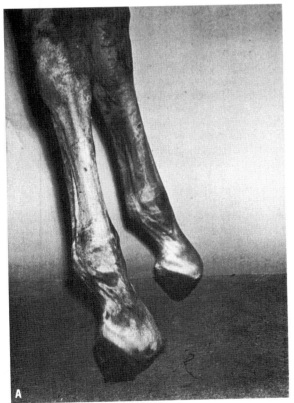
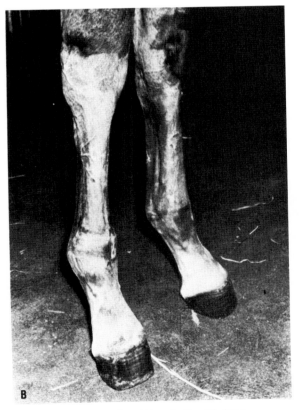

Figure 7.105   Stage 2 flexure deformity of distal interphalangeal deformity before (A) and after (B) deep digital flexor tenotomy.

shoeing still is recommended in chronic cases. An ultrasonically guided technique has also been described.[226]

Deep flexor tenotomy is indicated for severe long-standing cases of DDF contracture (Fig. 7.105), but in others, fibrosis and contraction of the joint capsule and associated ligaments does not permit proper realignment (Fig. 7.106). The cosmetic appearance following tenotomy is sometimes unsatisfactory, and the functional ability of the limb is often limited because of the drastic nature of the surgery. However, satisfactory cosmetic and functional results have been obtained following deep flexor tenotomy (Fig. 7.107). Performing the surgery more distally within the tendon sheath may give a better cosmetic result than the midmetacarpal approach.[54] However, wider separation of the transected tendon ends is of concern with later function. Successful treatment of five type 2 flexural deformities has been reported using inferior check desmotomy alone.[225] Corrective shoeing was also used in all cases. As a generalization, inferior check desmotomy should be attempted initially, even in severe cases. The same author described transection of the inferior check (accessory) ligament of the DDF tendon using an ultrasound-guided technique. A 7.5-MHz transducer was used to observe the dissection and isolation of the check ligament through a 1- to 1.5-cm incision and to check complete transection of the check ligament. The technique was reported effective in correcting flex-

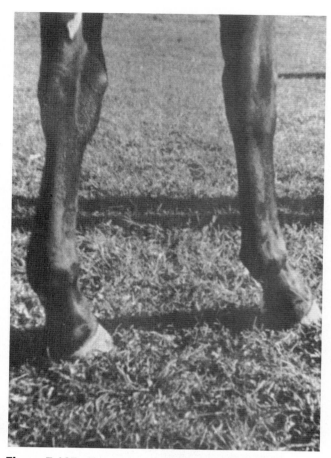

Figure 7.107 Horse 1 year after bilateral deep flexor tenotomy with good cosmetic results (the horse was also sound as a riding animal.)

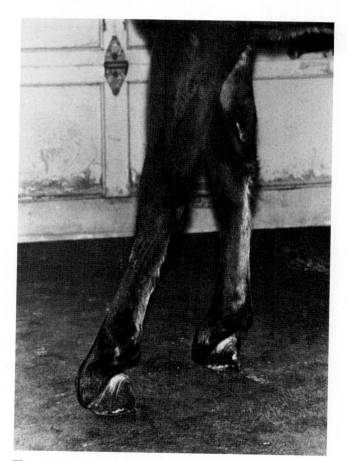

Figure 7.106 Severe flexure deformity of the distal interphalangeal joint not amenable to treatment.

ural deformity of the DIP joint as well as the metacarpophalangeal joint in all but three horses. The author also noted that check ligament desmotomy at a young age (median, 6 months) resulted in more horses with normal foot conformation than surgery completed at an older age (median, 12 months). The author felt that this technique reduced immediate postoperative wound morbidity. There is a smaller incision and reduced closure time because no subcutaneous sutures are used and subjectively less tissue swelling after surgery. An alternative to a tenotomy is a tendon-lengthening procedure. The actual functional differences between these two techniques is uncertain, and the cosmetic appearance does not appear to be significantly better after the tendon-lengthening procedure than after tenotomy.

Although the prognosis for full functional soundness is poor, tendon contracture following severe tendinitis can be treated by tenotomy to restore normal limb alignment.

The results of surgical treatment of flexural deformities of the fetlock joint are less predictable than those for flexure deformities of the DIP joint. A number of surgical treatments are available. If the SDF tendon is the most taut, either superficial flexor tenotomy or radial (superior) check ligament desmotomy may be performed. Superficial flexor tenotomy is simple and not

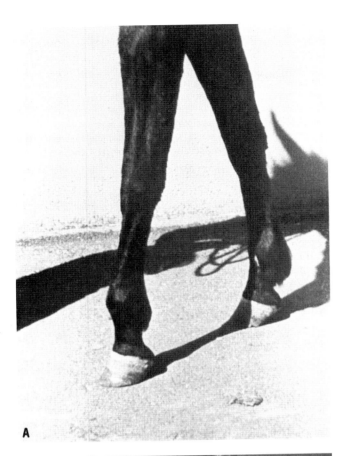

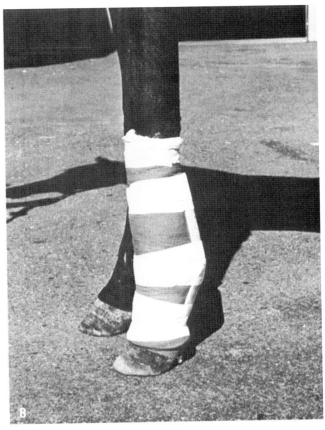

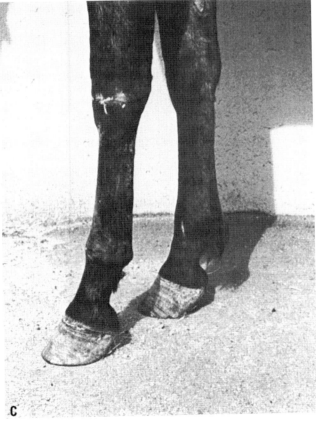

Figure 7.108   Flexure deformity of metacarpophalangeal joint before (A) and after (B) carpal (inferior) check ligament desmotomy and additional splinting. The splint was removed after 10 days with an excellent result (C).

as drastic as deep flexor tenotomy in terms of cosmetic appearance and postoperative functional ability.

However, in many instances, inferior (carpal) check ligament desmotomy has been most useful for the treatment of this condition when the DDF tendon seems the most taut on clinical examination. Following performance of the carpal check ligament desmotomy, a PVC splint is used to hold the fetlock in position as an adjunctive measure (Fig. 7.108). The author has had success with this technique, and it has been reported elsewhere.

Suspensory ligament desmotomy may be considered when the condition is refractory to the previous treatments (Fig. 7.109). The fact that cases of metacarpophalangeal flexural deformity respond to inferior check desmotomy does not imply that shortening of the DDF muscle–tendon unit is the primary event in such a deformity. Although the SDF musculotendinous unit may initiate flexural deformity of the metacarpophalangeal joint, the DDF muscle–tendon unit may shorten secondarily and become the structure that limits return of the fetlock to its normal position.[3] Rarely, the suspensory ligament may be the limiting structure.

In a report of 15 cases in 1985, horses with mild metacarpophalangeal joint flexural deformities were treated

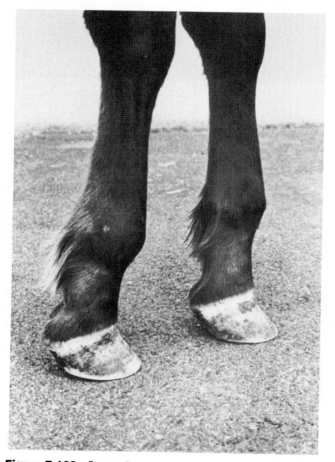

Figure 7.109 Severe flexure deformity of metacarpophalangeal joints that required sectioning of the carpal (inferior) check ligament, superficial digital flexor tendon, and branches of the suspensory ligament to return fetlock to normal position. (Courtesy of T. S. Stashak.)

with corrective trimming and shoeing. Those with moderate deformities were treated with desmotomy of the accessory ligament of the DDF tendon (inferior check ligament) and corrective shoeing, and desmotomies of the accessory ligaments of both DDF and SDF tendons were performed on severely affected horses, followed by corrective shoeing.[216] In this long-term study, four horses with mild lesions and four horses with moderate lesions returned to useful work. None of the horses with severe disease responded enough to withstand strenuous athletic training.

Suspensory ligament contracture may be a final secondary effect of a prolonged flexural deformity of the metacarpophalangeal joint. Probably more often, the failure to respond to other surgical procedures is due to fibrosis and contraction of the fetlock joint capsule, sesamoidean ligaments, and other associated structures in the region. Suspensory ligament desmotomy is a drastic final measure, and subluxation of the proximal interphalangeal joint is a possible sequel. This treatment method should only be performed as a last resort and after clear discussion with the owner.

Rupture of the Common Digital Extensor Tendon

Rupture of the common digital extensor tendon is usually bilateral and is generally present at birth or develops soon after birth.[6,137] Affected foals typically either have carpal flexural deformities with nominally extended fetlocks or have fetlock flexural deformities. (Sometimes flexural deformities may not be noted despite evidence of a ruptured extensor tendon.) The characteristic feature of this condition is the presence of swelling over the dorsolateral aspect of the carpus (Fig. 7.110). Depending on the amount of synovial fluid present in the synovial sheath of the common digital extensor tendon, it may or may not be possible to palpate the enlarged ends of the ruptured tendon. Commonly, the ruptured common digital extensor tendon is not recognized, and the problem is diagnosed as flexor tendon contracture.

Rupture of the common digital extensor tendon may be accompanied by contracture of the flexor tendons (Fig. 7.111). It is difficult to decide if the extensor tendon rupture occurs secondary to flexor contracture in these cases or if flexor contracture occurs secondary to the extensor tendon rupture. It is considered that most often the extensor tendon rupture is a primary condition, but I have observed extensor tendon rupture actually occurring when a fetlock flexure deformity was already present. Affected foals may have associated birth defects including prognathism, underdeveloped pectoral muscles, and incomplete ossification of the carpal bones.[137] The implication here is that the common digital extensor tendon rupture may be part of a complex of congenital defects.

TREATMENT

If associated contracture of the flexor tendons is not present, some foals recover spontaneously with stall rest. The use of protective bandaging is indicated to prevent abrasive damage to the dorsum of the fetlock. If the foal is knuckling over at the fetlock, the use of PVC splinting

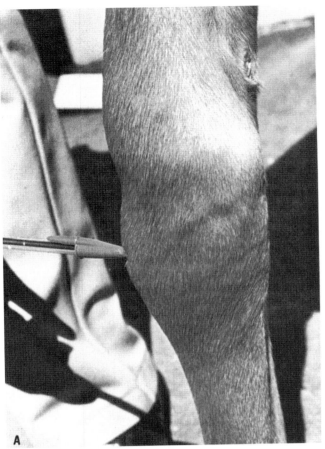

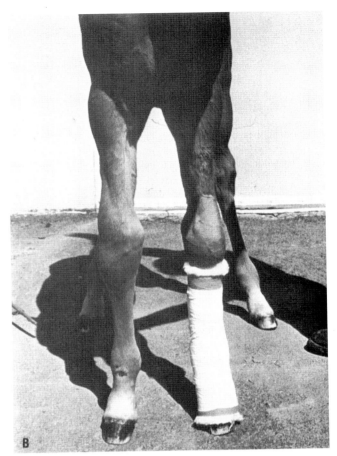

Figure 7.110 Rupture of the common digital extensor tendon. A. Note the bulge created by the swollen end of the distal part of the tendon. B. This patient had a carpal flexure deformity as well as knuckling over at the left fetlock, for which it was splinted.

is recommended (see the congenital flexure deformities section in this chapter). If delayed or incomplete ossification of the carpal bones is also present, tube casts (described above) should be applied. If there are associated fetlock flexure deformities that cannot be manually straightened and maintained in alignment with PVC splinting, full-length casts can be applied.

The prognosis for rupture of the common digital extensor unaccompanied by flexor tendon contracture is good. When contracture of the flexor tendons is also present, the prognosis is guarded.

Dorsal Subluxation of the Proximal Interphalangeal Joint in the Pelvic Limb

Dorsal subluxation of the proximal interphalangeal joint (pastern joint) in the pelvic limbs is a relatively rare disorder in young horses with straight legs. The condition usually occurs bilaterally and is recognized by the dorsal displacement of the proximal interphalangeal joint of the affected limb when it is non-weight-bearing. The subluxation is reduced as weight is borne by the limb, and an audible clicking sound often accompanies the reduction of the joint.[179]

The condition can cause lameness, but the severity of the lameness produced is inconsistent. The lameness may range from a stilted gait to one resembling that of a horse with azoturia.[114] It has also been suggested that dorsal subluxation of the proximal interphalangeal joint of the pelvic limb may represent a form of DDF tendon contracture.

Three cases have been described in one paper, and they were bilateral. Straighter than normal stifles and hocks were noted. A 5-month-old male Quarter Horse had radiographic changes of subluxation as well as minor periarticular spurring on the dorsoproximal aspect of the second phalanx. The heels were trimmed, and after 14 days without a response, bilateral tendinectomy of the medial head of the DDF was performed. Clinical improvement was seen 1 day after surgery, and at 10 months follow-up, the horse was sound. The second case was a 2-year-old female Arabian horse with a history of having had the problem for a year. It was also treated with bilateral tendinectomy of the medial head of the DDF tendon, as was a third case involving a unilateral subluxation problem.

The authors of this paper felt that the condition could possibly be caused by DDF tendon contraction with concomitant laxity of the SDF tendon. The proximal interphalangeal joint is normally prevented from dorsal subluxation through tension applied at the plantar insertions of the SDF tendon and the extensor branches

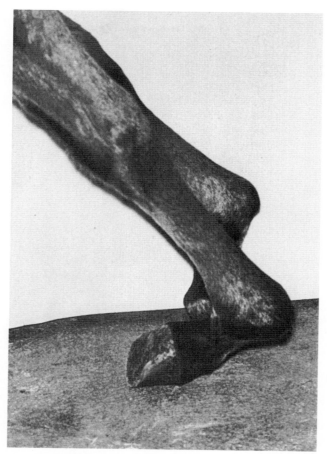

Figure 7.111 Severe fetlock flexure deformity associated with rupture of the common digital extensor tendon.

ular structure is a vestige of the third interosseous muscle rather than a true ligament.

Definitions

Tendinitis is inflammation of tendon and tendon muscle attachments. In the horse it refers specifically to inflammation of the flexor tendons due to excessive strain. The term "tendinitis," used correctly, applies to strain-induced inflammation involving tendon that is surrounded by paratendon and not tendon sheath. If the region of involved tendon is associated with a tendon sheath the term "tendosynovitis" is used (the term "adhesive tendosynovitis" could also be used). Tenosynovitis implies inflammation of the tendon sheath alone and is considered separately below. As noted above, inflammation of a ligament is referred to as "desmitis," and therefore, injury to the suspensory ligament is referred to as "suspensory ligament desmitis."

Tendinitis of the flexor tendons, tenosynovitis, suspensory desmitis, and desmitis of the inferior check ligament are discussed separately.

Tendinitis of the Flexor Tendons

Flexor tendinitis in general and tendinitis of the SDF tendon in particular are common causes of lameness in racehorses as well as other athletic horses. Lesions can range from minor tearing to complete tendon rupture. The SDF tendon of the forelimbs is the most frequently affected site. Similar lesions also occur in the DDF tendon, suspensory ligament, and carpal (distal accessory) check ligament.[78,79] Tendinitis results in high morbidity, with prolonged periods out of work. It has been estimated to affect at least 30% of the horses in training for the national hunt in Europe.[78] Knowledge of the pathogenesis is somewhat limited despite its clinical importance.

Lesions are generally localized to the core of the midmetacarpal region of the SDF in the forelimb and typically appear on ultrasound examination as an anechoic or hypoechoic core surrounded by tissue of normal appearance.[71] Standardbreds appear to have a higher incidence of injuries in the suspensory ligament and it is felt that this difference in predilection site may be explained by an analysis of the functional load distribution between the flexor structures of different gaits and in association with different locomotor demands.[230] At the gallop, as the forelimb contacts the ground, the fetlock is hyperextended, and the flexor tendons placed under very high tensile loads.[78] To maximize the energy stored, the tendons elongate to a point close to failure, and it is thought that this may account for the relatively high incidence of injury during athletic activity. Recent studies have shown that the strain magnitudes in the SDF tendon of a galloping Thoroughbred are about 16%.[189] In vitro studies have shown that with loading of an equine SDF tendon, there is a nonlinear toe region that represents straightening of crimps in the collagen fibers and strains of about 3%. This is elastically recoverable, and removal of the load results in reestablishment of the length and angle of the crimp.[32] Other investigators found that the crimp in the central region of the SDF tendon straightens before that in the peripheral area in older horses, suggesting that this region of the tendon is predisposed to fail-

of the suspensory ligament as well as some stability being provided by the fibrous layer of the joint capsule. The DDF muscle of the horse has three heads: the lateral head, the medial head, and the caudal tibial muscle. The small caudal tibial muscle and tendon are fused with the large lateral head and both pass through the tarsal canal. However, the medial head is smaller and more tendinous and goes past the tarsus to form a combined tendon of the DDF distal to the tarsus.

Traumatic Problems of Tendons and Ligaments

Strain

Strain has been defined as damage to a tendon or muscle caused by overuse or overstress.[1] Strain of a tendon can range from minor inflammation to disruption of the tendon or avulsion of the tendon from its bony attachment. There are various specific entities in the horse that could be classified as strains, and they are described separately. Tendinitis or tendosynovitis may range from a simple to a severe strain. Rupture of a tendon is obviously a severe strain. Stress injuries of the suspensory ligament are also classified as strains because this partic-

ure.[229] As loading takes the tendon beyond the nonlinear toe region, the tendon itself becomes more resistant to elongation, and a linear stress–strain relationship is seen up to the yield point when loss of linearity is seen, and it is probably associated with slippage of microfibrils and tropocollagen units. The entire tendon fails ultimately, and studies with the SDF tendon of the horse report that this occurs at a strain of 12 to 20%.[168,234] When this is compared with strain magnitudes recorded in a galloping Thoroughbred of about 16%, the safety margin at peak performance is very small, which is presumed to be a factor in the high incidence of SDF tendon injury.

There is a smaller cross-sectional area in the metacarpal region of the SDF tendon, and although it is likely that the metacarpal region contains proportionately more longitudinal load-bearing collagen fibers than other sites, this "stronger" composition is not enough to compensate for a smaller cross-sectional area.[36] Also comparison of collagen fibril populations in the SDF tendon of exercised and nonexercised Thoroughbreds has shown reduction in fibril diameter in the central region of the SDF tendon in association with exercise. This was considered evidence of microtrauma, as it implies that the region is weakened by the training regimen.[152] It was felt that repeated episodes of microtrauma may accumulate and eventually result in degenerative lesions and clinical tendinitis. Other work by this group in young Thoroughbreds with a specific 18-month exercise program confirmed that there was a significantly lower collagen fibril crimp angle and period length in the core region of the SDF tendon than in control horses. Crimp angle was also significantly lower in the central region than in the peripheral region in four of the five exercised horses. Separate research has shown that fibril bundles with a smaller crimp angle fail at a lower level of strain than those with a larger crimp angle, so these investigators felt that the results supported previous evidence that galloping exercise modifies normal age-related changes in crimp morphology in the core of the SDF tendon and that such changes indicate microtrauma and would be detrimental to tendon strength.[151] Although suspensory ligament desmitis and SDF tendinitis occur with approximately equal frequencies in the forelimbs of Standardbreds, MADs did not change significantly with exercise for either the DDF tendon or the suspensory ligament in young Thoroughbreds subjected to a treadmill exercise regimen. The authors concluded that between the trot and the gallop, loading of the suspensory ligament does not increase to the same extent as that of the SDF tendon. That only the SDF tendon shows evidence of microtrauma indicated to the authors that the SDF tendon is preferentially loaded at the gallop.[152] They did acknowledge that another possibility is that strain-induced microtrauma occurs in the suspensory ligament of the DDF tendon in response to training but at different sites. Central zone tissue from this SDF also has a significantly higher proportion of type III collagen than the peripheral zone of the SDF tendon.[23] The highest level of type III collagen was also found in the central zone tissue of the SDF tendon from older horses, and the authors felt that this may represent the early stages of a degenerative change. The SDF tendon has more type III collagen, more mature trifunctional collagen cross-link hydroxylysyl pyridinoline, lower total chondroitin sulfate–equivalent GAG content, smaller-diameter collagen fibers, and a higher cellularity than the DDF tendon.

Other studies in vivo have shown that the SDF tendon bears the load in the early part of the weight-bearing phase of gait, before the load is shared with the DDF tendon, and the rate of rise in load is greater in the SDF tendon.[159] Also, in an extended trot, the suspensory ligament is loaded preferentially in the initial part of the stance phase. Such differences in functional loading may explain the incidence of lesions in the SDF of racehorses and the suspensory ligament of trotters. Peak loads occur in the DDF only at the later stage of the gait cycle, and rate of loading is low, which may account for the low incidence of lesions in this tendon.

Goodship et al.[79] pointed out that when postmortem tendons are stretched to rupture in the laboratory they often show a characteristic pattern of failure, with the central fibers failing first, just as in clinical injuries. It has been suggested that the central core of the tendon undergoes degeneration which then predisposes the tendon to subsequent breakdown, but factors responsible for such changes are poorly understood. It is not uncommon to find a discoloration in the central core of otherwise apparently normal tendons, and it has been suggested that this may represent an early lesion that cannot be detected by current diagnostic procedures. An increase in core temperature of the tendon during high-intensity exercise has been suggested as a factor.[232,233] In vivo studies have shown that the central core of the SDF tendon has a temperature rise to about 45°C during a 7-minute gallop, whereas the temperature on the surface of the tendon is some 10°C lower.[235] It was suggested that local thermal effects result in cell death or impaired metabolism of tenocytes in the central core of tendons, used in storage of elastic energy. These authors also feel that the peak temperatures recorded in vivo are above those reported to have caused fibroblast death in vitro.[232] Goodship et al.[232] have suggested that these temperatures in the core of the tendon could cause cell necrosis followed by a repair process, resulting in increased type III collagen and an elevated GAG content (the latter two events have been reported by Birch et al.[22]).

It has often been stated that tendons in general and the SDF tendon in particular have a poor blood supply and so factors that could cause hypoxia could be critical. Reperfusion injury has also been suggested as a possible factor.[78]

People have debated in the past whether tendinitis of the SDF tendon results from a single episode in which nonphysiologic strain is suddenly imposed upon a normal tendon or from multiple episodes of submaximal strain sustained during athletic performance that induced microdamage in tendon structure that predisposed the tendon to mechanical failure. Work accumulates indicating that microdamage is a real primary phenomenon. In an ideal world, definition of training regimens that do not adversely affect central region crimp morphology, collagen type change, collagen fibril diameter, and heat-induced necrosis as well as identification of individuals that are less susceptible to these effects would assist in preventing SDF tendinitis.

Following injury, the repair process in tendon follows the same basic pattern seen in other tissues in the body.

After fibril disruption, there is hemorrhage and formation of intratendinous hematoma with resulting swelling and inflammation. After the initial inflammatory process and removal of damaged tissue by cells of the body, scar formation occurs. In the new scar tissue, the collagen initially is immature and arranged in a haphazard architecture composed predominantly of type III collagen and with small diameter fibrils. With maturation, fibril diameter increases as do the number of stable chemical cross-links together with the proportion of type I collagen. However, this process takes weeks to months to complete, and the original strength of the tendon is never restored.[79] The initial haphazard arrangement of collagen fibers may be modified as functional loading is restored, resulting in a return toward parallel alignment.

The author finds it interesting that microdamage preceding macrodamage in tendons so parallels what we feel is happening in articular cartilage and bone of the equine athlete.

DIAGNOSIS

Diagnostic advances, particularly with ultrasonography, have greatly enhanced our ability to diagnose and define the extent of damage in tendon and ligament injuries. However, the basic clinical evaluation remains an essential part of the lameness diagnosis and prognosis. Typically the horse with flexor tendinitis is presented because of local signs of swelling, distension, thickening, and heat with lameness. Astute grooms will notice localizing signs before any lameness has been observed. Severe tendon injuries are easily recognized clinically. Swelling, heat, and pain on palpation are apparent after exercise. Lameness varies from mild to moderate and generally resolves in a few days with rest and appropriate therapy. Subclinical tendon injuries are less easily recognized and require careful diligent observation of the tendons after exercise. If there is major disruption of tendon fibers, the fetlock cannot be "dropped."

The chronic stage is manifested by fibrosis and hard swelling on the palmar or plantar aspect (Fig. 7.112). The use of diagnostic ultrasonography enables accurate determination of the extent and location of the lesions. Tendonography has been used (single- or double-contrast studies) for further definition of change within the tendon sheaths, but ultrasonography has superseded most of these studies. In the case of pathologic change within a tendon sheath, diagnostic tenoscopy is the main diagnostic modality above and beyond ultrasonography. Technical details on ultrasonography of tendons and ligaments is beyond the scope of this chapter. The general principles of ultrasonography of the suspected areas include transverse and longitudinal–linear ultrasound scans. The size of both the tendons and the lesions can be measured. Loss of the normal intense echogenicity can be caused by fibrillar disruption and inflammatory processes (hemorrhage, edema, and cellular infiltration in the early stages). The reader is referred to texts on ultrasonography[163] and Chapter 4 for more information.

A consistent relationship between the ultrasonographic and histologic findings was demonstrated in a series of injured SDF tendons compared with normals.[121] The echogenicity of lesions, the distinctness of their de-

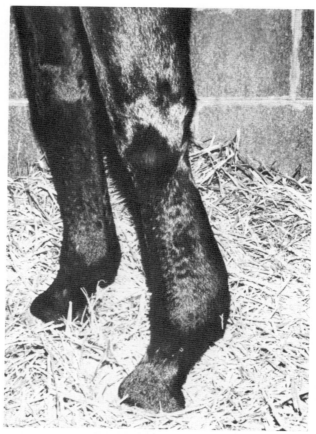

Figure 7.112 Tendinitis of the superficial digital flexor tendon ("bowed tendon").

lineation from the surrounding tissue, and presence and arrangement of the linear echoes were useful features for assessing the ultrasonogram. Acute lesions were anechoic, a complex mixture of anechoic and hypoechoic, or diffusely hypoechoic. These appearances represented hemorrhage, fibrolysis, and early granulation tissue. Fibroplasia and granulation tissue produced well- to moderately well–defined hypoechoic lesions. Chronic fibrosis was characterized by heterogeneously echogenic areas that were poorly defined from the surrounding tissue and had irregularly arranged linear echoes on longitudinal images. Intratendinous scar formation resulted in multiple hyperechoic foci. Extensive peritendinous lesions were readily apparent on ultrasonographs, but intertendinous adhesions were more difficult to assess and produced dual definition of the borders between the SDF and DDF tendons.

In another study, six horses with acute (≤2 weeks), six with healing (>2 weeks and ≤1 year), and six with chronic inactive ("set") bowed tendons (>1 year) were evaluated. The lesion and the tendon were measured every 2 cm throughout the length of the SDF tendon and were characterized ultrasonographically at each location.[164] The tendons were subsequently evaluated grossly and histopathologically at each of the previously scanned locations and the findings compared. There was excellent correlation between the location, extent, size, and ultrasonographic characterization of the lesion and its gross and histopathologic appearance. Anechoic areas (type IV) represented areas of recent hemorrhage. The hypoechoic areas (types II and III) corresponded to areas of granulation tissue and immature fibrous tissue. Areas of maturing fibrous tissue with collagen (type I) were more echogenic. Details of grading of lesions and quantitative assessment are provided by Genovese and Rantanen.[70] Another study showed that quantitative sonographic assessment using a systematic routine evaluation can provide objectivity for clinical information and improve the ability to render an accurate prognosis.[69] It has also been recognized that the mean gray scale of the DDF tendons and accessory ligament is significantly reduced when a horse is non-weight-bearing compared with when weight-bearing (the density of the suspensory ligament is not).[140] This obviously needs to be noticed when one is making quantitative assessments of density. The technique needs to be consistent, as minor changes in transducer placement and tilt can result in marked changes in gray-level statistics.

TREATMENT

Treating tendinitis of the SDF tendon can be extremely frustrating because of the difficulty in restoring previous structure and function of the tendon. Even when healing has occurred, there is the potential for reinjury, and loss of function remains. As with any condition that does not have a consistently successful treatment, a wide variety of treatments are used to try to modulate repair and enhance the rate and quality of repair after an acute injury. The goals of therapy for acute tendinitis are to decrease inflammation, to minimize scar tissue formation, and to promote restoration of normal tendon structure and function.

Experimental models of injured ligaments have shown that ice application decreases inflammation in injured ligamentous tissue while causing increased subcutaneous swelling, but the latter response can be handled satisfactorily with pressure bandaging.[56] Bandaging is used between treatments. This regimen can be followed by immobilization using either a plaster cast or soft casting (Jello cast), depending on the severity of the case. Initial therapy is aimed at decreasing inflammation and edema. It is important to reduce inflammation in the collagen fibers and matrix that surround the initial lesion. This is usually accomplished with a combination of local and systemic anti-inflammatory treatments. Cold hydrotherapy, ice packs, or an ice-water slurry is used to minimize hemorrhage and edema (which can exacerbate fiber disruption and later scarring). Ice-water slurries appear to deep-cool tissues more rapidly than ice or cold water alone. Cold application is generally done in the first 48 hours after injury, three to four times a day for no longer than 30 minutes. Longer exposure to cold has been shown to cause reflex vasodilation.

Topical medications that have been used include DMSO. Use of this medication is logical because of its antiedema and free radical scavenging properties as well as vasodilatory properties. The systemic NSAID used most commonly is phenylbutazone, although Banamine may be used initially because of its more immediate effect. Corticosteroids have been used systemically and locally. Although they have potent anti-inflammatory effects and therefore have potential benefit, studies have shown steroids to be detrimental to tendon repair by inhibiting fibroplasia as well as collagen and GAG synthesis.[84] In addition, injection of corticosteroids into normal tendons has been shown to cause collagen fiber necrosis, cellular death, and dystrophic calcification, and their use should probably be avoided.

Complete rupture of the SDF tendon is a career-ending event. Future gliding function is of minimal consequence, and a cast would be applied for 4 to 6 weeks, followed by support bandaging and a slow return to walking. It usually takes 10 to 12 weeks before the tendon is strong enough to accommodate pasture exercise.[148] Less severe tendon injuries are generally simply supported with a bandage. An obviously important part of treating tendinitis is rest, but appropriate return to exercise can help stimulate collagen fiber alignment. Slight tension on an injured tendon in the early phase of healing may help align fibrous strands in the early inflammatory coagulum and promote proper alignment of new collagen as well as inhibit adhesion formation.

Other medical treatments used in the management of tendinitis include HA and PSGAGs. Evidence for the value of HA is controversial. A clinical study of 81 tendon injuries assessed by clinical examination, thermography, diagnostic ultrasonography, and radiography and followed up from 3 to 10 months (the medication was injected into the damaged part of the tendon) found 77.8% recovered, 12.4% improved, 4.9% unsuccessful, and 4.9% recurrence. The authors concluded that they had a practical and successful therapy that might be superior to conventional methods.[87] On the other hand, controlled data have not demonstrated efficacy. A controlled study using collagenase-induced superficial flexor tendinitis in horses and 40-mg injections of sodium hyaluronate subcutaneously over an area 3.5 cm proximal to, and 3.5 cm distal to, the measured midpoint of the treatment limb 24 hours after collagenase injection did not reveal significant benefits of treatment. Horses were evaluated clinically, ultrasonographically, and the tendons were evaluated biomechanically and biochemically. There were, however, trends toward less lameness in treated limbs and better healing on ultrasonographic examination in control limbs.[59]

In another experiment with collagenase-induced SDF tendinitis and sequential intratendinous administration of HA, no significant differences in size of tendon lesions, tendon enlargement, lameness, or tendon healing were detected between tendons that received HA and control tendons.[62] In another study in which adhesion formation between the DDF tendon and tendon sheath in the pastern region and collagenase-induced tendinitis induced in the deep flexor tendon, 120 mg of sodium hyaluronate injected into the tendon sheath improved tendon healing ultrasonographically, and there were considered to be fewer and smaller adhesions on gross pathologic examination in limbs treated with HA. HA and control limbs did not differ significantly in pullout strength. Histologically, the HA-treated DDF tendons had less inflammatory change.[63] In an experimental study in rabbits, high-molecular-weight HA injected IA produced more pronounced repair, with increased antiangiogenesis and less inflammatory response. Biochemical analysis revealed a mean higher value of type III collagen in the HA-treated cases.[227] HA has also been used to aid ligamentous healing.[228]

PSGAGs have been used in the treatment of tendinitis. They have to benefit the acute stages of tendinitis,[81] reducing inflammation and stimulating collagen synthesis by fibroblasts. The authors recommended treatment within 28 to 48 hours, administered either perilesionally (250 mg in 1 mL) or intramuscularly at a dose of 500 mg. They recommend treatment every 4 days up to seven doses, and this is combined with a graded exercise program. In a clinical trial, 90 horses were treated by 30 independent practices, and initial results were encouraging. Rapid reduction in pain and swelling is reported by the third injection, and most veterinarians reported that the drug provided a better than expected outcome. Obviously, more objective analysis is necessary.[81] Clinical evaluation in a small number of performance horses with injuries to the SDF tendon indicated that treatment with PSGAG was more successful in allowing horses to return to work than conservative or laser therapy, but fewer than 50% of the horses were able to race, and there was a higher injury recurrence rate with PSGAGs.[120] In a study by Redding, horses with collagenase-induced lesions were treated systemically with PSGAG in the acute phase and reexamined at 8 weeks. The tendons of the PSGAG-treated horses showed significantly greater improvement than those of nontreated controls.[163a] This drug may be effective if used in the acute phase of a tendon injury.

The most recent nonsurgical treatment is the use of β-aminoproprionitrile fumarate (BAPN; Baptan). It is hypothesized that BAPN treatment diminishes the number of immature collagen cross-links in the repair tissue, and this in turn promotes more rapid longitudinal organization of the collagen fibers within the tendon. Baptan is injected intralesionally. Use of the drug has been recommended between 10 and 30 days postinjury. Intralesional treatments are administered every other day for five treatments. A carefully designed exercise program is an important aspect of the drug's action because cross-linking is delayed for approximately 30 days while the collagen scar remodels along the lines of stress into axial alignment of the fibers. It has been stated that the result is an improved quality of repair. In one report, Baptan-treated horses were compared with a similar group of conventionally treated horses and analyzed. At least 80% of the Baptan-treated horses showed a 76 to 100% increase in echogenicity, with a return toward normal echogenicity and consistent axial alignment of fibers. In the control group only 29% attained the same quality of repair. It was stated that in addition to the return to normal echogenicity of the treated lesions at 20 weeks, there also was a consistent sonographic alignment of fibers.[148] Genovese reported that an intralesional injection of Baptan resulted in more rapid improvement in the ultrasonographic appearance of an injured tendon than other methods of therapy.[67] Affected tendons were injected every other day for 10 days and ultrasonographically evaluated over a 19-week period. The sonograms were evaluated by assigning a severity rating to the tendon lesion, which consisted of a quantitative assessment of lesion grade and size. At all time periods, the Baptan-treated tendons had a greater reduction in severity score than tendons treated by various other methods. Reef et

al. reported on the initial long-term results of horses with SDF tendinitis treated with intralesional Baptan in 1997. They concluded that the administration of 7 to 8 mg of Baptan intralesionally results in a statistically significant lower tendon cross-sectional area and a better fiber alignment score than those of placebo-treated tendons. The use of Baptan 1 to 3 months postinjury results in better quality tendon repair with an improved chance of the horse returning successfully to racing. Ninety-nine horses with a recent injury (1 to 4 months) to the SDF in one or both forelimbs were treated with a 7- or 8-mg dose of intralesional Baptan (84 horses) or placebo (15 horses). A horse was classified as a success (group 1) if the it had returned to racing and had completed at least five races within the 2.5 years following treatment. A horse was classified as a partial success if the horse returned to racing within 2.5 years following treatment of a tendon injury but raced fewer than five times. Long-term follow-up data indicated a more successful return to performance; more horses receiving Baptan returned to racing than those treated conservatively, and a greater number of these horses were able to race or compete at least five times without reinjury of the injured tendon or sustaining an injury to the contralateral tendon. Overall, the horses treated with the 7- or 8-mg dose of intralesional Baptan that returned to racing had more severe injuries than the placebo-treated horses that returned to racing. Also, the horses that were treated with Baptan and were successful at starting at least five more times had more severe injuries than the horses that received the placebo and were similarly successful.[165]

Although this treatment presents a novel approach to the management of tendinitis, some issues still need to be addressed to establish its long-term efficacy. The early Baptan-induced reduction in collagen cross-linking might render wound collagen more susceptible to enzymatic degradation and potentially favor the removal of collagen. A reduction in collagen content of the wound certainly would decrease the rate of gain of strength of the repair tissue and possibly slow the overall healing process. Stable cross-link formation depends on prior formation of reducible cross-links.[86,143] The effect that Baptan may have on the formation of stable cross-links and on the strength of the healed tendon, therefore, is an important issue, especially in the athlete. The wound recovery period after withdrawal of Baptan therapy should be investigated. The effect of Baptan on collagen type in the wound is another issue.

Electrical and electromagnetic stimulations have been proposed as treatment for tendon injury. In a controlled study on healing of surgically created defects in equine SDF tendons in the horse, exposure to pulsed electromagnetic field therapy for 2 hours daily significantly delayed the maturation of the tissue formed within the defect at postsurgical weeks 8 and 12 as determined by histologic examination; transformation to type III collagen was also delayed but not to a significant degree.[220] An in vitro whole-tendon culture study assessed the effect of direct current electricity on healing (rabbit deep flexor tendons). Tendons through which a continuous 7-μA current was passed at the repair site were compared with nonstimulated controls and the incorporation of [^{14}C]proline and its conversion to [^{14}C]hydroxyproline measured at 10 days. The mean [^{14}C]proline and

[^{14}C]hydroxyproline activities were 91 and 255% greater, respectively, in the stimulated group. The activity was also higher in the stimulated group by 42 days.[139] Histologic sections showed that intrinsic tenoblastic repair could be enhanced with electrical stimulation in vitro. As yet, the author is unaware of any such modality that has definitively demonstrated tendon repair enhancement. The use of ionizing radiation[61] and ultrasonic therapy[135,136] has also been described.

Low-level laser therapy (also called soft or cold laser therapy) has also been used. Experimental studies have not substantiated clinical claims of benefit. Kaneps et al. found no benefit from laser irradiation of skin and tendon wounds in horses.[100] Maar found that laser therapy for SDF tendinitis resulted in a 50% return to training, 30% return to racing, and 20% injury recurrence rate in a group of national hunt racehorses.[120] The differences were not statistically significant, but the results were not as favorable as those in a group of horses treated conservatively.

Rooney and Genovese published a clinical survey of the tendons of 1087 racehorses that they followed during a 9-month race meet. Thirteen percent of horses competing sustained a tendon injury, and 48% of horses with previously injured tendons reinjured their tendons.[172a]

Dyson reported on a study comparing the incidence of reinjury in horses with tendinitis of the SDF tendon and treated conservatively (controlled exercise), with intralesional sodium hyaluronate, with intralesional and systemic PSGAG, or by systemic administration alone of a PSGAG. The study also gave an opportunity to compare the rate of reinjury in horses used for different athletic purposes.[45] Fifty horses were treated conservatively and were advised to follow a controlled exercise program. This program did not start cantering exercise until 12 to 16 months after injury, depending on the ultrasonographic appearance of the tendons. Fifty horses (group B) were treated by intralesional injection of high-molecular-weight sodium hyaluronate (2 mL). Twenty horses (group C1) received intralesional PSGAG (500 mg) and seven intramuscular injections at 5-day intervals. Thirty horses (group C2) received seven intramuscular injections of PSGAG at 5-day intervals. Transverse and longitudinal images before treatment and at 3-month intervals after treatment until 12 to 15 months after treatment were made. The fiber pattern and longitudinal images were graded 9, 12, and 15 months after injury (grade 1 had 75 to 100% of fibers in parallel alignment; grade 2, 50 to 75% of fibers; and grade 3, less than 50%). There was no difference in the incidence of recurrence of SDF tendinitis in horses treated conservatively and those treated with either HA or PSGAG. There was a higher incidence of reinjury in horses with a previous tendon injury. The incidence of reinjury was directly related to tendon healing as graded ultrasonographically. The incidence of reinjury was highest in racehorses and in horses used for either 3-day event horse trials or dressage.

Surgical Techniques for the Treatment of SDF Tendinitis

The surgical technique of longitudinal tendon splitting was first advocated to promote vascularization and consequent healing to the injured tendon. The first technique involving a complete longitudinal incision was described by Asheim in 1964.[7] Good revascularization and regeneration of tendon tissue was reported. A percutaneous fanning technique was later developed to minimize the peritendinous adhesions noticed following Asheim's technique.[8,104,141,142] Favorable clinical results have been advocated, but the rationale of the technique was disputed by a study that showed that surgical splitting of normal tendons diminished the vascularity.[193,194] Ultrasonographic examination of tendons has shown that many cases of acute tendinitis have core lesions and these central core lesions persisted for several months. It was theorized that tendon splitting during the early phase of tendinitis would decrease the size of the core lesions and promote more rapid revascularization and subsequent repair of the injured area of the tendon. A study of tendon splitting on experimentally induced acute equine tendinitis revealed a significantly lower mean tendon lesion area ultrasonographically in the split tendons than in the controls at weeks 3, 4, and 8.[85] Mean lesion grade was lower in the split tendon at weeks 2, 3, 4, and 8. The findings suggested that during the time period of the study, tendon splitting results in a more rapid decrease in lesion size and superior repair tissue organization than in controls.[84] Histologic examination confirmed more normal collagen orientation and wave formation in the repair tissue than in the split tendons at weeks 4 and 8. A clinical study demonstrated that surgical splitting of acutely to subacutely injured tendons that contained core lesions led to a significant reduction in lesion size, tendon diameter, and lesion grade within 8 to 12 weeks after surgery. Long-term follow-up of many of these cases revealed that this early reduction in lesion area was followed by an ultimate decrease in tendon diameter and thus most likely a reduction in fibrous tissue deposition.[86] Another ultrasonographic and clinical study found a similar reduction in lesion size of 44% and a mean decrease in lesion grade of 0.9 by day 10 following ultrasonographically guided tendon splitting. Some 81% of the horses were able to return to performance, and 68% competed at the same level following surgery. Results such as this are impressive, considering that the tendinitis in this case was accompanied by grade 3 or 4 lesions that involved up to 80% of the cross-sectional area of the tendon.[4] It is hypothesized that splitting creates a communication between the tendon core and the surrounding peritendinous tissue that promotes more rapid resolution of inflammatory edema and enhances revascularization and collagen production within the area of injury. Any effect on the mechanical properties of the mature collagenous repair tissue remains to be determined.[84]

Bramlage first described transection of the accessory ligament (superior check) of the flexor tendon as a novel surgical treatment for tendinitis of the SDF tendon in 1986.[28] This technique has been described elsewhere.[129] The SDF tendon inserts in the palmar aspect of the second phalanx in this joint to the distal medial aspect of the radius through the superior check ligament. This bone–tendon–bone segment sustains most of the load that the entire musculotendinous unit experiences. Bramlage proposed that transection of the superior check ligament would allow the SDF muscle belly to assume a greater portion of the load and create a more extensive musculotendinous unit that would in turn serve to protect the repaired digital flexor tendon.

In a retrospective study of 62 Thoroughbreds, Bramlage found that 92% of the horses were able to train and race after surgery, and 66% started at least five races after the surgery.[29] Forty-eight percent of the horses that raced maintained or increased their average earnings per start, and 86% maintained their race class. That only 19% reinjured the tendon appeared to be significant, considering that most of the horses in this study were experiencing at least their second episode of tendinitis. The results compared favorably with those of a study published by Reef et al.,[166] who found that approximately 50% of the horses were able to return to their previous type of competition, although most competed in a lower class or were not performing as well in the same class. A more recent study[90] using stricter definitions of success found that 97 of 137 horses raced (71%) and 70 horses (51%) made more than five starts after surgery. However, average earnings decreased for 58% of horses. In a smaller study evaluating the long-term effects of superior check desmotomy and other treatments, 53% of flat race horses, 58% of steeplechasers, and 73% of hurdlers competed in five or more starts after surgery.[146a] Another study, done on 124 Thoroughbred racehorses, compared the effects of superior check ligament desmotomy (31 horses) with nonsurgical treatment (93 horses) and found no benefit of surgery over nonsurgical treatment in preventing recurrence of tendinitis.[73] Recurrent new injuries occurred in 66% of horses in the nonsurgical group and in 78% of the surgical group. Horses undergoing surgery were also 5.5 times more likely to develop suspensory ligament desmitis than nonsurgically treated horses.[73]

Results following superior check desmotomy are clearly superior in the Standardbred to those achieved in the Thoroughbred. Hawkins and Ross reported that 35 of 38 horses raced after surgery (92%) and 33 horses (87%) started more than five races, although tendinitis recurred in 6 horses.[83,173] Using a strict definition of success, 71% of horses started five or more times after surgery, without recurrence of tendinitis. Suspensory desmitis developed in 5 horses, all of which had bilateral check ligament desmotomy. In a second study in Standardbreds, 82% raced after superior check desmotomy and 69% competed in five or more races.[90] In that study, horses that raced before injury had a better prognosis. It seems clear that superior check desmotomy is beneficial in the Standardbred horse.

There are no controlled studies of superior check desmotomy in other horses, but Ross claimed that hunters, jumpers, event horses, and dressage horses seem to have a prognosis somewhere between that published for the Thoroughbred and Standardbred horse. In a study of 33 horses in which 22 were nonracehorses, tendon splitting under ultrasound guidance combined in some horses with superior check desmotomy resulted in 68% return to the previous level of competition.[4] A scientific study has been done to show that desmotomy of the accessory ligament and SDF tendon in cadaver limbs altered the accessory ligament's function in transferring load in the SDF musculotendinous unit away from the muscle belly. Decrease in the metacarpophalangeal joint angle also indicated that the accessory ligament contributed to the

support of this joint under load. Increased SDF strain after desmotomy supports the rationale initially provided for the use of this treatment in tendinitis. There was increased strain in the SDF tendon, but the authors pointed out that it may not represent the situation in vivo.[180]

Another colleague has described using anular ligament desmotomy combined with radial check ligament desmotomy to treat distal tendinitis of the SDF tendon.[188] This indication is relatively rare.

A technique of autologous tendon transplantation is no longer practiced.[51,82] Carbon fiber implantation has also been tried.[80,109,122]

Summary

Treatment options will continue for SDF tendinitis. The primary goals of treatment are to obtain a good quality of repair of the primary lesion and to maximize the elastic limit of the injured tendon so it is compatible with future competition. If ultrasonography of a tendon shows newly echogenic repair, good axial alignment of fibers, and very little peritendon fibrosis, the prognosis is better. Another positive situation is no more than two zones with a residual severity rating, and they should rate below 1.5.[148] Resolution of swelling in the tendon will often mimic ultrasonographic healing. Prognosis is based on the extent of the initial lesion as well as the response to treatment and the behavior of the tendon when loading takes place.[84] Techniques including severance of adhesions associated with tendinitis and tenosynovitis, carbon fiber implant, and implantation of other materials have been tried and failed. Clearly, no panacea is available for the treatment of tendinitis and tenosynovitis, a major cause of wastage in the athletic horse. We need to continue to find ways to reduce the incidence of the problem by appropriate conditioning (such a regimen has not been clearly established yet) and careful monitoring of the state of the tendons.

Rehabilitation

A carefully controlled rehabilitation program combined with regular ultrasound examination provides the best chance for an equine athlete to return to full performance following SDF tendon (or suspensory ligament or biceps tendon) injury.[75] The author outlined a controlled exercise program and noted (in preliminary comments) that evidence indicates that small changes in ultrasonographic parameters of size, echogenicity, and fiber pattern are associated with a relatively large change in parameters associated with biomechanical strength. Based on a suggested need for a minimum of 6 months to return substantially toward normal, any case of tendon or ligament damage can be presumed to require a minimum of 6 months of restricted athletic activity to allow sufficient time for most healing to occur. Human athletes have reported that tendinitis causes a relatively short period of pain, ranging from 3 to 8 weeks if rest is initiated, and it appears the same for equine athletes; therefore, clinical signs of lameness should be absent after a short period of rest and long before substantial tendon healing has occurred. Based on ultrasonographic findings and clinical experience with 2800 cases of tendon and ligament injury at the University of California at Davis,

Gillis mapped out an exercise protocol for tendon rehabilitation. Protocols are tailored according to whether the tendinitis is graded as mild, moderate, or severe. *Mild* tendinitis has a tendon cross-sectional area (CSA) that is less than 20% larger than the established normal range for the affected site in the SDF, or the CSA of the opposite limb at the same site, a core lesion less than 15% of the total tendon CSA, and an affected area less than 20% of the total length of the tendon. *Moderate* tendinitis exists when the tendon CSA is 20 to 35% larger than the established normal range of the affected site or the opposite SDF CSA, if a core lesion is 15 to 30% of the total tendon CSA, and if the affected area extends 20 to 35% of the length of the tendon. *Severe* tendinitis exists when the tendon CSA is more than 35% above the established normal range for the affected site or the opposite SDF CSA at the same site, if the core lesion is more than 30% of the total tendon CSA, and if the affected area extends more than 35% of the length of the tendon.

A period of stall confinement and hand walking is initiated. In general, horses of all grades are hand walked 15 minutes twice daily from 0 to 30 days. Those with mild and moderate lesions are hand walked for 40 minutes daily for 30 to 60 days, and severe cases, 30 minutes daily. From 60 to 90 days, mild cases ride at the walk for 20 to 30 minutes daily, moderate cases are hand walked 60 minutes daily, and those with severe lesions are hand walked 40 minutes daily.

A second ultrasonographic examination is made at 90 to 120 days, and the tendon lesion is graded good, fair, or poor with regard to healing progress. Horses with good and fair grades of lesion are ridden at walk 30 minutes daily from 90 to 120 days and 45 to 60 minutes daily at 120 to 150 days. Five minutes trotting every 2 weeks is added at 150 to 180 days for good-graded horses, fair cases are ridden at a walk 60 minutes daily, and the poor-progress horses are ridden at the walk 60 minutes daily. The rehabilitation program continues to be gauged to the progress of the horse and whether the tendon healing is good, fair, or poor. Cantering is added for 5 minutes every 2 weeks for 120 days for good and fair cases, whereas poor cases have a reevaluation and discussion of further treatment options. Good and fair cases continue to have a canter 5 minutes every 2 weeks from 210 to 240 days, and at 240 days, full flat work with no racing speed or jumping is instituted in both good and fair cases.

Exercise may be tailored to suit the behavior and training level of the horse. For example, a racehorse might be exercised in a controlled manner by ponying rather than being ridden. The increase in exercise is graduated to avoid fatigue or overload injury to the healing tendon. Although controlled exercise requires time, effort, and money, Gillis proposes that if coupled with accurate interpretation of regular clinical and ultrasonographic examination, it provides the best opportunity for successful resolution of tendon injury. This statement is supported by the results of a retrospective study of 50 Thoroughbred racehorses with SDF tendinitis.[77] Twenty-eight of 50 horses underwent a controlled exercise program. Six of 50 (with mild tendinitis) followed an abbreviated (3- to 5-month) rehabilitation schedule, and 16 of 50 were turned out in pasture to recuperate from tendon injury. Eight of the 16 horses turned out to pasture were retired without an attempt to return to

previous use, including 6 mares who became broodmares and 2 geldings. Forty-two horses were trained for racing following tendon injury. Of these, 26 of 42 were able to complete 5 (range, 5 to 40; average, 14) or more races. Of the 26 successful horses, 4 of 26 were previously unraced, 8 of 26 remained in the same race category, 12 of 26 decreased one or more categories, and 2 of 26 improved at least one category (claiming, allowance stakes, and graded stakes).

Several factors influence return to racing, including severity of tendon injury, injury to more than one limb, and type of rehabilitation. The limb affected was not a significant factor, except that horses with both forelimbs injured had a decreased return-to-racing rate of 2 of 7. The severity of the lesion was a significant factor. Six of 9 mild lesions, 16 of 27 moderate lesions, and 4 of 9 severe lesions healed sufficiently to allow return to use. The type of rehabilitation was significant. Of 16 of 50 horses kept in pasture, 8 were tried at racing and 2 of 8 succeeded. Of 28 of 50 horses kept in a controlled exercise regimen, 20 of 28 succeeded. Gillis concluded that successful cases usually require 8 to 9 months of rest and rehabilitation to return to their previous full workload. Shortening this period or advancing too quickly usually results in worsening the tendon lesions. The premise for use of controlled exercise is to reduce inflammation initially, maintain gliding function, and improve healing.

The need for controlled exercise has also been emphasized by Madison.[117] Although the author prescribed a protocol for exercise regimen, there were no data to validate it (or otherwise). The program consisted of 1 to 2 months of stall rest with gradually increasing amounts of hand walking, turnout in a small paddock at 3 months, continuing to turn out in small paddock with enforced light exercise (lounging or ponying) at 4 months, turnout on pasture continued in months 5 and 6, continued turnout on pasture in month 7, and return to riding at a walk and trot (Thoroughbreds) or jogging (Standardbreds) and initial return to race training at 8 months (fast work being introduced at 9 months or jumping in jumping horses being instituted at 9 months).

Prevention

Based on changes seen in tendon matrix associated with development, aging, function, and exercise, it has been hypothesized that immature tendon can respond to load by synthesizing and maintaining the integrity of matrix, while mature tendon has limited if any ability to do so. These authors considered exercise detrimental to the matrix, particularly with increasing age, possibly as a consequence of accumulated microdamage and localized fatigue failure. They suggested that controlled, programmed exercise of the young growing animal might possibly have beneficial effects on the development of tendon extracellular matrix and in turn condition it for the inevitable microdamage that occurs with exercise in the mature animal. At the same time, excessive exercise would be anticipated to be detrimental to tendon development, and it is suggested therefore that a safe "window" exists for the optimum development of good quality tendon matrix. Obviously the safe window needs to be further defined. It is a novel idea that providing optimal conditioning to a young subject may result in improved performance and reduced injury later.[183]

Tendinitis of the Deep Digital Flexor Tendon

Strain injuries of the DDF tendon (DDFT) in the metacarpal or metatarsal region are uncommon compared with injuries of the SDF tendon (SDFT), accessory ligament of the DDF tendon (ALDDFT), or suspensory ligament (SL) on the basis of both postmortem surveys[221] and ultrasonographic examinations.[71,166] Webbon described the incidence and gross pathologic features of tendon injuries at postmortem of 589 tendons in 206 horses: there were 34 DDFT abnormalities found, compared with 100 SDFT abnormalities. However, most of the DDFT abnormalities (23 tendons) were described as degenerative changes in the distal phalangeal region, and 21 of 23 were found in the forelimb. All but one of these lesions was below the proximal interphalangeal joint. Distal lesions of the DDFT as it crosses the flexor cortex of the navicular bone are a well-recognized postmortem finding and are sometimes considered part of the navicular syndrome. Because the DDFT is difficult to image in this location, there is relatively little documentation of this problem in clinical cases. Webbon also described five DDFTs with fraying on the dorsal surface caused by friction against new bone on the proximal sesamoid bone exposed through ulceration of the intersesamoidean ligament. Six cases of "stress-induced DDFT injuries" were also described and of these, four were at the level of the proximal sesamoid bones and two were in the phalangeal region.[224]

Genovese et al. described one case of DDFT injury in a 10-year-old jumping horse with primary lameness and distension of the DFTS.[71] Denoix and Azevedo[38a] documented lesions in the DDFT within the deep flexor tendon sheath (DFTS) but only gave brief clinical details and few objective data on the subsequent outcome. They also mentioned DDF tendinitis in association with desmitis of the ALDDFT.

The most definitive study of DDF tendinitis was in 24 cases with ultrasonographic evidence of tendinitis of the DDFT in the metacarpometatarsal region, seen over a 7-year period.[14] Affected horses generally had a history of sudden onset of mild-to-moderate lameness associated with filling of the digital flexor tendon sheath. The lameness was exacerbated by flexion of the distal limb in approximately half the cases. The DDFT was occasionally thickened and painful on palpation, but it was often difficult to appreciate enlargement of the DDFT within a distended digital sheath. Intrasynovial analgesia of the DFTS consistently improved the lameness in all cases. Regional four-point blocks also produced significant improvement, but there was a less consistent response to abaxial sesamoid nerve blocks. On ultrasound examination, 20 of 24 cases had small, distinct, often circular focal hypoechoic areas within the DDFT in the distal metacarpus/metatarsus, usually within the digital sheath and proximal to the proximal sesamoid bones. These hypoechoic areas tended to be localized and extended only a short distance proximodistally (usually less than 1 cm). The lesions were considered focal, rather than true "core" lesions seen in the SDFT, and could be easily missed if not carefully examined through the digital sheath. All cases had an increase in the amount of fluid in the DFTS. One of the authors had seen three cases with lesions in the DDFT in addition to osteomyelitis of the proximal sesamoid bones.

In the cases described in this series, the palmar anular ligament appeared ultrasonographically thickened in four cases. The relationship between desmitis of the anular ligament (AL) and tendinitis of the DDFT within the digital sheath remains unclear, but the authors recommended that in horses with clinical signs of AL syndrome, a careful ultrasonographic examination should be done to exclude the possibility of a concurrent DDFT injury that could in turn adversely affect the prognosis. In the 24 cases of DDF tendinitis, only 7 horses made a full recovery and returned to their intended athletic activity. The DDFT had returned to normal ultrasonographically in 2 of those 7 cases. Although the numbers were too small to permit statistical evaluation, the authors said that neither intrasynovial medication nor palmar AL desmotomy appeared to improve the prognosis markedly in horses with DDFT injuries.

Anular Ligament Desmitis

Anular ligament desmitis was initially described as constriction of the palmar (volar) or plantar anular ligament of the fetlock in the horse.[1,213] It has a classical appearance (Fig. 7.113). It was also described as a syn-

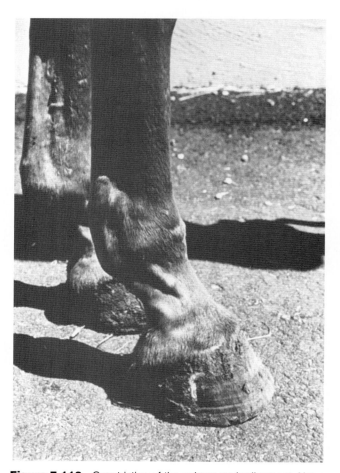

Figure 7.113 Constriction of the palmar anular ligament. Note distension of digital flexor tendon sheath above the anular ligament.

drome that responded to anular ligament desmotomy (ALD). The anular ligament of the fetlock joint extends transversely across the palmar/plantar aspect of the joint between the proximal sesamoid bones. The anular ligament creates with the intersesamoidean ligament an inelastic canal through which pass the superficial and DDF tendons. The fetlock canal is lined by synovial membrane of the digital sheath and serves to maintain the position and functional integrity of the flexors of the distal limb. Restriction of the free movement of the flexor tendons within the canal may result from enlargement of the tendons or from constriction by the anular ligament because of fibrosis. The resulting pressure can lead to tenosynovitis with distension of the digital flexor sheath, resulting in pain and persistent lameness. The same changes may also arise as a primary chronic digital sheath synovitis of unknown cause with excess production of synovia and a firm fibrous deposition at the proximal reflection of the sheath onto the flexor tendons.[71] The pathogenesis is traumatic (direct or indirect), but the clinical features of the condition are quite characteristic, and it has generally been treated by sectioning the anular ligaments of the fetlock joint as initially described by Adams[1,202] (Fig. 7.114).

A review of clinical and surgical findings of 49 equine fetlock palmar/plantar anular ligament (PAL) desmotomy patients at Colorado State University showed that ultrasonographic examination of the PAL and histologic evaluation of PAL biopsies in 24 of 40 cases revealed some changes that caused characterization of the syndrome a little differently than previously reported. Twenty-seven horses suffered lameness referable to a thickened PAL alone. The outcome of 24 of these horses was determined: 21 (87%) became sound and 3 (13%) were improved. Fifteen horses had tendinitis in addition to a thickened PAL. The outcome of 13 of these horses was determined: 5 (38%) became sound, 7 (54%) were improved, and 1 (8%) was not improved by ALD. ALD was also performed in 7 horses with septic processes involving the digital flexor tendons.

Ultrasonographic measurement from the external skin surface to the internal surface of the palmar anular ligament at the level of the apex of the proximal sesamoid bones yielded a mean thickness of 9.1 ± 2.3 mm

(normal, 3.6 ± 0.7 mm) and provided the most reproducible index of anular ligament thickening in affected horses. Ultrasonographically detectable tendon lesions and/or intrasynovial adhesions detected at surgery were negative prognostic signs. In all cases, tendon lesions consisted of focal-to-diffuse swelling seen ultrasonographically as areas of patchy hypoechogenicity and loss of a clear tendon margin outline. Anechoic tendon core lesions were not seen in these horses. Of the 11 group 2 horses with diagnostic ultrasound studies included in this investigation, 7 had SDFT lesions, and 4 had DDFT lesions. The fetlock PAL is not distinctly visible ultrasonographically unless it is thickened, and when it is thickened, its external surface can be difficult to detect. This was the reason for developing a technique in which the distance from the skin surface to the palmar–plantar surface was measured. Dik et al. reported that the skin over the anular ligament was 2 mm thick and that the normal anular ligament is too thin to measure. In their investigation, thickened anular ligaments measured 3 to 6 mm in thickness, resulting in a skin-through-anular-ligament measurement of 5 to 8 mm. Effusion within the digital sheath was present in 39 of 41 limbs and, therefore, of no prognostic significance. Only 1 of 7 (14%) horses with SDFT lesions detected ultrasonographically fully regained soundness, while 3 of 4 (75%) horses with ultrasonographically detectable DDFT lesions became fully sound (it is recognized that these lesions were different ultrasonographically from the typical lesion reported by Barr et al.). This study and another[72] appeared to support the conclusions of Adams in 1974 that the prognosis after ALD was favorable if the constriction of the palmar or plantar anular ligament was not accompanied by extensive changes in the tendon. It was also felt that the terms "stenosing desmitis," "tenosynovitis," or "tendinitis" might be more descriptive of the injury and effect than the word "constriction."

An open desmotomy technique was used in three limbs, and it resulted in an incisional infection in one case. The closed technique was done on 48 limbs in 44 horses,[201] and twice in 2 standing horses under local anesthesia. The most commonly reported postsurgical complication of horses without tendon injury was peri-incisional soft tissue swelling (7) that resolved in several days to several months, followed by peri-incisional fibrosis (1), dehiscence (1), and subcutaneous incisional infection that resolved with drainage and antimicrobial therapy (1). A tenoscopic technique for ALD has been described by Nixon.[144]

Histologic evaluation of biopsy specimens from the PAL demonstrated increased vascularity in a multifocal pattern of fibroblast hypercellularity and hyperplasia coupled with chronic inflammation and chondroid metaplasia as features of this desmitis.

Tenosynovitis of the carpal canal has been associated with constriction.[116]

Suspensory Ligament Desmitis

The suspensory ligament is predominantly a strong tendinous band containing variable amounts of muscular tissue.[46] It originates from the palmar carpal ligament and the proximal palmar surface of the third metacarpal bone in the forelimb and descends between the second

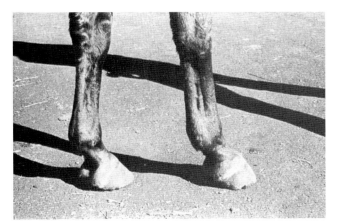

Figure 7.114   Two months after sectioning of the palmar anular ligament.

and fourth metacarpal bones. In the distal metacarpus it divides into two branches that insert on the proximal sesamoid bones. The extensor branches pass obliquely dorsad to join the common digital extensor tendon in the proximal phalangeal region. The suspensory apparatus is continued distally as the straight oblique cruciate and short distal sesamoidean ligaments. The suspensory ligament phylogenetically represents the median interosseous muscle and is also known as the interosseous muscle or proximal (superior) sesamoidean ligament. The percentage of muscle in each region has been determined.[234] Standardbreds had 40% more muscle in their suspensory ligament than did Thoroughbreds, and it has been suggested that this may be associated with biomechanical differences in gait between the two breeds or with genetic factors.[234] In vitro strength testing of the suspensory apparatus in training and resting horses suggests that there is an increase of strength with training. The absolute load to failure in a single load-to-failure compression test was higher in horses that had been in racehorse training, and failure in the trained group was usually by fracture of a proximal sesamoid bone. In the untrained group the suspensory ligament failed.[31]

Injuries to the suspensory ligament can be divided into three areas: 1) lesions restricted to the proximal one-third (proximal suspensory desmitis); 2) lesions in the middle one-third, sometimes extending into the proximal third (body lesions); and 3) lesions in the medial and/or lateral branch (branch lesions).

Proximal Suspensory Desmitis

Proximal suspensory desmitis (PSD) occurs in both the forelimb and the hindlimb and is diagnosed with a combination of clinical examination, ultrasonographic evaluation, and radiography.[42] Nuclear scintigraphy has also been used by some investigators. In acute cases, there may be localized heat in the proximal palmar metacarpal or plantar metatarsal area and, occasionally, slight edematous swelling in the region. Pain on palpation may be observed over the head of the suspensory ligament. In longer-term cases there are frequently no palpable abnormalities, although some enlargement of this region may be appreciated. Lameness may be acute or insidious in onset and vary in degree. It may be seen as severe after fast work. Lameness in forelimbs usually improves within a few days of rest but recurs when work is resumed, whereas hindlimb lameness is usually more persistent.[44] Flexion of the distal limb is positive in 50% of cases, whereas flexion of the hock accentuates the lameness in 85% of hindlimb cases. Forelimb lameness is often accentuated on a circle, especially when the lame limb is on the outside of the circle, and also may be worse on soft ground. It has been suggested that if local infiltration with a small volume of anesthetic (6 mL) is used, the risk of desensitizing the palmar outpouchings of the joint is far less than that of using the 20 mL used in the experimental study by Ford et al.[60a] Perineural anesthesia of the lateral palmar nerve performed just distal to the accessory carpal bone (and hence the medial and lateral palmar metacarpal nerves) should avoid the possibility of inadvertent injection into the palmar outpouchings of the capsule of the middle and carpometacarpal joint. The latter approach is preferred.

Local analgesic techniques are a critical part of the examination, and one must be aware of the relationship between the middle carpal/carpometacarpal joint in front and tarsometatarsal joint capsules with the proximal suspensory ligament.[60a] Palmar and palmar metacarpal (subcarpal) nerve blocks will usually elicit improvement, but it may be necessary to perform an ulnar nerve block or block a lateral palmar nerve below the accessory carpal bone to alleviate lameness. Similarly, false-negative responses to perineural analgesia of the plantar metatarsal nerves at the subtarsal level are sometimes obtained, but lameness can be improved with perineural analgesia of the tibial nerve. Because improvement in lameness associated with PSD is sometimes observed after intraarticular analgesia of the carpal or tarsometatarsal joints, the clinician must remain aware of alternate sources of pain.

Ultrasonographic abnormalities associated with PSD include 1) enlargement of the suspensory ligament in the median and/or transverse plane; 2) poor definition of one or more of the margins of the suspensory ligament, especially a dorsal margin; 3) a central hypoechoic area (well defined); 4) one or more poorly defined hypoechoic areas, central or more peripherally; 5) a larger area or areas of diffuse decreased echogenicity; and 6) small focal hyperechoic areas (usually in long-term cases) or combinations.[43] In the normal horse, the suspensory ligament is usually bilaterally symmetric, so comparison with the contralateral limb is helpful. With recent injury, the signs may be subtle but can become more obvious during the next 2 to 4 weeks. Details on the relative occurrence of ultrasonographic changes have been well described by Dyson.[42]

Radiographic abnormalities associated with PSD occur at the proximal aspect of the third metacarpal or metatarsal bones and include sclerosis of the trabecular pattern on a dorsopalmar projection, alteration of the trabecular pattern dorsal to the palmar or plantar cortex, and enthesiophyte formation on the palmar–plantar aspect of the bone on a lateromedial view. These radiographic abnormalities are seen more commonly in hindlimbs than forelimbs.[44] Radiographic examination is also useful to rule out an avulsion fracture of the palmar or plantar cortex of the third metacarpal (metatarsal) bone, a palmar cortical stress fracture, or other bony change. Radiographic abnormalities are rarely seen in acute PSD unless lameness represents recurrence of a previous injury.[42]

Many treatments have been used in the management of PSD. These include box rest and controlled exercise with or without local and/or systemic administration of PSGAG, local injection of corticosteroids, or an internal blister.[45] A report on 29 horses with PSD unassociated with any concurrent cause of lameness found that 86% resumed full work after box rest, and a controlled exercise program for a minimum of 2 months has been made.[43] Progressive "filling in" of lesions was detected by serial ultrasonographic examinations. Most horses with forelimb PSD were rested (box rest and controlled exercise) for 3 to 6 months, and it was felt that the speed of resolution of the lesions and the total convalescence time was proportional to the duration of lameness before instigation of treatment. The rate of ultrasonographic resolution of a lesion varies and has been suggested to relate to the chronicity of the lesion prior to institution of appropriate management.[42] Lesions identified soon after onset of lameness appeared to "heal" more quickly than longer-standing cases. Central hypoechoic lesions gradually decreased in size, became more echogenic, and in some cases ultimately had a relatively hyperechoic center. Twenty-five of the 29 horses mentioned above that resumed full work experienced no recurrent lameness associated with PSD in the follow-up period (3 to 30 months).

The prognosis for hindlimb PSD is much more guarded. In a study of 42 horses for which follow-up information was available for 2 years or more after diagnosis, only 6 (14%) returned to full athletic function with no detectable lameness for at least 1 year, including grand prix show jumping in advanced-level horse trials.[44] Tibial neurectomy was performed in 3 horses that had failed to respond to previous conservative therapy, enabling all to return successfully to full athletic function (horse trials and show jumping), and no problems have been encountered in the follow-up period of 1 year. It has been suggested that enlargement of the suspensory ligament within the bony confines of the second, third, and fourth metatarsal bones can cause pressure and secondary abnormalities of the adjacent plantar metatarsal nerve. Possibly, this compression may be the cause of persistent pain and lameness. Some preliminary postmortem data supports this, but larger numbers are required. It is logical to institute early diagnosis and therapy to reduce the size of the suspensory ligament and minimize inflammation.[46]

Newer treatments that have been used more recently for PSD include injection of bone marrow into the area and shock wave (lithotripsy) treatments. Neither technique has been published in refereed journals at the time of this writing.

Desmitis of the Body of the Suspensory Ligament

Lameness is usually less obvious with desmitis of the body of the suspensory ligament (SL), but there are more obvious localizing clinical signs of heat, pain, and swelling than with PSD. The condition is more common in the forelimbs than the hindlimbs and in all types of horses other than Standardbreds. In contrast to PSD and desmitis of the branch of the suspensory ligament, body lesions are far more common in racehorses than in other sport horses.

Diagnosis can usually be made on clinical signs, and local analgesics are not usually required. Ultrasonographic examination provides detailed assessment of the degree of structural damage and is particularly important when periligamentous soft tissue swelling makes palpation of the suspensory ligament itself difficult. Limitations in the value of ultrasonography to monitor repair of the ligament have been pointed out.[43] Fairly extensive hypoechoic areas persist for a long time despite resolution of clinical signs in many horses. Some horses may be able to return to work without recurrent clinical signs despite persistence of the lesions. However, there is still a relatively high incidence of recurrent suspensory ligament desmitis even with more than 12 months of rest, and this may be related to incomplete healing of the ligament. The incidence of persistent ultrasonographic change of the suspensory ligaments is much higher than

persistence of lesions in the SDF tendon.[43] In addition to examining the suspensory ligament, care should be taken to evaluate foot balance and shoeing, as well as the horse's conformation. Long pasterns or hyperextension of the fetlocks may predispose to suspensory ligament injury. Lesions of the suspensory body may be associated with a primary "splint" that impinges on the margin, resulting in localized desmitis; small splint fractures may have the same effect. Some distal-third splint fractures will heal, but the author prefers surgical removal, particularly in the acute stage. At the same time, it is critical to recognize that the degree of suspensory desmitis remaining will dictate the prognosis.

Suspensory ligament desmitis is managed in some horses by aggressive physiotherapy treatment such as water and ice or whirlpool boots, as well as the application of DMSO, correction of foot imbalance, and a rehabilitation program. Gillis et al.[76] reported that 117 of 173 SLD horses managed by controlled exercise were able to return to their intended use, whereas only 29 of 57 horses managed by 3 months of initial confinement followed by a pasture turnout were able to do so. Percutaneous ligament splitting has been used for central core lesions. Intralesional treatment with HA, corticosteroids, or PSGAG has produced variable results. Some authors advocate pin firing or the use of paints, particularly in Standardbreds. Suspensory body lesions have been reported to be relatively common in horses that race over fences. Also, injuries to the body of the suspensory ligament in event horses are less common than branch lesions, but they carry a guarded prognosis for return to full athletic function without recurrent injury. Recently, shock wave treatment has been used, but no controlled studies have been reported at the time of this writing.

Desmitis of the Branches of the Suspensory Ligament

Desmitis of the medial or lateral branches of the suspensory ligament occurs in both forelimbs and hindlimbs in all types of horses. The degree of lameness varies and can range from nondetectable to moderate. It is occasionally severe, depending on the extent of damage and its chronicity. Usually there is some enlargement palpable on the affected branch, with a variable degree of periligamentous soft tissue swelling and localized heat. There will be pain on pressure with palpation of its margins or over the apex of the proximal sesamoid bone. Sometimes palpation is difficult because of concurrent effusion in the digital flexor tendon sheath or fetlock joint. Suspensory ligament branch lesions can persist for a long time ultrasonographically, so clear identification of the current problem is difficult without previous ultrasound images for comparison. Because of the association between the branches and the distal aspect of the splint bones, radiographs should be done. Other lesions that can be seen on radiography include dystrophic mineralization within the ligament or small avulsion fractures of the abaxial or palmar surface of the proximal sesamoid bone. Ultrasonographic abnormalities include enlargement of the branch, poor definition of margins, change in shape (more oval), focal hypoechoic areas, a diffuse decrease in echogenicity, focal hyperechoic spots, periligamentous echodense material and irregularity in outline of the proximal sesamoid bones, or an avulsion fracture.

In some instances, there will be no ultrasonographic abnormalities despite palpable enlargement with associated soreness.

Treatment options are similar for desmitis of the body of the suspensory ligament. Usually, lameness resolves quite quickly with rest, unless considerable periligamentous adhesions develop.[46] Such a change warrants a guarded prognosis and is more common in hindlimbs. The author has done percutaneous splitting of the branch if there is a central core lesion. Controlled exercise programs and local and systemic anti-inflammatory treatments are recommended. Although lesions will improve to some extent during a 3- to 12-month period, quite often abnormalities persist for longer than 12 months. The total convalescent period depends on the severity of injury, but varies from 3 to 12 months. There is apparently a relatively high recurrence, especially in horses competing in 3-day events as opposed to 1-day events.[46]

There are some differences in treatment for suspensory desmitis in general between Thoroughbred and Standardbred racehorses. Pin firing and blistering as well as splitting tend to be used more in Standardbreds (at least in the body of the ligament) than in Thoroughbreds. Thoroughbred treatment revolves around anti-inflammatory management of the acute lesion followed by a controlled exercise program. Newer treatments with the injection of bone marrow and shock wave therapy have been advocated, but no controlled studies have been published at the time of this writing.

Desmitis of the Accessory Ligament of the Deep Digital Flexor Tendon (Inferior Check Ligament)

The ALDDFT (subcarpal or inferior check ligament) is direct continuation of the palmar carpal ligament and joins the DDFT in the midmetacarpus. It provides stability to the extended carpus,[99] and in the midstance phase of the stride, it shares tensile load with the DDFT.[105] Desmitis of the ALDDFT has been reported to be a fairly common injury in pleasure horses, ponies, and show jumpers and is less frequent in racehorses and event horses.[42] Brief reference was made to the ultrasonographic features of desmitis of the ALDDFT by Genovese et al.,[71] but the first definitive study was in 1991.[42] Desmitis of the ALDDFT was diagnosed in 27 horses. The first observed clinical sign in 4 horses was localized swelling in the proximal metacarpus. Twenty horses became lame suddenly during the work period, and most developed swelling within 24 hours of exercise. The injury was confirmed by ultrasonographic examination. There was palpable enlargement in the region in 24 horses at the time of diagnosis. In 1 horse there was a focal central hypoechoic lesion. The remaining 26 horses exhibited enlargement in the ALDDFT in transverse and/or median planes. Thirteen horses (48%) had overall diffuse decrease in echogenicity involving the entire cross section of the ligament and extending a variable distance proximodistally. Four of the 27 horses (15%) had a localized area of diffuse decrease in echogenicity only involving part of the cross section, and 7 horses (26%) had additional hypoechoic or anechoic regions. In 2 horses the ligament was predominantly hypoechoic or anechoic.

In follow-up, persistent local swelling was a consistent feature. Twelve horses (44%) resumed work within 5 months. Ten horses (37%) resumed full work without recurrence of clinical signs referable to the ALDDFT during the follow-up period (9 months to 4 years). In the 27 horses reported in the study, 18 (66%) were age 10 years or older, a much higher proportion of older horses than the normal hospital population. A separate in vitro mechanical study suggests that the clinical occurrence of desmitis of the ALDDFT of older horses could be due to fibrillar failure caused by differences in the material properties of the ligament. It was considered that there was failure of a number of fibers that either fail at lower forces or are subject to higher forces than the rest and that these differences in mechanical properties could result from age-related differences in the material properties of the accessory ligament of older horses, similar to alterations in collagenous tissue in other species.[15] It was also reported that adhesion formation between the ALDDFT and adjacent structures can occur but can be resolved by treating with phenylbutazone in an attempt to "stretch" adhesions; others have used local injection of sodium hyaluronate. It is strongly recommended that controlled exercise be used rather than pasture turnout, and lameness is resolved long before healing is complete. The horse's return to work should be based on the results of serial ultrasonographic appearance.

Another report[123] confirmed that ALDDFT desmitis appears to be more common in older horses used for jumping and that owners often did not initially recognize the seriousness of the injury. Ultrasonographic examination revealed either focal or generalized areas of decreased echogenicity. Adhesion formation around the dorsal compartment of the carpal sheath onto the abaxial margins of the SDFT was commonly found at follow-up. The long-term prognosis appeared guarded.

More recently, the use of desmotomy of the ALDDFT as a treatment was recommended. Dyson[43] and Van den Belt et al.[205a] found that of the chronic cases of desmitis (longer than 3 months), only 14 to 18% made a full recovery. This, coupled with the finding that there are age-related changes in the material properties of the ligament,[17] suggested that by relieving strain on the scar tissue with desmotomy, the risk of reinjury is reduced (the rationale is similar to desmotomy of the ALDDFT for SDF tendinitis). These authors propose that desmotomy of the ALDDFT could be used to treat chronic desmitis that does not improve clinically and ultrasonographically after 6 months. Severing the ligament would both relieve pain and lameness attributable to stretching of the affected tissue and prevent reinjury.[15] A kinematic and kinetic analysis after desmotomy showed that joint angles at midstance were not significantly different from those before surgery, and they felt that any instability of the limb after ALDDFT desmotomy does not cause changes in the locomotion of the horse or in the compensatory loading of other structures (changes were found in the second part of the stance phase at maximal extension of the distal interphalangeal joint). A histomorphologic and ultrasonographic study concluded that healing by scar tissue formation of ALDDFT 6 months after desmotomy restored a major part of functional strength, and although the scar tissue was inferior materially, there was an increase in the cross-sectional area of the

ALDDFT at the site of desmotomy and lengthening of the ALDDFT after desmotomy.[16] The author has used this technique on clinical cases.

Avulsion Fractures

Avulsion fractures may occur in association with tendinous insertions but are more common in association with ligaments. Avulsion fractures are discussed in Chapter 8. Their presence should be differentiated in cases of traumatic injury of tendons and ligaments. Examples of avulsion fractures include fracture of the extensor process of the distal phalanx (insertion site for common digital extensor tendon), avulsion at the origin of the suspensory ligament, avulsion of the proximal attachment of the peroneus tertius and avulsion of the proximal attachment of the distal sesamoidean ligaments.

Traumatic Tendon Rupture

Tendon rupture can occur in association with excessive stress. Although some loss of integrity may occur in association with tendinitis or tendosynovitis, complete rupture of the flexor tendons is not usually observed unless there is previous infection or degeneration. Some specific instances of complete traumatic rupture of tendons include rupture of the peroneus tertius and gastrocnemius and/or SDF tendon in the hindlimb. Severed tendons are discussed in a separate section. Disruption of the reciprocal apparatus has been reported.[181]

PATHOGENESIS

The peroneus tertius originates in common with the long digital extensor tendon from the extensor fossa of the distolateral femur and inserts on the dorsal surface of the proximal extremity of the third metatarsal bone, the calcaneus, and the fourth tarsal bone. It is an important part of the reciprocal apparatus, mechanically flexing the hock when the stifle is flexed. Rupture is associated with overextension of the hock. This may occur in association with struggling to free a trapped limb or in traumatic injury to the region. Generally the body of the peroneus tertius ruptures, but occasionally, an avulsion fracture occurs at its proximal attachment, particularly in younger horses (see Chapter 8 for more information).

The gastrocnemius and SDF tendons of the hindlimb are intimately associated with each other at their origin and near the tarsal insertion. Proximal to the point of the hock, the combined tendons are known as the common calcaneal tendon. Rupture of the gastrocnemius tendon may occur in one or both limbs in association with trauma due to strenuous effort. Incidents that may cause the problem include a fall with the hindlimbs flexed and underneath the body, being pulled up sharply and thrown back on the hocks, or making violent efforts to avoid slipping when going down a hill. The gastrocnemius muscle apparently ruptures before the SDF tendon. Rarely, both structures will rupture (rupture of common calcaneal tendon), and this injury is particularly serious.

Rupture of the extensor carpi radialis tendon may also occur, but it is rare. The condition is too uncommon to make a valid observation regarding the cause. The occurrence of rupture of the common digital extensor tendon in foals is discussed above.

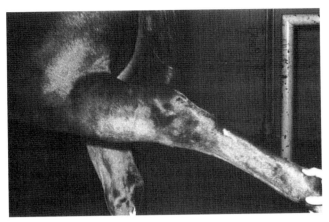

Figure 7.115 Rupture of the peroneus tertius demonstrated by simultaneous extension of the hock and flexion of the stifle.

DIAGNOSIS

The signs of rupture of the peroneus tertius muscle are classical. The hock joint does not flex as the limb moves craniad, and the distal limb tends to hang limp. The horse will bear weight, and pain is not a feature. On picking up the limb, the hock can be extended without extending the stifle (this cannot be done in a normal limb), and there is dimpling in the common calcaneal tendon (Fig. 7.115).

With gastrocnemius rupture, the hock is dropped so there is excessive angulation at the hock joint. If the entire common calcaneal tendon is ruptured, the horse cannot bear weight.

The signs of extensor carpi radialis rupture are more subtle, but careful observation of the gait will reveal that the carpus on the affected forelimb flexes more than the carpus of the normal limb. Consequently, the arc of the hoof in flight is significantly higher in the affected limb than in the sound limb. This is most noticeable at the trot. The problem is confirmed by palpation.

TREATMENT

Rupture of the peroneus tertius muscle is treated with rest. After stall rest for a month, the horse may be turned out to pasture. Most cases heal well, and surgical intervention is unnecessary.

Casting may be performed for a rupture of the gastrocnemius or the calcaneal (Achilles) tendon but cast sore problems are likely. The prognosis is guarded for gastrocnemius rupture and poor for calcaneal tendon rupture.

The management of disruption of the lateral head of the gastrocnemius muscle and SDF tendon muscle at their proximal attachments by use of a modified Thomas splint–cast combination in a 6-month-old female Warmblood horse has been described.[107] The intact medial head of the gastrocnemius muscle was the only portion of the caudal reciprocal apparatus that allowed weight bearing. In another report, a horse managed without external coaptation developed complete disruption of the caudal component of the reciprocal apparatus because of continued weight bearing in combination with further trauma, and at postmortem, the ruptured origins of the gastrocnemius and SDF muscles had contracted distally. The Thomas splint–cast combination has the advantages of stopping further injury and the potential for hemorrhage as well as allowing the ruptured muscle ends to be in closer apposition. Severe pressure sores as reported previously on the proximal portion of the tibia and calcaneus[167] are less of a problem because the modified Thomas splint limits excessive motion within the cast, because of the encircling portion of the splint in the inguinal region as well as the distal extension encircling the foot.

In the rare instances of rupture of the extensor carpi radialis muscle, treatment has not been attempted.[33] The animal is still usable. If treatment is considered warranted in an athletic horse, implantation of carbon fiber could be considered.

Degenerative Rupture of Tendons

Prior damage to a tendon can weaken it to the extent that spontaneous rupture can occur with normal tensile forces. Typical examples of this situation are rupture of tendons secondary to septic tenosynovitis, advanced navicular disease following palmar digital neurectomy, or a sequel to repair of severed tendons. Septic tenosynovitis (considered below) is associated with high levels of degradative enzymes as in septic arthritis. Rather than a rupture, it is probably more accurate to describe the process as dissolution.

Rupture of the DDF tendon has been associated with the deep flexor tendon being weakened by degeneration in proximity to the navicular bone. Following palmar digital neurectomy, the horse starts using the limb in a normal fashion, adhesions between the deep flexor tendon and navicular bone are broken down, and a weakened DDF tendon may rupture.[1] This may occur at a variable time following neurectomy. It is uncommon. In rare instances, rupture of the DDF tendon may occur in association with advanced navicular disease, even when neurectomy has not been performed. Rupture of the DDF tendon may also follow severe, longstanding suppurative navicular bursitis.

DIAGNOSIS

Loss of integrity of the tendon is recognized by the particular limb conformation and gait (these particular signs are discussed in the severed tendons section) (Fig. 7.116). These signs usually occur after other disease has been recognized.

TREATMENT

In most instances rupture due to degeneration is an indication for euthanasia.

Traumatic Rupture of the Suspensory Apparatus

This is a severe traumatic syndrome that may be due to rupture of the suspensory ligament, transverse fracture of both proximal sesamoid bones, or rupture of the distal sesamoidean ligaments. It occurs in racehorses.

PATHOGENESIS

The cause is considered to be extreme extension (dorsiflexion) of the fetlock while racing or jumping (steeplechase).

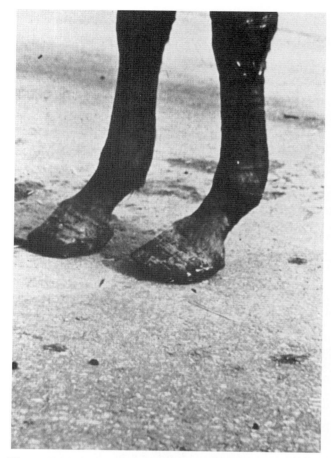

Figure 7.116 Case of degenerative rupture of deep digital flexor tendon. Note that the toe lifts off the ground with weight bearing.

DIAGNOSIS

The clinical appearance is characterized by lameness, swelling, and sinking of the fetlock. Diagnosis is confirmed by palpation and radiology (dorsal displacement of intact or fractured sesamoids). Compromise of the blood supply can lead to ischemic necrosis of both the soft tissues and the hoof, which becomes evident some days after the initial injury.

TREATMENT

Treatment is generally aimed at salvage for breeding. Immediate support of the fetlock is required in the form of a cast or a special splinting device.[223] Healing is slow and problematic. The treatment of choice is performing a fetlock arthrodesis.[27,205]

Severed Tendons

Traumatic division of the common and/or lateral digital extensor tendons of the forelimb and the long and/or lateral digital extensor tendons of the hindlimb is relatively common. In the forelimb, severance usually occurs between the fetlock and carpus; in the hindlimb, the tendons are usually severed just below the hock. The hindlimbs are more commonly affected. In one study on 50 horses suffering 53 extensor tendon lacerations, 89% involved the long and lateral digital extensors of the rear limbs.[19] Traumatic division of the digital flexor tendons usually occurs between the carpus and the fetlock.

Diagnosis

With a severed common digital or long digital extensor tendon, the horse is unable to extend the toe properly and may drag the toe or "knuckle over" on it. However, if the limb is set under the horse properly, weight can be borne normally. A horse that has severed the lateral digital extensor in the forelimb or hindlimb will not generally have a gait deficit. The degree of soft tissue damage associated with a severed tendon will depend on the case.

The clinical signs in terms of limb conformation and gait vary with cut flexor tendons, depending on the structures involved. If the SDF tendon only is cut, the fetlock will drop but not touch the ground (Fig. 7.117). If both SDF and DDF are cut, the fetlock will drop and the toe will come up into the air when weight is applied to the affected limb (Fig. 7.117). If both the flexors and the suspensory ligament are cut, the fetlock may rest on the ground. A laceration distal to the fetlock will usually involve the deep flexor tendon and the digital sheath, and in these cases, the toe turns up when weight is placed on the hoof. The type of laceration can vary from a clean cut of the tendon to marked tendinous damage (Fig. 7.118). There will also be variable damage to adjacent tissues. In some instances, a small clean cut may be all that is observed, which gives the impression of a minor wound until the animal moves and the tendons are assessed. If the wound has been present for some time, there may be extensive soft tissue swelling and infection. Septic tenosynovitis may also be present.

Treatment

There is no routine treatment protocol for these cases, but some general principles can be established. In all instances, there should be careful attention to surgical principles, with careful cleaning of the wound and debridement.

EXTENSOR TENDONS. With severed digital extensor tendons the wounds are cleaned, debrided, and sutured if amenable to primary closure. Debridement should include the removal of contaminated or unhealthy paratendon. If there is loss of tissue or infection, the wound is allowed to heal by granulation. In most cases, the ends of the digital extensor tendons are not sutured. Healing without suturing can generally be anticipated with severed extensor tendons. When healing is complete, normal function can be expected, but more than 6 months

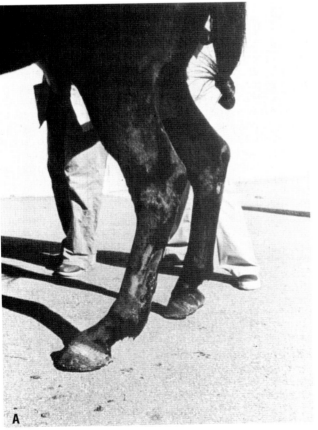
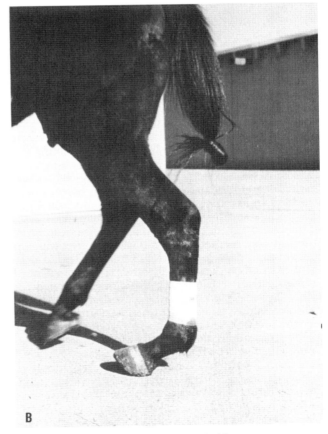

Figure 7.117 Clinical manifestations of severed digital flexor tendons. A. Severed superficial digital flexor tendon. B. Severed deep and superficial digital flexor tendons.

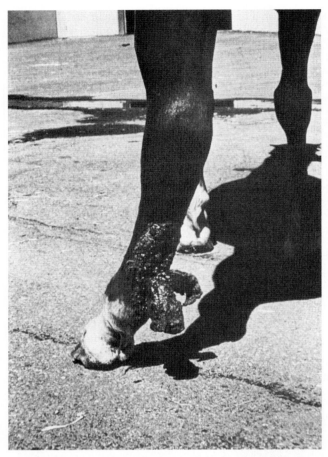

Figure 7.118 Severed deep and superficial flexor tendons, with distal tendons avulsed and hanging from wound.

may be required before full function is achieved. If the wound is clean and the cut has been sharp, primary repair can be performed but is rarely necessary. A cast or PVC pipe bandage splint can be used to immobilize the limb in the initial stages if excessive flexion or knuckling over is occurring. In other instances, casting or bandage splinting may not be necessary if suturing has not been performed and the animal has already compensated for the defect. If the lateral digital extensor tendon alone is cut, the cast or bandage splint is not necessary. If a cast is used, it can be removed in 2 weeks, after which a bandage splint may be used to prevent forward knuckling of the fetlock, which will interfere with continued healing. Generally, bandage splinting is continued for another 2 weeks. In some instances of severed digital extensor tendons, the use of a bandage and corrective shoe with an extended toe is an appropriate initial mode of treatment and an alterative to casting.

Wire cuts over the hock may involve the tarsocrural (tibiotarsal) joint, and septic arthritis may develop. Wounds in this region also may present problems with slow, second-intention healing if there is major loss of tissue.

FLEXOR TENDONS. The general results with flexor tendon lacerations are much less satisfactory.[64] If the laceration involves both flexor tendons and the suspensory ligament, euthanasia is probably indicated unless salvage of a very valuable animal is required. However, the value of the animal does nothing to enhance the success of anything attempted.

If a tendon cut is within the tendon sheath, it is particularly vital that the ends of the tendons remain in apposition to prevent nonunion and maximize intrinsic healing. Primary suturing of these wounds of the tendon in these cases is attempted, even in the presence of contamination, but the prognosis is appropriately worsened. If there is significant loss of tendinous material, the usefulness of repair must be questioned.

With a clean cut in the tendon outside the tendon sheath but where some contamination has occurred, I still prefer to suture the tendon, but very careful debridement is imperative, including the removal of any devitalized or contaminated paratendon.

In wounds that are more than a few hours old, with loss of tendon material and gross contamination present, a primary tendon closure is not usually appropriate. All hair is removed from the region, the wound is carefully cleaned, and wide debridement is performed. All devitalized tendon tissue is removed. If the wound is severely contaminated and debridement is less than satisfactory or if there is already established infection, suturing of the tendon ends should be delayed for 5 to 7 days (until the debridement phase of wound healing has produced a clean wound bed). Protocols for suturing tendons have been established, based on both experimental work and practical experience. Initial reports of the use of carbon fiber filaments were encouraging but experimentally have produced weaker repair and greater foreign body reaction and now are not used. Work at Colorado State University supports the use of large (No. 1 or 2), nonabsorbable suture, nylon or polypropylene being preferred. An alternative is No. 1 or 2 polydioxanone or polyglyconate.[20,145] These synthetic absorbable sutures are absorbed slowly and, in one report, were considered to withstand a larger maximum load than did tendon sutured with nylon.[94] Carbon fiber has been used but is not used now.[30,203,204]

The strongest repairs result from the use of a three-loop pulley, double-locking loop, or triple-locking loop suture pattern.[47,157] The locking loop suture pattern is illustrated in Figure 7.119. The disadvantage of the three-loop pulley pattern is that much of the suture material is exposed to the tissue surrounding the anastomosis site, and adhesions may result.[47] The three-loop pulley technique does have the greatest resistance to gap formation and its mode of failure differs in that it fails by suture pullout and then breakage, whereas the three-locking loop suture patterns fail by suture breakage.[47] In a model of gap healing in equine flexor tendon, nylon double-locking loop suture was preferred over double-locking loop with carbon fiber and controls, because of greater breaking stress, histologic maturity, biocompatibility, and the adequate functional and cosmetic outcome.[20]

Partial cuts in tendons are generally not sutured unless more than 75% of the tendon circumference has been transected. A partially crushed or severed tendon can swell, soften, and rupture from normal stresses at a later period. Debridement and other appropriate treatment to

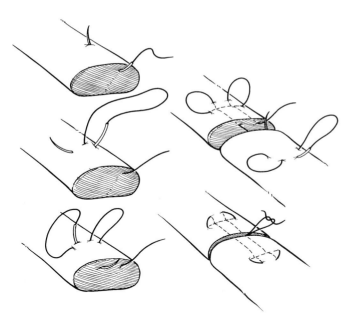

Figure 7.119   Diagram of locking-loop tendon suture.

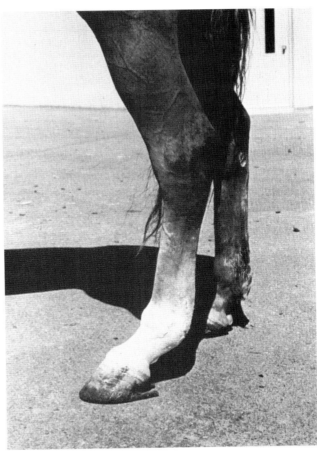

Figure 7.120   Patient with several flexor tendons (in which carbon was implanted) after removal of cast. Note the use of a shoe with extended heels. (Courtesy of A. S. Turner.)

rid the wound of infection should be performed, and the same support applied to the limb.

Whether tendons are sutured primarily or left to heal secondarily, postoperative support is necessary, and the method is generally the same in all cases. The biologic basis for immobilization is not simply to prevent tension on the anastomosis from causing dehiscence but also to allow revascularization to occur.[156] It has been suggested that active motion should not be attempted within 3 weeks. While mild, passive motion may help decrease adhesions, absence of more severe active motion is essential to healing in the early stages. The use of a cast is indicated for immobilization of the equine limb following severance of a digital flexor tendon. Minimizing gap formation in the early stages of tendon healing is very important.[146] The cast is used for 6 weeks, and when it is removed, either a fetlock supporting shoe or a shoe with trailers (depending on whether the SDF and/or DDF tendons are involved) is appropriate (Fig. 7.120). Following removal of the cast in the case of SDF tendon severance, the fetlock will drop but it will come up again with exercise.

Research has shown that beneficial effects can be associated with passive or active motion during healing. In one study, two groups of dogs had their flexor tendons severed and repaired within the digital sheath. Controlled passive motion was begun immediately in one group, while the second group had the limb immobilized.[65] The group that underwent passive motion had a significantly greater range of motion, strength of repair, and DNA content in the healed tendon. In the passive motion group, scanning electron microscopy of the repair tissue demonstrated that the epitendon proliferated, bridging the wound gap and providing the repair cells. The tendon healed without adhesions to the surrounding tissue, while the immobilized repair site had adhesions. Immobilization beyond 3 weeks resulted in a

significant reduction in tendon vascularity, and therefore the length of time that we immobilize should be reconsidered. Stress is also necessary at the repair site to develop any strength in the scar tissue bridging the ends. Mobilized tendons have greater strength than do immobilized tendons. A study in rabbits reported that flexor tendons have the intrinsic capacity to phagocytize all collagen and synthesize new collagen fibers, and thus clinical attempts to prevent or control the peripheral adhesions are valid, since these adhesions do not appear to be an essential component of the repair process.[119]

Another study implied that the duration of the daily controlled-motion interval is a significant variable insofar as postrepair flexor tendon function is concerned. The implication is that longer intervals or increased cycles improved healing, but the minimum duration or number of cycles necessary to achieve the improved healing response remains to be elucidated.[65] Another study concluded that higher frequency controlled passive motion accelerates tendon repair more than lower frequency controlled passive motion.[196] In considering tendon healing within a sheath, it has been shown that an irradiated, nonviable tendon could be healed when placed in the synovial cavity of a rabbit's knee joint, implying that tendon can be healed by cells present in the synovial fluid.[134]

Prognosis

The prognosis for fresh, uncomplicated cuts of digital extensor tendons is favorable. With infection or associated bone and joint damage, the prognosis becomes guarded. Follow-up in a retrospective study in 15 horses with extensor tendon lacerations that underwent treatment revealed that 47% returned to their intended use, 33% returned to limited use, 7% were used for breeding, and 13% were euthanized.[60] In another study, long-term follow-up (>1 year) of 40 horses with extensor tendon lacerations found that 73% returned to athletic soundness.[19] Time from injury to treatment did not correlate with outcome in one study reviewing outcomes of extensor tendon laceration in 22 horses.[95]

The prognosis for return to athletic use after flexor tendon laceration is generally considered guarded to poor, but two retrospective studies suggest that this may be overly pessimistic. In a retrospective review of 24 cases, Foland et al. reported that nearly 60% of horses returned to riding soundness after flexor tendon lacerations.[60] In a second study of 50 horses, 39 of 50 (78%) horses that were treated were still alive 1 year or more after injury.[198] Twelve of 16 horses that had one or the other flexor tendon transected survived, 13 of 16 horses that had both tendons transected survived, and 14 of 18 horses that had partial tendon disruption of one or both tendons survived. Of the 39 surviving horses, 27 horses returned to their original use, and 32 horses (82%) were sound for riding. Nine horses with one or both tendons transected were being used for athletic activity. Lacerated tendons were sutured in 16 horses, and 15 of these survived. Tendons were not sutured in 34 horses, and 24 of these survived.[198] When one tendon was transected (with or without partial transection of another tendon), 92% of the survivors could be ridden again, and 50% of them were used athletically. When both tendons were transected, 69% of the survivors could be ridden, and 23% were used in athletic activities (including ranch work, roping, dressage, cutting, harness driving, hunting/jumping, and competitive trail riding). The main cause of death associated with tendon laceration was wound infection. Lacerations that involved the flexor tendons and suspensory ligament are uncommon and are associated with a poorer prognosis; treatment may not be warranted except to salvage particularly valuable horses. The major cause of residual lameness was assumed to be restrictive adhesions. However, in most cases, this was not confirmed by diagnostic nerve blocks or ultrasonography.[197] In this latter study, the authors in general did not suture the tendon if it could not be apposed. Laceration involved the digital sheath in 16 horses, and 10 of these survived. They did not detect an association between tendon sheath involvement and outcome. Median duration of hospitalization time was 23 days. Taylor et al. did not find an association between time of injury to treatment, whereas Foland et al. suggested horses treated within 6 hours of injury had a better prognosis. Taylor et al. agreed that compared with primary suture repair, wound care followed by delayed suture repair of the tendon might be a better approach

to treatment of contaminated tendon lacerations. The authors noted that while no controlled passive motion is possible when a limb is immobilized with a cast, it is possible when a board or metal splint is used. In addition, these horses can be discharged from the hospital if their owners are capable of appropriate nursing care.[197] They did point out that when splints are used, it may be appropriate to increase the length of time that the limb is immobilized to compensate for any adverse effects that early movement may have on revascularization and tendon healing. The authors concluded that horses with transection of one tendon or partial disruptions of tendons had a good prognosis for return to intended use, while those with transection of both flexor tendons have a guarded prognosis for return to tendon use. They recommended primary suture repair or delayed primary suture repair of transected tendons followed by immobilization of the limb for 4 to 6 weeks and continued support for another 4 to 6 weeks.

Tenosynovitis

Tenosynovitis implies inflammation of the synovial membrane of the tendon sheath, but the fibrous layer of the tendon sheath is usually involved as well. The condition is manifested by distension of the tendon sheath due to synovial effusion. The condition has different causes and different clinical manifestations. The various types of tenosynovitis in the horse are classified here as follows: 1) idiopathic tenosynovitis, 2) acute tenosynovitis, 3) chronic tenosynovitis, and 4) septic (infectious) tenosynovitis. There is some overlap in this classification system, but it seems to be the most appropriate for an effective discussion of treatment.

Idiopathic Tenosynovitis

Idiopathic tenosynovitis may be defined as tenosynovitis with synovial effusion but without inflammation, pain, or lameness. The cause of the condition is vague, as indicated by its name. In some instances, foals are born with the condition,[206,211] and it is usually associated with the tendon sheaths of the extensor tendons as they pass over the carpus. In the adult, tendon sheath effusion without other signs typically develops insidiously, and the most commonly affected sites are the tarsal sheath, the digital flexor sheath, and the extensor tendon sheaths over the carpus.

Tenosynovitis of the tarsal sheath is also called "thorough-pin" (Fig. 7.121). The tarsal sheath encloses the DDF tendon of the hindlimb. Thorough-pin is a morphologic description of the swelling, and while most cases are idiopathic synovitis, the presence of other clinical signs may cause it to be classified in one of the other categories. The term "windpuffs" or "windgalls" has been used as a general term to describe synovial swelling of various joints and tendon sheaths that does not cause lameness, but it is most commonly used to describe tenosynovitis of the digital flexor tendon sheath.

PATHOGENESIS

The pathogenesis in newborn foals is unknown. In idiopathic tenosynovitis that develops with time, the

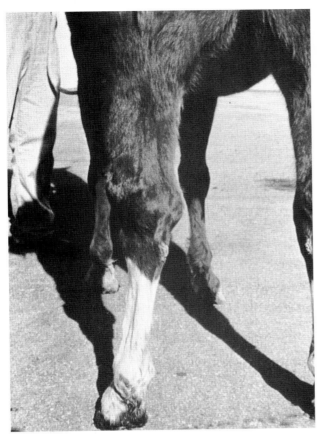

Figure 7.121 Thorough-pin.

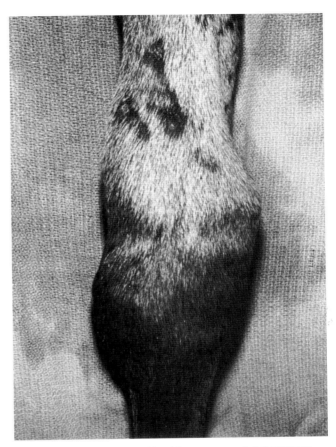

Figure 7.122 Tenosynovitis of the common digital extensor tendon sheath.

cause is presumed to be chronic low-grade trauma in many cases, but this is generally undefined. Conformation has been incriminated with tenosynovitis of the tarsal sheath.[207] Although it was stated that active inflammation is not necessary for synovial effusion, the same authors reported treatment of the problem with corticosteroids.[206] The presence of some pathologic change in the synovial membrane in these cases should be assumed. There is usually no previous history of injury or inflammation.

DIAGNOSIS

Distension of the tendon sheath due to effusion is the typical clinical presentation (Figs. 7.122 and 123). As stated above, there is no inflammation, pain, or lameness. The synovial fluid findings are unspectacular. The fluid varies from pale yellow and clear, through amber and clear, to amber and opaque. The average protein concentration is 2 to 2.5 mg/dL, and the leukocyte count is generally less than 600.[207] The mucin clot is fair to poor, indicating some dilution of mucin, which is probably associated with the increased volume of synovial fluid. Distension of the tarsal sheath may be confused with bog spavin or intertendinous calcaneal bursitis. Tenosynovitis of the digital sheath (wind puffs) manifests as distension that may be palpated between the suspensory ligament and the flexor tendons. Tendon sheath distension may also be palpated on the palmar or plantar

aspect of the pastern. Generally, the diagnosis of idiopathic tenosynovitis is made easily, but it is important to rule out septic and autoimmune problems in foals.

TREATMENT

These lesions are rather common and should be considered blemishes, as they are not causing a clinical problem. Treatment by synovial fluid aspiration and injection of a corticosteroid has been successful.[208] Our experience is that alleviation following steroid injection is often temporary. However, the use of bandaging following injection may improve the success rate. The use of orgotein (see the section, "Specific Diseases of Joints: Idiopathic Snyovitis (Bog Spavin and Articular Windpuffs)," in this chapter) is another option. Unless the presence of the blemish is of concern to the owner, no treatment is necessary. The application of a limb brace or sweat under cotton or bandage at the end of the day can be used if owners are particularly concerned. These measures will control the distension but will not cause permanent resolution. Distension will also become less evident with exercise. If lameness develops at any stage, the cause should be ascertained by appropriate examination.

Acute Tenosynovitis

Acute tenosynovitis is characterized by a rapidly developing effusion within a tendon sheath accompanied by heat, pain, and possibly lameness.

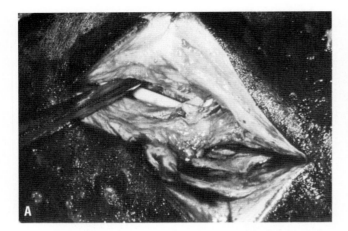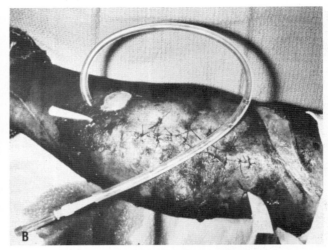

Figure 7.123 A. Septic tenosynovitis being explored. B. After closure with instillation of tubular ingress tube and Penrose drain.

PATHOGENESIS

There may be a history of trauma, but this is not always the case. The occurrence of tenosynovitis in the extensor sheath over the carpus has been associated with falling or hitting a jump with the carpus.[132] Direct trauma could be a cause in other sites as well. Acute tenosynovitis often develops in association with acute tendinitis (tenosynovitis). Other proposed causes include friction between opposing parietal and visceral layers of the synovial sheath, peritendinous pressure, or acute direct trauma to the tendon and its sheath.[218] In a report of 11 cases of tenosynovitis involving the tarsal sheath, 6 horses presented with either severe (4), moderate (1), or slight (1) lameness of sudden onset, and 2 with moderate lameness of gradual onset. Of the other 3, tarsal sheath distension occurred gradually in 1, without associated lameness. Reported accidents included kicks from horses (3 cases) and sudden onset after competition or training (2 cases).[41] Proposed causes of acute aseptic tenosynovitis in the digital flexor tendon sheath are direct trauma to the digital flexor tendon sheath and strain of a flexor tendon, suspensory ligament, or palmar/plantar anular ligament.[40] The proximal portion of the sheath is not protected by the anular ligament of the fetlock, and thus direct blunt trauma may cause sheath contusion and subsequent hemorrhage or herniation. In more complicated cases, SDF or DDF tendon or suspensory ligament injury may cause swelling of these structures, leading to relative stenosis of the fetlock canal and subsequent contusion of the digital flexor sheath. Overstretching or compression of the digital sheath may also cause friction between opposing parietal and visceral layers of the synovial sheath between the normal flexor tendon digital sheath attachments or in the intimate attachments between the superficial flexor tendon digital sheath and palmar/plantar or proximal digital anular ligaments. Wright and McMahon[237] recently described tenosynovitis associated with longitudinal tears of the digital flexor tendons in 20 horses. Nineteen defects involved the DDF tendon, and in 2 horses, the manica flexoria of the SDF was torn. Ultrasonography revealed nonspecific signs of chronic tenosynovitis but not the cause. Longitudinal tears of the deep flexor tendon should be considered in the differential diagnosis of tenosynovitis of the digital flexor tendon sheath.

DIAGNOSIS

Diagnosis is based on the presence of tendon sheath effusion accompanied by acute inflammatory signs. The presence of associated tendinitis should be differentiated with sonography. In tenosynovitis of an extensor tendon over the carpus, the differential diagnosis may include acute carpitis, hygroma, cellulitis, and synovial hernia. Acute septic tenosynovitis is usually characterized by a sudden onset of mild-to-severe lameness associated with warm painful effusion of the digital sheath. The distension is most prominent in the proximal portion of the digital sheath but is also palpable over the palmarodistal aspect of the pastern where the distal portion of the sheath protrudes between the proximal and distal digital anular ligaments. Ultrasonographic examination is important in these cases to define tendon lesions, particularly focal lesions of the DDFT in the case of a digital sheath problem. Ultrasonography is also useful, as well as radiology when there is distension of acute tenosynovitis of the tarsal sheath, as 6 of 11 cases reported by Dik and Merkens had associated bone abnormalities of the sustentaculum tali. Contrast arthrography is useful to delineate filling defects and other masses.[212] Unless there is an early response to treatment, tenoscopy may be included.

TREATMENT

Treatment includes rest and the use of cold hydrotherapy or ice packs initially. Astringent dressings and braces or sweats may be used at a later stage. Aspiration of fluid and injection of corticosteroids or orgotein may be used but should generally be reserved for cases that do not respond within a week. If no quick response to treatment occurs, then diagnostic tenoscopic examination may be useful, particularly in instances of tenosynovitis of the digital sheath or tarsal sheath.

The prognosis is favorable if the horse is rested, no damage to the tendon is present, and appropriate treatment is commenced immediately. With inappropriate treatment, chronic tenosynovitis may develop.

Chronic Tenosynovitis

Chronic tenosynovitis is characterized by a persistent synovial effusion and fibrous thickening of the tendon sheath. It is often accompanied by stenosis within the sheath or adhesions between the opposing parietal and visceral layers of the tendon sheath and the tendon.

PATHOGENESIS

The condition commonly follows acute tenosynovitis that has not resolved satisfactorily, but it can develop from trauma that is multiple and minor. Direct trauma and/or inflammation can lead to the formation of adhesions. Again, direct tendon damage may also be present.

DIAGNOSIS

The clinical signs include a persistent synovial effusion in the affected tendon sheath, generally accompanied by stenosis or adhesions within the sheath. One criterion for the diagnosis of chronic tenosynovitis is that compromised function is present. In other instances, the cases should be classified as idiopathic tenosynovitis. Inability to flex the carpus is the most common presenting complaint with chronic tenosynovitis of the extensor tendon sheaths of the carpus, and pain is not a major factor. Long-term tenosynovitis of the digital sheath may follow acute effusion that is not resolved completely, may result from persistent tendon and ligament injury, or can develop from multiple minor trauma such as recurrent overloading. Continuous irritation of the sheath may lead to diffuse or nodular thickening of the sheath wall. Adhesions reduce sheath capacity and elasticity or stenosis of the fetlock canal. The fluctuant swelling is usually cold and painless in chronic cases.[40] Ultrasonography is effective in demonstrating digital sheath synovial proliferation and adhesions as well as tendon or ligamentous injury. Arthroscopy is a suitable diagnostic and prognostic tool to assess digital sheath and associated flexor tendon abnormalities. It also provides an effective technique for resection of adhesions in solitary sheath wall proliferations.[126] As mentioned above, longitudinal tears of the digital flexor tendon should be considered in the differential diagnosis of tenosynovitis of the digital flexor tendon sheath.[236] The use of contrast radiography as well as tenoscopy can help define the condition in the case of chronic tenosynovitis of the tarsal sheath.

TREATMENT

As an initial treatment method, drainage and injection of corticosteroids or orgotein can be attempted. In clinical cases unresponsive to drainage and injection and where lameness is present, surgical exploration of the tendon sheath may be performed. This procedure has been generally restricted to carpal extensor tendon sheaths.[132,218] In a report of 15 horses with chronic tenosynovitis of the carpal extensor tendon sheath, the condition was seen most commonly in horses used for jumping, and penetration of the tendon sheath by thorns was the most common cause. Treatment involved surgical resection of the hyperplastic synovial membrane and adhesions within the tendon sheath with primary closure. When combined with early postoperative physiotherapy, this was found to be effective.[160] In most instances such debridement would be done arthroscopically now. Pathologic findings include rupture of the sheath, villous synovitis, granulation tissue formation, and adhesions.[132] Peripheral fibers of the tendon may also be affected. The tendon sheath most commonly affected is that of the extensor carpi radialis, digital flexor tendon sheath, and tarsal sheath.[132] Following exploration, the tendon sheath should be closed with synthetic absorbable sutures. In one report of 6 cases explored surgically, the result was satisfactory in 3.[132] In another series of two cases, both horses returned to racing.[218] Arthroscopic evaluation and treatment have been used increasingly in cases of chronic tenosynovitis of the tarsal sheath. In resection of solitary nodular perforations or minor adhesions, the results can be very beneficial. In 20 horses with longitudinal tears of the digital flexor tendon causing tenosynovitis, 11 horses became sound and returned to work.[236] If extensive resection of adhesions is required, the prognosis is guarded.

Septic (Infectious) Tenosynovitis

Septic tenosynovitis is characterized by marked synovial effusion, heat, pain, swelling, severe lameness, and suppurative synovial fluid.

PATHOGENESIS

As in septic arthritis, septic tenosynovitis can result from hematogenous, iatrogenic infection, or trauma (punctures and lacerations).[210] The severe inflammatory process causes fibrin deposition that can progress quickly to adhesion formation. In addition, lysosomal enzymes released by the inflammatory process can digest the tendon substance.

DIAGNOSIS

Septic tenosynovitis is recognized by severe lameness with associated tendon sheath effusion accompanied by heat, pain, and swelling. The diagnosis is confirmed by synovial fluid analysis. The fluid may be serosanguineous or purulent. Protein concentration will be above 3 g/dL, and the white cell count is generally above 30,000/mm^3. The temperature may be elevated.

If the clinical case has not been presented immediately the disease may already have progressed to the stage of degenerative tendon rupture.

TREATMENT

The principles of treatment are the same as those described for infectious arthritis. The use of parenteral broad-spectrum antibiotics is indicated, and synovial fluid aspiration with irrigation and drainage is usually appropriate. As discussed with infective arthritis, the author tends toward a more aggressive approach, including opening the tendon sheath and implanting irrigation devices and drains (Fig. 7.123). Adhesion formation is the most common reason for failure to return to athletic activity.

A retrospective study reviewed 25 horses with septic tenosynovitis treated over 7 years to determine clinical features of the disease and response to treatment.[91] Sepsis was located in the sheath of the digital flexor tendons in 22 horses, the extensor carpi radialis tendon in 1 horse, the long digital extensor tendon in 1 horse, and the common digital extensor tendon in 1 horse. Nine horses received only medical treatment, usually a combination of broad-spectrum parenterally introduced antibiotics (8 of 9 horses), NSAIDs (8 of 9 horses), or irrigation of the wound (4 of 9 horses). Fourteen horses were treated surgically with either transection of the palmar/plantar anular ligament of the metacarpometatarsal phalangeal joint (5 of 14 horses), lavage of the sheath after insertion of drains into the sheath (7 of 14 horses), or both (2 of 14 horses). All horses treated surgically were concurrently treated parenterally with broad-spectrum antibiotics and NSAIDs. Two horses with septic tenosynovitis were not treated and euthanized at the owner's request.

Five horses were euthanized before discharge from the hospital. Two horses (both treated medically) were lost to follow-up. Of 18 horses for which follow-up information was obtained 6 to 55 months after discharge, 5 were treated medically, 4 returned to their intended use (3 performance and 1 breeding), and 1 was being used for breeding rather than for performance as intended. Of the 13 horses treated surgically, 6 returned to their intended use (3 performance; 3 breeding), 3 were unable to return to their intended use (performance), and 4 horses used for performance prior to injury were retired for breeding. Overall, 18 of 23 horses (78%) for which long-term follow-up was available survived more than 6 months after discharge from the hospital. Ten of these (56%) returned to their intended use (6 performance; 4 breeding).[91] Although the small number of horses may have limited statistical power, no differences were seen between the results of medical and surgical treatment. Despite these data (and probably because of low numbers), the authors still choose to recommend a surgical approach in most cases. With regard to lavage of the sheath, a study in horses has revealed that 0.1% povidone iodine did not cause synovitis appreciably worse than that caused by balanced electrolyte solution. However, 0.5% povidone iodine and chlorhexidine lavage (0.5%) caused severe synovitis and should not be used for tendon sheath lavage.[11] In another report, survival following treatment of 14 cases of septic tenosynovitis was 100%.[176]

Laceration of a Tendon Sheath

An acute laceration of the tendon sheath should be managed similarly to an open joint injury. If the wound is clean and contamination is not obvious, suturing may be appropriate. If contamination has occurred, debridement and irrigation are performed. Primary closure is not generally recommended in these cases. The wounds can be left to granulate in, or delayed closure can be used. When delayed closure is used it is generally done between 4 and 6 days postinjury. Depending on the site,

cast immobilization is often appropriate in the initial healing stages. The cast is removed in 7 to 10 days, and a support wrap used. Radical debridement is necessary in severe wounds.

Luxation of Tendons

Luxation of the SDF tendon from the point of the hock is occasionally seen in the horse. The SDF tendon arises from the supracondylar fossa of the femur. Toward the distal third of the tibia, it winds around the medial surface of the gastrocnemius tendon to reach the point of the hock where it widens out, forming a cap over the tuber calcis. At this point the SDF tendon attaches the lateral and medial aspects of the tuber calcis by a strong band, together with the tarsal tendons of the biceps femoris and semitendinosus muscles. The function of these bands is to retain the SDF tendon in place on the summit of the tuber calcis.

PATHOGENESIS

Displacement of the SDF tendon results from a kick on the point of the hock or powerful muscle contraction of the hindlimb when the hock is flexed, as when a horse is pulled up suddenly at the gallop. One or both of the supporting bands may rupture, and the tendon slips to the side of the tuber calcis. The medial band appears to be the weaker of the two, and displacement occurs to the lateral side.[88]

DIAGNOSIS

The point of the hock is swollen, and there is excessive flexion of the hock joint. The displaced tendon may be palpated moving up and down the side of the calcaneus. It may regain its normal position on the point of the tuber calcis when the hock is extended but slips off again when the hock is flexed.

TREATMENT

Some form of surgical treatment is necessary to replace the cap of the superficial flexor tendon onto the tuber calcis and retain it in position. A number of methods have been tried without success. The use of a bone plate bent 180° to act as a tunnel over the SDF tendon has been described.[106] Conservative therapy with rest from 3 to 6 months was reported to produce a sound horse.[88] It may be that the tendon can become accommodated in its new position at the side of the calcaneus with fibrous tissue forming a channel. However, I feel that surgery should be attempted.

We have successfully operated by repairing the ruptured medial band and supplementing this repair with synthetic mesh. This technique has also been described in the literature.[177] Synthetic mesh was overlaid on the reconstructed tarsal ligament and sutured to the underlying tissues. A full-limb cast was applied, and removed 30 days after surgery. The horse withstood race training but did not return to a level of performance consistent with that prior to injury. (See Chapter 8, "Luxation of the Superficial Digital Flexor off the Point of the Hock," for details.)

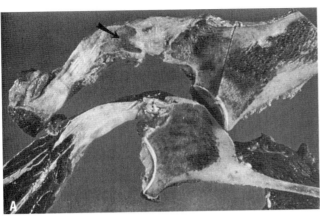

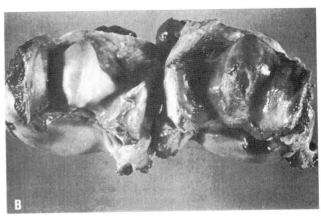

Figure 7.124 Ossification of biceps brachii tendon. A. Heterotopic bone formation in affected biceps brachii tendon (arrow). B. Damage to intertubercular (bicipital) groove of humerus caused by ossified tendon. Normal opposite humerus is depicted on the left. (Courtesy of T. S. Stashak.)

Tumors

Tumors in association with tendons or tendon sheaths are rare. Fibromas may be seen in tendons.[2] Multiple hemangiosarcomas in the tarsal synovial sheath have been reported.[209] Three sessile growths were excised from the sheath, and the horse returned to racing.

Tendon Ossification

Ossification of the biceps brachii tendon is a rare condition that develops in young horses.[133]

Pathogenesis

The cause is unknown. The biceps brachii has two fusiform regions of fibrocartilage within the tendon, in the area of the bicipital groove. Heterotropic bone appears to form in this region. These bony regions subsequently damage adjacent synovial membrane, bone, and cartilage and lead to chronic shoulder lameness.

Diagnosis

The condition presents as forelimb lameness with a shortened cranial phase. Muscle atrophy may be present around the shoulder, and extension and flexion of the shoulder may cause a painful response. Deep palpation over the point of the shoulder may elicit a painful response. Radiology confirms the presence of a calcified mass in the bicipital tendon in association with the bicipital bursa. The calcified mass causes damage to the intertubercular groove (Fig. 7.124).

Treatment

There is no reported treatment.

Synovial Ganglion, Hernia, or Fistula Associated with Tendon Sheath

Synovial ganglion associated with the common digital extensor sheath in the horse has been mentioned.[208] I

have not observed a synovial ganglion or hernia associated with a tendon sheath. Synovial fistulation can occur, usually between a tendon sheath and a joint.[110] This condition is confirmed by contrast radiography. If the fistula can be identified in a surgically accessible position, surgical repair can be performed.[110]

References

1. Adams OR. Constriction of the palmar (volar) or planter ligament in horses. Vet Med Sm Anim Clin 1974;69:327.
2. Adams SB, Fessler JF. Tendon fibromas in 2 horses. Equine Vet J 1982;14:95.
3. Adams SB, Santschi EM. Management of flexural limb deformities in young horses. Equine Pract 1999;21:9–14.
4. Allen AK. Experience with ultrasound-guided tendon puncture or splitting. In: Proceedings. 38th Annual Meeting of the American Association of Equine Practitioners, Orlando, FL, 1992;273–277.
4a. Amiel D, Frank C, Harwood F. Tendons and ligaments: A morphological and biochemical comparison. J Orthop Res 1984;1: 257–265.
5. Arnbjerg J. Changes in the distal phalanx in foals with deep digital flexor tendon contraction. Vet Radiol 1988;29:65–69.
6. Arnbjerg J, Smith M, Sonnichsen HV. Rupture of the common digital extensor in foals. Nord Vet Med 1970;22:452.
7. Asheim A. Surgical treatment of tendon injuries in the horse. J Am Vet Med Assoc 1964;145:447.
8. Asheim A, Knudsen O. Percutaneous tendon splitting. Proceedings. 13th Annual Meeting of the American Association of Equine Practitioners, New Orleans, LA, 1967;255–257.
9. Badame GF. A corrective appliance for contracted tendons in foals. Proceedings. 9th Annual Meeting of the American Association of Equine Practitioners, Lexington, KY, 1963;91–97.
10. Bailey AJ, Light ND, Atkins ED. Chemical cross-linking restrictions on models for the molecular organization of the collagen fiber. Nature 1980;288:408–410.
11. Baird AN, Scruggs DW, Watkins JP, Taylor TS. Effect of antimicrobial solution lavage on the palmar digital tendon sheath in horses. Am J Vet Res 1990;51:1488–1494.
12. Baker JR, Lindsay JR. Equine goiter due to excess iodine. J Am Vet Med Assoc 1968;153:1618.
13. Banes AJ, Enterline D, Bevin AG, Salisbury RE. Effects of trauma and partial devascularization on protein synthesis in the avian flexor profundus tendon. J Trauma 1981;21:505–512.
14. Barr ARS, Dyson SJ, Barr FJ, O'Brien JK. Tendinitis of the deep digital flexor tendon in the distal metacarpal/metatarsal region associated with tendinitis of the digital sheath in the horse. Equine Vet J 1995;27:348–355.

15. Becker CK, Sabelberg HHCM, Buchner HHF, Barneveld A. Long-term consequences of experimental desmotomy of the accessory ligament of the deep digital flexor tendon in adult horses. Am J Vet Res 1998;59:347–351.

16. Becker CK, Sabelberg CM, Buchner HF, Barneveld A. Effects of experimental desmotomy on material properties and histomorphologic and ultrasonographic features of the accessory ligament of the deep digital flexor tendon in clinically normal horses. Am J Vet Res 1998;59:352–358.

17. Becker CK, Sabelberg HH, Barneveld A. In vitro mechanical properties of the accessory ligament of the deep digital flexor tendon in horses in relation to age. Equine Vet J 1994;26:454–459.

18. Beeman GM. Factors that may influence club feet: Genetics, nutrition, stance and proper trimming and medical treatment. Equine Athlete 1990;3:9.

19. Belknap JK, Baxter GM, Nickel FA. Extensor tendon lacerations in horses: 50 cases (1982–1988). J Am Vet Med Assoc 1993;203:428.

20. Bertone AL, Stashak TS, Smith FW, et al. A comparison of repair methods for gap healing in equine flexor tendons. Vet Surg 1990;19:254–265.

21. Birch HL, Bailey AJ, Goodship AE. Macroscopic 'degeneration' of equine superficial digital flexor tendon is accompanied by a change in extracellular matrix composition. Equine Vet J 1998;30:534–539.

22. Birch HL, Bailey AJ, Goodship AE. Extracellular matrix changes in clinically normal equine superficial digital flexor tendons may account for subsequent tendon rupture. Proceedings. 32nd British Equine Veterinary Association Congress, Warwick, England, 1993.

23. Birch HL, Bailey JVB, Bailey AJ, Goodship AE. Age-related changes to the molecular and cellular components of equine flexor tendons. Equine Vet J 1999;31:391–396.

24. Blackwell RB. Response of acquired flexural deformity of the metacarpophalangeal joint to desmotomy of the inferior check ligament. Proceedings. 28th Annual Meeting of the American Association of Equine Practitioners, Atlanta, GA, 1982;107–112.

25. Bloom N, Fawcett DW. A Textbook of Histology. 10th ed. Philadelphia: WB Saunders, 1975.

26. Boyd JS. Congenital deformities in two Clydesdale foals. Equine Vet J 1976;18:161.

27. Bramlage LR. An initial report on a surgical technique for arthrodesis of the metacarpophalangeal joint in the horse. Proceedings. 27th Annual Meeting of the American Association of Equine Practitioners, New Orleans, LA, 1981;257–261.

28. Bramlage LR. Superior check ligament desmotomy as a treatment for superficial digital flexor tendinitis. Proceedings. 32nd Annual Meeting of the American Association of Equine Practitioners, Nashville, TN, 1986;365–369.

29. Bramlage LR, Rantanen NW, Genovese RL, et al. Long term effects of surgical treatment of superficial digital flexor tendinitis by superior check desmotomy. Proceedings. 34th Annual Meeting of the American Association of Equine Practitioners, San Diego, CA, 1988;655–656.

30. Brown MP, Pool RR. Experimental and clinical investigations of the use of carbon fiber suture in equine tendon repair. J Am Vet Med Assoc 1983;182:956.

31. Bukowiecki CF, Bramlage LR, Gabel AA. In vitro strength of the suspensory apparatus in training and resting horses. Vet Surg 1987;16:126–130.

32. Butler DL, Grood ES, Noyes FR, Zernicke RF. Biomechanics of ligaments and tendons. Exerc Sport Sci Rev 1978;6:125–181.

33. Catlin JE. Rupture of the extensor carpi radialis tendon. Vet Med Sm Anim Clin 1964;59:1178.

34. Collins SM. Discussion of Dr. Cosgrove's paper. Vet Rec 1955;67:965.

35. Cosgrove JSM. The veterinary surgeon and the newborn foal. Vet Rec 1955;67:961.

36. Crevier N, Pourcelot P, Denoix J-M, et al. Segmental variations of in vitro mechanical properties in equine superficial digital flexor tendons. Am J Vet Res 1996;57:1111–1117.

37. Crevier-Denoix N, Collobert C, Sanaa M, et al. Mechanical correlations derived from segmental histologic study of the equine superficial flexor tendon, from foal to adult. Am J Vet Res 1998;969–977.

38. Curtis SJ, Stoneham S. Effect of farriery treatment of hypoflexion tendons (severe digital hyperextension in a foal. Equine Vet Educ 1999;113–117.

38a. Denoix JM, Crevier N, Azevedo C. Ultrasound examination of the pastern. Proceedings. 37th Annual Convention of the American Association of Equine Practitioners, San Francisco, CA, 1991;363–380.

39. Diamant J, Keller N, Vaer E, et al. Collagen: Ultrastructure and its relation to mechanical properties as a function of aging. Proc R Soc Lond (B) 1972;180:293–315.

39a. DiCesare P, Hauser N, Lehman D, et al. Cartilage oligomeric matrix protein (COMP) is an abundant component of tendon. FEBS Lett 1994;354:237–240.

40. Dik KJ, Dyson SJ, Vail TB. Aseptic tenosynovitis of the digital flexor tendon sheath, fetlock and pastern anular ligament constriction. Vet Clin North Am Equine Pract 1995;11:151–162.

41. Dik KJ, Merkens HW. Unilateral distention of the tarsal sheath in the horse: A report of 11 cases. Equine Vet J 1987;19:307–313.

42. Dyson SJ. Desmitis of the accessory ligament of the deep digital flexor tendon: 27 cases (1986–1990). Equine Vet J 1991;23:438–444.

43. Dyson S. Proximal suspensory desmitis: Clinical, ultrasonographic and radiographic features. Equine Vet J 1991;23:25–31.

44. Dyson SJ. Proximal suspensory desmitis in the hindlimb. Equine Vet Educ 1995;7:275–278.

45. Dyson SJ. Treatment of superficial digital flexor tendinitis: A comparison of conservative management, sodium hyaluronate and glycosaminoglycan polysulfate. Proceedings. 43rd Annual Meeting of the American Association of Equine Practitioners, Phoenix, AZ, 1997;297–300.

46. Dyson SJ, Arthur RM, Palmer SE, Richardson D. Suspensory ligament desmitis. Vet Clin North Am Equine Pract 1995;11:177–215.

47. Easley KJ, Stashak TS, Smith FW, et al. Mechanical properties of four suture patterns for transected tendon repair. Vet Surg 1990;19:102–106.

48. Elliott DA. Structure and function of mammalian tendon. Biol Rev 1965;40:392.

49. Embertson RM. Congenital abnormalities of tendons and ligaments. Vet Clin North Am Equine Pract 1994;10:351–364.

50. Evans JH, Barbenel JC. Structural and mechanical properties of tendon related to function. Equine Vet J 1975;7:1.

51. Fackelman GE. Autologous tendon transplantation in the horse—The technique of its histologic evaluation. Schweiz Arch Tierheilkd 1973;115:231.

52. Fackelman GE. Flexure deformity of the metacarpophalangeal joints in growing horses. Comp Cont Educ Pract Vet 1979;1:S1.

53. Fackelman GE. The nature of tendon damage and its repair. Equine Vet J 1973;5:141.

54. Fackelman GE, Auer JA, Orsini J, von Salis B. Surgical treatment of severe flexural deformity of the distal interphalangeal joint in young horses. J Am Vet Med Assoc 1983;182:949–952.

55. Fackelman GE, Clodius L. Surgical correction of the digital hyperextension deformity in foals. Vet Med Sm Anim Clin 1972;67:1116.

56. Farry PJ, Prentice NG, Hunter AC, Wakelin CA. Ice treatment of injured ligaments: An experimental model. NZ Med J 1980;651:12–14.

57. Fessler JF. Tendon disorders of the young horse. Archives ACVS 1977;6:19.

58. Flecker RH, Wagner PC. Therapy and corrective shoeing for equine tendon disorders. Comp Cont Educ Pract Vet 1986;8:970–976.

59. Foland JW, Trotter GW, Powers BE, et al. Effect of sodium hyaluronate in collagenase-induced superficial digital flexor tendinitis in horses. Am J Vet Res 1992;53:2371–2376.

60. Foland JW, Trotter GW, Stashak TS, et al. Traumatic injuries involving tendons of the distal limb in horses: A retrospective study of 55 cases. Equine Vet J 1991;23:422–425.

60a. Ford T, Ross M, Orsini P. A comparison of methods for proximal palmar metacarpal anesthesia in horses. Vet Surg 1988;18:146–150.

61. Franks PW. The use of ionizing radiation for the treatment of injuries to flexor tendons and supporting ligaments in the horse. Equine Vet J 1979;11:106.

62. Gaughan EM, Gift LJ, DeBowes RM. The influence of sequential intratendinous sodium hyaluronate on tendon healing in horses. Vet Compar Orthop Traumatol 1995;8:40–45.

63. Gaughan EM, Gift LJ, Nixon AJ, Krook LP. Effects of sodium hyaluronate on tendon healing and adhesion formation in horses. Am J Vet Res 1001;52:764–773.

64. Gelberman RH, Manske PR, Akeson WH. Flexor tendon repair. J Orthop Res 1986;4:119–128.

65. Gelberman RH, Nunley JA, Osterman AL, et al. Influence of the protected passive mobilization interval on flexor tendon healing. A prospective randomized clinical study. Clin Orthop 1991;264: 190–196.

66. Gelberman RH, Vande Berg JS, Lundborg GN, Akeson WH. Flexor tendon healing and restoration of the gliding surface. J Bone Joint Surg [Am] 1983;65:70–80.

67. Genovese RL. Sonographic response to intralesional therapy with beta-aminoproprionitrile fumarate for clinical tendon injuries in horses. In: Proceedings. 38th Annual Meeting of the American Association of Equine Practitioners, Orlando, FL, 1992; 265–272.

68. Deleted in proof.

69. Genovese R, Longo K, Berthold B, Jorgenson J. Quantitative sonographic assessment in the clinical management of superficial digital flexor tendon injuries in Thoroughbred racehorses. Proceedings. 43rd Annual Meeting of the American Association of Equine Practitioners, Phoenix, AZ, 1997;285–290.

70. Genovese RL, Rantanen NW. The superficial digital flexor tendon. In: Rantanen NW, McKinnon AO, Eds. Equine Diagnostic Ultrasonography. Baltimore: Williams & Wilkins, 1998; 289–398.

71. Genovese RL, Rantanen NW, Hauser ML, et al. Diagnostic ultrasonography of equine limbs. Vet Clin North Am Equine Pract 1986;2:145–226.

72. Gerring EL, Webbon PM. Fetlock anular ligament desmotomy: A report of 24 cases. Equine Vet J 1984;16:113–116.

73. Gibson KT, Burbridge HM, Pfeiffer DU. Superficial digital flexor tendinitis in Thoroughbred racehorses: Outcome following nonsurgical treatment and superior check ligament desmotomy [abstract]. Am Coll Vet Surg 1997;25:7.

74. Getty R. Sisson and Grossman's The Anatomy of Domestic Animals, vol 1. 5th ed. Philadelphia: WB Saunders, 1975;431.

75. Gillis CL. Rehabilitation of tendon and ligament injuries. Proc Am Assoc Equine Pract 1997;43:306–309.

76. Gillis CL, Meagher DM, Balesdent A. Suspensory ligament desmitis and associated fractures. Proceedings. 40th Annual Meeting of the American Association of Equine Practitioners, Vancouver, Canada, 1994;187–188.

77. Gillis CL, Meagher DM, Peal RR, et al. Ultrasonographically detected changes in the equine superficial digital flexor tendon during the first month of race training. Am J Vet Res 1993;54: 1797–1802.

78. Goodship AE. The pathophysiology of flexor tendon injury in the horse. Equine Vet Educ 1993;5:23–29.

79. Goodship AE, Birch HL, Wilson AM. The pathobiology and repair of tendon and ligament injury. Vet Clin North Am Equine Pract 1994;10:323–349.

80. Goodship AE, Brown PN, Yeats JJ, et al. An assessment of filamentous carbon fibre for the treatment of tendon injury in the horse. Vet Rec 1980;106:217–221.

81. Goodship AE, Silver IA, Wilson AN. Treatment of tendinitis in horses [letter]. Vet Rec 1991.

82. Grant BD, Cannon HJ, Rose JA. Equine tendinitis: Results of eleven cases treated with autografts. J Equine Med Surg 1978;2: 509.

83. Hawkins JF, Ross MW. Transection of the accessory ligament of the superficial digital flexor muscle for the treatment of superficial digital flexor tendinitis in Standardbreds: 40 cases (1988–1992). J Am Vet Med Assoc 1995;206:674–678.

84. Henninger R. Treatment of superficial digital flexor tendinitis. Vet Clin North Am Equine Pract 1994;10:409–424.

85. Henninger RW, Bramlage LR, Bailey M, et al. Effects of tendon splitting on experimentally-induced acute tendinitis. Vet Compar Orthop Traumatol 1992;5:1–9.

86. Henninger R, Bramlage L, Schneider R. Short term effect of superior check ligament desmotomy and percutaneous tendon splitting as treatment for acute tendinitis. Proceedings. 36th Annual Meeting of the American Association of Equine Practitioners, Lexington, KY, 1990;539–540.

87. Hertsch B, Schmidt H, Tilkorn P. Ergebnisse der behandlung von Tendopathien des Pferdes mit hochmoleqularem NaHyaluronat. Pferdeheilkunde 1989;5:235–243.

88. Hickman J. Veterinary Orthopaedics. Philadelphia: JB Lippincott, 1964.

89. Hintz HF, Schryver HF, Lowe JE. Delayed growth response and limb conformation in young horses. Cornell Vet.

90. Hogan PA, Bramlage LR. Transection of the accessory ligament of the superficial digital flexor tendon for treatment of tendinitis: Long term results in 61 Standardbred racehorses (1985–1992). Equine Vet J 1995;27:221–226.

91. Honnas CM, Schumacher J, Cohen ND, et al. Septic tenosynovitis in horses: 25 cases (1983–1989). J Am Vet Med Assoc 1991;199: 1616–1622.

92. Deleted in proof.

93. Hutt FB. Genetic defects of bones and joints in domestic animals. Cornell Vet (Suppl) 1968;58:104.

94. Jann HW, Good JK, Morgan SJ, et al. Healing of transected equine superficial digital flexor tendons with and without tenorrhaphy. Vet Surg 1992;21:40–46.

95. Jansson N. Digital extensor tendon lacerations in horses: A retrospective evaluation of 22 cases. J Equine Vet Sci 1995;15: 537–540.

96. Jansson N, Sonnichsen HV. Acquired flexural deformity of the distal interphalangeal joint in horses: Treatment by desmotomy of the accessory ligament of the deep digital flexor tendon. A retrospective study. J Equine Vet Sci 1995;15:353–356.

97. Deleted in proof.

98. Johnson JH. Contracted tendons. Mod Vet Pract 1973;54:67.

99. Kainer RJ. Carpal joints. In: Stashak T, Ed. Adams' Lameness in Horses. 4th ed. Philadelphia: Lea & Febiger, 1987;24.

100. Kaneps AJ, Hultgren BD, Riebold TW, et al. Laser therapy in horses: Histologic response. Am J Vet Res 1984;45:581–582.

101. Kasper CA, Clayton HM, Wright AK, et al. Effects of high doses of oxytetracycline on metacarpophalangeal joint kinematics in neonatal foals. J Am Vet Med Assoc 1995;207:71–73.

102. Keeler RF, James LF. Failure of dietary supplementation to prevent abortions and congenital malformations of lathyrism and locoism in sheep. Can J Comp Med 1971;35:342.

103. Ketchum LD. Tendon healing. In: Hunt TK, Dunphy JE, Eds. Fundamentals of Wound Management in Surgery. New York: Appleton-Century-Crofts, 1979.

104. Knudsen O. Percutaneous tendon splitting—methods and results. Equine Vet J 1976;8:101.

105. Leach D, Harland R, Burko B. The anatomy of the carpal tendon sheath of the horse. J Anat 1981;133:301–307.

106. Leitch M. Personal communication, 1979.

107. Lescun TB, Hawkins JF, Siems J. Management of rupture of the gastrocnemius and superficial digital flexor muscles with a modified Thomas splint-cast combination in a horse. J Am Vet Med Assoc 213:1457–1459.

108. Lewandowski M. Proby operacyinego leczenia szczudiowwatosci pochodzenia sciegnowego przez przeciecie glowy sciegnisitej (caput tendineum). Med Weter 1967;23:321.

109. Littlewood HE. Treatment of sprained tendons in horses with carbon fiber implants. Vet Rec 1979;105:223.

110. Llewellyn HR. A case of carpal intersynovial fistula in a horse. Equine Vet J 1979;11:90.

111. Lochner FK, Milne DW, Mills EJ, Groom JJ. In vivo and in vitro measurement of tendon strain in the horse. Am J Vet Res 1980; 41:1929–1937.

112. Lokai MD, Meyer RJ. Preliminary observations in oxytetracycline treatment of congenital flexural deformities in foals. Mod Vet Pract 1985;66:237–239.

113. Lokai MD. Case selection for medical management of congenital flexural deformities in foals. Equine Pract 1992;14:23–25.

114. Lose MP. Correction of hind limb pastern subluxation. Mod Vet Pract 1981;62:156.

115. Lysholt B, Sonnichsen HV. Senestylfefod hos fol og plage. Nord Vet Med 1969;21:601.

116. Mackay-Smith MP, Cushing LS, Leslie JA. "Carpal canal" syndrome in horses. J Am Vet Med Assoc 1972;160:993–997.

117. Madison JB. Acute and chronic tendinitis in horses. Comp Cont Educ Pract Vet 1995;853–856.

118. Madison JB, Garber JL, Rice B, et al. Effect of oxytetracycline on metacarpophalangeal and distal interphalangeal joint angles in newborn foals. J Am Vet Med Assoc 1994;204:246–254.

119. Manske PR, Gelberman RH, Vande Berg JS, Lesker PA. Intrinsic flexor-tendon repair. A morphologic study in vitro. J Bone Joint Surg [Am] 1984;66:385–396.

120. Marr CM, Love S, Boyd JS, et al. Factors affecting the clinical outcome of injuries to the superficial digital flexor tendon in National Hunt and Point-2-Point racehorses. Vet Rec 1993;132:476–479.

121. Marr CM, McMillan I, Boyd JS, et al. Ultrasonographic and histopathological findings in equine superficial digital flexor tendon injury. Equine Vet J 1993;25:23–29.

122. McCullagh KG, Goodship AE, Silver IA. Tendon injuries and their treatment in the horse. Vet Rec 1979;105:54.

123. McDiarmid AM. Eighteen cases of desmitis of the accessory ligament of the deep digital flexor tendon. Equine Vet Educ 1994;6:49–56.

124. McGeadt PA. General discussion following Dr. Cosgrove's paper. Vet Rec 1955;67:967.

125. McIlwraith CW. Diseases of joints, tendons, ligaments and related structures. In: Stashak TS, Ed. Adams' Lameness in Horses. 4th ed. Philadelphia: Lea & Febiger, 1987;451–453.

126. McIlwraith CW. Fortschritte in der Arthroscopie. Pferdeheilkunde 1992;8:85–94.

127. McIlwraith CW, Fessler JF. Evaluation of inferior check ligament desmotomy for treatment of acquired flexor tendon contracture in the horse. J Am Vet Med Assoc 1978;294:293.

128. McIlwraith CW, James LF. Limb deformities in foals associated with ingestion of locoweed by mares. J Am Vet Med Assoc 1982;181:255.

129. McIlwraith CW, Robertson JT. Superior check ligament desmotomy (after Bramlage) In: McIlwraith & Turner's Equine Surgery: Advanced Techniques. 2nd ed. Baltimore: Williams & Wilkins, 1998;182–186.

130. McLaughlin BG, Doige CE. Congenital musculoskeletal lesions and hyperplastic goitre in foals. Can Vet J 1981;22:130.

131. Deleted in proof.

132. Mason TA. Chronic tenosynovitis of the extensor tendons and tendon sheaths of the carpal region in the horse. Equine Vet J 1977;9:186.

133. Meagher DM, Pool PR, Brown MP. Bilateral ossification of the tendon of the biceps brachii muscle in the horse. J Am Vet Med Assoc 1979;174:282.

134. Menon J, Frykman G, Swarm OJ. Role of synovial fluid cells in the healing of flexor tendons. Clin Orthop 1985;199:300–305.

135. Morcos MB, Aswad A. Histological studies of the effects of ultrasonic therapy on surgically split flexor tendons. Equine Vet J 1978;10:267.

136. Morcos MB, Aswad A. Treatment of two clinical conditions in racehorses by ultrasonic therapy. Equine Vet J 1978;10:128.

137. Myers VS, Gordon GW. Ruptured common digital extensor tendons associated with contracted flexor tendons in foals. Proceedings. 21st Annual Meeting. American Association of Equine Practitioners, Boston, MA, 1975;67–74.

138. Myers VS Jr, Lundvall RL. Corrective trimming for weak flexor tendons in a colt. J Am Vet Med Assoc 1966;148:1523.

139. Nessler JP, Mass DP. Direct current electrical stimulation of tendon healing in vitro. Clin Orthop 1987;217:303–312.

140. Nicoll RG, Wood AKW, Martin ICA. Ultrasonographic observations of the flexor tendons and ligaments of the metacarpal region of horses. Am J Vet Res 1993;54:502–506.

141. Nilsson G. A survey of the results of the tendon splitting operation for chronic tendinitis in the horse. Equine Vet J 1970;2:111.

142. Nilsson G, Bjorck G. Surgical treatment of chronic tendinitis in the horse. J Am Vet Med Assoc 1969;155:920–926.

143. Nimni ME. Collagen: Structure, function, and metabolism in normal and fibrotic tissues. Semin Arthritis Rheum 1983;13:1–64.

144. Nixon AJ. Endoscopy of the digital flexor tendon sheath in horses. Vet Surg 1990;19:266–271.

145. Nixon AJ, Stashak TS, Smith FW, Norrdin RW. Comparison of carbon fibre and nylon suture for repair of transected flexor tendons in the horse. Equine Vet J 1984;16:93–102.

146. Nystrom B, Holmlund D. Separation of tendon ends after suture of Achilles tendon. Acta Orthop Scand 1983;54:620.

146a. Ordidge RM. Comparison of three methods of treating superficial digital flexor tendinitis in the racing Thoroughbred by transection of its accessory ligament alone (proximal check ligament desmotomy) or in combination with either intralesional injections of hyaluronidase or tendon splitting. Proc Am Assoc Equine Pract 1996;42:164–167.

147. Owen JM. Abnormal flexion of the corono-pedal joint or "contracted tendons" in unweaned foals. Equine Vet J 1975;7:40.

148. Palmer SE, Genovese R, Longo KL, et al. Practical management of superficial digital flexor tendinitis in the performance horse. Vet Clin North Am 1994;10:425–481.

149. Parry DAD, Craig AS. Collagen fibrils during development and maturation and the contribution to the mechanical attributes of connective tissue. In: Nimni ME, Ed. Collagen, vol 2. Boca Raton, FL: CRC Press, 1988;1–23.

150. Parry DAD, Craig AS, Barnes GRG. Tendon and ligament from the horse: An ultrastructural study of collagen fibrils and elastic fibers as a function of age. Proc R Soc Lond (B) 1978;203:293–303.

151. Patterson-Kane JC, Firth EC, Goodship AE, Parry DAD. An age-related analysis of collagen fibril diameter distributions and collagen crimp patterns in superficial digital flexor tendons from a sample of wild ponies. Connect Tissue Res 1998 (in press).

152. Patterson-Kane JC, Firth EC, Parry DAD, et al. Effects of training on collagen fibril populations in the suspensory ligament and deep digital flexor tendon of young Thoroughbreds. Am J Vet Res 1998;59:64–68.

153. Patterson-Kane JC, Firth EC, Parry DAD, Goodship AE. Comparison of collagen fibril populations in the superficial digital flexor tendon in exercised and non-exercised Thoroughbreds. Equine Vet J 1997;29:121–129.

154. Patterson-Kane JC, Parry DAD, Goodship AE, Firth EC. Exercise-induced acceleration of collagen fibril crimp changes in the core regions of superficial digital flexor tendons from young Thoroughbreds. NZ Vet J 1997;45:135–139.

155. Patterson-Kane JC, Wilson AM, Firth EC, et al. Exercise-related alterations in crimp morphology in the central regions of superficial digital flexor tendons from young Thoroughbreds: A controlled study. Equine Vet J 1998;30:61–64.

156. Peacock EE, Van Winkle W. Wound Repair. 2nd ed. Philadelphia: WB Saunders, 1976;37–464.

157. Pennington DG. The locking loop tendon suture. Plast Reconstr Surg 1979;63:648.

158. Pettinger C, Adamson R. Antibiotic blockade of neuromuscular function. Annu Rev Pharmacol 1972;12:169–184.

159. Platt D, Wilson AE, Timbs A, et al. An investigation into the biomechanics of equine flexor tendon using an implantable microforce leaf. J Biomech 1991;24:449.

160. Platt D, Wright IM. Chronic tenosynovitis of the carpal extensor tendon sheaths in 15 horses. Equine Vet J 1997;29:11–16.

161. Prichard JT, Voss JL. Fetal ankylosis in horses associated with hybrid Sudan grass pasture. J Am Vet Med Assoc 1967;150:871.

162. Proctor DL. Surgical treatment of tendinitis. Proceedings. 4th Annual Meeting of the American Association of Equine Practitioners, Chicago, IL, 1958;111–120.

163. Rantanen NW, McKinnon AO. Equine diagnostic ultrasonography. Baltimore: Williams & Wilkins, 1998.

163a. Redding WR, Booth LC, Poole RR. Effects of polysulfated glycosaminoglycan on the healing of collagenase-induced tendinitis of the equine superficial digital flexor tendon. Vet Surg 1992;21:403.

164. Reef VB, Benson BB, Stebbins K. Comparison of ultrasonographic, gross, and histologic appearance of tendon injuries in performance horses. Proc Am Assoc Equine Pract 279.

165. Reef VB, Genovese RL, Davis WM. Initial long term results in horses with superficial digital flexor tendinitis treated with intralesional beta-aminoproprionitril fumarate. Proceedings. 43rd Annual Meeting of the American Association of Equine Practitioners, Phoenix, AZ, 1997;301–305.

166. Reef VB, Martin BB, Elser A. Types of tendon and ligament injuries detected with diagnostic ultrasound: Description and followup. In: Proceedings. 34th Annual Meeting of the American Association of Equine Practitioners, San Diego, CA, 1988; 245–247.

167. Reeves MJ, Trotter GW. Reciprocal apparatus dysfunction as a cause of severe hindlimb lameness in a horse. J Am Vet Med Assoc 1991;199:1047–1048.

168. Riemers MADJ, Schamhardt HC. In vitro mechanical properties of equine tendons in relation to cross-sectional area and collagen content. Res Vet Sci 1985;39:263–270.

169. Rigby BJ, et al. The mechanical properties of rat tail tendon. J Gen Physiol 1959;43:265.

170. Rodney JR. Forelimb contracture in the young horse. J Equine Med Surg 1977;1:350.

171. Rodney JR. Contracted foals. Cornell Vet 1966;56:173.

172. Rodney JR, Quddus MA, Kingsbury HB. A laboratory investigation of the function of the stay apparatus of the equine foreleg. J Equine Med Surg 1978;2:173.

172a. Rooney JR, Genovese RL. A survey and analysis of bowed tendon in Thoroughbred racehorses. Equine Vet Sci 1981;1:49–53.

173. Ross MW. Surgical management of superficial digital flexor tendinitis. Proceedings. 43rd Annual Meeting of the American Association of Equine Practitioners, Phoenix, AZ, 1997;291–296.

174. Rudolph R, Woodward M, Hurn I. Ultrastructure of active versus passive contracture of wounds. Surg Gynecol Obstet 1980;151: 396.

175. Sack WO, Mabel RE. Rooney's Guide to the Dissection of the Horse. Ithaca, NY: Veterinary Textbooks, 1977.

176. Schneider RK, Bramlage LR, Moore RM, et al. A retrospective study of 192 horses affected with septic arthritis/tenosynovitis. Equine Vet J 1992;24:436–442.

177. Scott EA, Breuhaus B, Gertsen KE. Surgical repair of dislocated superficial digital flexor tendon in a horse. J Am Vet Med Assoc 1982;181:171–172.

178. Deleted in proof.

179. Shiroma JT, Engel HN, Wagner PC, Watrous BJ. Dorsal subluxation of the proximal interphalangeal joint in the pelvic limb of three horses. J Am Vet Med Assoc 1989;195:777–780.

180. Shoemaker RS, Bertone AL, Mohammad LN, et al. Desmotomy of the accessory ligament of the superficial digital flexor muscle in equine cadaver limbs. Vet Surg 1991;4:245–252.

181. Shoemaker RS, Martin GS, Hillmann DJ, et al. Disruption of the caudal component of the reciprocal apparatus in two horses. J Am Vet Med Assoc 1991;198:120–122.

182. Sisson S, Grossman JD. The Anatomy of the Domestic Animals. 4th ed. Philadelphia: WB Saunders, 1953.

183. Smith RK, Birch LH, Patterson-Kane J, et al. Should equine athletes commence training during skeletal development? Changes in tendon matrix associated with development, aging, function and exercise. Equine Vet J 1999;S30:201–209.

184. Smith RKW, Zunino L, Webbon PM, Heinegard D. The distribution of cartilage oligomeric matrix protein (COMP) in tendon and its variation with tendon site, age and load. Matrix Biol 1997; 16:255–271.

185. Sonnichsen HV. Desmotomia capitis tendinei. Vet Annual 1977; 17:133.

186. Sonnichsen HV, Christiansen FR. Desmotomia capitis tendinei. Proceedings. 11th Congress European Society of Veterinary Surgery, 1975;1–2.

187. Stashak TS. Adams' Lameness in Horses. 4th ed. Philadelphia: Lea & Febiger, 1987;593–595.

188. Deleted in proof.

189. Stevens PR, Nunamaker DM, Butterweck DM. Application of a Hall-effect transducer for measurement of tendon strains in horses. Am J Vet Res 1989;50:1089–1095.

190. Stromberg B. The normal and diseased superficial flexor tendon in racehorses. A morphologic and physiologic investigation. Acta Radiol (Suppl) 1971;305:5.

191. Deleted in proof.

192. Stromberg B, Tufvesson G. An experimental study of autologous digital tendon transplants in the horse. Equine Vet J 1977;9:231.

193. Stromberg B, Tufvesson G. Lesion of the superficial flexor tendons in racehorses. A microangiographic and histopathologic study. Clin Orthop 1969;62:113.

194. Stromberg B, Tufvesson G, Nilsson G. Effect of surgical splitting on vascular reactions in the superficial flexor tendon of the horse. J Am Vet Med Assoc 1974;164:57–60.

195. Stromberg B, Wiederhielm CA. Viscoelastic description of a collagenous tissue in simple elongation. J Appl Physiol 1969;26:857.

196. Takai S, Woo SL, Horibe S, et al. The effects of frequency and duration of controlled passive mobilization on tendon healing. J Orthop Res 1991;9:705–713.

197. Taylor D, Pascoe JR, Honnes CM, Hoffman AG. Management of flexor tendon lacerations in horses. Comp Cont Educ Pract Vet 1997;19:238–246.

198. Taylor DS, Pascoe JR, Meagher DM, Honnes CM. Digital flexor tendon lacerations in horses: 50 cases (1975–1990). J Am Vet Med Assoc 1995;206:342–346.

199. Thompson KN, Cheung TK, Silberman M. The influence of toe angle on strain characteristics of the deep digital flexor tendon, superficial flexor tendon, suspensory ligament, and hoof wall. Equine Athlete 1992;5:1 and 6.

200. Trout DR, Lohse CL. Anatomy and therapeutic resection of the peroneus tertius muscle in a foal. J Am Vet Med Assoc 1981;179: 247.

201. Turner AS, McIlwraith CW. Techniques in Large Animal Surgery. Philadelphia: Lea & Febiger, 1982.

202. Turner AS, McIlwraith CW. Techniques in Large Animal Surgery. 2nd ed. Philadelphia: Lea & Febiger, 1989;156–160.

203. Valdez H, Clark RG, Hanselka DV. Repair of digital flexor tendon lacerations in the horse, using carbon fiber implants. J Am Vet Med Assoc 1980;177:427.

204. Valdez H, Coy CH, Swanson T. Flexible carbon fiber for repair of gastrocnemius and superficial digital flexor tendons in a heifer and gastrocnemius tendon in a foal. J Am Vet Med Assoc 1982; 181:154.

205. Valdez H, McLaughlin SA. Arthrodesis of the fetlock joint with dynamic compression plates. J Equine Med Surg 1979;3:421.

205a. Van den Belt AJM, Becker CK, Dik KJ. Desmitis of the accessory ligament of the deep digital flexor tendon in the horse: Clinical and ultrasonographic features. A report of 24 cases. Zentralbl Veterinarmed A 1993;40:492–500.

206. Van Pelt RW. Idiopathic tenosynovitis in foals. J Am Vet Med Assoc 1969;155:510–517.

207. Van Pelt RW. Inflammation of the tarsal synovial sheath (thoroughpin) in horses. J Am Vet Med Assoc 1969;155:1481–1488.

208. Van Pelt RW. Tenosynovitis in the horse. J Am Vet Med Assoc 1969;154:1022.

209. Van Pelt RW, Langham RF, Gill HF. Multiple hemangiosarcomas in the tarsal synovial sheath of a horse. J Am Vet Med Assoc 1972;161:49.

210. Van Pelt RW, Riley WE Jr. Treatment of bilateral septic tenosynovitis in a foal. J Am Vet Med Assoc 1971;159:1032.

211. Van Pelt RW, Riley WE Jr, Tillotson PJ. Tenosynovitis of the deep digital flexor tendon in horses. Can Vet J 1969;10:235.

212. Verschooten F, De Moor A. Tendinitis in the horse: Its radiologic diagnosis with air-tendograms. J Am Vet Radiol Sci 1978;19:23.

213. Verschooten F, Picavet T-M. Desmitis of the fetlock anular ligament in the horse. Equine Vet J 1986;18:138–142.

214. Vogel KG, Heinegard D. Characterization of proteoglycans from adult bovine tendon. J Biol Chem 1995;260:9298–9306.

214a. Vogel KG, Sande AD, Bogany G, Robbins JR. Aggrecan in bovine tendon. Matrix Biol 1994;14:171–179.

215. Wagner PC, Grant BD, Kaneps AJ, Watrous BJ. Long-term results of desmotomy of the accessory ligament of the deep digital flexor tendon (distal check ligament) in horses. J Am Vet Med Assoc 1985;187:1351–1356.

216. Wagner PC, Shires MG, Watrous BJ, et al. Management of acquired flexural deformity of the metacarpophalangeal joint in Equidae. J Am Vet Med Assoc 1985;187:915–918.

217. Wagner von Matthiessen PC. Case selection and management of flexural limb deformities in horses: Congenital flexural limb deformities, part II. Equine Pract 1994;16:7–11.

218. Wallace CE. Chronic tendosynovitis of the extensor carpi radialis tendon in the horse. Aust Vet J 1972;48:585.

219. Deleted in proof.

220. Watkins JP, Auer JA, Morgan SJ, Gay S. Healing of surgically created defects in the equine superficial digital flexor tendon: Ef-

fects of pulsing electromagnetic field therapy on collagen-type transformation and tissue morphologic reorganization. Am J Vet Res 1985;46:2097–2103.

221. Webbon PM. A histological study of macroscopically normal equine digital flexor tendons. Equine Vet J 1978;10:253.
222. Webbon PM. A postmortem study of equine digital flexor tendons. Equine Vet J 1977;9:61.
223. Webbon PM. Equine tendon stress injuries. Equine Vet J 1973; 5:58.
224. Webbon PM. The racing performance of horses with tendon lesions treated by percutaneous tendon splitting. Equine Vet J 1979; 11:246.
225. Wheat JD, Pascoe JR. A technique for management of traumatic rupture of the equine suspensory apparatus. J Am Vet Med Assoc 1980;176:205.
226. White NA II. Ultrasound-guided transection of the accessory ligament of the deep digital flexor muscle (distal check ligament desmotomy) in horses. Vet Surg 1995;24:373–378.
227. Whitehair KJ, Adams SB, Toombs JP, et al. Arthrodesis for congenital flexural deformity in the metacarpophalangeal and metatarsophalangeal joints. Vet Surg 1992;22:228–233.
228. Wiig ME, Amiel D, VandeBerg J, et al. The early effect of high molecular weight hyaluronan (hyaluronic acid) on anterior cruciate ligament healing: An experimental study in rabbits. J Orthop Res 1990;8:425–434.
229. Williams IF, Heaton A, McCullagh KG. Cell morphology and collagen types of equine tendon scar. Res Vet Sci 1980;28:302.
230. Wilmink J, Wilson AM, Goodship AE. Functional significance of the morphology and micromechanics of collagen fibers in relation to partial rupture of the superficial digital flexor tendon in racehorses. Res Vet Sci 1992;53:354–359.
231. Wilson AM. The effect of exercise intensity on the biochemistry, morphology and mechanical properties of tendon. PhD thesis, Bristol, England, University of Bristol, 1991.
232. Wilson AM, Goodship AE. Exercise-induced hyperthermia as a possible mechanism for tendon degeneration. J Biomech 1994; 27:899–905.
233. Wilson AM, Goodship AE. Historrhexis energy losses in the equine superficial digital flexor tendon during exercise produce a local temperature sufficient to damage fibroblasts in vitro. Proceedings. 38th Annual Meeting of the Orthopaedic Research Society, 1992;679.
234. Wilson AM, Goodship AE. Mechanical properties of the equine superficial digital flexor tendon. J Biomech 1991;24:474.
235. Wilson DA, Baker GJ, Pijanowski DJ, et al. Composition and morphologic features of the intraosseous muscle in Standardbreds and Thoroughbreds. Am J Vet Res 1991;52:133–139.
236. Wright AK, Petrie L, Papich MG, et al. The effect of high dose oxytetracycline on renal parameters in neonatal foals: Recommended dose for treatment of flexural limb deformities. In: Proceedings. Annual Meeting of the American Association of Equine Practitioners, San Antonio, TX, 1993;38:297–298.
237. Wright IM, McMahon PJ. Tenosynovitis associated with longitudinal tears of the digital flexor tendons in horses: A report of 20 cases. Equine Vet J 1999;31:12–18.
238. Yovich JV, Stashak TS, McIlwraith CW. Rupture of the common digital extensor tendon in foals. Comp Cont Educ Pract Vet 1984; 5373.

DISEASES OF BURSAE AND OTHER PERIARTICULAR TISSUES

Anatomy and Physiology

A bursa is a closed sac lined with a cellular membrane resembling a synovial membrane, which is interposed between moving parts or at points of unusual pressure

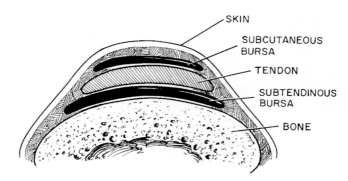

Figure 7.125 Diagram of synovial bursa and various positions in which it may occur.

such as between bony prominences and tendons. According to position, they have been classified as subcutaneous, subfascial, subligamentous, submuscular, and subtendinous bursae[12] (Table 7.3 and Fig. 7.125). There are also two types of bursae on the basis of their method of formation: congenital bursae, which develop before birth and are located in a constant position, and acquired bursae, which are formed after birth and generally develop subcutaneously over bony prominences such as the olecranon tuberosity or tuber calcis.

There is a relationship between bursal type and bursal position. Congenital, or true, bursae are associated with deep structures (beneath deep fascia, muscles, or tendons). Subcutaneous bursae grow as a result of mechanical effects in postnatal life and might therefore be termed "reactive" or "functional." Movement of the skin causes tearing of the subcutaneous connective tissue and leads to formation of a gap that becomes filled with fluid so that only a few fibrous elements remain within the bursa when it is finally formed.[12] Fluid exudate accumulates in the subcutaneous tissue and becomes encapsulated by fibrous tissue to form this acquired, or false, bursa.

There is some confusion about the nomenclature of subcutaneous bursae, depending on whether they are above or below the superficial fascia. This positional difference has been used to classify them as either functional or pathologic.[12] For simplicity, it is more convenient to consider all bursae above the deep fascia subcutaneous, to consider them all acquired, and to classify them as functional or pathologic on the basis of their clinical signs.

Histologically, the walls of the true bursae are lined with connective tissue membrane that is practically identical to the synovial membrane of joints and may be classified as areolar, fibrous, or adipose as the synovial membrane of joints is classified. Acquired bursae are considered structurally identical to true bursae, but the structure depends on the stage of development. Superficial bursae do contain synovial-like fluid, but this fluid differs from joint synovial fluid in viscosity and mucin clot, which suggests differences in HA quantity or quality. In addition, bursae react less intensely than joints to specific disease stimuli on the basis of synovial fluid analysis in traumatic and septic bursitis.[2,13]

Several bursae may exist at different tissue levels in the same part of the body; a good example are those over

Table 7.3 EXAMPLES OF BURSAE OF CLINICAL SIGNIFICANCE

Bursa	Position	Significance or Clinical Condition
Subcutaneous		
Olecranon bursa	Over olecranon tuberosity	Capped elbow
Subcutaneous calcaneal bursa	Above tuber calcis on plantar aspect of superficial digital flexor tendon	Capped hock
Subligamentous		
Atlantal bursa	Between ligamentum nuchae and rectus capitis dorsalis major muscle	Poll evil
Supraspinous bursa	Beneath ligamentum nuchae and over third and fourth thoracic vertebrae	Fistulous withers
Subtendinous		
Bicipital bursa (bursa intertubercularis)	Under tendon of biceps brachii muscle on the central ridge of the bicipital groove of the humerus; bursa extends around tendon	Bicipital bursitis
Bursa of extensor carpi radialis	Beneath extensor carpi radialis tendon and on the third carpal bone	To be avoided during carpal arthrotomy
Navicular bursa (bursa podotrochlearis)	Between navicular bone and deep digital flexor tendon	Involved in navicular disease, septic bursitis
Bursa of long digital extensor	Beneath common origin of long digital extensor and peroneus tertius muscles and over lateral surface of tibia	Communicates with lateral femorotibial joint
Intertendinous calcaneal bursa	Between gastrocnemius and superficial digital flexor tendons	Intertendinous calcaneal bursitis (deep capped hock)
Subtendinous calcaneal bursa	Beneath insertion of gastrocnemius tendon on tuber calcis	Subtendinous calcaneal bursitis (deep capped hock)
Cunean bursa	Between cunean tendon (medial tendon of tibialis cranialis muscle) and distal tarsal bones	Cunean bursitis
Bursa under common digital extensor at the fetlock and pastern joints	Beneath the common digital extensor tendon at level of fetlock and pastern joints	Bursal fistula

the tuber calcis, where intertendinous and subtendinous bursae may be present. In this instance, the two deeper bursae are congenital, and the upper one is acquired. Certain bursae may communicate with the joint, and these have been described as diverticula of that associated joint. An example of this is the bursa beneath the long digital extensor tendon that communicates with the lateral femorotibial joint capsule. This bursa is clinically significant because it provides a means of injecting the lateral femorotibial joint space, for which direct entry can be difficult.[11] There are many bursae in the horse. One early paper listed 77 bursae in the horse, and others may form in addition to these. Examples of some bursae that are of clinical significance are given in Table 7.3.

Bursitis

Bursitis is defined as an inflammatory reaction within a bursa. This may range from a mild inflammatory reaction to septic bursitis. Most instances of bursitis are of irritative or traumatic origin. Bursitis can also be classified as true or acquired, and this relates to the classifications of bursae discussed in the previous section. True bursitis is inflammation that develops in a congenital or natural bursa (deeper than the deep fascia). Examples include trochanteric bursitis and supraspinous bursitis (fistulous withers). Acquired bursitis has been defined as a bursa that develops as a result of trauma where a natural bursa is not normally present.[1] This definition has obvious defects because all subcutaneous bursae grow as a result of mechanical effects in postnatal life and, in many instances, may be functional rather than pathologic.[12] A better definition of acquired bursitis is the development of a subcutaneous bursa and/or inflammation of that bursa.

As with other entities of synovitis, bursitis may manifest as an acute inflammation or in a chronic form. Examples of acute bursitis include bicipital bursitis and trochanteric bursitis in the early stages. Chronic bursitis may follow the acute form but is more frequently due to the development of an acquired bursa as a result of repeated injuries that subsequently becomes clinically unacceptable. Examples of this type of bursitis include capped elbow, capped hock, and carpal hygroma. The condition is characterized by the accumulation of excessive bursal fluid and thickening of the bursal wall by fibrous tissue. Fibrous bands or septa may form within the bursal cavity, and generalized subcutaneous thickening usually develops. These bursal enlargements develop as cold, painless swellings, and unless they become greatly enlarged, they do not severely interfere with function. If they become infected (particularly in the elbow or carpus), they may enlarge and rupture. The lesion is then characterized by exuberant granulation tissue, discharging sinuses, and excessive fibrous tissue formation.

Bursitis can be classified as traumatic or septic.

Traumatic Bursitis

Most cases of bursitis fall under this classification. This group includes bicipital, trochanteric, and cunean bursitis as well as bursitis associated with the olecranon (capped elbow, shoe-boil), hock (capped hock), and carpus (carpal hygroma).

PATHOGENESIS

The trauma that causes the bursitis can either be direct or associated with racing stresses. Bicipital bursitis may be associated with a direct injury to the point of the shoulder.[9] Trochanteric and cunean bursitis occur typically in Standardbred racehorses and are associated with racing stresses. Trochanteric bursitis is a poorly defined entity but is commonly considered to arise secondarily to hock lameness, and presumably the change in gait due to the primary lameness causes abnormal stresses in the region of the trochanteric bursa. Cunean bursitis usually occurs in conjunction with inflammation of the distal tarsal and/or tarsometatarsal joints and is referred to as cunean tendon bursitis–tarsitis.[4] Direct trauma is the cause of the other traumatic bursitis entities. Olecranon bursitis is an acquired bursitis caused by the shoe on the foot of the affected limb traumatizing the point of the olecranon during motion or when the horse is lying down. Bursitis of the hock (traumatic calcaneal bursitis) is usually associated with trauma from the horse kicking a wall or trailer gate. Direct trauma is also associated with carpal hygroma.

DIAGNOSIS

Bicipital, trochanteric, and cunean bursitis manifest as lameness. Localizing pain to palpation is usually present with bicipital bursitis and sometimes present with trochanteric bursitis.[10] Cunean bursitis requires local analgesic blocking to define, although there are certain characteristic clinical signs. The other bursitis entities are characterized by local fluctuant swelling in the region (Fig. 7.126). The relative amount of fluid and thickened soft tissue varies with the stage of the condition. Bicipital tendons and bursae of the horse can be imaged ultrasonographically, and this has upgraded considerably how much we can define pathologic change in this area. Tendinitis is commonly diagnosed in addition to bicipital bursitis in the same patient. Diagnosis of bicipital bursitis is confirmed by a positive response to local analgesia, with assistance from radiography, diagnostic ultrasound, and in some cases nuclear scintigraphy.[8]

TREATMENT

The treatment methods vary considerably. Rest has been the preferred method of treatment with bicipital bursitis. However, Gillis reported that 3 of 14 horses treated with pasture turnout returned to use (horses with biceps tendinitis), whereas 8 of 16 horses treated with controlled exercise were able to do so.[6] Cold applications in the acute stage and counterirritation during later stages have been used. Surgical treatment may be indicated when external trauma is the cause. Both incisional and arthroscopic approaches have been described for removal of bone fragments and for performing synovectomy.[8] Three cases of bicipital bursitis needing surgical exploration and debridement of necrosis and enthesiophytes had favorable results.[8] Treatments for cunean tendon bursitis–tarsitis include cunean tenectomy, rest,

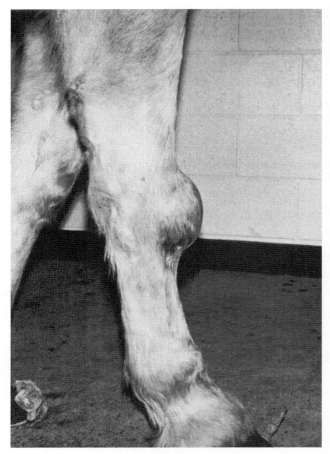

Figure 7.126   Carpal hygroma.

local corticosteroid injections or phenylbutazone, and there is no statistical difference in the results of surgical and nonsurgical treatments.[5] The use of HA has been advocated for the treatment of biceps brachii tendinitis and intertubercle bursitis.[7] An arthroscopic approach to the intertubercular (bicipital) bursa has been described and provides a better alternative to surgical incision of this area.[11a]

With bursitis associated with the elbow, hock, or carpus, the first principle of treatment is prevention of further trauma to the region (not always easy or possible). Local injection of corticosteroids and pressure bandaging have been used with variable results. Orgotein may be used in place of corticosteroids. In refractory cases, the implantation of Penrose drains[14] for a period of 10 days to 2 weeks allows fluid drainage and acts to enhance fibrosis and obliteration of the cavity. If this method fails, injection of the cavity with an iodine compound or incision into the cavity and packing it with gauze soaked in Lugol's iodine is recommended as an alterative. The range of treatments reflect the fact that no one treatment is a panacea. Surgical excision of the mass and primary closure is the final treatment of choice. Results of this treatment can be good if adjunctive immobilization of the region is also performed. Based on a report of two cases of chronic calcaneal bursitis with osteolytic lesions on the tuber calcanei, the prognosis for athletic activity is guarded.[1a]

Septic Bursitis

The term "septic bursitis" is restricted to bursitis that originates with deposition of infection in the bursa. The classic example is septic navicular bursitis following nail penetration. Supraspinous bursitis (fistulous withers) may be considered a septic bursitis when it is associated with *Brucella abortus* infection, for instance. This group does not include cases of traumatic bursitis that become secondarily infected.

PATHOGENESIS

Septic navicular bursitis is usually associated with penetration by a nail or similar foreign body through the frog. Establishment of infection in the region of the navicular bursa causes severe lameness, and the septic process can rapidly involve the neighboring navicular bone and DDF tendon. Septic bursitis of the supraspinous bursa can be acquired by a systemic (occasionally) or a local route.

CLINICAL SIGNS

Septic navicular bursitis is characterized by severe lameness that is usually associated with recognition of foreign body penetration of the hoof. Drainage above

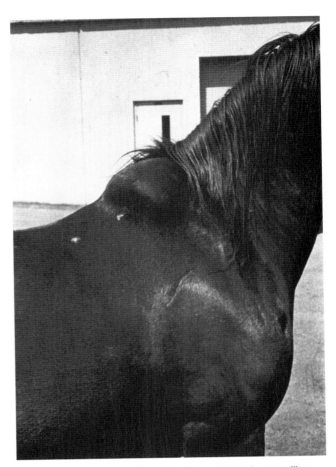

Figure 7.128 Supraspinous bursitis manifested as swelling over the withers.

the bulbs of the heel may develop. Septic bursitis can occur over the point of the hock (Fig. 7.127). Fistulous withers is characterized by swelling over the withers with or without drainage (Figs. 7.128 and 7.129).

TREATMENT

The principle of treatment for septic bursitis involves surgical drainage with removal of infected and necrotic tissue. In both examples given here, the surgical techniques are radical, and the prognosis for complete recovery is guarded.[3] More recently, cases of septic navicular bursitis have been treated successfully using arthroscopy, and surgical morbidity is minimal.[15] Cases of septic bicipital bursitis have also been treated successfully with surgery.[8]

Bursal Fistula

As described in the section on joints, intersynovial fistulae may develop between a bursa and a joint or tendon sheath. The typical site of occurrence for this problem involves the bursae under the common digital extensor tendon at the level of the fetlock joint (over the dorsal

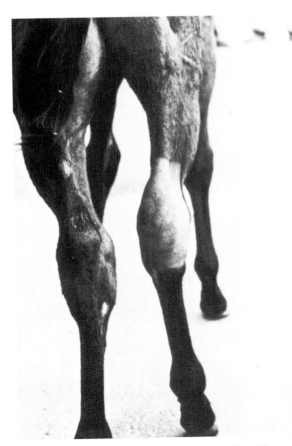

Figure 7.127 Septic calcaneal bursitis.

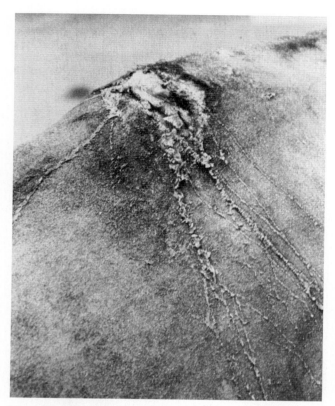

Figure 7.129 Supraspinous bursitis with drainage from the withers.

capsule of the fetlock joint) or at the level of the pastern joint where the common digital extensor tendon unites with the branches of the suspensory ligament. These bursae may develop fistulae with the fetlock and coffin joints, respectively.

References

1. Adams OR. Lameness in Horses. 3rd ed. Philadelphia: Lea & Febiger, 1974.
1a. Bassage LH, Garcia-Lopez J, Currin EM. Osteolytic lesions of the tuber calcanei in two horses. J Am Vet Med Assoc 2000;217: 710–716.
2. Canoso JJ, Yood RA. Reaction of superficial bursae in response to specific disease stimuli. Arthritis Rheum 1979;22:1361.
3. Frank ER. Veterinary Surgery. 7th ed. Minneapolis: Burgess Publishing, 1964.
4. Gabel AA. Diagnosis, relative incidence and probable cause of cunean tendon bursitis-tarsitis of Standardbred horses. J Am Vet Med Assoc 1979;175:1079.
5. Gabel AA. Treatment and prognosis for cunean tendon bursitis-tarsitis of Standardbred horses. J Am Vet Med Assoc 1979;175: 1086.
6. Gillis CL. Biceps brachii tendinitis and bicipital bursitis. Proceedings. 42nd Annual Meeting of the American Association of Equine Practitioners, Denver, CO, 1996;276–277.
7. Gillis CL, Batistis NJ. Biceps brachii tendinitis and bicipital (tubercular bursitis). In: Robinson NE, Ed. Current Equine Therapy IV. Philadelphia: WB Saunders, 1996;12–14.
8. Grant BD, Peterson PR, Bohn A, Rantanen NW. Diagnosis and surgical treatment of traumatic bicipital bursitis in the horse. Am Assoc Equine Pract 1992;38:349–355.
9. Hawe C, McDiarmid AM. Tendinitis of the biceps brachii and intertubercle (bicipital) bursitis in a Thoroughbred racehorse. Equine Vet Educ 1999;11:60–62.
10. McDiarmid AM. Equine bicipital apparatus—Review of anatomy, function, diagnostic investigative techniques and clinical conditions. Equine Vet Educ 1999;11:63–68.
11. McIlwraith CW, Blevins WE. Unpublished data, 1978.
11a. Norris-Adams M, Turner TA, Endoscopy of the intertubercular bursa in horses. J Am Vet Med Assoc 1999;214:221–225.
12. Ottaway CA, Worden AN. Bursae and tendon sheaths of the horse. Vet Rec 1940;52:477.
13. Van Pelt RW, Riley WF Jr. Traumatic subcutaneous bursitis (capped hock) in the horse. J Am Vet Med Assoc 1968;153: 1176.
14. Van Veenendaal JC, Speirs VC, Harrison I. Treatment of hygromata in horses. Aust Vet J 1981;57:513.
15. Wright IM, Phillips TJ, Walmsley JP. Endoscopy of the navicular bursa. A new technique for the treatment of contaminated and septic bursae. Equine Vet J 1999;31:5–11.

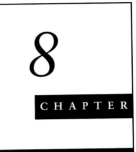

CHAPTER 8

Lameness

Part I

THE FOOT

Ted S. Stashak

LAMINITIS

Laminitis has been defined as inflammation of the sensitive laminae of the foot.[2] However, this is a gross oversimplification of a complicated, interrelated sequence of events that results in varying degrees of breakdown of the interdigitation of the primary and secondary epidermal and dermal laminae in the foot. If the loss of interdigitation is severe enough, rotation and/or distal displacement of the distal phalanx may follow. It is suggested that a more appropriate term for laminitis may be acute laminar degeneration.[59] It is believed that rotation of the distal phalanx results from a combination of laminar degeneration primarily in the dorsal hoof wall and the pulling forces of the deep digital flexor tendon (Fig. 8.1). If the laminae degeneration is extensive, involving the circumference of the hoof wall, the distal phalanx has a tendency to sink (Fig. 8.2).

Although numerous mechanisms for the laminar degeneration have been proposed, the pathogenesis of laminitis remains unknown.[9] However, the result of the disease process is thought to include hypoperfusion of the digit, leading to ischemia, necrosis, and edema of the laminae.[39,58,74] Affected horses are often in severe pain and sometimes must be destroyed because of extensive damage to the laminae. Notably, laminar degeneration can be associated with systemic metabolic disorders involving the cardiovascular, renal, endocrine, coagulation, and acid-base status.[5,36,42,95]

Etiopathogenesis

Proposed causes for acute laminitis include endotoxin-induced microthrombosis, alterations in vascular dynamics either by shunting of laminar blood flow through arteriovenous anastomoses (AVAs) or by vasoconstriction and edema, and activated lamellar enzyme destruction of the basement membrane.

Endotoxin-Induced Microthrombosis

Support for this theory was based on studies in horses given a laminitis-inducing starch ration. In these studies, investigators found an increase in lactic acid–producing bacteria, a decrease in pH, a decrease in the number of gram-negative bacteria, and an increase in endotoxin in the cecal contents. Additionally, evidence of cecal mucosal damage was found, and endotoxin was detected in the circulation of 85% of horses developing laminitis.[32,60]

The link between endotoxemia, coagulation dysfunction, and the formation of microthrombi in the laminae is unclear.[23,58] Although there is histologic evidence of thrombosis in the laminae of horses with severe laminitis, there are conflicting reports regarding the relation between coagulation dysfunction and the development of acute laminitis. Laboratory indices of coagulation are not significantly changed during the earliest signs of laminitis, and only mild periodic fluctuations in coagulation parameters and platelet numbers have been observed as horses progress to Obel grade 3.[61,76] In contrast, in one study done in ponies, an accumulation of platelets was found in the soft tissue distal to the coronary band, whole blood recalcification time was shortened, and a variable number of microthrombi were present in the dermal veins when the ponies became lame.[95]

The results of these studies and the fact that acute laminitis has not been caused by administration of endotoxin to previously healthy horses suggest that the proposed role of endotoxin as a triggering mechanism in the development of acute laminitis remains speculative.[38,58]

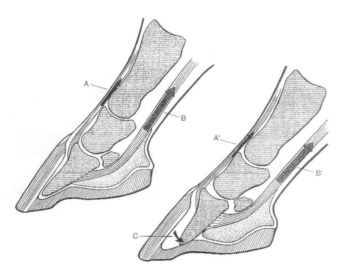

Figure 8.1 Arrows indicate the various forces thought to contribute to rotation of the distal phalanx. Left: A, extensor tendon; B, deep digital flexor tendon. Right: Pull of the deep digital flexor tendon (B') overrides the pull of the extensor tendon (A'), resulting in rotation of the distal phalanx C.

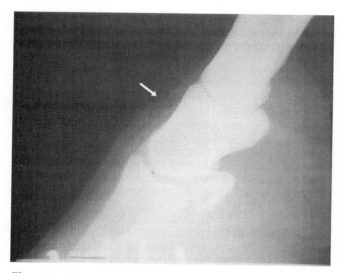

Figure 8.2 Lateral view of a sinker. Note the distal phalanx is at the same level as the shoe and a cleft can be seen at the coronet band (arrow).

However, although there seems to be a direct causal relation between endotoxemia and laminitis, clinically horses that exhibit signs of endotoxemia seem at greater risk to develop laminitis.[97,98] Also, a strong relation between certain disease processes and the development of endotoxemia and laminitis seems to exist. Disease processes often associated with endotoxemia are gastrointestinal problems, metritis, retained placenta, and grain overload. In one study, 55% of the horses that developed laminitis had gastrointestinal problems.[44]

Alterations in Vascular Dynamics
SHUNTING THROUGH ARTERIOVENOUS ANASTOMOSES

Shunting of blood through AVAs results in laminar capillary hypoperfusion. In scanning electron microscopic studies of corrosion casts of the microcirculation of the dermal laminae, more than 500 AVAs/cm^2 were found in the dermal laminae, which may provide a low-resistance conduit connecting the arterial and venous systems in the laminar region (Fig. 8.3).[74] Vasodilator substances released from organs remote to the foot or to neuronal influences may cause prolonged dilation of AVAs, and blood flow bypasses the dermal capillary beds, resulting in laminar capillary hypoperfusion and ischemic necrosis of the epidermal laminae (Fig. 8.4).

VASOCONSTRICTION AND PERIVASCULAR EDEMA

Distal limb preparations in ponies and horses have allowed investigators to quantify blood flow to and from the digit; measure arterial, venous, and capillary pressures; and evaluate capillary permeability by measuring lymph flow and the relative concentrations of protein in plasma and lymph in the digit.[3,11,82] The results of these studies indicated that the dermal microvascular beds of a horse's digit are extremely permeable to protein, which would tend to favor edema formation.

With the use of more refined techniques,[3] significant increases in digital venous, capillary, and tissue pressures and postcapillary resistance to blood flow were observed in horses with Obel grade 1 laminitis, 16 to 20 hours after carbohydrate overload.[58] Similar changes in capillary and tissue pressures were obtained after horses were administered a black walnut extract.[27] However, no change in the microvasculature permeability within the foot was observed. These findings suggest an increase in the number of capillaries being perfused and an increase in the hydrostatic pressure within these capillaries, and this could result in the increased movement of fluid from the vascular compartment into the interstitial tissue.[58]

Further studies found the initial hemodynamic response during the onset of acute laminitis after either carbohydrate overload or administration of black walnut extract is digital venoconstriction.[46,59] Constriction of the digital veins is believed to increase capillary pressures within the digital microvasculature, which forces fluid out into the tissues of the foot. The resulting increased interstitial fluid volume causes increased tissue pressure within the noncompliant foot, producing a situation analogous to compartment syndrome. As tissue pressure increases, it further reduces the digital blood flow, resulting in pressure necrosis or ischemia of the tissues (laminae) of the foot. In contrast to this hypothesis, however, nuclear scintigraphic studies of digital circulation in horses with starch-induced laminitis showed increased blood flow caused by increased capillary flow and/or increased arteriovenous shunting.[89] Conversely, horses with black walnut (*Juglans nigra*)–induced laminitis had decreased laminar perfusion at the onset of laminitis and then had increased perfusion 72 hours later, which were demonstrated with nuclear scintigraphy.[31] Dilation of AVAs in the dermal microcirculation is compatible with these studies.

Currently, the cause of laminitis has been suggested to involve a malfunction in endothelium-mediated vaso-

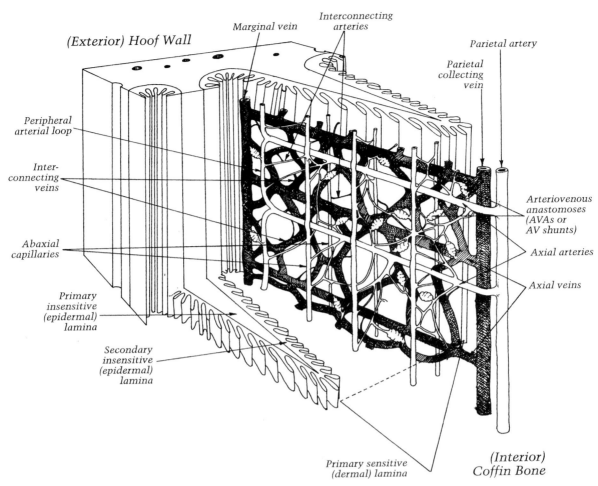

(Exterior) Hoof Wall

Peripheral
arterial loop

Inter-
connecting
veins

Abaxial
capillaries

Primary
insensitive
(epidermal)
lamina

Secondary
insensitive
(epidermal)
lamina

Marginal vein

Interconnecting
arteries

Parietal artery

Parietal
collecting
vein

Arteriovenous
anastomoses
(AVAs or
AV shunts)

Axial arteries

Axial veins

Primary sensitive
(dermal) lamina

(Interior)
Coffin Bone

Figure 8.3 Microcirculation of the sensitive (dermal) laminae. (Reprinted with permission from Pollitt CC, Molyneux GS. A scanning electron microscopical study of the dermal microcirculation of the equine foot. Equine Vet J 1990;22:79–87.)

dilation, leading to enhanced vasoconstriction through the L-arginine–nitric oxide (NO) pathway.[8,15,37,48] Endothelial cells can be stimulated by several agents, such as acetylcholine and bradykinin, to release endothelium-derived relaxing factor (EDRF), more recently identified as NO. NO is a vasodilating agent causing adjacent smooth muscle cells to relax. Damage to the endothelium from any cause could potentially inhibit the NO pathway, disrupting the balance between vasodilation and vasoconstriction.[50,55,88]

It has been suggested that only by understanding the factors affecting capillary and arteriovenous anastomotic flow in the hoof will it be possible to determine the various vascular mechanisms involved in acute laminitis.[81] It is also plausible that the digital vascular changes may vary with the inciting cause of laminitis and with time during the development or prodromal stages of acute laminitis.[7]

ACTIVATED ENZYME DESTRUCTION OF THE BASEMENT MEMBRANE

In this theory, dilated lamellar vessels carry circulating laminitis trigger factors that activate lamellar en-zymes. These activated enzymes lyse the basement membrane (BM) attachments between the hoof wall and the distal phalanx.[71] Because the BM is believed to be the key structure bridging the epidermis of the hoof to the connective tissue of the distal phalanx, it follows that loss of the BM would result in movement of the distal phalanx characteristic of laminitis. Evidence for vasodilation during the developmental phase of carbohydrate overload–induced laminitis has been supported by experiments.[73,82,89] Activated metalloproteinases (MMPs 2 and 9) capable of destroying the lamellar BM attachments have been isolated from normal lamellar tissues and were increased in lamellar tissues of horses affected by laminitis.[73,75] *Streptococcus bovis*, the principal microorganism responsible for the rapid fermentation of carbohydrate to lactic acid in the hindgut of horses, has been shown to activate equine hoof MMP and to cause lamellar separation.[71] It is proposed that an *S. bovis* trigger factor may be the "missing link" connecting events in the hindgut of the horse with the development of laminitis.[71] An additional feature of damage to the BM is the loss of dermal capillaries.[71] The loss of these capillaries may explain why resistance to blood flow was increased 3.5 times in horses during early laminitis.[3] It is also pro-

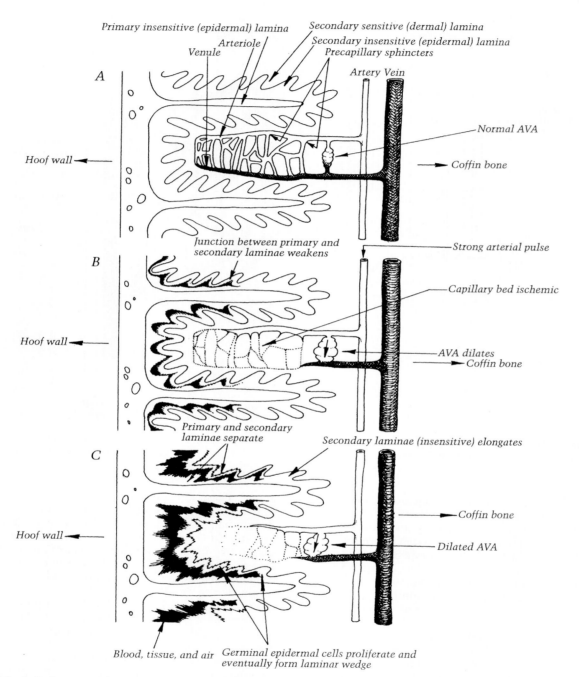

Figure 8.4 A. During normal function, the AVAs open and close periodically, allowing blood to flow through the capillary bed. Optimum blood flow maintains the health of the dermal and epidermal cells and the strength of the bond between the coffin bone and the hoof wall. B. As laminitis develops, the AVAs can remain dilated for long periods, which shunts (diverts) the blood away from the capillary bed. Deprived of necessary nutrients, the epidermal cells deteriorate. C. As laminitis progresses, the primary and secondary laminae separate, and the hoof wall tears away from the sensitive laminae overlying the coffin bone. Without its supportive attachment, the coffin bone can rotate or sink in the hoof capsule.

posed that this increased resistance to blood flow may cause the pounding digital pulse and may answer why blood bypasses the capillary bed through the dilated AVAs.

Histopathology

Midhoof wall lamellar sections from horses euthanized 48 hours after the administration of alimentary carbohydrate overload revealed disintegration of the basement membrane and a failure of its attachment to basal epidermal cells.[70] This is thought to be one of the earliest pathologic events to occur in acute laminitis and may be the change that results in loss of the laminar interdigitation. The histopathologic grades 1 to 3 correlated well with lameness degree at the time of euthanasia.

Microscopic evaluation of chronically affected digits reveals hyperplasia of the epidermal laminae to the point that it creates a wedge of tissue of sufficient magnitude that it forces the epidermal and dermal laminae apart (Fig. 8.5). An epidermal growth factor–mediated response may be involved in hyperplastic epidermal response.[35] It is hypothesized that this wedge of tissue is, in part, the reason the rotation persists once it has occurred chronically.[80]

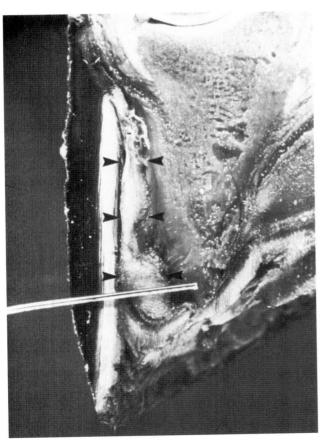

Figure 8.5 Sagittal section of the hoof wall of a horse with rotation of the distal phalanx. The metal probe is pointing to the site of penetration at the sole. Note the wedge of tissue that separates the white line from the dermal lamina (arrows).

Predisposing Factors

Predisposing or risk factors for the development of laminitis in horses include inflammatory conditions of the gastrointestinal tract, grain overload, grazing on grass during certain months of the year, retained placenta or metritis, pleuropneumonia, endotoxemia or sepsis, Cushing's disease (pituitary pars intermedia dysfunction [PPID]), prolonged weight bearing on one limb, and exposure to black walnut wood shavings.[32,44,54,69,85,87] Under certain climatic conditions (cold nights, sunny days), grasses can manufacture high concentrations of fructan (soluble fructose polymer) sufficient to trigger hindgut fermentation and lactic acid production in horses, resulting in grass founder.[54] Other less common predisposing factors include trimming hooves too short, exercising on hard surfaces, administering large doses of corticosteroids, feeding a diet containing estrogens, and allergic reactions to certain medications.[7,30] Ponies seem to be particularly susceptible.

Although no association between age, breed, sex, and weight has been established for the development of acute laminitis, horses younger than 1 year old seem at less risk to develop support limb laminitis no matter what the cause of the lameness in the contralateral limb.[69] Also, horses with chronic laminitis tend to be older, and more mares are affected.[7] In a study done on 33 horses with duodenitis or proximal jejunitis, horses that weighed more than 550 kg were more than twice as likely to develop bilateral laminitis than were horses that weighed less than 550 kg.[18] In another study, body weight of horses that had distal displacement of the distal phalanx (sinkers) and survived (mean, 384 kg) was less than the body weight of horses that had this condition and did not survive (mean, 473 kg).[10] In another study done on 35 horses to evaluate the outcome of deep digital flexor tenotomy for chronic laminitis, investigators found no correlation between body weight and outcome.[26]

Clinical Signs

Acute Laminitis

Acute laminitis may be subdivided into subacute (mild form), acute (severe form), and refractory (unresponsive). Subacute laminitis is a mild form of the disease with less severe clinical signs. It may be seen in horses that are worked on hard surfaces (road founder), those with hooves that are trimmed too short, and those that are exposed to black walnut wood shavings.[7] Signs of subacute laminitis often resolve quickly without permanent laminar damage, and rotation of the coffin bone usually does not occur. With the acute form of laminitis, the clinical signs are more severe, the disease does not respond as rapidly to treatment, and coffin bone rotation (movement) is more likely to occur.[7] Horses with refractory laminitis are those with acute laminitis that either does not respond or responds minimally to therapy within 7 to 10 days.[7] Refractory laminitis is believed to indicate severe laminar degeneration and inflammation and usually has a poor prognosis for recovery.

With acute laminitis, the clinical signs are often a delayed response to the inciting cause. Once clinical signs of laminitis are present, the clinical course of the disease is probably related to the quantity of laminar damage that has occurred. Horses with minimal laminar damage have milder signs and usually respond quickly to therapy. Horses with extensive laminar damage have more severe signs and either respond less quickly or not at all to medical therapy.

The subacute form of laminitis can be difficult to diagnose in some cases. Clinical signs of mild acute laminitis include moderately increased digital pulses; treading of the feet (lifting feet incessantly every few seconds); mild lameness, detected when the horse is circled; and pain, detected over the toe region with hoof testers. Horses with subacute laminitis usually have only minor laminar damage. If these horses are treated early, they recover completely, and the disease does not progress to the more severe acute laminitis.

The acute (severe form) of laminitis most commonly affects both front feet, but all four feet or one foot may be involved. When the two front feet are involved, the back feet are carried well up under the body, and the front feet are placed forward with the weight on the heel of the foot (Fig. 8.6). If all four feet are affected, the horse tends to lie down for extended periods. When standing, the horse often carries its hindfeet well up under it and places the forefeet caudally so that there is a narrow base of support. If a single foot is involved, as a result of supporting weight on that limb (support limb laminitis), the horse begins shifting weight to the opposite limb, giving one the impression that the condition that leads to the selective weight bearing is improving. Additionally, some horses exhibit anxiety, muscle trembling, increased respiration, and variable elevation in rectal temperature. On palpation, heat may be present over the hoof wall and the coronary band. An increased bounding digital pulse is evident. In acute laminitis cases, hoof tester pain may be elicited over the toe region or may not be elicited at all.

Obel clinically characterized and graded the severity of lameness by the following criteria[63]:

Grade 1: At rest the horse alternately and incessantly lifts the feet, often at intervals of a few seconds. Lameness is not evident at a walk, but a short stilted gait is noted at a trot.
Grade 2: The horse moves willingly at a walk, but the gait is stilted. A foot can be lifted off the ground without difficulty.
Grade 3: The horse moves very reluctantly and vigorously resists attempts to have a foot lifted off the ground.
Grade 4: The horse refuses to move and will not do so unless forced.

Chronic Laminitis

Chronic laminitis is a continuation of the acute stage, and it begins at the first sign of movement (displacement) of the coffin bone in the hoof capsule. Chronic laminitis may be divided into early chronic, chronic active, and chronic stable.[42,45] The early chronic stage begins at the first sign of movement of the coffin bone (laminar thickening, rotation or distal displacement). It may take days to months. Some cases resolve with minimum displacement, whereas others continue to displace and, in some cases, distally displace or slough the hoof capsule over time. In the chronic active stage, the coffin bone is rotated, remains unstable, and may have penetrated the sole (Fig. 8.7). Foot abscesses are common. In the chronic stable stage, the coffin bone becomes stable, the hoof and sole begin to regrow, and there is usually steady clinical improvement. Alterations in hoof growth include a dishing of the dorsal hoof wall (Fig. 8.8), a dorsal converging of the hoof wall rings (Fig. 8.9), a seedy toe (Fig. 8.10), and a dropped sole (Fig. 8.11). All these changes are presumed a result of altered vascular supply and a loss of laminar interdigitation. Hoof tester response can

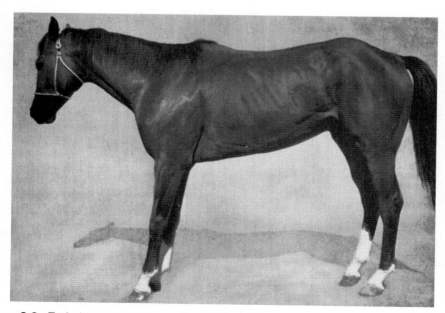

Figure 8.6 Typical stance of a horse with acute laminitis. Note the forefeet are camped out in front.

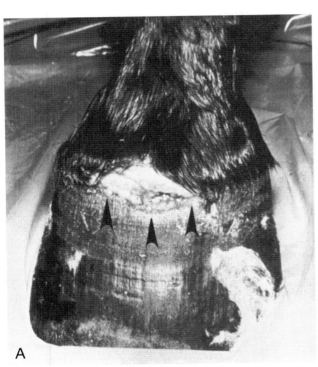

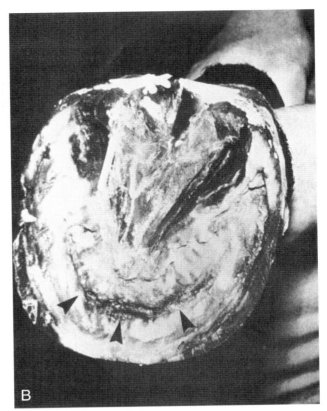

Figure 8.7   A. Severe laminitis with rotation of the distal phalanx and separation at the coronary band (arrows). B. Same horse.

Note the semicircular separation of the sole just dorsal to the apex of the frog (arrows).

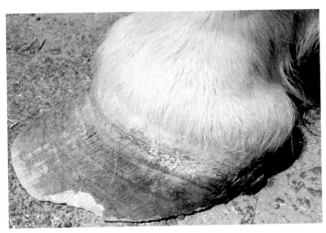

Figure 8.8   Dishing of the dorsal hoof wall.

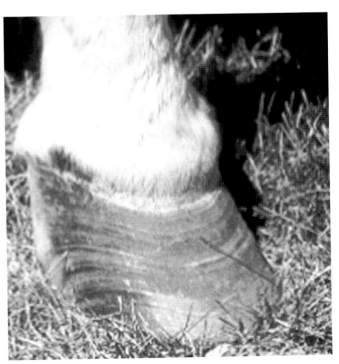

Figure 8.9   Chronic stable laminitis. Note the spaces between the rings at the heel are wider than those at the toe.

be variable during the chronic phases, presumably because of tissue death and subsequent loss of sensation once laminar shearing has occurred.

Rotation of the distal phalanx can vary from severe to mild. Severe rotation may result in separation of the coronary band over the extensor process region, and serum oozes out through this defect (Fig. 8.7A). Examination of the solar surface of the foot may reveal a semicircular separation of the sole just dorsal to the apex of

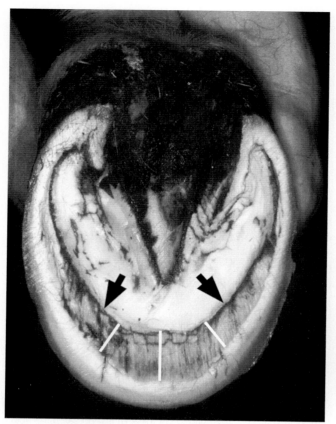

Figure 8.10 "Seedy toe." Note the increased width of the white line (white lines). Arrows point to the sole overlying the perimeter of the distal phalanx.

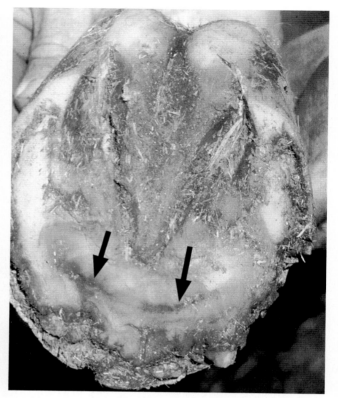

Figure 8.11 Dropped sole. Note the discoloration of the sole dorsal to the apex of the frog (arrows). This discolored area corresponds to the dorsal perimeter of the distal phalanx.

the frog (Fig. 8.7B), indicating that the tip of the distal phalanx is beginning to penetrate the sole.

Horses with chronic laminitis often assume a saw-horse stance, preferring to pivot on the hindlimbs and unweight the forelimbs. At a walk, they may land on the heel, followed by an exaggerated toe slap. This is to be expected, since the distal phalanx is not in normal alignment within the hoof wall or sole.

With seedy toe, enough separation of the white line may occur to allow infection to penetrate the laminae (Fig. 8.10). In humid climates, an infection similar to thrush may invade the flaky sole in chronic laminitis and destroy all protection of the distal phalanx.

Horses with distal displacement of the distal phalanx (sinkers) are usually severely lame. These patients generally stand with their limbs vertical to the ground instead of camped forward. A depression or cavitation may be palpable at the top of the hoof capsule. In some cases, serum may drain from an opening at the coronary band. In a case-control study of risk factors for the development of laminitis in the contralateral limb in horses with lameness, it was found that horses that develop support limb laminitis seem to have a greater risk of distally displacing their distal phalanx rather than of rotating their distal phalanx.[69] One of the earliest and most reliable signs of sinking was a palpable cavitation (depression) of the coronary band. Additionally, the duration of lameness was important. The median duration of lameness was 6.5 days in the control group (horses that did not

develop laminitis) and 40 days in the laminitis group. It was also noted that horses that were recumbent for several hours during a day were less likely to develop laminitis.

Horses with pituitary pars intermedia dysfunction (PPID) often have repeated bouts of laminitis. Other signs seen with the condition include polydypsia and polyuria, poor-quality hair coat, and long curly hair coat (hirsutism) that fails to shed normally in the summer months. Horses may appear obese and have a thick "cresty" neck.[57a,78a] In one report, the average age in years for horses affected with PPID was 19 to 20 (range, 15 to 40).[78a]

Diagnosis

The diagnosis of laminitis is based on clinical signs and radiography, and only occasionally is diagnostic local anesthesia used. Local anesthesia of the palmar nerves at the abaxial surface of the proximal sesamoid bone region or a pastern field block should eliminate the lameness in horses with acute laminitis (see Fig. 3.92). Occasionally, however, a horse with chronic laminitis will not block out completely with foot desensitization. This may result from remaining upper limb muscle pain.[45]

Radiographs should be taken at the first sign of acute laminitis to serve as a baseline for subsequent radiographic comparisons and to determine if preexisting radiographic changes suggestive of previous laminitis are present. A metal object can be taped to the dorsal hoof wall to help identify it and a thumbtack can be placed at the apex of the frog if the use of frog support is planned (Fig. 8.12). Early radiographic signs suggestive of laminitis include mild bony reaction along the dorsal aspect of the distal phalanx (P3) (Fig. 8.13) and widening of the distance between the distal phalanx and the dorsal hoof wall (Fig. 8.14).[53,64] This distance should be less than 18 mm (mean, 14.6 mm) in normal horses or less than 30% of the palmar length of the distal phalanx measured from the tip of the bone to its articulation with the navicular bone.[53] Thickness of the soft tissue should be divided by the palmar (solar) cortical length of the distal phalanx to correct for effects of radiographic magnification. An increase in this distance suggests hemorrhage, laminar swelling, and edema. In a radiographic study done on clinically normal Mammoth donkeys, a periosteal reaction on the dorsal surface of P3 was found; it was also noted that the mean distance from the dorsal aspect of P3 to the hoof wall were 22 to 23 mm for the forefeet and 20 to 21 mm for the hindfeet.[93] Palmar or plantar rotation of the distal phalanx away from the dor-

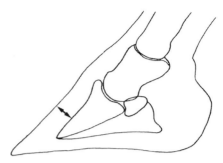

Figure 8.14 Measurement of the distance between the dorsal surface of the distal phalanx and the dorsal hoof wall.

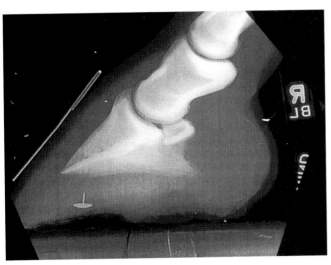

Figure 8.12 Lateral view of a metal object taped to the dorsal hoof wall and a thumbtack placed at the apex of the frog.

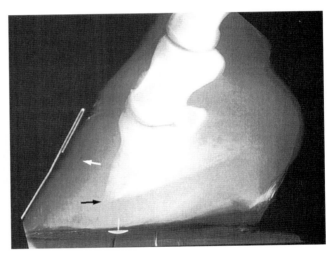

Figure 8.15 Lateral view of palmar rotation of the distal phalanx. Note the gas line (white arrow), the resorption of the tip of the distal phalanx, and the bone reaction on the dorsal surface of the distal phalanx (black arrow).

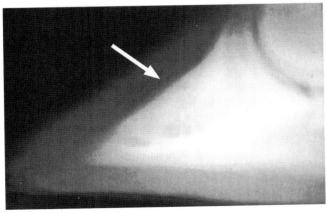

Figure 8.13 Arrow indicates bone reaction on the dorsal surface of the distal phalanx.

sal hoof wall confirms the diagnosis of laminitis (Fig. 8.15). The mean palmar and plantar rotation of the distal phalanx in normal horses is reported to be 0.5 ± 1.3 and less than 4°. If no abnormalities are detected on initial radiographs, but clinical signs of laminitis do not subside in 10 to 14 days, rotation or distal displacement of the distal phalanx is likely to occur.[7] Serial radiographs, therefore, should be taken to monitor the progression of the disease and to determine the success of selected treatments.

With distal displacement of the coffin bone, radiographs may show a soft tissue separation (seen as a parallel line) along the coronary band on the dorsopalmar and lateral views (see Figs. 8.2 and 8.16). On the lateral radiographic view, one can make an estimate of the displacement by measuring the distance from the coronary band to the proximal limits of the extensor process. A metal object can be placed at the coronary band to help identify it. An objective radiographic method to determine whether a horse has "sunk" within the hoof wall has not been developed. Additionally, distal displacement and rotation of the distal phalanx can occur concurrently, making objective assessment of both difficult radiographically. In one study, results of radiographic

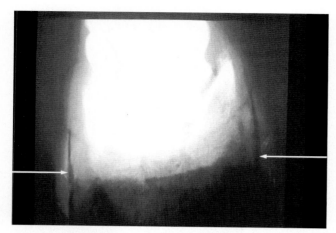

Figure 8.16 Dorsopalmar view of a "sinker." Note the separation at the coronet band (arrows).

evaluation suggested that laminitis of the contralateral limb (support limb) in horses with unilateral lameness often initially results in distal displacement of the distal phalanx (sinking) rather than in rotation.[69]

Digital venograms[45] and vascular perfusion casts[41] have been used to identify perfusion deficits, which, if present, usually indicate a poor prognosis. Digital venograms may be performed either with the horse standing or recumbent. A tourniquet is applied in the midmetacarpal region, and after appropriate skin preparation, 30 mL of intravenous contrast material is injected into a digital vein. Lateral and dorsopalmar radiographs are then taken.[45] After the study, the tourniquet is removed and a bandage is applied.

Diagnosis of PPID (Cushing's disease) is made from the clinical signs, laboratory findings, and endocrine function tests. Since PPID is the only cause of hirsutism in the horse, this finding appears as accurate as laboratory diagnosis for the condition. If hirsutism is not present, then laboratory findings are important. Evidence of either absolute or relative neutrophilia with lymphopenia is suggestive. Persistent hyperglycemia is also indicative of a possible PPID. Endocrine function tests include adrenocorticotropic hormone (ACTH) stimulation and dexamethasone suppression. Resting plasma ACTH concentrations appear valuable in the diagnosis of pituitary-dependent hyperadrenocorticism. Values in affected horses are typically 6 times greater than in normal horses.

Treatment Goals

Treatment regimens for acute laminitis are primarily based on the experience and results of retrospective studies. The goals of treatment are 1) to prevent the development of laminitis, 2) to reduce the pain or hypertension cycle, 3) to reduce or to prevent permanent laminar damage, 4) to improve dermal laminar capillary hemodynamics, and 5) to prevent movement of the distal phalanx.[7] Acute laminitis should be considered a medical emergency, and treatment should be initiated as soon as possible, preferably before clinical signs develop.

Prevention

Since many of the disease conditions that are thought to predispose horses to laminitis are associated with circulating endotoxin and infectious processes, combating the effects of endotoxemia and sepsis is important.[7] Recommended treatments include intravenous fluids (if needed), parenteral antimicrobials, flunixin meglumine, and hyperimmune serum or plasma. Additional laminitis-preventative measures include the administration of anti-inflammatory drugs (nonsteroidal anti-inflammatory drugs [NSAIDs]), vasodilators, heparin, oral acetylsalicylic acid (aspirin), and placement of the horse in a sand stall. In some cases, corrective trimming and shoeing may be indicated. Many treatments used to prevent laminitis are also used to treat laminitis once clinical signs develop.

Feeding an oral antibiotic (virginiamycin) to horses on a high-grain and pellet feed diet has also been proposed as a preventive measure. Feeding virginiamycin at 4 to 8 g/kg for 12 days resulted in a normal fecal pH and low blood D-lactate concentrations.[83] Intragastric mineral oil is often administered to grain overload cases. Mineral oil not only acts as a bulk laxative but also coats the intestinal wall, which may inhibit the absorption of endotoxins.

Anti-inflammatory Therapy

Nonsteroidal Anti-inflammatory Drugs

Phenylbutazone is the most common NSAID used to treat acute laminitis. Initially, it is often administered at 4.4 mg/kg orally or intravenously (IV) every 12 hours for 3 to 4 days. The dose is then gradually decreased to 2.2 mg/kg during the next 7 to 10 days or as long as needed. One study documenting the expressed pain relief effects of phenylbutazone in horses with chronic laminitis found that phenylbutazone resulted in gradual improvement in the load distribution profile, which reached plateau between the third and the fourth day.[38] Phenylbutazone is believed important for treating any form of laminitis because of its potential to reduce inflammation, edema, and pain within the digit, thus preventing progressive laminar damage. It also seems more effective in controlling digital pain than flunixin meglumine.[7] Flunixin meglumine (1.1 mg/kg IV every 12 hours or 0.25 mg/kg IV every 8 hours) may also be used alone or with phenylbutazone at the lower dose if the horse has clinical signs suggestive of endotoxemia or sepsis.[24,84]

Ketoprofen is thought to work similarly to flunixin meglumine and probably can be used interchangeably.[56] Ketoprofen (2.2 mg/kg IV every 12 hours) acts on both the lipoxygenase and the prostaglandin pathways of the arachidonic acid cascade and, therefore, may reduce inflammation more effectively than flunixin meglumine or phenylbutazone.[57] Ketoprofen at a dose of 3.63 mg/kg was found to reduce hoof pain to a greater extent than at a dose of 2.2 mg/kg. The higher dose of ketoprofen was also found to be more potent than phenylbutazone (at a dose of 4.4 mg/kg) in horses with chronic foot pain.[68]

Dimethyl Sulfoxide

A free radical scavenger and potent anti-inflammatory agent that may prevent reperfusion injury of ischemic tissues is dimethyl sulfoxide (DMSO, 0.1 g/kg IV every 12 hours for 2 to 3 days).[14] Although no studies have documented the efficacy of DMSO in treating acute laminitis, clinical impressions dictate its continued use.

Antiendotoxin Therapy

Treatments are aimed at the primary disease process and the endotoxemia.[7] Antiendotoxin therapies include parenteral antimicrobials, flunixin meglumine, ketoprofen, and hyperimmune antiendotoxin serum or plasma. Whether one or all of these medications are used depends on the severity of the primary disease process and the concurrent endotoxemia. The efficacy of these treatments is unknown. Antiendotoxin therapy use is supported in a study that documented a potential decrease in dermal laminar blood flow and a decrease in palmar digital artery blood flow after administration of low doses of endotoxins.[51]

Vasodilator Therapy

The goal of vasodilator or antihypertensive therapy is to improve laminar perfusion.

Acepromazine

Doses of acepromazine of 0.01, 0.02, 0.04, and 0.066 mg/kg IV have been shown to improve blood flow to the digit in standing, healthy horses.[46,49,52] With an acepromazine dose of 0.055 mg/kg IV, an improved blood flow rate and an actual increase in the diameter of the metatarsal artery have also been documented experimentally in standing horses.[92] In another study, acepromazine (0.066 mg/kg IV) significantly increased blood flow to the digit, but not to the laminae.[52] This is in contrast to a study that found an increase in the laminar blood flow in horses treated intravenously with acepromazine.[1] Clinically, acepromazine is usually given to horses at doses between 0.03 and 0.06 mg/kg intramuscularly (IM) every 6 to 8 hours for 3 to 5 days and, in some cases, weeks. The dose and the duration of treatment are adjusted in accordance with the alteration in the intensity of the digital pulses. As the digital pulses diminish, so does the dose and frequency of administration of acepromazine. Reduction in dose and frequency is done slowly, however. Acepromazine treatment also reduces anxiety, and horses appear to lie down more readily. For horses with acute laminitis, some researchers have advocated forced recumbency to reduce biomechanical strain on the laminae.[94]

Isoxsuprine

Isoxsuprine hydrochloride at 1.2 mg/kg every 12 hours orally is recommended. Acepromazine is used initially in nearly all horses with acute laminitis. Then, once clinical signs of improvement occur, vasodilator therapy is continued with isoxsuprine. One study evaluating the effects of oral isoxsuprine on blood flow to the digit or laminae could not identify an effect in healthy horses compared with control subjects.[52] It was proposed that the apparent clinical benefit of isoxsuprine in horses with ischemic conditions of the hoof may be the result of a different mechanism than improved perfusion or that the drug is only beneficial in horses with ischemic conditions of the hoof. Also, the duration of the study (10 days) may have been too short to detect an increase in blood flow, since it has been reported that 3 to 4 weeks of treatment is required before a clinical benefit is observed in horses.[90] That is why I initiate isoxsuprine treatment in conjunction with acepromazine within a few days after the first signs of laminitis. In another study in which thermography was used, investigators found that isoxsuprine administration caused an increase in skin surface temperature of the forelimbs in horses.[22]

Pentoxifylline

Pentoxifylline has been reported to improve circulation and oxygen delivery.[6,21] The results of one study indicated that oral dosing of pentoxifylline at 4.4 mg/kg every 8 hours did not cause a measurable increase in palmar digital or laminar blood flow in healthy horses.[52] In another report, oral absorption of pentoxifylline was found to be poor and erratic and may have been affected by food consumption at the time of dosing.[19]

Nitroglycerin

Nitroglycerin ointment applied topically to the pastern region subjectively reduced bounding pulses and lameness in ponies.[28,37] Two percent (2%) glyceryl trinitrate (GTN) ointment was applied once daily to the pasterns (clip hair) as a patch; each aliquot (1-inch bead) of paste was positioned over the digital vessels and secured in place with elastic adhesive tape (Fig. 8.17). GTN was administered at an initial dose of 60 mg (0.3 mg/kg per day) for 2 days. If the blood pressure decreased and the lameness improved, it was reduced to 40 mg (0.02 mg/kg per day) for 2 days and then to 20 mg (0.01 mg/kg per day) for an additional 2 days. Because GTN ointment is readily absorbed through the skin, it is advisable to use rubber gloves when applying it. At the time of this writing, GTN is being used routinely in clinical cases, but usually in conjunction with other treatments; therefore, accurate assessment of therapeutic effects are not clear.

Anticoagulant Therapy

Aspirin

Aspirin at 10 to 20 mg/kg orally every other day has been shown to inhibit platelet aggregation by increasing thromboxane synthesis.[12] The decreased platelet aggregation theoretically should minimize microthrombosis within the laminae, even when perfusion is sluggish. This dose of aspirin has minimal anti-inflammatory properties and no known side effects, and it can be used safely in combination with other NSAIDs, such as phenylbutazone and flunixin meglumine.[7]

Heparin

At doses of 40 to 80 IU/kg IV or subcutaneously (SC) every 8 to 12 hours, heparin has been shown to prevent

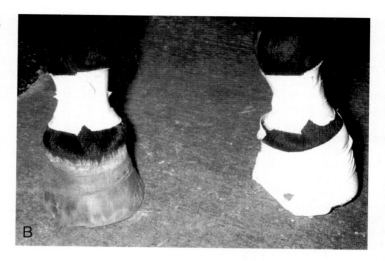

NITRO-BID® OINTMENT 2%
(nitroglycerin ointment USP)

| ½" | 1" | 1½" | 2" | 2½" |

DOSE MEASURING APPLICATOR

A

B

Figure 8.17 A. Dose-measuring applicator for nitroglycerin. B. Dose applicators held in place in the pastern region by elastic tape.

laminitis experimentally in horses with carbohydrate overload.[20,43] One retrospective study did not find a benefit of heparin in preventing laminitis in horses with diseases of the small intestines.[13] In another study in which horses with duodenitis and/or proximal jejunitis were evaluated, laminitis was found to be significantly reduced when horses received heparin prophylaxis.[18] Currently, we are using heparin primarily as a preventive measure in horses at a high risk for developing laminitis.

Miscellaneous Medical Treatments

Methionine and Biotin Supplements

Dietary supplementation of methionine and biotin to improve the quality and quantity of hoof growth may also be used to treat laminitis. Supplementation of dietary biotin at a dose of 15 mg/day has been shown to increase growth rates and hardness of hooves in normal horses.[16] Supplementation of biotin is probably unimportant in the initial treatment of acute laminitis, but it may be useful in the long-term management of horses recovering from laminitis.[7]

Thyroid Hormone Supplements

Although no scientific basis of support exists for its use, thyroid hormone supplements are still used in some horses suffering from chronic laminitis. Either iodinated casein or direct oral replacement is recommended. Of the two, direct oral replacement with 6 to 10 of the 5-grain thyroid tablets per 450 kg is preferred.[2] This treatment seems most beneficial in horses with a hypothyroid phenotype (large cresty neck, with fat deposits over the rump and back) or in horses that gain weight rapidly.[34] It has been reported that the hormone not only reverses the signs of laminitis but also maintains the laminae in a sound state.[46]

Dopamine Agonists or Serotonin Antagonists

Horses with PPID (Cushing's disease) that exhibit laminitis are often refractory to routine treatment. Medical management of these cases involves the use of either dopamine agonists or serotonin antagonists. Bromocrip-

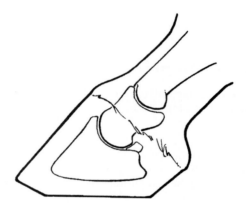

Figure 8.18 Rockering the toe of the hoof.

tine and pergolide are the two most commonly used dopamine agonists. The dose of pergolide is 1 to 5 mg/horse. The clinical response usually takes 3 to 4 weeks. Cyproheptadine inhibits ACTH secretion from the pars intermedia through the antiserotonin pathway. Doses range from 0.25 mg/kg daily; some horses require 0.36 mg/kg 2 times a day before changes in the clinical signs are observed. In horses requiring high doses, it is recommended that the dose be reduced after 30 days as long as the clinical response remains favorable. One study found that PPID horses treated with cyproheptadine were more likely to show improvement in the laminitis than those treated with pergolide.

Hoof Care or Corrective Trimming, Confinement, and Shoeing

Trimming and Confinement

The only trimming that should be done at the first examination of an acute laminitis case is to rocker (bevel) the toe of the hoof wall to approximately 15 to 20° (Fig. 8.18). This can be done with hoof nippers or a rasp.[65] Hoof testers are used to determine how far back from the toe the rocker should extend into the sole. The rocker is begun dorsal to the painful region in the sole. Rock-

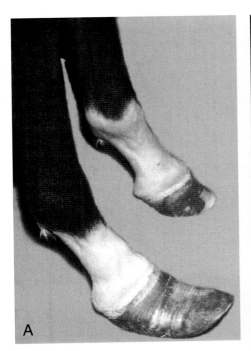

ering the toe is done to reduce weight-bearing forces on the dorsal hoof wall, thus reducing the continued laminar tearing and decreasing the leverage required for breakover. It also reduces the tension on the deep digital flexor tendon (DDFT) during breakover and exposes the back of the foot to weight bearing, which is generally the least painful region of the foot. In cases of severe laminitis, trimming is delayed until the horse is comfortable enough to withstand the procedure.

Horses with acute laminitis should be placed in a stall bedded with dry sand (a depth of 6 inches is best) or soft bedding to minimize concussion in the feet and to reduce leverage forces required for breakover. Straw can be added to dry sand bedding to encourage recumbency. Horses that prefer to remain recumbent should be allowed to do so, and if pressure sores begin to develop, a horse blanket can be used to protect these sites. Forced exercise is contraindicated.

A common problem after foot regrowth in cases of severe laminitis is abscess recurrence, pedal osteitis (nonseptic and septic), and abnormal hoof growth (Figs. 8.8 and 8.10). Abscesses should be drained, osteomyelitis is debrided as needed, and the foot is protected. At least one report has questioned the value of debriding the sole

of laminitic horses with abscessed feet.[65] In this report, horses that had the sole removed around the abscess site had their distal phalanx remain unstable for a longer period, and they had more setbacks than horses that did not have this procedure performed. Also, horses that had their feet soaked in the epsom salts and Betadine solution 3 to 4 times a day progressed slower and had more bouts of recurrent pain than the horses that were not treated with soaking. The most common microorganism cultured from the distal phalanx of horses with laminitis is *Staphylococcus*. Distal-limb vascular perfusion or medullary bone perfusion may be helpful in the treatment of osteomyelitis of the distal phalanx. Also, the topical application of sugardine (mixture of Betadine and sugar) as a dressing has been recommended.

Horses that have rotated their distal phalanx and are chronic and stable should have the feet trimmed to realign the hoof capsule with the distal phalanx (Fig. 8.19). The toe may be squared off or rockered to enhance breakover.

Foot Support

Support of the frog can be maintained with pads (e.g., Lily pads or Thera-Flex pads), thermoplastic frog sup-

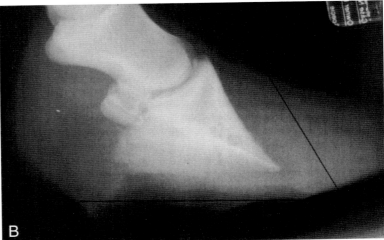

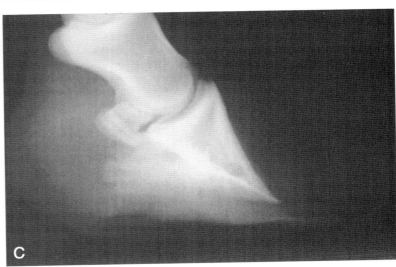

Figure 8.19 A. Chronic stable laminitis. The left forefoot has been trimmed. B. Lateral view of the left forefoot of the horse. The lines indicate the hoof wall and sole to be removed. C. Lateral view of the left forefoot after trimming.

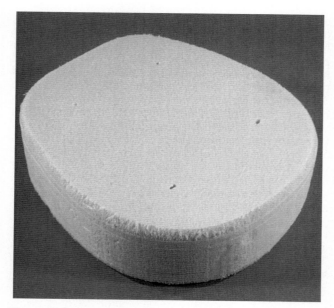

Figure 8.20 Styrofoam pad, 2 inches thick (Equine Digit Support System, Inc., Columbia Falls, MT).

port, 3M custom foam, roll gauze, or a roll of Vetwrap. One study comparing phenylbutazone, Lily pads, and trimming on expressed pain in horses with chronic laminitis found that Lily pads did not reduce expressed pain and that, in some cases, they increased the pain significantly.[40]

Alternatively, a 2-inch-thick Styrofoam pad, which is roughly the diameter of the bottom of the foot, can be used to provide support to the frog and to the caudal one-half to two-thirds of the foot underlying the distal phalanx (Fig. 8.20).[66,67] Before the Styrofoam pad application, the toe 1¼-inch in front of the frog is slightly rockered to enhance breakover (Fig. 8.18). Duct tape is then used to attach the pad to the bottom of the foot, after which the horse is allowed to bear weight on the limb. After 24 to 48 hours, the pad compresses to a thickness of ¾ inch. It is then removed. Hoof testers are then used to identify the painful regions on the sole after which the compressed pad is trimmed to fit the foot so it is ⅜ inch behind the painful region. The compressed pad is then attached to the foot with tape, and a new Styrofoam pad is applied on top of it as previously described. This process is repeated and continued until the horse is comfortable and stabilized. Generally, horses with acute laminitis require 3 to 4 compressed layers of Styrofoam trimmed and fitted to the caudal sole of the foot before they are comfortable. After the horse becomes comfortable, it can be placed in the Equine Digit Support System (EDSS) shoeing (discussed under "Shoes," below).[67] Generally, corrective shoeing is only considered after acute digital pain and inflammation have subsided.

Shoes

Therapeutic shoeing plays an important roll in the treatment of laminitis. The types of shoes that are used most commonly include heart bar shoes (nonadjustable

and adjustable), reverse shoes with pads, egg bar shoes, shoes with pads, elevated heel shoes, and EDSS shoes.[17,29,33,67,96] Plastic shoes have also been advocated.

The heart bar shoe is basically a bar shoe with an extended V-shaped frog plate (Fig. 9.81). It is designed to apply pressure to the frog, thus supporting the distal phalanx. To be effective, it should extend dorsally (forward) to cover at least the caudal two-thirds of the length of the distal phalanx. This shoe is difficult to make and apply properly, and it has received mixed reviews with regard to its benefit in the treatment of laminitis. In one study, however, it was shown that heart bar shoes improve blood flow though the dorsal artery to the dorsal laminae of the foot in in vitro studies.[72] Presently, we find limited use for this shoe.

Elevating the heel decreases the pull of the DDFT and appears to improve the blood flow to the dorsal laminae though the dorsal artery of the foot.[72] An 18° heel wedge has been recommended (Figs. 8.21 and 8.22).[77] Elevating the heels should minimize the physical tearing of the susceptible laminae during the acute stage of the disease and thus potentially decrease the amount of movement of the distal phalanx within the hoof wall.

The EDSS shoes can be applied once the acute case of laminitis has stabilized.[67] A major objective when applying these shoes is to transfer the weight bearing to the palmar aspect of the foot underlying the distal phalanx. These weight-bearing structures include the sole, frog, and bars. For this to be done, the foot is trimmed, to derotate it, from the widest part of the foot back to the heels (Fig. 8.23). Lateral radiographs are taken to document the degree of rotation and to determine the amount of heel to be removed to provide a normal alignment of the sole and distal phalanx. After hoof preparation, hoof testers are applied to identify the painful regions of the foot. Painful regions are usually found in the dorsal one-third of the sole dorsal to apex of the frog. After this, a

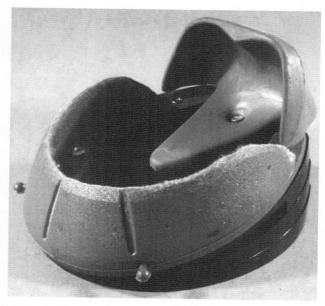

Figure 8.21 Redden boot with ultimate wedge set (obtained from R. F. Redden, Box 507, Versailles, KY 40383).

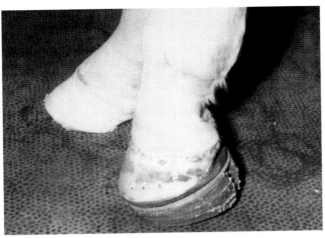

Figure 8.22 Elevated heel shoe. Three 6° wedge pads have been applied to the bottom of the shoe.

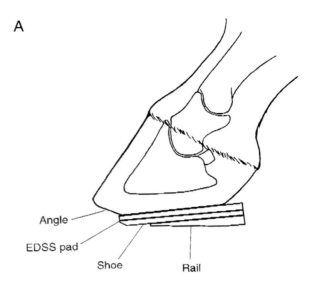

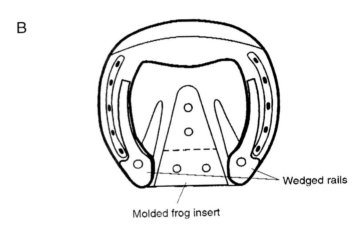

Figure 8.24 Application of the EDSS shoe plus rails and frog pad. A. Lateral view. Note the heel elevation as a result of the rails and the rockering of the pad. B. Bottom view. Note the frog pad and the placement of the wedged rails. (Based on Ovnicek G. New Hope for Soundness: Seen Through the Window of Wild Horse Hoof Patterns. Columbia Falls, MT: Equine Digit Support System, Inc., 1997.)

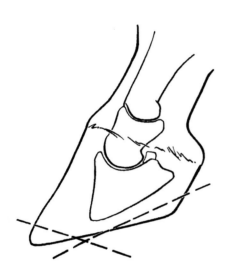

Figure 8.23 Hoof is trimmed to derotate it.

two-part impression material is applied to the bottom of the foot and allowed to dry. Once dry, the impression material is trimmed so as not to apply pressure to the painful regions of the foot identified with hoof testers. Then the trimmed impression material is replaced in the palmar aspect of the foot, after which an EDSS pad, molded frog insert, and shoe are applied. The EDSS shoes have holes drilled into them to accept three different elevations of wedge rails. These rails elevate the heels and reduce the tension on the DDFT (Fig. 8.24). The selected rail elevation is determined by the horses comfort. In most cases, the wedge rails return the distal phalanx to no more than 5° above normal. The horse is reshod when the hoof has sufficiently grown and requires trimming. Radiographs should be taken after each trimming session.

Surgical Treatment

Carpal Check Ligament Desmotomy

Some researchers have advocated carpal check ligament desmotomy to decrease the tension of the DDFT, thus reducing subsequent tearing of the laminae.[45] It may be a useful procedure in horses with low-grade mild chronic laminitis.

Deep Digital Flexor Tendon Tenotomy and Derotation of the Distal Phalanx

DDFT tenotomy has been recommended to help relieve the pain in horses with chronic laminitis that have not responded to other forms of therapy.[25,45,47,91] The procedure seems most effective in chronic laminitis cases and least effective in cases of acute laminitis, those with distal displacement of the distal phalanx (sinkers), and those with evidence of distal phalangeal disease.[91] A combination of DDFT tenotomy and derotation of the

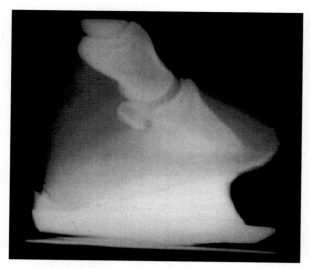

Figure 8.25 Lateral view of subluxation of the coffin joint after DDFT tenotomy. (Courtesy of Dr. F. W. Nickels.)

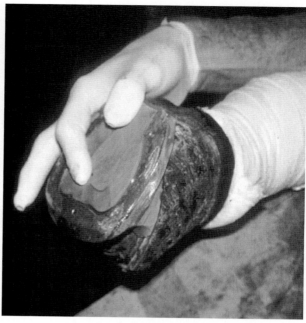

Figure 8.26 Two-part impression material is being used to hold the shoe away from the hoof. (Courtesy of Dr. F. W. Nickels.)

distal phalanx is recommended and can offer even penetrated laminitic horses a chance for full recovery.[78]

DDFT tenotomy in the midmetacarpal region is the preferred technique. The tenotomy can be done in the standing sedated horse (most common) or under general anesthesia, and it can be repeated. The foot is derotated so a normal alignment of the sole and distal phalanx exists (Fig. 8.23). The procedure, if done properly, reestablishes the weight-bearing forces of the hoof underneath the distal phalanx. Radiographs are necessary to assist in the derotation procedure. Once the radiographs have been taken and the amount of heel to be removed is determined, the foot is trimmed from the widest part of the hoof palmar, so that the frog, bars, and sole are loaded equally. Because DDFT tenotomy causes subluxation of the coffin joint and hyperextension of the digit, an extended heel shoe is often used for palmar heel support (Fig. 8.25). Alternatively, an EDSS shoe with wedge rails (our preference) can be used (Nickels FA, personal communication, 1999).[67,78] The shoe is held to the foot with hoof acrylic or cast material or nails in a position to support the palmar foot region and to create breakover just dorsal to the apex (tip) of the frog. A two-part impression material is applied to the bottom of the foot underlying the distal phalanx and, in some cases, is used to help hold the shoe away from the hoof to derotate the foot properly (Fig. 8.26). Wedge rails (medium height most common) are applied to the shoe to elevate the heels, thus preventing the subluxation of the coffin joint that occurs after DDFT tenotomy (Fig. 8.27). The rails also reduce the stress on the DDFT while it heals and maintains the weight-bearing load in the heel region (Nickels FA, personal communication, 1999).[78] The rails are left on for at least 4 months, after which a smaller wedge rail is used for another 2 to 3 months (Nickels FA, personal communication, 1999). The horse is reshod when the hoof has sufficiently grown and requires trimming.

Complications associated with the tendon healing site include swelling, pain, fibrosis, and, occasionally, tendon contracture.[62] The use of support bandages for at

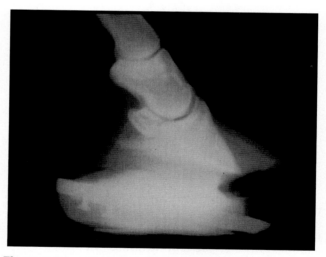

Figure 8.27 Lateral view of the use of the rails to prevent subluxation of the coffin joint after DDFT tenotomy. (Courtesy of Dr. F. W. Nickels.)

least 8 weeks reduces the local swelling and excessive fibrosis and ensures a more cosmetic and functional result. Stall rest and controlled exercise are important during the healing period. Ultrasound may be used during the healing period to document its progress. Tendon contracture after tenotomy is usually a result of passive constriction of the scar as a result of unweighting the limb because of chronic pain. Recurring infection of the digit is often the cause for the recurrent pain, and prompt, aggressive treatment often can reduce this complication.[62]

DDFT tenotomy in the pastern region has also been used, and general anesthesia is recommended.[4] An extended heel shoe is needed after this surgery for a period of 8 to 12 weeks. Although the initial reports of the outcome of this procedure were favorable, our limited experience with it did not result in a favorable outcome. As a result, we rarely see an indication for doing the tenotomy in the pastern region.

One study evaluating the effect of DDFT tenotomy as a treatment for chronic laminitis in 35 horses (midmetacarpal, 30 horses; pastern, 5 horses) found that 27 of 35 (77%) horses were alive 6 months after surgery and that 19 of 32 (59%) horses were alive for at least 2 years. Of the horses that were living at 2 years, their average survival time was 4.5 years. Body weight and Obel grade of lameness had no effect on the 6-month or 2-year survival rate. Of the horses in this study, 10 became sound enough for light riding, and there was no correlation between the Obel grade of lameness and the degree of rotation and the ability to be ridden.[25,26] Another study evaluating the effect of DDFT tenotomy in the midmetacarpal region of 9 horses with severe laminitis with complications such as intense pain, rotation of more than 15°, penetration of the sole, and/or evidence of infection of the sole or distal phalanx, found 9 of 9 horses were still alive.[62] Six of the nine horses have survived more than 1.5 years, and the other three are convalescing. Four of the nine horses were able to be used for pleasure riding.

Hoof Wall Resection

Removal of the dorsal hoof wall is not recommended in horses with acute laminitis. Dorsal hoof wall resection is reserved for horses with chronic laminitis when there is a physical separation between the insensitive and the sensitive laminae (Fig. 8.28).[7,45] The value of hoof resection has been questioned, and documentation of a clear benefit is lacking.

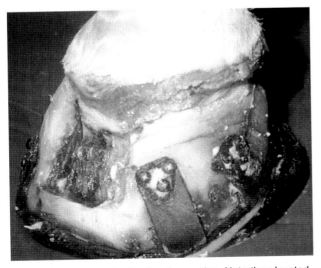

Figure 8.28 Extensive hoof wall resection. Note the elevated heel shoe is held in place by sheet metal screws that are placed through holes in metal extensions. The metal extensions were welded to the shoe. The hoof wall below the coronet band also had to be resected.

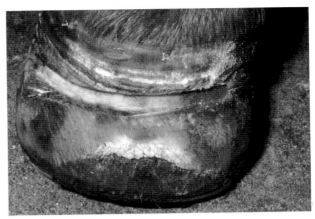

Figure 8.29 Chronic laminitis for which coronary grooving was used. (Courtesy of Dr. G. M. Baxter.)

Coronary Grooving

Coronary grooving (Fig. 8.29) has been advocated to promote dorsal hoof wall growth in horses with chronic laminitis that are exhibiting abnormal (slower) growth in this region.[79] In this technique, a motorized rotary burr is used to create a 20-cm-wide groove in the hoof wall parallel to the coronary band. The groove is begun 1.5 cm distal to the hair–periople junction and extends from the center of the lateral quarter to the center of the medial quarter. The groove is deepened until the soft translucent horn is reached. Sedation is usually all that is needed. As an alternative, a hoof rasp can be used to create this groove (Ovnicek G, personal communication, 1998). In a controlled study in which the effect of coronary grooving and no grooving in horses with chronic laminitis that had abnormal hoof growth was evaluated, investigators found a significant increase in the dorsal hoof wall growth compared with that of control subjects. The grooving was done in conjunction with corrective trimming.[79] It was hypothesized that grooving the dorsal hoof wall relieves the external pressure on the dorsal coronary corium and restores the blood supply, thus promoting hoof wall growth. Although the grooving technique increased hoof wall growth, no difference existed in clinical improvement between the groups.

Prognosis

Predicting the prognosis and survival of horses with acute laminitis can be difficult. It has been reported previously that the amount of rotation of the distal phalanx can be used to predict the prognosis of horses with laminitis.[86] It was found that the majority of horses with less than 5.5° rotation returned to former athletic function, whereas those with more than 11.5° rotation lost their use as performance animals, although some could be used for breeding. In another study, the degree of rotation or distal displacement of the distal phalanx observed on radiographs did not correlate with the outcome of the horses.[44] The clinical assessment of lameness severity based on Obel grades 1 to 4 was a more reliable means of determining the final outcome. It was recommended that lameness severity take precedence over radiographic findings in predicting the prognosis of horses with laminitis. This suggests that lameness severity in horses with laminitis probably correlates with the severity or quantity of permanent laminar damage that has or is likely to occur. In another study, body weight, Obel grade of lameness, and degree of distal phalangeal rotation did not appear to be factors in the survival of horses with chronic laminitis that had a DDFT tenotomy.[26]

The response to therapy may also be a predictor of the quantity of laminar damage that has occurred and, thus, the probability of resolving the problem.[9] The quicker a horse responds to appropriate therapy, the less laminar damage occurs and the better the prognosis for recovery from the episode of laminitis. Horses that recover from laminitis, however, seem more susceptible to recurrent episodes of laminitis.

It has been suggested that digital venograms are helpful in defining disruption of the vascular architecture and, therefore, may be of help in determining prognosis, especially early in the course of the disease.[45] A tourniquet is applied after the limb is prepared, and 30 mL of intravenous contrast medium is injected into the digital vein. I have no experience using this technique for the assessment of chronic laminitis cases.

Owners should be informed that the damage to the laminae is not completely reversed, only repaired, and thus affected horses are more likely to develop laminitis again than horses that have not had previous laminitis.

References

1. Adair HS, Goble DO, Shires GM, Sanders WL. Evaluation of laser Doppler flowmetry for measuring coronary band and laminar microcirculatory blood flow in clinically normal horses. Am J Vet Res 1994;55:445–449.
2. Adams OR. Lameness in Horses. Philadelphia: Lea & Febiger, 1974:247.
3. Allen D, Clark ES, Moore JN, Prasse KW. Evaluation of equine digital Starling forces and hemodynamics during early laminitis. Am J Vet Res 1990;51:1930–1934.
4. Allen D, White NA, Foerner JF, Gordon BJ. Surgical management of chronic laminitis in horses: 13 cases (1983–1985). J Am Vet Med Assoc 1986;189:1604–1606.
5. Amoss MS, Hood DM, Miller WG, et al. Equine laminitis II. Elevation in serum testosterone associated with induced and naturally occurring laminitis. J Equine Med Surg 1979;3:171.
6. Aviado DM, Porter JM. Pentoxifylline: A new drug for treatment of intermittent claudication. Pharmacotherapy 1984;4:297–307.
7. Baxter GM. Acute laminitis. Vet Clin North Am Equine Pract 1994;10(3):627–642.
8. Baxter GM. Alteration of endothelium-dependant digital vascular responses in horses given low dose endotoxin. Vet Surg 1995;24:87–96.
9. Baxter GM. Diagnosing and treating acute laminitis: Symposium on acute laminitis. Vet Med 1996;91:940–952.
10. Baxter GM. Equine laminitis caused by distal displacement of the distal phalanx: 12 cases (1976–1985) J Am Vet Med Assoc 1986;189:326–329.
11. Baxter GM, Laskey RE, Tackett RL, et al. In vitro reactivity of digital arteries and veins to vasoconstrictive mediators in healthy horses and in horses with early laminitis. Am J Vet Res 1989;50(4):508–517.
12. Baxter GM, Moore JN. Effect of aspirin on ex vivo generation of thromboxane in healthy horses. Am J Vet Res 1987;48:13–16.
13. Belknap JK, Moore JN. Evaluation of heparin for prophylaxis of equine laminitis: 71 cases (1980–1986). J Am Vet Med Assoc 1989;95:505–507.
14. Blythe LL, Craig AM, Christensen JM, et al. Pharmacokinetic disposition of dimethyl sulfoxide administered intravenously to horses. Am J Vet Res 1986;47:1739–1743.
15. Bryant CE, Elliott J. Nitric oxide: Friend or foe? Equine Vet Educ 1994;6:59–64.
16. Buffa EA, Van Den Berg SS, Verstraete FJM, Swart NG. Effect of dietary biotin supplement on equine hoof horn growth rate and hardness. Equine Vet J 1992;24:472–474.
17. Chapman B, Platt GW. Laminitis. Proc Am Assoc Equine Pract 1984;13:129.
18. Cohen ND, Parson EM, Seahorn TL, et al. Prevalence and factors associated with laminitis in horses with duodenitis/proximal jejunitis: 116 cases (1985–1991). J Am Vet Med Assoc 1994;204:250–254.
19. Crisman MV, Wilcke LS, Correll LS, et al. Pharmacokinetic disposition of intravenous and oral pentoxifylline in horses. J Vet Pharmacol Ther 1993;16:23–31.
20. Darien BJ. Heparin therapy: Rationale and clinical indications. Comp Cont Educ Pract Vet 1993;15:1273–1276.
21. Dettelbach HR. Clinical pharmacology of pentoxifylline with special reference to its hemorheologic effect for the treatment of intermittent claudication. J Clin Pharmacol 1985;25:8–26.
22. Deumer J, de Haan F, Tulp MTM, et al. Effect of an isoxsuprine–resin preparation on blood flow in the equine thoracic limb. Vet Rec 1991;129:427–429.
23. Duncan SG, Meyers KM, Reed SM, Grant B. Alterations in coagulation and hemograms of horses given endotoxins for 24 hours via hepatic portal infusions. Am J Vet Res 1985;46:1287–1293.
24. Dunkle NJ, Bottoms GD, Fessler JF, et al. Effects of flunixin meglumine on blood pressure and fluid compartment volume changes in ponies given endotoxin. Am J Vet Res 1985;46:1540–1544.
25. Eastman TG, Honnas CM, Hague BA, Moyer W. Deep digital flexor tenotomy as a treatment for chronic laminitis in horses: 37 cases. Proc Am Assoc Equine Pract 1998;44:265–266.
26. Eastman TG, Honnas CM, Hague BA, Moyer W, et al. Deep digital flexor tenotomy as a treatment for chronic laminitis in horses: 35 cases (1988–1997). J Am Vet Med Assoc 1999;214:517–519.
27. Eaton SA, Allen D, Eades SC, Schneider DA. Equine digital Starlings forces and hemodynamics during early laminitis induced by an aqueous extract of black walnut (Juglans nigra). Am J Vet Res 1995;56:1338–1344.
28. Elliot J. Nitric oxide and equine laminitis: Topical speculation or scientific fact? Equine Vet J 1996;28:1–2.
29. Eustace RA, Caldwell MN. Treatment of solar prolapse using the heart bar shoe and hoof wall resection technique. Equine Vet J 1989;21:370–372.
30. Eyre P, Elmes PJ, Strickland S. Corticosteroid potentiated vascular responses of the equine digit: A possible pharmacologic basis for laminitis. Am J Vet Res 1979;40:135.
31. Galey FD, Twardock AR, Goetz TE, et al. Gamma scintigraphic analysis of the distribution of perfusion of blood in the equine foot during black walnut (Juglans nigra)-induced laminitis. Am J Vet Res 1990;51:688–695.
32. Garner HE, Moore JN, Johnson JH. Changes in cecal flora associated with the onset of laminitis. Equine Vet J 1978;4:249–252.
33. Goetz TE. Anatomic, hoof and shoeing considerations for the treatment of laminitis in horses. J Am Vet Med Assoc 1987;190:1323–1332.
34. Goetz TE. The treatment of laminitis in horses. Vet Clin North Am Equine Pract 1989;5:73–108.
35. Grosenbaugh DA, Hood DM, Amoss MS, Williams JD. Characterization and distribution of epidermal growth factor receptors in equine hoof wall laminar tissue: Comparison of normal horses and horses affected with chronic laminitis. Equine Vet J 1991;23:201–206.
36. Harkema JR, Robinson NE, Scott JB. Cardiovascular, acid-base, electrolyte and plasma volume changes in ponies developing alimentary laminitis. Am J Vet Res 1978;39:741.
37. Hinckley KA, Fearn S, Howard BR, Henderson IW. Nitric oxide donors as treatment for grass induced acute laminitis in ponies. Equine Vet J 1996;28:17–28.
38. Hood DM. Endotoxemia as a direct cause of laminitis. Proc Am Assoc Equine Pract 1995;41:245–247.
39. Hood DM, Amoss MS. Equine laminitis-radioisotopic analysis of the hemodynamics of the foot. J Equine Med Surg 1978;2:439–444.
40. Hood DM, Beckham AS, Chaffin MK, et al. Comparison of phenylbutazone, Lily pads and trimming on expressed pain in horses with chronic laminitis. Proc Am Assoc Equine Pract 1995;41:248–250.

41. Hood DM, Grosenbough DA, Slater MR. Vascular perfusion in horses with chronic laminitis. Equine Vet J 1994;26:191–196.

42. Hood DM, Stephens KA. Pathophysiology of equine laminitis. Comp Cont Educ Pract Vet 1981;3:454.

43. Hood DM, Stephens KA, Amoss MS. Heparin as a preventative for equine laminitis. Proc Am Assoc Equine Pract 1982;2:146–149.

44. Hunt RJ. A retrospective evaluation of laminitis in horses. Equine Vet J 1993;25:61–64.

45. Hunt RJ. Diagnosing and treating chronic laminitis in horses. Vet Med 1996;91:1025–1032.

46. Hunt RJ. Pathophysiology of acute laminitis. Comp Cont Educ Pract Vet 1991;13:1003–1010.

47. Hunt RJ, Allen D, Baxter GM, et al. Mid-metacarpal deep digital flexor tenotomy in the management of refractory laminitis in horses. Vet Surg 1991;20:15–20.

48. Hunt RJ, Allen D, Moore JN. Effect of endotoxin on equine digital hemodynamic and starlings forces. Am J Vet Res 1990;51:1703–1707.

49. Hunt RJ, Brandon CI, McCann ME. Effects of acetylpromazine, xylazine and vertical load on equine digital blood flow. Am J Vet Res 1994;55:375–378.

50. Ignarro LJ, Byrns RE, Buga GM, Wood KS. Endothelium-derived relaxing factor from pulmonary artery and vein possess pharmacologic and chemical properties identical to those of nitric oxide radical. Circ Res 1987;61:866–879.

51. Ingle-Fehr JE, Baxter GM. Evaluation of digital and laminar blood flow in horses given a low dose of endotoxin. Am J Vet Res 1996;59:192–196.

52. Ingle-Fehr JE, Baxter GM. The effect of oral isoxsuprine and pentoxifylline on digital and laminar blood flow in healthy horses. Vet Surg 1999;28:154–160.

53. Lindford RL, O'Brien TR, Trout DR. Qualitative and morphometric radiographic findings in the distal phalanx and digital soft tissues of sound Thoroughbred racehorses. Am J Vet Res 1993;54:38–51.

54. Longland A, Cairns A. Sugars in grass—an overview of sucrose and fructan accumulation in temperate grasses. Proceedings. Dodson and Horrell International Research Conference on Laminitis, Stoneleigh, Warwickshire, England, 1998, 1–3.

55. Luscher TF, Haefeli WE. L-Arginine in the clinical arena: Tool or remedy? Circulation 1993;87:1746–1748.

56. MacAllister CG, Morgan SJ, Boine AT, et al. Comparison of adverse effects of phenylbutazone, flunixin meglumine and ketoprofen in horses. J Am Vet Med Assoc 1993;202:71–76.

57. Merrit AM, Mackay RJ, Burrow JR, et al. Ant-endotoxin effect of ketoprofen in horses. Proceedings of the Fourth Colic Symposium, Athens, Georgia, 1991, 56.

57a. Messer NT. How to diagnose equine pituitary pars intermedia dysfunction. Proc Am Assoc of Equine Pract 1999;45:145–147.

58. Moore JN, Allen D. The pathophysiology of acute laminitis. Vet Med 1996;91:936–939.

59. Moore JN, Allen D, Clark ES. Pathophysiology of equine laminitis. Vet Clin North Am Equine Pract 1989;5:67–71.

60. Moore JN, Garner HE, Berg JN, Sprouse RF. Intracecal endotoxin and lactate during the onset of acute laminitis: A preliminary report. Am J Vet Res 1979;40:722.

61. Moore JN, Garner HE, Coffman JR. Haematological changes during development of acute laminitis hypertension. Equine Vet J 1981;13(4):240–242.

62. Nickels FA. Deep digital flexor tenotomy: A personal perspective. Proceedings of the Thirteenth Annual Bluegrass Laminitis Symposium, Louisville, KY, February 28–March 2, 1999, 67–70.

63. Obel N. Studies on the Histopathology of Acute Laminitis. Uppsala, Sweden: Almqvist and Wiksells Boktryckteri AK, 1948.

64. O'Grady S. A practical approach to treating laminitis. Vet Med 1993;88:867–875.

65. Ovnicek G. Life cycle of laminitis: Part I. Anvil, February 1999.

66. Ovnicek G. Life cycle of laminitis: Part II. Anvil, March 1999.

67. Ovnicek G. New Hope for Soundness: Seen Through the Window of Wild Horse Hoof Patterns. Columbia Falls, MT: Equine Digit Support System, Inc., 1997:32–40.

68. Owens JG, Kamerling JG, Stanton SR, Keowen ML. Effects of Ketofen and phenylbutazone on chronic hoof pain and lameness in horses. Equine Vet J 1995;27:296–300.

69. Peloso JG, Cohen ND, Walker MA, Watkins JP. Case-control study of risk factors for the development of laminitis in the contra-lateral limb in Equidae with unilateral lameness. J Am Vet Med Assoc 1996;209:1746–1748.

69a. Perkins G, Lamb S, Erb HN, et al. Plasma adrenocorticotropin (ACTH) concentrations and clinical response in horses treated for equine Cushing's disease with cyproheptadine or pergolide. Proceedings of the 19th Annual American College of Veterinary Internal Medicine Forum, Denver, CO, 2001, 851.

70. Pollitt CC. Basement membrane pathology: A feature of acute equine laminitis. Equine Vet J 1996;28:38–46.

71. Pollitt CC. Equine laminitis: A revised pathophysiology. Proc Am Assoc Equine Pract 1999;45:188–192.

72. Pollitt CC. Horse foot studies [video]. School of Veterinary Sciences, University of Queensland, Australia, 1992.

73. Pollitt CC, Davies CL. Equine laminitis: Its development post alimentary carbohydrate overload coincides with increased sublamellar blood flow. Equine Vet J Suppl 1998;27:125–132.

74. Pollitt CC, Molyneux GS. A scanning electron microscopic study of the dermal microcirculation of the equine foot. Equine Vet J 1990;22:79–87.

75. Pollitt CC, Pass MA, Pollitt S. Batimastat (BB-94) inhibits matrix metalloproteinases of equine laminitis. Equine Vet J Suppl 1998;27:119–124.

76. Prasse KW, Allen D, Moore JN, Duncan A. Evaluation of coagulation and fibrinolysis during the prodromal stages of carbohydrate-induced acute laminitis in horses. Am J Vet Res 1990;51:1950–1955.

77. Redden RF. 18° elevation of the heel as an aid to treating acute and chronic laminitis in the equine. Proc Am Assoc Equine Pract 1992;37:375–379.

78. Redden RF. Shoeing the laminitic horse. Proc Am Assoc Equine Pract 1997;43:356–359.

78a. Reed SM. Pituitary adrenomas: Equine Cushing's disease. In: Reed SM, Bayly WM, Eds. Equine Internal Medicine. Philadelphia: WB Saunders, 1998;912–915.

79. Ritmeester AM, Ferguson DW. Coronary grooving promotes dorsal hoof wall growth in horses with chronic laminitis. Proc Am Assoc Equine Pract 1996;42:212–213.

80. Roberts ED, Ochoa R, Haynes PF. Correlation of dermal-epidermal laminar lesions of the equine hoof with various disease conditions. Vet Pathol 1980;17:656.

81. Robinson NE. Digital blood flow, arteriovenous anastomosis and laminitis. Equine Vet J 1990;2:381–383.

82. Robinson NE, Scott JB, Dabney JM, Jones GA. Digital vascular responses and permeability in equine alimentary laminitis. Am J Vet Res 1976;37:1171–1176.

83. Rowe JB, Lees MJ, Pethick DW. Prevention of acidosis and laminitis with grain feeding in horses. J Nutr 1994;124:2742S–2744S.

84. Semrad SD, Hardee GE, Hardee MM, Moore JN. Low dose flunixin meglumine: Effects on eicosanoid production and clinical signs induced by experimental endotoxemia in horses. Equine Vet J 1987;19:201–206.

85. Sprouse RF, Garner HE, Green EM. Plasma endotoxin levels in horses subjected to carbohydrate induced laminitis. Equine Vet J 1987;19(1):25–28.

86. Stick JS, Jann HW, Scott EA, et al. Pedal bone rotation as a prognostic sign in laminitis in horses. J Am Vet Med Assoc 1982;180:251–253.

87. Swanson TD. Lameness of the equine foot. Proceedings of the Ninety-Second Annual Conference of the Colorado Veterinary Medicine Association, Snowmass, CO, 1998, 29–35.

88. Tanner FC, Noli G, Boulanger CM, et al. Oxidized low-density lipoproteins inhibit relaxation of porcine coronary arteries: Role of scavenger receptor and endothelium-derived nitric oxide. Circulation 1991;83:2012–2020.

89. Trout OR, Hornoff WJ, Linford RL, et al. Scintigraphic evaluation of the digital circulation during the development and acute phases of equine laminitis. Equine Vet J 1990;22:416–421.

90. Turner AS, Tucker CM. The evaluation of isoxsuprine hydrochloride for the treatment of navicular disease: A double blind study. Equine Vet J 1989;21:338–341.

91. Turner TA. Use of deep digital flexor tenotomy in the management of laminitis. Proc Am Assoc Equine Pract 1992;38:11–12.

92. Walker M, Geiser D. Effects of acetylpromazine in the hemodynamics of the equine metatarsal artery as determined by two-dimensional real-time and pulsed Doppler ultrasonography. Am J Vet Res 1986;47:1075–1078.

93. Walker M, Taylor T, Slater M, Hood D, et al. Radiographic appearance of the feet of Mammoth donkeys and the findings of subclinical laminitis. Vet Radiol Ultrasound 1995;36:32–37.
94. Wattle O, Ekfalck A, Funkquist B, Obel N. Behavioral studies in healthy ponies subjected to short-term forced recumbency aiming at an adjunctive treatment in an acute attack of laminitis. Zentralbl Veterinarmed A 1995;42:62–68.
95. Weiss DJ, Geor RJ, Johnston G, Trent AM. Microvascular thrombosis associated with onset of acute laminitis in ponies. Am J Vet Res 1994;55(5):606–612.
96. White NA, Baggett N. A method of corrective shoeing for laminitis in horses. Vet Med Small Anim Clin 1983;5:775–778.
97. White NA, Tuler DE, Blackwell RB. Hemorrhagic fibrinonecrotic duodenitis proximal jejunitis in horses: 20 cases. J Am Vet Med Assoc 1987;190:311–318.
98. Yelle M. Clinicians guide to equine laminitis. Equine Vet J 1986; 8:156–158.

NAVICULAR SYNDROME (NAVICULAR DISEASE OR NAVICULAR REGION PAIN)

Navicular syndrome remains one of the most controversial and common causes of intermittent forelimb lameness in horses between 4 and 15 years of age.[1,29,49,57] It is estimated that the syndrome is responsible for one-third of all chronic forelimb lameness in horses.[8] In North America, male Quarter Horses and Thoroughbreds, particularly geldings, seem at greatest risk, whereas the syndrome is rarely diagnosed in ponies or Arabian horses.[29] Although the hindlimbs can be affected, it is predominantly considered a problem of the forelimbs.

The syndrome has been shown to have a hereditary predisposition, which is perhaps related to conformation.[32] Factors such as faulty conformation, hoof imbalance, improper or irregular shoeing, and exercise on hard surfaces are believed to predispose and to aggravate the condition.[39,49,57] The exact cause remains unclear, although two schools of thought prevail: One is that it is a vascular problem, and the other is that it is of a biomechanical origin.[28]

Although not all would agree, the term "navicular syndrome" should be used to describe the complex etiologies and pathogenic mechanisms involved in the production of clinical signs associated with the navicular region, in that the term "disease" implies a known cause and a specific treatment.[39] Note that not all lameness associated with the palmar aspect of the hoof should be labeled the navicular syndrome and that this term should be reserved for chronic bilateral forelimb lameness that fit a specific set of diagnostic criteria.[49] In my opinion, pain elicited with hoof tester pressure over the central and, occasionally, the cranial one-third of the frog remains an important diagnostic criteria.

Etiology

Interruption of the blood flow to and from the navicular region has been proposed as a contributing factor in the development of navicular syndrome.[8,9,28] Thrombosis of the navicular arteries within the navicular bone, partial or complete occlusion of the digital arteries at the level of the pastern and fetlock, and a reduction in the distal arterial blood supply as a result of atherosclerosis of these vessels, resulting in ischemia, were thought to be the cause of navicular syndrome.[16,30] These opinions, however, lack support. Attempts to induce the navicular

syndrome by ligation of the medial palmar digital arteries,[48] by bilateral ligation of the palmar digital arteries,[30,42] by bilateral neurectomy and ligation of the digital arteries,[44] and by occlusion of the ramus navicularis arteries and branches[41] failed to produce lasting clinical radiographic or pathologic changes of navicular syndrome.

Further refuting the interruption of blood flow hypothesis are other studies in which the following are used: fluorescent bone-labeling techniques and microradiography in navicular syndrome cases, which have shown an increased rate of bone remodeling and increased vascularization.[30,33] The increased vascularization was a combination of active arterial hyperemia and passive venous congestion. The increased vascularity is seen primarily under the palmar flexor cortex, and the central and peripheral blood vessels are more dilated. Obstruction of the venous outflow results in congestion, increased bone marrow pressure, and pain.[39,51] Proponents of biomechanics as a cause of navicular syndrome believe that the degenerative changes observed within the navicular bone result from nonphysiologic forces exerted on the navicular bone and its supporting ligaments.[4,28,33,39,53] Tension acting through the deep digital flexor tendon (DDFT) is believed important because it compresses the navicular bone dorsally against the distal and the middle phalanges. While the horse walks, the peak forces on the navicular bone approximate $0.67 \times$ body weight and occur during 70 to 75% of the stance duration. When the horse moves at a slow trot, the peak compressive forces of the DDFT on the navicular bone are approximately $0.77 \times$ body weight and occur at approximately 65 to 70% of the stance phase duration.[39] In an in vitro study, done in normal horses, pressure-sensitive film was used to document contact load between the articulations of the navicular bone and the distal and the middle phalanges when the horse's limbs were placed in dorsiflexion (extension). In this study, researchers found that the contact load increased significantly on the articulations between these bones when the phalanges were extended as occurs during the stance phase of the stride.[4] Additionally, the navicular ligaments are tensed in the normal horse as the hoof breaks over at the end of the stance phase. These ligaments are under excessive tension and possibly compression when the hoof-pastern axis is broken backward as with a long toe and an underrun heel conformation.[4,28] Also, the forces applied to the navicular region are influenced by body weight, conformation, and use. Factors such as excessive body weight, small feet, upright pastern angles, hoof imbalances, and work on hard surfaces are likely to increase the forces per unit area of the hoof and bone.

In a proposed unifying theory of the pathogenesis of navicular syndrome, faulty conformation and hoof imbalance resulting in abnormal biomechanical forces are considered the main etiologic factors in this biomechanical disorder.[39] In a majority of horses, these forces fall within normal range. With minor conformational abnormalities and hoof imbalances, these forces remain in physiologic ranges, which serve to stimulate remodeling of the navicular bone and probably the supporting ligaments and DDFT. When the conformational abnormalities are severe, nonphysiologic forces exerted primarily on the distal third of the flexor cortex of the navicular bone begin the pathologic process that affects fibrocartilage and underlying bone and marrow cavities. The resultant pathologic changes in the navicular bone are essentially the same changes as those seen grossly and microscopically with bone spavin and high ringbone. The microscopic changes include focal degeneration, cartilage erosion, subchondral bone sclerosis, focal areas of lysis, fibrous ankylosis of the opposing surfaces at the site of subchondral bone destruction, edema, congestion, and fibrosis in the marrow spaces.[37,39] Biomechanical factors in high-load and low-motion joints (small tarsal and pastern joints) are also similar. In the case of the navicular bone, the high load is believed to be generated by a taut DDFT against the distal border of the navicular bone. Excessive body weight and conformational abnormalities, including hoof imbalances, exacerbate these forces. Scanning electron microscopy studies of the distal sesamoid bone and DDFT in navicular disease horses identified fraying of collagen fibers in the DDFT and fissuring of the fibrocartilage on the flexor surface of the navicular bone. Both these changes seem consistent with repeated microtrauma.[14,67]

Histologic studies of the distal interphalangeal (DIP) joint and navicular region in normal horses, of varying ages and breeds, revealed areas of high stress in the articular cartilage of the distal phalanx and navicular bone and in the distal sesamoidean impar ligament (DSIL) and the DDFT.[4] Evidence of high-stress areas in the DSIL and the DDFT was indicated by an increase of safranin O binding of secreted proteoglycans in aged horses compared with younger horses. In another study, these stress indicators were more obvious in horses exhibiting signs consistent with navicular syndrome than was seen in normal horses.[5]

Pain presumably comes from within the bone and from sprain and strain of the surrounding supporting soft tissue structures. Using intraosseous venography in human patients, researchers demonstrated that venous drainage of marrow spaces below lesions of degenerative joint disease is sluggish and that pain is associated with dilated vessels in the subchondral spongiosa.[39] When bone marrow pressure exceeds 40 mm Hg in human patients, they experience pain even in resting positions. Horses with navicular syndrome also have impaired venous drainage[39,51] and have bone marrow pressures exceeding 50 mm Hg, which is higher than is seen in normal control subject horses.[37,51] Therefore, it is logical to envision that venous distension from venous hypertension seen in navicular syndrome is the cause of bone pain. The cause of venous hypertension appears to be from fibrosis in the marrow cavity, which retards venous drainage. Edema is seen histologically and is probably a consequence of active hyperemia and of subsequent leakage from capillaries associated with active bone remodeling.[39]

Pain from sprain and strain of supporting ligaments and the DDFT is also logical. Evidence of enthesiophyte formation on the proximal extremities and on the distal border of the navicular bone has been documented.[28,49] Radiographic evidence of avulsion fracture at the distal border of the navicular bone where the impar ligament attaches may represent a true fracture or the development of an enthesiophyte.[62] Enthesiophytes develop in torn soft tissue attachments to bone. It is generally be-

lieved that these sites, while actively healing, are a source of pain and, once healed, are no longer painful. Tendinitis of the DDFT as it courses over the navicular bone has also been documented radiographically as well as with ultrasound. This also could be the source of pain in some cases. In a histologic study done in normal horses and horses diagnosed with navicular syndrome, they found that the DSIL and the DDFT normally do not stain with safranin O as the fibroblasts do not secrete proteoglycans unless the cells are stressed.[4] Although they found increased staining with safranin O as horses aged, the increase in staining was far greater in horses exhibiting signs of navicular syndrome.

The proposed unifying concept[39] still has some appeal from a clinical standpoint because it explains why there may be similar radiographic and gross pathologic findings in asymptomatic horses and horses with early signs of the navicular syndrome.[39] It is highly likely that the early changes of the navicular bone of asymptomatic horses represents successful remodeling in face of compressive forces, although pain may have been present during part of this remodeling process. On the other hand, nonphysiologic sustained forces that trigger the sequence of events, which result in navicular bone pain, really represent the onset of the clinical disease.

History and Clinical Signs

Horses with navicular syndrome usually have a history of progressive, chronic, unilateral, or bilateral forelimb lameness, which may have a subtle (most common) or an acute onset. The syndrome is usually bilateral, but the lameness may appear unilateral.[49] An incidence of asymmetric lameness of greater than 95.5% has been reported.[68] The horse may tend to point one forelimb or to alternate pointing each forelimb. In one study, approximately 60% of the horses with navicular syndrome presented with this finding.[68] Asymmetry in the extensor muscles with atrophy of the muscles associated with a lame limb is commonly observed in horses with chronic histories of lameness (Fig. 8.30).[49] This was observed in approximately 75% of the cases in one study dealing with navicular syndrome.[68]

Various abnormalities of the hoof can be associated with navicular syndrome. For example, heels may be low, underrun, or collapsed with a broken back hoof-pastern axis (Figs. 8.31 and 8.32). Medial to lateral hoof imbalance may also be an initiator of the navicular syndrome, and a range of incidence between 33 and 45% has been reported (Fig. 8.33 and see Fig. 3.12).[57,68] One forefoot may also be smaller and more upright than the other, and the heels in one or both forefeet may be contracted. Hoof atrophy is a result of disuse, and it is usually seen in the hoof of the limb with the greatest lameness.[49,68] Of the navicular syndrome cases, 80 to 90% have one hoof narrower than the counterpart.[30,68] In a study evaluating the clinical features of 118 horses with navicular syndrome, broken back hoof-pastern axis had an incidence of 71.2%.[68] This conformation tends to exaggerate the tension on the DDFT, which causes increased pressure on the navicular bone, and probably places the perinavicular ligaments under tension also. Angular limb deformities, either valgus or varus, associ-

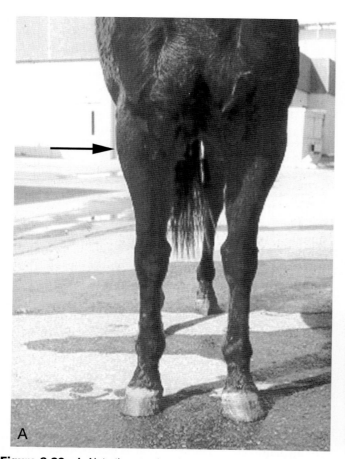

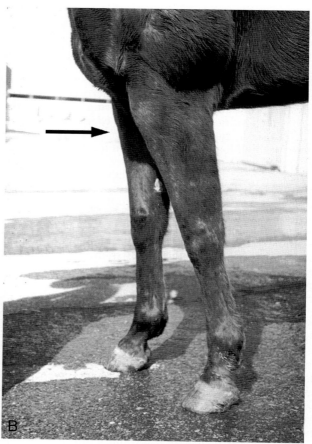

Figure 8.30 A. Note the atrophy of the extensor carpi radialis muscle (arrow) of the right forelimb. B. Lateral view of the same horse as in A. Note flattening (atrophy) of the extensor carpi radialis muscle (arrow).

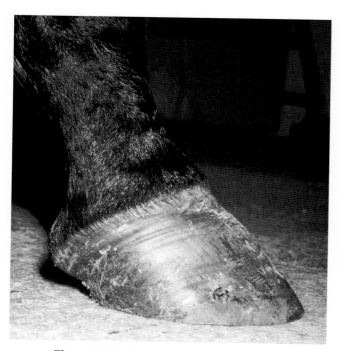

Figure 8.31 Long toe and low underrun heel.

ated with the carpus and fetlock region have been observed in a small percentage of cases. The significance of this finding in navicular syndrome cases is unclear. Possibly, the shift in axial compressive forces, either lateral or medial, can influence hoof wall development, resulting in mediolateral hoof imbalance, which places abnormal stresses on the navicular region.

At exercise, most horses with navicular syndrome exhibit mild to moderate lameness, and only occasionally is severe lameness encountered. Generally, the longer the duration, the more severe the lameness. While walking or trotting, horses with navicular syndrome tend to land toe first and may occasionally stumble. In one study, the toe-first ground contact was seen with a frequency of 96.7%.[30] At a trot, horses with bilateral navicular syndrome tend to have a stiff shuffling gait and to carry their head and neck rigidly. Owners often misinterpret these signs as being indicative of shoulder pain. When the horse is circled in either direction, the lameness is usually exaggerated in the limb that is on the inside of the circle. The horse may hold its head and neck to the outside of the circle in an effort to reduce the amount of weight carried on the inside limb. A sharp turn may cause a sudden exaggeration in lameness on the inside limb, and this exaggerated lameness might be misinterpreted as shoulder pain.[49]

Occasionally, a horse with severe navicular bone pathology coupled with DDFT damage lands on its heels first, tipping its toe up off the ground as weight is applied to the limb. This action is seen only rarely in horses with navicular syndrome, but when it does occur, because of navicular syndrome, one can assume that the horse's DDFT is severely damaged. Confirmation of severe damage to the DDFT is reason for euthanasia.[49]

A thorough systematic examination of the hoof with hoof testers is essential for the clinical diagnosis of navicular syndrome. First, the sole is examined. Because the horse with heel pain tends to land on the toe first, it can bruise the sole at the toe, resulting in painful withdrawal when hoof testers are applied in the toe region. Painful withdrawal to intermittent hoof tester pressure over the central and, occasionally, the cranial third of the frog is still, in my opinion, important for the clinical diagnosis of navicular syndrome (Fig. 8.34). When hoof testers are applied, rather than simply applying lateral (shearing pressure) across the frog, it is important that the navicular region itself be compressed.[49] Occasionally, horses with thick soles and hard frogs do not respond to hoof tester pressure (see Fig. 3.3). In these horses, one must rely on other clinical findings. Contrary to my opinion regarding the value of hoof testers being important in the diagnosis of navicular syndrome is the findings in one study done to evaluate the predictive value of diagnostic tests for navicular pain.[59] In that study, 19 of 42 (45%) horses with navicular region pain and 19 of 38 (50%) horses with palmar heel pain, identified by the criteria used, responded positively to hoof tester pressure over the central third of the frog. Pain elicited with hoof tester pressure over the cranial third of the frog may indicate pain from the subchondral bone or pain associated with the attachment of the DDFT to the distal phalanx.[52]

Many horses with navicular syndrome react positively to a phalangeal flexion test because the test exacerbates the lameness.[68] Although it has not been established why this occurs, it may be that the navicular bone becomes compressed between the middle and the distal phalanges and that tensional stresses increase in the soft tissues supporting the navicular bone. One study found that distal limb flexion was sensitive (88%) for navicular region pain (NRP) but that the specificity for detecting only NRP was low (13%).

Two types of wedge tests have been recommended to aid in the diagnosis of navicular syndrome.[57] To perform the frog wedge test, one places a wedge of wood under the palmar two-thirds of the frog and forces the horse to stand on that foot for 60 seconds (see Fig. 3.20). If this exacerbates the lameness, navicular bursitis could possibly be the problem. One performs the toe extension test by elevating the toe of the hoof with the wedge of wood and forcing the horse to stand on the limb for 60 seconds (see Fig. 3.21). Exacerbation of the lameness may indicate tendinitis of the DDFT or desmitis of the support ligaments. If one looks at the biomechanical effect of the wedge tests, however, both tests probably apply compressional forces to the navicular bone region also. One study found that the frog wedge and toe wedge tests had a sensitivity of 76 and 55%, respectively. The specificity for identifying NRP only, however, was low (26 and 42% for the frog wedge and toe wedge tests, respectively).[59]

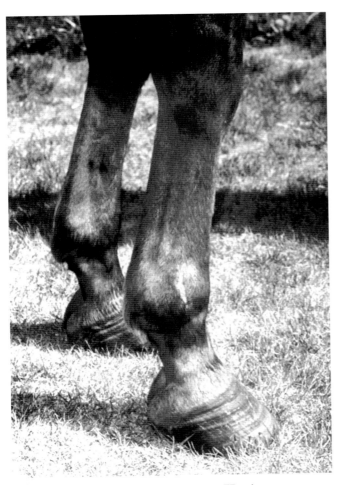

Figure 8.32   Broken back FP axis.

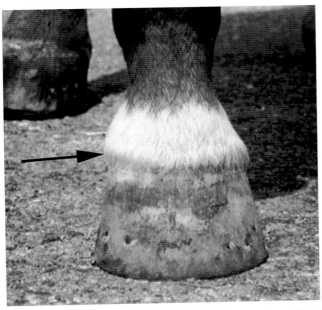

Figure 8.33   Medial lateral imbalance. Note that the lateral hoof wall (arrow) is taller than the medial hoof wall.

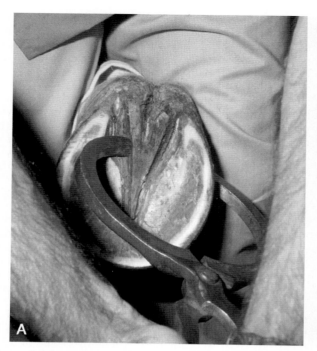 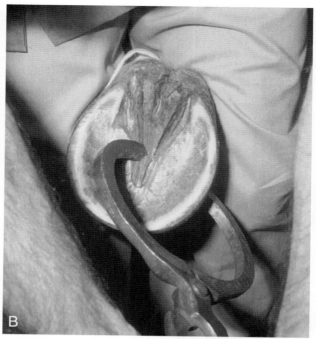

Figure 8.34 A. Application of the hoof testers to apply pressure over the central one-third of the frog. Note the testers are placed at a slight oblique angle. This placement is important, particularly for low-heeled horses, for it allows the examiner to apply pressure to the navicular region. If the tester is applied perpendicular to the long axis of the hoof, the frog will be sheared rather than compressed. B. Application of the hoof tester over the cranial one-third of the frog. Pain elicited from this site may be from the attachment of the DDFT to the distal phalanx or from subchondral bone pain from the distal phalanx.[52]

Diagnostic Procedures

Perineural anesthesia of the palmar digital nerve (i.e., palmar digital nerve blocks [PDNBs]) axial and distal to the proximal limits of the collateral cartilages is believed to be important in localizing the site of pain to the palmar aspect and the bottom of the foot region (see Fig. 3.91). Blocking the nerves distal to the proximal limits of the collateral cartilage is done to avoid desensitizing dorsal nerve branches that may be present close to the proximal limits of the collateral cartilages. Horses affected with navicular syndrome should show a significant improvement (80 to 90%) in their lameness.[49] This block is not specific for navicular region pain, however. In a study done to clarify the predictive value of various tests for navicular region pain, the PDNB had high predicative value, but its ability to detect only the disease in question (specificity) was 0%.[59] Further demonstrating the lack of specificity of the PDNB was a study done with scintigraphy to investigate the site of lameness in 164 horses that blocked out with a PDNB, but that had negative or equivocal radiographic changes.[43] In that study, causes of lameness included

1. Stress reaction or stress fracture of the distal phalanx (41 cases, primarily racehorses)
2. Subchondral trauma or remodeling of the DIP joint (20 cases, primarily in nonracehorses)
3. Navicular syndrome (39 cases) and a combination of navicular syndrome and subchondral trauma of the DIP joint (19 cases) (for a total 58 cases)
4. Osteoarthritis of the phalangeal joints (13 cases)

5. Soft tissue inflammation (6 cases)
6. Laminitis (4 cases)
7. Distal phalanx wing fractures (4 cases)
8. Dorsal distal phalanx (P-3) trauma (3 cases)
9. Midsagittal proximal phalanx fractures and collateral cartilage injury (2 cases each)
10. Proximal middle phalanx trauma, navicular bone fracture, distal phalanx solar margin fracture, and an extensor process fracture (1 case each)

In a study done to evaluate the effects of PDNBs on kinematic gait analysis in horses with (7 horses) and without (5 horses) navicular disease, investigators found that in normal horses the only significant change was an increase in the maximum extension of the fetlock joint at the midstance phase of the stride. In horses with navicular disease the mean maximal extension of the fetlock during the stance phase of the stride and the maximum flexion of the carpal joint during the swing phase of the stride were significantly increased after PDNB. Interestingly, the total stance phase, cranial stance phase, and breakover duration were significantly shorter.[23] In another study evaluating the affect of PDNBs on experimentally induced coffin joint synovitis, investigators found a significant reduction in lameness 15 minutes after the administration of 3 mL of local anesthetic placed subcutaneously over the lateral and medial palmar digital nerves just proximal to the heel bulbs.[27a] Their conclusion was that PDNBs done as described in this report could not differentiate coffin joint pain from navicular pain or sole pain or other causes of palmar heel pain. It is for this reason that we recommend the

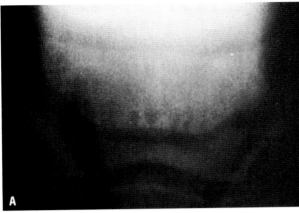
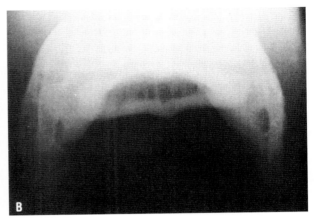

Figure 8.35   A. DP view of the elongated foramina. B. Skyline (pedal upright) view of enlarged foramina, osteosclerosis of the marrow cavity, and a thick flexor cortex (same horse as in A).

administration of no more than 1 to 1.25 mL of local anesthetic and that the block be performed distal and axial to the proximal limits of the collateral cartilages (see Fig. 3.91).

It has been suggested that intrasynovial anesthesia of the DIP joint may be helpful in distinguishing between problems associated with the DIP joint and those involving the navicular region (see Fig. 3.98). Investigators, however, have demonstrated a lack of specificity of intrasynovial anesthesia of the DIP joint and found that it can eliminate lameness associated with pain in the navicular region (navicular bone, navicular ligaments, and navicular bursa).[6,7,15,38] The probable reason for this lack of specificity is that sensory nerves supplying this region are located subsynovially in the DIP joint and that local anesthetics are passively diffused into the navicular bursa. In one study, DIP joint anesthesia improved lameness in 92% of the horses diagnosed with navicular syndrome.[68] Researchers in another study evaluated the effect of intraarticular anesthesia in the DIP joint on lameness associated with amphotericin-induced navicular bursitis and found a significant reduction in lameness 5 to 30 minutes after the anesthetic was injected.[38] In a different clinical study, an attempt was made to differentiate navicular region pain from other forms of palmar heel pain.[58] In this study, 80 horses with palmar heel pain who received a PDNB were placed into two groups on the basis of their response to both DIP joint and navicular bursa anesthesia. Horses that were significantly improved by both blocks were considered to have navicular region pain, and all others were considered to have other causes of palmar heel pain. Of the 80 horses, 40 had navicular region pain. When various diagnostic tests (e.g., hoof tester, distal-limb flexion, and frog and toe wedge tests) were compared between the groups, a difference was found. It was thought that the DIP joint block was the single best diagnostic test.[58] A more recent experimental study evaluating the affect of intrasynovial anesthesia of the DIP joint on set screw–induced solar pain found that analgesia of the joint resolved the lameness.[47] On the basis of the results of the investigation, the authors questioned the value of anesthesia of the DIP joint to localize pain to this joint or to the navicular region. They also concluded that sole pain should be considered a cause of lameness when the lameness is abolished by diagnostic analgesia of the DIP joint. In another study,[47a] investigators found that lameness created by the set screw pressure in the heel region was less likely to be attenuated by the injection of the local anesthetic in the DIP joint than was lameness created by a set screw placed in the toe region. Attenuation of lameness was more effective with 10 mL than with 6 mL of local anesthetic solution. The attenuation of lameness was increased over time. They suggested that the use of 6 mL or less of local anesthetic in the DIP joint may help to distinguish between pain arising from the DIP joint or the navicular region and pain arising from the heel of the foot.

Radiographic Examination

Important in the diagnosis of navicular syndrome is radiographic examination of the navicular bone. A minimum of three radiographic views (dorsopalmar [DP] 60°, lateromedial [LM], palmaroproximal-palmarodistal oblique) should be done, and high-quality images are required. Radiographic findings compatible with the diagnosis of navicular syndrome include 1) alterations in the distal foramina, 2) cystic changes, 3) elongation and enthesiophyte formation at the proximal and distal borders of the navicular bone, 4) flexor cortex defects, i.e., loss of corticomedullary distinction, and 5) small calcification of the flexor surface of the navicular bone.[22] Chip fractures and osseous bodies in the impar ligament have also been described.[40,62]

Abnormal foramina, which are best evaluated on the DP view, were seen in only 40% of horses with navicular syndrome and in 11% of normal horses[22] (Fig. 8.35). Thus, it is generally accepted that enlarged foramina by themselves are not a conclusive radiographic indication of navicular syndrome. On the other hand, cystic changes in the navicular bone have been associated histologically with changes in blood supply and probably should be considered a significant radiographic change (Fig. 8.36).

Elongation of the navicular bone's flexor cortex is a common finding. In normal horses, 55% had elongation distally and 30% had elongation proximally.[22] Enthesio-

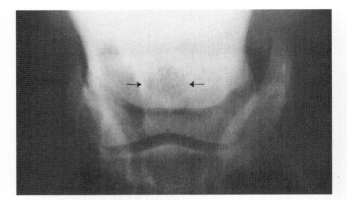

Figure 8.36 Large cyst in the navicular bone.

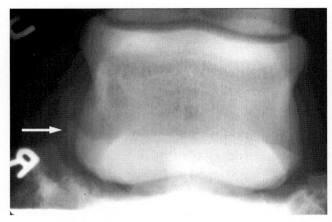

Figure 8.37 Enthesiophyte (arrow) on the proximal lateral border of the navicular bone.

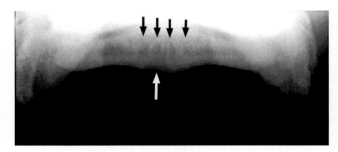

Figure 8.38 Sclerosis in the medullary cavity, enlarged foramina (black arrows), and a defect in the flexor cortex (white arrow).

phytes of the proximal bone border and calcification of the impar ligament represent injuries to the attachments of the navicular bone ligaments (Fig. 8.37). It is likely that there is pain while enthesiophytes are forming, and it is believed that the pain subsides when healing is complete.

Defects in the navicular bone flexor cortex are often associated with other navicular bone changes, such as sclerosis of the medullary cavity, thickening of the flexor cortex, and loss of corticomedullary distinction (Fig. 8.38). Flexor cortex defects were seen in less than 1%

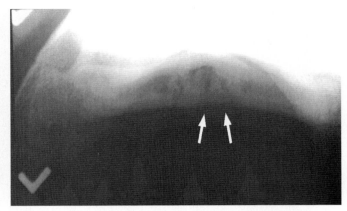

Figure 8.39 Loss of corticomedullary distinction, extensive sclerosis of the marrow cavity, and a defect in the flexor cortex (arrows).

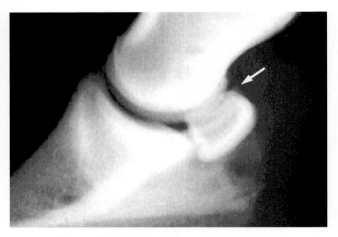

Figure 8.40 Periarticular osteophyte (arrow).

of horses and, therefore, if present, should be considered important indicators of navicular syndrome. Loss of corticomedullary distinction with sclerosis of the spongiosa is an important radiographic finding (Fig. 8.39). These changes are seen in up to 80% of horses with navicular syndrome but in less than 16% of normal horses.[22]

Small calcifications of the flexor cortex of the navicular bone are an indication of degeneration, fibrillation, and possibly adhesions of the flexor cortex to the DDFT. Less than 2% of normal horses had such calcifications, which is in contrast to 32% of horses with navicular disease.[22] Periarticular osteophytes at the articular border adjacent to the middle phalanx is probably a sign of arthrosis of the DIP joint and should not be considered a primary radiographic sign of navicular syndrome (Fig. 8.40).

Chip fractures of the distal border of the navicular bone and osseous bodies associated with the impar ligament have been reported as radiographic findings associated with navicular disease[40,62] (Fig. 8.41). The processes by which bone tissue may develop in the impar ligament include ossification secondary to ligamentous damage, separate centers of ossification, and ossification of cartilage particles in adjacent synovial tissue.[40] Chip

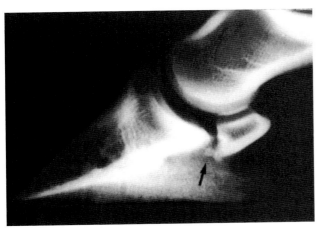

Figure 8.41 Osseous fragment in the impar ligament (arrow). (Courtesy of Dr. Barbara Kaser-Hotz.)

fractures and osseous bodies are often associated with other radiographic findings of navicular disease.[62]

Researchers evaluating the frequency of radiographic monitoring of navicular disease in 205 horses found that the optimum interval for reexamination was at least 1 year.[25] In another study in which radiographic measurements from the LM projection of the foot in horses with navicular disease were evaluated, researchers compared three groups: Group 1 consisted of 143 normal horses (control); group 2 consisted 60 horses with clinical signs of navicular disease only; and group 3 consisted of 161 horses with clinical signs and radiographic changes consistent with a diagnosis of navicular disease.[65] In this study they found an enlargement of the navicular bone in a proximodistal and DP direction in group 3 horses compared with control subjects. Additionally, a slight enlargement of the distal phalanx was seen in group 2 and 3 horses compared with control subjects. All horses 4 years and older had an increased length of the hoof in the DP direction and a decrease of the cranial angle of the hoof.

Although radiography is considered an important diagnostic tool, it is not particularly effective or sensitive in defining the pathologic changes, unless they are advanced, of the distal sesamoid bone of horses with navicular syndrome. Scanning electron microscopy of the distal sesamoid bones in 49 cases of navicular disease revealed severe pathologic changes in horses that had only slight radiographic changes.[14]

Navicular Bursography

Important information regarding pathologic changes associated with the fibrocartilage on the flexor surface of the navicular bone and the DDFT can be obtained with navicular bursography.[60] Ninety-seven horses presenting with palmar heel pain were evaluated by navicular bursography. A dosage of 3 mL of a 1:1 mixture of a contrast material and a local anesthetic was injected in the navicular bursa by use of radiographic documentation. Findings included 1) normal flexor fibrocartilage in 13% of cases, 2) thinning or erosions of the flexor fibrocartilage in 69% of cases, 3) complete focal loss of

the dye column representing adhesion of flexor to the bone in 8% of cases, 4) focal filling of the flexor cortex with contrast in 2% of cases, and 5) fibrillation of the flexor tendon in 21% of cases. When horses were separated into clinical groups, NRP or palmar foot pain (PFP), according to the criteria described,[59] the following comparisons were made.[59] Horses with normal flexor fibrocartilage were more likely to have NRP (8 of 97) than PFP (5 of 97). Horses with flexor cartilage thinning or erosions were more likely to have PFP (38 of 97) than NRP (29 of 97). All horses with flexor surface adhesions had NRP. Horses with tendon fibrillation were also more likely to show PFP (14 of 97) than NRP (6 of 97). Navicular bursography identified pathology in the flexor cortex of the navicular bone 60% more often than did plain radiography.

Scintigraphy

Because it identifies early alterations in bone metabolism, scintigraphy (nuclear imaging) can be used to detect early pathologic changes in the navicular bone (Fig. 8.42), making it unnecessary for clinicians to rely on radiographic changes. Scintigraphy is probably most useful for cases in which radiographic changes have not developed or are equivocal.[43,55] In one scintigraphic study, researchers evaluating the uptake in the navicular area of horses with lameness isolated to the foot by perineural anesthesia of the palmar digital nerves found a significantly greater uptake in the navicular bone of seven affected horses compared with seven control horses.[24] Also, images taken after 1 hour were as good

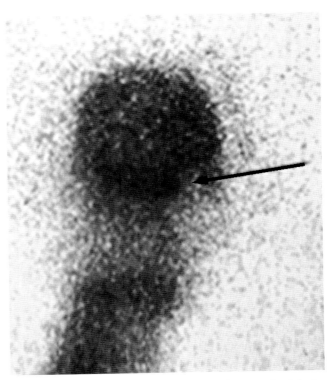

Figure 8.42 Nuclear scintigraphy showing increased uptake in the navicular bones (arrow).

at differentiating affected horses from control horses as images obtained between 2 and 4 hours after injection. It was concluded that a substantial number of horses with clinical signs of PFP had increased scintigraphic uptake within the navicular bone 1 to 4 hours after injection of ^{99m}Tc-methylene diphosphonate and that the palmar view bone phase images were more sensitive than the lateral views.

Computed Tomography

Computed tomography may have some promise in the future. In one study of the navicular bone in 67 forelimbs of horses, computed tomography exhibited an improved ability to evaluate the wings, articulation and flexor surfaces, and associated ligaments of the navicular bone, compared with plain radiography.[54]

Magnetic Resonance Imaging

Magnetic resonance imaging has been used to image the forefeet of a limited number of horses. Reportedly, the images accurately depicted normal and pathologic structures in the foot and were precise for detecting degenerative changes in the navicular bone and other structures of the foot.[13]

Treatment

Because many horses with navicular syndrome are managed with various treatment options, definitive assessment of the efficacy of a specific treatment on outcome is difficult. Additionally, the success of a treatment probably depends on several factors, including when treatment was initiated and the use of the horse and its conformation. Treatment of early cases of navicular syndrome with minimal radiographic changes can be rewarding. With chronic cases that have radiographic changes, at best we can hope to prevent the progression of the syndrome and manage the horse so it can continue to perform. Treatment usually involves variable periods of rest, corrective trimming and shoeing, drugs to improve blood flow, anti-inflammatory agents, and recently, drugs specific for the treatment of arthritis.[49,56,57]

Rest and Controlled Exercise

Rest is important to allow time for soft tissue inflammation to subside, to allow the horse to acclimate to corrective trimming and shoeing, and to allow the navicular bone to begin the remodeling process. Although the rest period varies for individual cases, generally a period of complete rest for 3 weeks followed by controlled exercise is recommended. During the rest period, the horse is confined to a box stall with access to only a small run. Medical treatments as well as corrective trimming and shoeing are begun at this time. In week 4, controlled exercise in which the horse is walked 10 minutes two times a day, 4 to 5 days a week, with a rider on its back can be initiated. In week 5, the horse is exercised at a walk for 5 minutes (warm up), at a trot for 5 minutes, and at a walk for 5 minutes (cool down) twice daily. At week 6, the warm up and cool down remains the same, but the trotting exercise can be increased to 10 minutes if the horse is not lame. This exercise regimen is done

until recheck examination at the end of the 6 weeks. At 6 weeks, a decision is made regarding further exercise and continued treatment. It has been shown that 15 minutes of exercise at a trot increases the blood flow to the foot by 15%.[26]

Corrective Trimming and Shoeing

Most would agree that corrective trimming and shoeing is the basis for treatment for navicular syndrome; many horses respond favorably to this without need for further medical or surgical therapy. In one study, improvement in clinical signs within 3 months of initiation of treatment was seen, and 86% of the horses remained free of lameness for 1 year.[57] In another study, 73% (22 of 30) of the horses exhibiting signs of navicular syndrome improved one grade in lameness 6 weeks after corrective trimming and shoeing; no long-term follow-up was available.[36] The aims of trimming and shoeing are to 1) restore normal foot balance, 2) correct foot problems such as shearing of the quarters and heels, underrun heels, and heel bulb contraction, 3) reduce biomechanical forces on the navicular region, and 4) protect the injured region.

For these four aims to be accomplished, the trimming and shoeing principles to achieve natural balance, outlined by Ovnicek[34] 1997, are recommended. First, only the loose flaky sole (exfoliating epidermis) is removed down to the deeper nonexfoliating epidermis referred to as the sole plane (where the sole becomes like wax). Second, the frog is trimmed of loose undermined epidermis, thus exposing the true apex of the attached frog and the firm sole. The transition zone between the attached frog and sole is identified by a color difference; the frog is darker and the sole is lighter in color.[36] Third, a trans-

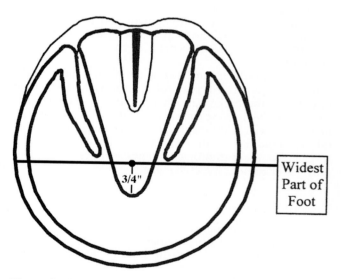

Figure 8.43 Natural balance trimming technique. A TL is drawn at the widest part of the foot. The TL is usually ¾ inch palmar to the trimmed apex of the frog; the bars often end here. Note that the heels terminate close to the widest part of the frog. (Reprinted with permission from Ovnicek G. New Hope for Soundness: Seen Through the Window of Wild Horse Hoof Patterns. Columbia Falls, MT: Equine Digit Support System, Inc., 1997.)

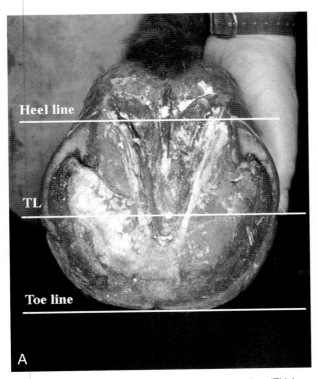
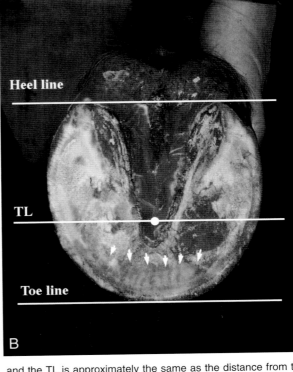

Figure 8.44 A. Foot prior to trimming. A transverse line (TL) is drawn at the widest part of the foot for reference. Note how far forward the heels are. The distance between the heels (heel line) and the TL is approximately the same as the distance from the toe (toe line) to the TL. B. The same hoof as in A after trimming. Note the toe callus (arrows).

verse line (TL) is drawn at the widest part of the foot (Fig. 8.43). This TL is usually close to a reference point ¾ of an inch palmar to the apex of the trimmed frog. This point on the frog is often where the bars end (Fig. 8.43). Fourth, beginning at the TL, one should trim the wall flat toward the heels, so the heels terminate at the widest part of the frog (Figs. 8.43 and 8.44). This generally requires removing the heel so that the hoof wall is approximately ⅟₁₆ to ⅛ inch from the sole plane at the deepest part at the quarters. Each side of the hoof wall is prepared so that the sole plane depth to the ground surface is equal. The sensitive sole at the heels should not contact the ground. Fifth, the foot is trimmed forward from the TL to the toe, so that there is approximately 1/16 inch of sole clearance. The sole callus inside the white line is left intact. This modified sole is believed important for the support of the distal phalanx (Ovnicek G, personal communication, 1998) (Fig. 8.44). The horse should then be walked on a hard flat surface to assess DP and LM dynamic balance. If necessary, further trimming to correct the imbalance is done. In cases in which the horse still has a broken backward foot pastern (FP) axis or has a tendency to land toe first, the heel may have to be elevated when a shoe is applied. Elevating the heel can establish a normal FP axis and a heel-first contact at a walk. Heel elevation can be accomplished with wedge shoes, wedge pads, or wedge rails added to the Equine Digital Support System (EDSS) shoe. The advantage of the EDSS is that there are three heights of wedge rails to select from, and they are easy to apply and remove from the shoe.

The shoe should be applied to enhance (ease) breakover. Breakover has been defined as the most dorsal location of the solar aspect of the hoof capsule that contacts the ground during weight bearing, and it is the last part of the hoof capsule to leave the ground in the caudal phase of the stride.[36] If a modified keg shoe or a world racing plate is used, the breakover should be between 1 (small feet) and 1½ inches (large feet) dorsal to the apex of the frog, and the shoe should extend to the end of the frog[34] (Fig. 8.45). If a Natural Balance Shoe is used, the distance from the frog apex to the inside border of the shoe should be ⅛ to ¼ inch for small shoes, ¼ to ⅜ inch for medium shoes, and ⅜ to ½ inch for large shoes (Fig. 8.46).

Alternatively, a lateral radiograph of the foot can be taken to define the breakover point of the shoe in relation to the location of the distal phalanx.[35,36] For this to be done, the tip of the frog and the sole is trimmed until the true apex of the frog is identified as it attaches to the sole plane. A thumbtack is then placed at the apex of the frog, and a metal object (e.g., wire or horseshoe nail) is taped to the dorsal hoof wall. The metal object should extend to the cornet band with the proximal aspect of the wire being placed at the most distal hair follicles.[36] The horse is then placed on wood blocks (placement of all four limbs is recommended) so both forelimbs are bearing weight equally, and the forefeet are positioned so the metacarpi and metatarsi are perpendicular to the ground. A lateral radiograph is then taken with both heel bulbs being parallel to the x-ray beam.[36] Breakover of the shoe, dorsal to the tip of the distal pha-

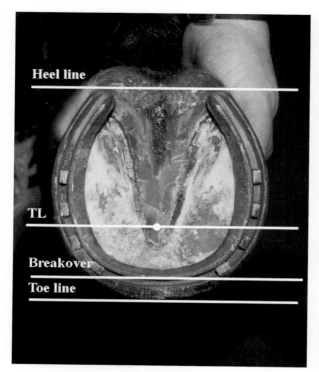

Figure 8.45   Same horse as in Figure 8.44 after a shoe is applied. Note the relations of the various lines and the position of breakover.

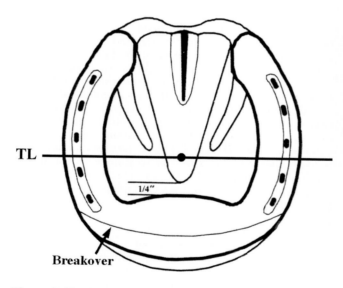

Figure 8.46   Application of a Natural Balance Shoe. (Reprinted with permission from Ovnicek G. New Hope for Soundness: Seen Through the Window of Wild Horse Hoof Patterns. Columbia Falls, MT: Equine Digit Support System, Inc., 1997.)

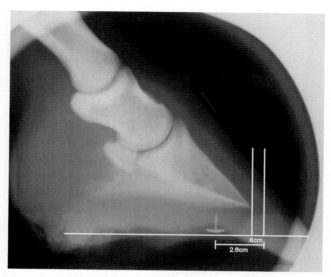

Figure 8.47   Lateral radiograph of the foot with radiographic markers in place. Note the measured distance from the tip of the distal phalanx dorsal is 0.6 cm, which is the desired breakover point in this horse. Also note that the measured distance from the thumbtack to the desired breakover point dorsal to the distal phalanx is 2.8 cm. This 2.8-cm distance is the measurement the farrier uses to determine breakover point on the sole.

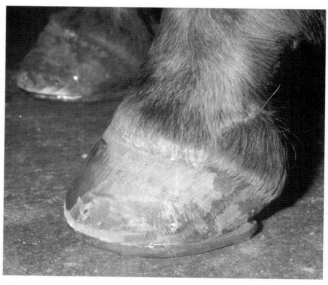

Figure 8.48   Same horse as in Figure 8.44. Note the shoe placement in relation to the trimmed hoof. Also note that the dorsal hoof wall is not trimmed back to the shoe, but rather the flare was removed from the dorsal hoof wall, and the remaining hoof wall was undercut toward the shoe.

lanx, is 0.4 cm for horses weighing 200 to 300 kg, 0.5 cm for horses weighing 300 to 400 kg, 0.6 cm for horses weighing 400 to 500 kg, and 0.7 cm for horses weighing 500 to 600 kg.[36] The distance from the thumbtack to the designated point of breakover dorsal to the tip of the distal phalanx is measured on the radiograph (Fig. 8.47). This measured distance is then transferred to the bottom of the horse's foot with the thumbtack as the reference point, and it is used by the farrier to locate the breakover point of the shoe dorsal to the apex of the frog.

When finishing the foot, remove only the flares that are obvious and undercut the remaining hoof wall left over the shoe (Fig. 8.48). Do not rasp the dorsal hoof

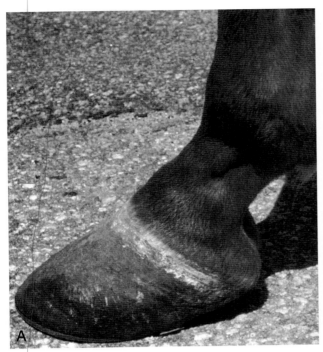
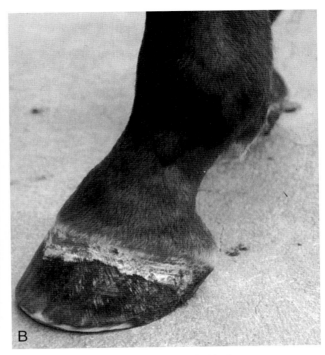

Figure 8.49   A. Severely distorted hoof with a long toe and underrun heel. B. Hoof (same as in A) after trimming.

wall from the center of the toe back to the shoe. In extreme cases with long toes and underrun heels, trimming, following the guidelines described, effectively redistributes the weight-bearing forces to under the distal phalanx (Fig. 8.49). Once the shoe is applied, the horse is walked again on a flat hard surface to assess dynamic balance and heel-first contact.

Egg bar shoes may be recommended in some cases in which the hoof capsule is unstable because of shearing, in which a large horse has small feet, or in which the horse's heels are severely underrun or collapsed. The egg bar shoe increases the surface area of contact and increases the stability of the hoof. The shoe should be applied so it is clearly visible at the quarters and extends palmarad to cover the heels[49,57] (see Fig. 9.78). To allow for heel expansion, one should not use nails past the bend in the quarters. (For more information the reader is referred to Chapter 9.)

Pads may be necessary for the first shoeing in some horses that have painful responses to hoof tester pressure over the central third of the frog or that have excessive sole pain. In some cases, we recommend applying a frog pad and a two-part impression material under the pad to create diffuse frog pressure that promotes heel expansion (Fig. 8.50). The two-part impression material is placed over the frog and in the sulci. Rolling, rockering, or squaring the toe of the shoe enhances breakover, thus reducing the stress on the DDFT. Note that although adjustment in the horse's hoof angles can be made rather drastically, the response might be immediate or gradual.

In most cases improvement in clinical signs after corrective trimming and shoeing is seen within 6 weeks; in some horses, however, it may take 2 to 3 months. Achieving a normal hoof confirmation takes months,

and in some cases, the run under heels may be past the point of return. Additionally, corrective trimming and shoeing is most beneficial when performed correctly at the earliest onset of clinical signs.[9]

Medical Treatments

Nonsteroidal Anti-inflammatory Drugs

Although many nonsteroidal anti-inflammatory drugs (NSAIDs) can be used in the treatment of navicular syndrome, phenylbutazone is by far the most commonly selected. As with other NSAIDs, phenylbutazone reduces pain by inhibiting the enzyme cyclooxygenase and the subsequent synthesis of prostanoids. It also inhibits platelet aggregation, thus improving blood flow. Phenylbutazone may be necessary for pain relief if the horse is severely lame or if it is to continue working through the initial treatment period. Phenylbutazone is also beneficial to allow pain-free adjustment to new shoes and hoof angles. Generally, it is recommended that 4.4 mg/kg be given orally for 7 to 10 days along with stall rest. This appears to break the pain cycle effectively and allows for adjustment to corrective trimming and shoeing.[49] In some cases, phenylbutazone is used to manage pain associated with eventing the horse.

Corticosteroids

Corticosteroids may prove beneficial as adjunctive therapy in the treatment of navicular syndrome. They can be injected into the DIP joint or the navicular bursa. I prefer intrasynovial treatment of the DIP joint as an alternative treatment and, for those cases that yield no

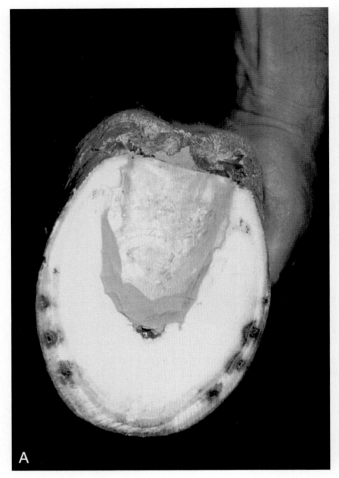

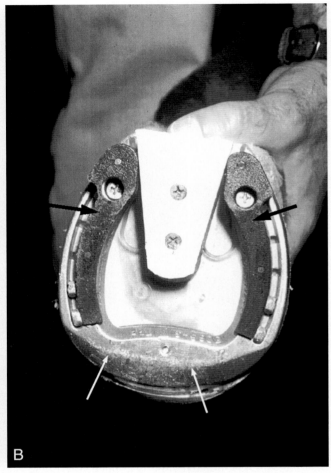

Figure 8.50   A. Two-part impression material applied to the frog and the sulci. B. The frog insert on the pad and an EDSS shoe. White arrows point to the breakover point on the shoe. A set of rails (black arrows) was added to elevate the heels and to cause a heel-first contact at a walk.

favorable response to initial treatment with corrective trimming and shoeing, isoxsuprine and phenylbutazone. Generally, the decision for their use is made at the 6-week or 3-month follow-up. If sufficient improvement is not seen in the lameness, intrasynovial anesthesia of the DIP joint is done to assess improvement. If the lameness is improved by 70 to 90%, I offer the client the option of intraarticular treatment of the DIP joint with either betamethasone, 6 mg/joint or methylprednisolone acetate, 100 mg/joint. At this point the agent I prefer is betamethasone.

Although improvement in lameness has been seen in the majority of cases after this treatment, the duration tends to be variable, lasting anywhere from 3 to 12 weeks. In some cases, intrasynovial injection of sodium hyaluronate is included. This is done at the time of steroid treatment or 3 weeks after treatment. Delaying the hyaluronic acid intrasynovial injection, in my experience, seems to prolong the beneficial effects of intrasynovial corticosteroid treatment.

Intrabursal injection of 40 mg of methyl prednisolone or triamcinolone has also been recommended.[63] The needle placement (injection) should be monitored by radiography or fluoroscopy, and horses are rested for 3 days after which they can be returned to work. Long-term follow-up on 148 navicular disease cases in which the horses had received intrabursal injections revealed an immediate beneficial effect in 80% and no effect in 20%. In those cases that did respond favorably, the effect of the injection lasted less than 1 month in 14% of cases, 1 month in 6% of cases, and 2 months in more than 60% of cases. Although not considered a cure, this approach can be used to provide short-term relief from pain in cases that have not responded to more conventional treatment.

Hemorheologic Agents

Isoxsuprine hydrochloride is commonly used in the treatment of navicular syndrome. It is a β-adrenergic agent with both vasodilatory and rheologic properties. In a trial, horses with navicular syndrome that were treated with isoxsuprine showed significantly greater improvement than horses treated with a placebo.[56] Various dose regimens have been evaluated, and no dose-related response was identified in horses treated with higher doses up to 1.8 mg/kg of isoxsuprine.[56] Currently, isoxsuprine is being administered orally at 0.66 mg/kg twice daily for 3 weeks, followed by 0.66 mg/kg once daily for 2 weeks, followed by an every other day dosing.[56] Typically, horses will have palpably warmer extremities because of the drug's vasodilatory effect. Reported success rates range from 40 to 87%, with the best results occurring in horses affected less than 1 year.[57] The improvement in clinical signs can persist for as long as 1 year after isoxsuprine is discontinued, especially when foot problems are corrected. In some cases (many that I deal with), however, isoxsuprine therapy is continued year round but at a lower dose. Continuous treatment with isoxsuprine is used in horses that perform year round and then, when they are taken off the drug, show signs of pain. Adverse side effects have not been reported in the horse given isoxsuprine per os, although the drug has not been proved safe for use in pregnant mares. At this time, isoxsuprine is considered a masking agent by the American Horse Show Association and should be discontinued 96 hours before the horse is shown or raced. The beneficial response to therapy with isoxsuprine is probably because of its ability to improve blood flow to the navicular region and its rheologic effects.

Pentoxifylline and propentofylline are synthetic xanthene derivatives that have been used in the treatment of navicular syndrome.[11,27] The hemorheologic agents act by altering the physical characteristics of the blood: 1) increasing erythrocyte flexibility, thereby easing blood flow through capillaries; 2) decreasing fibrinogen; 3) preventing aggregation of red cells and platelets, which decrease blood viscosity; and 4) inhibiting the action of inflammatory cytokines. A horse study in which researchers evaluated the pharmacokinetics of pentoxifylline identified erratic absorption and bioavailability after oral administration.[11] Results of a clinical trial assessing propentofylline in the treatment of navicular syndrome indicated a significant improvement in lameness, but none of the horses was completely sound within the 6 months of the study. Propentofylline was administered at 7.5 mg/kg twice daily for 6 weeks.[27]

Metrenperone, a vasoactive drug with S2 and α_1-antagonistic properties, has been used to treat horses with navicular syndrome. In a trial comparing the effect of metrenperone (60 horses) and isoxsuprine (40 horses) in the treatment of navicular syndrome, long-term follow-up (1 to 5 years) found that isoxsuprine was a better treatment.[64]

Sodium Hyaluronate

Sodium hyaluronate (HA) has been used in the treatment of some horses with navicular syndrome. Both intrasynovial (20 mg) and intravenous (40 mg) routes have been used. Although intrasynovial injection of the navicular bursa can be done, the intrasynovial injection of the DIP joint is most common. HA can be injected intrasynovially at the same time as the corticosteroid, or its use can be delayed for 3 to 4 weeks, depending on the type of steroid injected and the response to treatment. More than one intrasynovial injection of HA may be required. Anecdotally, reports indicate some benefit to intravenously administered HA in the treatment of navicular syndrome in some horses.

Polysulfated Glycosaminoglycans

Polysulfated glycosaminoglycans (PSGAGs) have been used in patients with navicular syndrome and, when administered intramuscularly in at least one trial, showed documented benefit.[10] In this double-blind study, seven horses received 500 mg of PSGAG intramuscularly at 4-day intervals for seven treatments, and eight horses received saline as a placebo. The conclusion was that there was an improvement in the lameness associated with navicular syndrome in horses receiving PSGAG with clinical signs of less than 12 months duration, compared with control horses. PSGAG has also been used intrasynovially as well as orally for the treatment of navicular syndrome, but no controlled studies have yet been reported.

Nutraceutical

The clinical efficacy of a chrondromodulatory nutraceutical has been evaluated in the treatment of 10 horses with navicular syndrome.[18] The trial was double blinded, placebo controlled (5 horses), and randomized. The nutraceutical was composed of 9 g of glucosamine HCl, 3 g of purified sodium chondroitin sulfate, and 600 mg of manganese ascorbate and was given orally twice daily for 56 days. Statistically significant improvement (clinical and owner assessed) was observed in the treatment group compared with the control group.

Surgical Treatments

Surgery is usually reserved for cases of navicular syndrome that have not responded to more conservative treatments. Three surgical treatments are currently available: palmar digital neurectomy, navicular suspensory desmotomy, and desmotomy of the carpal check ligament.

Palmar Digital Neurectomy

The most commonly performed surgical technique for navicular syndrome is palmar digital neurectomy. The procedure desensitizes the caudal one-third to one-half of the palmar foot region and the sole extending dorsally to the toe. It should be done in conjunction with corrective hoof trimming and shoeing to reduce abnormal forces on the foot, thus slowing the progression of the degenerative changes associated with the navicular syndrome.[49]

In all cases in which palmar digital neurectomy is considered, a low palmar digital nerve block should be performed first. The degree of response to the nerve block is similar to the pain relief achieved by a neurectomy. Some horses have additional nerve branches supplying the navicular region, and if these nerves are not identified and transected, the response to neurectomy will be less than optimal. Various methods of palmar digital neurectomy have been described, including "guillotine" technique (sharp transection of the nerve and a segment of the nerve is removed), cryoneurectomy, laser neurectomy (CO_2 and neodymium:yttrium-aluminum-garnet [Nd:YAG]), neurectomy "stripping" technique (8 to 10 cm of the nerve is removed), epineural (perineural) capping, silicone capping, cyanoacrylate glue capping, the injection of neurotoxic agents, radioactive ligature, and intramedullary anchoring of the nerve.[3,12,17,19–21,31, 45,49] All share common goals in that they attempt to reduce the incidence of neuroma formation and axonal regrowth, resulting in reinnervation.

In a study done on 57 horses and in which the long-term results of palmar digital neurectomy (guillotine, 10 horses and transection; electrocoagulation, 47 horses) were documented, researchers found complications in 34% (17 of 50) of the horses for which follow-up information was obtained.[21] Recurrence of heel pain was the most common complication (14 horses), and palpable neuromas were detected in 3 horses. One year after neurectomy, 74% of the horses were sound; this decreased to 63% after the second year. In a study comparing techniques of palmar digital neurectomy (guillotine, perineural capping, CO_2 laser transection, or CO_2 coagulation), researchers found the guillotine technique resulted in a longer duration of cutaneous desensitization of the heels and less neuroma formation, compared with the other techniques. Horses in this study were followed for as long as 360 days.[12] In another study evaluating five techniques (noncontact Nd:YAG laser transection, sapphire-tip contact Nd:YAG laser transection, guillotine transection, cryoepineural capping, and cyanoacryl glue capping) for palmar digital neurectomy in horses, researchers found that the noncontact Nd:YAG technique had the lowest composite neuroma scores and hence was judged to be the superior technique.[31] Anecdotally, the palmar digital neurectomy "stripping" technique, where part (8 to 10 cm) of the nerve is removed, is supposed to offer the advantage of a lower incidence of nerve regeneration and painful neuroma formation.[3] Unfortunately, the number of cases, successes and failures, was not reported. Good results have been reported with the modified "Lose" neurectomy technique. In this technique, the distal end of the palmar digital nerve is drawn through a tunnel created under the digital artery and inserted in the medullary cavity of the proximal phalanx.[19] Results of follow-up on 28 horses for a period of 1.5 to 11 years revealed that 96% (27 of 28) of the horses were completely sound with no evidence of neuroma formation or reinnervation after neurectomy with the modified "Lose" technique.

Navicular Suspensory Desmotomy

Navicular suspensory desmotomy has been advocated by some as a treatment for navicular syndrome.[2,66,68] In a review of 118 horses suffering from navicular syndrome that were treated with navicular suspensory desmotomy, 76% were sound at 6 months, and 43% were sound after 36 months.[69] All of the following were associated with a diminished response: the presence of flexor cortex defects, proximal border enthesiophytes, mineralization of the DDFT, and medullary sclerosis. In a retrospective study on 22 horses with navicular syndrome that had navicular suspensory desmotomy, 15 of 21 horses that were available for follow-up were performing at their intended use.[66] Unfortunately, this study did not describe the duration of follow-up.

Carpal Check Ligament Desmotomy

Carpal check ligament desmotomy has been used in selected cases of navicular syndrome in which dorsal pal-

mar hoof imbalance (either broken forward or broken backward axis) seems a factor. In one study, four horses with navicular syndrome and with broken FP axes were treated with carpal check ligament desmotomy; all horses returned to full use, and the surgery made it possible to align the hoof pastern axis after surgery.[61]

Acupuncture

Acupuncture has been used for the treatment of navicular syndrome.[46] The treatment consists of the insertion and manipulation of needles in prescribed acupuncture points. Although some points suppress pain, others reportedly regulate blood flow. Although anecdotal comments estimate that 40 to 50% of horses with navicular syndrome improve with this treatment, in one controlled study in which electroacupuncture was used, researchers found no significant difference between treatment (10 horses) and control (10 horses) groups.[50]

References

1. Ackerman N, Johnson JH, Dorn CR. Navicular disease in the horse: Risk factors, radiographic changes and response to therapy. J Am Vet Med Assoc 1977;170:183.
2. Bell BTL, Bridge IS, Sullivan STK. Surgical treatment of navicular syndrome in the horse using navicular suspensory desmotomy. N Z Vet J 1996;44:26–30.
3. Black JB. Palmar digital neurectomy: An alternative surgical approach. Proc Am Assoc Equine Pract 1992;38:429–432.
4. Bowker RM, Atkinson PJ, Atkinson TS, Haut RC. Effect of contact stress in bones of the distal interphalangeal joint on microscopic changes in articular cartilage and ligaments. Am J Vet Res 2001; 62(3):414–424.
5. Bowker RM, Bidwill LA, Natchek KA. Relationship of palmar foot to stress at the insertion of the impar ligament and the deep digital flexor tendon: Histomorphological evidence. Unpublished manuscript.
6. Bowker RM, Linder K, Van Wulfen KK, et al. Distribution of local anesthetics injected into the distal interphalangeal joint and podotrochlear bursa: An experimental study. Pferdeheilkunde 1996;12:609–612.
7. Bowker RM, Rockershouser SJ, Vex KB, et al. Immunocytochemical and dye distribution studies of nerves potentially desensitized by injection onto the distal interphalangeal joint or the navicular bursa of horses. J Am Vet Med Assoc 1993;203:1707–1714.
8. Colles CM. Navicular disease and its treatment. In Practice 1982; 4:29–35.
9. Colles CM, Hickman J. The arterial supply of the navicular bone and its variations in navicular disease. Equine Vet J 1977;25: 150–154.
10. Crisman MV, Furr MO, Ley WB, et al. Evaluation of polysulfated glycosaminoglycan for the treatment of navicular disease: A double blind study. Proc Am Assoc Equine Pract 1993;39:219–220.
11. Crisman MV, Wilcke JR, Correll LS, Irby MH. Pharmacokinetic disposition of intravenous and oral pentoxifylline in horses. J Vet Pharmacol Ther 1993;16:23–31.
12. Dabareiner RM, White NA, Sullins KE. Comparison of current techniques for palmar digital neurectomy in horses. Proc Am Assoc Equine Pract 1997;43:231–232.
13. Denoix JM, Crevier N, Roger B, et al. Magnetic resonance imaging of the equine foot. Vet Radiol Ulrasound 1993;34:405–411.
14. Drommer W, Damsch S, Winkelmeyer S, et al. Scanning electron microscopy of the sesamoid bone and deep flexor tendon of horses with navicular disease. DTW 1992;99:235.
15. Dyson S. Comparison of responses to analgesia of the navicular bursa and intraarticular analgesia of the distal interphalangeal joint in 102 horses. Proc Am Assoc Equine Pract 1995;41:234–239.
16. Fricker C, Reik W, Hugelshoter F. Occlusion of the digital arteries—A model for pathogenesis of navicular disease. Equine Vet J 1982;14:203–207.

17. Fubini SL, Cummings JF, Todhunter RJ. The use of intraneural doxorubicin in association with palmar digital neurectomy in 28 horses. Vet Surg 1988;17:346–349.

18. Hanson RR, Hammad WR. Evaluation of the clinical efficacy of a nutraceutical in the treatment of navicular syndrome: A double-blinded placebo-controlled randomized clinical trial [abstract]. Proceedings of the 7th Annual American College of Veterinary Surgeons Symposium, Orlando, FL, October 16–19, 1997, Large Animal Proceeding, 9.

19. Harris JM, Kennedy MA. Modified posterior digital neurectomy for management of chronic heel pain in horses. Proc Am Assoc Equine Pract 1994;40:99–100.

20. Haugland LM, Collier MA, Panciera RJ, et al. The effect of CO_2 laser neurectomy of formation and axonal regeneration. Vet Surg 1992;21:351–354.

21. Jackman BR, Baxter GM, Doran RE, et al. Palmar digital neurectomy in horses. 57 cases 1984–1990. Vet Surg 1993;22:285–288.

22. Kaser-Hotz B, Ueltschi G. Radiographic appearance of the navicular bone of sound horses. Vet Radiol Ultrasound 1992;33:9–17.

23. Keegan KG, Wilson DJ, Frankeny RL, et al. Effects of anesthesia of the palmar digital nerves on kinematic gait analysis in horses with and without navicular disease. Am J Vet Res 1997;58:218–223.

24. Keegan KG, Wilson DA, Lattimer JC, et al. Scintigraphic evaluation of ^{99m}Tc-methylene diphosphonate uptake in the navicular area of horses with lameness isolated to the foot by anesthesia of the palmar digital nerves. Am J Vet Res 1996;57:415–421.

25. Keller H, Grundmann S. Radiographic monitoring of navicular disease. Tierarztl Prax 1995;23:46–52.

26. Kirker-Head CA, et al. Proceedings of the International Symposium on Pod, Germany, 1993.

27. Kirker-Head CA, Fackelman GE, Hoogasian JJ. Studies on propentofylline for the treatment of navicular disease. J Equine Vet Sci 1993;13:239–249.

27a. Lane Easter J, Watkins JP, Stephens SL, et al. Effects of regional anesthesia on experimentally induced coffin joint synovitis. Proc Am Assoc Equine Pract 2000;46:214–216.

28. Leach DH. Treatment and pathogenesis of navicular disease ("syndrome") in horses. Equine Vet J 1993;25:477–481.

29. Lowe JE. Sex, breed and age incidence of navicular disease. Proc Am Assoc Equine Pract 1976;20:37.

30. MacGregor CM. Studies on the pathology and treatment of equine navicular disease. PhD Thesis, University of Edinburgh, 1984.

31. Martin F, Tulleners E, Habecker P, et al. Evaluation of five techniques for performing palmar digital neurectomy in horses [abstract]. Proceedings of the 7th Annual American College of Veterinary Surgeons Symposium, Orlando, FL, October 16–19, 1997, Large Animal Proceeding, 25.

32. Numans SR, Van der Watering CC. Navicular disease: Podotrochilitis chronica asceptica podotrochlosis. Equine Vet J 1973;5:1–7.

33. Ostblom L, Lund C, Melsen F. Histological study of navicular bone disease. Equine Vet J 1982;14:199–202.

34. Ovnicek G. New Hope for Soundness; Seen Through the Window to Wild Horse Hoof Patterns. Colombia Falls, MT: Equine Digit Support Systems, Inc., 1997.

35. Page BT, Bowker RM, Ovnicek G. Breakover of the hoof and its effect on structures and forces within the foot. Submitted to Equine Vet J 1999.

36. Page BT, Bowker RM, Ovnicek G, et al. How to mark the hoof for radiography to locate the distal phalanx and determine breakover. Proc Am Assoc Equine Pract 1999;45:148–150.

37. Pleasant RS, Baker GJ, Foreman JH, et al. Interosseous pressure and pathologic changes in horses with navicular disease. Am J Vet Res 1993;54:7–12.

38. Pleasant RS, Moll HD, Ley WB, et al. Intra-articular anesthesia of the distal interphalangeal joint alleviates lameness associated with the navicular bursa in horses. Vet Surg 1997;26:137–140.

39. Pool RR, Meagher DM, Stover SM. Pathophysiology of navicular disease. Vet Clin North Am Equine Pract 1989;5:109–129.

40. Poulos P, Brown A. On navicular disease in the horse. A roentgenological pathoanatomic study. Part I. Evaluation of the flexor control eminence. Vet Radiol Ultrasound 1989;30(2):50–53.

41. Rijkenhuizen ABM, Nemeth F, Dik KJ, et al. The effect of artificial occlusion of the ramus navicularis and its branching arteries on

42. the navicular bone in horses. An experimental study. Equine Vet J 1989;21:425–430.

42. Rijkenhuizen ABM, Nemeth F, Dik KJ, et al. The effect of unilateral resection of segments of both palmar digital arteries on the navicular bone in ponies. An experimental study. Equine Vet J 1989;21:413–417.

43. Ross MW. Observations in horse with lameness abolished by palmar digital analgesia. Proc Am Assoc Equine Pract 1998;44:230–232.

44. Said AH, Khamis Y, Mafouz MF, et al. Clinicopathological studies on neurectomy in equids. Equine Vet J 1984;16:442–446.

45. Schneider RK, Mayhen GI, Clarke GL. Effects of cryotherapy on the palmar and plantar digital nerves in the horse. Am J Vet Res 1985;46:7–12.

46. Schoen AM. Navicular disease. In: Schoen AM, Ed. Veterinary Acupuncture Ancient Art to Modern Medicine. Goleta, CA: American Veterinary Publications, Inc., 1994;520–528.

47. Schumacher J, Schramme M, DeGraves F, et al. Abolition of lameness caused by experimentally induced solar pain in horses after analgesia of the distal interphalangeal joint. Proc Am Assoc Equine Pract 1999;45:193–194.

47a. Schumacher J, Schramme M, Schumacher J, et al. The effect of volume of local anesthetic administered into the coffin joint on solar toe and heel pain. Proc Am Assoc Equine Pract 2000;46:27–28.

48. Scott EA, Thrall DE, Sandler GA. Angiography of the equine metacarpus and phalanges. Alterations with medial palmar artery and medial palmar digital artery ligation. Am J Vet Res 1976;37:869–873.

49. Stashak TS. Navicular syndrome (navicular disease). In: White NA, Moore JN, Eds. Current Techniques in Equine Surgery and Lameness. 2nd ed. Philadelphia: WB Saunders, 1998;537–544.

50. Steiss JE, White MA, Bowen JM. Electroacupuncture in the treatment of chronic lameness in horses and ponies: a controlled clinical trial. Can J Vet Res 1989;53:239–243.

51. Svalastoga E, Smith M. Navicular disease in the horse: The subchondral bone pressure. Nord Vet Med 1983;35:31–37.

52. Swanson TD. Navicular syndrome. Proceedings of the Colorado Veterinary Medicine Association, Snowmass, CO, September 1998.

53. Thompson KN, Rooney JR, Petrites-Murphy MB. Considerations on the pathogenesis of navicular disease. J Equine Vet Sci 1991;11:4–8.

54. Tietje S. Computed tomography of the navicular bone region in the horse: A comparison with radiographic documentation. Pferdeheilkunde 1995;11:51–61.

55. Trout DR, Hornof WJ, O'Brien TR. Soft tissue- and bone-phase scintigraphy for diagnosis of navicular disease in horses. J Am Vet Med Assoc 1991;198:73–77.

56. Turner AS, Tucker CM. The evaluation of isoxsuprine hydrochloride for the treatment of navicular disease: A double blind study. Equine Vet J 1989;21:338–341.

57. Turner TA. Diagnosis and treatment of navicular disease in horses. Vet Clin North Am Equine Pract 1989;5:131–143.

58. Turner TA. Differentiation of navicular region pain from other forms of palmar heel pain. Pferdeheilkunde 1996;12:603–606.

59. Turner TA. Predictive value of diagnostic tests for navicular pain. Proc Am Assoc Equine Pract 1996;42:201–204.

60. Turner TA. Use of navicular bursography in 97 horses. Proc Am Assoc Equine Pract 1998;44:227–229.

61. Turner TA, Rosenstein D. Inferior check desmotomy as a treatment for caudal hoof lameness. Proc Am Assoc Equine Pract 1992;38:157–163.

62. Van de Watering CC, Morgan JP. Chip fractures as a radiologic finding in navicular disease of the horse. J Am Vet Radiol Soc 1975;16:206–210.

63. Verschooten F, Desmet P, Peremans K, et al. Navicular disease in the horse: The effect of controlled intrabursal corticoid injection. J Equine Vet Sci 1990;10:316–320.

64. Verschooten F, Ooms LAA, Desmet P, et al. Metrenperone treatment of navicular disease in horses compared with isoxsuprine: A clinical study. J Equine Vet Sci 1990;10:230–233.

65. Verschooten F, Roels J, Lampo P, et al. Radiographic measurements from the lateromedial projection of the equine foot with navicular disease. Res Vet Sci 1989;46:15–21.

66. Watkins JP, McMullan WM, Morris EL. Navicular suspensory desmotomy in the management of navicular syndrome: A retrospective analysis. Proc Am Assoc Equine Pract 1993;39:261–262.

67. Winkelmeyer S. Histological and scanning electron microscopical findings in deep flexor tendons and the distal sesamoid bone of horses. Correlations with a clinical diagnosis of navicular disease. Tierarztl Hochschule 1989;191.
68. Wright IM. A study of 118 cases of navicular disease: Clinical feature. Equine Vet J 1993;25:488–492.
69. Wright IM. A study of 118 cases of navicular disease: Treatment by navicular suspensory desmotomy. Equine Vet J 1993;25:501–509.

NAVICULAR (DISTAL SESAMOID) BONE FRACTURES

Fractures of the navicular bone are an uncommon cause of lameness in horses[1,8,11] and have been reported in many breeds of horses and in horses used for various purposes.[3,11] Such fractures have been classified as avulsion (chip) fractures,[13,17,19] simple complete fractures (transverse or oblique),[19,20] comminuted complete fractures,[19] and congenital separation (nonfusion) bipartite and tripartite sesamoid bones.[9] (The latter is not considered a true fracture and is covered only in the Chapter 4, Part I, "Radiology." Complete fracture can occur after acute trauma or secondary to severe bone demineralization–associated navicular syndrome or from osteomyelitis of the navicular bone after sepsis from a puncture wound of the navicular bursa (pathologic fracture).[3,8,15] Avulsion fractures are often associated with the navicular syndrome.[3,19] The forefeet seem at a greater risk for fracture.[3,7,11] In one report, 22 of 25 fractures of the navicular bone were in the forelimbs,[7] and in another, 15 of 17 were in the forelimbs.[11]

Avulsion (chip) fractures usually involve the distal border of the navicular bone (see Fig. 8.41). They are considered uncommon and are frequently associated with other radiographic signs of navicular syndrome.[19] Fracture fragments range from rectangular to ellipsoidal and usually measure from 0.2 to 1.2 cm in transverse

dimension.[19] Van der Watering[19] reported on 50 cases of chip fractures of the distal navicular bone that were detected in a review of more than 400 radiographic cases of navicular disease in the horse. All except three of these cases were associated with other radiographic signs of navicular disease. The fractures were most frequently observed in horses 5 to 9 years of age, which is similar to that seen in navicular syndrome cases.

Simple complete fractures may be vertical, slightly oblique, or transverse.[10,19,20] The vertical and slightly oblique fractures usually occur close to the central eminence (sagittal ridge) of the navicular bone, either lateral or medial to it. Generally, these fractures are not displaced, but they are usually slightly separated so an obvious fracture line exists on the radiograph (Fig. 8.51). With simple complete fractures, the forelimb is most frequently affected, although these fractures have also been reported in the hindlimbs.[3,5,9,11] It is considered an uncommon fracture with a relative incidence of 6 of 1000 hospitalized horses in one report[6] and 3 of 150 hospitalized horses in another report.[19] Rupture of the distal sesamoidean (impar) ligament and fracture of the navicular bone in the hindlimb have been reported in one case.[5]

Comminuted complete fractures are more uncommon than simple complete fractures.[19] With comminuted fractures, there may be some dorsal and ventral displacement of the fracture.[6] In one report, the fractures were comminuted in only 3 of 18 horses with complete navicular bone fractures.[3]

Etiology

Avulsion or Chip Fractures

Because avulsion or chip fractures are frequently associated with severe radiographic signs of navicular syn-

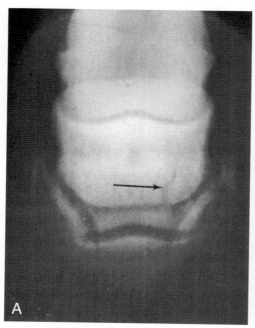
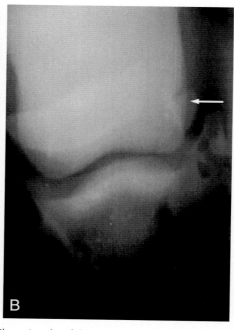

Figure 8.51 A. Fracture of the navicular bone (arrow). B. A dorsal palmar view identifying a significantly displaced fracture of the extremity of the navicular bone (arrow). This type of fracture is uncommon in my experience.

drome, it is easy to assume that the pathologic changes occurring at the distal border of the navicular bone may predispose to this type fracture.[19] The forefeet are more commonly involved with these fractures.

Simple and Comminuted Complete Fractures

Simple and comminuted complete fractures of the foot (primarily seen in the hindfeet) may be caused by acute trauma (concussion) or may be secondary to severe pathologic bone changes associated with navicular disease (almost exclusively the forefeet).[3] Adams[1] described a complete navicular bone fracture occurring after a neurectomy was performed in a case in which there was severe demineralization and flexor surface navicular bone changes on radiographic examination.

Clinical Signs

The lameness and clinical signs associated with avulsion fractures are identical with those seen with navicular syndrome, but there may be a history of acute exacerbation of the lameness that at one time responded to rest. With complete fracture, the lameness is usually acute from the onset and is severe. One study evaluating the outcome of horses with complete fractures of the navicular bone found that most horses were severely lame, but the degree of lameness decreased with time. Five horses that were only mildly lame (grade 2 of 5) at a trot were examined at a mean time of 90 days after the onset of lameness (range, 30 to 150 days).[11] In another study, the mean duration of lameness before presentation was 4.3 months.[3]

Although the palmar or plantar digital nerves supply sensory innervation to the navicular region, perineural anesthesia of these nerves may not totally eliminate the lameness, and regional anesthesia at a more proximal level may be required.[11] The reason for this may be that the navicular bone articulates with the distal interphalangeal joint and that fracture of the bone may cause articular pain that is not completely eliminated by palmar or plantar digital regional anesthesia. Intraarticular anesthesia of the distal interphalangeal joint should eliminate the lameness associated with navicular bone fracture.[2]

Diagnosis

Radiographic examination is needed to make the diagnosis (Fig. 8.52). Care is taken not to confuse the lines from the lateral sulci of the frog that cross the navicular region with a fracture. If the line extends beyond (above or below) the navicular bone, it is not a fracture. When in doubt, retake the radiograph at a slightly different angle. Careful packing of the foot can eliminate the line artifacts in most cases. (Refer to Chapter 4 for details.) Navicular bone fractures must be differentiated from congenital separation (nonfusion).[11] Radiographically, bipartite and tripartite navicular bones are symmetric, with smooth edges, and have a wide radiolucent region[14] (Fig. 8.52). They are often bilateral also; therefore, the opposite navicular region should be imaged.

Avulsion fractures can be difficult to identify on radiographs, and close scrutiny is required. Complete sim-

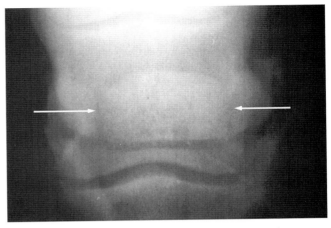

Figure 8.52 Bipartite navicular bone (arrows).

ple fractures are typically located in the sagittal plane medial or lateral to the midline.[15] It has been suggested that this site is the weakest and most exposed area of the bone.[20] To my knowledge, there have not been any biomechanical studies of this region to support this claim. The foot in all cases is trimmed and thoroughly cleaned to decrease the chance of artifactual duplication on radiographs.

Treatment

Avulsion fractures treatment is similar to that described for navicular syndrome. (Refer to "Navicular Syndrome" in Part I of this chapter.) Complete navicular bone fractures have been treated by rest, by rest and corrective shoeing (with or without heel elevation), or by external coaptation aimed at reducing hoof expansion.[3,8,11] The duration of stall rest is important, and a minimum of 6 months is recommended. One study documenting the outcome of complete navicular bone fractures found that a minimum of 6 months of stall rest was necessary before there was resolution of clinical signs.[11] In another study in which a 12° heel elevation shoeing technique was used to reduce tensional and compression forces on the navicular bone, it was found that a 4-month rest period was adequate.[18] The 12° heel elevation is achieved by use of four 3° wedge pads and a flat shoe. The horse is reshod every month, and at that time one pad is eliminated so that by 4 months the horse is shod normally without heel elevation. During this shoeing period, the horse is not exercised for 60 days and is confined to a box stall; after this 60-day interval, the horse can be hand walked for short periods (15 minutes daily). Hand walking exercise is continued for 4 months, at which time the lameness is evaluated after a flat shoe is placed. Palmar or plantar digital neurectomy has also been performed to relieve pain in cases that have not responded to conservative treatment.[3,11] In all cases in which neurectomy is considered, perineural anesthesia of the palmar digital nerves should be done to evaluate the potential effectiveness of neurectomy. Additionally, prolonged rest after the neurectomy should be considered to allow the fracture to heal and to prevent further damage to the surrounding structures.[4,6,9,16] Interfragmentary fixation with a single cortical bone screw placed in lag fashion was reported to be successful in 4 of 5 horses, but the follow-up period was short.[12]

The navicular bone is notoriously slow to heal. Follow-up radiography on 17 horses with complete navicular bone fractures revealed increases in the width of the fracture gap for up to 4 months after injury.[11] In one report,[2] the radiographic appearance of the fracture gap did not change over a period of 9.5 years, and in another report,[20] an uncalcified fibrous bone union was seen at necropsy 6 months after injury. Failure of an osseous union may be caused by constant motion at the fracture site.[11] The navicular bone is attached to the distal end of the proximal phalanx by the collateral distal sesamoid ligaments and to the distal phalanx by the impar ligament. During weight bearing the navicular bone is loaded between the distal and middle phalanx and the deep digital flexor tendon (DDFT). A combination of the attachments and loading forces presumably serve to distract the fracture fragments.[11] Also, the navicular bone is located between two synovial spaces, and synovial fluid may inhibit healing.[14] Additionally, the lack of periosteum and of poorly formed endosteum may contribute to poor fracture healing. Chronic lameness may result from poor fracture healing and the adhesions that develop between the DDFT and the navicular bone.[11] Although the navicular bone has poor healing qualities, in one case, satisfactory bone union has been reported after a 13-month rest period.[6]

Prognosis

The prognosis is considered poor for return to athletic performance. In one report, 3 of 6 horses treated with stall rest only or with stall rest and external coaptation and 2 of 4 horses treated with stall rest and corrective shoeing returned to their intended use.[11] In horses that did return to performance, a minimum of 6 months of stall rest was required before there was a resolution of clinical signs. Also, only 1 of 5 horses that underwent neurectomy returned to its intended use. In another report, 3 of 7 horses treated with rest returned to performance, and 4 remained lame. Of the 7 horses, 6 were treated with neurectomy: 2 of the 6 were sound for light riding, 2 were sound for 1 year only, and 2 remained lame.[3] Using the 12° elevated heel shoeing technique appears most promising at this time.[18] In this study, 4 of 4 horses with navicular fracture became serviceably sound for riding, and 2 of 4 returned to competition. Although these horses were sound for use, complete radiographic healing did not occur in any case.

References

1. Adams OR. Lameness in Horses. 3rd ed. Philadelphia: Lea & Febiger, 1974.
2. Arnbjerg J. Spontaneous fracture of the navicular bone in the horse. Nord Vet Med 1979;31:429–435.
3. Baxter GM, Ingle JE, Trotter GW. Complete navicular bone fractures in horses. Proc Am Assoc Equine Pract 1995;41:243–244.
4. Fessler JF, Amstutz CC. Fracture repair. In: Oehme FW, Prier JE, Eds. Textbook of Large Animal Surgery. Baltimore: Williams & Wilkins, 1974;296.
5. Frecklington PJ, Rose RJ. An unusual case of fracture of the navicular bone in the hind limb of a horse. Aust Vet Practitioner 1981; 11:57–59.
6. Freudenberg GFR. Über Spontanfrakturen des Strahlbeins beim Pferd. DTW Dtsch Tierarztl Wochenschr 1959;66:57.
7. Hertsch B, Konigsmann D. Sagittal fracture of the equine navicular bone. Contribution to diagnosis and treatment. Pferdeheilkunde 1993;9:3–13.
8. Honnas CM. Fractures of the distal sesamoid bone. In: Auer JA, Ed. Equine Surgery. Philadelphia: WB Saunders, 1992;992–993.
9. Johnson JH. The foot. In: Mansmann RA, McAllister ES, Eds. Equine Medicine and Surgery. 3rd ed. Santa Barbara, CA: American Veterinary Publications, 1982;1044.
10. Kaser-Hotz B, Ueltschi G, Hess N. Navicular bone fracture in the pelvic limb in two horses. Vet Radiol Ultrasound 1991;32: 283–285.
11. Lillich JD, Ruggles AJ, Gabel AA, et al. Fracture of the distal sesamoid bone in horses: 17 cases (1982–1992). J Am Vet Med Assoc 1995;207:924–927.
12. Nemeth F, Dik KJ. Lag screw fixation of sagittal navicular bone fractures in five horses. Equine Vet J 1985;17:137.
13. Numans SR, van der Watering CC. Navicular disease. Podotrochlitis chronica aseptica podotrochlosis. Equine Vet J 1973;5:1.
14. Reeves MJ. Miscellaneous conditions of the equine foot. Vet Clin North Am Equine Pract 1989;5:221–242.
15. Rick MC. Navicular bone fractures. In: White NA, Moore JN, Eds. Current Practice of Equine Surgery. Philadelphia: JB Lippincott, 1990;602–605.
16. Schleiter RH, Dettz O. Spontanfrakturen des Strahlbeines und Strahlbein-Luxation beim Pferd. Berl Munch Tierarztl Wochenschr 1957;70:409.
17. Smythe RA. Fractures of the navicular bone. Vet Rec 1961;73: 1009.
18. Turner TA. How to treat navicular bone fractures. Proc Am Assoc Equine Pract 1997;43:370–371.
19. Van De Watering CC, Morgan JP. Chip fractures as a radiologic finding in navicular disease of the horse. J Am Radiol Soc 1975; 16:206.
20. Vaughn LC. Fractures of the navicular bone. Vet Rec 1961;73:95.

SHEARED HEELS OR QUARTERS

Sheared heels and quarters are descriptive terms for the structural breakdown that occurs between the heel bulbs and the hoof capsule with a disproportionate use of one heel and or quarter.[2,3] Either the lateral or the medial heel or quarter may be out of balance and result in the overuse of one heel or quarter (see Figs. 3.12, 3.13, and 8.53). The degree of damage and lameness is proportional to the duration and degree of the foot imbalance.[1–3] This shearing of the heel or quarter can result in a chronic heel soreness (similar to navicular syndrome), hoof cracks in the heel bar or quarter, and deep thrush in the central sulcus of the frog. It may also initiate navicular syndrome.[3]

Etiology

Improper trimming and shoeing so that one heel and quarter is left longer than the other is a common cause of this condition.[1,3] This can be done easily because a right-handed farrier, when rasping, tends to remove slightly more heel and quarter off of the lateral side of the left forefoot and the medial side of the right forefoot.[1,3] Because the heels and quarters are a different length and height, the foot is said to be out of medial-lateral (ML) balance, and a disproportionate force is applied to the longer side during weight bearing. This creates an abnormal shearing force between the heel bulbs and the quarters, which results in structural breakdown. Horses with long toes and short heels are thought to be more suscepti-

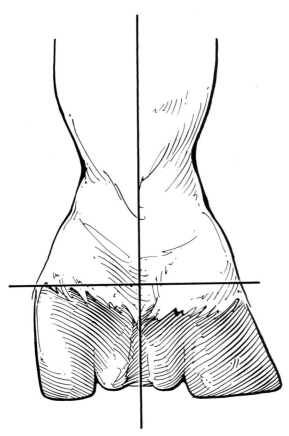

Figure 8.53 Sheared heels. Notice the left heel bulb is higher than the right. The hoof wall is straighter on the affected side (left side) while the hoof wall associated with the lower heel (right side) is flared. At exercise, the left heel contacts the ground first, causing a proximal displacement of the heel bulb.

is an abnormal flare to the hoof wall opposite the affected side (see Fig. 8.53). The differential height in the heel bulb or quarter is best viewed from behind, either when a horse is standing on a hard, flat surface or when the limb is handheld and viewed directly (see Fig. 3.12). The accentuated flare opposite the affected side can be noticed while the horse is viewed from the front or from above at the shoulder level. The hoof wall can also be rolled under in severe chronic cases. This hoof conformation may also be seen with a diagonal imbalance of the hoof.[5]

In horses viewed from the rear as they are walked on a smooth, hard surface, the heel of the affected side usually contacts the ground surface first, and a proximal displacement of that heel bulb occurs (see Fig. 8.53). Most frequently, horses break over in the short-toe region opposite the flare of the unaffected side. The lameness can be variable and depends on the degree of damage from the shearing effect. Horses with a diagonal imbalance usually land on the lateral toe and quarter and then load the medial heel and quarter.[5]

On palpation, an important finding is the loss of structural integrity between the heel bulbs.[2] On manipulation, the heel bulbs can be separated more easily and can be displaced in opposite directions (Fig. 8.54). Manipulation can be painful. Since hoof testers frequently indicate pain similar to that observed in navicular syndrome and perineural anesthesia of the palmar digital nerves may alleviate the lameness, this condition must be differentiated from navicular syndrome and diagonal hoof imbalance.[5] Radiographs should be taken to rule out the possibility of any bony structure involvement.

ble to the development of sheared heels.[6] This heel conformation is still commonly seen in racing Thoroughbreds in North America. Another situation in which this may occur is when corrective trimming is used in an attempt to alter conformational defects in young horses.[3] For instance, if the lateral heel and quarter are lowered and the medial heel and quarter are raised with a shim placed between the shoe and the hoof wall, a disproportionate force will be applied to the medial quarter of the heel during weight bearing.[3] This can result in shearing of the heels and quarters. Heel calks ("stickers") can further exaggerate the slightest imbalance in the heels and result in a shearing effect.[3]

A diagonal hoof imbalance can also result in an overload of one heel, which produces a shearing effect. In this condition, the hoof lands on one corner, and weight bearing then loads the diagonal corner. Horses with diagonal imbalance usually land on the lateral toe or quarter region and then overload the medial heel or quarter.[5] The overloading of one heel or quarter can result in a proximal displacement of the region.

Clinical Signs and Diagnosis

Visually, the heel bulb or quarter on the affected side is usually higher, the hoof wall is straighter, and there

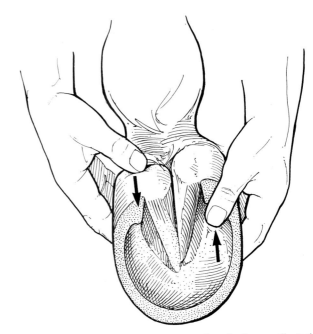

Figure 8.54 On palpation, the heel bulbs of a horse affected with sheared heels may be separated more easily and displaced in opposite directions. This increased movement is caused by a loss of structural integrity between the heel bulbs, and manipulation is often painful.

Treatment

Treatment is directed toward bringing the foot, heels, and quarters back into balance and alleviating the pain. The selection of treatment depends on the severity of the shearing and the degree of hoof wall distortion.[1-3] Mild cases usually respond to trimming of the longer heel or quarter and to allowing free exercise. If the horse is to perform, a full bar shoe is recommended for stability.[1,2] Since low heels and long toes are thought to predispose horses to sheared heels, the foot should be trimmed to balance it naturally.[4] (Refer to Chapter 9, "Medial-Lateral Balance," for details.) Using the live (nonexfoliating) sole as a guide to correct the ML imbalance is a relatively new concept that merits consideration. The exfoliating sole is carefully removed until the live (nonexfoliating) sole is encountered (waxy-like sole); then the hoof wall is trimmed to an equal distance or height to the live sole.[4] Refer to Chapter 9, "Medial-Lateral Balance," for more information.

More exaggerated cases require an additional trimming and more resets of the shoe to achieve balance. In these cases, the affected heel is displaced sufficiently proximad that a single trimming cannot restore the foot to balance. For treatment, the affected side is trimmed from the heel through the quarter to create a space when the shoe is applied (Fig. 8.55). Body weight and time force the heel back into alignment. Because these horses frequently exhibit considerable instability between their heels, a full bar shoe is recommended, and in some, it may be required for the rest of the animal's athletic career. Another approach that reportedly brings about rapid resolution of the hoof distortion involves trimming the feet, after which the foot is soaked in hot water for 15 minutes. Then a Lily pad and moist bandages are applied, and the horse is placed in a well-bedded stall for 12 to 24 hours.[7] After this period, the feet are reevaluated and balanced, and a shoe is applied.

In severe cases in which considerable structural damage to the heel bulb or quarter cracks have developed, a diagonal-bar shoe can be added to the full bar shoe. This is applied to the affected side to provide more protection and stability.[3]

If the hoof wall on the affected side begins to curl under, the horse can be shod full to the affected side in an attempt to encourage hoof wall growth to that side and a more normal alignment with the limb (see Fig. 9.65).[3]

Foals with sheared heels are best treated with corrective trimming of the heels or quarters and rounding the toe to encourage proper breakover. This should be done early to prevent possible damage to developing bones. But shoes should probably not be applied before 8 to 9 months of age.[3]

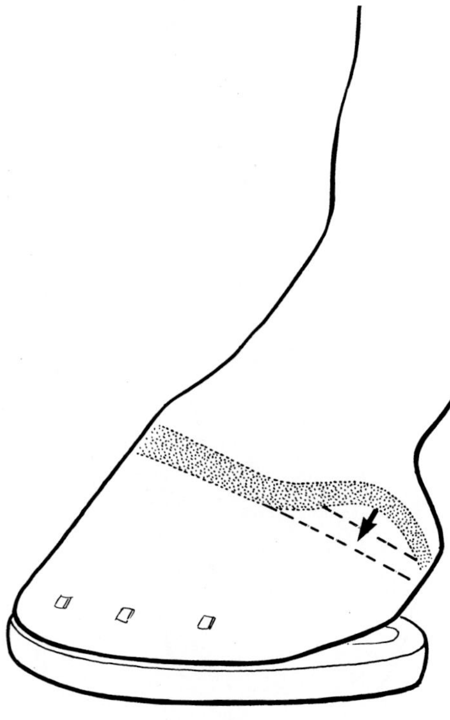

Prognosis

Prognosis is considered good for mildly affected horses. Horses presenting with severe exaggeration of this condition may require several shoe resets to bring the foot back into balance. The "hot-water" soaking method may decrease the time needed to correct the hoof deformity.[7] In cases with severe structural damage, the heel may require the added support of a full bar shoe for the rest of the animal's life.

References

1. Johnson JH. The foot. In: Mansmann RA, McAllister ES, Eds. Equine Medicine and Surgery. 3rd ed. Santa Barbara, CA: American Veterinary Publications, 1982;1044.
2. Moyer W. Diseases of the equine heel. Proc Am Assoc Equine Pract 1979;25:21.
3. Moyer W, Anderson JP. Sheared heels: Diagnosis and treatment. J Am Vet Med Assoc 1975;166:53.
4. Ovnicek G. Recognizing hoof deformity. In: Ovnicek G. New Hope for Soundness: Seen Through the Window of Wild Horse Hoof Patterns. Columbia Falls, MT: Equine Digit Support Systems, Inc., 1997;13-18.
5. Page B, Anderson GF. Diagonal imbalance of the equine foot: A cause of lameness. Proc Am Assoc Equine Pract 1992;38:413.
6. Rooney JR. Sheared heels. Mod Vet Pract 1977;58:708-709.
7. Snow VE, Birdsall DP. Specific parameters used to evaluate hoof balance and support. Proc Am Assoc Equine Pract 1991;37:299.

PEDAL OSTEITIS

With two recognized classifications, nonseptic and septic,[1,3] pedal osteitis (PO) is an inflammatory condition of the foot that results in demineralization of the distal phalanx. Radiographically, PO appears as a focal or a diffuse radiolucency or as new bone formation.[3,9,10,13] However, because the distal phalanx does

Figure 8.55 Corrective trimming and shoeing of a horse affected with sheared heels. The affected side is trimmed from the heel through the quarter to create a space between the hoof wall and the full bar shoe. The stippled area indicates the level of the coronary band. The arrow is pointing to where the coronary band should be.

not have a medullary cavity, inflammation of this bone is referred to as osteitis rather than osteomyelitis.[4]

Etiology

Nonseptic PO is a poorly defined disorder of the distal phalanx that may occur as a primary condition or that may develop from a secondary cause.[1] Primary PO is usually associated with severe or chronic sole bruising, resulting from repeated concussion during exercise on hard surfaces.[9,13] It is believed that the bone and the vascular channel changes result from pressure on and hyperemia of the solar lamina.[9] Secondary PO is the most common, and it can be a caused by persistent corns, laminitis, puncture wounds, bruised soles, and conformational faults.[1] Regardless of the cause, the disorder is typically associated with persistent, generally chronic, inflammation of the foot.[13] Histologically, nonseptic PO appears as a solar variant of laminitis, affecting epidermal and corial laminae of the distal wall and sole, primarily in the toe and the wing regions.[11]

Septic PO usually develops from introduction of environmental microbes, either into the soft tissues of the foot, with subsequent extension of infection into the distal phalanx, or from direct introduction of the microbes into the distal phalanx (e.g., deep penetrating wound).[5] Causes of septic PO include chronic severe laminitis, subsolar abscesses (most common), solar margin fractures, deep hoof wall cracks, avulsion hoof injuries, and penetrating wounds of the foot.[2,4,8] If soft tissue injury or infection is the cause, it is usually a while before the distal phalanx becomes involved. A sequestrum may develop in the distal phalanx as the osseous infection progresses.[6] In a review of 63 horses treated for septic PO, researchers found that subsolar abscess initiated 56%, solar margin fractures initiated 25%, and penetrating wounds initiated 13% of the cases.[8] In that study, subsolar abscesses were caused by bruising, wet or dry weather cycles, white line disease, or other events that compromised the keratinized barrier of the hoof. In another study in which the outcome in 18 horses with septic PO was reviewed, researchers found that of 9 cases in which there was follow-up, 7 were caused by penetrating objects, 1 was caused by deep hoof wall cracks, and 1 was caused by hoof avulsion.[2]

Clinical Signs

Nonseptic PO most commonly affects the forelimbs, and the condition can be either unilateral or bilateral. The severity of the lameness varies and depends on the cause and degree of injury. Lameness may be accentuated after exercise and after the horse has recently been trimmed and shod.[9] Hoof tester examination often reveals a focal or a diffuse region of increased sensitivity when pressure is applied to the sole and to the hoof wall. Perineural anesthesia of the palmar digital nerves usually eliminates the lameness, unless the dorsal surface of the distal phalanx is involved. In the latter case, the block must be done higher.

Septic PO most commonly affects the forelimbs. In one study reviewing the outcome of 63 cases of septic

PO, researchers found that the forelimbs were affected twice as much as the hindlimbs.[8] In another study, 11 of 18 cases presented with septic PO in the forefeet.[2] The degree of lameness, although variable and sometimes intermittent, is usually greater than that seen with nonseptic PO. Lameness grades ranging from 2 to 4.5 of 5 are common.[2] In one study evaluating septic PO, researchers found that 53% of the horses presented with lameness grade 4 of 5, 33% presented with lameness grade 3 of 5, and the average duration of lameness before presentation was 18.5 days.[8] On palpation, increases in temperature and prominent digital pulses can often be felt in the affected foot compared with the other feet. Increased digital pulses were found in 14 of 18 cases of septic PO in one study.[2] Hoof tester examination may be beneficial for localizing the site of pain as well as for promoting abscess drainage in some cases. Perineural anesthesia of the palmar digital nerves may not eliminate the lameness in horses with septic PO. Minimal or no response to palmar digital nerve block was seen in 5 of 5 cases of septic PO in which diagnostic anesthesia was used. All 5 cases were sound after an abaxial proximal nerve block.[2]

Diagnosis

Radiographic assessment of the distal phalanx for the presence of nonseptic PO should include at least three views: 65° dorsopalmar and the medial and the lateral oblique projections.[12] The radiographic signs associated with nonseptic PO include demineralization, widening of the nutrient foramina at the solar margin, and irregular bone formation along the solar margins of the dorsal surface of the distal phalanx[13] (Fig. 8.56). Osseous proliferation of the solar margin of the distal phalanx is thought to develop secondary to prolonged inflammation. Radiographs alone should not be used to make the diagnosis, since some unaffected horses will have similar changes. In one study done on 31 normal horses to evaluate the range of radiographic changes observed in the distal phalanx, researchers found that there was a large degree of variation in the number and size of the vascular channels and that the solar border of the distal phalanx appears more regular on the oblique projections than on the 65° dorsopalmar projection.[12] The degree of roughening can also vary from the medial to the lateral, and

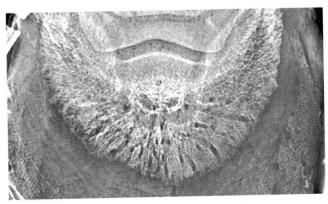

Figure 8.56   Horse with a nonseptic PO.

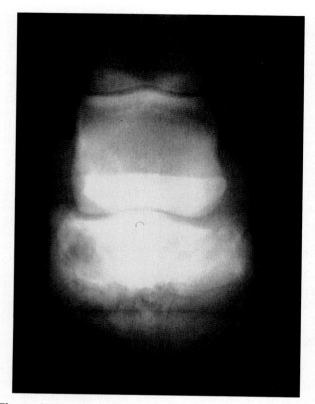

Figure 8.57 Horse with septic PO. Note the bone lysis (arrows) and the indistinct bone margins.

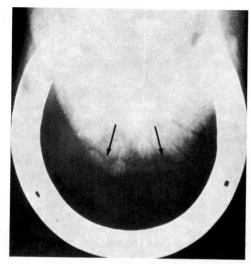

Figure 8.58 Septic PO associated with solar margin fractures. This condition resulted from a puncture wound to the foot that caused a subsolar abscess.

the lateral border usually appears more roughened when a variation exists.[12] Care should also be taken not to confuse the normal notch (crena) of the toe of the distal phalanx. Roughened ridged areas along the solar border of the distal phalanx may appear anywhere from the toe to the lateral wings. These ridges are not normally smooth because of vascular patterns in the bone, and when vascular patterns are present, careful evaluation must be made. The conclusion from the study was that the diagnosis of diffuse PO with radiographs alone was tenuous and that the diagnosis of PO should be made only when physical signs concur with the radiographic findings.[7,12] In a scintigraphic study evaluating the distal limb changes in horses whose lameness were blocked out with palmar digital nerve blocks, researchers found that changes associated with PO were uncommon and suggested that the condition may be overdiagnosed.[14]

Radiographic signs of septic PO are usually straightforward. Generally, there is a loss of trabecular detail, with indistinct margins fading into the surrounding bone.[12,15] Marginal sclerosis is rarely observed in cases in which sequestra develop[8] (Fig. 8.57). Radiographic examination of 18 horses diagnosed with septic PO revealed discrete osteolysis at the margins of the distal phalanx in 13 of 18 cases; gas density in adjacent bone on two different radiographic projections in 15 of 18 cases; decrease in bone density, focal in 9 of 18 and diffuse in 3 of 18; generalized roughening of the solar margin of the distal phalanx in 7 of 18; and widening of the vascular channels in 13 of 18.[2] In this study, sequestra were identified in 4 horses, and a solar margin fracture and a plan-

tar eminence fracture were observed in 1 horse each (Fig. 8.58 and Fig. 8.61).

Treatment

Treatment of nonseptic PO depends on the cause, the use of the horse, and environmental factors. If severe or chronic solar bruising is the primary cause, treatment is aimed at reducing the inflammation and minimizing the concussion to the foot.[9] Rest, the administration of nonsteroidal anti-inflammatory drugs (NSAIDs), and the avoidance of exercise on hard rocky surfaces are logical and often helpful but may not provide a long-term solution.[9] The application of protective shoes may be all that is needed. A handmade, wide-web, egg-bar shoe whose solar surface is deeply concave is most useful.[9] This shoe keeps the injured sole from contacting the ground and prevents pressure from being applied to it. The toe of the shoe can be squared to enhance breakover. Alternatively, full pads can be applied to reduce concussion and to protect the injured sole. (Refer to Chapter 9 for more information.) In horses in which the sole is thin and soft, the sole can be medicated topically with equal parts of phenol, formalin, and iodine to toughen them. If pathologic fracture of the distal phalanx is associated with PO, a prolonged convalescence will be required. Rest and avoiding exercise on hard rocky surfaces are indicated until the lameness subsides. Exercising on softer track surfaces, such as wood chips, or swimming the horse to maintain fitness may allow the horse to continue training until the lameness resolves. The primary cause should always be treated first. Palmar digital neurectomy is only recommended in cases that do not respond to more conservative measures. The effectiveness of the neurectomy should be documented by perineural anesthesia of the palmar digital nerves prior to performing the neurectomy.

Treatment of septic PO involves surgical debridement of the tract, if present, and the removal of infected bone.

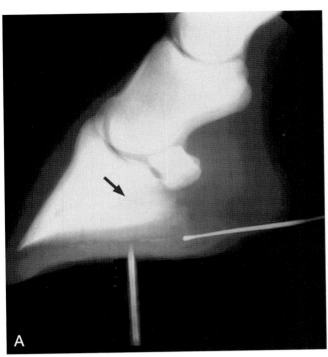

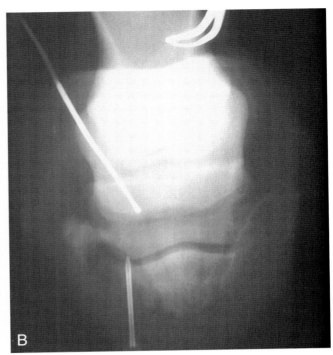

Figure 8.59   A. Lateral view showing two markers in place. The bone lysis is barely seen in this view (arrow) B. Dorsopalmar view showing the markers in place. These two views and the markers are used to document the lesion location in the distal phalanx for the surgical approach.

If the solar surface of the distal phalanx is involved, the procedure can be done while the horse is standing. If the infection is deep seated in the distal phalanx, general anesthesia is recommended. In all cases the foot should be cleaned and prepared aseptically for the procedure. A tourniquet should be applied in the midpastern region. If the procedure is done in the standing horse, appropriate sedation and perineural anesthesia at the proximal sesamoid bones are used. In cases in which there is no draining tract, metal markers or probes can be used to guide the exploration. At least two radiographic views are recommended to document the location of the abscess (Fig. 8.59) In most cases, the abscess is approached through the sole, and a 1- to 2-cm opening with a sterile hoof knife or scalpel blade is used. The debridement is continued until all the infected bone is removed. Infected bone appears grayer and is softer than the normal soft bone of the normal distal phalanx. Some have recommended radiographic monitoring to document complete removal of the infected bone.[2] A sample of bone should be taken and submitted for culture and sensitivity. Once curettage is complete, the tract is packed with gauze soaked in dilute povidone iodine, and a protective bandage is applied. Duct tape can be applied to the bottom of the bandage to make it waterproof. Alternatively, a plastic or rubber boot can be applied to protect the bandage. Dressings are changed daily until the exudative response is no longer apparent. Usually at this time, a healthy bed of granulation tissue is forming. Bandage changes can be done every 3 to 4 days. A shoe with a removable metal plate (refer to Chapter 9 for a discussion of treatment plates) can be applied. A broad spectrum is recommended and continued until a healthy bed

of granulation tissue forms and the exudative process has ceased. In one study in which researchers evaluated the outcome of cases with septic PO, they found that most of the bacterial isolates were sensitive to metronidazole, and therefore, they recommended its use in all cases.[2] In another study, researchers found that as much as 24% of the distal phalanx could be removed without long-term adverse effects.[4]

Prognosis

The prognosis for nonseptic PO is good if the condition is primary and of a relatively short duration and the horse's environment can be controlled. The prognosis is unfavorable if the disease is chronic and the horse must continue to compete on hard surfaces. The prognosis for secondary causes of nonseptic PO depends on the response of the primary to treatment.

The prognosis for septic PO appears good if the infection is controlled. Of 33 cases of septic PO in which follow-up was available, all 33 horses returned to their intended use.[8] Other studies had similar results. In one study, 7 of 9 horses returned to their intended use,[4] and in another, 17 of 18 had a favorable outcome despite a high incidence of sequestra and fractures.[2]

References

1. Chaffin MK. Pedal osteitis. In: White NA, Moore JN, Eds. Current Techniques in Equine Surgery and Lameness. 2nd ed. Philadelphia: WB Saunders, 1998;530–531.
2. Cauvin ERJ, Munroe GA. Septic osteitis of the distal phalanx: Findings and surgical treatment in 18 cases. Equine Vet J 1998; 30:512–519.

3. DeBowes RM, Yovich JV. Penetrating wounds, abscesses, gravel, and bruising of the equine foot. Vet Clin North Am Equine Pract 1989;5:179–194.
4. Gaughn EM, Rendano VT, Ducharme NG. Surgical treatment of septic pedal osteitis in horses: Nine cases (1980–1987). J Am Vet Med Assoc 1989;195:1131–1134.
5. Honnas CM. Standing surgical procedures of the foot. Vet Clin North Am Equine Pract 1991;7:695–722.
6. Honnas CM, Peloso JG, Carter GK, et al. Diagnosing and treating septic conditions of the equine foot. Vet Med 1994;89:1060–1071.
7. Johnson JH. The foot. In: Mansmann RA, McAllister ES, Eds. Equine Medicine and Surgery. 3rd ed. Santa Barbara, CA: American Veterinary Publications, 1982;1041.
8. Lindford S, Embertson R, Bramlage L. Septic osteitis of the third phalanx: A review of 63 cases. Proc Am Assoc Equine Pract 1994; 40:103.
9. Moyer W. Non-septic pedal osteitis: A cause of lameness and a diagnosis. Proc Am Assoc Equine Pract 1999;45:178–179.
10. Moyer W. Traumatic pedal osteitis (TPO) in racehorses. Proc Am Assoc Equine Pract 1988;34:417–419.
11. Pool RR. Gross, histologic and ultrastructural pathology of disorders of the distal extremity. Proceedings of the 13th Bain-Fallon Memorial Lectures, 1991;25–31.
12. Rendano VT, Grant B. The equine third phalanx: Its radiographic appearance. Am J Vet Radiol Soc 1978;19:125–135.
13. Reeves MJ, Yovich JV, Turner AS. Miscellaneous conditions of the equine foot. Vet Clin North Am Equine Pract 1989;5:221–242.
14. Ross MW. Observations in horses with lameness abolished by palmar digital analgesia. Proc Am Assoc Equine Pract 1998;44: 230–232.
15. Waters JW, Lebel JL, Park RD. Morphometric analysis of radiographic changes in the distal phalanges of Quarter horses with lower leg lameness. Am J Vet Radiol Soc 1978;19:60.

SUBCHONDRAL BONE CYSTS OF THE DISTAL (THIRD) PHALANX

Subchondral bone cysts of the distal (third) phalanx are uncommon and can affect horses of various breeds and all ages.[4,5,8,9] Affected horses are usually intermittently lame, and the forelimbs are more frequently affected than the hindlimbs. Verschooten and DeMoor[8] reported on 15 cases of subchondral bone cysts involving the distal phalanx, 14 of which were located in the forelimb. In another study, cysts in the distal phalanx were in the forelimbs in 27 of 28 cases.[2] Other terms such as subchondral cysts,[3,5] periarticular subchondral bone cysts,[3,4] and bone cysts[1] have been used as synonyms to describe the radiolucent area of bone located adjacent to the articular surface.[9] In the strictest sense, however, these lesions are not typical of cysts because they are not lined with a distinct membrane. Another interesting feature is that the communication with the adjacent joint space is also variable.[5,8,9] Subchondral bone cysts have been reported to affect other longbones,[4,5] smaller articular bones,[9] and the navicular bone.[3] For more information, refer to Chapter 7, "Osteochondrosis."

Etiology

The cause of subchondral bone cysts is unclear, although there are several proposed theories. One theory holds that infection is a plausible cause,[5] but the clinical observations do not support this. In horses in which the lesions communicate with the joint, there is no infectious arthritis. Also, cysts that have been monitored radiographically for years do not have a tendency to expand, and no evidence of infection has been found on histopathologic examination.[4,5,9]

Another theory holds that trauma is the most likely cause.[4,5,8,9] The fact that horses perform for years before a cyst is diagnosed supports this theory.[9] It is proposed that damage to the articular joint cartilage through repeated stress may allow joint fluid to pass through an opening to the subchondral bone.[8] Although subchondral bone cysts in humans develop in bone adjacent to osteoarthritic joints,[6] this does not seem the case in the horse.[8] Alternatively, subchondral bone may be weakened from a vascular accident or a previous infection to allow the synovial fluid to break through the normal cartilage when under pressure.[8] Histopathologic examination does not support this because no bone necrosis has been observed.[4,5,9] Additionally, subchondral bone cysts do not always communicate with the joint.[8,9] The basic question as to whether the lesion develops in normal bone or whether a preexisting lesion exists remains unanswered.

Another theory that merits comment holds that an osteochondrosis lesion precedes the development of a bone cyst. This has been discounted by some because older horses are affected.[8,9] However, it is conceivable that an osteochondrosis lesion remains quiescent for prolonged periods and that recent trauma may be sufficient to cause a cleavage in the articular surface and a bone cyst to develop. Histopathologic studies have not been enlightening, and various cell types and collagen stroma have been described.[4,5,8,9]

Signs

A history of an acute onset of lameness with a chronic course of intermittent lameness is common. Often, lameness subsides with rest and recurs with exercise. It is conjectured that the intermittence may be caused by reinjury of the cartilage roof of the cyst. At exercise, variable degrees of lameness are noticed. The digital pulse rate often is elevated, and the phalangeal flexion test is usually positive.[2] Hoof tester examination is not reliable for identification of this problem. Usually, large cysts that extend to the solar surface of the distal phalanx are responsive to hoof tester examination, whereas deep-seated cysts within the bone will not respond to hoof tester pressure. Although perineural anesthesia of the palmar digital nerve at the midpastern will remove the lameness in some cases, perineural anesthesia performed at the base of the sesamoid bones is more reliable. A pastern ring block is also helpful, and in most cases, intrasynovial anesthesia of the coffin joint removes the lameness if the cyst is subchondral and communicates with the joint.[8]

Diagnosis

Variable sizes of cystic lesions are identified radiographically within the body of the distal phalanx (Fig. 8.60). Arthrographic[9] and morphologic studies[4,5] indicate that the communication between the cyst and the joint is variable. Analysis of the synovial fluid in these cases is unrewarding.[9] In one study, researchers found that in 18 of 27 cases the cyst was located central in the distal phalanx and that communication with distal interphalangeal joint was observed in all cases.[2]

Treatment

Recommended treatments of subchondral bone cysts have included 1) enforced rest, 2) complete stall rest followed by increasing exercise,[4,5] 3) surgical curettage,[1,9] and 4) surgical curettage and packing the cyst with an autogenous bone graft.[7] Although the results in all these cases have been variable, surgical curettage with or without a bone graft seems the best method.

Prior to surgery, enough radiographic views should be taken to ensure the cyst's exact location. The day before surgery, the foot is trimmed, the sole and frog are pared out, and the hair is clipped from the coronet to above the fetlock. The outer hoof wall should be rasped smooth over the area proposed for surgical entry. After the hoof wall is scrubbed with povidone iodine soap the foot is soaked in a povidone iodine solution for 15 minutes, after which it is placed in an antiseptic bandage.

On the following day, the horse is anesthetized and placed in lateral recumbency, with the lesion uppermost, and a pneumatic tourniquet is applied. An Esmarch bandage can precede the tourniquet application to remove all the blood from the limb. After aseptic preparation of the hoof, the surgeon applies a sterile adhesive plastic drape. The foot should be thoroughly dried before the adhesive drape application. The foot is further isolated with drapes of the surgeon's choice. A hole is made in the hoof wall (epidermal lamina) with a trephine or air drill over the cyst. Radiographic documentation can be used if the surgeon is unsure of the exact location. The dermal laminae are then incised with the scalpel blade, and the cyst is penetrated with a small curette. Again, radiographic monitoring may be helpful. Once the cyst is identified, it is curetted until healthy bleeding bone is encountered. A definite difference between the soft cystic bone and the hard normal bone can be appreciated. After curettage is complete, a 16-gauge needle may be used to make holes in the normal bone to stimulate more rapid healing.[9] Care should be taken so the coffin joint is not penetrated during the curettage. The remaining cavity is flushed and packed with autogenous bone graft or with gauze soaked in dilute povidone iodine solution after which a sterile dressing is applied. Alternatively, the cavity can be packed with cancellous bone to enhance healing.[1,7]

Postoperatively, the bandage is changed daily for the first week. The povidone iodine soaked gauze is removed and replaced. This should be done aseptically. After a week or so the bandage is changed every third to fourth day until the granulation tissue that forms approximates the epidermal laminae. As healing progresses the povidone iodine packs are made smaller and are placed more loosely in the bone cavity. The foot must be protected and the horse rested until the hoof wall defect disappears at the solar surface.

Prognosis

Good results have been achieved at our clinic and at others in a limited number of cases with the surgical

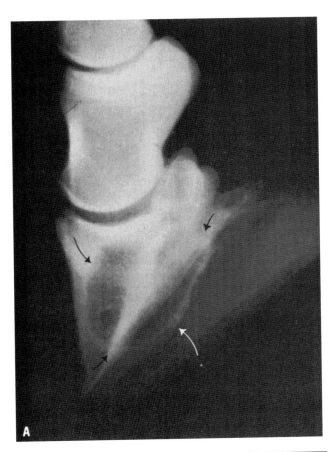
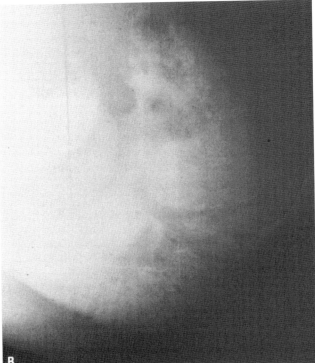

Figure 8.60   A. Large cyst involving the distal phalanx (arrows). B. An oblique view of the distal phalanx. Multiple small cysts involving the palmar process of the distal phalanx are present.

technique described, without packing the cyst with a bone graft. However, a local infection has been a consistent complication in three separate cases. The infection can be observed early or late when the hole in the hoof wall reaches the solar surface.[9] All cases have responded to systemic and local therapy. In most, there is radiographic evidence of the cysts filling in between 30 and 90 days, postoperatively.[4,8] In the one report that used an autogenous bone graft to pack the remaining cyst cavity, the horse returned to race training after 6 months.[7]

References

1. Evans LH, Jenny J. Surgical and clinical management of subchondral "bone cysts". Proc Am Assoc Equine Pract 1970;16:195.
2. Haack D, Hertsch B, Baez C. Cyst like defects in the coffin bone of horses. Pferdeheilkunde 1988;4:143–148.
3. Merriam JG, Johnson JH. Subchondral cysts of the navicular bone as a cause of lameness. Vet Med Small Anim Clin 1974;69:873.
4. Pettersson H, Reiland S. Periarticular subchondral "bone cysts" in horses. Proc Am Assoc Equine Pract 1968;14:245.
5. Pettersson H, Sevelius F. Subchondral bone cysts in the horse: Clinical study. Equine Vet J 1968;1:75.
6. Landells JW. Bone cysts in osteoarthritis. J Bone Joint Surg 1953; 35B:643
7. Stanek C, Edinger H. Surgical treatment of a subchondral bone cyst of the third phalanx in a Standardbred gelding by use of an autogenous bone graft. Wien Tierarztl Monatsschr 1990;77:198–202.
8. Verschooten F, DeMoor A. Subchondral cystic and related lesions affecting the equine pedal bone and stifle. Equine Vet J 1982;14:471.
9. Wagner PC, et al. Surgical management of subchondral bone cysts of the third phalanx in the horse. Equine Pract 1982;4:9.

FRACTURES OF THE DISTAL (THIRD) PHALANX (PEDAL BONE, OS PEDIS, COFFIN BONE)

Fractures of the distal (third) phalanx are uncommon.[2,25,31,32] In racehorses, the injury is usually associated with exercise on hard tracks, and the forefeet, particularly the left forefoot, seem predisposed in horses who race counterclockwise.[31,32] Two retrospective studies indicate that the incidence of fractures of the distal phalanx is 7 in 2,166 cases[32] presented for forefoot problems; another report identified 65 in 20,638 cases admitted to a hospital.[31] Of the 65 cases of distal phalanx fracture, 57 were in the forelimbs; 57 of 65 (89.5%) fractures affected the lateral wing of the left distal phalanx or the medial wing of the right distal phalanx; and 53 of 65 (82%) fractures entered the coffin joint.[31] Although all breeds and classes of horses are affected, a higher incidence has been observed in racing breeds, and at least two reports identified an increased incidence for Thoroughbred and Standardbred horses.[31,32].

Although distal phalanx fractures can assume various configurations, there are basically seven types of fractures that affect the distal phalanx. Type 1 fractures are nonarticular oblique palmar or plantar process (wing) fractures (Fig. 8.61) and are reported to be the second[31,32] and fourth[15] most common types. Type 2 fractures are articular oblique palmar or plantar process (wing) fractures (Fig. 8.62) and are the most common type.[31] Type 3 fractures are sagittal articular fractures

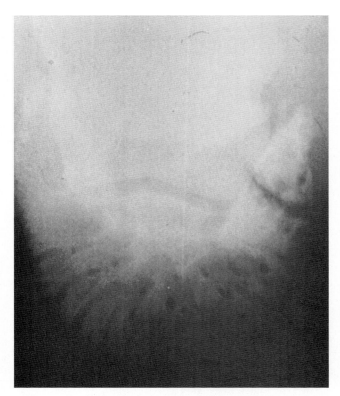

Figure 8.61 Dorsal palmar view of a type 1 nonarticular fracture of the distal phalanx.

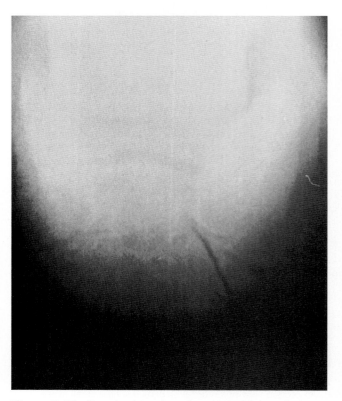

Figure 8.62 Dorsal palmar view of a type 2 oblique articular fracture of the distal phalanx.

that roughly divide the distal phalanx into two separate halves (Fig. 8.63); these fractures are uncommon and represent 3 to 4% of fractures of the distal phalanx.[12,31] Type 4 fractures are articular fractures involving the extensor process. They occur most frequently in the forelimbs and occasionally occur bilaterally.[12,33] For more information, refer to "Extensor Process (Type 4) Fractures of the Distal (Third) Phalanx" in this chapter. Type 5 fractures are comminuted articular and nonarticular fractures (Fig. 8.64). Type 6 fractures are nonarticular solar margin fractures of the distal phalanx (Fig. 8.65). These were reported to be the most common fracture

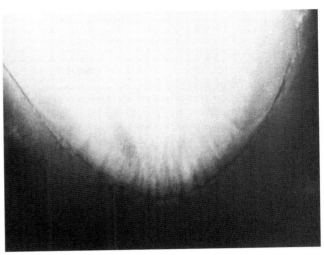

Figure 8.65   Dorsal palmar view of type 6 nonarticular solar margin fracture of the distal phalanx.

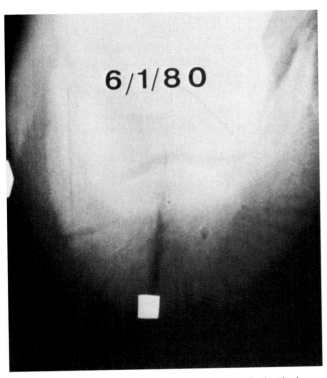

Figure 8.63   Dorsal palmar view of a type 3 sagittal articular fracture of the distal phalanx.

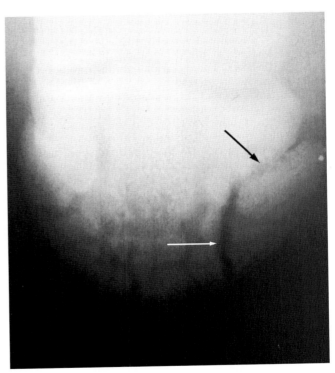

Figure 8.66   Dorsal palmar view of a type 7 nonarticular fracture of the palmar process of the distal phalanx (arrows).

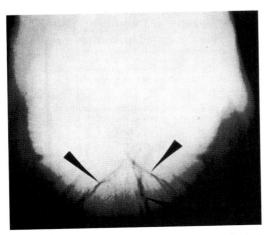

Figure 8.64   Dorsal palmar view of a type 5 comminuted articular fracture of the distal phalanx.

type in one study.[13] Type 7 fractures are most commonly seen in foals; they are nonarticular fractures of the palmar or plantar process of the distal phalanx. The fracture begins and ends at the solar margin, and they are either triangular or oblong (Fig. 8.66).[12,18,35] One study of 32 Thoroughbred foals (3 to 32 weeks of age) identified type 7 fractures in 19%.[18] Initially, these fractures were thought to represent osseous bodies; however, histologic findings in this study were consistent with a fracture.

Etiology

Trauma seems the predominant cause of fracture of the distal phalanx. Type 2 fractures in racing breeds affect the left lateral and the right medial processes; this is thought to be a direct result of the selective trauma to these regions during counterclockwise racing.[31,34] Type 3 midsagittal articular fractures are believed to result from direct trauma to the hoof from kicking a solid object.[31] Type 6 solar margin fractures may be related to the shape and location of the solar margin within the hoof and the tremendous forces the distal phalanx undergoes during weight bearing and work.[13] These fractures are also commonly seen with laminitis pedal osteitis (PO). Type 7 fractures seen in foals are thought to occur either as a result of compression on the solar or the dorsal cortex of the distal phalanx during weight bearing or as a result of tension forces generated by the deep digital flexor tendon (DDFT).[18] In a study done to evaluate the effect of hoof trimming on the occurrence of distal phalangeal palmar process fractures (type 7) in foals, researchers found that excessive trimming of the heels, sole, and frog did not affect the occurrence of these fractures.[20] Occasionally, the distal phalanx may be fractured as a result of the penetration of a foreign body through the sole.[9] The distal phalanx also may be fractured as the result of trauma to a large sidebone (Fig. 8.67). In such a case, the phalanx may break through one of the lateral processes.

Although trauma is regarded as the primary cause of fractures of the distal phalanx, other factors such as stone bruises, hard surfaces, improper shoeing, infectious conditions, and nutritional deficiencies have been implicated.[1,6,26,27,29,32] Type 6 solar margin fractures can develop as a result of trauma or can be secondary to laminitis or PO.[15] Type 5 comminuted fractures can develop secondary to septic osteitis with or without sequestra formation.[4]

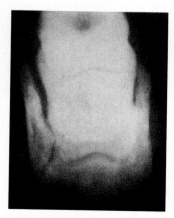

Figure 8.67 Fracture of the distal phalanx through one of the lateral wings. This horse had large sidebones. A cow stepped on the horse's foot, causing fracture of the distal phalanx on the left side. (Reprinted with permission from Gillette EL, Thrall DE, Lebel JL, Eds. Carlson's Veterinary Radiology. 3rd ed. Philadelphia: Lea & Febiger, 1977.)

Signs

Generally, the clinical signs during the acute phases are similar for all types of fractures of the distal phalanx, and a history of acute onset of a moderate to severe lameness is common.[5,11,22] In some cases, the lameness worsens within the first 24 hours after injury, presumably because of increased pressure within the hoof capsule secondary to inflammation and swelling. The degree of lameness is generally severe (grades 4 to 5 of 5); exceptions to this are type 6 and 7 fractures. Lameness associated with type 6 fractures varies, depending on the presence or absence of an underlying lesion associated with the distal phalanx. In the absence of an underlying lesion, most horses with a solar margin fracture exhibit a mild to moderate lameness.[13] Also, type 7 fractures generally result in a mild (grades 1 to 2 of 5) lameness.[20] In all cases, if the fracture has been present for some time, signs of lameness usually are diminished.

On palpation, an increased digital pulse may be felt, and if the fracture is paramedian, the pulse may increase most on the affected side.[5] An increase in temperature of the affected foot may also be appreciated. With articular fractures, coffin joint effusion may be observed and may be palpable dorsal and proximal to the coronet band. If the articular fracture is acute, swelling and edema may also be present in the region of the coronary band. Hoof tester examination usually reveals pain over the sole region, and focal pressure over the fracture site usually induces a obvious painful response. A negative hoof tester response, however, does not rule out the presence of a distal phalanx fracture.[14,19] Perineural anesthesia of the palmar or plantar digital nerves may aid in localizing the lameness to the foot region, and coffin joint synovial fluid analysis can help confirm an intraarticular fracture. Generally, regional anesthesia is not necessary to diagnose type 2 and 3 fractures because the clinical signs are sufficient to localize the pain to the foot region.

Differential diagnoses include sole bruising, PO, puncture wounds, foot abscesses, laminitis, navicular syndrome, and septic arthritis.

Diagnosis

Radiographic examination (30° dorsopalmar or dorsoplantar, 65° dorsoproximal-palmarodistal, lateral, and both obliques) are used to confirm the diagnosis and to document the type and location of the fracture.[23] In some cases it may be necessary to take special views of the palmar or plantar processes to identify the fracture. Solar margin fractures are most easily identified on the 65° dorsoproximal-palmarodistal projection with a radiographic technique with approximately one-half the exposure needed to evaluate the navicular bone.[12] A fracture of the distal phalanx may not be seen on the initial radiographic examination because of the insufficient time for resorption of the bone along the fracture line and because of the castlike effect of the hoof wall, which prevents the fragments from distracting.[12] In such a case, radiographs should be repeated in 10 to 12 days. This is usually sufficient time for bone resorption along the fracture line to occur, making the identification of a fracture more likely.

Alternatively, nuclear scintigraphy can be used to help identify radiographically occult fractures of the coffin bone. In a scintigraphic study done to evaluate fractures of the distal phalanx in 27 horses, researchers found that the palmar scintigraphic views had evidence of focal areas of increased ^{99m}Tc-methylene diphosphonate (MDP) uptake that corresponded to fracture line location on radiography.[22] Lateral views of the distal phalanx, on the other hand, had a diffuse pattern of uptake. An association between the duration of the fracture and the intensity of the uptake was also identified. All fractures of less than 10 days duration had intense focal uptake, whereas fractures of less than 3 months duration most often had increased uptake. As time passed, the uptake became less intense and more diffuse. In this study, 3 horses with fractures not evident on radiographic examination had focal evidence of ^{99m}Tc-MDP uptake on scintigraphy. In all cases, increased uptake of the radionuclide was evident 25 months after injury. It was concluded that bone phase scintigraphy can identify acute distal phalangeal fractures before they are visible on radiography and may be of benefit in assessing convalescent time.

Treatment

Nonarticular Fractures (Types 1, 5, 6, and 7)

Treatment of types 1 and 5 fractures is aimed at immobilizing the fracture and preventing expansion of the hoof wall. To do this, the distal phalanx can be immobilized by the use of a full bar shoe with quarter clips (Figs. 8.68 and 8.69). The bar should be placed on the shoe so that it is recessed from the frog and no frog pressure results. The quarter clips should be welded to or drawn on the outside of the branches of the shoe near the junc-

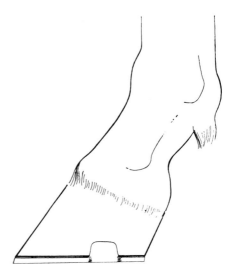

Figure 8.69   Side view of shoe used for distal phalanx fracture, showing quarter clip in place.

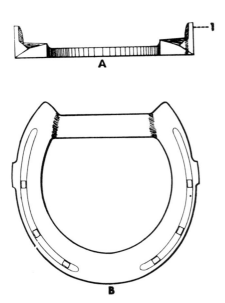

Figure 8.68   Full bar shoe used in case of fracture of the distal phalanx. A. Rear view of shoe showing quarter clips (1). B. Ground surface view of the shoe, showing full bar and quarter clips welded to shoe.

tion of the heel and quarters. This prevents the quarters from expanding and, when combined with the bar to prevent frog pressure, reduces movement of the phalanx. The foot should be kept in this type of shoe for 6 to 8 months, with the shoe reset every 4 to 6 weeks. After clinical relief of the symptoms, the horse should be shod either with quarter clips or with a bar shoe to prevent hoof wall expansion. Some horses require continued use of bar shoes with quarter clips to ensure working soundness. The affected horse should not be worked for approximately 8 to 10 months, and in some cases, 1 year of rest may be advisable if symptoms do not disappear. Alternatively, the foot can be placed in a continuous rim-type shoe or a Klimesh contiguous clip shoe (refer to Chapter 9 for more information), or it can be confined in fiberglass hoof tape (Figs. 8.70 and 8.71).[3,15,17,24,32] All of these approaches appear to effectively prevent the expansion of the hoof wall during weight bearing. One case of a comminuted frontal plane fracture was treated successfully by the application of a 3° wedge pad to the bottom of the foot, after which fiberglass hoof tape was applied to restrict hoof expansion and to hold the wedge in place. The heel wedge was used to prevent tension in the DDFT from causing distraction of the fracture.[3]

Treatment of type 6 solar margin fractures depends on whether the condition is primary or secondary to a chronic foot disorder (e.g., laminitis or PO). Primary causes of solar margin fractures are treated with wide-web shoes, pads, and stall or paddock rest for 4 to 12 months.[13] Strict immobilization with bar shoes and quarter clips is not necessary. Prolonged rest seems necessary to ensure the best fracture healing. If the cause is secondary, then treatment is directed at the underlying cause initially, followed by management of the solar margin fracture.[13]

Type 7 nonarticular fractures in foals usually heal satisfactorily when the foal is confined for 6 to 8 weeks. Exercise should be restricted until radiographic evidence of bony union is evident, which is usually observed at approximately 8 weeks after the diagnosis.[20] Applica-

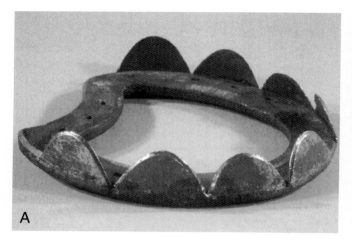

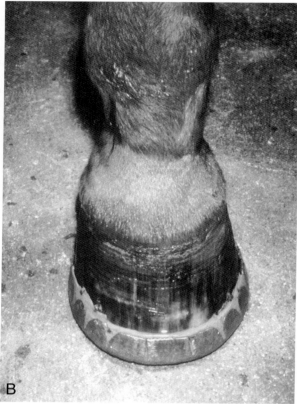

Figure 8.70 A. Contiguous slip shoe. B. Contiguous clip shoe after it has been placed on the foot. It is held in place with acrylic.

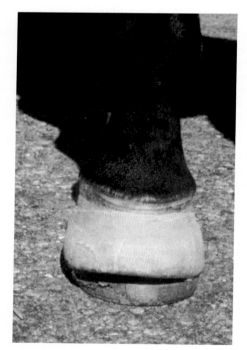

Figure 8.71 Fiberglass hoof tape. (Courtesy of Dr. Gayle Trotter.)

tion of restrictive external coaptation (e.g., bar shoe, or acrylic) to the hoof is not recommended because of the severe heel contraction that can occur and the potential for the hoof to slough.[35]

If the fracture has been caused by a puncture wound or is secondary to a septic osteitis or if a sequestrum is present, then treatment includes debridement of the infected bone, ventral drainage of the infected area, and support of the hoof with shoes, clips, and a sole treatment plate. Cancellous bone may be packed into the bone defect after debridement to enhance healing.[21]

In some cases of persistent lameness resulting from fracture of the distal phalanx, neurectomy of the palmar digital nerves may afford enough relief so that the horse can be returned to full use. The success of this operation can be determined beforehand by blocking the palmar digital nerves with a suitable local anesthetic.

Articular Fractures (Types 2 and 3)

Foals less than 6 months of age should be treated with stall confinement.[35] Treatment that restricts the expansion of the hoof is unnecessary and may result in severe hoof contraction. Foals should be confined for 6 to 8 weeks, and their exercise should be restricted until bony union of the fracture is observed radiographically. Fracture healing should be evident by 8 weeks and complete by 15 weeks or less.

Horses 6 months of age and older with types 2 and 3 articular fractures can be treated conservatively or surgically. Conservative treatment consisting of rest and the application of bar shoes with clips, complete rim-type bar shoes, fiberglass hoof tape, or encircling wires around the hoof and the application of a foot board and hoof acrylic to limit the hoof expansion during weight bearing has been recommended.[12,27,30,34] Regional anesthesia at the level of the proximal sesamoid bones aid in the application of a shoe. Many horses walk comfortably shortly after the hoof has been immobilized because the fracture becomes stable.[12] Bony union usually begins at the solar margin and progresses proximad toward the articular surface of the distal phalanx.[12] Generally, 6 to 12 months are needed for complete bony union to be achieved.[12,27,34] Even after the fracture appears healed radiographically, the horse should continue to be shod with a bar shoe during its remaining athletic career because refracture has been reported after shoe removal. Although conservative treatment of these articular fractures does not compress the fracture or ensure accurate anatomic reduction of the articular surface, most of the fractures heal after immobilization and rest. In some cases, however, residual degenerative joint disease (DJD) of the distal interphalangeal joint from these fractures may limit future athletic endeavors.[14] Nevertheless, approximately 50% of the horses with these types of fractures return to soundness with conservative treatment.[12,15,27,31,34] Horses younger than 3 years of age appear to have a better prognosis for return to performance, presumably because of a greater potential for healing.[27]

Horses 3 years and older with fresh (less than 5 days duration) types 2 and 3 articular fractures that are close to the midline are considered candidates for internal fixation with a single lag screw.[5,8,10,17,28] Fractures older than 5 days fill with fibrous tissue, making it difficult to reduce the fracture. Also, for internal fixation to be considered an option, the smaller fragment must have enough bone substance to hold a screw and not split when the screw is tightened.[14] A major risk with this procedure is the possibility of infection developing around the implant. If the infection extends to the fracture line and into the coffin joint, it may render the horse useless, and euthanasia may be indicated.[14]

The day before surgery the hoof should be trimmed and balanced with its wall lightly rasped and cleaned, after which the foot is placed in a povidone iodine–soaked bandage for 24 hours before surgery. Some have advocated applying a bar shoe with quarter clips to the foot prior to surgery.[17] The rationale is to prevent foot expansion immediately after recovery from surgery. Broad-spectrum antimicrobial drugs are administered prior to surgery and continued for at least 5 to 7 days. The surgeon determines the correct position for screw placement either before or at surgery by obtaining radiographs of the foot once radiographic markers have been applied to the hoof wall (Fig. 8.72).[17] Generally, multiple radiographs are required. Alternatively, fluoroscopy can be used during the surgery to determine the proper screw location. The correct site for screw placement is midway between the articular surface and the solar canal.[7,8] Once this location is identified, the surgeon applies a tourniquet to the distal limb. The screw can be placed freehand or with the aid of a C-clamp applied across the hoof wall.[16] When the screw is placed freehand, a small tre-

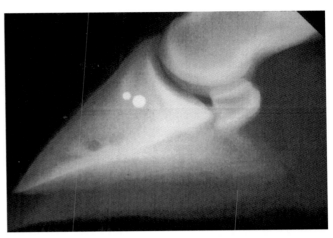

Figure 8.72 Radiographic markers are placed in the hoof to identify the correct position for screw placement.

phine (10 mm) or drill hole is made in the hoof wall to the surface of the distal phalanx. The depth of the outer hoof wall to the distal phalanx is determined, and this distance is doubled and subtracted from a measurement of the width of the hoof at that location. This calculation can provide an approximate estimate of the screw length.[5] A Kirschner wire can be directed through the distal phalanx to determine if the proper location and direction for screw placement have been selected. A 4.5- or 5.5-mm glide hole is drilled to the fracture gap under radiographic or fluoroscopic guidance. If the fracture is significantly displaced, the halves of the distal phalanx can be manipulated from the articular surface to improve the reduction prior to making the thread hole (Fig. 8.73).[5] An appropriate diameter pilot hole is then drilled and tapped. Care is taken not to drill too far and penetrate the laminae on the opposite side. The glide hole is countersunk to allow the screw head to be seated flush with the bone. The depth of the hole is measured, and a screw approximately 5 mm shorter than the drilled hole is selected and inserted.[15] The screw should not be overtightened because the threads easily strip in the soft bone (Figs. 8.74 and 8.75). After surgery, the trephine hole is packed with sterile gauze sponges soaked with antibacterial solution or with a dilute antiseptic solution, and a protective sterile waterproof bandage is applied to the foot. Initially, bandages are changed daily or every other day until a healthy bed of granulation tissue is seen; this granulation usually appears in approximately 2 weeks. At this time, the tissue in the trephine hole can be desiccated and prompted to cornify by application of a solution containing equal parts of 10% formalin and 7% iodine.[14] An alternative approach to managing the trephine hole is to pack it with an autogenous bone graft.[14] It is thought that the bone graft may form a scaffold and cells for the formation of granulation tissue. A bar shoe with clips or a rim shoe should be applied to the foot to provide additional support for healing.

Horses should be confined to box stall rest for 2 months, then to box stall rest with hand walking for 2 months. At 4 months, if the horse is sound, paddock exercise is allowed for 2 more months.[5] Radiographs at this time should show a healed fracture. Complete frac-

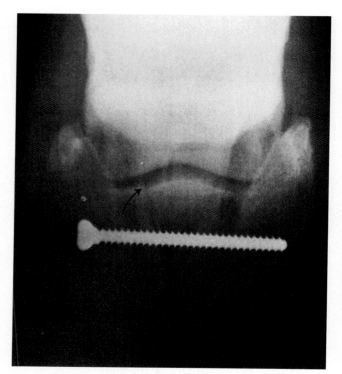

Figure 8.73 An ASIF cortical bone screw was used to repair this sagittal articular fracture of the distal phalanx. Unfortunately, a step in the articular surface remains (arrow). This will most likely result in degenerative joint disease of the coffin joint. (Courtesy of Dr. John Yovich.)

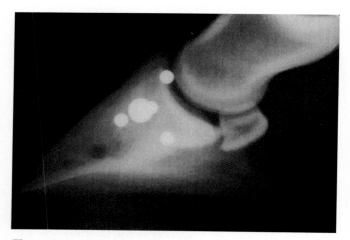

Figure 8.74 Lateral view of markers and ASIF cortical screws in place.

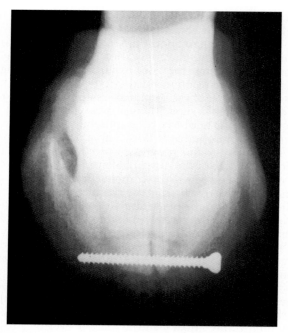

Figure 8.75 Dorsal palmar view of an ASIF cortical bone screw in place. Note the bone lysis adjacent to the head of the screw.

ture healing can be expected in 6 to 12 months, and the screw may have to be removed if lameness persists or if infection around the implant is evident.[15,26,27]

Pettersson[27] reported on 11 cases of articular fracture that were successfully treated by internal fixation. Others, however, have expressed concerns with this technique because of the increased chance of infection[31] and the possibility of creating a permanent step in the articular surface that would be undesirable (Fig. 8.73).[34] Al-

though internal fixation may improve the odds of fracture healing, particularly at the articular margin, it does not ensure that healing will occur.[5] Since distal phalanx fractures that have healed by both conservative treatment and internal fixation have refractured after the horses have returned to racing, it is recommended that performance horses be maintained in corrective shoes to prevent hoof wall expansion while competing.[31]

Prognosis

Nonarticular Fractures (Types 1, 5, 6, and 7)

The prognosis for type 1 nonarticular and oblique palmar or plantar process fractures seems good for all ages of horses if sufficient rest is given.[19,20,31] For type 5 comminuted fractures, insufficient data are available at the time of this writing to establish a prognosis. However, one horse with a comminuted frontal-plane nonarticular fracture of the distal phalanx became sound at paddock exercise at 7 months after the injury and returned to performance after 12 months.[3] For type 6 solar margin fractures, the prognosis depends on the severity of the primary disease.[5,13] In one report, 6 of 9 horses returned to soundness.[13] For type 7 nonarticular fractures in foals, the prognosis seems excellent for return to performance, and fracture healing is expected in approximately 8 weeks.[20,35]

Articular Fractures (Types 2 and 3)

For type 2 palmar or plantar process fractures treated conservatively (bar shoes and 6 months rest), a delay in performance training for 1 year results in soundness in approximately 50% of horses.[12,31,35] Scott et al.[31] found a correlation between the period of confinement of horses treated by conservative shoeing and the prognosis. Eight horses with a favorable outcome were confined to stall rest for a mean period of 6.4 months, 6 horses had a limited response to conservative therapy when only confined for an average of 5.5 months, and 7 horses experienced an unfavorable response for an average of 4.4 months. Since the outcome was independent of age, this is somewhat contrary to Pettersson's[27] finding in which a good prognosis for intraarticular fractures was expected in horses younger than 3 years of age and a guarded prognosis could be expected for horses older than 3 years of age. Moreover, 2 of 6 horses were euthanatized because of persistent chronic lameness 12 months after the fracture occurred.[27] The others were relegated to breeding status.

Variable results have been obtained from internal fixation of type 3 sagittal articular fractures.[14,26,27,31] Pettersson[26,27] reported that 11 of 11 horses older than 3 years of age with sagittal articular fractures of the distal phalanx treated with internal fixation became sound. Another report indicated favorable results in 2 of 5 cases in which lag screws were used. However, 1 horse refractured the distal phalanx after it was put back into training and the corrective shoe had been removed.

References

1. Adams OR. Lameness in Horses. 3rd ed. Philadelphia: Lea & Febiger, 1974.
2. Alexander JT, Rooney JR. The biomechanics, surgery and prognosis of equine fractures, 1967–1972. Proc Am Assoc Equine Pract 1972;18:219.
3. Anderson BH, Turner TA, Kobluk CN. Treatment of a comminuted frontal-plane fracture of the distal phalanx in a horse. J Am Vet Med Assoc 1996;209:1750–1752.
4. Baird AN, Seahorn TL, Morris EL. Equine distal phalangeal sequestration. Vet Radiol 1990;31:210–213.
5. Bertone AL. Fractures of the distal phalanx. In: Nixon AJ, Ed. Equine Fracture Repair. Philadelphia: WB Saunders, 1996; 146–152.
6. Dubs B, Nemeth F. Therapy and prognosis of pedal bone fractures. Schweiz Arch Tierheilkd 1972;114:423.
7. Fackelman GE. Sagittal fractures of the first phalanx (P1) in the horse: Fixation by the lag screw principle. Vet Med Small Anim Clin 1973;68:622.
8. Fackelman GE, Nunamaker DM. Manual of Internal Fixation in the Horse. New York: Springer-Verlag, 1982;61.
9. Febbl L. Suppurative osteomyelitis of the pedal bone in a Thoroughbred horse. Mil Med 1973;138:220.
10. Fessler JF, Amstutz HE. Fracture repair. In: Oehme FW, Prier LE, Eds. Textbook of Large Animal Surgery. Baltimore: Williams & Wilkins, 1974;294.
11. Heitsch VB. Diagnosis and treatment of pedal bone fractures. DTW Dtsch Tierärztl Wochenschr 1972;798:524.
12. Honnas CM, O'Brien TR, Linford RL. Distal phalanx fractures in horses: A survey of 274 horses with radiographic assessment of healing in 36 horses. Vet Radiol 1988;29:98–100.
13. Honnas CM, O'Brien T, Linford RL. Solar margin fractures of the equine distal phalanx. Proc Am Assoc Equine Pract 1987;33:399–410.
14. Honnas CM, Trotter GW. The distal interphalangeal joint. In: White NA, Moore JN, Eds. Current Techniques in Equine Surgery and Lameness. 2nd ed. Philadelphia: WB Saunders, 1998;389–397.
15. Honnas CM, Vacek JR, Schumacher J. Diagnosis and treatment of articular fractures of the equine distal phalanx. Vet Med 1992;87:1208–1214.
16. Hunt RJ, Kobluk CN, Steckel R. Diseases of the foot. In: Kobluk CN, Ames TR, Geor IJ, Eds. The Horse: Diseases and Clinical Management. Philadelphia: WB Saunders, 1955;682–684.
17. Johnson JH. The Foot. In: Mansmann RA, McAllister ES, Eds. Equine Medicine and Surgery. 3rd ed. Santa Barbara, CA: American Veterinary Publications, 1982;1042.
18. Kaneps AJ, O'Brien TR, Redden RF, et al. Characterization of osseous bodies of the distal phalanx of foals. Equine Vet J 1993;25:285–292.
19. Kaneps AJ, O'Brien TR, Redden RF, et al. Characterization of osseous bodies of the distal phalanx of foals. Proc Am Assoc Equine Pract 1992;38:283–284.
20. Kaneps AJ, O'Brien TR, Willits NH, et al. Effect of hoof trimming on the occurrence of distal phalangeal palmar process fractures in foals. Proc Am Assoc Equine Pract 1995;41:251–252.
21. Kasari TR, Taylor TS, Baird AN, et al. Use of autogenous cancellous bone graft for treatment of osteolytic defects in the phalanges of three cattle. J Am Vet Med Assoc 1992;201:1053–1057.
22. Keegan KG, Twardock AR, Losonsky JM, et al. Scintigraphic evaluation of fractures of the distal phalanx in horses: 27 cases (1979–1988). J Am Vet Med Assoc 1993;202:1993–1997.
23. Khokhlov AL. Roentgenodiagnosis and classification of fractures of the phalanx. Veterinarian 1966;43:84.
24. Moyer W, Sigafoos R. Treatment of distal phalanx fractures in racehorses using a continuos rim-type shoe. Proc Am Assoc Equine Pract 1988;34:325–328.
25. Peitel M. Frequency of fractures of the extremities in horses and cattle and resultant economic loss. Wien Tierärztl Monatsschr 1971;58:158.
26. Pettersson H. Conservative and surgical treatment of fractures of the third phalanx. Proc Am Assoc Equine Pract 1972;18:183.
27. Pettersson H. Fractures of the pedal bone in the horse. Equine Vet J 1976;8:104.
28. Rose RJ, Rose RJ, Taylor BJ, Bellenger CR. Internal fixation of fractures of the third phalanx in the three horses. Aust Vet J 1979;55:29–32.
29. Rooney JR. Biomechanics of Lameness in Horses. Baltimore: Williams & Wilkins, 1969.
30. Schedle J, Hofmann R. Diagnosis and conservative treatment of intra-articular sagittal fracture of the equine pedal bone. Wien Tierärztl Monatsschr 1983;70:15–19.
31. Scott EA, McDole M, Shires MH. A review of third phalanx fractures in the horse. Sixty-four cases. J Am Vet Med Assoc 1979;174:1337.
32. Weaver AD. Fracture of the equine pedal bone. Equine Vet J 1969;1:283.
33. Yovich JV. Fractures of the distal phalanx in the horse. Vet Clin North Am Equine Pract 1989;5:145–160.
34. Yovich JV, Hilbert BJ, McGill CA. Fractures of the distal phalanx in horses. Aust Vet J 1982;59:180.
35. Yovich JV, Stashak TS, DeBowes RM, et al. Fractures of the distal phalanx of the forelimb in eight foals. J Am Vet Med Assoc 1986;189:550–553.

EXTENSOR PROCESS (TYPE 4) FRACTURES OF THE DISTAL (THIRD) PHALANX

Fractures of the extensor process of the distal (third) phalanx occur most frequently in the forelimbs and, occasionally, are bilateral. In one report, 21 of 23 of the extensor process fractures involved the forelimbs.[10,18] In another report, 6 of 9 extensor fractures involved the forelimbs.[15] They may be displaced or nondisplaced and are almost as common as type 2 fractures of the distal phalanx.[10] The fragment size varies from small, with little articular involvement, to large, with greater articular

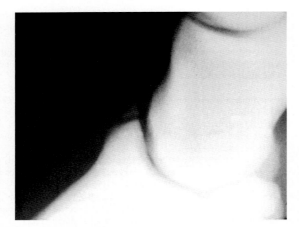

Figure 8.76 Small extensor process fracture.

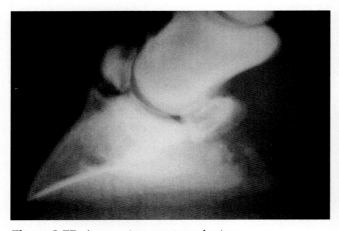

Figure 8.77 Large extensor process fracture.

involvement (Figs. 8.76 and 8.77).[2] Although uncommon, the condition may be accompanied by buttress foot, which is produced by periosteal new bone growth[1,19] (see "Pyramidal Distortion of the Hoof and Dorsal Pastern Region" in this chapter).

In a review of distal phalangeal fractures, researchers found that 23 of 79 cases involved the extensor process.[18] In another review of 65 cases of distal phalangeal fractures, researchers found that 4 horses sustained fractures of the extensor process.[21] Although various breeds are affected, male horses tend to be overrepresented with the large extensor process fractures.[5,18,21] This apparent sex predisposition may be related to a willingness to pursue treatment in nonbreeding animals.[5]

Etiology

In many cases, the etiology remains speculative. Trauma has been implicated. Excessive tension on the common digital extensor tendon may result in an avulsion fracture. Overextension of the coffin joint, resulting in contact of the extensor process with the middle phalanx and trauma to the dorsal aspect of the foot, has also been proposed as a cause.[12,23] Also, degenerative

joint disease (DJD) of the coffin joint can result in the development of an osteophyte on the extensor process, which may fracture as a result of overextension (Fig. 8.78).

The development of a separate center of ossification or an osteochondrosis lesion of the extensor process has also been proposed.[12,18,21,23] Small mineralized frag-

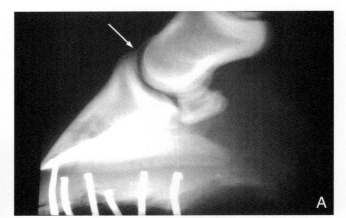

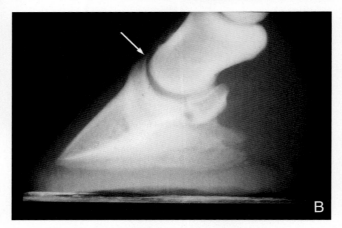

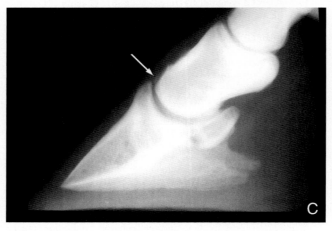

Figure 8.78 A. Lateral view of the distal phalanx, indicating osteophyte development of the extensor process (arrow). B. Same view 7 months later. Note the lengthening of the osteophyte (arrow). C. Presentation 4 months later. An extensor process fracture is present (arrow).

ments proximal to the extensor process can be observed radiographically as an incidental finding in horses that are clinically normal.[12] These fragments are often seen bilaterally and are thought to result from a developmental problem. Also large extensor process fractures

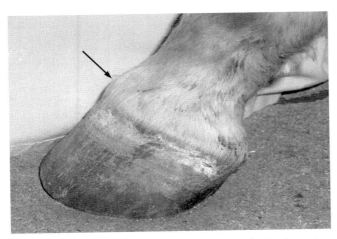

Figure 8.79   Lateral view showing coffin joint effusion (arrow) associated with an extensor process fracture.

are thought to result from a developmental disorder (Fig. 8.77) Supporting this theory is the development of clinical signs in relatively young horses and an apparent male sex predisposition.[5] One case report described subchondral bone cysts in association with an extensor process fracture.[22] Radiographically, a common feature of large extensor process fractures is lucency and cavitation of the fracture line, which is similar to that described in that case report.[5]

Signs

Distension of the coffin joint dorsal and proximal to the coronet band may be observed with articular fractures (Fig. 8.79). If the fragment is large, chronic, and associated with new bone formation at the fracture site, it can result in enlargement of the coronet band and abnormal growth of the hoof wall. The abnormal hoof growth is usually centered at the middorsal aspect of the hoof. As the hoof grows, it develops a V or triangular shape called a buttress foot. The abnormal hoof shape eventually extends from the coronet band to the ground surface as the hoof grows (Fig. 8.80).

The lameness is variable and depends on the cause, the size of the fragment, the extent of articular involve-

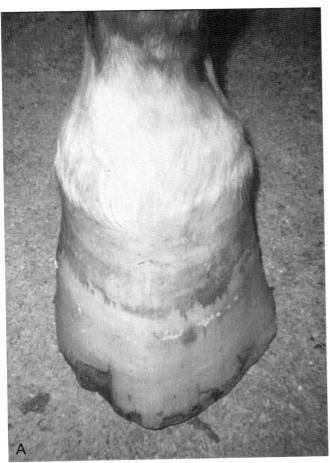
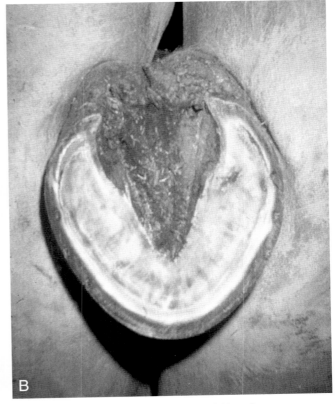

Figure 8.80   A. Dorsal view. Note the pyramidal shape of the hoof. B. Solar view of the front hoof. Note the triangular shape.

ment, the degree of fragment instability and synovitis, and the amount of DJD.[5,10,21] Small developmental or traumatically induced fractures may not cause lameness. If a lame horse has a small fragment of the extensor process, the fragment's contribution to lameness needs to be clarified.[7] Generally, however, a mild to moderate (1 to 3 on a scale of 5) lameness is observed.[15] Digital pressure just dorsal to the coronet band can reveal coffin joint effusion and pain on pressure if a large acute fracture is present. Phalangeal flexion usually elicits a painful response and may exacerbate the lameness.

Perineural anesthesia of the palmar digital nerves at the proximal sesamoid bones, a pastern ring block, or intrasynovial anesthesia of the coffin joint removes lameness in most cases (see Fig. 3.92).

Diagnosis

Extensor process fractures are best visualized on lateromedial radiographic projections, although the fracture can also be evaluated on the dorsopalmar view (Figs. 8.76 to 8.78). The oblique radiographic projections should also be taken to aid in the assessment of arthritic changes in the distal interphalangeal joint.

Treatment

It is generally accepted that surgery is indicated for any extensor process fracture with an articular component unless advanced DJD has developed.[9,12,14] Conservative treatment with prolonged stall rest has received mixed reviews and often horses do not become sound because the extensor process fracture does not heal.[10,18] An additional benefit to surgery is a shortened convalescent period.[6,8,16,17] One report on seven cases indicates that small acute extensor process fractures may be successfully treated with a fibrin adhesive.[4]

Arthroscopy through a dorsal lateral approach is the preferred technique for removal of small extensor process fractures. Using arthroscopy allows for a thorough evaluation of the dorsal aspect of the coffin joint, a more cosmetic outcome, and a shorter recovery time, compared with the incisional approach.[12,14] Usually, a partial synovectomy and careful probing are needed to adequately expose the fracture. Additionally, extension of the distal limb facilitates visualization of the fragment. The removal of hindlimb extensor process fractures is more difficult than for the forelimb because of the inability to position the coffin joint in full extension.

Postoperatively, an elastic bandage is applied to the distal extremity, including the foot. Bandages are changed at 3- to 4-day intervals for 2 weeks, at which time the sutures are removed. Stall confinement with increasing periods of hand walking exercise is begun at 2 weeks and continued until free exercise is allowed at 3 to 4 months. The administration of polysulfated glycosaminoglycans intramuscularly and/or the administration of a corticosteroid in combination with hyaluronic acid intrasynovially may benefit some horses that are mildly lame, postoperatively.[11] In one report, 14 of 16 of the horses that were lame from small extensor process fractures returned to soundness 10 weeks after the fragments were removed arthroscopically.[3] In this same report, 5 horses with extensor process fractures that were not lame had the fragment removed arthroscopically to avoid further damage to the coffin joint and to encourage the production of normal synovial fluid. All 5 of these horses were sound 14 days after surgery. In another report, 8 of 9 horses with extensor process fractures that were treated with arthroscopy had total resolution of their lameness and returned to their intended use.[15]

Large extensor process fractures (less than 1 cm) have been successfully treated with arthrotomy and lag screw fixation or fragment removal.[1,5,8,13,20] In either case, preoperative preparation includes clipping the hair in the pastern region and thorough cleaning of the hoof, after which the foot is placed in a povidone iodine bandage.[1,6,8] Broad-spectrum antimicrobials and phenylbutazone are recommended. A midline incision is made over the center of the common digital extensor tendon, just proximal to the coronary band. The common digital ex-

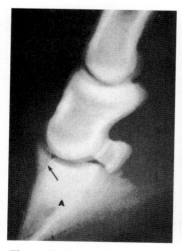 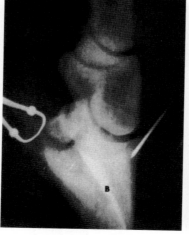 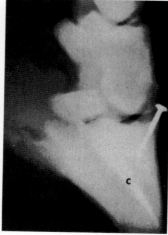

Figure 8.81 A. Large fracture (arrow) of extensor process of distal phalanx. B. Steinmann pins provide guide to check angulation for drilling. C. ASIF navicular screw in place.

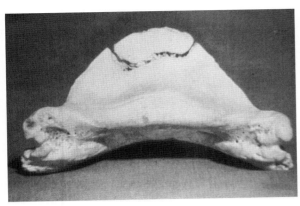

Figure 8.82 Dried bone specimen. Palmar view of the distal phalanx with a fracture of the extensor process. Note the width of the extensor process.

tensor tendon is incised longitudinally and separated with Gelpi retractors to expose the fragment. If internal fixation is used, a small Steinmann pin can be inserted through the fragment into parent bone to act as a radiographic marker for the placement of the screw (Fig. 8.81). If the fragment is to be removed, the tendinous attachments are separated from the fractured extensor process with an elevator, after which the fragment can be split sagittally with an osteotome. Sagittal splitting of the fragment into two or three smaller pieces greatly facilitates removal of large fragments (Fig. 8.82). Oschner grasping forceps or rongeurs are used to provide traction for removal of the fragment (Fig. 8.83). The tendon and subcutaneous tissues are sutured with simple interrupted sutures of 2-0 synthetic absorbable suture. The skin is then apposed with 2-0 synthetic monofilament nonabsorbable sutures, with a simple interrupted pattern.

Postoperatively, if the fragment was removed, the foot and pastern region are maintained in a bandage for 2 to 3 weeks, and the horse is confined to a box stall for at least 6 weeks. In one report the mean recovery time before returning to work was 7.5 months with a range of 2 to 4 months.[5] If internal fixation was used, the foot is placed in a cast that extends to proximal metacarpus for 4 weeks. After cast removal the horse is confined in a box stall for an additional 4 weeks. The horse should not be worked for at least 6 months.

Prognosis

The prognosis for small extensor process fractures treated by arthroscopic removal appears good. Two reports identified that 88% of the horses treated by this method returned to soundness.[3,15] The prognosis for large extensor process fractures treated by internal fixation also appears good in the small number of cases reported. Three of four cases treated with lag screw fixation achieved soundness.[8,20] Removal of chronic large extensor process results in a fair prognosis. In one report, 8 of 14 horses returned to their intended use.[5] A guarded prognosis is given if DJD of the distal interphalangeal joint is present.

References

1. Adams OR. Lameness in Horses. 3rd ed. Philadelphia: Lea & Febiger, 1974; 241.

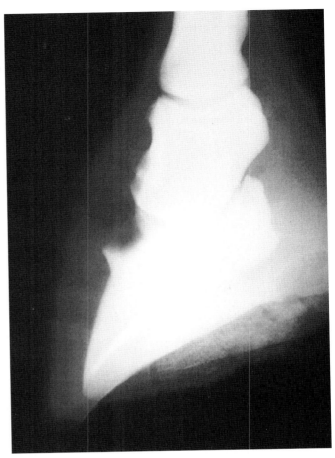

Figure 8.83 Lateral radiograph after a large extensor process was removed.

2. Bertone AL. Fractures of the distal phalanx. In: Nixon AJ, Ed. Equine Fracture Repair. Philadelphia: WB Saunders, 1996; 146–152.
3. Boening KJ, vonSaldren FC, Leendertse IP, et al. Diagnostic and surgical arthroscopy of the equine coffin joint. Proc Am Assoc Equine Pract 1989;34:311–317.
4. Brem R, Cronau PF, Fister D, et al. Fixation von knochen-fragmenten mit dem febrinkleber beim pferd am beispiel der fraktur des processus extensorius und des os carpi accessorium. Pferdeheilkunde 1986;2:261–266.
5. Dechant JE, Trotter GW, Stashak TS, et al. Removal of large fragments of the extensor process of the distal phalanx via arthrotomy in horses: 14 cases (1992–1998). J Am Vet Med Assoc 2000;217: 1351–1355.
6. Duncan DB, Dingwall JS. Surgical removal of avulsed portions of the extensor process of the third phalanx in the horse. J Am Vet Med Assoc 1971;159:201.
7. Dyson SJ. Lameness due to pain associated with the distal interphalangeal joint: 45 cases. Equine Vet J 1991;23:128–135.
8. Haynes PF, Adams OR. Internal fixation for repairs of fractured extensor process in the horse. J Am Vet Med Assoc 1974;164:61.
9. Honnas CM. Fractures of the extensor process. In: Auer JA, Ed. Equine Surgery. Philadelphia: WB Saunders, 1992;994–995.
10. Honnas CM, O'Brien TR, Linford RL. Distal phalanx fractures in horses: A survey of 274 horses with radiographic assessment of healing in 36 horses. Vet Radiol Ultrasound 1988;29:98–107.
11. Honnas CM, Trotter GW. The distal interphalangeal joint. In: White NA, Moore JN, Eds. Current Techniques in Equine Surgery and Lameness. 2nd ed. Philadelphia: WB Saunders, 1998;389.

12. Honnas CM, Vacek JR, Schumacher J. Diagnosis and treatment of articular fractures of the equine distal phalanx. Vet Med 1992; 87:1208–1214.
13. MacLellan KNM, MacDonald DG, Crawford WH. Lag screw fixation of extensor process fracture in a foal with a flexural deformity. Can Vet J 1997;38:226–228.
14. McIlwraith CW. Other uses of arthroscopy in the horse. In: McIlwraith CW, Ed. Diagnostic and Surgical Arthroscopy in the Horse. 2nd ed. Philadelphia: Lea & Febiger, 1990;219–223.
15. Miller SM, Bohanon TC. Arthroscopic surgery for the treatment of extensor process fractures of the distal phalanx in the horse. Vet Comp Orthop Traumatol 1994;7:2.
16. Numans SR, Wintzer HF. Surgical treatment of apophysial and chip fractures. Berl Munch Tierarztl Wochenschr 1961;74:205.
17. Pettersson H. Conservative and surgical treatment of fractures of the third phalanx. Proc Am Assoc Equine Pract 1972;18:183.
18. Pettersson H. Fractures of the pedal bone in the horse. Equine Vet J 1976;8:104–109.
19. Rooney JR. Ringbone versus pyramidal disease. Equine Vet Sci 1981;1:23.
20. Rose RJ, Taylor BJ, Bellenger CR. Internal fixation of fractures of the third phalanx in three horses. Aust Vet J 1979;55:29–32.
21. Scott EA, McDole M, Shires MH. A review of third phalanx fractures in the horse: sixty-five cases. J Am Vet Med Assoc 1979;174: 1337–1343.
22. Scott EA, Snyder SP, Schmotzer WB, et al. Subchondral bone cysts with fractures of the extensor process in a horse. J Am Vet Med Assoc 1991;199:595–597.
23. Yovich JV. Fractures of the distal phalanx in the horse. Vet Clin North Am Equine Pract 1989;5:145–160.

PYRAMIDAL DISTORTION OF THE HOOF AND DORSAL PASTERN REGION (PYRAMIDAL DISEASE OR BUTTRESS FOOT)

Pyramidal distortion of the hoof and the distal dorsal pastern region can result from a large chronic extensor process fracture (most common) or from a phalangeal exostosis involving the extensor process of the distal phalanx and the distal middle phalanx.[2,5] For more information regarding large extensor process fractures, refer to that section in this chapter. If phalangeal exostosis is the cause, it usually represents an advanced form of low ringbone.[3] The exostosis can cause an enlargement at the coronary band at the center of the hoof (Fig. 8.84) or, in chronic cases, cause a triangular (pyramidal) distortion of the dorsal hoof wall[3,5] (see Fig. 8.79).

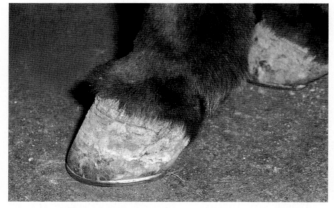

Figure 8.84 Lateral view of a horse with low ringbone. Note the extensive swelling dorsal to the coronet band.

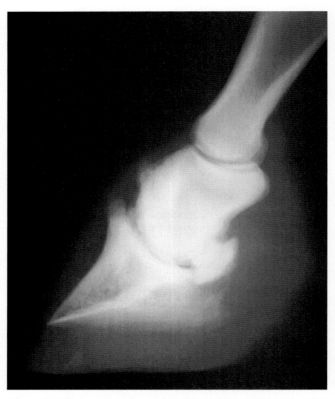

Figure 8.85 Low ringbone that led to pyramidal distortion of the hoof wall.

Etiology

Excessive strain of the attachments of the long or common digital extensor and the extensor branch of the suspensory ligament as these attachments insert on the extensor process of the distal phalanx is a proposed cause. The strain can result in a reactive periosteitis and a subsequent exostosis (Fig. 8.85). The phalangeal exostosis could also result from external trauma.

Horses with high heels and short toes and horses that move with limbs lifted high in a short and rapid manner (a "trappy gait"), such as the Paso Fino, seem predisposed to this problem. It has been suggested that the rapid angular acceleration of the foot in high-heeled horses may be responsible for tearing the soft tissue insertions at the extensor process.[6]

Signs and Diagnosis

An enlargement in the dorsal pastern region is often seen proximal to the coronary band (Fig. 8.84). The hair in the region may also have a tendency to stand upright, and the foot of the affected limb is smaller than that of the unaffected limb. Digital pressure over the site may elicit a painful response, particularly in the earlier stages of the disease. The signs of lameness are not specific, but the horse often "points" the affected foot.[1] At exercise, the cranial phase of the horse's stride is usually shortened, and reduced extension of the fetlock during the stance phase is evident. The phalangeal flexion test is often painful, and it may exacerbate the lameness. In chronic cases, the shape of the dorsal hoof wall changes to a pyramidal shape that extends from the coronary band distal to the weight-bearing surface (see Fig. 8.80). Radiographs reveal variable changes in the middle and distal phalanges and, in some cases, the coffin joint (Fig. 8.85).

Treatment

No treatment is of particular value in relieving the proliferative exostosis (low ringbone). In early cases with a reactive periosteitis, intralesional injection of corticoids and immobilization of the distal extremity may be of some help.[1] Nonsteroidal anti-inflammatory treatment is also logical. Palmar digital neurectomy in the proximal pastern region may also relieve some signs of lameness in chronic cases and allow limited use of the horse. Corrective trimming and shoeing is aimed at easing breakover (refer to trimming and shoeing subsection under "Navicular Syndrome"). Additionally, it has been suggested that rasping the dorsal hoof wall from just below the coronary band to the toe may relieve pressure and pain temporarily.[4] However, this approach has little effect on the progress of the disease process. Radiation therapy has also been suggested to reduce the development of the exostosis.[4]

If a large extensor process fracture is the cause, the extensor process fragment can be excised surgically (refer to "Treatment of Extensor Process Fractures" in this chapter) (see Figs. 8.77 and 8.82).

Prognosis

The prognosis is unfavorable in all cases of periosteitis (low ringbone) and fair for the surgical removal of large extensor process fractures.

References

1. Adams OR. Lameness in Horses. Philadelphia: Lea & Febiger, 1974.
2. Dechant JE, Trotter GW, Stashak TS, et al. Removal of large fragments of the extensor process of the distal phalanx via arthrotomy in horses: 14 cases (1992–1998). J Am Vet Med Assoc 2000;217:1351–1355.
3. Frank ER. Pyramidal disease. North Am Vet 1935;16:34.
4. Johnson JH. The foot. In: Mansmann RA, McAllister ES, Eds. Equine Medicine and Surgery. 3rd ed. Santa Barbara, CA: American Veterinary Publications, 1982;1033.
5. Park A. Chronic foot injury and deformity. In: White NA, Moore JN, Eds. Current Techniques in Equine Surgery and Lameness. 2nd ed. Philadelphia: WB Saunders, 1998;534–537.
6. Rooney JR. Ringbone versus pyramidal disease. Equine Vet Sci 1981;1:23.

PENETRATING WOUNDS OF THE FOOT

Penetrating wounds of the foot are commonly seen in equine practice. The injury is often sustained by the horse stepping on (bottom of foot) or contacting (coronet band) a sharp object. Although any deep puncture wound of the foot can be potentially serious, those that penetrate the frog region or coronary band and involve vital structures (deep digital flexor tendon [DDFT] or digital sheaths, navicular bone or bursa, and the distal

phalanx and the distal interphalangeal [coffin] joint) can be career and life threatening. Early identification of the involvement of a vital structure, aggressive medical treatment, and early surgical intervention has much to do with the success of the outcome.[1,5,11,13,17]

Penetrating wounds of the foot have been classified according to their depth and location.[14] Superficial wounds penetrate only the cornified tissue and do not invade the corium; the result is often a subsolar abscess. Deep wounds are separated further into three types, all of which penetrate the germinal epithelium. Type I penetrates the sole corium, possibly resulting in septic osteitis, fracture of the distal phalanx, or digital cushion abscess. Type II penetrates the corium deep to the frog, potentially resulting in a septic deep digital flexor tendinitis, navicular bursitis, distal interphalangeal joint septic arthritis, abscess of the digital cushion, septic osteitis of the distal phalanx or navicular bone, or fractures of the distal phalanx. Type III penetrates the coronary band, potentially resulting in septic osteitis of the distal phalanx, septic chondritis of the collateral cartilage, or septic arthritis of the distal interphalangeal joint (Fig. 8.86).

Clinical Signs and Diagnosis

The clinical signs may vary, depending on the depth (superficial versus deep), location of the injury (sole versus coronary band), and chronicity of the injury. Although superficial wounds that do not penetrate the dermis may be asymptomatic for a few days until a subsolar abscess develops, deep wounds involving the dermal lamina generally result in acute localizing signs of lameness. Also, wounds in the frog region that involve vital structures usually become rapidly symptomatic. Horses are often seen pointing the foot, and when they walk, selective weight bearing (landing on the toe if the heel region is involved) may be seen before inflammation and infection become widespread. On palpation, the hoof is often warmer than normal and a prominent digital pulse can usually be palpated.[10,14] Careful examination of the sole (visual, hoof tester, and probing) and coronary band is important. One study suggested that any penetrating wound of the foot deeper than 1 cm should be considered serious. The approximate depth of a perpendicular penetration before vital structures become involved is 1 cm for the sole, 1.5 cm for the frog, and 1.2 cm for the hoof wall.[10]

If a foreign body is present in the bottom of the foot, it should be left in place while a radiograph is taken; however, care should be taken so it is not driven deeper into tissue (Fig. 8.87). If a wound is not obvious, careful application of hoof testers may be helpful in identifying focal pain, which, in turn, may indicate a site of penetration. If the sole is thick and firm, trimming may have to precede hoof tester examination. Once a focal site of pain is found in the sole or frog, it is then pared with a hoof knife. If the injury is acute (before infection) and involves the sole, all that may be seen is a crack or small hole. Generally, puncture wounds of the sole appear black at the entry site (Fig. 8.88). Wounds that penetrate the frog can be particularly difficult to identify because the tissues being softer and more elastic than the sole tend to collapse and fill in the tract. More complete par-

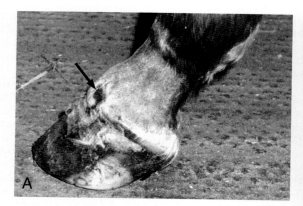
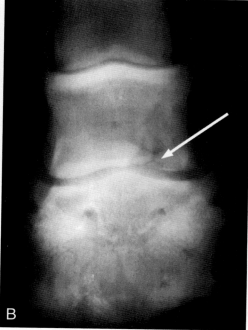

Figure 8.86 A. A penetrating wound of the dorsal lateral coronary band of 1-week duration (arrow). B. A radiograph identifying an articular fracture of the distal lateral middle phalanx (arrow) and septic osteitis. The coffin joint was also infected.

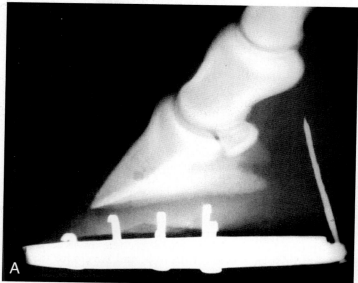
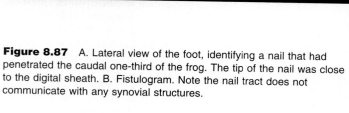
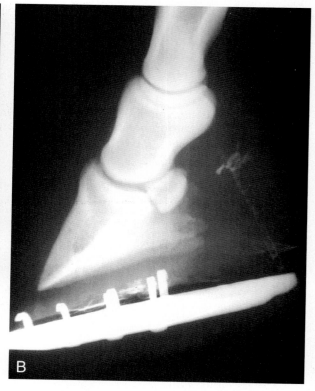

Figure 8.87 A. Lateral view of the foot, identifying a nail that had penetrated the caudal one-third of the frog. The tip of the nail was close to the digital sheath. B. Fistulogram. Note the nail tract does not communicate with any synovial structures.

ing of the frog is required in some cases to visualize a tract (Fig. 8.89). Sterile probing of the tract can be helpful to identify depth and direction of the injury (Fig. 8.90A). Care should be taken, however, not to push the probe deeper than the depth of the wound. While the probe is in place, a radiograph can be taken (Fig. 8.90B).

If infection is present but localized, paring of the sole and frog to thin them may allow pus to drain from a puncture site. Occasionally, gentle pressure with the thumbs or hoof testers may be required to visualize the pus. Additionally, walking the horse after the sole is pared may cause sufficient pressure that a subsolar ab-

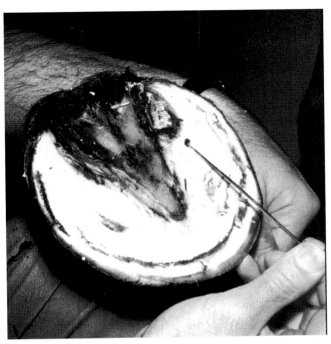

Figure 8.88   Penetrating wound of the sole. The metal probe is in the defect.

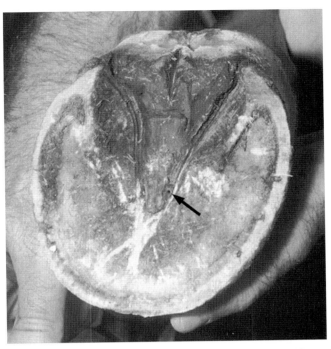

Figure 8.89   Hole in the lateral sulcus (arrow) became evident after this region was pared with a hoof knife.

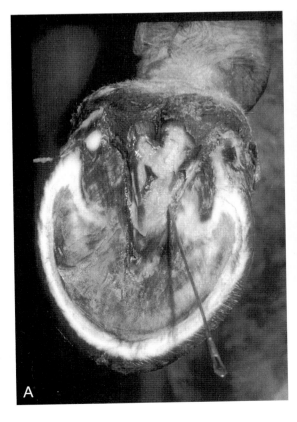

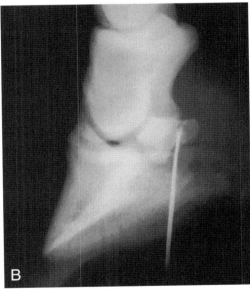

Figure 8.90   A. Probe placed in the penetrating wound of the sulcus to identify the depth and direction of the injury. B. Lateral slightly oblique view of the foot, indicating that there is a high probability that the navicular bursa was penetrated.

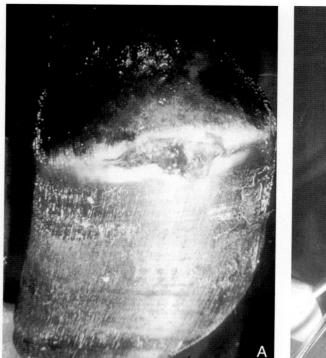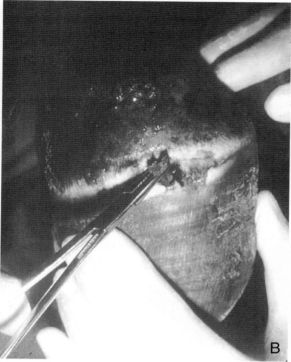

Figure 8.91   A. Penetrating wound of the hoof wall at the coronet band. B. A wood splinter is being removed from a penetrating wound at the coronet band.

scess may begin to drain. This approach is generally of little benefit if the frog or white line is involved. In these cases, gentle sterile probing of the tract may be helpful. Once the infection becomes diffuse (e.g., subsolar abscess), hoof tester examination is generally less beneficial in identifying the site of penetration. Careful paring of the sole and probing of the tract (e.g., dark spots or cracks) may be most helpful. Perineural regional anesthesia facilitates paring out a tract or probing the depth of the tract.

Palpation of the coronary band for heat, pain, and swelling may also be helpful in identifying the location of a penetrating wound to the white line (see "Penetrating Wounds of the White Line" in this chapter for more information) and of the coronary band. A penetrating wound of the coronary band can be overlooked if the hair is long or if local swelling and wound drainage is not present. Once identified, a wound at the coronary band should be carefully probed and explored because they are often caused by a wood splinter (Fig. 8.91).

Heat, pain, and swelling of one heel bulb and a pounding digital pulse may indicate migration of a subsolar abscess (Fig. 8.92). Swelling of the digital sheaths and distal interphalangeal joint may indicate a septic arthritis. If infection is suspected, a sample of synovial fluid should be taken for analysis. An elevated white blood cell count (more than 30,000) with neutrophilia, a pH less than 6.9, and an elevated protein (more than 4.0 g/dL) are highly suggestive of a septic process.[15]

Radiographic examination can be helpful in identifying a subsolar abscess (Fig. 8.93) and involvement of vital structures (Fig. 8.94). Although a radiograph with

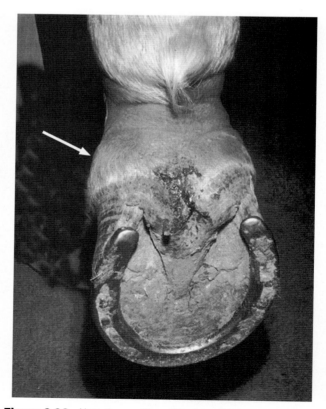

Figure 8.92   Note the swelling of the lateral heel bulb region (arrow). This horse had a subsolar abscess.

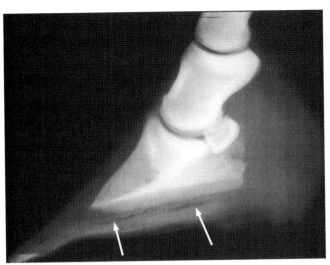

Figure 8.93 Lateral view of the foot. Note the gas (dark) line below the distal phalanx (arrows), indicating a subsolar abscess.

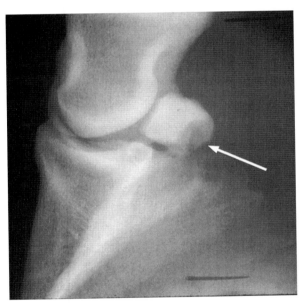

Figure 8.94 Lateral view of the foot. Note the bone lysis (arrow) associated with the navicular region.

a sterile metal probe placed in a tract or with a foreign body in place may provide important information regarding depth and direction of the injury, this approach is limited in its ability to identify an abscess cavity or extension of the injury into a synovial structure. A fistulogram in these cases is most often definitive (Fig. 8.95). At least two radiographic views at right angles to each other should be evaluated to assess the spatial relationship of the probe in relation to vital structures. Although a fracture of the distal phalanx or navicular bone can often be identified shortly after injury, bone changes secondary to infection and inflammation are often not observed for a period of 2 to 3 weeks after injury.[12] Radiographic changes consistent with septic osteitis of the

distal phalanx include bone lysis, irregular margins, increased vascular channel size, and bone sequestrum formation (Fig. 8.96).When a puncture wound involves the navicular bone, a skyline (tangential) view of the flexor surface of the navicular bone should be taken.

Treatment

Superfical Puncture Wounds

Treatment of superficial penetrating wounds that do not involve vital structures (bone, tendon, or synovial cavities) is generally uncomplicated. Effective treatment involves providing adequate drainage, removal of infected and necrotic tissues, and protecting the site from contamination (Fig. 8.97). The majority of cases can be treated while the horse is standing. If the frog and sole are hard, the foot (after the initial drainage) can be placed in a poultice for 12 to 24 hours to soften it, after which the sole or frog can be further debrided.[14] Although small local abscesses can be debrided effectively without perineural anesthesia, more extensive infection may require perineural anesthesia of the digital nerves at the base of the sesamoid bones and, of course, more extensive debridement. Drainage is established by removal of the undermined sole with a sharp hoof knife or a hoof groover (Fig. 8.98). Underlying necrotic or infected tissue can be removed with the aid of a standard curette or a nail hole curette. However, one should avoid disrupting the corium in the affected area because it will prolong wound healing.[14] For the superficial localized infection, antiseptic dressing and foot protection are usually all that is needed. For more extensive superficial infections, local periodic flushing with a sterile polyionic salt antiseptic solution and foot protection may be required. Although hyperosmotic treatment with foot soaks or topical application to the wound to draw out infection is commonly used, the value of this approach is yet to be clearly identified. Therefore, the use of this treatment is by personal choice. In either case the wound should be dressed daily until it is dry.

Protection of the foot is accomplished with bandages, bandages with duct tape, and bandages with an easy boot, and in some cases, a treatment plate may be applied to a shoe (Fig. 8.98). Nonsteroidal anti-inflammatory drugs (NSAIDs) are also often used at low doses and only as needed. Astringents such as 2% formalin, 2% phenol, or 7% or 3.5% strength Tincture of Iodine can be applied to the wound as a drying agent. Horses with resolving lesions may be shod with pads.

Deep Puncture Wounds

Wounds that penetrate the corium and bone or synovial structures should be treated promptly. Broad-spectrum antimicrobials, NSAIDs, and tetanus prophylaxis are indicated. Immediate debridement is recommended. Unfortunately, many horses are presented after infection has become established. Superficial curettage with local flushing of a deep wound is generally unsuccessful. For proper treatment, general anesthesia is usually required; and one should prepare the hoof and sole by trimming and rasping and performing standard surgical preparation. A tourniquet is placed at the midcannon bone re-

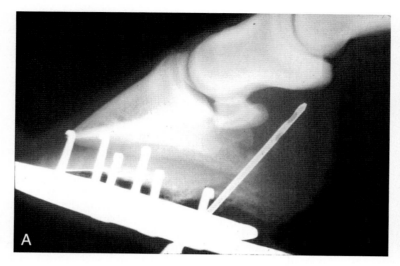

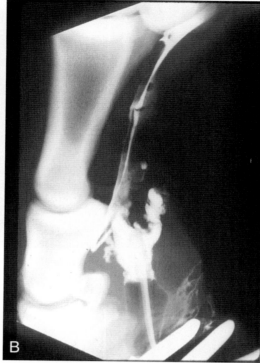

Figure 8.95 A. Probe placed in a penetrating wound in the foot. The tip of the probe is close to the digital sheath. B. Fistulogram reveals that the digital sheath was penetrated. Note the contrast material is going proximal in the digital sheath.

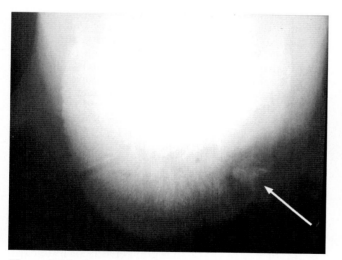

Figure 8.96 Bone sequestrum (arrow) and septic osteitis of the distal phalanx that resulted from a penetrating wound to the foot.

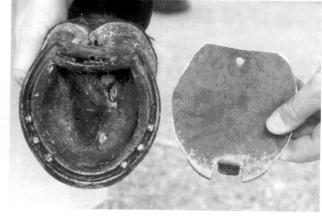

Figure 8.97 Treatment plate shoe. The metal plate on the right can be attached to the shoe to protect the bottom of the foot from contamination and pressure.

gion to reduce bleeding. Wounds that penetrate the distal phalanx should be opened, and the distal phalanx should be curetted until healthy bone is visualized. If osteomyelitis is established or if a sequestrum is present, it should be surgically treated in the same fashion, except that a tissue sample should be taken for culture and sensitivity. It is reported that as much as 24% of the distal phalanx can be removed and function of the foot can be normal.

Wounds that penetrate the navicular region should be carefully dissected to their depth. If the navicular bursa has been penetrated, a "street nail" operation is performed by creating a window into the DDFT.[7,11] A com-

munication between the distal interphalangeal joint or digital sheath and navicular bursa can be identified at this time by injecting sterile polyionic salt solutions into the joint from a dorsal location or into the digital sheath from a proximal site. If the joint is involved, fluid may be seen coming through and opening in the impar ligament. If the digital sheath is involved, fluid will be seen to flow from the opening in the navicular bursa. After the identification of a communication with either synovial structure, 1 to 2 L of sterile polyionic fluid followed with 1 L of 10% dimethyl sulfoxide (DMSO) solution should be flushed through the synovial cavity. Intrasynovial injection of a broad-spectrum antimicrobial is also appro-

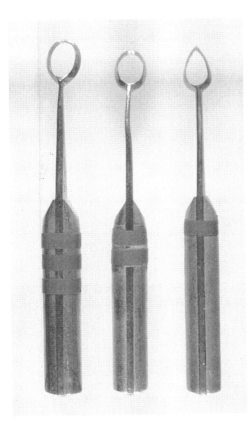

Figure 8.98 Hoof groovers.

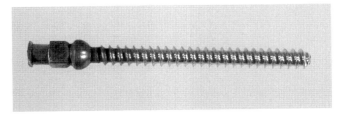

Figure 8.99 Centrally cannulated 5.5-mm ASIF cortical bone screw with a needle hub welded in place.

priate. If the infection is chronic and osteomyelitis of the navicular bone is present, curettage until healthy bone is visualized is indicated. Although packing the curetted navicular bone with cancellous grafts or methyl methacrylate has been used on a limited basis, too few cases have been done to make strong recommendation for this approach.[3,4,6] However, antibiotic-impregnated poly-methylmethacrylate (AI PMMA) beads can be packed in the wound for short-term postoperative treatment. The beads are removed and replaced at bandage changes and are used until a healthy bed of granulation tissue develops and all evidence of infection is gone. The AI PMMA allows the antibiotic to elute out, providing a high concentration of antibiotic locally.

Additionally, either medullary bone perfusion or intravascular perfusion of an antibiotic can be used to increase the level of antibiotic locally. With medullary bone perfusion, a 5.5-mm centrally cannulated ASIF (Association for the Study of Internal Fixation) bone screw can be used. The screw is modified by replacement of the screw head with a standard needle hub from a stainless-steel udder infusion cannula. The needle hub is welded on the cannulated screw (Fig. 8.99). A tourniquet is placed at the fetlock region, and after aseptic preparation, the surgeon makes a stab incision in the distal third of P1 (dorsal, lateral, or medial), after which the cannulated 5.5-mm screw is placed in the marrow cavity by use of standard techniques. A 60-mL syringe and an intravenous extension set are needed. The antimicrobial (usually an aminoglycoside) is diluted in 55 mL of sterile solution and injected over a 10-minute period. Alterna-

tively, intravenous digital perfusion can be done.[16] This can be accomplished by placing an intravenous 20- to 22-gauge 1-inch catheter into the lateral or medial palmar or plantar vein at the level of the proximal sesamoid bone. A heparinized extension set is attached to the catheter, and the catheter and extension set are secured to the skin with super glue, after which they are taped in place. An Esmarch bandage is then distally to proximally applied and ends at a pneumatic tourniquet at the midmetacarpal or midmetarsal region. The tourniquet is inflated, and the Esmarch bandage is removed. The digit is then perfused with 60 mL of a balanced electrolyte solution containing 125 to 250 mg of amikacin or 100 to 300 mg of gentamicin (adult) or 10 to 12 mL of balanced electrolyte solution containing 50 mg of amikacin or gentamicin (foal). The injection of the perfusate is done over 1 minute, after which the extension set is occluded. After 30 minutes the tourniquet and catheter are removed. Either procedure increases the antibiotic levels in the osteomyelitic bone and the infected synovial cavity.[8,19] Experimental studies in which 125 mg of amikacin was used for intravenous vascular digital perfusion resulted in mean peak synovial fluid concentrations of the drug 25 to 50 times the minimum inhibitory concentration for most pathogens. The antimicrobial was also delivered to the tissue of the digit.[8] In all cases, systemic broad-spectrum antimicrobials should be used until the results of culture and sensitivity are available. The results of Gram stain, culture, and sensitivity should guide the clinician in the choice of broad-spectrum antimicrobial. A penicillin and aminoglycoside combination is a good selection while you are awaiting culture and sensitivity analysis.

After debridement, lavage, and perfusion, if indicated, gauze sponges soaked in a dilute antiseptic is packed tightly in the wound, and a waterproof bandage is applied. The bandage is changed daily until a healthy bed of granulation tissue develops. Then, a shoe with a treatment plate can be applied. The practice of soaking the foot in a bucket of water with or without antiseptics to lavage the deep wounds of the foot cannot be recommended.[9]

Penetrating wounds of the coronary band can be managed in a similar fashion as just described. There is often a separation in the coronary band at the puncture site (see Fig. 8.91A). Curved hemostats or a probe can be used to explore and palpate the wound. Since these wounds are commonly caused by a stub of wood that penetrates the coronet and breaks off, it may be removed with hemostats. Penetration of a synovial structure (coffin joint most commonly) must be ruled out. This is done by placing a needle in a site in the synovial structure remote to the injury (a synovial fluid sample can be obtained for cytology and culture), after which sterile fluid is injected with pressure. Fluid coming from the wound indicates the synovial cavity was entered. Radiographs should be taken, and in some cases, a contrast study should be done.

Prognosis

Generally, a good prognosis can be expected for deep puncture wounds that do not involve vital structures, and a poor prognosis is expected for those that involve vital structures that have not been treated early and aggressively. In a retrospective study of 50 cases with deep puncture wounds of the foot, 95% (21 of 22) of horses with deep puncture wounds outside the frog or frog sulci regained full athletic soundness.[18] In the same study, only 50% (14 of 28) of horses receiving deep puncture wounds in the frog region fully recovered from the injury. However, of the horses that were operated within a few days after injury to the frog region, 80% (4 of 5) returned to full function. In another study on horses with puncture wounds into the navicular bursa, 32% (12 of 38) could return satisfactorily to function.[18] The most common reason for failure is osteomyelitis of the navicular bone, rupture of the DDFT, and septic arthritis of the distal interphalangeal joint. An improved outcome is seen in horses sustaining puncture wounds of the navicular region if they are operated on within a few days after injury. Follow-up on 9 cases of septic osteitis revealed that 7 of 9 horses returned to intended use within 12 weeks after surgery.[2]

References

1. DeBowes RM, Yovich JV. Penetrating wounds, abscesses, gravel, and bruising of the equine foot. Vet Clin North Am Equine Pract 1989;5:179–194.
2. Gaughan EM, Rendano VT, Ducharme NG. Surgical treatment of septic pedal osteitis in horses: Nine cases (1980–1987). J Am Vet Med Assoc 1989;195:1131–1134.
3. Hickman J, Kold SE, Ellis DR, et al. Use of bone cement in two orthopedic cases. Equine Vet J 1984;16:543–545.
4. Honnas CM, Crabill MR, Mackie JT, et al. Use of autogenous cancellous bone grafting in the treatment of septic navicular bursitis and distal sesamoid osteomyelitis in horses. J Am Vet Med Assoc 1995;206:1191–1194.
5. Honnas CM, Meagher DM, Lindford RL. Surgical management of difficult foot problems in the horse: Current concepts. Proc Am Assoc Equine Pract 1988;34:249.
6. Markel MD, Meagher DM, Ford TS. Use of cancellous bone graft in the treatment of navicular bone osteomyelitis in a foal. J Am Vet Med Assoc 1985;187:278–280.
7. McIlwraith CW, Robertson JT. Street nail procedure. In: McIlwraith & Turner's Equine Surgery: Advanced Techniques. 2nd ed. Baltimore: Williams &Wilkins, 1998;209–212.
8. Murphey ED, Santschi EM, Papich MG. Local antibiotic perfusion of the limb of horses. Proc Am Assoc Equine Pract 1994;40: 141–142.
9. Parks AH. Equine foot wounds: General principles of healing and treatment. Proc Am Assoc Equine Pract 1999;45:180–187.
10. Pascoe JR. Difficult foot wounds. Proceedings of the 12th Bain-Fallon Memorial Lectures, 1990;12:33.
11. Richardson GL. Surgical management of penetrating wounds to the equine foot. Proc Am Assoc Equine Pract 1999;45:198–189.
12. Richardson GL, O'Brien TR. Puncture wounds into the navicular bursa of the horse: Role of radiographic evaluation. Vet Radiol Ultrasound 1985;26:203.
13. Richardson GL, O'Brien TR, Pascoe JR, et al. Puncture wounds of the navicular bursa in 38 horses: A retrospective study. Vet Surg 1986;15:156–160.
14. Richardson GL, Pascoe JR, Meagher D. Puncture wounds of the foot in horses: Diagnosis and treatment. Comp Cont Educ Pract Vet 1986;8:S379–S387.
15. Ritta-Mari T, Bramlage LR, Gabel AD. Sequential clinical and synovial fluid changes associated with infectious arthritis in the horse. Equine Vet J 1989;21:325.
16. Santschi EM, Adam SB, Murphey ED. How to perform equine intravenous digital perfusion. Proc Am Assoc Equine Pract 1998; 44:198–201.
17. Stashak TS. Avulsion and penetrating injuries of the foot. Proceedings of the 20th Bain-Fallon Memorial Lectures, Hamilton Island, Queensland, Australia, July 26–31, 1998:245–256.
18. Steckel RR, Fessler JF, Huston LC. Deep puncture wounds of the equine hoof: A review of 50 cases. Proc Am Assoc Equine Pract 1989;35:67.
19. Whitehair KJ, Bowersock TL, Blevins WE, et al. Regional limb perfusion for antibiotic treatment of experimentally infected septic arthritis. Vet Surg 1992;21:367–373.

QUITTOR (INFECTION AND NECROSIS OF THE COLLATERAL [UNGUAL] CARTILAGE)

Quittor is a chronic purulent inflammation of a collateral cartilage of the distal phalanx, characterized by cartilage necrosis and multiple fistulous draining tracts proximal to the coronary band. The forelimbs and the lateral cartilages are most commonly affected (Fig. 8.100).[1,4,6] One study done on 16 horses with necrosis of the collateral cartilages of the distal phalanx found that 14 of 16 cases involved the lateral cartilage.[4]

Etiology

Infection with subsequent necrosis of the collateral cartilages results from injury to the collateral cartilage itself or to the soft tissue overlying collateral cartilage. Injuries that can result in quittor include penetrating wounds and lacerations over the affected cartilage, external blows resulting in bruising and damage to the circula-

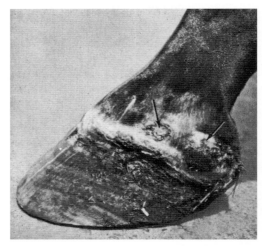

Figure 8.100 Clinical appearance of typical quittor. Arrows point to two draining tracts. This patient was cured through the surgical procedure described, making an elliptical incision above the coronary band.

tion of the collateral cartilage (e.g., interference), foot abscesses, chronic ascending infections of the white line (gravel) in the quarters, and hoof cracks that are deep enough that infection becomes localized in the collateral cartilages.[1,4]

Signs

Quittor is characterized by the formation of abscesses in the collateral cartilages that break open and drain just proximal to the coronet band. A history of recurrent drainage from fistulous tracts overlying the affected cartilage and intermittent severe lameness is common. Swelling, heat, and pain when pressure is applied above the coronary band over the affected cartilage and pain when hoof testers are applied to the affected quarter are also common. The degree of lameness is usually related to the patency of the fistulous tract draining the abscesses.[4] As pressure in the abscess builds, the lameness increases, and the horse may exhibit an acute non-weight-bearing lameness. Once the abscess breaks open and drains, the lameness subsides. Chronic inflammation of the involved collateral cartilage may result in permanent damage and deformity of the foot and cause persistent lameness.

Diagnosis

The diagnosis of quittor is based on a history of recurrent swelling, the affected collateral cartilage and the presence of one or more fistulous tracts proximal to the coronet band, and intermittent lameness. Swelling and pain over the affected cartilage supports the diagnosis. Quittor should be differentiated from shallow abscesses and ascending infection of the white line ("gravel").

The drainage tract associated with gravel is located at or just proximal to the coronary band, and the inflammatory process usually is localized. With quittor there may be multiple fistulous tracts, the swelling is usually more diffuse, and it is located more proximally over the collateral cartilages.[2,3,5]

Radiographs can be helpful to rule out bone involvement. The depth and dimension of these fistulous tracts can be elucidated with fistulography or the placement of a sterile flexible metal probe in the tract (Fig. 8.101).

Treatment

The treatment of choice is surgical excision of the fistulous tracts and necrotic cartilage.[1,5] Because of the limited blood supply to the cartilage, medical management with systemic antibiotics, foot soaks, and injection of the fistulous tracts with antiseptics or escharotics and enzymes is generally less effective and frequently prolongs the inevitable decision for surgery.[4] Prior to surgery, the hair in the pastern region is clipped, and the hoof is trimmed, rasped, scrubbed, and then placed in a povidone iodine–soaked bandage. At surgery, the foot is held in rigid extension by the placement of wires through holes drilled through the white line in either side of the hoof wall. Traction is then applied to the hoof. Extending the foot tenses the joint capsule and retracts it from

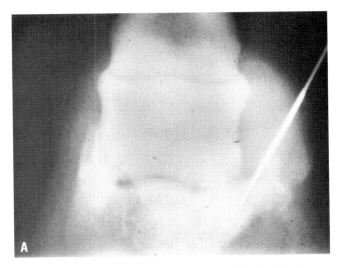
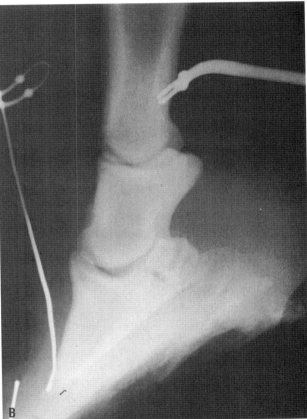

Figure 8.101 Sterile probes can be used to identify the depth and location of a tract.

the surgical dissection plane, thus reducing the chances of inadvertent penetration of the distal interphalangeal joint.[2,4] A tourniquet is also recommended.

Adams[1] described a technique of elliptic incision dorsal to the coronet that is effective in treatment of this condition and that heals it rapidly. However, the method by which deep-seated necrosis of the cartilage located below the coronary band is handled is not described, particularly with reference to how to establish ventral

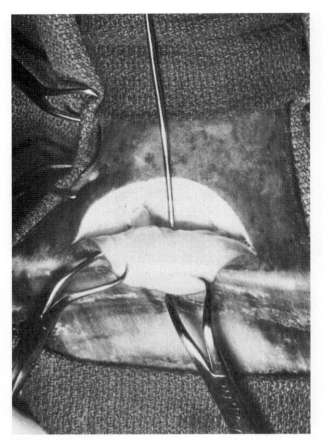

Figure 8.102 Curved incision made just proximal to the coronary band. A sterile probe was used to identify the tract.

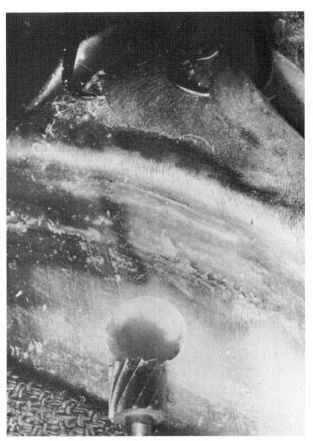

Figure 8.103 Hole made through the horny layer of the hoof wall down to the vascular layer at the distal limits of the tract.

drainage. For that reason I prefer to make a curved incision beginning just dorsal to the coronary band over the diseased collateral cartilage (Fig. 8.102). The flap is dissected distad to expose the collateral cartilage, and a sterile probe is used to identify the draining tract. Necrotic cartilage is recognized by its dark blue or reddish blue appearance. All of the necrotic soft tissue and cartilage is excised until only clean margins remain. If the necrotic cartilage extends to or below the coronary band, a hole is drilled in the hoof wall over the ventralmost limits of the necrotic cartilage to provide drainage (Fig. 8.103). Only in advanced cases is the entire cartilage removed.[2] If all of the necrotic tissue is removed and clean margins are evident, the elliptical incision can be closed primarily. Then the foot and pastern region are protected with application of either a bandage or a cast of the lower limb. If a cast is used, it removed in 10 to 14 days.[2] If there is question as to whether all the infected tissue has been removed, a multifenestrated polyethylene tube can be placed in the wound and sutured to the limb proximally. The remaining tract is then packed with an antiseptic-soaked 4 × 4 sponge, the top of the skin flap is incised so an opening remains at its top, and the flap is sutured (Fig. 8.104). The foot and sole can be either bandaged or placed in a protective boot. In either case, the surgical site is protected with sterile bandages. On the following day the bandage is removed, and the wound is flushed with a dilute povidone iodine solution. This is continued daily until all evidence of infection is gone. Antiseptic packing through the hole in the hoof wall is continued until infection is abated. In cases in which the necrotic cartilage does not extend to or below the coronary band and good ventral drainage can be achieved without drilling a hole, the flush system is applied, and the remaining drain tract is packed directly. Most cases I have treated have required drilling the hoof wall either to establish drainage or to remove necrotic cartilage at that depth. In all situations, incisions or excision of the coronary band should be avoided. Antiseptic flushes are usually continued for 2 to 3 days, after which the flush tube is removed. The packing is continued with smaller amounts of gauze until one is assured that no infection remains. Sutures are removed on day 14, and the remaining hole in the hoof wall is filled with acrylic as soon as a firm cornified layer develops. If acrylic is placed in the hole prior to this time, the exothermic (heat) reaction results in necrosis of the sensitive laminae and infection. Most frequently, acrylic can be placed in the hoof wall within a 4- to 6-week period after the initial surgery. Exercise can usually be begun in approximately 2.5 to 3 months.

Prognosis

The prognosis for acute and subacute cases after complete excision of the necrotic cartilage is good. Secondary

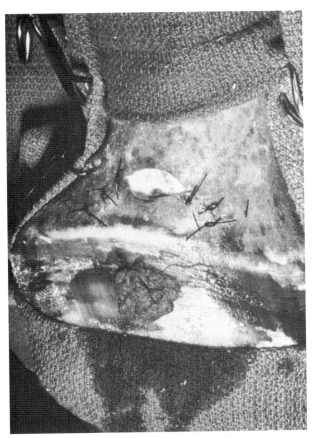

Figure 8.104 After the tract has been debrided, the skin is sutured, leaving a small opening at the top. The tract is packed with gauze soaked in Betadine solution.

complications, such as osteomyelitis of the distal phalanx, septic arthritis of the distal interphalangeal joint, or infection of the digital cushion or other soft tissues in the foot, reduce the prognosis appropriately.[2,4] One study documenting the outcome of 16 horses treated for necrosis of the collateral cartilage of the distal phalanx found that horses with drainage of less than 1-month duration had a better prognosis for return to soundness than horses with drainage of longer than 1-month duration prior to the initiation of treatment.[4]

References

1. Adams OR. Lameness in Horses. 3rd ed. Philadelphia: Lea & Febiger, 1974.
2. Honnas CM. Surgical treatment of selected musculoskeletal disorders of the forelimb. In: Auer JA, Ed. Equine Surgery. Philadelphia: WB Saunders, 1992;986–989.
3. Honnas CM, Meagher DM, Linford RL. Surgical management of difficult foot problems in the horse. Proc Am Assoc Equine Pract 1988;34:249.
4. Honnas CM, Ragle CA, Meagher DM. Necrosis of the collateral cartilage of the distal phalanx in horses: 16 cases (1970–1988). J Am Vet Med Assoc 1988;193:1303.
5. Johnson JH. The foot. In: Mansmann RA, McAllister ES, Eds. Equine Medicine and Surgery. 3rd ed. Santa Barbara, CA: American Veterinary Publications, 1982;1052.
6. Prolic I. Treatment of quittor. Veterinaria (Sarajevo) 1962;11:27.

GRAVEL (ASCENDING INFECTION OF THE WHITE LINE)

Gravel is the layman's term for what supposedly is a migration of a piece of gravel from the white line proximad to the coronet band, where it is discharged as through a small abscess.[6] This does not occur; what does happen is that an opening in the white line permits infection to invade the laminae, which results in the development of a submural abscess. The abscess follows the line of least resistance and eventually breaks and drains at the coronary band.

Etiology

A wound or crack in the white line or a separation in the white line ("seedy toe") and a subsolar abscess adjacent to the white line may predispose the horse to this condition.

Signs and Diagnosis

Lameness similar to that observed with subsolar abscesses or a penetrating wound to the foot may be observed in horses with ascending infections of the white line.[1] Moderate to severe lameness usually appears 1 or 2 days before drainage at the coronet band occurs. The condition, however, may go undiagnosed until drainage at the coronet band is observed. Signs of lameness may also vary according to the severity of the infection and location of the site of infection. The horse may modify its gait and selectively bear weight according to the location of the abscess. Hoof tester examination can help determine the approximate location of the ascending infection before it breaks out at the coronet band. If the hoof tester examination localizes pain to the hoof wall, careful examination of the white line and sole in the painful region should be done. Before examination of the sole and white line, the hoof should be trimmed lightly. Exploring any black areas (black spots) with a flexible metal may reveal the site where the laminae was penetrated (Fig. 8.105). Each of these dark sites should be probed to their depth. If the probe enters the laminae and exudate is observed, this is likely the site of the original wound. Diagnostic anesthesia may be helpful in some cases to verify the location of the lameness to the foot. When the condition has been present for some time, drainage at the coronary band is noted.

The diagnosis is often not made until the abscess breaks out at the white line. It is important that this condition be distinguished from quittor (necrosis of the collateral cartilages of the distal phalanx).[5] The tract associated with an ascending infection of the white line is superficial and usually breaks out just proximal to the coronet band. In contrast, draining tracts associated with quittor erupt from deep in the collateral cartilage. They may be multiple and are usually located 1 to 2 cm proximal to the coronet band. Fistulograms can be helpful in determining if the tract is deep or superficial.[4]

Treatment

If an ascending infection of the white line is suspected but cannot be confirmed, then soaking the foot in con-

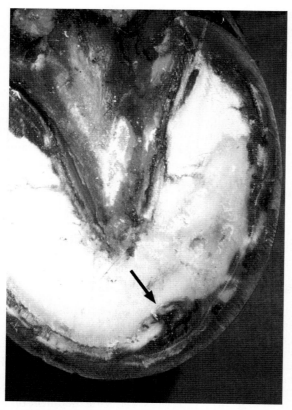

Figure 8.105 Darkened region on the white line, indicating a penetrating wound at that site (arrow).

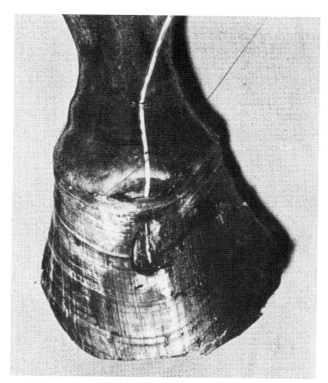

Figure 8.106 Oblong hole made in the dorsal surface of the hoof wall to remove the involved tissue and provide good drainage.

centrated magnesium sulfate (Epsom salts) solution may draw the infection to the surface. When the abscess comes to a "head" just proximal to the coronet band, drainage can be established by lancing the abscess.[2–4] If a draining tract is present at the time of presentation, maintenance of the drainage by flushing the tract with dilute povidone iodine solution and local wound care may be all that is needed.

If the site of infection at the bottom of the foot can be identified, it should be opened and enlarged to allow for ventral drainage. The tract can be debrided with a small bone curette if needed. The drainage hole at the white line should be large enough that the deeper tissues heal in advance of the more superficial tissues.[4] The infection usually resolves with soaking the foot in magnesium sulfate solution and irrigating the tract with povidone iodine. Bandaging the foot or placement of a protective boot to prevent contamination of the openings in the hoof should be done. If the drainage persists for longer than 7 to 10 days, a radiographic examination should be done, followed by a fistulogram to determine if a foreign body is present or if the collateral cartilage is involved.

In more chronic cases with a long-term history of drainage at the coronary band that has resulted in considerable undermining of the hoof wall, it may be helpful to create a circular hole in the hoof wall midway between the solar surface and the coronary band (Fig. 8.106). This allows better access to clear the tract more thoroughly of necrotic and infected tissue and to provide

better drainage.[1] In some cases, a trephine hole placed at the lowest point of infected tract in the hoof wall can be used to provide drainage.[7] Bandaging to protect the foot from contamination should follow until all signs of infection have disappeared. Soaking the foot in supersaturated solutions of Epsom salts and antiseptic agents has been traditional. Systemic antibiotics may be required if the infection involves the regional soft tissue of the pastern. If a hoof wall resection has to be done, a shoe with large clips drawn on either side of the resected area of the wall helps stabilize the hoof and prevent the development of a chronic hoof defect.[7]

Once the infection has resolved, a shoe with a pad can be applied to protect the sole of the hoof from dirt and manure being packed into the hole. Prosthetic hoof wall material can be applied to the circular hole in the hoof wall after it has become cornified and all signs of infection are gone.

Prognosis

The prognosis is generally favorable if the condition is diagnosed early and adequate drainage and wound care have been provided. The prognosis is guarded if the condition becomes chronic and extensive hoof wall undermining has occurred. Even in these cases, if the horses are properly cared for, they will return to complete soundness. The prognosis is even more guarded if contamination of the sensitive lamina is secondary to separation of the white line from chronic laminitis.[4]

References

1. DeBowes RM, Yovich JV. Penetrating wounds, abscesses, gravel, and bruising of the equine foot. Vet Clin North Am Equine Pract 1989;5:179–194.
2. Honnas CM. Standing surgical procedures of the foot. Vet Clin North Am Equine Pract 1991;7:695–722.
3. Honnas CM, Meagher DM, Lindford RL. Surgical management of difficult foot problems in the horse: Current concepts. Proc Am Assoc Equine Pract 1988;38:249.
4. Honnas CM, Peloso JG, Carter KG, et al. Managing two infectious diseases of the horse's foot. Vet Med 1994;89:891–896.
5. Honnas CM, Ragle CA, Meagher DM. Necrosis of the collateral cartilage of the distal phalanx in horses: 16 cases (1970–1985). J Am Vet Med Assoc 1988;193:1303–1307.
6. Johnson JH. The foot. In: Mansmann RA, McAllister ES, Eds. Equine Medicine and Surgery. 3rd ed. Santa Barbara, CA: American Veterinary Publications, 1982;1038.
7. Meagher DM. Ascending infection under the hoof wall (gravel). In: Smith BP, Ed. Large Animal Internal Medicine: Diseases of Horses, Cattle, Sheep, and Goats. Philadelphia: Mosby-Year Book, 1990; 1178.

OSSIFICATION OF THE COLLATERAL CARTILAGES OF THE DISTAL PHALANX (SIDEBONES)

Ossification of the collateral cartilages of the distal phalanx is common in some breeds of horses. The forefeet seem to be more commonly involved than the hindfeet, and the clinical significance of the condition is questionable.[4,5,8,14,15] Female horses seem more susceptible to the development of this condition, and the lateral cartilage often shows more ossification than the medial cartilage.[1,12] The cartilage ossification can begin at the base of the cartilage or can originate as a separate area in the center of the cartilage.[3,7,8] In either case, the palmar part of the cartilage is likely to be spared from the ossification process.[12]

In a radiographic study done on 462 Finnhorses, 80% had evidence of sidebones, and large sidebones or separate centers of ossification were significantly more common in females than in males.[13] Although the incidence of larger sidebones was lower in young females (1 to 3 years) than older females (4 to 6 years), there was no significant increased incidence when 4- to 6-year-old horses were compared with horses older than 6 years of age. In another study, researchers found that 10% of Warmblood horses and 80% of Draft horses had ossification of the cartilages of the distal phalanx and that the ossification was more extensive in the draft horses than in the Warmblood horses.[15] Also, the lateral and the medial cartilages were ossified equally in Draft horses, but the lateral cartilages were more commonly involved in Warmbloods. In this same study it was concluded that ossification of the cartilages had no clinical significance.

Etiology

The specific causes of sidebones are not clear.[13] It has been suggested that the tendency to develop sidebones is partly hereditary in certain horse breeds in Australia, Finland, and Sweden.[9,13,15] Hoof concussion causing trauma to the cartilage, poor conformation, particularly base narrow, and poor trimming and shoeing have also been proposed as causes.[14] One study documenting the incidence of sidebones in Finnhorses found that few horses were base narrow and that most horses were base wide and toed out.[13] Another study concluded that ossification of the cartilages was neither the cause nor the result of conformational adaptations of the front feet.[11] It has also been suggested that prolonged exercise or racing may have some preventative influence on the development of ossification of the collateral cartilages.[10]

Signs

Lameness resulting from sidebones is considered rare, and the clinical significance of ossification being present is questioned.[5] One study found no correlation between the extent of ossification of the collateral cartilages and the onset of lameness.[15] Furthermore, in spite of the development of large sidebones in many Finnhorses, most horses performed satisfactorily without lameness.[13]

Visually, an enlargement of the lateral and medial dimensions of the pastern region may be recognized if the ossification process is extensive (Fig. 8.107). If the ossification involves the proximal extent of the cartilage, palpation will reveal an obvious firmness to the cartilage. Rarely is pain elicited with digital pressure, but if it is, the sidebone may be contributing to the lameness. Sidebones may accompany other lamenesses associated with the

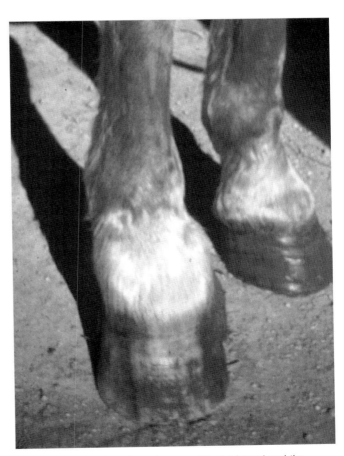

Figure 8.107 Note the enlargement in the lateral and the medial dimension of the right pastern region of this horse. The cause of the enlargement was ossification of the sidebones.

caudal heel region (e.g., navicular syndrome) and may be mistaken for the cause. On the other hand, pain in the caudal heel region may originate from the axial projections of the ungual cartilages that extend toward the midline and have an abundant sensory nerve supply.[2]

Diagnosis

The diagnosis of sidebones as the cause of lameness should not be made unless pain is present over the involved cartilage or cartilages. If sidebones are truly the cause of lameness, a palmar digital nerve block just above the collateral cartilage on the affected side should relieve signs of lameness.

Radiologic examination reveals the extent of the ossification of the cartilage or cartilages (Fig. 8.108). Occasionally, a sidebone may appear fractured; however, the radiolucent defect must be differentiated from the junction between a separate ossification center and that part of the cartilage that is ossifying from the palmar process of the distal phalanx.[7,12] In a radiographic study done on 462 Finnhorses, all of the radiolucent lines except one were located in the middle or distal part of the ossified cartilage.[13] A fracture in the ossified cartilage is painful but rare.[4,8]

Treatment

If the sidebones are suspected as the cause of lameness, rest and the administration of NSAIDs are logical treatment. It is suggested that the horse be trimmed to balance the feet naturally and that a shoe be applied to enhance breakover. (Refer to Chapter 9 for details.)

A fractured sidebone reportedly causes more acute signs of lameness.[4,8] However, one must not confuse

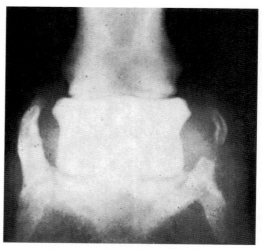

Figure 8.109 Sidebones. On the left, note the large sidebone. On the right, note the separate ossification center in the sidebone. This should not be confused with fracture of the sidebone, which is sometimes surgically removed. This type of ossification does not require surgical removal.

proximal fractures of sidebones with separate ossification centers (Fig. 8.109). Small proximal fragments can be surgically removed, but no attempt should be made to remove large proximal fragments.[6]

Prognosis

The prognosis is difficult to predict, since this condition rarely causes lameness.

References

1. Bengtsson G. Hovbroskforbining inom svenska kallblodraser. Sbensk Veterimartidning 1983;35:37–41.
2. Bowker RM, Van Wulfin K, Springer SE, et al. Functional anatomy of the cartilage of the distal phalanx and digital cushion in the equine foot and a hemodynamic flow hypothesis of energy dissipation. Am J Vet Res 1998;59:961–968.
3. Butler JA, Colles CM, Dyson SJ, et al. Distal phalanx. In: Clinical Radiology of the Horse. Oxford: Blackwell Scientific Publications, 1993;25–47.
4. Colles CM. Diseases and injuries of the horse's foot. In: Hickman J, ed. Equine Surgery and Medicine. London: Academic Press, 1986; 221–223.
5. Johnson JH. The foot. In: Mansmann RA, McAllister ES, Eds. Equine Medicine and Surgery. 3rd ed. Santa Barbara, CA: American Veterinary Publications, 1982;1052.
6. Lundvall RL. Surgical removal of fractured sidebones. Proc Am Assoc Equine Pract 1965;11:319–322.
7. Lebel JL. Lameness in horses. In: Gillette EL, Thrall DE, Lebel JE, Eds. Carlson's Veterinary Radiology. 3rd ed. Philadelphia: Lea & Febiger, 1977;415–461.
8. McNeel SV. The phalanges. In: Thrall DE, Ed. Textbook of Veterinary Diagnostic Radiology. 2nd ed. Philadelphia: WB Saunders, 1994;190–213.
9. Robertson WAN. The hereditary character of sidebone. Vet Rec 1932;12:83–90.
10. Ruohoniemi M, Laukkanen H, Ojala M, et al. Effects of sex and age on the ossification of the collateral cartilages of the distal phalanx of the Finnhorse and the relationships between ossification and body size and type of horse. Res Vet Sci 1997;62:34–38.
11. Ruohoniemi M, Raekallio M, Tulamo RM, Salonius K. Relationship between ossification of the cartilages of the foot and confor-

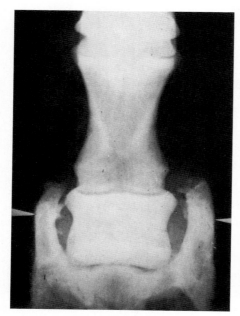

Figure 8.108 Ossification of collateral cartilages of the distal phalanx (sidebar).

mation and radiographic measurements of the front feet in Finn-horses. Equine Vet J 1997;29:44–48.

12. Ruohoniemi M, Ryhanen V, Tulamo RM. Radiographic appear-ance of the navicular bone and distal interphalangeal joint and their relationship with ossification of the collateral cartilages of the distal phalanx in Finnhorse cadaver forefeet. Vet Radiol Ultra-sound 1998;39:125–132.
13. Ruohoniemi M, Tulamo RM, Hackzell M. Radiographic evalua-tion of ossification of the collateral cartilages of the third phalanx in Finnhorses. Equine Vet J 1993;25:453–455.
14. Schneider RK, Stickle RL. Orthopedic problems of the foot. In: Current Therapy in Equine Medicine. 2nd ed. Philadelphia: WB Saunders, 1987;282–289.
15. Verschooten F, van Waerebeek B, Verbeeck J. The ossification of cartilages of the distal phalanx in the horse: An anatomical, experi-mental, radiographic and clinical study. J Equine Vet Sci 1996;16: 291–305.

SOLE BRUISES AND CORNS

A bruise results from the rupture of blood vessels in the dermis (corium or sensitive tissue) beneath the sole, frog, or hoof wall. With time the hemorrhage spreads into the deep layers of the epidermis and becomes visible as the hoof grows. Accordingly, the discoloration associated with a sole bruise is most often seen several weeks after injury, whereas the same injury occurring in the hoof wall may take months before it is apparent (Fig. 8.110).[7] Logically, bruises are most visible when the hemorrhage is superficial and the hoof is nonpigmented. It is likely that the inflammatory response and increased subsolar pressure cause the pain associated with the injury. The rest of the discussion focuses on the bruising of the tissues of the bottom of the foot.

Horses with flat feet, thin soles, and soft soles seem predisposed to bruising.[1] Also, horses that are barefoot, that have their hoof wall trimmed too short, or that have their hoof wall worn so that the sole protrudes below the hoof wall are likely to bruise their soles. A "corn" is a bruise that involves the tissues of the sole at the angle formed by the wall and the bar (Fig. 8.111).[2] This site is often referred to as the "seat" of the corn. Corns occur most frequently on the inner angle of the forefeet and

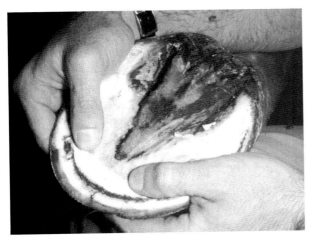

Figure 8.110   This horse had a sole bruise. Note the discoloration in the sole. Thumb pressure resulted in a painful response.

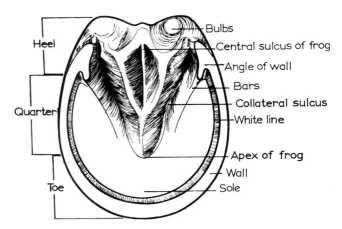

Figure 8.111   Normal forefoot showing structures.

are rarely found in the hindfeet. This may be because the forefeet bear more weight than the hindfeet. If the bruised site becomes infected, an abscess may develop.

Etiology

Trauma to the sole is the cause of sole bruising. Horses housed in muddy pens in freezing conditions, whether shod or not, often bruise their soles when the lumpy mud freezes hard. Also, horses that are barefoot and housed in rocky paddocks or pastures also are susceptible to bruising. Trimming of the hoof wall to short and the sole to thin can also cause sole bruising. Also, flat-footed horses that have repeated concussion to the sole adjacent to the white line because the sole contacts the inner aspect of the shoe often develop sole bruises.[4] Shoeing that concentrates weight bearing on the sole is likely to cause bruising also.

Corns are usually caused by pressure from horseshoes or when a stone becomes wedged between the shoe and the sole. Also, when shoes are left on the feet too long, the heels overgrow the shoe, resulting in selective pressure on the sole at the angle of the wall and the bar, which can result in a corn. Additionally, if the farrier bends the inside branch of the shoe toward the frog, to prevent pulling or stepping off the shoe, this practice can result in direct pressure to the sole at the angle, and repeated concussion leads to bruising.[5,6] The application of a shoe that is one-half to one full size too small for the foot also increases the pressure on the sole area at the angles.[6] Heel calks enhance this effect. Corns are rare among horses that are used barefooted.

Signs and Diagnosis

The signs associated with a bruised sole and a corn are similar, but sole bruises occur in the toe or the quarter regions rather than at the angle of the wall and bar. Occasionally, the frog can be bruised also.[7] Bruised sole or corns may be of dry, moist, or suppurating types. Dry bruises appear as red (old hemorrhage) stains. Moist bruises occur when serum accumulates beneath the injured epidermis. Suppurating bruises are infected bruises that may involve the sensitive lamina.

The horse will show varying degrees of lameness, depending on the severity and type of the bruise or corn, and the attitude of the lameness and foot placement will vary according to the location of the bruise or corn. If the bruise is acute or infected, the hoof may appear warmer, and an increased digital pulse may be felt.[7] Hoof testers often identify a site of pain unless the lesion is underneath the shoe at the white line. Perineal anesthesia may be required in some cases to exclude other sources of pain causing lameness. If the pain is localized to the foot region, the shoe should be removed, after which the exfoliating (flaky) sole is pared away with a hoof knife. Where acute bruises may not be readily apparent, because the hemorrhage has not migrated far enough distally, chronic bruises are usually visible as a "stippled," reddened region. In some cases the discoloration may be bluish, especially if a sole abscess is developing.

Acute bruises may not be evident radiographically unless a serum pocket or abscess has developed. On the other hand, chronic bruising may cause demineralization, increased vascular channels, and irregularity of the solar margin of the distal phalanx.[7]

Treatment

Many bruises resolve if the source of the trauma is removed. The horse should be rested from heavy work, especially if its soles are abnormally thin. When possible, the environment of the horse should be changed so that it is not worked on rough ground. If the horse must be used, the sole can be protected with a full pad applied under the shoe. Care is taken so pressure is not applied to the bruised site. Additionally, light paring of the sole overlying the bruise often relieves the pressure and makes the horse more comfortable.[7] NSAIDs are used as needed.

If the bruise abscesses, removing the diseased sole should drain it. The foot then should be soaked daily in antiseptic solution, after which the wound is dressed with an antiseptic ointment and the foot is protected with a bandage until a healthy bed of granulation tissue develops. A treatment plate can then be applied to the shoe to provide access to the defect and to protect the sole. (See Fig. 8.98.) For more information about treatment plates the reader is referred to Chapter 9.

In cases in which shoeing is the cause, removal of the shoe may be all that is necessary. To prevent shoes from causing corns, one must ensure that the heels of the shoe extend well back on the buttresses and fit full on the wall at the quarters and heels. Heel calks increase the chance of corns if a horse is shod too short at the heels or if the shoe is left on too long.[4] Removal of some of the tissue over the bruise helps relieve pressure, but sensitive tissue should not be exposed. The horse should be rested and should not be reshod until symptoms disappear.

If the horse must be used for some reason, the wall and bar in the region of the corn should be removed to prevent pressure by the shoe. A full support shoe can be applied to allow the frog to absorb the concussion that would normally be distributed to the corn area (Fig. 9.79).

Another option is to apply a wide-web shoe that has been made concave at the damaged region. This effectively decreases the pressure on the bruised site.[3,4] In cases in which it is difficult to place the wide-web shoe, a ¼-inch plastic rim can be applied and cut out over the region of the affected sole.[5]

Prognosis

The prognosis is good for horses suffering from a single traumatic episode and with horses with good foot conformation. The prognosis is guarded in horses with poor hoof conformation that are continually worked on hard ground. Many of these cases become chronic, which eventually may cause osteitis of the distal phalanx.

References

1. DeBowes RM, Yovich JV. Penetrating wounds, abscesses, gravel, and bruising of the equine foot. Vet. Clin North Am Equine Pract 1989;5:179–194.
2. Johnson JH. The foot. In: Mansmann RA, McAllister ES, Eds. Equine Medicine and Surgery. 3rd ed. Santa Barbara, CA: American Veterinary Publications, 1982;1039.
3. Moyer W. Therapeutic principles of diseases of the foot. Proc Am Assoc Equine Pract 1981;27:453.
4. Moyer W. Corrective shoeing. Vet Clin North Am Large Anim Pract 1980;2:3–24.
5. Moyer W. Diseases of the equine heel. Proc Am Assoc Equine Pract 1979;25:21.
6. Moyer W, Anderson T. Lameness caused by improper shoeing. J Am Vet Med Assoc 1975;166:47.
7. Parks A. Foot bruises: Diagnosis and treatment. In: White NA, Moore JN, Eds. Current Techniques in Equine Surgery and Lameness. 2nd ed. Philadelphia: WB Saunders, 1998;528–529.

CANKER

Equine canker is a chronic hypertrophic, moist pododermatitis of the epidermal tissues of the foot that has a characteristic fetid odor.[2,5,8] Historically, the disease was primarily observed in the hindfeet of Draft breeds; however, in recent reports there was no predilection for the hindfeet, and light breeds were also affected.[9] Although the cause of the disease is unknown, anaerobic gram-negative bacterial rods are consistently observed within epithelium.[7,9] The infection results in abnormal keratin production or dyskeratosis, which is seen as filamentous fronds of hypertrophic horn.[5] In time, the infection can spread from the frog region to involve the sole and hoof wall.[5] The disease is most commonly seen in semitropical areas of the southern states and in the humid environment of the Midwest. Canker may be misdiagnosed as "thrush," particularly in the early course of the disease, and unfortunately, the disease seems to flourish in the face of treatment aimed at resolving thrush.[8] The distinguishing feature of thrush being primarily the loss of frog tissue can be readily differentiated from the proliferative nature of canker.[8]

Etiology

The exact cause of canker is unknown, but affected horses often have a history of being housed either on moist pastures year round or in wet unhygienic conditions.[4,5,7] Horses standing in urine, feces, or mud-soaked bedding appear to be at risk.[5] The causative anaerobic gram-negative organisms are thought to be *Fusobacterium necrophorum* and one or more *Bacteroides* spp.[8]

Signs and Diagnosis

Lameness usually is not present in early stages of the disease because the superficial epidermis is primarily involved. Since neglect of the feet is a contributing cause, however, the disease may not be detected until it is well advanced and the corium may become involved, which can cause lameness. Examination of the foot usually reveals a fetid odor, and the frog, which may appear intact, has a ragged proliferative filamentous appearance. The epidermal tissue of the frog is usually friable and may have a white, cottage-cheese–like appearance.

The diagnosis is made with the physical findings of a moist exudative pododermatitis with characteristic hypertrophic filamentous fronds. It is confirmed with the histologic findings of hyperplastic epidermis with multifocal areas of intracellular edema.[6]

Treatment

Three essential components seem successful in the treatment of canker: early recognition of the problem, superficial debridement of the lesion to allow effective application of a topical antimicrobial agent, and maintenance of a clean dry environment for the foot. The misdiagnosis of canker as "thrush" early in the course of the disease can significantly delay the beginning of effective treatment, thus delaying the resolution of the problem before it becomes chronic. Both superficial and radical debridement have been used in the treatment of canker. Superficial debridement has been associated with a better outcome, however.[9] In this study,[9] done on 14 horses diagnosed with canker, 7 of 7 with superficial debridement of the lesion recovered, whereas only 4 of 7 with radical debridement of the lesion recovered. Because of this it is recommended that only the grossly abnormal tissue be debrided.

Successful treatment of canker in 5 horses by use of parenteral procaine penicillin has been described.[3] Tetracyclines have also been reported useful in the treatment of canker.[3] Superficial debridement and systemic administration and topical application of chloramphenicol to the diseased site resulted in complete resolution of canker in 7 horses.[9] Topical metronidazole has also been shown to be effective. In a report on 8 horses diagnosed with canker, all cases resolved with superficial debridement of the lesion and topical application of 2% metronidazole ointment.[8] The ointment was applied daily, and the feet were bandaged until the disease resolved. Treatment periods ranged from 2 to 8 weeks, with a mean treatment period of 4.6 weeks. The advantages to the use of metronidazole over chloramphenicol are lower cost and that there is no known human health risks associated with long-term use of metronidazole. Debridement and the topical application of ketoconazole, rifampin, and DMSO was reported to be successful in the treatment of one case of recurrent canker in a Shire mare.[6] Besides

dressings and bandaging until the lesion is healed, the horse should be kept in clean, dry surroundings.

Prognosis

The prognosis is favorable for complete resolution of the problem if treatment is instituted early in the course of the disease. For the best results the lesion should be superficially debrided of all abnormal-appearing tissue, followed by the topical application of metronidazole, after which the site is protected with a bandage. With use of this approach, 7 of 7 cases of canker were resolved.[8] Alternatively, a mixture of ketoconazole, rifampin, and DMSO may be used.[6]

References

1. Banic T, Skusek F. Experiences in the treatment of canker of the foot. Berl Munch Tierarztl Wochenschr 1960;73:186.
2. Bjorck G, Nilsson G. Chronic progressive pododermatitis in the horse. Equine Vet J 1971:2:65.
3. Mason TH. Penicillin treatment of foot canker. J S Afr Vet Assoc 1962;23:223.
4. Prescott CW. Canker in the hoof of a horse. Aust Vet J 1970;46:449–451.
5. Reeves MJ, Yovich JV, Turner AS. Miscellaneous conditions of the equine foot. Vet Clin North Am Equine Pract 1989;5:221–242.
6. Sherman K, Ginn PE, Brown M. Recurring canker in a shire mare. J Equine Vet Sci 1996;16:322–323.
7. Steckel RR. Puncture Wounds, Abscesses, Thrush, and Canker: Current Therapy in Equine Medicine. 2nd ed. Philadelphia: WB Saunders, 1987;269.
8. Wilson DG. Topical metronidazole in the treatment of equine canker. Proc Am Assoc Equine Pract 1994;40:49–50.
9. Wilson DG, Calderwood-Mays MB, Colahan PT. Treatment of canker in horses. J Am Vet Med Assoc 1989;194:1721–1723.

THRUSH

Thrush is a degenerative condition of the frog involving the central and lateral sulci, which is characterized by the presence of a black necrotic exudate in the affected areas and a foul odor. The hindlimbs are most frequently involved.[1,4] If the infection becomes chronic, it may extend to involve the dermal laminae and cause lameness. In severe cases, the infection may undermine the sole and result in swelling of the distal limb (cellulitis or phlegmon) and lameness.[4]

Etiology

Contributing factors for thrush are wet, unhygienic stable conditions, especially when horses stand in urine and manure-soiled bedding; neglect of daily foot care; and lack of exercise.[4] Inadequate or improper trimming and shoeing, which promotes long contracted heels and deep sulci, appears to increase the risk of infection. Although no specific organisms have been identified as the cause, *Fusobacterium necrophorum* is commonly isolated.

Signs and Diagnosis

An increased amount of moisture and a black discharge in the sulci of the frog are symptoms of thrush.

This discharge, which varies in quantity, has an offensive odor.[3] When the affected sulci are cleaned, they are deeper than normal and may extend into the sensitive tissues of the foot, causing the horse to flinch when they are cleaned. The frog may also be undermined, and large areas can be detached from the underlying frog. Lameness is present in severe cases that involve the corium, and swelling of the distal limbs may be seen.

The diagnosis is based on the odor and physical characteristics of the black discharge in the sulci of the frog. The condition should be differentiated from canker.

Treatment

Prevention by providing adequate, clean, dry bedding and daily foot care is preferable. This, of course, is most important for horses confined to a stall for prolonged periods. Proper hoof trimming and shoeing is also important.

Early cases usually respond to debridement of the diseased tissue and the topical application of an astringent with or without foot bandages.[3] Astringents that can be used include copper sulfate, equal parts of phenol and 7% iodine, tincture of iodine, and 10% formalin. Alternatively, the foot can be packed with "sugardine" (Betadine and equal parts of white sugar) or with cotton soaked in 10 to 15% sodium sulfapyridine solution. These treatments should be repeated until the infection is controlled. The horse should be kept in a dry, clean stall or in a dry yard. Repeated trimming of the frog may be required before the infection is controlled.

Severe cases of thrush are treated the same as acute cases, except that debridement of the diseased undermined tissue is more extensive. Also, some horses may benefit from daily soaking in supersaturated solutions of magnesium sulfate, after which an astringent is applied and the foot is protected in a sterile bandage.[2] Once the infection seems under control, the foot can be protected by applying a CVP gasket pad (refer to Chapter 9 for more information).

Prognosis

The prognosis is good if the disease is diagnosed early, before the foot has suffered extensive damage. The prognosis is guarded if there is extensive involvement of the corium.

References

1. Adams OR. Lameness in Horses. 3rd ed. Philadelphia: Lea & Febiger, 1974.
2. Johnson JH. The foot. In: Mansmann RA, McAllister ES, Eds. Equine Medicine and Surgery. 3rd ed. Santa Barbara, CA: American Veterinary Publications, 1982;1033.
3. Parks A. Chronic foot injury and deformity. In: White NA, Moore JN, Eds. Current Techniques in Equine Surgery and Lameness. Philadelphia: WB Saunders, 1998;534–536.
4. Reeves MJ, Yovich JV, Turner AS. Miscellaneous conditions of the equine foot. Vet Clin North Am Equine Pract 1989;5:235–236.

WHITE LINE DISEASE

Refer to Chapter 9 for a discussion of this subject.

KERATOMA

A keratoma is an uncommon condition of the hoof that is characterized by keratin-containing tissue growing between the hoof wall and the distal phalanx. Although the term implies a neoplastic process, histologic examination reveals abundant keratin, squamous epithelial cells, occasional granulation tissue, and inflammatory cells.[2,4,11] The growth usually begins near the coronet band, but it may extend to the solar surface anywhere along the white line.[3] A visible deviation of the coronary band and/or hoof wall is often present, and the most commonly affected areas of the foot are the toe and quarter.[11] Occasionally, a keratoma may be located at a focal site between the coronary band and sole.[8] Lameness and the radiographic changes are thought to arise from the growth of the keratoma and the subsequent pressure that is applied to the sensitive lamina and distal phalanx.[10,11] Keratomas have been observed in horses ranging from 2 to 20 years of age, and they should be differentiated from other growths that can occur in the hoof, such as squamous cell carcinoma, canker, and melanoma.[1,6,7,11,12]

Etiology

Trauma and chronic irritation in the form of sole abscesses or direct hoof injury are the cause in the majority of cases.[10] A keratoma can develop, however, without a history of previous injury, and the initiating cause often cannot be determined.[2,5,12]

Clinical Signs and Diagnosis

A history of a slow onset of intermittent lameness is common. The lameness is often seen before the distortion at the coronet band and hoof wall becomes obvious. Moderate to severe lameness is commonly observed at presentation.[2,5,11] The coronet band and hoof wall may be abnormally shaped, and close examination of the foot may be necessary to identify any abnormality. In those cases in which the growth has extended from the coronet band to the sole, a bulge in the hoof wall and a deviation in the white line toward the center of the foot may be seen (Fig. 8.112).[10] In some cases, a fistulous tract may develop in the sole or hoof wall, mimicking a subsolar abscess.[2,6,11,14] Hoof tester examination often elicits a painful response when pressure is applied over the lesion. Although perineural anesthesia of the palmar digital nerves at or below the level of the collateral cartilages often improves the signs of lameness, an abaxial sesamoid block is usually needed to eliminate the lameness.

Radiographically, the lesion may appear as a discrete semicircular defect in the distal phalanx (Fig. 8.113).[3] In one study that reported on 7 cases of keratoma, however, only 3 of 7 horses showed this radiographic sign.[11] The radiographic signs of a keratoma can usually be differentiated from septic bone lysis because of the smooth borders and lack of a sclerotic margin. Ultrasonographic imaging of a keratoma has been reported, and a hypoechoic, well-delineated soft tissue mass between the hoof wall and the articulation of the distal and middle phalanges was seen.[13] Only keratomas originating near the coronary band can be imaged ultrasonographically.

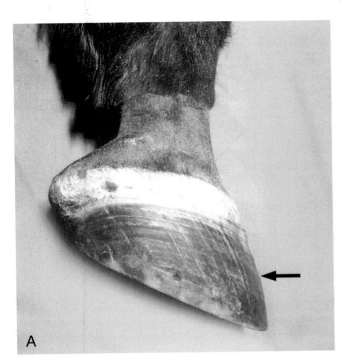

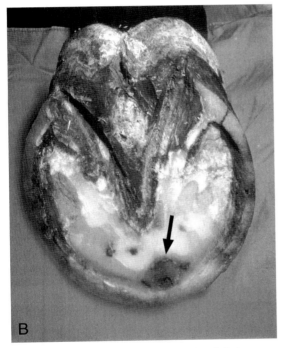

Figure 8.112 A. Dorsal bulge in the hoof wall that can occur with an extensive keratoma (arrow). B. Note the inward deviation of the white line caused by the keratoma (arrow).

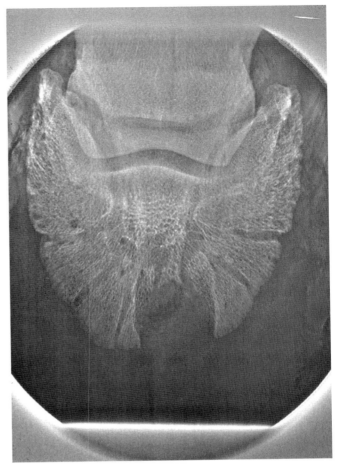

Figure 8.113 Dorsal palmar view of the distal phalanx. Note the defect in the distal phalanx.

Treatment

Treatment involves complete surgical removal of the abnormal growth. Incomplete removal frequently results in a high incidence of recurrence.[11] Surgery may be performed with the patient under general anesthesia or with the patient standing and under regional anesthesia and

sedation. The decision is made according to the patient's temperament and the extent of the lesion. In all cases, a tourniquet placed at the level of the fetlock is advised.

Two methods of gaining access to the abnormal tissue have been described. In one method a hoof wall flap can be created by making two parallel vertical cuts in the hoof wall down to the sensitive lamina on either side of the keratoma.[10] A third cut is made distally at the base of the mass, and a final cut can be made proximal to the mass (Fig. 8.114). The hoof wall cuts can be made with a motorized burr (my preference), a cast cutting saw, or an osteotome. The hoof wall is then grasped distally and reflected proximad to expose and remove the abnormal tissue. Care is taken to avoid damaging the coronet band. After the mass is removed, the soft tissue and bone are debrided to leave healthy margins (Fig. 8.115). The remaining defect is packed with gauze sponges soaked in dilute povidone iodine, and the foot is wrapped in a sterile bandage in such a way as to make the bandage impervious to environmental contamination. The hoof wall must be stabilized shortly after surgery. Hoof stabilization can be accomplished by application of a bar shoe with large clips drawn on either side of the defect. The clips help prevent independent movement of the two portions of the hoof wall. Drawing clips is usually adequate

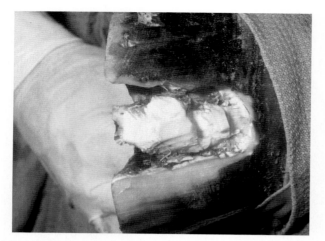

Figure 8.114 Distal, lateral, medial, and dorsal cuts have been made in the hoof wall with an air drill to expose the keratoma.

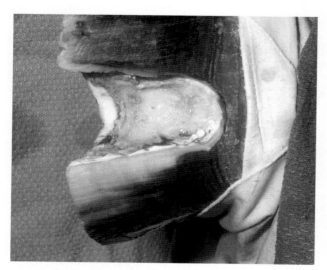

Figure 8.115 The keratoma has been removed, and the soft tissues and bone have been debrided.

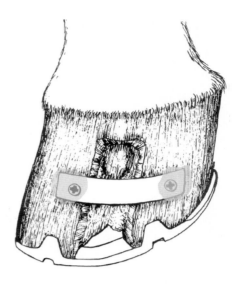

Figure 8.116 Metal strip being used to span the defect in the hoof wall and a clipped shoe. The metal strip is attached to the hoof wall with screws, and acrylic (gray) is placed over the top of the screws.

when the hoof defect is small and located distally. If the hoof wall resection extends proximad toward the coronet, a metal strip that spans the defect can be attached to the hoof wall with ⅜- to ¼-inch sheet metal screws to further stabilize the foot (Fig. 8.116).[8,9] Without the metal strip the proximal portion of the resected hoof wall may become unstable, resulting in the development of exuberant granulation tissue and pain.[2] The screws can be covered with hoof acrylic to prevent them from backing out. The shoe is reset at 6- to 8-week intervals, and this process is continued until the hoof wall reaches the ground. The metal strip is left in place as the hoof grows and reaches the weight-bearing surface.[6]

A second method used to gain access to the keratoma is to make a hole in the hoof wall with a large Galt trephine. This technique can be done while the patient is standing and sedated. The location of the keratoma must be documented. This can be done by gross observation and can be confirmed by radiographic documenta-

tion with metal objects used as markers. Multiple trephination can be done to adequately expose the lesion. The major advantage to this approach is relative lack of disruption of the hoof wall. Additional stabilization of the hoof wall is usually unnecessary.[5]

Postoperatively, bandages are changed every 3 to 4 days, and bandage protection is continued until the defect is completely cornified. This usually takes 2 to 3 weeks.[6] Gradually increasing the concentration of iodine applied to the surface of the defect may be used to enhance cornification.[9] Once a firm cuticle is formed, the defect in the hoof wall may be filled with polymethylmethacrylate.[5] The stabilizing shoe should be maintained until the hoof defect has grown out distally in the hoof wall. This process occurs generally over a period of 6 to 12 months. Stall rest is recommended until the hoof defect is healed enough to allow hoof reconstruction. Hoof wall reconstruction can be accomplished with a polymethyl methacrylate resin that may allow for a faster return to performance.[5] The acrylic is applied when the exposed laminar tissue is completely cornified and there is no evidence of lameness or radiographic changes in the defect.[5]

Prognosis

The prognosis is good for a return to performance if the abnormal tissue is completely removed.[2,5] In one study, 6 of 7 horses were sound 1 year after surgery with no recurrence of the keratoma.[11] Adequate stabilization of the hoof defect and complete removal of the lesion are most important to the outcome.

References

1. Berry CR, O'Brien TR, Pool RR. Squamous cell carcinoma of the hoof wall in a stallion. J Am Vet Med Assoc 1991;199:90–92.

2. Chaffin MK, Carter GK, Sustaire D. Management of a keratoma in a horse: A case report. J Equine Vet Sci 1989;323–326.
3. Frisbee DD, Trotter GW. Keratomas. In: White NA, Moore JN, Eds. Current Techniques in Equine Surgery and Lameness. 2nd ed. Philadelphia: WB Saunders, 1998;531–533.
4. Hamir AN, Kunz C, Evans LH. Equine keratoma. J Vet Diagn Invest 1992;4:99–100.
5. Helms J, Pleasant RS, Modransky PD. Management of a keratoma in a horse. Equine Pract 1994;16:35–38.
6. Honnas CM. Keratomas of the equine digit. Equine Vet Educ 1997; 9:203–207.
7. Honnas CM, Liskey CC, Meagher DM, et al. Malignant melanoma in the foot of a horse. J Am Vet Med Assoc 1990;197:756–758.
8. Honnas CM, Meagher DM, Linford RL. Surgical management of difficult foot problems in the horse: Current concepts. Proc Am Assoc Equine Pract 1988;34:249–262.
9. Honnas CM, Peloso JG, Carter GK, et al. Surgical management of incomplete avulsion of the coronary band and keratomas in the horse. Vet Med 1994;89:984–988.
10. Johnson JH. The foot. In: Mansmann RA, McAllister ES, Eds. Equine Medicine and Surgery. 3rd ed. Santa Barbara, CA: American Veterinary Publications, 1982;1039.
11. Lloyd KCK, Peterson PR, Wheat JD, et al. Keratomas in horses: Seven cases (1975–1986). J Am Vet Med Assoc 1988;193: 967–970.
12. Reeves MJ, Yovich JV, Turner AS. Miscellaneous conditions of the equine foot. Vet Clin North Am Equine Pract 1989;5:221–242.
13. Seahorn TL, Sams AE, Honnas CM, et al. Ultrasonographic imaging of a keratoma in a horse. J Am Vet Med Assoc 1992;200: 1973–1974.
14. Wagner PC, Balch-Burnett O, Merritt F. Surgical management of keratomas in the foot of the horse. Equine Pract 1986;11–14.

SELENIUM TOXICOSIS

Selenium toxicosis of horses has been classically divided into three categories: an acute form, a subacute form with horses exhibiting blind staggers, and a chronic form of the alkali disease type.[2,7,8] The acute form results when a horse rapidly consumes large quantities of selenium. The single minimum lethal dose of sodium selenite for the horse is 3.3 mg/kg.[12] Signs of acute selenium toxicosis include severe dyspnea, diarrhea, incoordination, prostration, and death within a few hours after ingestion of toxic levels.[6,8] Blind staggers was thought at one time to be a subacute form of selenium toxicosis caused by selenium's effect on the liver and brain. Presently, the symptom of blind staggers is thought to be caused by an alkaloid in selenium accumulator plants rather than from high levels of selenium intake.[9] Brittle dry hair, alopecia, abnormal hoof wall growth, and lameness are characteristic of the chronic form (alkali disease).[4,11] These changes in the hair and hooves reflect selenium's ability to bind the sulfur-containing amino acids methionine and cystine, which affects cell division and growth.[10] Further discussion of this subject is limited to the chronic (alkali) form of the disease (see Chapter 5, Selenium Toxicity, for more details).

Etiology

Chronic selenium toxicosis usually occurs after ingestion of a ration containing at least 5 to 10 ppm of selenium (dry matter).[14] The tolerance limits for oral ingestion of selenium-containing feed is 5 ppm.[3] Potential sources of foraged selenium are from secondary selenium accumulator plants or from grains grown in seleniferous regions.[7,8,11] Seleniferous regions in the United States exist in California, Colorado, Idaho, Kansas, Montana, Nebraska, New Mexico, Oregon, South Dakota, Utah, and Wyoming.[5] Similar areas also exist in western Canada, Mexico, Colombia, Ireland, Israel, and South Africa.[15] Three major plant groups extract selenium from the soil. Obligate accumulators require high selenium soil to grow and hence are called indicator plants. They can accumulate as much as 100 times the selenium levels found in other plants and may contain levels of 10,000 ppm even in soils containing only moderate amounts of selenium.[14] Plants in this group include species of *Astragalus* (milk vetches), *Haplopappus*, *Machaeranthera*, and *Stanleya* (prince's plume) (Fig. 8.117, A and B). These plants are generally unpalatable and therefore are rarely a cause of selenium toxicity. The plants may be ingested during the first spring growth, however, when they appear green and lush.[14] Facultative or secondary accumulators do not require increased levels of selenium in the soil to grow. When selenium is present, however, these plants may accumulate as much as 25 to 100 ppm of selenium (dry matter), compared with other plants in the same area. Important species in this group include *Aster*, *Atriplex* (four-winged salt brush), *Agropyron* (wheat grass or bluestem), *Castilleja*, *Comandra*, *Gutierrezia sarothral* (broomweed, snakeweed, or matchweed), *Grindelia squarrosa* (gumweed), *Machaeranthera*, and *Sideranthus*. These plants are common causes of selenium toxicosis.[14] Passive accumulators passively accumulate selenium if it is present. Cereal grains, grasses, alfalfa, and weeds from seleniferous soil may contain more than 5 ppm of selenium, which is above the tolerance limits.[3,10] Chronic poisonings from selenium salts have also been reported in animals drinking water containing 0.5 to 2.0 ppm of selenium.[6] Additionally, diets low in sulfur (less than 0.05%) may be a factor predisposing animals to selenium toxicosis.[13]

Signs and Diagnosis

Horses with chronic selenium toxicosis exhibit weight loss, hair loss, and lameness in all four limbs caused by defective hoof wall growth.[7,12,19] The hair coat is usually dull, short, and brittle, and the tail hairs and mane may be short (Fig. 8.118). There is no pruritus or skin lesions associated with the hair loss, nor is there a change in the coat color with the new hair growth.[4,19] The coronary band is often painful to palpation, and the band may separate, after which necrotic material exudes from the defect.[4] In severe cases, the hooves circumferentially detach from the coronary band region, and the hoof walls may slough. In less severe cases, horses develop uniform circumferential transverse fissures or cracks parallel to the coronet band in the hoof wall. These fissures may extend down to the sensitive lamina (Fig. 8.119). When the fissure has extended approximately halfway down the hoof wall, the lower portion of the hoof frequently overrides the new hoof.[16] In some cases, subsolar abscesses may also be present. Congenital hoof wall defects have been reported in foals born to mares ingesting toxic levels of selenium.[1] Radiographs usually indicate no changes in the deep hoof wall structures.

Although the diagnosis can be made from the clinical signs alone, samples of feed, serum, or tissues can be

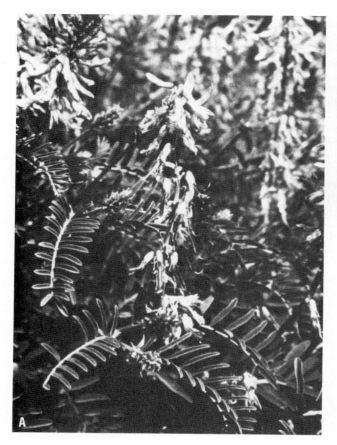

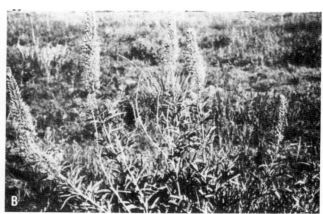

Figure 8.117   Two examples of selenium indicator plants. A. Prince's plume (*Stanleya pinnata*). B. Two-grooved milk vetch (*Astragalus bisulcatus*). (Courtesy of Dr. A. P. Knight.)

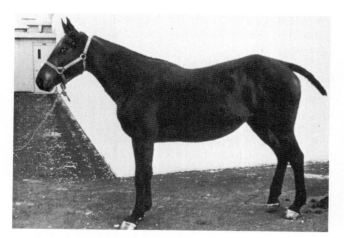

Figure 8.118   This horse presented with progressive hair loss and lameness. On physical examination, a dull, dry hair coat, loss of tail and mane hairs, and lameness were present, and transverse hoof wall cracks were evident on all four feet. These signs are consistent with selenium toxicosis.

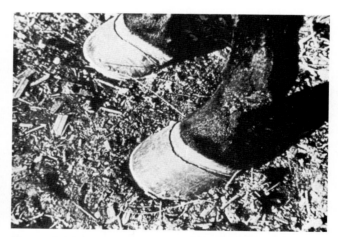

Figure 8.119   Transverse cracks in the hoof walls are often seen with chronic selenium toxicosis. If these cracks extend down to the sensitive lamina, horses often become lame.

taken to measure selenium levels and confirm a diagnosis. Horses being fed selenium at more than 5 ppm on a dry-matter basis for prolonged periods are susceptible to toxicosis.[1] Serum selenium levels of 1 to 5 ppm are consistent with a diagnosis of chronic selenosis.[4] How-ever, horses must still be consuming the high selenium diet for serum values of selenium to be diagnostic. If the horse is no longer on seleniferous feed, tissues levels of selenium are best used to detect selenium toxcity.[18] A hoof wall sample containing 5 to 20 ppm of selenium is considered diagnostic of chronic selenium toxicity.[2,7] Hair samples may not be reliable, as the level of selenium in different parts of the mane and tail are variable.[18] Hepatic and renal levels of 4 to 25 ppm or higher are consistent with a diagnosis of selenium toxicity.[1]

Treatment and Prevention

Treatment of chronic selenium toxicity is aimed at reducing the intake of selenium and treatment of the feet if necessary. Horses with chronic selenium toxicity should be removed from the dietary source of selenium and provided with a balanced, high-protein, low-selenium ration. A protein diet rich in the sulfur-containing amino acids cysteine and methionine helps counteract selenium's effect.[10] If foot abscesses are present, they should be opened and drained, and the feet should be placed in antiseptic bandages until they are healed. Horses that slough their hooves distal to the transverse fissures also must be maintained in antiseptic hoof bandages or treatment boots until the keratinized layer forms. After the hoof wall defects have completely keratinized, they can be filled with an acrylic.[7]

Prevention of chronic exposure to selenium can be accomplished by restricting dietary concentration of selenium, on a dry-matter basis, in the ration to less than 5 ppm. Therefore, if feedstuffs are high in selenium, they can be blended with feed grown in low-selenium soils to achieve a ration with less than the toxic level of selenium. Horses that must be pastured in areas with a high concentration of selenium can have their diet supplemented with a high-quality source of protein, such as alfalfa hay, that is also high in sulfur-containing amino acids.[1] High-protein diets seem protective against the development of selenosis. Pretreatment with copper is effective in preventing selenium toxicity in all species; and the mechanism of this protection is unknown.[1,17] Using organic or inorganic arsenic or naphthalene also appears to have a protective effect.[2,3,7] Salts containing 40 ppm arsenic and 5 ppm inorganic arsenic, placed in the drinking water, are useful to prevent selenium toxicosis.[7] Cattle and horses have been treated for selenium toxicity with 4 to 5 g of naphthalene orally for 5 days, without for 5 days, and then with the dose for 5 more days.[7]

Prognosis

The prognosis for the chronic form of the disease appears good provided the treatment of the feet is successful. In some cases, 8 to 10 months pass before the affected horse can be ridden.

References

1. Blood DC, Radostitis OM, Henderson JA. Veterinary Medicine. 6th ed. London: Bailliere Tindall, 1983;1102–1104.
2. Buck WB, Osweller GD, van Gelder GA. Clinical and Diagnostic Veterinary Toxicology. 2nd ed. Dubuque, IA: Kendall/Hunt, 1986; 345–354.
3. Clarke EGC, Clarke ML. Veterinary Toxicology. Baltimore: Williams & Wilkins, 1975;95.
4. Crinion RAG, O'Connor JG. Selenium intoxication in horses. Ir Vet J 1978;32:81–86.
5. Edmondson AJ, Norman BB, Suther D. Survey of state veterinarians and state veterinary diagnostic laboratories for selenium deficiency and toxicosis in animals. J Am Vet Med Assoc 1993;202: 865–872.
6. Harr JR, Muth OH. Selenium poisoning in domestic animals and its relationship to man. Clin Toxicol 1972;5:175–186.
7. Hultine JD, Easley KJ. Selenium toxicosis in the horse. Equine Pract 1979;1:57.
8. Fowler ME. Diseases caused by chemical and physical agents. In: Catcott EJ, Smithcors JE, Eds. Equine Medicine and Surgery. 2nd ed. Wheaton, MD: American Veterinary Publications, 1978;208.
9. James LF, Smart RA, Shupe JL, et al. Suspected phytogenic selenium poisoning in sheep. J Am Vet Med Assoc 1982;180: 1478–1481.
10. Knight AP. Selenium toxicosis. In: Lewis LD, Ed. Equine Clinical Nutrition: Feeding and Care. Baltimore: Williams and Wilkins, 1995;473–479.
11. Knott SG, McCray CWR. Selenium poisoning in horses in North Queensland. Queensland J Agri Sci 1958;15:43.
12. Miller QT, Williams KT. Minimum lethal dose of selenium of sodium selenite for horses, mules, cattle and swine. J Agri Res 1940; 60:163–167.
13. Pope AL, Moir RJ, Somers M, et al. The effect of sulphur on ^{75}Se absorption and retention in sheep. J Nutr 1979;109:1448–1455.
14. Reeves MJ, Yovich JV, Turner AS. Miscellaneous conditions of the equine foot. Vet Clin North Am Equine Pract 1989;5:239–241.
15. Rosenfeld I, Beath OA. Selenium: Geobotany, Biochemistry, Toxicity and Nutrition. New York: Academic Press, 1964;141–213.
16. Subcommittee on Selenium. Selenium in Nutrition. Washington, DC: National Research Council, National Academy of Sciences, 1983;109.
17. Smith HA, Jones TC, Hulnt RD. Veterinary Pathology. 4th ed. Philadelphia: Lea & Febiger, 1972;901–904.
18. Stowe HD. Effects of copper pretreatment upon the toxicity of selenium in ponies. Am J Vet Res 1980;41:1925–1928.
19. Traub-Dargatz JL, Knight AP, Hamar DW. Selenium toxicity in horses. Comp Cont Educ Pract Vet 1986;8:771–776.

AVULSION INJURIES OF THE FOOT REGION

Avulsion of the foot region is an uncommon injury that may seriously limit function, and in some cases euthanasia may be advised (Fig. 8.120). The avulsion may be complete where the tissue is totally removed, or it may be incomplete where a border remains intact. It may involve the hoof wall, the coronary band, the pastern region, and the sole and structures deep to the hoof capsule (e.g., distal phalanx) (Fig. 8.121). Generally, the deeper the avulsion and the more complete it is, the more serious the injury. Even with significant loss of germinal tissue, however, the foot has the capacity to heal, although it heals slower than other tissues, with complete reformation of hoof wall structures if it is treated properly for a long enough period.[3,7] Because the foot region has limited ability for wound contraction, the wound heals primarily by epithelialization and reformation of the corium.[6] These processes require a healthy bed of granulation tissue and a stable clean environment to reach an ideal conclusion. If the granulation tissue remains infected and becomes fibrous or if excessive motion is present, a permanent hoof defect may remain. In some cases, improved healing can be achieved in older wounds by periodically debriding the granulation surface, which stimulates new capillary formation.[1] If proper wound care follows, some of these older wounds heal completely.

Although avulsion injuries of the coronary region, complete or incomplete, may result in deformities or per-

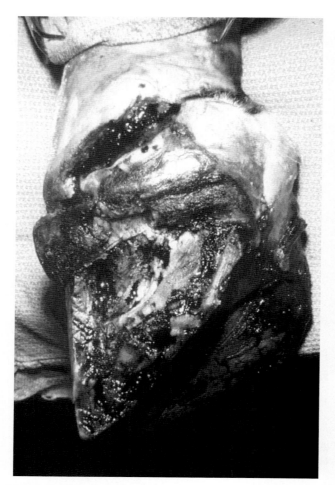

Figure 8.120 Extensive avulsion injury of the hoof wall and coronet band that may limit function.

manent hoof wall defects, the majority, if treated properly initially, will heal without problems (Fig. 8.122).[1,2,7] If a horn (epidermal) spur develops as a result of complete avulsion or partial avulsion, it usually remains painful until surgical treatment is employed (Fig. 8.123). Neither partial loss of the distal phalanx or digital cushion nor collateral cartilages seems a serious detriment to future soundness. Involvement of the deep digital flexor tendon (DDFT), although serious, can result in pasture soundness and, in some cases, riding soundness if treatment is not delayed.[7] On the other hand, treatment delay often results in degenerative changes within the tendon, and necrotic tendinitis may follow. Infection naturally accelerates this degeneration process and duly alters the prognosis. Other complications that may arise from these injuries include osteomyelitis and fracture of the distal phalanx, septic arthritis of the coffin joint, and septic tenosynovitis of the digital sheath. Even if these complications are not present, the horse may remain permanently lame simply because of the volume of tissue loss. Although the time required for healing depends on the size and extent of the avulsion injury and the method of treatment, generally, 3 to 5 months are needed for healing of a complete avulsion, whereas incomplete avulsions that are reconstructed surgically usually heal in 3

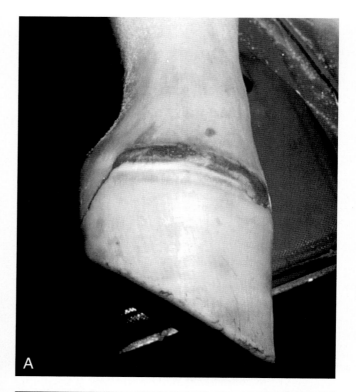

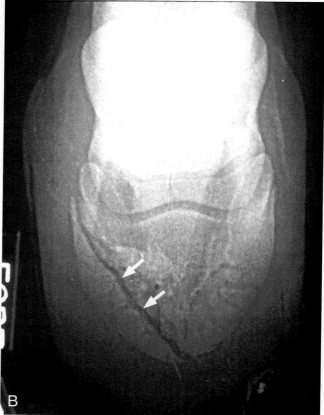

Figure 8.121 Incomplete avulsion injury of the hoof wall that involved the distal phalanx. A. Avulsion injury. B. Dorsal palmar view identifying the involvement (fracture) of the distal phalanx (arrows).

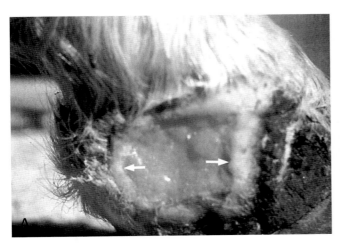

Figure 8.122 A. Complete avulsion injury of the foot of 2 weeks duration. Note the wound is filled with granulation tissue. The white tissue at the periphery represents epithelialization

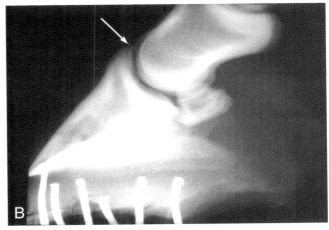

(arrows). B. One and half years later. Even though the hoof wall did not appear normal, this horse remained sound but required a bar shoe. (Courtesy of Dr. W. A. Aanes.)

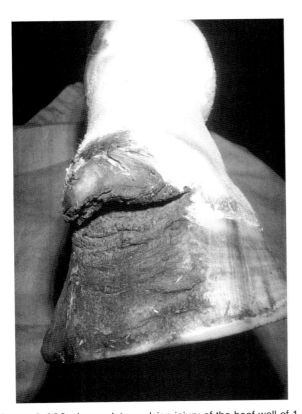

Figure 8.123 Incomplete avulsion injury of the hoof wall of 1 year duration. This horse was lame at presentation, and pressure applied upward on the horny projection elicited a painful response. Historically, when the projection was removed the horse became sound.

to 4 weeks.[2] Even when healing is complete, soundness may not return for many months, and in some cases, a year may be required. Because the duration to final outcome is so long, it is difficult to prognosticate on many of these cases at the onset of treatment.[5]

Etiology

Incomplete avulsion of the hoof wall of the heel can be caused by vertical tears of the hoof wall, infection and subsequent separation between the epidermal and the dermal laminae, kicking or stepping on sharp objects, continued foot imbalance, and improper shoe removal where nails are torn out of the heel and quarter regions.[5] Other avulsions of the foot and pastern region are usually caused by laceration from sharp objects. The horse either steps on or kicks at a sharp object or the foot becomes entrapped, resulting in the avulsion.

Clinical Signs and Diagnosis

The degree of lameness usually varies with the duration, extent, and location of the avulsion injury. Excessive contamination caused by the foot's distal location may result in infection if proper treatment is not employed.

Moderate lameness is usually seen with the acute superficial injury that does not involve deeper vital structures. However, palpation may cause considerable pain and render the animal non-weight bearing. More extensive avulsion injuries usually cause non-weight-bearing lameness (Fig. 8.121). If the injury involves the digital vessels, hemorrhage may be excessive, resulting in shock. Often these horses are quite nervous, making it tempting to sedate or tranquilize the horse before a thorough physical is performed. Gentle manipulation of the foot and phalanges can provide important information regarding the status of support structures. Where laxity and instability of a joint indicate loss of collateral ligament support, a sucking noise may indicate an open joint. More discriminating palpation is performed after the region has been cleaned and antiseptically prepared.

For the chronic avulsion injury, varying degrees of lameness are seen. If the wound is healing without problems, lameness usually subsides with time. If lameness is persistent, however, look for the cause. This often requires radiographic examination; in some cases, ultrasound examination may be helpful to assess soft tissue involvement. If a portion of the wound remains unhealed and drainage is present or, historically, drainage or pus is seen periodically, infection deep to the site is most likely the problem.

Although the diagnosis of avulsion injury is straightforward, the involvement of deeper structures must be identified. Prior to a more complete examination of the wound, the hair is clipped from the surrounding region, and the wound site is cleaned with an antiseptic scrub, after which it is rinsed with a mild antiseptic sterile salt solution. If the avulsion extends to the sole, the sole may be trimmed and cleaned in a similar fashion. Loose pieces of dead tissue and debris are removed during this cleaning process. Once complete, the wound can be palpated digitally after a sterile glove has been applied. Further manipulation of the foot and phalanges at this time may be helpful to identify an open synovial structure, torn support structure, or a fracture. A sterile probe can be used for palpation of a small opening. If there is any question that a synovial structure is involved a needle should be placed in a site in the synovial cavity remote to the site of injury. Then sterile fluid is injected under pressure. Fluid flowing from the wound confirms that the synovial cavity was penetrated.

Because fracture of the distal and middle phalanges may accompany these injuries, radiographic examination should be performed on all cases in which deep avulsion injuries are present or in which draining tracts have developed during the healing process. Additionally, contrast radiographic studies of draining tracts may be helpful in identifying openings in synovial structures.

Treatment

Incomplete Avulsion (Coronary Band Not Involved)

Incomplete avulsion of the hoof wall at the heel and quarter without involvement of the coronary band can be managed with the horse either standing for limited involvement or in recumbency under general anesthesia for a larger avulsion. Although a sharp hoof knife and nippers can be used to excise these undermined regions, I prefer to use a handheld electric drill to burr the hoof wall at its attachments. Using this method allows a more discrete removal of the hoof wall without a tearing of healthy hoof wall from the dermal laminae. Using a hoof knife or nippers may result in tearing of healthy tissues. Additionally, the burring procedure allows the surgeon to debride the infected underlying tissues superficially. The dorsal attachment of the unaffected hoof wall can be beveled flush to the wound so that there is little tendency for it to be snagged, resulting in further separation (Fig. 8.124). All crevices within the wound are debrided until only healthy tissue remains. After debridement is completed, the wound is lavaged with a mild antiseptic sterile salt solution delivered under pressure to achieve at least 7 psi. After this, an antiseptic or antibiotic dressing is applied to the wound, which is protected by a sterile bandage. Bandages are changed at 2- to 4-day intervals, at which time the wound is cleaned, retreated, and protected in a similar fashion. Alternatively, a rubber or plastic boot can be used instead of a bandage.

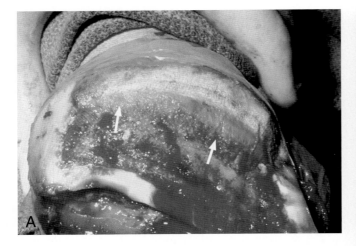

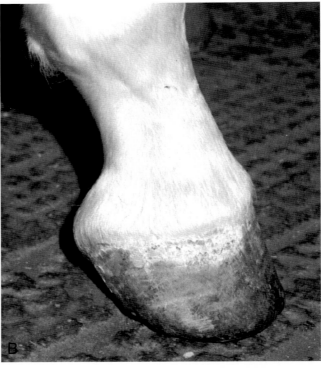

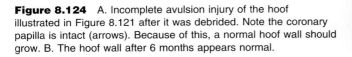

Figure 8.124   A. Incomplete avulsion injury of the hoof illustrated in Figure 8.121 after it was debrided. Note the coronary papilla is intact (arrows). Because of this, a normal hoof wall should grow. B. The hoof wall after 6 months appears normal.

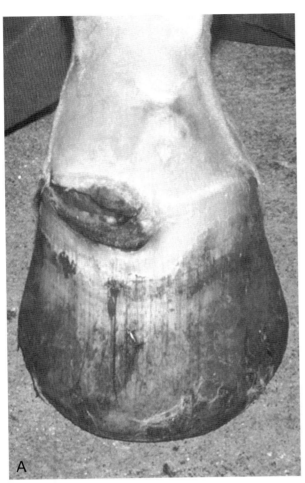

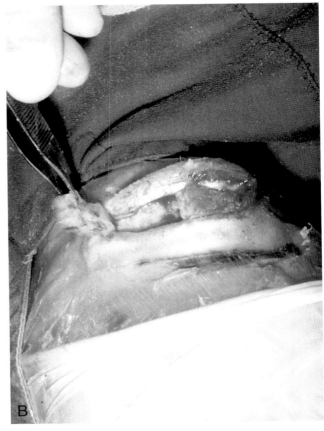

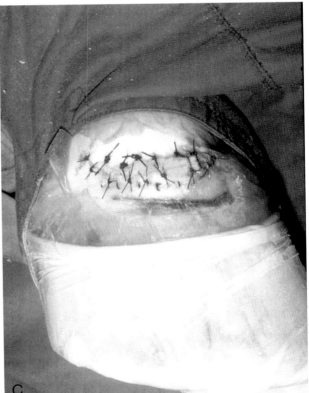

Figure 8.125 A. Incomplete avulsion injury of 3 weeks duration. B. Granulation tissue is being removed with forceps. C. The flap of skin and the hoof wall are sutured in place. A cast was then applied.

Sterile dressings are still applied to the wound surface. Protection from contamination and the application of antiseptics and antibiotics are continued until exposed tissues become keratinized. After this, a full support shoe (egg bar or heart bar shoe) is applied to provide hoof wall stability, and a hoof acrylic can be used to fill the deficit until the hoof wall grows to approximate the solar margin.

Incomplete Avulsion (Coronary Band Involved)

Incomplete avulsion of the coronary band alone or of the coronary band and the hoof wall is generally best managed by suture, although in some cases loss of blood supply requires excision of the separated tissue, thus converting it to a complete avulsion. The treatment for this latter situation is covered under the heading, Complete Avulsion. The acute incomplete avulsion injury of the coronary band and a small portion of the hoof wall may be treated acutely if a good blood supply exists. The hoof wall adjacent to the defect is thinned with a hoof rasp, and the separated piece of hoof wall is thinned with a motorized burr to allow suturing. After debridement and cleansing, sutures of 0 or 1 monofilament nylon are placed through the hoof wall into the separated horn in an interrupted vertical mattress pattern to appose them. After this, the coronary band and tissues in the pastern region are apposed with 2-0 monofilament nylon in an interrupted vertical mattress suture pattern. If the blood supply is questionable or if excessive contamination exists, delayed primary closure may be selected.[4,6] Usually, granulation tissue must be removed before the tissues are sutured. If left untreated, these incomplete avulsion injuries of the coronary band remain elevated, eventually producing a horny spur at the distal extremity of the avulsion, while the remaining underlying tissue heals by scarring and epithelialization. Invariably, these avulsions protrude above the skin and hoof wall surface, making them susceptible to further trauma, and generally, they are painful to palpation (Fig. 8.125A). If the avulsed tissue is removed, a hoof wall defect may remain. Therefore, surgical reconstruction is recommended. After thinning the hoof wall adjacent to the defect, the surgeon contours and thins the horny spur with a handheld electrical drill and burr until it fits into the hoof wall defect. Scarred tissue is then excised (debulked) from underneath the avulsed skin flap and within the wound so that the flap lays flat (Fig. 8.125B). A thin (1.5 mm) piece of hoof wall and skin is removed from all edges of the wound before suturing. Suture apposition is as previously described (Fig. 8.125C). If the coronary band has been destroyed, making it difficult to identify, yet proliferative hoof that causes pain and lameness continues to be produced, the proliferative hoof can be completely excised. Often this results in a granulating wound proximal to the coronary band that can be skin grafted at an appropriate time (Fig. 8.126).

When the avulsion injury extends from the solar surface proximad through the coronet, the majority of the hoof wall is removed to within 1 cm of the coronary region, and the coronary band and soft tissues are sutured (Fig. 8.127). Accurate approximation of the coro-

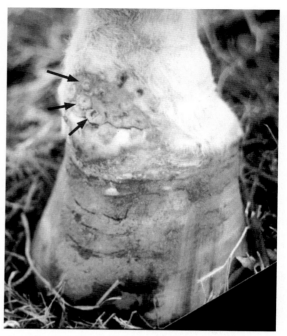

Figure 8.126 This is the same horse as in Figure 8.123 4 weeks after the proliferative horn has been removed. A punch skin graft (arrows) was done 2 weeks after surgery.

nary band is important. If the entire avulsion injury is sutured, a semiocclusive dressing is applied to the wound and held in place with elastic gauze. If an open wound remains, a topical antiseptic or antibiotic is applied prior to wound dressing. A lower limb cast is then applied for 2 to 3 weeks, after which bandages are maintained for as long as 6 weeks, postoperatively. Generally, systemic antibiotics are not required unless a question exists regarding the blood supply or the cleanliness of surgery. In cases in which a portion of the hoof wall was excised, a full-support shoe should be applied to provide stability. This is done shortly after the cast is removed. Acrylic can be used when keratinization of the entire wound is complete.

Complete Avulsion

Complete avulsion injury of the hoof, including some tissues in the pastern region, may be managed by bandaging alone if the injury site does not appear unstable during movement. If the wound is unstable or a large defect is present, cast application is recommended as soon as you are sure that infection will not be a problem. Casts are usually left in place for 2 to 3 weeks. In some cases, two to three cast changes are required before the wound is completely healed. The more stable these wounds remain, the better the chance a complete reformation of the hoof wall will occur. For the acute injury involving deeper structures, the decision for cast application should be delayed until such time you are assured

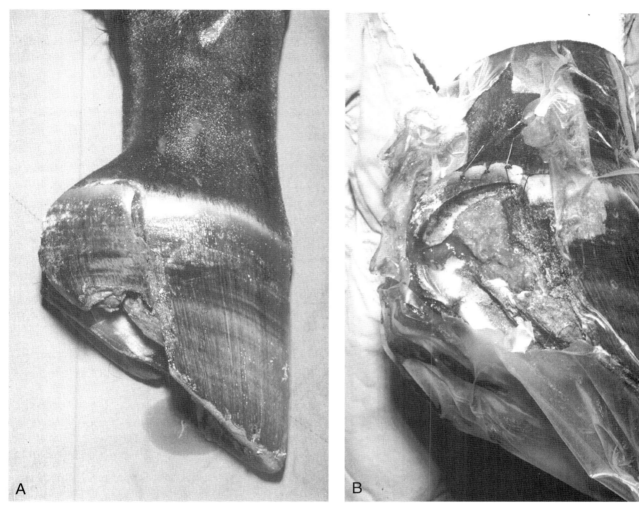

Figure 8.127   A. Incomplete avulsion injury that involves the coronet band. B. After debridement and surgical reconstruction. Note the hoof wall distal to the repair site has been removed.

that infection is not going to be a problem and that a good blood supply exists. Debridement, including that of necrotic lacerated ungual cartilage and of the distal phalanx, if it has been involved and appears abnormal or has been fractured, is important. All soft tissues and support structures should be assessed. If the injury has entered a synovial cavity, adequate drainage should be afforded, the cavity should be flushed with 1 to 3 L of sterile salt solution followed by a liter of 10% DMSO, after which a broad-spectrum antibiotic is administered intrasynovially. Additionally, broad-spectrum antibiotics are administered systemically. The injury should be protected in a sterile bandage until healthy tissue is formed. At this time, a cast can be applied. If the wound is chronic and already infected, cast application should be delayed until the infection is under control. Bandages are changed as often as necessary during this period. Additionally, periodic debridement of the wound, particularly if dense fibrogranuloma or a dense scar has formed within the wound, can be helpful in restimulating the healing process.

Occasionally, a chronic complete avulsion injury of the hoof wall will develop a keratomatous growth (horny spur) after it heals. If the spur extends proximad to the hoof wall, it can irritate the pastern region during movement and cause lameness. In some cases, periodic removal of the keratomatous growth may render the horse pain free (Fig. 8.128). Alternatively, surgical excision of the horny growth and suture apposition of adjacent soft tissue, after the soft tissues have been mobilized by undermining, can be done. If surgical excision is elected, a cast should be applied for 2 to 3 weeks, after which bandages are recommended for at least 6 weeks.

Prognosis

Generally, incomplete superficial avulsion injuries of the hoof wall alone or of the hoof wall and the coronary band, if the injuries are sutured, result in a functional and, in many cases, a cosmetic result. Prognosis for deeper avulsion injuries may have to be withheld until complete healing has occurred. Complications such as fracture of the distal phalanx, osteomyelitis, septic ar-

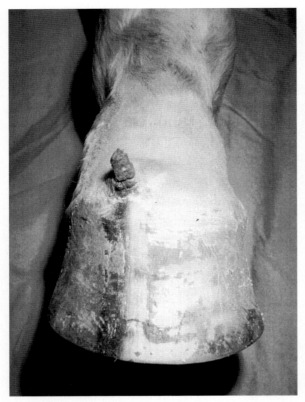

Figure 8.128 Keratomatous growth just proximal to the coronet band that developed after an avulsion injury. When the growth was present, the horse was lame. The spur of horn could be removed with a hoof nipper, and this returned the horse to soundness. The removal of the growth periodically would eliminate the pain.

thritis, and potential degenerative joint disease (DJD) of a damaged pastern joint and their implications in the prognosis should be discussed with the client at the onset of treatment.

References

1. Fessler JF. Surgical management of equine foot injuries. Mod Vet Pract 1971;52:41.
2. Markel MD, Richardson GL, Peterson PR, Meagher DM. Surgical reconstruction of chronic coronary band avulsion in three horses. J Am Vet Med Assoc 1987;190:687–688.
3. Park AH. Equine foot wounds: General principles of healing and treatment. Proc Am Assoc Equine Pract 1999;45:180–187.
4. Stashak TS. Avulsion and penetrating wound of the hoof. Proceedings of the 20th Bain-Fallon Memorial Lectures, Hamilton Island, Queensland, Australia, July 26–31, 1998;245–256.
5. Stashak TS. Management of lacerations and avulsion injuries of the foot and pastern region and hoof wall cracks. Vet Clin North Am Equine Pract 1989;5:195–220.
6. Stashak TS. Wound management and reconstructive surgery of problems associated with the distal limbs. In: Equine Wound Management. Philadelphia: Lea & Febiger, 1991;193–202.
7. Steckel RR, Fessler JF. Surgical management of severe hoof wounds in the horse: A retrospective study of 30 cases. Comp Cont Educ Pract Vet 1983;5:S435.

TOE CRACKS, QUARTER CRACKS, HEEL CRACKS (SAND CRACKS)

Cracks in the wall of the hoof, starting at the bearing surface of the wall and extending to a variable distance up the hoof wall, or cracks originating at the coronary band as the result of a defect in the band and extending downward are identified as toe, quarter, or heel cracks, depending on their location in the hoof wall. They may occur in either the forefeet or the hindfeet.

Quarter cracks and heel cracks are usually the most severe because they often involve the sensitive laminae. Affected horses are usually lame, and hemorrhage after exercise may be noticed. Infection is commonly observed.

Etiology

Excessive growth of the hoof wall, causing a splitting of the wall, from lack of trimming of the feet is a common cause. Injury to the coronary band, producing a weak and deformed hoof wall, leads to cracks originating at the coronary band. Weakening of the wall caused by excessive drying or excessively thin walls also causes hoof cracks.

Moisture is the key to flexibility of the hoof wall and sole. The normal hoof wall contains approximately 25% water; the sole, approximately 33%, and the frog, approximately 50%. If the foot is allowed to dry, it becomes brittle and thus more susceptible to cracking.

Signs

The presence of the split in the wall is obvious. Lameness may not be present, but it becomes evident if the crack extends into the sensitive tissues, allowing infection to gain access to these structures. An exudate under the cracks or suppurative inflammation of the laminae may be present, depending on the size of the opening into the sensitive tissues. The location of the crack is obvious. Variable lesions are found above the coronary band in those cases in which the crack is caused by injury of the band. Lesions may result from lacerated wounds or from other causes, such as overreaching and interfering.

Diagnosis

The diagnosis is based on the presence of the crack, which is easily identified. The crack is classified according to its location.

Hoof testers can be used to verify that the pain resulting in the lameness is associated with the crack in the hoof wall. Perineural anesthesia can also be helpful in some cases in determining how much the hoof crack contributes to the horse's lameness. Bleeding from the hoof wall crack after exercise indicates that the crack has extended down to the sensitive laminae. Pus exudes from the infected hoof when pressure is applied.

Treatment

For a discussion of the treatment options, the reader is referred to the section entitled Cracks in Chapter 9.

VERTICAL TEARS OF THE HOOF WALL

Vertical tears of the hoof wall can be difficult to recognize and are an ill-defined entity.[1] They occur most frequently at the medial quarter and heel and are caused by tearing of the hoof wall from the underlying soft tissue of the hoof.

Etiology

Although the cause is unknown, it occurs most frequently in 2- to 3-year-old Thoroughbreds with small feet for their size. Commonly, these horses also have long toes, underrun heels, thin walls, and flat soles. At necropsy, a loss of the normal attachment occurs between the laminae that may extend to the solar surface, and hemorrhage is usually present.[3] It appears like a focal acute laminitis without rotation of the distal phalanx.[3]

Clinical Signs and Diagnosis

Visually, one can often see hemorrhage through the hoof wall in white-footed horses (Fig. 8.129).[1] Although the degree of lameness can range from mild to severe, it is usually mild but sufficient to affect performance. It is more difficult to appreciate lameness on soft surfaces, but when the horse is trotting on hard surfaces, shortening in the stride is obvious. On hoof tester examination, pain is present, and an obvious lack of hoof wall strength is noticed.[1] Prolonged hoof tester application either causes or exacerbates a lameness. Unilateral perineural anesthesia of the palmar digital nerve usually relieves the signs of pain and lameness.

Treatment

The treatment can be difficult to attain quickly, because the foot so often is underrun and small, and a thin wall exists. Because a vertical tear remains until the hoof wall has grown to the solar surface, the initial treatment is aimed at corrected trimming and providing stability to the foot so that tearing will not continue.[1,2] Relief of

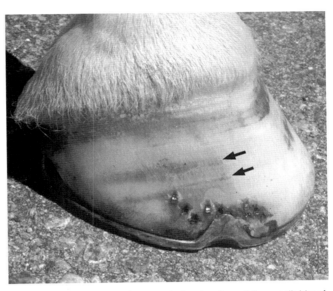

Figure 8.129 Hemorrhage and discoloration of the medial hoof wall that can occur with vertical tears of the hoof wall.

pain can usually be provided by 1) correcting any shoeing disorder that exists (poorly placed shoe or a shoe that is too small) and 2) using steel training plates with quarter clips to provide hoof wall stability.[1,2] The foot should be shod as flat as possible, so calks and toe grabs are not used.

Prognosis

The prognosis should be good if the proper corrective trimming and shoeing is done and the owner-trainer continues to treat the problem.

References

1. Moyer W. Disease of the equine heel. Proc Am Assoc Equine Pract 1979;25:21.
2. Moyer W, Anderson J. Sheared heels: Diagnosis and treatment. J Am Vet Med Assoc 1975;166:53.
3. Rooney JR. Autopsy of the Horse. Baltimore: Williams & Wilkins, 1970.

Part II

THE PASTERN

Ted S. Stashak

DEGENERATIVE JOINT DISEASE OF THE PROXIMAL INTERPHALANGEAL (PASTERN) JOINT (HIGH RINGBONE)

The term *high ringbone*, used to describe degenerative joint disease (DJD) of the proximal interphalangeal joint (PIPJ) has been somewhat confusing. Historically, *ringbone* was used to describe any bony enlargement of the

phalanges in the pastern region below the fetlock joint, which may lead to osteoarthritis.[1,24] If the bony enlargement was associated with the distal proximal phalanx (PP) and the proximal aspect of the middle phalanx with or without PIPJ involvement, it was classified as *high ringbone*. If the bony enlargement was associated with the distal aspect of the middle phalanx and the proximal aspect of the distal phalanx with or without distal interphalangeal joint (DIPJ) involvement, it was classified as *low ringbone*.[1,24] *Low ringbone* has already been discussed; for more information, therefore, the reader is referred to "Pyramidal Distortion of the Hoof and Dorsal Pastern Region" in this chapter. Since *ringbone* is purely a descriptive term for bony enlargement of the pastern region, it has been suggested that it be replaced by more specific terms that describe the anatomic site involved and the pathologic process.[6]

Ringbone has also been classified as *articular* (involving the joint surface) or *periarticular* (involving the structures at the perimeter of the joint and including the adjacent phalanges). Supporting the distinction between *articular* and *periarticular* is a limited study done in young horses (younger than 4 years) in which histologic examination of the diseased PIPJ revealed that periarticular changes preceded the development of articular cartilage changes.[13] Unlike osteochondrosis, in which the disease process is centered at the osteochondral junction, the earliest changes seen in these young horses occurred in the superficial layer of the cartilage. Subchondral bone cyst formation and bone sclerosis occurred secondary to the cartilage degeneration in a pattern consistent with DJD.[13] On radiographic examination, the two forms can be distinguished in a small number of cases. In these, periarticular bone proliferation precedes articular changes, which include marginal osteophyte formation and narrowing of the joint space.[30] Most cases, however, present with joint involvement and periarticular pathology. Therefore, it is suggested that the distinction between articular and periarticular is probably inappropriate in most cases.[17] Further supporting this is the difficulty in differentiating between the articular and the periarticular forms of the disease at necropsy, when the condition becomes chronic.[24] Therefore, in this section, DJD of the PIPJ includes both articular and periarticular forms of the disease. DJD has also been described as osteoarthritis or osteoarthrosis.[19,30]

DJD (arthrosis) of the PIPJ is an important and common cause of lameness in virtually all breeds and ages of horses.[23] In one study, the disease represented the most common reason for insurance claims for musculoskeletal disorders among horses insured in Sweden.[2] Horses older than 5 years seem at greater risk.[6,16] The forelimbs are affected more frequently than the hindlimbs except when proximal palmar or plantar eminence fracture of the middle phalanx result in osteoarthrosis or when osteochondrosis (OC) is the cause. In the latter two, the hindlimbs are involved more frequently.[1,30] A higher incidence of the disease has also been identified in geldings compared with stallions and mares.[6] The possibility of a hormonal imbalance in geldings was proposed as the cause.

Etiopathogenesis

The causes for DJD of the PIPJ are varied. They include OC and selective weight bearing in horses younger than 4 years, various forms of trauma, septic arthritis, conformation defects, and heredity.[1,11–13,30]

When OC is the cause, it is usually seen in horses younger than 3 years of age, the hindlimbs are involved most frequently, and more than one joint can be affected.

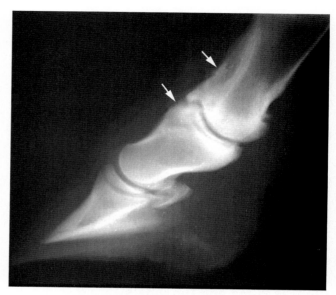

Figure 8.130 Laceration to the pastern region several months before presentation for a lameness workup. Note the osseous changes associated with the middle phalanx, the PIPJ, and the distal PP (arrows). (Courtesy of Dr. Paul Foy.)

In one study, 6 horses diagnosed with OC had 9 PIPJs involved.[30] The reason the distal end of the PP is affected most commonly with OC is unknown. Selective excessive weight bearing in horses younger than 4 years of age has also been shown to be a cause of this condition.[7] In a limited study done in 6 young Thoroughbred horses, DJD of the PIPJ developed in the contralateral support limb after severe lameness in the opposite rear limb.[7]

In older horses the condition often occurs from various forms of trauma to the periarticular soft tissues and the PIPJ itself. The trauma may cause pulling or tearing of the periosteal attachments of the extensor tendons, ligaments, and joint capsule, resulting in periostitis and new bone formation. If the soft tissue injury is severe enough to cause joint instability or subluxation, direct cartilage damage and DJD may follow. Whether primary synovitis is a distinct entity involving the PIPJ is unknown.[17] Because the PIPJ is a low-motion, high-load joint, the articular cartilage and subchondral bone are placed under a greater workload, making these structures more susceptible to injury from nonphysiologic loading.[20] Interestingly, the articular lesions associated with DJD of the PIPJ resemble experimental lesions induced in immobilized joints placed under sustained pressure.[29] In the performance horse the injury may be a result of an imbalance between a repetitive microtrauma sustained in athletic performance and an adaptive repair mechanism of the skeletal tissue, or it may result from a single event.[1,20] Direct blows to the region and lacerations into or at the margin of the PIPJ or involving the collateral ligaments with or without the development of septic arthritis have also been implicated as a cause (Fig. 8.130).[1,28] Various fractures of the phalanges involving the PIPJ can cause DJD also.

Conformational defects can result in abnormal forces being applied to the PIPJ and the periarticular soft tissue support structures, which can cause DJD. In a limited study done in young horses that had not participated in any strenuous exercise, faulty conformation was believed to be the cause of DJD of the PIPJ.[7] Poor conformation may predispose to pulling or tearing of the collateral ligaments, joint capsule, and tendon insertions. Horses that are base-narrow and toe-in or toe-out are thought to be predisposed to osteoarthrosis on the lateral side of the joint, whereas horses that are base-wide and toe-in or toe-out are believed to be predisposed to injury and arthrosis on the medial side of the joint because the foot and limb conformation exerts greater stress on these regions.

The condition is considered inheritable by some,[26] but it is probably inheritable through poor conformation. Pasterns that are overly upright may result in increased concussion to the PIPJ.[1] Osteoarthrosis may result from abnormal joint surface shape (uneven spacing of the articular surfaces of the pastern joint and insufficient height of the intermediate ridge dividing the proximal articular surface of the middle phalanx), which can result in abnormal stress.[12]

Although the pathogenesis for use-related osteoarthrosis of the PIPJ is undetermined, the following appears logical. Injury to periarticular soft tissues results in pain and healing by fibrosis. It is proposed that the pain and periarticular fibrosis further limit the motion of the PIPJ, causing a sustained loading of a small area of the joint surface and subchondral bone.[20] The focal loading results in cartilage cell death and remodeling of the subchondral bone. The subchondral bone then responds by recruiting bone-remodeling units, and in an attempt to relieve pressure, cysts are formed. Osteogenic granulation tissue arising from the cystic sites of the subchondral bone penetrates the necrotic cartilage and merges with the granulation tissue from the opposite surface. Fibrous ankylosis is followed by bony ankylosis. If the bony bridges are strong enough to maintain joint stability, the process progresses to involve more of the joint surface.

Clinical Signs

Variable enlargement of the pastern region may be evident visually as well as on palpation. The swelling may be focal or diffuse (Figs. 8.131 and 8.132). On palpation, heat and pain with firm digital pressure may be appreciated, depending on how acute the injury is. Additionally, the affected pastern joint region may feel larger, particularly the dorsolateral and dorsomedial surfaces, than the contralateral joint. Lameness is also variable and is usually exacerbated at a trot, at exercise on an uneven surface (e.g., slope), or by circling at a trot (increased lameness is seen when the affected limb is on the inside of the circle). In some cases during foot flight, an exaggerated extension of the toe may be seen before foot placement.[28] In most cases, there is pain on flexion and rotation of the pastern region, unless the joint has undergone ankylosis. The lameness completely blocks out with a pastern ring block and may only partially block out with perineural anesthesia of the palmar or plantar digital nerves at the base of the proximal sesamoid bones. Intrasynovial anesthesia only blocks out the intraarticular pain.

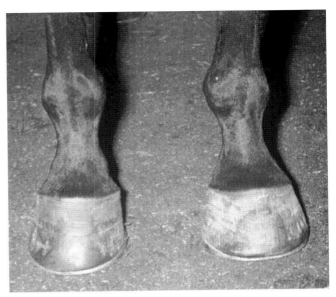

Figure 8.131   Focal swelling on the medial side of the right fore pastern region that can be seen in some early cases of DJD of the PIPJ.

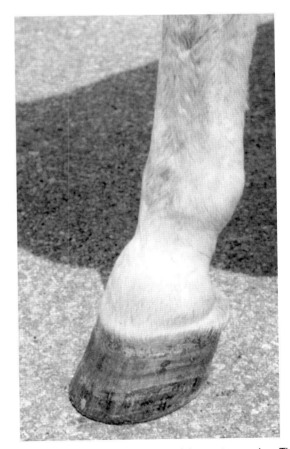

Figure 8.132   Diffuse enlargement of the pastern region. This horse had advanced radiographic changes consistent with DJD of the PIPJ.

Diagnosis

A diagnosis of DJD of the PIPJ can usually be confirmed with a radiographic examination. In early acute cases, however, only soft tissue swelling may be present, and radiographic examination may appear normal. In these cases, repeat radiographic examination is recommended in 3 to 4 weeks. At this time, the evidence of periostitis (periarticular new bone) and peripheral osteophyte formation may be present (Fig. 8.133). In some cases, periostitis may precede evidence of articular involvement.[30] Alternatively, nuclear scintigraphy can be

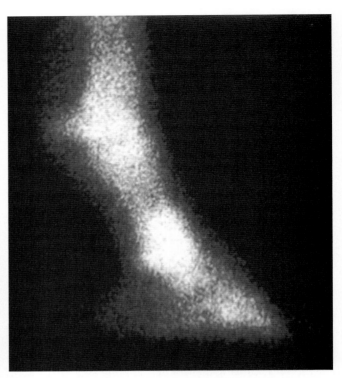

Figure 8.134 Nuclear scintigraphy. Note the increased uptake (white area) associated with the PIPJ region.

done in the early acute case to help confirm the region involved (Fig. 8.134).

Radiographs taken of young horses with OC resulting in DJD of the PIPJ are characterized by a narrowing of the joint space, marginal osteophytosis, and periarticular bone proliferation (Fig. 8.135). Additionally, diffuse subchondral lucencies can be present in the subchondral bone at the distal end of the PP (Fig. 8.136).[30] The opposite pastern region should also be radiographed for comparison.

Radiographic findings in the pastern of a horse sustaining fracture are obvious. Periarticular new bone growth associated with wire cuts is usually limited to the site of trauma unless the joint was invaded and the DJD results from the joint trauma or from a septic arthritis (see Fig. 8.130).

The most common radiographic findings in a study done on 196 horses (262 joints) with chronic osteoarthrosis of the PIPJ were as follows:

1. Joint space narrowing or collapse (83.6%) (Fig. 8.136)
2. Osteophyte formation (65.6%) (Figs. 8.133, A and C, and 8.137)
3. Subchondral bone sclerosis (64.9%) (Fig. 8.136)
4. Periosteal or periarticular bony proliferation (62.2%) (Fig. 8.138)
5. Deformity of the joint space (51.2%)
6. Bone atrophy (13%)
7. Synovial osteochondroma (5.7%)
8. Subchondral bone cysts (4.2%) (Figs. 8.136 and 8.139)
9. Joint capsule ossification (3.8%)[6]

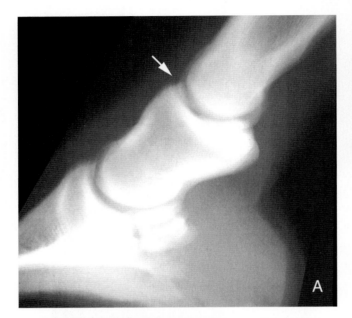

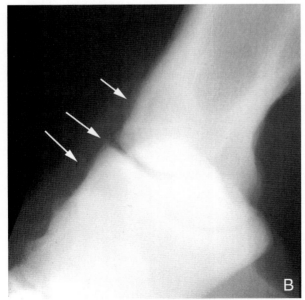

Figure 8.133 A. Lateral view of an osteophyte (arrow) at the dorsal articular margin of the DIPJ. B. Oblique view. Note the proliferative exostosis (upper and lower arrows) and osteophytes (middle arrow).

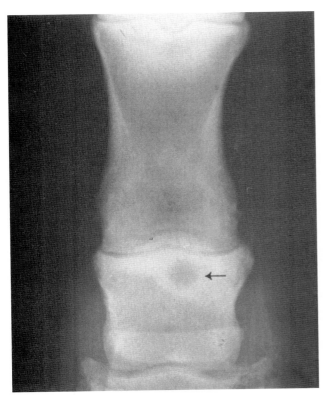

Figure 8.135   Dorsal plantar view of a horse with DJD of the pastern joint. The degenerative process is characterized by narrowing of the joint space, subchondral lucencies and sclerosis, and a large osteochondrosis lesion in the proximal extremity of the middle phalanx (arrow).

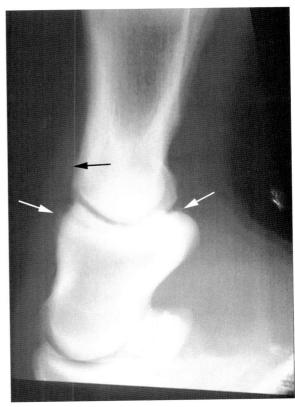

Figure 8.137   Lateral view of osteophyte formation. Note the development of the osteophytes on the dorsum and plantar articular margins (white arrows) and the proliferative exostosis (black arrow).

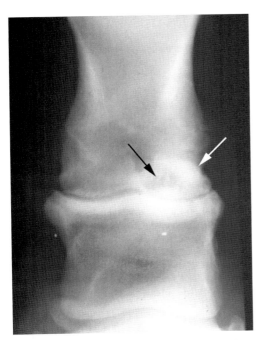

Figure 8.136   Joint space collapse and narrowing. Sclerosis (white arrow) and subchondral cyst formation (black arrow) are also seen.

Ultrasonography can also be used to evaluate the soft tissue support structures in the pastern region. One study found that injury to the branches of the superficial digital flexor tendon and the desmitis of the oblique distal sesamoid ligament were common.[22] Injury to the axial palmar ligament of the PIPJ has also been documented.[5]

Treatment

Conservative management involves rest, anti-inflammatory therapy, trimming and shoeing, and controlled exercise. Stall confinement and rest from exercise are important to prevent further trauma, reduce inflammation, particularly for the acute injury, and allow healing to occur.[7,28] Rest periods may extend from weeks to months. Prolonged rest for 3 to 7 months in foals and weanlings (younger than 7 months of age) with early signs of DJD may allow some horses to heal completely and to perform at their intended use.[7]

Anti-inflammatory treatments are often only palliative but may allow continued use for some time. Phenylbutazone administered orally at 2.2 mg/kg every 24 hours for 10 to 14 days with rest is recommended for the acute injury. Phenylbutazone is then administered as needed. For chronic cases, phenylbutazone administered before performance, during the days the horse is performing, and after performance may allow some horses

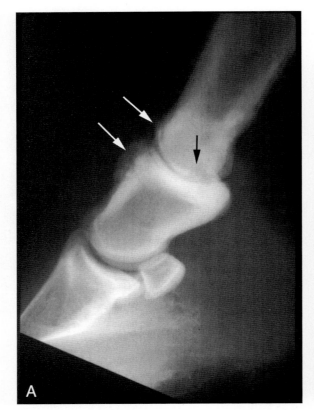

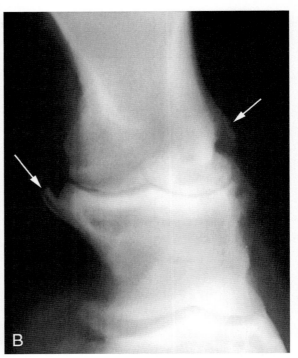

Figure 8.138 A. Lateral view of periosteal or periarticular bony proliferation. Note the extensive periosteal and periarticular bone reaction (white arrows) and subchondral bone cyst (black arrow).

B. Oblique view. Note the periarticular enthesiophyte (arrows), subchondral bone sclerosis, cyst formation, and joint space narrowing.

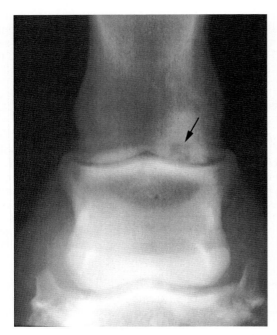

Figure 8.139 Dorsoplantar view of subchondral bone cyst (arrow) and sclerosis. This is the same horse as in Figure 8.133, 6 months later.

to perform relatively pain free for prolonged periods. Orgotein injections every other day intramuscularly for 12 treatments has been reported to be effective for some horses.[28] Adequan injections (intramuscular) at weekly intervals for 4 to 6 treatments and hyaluronic acid (HA) administered intravenously at weekly intervals for 4 treatments may also be affective. A combination of a steroid and HA injected intraarticularly into the affected PIPJ may eliminate the progression of the disease in acute cases with minimal articular changes and reduce signs of lameness in more chronic cases. Cold therapy in the form of an ice-water slurry applied twice daily for 30 minutes for 2 to 3 days may help reduce the inflammation in the region. Dimethyl sulfoxide (DMSO) and a steroid placed under a sweat wrap can also reduce inflammation.

The feet should be trimmed and balanced, and shoes that enhance breakover and provide good lateral and medial support should be applied. (Refer to Chapter 9 for more information.) Controlled exercise (hand walking) for 5 minutes twice daily for 5 days a week can begin if considerable improvement in the lameness is observed after the rest period. Hand walking duration can be increased by 2.5 minutes/week until recheck at 6 weeks. The decision for increasing exercise is made at that time. In some cases, the rest period and controlled exercise may extend for 3 to 4 months before riding exercise. In some, the condition may not be responsive or eventually become unresponsive to conservative treatment. In a small number, the disease process is so advanced that spontaneous ankylosis occurs.

Surgical treatment for DJD of the pastern joint consists of arthrodesis, which is aimed at eliminating any motion of the pastern joint, thereby decreasing pain and lameness. Although various techniques for surgical fusion (arthrodesis of the pastern joint) have been used,[1,3,8–10,15,25,31,32] a technique consisting of removal of the articular cartilage by curettage or with an air drill and burr and the internal fixation with screws (two 5.5-mm, or three 4.5-mm, or a combination of 4.5- and 5.5-mm screws) (Fig. 8.140 and 8.141)[10,15,25,30–33] or with a bone plate (Fig. 8.142),[8] followed by external immobilization with a cast for 3 to 5 weeks, is preferred.[14] In a comparative study done to evaluate the tensile breaking strength (TBS) and holding power (HP) of 4.5-mm cortical screws and 5.5-mm cortical screws in adult equine metaphyseal bone, researchers found that the TBS for 5.5-mm screws was superior (5.5 mm = 1391.4 kg and 4.5 = 832.7 kg) and that the HP of the 5.5-mm screws was approximately 50% greater than achieved with 4.5-mm screws.[34] On the basis of these data, it would appear that two 5.5-mm screws should provide comparable fixation strength to that of three 4.5-mm cortical screws.[33] Although cancellous bone grafting in conjunction with internal fixation has been recommended,[32] bone grafting does not appear necessary for a successful outcome. Bilateral forelimb and hindlimb arthrodeses have been performed successfully.[4,23,25,35]

In a study done to compare cruciate placement of compression screws and parallel placement of compression screws for arthrodesis, researchers found that parallel screw placement was superior.[10] The region was stronger with three parallel screws; it was easier to apply, provided better alignment of the proximal and middle phalanges, and was prone to less error in screw placement.[10] Crisscross screw placement may have some advantage for arthrodesis of pastern joints when lateral and medial caudal eminences of the middle phalanx are fractured.[10] These fractures have been handled successfully, however, with parallel screwing techniques and bone plates.[15] In another study comparing various techniques for pastern arthrodesis (two screws cruciate pattern, three parallel screws, three converging screws, and a T-plate) in 35 horses, the technique used did not influence the success rate.[4]

Although the technique for arthrodesis has been adequately described,[3,4,8–10,14,15,18,25,31,32] a few comments may help avoid complications. Adherence to the principles of arthrodesis, including complete removal of the articular cartilage, close apposition of the bone surfaces, and stable internal fixation, are most important to the outcome. The surgeon should avoid extensive elevation of the extensor tendon from the dorsal surface of the middle phalanx; if it is elevated extensively, the proliferative exostosis that results may extend to affect the coffin joint. The collateral ligaments should be incised just enough to gain adequate exposure of the palmar or plantar joint surfaces for cartilage removal. In one study in which 2 of 10 horses did not have the collateral ligaments cut to gain access to the entire PIPJ surface, researchers found that the joint space was still visible and there was considerable periosteal reaction on radiographic examination 5 months postoperatively.[27] In cases of excessive

periarticular bone proliferation, a chisel or osteotome is required to open the joint adequately. To avoid the potential complication of having the distal end of the PP fracture off when a shelf is made for screw placement on the dorsal distal phalanx,[15] one can use an air drill and a medium fluted burr to create individual grooves in the PP for screw placement (Fig. 8.140). After this, I prefer to make the center glide hole (for the three-screw technique) and the lateral glide hole (for the two-screw technique) through the PP and then thread hole in the middle phalanx before the cartilage is removed so good joint alignment can be assured after the cartilage is removed. Next, I drill the other two holes for three-screw technique or one hole for the two-screw technique through the distal PP. It is also helpful to the level of the grooves on the dorsal distal surface of the PP from the lateral and medial radiographs so that sufficient bone remains to support the screw fixation. For this, a line can be drawn on an overlay of acetate placed on a lateral medial radiographic view, and the correct placement and length of the screws can be estimated. Alternatively, a combined aiming device can be used for more accurate hole placement in the PP.[33] The cartilage can be removed by curettage (my preference) or with an air drill and a medium-sized fluted burr. If an air drill is used to remove the cartilage, care should be taken not to destroy the normal contour of the joint. The cartilage in the palmar or plantar recesses of the joint can be removed with a smaller curet or bur. After the cartilage is removed, the joint should be thoroughly lavaged to remove cartilage and, in some cases, bone fragments. One should avoid drill penetration of the palmar or plantar surface of the middle phalanx because damage to the deep digital flexor tendon (DDFT), suspensory ligament (SL) of the navicular bone, or the navicular bone itself may result (Fig. 8.141). The palmar cortex of the middle phalanx is felt, during drilling, as an increased bone density (resistance). The density of the middle phalanx seems sufficient to support interfragmental compression without penetrating this palmar or plantar cortex. If a bone plate is used, it should be placed as proximal as possible on the middle phalanx so that the extensor process of the distal phalanx does not contact it when the joint is extended (Fig. 8.142).[4] If a tourniquet is used, it should be released after the extensor tendon is sutured and before the subcutaneous tissue is apposed.

After surgery, the limb is immobilized in a lower limb (just below the carpus or tarsus) cast. The foot must be included in the cast. After the stockinette is applied, and a ring of ¼-inch orthopedic felt is placed just below the carpus or tarsus and secured in place with tape, cast foam may be applied. The foot is cast in as normal a position as possible.

The cast is removed in 3 to 8 weeks, depending on the reason for the operation and the technique used. Generally, phalanx fractures that require pastern arthrodesis require longer casting periods. If DJD of the PIPJ is the problem and 5.5-mm screws or a bone plate is used, the cast can be removed in 3 weeks. After the cast is removed, stall confinement is recommended for another 8 weeks, and hand walking exercise can begin after this time. Free exercise can usually begin after 4 to 6 months, but each case is assessed individually. Contrary to other reports, a year of convalescence may be

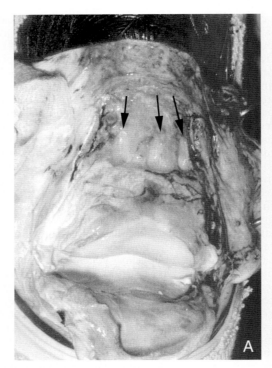 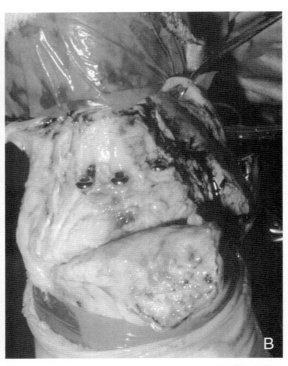

Figure 8.140   Intraoperative view of an exposed DIPJ. A. An air drill with a large fluted burr attached was used to create the grooves in the distal end of the PP for screw placement (arrows). B. Screw heads are seen after their placement.

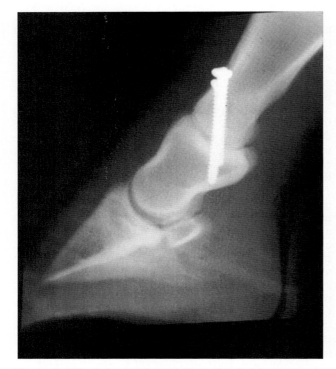

Figure 8.141   Lateral radiograph illustrating that the screw threads did not penetrate the plantar cortex.

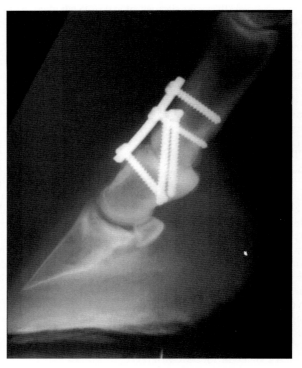

Figure 8.142   Lateral view showing the use of a bone plate and screws for arthrodesis of the PIPJ. Note the distal plate screw is placed at the proximal extent of the middle phalanx well away from the extensor process.

required before horses are able to resume full serviceability.[4,15]

Complications that were identified in a retrospective study on 21 cases in which arthrodesis was achieved by interfragmental screw compression include 1) implant breakage in 2 cases and a bent screw in 1 case and 2) fracture of the dorsal distal portion of the PP, which resulted from a technical error in which the dorsal shelf of the PP was too small to support the weight bearing.[15] Infection and loosening of the implants in 1 of 22 cases have also been reported.[25] Other complications include exuberant periosteal callus, laminitis, toe elevation, DJD of the DIPJ, and navicular abnormalities.[15,23,25]

Prognosis

With the advent of arthrodesis of the PIPJ with lag screw fixation or bone plate application, the prognosis is greatly improved.[4,8,15,25] In one report in which the three parallel screw technique was used on clinical cases, 16 of 22 horses resumed full service, 3 of 22 horses were used for breeding, and 3 of 22 horses had unsatisfactory results (1 became infected, 1 broke screws, and 1 developed DJD in the coffin joint).[25] In another report, 16 of 21 horses became serviceable, 4 of 21 horses remained unserviceable, and 1 of 21 horses died from unrelated causes.[15] The prognosis for arthrodesis is less predictable in the forelimb, as problems may later develop in the navicular and coffin joint regions.[15] In a retrospective study on 64 horses treated for pastern arthrodesis, 65% of horses with arthrodesis in the forelimb and 82% of horses with arthrodesis in the hindlimb returned to intended use.[21] This is in contrast to a study done on 35 horses in which success rates for forelimb was 46% and for hind limb was 83% after pastern arthrodesis.[4] A successful outcome was also reported in 4 of 6 horses with bilateral pastern arthrodesis.[4]

References

1. Adams OR. Lameness in Horses. 3rd ed. Philadelphia: Lea & Febiger, 1974;359.
2. Bergsten G. Frequency of diseases of the locomotor system among insured horses in Sweden, 1973–1981. Svensk-Veterinartidning 1983;35:14–20.
3. Caron JP, Fretz PB, Bailey JV, Barber SM. Proximal interphalangeal arthrodesis in the horse. A retrospective study and a modified screw technique. Vet Surg 1990;19:196–202.
4. Colahan PT, Wheat JD, Meagher DM. Treatment of middle phalangeal fractures in the horse. J Am Vet Med Assoc 1981;178:1182.
5. Denoix JM. Ultrasound examination of the pastern in horses. Proc Am Assoc Equine Pract 1990;36:363–380.
6. El-Guindy MH, Ali MA, Samy MT. Chronic osteoarthrosis in the equine proximal interphalangeal joint. Equine Pract 1986;8:6–15.
7. Ellis DR, Greenwood ES. Six cases of degenerative joint disease of the proximal interphalangeal joint of young Thoroughbreds. Equine Vet J 1985;17:66–68.
8. Fackleman GE, Nunamaker DM. Manual of Internal Fixation in the Horse. New York: Springer-Verlag, 1982;74.
9. Fessler JF, Amstutz HE. Fracture repair. In: Oehme FW, Prier JE, Eds. Textbook of Large Animal Surgery. Baltimore: Williams & Wilkins, 1974;260.
10. Genetzky RM, Schneider EJ, Butler HC, Guffy MM. Comparison of two surgical procedures for arthrodesis of the proximal interphalangeal joint in horses. J Am Vet Med Assoc 1981;179:464–468.
11. Haakenstad LH. Investigations on ringbone. Nord Vet Med 1954;7:1.
12. Haakenstad LH. Chronic bone and joint disease in relation to conformation in the horse. Equine Vet J 1969;1:248–260.
13. Hoffman KD, Pool RR, Pascoe JR. Degenerative joint disease of the proximal interphalangeal joints of the forelimbs of two young horses. Equine Vet J 1984;16:138–140.
14. Johnson JE. Ringbone: Treatment by ankylosis. Proc Am Assoc Equine Pract 1974;20:67.
15. Martin GS, McIlwraith CW, Turner AS, et al. Long-term results and complications of proximal interphalangeal arthrodesis in horses. J Am Vet Med Assoc 1984;184:1136–1140.
16. Mackay-Smith MP. Pathogenesis and pathology of equine osteoarthritis. J Am Vet Med Assoc 1962;141:1246–1252.
17. McIlwraith CW, Goodman NL. Conditions of the interphalangeal joints. Vet Clin North Am Equine Pract 1989;5:161–178.
18. Milne DW, Turner AS. An Atlas of Surgical Approaches to the Bones of the Horse. Philadelphia: WB Saunders, 1979;31.
19. Olsson GE. Degenerative joint disease (osteoarthrosis). A review with special reference to the dog. J Small Anim Pract 1971;12:333–342.
20. Pool RR, Meagher DM. Pathologic findings and pathogenesis of racetrack injuries. Vet Clin North Am Equine Pract 1990;6:1–30.
21. Ray CR, McIlwraith CW, Trotter GW, et al. Arthrodesis of the proximal interphalangeal joint: A retrospective study of sixty-four horses. Proceedings of the Colorado Veterinary Medicine Association, Breckenridge, CO, September 1993.
22. Reimers JM. Ultrasonography of the pastern: 1. Anatomy and pathology. 2. Outcome of the selected injuries in racehorses. Proc Am Assoc Equine Pract 1997;43:123–126.
23. Rick MC, Herthel D, Boles C. Surgical management of middle phalangeal fractures and high ringbone in the horse: A review of 16 cases. Proc Am Assoc Equine Pract 1987;32:315–321.
24. Rooney JR. Ringbone vs pyramidal disease. Equine Vet Sci 1981;1:23.
25. Schneider JE, Carnine BL, Guffy MM. Arthrodesis of the proximal interphalangeal joint in the horse: a surgical treatment for high ringbone. J Am Vet Med Assoc 1978;173:1364–1369.
26. Stecher RM. Discussion of osteoarthritis. J Am Vet Med Assoc 1962;141:1249.
27. Steenhaut M, Verschooten F, De Moor A. Arthrodesis of the pastern joint in the horse. Equine Vet J 1985;17:35–40.
28. Swanson TD. Degenerative disease of the proximal interphalangeal joint in performance horses. Proc Am Assoc Equine Pract 1989;34:392–397.
29. Trias A. Effect of persistent pressure on the articular cartilage. An experimental study. J Bone Joint Surg 1961;43B:376–386.
30. Trotter GW, McIlwraith CW, Norrdin RW, et al. Degenerative joint disease with osteochondrosis of the proximal interphalangeal joint in young horses. J Am Vet Med Assoc 1982;180:1312–1318.
31. von Salis B. Arthrodesis of the pastern joint in horses. Tijdschr Diergeneeskd 1973;98:1030.
32. von Salis B. Internal fixation in the equine: Recent advances and possible application in private practice. Proc Am Assoc Equine Pract 1972;18:193–218.
33. Wilson DG, Crawford WH. The use of a combined aiming device for pastern arthrodesis in horses. Vet Compar Orthop Traumatol 1991;4:59–61.
34. Yovich JV, Turner AS, Smith FM. Holding power of orthopedic screws in equine third metacarpal and metatarsal bones: Part II. Adult horse bone. Vet Surg 1985;14:230–234.
35. Yovich JV, Stashak TS, Sullins KE. Bilateral pastern arthrodesis in a horse. Equine Vet J 1986;18:79–81.

LUXATION AND SUBLUXATION OF THE PROXIMAL INTERPHALANGEAL (PASTERN) JOINT

Luxation and subluxation of the PIPJ, although uncommon, occur in the forelimbs and hindlimbs.[2,7,9] Complete luxations usually occur in a lateral or a medial plane and are often associated with external trauma. They can present with the PIPJ either open or closed,

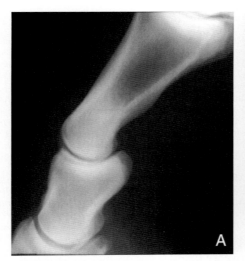 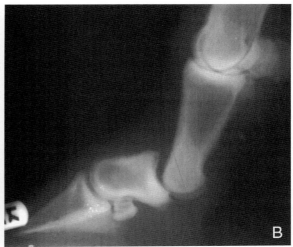

Figure 8.143 A. Lateral view of a dorsal subluxation of the PIPJ. B. Lateral view of a plantar subluxation of the PIPJ.

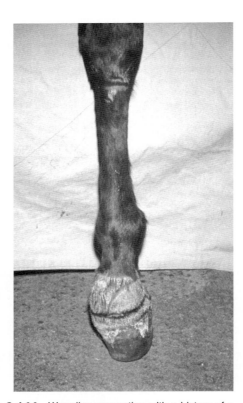

Figure 8.144 Weanling presenting with a history of a subluxation of the PIPJ in a lateral and a medial plane of several weeks duration. (Courtesy of Dr. Gayle Trotter.)

Etiology

Lateral and medial complete luxations or subluxations of the PIPJ are often caused by severe trauma, resulting in joint capsule and ligamentous tearing (e.g., distal limb caught fast and the horse struggles and falls), lacerations (Fig. 8.145), and a uniaxial condylar fracture of the distal end of the PP[2,8] (see Fig. 8.169).

Dorsal subluxations are thought to be secondary to flexure deformities or contracture and may occur acutely secondary to collateral ligament injury.[1] It is believed that a form of DDFT contracture was responsible for dorsal subluxation in the pelvic limbs of 3 horses (ages 5 months, 2 years, and 4 years).[10] Also, Thoroughbred racehorses that have sustained an injury to the soft tissue support structures of the fetlock region may secondarily develop a dorsal subluxation of the pastern joint that has been described as "Thoroughbred ringbone."[4] Dorsal subluxation may also occur after desmotomy of the SL in treating cases of severe flexure deformities of the fetlock joint, and it may occur secondary to injury to the SL and its branches.[4]

Palmar or plantar subluxations often result from an acute trauma that causes an overextension of the PIPJ. The trauma either causes tearing of the palmar or plantar soft tissue support structures (joint capsule, superficial distal sesamoidean ligament, and the insertion of the superficial digital flexor tendon) or results in a fracture of the proximal palmar or plantar eminences of the middle phalanx (P2). Palmar subluxation is most common and has been seen in foals and weanlings that have jumped from heights such as from the back of a pickup truck and in foals with flexor tendon laxity that overexert themselves during free exercise.[5]

Clinical Signs

The clinical signs associated with complete luxation caused by tearing of the collateral ligament or fracture is obvious. These horses are usually non-weight-bearing,

and the forelimbs seem at a greater risk for the injury.[9] Generally, only one limb is involved.

On the other hand, subluxations are most often either dorsal, palmar, or plantar and may involve one or both limbs (Fig. 8.143). The terms *dorsal*, *palmar*, and *plantar* refer to the subluxation of the PP relative to the position of the middle phalanx. Subluxation of the PIPJ in a lateral or medial plane can also occur (Fig. 8.144).

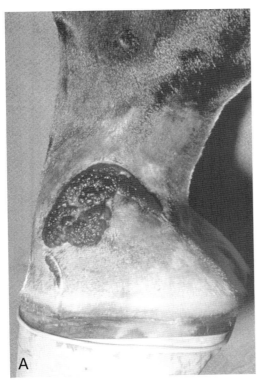

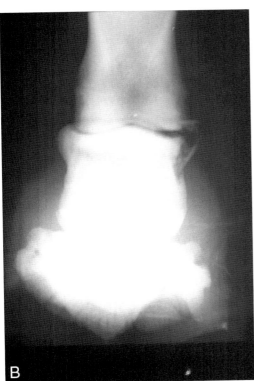

Figure 8.145 A. Laceration of the pastern region that entered the PIPJ. On manipulation, a lateral instability could be appreciated. B. Lateral view. Note subluxation of the PIPJ and the fractures associated with the region of trauma.

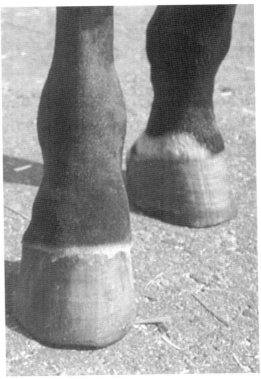

Figure 8.146 Note the diffuse swelling in the pastern region of the right forelimb. On manipulation, instability of the PIPJ could be appreciated. Stress radiographs revealed a subluxation of the PIPJ.

and a limb deformity associated with the pastern region is present. The PIPJ may be open or closed. Some horses with a subluxation of the PIPJ in a lateral or medial plane present either with diffuse swelling of the pastern region or with an obvious angular limb deformity (Figs. 8.144 and 8.146).

A horse may have an intermittent dorsal subluxation of the PIPJ and not be lame. In these, the subluxation is recognized by a dorsal swelling in the pastern region when the affected limb is non-weight-bearing. The subluxation is reduced when weight is borne on the affected limb. An audible clicking sound often accompanies the reduction of the joint. When the pelvic limbs are involved, the condition is often associated with an upright conformation (straighter than normal hocks and stifle angles).[10] The lameness may vary in these cases from a stilted gait to one resembling that of a horse with azoturia.[6] With persistent dorsal subluxation, a swelling over the dorsal surface of the pastern region is often evident, and the fetlock may appear slightly more extended (dropped) compared with the contralateral unaffected limb. At first glance a dorsal swelling may appear similar to ringbone; on closer observation, however, an abnormal alignment between the proximal and the middle phalanx is evident. Lameness is variable and inconsistent in these cases.

Signs of palmar or plantar subluxation present a somewhat reversed picture, in which the dorsal surface of the pastern region appears concave (dished out) rather than straight or convex as would appear with dorsal subluxation, and the swelling is most prominent on the flexor surface of the pastern region. These horses are usually lame shortly after the subluxation occurs; as time passes, the lameness generally subsides. In chronic cases, the heel bulbs may contact the ground, and a sinking in the pastern is noted while the horse is walking.

On manipulation of the pastern, instability and pain may be identified with flexion and rotation of the phalanges. In acute cases, heat and swelling are evident, and the misalignment of the phalanges can often be appreciated. Diagnostic anesthesia is generally not required.

Diagnosis

The diagnosis can usually be made from the physical examination alone, but radiographs should be taken to confirm the diagnosis and differentiate lesions associated with DJD and concurrent fracture of the proximal and middle phalanges. Stress films can also be taken to identify the degree of subluxation and to identify if the pastern joint can be reduced in normal alignment.

Treatment

Although it has been reported that recent fractures resulting in luxation may be treated with cast immobilization alone or cast immobilization and internal fixation of the fracture fragment with screws,[3,7,8] it is generally accepted that arthrodesis of the PIPJ with screws alone and/or screws and a bone plate results in a better outcome. Unlike luxations of the metacarpophalangeal (MCP) or metatarsophalangeal (MTP) (fetlock) joint, luxations of the PIPJ caused by rupture of the collateral ligaments do not respond as well to casting alone in my experience. Although the collateral ligament heals, a subluxation usually results, which eventually requires surgical arthrodesis. For more information on the technique for arthrodesis of the PIPJ, refer to treatment of DJD of the PIPJ.

Horses with chronic dorsal subluxation with no apparent lameness may be treated conservatively. Cases with acquired intermittent dorsal subluxation of the pelvic limb PIPJs, caused by excessive tension of the DDFT, have been treated successfully. Transection of the medial head of the DDFT allows enough length gain in the DDFT to correct the subluxation.[10] The approach is made medial between the DDFT and the SL at the level of the proximal third of the third metatarsal bone, and a 2.5-cm segment of the tendon is removed. Alternatively, it has been suggested that surgical transection to the accessory ligament of the DDFT may be of benefit.[6] However, since this structure is commonly absent in horses and, when present, is thin,[3] it would seem unlikely that transection of this structure would provide much relief.[10] Although transection of the straight distal sesamoidean ligament (DSL) for the treatment of dorsal subluxation caused by contraction of this structure has been suggested,[4] the technique was not successful in the treatment of one chronic case treated by us. Arthrodesis of the PIPJ has been used successfully for dorsal and palmar or plantar subluxations.[1,5,7,9] In most cases, the subluxation is best treated surgically by arthrodesis early before

scar tissue healing occurs. Treating early allows for better and easier alignment of the joint. Although internal fixation with screws alone has been used successfully for treatment, the use of a bone plate or plates and screws placed transarticularly is recommended (see Fig. 8.142). Additionally, the bone plate may be used to help align the joint in chronic cases.

Prognosis

Although there are only a few reports on long-term follow-up, the prognosis for luxation and subluxations treated early by arthrodesis in which good reduction and stabilization of the PIPJ are achieved seems good.[1,5,7,9] Convalescence for as long as a year may be required before the horse may return to performance. Three cases of bilateral acquired pelvic limb intermittent dorsal subluxation treated by tendonectomy of the medial head of the DDFT responded favorably to the treatment, and the subluxation resolved between 1 and 7 days postoperatively.[10] Long-term follow-up (10 months) on one case found the horse to be free of lameness in the pelvic limbs.

References

1. Adams P, Honnas CM, Ford TS, et al. Arthrodesis of a subluxated proximal interphalangeal joint in a horse. Equine Pract 1995;3: 26–31.
2. Colahan PT, Wheat JD, Meagher DM. Treatment of middle phalangeal fractures in the horse. J Am Vet Med Assoc 1981;178: 1182.
3. Getty R, Ed. Sisson and Grossman's The Anatomy of the Domestic Animals. 5th ed. Philadelphia: WB Saunders, 1975;358–360, 450–452.
4. Grant BD. The Pastern Joint. In: Mansmann RA, McAllister ES, Eds. Equine Medicine and Surgery. 3rd ed. Santa Barbara, CA: American Veterinary Publications, 1982;1055.
5. Harrison LJ, May SA. Bilateral subluxation of the pastern joint in the forelimbs of a foal. Vet Rec 1992;131:68–70.
6. Lose MP. Correction of hindleg pastern subluxation. Mod Vet Pract 1981;62:156.
7. Martin GS, McIlwraith CW, Turner AS, et al. Long-term results and complications of proximal interphalangeal arthrodesis in horses. J Am Vet Med Assoc 1984;184:1136–1140.
8. Schneider JE, Carnine BL, Guffy MM. Arthrodesis of the proximal interphalangeal joint in the horse. A surgical treatment for high ringbone. J Am Vet Med Assoc 1978;173:1364.
9. Steenhaut M, Verschooten F, De Moor A. Arthrodesis of the pastern joint in the horse. Equine Vet J 1985;17:35–40.
10. Shiroma JT, Engel HN, Wagner PC, et al. Dorsal subluxation of the pelvic limb of three horses. J Am Vet Med Assoc 1989;195: 777–780.

FRACTURES OF THE MIDDLE (SECOND) PHALANX (P-2)

Fractures of the middle phalanx occur most commonly in the hindlimbs of middle-aged (4 to 10 years) western performance horses used for cutting, roping, barrel racing, pole bending, and reining.[1,2,4,7,16] Although the fracture is common in Quarter horses, most breeds are affected, and foals can sustain these fractures as well.[4–6] In a retrospective study on 47 horses, the Quarter horse represented 54% of the breeds affected, western stock performance was the most common activity during the injury, and the hindlimbs were affected 3 times more frequently than were the forelimbs.[4,5] In two smaller studies, 8 of 10 horses with comminuted fracture had the forelimb involved, and in another, 4 of 4 adults had the forelimb involved.[5,6] When foals sustain a fracture of the middle phalanx, it usually involves the physis, and subluxation of the PIPJ is common.[6] Various fractures can affect the middle phalanx, including 1) osteochondral (chip) fractures, 2) palmar or plantar eminence fractures (nonarticular/articular), 3) axial fractures, and 4) comminuted fractures.[1,2,4,7,13,14,21–24]

Osteochondral fractures involving the PIPJ are uncommon. Thoroughbred and Standardbred racehorses and hunters and jumpers seem at increased risk.[12,20] The fracture can either be dorsal (most common) or palmar or plantar, and most involve the middle phalanx either lateral or medial to the midline and can involve either eminence.[13,14,19,20,25,26] Generally, the palmar or plantar fractures do not involve the attachments of the distal sesamoidean ligaments or the superficial digital flexor tendon and, therefore, do not become distracted (Fig. 8.147). Occasionally, multiple fragments appear on the proximal palmar border of the middle phalanx that appear to be avulsion fractures (Fig. 8.148). Despite the size of the fragments, the development of DJD appears slow. Nevertheless, lameness does occur in some cases, and fragment removal is recommended.[14,20] Radiographic examination of the opposite PIPJ should be done because palmar or plantar eminence fractures have been reported to occur bilaterally.[13] Osteochondral fractures involving the DIPJ are uncommon and may be caused by use-related trauma or may be associated with a penetrating wound (Fig. 8.149).[20,23]

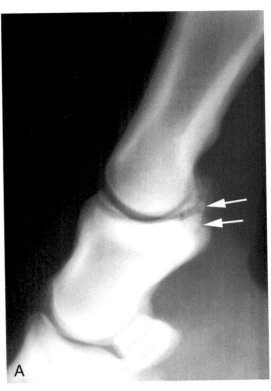

A

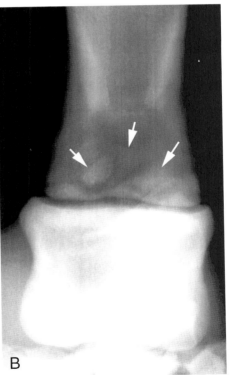

B

Figure 8.148 A. Lateral view of multiple palmar eminence fractures (arrows). B. Dorsopalmar view. Note the multiple fragments (arrows).

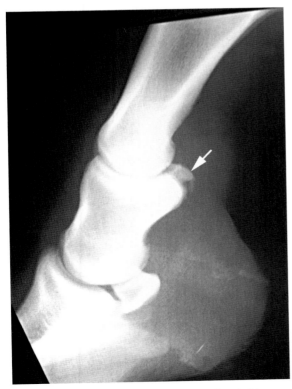

Figure 8.147 Lateral view of palmar osteochondral fragment involving the PIPJ (arrow).

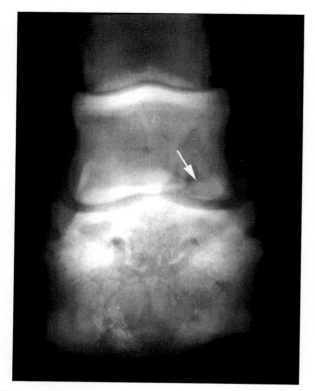

Figure 8.149 Dorsopalmar view of an osteochondral fragment on the distal aspect of the middle phalanx of the DIPJ (arrow), a result of a penetrating wound to the coronet band.

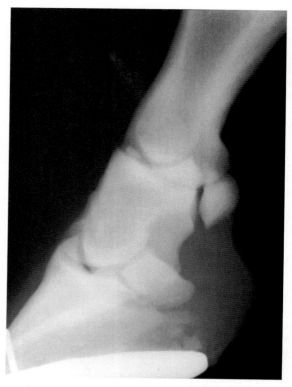

Figure 8.150 Oblique view of a uniaxial plantar eminence fracture of the middle phalanx.

Palmar or plantar eminence (wing) fractures involving the PIPJ occur frequently. The fracture can be either uniaxial (involving one eminence) or biaxial (involving both eminences) (Fig. 8.150). Although uniaxial fractures do not result in subluxation of the PIPJ, biaxial fractures can cause a subluxation. Biaxial fractures require external immobilization prior to transport to a surgical facility. Palmar or plantar nonarticular eminence fractures are uncommon (Fig. 8.151).

Simple axial fractures of the middle phalanx occur rarely.[14] A misdiagnosis of this fracture can easily be made if the central sulcus of the frog is prominent and if it is filled inadequately with packing material prior to the radiographic examination (Fig. 8.152). To make the diagnosis, one should see the fracture on at least two radiographic views. This type fracture may precede a comminuted fracture under an appropriate stress.[8]

Comminuted fractures are the most common fracture involving the middle phalanx. Although they most frequently involve the PIPJ, they may extend distally to involve the distal interphalangeal (coffin) joint.[1,2,4,7,21,22] If the fracture involves the PIPJ only, it is referred to as uniarticular; if the fracture extends distad to involve the DIPJ, it is referred to as a biarticular fracture (Fig. 8.153). Rarely, the navicular bone is also fractured.[14] In one report, comminuted fractures were encountered 4 times more frequently than palmar or plantar eminence fractures, and osteochondral or simple axial fractures were not described.[4] Comminuted fractures require external immobilization prior to transport to a surgical facility.

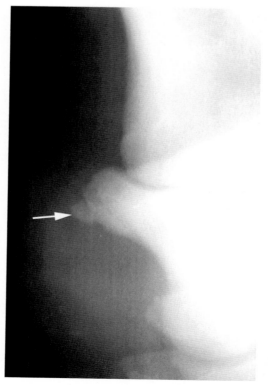

Figure 8.151 Oblique view of a nonarticular palmar eminence fracture of the middle phalanx (arrow).

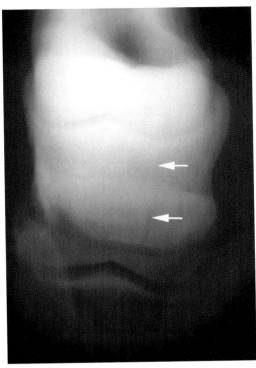

Figure 8.152 Dorsopalmar view of what appeared to be a sagittal fracture of the middle phalanx (arrows). The fracture was not seen on other radiographic views. After the sulcus of the frog was packed properly, the line disappeared.

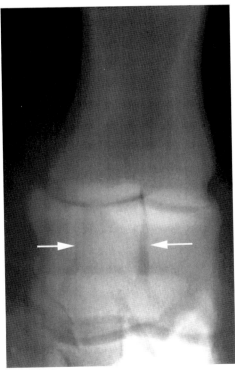

Figure 8.153 Dorsoplantar view of a comminuted biarticular fracture of the middle phalanx (arrows). Note that the fracture extends into the DIPJ.

Etiology

Osteochondral fractures result either from use or direct trauma to the site (e.g., a penetrating wound) or, occasionally, from avulsion resulting from tearing of soft tissue attachments (see Fig. 8.148). Palmar or plantar eminence fractures that involve the PIPJ may result from compression and the twisting that occurs with sudden stops and short turns, or they can occur during joint overextension that results in excessive tension of the superficial digital flexor tendon and distal sesamoidean ligaments, causing an avulsion of the eminence or eminences.[12,14] Nonarticular palmar or plantar eminence fractures are avulsion-type fractures (Fig. 8.151). The cause of simple axial fractures is unknown, but repeated trauma might be the cause. It is conjectured that these axial fissure fractures may precede the development of a comminuted fracture.[8] Comminuted fractures are thought to result from external trauma or a combination of compression and torsion (twisting) forces that occurs with sudden stops, starts, and short turns.[1,2,4,7,10] Horses shod with heel calks are believed to be more prone to such fractures because the calks grip the ground, preventing the normal rotation of the foot and phalanges when the horse is rapidly changing directions.[1,2] Although western stock performance was the most common activity reported in one study at the time of injury to the middle phalanx, a sizable group sustained these fractures during light work or unrestrained paddock exercise.[4] These fractures have also occurred in horses turned out for exercise after long-term confinement to a stall.[10] A history of lameness in the affected limb may be given prior to the development of a comminuted fracture, suggesting that all these fractures are not a single-event injury.[8]

Clinical Signs

The clinical signs associated with osteochondral, nonarticular palmar or plantar eminence, and simple axial fractures are variable. A history of an acute onset of lameness may be given for some, but for others, the onset of lameness cannot be pinpointed. Lameness that waxes and wanes with exercise is common for osteochondral and nonarticular eminence fractures. Generally, fetlock or phalangeal flexion and phalangeal rotation are painful. Circling at a trot usually exacerbates the lameness. For osteochondral fractures, diagnostic anesthesia, either a basisesamoid nerve block or an intrasynovial anesthesia of the PIPJ or DIPJ, may be needed to verify whether the lesion seen radiographically is the cause of lameness. For nonarticular eminence fractures, a basisesamoid block eliminates the lameness. Because of the risk of the fracture becoming displaced when the horse bears weight on the anesthetized digit, diagnostic anesthesia is contraindicated if an axial fracture is suspected.

A history of acute onset of severe lameness, painful withdrawal with or without, and instability on manipulation of the pastern region is common for articular eminence and comminuted fractures. In some, a history that a "pop" was heard just before the onset of severe lameness is revealed. Occasionally, a history of lameness in the affected limb is given before the development of a comminuted fracture. Although these fractures present with non-weight-bearing lameness, initially the lameness may quickly subside with the uniaxial eminence fracture, resulting in a misdiagnosis of soft tissue injury (e.g., ligament damage). With comminuted and biaxial fractures, the lameness generally remains severe.

On gross observation, obvious swelling is usually present just above the coronary band in cases of comminuted fractures. With articular eminence fractures, the swelling is less evident and may not be apparent. Swelling is usually not evident with osteochondral, nonarticular eminence, and simple axial fractures.

On palpation, varying degrees of swelling are appreciated. Fetlock and phalangeal flexion and rotation usually result in a painful response, particularly for the biaxial articular eminence and comminuted fractures. In some cases, crepitation may be appreciated with biaxial eminence fractures and comminuted fractures. Instability of the phalanges is usually prominent with comminuted fractures. Crepitation or instability is generally not appreciated with uniaxial eminence fractures. In some cases, direct palpation of the fractured eminence causes movement of the fracture and pain.

Diagnosis

A definitive diagnosis requires a complete radiographic examination. Four views, dorsopalmar (DP), lateromedial (LM), dorsopalmar-lateromedial oblique (DPLMO), and dorsopalmar-mediolateral oblique (DPMLO), are recommended. These projections should be taken so that fracture location and configuration can be appreciated (Fig. 8.154). Additionally, these views identify if the DIPJ is involved with comminuted fractures. The radiographs are examined carefully and systematically, as the fracture configuration has considerable bearing on the treatment method selected and the prognosis for future soundness. Computed tomography (CT) of comminuted middle phalangeal fractures has been shown to be most helpful in defining the fracture configuration.[18] CT has an advantage, in that it allows the production of cross-sectional images, resulting in spatial separation of superimposed structures seen on survey radiographs.

Treatment

Osteochondral fractures associated with the PIPJ that result in lameness are best treated by surgical removal. Although open approaches have been described,[13,20] the use of the arthroscope is preferred.[14,19,23] Dorsal and palmar or plantar fragments can be removed by arthroscopy, although the maneuverability of the instrumentation is somewhat limited in the dorsal approach because of the extensor tendon attachment immediately distal to the joint.[14,19] The palmar or plantar recess of the PIPJ is larger, which makes surgical manipulation easier. Osteochondral fractures involving the DIPJ are best managed by arthroscopy.

Uniaxial or biaxial eminence fractures of the middle phalanx that involve the PIPJ can be treated by casting alone, internal fixation with the lag screw principle, or arthrodesis of the joint followed by cast application.[7,21,22] Casting can be used for periods of 8 to 12 weeks in selected cases in which only pasture or breeding soundness is desired and in which economic constraints dictate this approach. Although some have recommended casting these fractures with full limb casts,[7] a lower limb (half) cast that includes the hoof and extends to the proximal limits of the metacarpus or metatarsus is all that is needed. The limb should be cast with the phalanges in a relaxed position in alignment. A lateral radiograph documents phalangeal alignment and fracture reduction. In some cases, the phalanges must be placed in slight flexion to achieve fracture reduction. If the limb is cast with the phalanges in an extended position, it can, in some cases, distract the eminence fragment(s) away from parent bone. Casting the limb with the phalanges in a relaxed position and, in some cases, slight flexion not only serves to reduce the fracture but also focuses the axial forces on the normal proximal dorsal border of the middle phalanx rather than on the center of the bone close to where the fracture is. The limb is cast in this position for 3 weeks with a cast that incorporates the foot. At the 3-week cast change, the phalanges are placed in a somewhat relaxed position, but this time the toe is extended slightly dorsad. Usually, 3 weeks is a sufficient period for enough healing to occur so that the fracture site will not become separated. At the 6-week cast change, radiographs are taken to assess fracture healing, and the limb is recast at this time in a more extended position. Cast application is continued until fracture healing is evident (usually 8 to 10 weeks). Once fracture healing is documented, the cast is removed while the horse is standing and sedated. After cast removal, a pressure support bandage is applied and continued for an additional 3 weeks. Exercise is permitted according to the horse's capabilities. This technique has been used successfully in numerous cases in which breeding or pasture soundness was desired. Additionally, it has been used in a few cases that have resumed performance.

Internal fixation of articular uniaxial palmar or plantar eminence fractures has been reported to be successful in returning some horses to athletic performance, but it depends on the duration and displacement of the fracture.[4,11,12,21] Generally, acute fractures that are not displaced have the best outcome with use of this approach. Lag screw fixation can be performed through a stab incision made either between the flexor tendons and the palmar digital neurovascular plexus or by splitting longitudinally the branch of the superficial digital flexor tendon over the proximal extremity of the fragment. Needles can be used to identify the PIPJ and the dorsal and palmar or plantar bone surfaces. Radiographic monitoring or fluoroscopy is used to identify the spacial relation for screw placement. If any question exists, a small drill bit can be used to drill the proposed site for screw placement, after which radiographs are taken. If fluoroscopy is used there is no need to predrill the hole with a small drill bit. The drill hole is made in a distal axial direction. The principle of interfragmentary compression is used, but countersinking is not necessary. After suture closure, a cast is applied to protect the limb during recovery. The cast can be removed in 14 to 21 days, depending on the degree of fracture stability achieved. Horses are stalled for 6 weeks and controlled hand walking exercise is begun after that time. A total rest period of approxi-

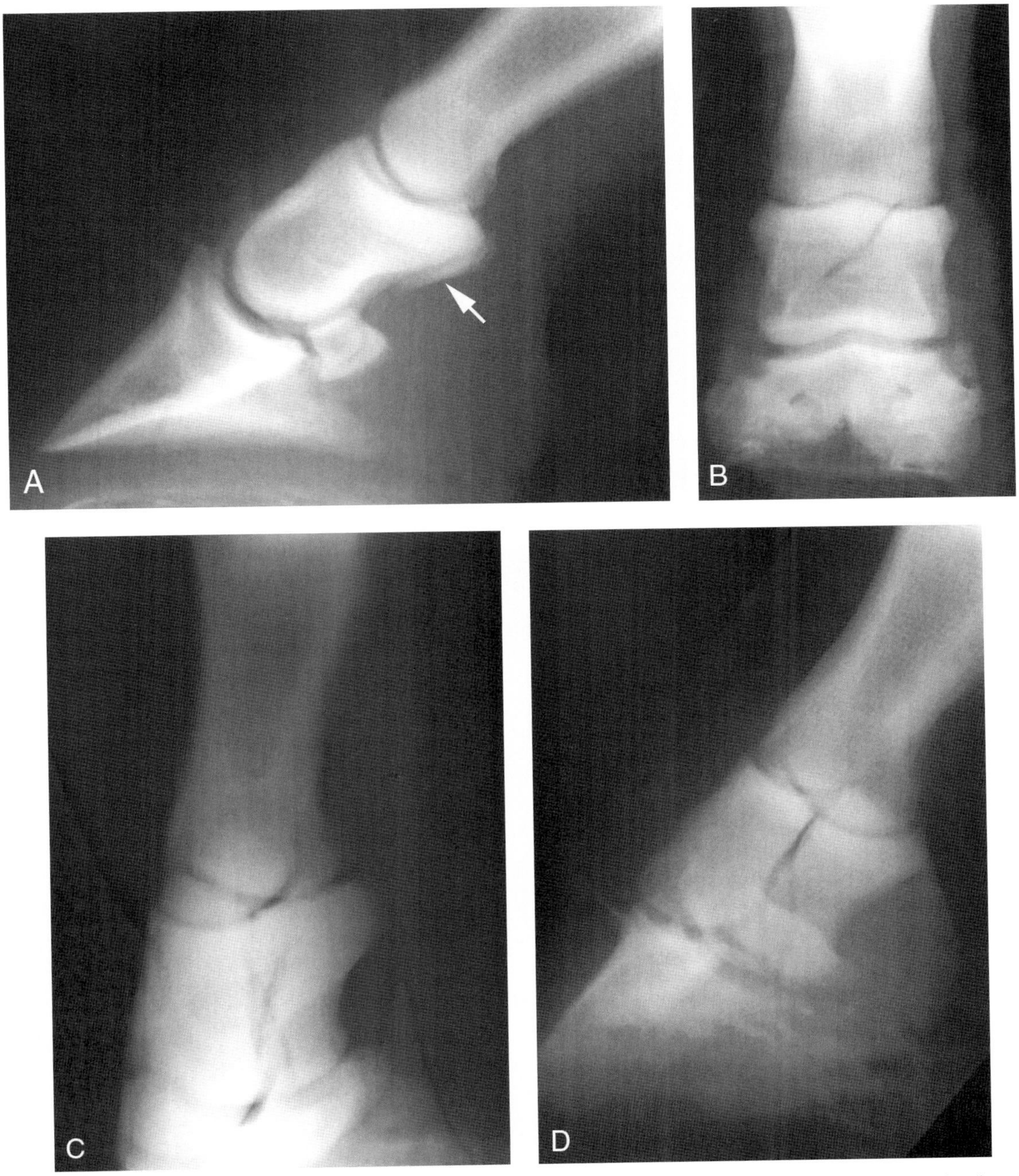

Figure 8.154 Substantiation of the necessity of four radiographic views to identify the fracture configuration. A. Lateral view indicating a possibility of plantar eminence fracture (arrow).

B. Dorsoplantar view indicating that the fracture involves the PIPJ. C and D. Oblique views indicating that the fracture is comminuted and biarticular.

mately 12 to 16 weeks is recommended before free exercise is begun. Riding exercise may begin in 9 to 12 months. Although these eminence fractures are occasionally lagged back into place, performing arthrodesis of the PIPJ most commonly treats these fractures.

Surgical arthrodesis of the PIPJ is our preference for treatment of most uniaxial or biaxial eminence fractures. Even with stable interfragmentary compression of the fragment, i.e., of several days duration and minimally displaced, we have observed DJD develop later, requir-

ing pastern arthrodesis (Fig. 8.155). For uniaxial fractures, pastern arthrodesis is most commonly accomplished with transarticularly placed screws. The use of two or three 5.5-mm cortical screws placed in a lag fashion is recommended. The 5.5-mm screws provide more stable fixation than do the 4.5-mm screws. For the discussion of the technique of arthrodesis with transarticular screws, the reader is referred to treatment of DJD of the PIPJ above. The only differences are that we place the screws in such a fashion as to avoid the fracture plane

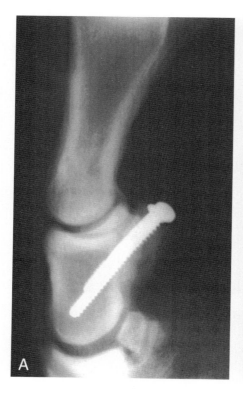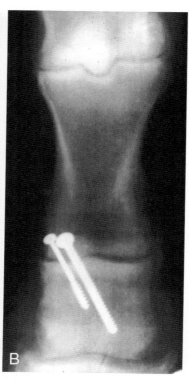

Figure 8.155 Plantar eminence fracture treated by lag screw fixation 4 months earlier. A. Lateral view. B. Dorsoplantar view. Note the periarticular and articular margin changes on the lateral and medial margins of the joint. Because of persistent lameness, a pastern arthrodesis was performed.

and, in some cases, we lag the fracture fragment back into place prior to performing the arthrodesis (Fig. 8.156). Pastern arthrodesis by dorsal plate application is preferred for biaxial fractures.[3,6] Generally, two 4- to 5-hole narrow dynamic compression plates (DCPs) are placed on either side of the midline for adult horses. The palmar or plantar eminence fractures are stabilized by lag screw fixation with the distal plate screws. For adults, 4.5-mm DCPs are used, and for foals, generally, 3.5-mm DCPs are used. Other plate configurations include single broad DCP, T-plates, and Y-plates. When a single broad or narrow DCP is used, a separate screw independent of the plate can be placed to lag one of the fractures. Unfortunately, the thin profile of the T-plate often precludes its use in adult horses.[14] Recently, a Y-plate has been developed for the treatment of comminuted middle phalanx fractures, and it may have some use for biaxial eminence fractures also.[9] See the "Comminuted Fractures" for more discussion on the Y-plate.

Comminuted fractures can be treated with casting alone, similar to that previously described for eminence fractures. They can also be treated with casting and transfixation pins placed through the diaphysis of the middle or the distal third of the metacarpus or metatarsus; with internal fixation screws only; or with one or two bone plates placed dorsally to bridge the PIPJ, with or without transfixation pins.

The use of casts with or without transfixation pins is relegated for some severely comminuted fractures that cannot be adequately reduced or stabilized by internal fixation and breeding soundness is acceptable or there are economic constraints and/or euthanasia is not an option. Because comminuted fractures are so unstable, wires are placed through the perimeter of the hoof wall

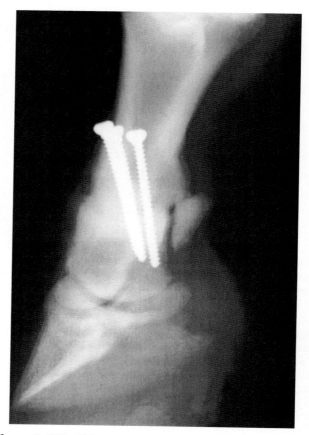

Figure 8.156 Oblique view of placement of screws to miss the fracture plane.

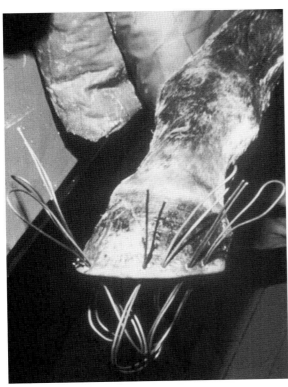

Figure 8.157   Wires being placed through the hoof wall to apply traction.

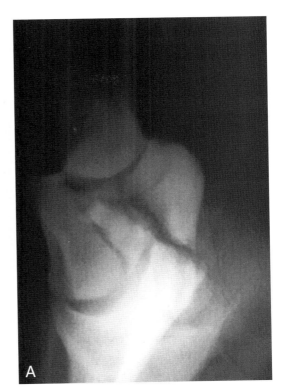

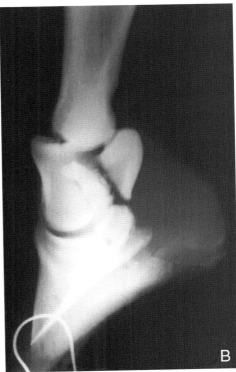

Figure 8.158   Lateral view of a comminuted biarticular fracture of the middle phalanx. A. Before tension was applied. B. After tension was applied. Note that the fractures have been partially reduced and the alignment of the PIPJ is improved.

to apply traction to the phalanges and to reduce the fracture fragments (Fig. 8.157). Radiographs are taken to document that fracture reduction has been achieved (Fig. 8.158). After this, a lower limb cast that incorporates the hoof is applied. Some comminuted middle phalangeal fractures have been treated successfully with this approach (Fig. 8.159).

In the most severely comminuted unstable fractures the use of centrally threaded positive profile transfixation pins is preferred to reduce the chance of fracture collapse within the cast. A suitably sized drill and tap are used to make the holes and threads for pin placement (Fig. 8.160). After pin placement, a lower limb cast that incorporates the foot and pins that extends to the proximal metacarpus or metatarsus is applied. Hoof acrylic is often used to further secure the pins to the cast (Fig. 8.161). The transfixation pins reduce the chance of fracture collapse within the cast by transferring the weight from the fracture site to the bottom of the cast to the pins placed in the diaphysis of the metacarpus or metatarsus. A complication of using a transfixation cast is the development of a ring sequestrum 3 to 6 weeks after the cast is applied (Fig. 8.162). Placing the pins too far proximally can result in fracture through the pinhole site, even while the cast is still in place. An alternative to the transfixation cast is an external fixator, which uses a series of large transfixation pins placed through the metacarpus or metatarsus and incorporates side connecting bars to a foot plate.[15] In our hands, this device has been difficult and time consuming to apply and has resulted in fracture of the metacarpus or metatarsus post-

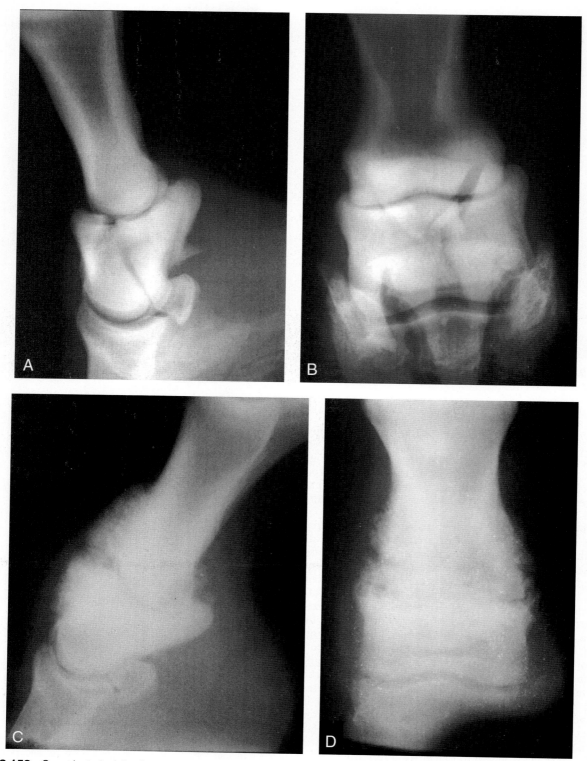

Figure 8.159 Comminuted minimally displaced biarticular fracture of the middle phalanx that was treated successfully with cast application. A and B. Fracture at presentation. C and D. Fracture site at 6-month follow-up. Note that there is little radiographic evidence of DJD involving the DIPJ. This horse was pasture sound at this time.

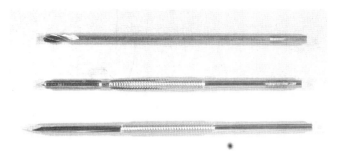

Figure 8.160 Drill (top), a centrally threaded positive profile tap (middle), and a positive profile centrally threaded pin (bottom) used for the application of transfixation pins. (Courtesy of IMEX Veterinary Inc., Longview, TX.)

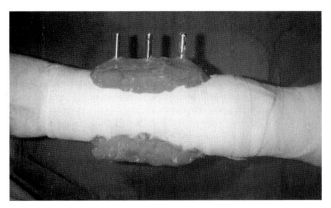

Figure 8.161 Application of hoof acrylic around transfixation after cast had been applied. The pins are then cut to the level of the acrylic. A cotton bandage is applied to the opposite limb to protect it during recovery from anesthesia.

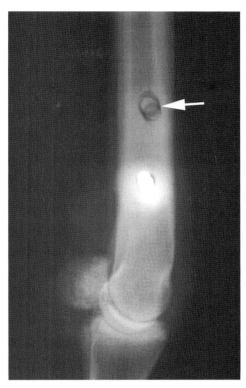

Figure 8.162 Development of ring sequestra in upper pin tract (arrow). Also note the bone lysis surrounding the distal pin.

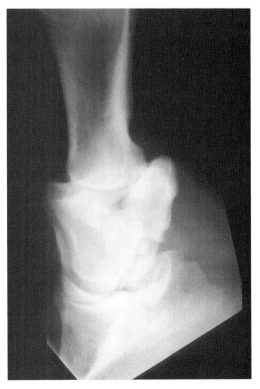

Figure 8.163 Same horse as in Figure 8.151, months after treatment with transfixation pins and a cast. At 1-year follow-up, this stallion was breeding successfully and appeared pain free except during cold weather.

operatively. In cases in which casting alone or casting with transfixation pins is used, the damage to the PIPJ surface is, with time, usually sufficient to create fusion (Fig. 8.163).

The use of dorsal plate application combined with pastern arthrodesis is recommended for optimal return to performance. Plate configurations used to reduce and stabilize the fracture include single broad DCP, a single or a double narrow DCP, a T-plate, or a specially designed Y-plate.[3,5,6,9,15,17] The thin profile of the T-plate often precludes its use; therefore, narrow DCPs are usually preferred. After exposure of the PIPJ, the cartilage is removed from the joint surfaces, and the fracture configuration is visualized to determine the best placement of implants. The clinician then reduces and stabilizes the palmar or plantar eminence(s) with a lag screw placed through the distal plate hole. The plate should be placed as far proximally in the middle phalanx as possible so that impingement of the extensor process of the distal phalanx is avoided during phalangeal extension (Fig. 8.164).[6] Individually placed lag screws independent of the plate can also be placed to provide added strength to the repair. Recently, a biomechanical study was done to compare double-plate and Y-plate fixation of the comminuted fractures.[9] The conclusion was that the Y-plate was as affective as the double-plate configuration and

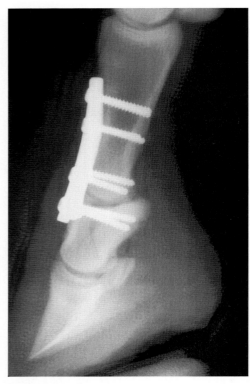

Figure 8.164 Two plates were used to treat this comminuted biarticular middle phalanx fracture. Note that the distal hole screws are placed proximal in the middle phalanx to avoid impingement of the extensor process during phalangeal extension.

that the Y-plate may provide increased stability by allowing the proximal fragments of the middle phalanx to be stabilized by three screws placed through the plate.

Prognosis

The prognosis for osteochondral (chip) fractures treated surgically seems good for return to full serviceability.[13,14,19,20] If arthrotomy is used, it is important to avoid further damage to the support structures (ligaments and tendons) that may increase the chances of the development and progression of a periostitis and DJD. In one study, 4 of 5 cases with osteochondral fragments (3 involved the PIPJ and 2 involved the DIPJ) treated by arthrotomy returned to their intended use.[20] Although there are only few reports in which arthroscopy is used for the removal of these osteochondral fragments, it would appear that it is a superior approach.[14,19,23]

The prognosis for uniaxial fractures or palmar or plantar eminence fractures treated by arthrodesis seems good for return to performance and is similar to that expected for pastern arthrodesis used for treatment of DJD of the pastern joint.[11] For biaxial eminence fractures repaired by arthrodesis, the prognosis is fair for return to performance, particularly for fractures involving the hindlimbs.[4,11] The use of bone plates for repair of biaxial fractures may improve the prognosis for return to function.[6]

The prognosis for axial fractures appears guarded for freedom from lameness because of the proliferative bone, particularly at the articular margins, that may develop from the initial trauma.[14]

For comminuted fractures involving the PIPJ only, a good prognosis can be given for pasture soundness, and a guarded to poor prognosis can be given for return to athletic performance. One report identified a 30% chance of returning to athletic performance.[4] Horses that had sustained comminuted biarticular fractures were reported to have a 50% survival rate and a slightly greater than a 1 to 10 chance of return to athletic performance with casting alone. Surgical intervention in these cases did not improve the survival rate, but it increased the chance of return to athletic function by a 1 to 4 margin.[4] In general, the prognosis for hindlimb fractures was reported to be better, no matter what treatment is applied.[1,2,7,21,24] In one report, 20% of the horses with hindlimb injuries resumed athletic function, whereas only 9% resumed function after forelimb involvement.[4]

The use of bone plates in the treatment of these comminuted fractures has increased the chances of survival and a return to athletic function. In one report, 7 of 8 horses with forelimb involvement were alive at follow-up 2 years postinjury, and 4 of 7 horses were being ridden. Of the 2 horses with hindlimb involvement, 1 was being ridden, and 1 was lost to follow-up.[5] In another report, 2 of 3 mature horses with comminuted fractures that involved the forelimbs returned to athletic performance, and 2 of 3 foals with physeal fractures also performed.[6]

In all cases, the prognosis is appropriately decreased if the horse develops support limb laminitis or has sustained a fracture of the navicular bone associated with a comminuted biarticular fracture.

References

1. Adams OR. Lameness in Horses. 3rd ed. Philadelphia: Lea & Febiger, 1974;359.
2. Adams OR. Lameness in rodeo horses. Vet Scope 1962;7:8.
3. Bukowieki CF, Bramlage LR. Treatment of a comminuted middle phalangeal fracture in a horse by use of a broad dynamic compression plate. J Am Vet Med Assoc 1989;194:1731.
4. Colahan PT, Wheat JD, Meagher DM. Treatment of middle phalangeal fractures in the horse. J Am Vet Med Assoc 1981;178:1182.
5. Crabill MR, Watkins JP, Schneider RK, et al. Double-plate fixation of comminuted fractures of the second phalanx in horses: 10 cases (1985–1993). J Am Vet Med Assoc 1995;207:1459.
6. Doran RE, White NA, Allen D. Use of a bone plate for treatment of middle phalangeal fractures in horses: Seven cases (1979–1984). J Am Vet Med Assoc 1987;191:575–578.
7. Fessler JF, Amstutz HE. Fracture repair. In: Oehme FW, Prier JE, Eds. Textbook of Large Animal Surgery. Baltimore: Williams & Wilkins, 1974;296.
8. Gabel AA, Bukowiecki CF. Fractures of the phalanges. Vet Clin North Am Large Anim Pract 1983;5:233–260.
9. Galuppo LD, Stover SM, Willits NH. A biomechanical comparison of Double-plate and Y-plate fixation for comminuted equine second phalangeal fractures. Vet Surg 2000;29:152–162.
10. Honnas CM. Surgical treatment of selected musculoskeletal disorders of the forelimb. In: Auer JA, Ed. Equine Surgery. Philadelphia: WB Saunders, 1992;986–989.
11. Martin GS, McIlwraith CW, Turner AS, et al. Long-term results and complications of proximal interphalangeal arthrodesis in horses. J Am Vet Med Assoc 1984;184:1136.
12. McIlwraith CW, Goodman NL. Conditions of the interphalangeal joints. Vet Clin North Am Equine Pract 1989;5:161–178.

13. Modransky PD, Grant BD, Rantanen NW, et al. Surgical treatment of a palmar midsagittal fracture of the proximal second phalanx in a horse. Vet Surg 1982;11:129.

14. Nixon AJ. The phalanges and metacarpophalangeal joint. In: Auer JA, Stick JA, Eds. Equine Surgery. 2nd ed. Philadelphia: WB Saunders, 1999;792–794.

15. Nunamaker DM, Richardson DW, Butterweck DM, et al. A new external skeletal fixation device that allows immediate full weightbearing application the horse. Vet Surg 1986;15:345–355.

16. Rick MC. Fractures of the middle phalanx. In: White NA, Moore JN, Eds. Current Practice of Equine Surgery. Philadelphia: JB Lippincott, 1990;606–609.

17. Rick MC, Herthel D, Boles C. Surgical management of middle phalangeal fractures and high ring bone in horses: A review of 16 cases. Proc Am Assoc Equine Pract 1986;32:315–321.

18. Rose PL, Seeherman H, O'Callaghan M. Computed tomographic evaluation of comminuted middle phalangeal fractures in the horse. Vet Radiol Ultrasound 1997;38:424–429.

19. Schneider RK, Ragle CA, Carter BG, et al. Arthroscopic removal of osteochondral fragments from the proximal interphalangeal joint of the pelvic limbs in three horses. J Am Vet Med Assoc 1994;205:79.

20. Torre F. Osteochondral chip fractures of the palmar/plantar aspect of the middle phalanx in the horse: 5 cases (1991–1994). Pferdeheilkunde 1997;13:673–678.

21. Turner AS. Fractures of specific bones. In: Mansmann RA, McAllister ES, Eds. Equine Medicine and Surgery. 3rd ed. Santa Barbara, CA: American Veterinary Publications, 1982;1012.

22. Turner AS, Gabel AA. Lag screw fixation of avulsion fractures of the second phalanx in the horse. J Am Vet Med Assoc 1975;167:306.

23. Vail TB, McIlwraith CW. Arthroscopic removal of an osteochondral fragment from the middle phalanx of a horse. Vet Surg 1992;21:260–272.

24. von Salis B. Internal fixation in the horse. Proc Am Assoc Equine Pract 1972;18:193–218.

25. Watkins JP. Fractures of the middle phalanx. In: Nixon AJ, ed. Equine Fracture Repair. Philadelphia: WB Saunders, 1996;129.

26. Welch RD, Watkins JP. Osteochondral fracture of the proximal palmar middle phalanx in a Thoroughbred. Equine Vet J 1991;23:67–69.

FRACTURES OF THE PROXIMAL (FIRST) PHALANX (P-1)

Fractures of the proximal (first) phalanx (PP) occur frequently and are broadly categorized into noncomminuted and comminuted fractures.[13] Noncomminuted (excluding the osteochondral fracture) and comminuted fractures occur commonly in horses.[1–3,7,8,24] Fracture configurations range from small fissures that enter the MCP or MTP joint to highly comminuted fractures affecting both cortices and the proximal and distal joint surfaces (Figs. 8.165 and 8.166).[3,7,8,24] Although it is uncommon for the PP fractures to be open,[9,23] one study found that 5 of 30 comminuted fractures were open at the time of presentation.[16] The most common noncomminuted fracture involving the PP, the osteochondral fracture of the proximal dorsal articular margin, is covered in the section dealing with the fetlock in this chapter.

Noncomminuted PP fractures have been classified into six types:

1. Midsagittal, including short (less than 30 mm) and long (greater than 30 mm); proximal incomplete fractures; and complete midsagittal fractures that exist out of the lateral cortex or involve both joint surfaces (Figs. 8.165 and 8.167)

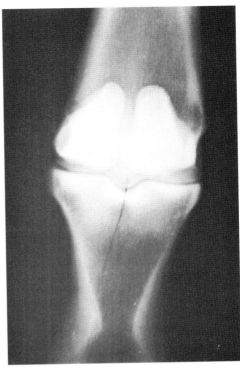

Figure 8.165 Long incomplete midsagittal fracture of the PP.

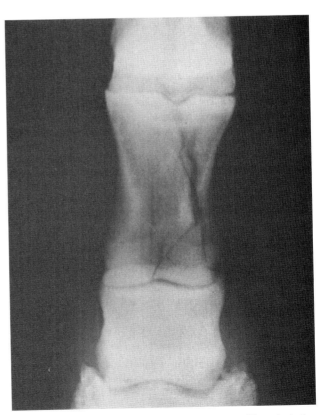

Figure 8.166 Comminuted fracture of the PP with a strut of intact bone on one side that extends from the fetlock joint to the PIPJ.

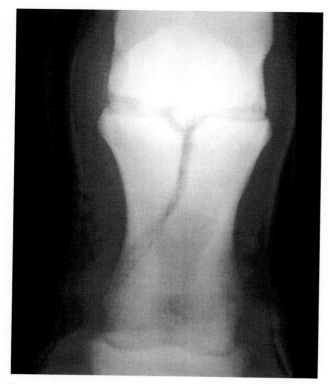

Figure 8.167 Midsagittal complete fracture of the PP that exits out the lateral cortex. Note that the radiograph was taken through a cast, which was applied prior to transport to Colorado State University.

2. Dorsal fractures; oblique fractures extending dorsad, which can be either incomplete or complete, exiting the dorsal cortex; or complete fractures extending distad from the MCP or MTP to the PIPJ (Fig. 8.168)
3. Distal joint fractures (Fig. 8.169)
4. Palmar or plantar eminence fractures (Fig. 8.170) (refer to disease of the fetlock for more discussion)
5. Physeal fractures
6. Oblique or transverse diaphyseal fractures (Fig. 8.171)[5,6,12,14,15]

A seventh type of fracture that has not been described previously is the dorsal avulsion fracture (Fig. 8.172). This fracture is uncommon in my experience. Possibly, this avulsion fracture should be added to the dorsal fracture type 2 classification in the future. Of these seven fracture types, the midsagittal is the most common and may be present in the contralateral limb in a small percentage of the cases.[6,15] The contralateral limb was affected in 3 of 49 horses in one study and in 3 of 119 horses in another study.[6,22]

Noncomminuted PP fractures are more commonly seen in racing Thoroughbreds, Standardbreds, and hunters and jumpers, and comminuted fractures are most common in the western performance (cutting and barrel racing) horses, racing Thoroughbreds, and Standardbreds.[1,9,16,24] Interestingly, in one report, 27% of the horses sustained the comminuted fracture while at pasture, and a smaller percentage developed the fracture

while being used for showing or pleasure riding.[16] Noncomminuted fractures in racehorses most commonly affect the hindlimbs in Standardbreds and the forelimbs in Thoroughbreds.[6,16,22] A slightly higher incidence of left forelimb involvement has been identified in racing Thoroughbreds that sustain comminuted fractures.[16]

Etiology

It appears that a combination of longitudinal compression in conjunction with asynchronous lateral to medial rotation of the PP or of twisting of the PP in relation to the third metacarpal or third metatarsal bone is the cause.[1,21] Probably two situations exist. During the weight-bearing phase, the convex sagittal ridge of the distal end of the third metacarpal or the third metatarsal bone comes to fit in congruity with the concave groove in the proximal surface of the PP. If the alignment is not perfect, the convex sagittal ridge acts as a wedge to create the fracture.[8] Such would be the case when the horse is required to make quick turns. Also, as the limb goes to the flexed position, there is a lateral to medial rotation of the PP around its long axis.[21] In this case, if the rotary movement is accelerated, as it would be if the foot slips, a fracture may result. Factors such as shoeing the horse with heel calks, which are needed to make rapid turns, tend to fix the foot and phalanges fast, allowing the third metacarpal or the third metatarsal bone to twist in relation to these structures, thus resulting in a fracture.[1]

Type 1 PP fractures in the forelimb tend to be oriented lateral to the midline of the PP. This may be the result of a smaller lateral articular surface of the PP in the forelimb than in the hindlimb. The consequent position of the center of the sagittal groove lateral to the midline thus dictates that fractures propagate down that side of the bone.[6] Sagittal fractures that extend distad or medial to the midline are approximately twice as common in the hindlimbs than in the forelimbs. This may be because the proximal articular surface in the hindlimb slopes distad laterally more than the distal joint surface in the forelimb.[6] The dorsal avulsion nonarticular fracture is believed to result from excess tension of the extensor tendon created during flexion of the fetlock and the phalanges.

Clinical Signs

The clinical signs associated with PP fracture are variable and depend on the type of fracture. Whereas the noncomminuted fracture often results in a lameness grade 3 to 4 (on a scale of 5) or may even be subtle with incomplete short midsagittal fractures, particularly after a long period of rest, the comminuted fracture results in a non-weight-bearing lameness.[22] In any case, there is usually a history of acute onset of lameness, and the horse may show signs of physical distress, such as sweating.[6] Visual observation reveals that the pastern region is obviously swollen with comminuted fractures because of the attendant hemorrhage and edema associated with the soft tissues. The swelling associated with the noncomminuted fracture, on the other hand, is usually less profound and may take hours or days before it is appar-

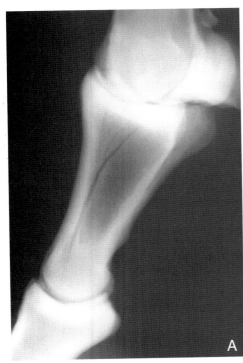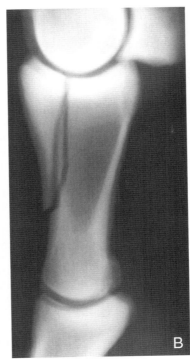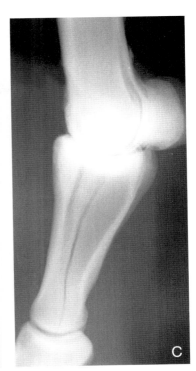

Figure 8.168 A. Oblique view of an incomplete dorsal fracture of the PP. B. Lateral view of a complete dorsal fracture of the PP that exits the dorsal cortex. C. Lateral view of a complete dorsal fracture of the PP that enters the fetlock joint. (Courtesy of Dr. Julie Dechant.)

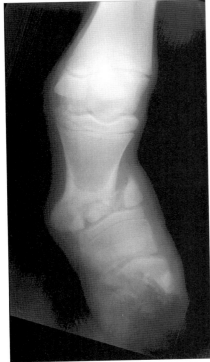

Figure 8.169 Condylar fracture of the PP that enters the PIPJ. Note the subluxation of the PIPJ, leading to a malalignment of the phalanges.

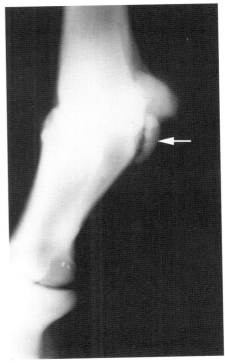

Figure 8.170 Oblique view of a plantar eminence of the PP (arrow).

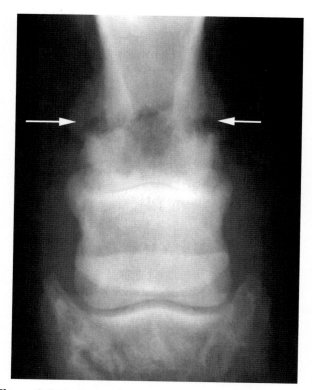

Figure 8.171   Dorsopalmar view of a healing transverse fracture of the distal PP (arrows). This fracture had been treated by external coaptation.

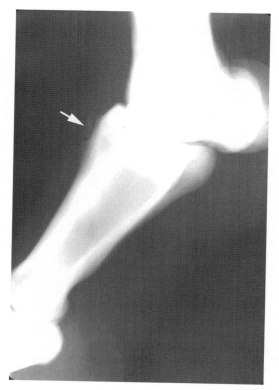

Figure 8.172   Lateral view of a nonarticular avulsion fracture at the attachment of the extensor tendon to the PP (arrow).

ent.[6] Fetlock synovial distension (effusion) is commonly seen with incomplete midsagittal fractures.[22] An angular limb deformity of the pastern region is commonly observed with displaced distal condylar PP fractures that enter the PIPJ. The limb deformity develops as a result of the lateral or medial subluxation of the PIPJ. On palpation and manipulation, a painful response is elicited with flexion and rotation of the phalanges in cases of noncomminuted fracture. For comminuted fracture, crepitation and instability are obvious.

If a noncomminuted fracture is suspected, radiographs should be taken immediately. Perineural anesthesia or exercise to establish lameness is contraindicated because it may result in dehiscence of the fracture and lessen the prognosis for athletic performance in the future.

Nonarticular avulsion fracture of the PP usually presents with a history of mild intermittent lameness that increases with exercise. Swelling at the proximal dorsal limits of the PP, although mild, is usually apparent. Digital pressure applied over the swelling generally elicits pain if the condition is acute. Fetlock or phalangeal flexion is usually painful.

Diagnosis

Radiographs are taken to characterize the type of fracture and to indicate if internal fixation is required. If the horse has to be transported a short distance for radiographic examination, a tight-fitting bandage splint should be applied. Most horses protect their limbs well because of the extreme pain. On the other hand, a cast or an effective splint is indicated for horses that must be transported for long distances and for all horses that have sustained a comminuted fracture.

The radiographic examination should include at least four views, the DP, the LM, the DPLMO, and the DPMLO, to confirm the diagnosis and to gain a full appreciation of the fracture configuration. With some, there is a duplication of the fracture line on the dorsal and the palmar or plantar or lateral and medial surfaces at different sites that may give the impression that there is more than one fracture[8] (see Fig. 8.98). This occurs because the fracture lines are not superimposed on the radiographic view.[6] Also, the variable location of the nutrient foramen in the PP of the forelimbs of Standardbreds may occasionally be misinterpreted radiographically as a fracture.[13] The radiographic appearance of the foramina occurs in three patterns; they are located either in the dorsal cortex or in the palmar cortex, or they are absent. In 55% of cases in Standardbreds, the foramina are bilaterally asymmetric.[13] Dorsal nutrient foramina are most frequently misdiagnosed as a fracture because of the length of the radiolucent line in a vertical direction in the dorsal cortex. Palmar foramina generally course transversely to the long axis of the bone and are less readily mistaken for a fracture.

Treatment

Noncomminuted Fractures

Type 1 incomplete fractures can receive conservative treatment, consisting of pressure bandaging and stall rest for 6 to10 weeks followed by a gradual return to normal exercise over the next 6 weeks.[6] Generally, these fractures heal with a periosteal callus over the dorsal aspect of the fracture site, but this does not appear to limit function.[6,15] A risk of treating these fractures conservatively, however, is the chance that they can dehisce to become complete fractures. One study found that this happened in 3 of 85 cases that initially presented as type 1 short (less than 30 mm) incomplete fractures.[6] Presently, midsagittal incomplete fractures in horses that have sustained acute long (greater than 30 mm) fractures and that are to be used for racing are treated with lag screw fixation placed through stab incisions, followed by external coaptation.[7,8,12] Two to three screws are generally used, depending on the length of the fracture, and radiographic monitoring is recommended to make sure the MCP or MTP joint is not entered and to document that the fracture is compressed (Fig. 8.173). The cast, if used, is generally left in place for 10 to 14 days. Others prefer bandage support for recovery.[18] Interestingly, one retrospective study indicated that all incomplete midsagittal fractures greater than 15 mm were treated surgically.[22] Chronic long midsagittal fractures that are diagnosed 4 to 6 weeks after the onset of lameness are generally treated with stall confinement and bandaging.[15]

Complete acute midsagittal fractures that extend distad from the fetlock joint to involve the PIPJ or that exit the lateral cortex are best treated by internal fixation and coaptation. Internal fixation has been accomplished by lag screw fixation or by the use of a neutralization plate.[6,15] Presently, we recommend lag screw fixation through stab incisions. Needles placed in the MCP or MTP joint (fetlock) and PIPJ and radiographic monitor-

ing help define the placement of screws. Generally, three to five screws are used, depending on the length of the fracture, and the cast is left in place for 3 to 4 weeks (Fig. 8.174). Bandaging and/or external coaptation has been used alone in cases in which breeding soundness is the objective and/or in which there are economic constraints.[6] Generally, horses treated conservatively take approximately 4 months to become free of pain and lameness but invariably develop considerable exostosis at the fracture healing site and secondary DJD that may cause lameness when they resume work.[6,15] Healing time for horses treated surgically is reduced approximately 2 months, and less callus formation and DJD result.[12]

Type 2 dorsal oblique incomplete or complete nondisplaced PP fractures can be treated by rest and bandaging as described for type 1 fractures or by internal fixation with the lag screw principle (Fig. 8.175). Needles placed in the MCP or MTP joint help determine the proper placement of the screws through stab incisions. Alternatively, an arthroscope can be inserted into the fetlock joint to visualize the dorsal articular margin and to debride damaged cartilage if needed.[18] After internal fixation, a cast can be applied and kept in place for 2 to 3 weeks. Alternatively, some prefer to recover the horse in a bandage.[18] Complete dorsal fractures that extend into the PIPJ are best treated by lag screw fixation placed through stab incisions and external coaptation (Fig. 8.176).[5] Needles placed in the MCP or MTP joint and PIPJ help guide the placement of 3 to 4 screws. Generally, the cast is removed in 3 weeks.[5] After surgical treatment, fracture healing and return to training can be expected 1 to 3 months earlier than with nonsurgical treatment. Lag screw fixation of nondisplaced fractures may be in-

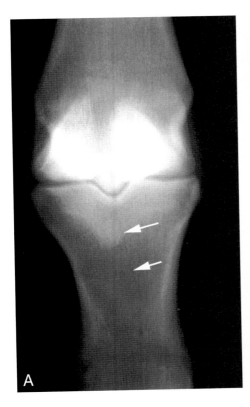
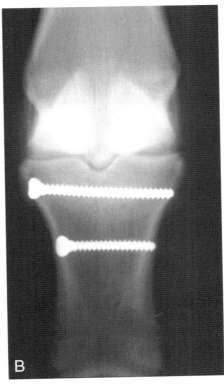

Figure 8.173 Dorsopalmar view of a long midsagittal incomplete fracture of the PP that was treated by lag screw fixation. A. Fracture before surgery (arrows). B. Two screws placed in lag fashion were used to repair this fracture.

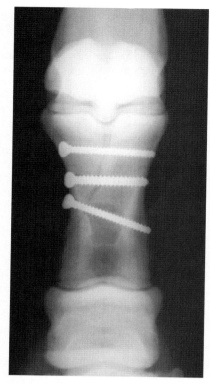

Figure 8.174 Same horse as in Figure 8.167 after fracture repair with three screws placed in lag fashion. At 6-year follow-up, this horse had returned to its intended use and was still performing successfully.

dicated in some horses to reduce the length of the convalescent period.[12]

Type 3 distal articular PP fractures occur almost exclusively in the hindlimbs and seem more common in foals[15] (see Fig. 8.169). The acute fracture is generally best treated by lag screw fixation placed through stab incisions, after which external coaptation is applied. The cast is usually removed in 2 to 3 weeks. If the fracture is chronic, then arthrodesis of the PIPJ is recommended. (Refer to treatment of DJD of the PIPJ above for more information regarding the techniques for arthrodesis.)

Treatment of type 4 palmar or plantar eminence fractures is covered under diseases of the fetlock region.

Type 5 physeal fractures are usually Salter-Harris type 2 fractures and are most common in weanlings.[15] Minimally displaced fractures are generally best treated conservatively with stall confinement and bandage support. In one report (4 cases), all type 5 fractures healed with a moderate degree of malunion, but the PP remodeled so that a normal hoof-pastern axis was maintained.[15] If the fracture results in considerable limb deformity and cannot be reduced, internal fixation may be required. If the PIPJ becomes subluxated as a result of the injury and the fracture is chronic, then a pastern arthrodesis may have to be performed to align the phalanges.

Type 6 oblique or transverse PP fractures are uncommon and do not affect the physis or articular margins. Stabilization of the fracture with lag screws placed through stab incisions has been described.[15] Alternatively, these fractures, if minimally displaced, heal with external coaptation (see Fig. 8.171).

Type 7 avulsion PP fractures appear to respond favorably to rest, bandaging, controlled exercise, and treatment with nonsteroidal anti-inflammatory drugs

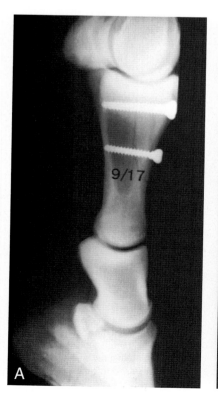
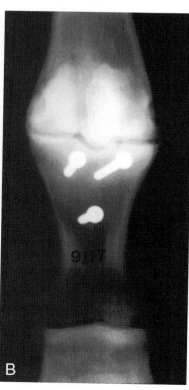

Figure 8.175 Same fracture as in Figure 8.168 after treatment with lag screw fixation. A. Lateral view after surgery. B. Dorsopalmar view of screw placement.

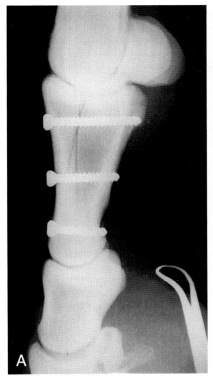
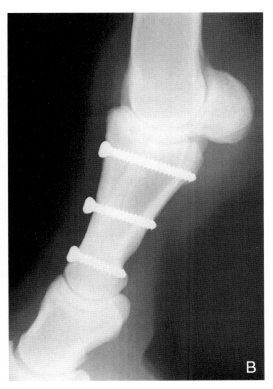

Figure 8.176   Same horse as in Figure 8.168C. A. Lateral view taken intraoperatively. Three 5.5-mm AO/ASIF cortical bone screws were used to create interfragmentary compression. B. Follow-up at 12 weeks after operation. (Courtesy of Dr. Julie Dechant.)

(NSAIDs). Rest periods extend from 6 weeks to 3 months, depending on the horse's response. Hand walking exercise begins when the horse is no longer painful to fetlock and phalangeal flexion; this is usually at 3 to 4 weeks postinjury. Return to performance generally occurs between 3 and 4 months postinjury.

Comminuted Fractures

Prior to referral for possible surgical repair, initial treatment should be aimed at providing adequate support and counterpressure to prevent further bony damage and reduce soft tissue swelling.[3,4] To avoid the bending forces of the MCP or MTP joint, one should align the dorsal cortices of the PP with the long axis of the metacarpus or metatarsus and splint or preferably cast in that position.[4] This position neutralizes the bending forces at the fracture site within the PP. Most comminuted fractures disrupt both joint surfaces (see Figs. 8.166 and 8.176). The objective for treatment of these cases is usually to preserve the horse for breeding purposes.[12] Ideally, the articular congruity of the joint(s) is restored and the fracture can be stabilized to maintain bone length.

Methods for treatment of comminuted fractures include 1) closed reduction and external coaptation, 2) closed reduction, skeletal transfixation, and external coaptation, 3) closed reduction followed by lag screw fixation through stab incisions with or without skeletal transfixation and external coaptation, 4) open reduction followed by lag screw fixation and external coaptation,

and 5) open reduction followed by lag screw fixation and the application of a neutralization plate and external coaptation.[12,15,18–20] Selection of treatment method depends on the configuration of the fracture, intended use of the horse, and economic constraints. A complete radiographic series should be assessed to define the fracture configuration and the possibility of treatment or humane destruction. If surgery with internal fixation is the choice, at least two criteria should be met: 1) the implants should allow reapposition of the joint surfaces, especially the proximal joint surface; and 2) the implants should provide longitudinal stability of the PP.[6] If either of these criteria cannot be met, then external skeletal fixation should be used alone or in combination with internal fixation.[12] Regardless of the treatment selected, the vascular supply to the region and the integrity of the skin overlying the fracture site should be evaluated by means of physical examination. If a question still exists regarding the vascular supply, thermography, nuclear scintigraphy, or both may be helpful.

Horses with an intact cortex (strut of intact bone on one side of the fractured PP that extends from the proximal to the distal joint surface) have a significantly greater chance of survival than do horses without an intact strut of bone (see Fig. 8.166). In one study reviewing the outcome of cases of comminuted PP fracture, researchers found that 57% of the horses with an intact strut of bone were alive more than 1 year after treatment, whereas only 23% of horses without an intact strut of bone were alive at 1 year.[16] The intact strut of bone provides longitudinal stability to the fracture site as well as a solid piece of bone to which to lag the fractured fragments.

The use of external coaptation in the form of a cast as the sole treatment for comminuted PP fractures can give satisfactory results in some cases.[12,16] In one study, 2 of 3 horses with comminuted fractures that were treated with cast alone had a satisfactory outcome.[16] Since the cast does not provide resistance to axial collapse of the PP, however, for a good outcome the fracture should be minimally comminuted and be stable or at least have one cortex of the fractured bone (strut) intact to prevent axial collapse. Healing of the fracture with minimal malunion is more likely in those cases in which both joint surfaces of the PP are in good alignment prior to the application of the cast.[16] Complications associated with using a cast alone for treatment of a highly comminuted and unstable PP fracture include 1) a high risk of axial collapse of the PP, which can result in pressure necrosis of the skin overlying the fracture, leading to an open fracture; 2) the development of support limb laminitis and deep digital flexor tendinitis below the MCP or MTP joint of the opposite limb because of continued pain at the fracture site; 3) excess callus formation and extensive DJD of both joints; 4) shortening of the pastern region; and 5) partial ankylosis of the fetlock joint, which may result in continued lameness.[6,12,18] Since the risk of development of these complications is high, it is difficult to recommend the use of a cast alone for the treatment of a highly comminuted unstable fracture.

External skeletal fixation should be considered for the repair of highly comminuted fractures that lack an intact bone strut and for those fractures that are open or have a severely compromised blood supply. Transfixation techniques reduce the collapse of the fracture within the cast by means of transcortically placed pins in the mid to distal portion of the third metacarpus or metatarsus.[17] Centrally threaded positive profile pins are preferred, and a suitably sized drill and tap are recommended for the best results (Fig. 8.177). Usually 2 to 3 pins are used. After the application of the pins, the limb is placed in traction to reduce the fracture and to align the articular surfaces. Wires placed through the solar margin of the hoof wall can be used to attach the foot to a traction device (e.g., ropes attached to a solid object) (see Fig. 8.157). Once the traction is applied, radiographs are taken to document the reduction of the fracture and the alignment of the articular surfaces. Then a lower limb cast that incorporates the foot and extends to the proximal metacarpus or metatarsus is applied. Hoof acrylic is then applied around the pins to further stabilize them in their position. Most horses walk comfortably after surgery with the transfixation casts. A complication of the transfixation pin cast is the potential for formation of ring sequestra around the pin holes, 3 to 6 weeks after their application, which may result in a fracture through the pin tract (see Fig. 8.162). Fracture through the pin tract has been uncommon in my experience. An alternative to the transfixation cast is the external skeletal fixator, which uses a series of large diameter transfixation pins through the third metacarpus or metatarsus and incorporates side-connecting bars to a foot plate.[19] In our hands, this external fixator has not been user friendly and has resulted in a fracture through the pin tracts shortly after the horse recovers from anesthesia.

The combination of internal fixation with lag screws placed through stab incisions and a transfixation pin cast can provide improved alignment of the joint surface and, in some cases, more stability to highly comminuted PP fractures (see Figs. 8.177, A to F). The lag screws are placed after the traction is applied. Internal fixation with lag screws placed through stab incisions followed by the application of a cast can be considered in less comminuted fractures, particularly those that have an intact strut of bone on one side.

Widely invasive open-reduction techniques used for the repair of highly comminuted PP fractures seem contraindicated at this time because of the unacceptable high postoperative infection rates.[12] In one retrospective study, H or Y incisions over the dorsum of the PP used for reduction and internal fixation of comminuted fractures resulted in a 55% infection rate.[16] It was thought that these open approaches contributed to the development of infection by further damaging the soft tissues and blood supply in an already compromised area and by prolonging the surgery time. The conclusion was that the surgical approach used should result in the least soft tissue damage and the shortest surgery time.[16]

Prognosis

Noncomminuted Fractures

Horses with noncomminuted PP fractures generally have a good prognosis for long-term survival.[14] The prognosis for performance noncomminuted fractures of the PP is believed to depend on the configuration of the fracture, the duration of the fracture to treatment, the fracture length, the method of treatment, the breed, and the intended use.[5,6,10,11,22] In one retrospective study done in racehorses, a significantly lower percent of horses returned to racing after repair of complete midsagittal fractures that extended into the PIPJ (46%) than after repair of short incomplete midsagittal fractures (71%), long incomplete midsagittal (66%), or complete fractures that extended to the lateral cortex (71%).[11] The time from fracture to repair did not affect the outcome. Additionally, the median number of races and the median fastest race times before and after surgery were not significantly different.[11] In another retrospective study done in Standardbred racehorses, researchers found that 89% of the horses returned to racing, but at significantly decreased performance level.[22] In this study, fractures longer than 15 mm were treated surgically; fractures between 15 and 30 mm long and fractures longer than 45 mm did affect racing times adversely.[22] In another study done on young Thoroughbred racehorses, 70% of the horses treated conservatively for short incomplete midsagittal fractures raced (15 won or placed), and 65% of the horses treated conservatively for long incomplete midsagittal fractures raced.[6] None of the horses treated conservatively for complete midsagittal fractures or type 2 and 3 fractures raced. Of the horses treated surgically for type 1 incomplete and complete midsagittal fractures, 46% returned to performance and 38% were retired immediately after surgery.

Type 2 dorsal fractures, either oblique (exiting the dorsal cortex) or complete (extending distad to enter the PIPJ), that are treated by lag screw fixation appear to

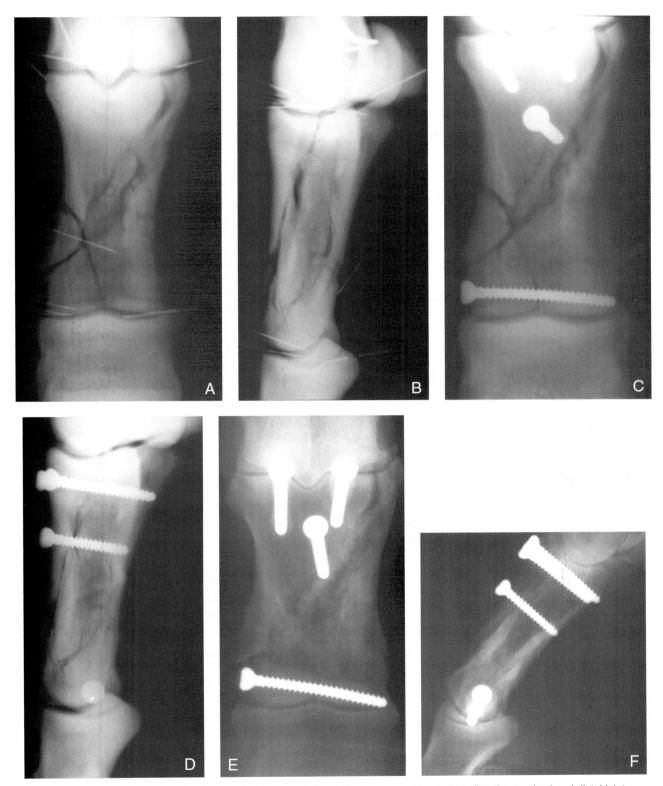

Figure 8.177 Highly comminuted PP fracture that lacks a strut of bone and was treated by means of lag screws placed through stab incisions, with transfixation pins, and with cast application. A. Dorsopalmar view at surgery. Note that many needles were placed in the fetlock and PIPJ to act as references. The limb was placed under traction to reduce the fracture. B. Lateral view. C and D. Four screws were used to align the proximal and distal joint surfaces. After this, transfixation pins were placed and a cast was applied. E and F. Three-month postoperative views just before the horse was sent home. The fracture is healing and disuse osteopenia is obvious. At 13-month follow-up, this horse seemed pain free at pasture and was being used as a brood mare.

have favorable prognosis for return to performance.[5,15] In one report, two middle-aged horses with complete dorsal fractures that were treated surgically returned to performance 9 and 13 months postoperatively.[5] Both horses exhibited mild lameness after exercise, but both horses had radiologic evidence of DJD of their fetlock joints prior to surgery.

As for types 3, 5, and 6 fractures, too few cases have been reported to predict a prognosis.

Comminuted Fractures

The prognosis for horses sustaining comminuted PP fractures depends on the configuration of the fracture and the treatment approach selected. Horses with highly comminuted fractures without an intact strut of bone extending from one joint surface to the other have a guarded prognosis for survival. In one study done on horses with comminuted PP fractures, 57% of the horses that had an intact strut of bone were alive more than 1 year after treatment, whereas only 23% of horses without an intact strut of bone were alive at 1 year.[16] The prognosis for horses treated by widely invasive surgical approaches with internal fixation is poor for long-term survival. In one study, the most common reasons for euthanasia after surgical repair were infection and persistent lameness.[16] In this same study, researchers found that an invasive surgical approach resulted in an unacceptably high infection rate (55%). As a result of this, they recommended surgical techniques that were less invasive.

References

1. Adams OR. Lameness in Horses. 3rd ed. Philadelphia: Lea & Febiger, 1974;259.
2. Barr ARS, Deny HR, Waterman AE, et al. Proximal phalangeal fractures in the horse. Vet Compar Orthop Traumatol 1988;2:86–90.
3. Bowan KF, Fackleman GE. The management of comminuted fractures in the horse. Comp Cont Educ Pract Vet 1980;2:98.
4. Bramlage LR. Current concepts of emergency first aid treatment and transportation of equine fracture patients. Comp Cont Educ Pract Vet 1983;5:S564.
5. Dechant JE, MacDonald DG, Crawford WH. Repair of complete dorsal fracture of the proximal phalanx in two horses. Vet Surg 1998;27:445–449.
6. Ellis DR, Simpson DJ, Greenwood RES, et al. Observations and management of fractures of the proximal phalanx in young Thoroughbreds. Equine Vet J 1987;19:43–49.
7. Fackleman GE. Sagittal fractures of the first phalanx (P1) in the horse. Vet Med Small Anim Clin 1973;68:622.
8. Fackleman GE, Nunamaker DM. Comminuted fractures of the first phalanx. In: Fackelman GE, Nunamaker DM, Eds. Manual of Internal Fixation in the Horse. New York: Springer-Verlag, 1982;86.
9. Fessler JF, Amstutz HE. Fracture repair. In: Oehme FW, Prier JE, Eds. Textbook of Large Animal Surgery. Baltimore: Williams & Wilkins, 1974;297.
10. Gabel AA, Bukowiecki CF. Fractures of the phalanges. Vet Clin North Am Large Anim Pract 1983;5:233–242.
11. Holcombe SJ, Schneider RK, Bramlage LR, et al. Lag screw fixation of noncomminuted sagittal fractures of the proximal phalanx in racehorses: 59 cases (1973–1991). J Vet Med Assoc 1995;206:1195–1199.
12. Honnas CM. Fractures of the proximal phalanx. In: Auer JA, Ed. Equine Surgery. Philadelphia: WB Saunders, 1992;998–1002.
13. Losonsky JM, Kneller SK. Variable locations of nutrient foramina of the proximal phalanx in forelimbs of Standardbreds. J Am Vet Med Assoc 1988;93:671.
14. Markel MD. Fractures of the proximal phalanx. In: White NA, Moore JN, Eds. Current Practice of Equine Surgery. Philadelphia: JB Lippincott, 1990;610–617.
15. Markel MD, Richardson DW. Noncomminuted fractures of the proximal phalanx in 69 horses. J Am Vet Med Assoc 1985;186:573–589.
16. Markel MD, Richardson DW, Nunamaker DM. Comminuted first phalanx fractures in 30 horses: Surgical vs nonsurgical treatments. Vet Surg 1985;14:135.
17. McClure SR, Watkins JP, Bronson DG, et al. In vitro comparison of the standard short limb cast and three configurations of short limb transfixation casts in equine forelimbs. Am J Vet Res 1994;55:1331.
18. Nixon AJ. The phalanges and metatarsophalangeal joint. In: Auer JA, Stick JA, Eds. Equine Surgery. 2nd ed. Philadelphia: WB Saunders, 1999;796–801.
19. Nunamaker DM, Richardson DW, Butterweck DM, et al. A new external skeletal fixation device that allows immediate full weight bearing: Application in the horse. Vet Surg 1986;15:345.
20. Richardson DW, Nunamaker DM, Sigafoos RD. Use of an external skeletal fixation device and bone graft for arthrodesis of the metacarpophalangeal joint in horses. J Am Vet Med Assoc 1987;191:316–321.
21. Rooney JR. Biomechanics of Lameness. Baltimore: Williams & Wilkins, 1969.
22. Tetens J, Ross MW, Lloyd JW. Comparison of racing performance before and after treatment of incomplete, midsagittal fractures of the proximal phalanx in Standardbreds: 49 cases (1986–1992). J Vet Med Assoc 1997;210:82–86.
23. Trum BF. Fractures. Vet Bull Suppl Army Med Bull 1939;33:118.
24. Turner AS. Fractures of specific bones. In: Mansmann RA, McAllister ES, Eds. Equine Medicine and Surgery. 3rd ed. Santa Barbara, CA: American Veterinary Publications, 1982;1011.

DESMITIS OF THE DISTAL SESAMOIDEAN LIGAMENTS

Although desmitis of the distal sesamoidean ligaments (DSLs) is an uncommon cause of lameness, in my experience it has been reported to be a reasonably common injury in horses that jump (e.g., event horses, show jumpers, field and show hunters, steeplechasers, and timber race horses), racehorses, and horses that are ridden for pleasure.[2,3,6,7,9,11] In one study, Thoroughbred and Thoroughbred crossbreds were the most frequently affected breeds, and the forelimbs were most commonly involved.[7] There also seems to be an equal distribution of the injury between the right and the left limbs, and the injury can occur bilaterally in the forelimbs.[7] Desmitis of the DSLs has also been diagnosed with some frequency in the Norwegian Dole horse, and it has been referred to as a "volar ringbone."[6]

There are four DSLs: the straight (superficial), the paired oblique (middle), the paired cruciate (deep), and the paired short (Fig. 1.13). All of the ligaments originate from the base of the proximal sesamoid bones and intersesamiodean ligament. The straight ligament attaches distally to scutum medium at the proximopalmar aspect of the middle phalanx. The paired oblique ligaments attach to a triangular rough region on the PP, forming a V shape as they travel distally and axially to become a single band just before insertion on the distal third of the PP.[5] The paired cruciate ligaments attach distally to the contralateral eminence of the proximal extremity of the PP. The paired short ligaments attach at the proximal articular margins of the MCP or MTP joint. For more information regarding the anatomy of the DSLs, refer to Chapter 1.

Before the routine use of ultrasound, the diagnosis of desmitis of the DSLs relied on physical finding and, to some degree, radiologic evidence of a problem. Physical findings were often difficult to interpret because of the numerous soft tissue structures in the region. Radiographic evidence included enthesiophyte formation or avulsion fracture at the attachments of the individual ligaments (Figs. 8.178 and 8.179). Since the distal attachments of the DSLs are different, the radiographic signs of each are distinctive. Occasionally, all three ligaments rupture, resulting in loss of the suspensory apparatus (see "Traumatic Rupture of Suspensory Apparatus" in this chapter). With the use of ultrasonography, the involvement of the individual DSLs has been more clearly defined.[3,5,10,11] Although the injury can involve any one of the four ligaments, the body of the oblique DSL seems affected most frequently.[4,10] Generally, desmitis is recognized as having an acute onset involving one branch, but both branches can be affected occasionally.[4,10] Basilar sesamoid fracture, desmitis of the ipsilateral branch of the suspensory ligament in the same limb, and fracture of the proximopalmar aspect of the PP have been associated problems in more chronic cases (Fig. 8.180).[3,4] Desmitis of the straight DSL only has been identified on ultrasound examination in the forelimbs on rare occasions. Concurrent injury to the straight and oblique DSL has also been seen in flat racing Thoroughbreds.[3]

Although Adams[1] described desmitis of DSLs as a secondary disorder that is rarely the primary cause of lameness, this clearly is not the case.[3,4,10]

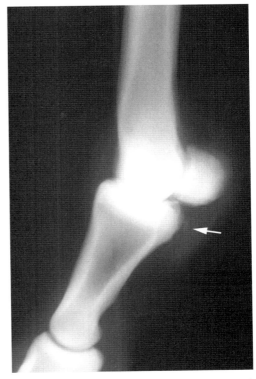

Figure 8.179 Lateral view of an avulsion fracture that is probably associated with the cruciate DSL (arrow).

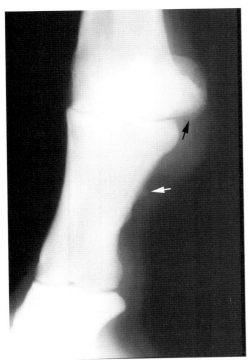

Figure 8.178 Oblique view of enthesiophyte formation associated with attachment of the oblique DSL (white arrow). Note the enthesiophyte at the base of the proximal sesamoid bone (black arrow).

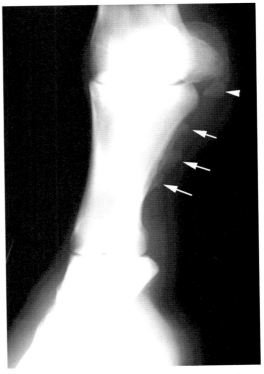

Figure 8.180 Oblique view of enthesiophyte formation associated with the oblique DSL (white arrows) and an avulsion fracture of the base of the proximal sesamoid bone (arrowhead).

Etiology

The DSLs being a functional continuation of the more proximally located SL are an important part of the suspensory apparatus that provides resistance to extension of the MCP or MTP joint during the stance phase. Hyperextension of the MCP or MCT joint can result in supraphysiologic strains in the suspensory apparatus, which may lead to failure of the DSLs. Although the DSLs in total provide this functional counter resistance to extension, each ligament has a separate function that most likely accounts for the specific injuries that occur to these structures.[10]

The straight DSL, being the only unpaired ligament, participates in the sagittal stabilization of the MCP or MTP joint and PIPJ, and therefore it would most likely be injured during hyperextension.[10] Interestingly, injury to the ligament is uncommon.[4,10] The paired oblique DSLs play a prominent role in the limitation of rotation and abaxial movements of the MCP or MTP joint.[10] Injuries to the oblique DSLs being more commonly unilateral probably result from asymmetric loading caused by abnormal conformation, lateral or medial foot imbalances, missteps, or poor footing. The asymmetric forces create tension on one side and compression on the other. The tension side realizes higher strains and is at risk of injury.[10]

Signs

Horses with acute desmitis often present with a sudden onset of lameness. Visually, a slight increase in swelling of the palmar or plantar surface of the pastern region may be present as a result of digital sheath effusion (Fig. 8.181). The effusion is most commonly seen in cases of

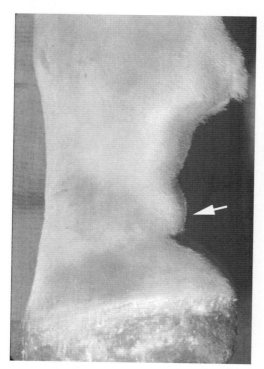

Figure 8.181 Digital sheath effusion (arrow) that may be associated with desmitis of the DSL.

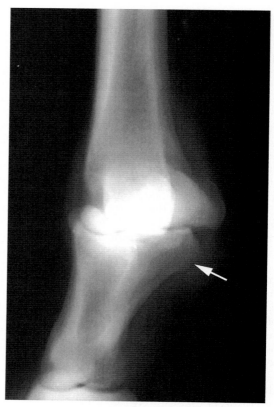

Figure 8.182 Oblique view of enthesiophyte formation probably associated with the short DSL (arrow).

less than 3 weeks duration.[7] On palpation, heat and pain with digital pressure are common with acute injuries.[10] In one study, 21 of 39 cases demonstrated pain on deep pressure over the respective bases of the proximal sesamoid bones.[7] Digital palpation lateral or medial and dorsal to the flexor tendons midway between the heel bulbs and the proximal sesamoid bones may also result in pain, and in some cases, firm swelling can be appreciated (Fig. 8.182). The foot is held off the ground, and the MCP or MTP joint is flexed so that the flexor tendons are relaxed. Flexion allows for a more accurate application of the digital pressure to the suspected area. In one study, 17 of 39 horses had firm swelling palpable in the region of the middle DSL.[7] Fetlock and phalangeal flexion is commonly painful and increases the lameness when the flexion is performed for 30 seconds. In one study, 39 of 39 horses with DSL desmitis exhibited an increased lameness after the test.[7] Digital pressure over the sensitive region for 30 seconds often results in increased signs of lameness also.[10] Contrary to this, one study found that direct digital pressure to the DSLs occasionally resulted in an increase lameness at a trot.[7] If there are any questions, this response should be compared with that of the opposite limb.

Although the clinical findings may direct the examiner to the palmar or plantar region as a site of pain or lameness, perineural anesthesia of the palmar digital nerves just below the level of the collateral cartilages should be performed to rule out coexistent involvement of the bottom of the foot.[7] This can be followed by perineural anesthesia of the palmar nerve at the base of the sesamoid bone, which should eliminate the lameness. Refer to Chapter 3, "Perineural Anesthesia," for more information.

Diagnosis

Radiographic evidence of desmitis of the DSLs include 1) enthesiophyte (proliferative bone) formation, 2) avulsion fractures (bone fragments), and 3) dystrophic mineralization (radio-opaque densities) within one of the DSLs.

Enthesiophyte (proliferative bone) formation at the attachment of the oblique DSL is a common finding (see Figs. 8.178 and 8.180). The changes are usually seen on the middle, medial or lateral, or palmar or plantar aspect of the PP. In one study these proliferative changes were observed on the medial and lateral aspect of the PP in 31 of 39 horses and on the medial or lateral aspect only in 7 of 39 horses diagnosed with desmitis of the DSLs.[7] This same report also revealed a high incidence of coexistent problems in either the same or the contralateral limb. Based on the radiographic changes present at the time of diagnosis in this study, it would appear that the DSL desmitis was chronic and that the other injuries may have occurred as compensatory result of the original lameness. Possibly, this is the reason these proliferative changes have been reported as an incidental finding on radiographic examination.[1,3,4,8] Interestingly, one report found little correlation between the radiographic change and the ultrasonographic abnormalities in the oblique DSL.[4] Enthesiophyte formation at the proximal extent of the PP and at the base of the proximal sesamoid bone are also believed to be evidence of injury to the cruciate or short DSL (see Fig. 8.178).

Fractures of the base of the proximal sesamoid bone can involve the DSLs.[3,4] Fragments from either the dorsal aspect of the base of the proximal sesamoid bone or proximal palmar or plantar articular margin of the PP typically involve the short DSL[10] (see Figs. 8.179 and 8.180). Although these fragments are believed to be avulsion fractures, it is possible that some are secondary centers of ossification. Rounded osteochondral fragments are seen occasionally in screenings at yearling sales and in prepurchase examination without evidence to suggest that they are of clinical significance.[10] In those cases in which these fragment are believed to be of clinical significance, intraarticular anesthesia of the MCP or MTP joint should eliminate the lameness.[10] Theses fragment have also been observed on the nonarticular proximal extremity of the PP (see Fig. 8.179). More severe fractures of the base of the sesamoid bones occur in horses that compete at speed. The fracture fragments may involve the oblique or cruciate and short DSLs (Fig. 8.180).[10]

Dystrophic mineralization (radio-opaque densities) associated with the DSLs is also seen on radiographic examination. In one study, 24 of 39 cases showed evidence of this radiographic change at the base of the medial and lateral sesamoid bones.[7] The medial or lateral sesamoid bone was involved in 7 of 39 cases.

Sonographic evidence of acute desmitis of the DSLs is manifested by a diffuse increase in ligament size, fiber disruption, and periligamentous fluid surrounding the affected ligament.[4,10,11] The anechoic space between the ligament and the superficial digital flexor tendon is often reduced in size with desmitis of the oblique DSL.[4] Chronic sonographic changes may include varying degrees of the acute changes within the ligament and occasionally reveal hyperechoic areas consistent with dense scar tissue formation. Chronic injuries often have less distinct margins because of the healing by scar tissue, and occasionally, areas of dystrophic calcification can be seen.[10] Periosteal proliferation in areas of ligament attachments may appear as irregular contours in the bone surface.[10] When imaging the straight DSL, the ligament should be placed under tension to minimize artifacts.[5] For more information regarding the technique of ultrasound examination, refer to Chapter 4.

Treatment

For the acute case, rest, cold therapy, pressure or support wraps, administration of NSAIDs, corrective trimming and shoeing, controlled exercise, and a gradual return to work are recommended.[7,8] Stall rest for a period of 6 weeks is generally recommended. Cold therapy in the form of an ice-water slurry applied for 30 minutes 3 times daily for the first 48 hours after the acute injury seems most beneficial. Pressure or support bandages are applied in between the cold treatments and maintained from 3 to 5 weeks or as needed. Warm therapy can begin after 48 hours. NSAIDs are administered for 2 to 3 weeks. The feet should be balanced and shod with the natural balance shoeing techniques. (Refer to Chapter 9 for more information on the natural balance shoeing.) Controlled exercise in the form of hand walking is begun between 2 and 3 weeks postinjury, depending on the severity of the condition. Generally, hand walking exercise for 5 minutes twice daily, 5 days a week, increasing 2.5 minutes/week, is recommended. One should monitor the region of injury closely by palpation for heat and pain. Clinical evaluation at 6 weeks is recommended, and if the horse has improved, the controlled exercise can be increased and access to a small run may be allowed. Reevaluation with ultrasound is recommended at 3 months postinjury. Further controlled or free exercise recommendations are made, depending on the ultrasound findings. Generally, it takes 4 to 6 months for the desmitis to clear; occasionally, a year or more convalescence may be required before the horse becomes serviceable.[7] As with any musculoskeletal disorder, an informed thoughtful owner usually successfully manages these problems, whereas the anxious owner or trainer pushes the horse too fast, resulting in recurrence of the problem.

The chronic injury is treated in much the same way. Treatment can be modified, depending on the clinical, radiographic, and ultrasonographic findings.

Prognosis

The prognosis varies, depending on the degree of the injury and the intended use of the horse. Generally, the prognosis is guarded for the performance horse because of the high probability of reinjury.[1,4,7,10] Also, when desmitis of the DSLs is combined with other skeletal problems (e.g., DJD of the PIPJ, navicular syndrome, proximal sesamoidean ligament desmitis, or fracture of the proximal sesamoid bone), the prognosis is worsened.[8]

References

1. Adams OR. Lameness in Horses. 3rd ed. Philadelphia: Lea & Febiger, 1974;223.
2. Bukowiecki CF, Bramlage LR, Gavel AA. Proximal sesamoid bone fractures in horses: Current treatments and prognoses. Comp Cont Educ Pract Vet 1985;12:684–698.
3. Denoix JM, Crevier N, Azevedo C. Ultrasound examination of the pastern. Proc Am Assoc Equine Pract 1991;37:363–380.
4. Dyson SJ, Denoix J-M. Tendon sheath and ligament injuries in the pastern. Vet Clin North Am Equine Pract 1995;11:217–233.
5. Gillis C. Soft tissue injuries to the palmar aspect of the pastern. In: White NA, Moore JN, Eds. Current Techniques in Equine Surgery and Lameness. 2nd ed. Philadelphia: WB Saunders, 1998; 338–340.
6. Haakenstad LH. Chronic bone and joint disease in relation to conformation in the horse. Equine Vet J 1969;1:248.
7. Moyer W. Distal sesamoidean desmitis. Proc Am Assoc Equine Pract 1982;28:245–251.
8. Moyer W, Raker CW. Diseases of the suspensory apparatus. Vet Clin North Am Large Anim Pract 1980;2:61–80.
9. Parente EJ, Richardson DW, Spencer P. Basal sesamoidean fractures in horses: 57 cases (1980–1991). J Am Vet Med Assoc 1993; 202:1293–1297.
10. Redding R. Distal sesamoidean ligament injuries and desmitis of the inferior check ligament. Proceedings of the Dubai International Symposium, Arab Emerites, March 27–30 1996;1:227–240.
11. Reef VB. Ultrasonic evaluation of tendons and ligaments. In: White NA, Moore JN, Eds. Current Practice of Equine Surgery. Philadelphia: JB Lippincott, 1990;425–435.

RACHITIC RINGBONE

Rachitic ringbone is described as a fibrous tissue enlargement of the pastern region of young horses. The disease usually develops before the horse reaches 2 years of age and is most common between 6 and 12 months of age. Deficiencies in calcium, phosphorus, and vitamins are believed to be the cause. Clinically, the fibrous swelling resembles new bone growth caused by DJD of the PIPJ, but there are no bone or joint changes. For more information, refer to *Adams' Lameness in Horses*, Chapter 8, fourth edition.[1]

Reference

1. Stashak TS. Lameness. In: Stashak TS, ed. Adams' Lameness in Horses. 4th ed. Philadelphia: Lea & Febiger, 1987;568.

Part III

THE FETLOCK

Alicia L. Bertone

OSTEOCHONDRAL (CHIP) FRACTURES OF THE PROXIMAL (FIRST) PHALANX IN THE METACARPOPHALANGEAL OR METATARSOPHALANGEAL (FETLOCK) JOINT

Osteochondral fractures of the proximal end of the proximal phalanx are relatively common in the forelimb of the horse, particularly the racehorse. Most fractures of this type involve the dorsal surface of the proximal eminences, just medial or lateral to the digital extensor tendon. The left forelimb and medial eminence are affected more often than the right forelimb and lateral eminence. Other regions are not so commonly involved. Concussion and overextension of the joint are factors in the production of these fractures. Chip fractures from the distal end of the third metacarpal or metatarsal bone also occur but are less common.

Other less frequently occurring fractures of the proximal phalanx include fractures of the lateral and medial eminences of the proximopalmar (or proximoplantar) surfaces and avulsion fractures of the midproximal palmar articular margins just below the sesamoid bone. These fractures can be successfully removed with a good prognosis (about 70%) of return to performance.[1,5,9] Fractures of the proximopalmar (or proximoplantar) surfaces are also associated with complete or partial tearing of the collateral ligament of the fetlock joint and traumatic subluxation, which induce the intraarticular fracture. Careful evaluation of the joint is indicated to identify this more complex injury.[6]

Causes

Trauma is the cause of these chip fractures in the horse. From the appearance of the fractures, it seems that excessive overextension of the joint is probably involved (Fig. 8.183). Overextension places stress on the dorsal aspect of the proximal end of the proximal phalanx as it is pressed against the third metacarpal bone. Limb fatigue is a factor in overextension of the fetlock joint, noted at the end of races when the back of the fetlock may contact the ground (running down). Why the fracture occurs most frequently medial to the midline is not fully understood (Fig. 8.184). However, it may be because the medial tuberosity on the proximal dorsal border of the proximal phalanx is more prominent and extends slightly more proximad than its lateral counterpart.

Signs

Signs of chip fractures in the fetlock joint are similar to those of "osselets." Synovitis of the fetlock joint, indicated by distension of the joint capsule (between the suspensory ligament and the palmar or plantar surface of the cannon bone), is commonly found. Horses often present with a history of lameness that increases after exercise, and a workout or a race may cause the horse to be markedly lame. After prolonged rest, the horse may seem to be sound, only to go lame again when returned to training. Occasionally, there may be a history of acute lameness followed by dramatic relief when a chip that was caught in the joint is dislodged.

Some horses, particularly those with chronic chip fractures, have only a small amount of swelling or lameness to indicate that there is a chip fracture. There may be fibrous enlargement on the dorsal surface of the fetlock joint that is easily palpated. However, dorsal swelling is also often seen in osselets. It is difficult to produce pain in the affected region by digital pressure, but some heat may be detected over the dorsal surface of the joint. Flexion of the affected fetlock will often elicit pain. If the examiner is unsure of this response, it should be compared to the opposite fetlock. Lameness is most obvious at the trot during the stance phase. A fetlock flexion test done for 30 seconds usually exacerbates the lameness.

In most cases it is not necessary to use local anesthesia to identify chip fractures within the fetlock. If the examiner is suspicious that the fetlock is involved, radiographs should be taken. However, if confusion exists regarding the contribution of the fetlock to the lameness, either intrasynovial anesthesia of the fetlock (preferred) or a low four-point nerve block (proximal to the fetlock) can be performed (see Chapter 3).

Diagnosis

Diagnosis cannot be made without radiographic examination. The lateral radiograph is most diagnostically revealing. Oblique radiographs should be taken to determine if the chip is on the medial or lateral side of the midline (Fig. 8.185). This is important because the surgical positioning of the arthroscope is opposite of the chip fracture. The contralateral fetlock should be radiographed because bilateral fractures are not uncommon and clinical signs may not appear until the horse is back in training.[1–3,7,10] Acute proximal eminence fractures show increased activity on a nuclear bone scan, but nuclear scintigraphy is not usually necessary for diagnosis (Fig. 8.186).

Treatment

Proximal Dorsal Osteochondral (Chip) Fractures of the Proximal Phalanx

Arthroscopic removal of chip fractures is the treatment of choice for the greatest chance of a quick return to full performance (Fig. 8.185, B and C). Arthroscopic evaluation permits removal of multiple fragments, visualization of the entire joint, and surgical treatment of lesions that may not have been identified on radiographs. Lesions commonly seen in association with proximal phalanx chip fractures include proliferative synovitis of the dorsal metacarpal synovial pad (32% had chip fractures) and cartilage erosion of the metacarpal condyle.[3,7]

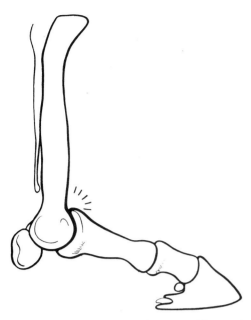

Figure 8.183 Mechanism of chip fractures of the proximal phalanx. (Courtesy of W. Berkeley.)

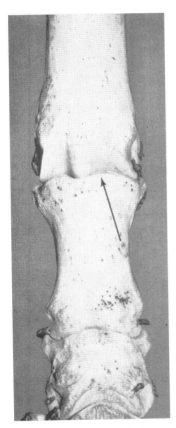

Figure 8.184 The equine metacarpophalangeal joint revealing the most common region of fractures of the proximal phalanx medial to the midline (arrow). These fractures occur less commonly lateral to the midline on the proximal phalanx. (Reprinted with permission from Adams OR. Chip fractures into the metacarpophalangeal (fetlock) joint. J Am Vet Med Assoc 1966;148:360.)

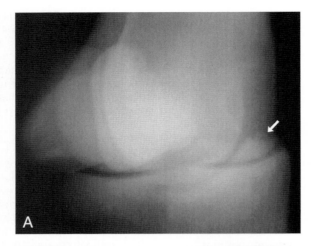

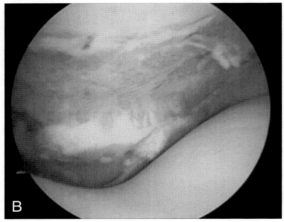

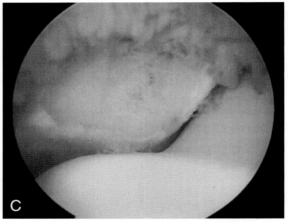

Figure 8.185 A. Dorsopalmar lateromedial oblique view of a typical nondisplaced traumatic osteochondral fragment (chip fracture) of the dorsomedial eminence (arrow) in a 2-year-old racehorse. B. Arthroscopy reveals a fresh dorsomedial eminence first phalanx chip fracture in a racing Thoroughbred. C. Arthroscopic examination after removal of the fragment and debridement of the damaged cartilage. Note that there is little scoring of the articular condyle cartilage.

It is recognized that many of small nondisplaced fractures can be treated successfully with adequate rest for 120 days.[5] If training continues, the fragments often displace and cause adjacent articular cartilage erosion (Fig. 8.185C). Arthrotomy for fragment removal from the dorsal fetlock has been abandoned in favor of arthroscopy, because arthroscopy offers improved access to the joint and arthrotomy is associated with complications of wound healing at the dorsal fetlock joint. Incisional complications with arthrotomy are further exaggerated when the joint has been treated with corticosteroids before surgery, and a significant number of horses with proximal phalanx fracture are given corticosteroids.[5]

If surgical removal of the bone fragment is elected, the exact location of the chip must be established (most chips are located medial to the midline). All other joints that have soreness or effusion on physical examination should be radiographed to determine if silent chip fractures are present. Carpal or contralateral fetlock chip fractures are common and are usually removed during the same surgical procedure.

General anesthesia is administered, and the area of incision is prepared for aseptic surgery. Dorsal recumbency is preferred by many surgeons, because it permits multiple joint access without repositioning the horse and it decreases hemorrhage into the joint during surgery. The hair is clipped from the coronary band to the carpus.

The area of incision is shaved and scrubbed, and skin antiseptics are applied. Tourniquets are not necessary for dorsal phalanx fragments. A self-adhering sterile plastic adhesive drape is placed over the incision site to prevent fluid from soaking through and contaminating the area. The area is then further prepared by placing additional sterile drapes in a routine fashion. The surgeon, of course, uses sterile gloves and instruments. The arthroscope portal is made to the side of the common digital extensor tendon in the center of the distended dorsal pouch adjacent to the extensor tendon.[8]

A small skin incision is made, and the joint is distended with a balanced electrolyte solution. Then the arthroscope is inserted into the joint on the side opposite the fragment along with the trocar and cannular. The joint is explored and the fracture located. The site of the instrument portal is identified with a marker needle and is created with a stab incision through the skin, fascia, and fibrous and synovial layers of the joint capsule on the same side and proximal to the fragment.

Most fragments require forcible elevation before grasping with rongeurs for removal. The fragments are usually attached to the joint capsule, which should be cleanly and sharply dissected to minimize trauma. Resection of the dorsal synovial pad is performed with a sharp scalpel or scissors, and articular cartilage injury is debrided with a curette to healthy subchondral bone. The

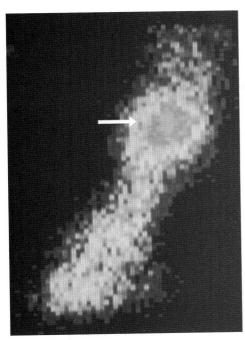

Figure 8.186 Oblique nuclear scintigram of the same horse shown in Figure 8.185, demonstrating the increased uptake of technetium in the bone of the proximal first phalanx (arrow). Nuclear scintigraphy is sensitive to bone trauma but nonspecific for the site and structure of the disease. A condylar injury in the distal metacarpus may have a similar appearance; thus a radiograph is required for diagnosis.

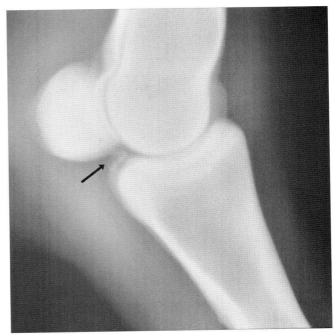

Figure 8.187 Lateral view demonstrating a plantar eminence osteochondral fragment (arrow) that, owing to its location and shape, is most likely developmental rather than traumatic in origin. These fragments are common, are often cashew shaped, and conform to the proximal eminence of the first phalanx. This fragment is articular, but nonarticular fragments also occur.

joint is flushed liberally with a balanced electrolyte solution to remove any bone or cartilage debris. An intraoperative radiograph or fluoroscopic image is taken to confirm that the fragment was removed and that no free-floating fragments exist.

The surgeon then closes the skin with 2-0 monofilament suture material using a simple interrupted pattern. A sterile bandage is placed over the incisions, and the limb is placed in a strong supportive wrap, which includes the hoof and extends to just below the carpal joint. The supporting wrap is left in place for 1 to 3 days, after which it is replaced by a pressure bandage. Pressure bandaging is used until the sutures are removed. Horses are usually confined for 30 days. Between 2 and 4 months' rest is recommended before training is resumed, depending on the degree of joint damage and cartilage debridement.

Fractures of the Proximal Palmar Eminence of the Proximal Phalanx

Fractures of the medial and lateral eminences of the proximal phalanx are not common and should not be confused with osteochondral fragmentation of this site in young growing horses, which is debated to be part of the osteochondrosis syndrome (Fig. 8.187).[4] Osteochondral fragmentation of the caudal eminences of the proximal phalanx occurs in approximately 5% of Standardbreds and Thoroughbreds without any clinical signs. Fragments are not usually a source of lameness until the

horse undergoes aggressive training. If clinical signs occur, they are mild and consist of a high-performance lameness, joint effusion, and mild soreness to flexion. Fractures of the caudal eminence of the proximal phalanx, however, are usually associated with fetlock joint swelling, lameness, and soreness to direct pressure over the eminence. Joint flexion usually markedly worsens the lameness. Stability of the joint should be assessed in these horses to determine if collateral ligament damage has also occurred.

Horses may respond to stall rest of at least 90 days, but reinjury may occur. Bony healing is not seen in conservatively treated cases, because the fracture is distracted by the distal sesamoid ligament insertions. Nuclear scintigraphy can be used to distinguish fractures from incidental caudal eminence fragments. Fractures that continue to be a source of pain or are large enough to anchor to the parent bone with a bone screw can be treated surgically (Fig. 8.188). If the fracture has an articular component and is to be removed, arthroscopic removal is possible; but dissection outside the joint capsule is required. Alternatively or for fractures without an articular component, an incision can be made directly over the fragment, which can be removed with sharp dissection. If a compression screw fixation is required, intraoperative monitoring with fluoroscopy or radiographs is needed for proper screw placement. After internal fixation, a cast should be applied for recovery from anesthesia and removed within 48 hours, after which support pressure wraps are applied. To allow bone healing and repair of the distal suspensory injury, 6 months' rest is

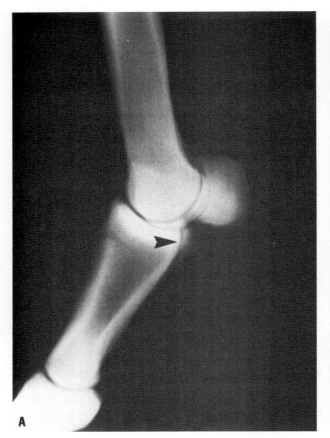
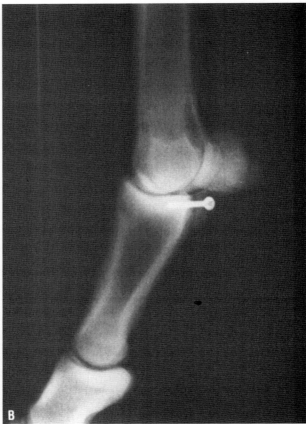

Figure 8.188 A. An articular fracture off of the proximal palmar eminence of the proximal phalanx. B. One bone screw was used to repair this fracture. (Courtesy of T. S. Stashak.)

recommended in these cases. When the chip fracture has been removed, bandaging alone can be used for postoperative care.

If collateral ligament injury or instability is noted in the joint, cast support should continue for 1 to 2 months, depending on the severity of the injury, to support healing of the ligament and minimize the development of degenerative joint disease (DJD). Suturing the ligament and removing the caudal eminence of a proximal phalanx fracture is not necessary for breeding soundness or light athletic soundness. The degree of the proximal phalanx fracture displacement and of the collateral ligament avulsion determine if surgery is needed to maximize joint health during healing; such surgery is performed before placing the cast.

Prognosis

The prognosis is usually good to excellent for treatment of proximal dorsal chip fractures, but it somewhat depends on the size and number of fractures, the duration of the fractures, the use of injected steroids, the amount of concomitant articular cartilage damage, and the degree of DJD (Fig. 8.189). Several reports indicate a good prognosis for return to athletic performance, including racing; the prognosis is good to excellent (about 80%) with arthroscopic surgery to remove the fragment.

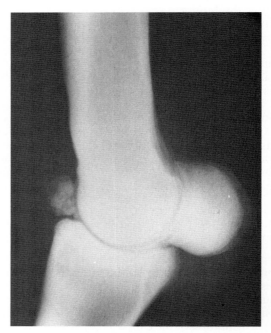

Figure 8.189 The large osteochondromatosis in the fetlock resulted in lameness; after surgical removal, the horse became sound. (Courtesy of T. S. Stashak.)

The presence of other fetlock lesions noted at arthroscopic surgery decreased the prognosis in racing Thoroughbreds, but success was still good (greater than 70% return to racing).[1,2,7,10]

Small acute, nondisplaced fetlock chip fractures usually have a good prognosis with conservative treatment. Arthroscopic surgical removal may still be elected in these cases, because the convalescence is shorter after surgical removal (often less than 30 days) than for the bone to heal (90 to 120 days) and the risk of fracture displacement or refracture is eliminated. Factors that lower the prognosis include extreme large size of the fragment, chronicity, the degree of synovitis/capsulitis, and the amount of DJD present. Standardbred racehorses often have chronic joint changes associated with dorsal proximal phalanx fractures.

The prognosis for proximal palmar fractures requiring compression screw fixation depends on the degree of initial trauma at the time of fracture. Often this will not be fully appreciated until the radiographs are taken 3 to 4 months after surgery.

References

1. Adams OR. Chip fractures of the first phalanx in the metacarpophalangeal (fetlock) joint. J Am Vet Med Assoc 1966;148:360.
2. Colon JL, Bramlage LR, Hance SR, Embertson RM. Qualitative and quantitative documentation of the racing performance of 461 Thoroughbred racehorses after arthroscopic removal of dorsoproximal first phalanx osteochondral fractures (1986–1995). Equine Vet J 2000;32(6):475.
3. Dabareiner RM, White NA, Sullins KE. Metacarpophalangeal joint synovial pad fibrotic proliferation in 63 horses. Vet Surg 1996;25:199–206.
4. Grondahl AM. Incidence and development of ununited proximoplantar tuberosity of the proximal phalanx in Standardbred trotters. Vet Radiol Ultrasound 1992;33(1):18.
5. Haynes PF. Disease of the metacarpophalangeal joint and metacarpus. Vet Clin North Am Large Anim Pract [Special Edition: Symposium on Equine Lameness] 1980;2:33.
6. Hubert J, Williams J, Moore RM. What is your diagnosis? Avulsion fracture of the medial plantar eminence of the first phalanx; subluxation of the metatarsophalangeal joint resulting from avulsion of the insertion of the medial collateral ligament. J Am Vet Med Assoc 1998;213(2):203.
7. Kawcak CE, McIlwraith CW. Proximodorsal first phalanx osteochondral chip fragmentation in 336 horses. Equine Vet J 1994;26(5):392.
8. McIlwraith CW. Fetlock fractures and luxations. In: Nixon AJ, Ed. Equine Fracture Repair. Philadelphia: WB Saunders 1996;153.
9. Pettersson H, Ryden G. Avulsion fractures of the caudoproximal extremity of the first phalanx. Equine Vet J 1982;14(4):333.
10. Yovich JV, McIlwraith CW. Arthroscopic surgery for osteochondral fractures of the proximal phalanx of the metacarpophalangeal and metatarsophalangeal (fetlock) joints in horses. J Am Vet Med Assoc 1986;188(3):273.

FRACTURES OF THE PROXIMAL SESAMOID BONES

Fractures of the proximal sesamoid bones are common injuries in racing Thoroughbreds, Standardbreds, and Quarter Horses[2,3,17,21] and are the most common fatal fracture in racing Thoroughbreds and Quarter Horses.[12] These fractures take a variety of forms, including apical, abaxial (articular and nonarticular), midbody, basilar (articular and nonarticular), sagittal, and comminuted (see Fig. 7.40). The forelimbs are most frequently affected in the Thoroughbred (right forelimb) and Quarter Horse, whereas the hindlimbs are most frequently affected in the Standardbred (left hindlimb). Most of these fractures distract as a result of the pull of the suspensory ligament proximally and the distal sesamoid ligaments distally.

Fractures of the apical portion of the sesamoid bone are by far the most common, making up more than 88.1% of sesamoid fractures. Sesamoid fractures are most common (53.4%) in 2-year-olds, followed by 3-year-olds (23%). Apical fractures are frequently articular, are singular, are rarely comminuted, and usually involve less than one-third of the bone (Fig. 8.190). In Standardbreds, apical fractures occur more frequently on the lateral sesamoid bones of the left hindlimb (42.8%) than on the right hindlimb (36.6%), whereas a more equal distribution is observed in Thoroughbreds.

Basilar fractures are less common than apical fractures (6% of sesamoid fractures in Standardbreds) and represent avulsion fractures associated with the distal sesamoid ligaments and may be comminuted. Basilar fractures are more common in the Thoroughbred than in the Standardbred and can be small articular, transverse articular, or nonarticular (Figs. 8.191 to 8.193). Nonarticular displaced basilar sesamoid fractures are removed only if they are associated with recurrent pain. These fractures are usually associated with a distal sesamoid ligament injury.

The abaxial fracture is an uncommon sesamoid fracture (3%) in Standardbreds but may be more common in Thoroughbreds and Quarter Horses (Fig. 8.193).[19,21] This fracture can be either articular or nonarticular. Abaxial fractures can be difficult to diagnose and may require an additional tangential projection on the radiographic examination to identify their exact location or can be identified on the craniocaudal view.[3,16]

The midbody transverse fracture is seen most frequently in the Thoroughbred, older Standardbred (mean age 6.5 years), and young foal (under 2 months). This fracture roughly separates the bone into equal portions and invariably enters the fetlock joint. Because of the distractive forces of the suspensory ligament proximally and the distal sesamoid ligament distally, most of these fractures tend to separate. Infrequently, they remain in apposition but may separate later. If both sesamoid bones are fractured, they usually become distracted and the suspensory support apparatus is lost (Fig. 8.194).

Causes

The cause of proximal sesamoid bone fractures is excessive tensile forces and direct blunt trauma to the bone. At the end of a race, fetlock extension is greatest because of fatigue of the digital flexor muscles that support the fetlock. This hyperextension maximally loads the sesamoid bones. When the sesamoid bone can no longer withstand the distraction forces applied to it by the suspensory ligament and distal sesamoid ligaments, the bone fails. This muscle fatigue factor is most clearly illustrated when young foals that are placed on pasture fracture their sesamoid bones while running to keep up with their dams.[7,11]

Other factors such as poor conditioning, improper trimming and shoeing, and poor conformation create ad-

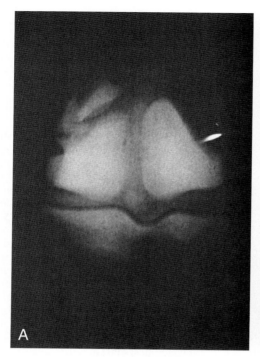
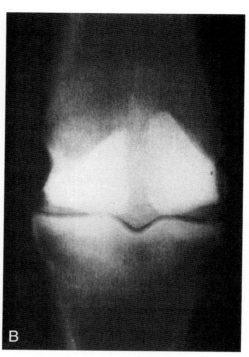

Figure 8.190 A. A comminuted fracture of the apical portion of the sesamoid bone. This type of fracture is uncommon. B. The same sesamoid bone after the fragment was removed. (Courtesy of T. S. Stashak.)

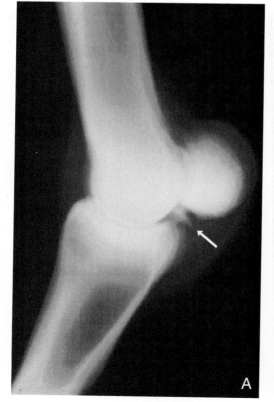
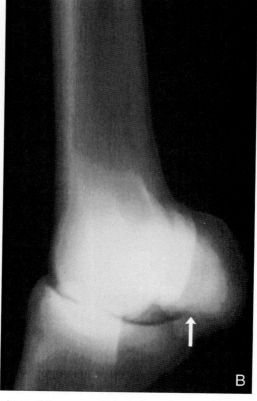

Figure 8.191 A. Typical articular displaced basilar sesamoid fracture (arrow) in a racing Thoroughbred. The articular component is wider than the nonarticular component. B. Note the defect at the base of the sesamoid bone (arrow) after arthroscopic removal of the fragment. This horse returned to racing.

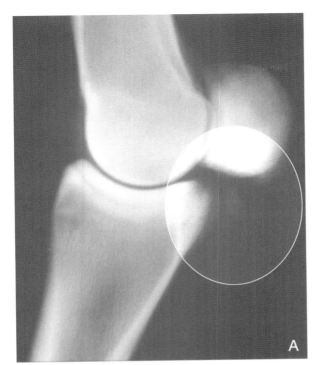

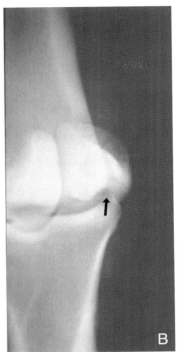

Figure 8.192   A. A nonarticular displaced basilar sesamoid fracture (oval). B. Note the defect at the base of the sesamoid bone (arrow) after surgical removal of the fragment through a small ligamentous separation approach to the base of the sesamoid.

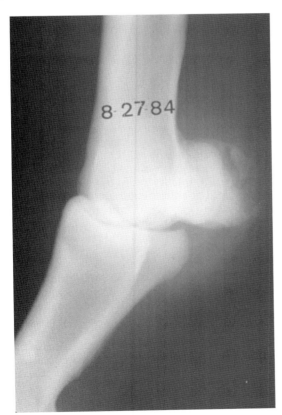

Figure 8.193   An abaxial nonarticular fracture of the proximal sesamoid bone.

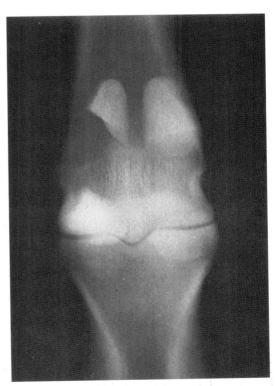

Figure 8.194   Dorsopalmar view of the fetlock of a horse that sustained transverse fractures of the proximal sesamoid bones. The apical fragments are displaced proximally. (Courtesy of T. S. Stashak.)

ditional stresses on this bone. Unequal tension applied to the sesamoid bone as the foot strikes the ground in an unbalanced position may also be a causal factor.

During training, these bones rapidly remodel, which initially decreases bone porosity and increases bone trabecular width and mineralizing surface, thereby enhancing the bone's ability to withstand stress.[26] The suspensory ligament also increases in strength with training until it exceeds the strength of the bone, making bone failure the method of suspensory breakdown in racing or heavily training racehorses.[6] The vascular pattern of the sesamoid bones may be implicated in site selection of fractures, because the orientation and distribution of vessels parallel the radiographic lucencies seen in horses with sesamoiditis and correspond to the configuration of apical fracture patterns.[22]

Direct trauma to the sesamoid bone can cause comminuted fractures and midbody fractures. Direct trauma can occur if the fetlock hits the ground in an athletic event or at the time of a uniaxial sesamoid fracture. It is also possible that a hindlimb could clip the sesamoid, causing fracture and often a wound. The medial sesamoid bone is reported to be the most frequently involved when interference is the cause.[1]

The sesamoid bones also undergo marked bone resorption when the fetlock is immobilized and pathologic fracture after cast removal has been reported in adult horses.[13]

Signs

The medial and/or lateral sesamoid bones may be fractured. Lameness is quite pronounced in acute stages: The horse is reluctant to bear weight on the limb and will not permit the fetlock to descend to a normal position during weight bearing. Swelling, heat, and pain are marked in the fetlock region. Tendosynovitis or suspensory desmitis may confuse the diagnosis if radiographs are not taken. The horse evidences pain when pressure is applied to the affected bone or bones. Descent of the fetlock during weight bearing causes pain. Observation of the gait reveals that the fetlock is held rigid so that it cannot descend as much as the opposite normal fetlock.

The fracture in the bone may occur in any area of the sesamoids, but proximal fractures are more common than distal fractures; proximal fractures also are more amenable to treatment (Figs. 8.190, 8.195, and 8.196). Desmitis of the suspensory ligament and distal sesamoid ligaments may occur concurrently with fractured sesamoids. After 1 to 2 weeks' rest, lameness at the walk and trot may not be obvious, but joint effusion persists.

A history of galloping to exhaustion in an attempt to keep up with the dams is common for young foals under 2 months of age that have sustained fractures of their sesamoid bones. These fractures often occur in foals that have been confined to a box stall for several days and then are turned out for free exercise with the dams.

Diagnosis

Diagnosis is based on radiologic examination of the affected fetlock and the physical changes described. If a

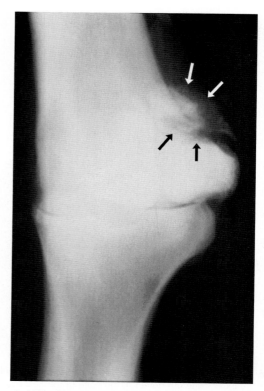

Figure 8.195 Chronic apical sesamoid fracture demonstrating chronic fibrous union (black arrows) and enthesiophyte formation (white arrows) after conservative management (stall rest) followed by return to training.

fetlock joint is severely swollen and the horse shows pain when pressure is applied over the sesamoid bone(s), radiographs should be taken to rule out the possibility of fracture. Cases of tendosynovitis should be radiographed to eliminate the possibility of fractured sesamoid bones accompanying this condition. Sesamoiditis may cause similar signs, but radiographs will show no fracture and joint effusion will not be a prominent feature.

Because the radiodensity and contrast may be poor in radiographs taken in very young foals (because of limited ossification), good-quality radiographs and close scrutiny are required for the diagnosis. In some cases, the fracture cannot be diagnosed immediately and may require a few weeks before it becomes apparent. This is also true for hairline nondisplaced fractures that occur in adults. These fractures may be difficult to differentiate from increased vascular channels associated with chronic sesamoiditis.[8,9] Nuclear scintigraphy can be helpful in making the diagnosis in these situations.

Standard radiographic views should include the dorsopalmar (DP), the lateral medial (LM), and oblique projections. Occasionally, the flexed LM may demonstrate lesions that are not detectable on the other standard projections, and estimation of reduction potential of midbody fractures can be made. The addition of the skyline projection of the abaxial surface of the sesamoid bone is helpful in some cases to identify the exact location of fractures on the abaxial surface.[16]

The radiographs should be closely examined for any signs of DJD associated with the fetlock and incomplete

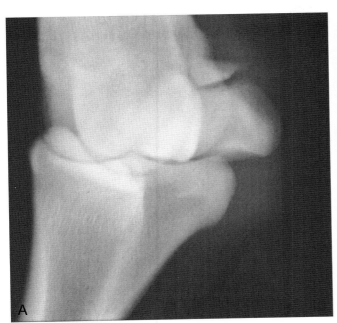
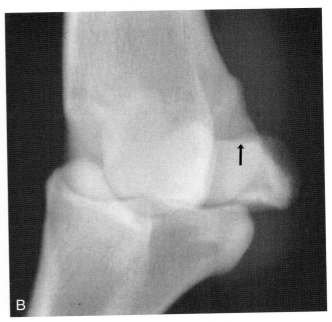

Figure 8.196   A. A typical minimally displaced fresh apical sesamoid fracture in a racing Standardbred that can be removed arthroscopically or by arthrotomy with an excellent chance of return to racing. B. After fragment removal, the suspensory ligament will reattach with fibrous tissue to the flat bed of the sesamoid bone (arrow).

fractures that may be confused with increased interosseous vascular channels. The fracture can be differentiated from the vascular canals by the following criteria: 1) the fracture usually extends to the margin of the abaxial surface of the proximal sesamoid bone, whereas the increased vascular canal does not, and 2) the fracture line frequently runs in a different direction or plane from the vascular canal. If an incomplete sesamoid bone fracture is suspected, a repeat radiograph should be taken after 2 to 4 weeks of stall rest, or nuclear scintigraphy can be performed. This will permit better evaluation of the fracture line, because it allows sufficient time for lysis of the bone to occur. Furthermore, a better appreciation for the fibro-osseous disruption can be made at this time. It should be reemphasized that if these horses are allowed to exercise, they run a great risk of distracting the fracture and worsening the prognosis. Ultrasonography should be performed on all apical and basilar fractures to identify if an injury has occurred to the supportive ligaments.

Treatment

The selection of treatment of a sesamoid bone fracture is based on the location of the fracture and the intended use of the animal. Treatments include stall rest, cast application, surgical excision, lag screw fixation, circumferential wiring, and bone grafting.

In general, most horses not intended for performance and relegated to breeding do not require surgery; and simple support bandaging, splinting, or casting with stall rest is sufficient.[1] For more severe injuries with partial collapse of the suspensory apparatus (identified as a dropped fetlock on weight bearing), use of a splint that places the horse on the toe and relieves suspensory tension (e.g., the Kimzey leg saver) should be used to support fetlock joint ankylosis in a more normal position. The splint can be worn for 2 to 3 months, depending on the severity of the injury.

Stall rest (with or without soft cast or external coaptation) for 3 to 4 months has been successful to obtain fibrous or partial bony union; but management is prolonged, and if casting is used, weakening of the bone is anticipated (Fig. 8.195).[13] This prolonged period is needed because the sesamoid bones heal so slowly. The delayed healing may result from limited periosteal covering and the extensive ligamentous attachments that cause distraction and movement. Most fractures that are treated conservatively heal by a weak fibrous union, and the fracture line will be observed on radiographic examination for a long time. (A portion of these fractures that have apparently healed will eventually separate, resulting in pain.) Generally, the conservative approach should be used for horses that are not going to be used for performance in the future and for young foals without distraction of fracture fragments.

Surgical treatment of sesamoid bone fractures (if indicated) in a horse intended for performance appears to be beneficial and is preferred for the most rapid return to performance with the least risk of future DJD or sesamoid reinjury. Surgical removal or stabilization may promote earlier union and bony union and reduce the risk of secondary DJD within the fetlock joint.

Apical, articular abaxial, and basilar fractures involving less than one-third of the sesamoid bone are best treated by surgical removal of the fragment (Figs. 8.190, 8.191, 8.196 to 8.198).[3,4,17–20] Nonarticular abaxial fractures may require removal, but horses will often perform successfully without surgery. Midbody transverse fractures affecting the middle third and basilar transverse

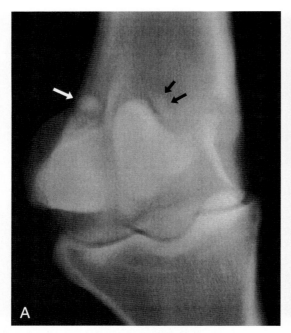
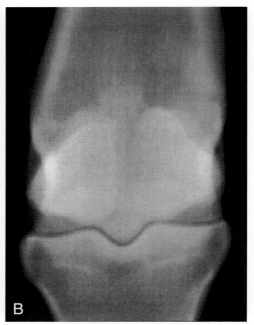

Figure 8.197 A. A small, completely articular sesamoid fracture (white arrow) and articular abaxial sesamoid fracture (black arrows). B. The fractures were removed arthroscopically to permit adequate soft tissue healing and return to training in as little as 3 weeks. The short convalescence was acceptable because the suspensory ligaments were uninjured and removal did not require any ligament dissection.

fractures of the proximal sesamoid bones have been treated successfully with lag screw fixation (Fig. 8.199) or circumferential wiring to provide postoperative bone compression and immobilization.[3,10,14,25]

Autogenous cancellous bone grafting and cast immobilization have been used with some degree of success in both experimental situations and on a limited number of clinical cases,[15] but most surgeons prefer to combine autogenous cancellous bone grafting with internal fixation of the fracture for the best and fastest results. Internal fixation offers the advantage of earlier removal from the cast and earlier weight bearing.

Fractures through the bodies of both sesamoid bones are a common cause of breakdown in the racing horse (Fig. 8.194).[12] Because the suspensory apparatus is lost and distal limb vascular supply may be disrupted, these horses may be humanely euthanized. However, animals with breeding potential or sentimental value can be salvaged by arthrodesis of the fetlock (see "Traumatic Rupture of the Suspensory Apparatus" in this chapter).

Surgery is easily performed with the horse in lateral or dorsal recumbency under general anesthesia. For large fractures, fresh fractures, or fractures removed by arthrotomy rather than arthroscopy, a tourniquet should be used to control hemorrhage. An Esmarch bandage, used to force blood from the limb before the tourniquet is applied, will give one an almost bloodless field. An Esmarch bandage may be fashioned from a piece of rubber inner tubing, approximately 2 inches wide, or other suitable material.

Surgical removal of apical sesamoid fractures can be performed by arthroscopy or arthrotomy through the palmar–plantar recess of the fetlock joint. Arthroscopy offers the advantage of rapid return to performance for small articular fractures without suspensory involvement (3 weeks) and the ability to remove more than one fracture from a joint with minimal incisional morbidity. Dorsal proximal phalanx fractures or biaxial sesamoid fractures may occur simultaneously. Dorsal recumbency offers the advantage of not having to move the horse to gain access to multiple sites or limbs for surgery, less bleeding, and passive flexion of the joint to enhance visualization and decrease tension of the suspensory ligament. Apical and articular abaxial fractures on both sesamoids can be removed from one arthroscopic portal.

Hemorrhage can limit visualization in fresh fractures that require dissection of the suspensory ligament (apical, articular abaxial, and basilar fractures). Use of electrocautery probes for transection of the ligament may enhance precision of separation and lessen hemorrhage.[4] For classical apical fractures that involve a suspensory ligament but are smaller than one-third the length of the bone, arthrotomy or arthroscopy is a valid surgical approach. The arthrotomy can be made small, and this joint location heals well. When the fragment is in the apex of the bone, the incision should be made between the suspensory ligament and the palmar or plantar surface of the cannon bone (Fig. 8.196). Flexion of the fetlock reduces tension on the suspensory ligament and flexor tendons for better visualization of the fracture. This enables one to retract the suspensory ligament so that the apex of the sesamoid bone can be seen. The fragment should be gently but sharply dissected away from the rest of the bone. The fragment can be grasped with a small pair of rongeurs to permit dissection of the fibrous attachments from the bone. After the fragment is removed, tissue fragments are removed and the bone is smoothed with a curette.

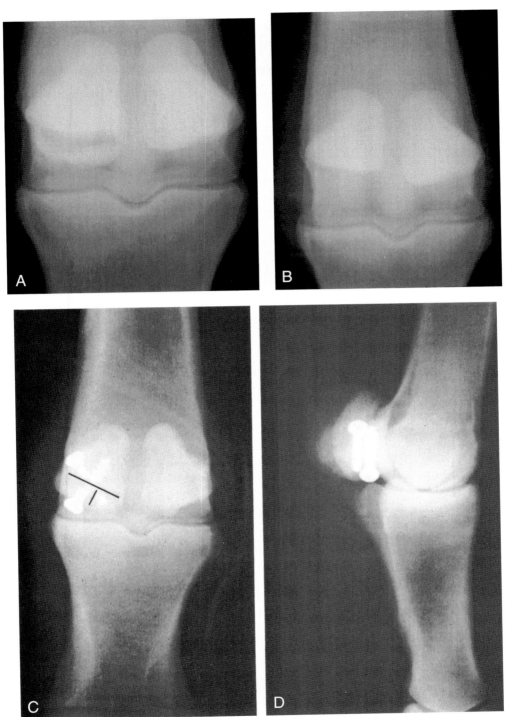

Figure 8.198 A. A relatively large, complete comminuted fracture of the base of the lateral sesamoid in a racing Thoroughbred. B. After fragment removal. This type of fragment can be removed arthroscopically with a fair to good prognosis for return to riding soundness. C and D. Alternatively, a double transfixation screw technique can be used to secure both distal fragments. (Panels C and D are provided courtesy of T. S. Stashak.)

A layer of simple interrupted sutures should be placed in the fibrous joint capsule and adjacent tissues with 2-0 synthetic absorbable suture with swaged-on taper-point needle. A second layer of simple interrupted sutures should be placed in the subcutaneous tissues, and the skin closed with a noncapillary, nonabsorbable plastic suture. The skin incision should be protected with a non-adherent sterile dressing, and the limb should be heavily wrapped in supporting elastic bandages. Casting or splinting is recommended for midbody fractures and

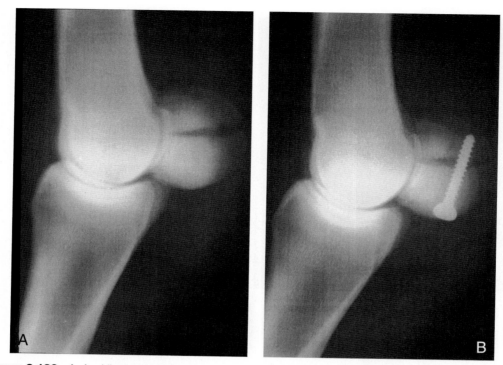

Figure 8.199 A. A midbody sesamoid fracture. B. Postoperative view showing a single cortical transfixation screw stabilizing the fracture. A bony union resulted.

comminuted fractures and if clinical evidence of suspensory disruption accompanies the sesamoid fracture. After 10 to 14 days, the horse should be walked daily. Supporting wraps should be kept on for a minimum of 30 days; they are especially important during the 2 weeks after surgery to prevent swelling. Reattachment of the suspensory ligament is slow; and for large fractures, 4 to 6 months may be required before allowing the horse to return to training.

For basilar fractures, the arthroscope is similarly placed in the fetlock recess, but the instrument portal must be made into the distal fetlock recess so that instruments can be placed parallel to the base of the sesamoid. These fractures are more difficult to remove because of the extent of ligamentous structure attached to the bone. The axial fragment is often separated from the abaxial fragment and can get lost in the ligament and joint capsule. An intraoperative radiograph is strongly encouraged to confirm complete removal of the fracture. If the fragment cannot be completely removed by arthroscopy owing to hemorrhage or migration of the fragment, the distal instrument portal can be enlarged to allow direct removal by arthrotomy. Blunt dissection in between distal sesamoid ligaments can retrieve most fragments. Avoid entrance into the synovial sheath with this incision, and close the soft tissues meticulously.

Abaxial fragments that lie entirely on the basilar aspect (nonarticular) of the sesamoid bone cannot be reached by any arthroscopic approach and must be removed by incision directly over the fragment. Most of these fractures do not need to be removed and heal by fibrous union. Removal of the fragment allows direct healing of the torn ends of the suspensory ligament to the bone, rather than a fibrous union between bone.

Removal of nonarticular basilar sesamoid fractures is made on the palmar or plantar aspect of the fetlock on the side of the superficial flexor tendon just distal to the fetlock anular ligament. There is a depression palpable at the base of the sesamoid. The distal sesamoid ligaments are bluntly dissected, and the fragment is located with a needle and radiographic imaging, if necessary. Once the fragment is located it can be shelled out with a sharp curette or elevator to avoid cutting the distal sesamoid ligament fibers. In most instances, nonarticular basilar sesamoid fractures do not require removal and heal with a fibrous union. Chronic pain from recurring tearing of the fibrous tissue can occur, and removal seems to improve the outcome. Entering the tendon sheath with an incision should be avoided because postoperative complications with synovial fluid leakage and chronic sheath distension can result. Careful closure and anatomic reapposition of soft tissues are recommended, and support of the incision in a splint or cast for 5 to 7 days is suggested.

When a sesamoid fracture involves one-third or more of the sesamoid bone, it may be repaired with a bone screw, using an ASIF (Association for the Study of Internal Fixation) cortical screw and a lag technique. A large basal fragment may be split in two pieces, and these fragments can sometimes be fixed into position by bone screws (Fig. 8.199). The incision is made directly over the region for drilling, as described above for approach to nonarticular basilar fractures. All structures are dissected away from the palpable depression at the base of the bone to expose the location to seat the screw. To evaluate the progress of the operation properly when placing the bone screws, open the palmar or plantar recess of the joint capsule between the suspensory ligament and the bone. The approximation of the fragments can be monitored through the incision in the palmar or plantar reflection of the joint capsule by visualizing the fracture, and bone graft can be placed from the joint surface. Fluoroscopic or radiographic examination is necessary to confirm the drilling angulation. A small 2-0 marker drill bit can be placed axial to the projected site for the screw and left in place for the radiograph and to maintain fracture reduction. Distraction of the fracture can make overdrilling to obtain compression difficult. Drilling the bone should be done at a slow speed to avoid thermal necrosis caused by the drill. Care should be taken not to drill through the proximal portion into the suspensory ligaments, since this may result in dystrophic calcification of this ligament. It is necessary to study the approach and to be thoroughly acquainted with the anatomy involved before placing the screw.

If the fracture is of some duration, the distal fragment may be demineralized and easily fractured. One should exercise caution when tightening the screw to make sure that the fragment does not split as a result of demineralization or excessive pressure. The cancellous bone in the sesamoids is quite soft, and care must be used not to strip the threads in the cancellous and cortical bone. The cortex on the sesamoid bone is quite thin and can also be easily damaged (Fig. 8.199). Usually, a single 4.5-mm cortical bone screw is selected although one or two 3.5-mm cortical screws have been successful. Placement of the screws from proximal to distal has been described for fractures with a large abaxial component. Casting is recommended, because of the high forces at the fracture site that can bend or cause the screw to cyclically fail, particularly if anatomic reduction was not complete. Bone graft can be inserted into the fracture site just before tightening the screw. Bony union is expected within 6 months and return to training at about 9 months.

The screw does not need to be removed, even if it breaks, as long as it is not infected. This surgery is technically challenging and care must be taken to cover the foot well, but not with bulky drapes, or the correct angle of the drill cannot be achieved. I use several layers of sterile gloves and adhesive plastic over the foot.

Ideally for use of screw fixation repair, the fragment should be in one piece and should involve at least 30% of the bone. Fractures approaching half of the bone volume are the most favorable. If the fragment is split, the prognosis is less favorable, and additional fragments may make the operation impractical. Circumferential wiring, which may contain these fragments and enhance the chance of bony union, could be elected as an alternative.

An alternate approach to internal stabilization of sesamoid fractures that involve more than one-third of the bone is circumferential and transfixation wiring. Two incisions are required to place the wire. A palmar or plantar pouch arthrotomy is made to expose the articular surface and apex of the sesamoid bone, and another incision is made into the digital tendon sheath through the anular ligament. A small 2-mm drill hole is made from lateral to medial across the apex of the sesamoid, and a 16-gauge needle is passed through the distal sesamoid ligaments parallel to the base of the sesamoid bone, both to exit into the tendon sheath. An 18-gauge, 40-cm wire

is passed through the needle and drill hole, tightened, and twisted on the lateral side. The fracture can be held in reduction at wire tightening with bone reduction forceps.

Researchers are investigating ways to minimize wire breakage before adequate fracture healing, including the use of two wires or other braided materials not as susceptible to cyclic failure. Wire migration after breakage occurs and usually necessitates removal. Casting for a minimum of 30 days is recommended to reduce risk of wire breakage. Initial breaking strength of the circumferential wiring technique is similar to[25] or greater than[23] that of the screw technique; however, in vivo studies of cyclic failure have not been performed. I prefer the screw technique, because it does not enter the tendon sheath, place foreign material into the tendon sheath, or require implant removal even if implant failure occurs. In addition, if the screw does not work (i.e., cannot achieve compression or is malpositioned), a wire can subsequently be placed.

When fractures of both bodies of the sesamoid have occurred and the suspensory apparatus is lost, early treatment is required for a successful outcome. Even with early treatment, the initial soft tissue trauma may be severe enough that the blood supply to the foot is lost.[5] Management of such injuries is directed toward the support and immobilization of the fetlock joint for a sufficient period to stabilize soft tissue destruction; then consideration is given to surgical arthrodesis or conservative ankylosis by soft tissue fibrosis (see "Traumatic Suspensory Rupture").

A major complication to this breakdown injury is support limb laminitis in the contralateral weight-bearing limb. This will often be first recognized as increased weight bearing on the affected limb and is erroneously recorded as a good sign. In most cases, the laminitis occurs between the third and fourth week after injury. To reduce the chances of this laminitis, the contralateral hoof support should be maintained and analgesics should be administered to increase the weight bearing on the traumatized limb and decrease the stress to the contralateral weight-bearing limb.

Fractures of the sesamoid that occur in conjunction with fracture of the metacarpal or metatarsal condyle are serious injuries that should be identified on the radiograph. The prognosis for returning to racing, even with repair of the condylar fracture, is not good.[2] These fractures are usually sagittal and axial and occur with extreme pulling on the intersesamoid ligament when the condylar fracture displaces. The fractures indicate significant soft tissue injury to the fetlock joint and that DJD is likely to ensue.

Prognosis

The reported prognoses are as follows:

- Apical sesamoid fractures: good to excellent (88% of Standardbreds return to racing)[24]
- Abaxial fractures: good (71% of Thoroughbreds and Quarter Horses return to racing)[19]
- Basilar fractures: fair (50 to 60% of Thoroughbreds return to racing)[18]

• Midbody fractures repaired by either lag screw fixation or circumferential wiring: fair (50 to 60% of horses return to performance)[10,14]

Conservative management reports are not available for comparison, but generally it is presumed that the prognosis is guarded for a basilar or midbody fracture that is not treated but heals on its own. Most of these joints develop significant DJD and restricted range of motion. If both sesamoids are fractured, the prognosis is less favorable owing to the loss of suspensory support.

The prognosis for treatment of fractures of the sesamoid bones that result in loss of the suspensory apparatus is poor and should be considered only for salvage of valuable breeding stock and for horses of great sentimental value.

In all cases, however, the prognosis can be made only after thorough radiographic evaluation of the fetlock joints for signs of DJD and evaluation of the suspensory ligament as a source of pain from desmitis.

References

1. Adams OR, ed. Lameness in Horses. 3rd ed. Philadelphia: Lea & Febiger, 1974.
2. Bassage LH, Richardson DW. Longitudinal fractures of the condyles of the third metacarpal and metatarsal bones in racehorses: 224 cases (1986–1995). J Am Vet Med Assoc 1998;212:1757.
3. Bertone AL Fractures of the proximal sesamoid bones. In: Nixon AJ, ed. Equine Fracture Repair. Philadelphia: WB Saunders, 1996; 16:163.
4. Boure L, Marcoux M, Laverty S, Lepage OM. Use of electrocautery probes in arthroscopic removal of apical sesamoid fracture fragments in 18 Standardbred horses. Vet Surg 1999;28:226.
5. Bramlage LR. First aid and transportation of fracture patients. In: Nixon AJ, Ed. Equine Fracture Repair. Philadelphia: WB Saunders, 1996;36–43.
6. Bukowiecki CF, Bramlage LR, Gabel AA. In vitro strength of the suspensory apparatus in training and resting horses. Vet Surg 1987; 16:126.
7. Ellis DR. Fractures of the proximal sesamoid bones in Thoroughbred foals. Equine Vet J 1979;11:48.
8. Grondahl AM, Gaustad G, Engeland A. Progression and association with lameness and racing performance of radiographic changes in the proximal sesamoid bones of young Standardbred trotters. Equine Vet J 1994;26:152.
9. Hardy J, Marcoux M, Breton L. Clinical relevance of radiographic findings in proximal sesamoid bones of two-year-old Standardbreds in their first year of race training. J Am Vet Med Assoc 1991; 198:2089–2094.
10. Henninger RW, Bramlage LR, Schneider RK, Gabel AA. Lag screw and cancellous bone graft fixation of transverse proximal sesamoid bone fractures in horses: 25 cases (1983–1989). J Am Vet Med Assoc 1991;199(5):606.
11. Honnas CM, Snyder JR, Meagher DM, Ragle CA. Traumatic disruption of the suspensory apparatus in foals. Cornell Vet 80: 123,1990.
12. Johnson BJ, Stover SM, Daft BM, et al. Causes of death in racehorses over a 2-year period. Equine Vet J 1994;26:327.
13. Malone ED, Anderson BH, Turner TA. Proximal sesamoid bone fracture following cast removal in two horses. Equine Vet J 1997; 9:185.
14. Martin BB, Nunamaker DM, Evans LH, et al. Circumferential wiring of mid-body and large basilar fractures of the proximal sesamoid bone in 15 horses. Vet Surg 1991;20(1):9.
15. Medina LE, et al. Am Assoc Equine Pract 1980.
16. Palmer SE. Radiography of the abaxial surface of the proximal sesamoid bones of the horse. J Am Vet Med Assoc 1982;181:264.
17. Parente EJ, Richardson DW, Spencer P. Basal sesamoidean fractures in horses: 57 cases (1989–1991). J Am Vet Med Assoc 1993; 202:1293.
18. Southwood LL, McIlwraith CW. Arthroscopic removal of fracture fragments involving a portion of the base of the proximal sesamoid bone in horses: 26 cases (1984–1997). J Am Vet Med Assoc 2000; 217(2):236.
19. Southwood LL, Trotter GW, McIlwraith CW. Arthroscopic removal of abaxial fracture fragments of the proximal sesamoid bones in horses: 47 cases (1989–1997). J Am Vet Med Assoc 1998; 213(7):1016.
20. Spurlock GH, Gabel AA. Apical fractures of the proximal sesamoid bones in 109 Standardbred horses. J Am Vet Med Assoc 1983; 183:76.
21. Torre, K., Motta M. Incidence and distribution of 369 proximal sesamoid bone fractures in 354 Standardbred horses (1984–1995). Equine Pract 1999;21(8):6.
22. Trumble, TN, Arnoczky SP Stick JA, Stickle RL. Clinical relevance of the microvasculature of the equine proximal sesamoid bone. Am J Vet Res 1995;56:720.
23. Wilson DA, Keegan KG, Carson WL. An in vitro biomechanical comparison of two fixation methods for transverse osteotomies of the medial proximal forelimb sesamoid bones in horses. Vet Surg 1999;28:355.
24. Woodie JB, Ruggles AJ, Litsky AS. In vitro biomechanical properties of 2 compression fixation methods for midbody proximal sesamoid bone fractures in horses. Vet Surg 2000;29:358.
25. Woodie JB, Ruggles AJ, Bertone AL, et al. Apical fracture of the proximal sesamoid bone in Standardbred horses: 43 cases (1990–1996). J Am Vet Med Assoc 1999;214(11):1653.
26. Young, DR, Nunamaker DM, Markel MD. Quantitative evaluation of the remodeling response of the proximal sesamoid bones to training-related stimuli in Thoroughbreds. Am J Vet Res 1991; 52:1350.

SESAMOIDITIS

Sesamoiditis is observed frequently in racing horses and hunters and jumpers that are between 2 and 5 years of age.[5-7] The condition is characterized by pain associated with the proximal sesamoid bones and insertions of the suspensory ligament, resulting in lameness. The pain is thought to result from inflammation at the interface of the suspensory ligament and distal sesamoid ligaments with the proximal sesamoid bone. Primary disease of the suspensory ligament or distal sesamoid ligament can also accompany this condition. Pain, heat, and inflammation can be clinically detected at the insertion of the ligament during the active stages of the disease process, but marked lameness and limitations in performance can also occur without any clinically detectable signs.[1,3]

Radiographs can reveal a range of changes from accelerated early remodeling response in the bones (increased size and number of vascular channels) to marked proliferation of bone along the abaxial margin of the sesamoid and increased bone density of the sesamoid. The suspensory ligament and the distal sesamoid ligaments may also be affected and show calcified areas. Demineralization of the sesamoid bone(s) may result from inflammation and impaired blood supply (Fig. 8.200).[7] The increased bone production is thought to result from inflammation from tearing of the attachments of either the suspensory ligament or the distal sesamoid ligament (Fig. 8.201). It is also possible to see radiographic changes that indicate chronic sesamoiditis in sound performing horses, suggesting that some horses are able to repair the injury and regain suspensory strength.[3]

Causes

Any unusual strain to the fetlock region may produce sesamoiditis. Although most common in racehorses,

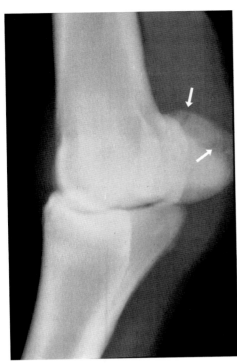

Figure 8.200   Typical findings in sesamoiditis. Note the osteolysis along a vascular channel and bone proliferation at the abaxial edge of the lesion (arrows).

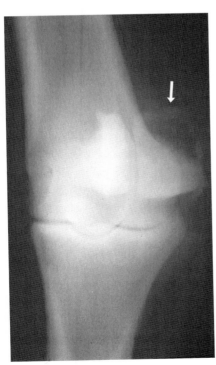

Figure 8.201   Aggressive sesamoiditis can result in bone proliferation into the suspensory ligament (arrow).

hunters, and jumpers, it can affect any type of horse. It is caused by injury to the attachment of the suspensory ligament to the sesamoid bones. This injury may alter the blood supply to the sesamoid bone(s). Injury to the distal sesamoid ligaments may also occur at their attachment to the basilar portion of the sesamoid bones.

The sesamoid bones have a substantial intraosseus blood supply, which enters the midportion of the bone through multiple abaxial channels that correspond to the channels that enlarge in sesamoiditis, indicating bone resorption. This may represent the initiation of the re-modeling response to bone stress of training or may reflect an increase in blood flow as a result of inflammation and injury to the suspensory ligament or both.[9] The sesamoid bones undergo intense remodeling in response to training,[10] and the progression of radiographic changes correlate with bone response to remodeling and injury. Note that several studies have categorized radiographic changes in the sesamoid bones of young (2- and 3-year-old) racehorses and discovered that many horses have an increased size and number of vascular channels but no lameness.[3,4] This supports the idea that remodeling is a normal response to training and that only if the stresses exceed the bones' capability to strengthen themselves would microfracture and damage occur. Although radiographic vascular changes of bone remodeling in these studies were not associated with sesamoid fracture, the vascular structures coursed along known lines of fracture in adult racehorses.

The sesamoids bones have an extensive sensory nerve supply, which may explain the pain associated with trabecular bone injury.[2]

Signs

Symptoms of this condition are similar to those caused by fracture of the sesamoid bone. In the early stage, minimal swelling is observed, but increased heat may be felt over the abaxial surface of the sesamoid bone. As the disease progresses, a visible enlargement of the soft tissues overlying the palmar surface of the fetlock can be seen as fibrosis of the injured suspensory ligament becomes apparent. On palpation, pain withdrawal can usually be elicited by placing pressure over the abaxial surfaces of the sesamoid bone. In more advanced cases, pain may be elicited by applying pressure over the branches of the suspensory ligament and possibly the distal sesamoid ligament as well. Flexion of the fetlock is also painful.

At exercise, the lameness varies considerably among horses and depends on the acuteness of the injury and its degree. In general, the lameness is most evident during the first part of exercise and is more exaggerated when the horse is exercised on hard surfaces. On close observation, a reduction in extension of the fetlock can noticed, and a fetlock flexion test usually exacerbates the lameness.[8] Perineural anesthesia and/or intrasynovial anesthesia are used infrequently to diagnose sesamoiditis. Horses respond to a distal metacarpal nerve block but not to an intraarticular fetlock block, locating the lameness to the periarticular structures.

Diagnosis

The radiologic changes of true sesamoiditis have been described as bony changes on the abaxial surface or basilar region with increased radiodense buildup, increased number and irregularity of the vascular channels, and increased coarseness and mottling of the bone trabeculation (Figs. 8.200 and 8.201). In acute cases, radiographs may have to be taken approximately 3 weeks after onset of the condition to determine if the sesamoid bones have undergone bony changes. The condition may also occur with tendosynovitis, fracture of the sesamoid bones, and injury to the suspensory ligament, from which it must be differentiated. Careful radiographic interpretation of the mottled trabecular pattern seen in the proximal sesamoid bone is necessary to differentiate the condition from a fracture. An incomplete fracture can be differentiated from the coarse vascular canals, because the fracture usually extends to the abaxial surface and the vascular canals do not. Also, the fracture line frequently runs at different angles from the vascular channels.

Nuclear scintigraphy indicates increased radioactivity in the region of the sesamoid bones but usually not fracture activity. Ultrasound of the suspensory and distal sesamoid ligaments may not be useful, because many horses have no abnormalities in the ligaments in the acute phases of sesamoiditis.

Treatment

If heat, pain, and swelling are detected at the bone or suspensory insertion, then efforts should be made to reduce the inflammation. Alternating cold and hot packs, as well as antiphlogistic packs, should be used. Rest from performance until soundness at the trot is achieved and then slow convalescent exercise allow the bone to continue to remodel and strengthen. It is important to keep the exercise below a level that would reinjure the bone. Similar to other suspensory ligament injuries, convalescence is long (6 to 8 months), and injury often recurs when the horse returns to full work.

In chronic stages, firing and blistering have been used, but with only limited success. Radiation (x-ray and γ-ray), laser heat, shock wave therapy, and a balanced mineral diet are considered by some clinicians to be valuable therapy for sesamoiditis as well as for the treatment of calcification in the suspensory ligament.

Prognosis

The prognosis for return to full athletic performance is guarded to unfavorable, depending on the amount of periosteal reaction and new bone growth that occurs on the sesamoid bones and the extent of injury to the suspensory ligament and to the distal sesamoid ligaments.

References

1. Clayton HM. Cinematographic analysis of the gait of lame horses II: Chronic sesamoiditis. Equine Vet Sci 1986;6:310.
2. Cornelissen BP. The proximal sesamoid bone of the horse; vascular and neurologic characteristics. Tijdschr Diergeneeskd 1998;15:123.
3. Grondahl AM, Gaustad G, Engeland A. Progression and association with lameness and racing performance of radiographic changes in the proximal sesamoid bones of young Standardbred trotters. Equine Vet J 1994;26:152.
4. Hardy J, Marcoux M, Breton L. Clinical relevance of radiographic findings in proximal sesamoid bones of two-year-old Standardbreds in their first year of race training. J Am Vet Med Assoc 1991;198:2089.
5. Nemeth F. The pathology of sesamoiditis. Tijdschr Diergeneeskd 1973;98:1003.
6. Nemeth F. Sesamoiditis in the horse. Tijdschr Diergeneeskd 1973;98:994.
7. O'Brien TR, et al. Sesamoiditis in the Thoroughbred: A radiographic study. J Am Vet Radiol Soc 1971;12:75.
8. Stashak TS. Sesamoiditis. In: Stashak TS, ed. Adams' Lameness in Horses. 4th ed. Philadelphia: Lea & Febiger, 1987;582.
9. Trumble TN, Arnoczky SP, Stick JA, Stickle RL. Clinical relevance of the microvasculature of the equine proximal sesamoid bone. Am J Vet Res 1995;56:720.
10. Young DR, Nunamaker DM, Markel MD. Quantitative evaluation of the remodeling response of the proximal sesamoid bones to training-related stimuli in Thoroughbreds. Am J Vet Res 1991;52:1350.

OSTEOMYELITIS OF THE AXIAL BORDER OF THE PROXIMAL SESAMOID BONES

Osteomyelitis of the axial border of the proximal sesamoid bones is an uncommon cause of lameness in horses. It is presumably an injury to the attachment of the intersesamoid ligament and seeding with bacteria from intraarticular injections may be associated with the condition (Fig. 8.202). In one report on seven cases, three affected horses had a septic tenosynovitis of the digital sheath

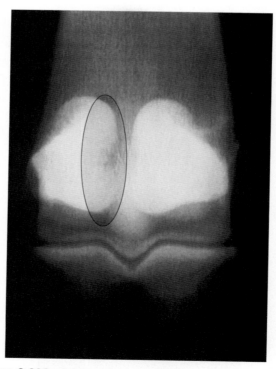

Figure 8.202 Axial margin sesamoiditis (oval) is often a result of an injury to the intersesmoidean ligament and may harbor bacteria and an osteomyelitis, particularly if preceded by an intraarticular injection.

and two of the seven had a fetlock septic arthritis (Stashak TS, personal communication).[1] In some cases, even though the clinical signs and radiographic lesions suggest sepsis, histologic studies of the lesions reveal infarction and necrosis, not purulent inflammation.

In this condition, horses are quite lame at the walk. In one report, lameness was 2 to 5/5 (mean 4/5).[1] Radiographs usually reveal bone lysis at the attachment of the intersesamoid ligament, primarily at the midbody and apical regions (Fig. 8.202). Some lesions appear cystic, whereas others appear to erode the axial border more diffusely. In one report, evidence of acute, subacute, and chronic reparative osteomyelitis was seen on the proximal sesamoid bones in 10 fetlocks of affected horses.

Surgical access to the area is possible from the palmar–plantar fetlock joint and digital sheath using arthroscopy. Any abnormal bone and ligament is debrided, and samples are submitted for culture and sensitivity. After debridement, the sheath and joint are flushed with a sterile balanced electrolyte solution, followed by 1 liter of 10% dimethyl sulfoxide (DMSO) and a broad-spectrum antimicrobial, which is instilled in the synovial cavities (see Chapter 7). The prolonged administration (6 to 12 weeks) of broad-spectrum antimicrobials is also recommended (Stashak TS, personal communication).

Although the prognosis for return to performance is considered poor,[1] using the approach described under "Treatment" can result in pasture soundness and, less commonly, return to intended use. If the intersesamoid ligament is damaged extensively the prognosis for return to performance remains poor.

Reference

1. Wisner ER, O'Brien TR, Pool RR, et al. Osteomyelitis of the axial border of the proximal sesamoid bones in seven horses. Equine Vet J 1991;23:383.

TRAUMATIC ARTHRITIS OF THE METACARPOPHALANGEAL (FETLOCK) JOINT (OSSELETS)

See Chapter 7.

FETLOCK SUBCHONDRAL BONE CYSTS

Fetlock subchondral bone cysts occur most commonly on the weight-bearing surface of the metacarpal condyle (Fig. 8.203) and less commonly on the weight-bearing surface of the proximal (first) phalanx. Cysts of the distal metacarpus that open into the fetlock joint occur in young horses and are considered part of the developmental osteochondrosis syndrome.[1]

Causes

Developmental bone cysts are considered part of the developmental orthopedic diseases that occur during growth and the conversion of cartilage to bone (see Chapter 7 for further details). Proximal phalanx cysts may be traumatically induced. Injury to the articular cartilage and underlying subchondral bone from high impact may allow synovial fluid to enter the fissure and

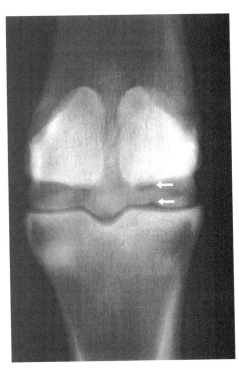

Figure 8.203 A distal third metacarpal subchondral bone cyst that opens into the fetlock joint.

increase intraosseus pressure. I have seen several of these develop in mature working horses in which the cyst is not initially apparent on radiographs but develops 30 to 60 days after injury. Typically, the lameness and joint inflammation improve as the cyst matures.

Signs

The average age of horses with clinical signs is 18 months, although such cysts may develop before onset of clinical signs. Also proximal phalanx cysts can develop in horses of any age from trauma. Moderate lameness is a feature of the disease that includes soreness to fetlock flexion in most cases and fetlock joint effusion in about 50% of the cases. In my experience, the clinical signs of first phalanx cysts are an acute onset of lameness and joint heat and effusion with marked soreness to fetlock flexion in a working horse.

Diagnosis

The diagnosis is made by radiographic evaluation of the joint (Fig. 8.203). In their early development, the cysts may not be apparent on radiograph; thus follow-up radiographic examination is recommended if clinical signs referable to the joint persist. Nuclear scintigraphy identifies a focal area of increased uptake in the bone as the cyst is developing and for several months after it has formed. Chronic cysts may not have significant bone turnover above the surrounding condyle and may appear quiet on nuclear scan.

Treatment

Surgical debridement of metacarpal cysts by an arthroscopic approach is the preferable treatment if the diagnosis is made before significant signs of DJD have developed. The arthroscope is inserted in the dorsal pouch on the side opposite the lesion, and the limb is flexed to expose the cyst. A small curette is directed into the cyst from an ipsilateral dorsal approach to remove contents and debride the cartilage edges. Some cysts cannot be reached by arthroscopy because the joint cannot be maximally flexed with the arthroscope in place. In these cases, the arthroscope can be removed, the limb forcibly flexed, and a small arthrotomy made directly over the cystic opening into the joint.

Proximal phalanx cysts cannot be reached by an articular approach, because the weight-bearing surface is fully articulating and cannot be exposed by altering joint position. These cysts can be surgically debrided from an extraarticular approach. A small 2.7-mm drill bit is directed to enter the cyst from the dorsal surface of the first phalanx. Radiographic or fluoroscopic control is required to ensure entrance into the cyst and to avoid the joint (Fig. 8.204). The cyst can be decompressed and debrided from this approach.

Relieving the intraosseus pressure has the immediate effect of improving lameness in early cases and can produce dramatic clinical improvement. Some articular cartilage damage is expected to remain and an adequate rest period is recommended for cartilage healing. Use of postoperative systemic medication and follow-up intraarticular medication to support joint healing is indicated (see Chapter 7).

Prognosis

The prognosis for return to performance appears to be good. In one report, surgical treatment of third metacarpal subchondral cystic lesions allowed 80% of horses (12/15) to return to their intended use.[1] However horses intended for elite performance—such as racing or national-level competition for cutting, western riding, or three-day eventing—are unlikely to stay sound in my opinion. Follow-up radiographs assist with this prognosis, because osteophyte formation and signs of DJD develop 1 to 2 years after the onset of clinical signs.

The prognosis for proximal phalanx cysts is, in my opinion, slightly lower than metacarpal cysts, particularly if they are traumatically induced. Horses usually dramatically improve in lameness after surgery and usually become sound to the trot, but lameness can recur when returned to heavy training.

Reference

1. Hogan PM, McIlwraith CW, Honnas CM, et al. Surgical treatment of subchondral cystic lesions of the third metacarpal bone: Results in 15 horses (1986–1994). Equine Vet J 1997;29(6):477–482.

TRAUMATIC RUPTURE OF THE SUSPENSORY APPARATUS

Traumatic rupture of the suspensory apparatus with or without fractures of both proximal sesamoid bones is a common cause of acute breakdown in the racing Thoroughbred and often results in humane destruction of the animal.[1,4] Proximal luxations of the sesamoid bone without fracture can also occur with traumatic rup-

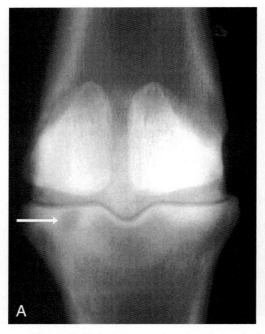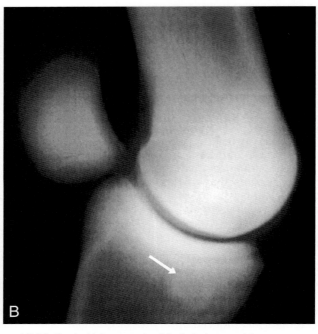

Figure 8.204 Intraoperative view demonstrating a drill bit directed into a proximal first phalanx cyst to decompress the cyst and allow a portal for curettage.

ture of the distal sesamoid ligament. Transverse or comminuted fractures of the proximal sesamoid bones can result in distraction of these bones. The apical portions are drawn proximally by the pull of the sesamoid ligament, whereas the basilar fragments remain attached to the distal sesamoid ligaments (Fig. 8.194). Occasionally, open luxation of the fetlock joint can occur. Besides the severe trauma sustained by the supporting soft tissues and bone, the adjacent digital arteries are frequently damaged sufficiently to result in ischemic necrosis of the hoof. Treatment of traumatic rupture of suspensory apparatus should be considered only as a salvage for valuable breeding horses or for animals with great sentimental value.[1]

Causes

The extreme overextension of the fetlock is the likely cause for disruption of the suspensory apparatus. Preexisting pathology of the bones or suspensory ligament do not have to be present for this catastrophic failure to occur. However, an abnormal finding in the suspensory ligament found on prerace inspection by a regulatory veterinarian was associated with a 3.4-fold increase in the risk of injury in future races, compared with a control population.[2] Factors that increase the strain on the flexor surface of the limb are expected to increase the risk of suspensory apparatus failure. Indeed, Thoroughbred horses racing with low toe grabs were 6.5 times more likely and those with full toe grabs were 15.6 times more likely to incur a fatal suspensory apparatus injury than horses without toe grabs.[5]

Signs

On gross observation, the affected fetlock will be swollen, and the horse is usually bearing its entire weight on the unaffected limb. The lameness will be obvious; and if the animal transfers its weight to the affected limb, the fetlock will sink to the ground. Palpation often reveals the proximal displacement of either the intact sesamoid bone or the apical fractured fragment. Immediate stabilization of the limb is critical to prevent rupture of the neurovascular bundles. The blood supply to the distal limb can be estimated by palpation of a pulse, the presence of distal bleeding, the use of Doppler devices,[3] or the intravenous injection of 5 g sodium fluorescein.[9] A Wood's ultraviolet lamp is required to document fluorescence of viable tissue if the injection of sodium fluorescein is used. The vascular supply is best evaluated after the horse has been treated for shock and the limb has been stabilized. The initial intense vasoconstriction can be interpreted as lack of blood supply.

Diagnosis

Radiographic examination usually reveals either the proximal displacement of the intact sesamoid bone or proximal displacement of the apical portions of the fractured sesamoid bones (Fig. 8.194). Associated swelling of the soft tissues is also quite evident and preexisting degenerative lesions within the sesamoid bones and fetlock joint may also be present.[10]

Treatment

Treatment should be considered for horses to be used for breeding or that have great sentimental value, because normal gait will not be achieved. Management of the horse on the race track is critical for success in treatment. Emergency crews must immediately restrain the horse and apply secure splints, such as the Leg Saver. Horses should then be moved to a surgical facility for radiographs. Immediate immobilization of the affected limb is required to decrease the chances of further injury to the soft tissue and vascular supply.

Maintaining the splint for 4 to 5 days before selecting the final treatment allows the horse to acclimate to the immobilization and recover from the trauma and allows the clinician to define the extent of skin necrosis and loss of vascular supply accompanying the injury. The arthrodesis procedure does not need to be done immediately, and evaluation of the soft tissue injury, the permanent deficit, and the risk of infection must be conducted to predict the outcome with surgery.

Various treatments that have been used successfully include casting, splinting, and fetlock arthrodesis (Figs. 8.205 to 8.207).[1,3,10] Casting and splinting are aimed at supporting and immobilizing the fetlock until the soft tissues have healed sufficiently to support body weight (ankylosis). A fetlock sling shoe can be used for partial breakdown injuries (Fig. 8.205). The Leg Saver splint is not as rigid as a cast, but allows cleaning and treatment of soft tissue injuries and is designed to assist with fetlock joint support in suspensory apparatus injuries (Fig. 8.206). Ankylosis can also be supported by use of an external fixator placed on the foot and metacarpus to fix the position of the joint during healing. Without other surgical stimulation, fusion will not be complete when

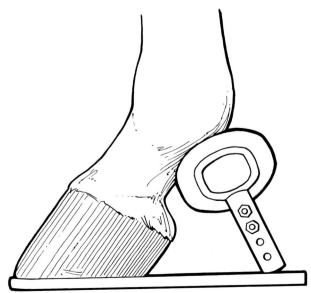

Figure 8.205 A Roberts, or fetlock, sling shoe. The height of the fetlock support can be adjusted. (Courtesy of T. S. Stashak.)

A   B

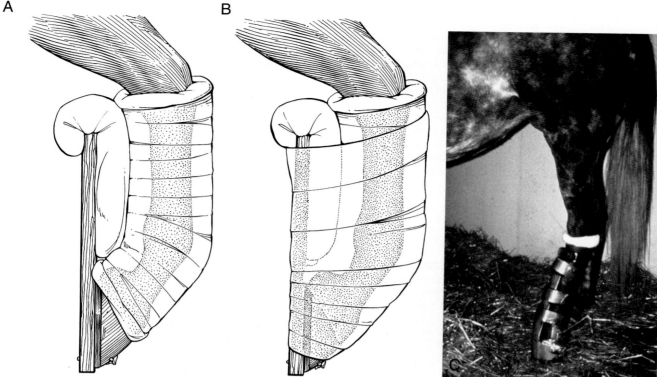

Figure 8.206 A. A heavily bandaged limb with the padded splint brought up to approximate the palmar aspect. B. Complete bandage splint. (Panels A and B are reprinted with permission from Wheat HD, Pascoe JR. A technique for management of traumatic rupture of the equine suspensory apparatus. J Am Vet Med Assoc

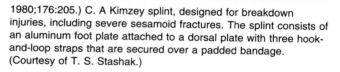

1980;176:205.) C. A Kimzey splint, designed for breakdown injuries, including severe sesamoid fractures. The splint consists of an aluminum foot plate attached to a dorsal plate with three hook-and-loop straps that are secured over a padded bandage. (Courtesy of T. S. Stashak.)

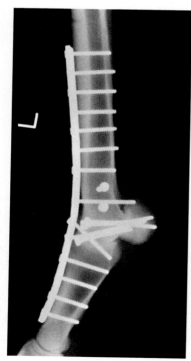

Figure 8.207 Surgical arthrodesis of a fetlock joint with plates and screws to correct a breakdown injury.

the external fixator is removed, and continued coaptation is usually necessary.

Arthrodesis with implants and bone graft can be used to achieve a pain-free stable fusion of the fetlock joint, if the soft tissues are intact and risk of infection is minimal (Fig. 8.207). Since support limb laminitis of the foot of the unaffected limb is a common sequela to this injury, the supporting foot should be supported to distribute loading along the sole (see "Laminitis" in this chapter).

Although casting the limb in flexion can support and immobilize the fetlock until healing has occurred, it is usually associated with severe pressure sores on the back of the sesamoids, which may result in septic osteomyelitis requiring euthanasia.[10] Casting is also expensive and labor intensive, owing to the multiple changes under general anesthesia and the prolonged duration for fusion. After 8 weeks in a cast, the limb is supported in a bulky bandage and a special shoe is applied to elevate the heel. The height of the heel is gradually lowered in increments over 4 weeks, until finally only a wedge is required. The support bandages are usually required for at least an additional 3 weeks after the cast is removed, but they also may be needed for longer periods if pressure sores persist.

Unfortunately, many horses succumb to supporting limb laminitis during the fusion process. Other methods of supporting the limb with weight bearing on the toe (splints) and with sling support shoes can achieve success, but continual monitoring and aftercare are required for an extended duration (Fig. 8.205). Of 25 cases managed conservatively, 15 survived. Complications were similar to the surgical techniques and included pressure sores, osteomyelitis, avascular necrosis, and supporting limb laminitis.[8]

Surgical arthrodesis of the fetlock should be considered in acute cases with intact skin that have not developed wounds during the initial management of the soft tissues and in chronic cases that fail to fuse or that develop chronic joint pain (Fig. 8.207). The goals of surgical arthrodesis are to stabilize the joint rigidly in a neutral position, support osteoinduction, and provide comfort during the healing process. The most popular method is the use of a single 14-hole broad plate secured with 5.5- and 4.5-mm cortical screws spanning the dorsal surface of the metacarpus, fetlock joint, and proximal phalanx. If the suspensory apparatus is disrupted, the palmar tension band must be reestablished or the plate will bend when loaded. The palmar tension band can be reestablished by securing dorsal 4.5-mm cortical screws into the sesamoid bones adjacent to the plate for avulsions proximal to the sesamoid bones or into the apex of the sesamoid bones. For injuries without intact sesamoid bones and for disruption of the distal sesamoid ligaments, a tension band wire must be placed around the palmar surface of the joint.[1]

In this technique, the horse is placed in lateral recumbency with the affected limb up so that a dorsolateral approach can be made through the lateral digital extensor tendon. The fetlock joint is exposed through an incision that extends from the proximal cannon bone to the coronary band and from under the periosteum. The tissues are reflected medially as one layer to expose the dorsal surface. The plate is contoured to 15° extension and should engage as much of the metacarpus as possible without ending at the top of the cast. To remove all articular cartilage in the fetlock joint, the joint is luxated by transection of the collateral ligament. An osteotomy of the lateral condyle can also be performed to gain joint access. Subchondral drilling of the metacarpal condyle can be performed if desired to expose osteogenic cells to the joint surface.

A bone plate is then conformed to the dorsal surface of the proximal phalanx and secured to it with four screws. The palmar tension band is then established by either placing the dorsal cortical screws into the sesamoid bones or by drilling a 2.0-mm hole through the metacarpus and proximal phalanx from lateral to medial and threading an 18-gauge wire in a figure-eight pattern behind the joint. Both these techniques are placed and ultimately secured in slight flexion so that extension tightens the palmar tension band.

If an osteotomy was performed, the condyle is now replaced and reattached by intrafragmental compression through the previously drilled holes. The tension band wire is tightened over the palmar or plantar aspect of the fetlock. The conformed bone plate is attached to the dorsal surface of the cannon bone. Soft tissues are apposed over a suction drain and plate, and the rest of the closure is performed in a routine manner.

A cast is applied that includes the foot and extends to just below the carpus or tarsus. The cast is removed in 14 days and reapplied only if required. Minimal coaptation is usually needed after cast removal, making the aftercare simple. With this technique, the functional length of the limb is slightly increased; but it takes only a short period for the animal to adapt. In most cases reported, the technique has provided a pain-free functional limb that can withstand weight bearing. Because the fetlock is fused, it cannot be flexed. Horses can be turned out after 4 months of healing. It will take 6 to 12 months for fusion to be complete.

The use of external fixation to immobilize the fetlock and subsequently allow ankylosis, or combined with bone graft to stimulate ankylosis, is an alternative to internal fixation for rupture of the suspensory apparatus. A transfixation device places three parallel 9.6-mm threaded transfixation pins in the metacarpus and attaches an aluminum foot plate with a tubular frame distally. The vertical bars are linked to the transfixation pins, using a filled polyurethane material that is poured into the tubular frame in liquid form. The dorsal fetlock joint is opened surgically to remove the articular cartilage and to place the bone graft. The construct provides rigid fixation of the fetlock joint for fusion and permits access to wounds and infected tissues. The fixator can be maintained for 6 to 8 weeks, but fracture through the pin tracts can occur.

In nine horses, four were successfully managed with this technique and two survived with fair results.[7] External fixation offers an advantage over internal fixation for treatment of suspensory apparatus ruptures with open wounds or infected ischemic soft tissues. Horses are comfortable in the frame, reducing the risk of supporting limb laminitis.

Techniques and materials to replace the suspensory apparatus have been investigated by placing a thick braided nonabsorbable material (aramid yarn) secured to the metacarpus with a screw, tunneled along the back of the fetlock joint and secured to the proximal phalanx with a screw.[6] The strength of the repair was significantly less than control limbs, with failure reported as fracture through the screw holes. The braided material induced significant granulomatous reaction in the tissues caudal to the joint. Other materials have not yet been evaluated.

Prognosis

The prognosis appears to be good for pasture and breeding soundness with preselection of cases. With arthrodesis, 32 of 54 horses with fusion of the fetlock survived and were eventually allowed unrestricted activity.[1] The prognosis is better for horses in which fetlock arthrodesis is elected as the primary treatment rather than as a last resort and is better for horses in which fusion is elected for osteoarthritis rather than rupture of the suspensory apparatus. The success rate increases if no signs of supporting laminitis are apparent at the time of surgery.

References

1. Bramlage LR. Fetlock arthrodesis. In: Nixon AJ, Ed. Equine Fracture Repair. Philadelphia: WB Saunders, 1996;17:172.
2. Cohen ND, Peloso JG, Mundy GD, et al. Racing-related factors and results of prerace physical inspection and their association with musculoskeletal injuries incurred in Thoroughbreds during races. J Am Vet Med Assoc 1997;211(4):454.

3. Haynes PF. Disease of the fetlock and metacarpus. Vet Clin North Am Large Anim Pract [Special Edition: Symposium on Equine Lameness] 1980;2:43.
4. Johnson BJ, et al. Equine Vet J 1994.
5. Kane AJ, Stover SM, Gardner IA, et al. Horseshoe characteristics as possible risk factors for fatal musculoskeletal injury of Thoroughbred racehorses. Am J Vet Res 1996;57(8):1147.
6. Major MD, Grant BED, White KK et al. Suspensory apparatus prosthesis in the horse. Part I: In vitro mechanical properties. Vet Surg 1992;21(2):126.
7. Richardson DW, Nunamaker DM, Sigafoos RD. Use of an external skeletal fixation device and bone graft for arthrodesis of the metacarpophalangeal joint in horses. J Am Vet Med Assoc 1987;191(3):316.
8. Snyder JR, Wheat JD, Bleifer D. Conservative management of metacarpophalangeal joint instability. Am Assoc Equine Pract 1986;357.
9. Stashak TS. Traumatic rupture of the suspensory apparatus. In: Stashak TS, Ed. Adams' Lameness in Horses. 4th ed. Philadelphia: Lea & Febiger, 1987;584–587.
10. Wheat HD, Pascoe JR. A technique for management of traumatic rupture of the equine suspensory apparatus. J Am Vet Med Assoc 1980;176:205.

LATERAL AND MEDIAL LUXATION OF THE METACARPOPHALANGEAL AND METATARSOPHALANGEAL JOINTS (FETLOCK LUXATION)

Lateral and medial luxation of the fetlock joint occurs uncommonly but is a recognized syndrome that can affect all ages and breeds of horses. Usually, either the lateral or the medial collateral ligament is ruptured, creating an obvious varus or valgus deformity of the fetlock region.[4,6] Occasionally, avulsion fracture associated with the insertion of these ligaments or joint capsule may occur and be noted on the radiograph proximal to the joint space (Fig. 8.208). Articular fractures of the palmar–plantar eminence may also accompany the luxation.[2] Both forelimbs and hindlimbs can be affected with luxation and the joint was open in half of 10 reported cases.[4,6] The diagnosis is quite obvious, because an angular deviation of the fetlock joint is present.

Occasionally, the luxation reduces spontaneously and only a lateral or medial swelling is noticed. Immediately after the injury, if the luxation is reduced, some horses will be minimally lame and appear sound at the walk. Reluxation can occur at any moment if the joint is not stabilized, until the swelling and pain begin to protect the joint. Physical manipulation of the fetlock in these cases clarifies the suspicion of luxation. Typically, the joint reluxates when it is flexed and abducted away from the side of injury.

Subluxations of the fetlock joint resulting from flexure deformity of the limb are covered in Chapter 7. Fetlock luxation resulting from traumatic rupture of the suspensory apparatus is covered in "Traumatic Rupture of the Suspensory Apparatus" in this chapter.

Causes

This injury frequently occurs when the horse steps in a hole or gets its foot caught between two immovable objects. The luxation results when the horse attempts to gain freedom. Owners frequently relate the history of finding the horse caught in this situation. Occasionally,

horses spontaneously luxate their fetlock during high-speed activities (e.g., racing, rodeo eventing) or after running into an object.[4]

Signs

The clinical signs are usually obvious and help differentiate this injury from fracture.[1] A varus angular deformity (outward deviation of the cannon bone and inward deviation of the digit) or valgus angular deformity (inward deviation of the cannon bone and outward deviation of the digit) is usually present. Sometimes, the luxation reduces spontaneously and the remaining evidence of its occurrence is lameness, joint instability, and swelling over the torn collateral ligament.

On palpation, the fetlock can be reduced and reluxated without the degree of pain or evidence of crepitation associated with fracture. Most frequently, the swelling is less than that observed with fracture and is located selectively over the lateral or medial surface. Although the digital vascular supply is rarely compromised, it should be carefully evaluated, particularly in open luxations.

Diagnosis

Generally, the diagnosis can be made by physical examination alone. However, radiographs should be taken to identify an avulsion fracture, intraarticular fractures, or damage to the articular surface that has entered into the subchondral bone (Fig. 8.208B). Radiographs are particularly important in young foals to rule out the possibility of growth plate fractures as a primary or a secondary cause of the angular deformity.

Treatment

Treatment of simple luxation of the fetlock can be rewarding. In most cases, the injury is limited to the supporting soft tissues; and after the luxation is reduced under anesthesia, good axial alignment can be maintained by casting or splinting the limb until healing occurs. Before applying the cast, needle drainage of any hematoma overlying the ruptured collateral ligament provides a better fit for the cast. This area should be clipped and shaved and aseptically prepared before percutaneous puncture and aspiration. Although centesis of the hematoma and cast application can be performed in the standing horse, general anesthesia and lateral recumbency are preferred. Reduction of the luxation is usually not difficult. A cast is applied that incorporates the foot and extends to just below the carpus or tarsus in the adult. Alternatively, a cast that does not encase the foot can be used. Casts or splints are maintained for 6 weeks with stall rest. After cast or splint removal, bandage support and limited exercise are recommended. Initially, the horse appears stiff, but it soon feels free to flex its fetlocks. Only slight swelling (thickening) will be noticed over the area of collateral ligament rupture, and a cosmetic blemish will remain.

Success can be achieved without suture of the collateral ligament, although several reports exist in the litera-

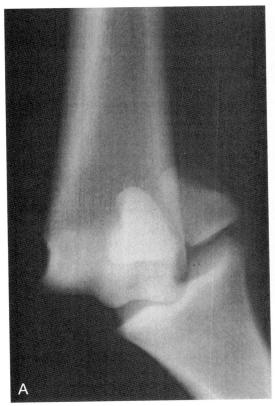

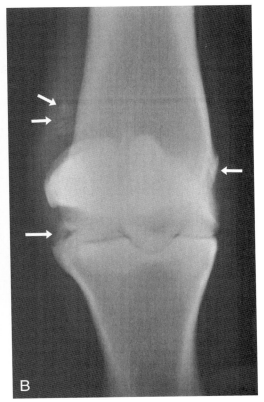

Figure 8.208 A. Subluxation of the fetlock joint with rupture of the lateral and medial collateral ligaments. (Courtesy of T. S. Stashak.) B. Craniocaudal view after reduction, demonstrating the classical bony lesions, including a plantar eminence fracture of the first phalanx (lower left arrow), a bone fragment attached to the proximal end of the displaced medial collateral ligament (upper left arrows), and a fracture at the origin of the lateral collateral ligament (right arrow).

ture for open repair. To repair the ligament, the end is located after surgical incision, debrided, and sutured.[6] Alternatively, a polypropylene mesh has been substituted for the ruptured ligament and incorporated into the healing under a cast.[5] Arthroscopic removal of the articular fractures should be elected if full athletic performance is a goal. For light riding soundness, it is not necessary if the fragments are small and from the palmar–plantar eminence.

Acute open luxations can also be handled successfully.[4] However, before immobilization, thorough debridement of all devitalized soft tissues, bone, and cartilage should be performed. Copious amounts of sterile balanced electrolyte solution are flushed through the joint with a needle placed in a site remote to the injury to remove the debris. It is important that all recesses within the joint capsule be thoroughly cleaned and debrided. Flushing may be completed with 1 liter 10% DMSO solution followed by the instillation of a broad-spectrum antimicrobial in the synovial cavity. If the joint is minimally contaminated and was treated immediately, a primary suture apposition of the soft tissues is recommended.

A sterile bandage that is thick enough to absorb and lift the drainage from the wound surface is applied. A lower limb cast is then applied similarly to that previously described. The cast is removed in 4 to 7 days, and the wound is reexamined. The decision is made at that time regarding the advisability of delayed primary closure or recasting over a sterile bandage and relying on secondary intention healing for wound closure. Casts are required in most cases for at least 6 weeks. During that time, the horse is confined to a dry box stall and treated with the appropriate broad-spectrum antibiotics and analgesics.

Chronic severe injuries such as traumatic rupture of the suspensory apparatus or luxation combined with extensive fracture can best be managed with surgical arthrodesis. In open fractures/luxations an external fixator may be necessary. Immediate bone grafting and removal of cartilage and damaged bone may need to be done (see "Traumatic Rupture of the Suspensory Apparatus" in this chapter) (Fig. 8.209).

Prognosis

The prognosis for simple luxation of the fetlock is good for breeding soundness but guarded for athletic performance. In one report, 7 of 10 horses, some with open luxations, could be used for breeding, and 1 horse was riding sound.[6] However, the final decision should be made regarding the outcome after follow-up radiographs are taken at 2 months. Immediate stabilization of the joint permits healing without the development of DJD. Lack of stabilization or unrecognized luxation results in osteoarthritis in horses allowed exercise.[3]

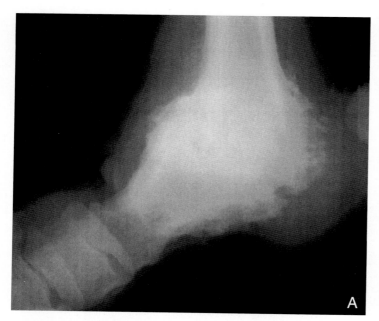

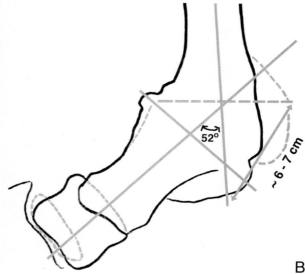

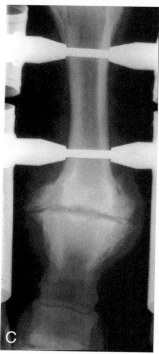

Figure 8.209   A. Chronic fetlock luxation with malunion ankylosis of the joint. B. Radiographic measurements for a wedge ostectomy to straighten the limb. C. Postoperative view demonstrating completion of the wedge ostectomy, straightening of the limb, and application of a Nunamaker transfixation pin and foot plate device.

Acute open luxations exposing the fetlock joint also respond well to early therapy, as described. However, one always has to be reserved in giving a good prognosis until joint infection and DJD from direct trauma have been ruled out as complications. The long-term outlook for return to serviceability depends totally on the degree of initial trauma sustained by the bone. Follow-up radiographs in 3 to 4 months can help one give a realistic prognosis.

References

1. Fessler JF, Amstutz HE. Fracture repair. In: Oehme FW, Prier JE, Eds. Textbook of Large Animal Surgery. Baltimore: Williams & Wilkins, 1974;260–339.
2. Moore RM, Weisbrode SE, Biller DS, et al. Metacarpal fracture associated with lymphosarcoma-induced osteolysis in a horse. J Am Vet Med Assoc 1995;207:208–210.
3. Simmon EJ, Bertone AL, Weisbrode SE. Instability-induced osteoarthritis in the metacarpophalangeal joint of horses. Am J Vet Res 1999;60(1):7.
4. Stashak TS. Lateral and medial luxation of the metacarpophalangeal and metatarsophalangeal joints. In: Stashak TS, Ed. Adams' Lameness in Horses. 4th ed. Philadelphia: Lea & Febiger, 1987;587–589.
5. Van der Harst MR, Rijkenhuizen AB. The use of polypropylene mesh for treatment of ruptured collateral ligaments of the equine metatarsophalangeal joint: A report of 2 cases. Vet Q 2000;22(1):57.
6. Yovich JV, Turner AS, Stashak TS, McIlwraith CW. Luxation of the metacarpophalangeal and metatarsophalangeal joints in horses. Equine Vet J 1987;19(4):295.

ANGULAR LIMB DEFORMITIES ASSOCIATED WITH THE METACARPOPHALANGEAL AND METATARSOPHALANGEAL JOINTS (FETLOCK DEVIATION)

An angular deformity refers to a deviation of a limb in the frontal plane defined by the joint or bone that is at the center (pivot point) of the deviation. If the limb distal to the pivot point is axial (medial), the deviation is varus. If the limb distal to the pivot point is abaxial (lateral), the deviation is valgus. For example, fetlock varus refers to an outward deviation of the distal part of the cannon bone and an inward deviation of the phalanges and is the most common deviation of this joint (Fig. 8.210A).[1,8] Valgus refers to the opposite situation, in which there is an inward deviation of the cannon bone and outward deviation of the phalanges, the most common deviation of the carpus. Varus deformities of the fetlock may develop independently of or in association with carpal valgus.

Angular limb deformities are being treated with increased frequency in foals of all breeds, because the surgical correction is effective and relatively simple. Metacarpophalangeal and metatarsophalangeal deviations are much less common than carpal deformity (12% of foal angular deformities).[1,8] Foals can either be born with angular deformity (congenital) or develop the angular deformity shortly after birth (acquired). The angular deformity of many foals straightens out on its own in a short period of time and does not require treatment. In others, the angular deformity either remains static or worsens, and these usually require treatment. Foals that are born with straight limbs and acquire an angular limb deformity as they mature most often require the assistance of a veterinarian. Some cases can present with multiple limb and joint involvement, such as carpus valgus and tarsus valgus or carpus valgus and fetlock varus.

Regardless of the situation, it is most important to correct the angular limb deformity well in advance of growth plate closure and early enough to prevent secondary changes to the joints and bones distal to it. Early treatment is particularly important for the fetlock because, unlike the carpus, treatment within the first 3 to 5 weeks of life is necessary for a successful outcome. The reason is twofold: 1) The growth of the distal end of the cannon bone rapidly slows at 90 days and is virtually nonexistent at 120 days and 2) the distal growth plate of the cannon bone accounts for only 5% of growth in the total length of the bone.[4] In general, the ideal time for treatment is within the first 30 days of life, because after 60 to 80 days the deviation will be virtually uncorrectable by conventional means.[8] Deviation present after closure of the growth plate requires a wedge ostectomy to regain axial alignment.[6]

Causes

The cause of angular limb deformity appears to be complex and multifactorial. The morphologic changes associated with angular deformity of the fetlock include the following:

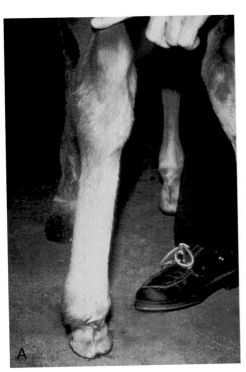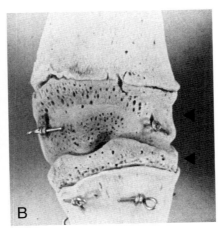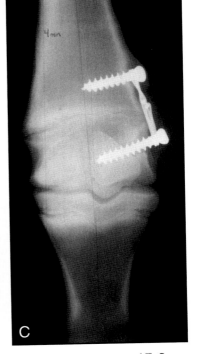

Figure 8.210 A. A 6-week-old foal with severe fetlock varus of the hindlimb. B. Dried bone specimen of the fetlock of a 3-month-old foal. Note the wedging of the epiphysis of the distal end of the metacarpus (upper arrow) and the proximal end of the proximal phalanx (lower arrow). (Panel B is provided courtesy of T. S. Stashak.) C. Postsurgical view demonstrating placement of the screw and wire for the transphyseal bridging technique.

- Asymmetric growth of the metaphysis of the cannon bone
- Wedging of the epiphysis
- Asymmetric longitudinal growth of the phalanges
- A degree of joint laxity, which may be present particularly in very young foals

Accompanying the asymmetric growth may be varying degrees of defective endochondral ossification.[9] Many of the factors for this entity are the same as those observed with angular limb deformity associated with the carpus (see "Angular Limb Deformities Associated with the Carpus" in this chapter).

Signs

To evaluate foals for angular limb deformity, it is necessary to get them on a clean, flat surface in a calm environment that allows visualization from all angles. When the limb is straight and weight bearing, an imaginary plumb line can be dropped through the center of the limb from the top to the bottom, dividing the limb into two halves. It will be clear if the foal has an angular deformity and, if so, whether it is valgus or varus. Rotational deformities, which often occur with angular deformities, can also be estimated; but they are not corrected by the treatments outlined in this chapter, and the owner should be so notified. All four limbs and all joints should be evaluated.

On visual observation, the degree of deviation and the pivotal point (center of deviation) can be roughly estimated. The foal should be exercised to gain an appreciation for any lameness and joint laxity. This can be difficult to appreciate with very active foals. In most cases, it is best to walk the mare slowly away from the foal and attempt to make this observation as the foal trots toward the dam. If a unilateral angular limb deformity of the fetlock is present, the examiner should pay close attention to the limb opposite the angular deformity. The affected limb should be palpated for heat and pain on pressure as well as for swelling. Manipulation by flexion, extension, and rotation is important to evaluate pain and joint laxity. Perineural anesthesia and intrasynovial anesthesia are rarely indicated in these cases.

Diagnosis

A good radiographic study is important to characterize the angular deformity and to identify morphologic changes within the bones and soft tissues. In general, the dorsal palmar, dorsal plantar, and lateral medial views will suffice in most cases. Cassettes (7 by 17 inches), should be used (see Chapter 4). The pivot point (axis of deviation) can be determined by placing an overlay of acetate or undeveloped x-ray film on the dorsal palmar radiograph. Two lines are drawn to bisect the cannon bone and the other line bisects the proximal phalanx. The point at which these lines intersect (axis of deviation) is referred to as the pivot point.

The pivot point is important to determine, because it helps identify the underlying cause of the angular defor-

mity. If the pivot point is located close to the growth plate (metaphyseal or epiphyseal side) then the probable cause of the angular limb deformity is asynchronous growth in the distal metacarpal metaphysis. If the pivot point is closer to the fetlock, then there may be wedging of the epiphysis or asymmetric growth of the proximal end of the proximal phalanx (Fig. 8.210B). The angle of deviation can also be calculated or measured with a protractor from this pivotal point.

The morphologic changes commonly observed on radiographic examination with angular deformities of the fetlock include the following:

- Metaphyseal flaring and metaphyseal sclerosis
- Widening of the growth plate
- Wedging of the epiphysis
- Asymmetric growth of the proximal phalanx, often associated with similar changes in the distal cannon bone area
- Osteochondrosis-like lesions of the cannon bone or proximal phalanx

Both the morphologic findings and the identification of the pivot point are important when deciding what course of treatment should be selected and for helping predict the eventual outcome.

Treatment

Congenital Form

Foals with the congenital form are born with the deformity. If it is mild to moderate, confinement of the mare and foal to a stall will allow rapid (within 7 to 10 days) correction of the deformity as the ligaments mature and strengthen. If the problem is severe, worsens within days, or does not improve, treatment should begin. Radiographs should be taken to determine if and how severe the delayed endochondral ossification is. The limb should be examined to see if it is manually reducible. If the deformity is reducible (as may occur in the carpus) and, therefore, attributed to ligamentous laxity, treatment consists of reducing the limb and applying sleeve casts for 10 to 14 days, until mineralization of the bones occurs (see "Carpal Angular Limb Deformity").

In the fetlock, congenital angular deformities are rarely reducible and thus, if severe or worsening, surgical intervention is required. It is unlikely that an angular deformity in excess of 5° in the fetlock will correct fully on its own with conservative management. Early intervention is recommended—surgical hemicircumferential transection of the periosteum (HCTP) and periosteal stripping (PS) by 1 or 2 weeks[2]—and, if significant deformity persists, transphyseal bridging (screw and figure-eight wire) by 1 month (Fig. 8.210C).[1] Diaphyseal deformities of the cannon bone can occur, usually in the hindlimb. Surgical intervention should include not only HCTP and PS just proximal to the distal metacarpal/metatarsal growth plate but also stripping of the diaphysis to stimulate bone modeling. To assist with correction of fetlock deformities, HCTP and PS can also be performed in the proximal phalanx growth plate.

Developmental Form

Foals with the developmental form acquire the condition during the first few months of life. Reducing exercise, feed intake, and body weight may improve mildly affected foals. Foals with more severe cases that worsen, and/or that don't improve with conservative management need surgery. For the carpus and hock, surgery is best performed between 1 and 4 months of age, but growth at the distal radius occurs up to 16 months, and correction can be achieved in older foals with screws and wires and periosteal stripping simultaneously. Surgery of the fetlock is best performed by 1 month of age because the distal third metacarpal/metatarsal growth plate is physiologically closed by 3 months.

Surgery for nonreducible angular limb deformity consists of HCTP and PS for most cases in which the foal is less than 1 month old and has a deformity that is less than 5°. This is a simple procedure performed on the shorter side just proximal to the growth plate. A small, cosmetic skin incision is made 3 cm proximal to the widest point of the fetlock (the growth plate) and then extended deep to bone. The periosteum is transected hemicircumferentially and elevated to release that side of the growth plate mechanically and to stimulate growth. It is theorized that the periosteum represents a restrictive fibroelastic tube that not only surrounds the diaphysis of the long bone but also connects the proximal and distal epiphysis, which places it under tension. For longitudinal bone growth to occur, the fibroelastic tube must stretch and grow in synchrony with the longitudinal bone growth. When the periosteum is transected hemicircumferentially, it reduces the tension at the growth plate, and rapid longitudinal bone growth will occur. This tension theory is substantiated by the fact that when the periosteum is transected horizontally to the long axis just up above the growth plate, a 5-mm gap appears as the periosteal edges separate.

The surgery for the fetlock is performed slightly more proximal to the growth plate than in the carpus, because of the wide perichondrium around the fetlock. If the perichondrium is elevated, more periosteal bone reaction occurs and slightly more blemish can result. Correction is best achieved in foals less than 1 month of age and can be performed in foals as young as several days of age. The ideal time is 2 to 4 weeks of life. Satisfactory correction is achieved in 75% of foals, and the surgery can be repeated if necessary in 30 to 45 days. The blemish is minimal and can be minimized by placing the incision just palmar–plantar to the lateral border of the limb.

One report noted race follow-up of affected foals compared with their siblings. Horses treated with distal metacarpal/metatarsal HCPT had fewer 2-year-old starts (1.09 versus 2.19) but did not have a significantly lower starting percentage compared with values for controls.[7]

For foals older than 1 to 2 months with fetlock angular deformities greater than 5° or with severe windswept conditions, transphyseal bridging can be performed either as the sole procedure or in conjunction with HCTP and PS. Windswept conditions (congenital angular limb deformity secondary to uterine malpositioning) may be particularly difficult to correct because the entire fetlock joint structure may be malformed, including a tighter joint capsule on the shorter side of the limb. Transphyseal bridging is performed on the longer side of the growth plate and arrests growth on that side. The growth plate is bridged by an implant (usually a screw and wire; sometimes with staples and plates) (Fig. 8.210C). The disadvantages of this technique include more blemish, the cost of the implants, the necessity to remove the implant when correction occurs (or the limb will overcorrect), and the need for the equipment. Success, however, is almost always complete. HCTP and PS are often not necessary when performing transphyseal bridging, but if there is concern about obtaining full correction, all procedures should be used.

Early correction of the angular deformity associated with the fetlock region is important because of the relatively short period of time with which rapid longitudinal growth from the growth plate occurs.[5] Furthermore, there is a limited gain in total length. An analysis of a series of foals treated by transphyseal bridging of the distal growth plate of the cannon bone indicated that after 60 to 80 days there is virtually no improvement in the angular deformity.[4] It was also shown that a maximum of 12° correction could be expected if the transphyseal bridging was performed at 14 days of age.[4] It can be construed that foals with deviations greater than 12° will not achieve complete correction from transphyseal bridging. Therefore, it is of utmost importance to have foals examined by the veterinarian as soon as the angular deformity is recognized.

Correctional management of the foal should occur simultaneously with surgical treatment and includes confined exercise, regular rasping of the hooves to balance the foot, and reduction of creep feeding to decrease the odds of physitis complicating the correction. Use of casts or splints to force the nonreducible limbs to grow straight can and have worked but are now less commonly elected. The reasons include the simplicity and success of the HCTP and PS and the difficult management of splints in foals. Pressure sores from the casts and splints may leave a worse blemish than the deformity or surgical scar, and the bandages used under the splints are expensive.

Initial confinement is recommended to control the forces on the growth plate. If these forces become excessive, as when the foal runs on pasture, the compression trauma to the medial side may be sufficient to arrest or delay the growth of the growth plate. This results in perpetuation or worsening of the angular deformity. On the other hand, focal physiologic axial compression forces focused on the medial aspect of the growth plate result in stimulation in long-bone growth, with eventual straightening. Therefore, stall confinement serves to shift the potential pathologic compressive forces into the physiologic range (see "Angular Limb Deformities Associated with the Carpus" in this chapter).

Corrective trimming balances the foot and assists in proper alignment of the limb. With a varus deformity of the fetlock, increased wear is noted on the lateral side (outside) of the hoof wall compared to the medial side. If this is allowed to remain, the compressive forces continue to be increased on the medial (inside) side of the growth plate. Trimming the foot to base level (balancing the foot) distributes the pressure more equally across the growth plate. Nutritional management should include good-quality alfalfa, a 2:1 calcium to phosphorus ratio, and free-choice balanced minerals and should restrict concentrates (see Chapter 5).

For foals that fail to respond and still have significant deformity or for foals older than 120 days, a wedge or step ostectomy can successfully manage the condition.[3,6] If, however, the deformity has persisted for years, subsequent malformation of the hoof and distal phalanges may be so extreme that correction of the fetlock angle may make the horse more lame. The following criteria are used to select foals for surgery:

- Older than 120 days
- Greater than 8° deviation of the limb
- Soundness not expected without treatment
- No lameness or DJD of the fetlock

The wedge osteotomy in all cases has been performed on the convex side. It is recommended that it be performed at least 4 cm proximal to the growth plate of the cannon bone to decrease the trauma to vital joint structures. After the osteotomy, internal fixation is achieved with bone plates, after which casts are applied for some period of time.[6] Out of 15 horses that received step ostectomy for permanent angular limb deformity, 12 survived with pain-free use of their limbs, three procedures were performed for fetlock angular limb deformity, the others for fracture malunion.[3]

Prognosis

The prognosis is good to excellent for straightening of the fetlocks in cases in which the angular limb deformity is mild (less than 5°) and the result of asymmetric growth of the distal/tarsal metaphysis in a young foal. The prognosis becomes guarded to poor for complete straightening of the angular deviation if it is severe (greater than 12°), the growth plate of the proximal phalanx is severely affected and the joint is malformed, a severe windswept condition exists, the foal is already 3 months of age, or osteochondrosis lesions are present.

References

1. Auer JA. Periosteal transection of the proximal phalanx in foals with angular limb deformities of the metacarpo/metatarsophalangeal area. J Am Vet Med Assoc 1985;187:496.
2. Auer JA, Martens RJ, Williams EH. Periosteal transection for correction of angular limb deformities in foals. J Am Vet Med Assoc 1982;18:459.
3. Bertone AL, Turner AS, Park RD. Periosteal transection and stripping for treatment of angular limb deformities in foals: clinical observations. J Am Vet Med Assoc 1985;187(2):145.
4. Bramlage LR. Step ostectomy: A surgical technique for correction of permanent angular limb deformities in horses. Am Assoc Equine Pract 1994;111.
5. Campbell JR, Lee R. Radiological estimation of differential growth rates of the long bones of foals. Equine Vet J 1981;13:247.
6. Fretz PB. Angular limb deformities in foals. Vet Clin North Am Large Anim Pract 1980;2:125.
7. Fretz PB, McIlwraith, CW. Wedge osteotomy as a treatment for angular deformity of the fetlock in horses. J Am Vet Med Assoc 1983;182:245.
8. Mitten LA, Bramlage LR, Embertson RM. Racing performance after hemicircumferential periosteal transection for angular limb deformities in Thoroughbreds: 199 cases (1987–1989). J Am Vet Med Assoc 1995;207(6):746.
9. Mitten LA, Bertone AL. Angular limb deformities in foals. J Am Vet Med Assoc 1994;204:717.

CONSTRICTION OF OR BY THE FETLOCK PALMAR–PLANTAR ANULAR LIGAMENT

Constriction of or by the fetlock anular ligament is a relatively common cause of lameness in performance horses. Although all breeds and uses of horses can be affected, sport horses, racehorses, Paso Fino, and Warmblood horses appear to be at a greater risk. In one report, desmitis of the fetlock anular ligament was diagnosed mainly in sport horses and less frequently in racehorses.[10] In an unpublished report on 49 horses taken to Colorado State University Veterinary Teaching Hospital for constriction of or by the fetlock anular ligament, Paso Fino and Warmblood horses were overrepresented (19 and 5 cases, respectively) compared to the rest of the hospitalized patients.[9] Of the horses presented, their uses included pleasure and pleasure show, western competition, untrained breeding stock, racing, endurance, and hunter/jumpers. The mean age at presentation was 8.6 years (range, 1 to 20 years). There was a significantly smaller portion of horses in the 2- to 4-year age group, and a significantly larger proportion of horses older than 10 years.

Anular ligaments are tough, fibrous, thickened, relatively inelastic parts of the fascial tendon sheath strategically located to support the tendons as they course around a joint and to provide a canal for them to glide through. They are lined with synovia and prevent displacement of the tendon, which would reduce its mechanical efficiency. Tendons lying within a tendon sheath and supported by an anular ligament can become enlarged from injury or infection. The anular ligament itself can also be injured, resulting in thickening (desmitis) and a reduction of the diameter of the canal.[8] As a result of either of these situations, compression of the tendon and pressure within the canal subsequently restricts the free gliding function of the tendon, inducing pain and possibly ischemia to the tissues within the canal (tunnel syndrome).

The condition can affect any limb. In a report of 49 horses, the condition was distributed evenly among all four limbs in Quarter Horses, Thoroughbreds, and Arabians; whereas it affected only the rear limb in Paso Fino and Warmblood horses.[9]

Causes

Constriction of or by the fetlock anular ligament usually occurs as a result of trauma and/or infection. The injury may involve the anular ligament primarily, resulting in inflammation and thickening (desmitis) of the structure and producing constriction without abnormalities in other structures within the fetlock canal. Alternatively, the condition may be associated with distal superficial digital flexor tendinitis (low bow). Because the anular ligaments are minimally elastic, swelling of the digital flexors, caused by fibrosis and associated tenosynovitis, can produce signs of constriction of the anular ligament. Inflammation and subsequent scar tissue enlargement often associated with a low flexor tendinitis (low bowed tendon) may extend to involve the palmar or plantar anular ligament, which also results in desmitis. Adhesions may form between the superficial flexor tendon and the anular ligament, further restricting motion. Tendinitis of the deep digital flexor tendon within the fetlock canal enlarges the tendon within the canal, inducing a tenosynovitis and producing the signs of anular ligament constriction. Wounds, such as wire cuts or nail punctures, can occur in the region of the palmar–plantar aspect of the fetlock, producing thickening tenosynovitis and constriction. One report on 49 horses presenting with signs of constriction of or by the anular ligament found that desmitis of the anular ligament was the cause of 55% of cases; tendinitis, of 31%; and sepsis, of 14%.[9]

Biopsies of anular ligaments from horses suffering with fetlock tunnel syndrome reveal an increase in thickness of collagen bundles, loss of parallel alignment of fibers, presence of fibroblastic nuclei, and increased number of blood vessels. This evidence indicates direct trauma and restructuring of the anular ligament.[10] Similar findings were reported in another study of 27 anular ligament biopsies taken from clinically affected horses.[9]

Signs

Horses often present with a history of lameness that increases with exercise, resolves with rest, and returns when put back into performance. The most notable feature of anular ligament constriction is swelling of the palmar–plantar soft tissues of the distal limb around the fetlock and a characteristic observable proximal border of the anular ligament (notching). This notching is caused by anular ligament constriction. In nearly all cases, there is distension of the digital tendon sheath proximal to the anular ligament (Fig. 8.211). Palpation

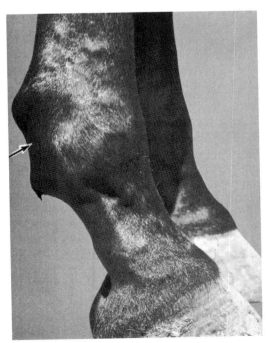

Figure 8.211 Constriction of the anular ligament. Note the notched appearance of the palmar aspect of the fetlock above the ergot. The upper swelling is caused by fluid distension of the flexor tendon sheath.

of the region usually reveals thickening at the junction of the superficial flexor tendon and the anular ligament.

The lameness is characterized by its persistence, failure to improve, pain on fetlock flexion, and worsening with exercise because of inflammation and increased constriction. Lameness is characterized by a decreased extension (dorsiflexion) of the fetlock during weight bearing and a shortened caudal phase to the stride. In the most severe cases, the horse is reluctant to place the heel on the ground and accentuates the cranial phase of the stride to compensate. Continued pressure may produces changes in the digital flexor tendons.[8]

Regional perineural anesthesia, first of the foot and subsequently of the distal metacarpus or metatarsus, eliminates the lameness and locates the source to the region of constriction. Direct anesthesia of the tendon sheath is usually not necessary but could be performed if a fluid sample is obtained for cytology or if the sheath is injected as a conservative treatment. Most horses improve slightly with anesthesia to the sheath; but other structures involved, such as the tendons and anular ligament, may still induce lameness. However, for horses that respond dramatically to tendon sheath anesthesia, arthroscopy of the tendon sheath, rather than simple anular ligament transection, is indicated.

Diagnosis

The physical findings and the results of diagnostic anesthesia provide a presumptive diagnosis. Ultrasonography is indicated to identify the structures involved and to assist with the selection of treatment. Normally, the anular ligament is thin (less than 2 mm) and cannot be distinguished without contrast agents, such as air tenograms. The distance from the skin surface to the palmar–plantar surface of the superficial digital flexor tendon is 3 to 4 mm for the forelimb and 3 to 5 mm for the hindlimb (Lowery J, personal communication). One study found that measurement from the external skin surface to the internal anular ligament surface was the most reproducible index of anular ligament thickening.[9] One report on 49 horses with constriction by or of the anular ligament found that the mean anular ligament thickness measured ultrasonographically was 9.1 mm (±2.3 mm).

A variety of lesions can be identified at ultrasound and can include core tendon lesions or tearing of the deep digital flexor tendon, superficial digital flexor tendinitis and fibrosis, tenosynovitis and synovial proliferation, adhesions, and thickening of the anular ligament. In 16 Warmblood horses with fetlock anular ligament constriction, 9 had thickening of the anular ligament and tenosynovitis, 3 were dominated by distension of the sheath, 3 had superficial digital flexor tendon injury, and 1 had marked synovial sheath proliferation.[3] In racehorses, superficial digital flexor tendinitis may be more commonly associated with fetlock anular ligament constriction.[5] In another report on 49 cases of fetlock anular constriction, 27 horses had thickening of the anular ligament and 15 had tendon injuries.[9]

Radiographic evaluation of the fetlock region should always be performed to evaluate bone involvement, particularly of the sesamoids. In lesions of wound or trauma origin, an osteomyelitis or sequestrum of the sesamoid bones necessitates additional treatment and reduces the prognosis for soundness or elimination of infection. In 38 cases of anular ligament constriction, 6 horses had proximal sesamoid bone abnormality and 12 horses had bone enthesiophytes at the attachment of the anular ligament (insertion desmopathy).[7] Radiography with the use of air tenograms allows the evaluation of the thickness of the anular ligament and the presence of adhesions, but this technique has generally been replaced by ultrasonographic evaluation.[11]

Treatment

Surgical resection of the palmar or plantar anular ligament is the most effective treatment.[1] Adjunctive surgical procedures to treat tendinitis, tendon core lesions, adhesions, and synovial proliferation simultaneously are indicated if the underlying conditions exist. These procedures include accessory ligament desmotomy of the superficial digital flexor tendon, tendon splitting, adhesiolysis, and synovial resection, respectively. Three approaches to performing transection of the anular ligament are described, and the decision to select one over the other depends on concomitant pathology, cost, and available surgical facilities. The three techniques are

open transection, tenoscopic release, and percutaneous transection.

The originally described open transection technique is rarely elected today unless septic tenosynovitis is present and open drainage, lavage, and release of the anular ligament are goals of therapy. Even in those instances, the sheath incision may be made proximal to the anular ligament and the actual transection still performed subcutaneously.[2,6] Limitations of open transection include incisional drainage and dehiscence, limited visibility compared to tenoscopy, and greater soft tissue morbidity.

To perform an open transection of the fetlock anular ligament, the horse is placed under general anesthesia; after proper surgical preparation of the area, an incision is made, preferably on the lateral edge of the superficial flexor tendon (Fig. 8.212) behind the digital vessels and nerves. The incision continues through the palmar or plantar anular ligament and through the digital tendon sheath. If inflammation has been present for some time, the ligament and the tendon sheath cannot be separated and no effort is made to do so. After the palmar or plantar ligament has been completely transected, the deep digital flexor tendon can be inspected for injury and sutured, if necessary, or tendon splitting of core lesions can be performed. Meticulous closure of the subcutaneous

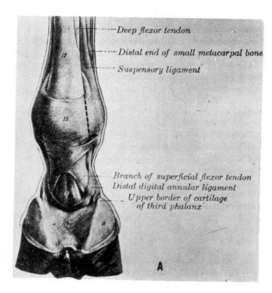
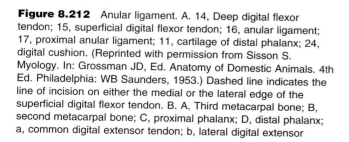
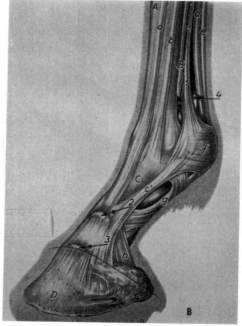

Figure 8.212 Anular ligament. A. 14, Deep digital flexor tendon; 15, superficial digital flexor tendon; 16, anular ligament; 17, proximal anular ligament; 11, cartilage of distal phalanx; 24, digital cushion. (Reprinted with permission from Sisson S. Myology. In: Grossman JD, Ed. Anatomy of Domestic Animals. 4th Ed. Philadelphia: WB Saunders, 1953.) Dashed line indicates the line of incision on either the medial or the lateral edge of the superficial digital flexor tendon. B. A, Third metacarpal bone; B, second metacarpal bone; C, proximal phalanx; D, distal phalanx; a, common digital extensor tendon; b, lateral digital extensor tendon; c, c', suspensory ligament; d, deep flexor tendon; e, superficial flexor tendon; f, anular ligament; g, superficial distal sesamoid ligament; h, ligament to cartilage of distal phalanx; i, joint capsule of metacarpophalangeal (fetlock) joint; 2, proximal interphalangeal (pastern) joint; 3, distal interphalangeal (coffin) joint; 4, tendon sheath of superficial and deep digital flexor tendons. (Reprinted with permission from Topographical Anatomical Diagrams of Injection Technique for Horses. Kansas City, MO: National Laboratories, 1972.)

tissues must be done, because the gaping sheath and fluid will be directly under the incision. The skin is then sutured with a noncapillary, nonabsorbable suture. Postoperative management is critical to prevent incisional leakage, dehiscence, and possible infection. A tight elastic bandage and strict stall confinement are recommended for 7 to 10 days. If synovial leakage is noted, immobilizing the limb in a boot (forelimb) or Leg Saver splint (hindlimb) will permit primary healing (Fig. 8.206C).[4]

To perform the percutaneous approach to transection, a small incision (1 to 2 cm long) is made at the proximal limits of the anular ligament down through the ligament to expose the tendon. A straight pair of Mayo scissors is then used to make a subcutaneous tunnel over the ligament and then to cut the ligament, leaving the overlying subcutaneous tissue and skin intact. (A curved blunt-tipped bistoury can be used instead of the Mayo scissors.) Suture closure in these cases is relatively quick, so there is less chance of incisional dehiscence.

The horse is put in a snug-fitting support wrap of elastic gauze and tape or medicated gauze bandage. Exercise can begin in 3 days with this approach, by hand walking the horse and gradually increasing exercise so that the adhesions will not unite the incised edges of the anular ligament. Antibiotics are optional, and nonsteroidal anti-inflammatory drugs (NSAIDs) are usually administered. This technique is inexpensive and can be performed standing, if necessary, but visibility of tendon or tendon sheath structures is not attained.

For endoscopic transection of the fetlock anular ligament, the horse is placed under general anesthesia and prepared as described earlier. The arthroscope portal is made distal to the fetlock joint on the side of the deep flexor tendon in the small space distal to the palmar anular ligament and proximal to the proximal digital anular ligament. A second portal proximal to the palmar anular ligament is made for insertion of a slotted cannula and, subsequently, a 90° knife used for the transection of the ligament under endoscopic guidance. The separation of the ligament is visible and ensures complete transection. The portals are closed routinely. The endoscopic approach offers the advantage of visualization of the sheath, synovium, and tendons (partially). Resection of adhesions, proliferative synovium, and tendon splitting can be performed as desired (Lowery J, personal communication). The disadvantages of the technique are cost and equipment requirements. Tenoscopy would be specifically recommended in horses with adhesions and synovial proliferation noted on ultrasound and in horses that respond dramatically to anesthesia of the digital sheath (Lowery J, personal communication).

Alternatively, the tendon sheath can be evaluated with the arthroscope through a different portal just proximal to the palmar anular ligament. Subsequently, the anular ligament can be transected by using this portal as the incision for the percutaneous method.

Prognosis

If the primary cause is desmitis of the palmar–plantar anular ligament and is not accompanied by extensive changes in the tendon (bowed tendon), the prognosis after surgical resection is good (84% returned to performance).[4,11] Another study found that 87% of horses with desmitis of the palmar–plantar ligament became sound after anular ligament resection.[9] If superficial digital flexor tendinitis is present, the tendinitis—not the constriction—appears to limit the performance. Standardbreds that underwent anular ligament desmotomy in addition to other surgical procedures for tendinitis improved and were able to race.[5] Of 13 horses with tendinitis and anular ligament desmitis treated by anular ligament resection, 38% became sound.[9]

References

1. Adams OR. Constriction of the palmar (volar) or plantar annular ligament in horses. Vet Med Small Anim Clin 1974;69(3):327.
2. Bertone A. Infectious tenosynovitis. Vet Clin North Am Equine Pract 1995;11(2):163–176.
3. Dik KJ, Van den Belt JM, Keg PR. Ultrasonographic evaluation of fetlock annular ligament constriction in the horse. Equine Vet J 1991;23(4):285–288.
4. Gerring EL, Webbon PM. Fetlock annular ligament desmotomy: A report of 24 cases. Equine Vet J 1984;16(2):113–116.
5. Hawkins JF, Ross MW. Transection of the accessory ligament of the superficial digital flexor muscle for the treatment of superficial digital flexor tendinitis in Standardbreds: 40 cases (1988–1992). J Am Vet Med Assoc 1995;206(5):674–678.
6. Honnas CM, Schumacher J, Cohen ND, et al. Septic tenosynovitis in horses: 25 cases (1983–1989). J Am Vet Med Assoc 1991; 199(11):1616.
7. Stanek C, Edinger H. Radiographic diagnosis of stricture of, or constriction by the annular ligament of the equine fetlock. Pferdeheilkunde 1990;6(3):125–128.
8. Stashak TS. Constriction of or by the palmar (volar) or plantar annular ligament. In: Stashak TS, Ed. Adams' Lameness in Horses. 4th ed. Philadelphia: Lea & Febiger, 1987;593–595.
9. Vail T, Stashak TS, Park RD, et al. Results and prognosis of desmotomy of the equine fetlock anular ligament (49 horses). Unpublished manuscript, 1993.
10. Vandenberg MJ, Rijkenhuizen ABM, Nemeth F. The fetlock tunnel syndrome: A macroscopic and microscopic study. Vet Q 1995; 17(4):138–142.
11. Verschooten F, Picavet TM. Desmitis of the fetlock annular ligament in the horse. Equine Vet J 1986;18(2):138–142.

Part IV

THE METACARPUS AND METATARSUS

Alicia L. Bertone

PERIOSTITIS AND FRACTURE OF THE DORSAL METACARPUS (BUCKED SHINS, SHIN SPLINTS, AND STRESS FRACTURE)

Periostitis and stress fracture of the dorsal surface of the third metacarpal bone constitute a spectrum of diseases that are commonly observed in young (2 to 3 years of age) fast-gaited horses. Although the greatest incidence is observed in young racing Thoroughbreds, it also affects young Quarter Horses and occasionally racing Standardbreds (Fig. 8.213). The hindlimbs are infrequently involved.[16]

Causes

Although there are different subdivisions of this disease (as described later), it appears that all clinical syndromes have a common pathogenesis. In young horses put in training, the metacarpal bone is exposed to new stresses. In younger horses (2 year olds), the metacarpal

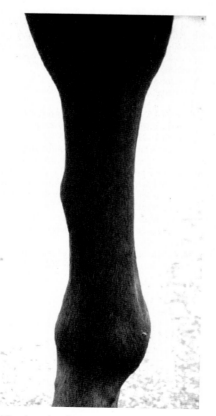

Figure 8.213 A racing Quarter Horse with the classical metacarpal profile of a dorsal cortical stress fracture.

bone is less stiff and, therefore, greater strains (bone movement) are put on the dorsal cortex during high-speed exercise than in older horses. These high strains may lead to low-cycle fatigue of the bone and subsequent bone pain (bucked shins, sore shins).[19] Dorsal metacarpal strain is even greater in the lead limb (the left limb in racing), correlating with the most common location of fracture.[6]

During normal maturation of the third metacarpal, horses aged 1 to 2 years are normally resorbing primary osteons and have greater amount of resorption cavities and incompletely filled secondary osteons than older horses. This bone structure is more susceptible to fatigue microdamage caused by training because of its higher porosity, fewer completed secondary osteons, and a lower proportion of circumferentially oriented collagen fibers.[28] In racing Quarter Horses put in training, the bone density of the medial and lateral dorsal metacarpus significantly decreased during the first 62 days of training, then significantly increased from day 104 to 244 of training.[7,15] Horses experienced fewer bone-related injuries when they had greater cortical mass in the lateral aspect of the third metacarpal at the commencement of training.[15]

The changing shape of the metacarpal bone during maturation[17] and training[5,24] is consistent with lower strains during high-speed exercise in older horses. The thickening of the dorsal cortex, including diffuse dorsal periosteal new bone seen particularly in horses in training, is likely a natural response to these demands on the bone to withstand stress without developing microfractures or dorsal cortical fractures (Fig. 8.214). This has been further confirmed by experimental exercise conditions that induced marked modeling (not remodeling) of the dorsal cortex, specifically subperiosteal bone formation at the mid-shaft of the third metacarpal bone. In addition, horses completing the full training program had greater mineral bone content despite a lighter body weight.[13] Foals significantly increase metacarpal bone mineral density with age, and lack of exercise retards the normal bone development.[3]

In summary, for horses in race training, high strains can induce low-cyclic fatigue of bone, resulting in microdamage or ultimate bone failure. The body responds with bone modeling, but microfracture damage may develop and cause pain. The majority (more than 80%) of 2-year-old racing Thoroughbreds[1] and many racing Quarter Horses[7] demonstrate dorsal cortical pain. It is estimated that about 12% go on to develop acute failure or dorsal cortical fracture, usually within 6 to 12 months of showing dorsal cortical pain.[17] Thoroughbred horses trained on dirt surfaces (instead of wood fiber)[14] and 2-year-old horses with faster works (15 m/sec)[1] had significantly greater incidence of dorsal metacarpal disease, further supporting this pathogenesis. The incidence of

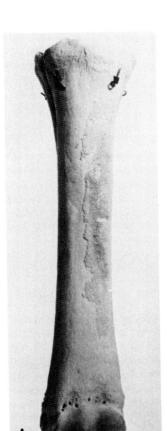

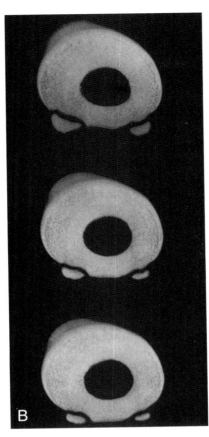

Figure 8.214   A. A macerated specimen of the right third metacarpal bone, illustrating a subperiosteal callus on the dorsal medial surface. B. Cross section through the third metacarpal bone of a horse with dorsal metacarpal disease. Note that the dorsal cortex is thicker than the palmar cortex. (Panels A and B are provided courtesy of P. F. Haynes.)

fatigue failure of the metacarpal dorsal cortex is greater in Thoroughbreds than in Standardbreds; this was not attributed to inherent differences in the mechanical properties of the bone but rather to gait differences and resultant bone stresses during training and racing.[18]

Signs

Early dorsal metacarpal disease is usually observed in young Thoroughbred racehorses (8 to 36 months of age) and occasionally in older horses that have not been strenuously trained or raced as 2-year-olds. The disease has an acute onset and is most obvious after intense exercise. There is usually minimal alteration of the horse's gait, particularly after short periods of rest. A visible convex swelling overlying the surface of the affected portion of the cannon bone is common (Fig. 8.213). On palpation, the dorsal cortex of the third metacarpal bone is acutely painful to pressure. Frequently, the horse will withdraw the limb in response to pain. Radiographs taken at this time are usually negative; however, fractures are occasionally observed as is a minimal amount of superficial cortical osteolysis.[16]

Subacute to chronic dorsal metacarpal disease invariably develops as a result of acute disease that is unresponsive to therapy or that has gone unrecognized. It is most frequently seen in horses 26 to 42 months of age.[16] At exercise, only mild degrees of gait deficit may be noticed. On palpation, varying degrees of pain may be elicited, but a more obvious enlargement is palpable on the dorsomedial cortex (Fig. 8.214). The pain response is typically more profound after strenuous exercise. As with earlier disease, the left limb is usually more severely affected. On radiographic examination, periosteal new bone formation is usually observed (Figs. 8.215 and 8.216).[16]

Dorsal metacarpal bone failure results in a fracture of the dorsal or dorsolateral cortex of the third metacarpal bone. It is usually observed in older horses (3 to 5 years of age) (Figs. 8.213 and 8.214). As with dorsal metacarpal disease, the lameness may not be prominent while the horse is rested. However, it is usually prominent after strenuous exercise. On palpation, a rather discrete painful area can be noted on the dorsolateral surface of the left third metacarpal (cannon) bone at the junction of its middle and distal third. Only rarely will the right third metacarpal bone be involved. Radiographs usually point to a cortical fracture on the dorsolateral surface (Figs. 8.213 and 8.215).[16]

Diagnosis

A tentative diagnosis of metacarpal periostitis or stress fracture can be made from the clinical findings and the age relationship. Little information is derived from local direct infiltration anesthesia of the painful area, because it provides only partial relief in the lameness. Median and ulnar nerve perineural anesthesia or proximal metacarpal regional anesthesia with a ring block is

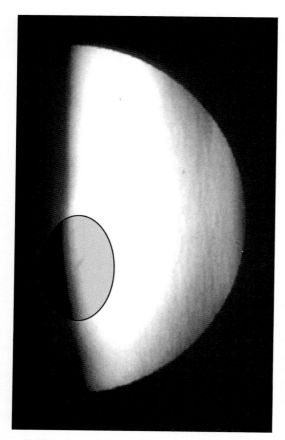

Figure 8.215 Lateral view demonstrating a classical dorsal cortical stress fracture extending from the dorsal cortex and coursing proximad toward the endosteal surface (tongue fracture) (arrow).

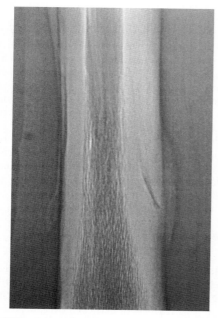

Figure 8.216 A long dorsal cortical metacarpal stress fracture with periosteal new bone formation around the fracture indicating chronicity and failure to heal.

required for total relief of pain, but this is rarely indicated.

Radiographs can assist with the diagnosis of dorsal cortical fracture. A series of four radiographic views should be taken: dorsopalmar (DP), lateral medial (LM), dorsopalmar, lateral medial oblique (DPLMO), and dorsopalmar, medial lateral oblique (DPMLO). The DPLMO and the LM views best identify dorsal medial bone proliferation. and the DPMLO and LM views best identify dorsal lateral cortical fractures. Horses continuing to train and race with sore shins can be screened for the development of fractures with radiographs.

In acute dorsal metacarpal disease, it is rare to see radiographic abnormalities. In subacute dorsal metacarpal disease, periosteal new bone formation (of reduced density compared to underlying cortex) and surface cortical bone resorption may be observed. In chronic disease, a thickening of the dorsomedial cortex with associated periosteal new bone formation is seen (Figs. 8.215 and 8.216). Occasionally, an endosteal response may be noted in the advanced cases.

Dorsal cortical fractures have a characteristic radiographic appearance and usually enter the cortex distally and progress proximad at a 35 to 45° angle. Most frequently, the fracture appears in radiographs as a straight or slightly concave fracture line (tongue fracture) (Figs. 8.215 and 8.216). Occasionally, it will proceed proximad to exit through the dorsal cortex (saucer fracture). Rarely, the fracture continues to enter the medullary canal. Multiple fractures may emanate from the distal site of the cortical entry (often termed fissure fractures). A periosteal callus is often present at the site of fracture and is a function of the chronicity of the disease. Endosteal proliferation is sometimes observed in fractures that are complete through the cortex. Repeated radiographs at 7- to 10-day intervals may be necessary to identify a fracture that is suspected but not observed on initial radiographic examination.[16]

Nuclear scintigraphy can provide information about the stage of disease in horses with dorsal cortical pain or with undiagnosed forelimb pain. This technique has a high sensitivity for identifying bone metabolism and turnover and allows detection of abnormalities in horses in the acute to subacute stages that are still in training. Racehorses may have bone scintigrams performed to determine if training should continue or to identify focal uptake that indicates impending fracture. In review of 121 bone scintigrams of racing Thoroughbreds with clinical history of dorsal metacarpal disease, horses without fracture (bucked shins) had a mild to moderate diffuse uptake of bone radiolabel, unlike the focal intense uptake typical of dorsal cortical fracture. Chronic fractures are less focal and intense because of surrounding bone remodeling but still appear relatively focal compared to early disease.[11]

Use of quantitative CT to measure bone mineral density and three-dimensional morphologic changes in the metacarpus may provide improvements in identifying risk factors or imminence of fracture.

Treatment

Early acute dorsal metacarpal disease usually responds to rest. Approximately half the horses with acute bucked shins can continue to train after 5 to 10 days of rest and anti-inflammatory analgesics. Hand walking, ponying, cold water hosing, and bandaging should continue until the dorsal cortex can be palpated without eliciting pain.

Speed and distance are introduced slowly, with constant monitoring of dorsal cortical pain. Initially, the daily galloping distance is reduced to 50%. If speed is increased, distance should be decreased.[17] The goal is to increase the stress to the dorsal surface of the metacarpal bone gradually, at a rate that allows this surface to model according to compressive demands without producing structural damage.

Subacute and chronic dorsal metacarpal disease can be the most difficult to treat. After an exacerbation, many horses may not be suitable for the modified training regimen described above and pain immediately returns with any sustained galloping. These horses may have marked periosteal new bone formation. More prolonged rest (generally 110 days) is usually necessary for bone remodeling of the new periosteal bone and remodeling of fatigued bone. Many horses are fired and turned out after an initial treatment period.

Dorsal cortical fractures in young horses may resolve with the conservative approach outlined above for subacute or chronic bucked shins. Convalescent periods may extend from 4 to 6 months, because fracture healing is slow at this site.[16] Older horses often do not respond as well to conservative treatment, and surgery is recommended. In either case, serial radiographic studies should be performed at least 30 to 45 days to assess bone healing.[16]

Several surgical procedures have been recommended for treatment of dorsal cortical metacarpal fractures, including placement of a unicortical or transcortical screw in lag fashion, placement of a neutral unicortical positional screw, and dorsal cortical drilling (Figs. 8.217 and 8.218). Transcortical screws are no longer recommended because of the expected differences in strain between the palmar and the dorsal cortices, the risk of fracture, and the risk of damage to the suspensory ligament. Placement of a dorsal unicortical screw in lag fashion can be technically difficult owing to the short depth of the cortex (about 22 mm) and the need for radiographic control, but it provides the best fracture stability. Placement of a neutral dorsal unicortical screw to help stabilize the fracture combined with dorsal cortical drilling is often elected for increased stability over dorsal cortical drilling alone. Cortical bone screws (4.5 or 3.5 mm) are used.

There is no consensus on the recommendation for screw removal. Many horses have and will race successfully with the dorsal cortical screw in place. However, reoccurrence of dorsal cortical pain may occur (regardless of the presence of a screw), and the screw will be presumed to be the cause. If any fracture occurs in this horse in the future, such as condylar fracture or complete metacarpal failure, the screw may be considered a cause. Many surgeons currently recommend removal of the screw after sufficient time of healing (2 months) (Fig. 8.218B). Selection of 4.5-mm cortical screws allow for easy removal with the horse standing.[2,4,9,25]

Fracture fixation is accomplished under general anesthesia with the aid of precise radiographic or fluoroscopic monitoring. A longitudinal incision is made be-

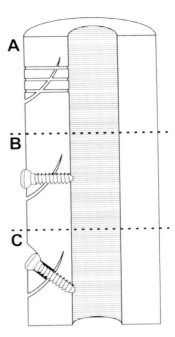

Figure 8.217 A. Dorsal cortical drilling (osteostixis) of a dorsal metacarpal stress fracture. B. Positional unicortical screw placement. C. Unicortical screw placement in lag fashion.

tween the common and lateral digital extensor tendons over the area of greatest swelling. The incision is continued down to the periosteum. Using the preoperative radiographs and anatomic landmarks as guides, the lesion position is estimated and marker needles are placed for intraoperative documentation. Once the precise position of the fracture is identified a 3.5- or 4.5-mm cortical screw is used. A single screw is placed to lag the outer dorsal cortex to the inner surface of the dorsal cortex (Fig. 8.218). The drill bit is placed at a right angle to the fracture line. The outer dorsal cortex is overdrilled to the fracture. The thread hole is drilled into the marrow cavity and tapped. Final radiographs document the appropriate length and position of the screw.

For neutral placement, the screw can be placed perpendicular to the surface of the bone, and no overdrilling is required. This procedure is technically easier, does not require radiographic monitoring, and places the head of screw flush with the bone.

Postoperative management includes bandaging for 2 to 4 weeks, hand walking after 2 weeks, stall rest for 6 weeks, screw removal at 8 weeks, hand walking for 2 weeks, and then limited turnout to 3 months. Light training can begin as early as 3 months. Greater than 95% of horses can return to racing in about 8 months.[4]

Osteostixis can be performed under general anesthesia or in the standing horse. Five to seven drill holes are made in a diamond pattern through the dorsal cortex into the marrow cavity. This procedure can be combined with unicortical screw application. Success for return to racing is similar (more than 80%) to that recently reported for screw fixation, and shorter durations for return to racing (4 to 6 months) are reported.[9] Clustered drill holes act as a stress concentrator and significantly

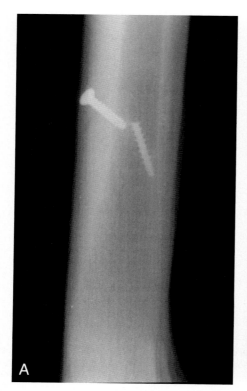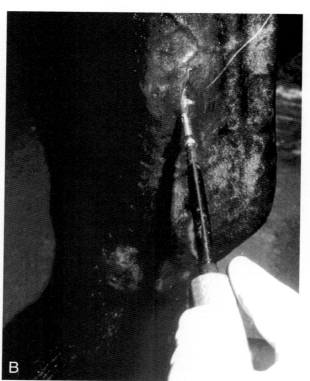

Figure 8.218   A. A singular cortical screw placed across a dorsal cortical stress fracture in lag fashion. The broken tap will remain in the medullary cavity and is not a clinical problem. B. These screws can be removed in the standing horse 2 to 4 months after surgery.

decrease the stress required for metacarpal failure in cadaver limbs, but catastrophic failure through the drill holes is not a reported complication of the procedure in vivo.[26]

Other adjunctive treatments have been recommended with or without surgical treatment, including electrical stimulation at the fracture, shock wave therapy, injection of osteogenic substances (sodium oleate), intralesional injection of steroids, thermocautery (pin firing), chemical vesication (blistering), needle drainage of the hematoma, and cryotherapy (point freezing). These treatments have met with different degrees of success, and no controlled studies have been performed. In all cases, no matter what the treatment, an adequate period of rest and a controlled exercise program are required.

In one study on Thoroughbred racehorses, distinct training strategies were used at different stables, and the allocation of exercise to breezing (15 m/sec), galloping (11 m/sec), and jogging (5 m/sec) was associated with lack of bucked shins for 1 year (survival of bucked shin syndrome). Survival was significantly reduced by allocation of exercise to breezing and increased by allocation to galloping. The study recommended that to reduce the incidence of bucked shins trainers should allocate more training effort to regular short-distance breezing and less to long-distance galloping.[1]

Prognosis

The prognosis is good to excellent for return to racing with surgical treatment of dorsal cortical fractures; re-

ports range from 80 to 98%. But this underestimates the loss of racing days of horses with sore shins that remain in training and recurrence of pain or fracture once subacute or chronic disease occurs. The impact of this syndrome, particularly in 2-year-olds, is evidenced by the following observation: If 2-year-old racing Thoroughbreds that have sore shins on palpation are not permitted to race for 6 weeks, significant improvements in predictable finishes occur.[8] Adjustment of training regimens may assist with prevention; and training on grass, wood fiber, or softer surfaces without toe grabs is recommended.

Other Stress Fractures of the Metacarpal

Although dorsal cortical stress fractures are by far the most common stress fractures in horses, particularly racehorses, other sites and variations within the metacarpus can occur. Dorsal cortical fractures may extend more proximal than the site of exit from the cortex, and fissure lines can sometimes be identified, most typically in the proximal metacarpus on other views. If a fracture line is noted on the craniocaudal view, a spiraling fracture or nondisplaced complete metacarpal fracture should be suspected. Fractures may be limited to the dorsal cortex and may respond to lag screw fixation. Detailed radiographic investigation should be performed to define the fracture and determine if confinement to an overhead wire or casting is recommended.[20,27,29] Similar fractures can occur in the metatarsus of the hindlimb.[20]

Incomplete fractures of the distal palmar condyle were reported in five racehorses. Nuclear scintigraphy or the 125° dorsoproximal-dorsodistal view was necessary to identify them. With rest, affected horses returned to their previous level of racing.[10]

Primarily in racing Standardbreds, stress fractures or focal intense radioactive label uptake on nuclear scintigraphy can occur in the proximal palmar aspect of the third metacarpus and is a recognized syndrome. Physical findings are subtle, but lameness can be blocked to the proximal metacarpus, and scintigraphy is diagnostic. Most horses have abnormal radiographs, although high-detail film and several projections may be needed to see the fracture. Rest resulted in a 64% return to previous level of performance.[12,21] Internal screw fixation in one case[22] and surgical drilling in another case[30] also resulted in success. Dorsomedial articular fractures of the third metacarpal bone can occur in racing Standardbreds. Lameness is abolished with intracarpal anesthesia. Periosteal new bone production can be seen near the distal aspect of the fracture on radiographs. All seven horses in one study healed and returned to soundness (one with internal fixation).[23]

References

1. Boston RC, Nunamaker DM. Gait and speed as exercise components of risk factors associated with onset of fatigue injury of the third metacarpal bone in 2-year-old Thoroughbred racehorses. Am J Vet Res 2000;61:602.
2. Cervantes C, Madison JB, Ackerman N, et al. Surgical treatment of dorsal cortical fractures of the third metacarpal bone in Thoroughbred racehorses: 53 cases (1985–1989). J Am Vet Med Assoc 1992;200:1997–2000.
3. Cornelissen BP, Vanweeren PR, Ederveen AG, et al. Influence of exercise on bone mineral density of immature cortical and trabecular bone of the equine metacarpus and proximal sesamoid bone. Equine Vet J 1999;31(Suppl):79.
4. Dallap BL, Bramlage LR, Embertson RM. Results of screw fixation combined with cortical drilling for treatment of dorsal cortical stress fractures of the third metacarpal bone in 56 Thoroughbred racehorses. Equine Vet J 1999;31:252.
5. Davies HM, Gale SM, Baker ID. Radiographic measures of bone shape in young Thoroughbreds during training for racing. Equine Vet J 1999;30(Suppl):262.
6. Davies HM, McCarthy RN, Jeffcott LB. Surface straining on the dorsal metacarpus of Thoroughbreds at different speeds and gaits. Acta Anat (Basel) 1993;146:148.
7. Goodman NL, Baker BK. Lameness diagnosis and treatment in the Quarter Horse racehorse. Vet Clin North Am Equine Pract 1990;6:85.
8. Griffiths JB, Steel CM, Symons PJ, et al. Improving the predictability of performance by prerace detection of dorsal metacarpal disease in Thoroughbred racehorses. Aust Vet J 2000;78:488.
9. Hanie EA, Sullins KE, White NA. Follow-up of 28 horses with third metacarpal unicortical stress fractures following treatment with osteostixis. Equine Vet J 1992;22(Suppl):5.
10. Kawcak CE, Bramlage LR, Embertson RM. Diagnosis and management of incomplete fracture of the distal palmar aspect of the third metacarpal bone in five horses. J Am Vet Med Assoc 1995;206(3):335–337.
11. Koblik PD, Hornof WJ, Seeherman HJ. Scintigraphic appearance of stress-induced trauma of the dorsal cortex of the third metacarpal bone in racing Thoroughbred horses: 121 cases (1978–1986). J Am Vet Med Assoc 1998;192:390.
12. Lloyd KE, Koblik P, Ragle C, et al. Incomplete palmar fracture of the proximal extremity of the third metacarpal bone in horses: Ten cases (1981–1986). J Am Vet Med Assoc 1988;192:798.
13. McCarthy RN, Jeffcott LB. Effects of treadmill exercise on cortical bone in the third metacarpus of young horses. Res Vet Sci 1992;52(1):28.
14. Moyer W, Spencer PA, Kallish M. Relative incidence of dorsal metacarpal disease in young Thoroughbred racehorses training on two different surfaces. Equine Vet J 1991;23:166.
15. Neilsen BD, Potter GD, Morris EL, et al. Changes in the third metacarpal bone and frequency of bone injuries in young Quarter Horses during race training—Observations and theoretical considerations. J Equine Vet Sci 1997;17:541.
16. Norwood GL, Haynes PF. Dorsal metacarpal disease. In: Mansmann RA, McAllister ES, Eds. Equine Medicine and Surgery. 3rd ed. Santa Barbara, CA: American Veterinary Publications, 1982;1110.
17. Nunamaker DM. Metacarpal stress fractures. In: Nixon AJ, Ed. Equine Fracture Repair. Philadelphia: WB Saunders, 1996;195.
18. Nunamaker DM, Butterweck DM, Black J. In vitro comparison of Thoroughbred and Standardbred racehorses with regard to local fatigue failure of the third metacarpal bone. Am J Vet Res 1991;52:97.
19. Nunamaker DM, Butterweck DM, Provost MT. Fatigue fractures in Thoroughbred racehorses: Relationships with age, peak bone strain, and training. J Orthop Res 1990;8(4):604.
20. Pilsworth RC. Incomplete fracture of the dorsal aspect of the proximal cortex of the third metatarsal bone as a cause of hind-limb lameness in the racing Thoroughbred: A review of three cases. Equine Vet J 1992;24:147.
21. Pleasant RS, Baker GJ, Muhlbauer MC, et al. Stress reactions and stress fractures of the proximal palmar aspect of the third metacarpal bone in horses: 58 cases (1980–1990). J Am Vet Med Assoc 1992;201(12):1918–1923.
22. Ross MW, Ford TS, Orsini PG. Incomplete longitudinal fracture of the proximal palmar cortex of the third metacarpal bone in horses. Vet Surg 1988;17(2):82–86.
23. Ross MW, Martin BB. Dorsomedial articular fracture of the proximal aspect of the third metacarpal bone in Standardbred racehorses: Seven cases (1978–1990). J Am Vet Med Assoc 1992;201(2):332–335.
24. Sherman KM, Miller GJ, Wronski TJ, et al. The effect of training on equine metacarpal bone breaking strength. Equine Vet J 1995;27:135.
25. Specht TE, Colahan PT. Osteostixis for incomplete cortical fracture of the third metacarpal bone. Results in 11 horses. Vet Surg 1990;19(1):34.
26. Specht TE, Miller GJ, Colahan PT. Effects of clustered drill holes on the breaking strength of the equine third metacarpal bone. Am J Vet Res 1990;51:1242.
27. Spurlock GH. Propagation of a dorsal cortical fracture of the third metacarpal bone in two horses. J Am Vet Med Assoc 1988;192:1587.
28. Stover SM, Pool RR, Martin RB, et al. Histological features of the dorsal cortex of the third metacarpal bone mid-diaphysis during postnatal growth in Thoroughbred horses. J Anat 1992;181:455.
29. Watt BC, Foerner JJ, Haines GR. Incomplete oblique sagittal fractures of the dorsal cortex of the third metacarpal bone in six horses. Vet Surg 1998;27:337.
30. Wright IM, Platt D, Houlton JE, et al. Management of intracortical fractures of the palmaroproximal third metacarpal bone in a horse by surgical forage. Equine Vet J 1990;22(2):142–144.

FRACTURES OF THE CONDYLES OF THE THIRD METACARPAL AND METATARSAL BONES (CONDYLAR FRACTURES, LONGITUDINAL ARTICULAR FRACTURES)

Fractures of the condyles of the third metacarpal and metatarsal bones occur most frequently in racing Thoroughbreds, less frequently in Standardbreds, and occasionally in Quarter Horses and Polo ponies.[2] Males are overrepresented (59% in one study and 75% in another) and the distribution of fractures is approximately one-third incomplete nondisplaced, one-third complete nondisplaced, and one-third complete displaced (Fig. 8.219).[16] In a study of 145 condylar fractures in mostly

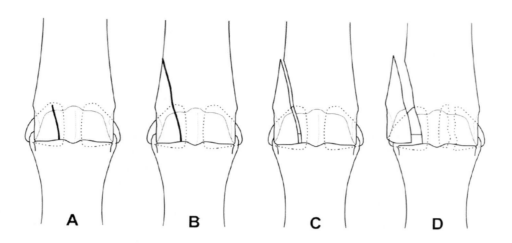

Figure 8.219 Condylar fractures. A. Incomplete. B. Complete nondisplaced. C. Complete separated. D. Complete displaced.

Thoroughbreds, forelimbs (81%) and the lateral condyle (85%) were more frequently involved. The right and left forelimbs were about equally involved. Most fractures (59%) were initiated in the middle of the condyle and extended a mean of 75 mm proximally to exit the cortex. Axial fractures and medial condylar fractures tend to be longer. Articular comminution can occur, usually at the palmar–plantar articular margin, and were identified in 15% of fractures. The axial fractures were more likely to have articular comminution (23%). Of the 145 fractures evaluated, 8 spiraled proximally. Concurrent lesions included proximal phalanx eminence fractures, sesamoid fractures, and sesmoiditis.[16]

In another study of 233 condylar fractures, Thoroughbreds were overrepresented and Standardbreds were underrepresented based on the hospital population. Standardbreds had more metatarsal condylar fractures. Medial metatarsal condylar fractures had a 25% chance of suffering a mid-diaphyseal fracture (Y fracture). In this study, the distribution of Thoroughbred condylar fractures was 66% in the forelimb and about 50% were complete. Approximately 79% of Thoroughbreds with incomplete lateral condylar fractures (77% treated surgically) returned to racing, whereas a significantly lower percentage (33%) of horses with complete lateral condylar fractures returned to racing (all treated surgically). About 80% of Standardbreds (six of seven were treated surgically) raced after treatment. In summary, return to racing in Thoroughbreds was significantly reduced with complete fractures, forelimb fractures, evidence of sesamoid fracture, or female sex (presumed retired for breeding).[2] Complete condylar fractures tend to be longer (mean 85 mm) than incomplete fractures (mean 57 mm).[11] Axial sesamoid fractures are associated with displaced lateral condylar fractures that disrupt the collateral ligament and avulse the intersesamoid ligament complex.[1,5]

Another report of 124 condylar fractures in Thoroughbreds corroborates the above findings. It was noted that 90% of condylar fractures occurred in 2- and 3-

year-olds and that most were acquired during training between April and October. A total of 17% of horses with displaced lateral condylar fractures returned to racing.[4] The variation in successful return to racing after displaced condylar fractures may be related to the duration of fracture before surgery. Destruction of the articular surface occurs quickly after a displaced fracture; therefore, immediate immobilization and repair are critical to a successful outcome.[9]

Condylar fractures of the hindlimb are more common in Standardbreds, are more likely to be medial, and generally do not exit the cortex. These fractures can propagate proximally or progress to a complete Y fracture, even with stall confinement.[9,10]

Causes

The cause of these fractures is trauma from high compressive loads, asynchronous longitudinal rotation of the cannon bone, and exercise on uneven surfaces. The risks of fatal condylar fracture in Thoroughbred racehorses are 7 and 17 times more likely if the horse is shod with low and regular toe grabs, respectively.[6] The toe grab changes the hoof angle and presumably places more stress on the suspensory apparatus and plants the foot more securely, likely altering the compressive and rotatory forces on the distal metacarpus.

Structural studies of the distal condyle of unexercised and exercised horses have demonstrated that the normal mineralized articular cartilage tends to cleave in the sagittal plane and that the main subchondral bone trabeculae are columnated and running in the sagittal direction with few mediolateral connections. Blood vessel canals lie inside the sagittally oriented structure. The sagittal column orientation provides maximum strength and protection in the sagittal plane in which the joint rotates but offers minimal resistance to fracture propagation in this plane.

The anatomic course of condylar fractures of the third metacarpal bone can be explained by the anisotropic structural arrangement of the mineralized tissues.[3] In horses in race training, densification (sclerosis) of the subchondral bone of the palmar–plantar surface of the condyles was identified by CT techniques,[13] and this correlated with linear defects in the mineralized cartilage and subchondral bone in the same region, with intense surrounding bone remodeling.[13]

In a histopathologic study on North American racehorses, similar palmar condylar cartilage fibrillation with underlying bone sclerosis and areas of bone necrosis were noted. Evidence of active bone remodeling was present around the sclerotic zones, and osteocyte necrosis was apparent as prominence of subchondral vessels and osteoclastic activity. Fragmentation lines, indicating matrix fragility and microfractures, were noted. This

area of the condyle was grossly flattened.[7] Similar microdamage, including microfractures in regions of osteoporosis and thinning of the zone of calcified cartilage, was seen histologically in the bone of lateral condylar fractures obtained from fatal injuries.[15] In an experimental study with controlled training exercise, bone density, particularly in the palmar condyle region, was significantly greater in horses undergoing high-intensity exercise.[12]

In summary, the palmar condyle is the site of maximum loading in racing, and the bone responds by increasing density (sclerosis). Bone fatigue failure occurs and, owing to the normal columnar arrangement of the bone trabeculae, propagates acute failure in the configuration seen in condylar fractures (Fig. 8.220).

Figure 8.220 A. Palmar subchondral nondisplaced cortical stress fracture seen in racehorses (arrow in circle). B. Palmar subchondral cortical bone lysis seen in racehorses (arrows). C. A Standardbred racehorse's condyle demonstrating the classical appearance of the lesions corresponding to collapse and necrosis of the subchondral bone with secondary distortion of the articular cartilage. D. Severe osteolysis, necrosis, and collapse of the subchondral bone with a complete ulcer through the articular cartilage seen in a racing Standardbred that was lame at the walk.

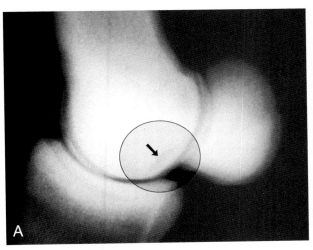
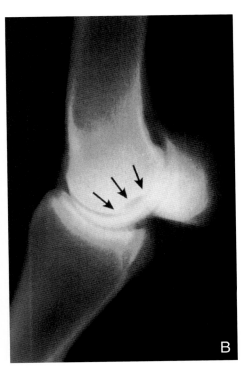
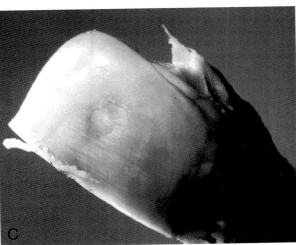
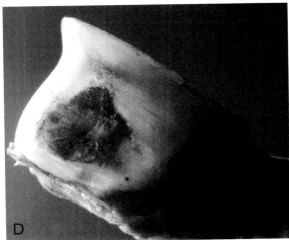

Signs

The clinical signs for nondisplaced incomplete fractures are a mild lameness that is exacerbated by exercise and the presence of little heat or swelling; with acute displaced fractures, there is severe lameness with heat, pain, and swelling. Incomplete nondisplaced fractures are often so subtle they are missed on physical examination but may be detected by screening radiographs or nuclear scintigraphy. However, fetlock joint effusion is always present, because all actual fractures originate at the articular surface. This is best seen in the palmar or plantar recess of the fetlock joint capsule. The external swelling on the lateral side of the large metacarpal or metatarsal bone depends on the degree of separation of the proximal end of the fragment and is readily palpated in displaced fractures. More swelling is observed with greater separation of the fracture fragment. The degree of pain associated with palpation and the amount of heat that is felt depend on the acuteness of the fracture. More heat is noted with acute displaced fractures. Fracture movement and crepitation may also be detected.

Increased lameness can be observed in a horse after it has been exercised and when it is circled to the affected side. Flexion and rotation of the fetlock usually result in sufficient pain to cause withdrawal of the limb. In acute displaced fractures, crepitation may be felt with rotation of the fetlock. When flexion tests are used in a horse with a fissure fracture, increased lameness is observed. If a fracture is suspected based on history, clinical signs, and joint effusion, radiographs should be taken immediately, without further lameness examination or joint manipulations, to decrease the risk of propagating the fracture or worsening the articular cartilage injury.

Diagnosis

Radiographs are recommended for suspected condylar fracture. Only if a fracture is not present can perineural anesthesia and intrasynovial anesthesia be considered. However, a small percentage of these fissure fractures are difficult to identify radiographically, so make certain that radiographs are closely scrutinized.

Diagnosis is made by examination of a standard series of radiographs (DP, LM, DPLMO, and DPMLO) plus a 125° caudocranial view, which provides a view that is tangential to the palmar surface of the condyle. Alternatively, this view can be taken palmar dorsal with the fetlock in flexion, although bone distortion occurs. Long cassettes should be used, so that the fetlock joint and the proximal cannon bone can be included in the study (Fig. 8.221). Close evaluation of the image should be done to rule out the possibility of other injuries. Lesions associated with condylar fractures include osteocondylar fractures of the proximal phalanx on the proximal border, fractures of the proximal sesamoid bone, degenerative joint disease (DJD) of the fetlock, palmar and plantar erosive lesions of the distal third metacarpal or metatarsal bone, suspensory ligament desmitis, and longitudinal fractures of the metatarsus. These associated lesions may influence the treatment recommendation and the prognosis.

Nuclear scintigraphy can be used to locate bone damage before fracture or to identify a fracture (Fig. 8.222).

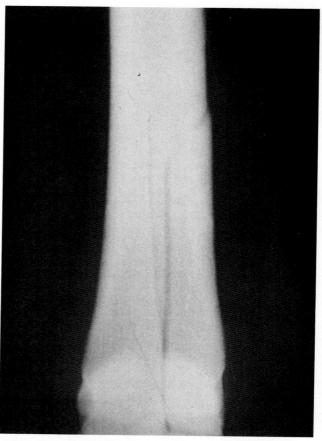

Figure 8.221 A fracture of the lateral condyle of the metatarsus that extends proximad to approximately the midmetatarsal region. (Courtesy of T. S. Stashak.)

Treatment

The recommended treatment of most condylar fractures is internal fixation with transcortical screws placed in lag fashion for best return to full athletic performance and the health of the fetlock joint (Fig. 8.141). Incomplete, nondisplaced fractures can be treated conservatively with successful return to racing, and surgery is not always required. The advantages of screw fixation include the following: the original fracture will not become further displaced; relatively short convalescence; reduced incidence of refracture at the same site; and primary bone healing, which decreases the chances of DJD of the fetlock. Articular alignment and minimal cartilage gap are maintained best when compression is used.

Arthroscopic evaluation of the articular alignment can be used, if necessary, for displaced fractures, particularly if other bone fragments need to be removed, such as proximal phalanx eminence fractures or comminution of the palmar fracture line. Articular damage can also be assessed and may affect the prognosis for displaced fractures, particularly those of more chronic duration (days to weeks).

Horses with incomplete fractures that are treated with a cast or support bandages should be confined to box stalls and observed closely over a period of 2 to 3 weeks

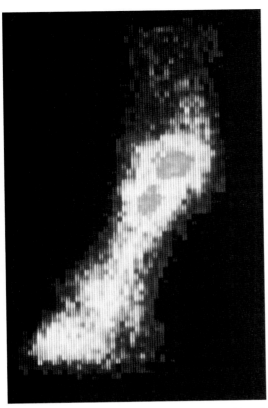

Figure 8.222 Nuclear scintigram of a racehorse with a dorsal first phalanx chip fracture and a condylar fracture, demonstrating two distinct areas of radiopharmaceutical uptake.

for any signs of increased pain and possible displacement. If bandages are used, they should be reset at least every other day for limb inspection and maximal support. For conservative management of nondisplaced fractures, stall rest for 2 months, followed by 30 days of hand walking, and then 30 days of light turnout are ideally recommended. Fractures in young horses can heal by 90 days, but the most articular edge of the fracture often requires additional time. Horses put in training at 90 days are at risk of articular osteolysis on return to training.

Internal fixation should be used for all complete condylar fractures (nondisplaced and displaced) in horses intended for athletic performance (Fig. 8.223). Immediate diagnosis and immobilization of the limb are critical preoperatively to enhance success. Surgery should be performed quickly, but does not need to be performed on an emergency basis. If the limb is immobilized in a cast or complete commercial splint, the horse can be safely transported and permitted to recover from the incident.

For surgery, the horse is positioned in lateral recumbency under general anesthesia with the affected limb up for a lateral condylar fracture. If a nondisplaced condylar fracture is present, the screws can be placed through strategically placed stab incisions in the skin. The location and spacing of the screws can be preplanned by measurements made on the radiographs; however, the first screw is always located in the condylar fossa, and subsequent screws are placed 1.5 to 2 cm proximal to the first screw. If comminution of the most proximal tip of the cortical fracture is evident on radiographs, placement of the most proximal screw can be omitted. Ideal screw placement is parallel to the joint with the first screw in the condylar fossa, engagement of both cortices without deposit of bone material in the opposing collateral ligament, and compression of the fracture so the fracture line is eliminated or barely identifiable on the immediate postoperative radiograph. Increased duration and displacement of the fracture reduce the success in obtaining the latter result. Intraoperative fluoroscopy (preferred) or radiography should be used as needed to obtain the best results.

To achieve interfragmentary compression, the depth of the glide hole can be estimated by measuring the width of the fracture fragment (Fig. 8.223). At least 5 mm should be added to the measurements to compensate for magnification and to ensure that the drill passes the fracture line. This is identifiable by the surgeon intraoperatively as a slight disruption in drill smoothness and adds further confidence that compression will achieved. The first screw is always the most distal screw.

Complete fractures or displaced fractures should be compressed with ASIF (Association for the Study of Internal Fixation) bone clamps before drilling to stabilize the fracture and initiate compression. The reduction of displaced condylar fractures can be a challenge, particularly in the cranial to caudal direction, which may not be apparent on craniocaudal radiographs taken at surgery. Arthroscopic inspection of the dorsal articular surface often reveals a 1- to 2-mm step in the cranial direction of the fractured component. For displaced fractures, an open incision the full length of the fracture, use of multiple bone clamps, and initially focusing the reduction on the most proximal portion of the fracture may help maximize reduction. The longer the duration of displaced fracture before surgery, the less likely perfect reduction will be achieved.

Screws are tightened distal to proximal and retightened to maximize compression. The head of the most distal screw is not countersunk, as it is placed in the condylar fossa, and countersinking of the most proximal screw may split the thin proximal portion of the fragment. The number of screws needed depends on the length of the fracture fragment. However, in most cases of condylar fracture, only two or three screws are required. If spiraling of the fracture was identified on radiographs, screws are placed in lag fashion across the fracture for as far as it is identified, and a cast is applied for recovery. This is particularly important for medial condylar fractures in the hindlimb. Final images of the repair should documented for the record and to ensure a satisfactory reduction and selection of implants.

Currently, most condylar fractures are repaired with 4.5-mm cortical bone screws. Some surgeons use 5.5-mm screws, but complications of screw pullout or bending has not been a problem with 4.5-mm screw repairs. Refracture after return to racing can occur (rarely), even with screws in place, and 5.5-mm screws may offer an advantage in this situation. Screw design does affect screw stiffness and strength in the equine distal condyle. Cortical screws (4.5 and 5.5 mm) with shafts were 30% (20-mm shaft) and 40% (25-mm shaft) stiffer and 60% (20-mm shaft) and 70% (25-mm shaft) stronger than

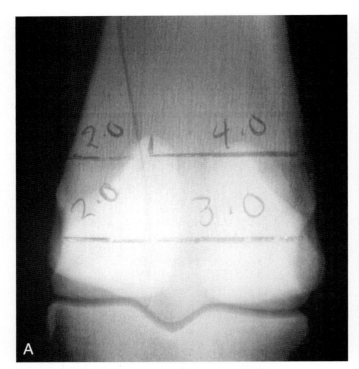

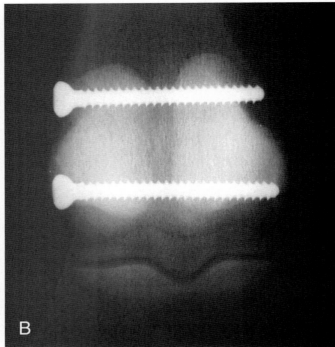

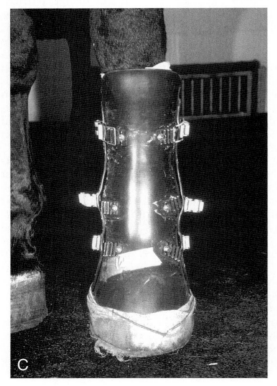

Figure 8.223 A. Preoperative view demonstrating the surgical plan for screw placement, spacing, and depth of the gliding hole. B. Postoperative view demonstrating immediate complete reduction of the fracture. The first screw is placed in the condylar fossa, and the screws do not exit the medial cortex. C. A half-limb immobilizing boot or a half cast is used. External coaptation does not need to be maintained after recovery from general anesthesia.

similar sized screws without shafts.[8] Their selection for use in condylar fractures may depend on availability and cost.

Casting is not usually performed for nondisplaced incomplete fractures or for complete fractures if a secure repair is obtained. Use of a complete boot or cast should be used if the repair was less than ideal, for displaced fractures, and for spiraling fractures. If a long spiraled fracture was repaired, a full limb cast is recommended, although it is not used by all surgeons because of the risks of complications during recovery with a full limb cast.[10] Horses are usually comfortable on the limb immediately after repair and walk in the stall without gait deficit when on low doses of phenylbutazone. Continued postoperative lameness is a red flag for problems, and radiographs should be obtained.

Postoperative exercise should be limited for at least 90 days. Stall rest confinement is recommended for this period, and after 6 weeks hand walking exercise can begin. Follow-up radiographs should be taken at that time; and if the healing is progressing normally, the horse can be turned out into a small paddock for an additional 90 days. If the radiographic follow-up shows good healing, the horse can be placed on pasture or in a large paddock. The training schedule depends on the type of fracture but could begin as early as 4 months or as late as 6 months. One study noted that horses were more likely to race if the fracture line could no longer be identified on the 2- to 4-month radiographs.[17]

Screws are generally not removed after healing has occurred unless residual lameness results that can be directly attributed to their presence. In a review of 233 cases of condylar fractures—most repaired by interfragmentary compression—screws were removed in only 20 cases. There appeared to be no consistent difference in the performance between this group and the group with screws in place.[2] The study noted that horses with screws placed closer to the joint had a lower rate of return to racing. Subchondral sclerosis was proposed as a cause for the pain. In general, removal of screws is not routinely performed for condylar fractures, except if screws are placed in the diaphysis as for medial condylar fractures of the metatarsus or for spiraling fractures. The screws can be easily removed with the horse under general anesthesia, and their location can be confirmed with marker needles and radiographs. In most cases, the screws can be removed through small stab incisions alone.

Prognosis

The general prognosis for athletic performance and return to racing is excellent for nondisplaced incomplete fractures, whether treated conservatively (82 and 87%, in two reports)[2,17] or after internal fixation (74 and 79%, in two reports) for forelimb fractures[2,17] and 93% for metatarsal fractures in one report.[2] Prognosis for athletic performance and return to racing is fair for complete displaced and nondisplaced fractures after internal fixation (58% in one report).[17] In two reports, 33% of horses with complete fractures (displaced and nondisplaced)[2] and 19% with displaced fractures[4] returned to racing. Rapid immobilization and repair of the displaced fractures probably dramatically affect outcome. In cases of complete displaced fractures, when there has been a delay in diagnosis and treatment, and/or when improper immobilization was selected, a guarded to poor prognosis can be expected.[11] Only 12 of 38 horses in one report were able to return to racing.[11] This prognosis is altered because of increased damage to the articular surface likely to result in DJD of the fetlock and irritation to the periosteum, resulting in increased callus formation. The prognosis for return to racing is considered poor for comminuted fractures or when there are subchondral erosive lesions in the palmar or plantar surface of the distal end of the cannon bone.[11]

References

1. Barclay WP, Foerner JJ, Phillips TN. Axial sesamoid injuries associated with lateral condylar fractures in horses. J Am Vet Med Assoc 1985;186:278.
2. Bassage LH, Richardson DW. Longitudinal fractures of the condyles of the third metacarpal and metatarsal bones in racehorses: 224 cases (1986–1995). J Am Vet Med Assoc 1998;212:1757.
3. Boyde A., Haroon Y, Jones SJ, et al. Three dimensional structure of the distal condyles of the third metacarpal bone of the horse. Equine Vet J 1999;31:122.
4. Ellis DR. Some observations on condylar fractures of the third metacarpus and third metatarsus in young Thoroughbreds. Equine Vet J 1994;26:178.
5. Greet TR. Condylar fracture of the cannon bone with axial sesamoid fracture in three horses. Vet Record 1987;120(10):223.
6. Kane AJ, Stover SM, Gardner IA, et al. Horseshoe characteristics as possible risk factors for fatal musculoskeletal injury of Thoroughbred racehorses. Am J Vet Res 1996;57:1147.
7. Norrdin RW, Kawcak CE, Capwell BA, et al. Subchondral bone failure in an equine model of overload arthrosis. Bone 1998;22:133.
8. Rahm C, Ito K, Auer J. Screw fixation in lag fashion of equine cadaveric metacarpal and metatarsal condylar bone specimens: A biomechanical comparison of shaft and cortex screws. Vet Surg 2000;29(6):564.
9. Richardson D. Specific fractures. In: Nixon AJ, Ed. Equine Fracture Repair. Philadelphia: WB Saunders, 1996;186.
10. Richardson DW. Medial condylar fractures of the third metatarsal bone in horses. J Am Vet Med Assoc 1984;185:761.
11. Rick MC, O'Brien TR, Pool RR, et al. Condylar fractures of the third metacarpal bone and third metatarsal bone in 75 horses: Radiographic features, treatments, and outcome. J Am Vet Med Assoc 1983;183:287.
12. Riggs CM, Boyde A. Effect of exercise on bone density in distal regions of the equine third metacarpal bone in 2-year-old Thoroughbreds. Equine Vet J 1999;30(Suppl):555.
13. Riggs CM, Whitehouse GH, Boyde A. Pathology of the distal condyles of the third metacarpal and third metatarsal bones of the horse. Equine Vet J 1999;31:140.
14. Riggs CM, Whitehouse GH, Boyde A. Structural variation of the distal condyles of the third metacarpal and third metatarsal bones in the horse. Equine Vet J 1999;31:130.
15. Stover SM, Deryck HR, Johnson BJ, et al. Lateral condylar fracture histomorphology in racehorses. Proc Am Assoc Equine Pract 1994;173.
16. Zekas LJ, Bramlage LR, Embertson RM, et al. Characterisation of the type and location of fractures of the third metacarpal/metatarsal condyles in 135 horses in central Kentucky (1986–1994). Equine Vet J 1999;31(4):304.
17. Zekas LJ, Bramlage LR, Embertson RM, et al. Results of treatment of 145 fractures of the third metacarpal/metatarsal condyles in 135 horses (1986–1994). Equine Vet J 1999;31:309.

FRACTURES OF THE THIRD METACARPAL/METATARSAL (CANNON) BONE

Fractures of the third metacarpal/metatarsal (cannon) bone occur at all ages, but more commonly in young horses, and in all breeds of horses. The metacarpus is particularly susceptible to fracture because of its distal location, and little soft tissue covers the bone to help absorb impact energy in blunt trauma.[19]

Although fractures of the cannon bone can assume a variety of configurations, ranging from a simple fissure to severe comminution, younger horses seem to sustain simpler fractures than adults, possibly because of more elastic, less brittle, and less shatter-prone bone. The fracture can occur anywhere along the bone length and can enter either the proximal or distal joint. Frequently, dis-

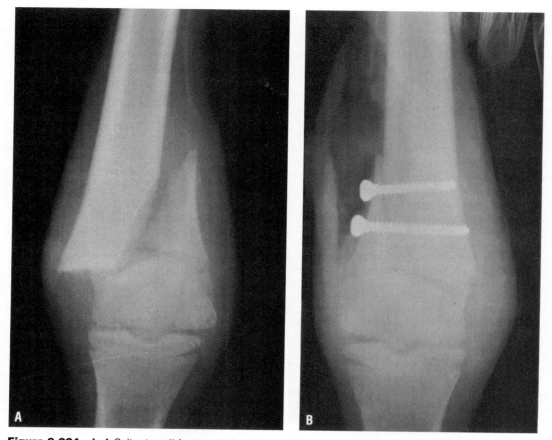

Figure 8.224 A. A Salter type II fracture in the distal metacarpus. B. Two bone screws were used to repair the fracture. (Courtesy of A. S. Turner.)

tal fractures that involve the growth plate, or rarely persistent proximal physes, in young animals will be of the Salter type II fractures (Fig. 8.224).[13] Also, because of the minimal soft tissue covering, the fractures are commonly open or become open soon after the injury occurs; and more than half of referred metacarpal/metatarsal fractures are open.[16] Concurrent fractures of the small metacarpal bones are common. (See also "Fractures of the Small Metacarpal and Metatarsal (Splint) Bones and Periostitis," "Fracture of the Dorsal Metacarpus" and "Periostitis and Fracture of the Dorsal Metacarpus" in this chapter). Once catastrophic failure occurs, fractures are treated as discussed below.

Causes

External trauma in any form can cause this fracture. Injuries frequently reported by clients include kicks; halter-breaking injuries; injuries associated with ground holes, fences, and cattleguards; slipping accidents; slipping on ice; and accidents associated with moving vehicles. In foals, the cause is often the result of the dam having stepped on the limb. Propagation of stress fractures, particularly the more uncommon stress fractures, and propagation of forces through screw or pin holes from other repairs can result in similar complete cannon bone failure. Preexisting bone abnormalities are not typi-

cally present, because the injury represents a singular overloading event on the metacarpus or metatarsus.

Signs and Diagnosis

Complete but nondisplaced fractures of the cannon bone secondary to direct trauma can occur and may be initially difficult to diagnose. The lameness may be nonspecific and variable. On gross observation, the cannon bone may be slightly enlarged; and heat, swelling of the soft tissues overlying the fracture, and pain on deep digital palpation are present. Swelling and pain are more diffuse than with stress fractures, and a wound at the site of impact is often present. Diagnosis may be delayed if soft tissue injury is evident, since the lameness may be attributed to this cause. As lameness persists or worsens, radiographs are usually taken, which may reveal fracture lines. If the horse is turned out, invariably complete bone failure occurs. If stall confinement is maintained, the diagnosis is often made from the second radiograph, on which a periosteal reaction can noted at sites of cortical exit and bone resorption of the fracture line widens the fractures.

In complete bone failure, the diagnosis of fracture of the cannon bone is obvious (Fig. 8.225). An angular limb deformity is present, along with a non-weight-bearing lameness. In all cases, these fractures should be immedi-

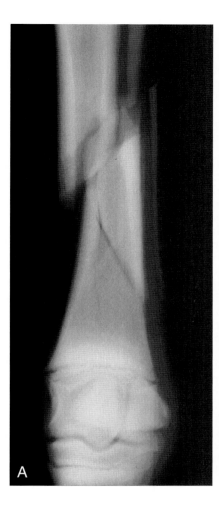
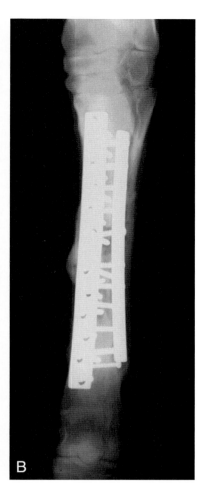

Figure 8.225 A. Open comminuted mid-diaphyseal fracture of the metatarsus in a 7-month-old weanling. B. Postoperative view demonstrating fracture repair with two broad dynamic compression plates on the dorsolateral and dorsomedial sides of the metacarpus. Additional screws were placed in lag fashion from outside the plate to secure the butterfly fragments.

ately supported and eventually radiographed to identify the type (simple versus comminuted) and location in relation to joint surfaces. The limb should not be manipulated excessively during physical examination, because it may lead to penetration of bone fragments through the skin.

If treatment is to be considered or further diagnosis is to be obtained, a cast or a polyvinyl chloride (PVC) full-limb splint should be immediately secured to the limb without moving the horse. Loss of lower limb control may panic the horse, resulting in further soft tissue injury and an open fracture. Splinting is critical because a poorly applied splint may actually do more harm than good. Cast material can be applied over a light padded bandage for transport to a facility where radiographs and a better cast can be applied.

Cast material is the easiest way to immobilize a limb above the carpus and tarsus. If cast material not available, PVC pipe cut in half to create a sleeve can be placed over a tight padded bandage and secured aggressively with nonelastic tape. In the forelimb, the splint should extend to the elbow; in the hindlimb, it can extend to the top of the hock with a heavily padded and taped bandage extending proximally to the stifle. Use of wooden boards, broom handles, etc. has not yielded good success in many cases. A more appropriate hind-

limb splint to suspend the tibia can be constructed from aluminum rods if time permits.

When placing the horse in the trailer for transport to a facility it is important to take into account whether a forelimb or hindlimb is affected. Because the horse has less control during braking than during acceleration, horses with forelimb fractures should face backward in the trailer.[2,3]

Radiographs can often be obtained through the cast material or PVC splint, particularly if euthanasia is likely and final confirmation of the severity is all that is needed for the decision. If, however, surgical repair is anticipated, a full series of highly detailed radiographs is needed and can be obtained under general anesthesia, either as a separate procedure or preferably, just before surgery.

Treatment

The selection of treatment of cannon bone fractures depends on the type of fracture (open versus closed; simple versus comminuted), the location of the fracture (articular versus nonarticular; proximal versus distal), the animal's age, the animal's intended use, the presence of wounds and/or vascular compromise, and cost.

The preferred treatment for most cannon bone fractures is internal fixation with one or two dynamic compression plates (DCPs), extending the length of the bone, combined with individual screws where appropriate (Fig. 8.225). This technique is recommended even for open fractures, particularly if the wound is minor (e.g., a puncture of the bone end through the skin) and the area was clipped, cleaned, and placed under an antiseptic wrap early in the process.

If the fracture includes quite proximal or distal comminution, severe comminution with extensive fissuring, extensive wounds, or vascular compromise, internal fixation alone is not the ideal method of repair; it may be necessary to include arthrodesis or external coaptation. Such severe fractures may heal with transfixation pins and external fixators or casts. These methods are more successful in foals, who undergo rapid healing and have low body weight. In adult horses, severe fractures have a guarded prognosis; but use of external coaptation, plating in the face of open wounds and vascular compromise, or sequential procedures have been successful in rare instances.

The basic principles of cannon bone fracture repair include the following:

- Reconstruct the fracture into two fragments (usually with lag screws) before applying the plates.
- Perform anatomic reduction of the fracture, particularly of the articular components.
- Place the plates at a 90° angle to each other on the tension band side of the cannon bone (dorsal or dorsolateral) and over the fragments.
- Stagger the plates.
- Fill all screw holes, if at all possible.
- Use 5.5-mm screws in the metaphyses and adjacent to the fracture ends for maximal pullout and bending strength, respectively.
- Lute the plates with antimicrobial-impregnated polymethylmethacrylate.
- Place autogenous bone graft in most cases.
- Do not end the plates at the top of the cast.
- Apply a cast for recovery and possibly longer.

The surgical approach to the metacarpus and metatarsus for bone plate application is through a flaplike incision. The flap should be large enough to allow coverage of the plates, and the suture line should not be directly over the plates. Dissection deep within the subcutaneous tissue ensures a good blood supply to the skin flap. The long or common digital extensor tendon is divided to assist with coverage of the plate at closure. The periosteum is incised and elevated so the bone plates can be placed in a subperiosteal fashion.

Two plates are used, except in small neonates (Fig. 8.225). Two narrow or one narrow and one broad DCP could be used in a foal or pony, depending on its size. Two broad DCPs are needed for most horses, even large weanlings and yearlings. The limiting factor is the size of the metacarpus and whether two broad plates can fit on the bone. In the classic metacarpal fracture with one large butterfly fragment, the fragment can be secured to the proximal bone with two 3.5-mm cortical bone screws. The heads of these screws are small and can be easily countersunk to allow placement under the plate if necessary.

After the fracture is reconstructed into two pieces, it can be reduced by a combination of traction and toggling. Use of muscle paralytics can be extremely helpful in this process; I routinely use them about 30 minutes before and during reduction to speed up this process. Reduction of a fresh fracture should be close to perfect. Reduction of more chronic fractures may be less secure because of eburnation of the fracture ends; pulverization of smaller fragments, which produces gaps; and contracture, which can occur quite quickly. The goal is to achieve the best possible anatomic reduction to minimize the gap that the fracture callus has to bridge and to produce the most interdigitation for inherent stability.

Once reduction is achieved, the plates are contoured. Usually one plate is placed dorsolateral and one dorsomedial, but combinations of dorsal and medial or dorsal and lateral are acceptable and may be necessary, depending on the fracture configuration. If a screw must cross the fracture line, it is best to angle it perpendicular to the fracture and to place it in lag fashion. It is important that the screws in the first plate do not interfere with the screws placed in the second plate.

Compression of the fracture may not be necessary if the reduction was difficult and once achieved, already compressed. Overcompression can displace the fracture. If a gap still exists, the DCP can be used to compress the fracture. First secure the plate to the most proximal bone, then secure the most distal screws on the distal bone. After all screws are placed, the plates can be loosened one at a time, and plate luting performed to fill the gaps under the plate and screw heads. This increases the strength of the plate–screw construct by threefold.[18]

If screws strip out in the process, 5.5- or 6.5-mm screws can be placed to regain construct strength.[21] Cancellous screws (6.5 mm) will fit through the plate, but cannot be angled, which limits their application. Cannulated screws are not usually selected because of their lower pullout strength.[7]

After plate luting, autogenous bone graft, which should have already been harvested, is placed into any gaps and around the fracture site. Graft can be obtained from the sternum in horses in dorsal recumbency and the tuber coxae for horses in lateral recumbency. The graft is expected to increase bone density in the screw holes during healing.[9]

The limb should be liberally lavaged and a radiographic image obtained to ensure appropriate repair and screw lengths. The incision should be rapidly closed to cover the plate securely, and a high half-limb cast is then applied. Suction drains are not usually used for metacarpal fractures because the soft tissue dissection and hemorrhage are not as great as with other long bone fractures, such as of the humerus or femur.

If the fracture is stable and the animal is young or small, the cast can be removed in 10 to 14 days after incisional healing is anticipated. Antimicrobials are discontinued after hemorrhage is thought to have ceased (24 to 72 hours). Horses should be willing to use the cast within 72 hours postoperatively, if not immediately.

Administration of morphine during general anesthesia provides 12 hours or more of analgesia and helps with the early postoperative pain. Use of phenylbutazone is typical, except in foals, in whom flunixin meglumine or ketoprofen is preferable or intramuscular α_2-agonists and narcotics (morphine) can be readministered as necessary. Typically, horses seem painful (tense, stationary, pawing) for 24 to 72 hours, after which dramatic relaxation and use of the limb usually begin.

Healing of the bone requires 2 to 3 months in foals and 4 to 12 months in adults, depending on the complications and severity of fracture. Stall rest should be anticipated for 4 months in foals and 6 months in adults, although hand walking can begin as soon as the fracture callous is bridging the fracture and other complications of implant failure have not occurred or have arrested. An unsuccessful outcome in foals may be the result of infection and nonunion or secondary complications, such as cast sores and osteonecrosis or severe tendon laxity. An unsuccessful outcome in adults is usually the result of laminitis of the supporting limb, infection, or sequestration of large fracture fragments and loss of repair stability as well as of other secondary complications that increase cost prohibitively.

Use of the interlocking nail system for the internal fixation of cannon bone fractures is not usually elected, because fractures are commonly comminuted and the interlocking nail system is not as strong as double plating in torsion.[12] The use of external fixators in adult fractures is not usually selected, because the external fixation ring constructs with 1/4-in. Steinmann pins are not stiff enough for repair of an unstable third metacarpal bone fracture in a mature animal.[6] Other unusual internal fixation methods have been reported to be successful and include use of an Ilizarov ring fixator in a metacarpal fracture in a foal[11] and use of a cortical allograft under two plates to replace a large portion of sequestered bone in a metatarsal fracture of a foal.[5]

In young foals with fractures that have extended into the growth plate, it may be necessary to bridge the growth plate with an implant to achieve stability of the fracture. In very young foals, from birth to 6 weeks, this may alter limb growth sufficiently to cause shortening or an angular limb deformity. Because the majority of the growth from the physis (growth plate) occurs before 2.5 or 3 months of age, there is little chance of altering or arresting growth after this age. Alignment of the limb is critical during repair, and closure of the distal growth plate to prevent asymmetric growth can be a goal in the repair. The slightly shorter cannon bone is often compensated for with fetlock angle and hoof growth.

The decision to remove the bone plates depends on the animal's age, its intended use, and whether draining fistulae are present. In general, horses that are to be used in athletic competition should have their plates removed in stages, 3 months apart. Many horses do well with the plates in place and finances and use of the horse determine if the plates should be removed. After plate removal, the limb is supported in a cast for a short period and exercise is initiated slowly. If draining fistulae are present, fracture healing should be complete before the plates are removed. Removing all plates and screws usually resolves the infection.

External coaptation alone has been used successfully to treat many cases of nondisplaced cannon bone fractures,[1,8] but this is not optimal for complete fractures. In complete fractures, the healed result is likely to be a malunion, if the horse survives the prolonged healing time and discomfort. Standard casts do not adequately decrease axial loading or movement of the fracture ends, even if applied up to the elbow or stifle. Axial alignment will be better than if a bandage had been used, but non-union or failure owing to secondary complications of a prolonged healing time and lameness are likely. Cast application often becomes as expensive as internal fixation, because of the multiple applications and prolonged healing time.

Simple distal fractures in foals may be successfully treated with casts, but internal fixation is still preferred for early weight bearing and reduction when there are secondary complications, such as poor reduction, tendon laxity, cast sores, and non-union. A full limb cast significantly reduces metacarpal bone strains by 7 to 84%. Use of a full-limb walking cast more consistently reduces metacarpal bone strains to 11% of baseline and neutralized bending and torsional forces.[4] A half-limb cast or half-limb transfixation pin cast does not significantly reduce metacarpal bone strain, as it does on the phalanges; therefore, it probably does not provide adequate immobilization or load sharing for metacarpal fractures.[20]

Casts in conjunction with transfixation pinning have been used successfully in a limited number of cases in foals and adults that have sustained proximal comminuted fractures of the cannon bone. Pinning provides significantly greater resistance than standard casts against the axial collapse of metacarpal fractures.[10] These fractures are so proximal that they are not amenable to routine techniques of internal fixation (e.g., bone plating). In most cases, two large-diameter pins (6 mm) are placed transversely from lateral to medial through the distal end of the radius, and two more pins are placed in a similar fashion below the fracture site in the third metacarpal bone. A full-limb cast is applied over the pins.

Divergent transfixation pins create a stronger configuration under torsional strain.[15] Holes drilled in the metacarpus significantly reduce the metacarpal strength over intact bone,[22] and centrally threaded, positive-profile transfixation pin designs provide greater strength over negative-profile pins and should not be self-tapped for maximal pullout strength and least bone damage on insertion.[17] A cast is then applied over and around the pins. With the new fiberglass casting materials available, a strong lightweight external support can be applied. The pins are used to further stabilize the extremely unstable comminuted fracture. Foals can be maintained in stall confinement, whereas adults may require slinging.

Other forms of coaptation, such as leg braces in many forms and splints, have been used to successfully treat cannon bone fractures in a limited number of cases. But these methods are not recommended as first-choice treatment.[8]

Open fractures associated with moderate to severe contamination and increased soft tissue inflammation may be treated by temporary casting or pin casting for periods of 7 to 10 days, after which internal fixation can be applied. This delayed approach is recommended only if reasonable stabilization of the fracture can be achieved. If the delayed approach is selected, the initial treatment should include clipping and shaving of the wound, a deep sample for culture sensitivity, complete debridement of devitalized soft tissue and bone, and thorough lavage with a mild antiseptic. A sterile bandage is applied with sufficient padding to lift and store any of the exudate that is formed. The carpus or tarsus is placed in slight flexion to reduce the axial compression and rotational forces, and a full-limb cast is applied with or without transfixation, depending on the duration of casting expected and consideration of interference with the planned internal fixation. Broad-spectrum antibiotics are begun and continued pending the results of the culture sensitivity.

After 3 to 4 days, the cast is removed and the wound is examined. Deep samples for culture sensitivity are retaken, further debridement and lavage may be performed if indicated, and a sterile bandage and cast are reapplied. Alteration in antibiotic therapy may be necessary if the results of sensitivity testing indicate it. Depending on the state of the wound, the cast is removed in 7 to 10 days and a final decision is made regarding the application of internal fixation.

If the wound is clean, then internal fixation can be attempted. If on the other hand, the wound is obviously infected, euthanasia may be advised. This delay provides sufficient time to determine if infection will be a problem before committing the client to the expense of internal fixation. The delay also allows the process of autodebridement to occur and minimizes the chances of local infection. If a plate was applied at the time of injury, the chances of the spread of infection to surrounding tissues are increased. Although plates are relatively nonreactive stainless steel, they are still foreign material and do harbor bacteria. This method may be successful in foals, but adults rarely survive.

If the fracture line extends into the nutrient foramen of the cannon bone, attempt at repair may be futile as ischemic necrosis and sequestrum may result.[19] Serial use of nuclear scintigraphy can detect loss of cortical bone vascularity, but does not predict successful healing. In the two cases reported, one case revascularized.[14]

Prognosis

The prognosis for successful treatment of third metacarpal and metatarsal bone fractures depends on the nature of the injury, the type of fracture, where the fracture occurred, and whether it is opened or closed so an individual assessment of each case is warranted. In a study of 25 complete fractures of the metacarpal or metatarsal bones of horses that were treated, age, sex, weight, and limb did not affect outcome; but case selection had already occurred. A total of 17 of 25 cases had an open fracture; non-union of an infected fracture was the most common cause of postoperative failure in 7 cases. In this study, 11 horses had no complications related to the surgical repair.

In general, transverse, slightly oblique and minorly comminuted (one butterfly fragment) fractures in the midcannon bone region in foals under 7 months of age have a good to excellent prognosis with internal fixation. Older horses with similar fractures would have a more guarded prognosis owing to their size and the risk of supporting limb laminitis but, in general, have a fair to good prognosis. Older horses with open, comminuted or articular fractures have a guarded to poor prognosis for recovery. Unfortunately, older horses have a greater risk of comminuted open fractures that involve the nutrient foramen.[16]

References

1. Bowman KF, Fackleman GE. Management of comminuted fractures in the horse. Comp Cont Educ Vet Pract 1980;11:298.
2. Bertone AL. Management of orthopedic emergencies. Vet Clin North Am Equine Pract 1994;10:603.
3. Bramlage LR. Fetlock arthrodesis. In: Nixon AJ, Ed. Equine Fracture Repair. Philadelphia: WB Saunders, 1996;172.
4. Brommer H, Back W, Schamhardt HC, et al. In vitro determination of equine third metacarpal bone unloading, using a full limb case and a walking cast. Am J Vet Res 1996;57:1386.
5. Cassotis NJ, Stick JA, Arnoczky SP. Use of full cortical allograft to repair a metatarsal fracture in a foal. J Am Vet Med Assoc 1997; 211:1155.
6. Cervantes C, Madison JB, Miller GJ, et al. An in vitro biomechanical study of a multiplanar circular external fixator applied to equine third metacarpal bones. Vet Surg 1996;25:1–5.
7. Colgan SA, Hecker AT, Kirker-Head CA, et al. A comparison of the Synthes 4.5-mm cannulated screw and the Synthes 4.5-mm standard cortex screw systems in equine bone. Vet Surg 1998;27: 540.
8. Fessler JF, Amstutz HE. Fracture repair. In: Oehme FW, Prier JE, Eds. Textbook of Large Animal Surgery. Baltimore: Williams & Wilkins, 1974;301.
9. Hanie EA, Sullins KE, Powers BE. Comparison of two grafting methods in 4.0-mm drill defects in the third metacarpal bone of horses. Equine Vet J 1992;24:387.
10. Hopper SA, Schneider RK, Johnson CH, et al. In vitro comparison of transfixation and standard full-limb cases for prevention of displacement of a mid-diaphyseal third metacarpal osteotomy site in horses. Am J Vet Res 2000;61:1633.
11. Jukema GN, Settner M, Dunkelmann G, et al. High stability of the Ilizarov ring fixator in a metacarpal fracture of an Arabian foal. Arch Orthop Trauma Surg 1997;116(5):287.
12. Lopez MJ, Wilson DG, Vanderby R, et al. An in vitro biomechanical comparison of an interlocking nail system and dynamic compression plate fixation of ostectomized equine third metacarpal bones. Vet Surg 1999;28:333.
13. Lumsden JM, Caron JP, Stickle RL. Repair of a proximal metatarsal Salter type-II fracture in a foal. J Am Vet Med Assoc 1993; 202(5):765.
14. Markel MD, Snyder JR, Hornof WJ, et al. Nuclear scintigraphic evaluation of third metacarpal and metatarsal bone fractures in three horses. J Am Vet Med Assoc 1987;191:75.
15. McClure SR, Watkins JP, Ashman RB. A in vitro comparison of the effect of parallel and divergent transfixation pins on the breaking strength of the equine third metacarpal bone. Vet Surg 1993;389.
16. McClure SR, Watkins JP, Glickman NW, et al. Complete fractures of the third metacarpal or metatarsal bone in horses: 25 cases (1980–1996). J Am Vet Med Assoc 1998;213:847.
17. Morisset S, McClure SR, Hillberry BM, et al. In vitro comparison of the use of two large-animal, centrally threaded, positive-profile transfixation pin designs in the equine third metacarpal bone. Am J Vet Res 2000;61:1298.
18. Nunamaker DM, Richardson DW, Butterweck DM. Mechanical and biological effects of plate luting. J Orthop Trauma 1991;5(2): 138.
19. Schneider RK, Jackman BR. Fractures of the third metacarpus and metatarsus. In: Nixon AJ, Ed. Equine Fracture Repair. Philadelphia: WB Saunders, 1996;179.
20. Schneider RK, Ratzlaff MC, White KK, et al. Effect of three types of half-limb casts on in vitro bone strain recorded from the third metacarpal bone and proximal phalanx in equine cadaver limbs. Am J Vet Res 1998;59:1188–1193.
21. Sedrish SA, Moore RM, Kelly K, et al. In Vitro pullout strength of screws inserted in adult equine third metacarpal bone after overdrilling a 4.5-mm threaded insertion hole. Vet Surg 1998;27: 143–149.
22. Seltzer KL, Stover SM, Taylor KT, et al. The effect of hole diameter on the torsional mechanical properties of the equine third metacarpal bone. Vet Surg 1996;25:371.

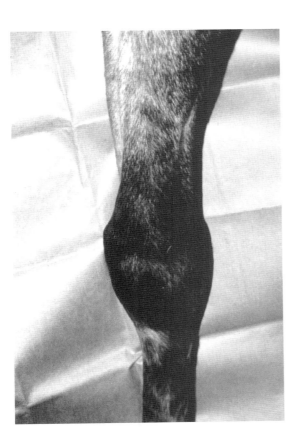

Figure 8.228 Bench knee conformation in which the cannon bone (metacarpus) is shifted toward the outside of the carpus. The condition may predispose horses to second metacarpal (inside) splints.

and osteoperiostitis. Either tearing of the interosseous ligament that binds a small metacarpal bone to the large metacarpal/metatarsal bone, external trauma, or healing of a transverse or longitudinal fracture are the causes. If the inflammation associated with the periosteum is sufficient, it will eventually result in ossification (prolif-erative exostosis) of the splint bone. The size of the splint usually depends on the degree of inflammation and the surface area involved. In any case, the splint generally assumes an elongated form, lying parallel to the small metacarpal bone.

The second metacarpal is more frequently involved because of the difference in its articulation with the car-pus. The second metacarpal is entirely articular and its articulation is flatter than that of the fourth metacarpal bone (see Figs. 4.51D and 4.52D). In Rooney-Prickett type A articulation, there is no measurable articulation between the third and second metacarpal bones or the second metacarpal bone articulates with the second car-pal bone alone. This configuration was rare in a survey of 100 horses at necropsy. Rooney-Prickett type B articu-lations accounted for 98.5% of metacarpals in which the second metacarpal articulated proximally with the second and third carpal bones.[3,6] When mechanical load tests were performed on ligamentous preparations of the carpus and metacarpus, it was noted that the carpal bones pushed the small metacarpal bones distad.[5]

It is proposed that excessive loading can lead to tear-ing of the interosseous ligament in the region that is most frequently affected. Metacarpal fusion progresses nor-mally with aging, and 78% of all horses 2 years old and older had two or more sites of fusion. The rate of meta-carpal fusion per horse per year appeared to be at least 10 times higher than the clinically evident rate, indicating that this process occurs subclinically in most horses.[3]

Conformation abnormalities that increase the stress on the small metacarpal bones also increase the incidence of this disease.[4] Offset carpi (bench knees) is an example of a conformational abnormality that predisposes the horse to splints on the medial small metacarpal bones (Fig. 8.228). Furthermore, horses that have a base-nar-row, toe-out conformation may experience external trauma to the splint bone by hitting it with the opposite limb (interference) (see Chapter 3). Improper shoeing and trimming can cause enough alteration in the foot flight that the horse may interfere as well. All can cause either a tearing of the interosseous ligament or a prolifer-ative periostitis of the second and/or third metacarpal bone. The fourth metacarpal bone may be affected by external blows (hitting objects or being kicked). A higher incidence of this type of injury has been observed in the fourth metatarsal bone.

Imbalanced nutrition or overnutrition in young horses has also been implicated in the development of splints.[4] Imbalances and deficiencies in calcium and phosphorus have been associated with an increased inci-dence of splints. However, no well-documented study has proven this to be true. In many cases, horses that are suspected of having a calcium and phosphorus imbal-ance are also growing rapidly. It may be that their in-creased weight causes sufficient compressive forces so that splints develop as a result of this rather than the imbalance.

Young horses that are poorly conformed, overweight, and vigorously overexercised have a greater chance of tearing the interosseous ligament before metacarpal fu-sion is complete and is stable.

Signs

The condition is most common in 2-year-old horses undergoing heavy training, but cases occasionally occur among 3- and 4-year-olds as well. Splints most often are found on the medial aspect of the limb, because the sec-ond metacarpal bone normally bears more weight than the fourth metacarpal bone and thus is more subject to stress. Lameness is usually most obvious in the trot. Heat, pain, and swelling over the affected region may occur anywhere along the length of the splint bone. Splints most commonly occur about 3 inches below the carpal joint (Fig. 8.227). One large swelling or a number of smaller enlargements may occur along the length of the splint bone at its junction with the third metacarpal or third metatarsal bone.

If new bone growth occurs near the carpal joint, it may cause carpal arthritis (knee splints). Extensive new bone formation on a splint bone may encroach on the suspensory ligament and cause chronic lameness unless it is removed. The existence of growths of this kind can be determined by palpation and radiographic and ultra-

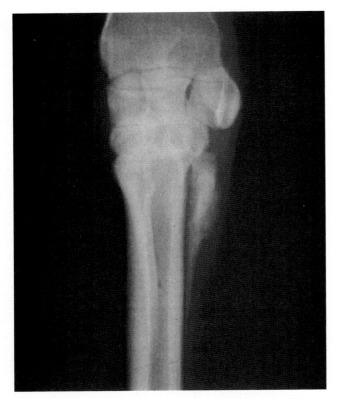

Figure 8.229 Periostitis of the splint bone. (Courtesy of T. S. Stashak.)

sound examination. Splint lameness becomes more marked with exercise on hard ground. In mild cases, no lameness may be evident in the walk, but lameness is exhibited during the trot. After the original inflammation subsides, the enlargements usually become smaller but firmer as a result of the ossification. The reduction in swelling is usually the result of resolution of fibrous tissue and not a decrease in size of the actual bone formation. In the early stages, the greatest bulk of the swelling is from inflammation, and this normally resolves to a much smaller size. Some cases of splints may not cause lameness.

Diagnosis

If the affected limb is examined carefully, the obvious signs will lead to a diagnosis. Heat, pain, and swelling over the regions mentioned, plus lameness, are enough to make the diagnosis. However the diagnosis should be confirmed with a radiograph (Fig. 8.229). Fracture of the splint bone can be confused with splints. Ultrasonographic examination can demonstrate concomitant injury to the suspensory and ligament impingement. In some cases, nuclear scintigraphy may be needed to confirm a blind splint. New bone growth resulting from trauma may occur on the third metacarpal or third metatarsal bones, close to the splint bone and may be mistaken for splints. Palpation and radiographs, however, show that these swellings are dorsal to the junction with the splint bones. This type of new bone growth is most often caused by interference.

Treatment

There are many recommended methods of treating splints, but all basically rely on the use of anti-inflammatory agents and rest for the acute phase and sometimes surgery for the more chronic stages. Counterirritation is still practiced for the chronic phases but is of unknown significance.

In the acute phase, inflammation and swelling are the hallmark of this disease. The administration of nonsteroidal anti-inflammatory drugs (NSAIDs) coupled with the application of hypothermia and pressure support wraps appears to be most beneficial to decrease the heat, pain, and swelling. Hypothermia can be attained with ice, ice and water packs, or whirlpool boots. Ice should be applied for 30 minutes two to three times a day for at least 2 to 3 days. Some clinicians recommend hand massage for 10 minutes after each treatment, after which a support bandage is applied. The application of dimethyl sulfoxide (DMSO)/Furacin or DMSO/steroid sweats is also logical. After the inflammation is gone, a mild liniment may be applied underneath the support wraps. Affected horses should be confined to a stall for 30 to 45 days and hand-walking exercise for 15 to 20 minutes twice a day should begin after the acute inflammation subsides.[4]

Intralesional corticosteroid can reduce inflammation and may help prevent excessive bone growth. Corticoid therapy should be accompanied by counterpressure bandage. In this case, the horse is generally rested longer than 30 days and should not resume training as rapidly as when counterirritation is used. However, the swelling may be considerably less. It is also true that a case of splints will heal without therapy, given adequate rest.[4]

If the splint results from interference, splint or shin boots (guards) may help prevent further trauma. If the reason the horse interferes is because of improper trimming and shoeing, they should be corrected. Intralesional injections of steroids may help, along with systemic administration of phenylbutazone to decrease the acute inflammation. Support wraps and stall rest may be required in acutely affected cases. If the proliferative bone is excessive, surgery may be indicated in a small percentage of cases.

Counterirritation in the form of pin firing, local injection of sclerosing agents, topical applications of blisters, and radiation is frequently used in subacute or chronic cases. The rationale for this treatment is that it converts a low-level inflammatory process into an acute one, which may accelerate the healing process. Pin firing or pin firing for splints is still performed, usually in racehorses. These techniques may be unacceptable for show horses because of the blemish that results. After firing, horses should be rested for at least 30 days.

Surgery to remove exostoses for medical or cosmetic reasons has resulted in fair to good success. In one study, 15 exostoses removed for cosmetics or lameness resulted in minimal recurrence of the bone proliferation.[2] In a larger study of 95 Standardbreds the splint bones were amputated to remove excessive bone callus. In horses with proximal splint bone removal in which the proximal portion was stabilized with screws or bone plates, horses were still limited in performance at 12 weeks.

Horses in which a subperiosteal removal of the exostosis was performed were sound at 12 weeks postoperatively.[7]

It is recommended that one retains the splint bone lever arm by reflecting the periosteum to prevent formation of excessive new bone and associated irritation of the suspensory ligament. In some cases, it is necessary to surgically remove a bony exostosis that interferes with the action of the suspensory ligament or the carpal joint or that is large enough to be hit repeatedly by the opposite foot. These will require care in dissection of the proximal structures, including ligaments of the palmar carpal support. If the bone growth has been caused by trauma from interference, the surgery will not be successful unless corrective shoeing or use of splint boots will stop the interference.

Prognosis

Prognosis is good to excellent for soundness, except for horses in which the exostosis is large and encroaches on the suspensory ligament or the carpal joint. Chronic recurring lameness can occur in horses that are not rested long enough, which can be 5 or 6 months. Surgery to remove the excess bone callus can successfully alleviate lameness and recurrence does not occur in most cases. Surgery may speed up the return to athletic soundness and improve blemish.

References

1. Adams OR. Lameness in Horses. 3rd ed. Baltimore: Williams & Wilkins, 1974;207.
2. Barber SM, Caron J, Pharr J. Metatarsal/metacarpal exostosis removal—A prospective study. Vet Surg 1987;16:82.
3. Les CM, Stover SM, Willits NH. Necropsy survey of metacarpal fusion in the horse. Am J Vet Res 1995;56:1421.
4. Ray C, Baxter GM. Splint bone injuries in horses. Comp Cont Educ Vet Pract 1995;17:723.
5. Rooney JR. Biomechanics of Lameness in Horses. Baltimore: Williams & Wilkins, 1969;143.
6. Rooney JR, Prickett ME. Foreleg splints in horses. Cornell Vet 1996; 56:259.
7. Welling EK. Evaluation of the efficacy of surgical intervention on middle and proximal splint bone injuries in 95 Standardbred horses. Vet Surg 1993;253.

FRACTURES OF THE SMALL METACARPAL AND METATARSAL (SPLINT) BONES

Fractures of the small metacarpal and metatarsal bones (splint bones) can occur anywhere along their length, but they are most commonly located at the distal third.[1,3,5–7,11] In most cases, fractures located at the distal third are simple fractures (Fig. 8.230), in contrast to fractures of the middle and proximal portion, which are often complicated by comminution, osteomyelitis, and bone sequestration (Figs. 8.230 and 8.231).[8,10,11]

Fractures of the distal part of a small metacarpal or metatarsal bone usually occur in older horses (5 to 7 years of age) and only rarely occur in horses under 2 years of age (Fig. 8.230).[3] This is thought to occur as a result of decreased pliability in the interosseous ligament and the strenuous training programs in older horses.[3] In contrast, younger horses tend to sustain damage to the

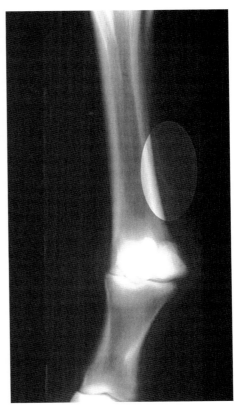

Figure 8.230 Fracture of the distal end of the splint bone. Note the chronic nonunion with ineffectual callous. Most horses with this condition have concomitant suspensory ligament injury.

interosseous ligament that supports the small metacarpal bones, resulting in splints. The forelimbs are more frequently involved than the hindlimbs, with the left forelimb with the lateral splint being affected more commonly in the hindlimb.[3,11] The relationship between suspensory ligament desmitis, sesamoiditis, and fetlock arthritis or arthrosis is more than casual. It would appear the enlarged fibrotic suspensory ligament decreases the absorptive capacity of the fetlock and creates a space-occupying mass that may cause the fracture and then further displace the fractured small metacarpal bone. It is assumed that the decreased ability to extend the fetlock contributes to the arthrosis.

Fractures of the proximal half of the small metacarpal or metatarsal bone are often comminuted, and osteomyelitis with or without sequestrum is a complicating feature. The lateral surface of these bones is most frequently involved and it is thought to result from direct trauma (Figs. 8.231 and 8.234).[2,8,10]

Causes

Fractures of the distal part of the small metacarpal/metatarsal bone result from external as well as internal trauma. External trauma can result from a kick from another horse, interference, direct blows from hitting another object, or puncture wounds. Internal trauma occurs from increased axial compression forces on these

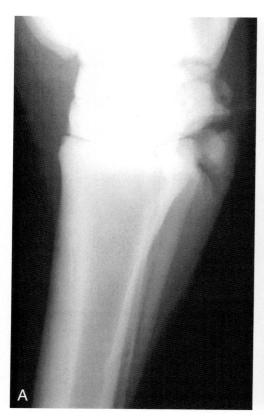
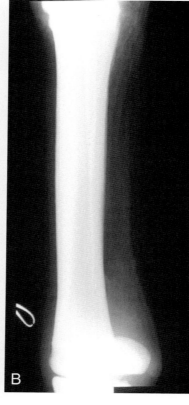

Figure 8.231 A. Comminuted articular fracture of the head of the fourth metatarsal (splint) bone in a horse that was severely lame. B. Postoperative view demonstrating complete extirpation of the fourth metatarsal bone. The horse became pasture sound but was not sound for athletic use.

bones during races or from pressure from the suspensory ligament or increased tension from the fascial attachments. It is conjectured that the increased incidence of left fourth metacarpal bone and right second metacarpal bone fractures observed in Thoroughbreds may be the result of increased weight bearing on the bones when they are racing in a counterclockwise direction. In contrast, the suspensory ligament and supporting fascia may put these bones under tension sufficient enough to cause fracture in the hindlimbs.[1,3,5-7,11] Since there is an increase in incidence of left second metatarsal bone and right fourth metatarsal bone, which is the tension side of the hindlimb in horses that run counterclockwise, it is logical to assume that tension created by the bowstring effect of the suspensory ligament or increased tension developed by the internal fascia may lead to fracture.

It is difficult to decide whether the incidence of suspensory ligament desmitis is caused by the fractured small metacarpal/metatarsal bones, which may cause irritation to the ligament, or if the swollen suspensory ligament becomes large enough to cause the fractures. Whichever the case, a higher incidence of suspensory ligament desmitis is noted in the forelimb in association with these fractures.[1,3,5-7,11]

More complicated fractures of the proximal part of the small metacarpal/metatarsal bones result from direct trauma, either from interference or direct blows to the surface. These fractures are often open initially, which frequently results in osteomyelitis. In some cases, there is no break in the skin initially, but the comminuted frac-

tures become sequestered and result in recurrent draining tracts.

Signs

On visual observation, swelling is usually a prominent feature of a proximal splint fracture, but it may not be present with a distal splint fracture. In general, the degree of swelling associated with the distal splint fracture depends on the acuteness of the fracture. The more acute the fracture, the more swelling. Associated swelling in the suspensory ligament as well as the fetlock joint may also be observed.

In the acute case, in both instances, horses will frequently point their foot. Trotting exercises may or may not cause lameness, but this totally depends on the acuteness and type of fracture that has resulted. Circling or fast work may be required to cause sufficient lameness to be observed.

On palpation, obvious features of an acute fracture are heat, pain, and swelling; in some cases, draining tracts will also be present. The pain and heat decrease with time. However, because callus formation is a frequent sequela to the nonsurgically treated fracture, the fracture site will eventually become enlarged. When only mild pain is evidenced on palpation yet the horse is quite lame, the limiting factors for this horse to resume performance may be associated with suspensory ligament desmitis or fetlock arthrosis.[1,3,5-7,11] To gain a full appreciation of the involvement of the small metacarpal/metatarsal bone, the limb is flexed so the full extent of the bone can be palpated. A thorough physical examination of the suspensory ligament should follow as well.

Diagnosis

A persistent swelling over the affected splint bone that exhibits heat and pain when pressure is applied should lead one to suspect fractured splint bone. Some fractured splint bones closely resemble the disease called splints. Some such fractures heal, but the bony swelling can be confused with splints. Radiographs are necessary for a positive diagnosis of a fractured splint bone and to differentiate among it, splints, and other soft tissue injury (Fig. 8.229). Direct infiltration anesthesia of the fractured small metacarpal/metatarsal may be used when there is a concomitant suspensory ligament desmitis or fetlock arthrosis. This approach helps define the contribution the fractured splint has in the lameness. This is particularly important in cases in which minimal pain is elicited on deep palpation of the bone but the horse is quite lame.

Radiographs should be taken in all cases to identify the fracture and its limits and to determine if sequestration and osteomyelitis exist in association with a complicated fracture (Fig. 8.233). Proximal fractures may extend toward or into the carpometacarpal joint (Figs. 8.231, 8.232, 8.234, 8.236 to 8.240).

Treatment

Small distal fractures of the splint bones are traditionally treated by removal of the distal fragment of the frac-

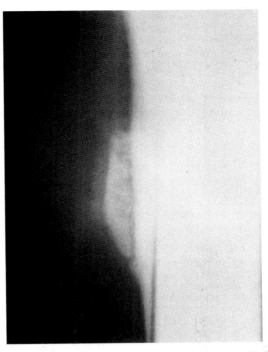

Figure 8.233 A sequestrum of the second metacarpal bone, which can be treated by surgical excision alone, without removal of the remaining distal segment of the small metacarpal bone. (Courtesy of T. S. Stashak.)

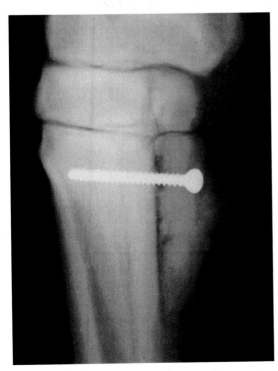

Figure 8.232 Healed comminuted fracture of the proximal second metacarpal bone (medial splint bone) in which the proximal fragment was secured with a screw during uninterrupted healing of the fracture.

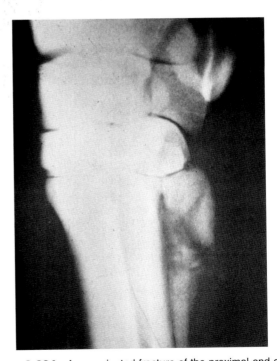

Figure 8.234 A comminuted fracture of the proximal end of the fourth metacarpal bone. This type of fracture usually requires internal fixation with a bone screw to hold it in place. (Courtesy of T. S. Stashak.)

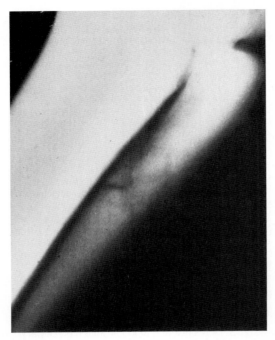

Figure 8.235   This proximal comminuted fracture of the fourth metatarsal bone was managed successfully by placing a full-limb cast for 4 weeks and then a support wrap for another 2 weeks. Free exercise was begun at 3 months. (Courtesy of T. S. Stashak.)

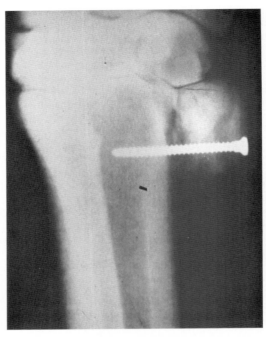

Figure 8.237   Internal fixation of the proximal comminuted fracture shown in Figure 8.234. (Courtesy of T. S. Stashak.)

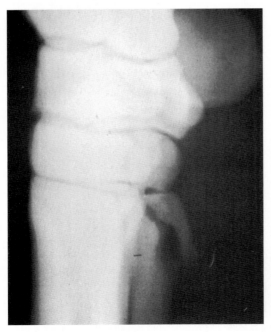

Figure 8.236   Fracture of the proximal end of the second metacarpal bone. (Courtesy of T. S. Stashak.)

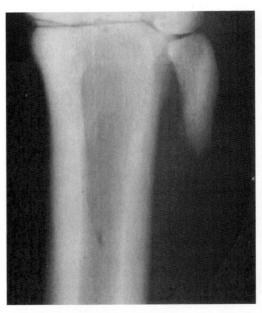

Figure 8.238   Avulsion of the proximal part of the fourth metacarpal bone after the distal end had been surgically excised. (Courtesy of T. S. Stashak.)

tured splint, but this approach is not universally recommended.[7,11] Up to two-thirds of the length of the splint can be removed without untoward sequelae; however, 80% of distal splint fractures heal spontaneously and are not usually the continued cause of lameness. Nonunion distal splint fractures were also not associated with lameness. In conclusion, surgical removal of these distal splint fractures is not necessary. At least 70% of horses with distal splint fractures have suspensory desmitis, which is generally agreed to be the cause of continued lameness.[11]

Closed nonarticular and nondistracted proximal comminuted fractures of the splint bones heal successfully with 2 to 4 months of rest (Figs. 8.232 and 8.235). In hindlimb lateral metatarsal fractures, the horses will be minimally lame, and training can continue after the acute inflammation is resolved (in about 30 days). Surgery may be necessary under the following conditions:

- If draining tracts develop
- If lameness and pain associated with the fracture are moderate to marked
- If exuberant bony callus impinges on the suspensory ligament
- If infection is present
- If follow-up radiographs show non-union or developing sequestra
- If a faster recovery and return to performance are desired

When surgery is required, it should be performed aseptically with the horse placed in lateral or dorsal recumbency.

Two surgical approaches have been successful: removal of the fractured fragments only and removal of the fracture and distal splint bone. If the fracture is in the proximal third of the bone, any contiguous piece of bone present should remain to stabilize the proximal component. In closed fractures in which more than two-thirds of the splint bone is to be removed, a small bone plate or screw can be used to stabilize the remaining proximal fragment (Figs. 8.232, 8.237, and 8.239).[4,10] If the proximal fragment is not anchored, excessive movement of the fragment may occur, resulting in interosseous desmitis, degenerative arthritis of the carpometacarpal articulation or tarsometatarsal joint, or avulsion of the proximal fragment. Screw fixation is less frequently successful (Figs. 8.232, 8.237, and 8.239). The lateral small metacarpal bone may be more predisposed to avulsion after fracture of its proximal part because of the major attachment of the lateral collateral ligament.

Open distal and middle fractures of the splint bone will often lead to draining tracts or sequestra so it is recommended that these be treated surgically with open removal of the fracture with or without the distal splint. The distal splint bone is left if it seems to provide some stability to the proximal fragment.

Open proximal fractures of the splint bones have a more guarded prognosis; but most require surgery owing to draining tracts, sequestra, infectious arthritis, and unstable proximal fragments. The fracture can be stabilized with bone plates[10] or extirpated completely[2] with 60% success (Fig. 8.231). It is possible to treat open comminuted fractures with antimicrobials and lavage of the wound, after which loose fragments can be removed with

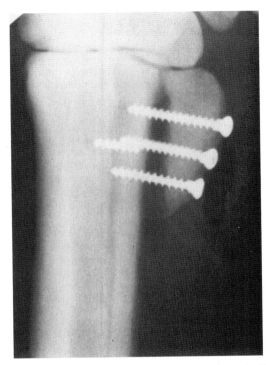

Figure 8.239   The avulsion of the splint bone shown in Figure 8.236 was treated with three screws. (Courtesy of T. S. Stashak.)

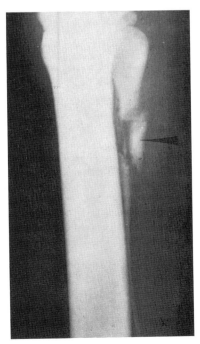

Figure 8.240   Fracture of the fourth metatarsal bone. Note the piece broken from the bone (arrow). (Courtesy of T. S. Stashak.)

a grasping forceps in the standing horse. This technique can be successful if the proximal fragment is not avulsed (displaced) and if septic arthritis has not occurred. Retained sequestra is a frequent consequence, resulting in recurrence of swelling and drainage, often months later. Open surgical treatment is optimal to address all damaged tissue and remove all fragments.

If surgery is required, the horse is anesthetized and placed in recumbency. An incision is begun just dorsal to the small metacarpal/metatarsal bone and made parallel to it. Once the dorsal border of the small metacarpal/metatarsal bone is identified, the periosteum is reflected for removal of the splint bone. If periosteal new bone has formed, it is often impossible to reflect the periosteum, and it is removed with the bone. The distal button is resected free from all surrounding tissue, and dissection between the splint bone and the large metacarpal/metatarsal bone can be made with a gouge or a chisel. Careful dissection of the axial portion of the bone from the suspensory ligament frees the fragment and allows it to be removed. A bone chisel is used to taper the distal portion of the proximal fragment. The wound edges are debrided and lavaged. Soft tissues are secured in apposition and closed.

If an open contaminated fracture is present, the bone fragments are removed and the area is liberally lavaged. The surgeon should change gloves before proceeding with removal of the rest of the splint bone. A small Penrose drain can be placed to exit the wound and be pulled in 48 hours. If the fragments are all removed and liberal lavage has been performed, the incision can be closed primarily.

If more than two-thirds of the bone is removed, the bone appears unstable, and active infection is not present, a small bone plate can be secured with 3.5-mm screws to the proximal portion of the splint and the cannon bone. If the fourth metatarsal bone is involved, bone plates may be abandoned for complete removal of the splint bone. If bone plate placement is thought to result in implant infection, the proximal portion can be left as is; if luxation occurs, it can be addressed at that time. This may allow adequate time for the wound to clean up and may decrease the chance of infection. Intraoperative radiographs should be taken to confirm the removal of all fragments and to assess the repair.

After surgery, a sterile pressure bandage is applied and changed as needed. Because the small metacarpal/metatarsal bone is located in the depression behind the cannon bone and because its removal creates an increased depression, it helps to apply several rolled-up gauze sponges to the depression to provide some direct pressure, minimizing swelling. Penrose drains are maintained under sterile bandages and are usually removed 2 days postsurgery. The bandage should be thick enough to absorb and lift the drainage material from the wound between bandage changes. For an optimal cosmetic end result, the bandages are maintained for a minimum of 6 weeks after surgery. The horse should be maintained in a box stall for at least a total of 6 weeks. Hand-walking exercise can begin about week 2 after surgery, and free exercise can begin after 6 weeks. Training is usually initiated after 2 to 3 months of rest and totally depends on the degree of soft tissue damage associated with the fracture site.

Prognosis

For distal splint bone fractures, the prognosis for return to performance depends on the severity of the suspensory desmitis, not on the radiographic healing of the fracture.[3] In a retrospective study of 34 cases of distal splint fractures without suspensory ligament desmitis, 75.3% of the horses returned to previous levels of performance; of the horses that also had suspensory ligament desmitis, only 50% returned to previous levels of performance.[9] In another series with an increased percentage of suspensory ligament desmitis, only 25% of the horses resumed previous levels of performance.[3]

The prognosis for comminuted closed splint bone fractures is good to excellent with or without surgery, particularly if the horse is used for performances other than racing.[4] The prognosis for open comminuted splint bone fractures is good to excellent with surgery if about one-third of the proximal splint remains. The prognosis for open comminuted fractures of the proximal splint is more guarded, and approximately 60% return to performance without lameness. Surgery is necessary in these cases or sequestration, osteomyelitis, and infectious arthritis persist.

References

1. Allen D, White NA. Management of fractures and exostosis of the metacarpals and metatarsals II and IV in 25 horses. Equine Vet J 1987;19:326.
2. Baxter GM, Doran RE, Allen D. Complete excision of a fractured fourth metatarsal bone in eight horses. Vet Surg 1992;21:273.
3. Bowman KF, Evans LH, Herring ME. Evaluation of surgical removal of fractured distal splint bones in the horse. J Vet Surg 1982;11:116.
4. Bowman KF, Fackleman GE. Surgical treatment of complicated fractures of splint bones in the horse. J Vet Surg 1982;11:121.
5. Doran R. Fractures of the small metacarpal and metatarsal (splint) bones. In: Nixon AJ, Ed. Equine Fracture Repair. Philadelphia: WB Saunders, 1996;200.
6. Doran R. Management of simple and complicated splint bone fractures in horses. Equine Pract 1994;16:29.
7. Dupreez P. Fractures of the small metacarpal and metatarsal bones (splint bones). Equine Vet Educ 1994;6:279.
8. Harrison LJ, May SA, Edwards GB. Surgical treatment of open splint bone fractures in 26 horses. Vet Rec 1991;128:606.
9. Jones RD, Fessler TF. Observations on small metacarpal and metatarsal fractures with or without associated suspensory desmitis in Standardbred horses. Can Vet J 1977;18:29.
10. Peterson PR, Pascoe JR, Wheat JD. Surgical management of proximal splint bone fractures in the horse. Vet Surg 1987;16:367.
11. Verschooten F, Gasthuys F, De Moor A. Distal splint bone fractures in the horse: An experimental and clinical study. Equine Vet J 1984;16:532.

LAMENESS ASSOCIATED WITH THE ORIGIN OF THE SUSPENSORY LIGAMENT

Lameness associated with the origin of the suspensory ligament occurs in about 5% of horses (36 of 1094 horses in one study and 31 of 638 horses in another) with a forelimb lameness and, therefore, is relatively un-

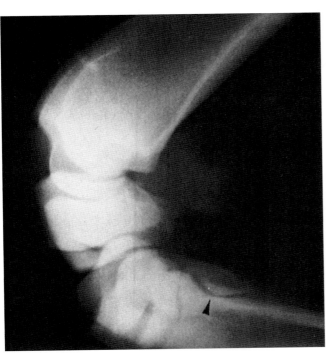

Figure 8.241 Lateral view of the carpus and proximal metacarpus. A saucer-shaped avulsion fracture (arrow) of the attachment of the suspensory ligament is present on the palmar aspect of the proximal end of the third metacarpal bone. (Courtesy of T. S. Stashak.)

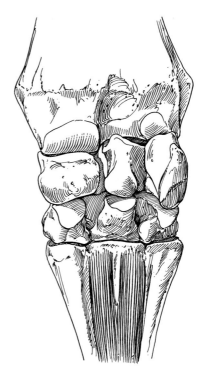

Figure 8.242 The attachments of the suspensory ligament at the proximal palmar surface of the third metacarpal bone. (Courtesy of T. S. Stashak.)

common.[3,10] It can be caused by a proximal suspensory ligament desmitis, torn Sharpey's fibers at the origin of the suspensory ligament, or an avulsion fracture of the origin of the suspensory ligament. Horses with high proximal suspensory ligament desmitis and an acute tear of Sharpey's fibers may present with similar signs as those described for blind splint and desmitis of the carpal (inferior) check ligament.[9]

In chronic cases of tearing at the origin of the suspensory ligament, radiographic evidence of bone resorption and surrounding sclerosis can be noted. With an avulsion fracture of the origin of the suspensory ligament either the lateral or medial branch may be involved in one or both limbs and are likely seen on radiographs or as a displaced piece of bone on ultrasound (Fig. 8.241). This lameness most frequently occurs in Standardbreds, hunters and jumpers, and polo ponies; but other breeds are affected as well.[10]

Causes

The suspensory ligament is primarily made up of dense white fibrous connective tissue. Proximally, the body of the suspensory ligament separates and attaches into two palmar depressions just distal to the carpometacarpal joint (Fig. 8.242). Overloading of the suspensory ligament may cause sprain trauma to any portion of the ligament, but origin injuries are seen more commonly in sport horses. Hyperextension of the carpus in conjunction with severe overextension of the metacarpophalangeal joint has been proposed to cause this lesion. Ob-

viously, the more severe the sprain trauma, the more severe the lesion. Working horses in deep, soft arenas or in eventing where there is excessive rotational movement of the limbs may be at greater risk.

Signs

Most horses with proximal suspensory ligament desmitis present with a history of intermittent lameness of several days' or weeks' duration that is exacerbated by resumed exercise. The onset may be acute or insidious. Generally, only in acute cases can heat and swelling be palpable on the proximal aspect of the limb (medial or lateral). In chronic, intermittent cases, physical findings are less obvious or may not be present to assist with a diagnosis. However, slight proximal swelling may be felt on the medial side between the suspensory ligament and deep digital flexor tendon in some cases.[11] In addition, firm digital pressure overlying the proximal suspensory ligament in these cases will usually elicit a nonfatigable painful response (Fig. 8.243). The lameness is generally mild to moderate (1 to 2 +/5) at a trot, and may be more obvious when the horse is circled at a trot with the affected limb on the outside of the circle. Lower limb flexion exacerbates 50% of forelimb origin of suspensory lamenesses and hock flexion exacerbates 85% of hindlimb origin of suspensory lamenesses.[4]

Horses with torn Sharpey's fibers at the origin of the suspensory ligament or avulsion fractures most frequently present with a history of acute onset of moderate to severe lameness. Horses sustaining a fracture of the

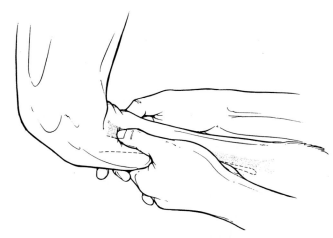

Figure 8.243 Location for digital palpation of the origin of the suspensory ligament.

origin of the suspensory ligament have often attained racing speeds in their workouts. Digital pressure at the origin of the suspensory ligament may induce a pain response and exacerbate the lameness (Fig. 8.243).

Diagnosis

Proximal suspensory injury (origin of suspensory ligament injury) occurs in both forelimbs and hindlimbs and is being recognized more frequently because of the better use of local anesthesia techniques and the advent of diagnostic ultrasonography and nuclear scintigraphy.[4] Pain withdrawal after selective digital palpation over the origin of the suspensory ligament should direct the examiner to this injury, but it may be absent in some cases.

A presumptive diagnosis of proximal suspensory ligament problems can be made from physical findings and the elimination of the lameness after direct infiltration of the origin of the suspensory ligament or perineural anesthesia. In the forelimbs, either direct infiltration of the origin of the suspensory ligament or perineural anesthesia of the lateral palmar nerve (preferred) just below the accessory carpal bone or of the ulnar nerve can be performed and usually eliminates the lameness (see Chapter 3). Because the distal extent of the carpometacarpal joint extends axial on either side of the small metacarpal bones for about 4 cm and because the carpometacarpal joint communicates with the middle carpal joint, intrasynovial anesthesia of the middle carpal joint may also eliminate lameness associated with the proximal suspensory ligament. Perineural analgesia of the palmar–plantar nerves and palmar–plantar metacarpal/metatarsal nerves (high four point) may not eliminate the lameness, since the blocks are often performed too distally. In the hindlimb, direct local infiltration of the origin of the suspensory ligament will eliminate lameness as will a tibial nerve block. In one study, lesions were created in the flexor tendons or proximal suspensory ligament of forelimbs with collagenase injection. Perineural anesthesia of the proximal metacarpus did not reliably abolish pain from suspensory desmitis, unless the ulnar

block was added.[8] Similar results were obtained with hindlimb blocks.[7]

Care must be taken when performing the ulnar nerve block or the lateral palmar nerve block just below the accessory carpal bone, because the carpal sheath is entered 68% of the time.[6] Care must also be taken when direct infiltration of the origin of the suspensory ligament of the forelimb is done, because the distal reflection of the carpometacarpal joint capsules that lie axial to the small metacarpal bone and extend distad for approximately 4 cm may be injected.

Radiographic examination may be negative for acute high suspensory ligament desmitis and torn Sharpey's fibers. However, bone sclerosis of the trabecular pattern of the proximal plantar cannon bone, alteration of the plantar subcortical trabecular pattern, and entheseophyte formation were noted in 23 of 47 horses diagnosed with hindlimb proximal suspensory desmitis.[2] Early bone resorption can occur at the origin of the heads of the suspensory ligament (Fig. 8.244). A fracture associated with the origin of the suspensory ligament can be observed on radiographic examination (Fig. 8.241).

Ultrasonographic examination is the only current method to determine damage to the origin of the suspensory ligament. Nuclear scintigraphy is a highly sensitive method for localizing an abnormality to that site, but the structure cannot be assessed. Ultrasound examinations should be performed every 60 days until the ligament has healed. Morphologic abnormalities of the suspensory ligament that are often identified include enlargement of the ligament (linear width and circumference),

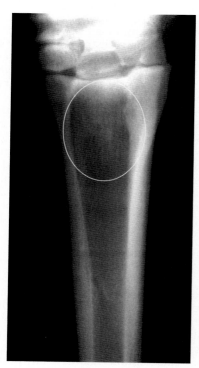

Figure 8.244 Craniocaudal view of the proximal metacarpus in a horse with origin of suspensory pain without ultrasound lesions. Note the bone resorption at both heads of the suspensory ligament origin (oval).

poor definition of margins, central or peripheral hypoechoic areas, diffuse reduction in echogenicity, hyperechogenic foci, and irregularity of the plantar cortex of the third metatarsal bone (entheseophyte formation).[3] Normally, the suspensory ligament is the most echodense structure in the palmar–plantar metacarpus/metatarsus.[12] Comparison to the contralateral limb should be performed, but the disease condition is bilateral in 18% of horses,[3] so standardized normals should also be used.

Nuclear scintigraphy is reportedly a highly sensitive (100%) but only fairly specific (41%) test for the detection of high suspensory injury.[5] In 21 horses in which nuclear scintigraphy was performed as part of the diagnosis of proximal suspensory injury, all revealed increased uptake of radiolabel. Only 67% of horses radiographed had an identified lesion (86% in hindsight). However, although scintigraphy was sensitive in identifying inflammation of the proximal aspect of the metacarpal/metatarsal region, no specific diagnosis of suspensory injury could be made without concurrent radiography. In comparison to horses with increased radiolabel uptake in a similar region without a diagnosis of high suspensory injury, the specificity of scintigraphy was 41%. Scintigraphy can help locate the suspensory ligament as a possible problem area and offers an advantage over direct infiltration of local anesthetic in that it does not affect the ultrasound image. Ultrasound and radiographic examination of the region should follow to document and specify the type of injury.

Treatment

Treatment for horses with a structural abnormality on ultrasound and on radiography consists of box-stall rest for 2 months followed by repeat ultrasound. Hand walking for 15 minutes twice daily for the first 4 weeks and for 20 minutes twice daily for the last 4 weeks can be performed[4] if the horses are sound at the walk, the origin lesion is not greater than 50% of the cross-sectional area, and straight hindlimb conformation is not present in a hindlimb injury. Trotting can begin after 8 weeks if the lesion is reasonably improved on ultrasound and the horse is sound at the trot in hand. A slow and controlled (saddle) or rein lunging exercise program can continue until 16 weeks, when another ultrasound is performed. If soundness has persisted and the lesion appears healed after 16 weeks, the horse's exercise can increase. Total healing time is about 8 months, and return to full competitive performance may not be possible for 1 year.

Recurrence of injury is greater in horses that have been inadequately rested. Balancing the foot, shoeing with egg bars, and using sport fetlock support bandages can improve the flexor surface support. Phenylbutazone is recommended for its anti-inflammatory effect. If pain returns after exercise has begun, a more prolonged convalescent period is required. The direct infiltration of corticosteroids into the site is not recommended, because it may delay the healing process. Use of oral glycosaminoglycans—systemic polysulfated glycosaminoglycans or systemic hyaluronic acid—may have some benefit, although unproven. Use of internal blisters, intralesional steroids, and mineralizing agents are contraindicated.

Prognosis

The prognosis is good (greater than 80%) for return to full work in sport horses with forelimb proximal suspensory ligament desmitis after 3 to 6 months' rest and controlled exercise.[4,10] For hindlimb lameness, only 14% of horses returned to full athletic function without detectable lameness in one study.[2] The presence of upright hindlimb (straight hock) conformation is overrepresented in horses with hindlimb suspensory injury and may predispose the suspensory ligament to injury and recurrence; hence the poor success for permanent resolution of soundness. Another proposed reason for the poor prognosis associated with hindlimb proximal suspensory ligament desmitis is the development of a compartmental syndrome, resulting from the limited space available between the prominent splint bones that the inflamed suspensory ligament has to expand into.[2]

Recurrence of proximal suspensory ligament desmitis also relates to use. In one study, dressage and show jumping horses had the highest recurrence rate (37% and 46%, respectively) compared to racehorses (27%), show hunters (19%), and field hunters (18%).[1] The larger the suspensory ligament lesion the greater the chance of recurrence. Generally, the recurrence of proximal suspensory ligament desmitis 1 year after successful treatment is low, but when it does occur the prognosis was guarded for return to performance. The prognosis is also reduced when proximal suspensory ligament desmitis is associated with other lesions, such as tendinitis of the superficial and deep digital flexor tendons or desmitis of the radial check ligament.[2]

The prognosis for avulsion fracture associated with the origin of the suspensory ligament appears good for uneventful recovery and return to full work after 3 to 6 months' rest and controlled exercise. A good blood supply is thought to be the reason that these fractures heal so readily.

References

1. Cowles RR, Johonson LD, Holloway PM. Proximal suspensory desmitis: A retrospective study. Proc Am Assoc Equine Pract 1994; 4:183–185.
2. Dyson SJ. Proximal suspensory desmitis in the hindlimb. Equine Vet J 1995;7:275.
3. Dyson SJ. Some observations on lameness associated with pain in the proximal metacarpal region. Equine Vet J Orthop 1992; 6(Suppl):43.
4. Dyson SJ, Arthur RM, Palmer SC, et al. Suspensory ligament desmitis. Vet Clin North Am 1995;11(2):177.
5. Edwards RB, Ducharme NG, Fubini SL, et al. Scintigraphy for diagnosis of avulsions of the origin of the suspensory ligament in horses: 51 cases (1980–1993). J Am Vet Med Assoc 1995;207: 608.
6. Ford TS, Ross MW, Orsini PG. A comparison of methods for proximal palmar metacarpal analgesia in horses. Vet Surg 1989;18: 146.
7. Keg PR, Barneveld A, Schamhardt HC, et al. Clinical and force plate evaluation of the effect of a high plantar nerve block in lameness caused by induced mid-metatarsal tendonitis. Vet Q 1994; 16(Suppl 2):S70.
8. Keg, PR, van den Belt AJ, Merkens HW, et al. The effect of regional nerve blocks on the lameness caused by collagenase-induced tendonitis in the midmetacarpal region of the horse: A study using gait analysis, and ultrasonography to determine tendon healing. Zentralbl Veterinarmed A 1992;39:349.

9. Marks D, MacKay-Smith MP, Leslie JA, Soule SG. Lameness resulting from high suspensory disease (HSD) in the horse. Am Assoc Equine Pract 1981;27:493–498.

10. Personett LA, McAllister ES, Mansmann RA. Proximal suspensory desmitis. Mod Vet Pract 1983;541–545.

11. Stashak TS. Lameness associated with the proximal palmar/plantar cannon bone region. In: Proceedings. 20th Bain-Fallon Memorial Lectures: Lameness and Ultrasound, 1998;295–302.

12. Wood AK, Sehgal CM, Polansky M. Sonographic brightness of the flexor tendons and ligaments in the metacarpal region of horses. Am J Vet Res 1993;54:1969–1974.

SPRAIN (DESMITIS) OF THE SUSPENSORY LIGAMENT

See Chapter 7.

DESMITIS OF THE CARPAL (INFERIOR) CHECK LIGAMENTS

See Chapter 7.

Part V

THE CARPUS

Alicia L. Bertone

ANGULAR LIMB DEFORMITIES ASSOCIATED WITH THE CARPUS (CARPUS VALGUS AND VARUS; MEDIAL AND LATERAL DEVIATION OF THE CARPUS)

Limb deformities in foals can be described as angular, flexural, or rotational. An angular deformity refers to a deviation of a limb in the frontal plane defined by the joint or bone that is at the center (pivot point) of the deviation. If the limb distal to the pivot point is axial (medial), the deviation is varus. If the limb distal to the pivot point is abaxial (lateral), the deviation is valgus. The most common angular limb deformity (ALD) in foals is carpus valgus, which refers to the outward deviation of the distal part of the cannon bone below the carpus[6,18,25] (Fig. 8.245). Most foals have some degree of more than one type of deformity.

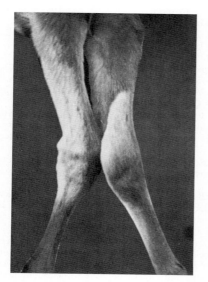

Figure 8.245   Knock knees in foal. (Courtesy of T. S. Stashak.)

Flexural deformities are a deviation of the limb in the sagittal plane such that the joint of origin is cranial or caudal to a plumb line drawn through the center of the limb from the side. This line should bisect the limb into cranial and caudal halves and then exit the fetlock joint and touch the caudal heel.[25] The deformity is named by the joint at the pivot point and its location relative to the plumb line—i.e., cranial (flexural deformity) or caudal (laxity deformity).

Rotational deformities are commonly seen in conjunction with angular deformities. The rotation occurs around a plumb line that bisects the limb from the front.[25] Rotations can be outward (toe out) or inward (toe in) and are often named by the joint at which the rotation starts or is most prominent. Rotational deformities are not usually associated with lameness, unless they are severe and produce limb interference. Most are considered conformational abnormalities.

Angular and flexural deformities are associated with a pathologic process (developmental orthopedic disease) and if untreated can produce permanent deformities associated with lameness or loss of athletic performance. Angular limb deformities are by far the most common. Combined with physeal dysplasia, they represented 72.9% of developmental orthopedic diseases treated in a foal crop of Irish Thoroughbreds ($n = 1711$) in which 248 were examined (4.24% of foal registrations).[1,3] Most of the animals with developmental orthopedic disease recovered (54% sold for expected value), but 27.5% sold for a lower than expected value and 18.7% were killed. In a survey that evaluated the reproductive performance of mares, ALD was the health problem most commonly reported in foals receiving unacceptable physical assessments.[20] Therefore, the impact of this condition in breeding operations is high.

Carpus valgus (knock kneed) refers to a deformity in which the metacarpus deviates laterad (outward) and the distal radius deviates mediad (inward). It represents by far the most common abnormality (Fig. 8.245).[25] Approximately 80% of deformities referred for surgery are carpal deviations (more than 80% valgus; 78% bilateral), and about 15% are fetlock deviations (usually

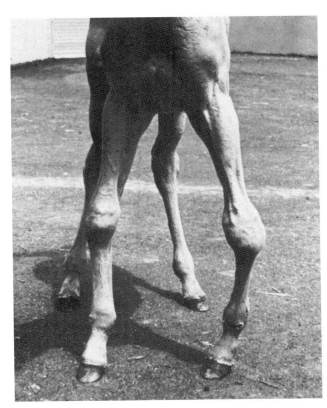

Figure 8.246   Carpus varus. (Courtesy of T. S. Stashak.)

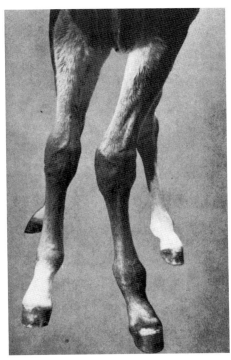

Figure 8.247   Limb deviation owing to uterine positioning. The right forelimb has a slight lateral deviation (varus) of the carpus, and the left forelimb has a severe medial deviation (valgus) of the carpus. Both limbs are bowed toward the same direction. (Courtesy of T. S. Stashak.)

varus) and less than 2% are distal tibial deviations (tarsus valgus or varus).[6,19] Carpus varus (bowlegged) refers to the opposite situation in which the distal metacarpus deviates mediad and the distal radius deviates laterad (Fig. 8.246). Angular limb deformities can result from asymmetric growth of the distal radial metaphysis or the distal radial epiphysis, from incomplete development of the cuboidal bones and proximal second and fourth metacarpal bones, or from joint laxity.[18,25]

Angular limb deformities are being treated with increasing frequency in foals of all breeds, particularly Thoroughbreds. In a report from one surgical practice, 199 Thoroughbred foals were treated with surgery for ALD in a 2-year period,[19] which represents only a fraction of the total surgeries performed for this condition nationwide. Reasons for this include the availability of simple, highly successful surgical procedures and an excellent prognosis for straightening the limbs. The incidence of ALD is probably not breed specific, because reports reflect the type of horse seen in the practice and the sex distribution is approximately equal.[10,19]

Foals either are born with deviated limbs (congenital) or develop ALD within several weeks to months after birth (acquired) (Fig. 8.247).[25] Congenital deformity should be immediately assessed in terms of severity, degree of immaturity of skeletal development, and whether the limb can be manually reduced. Most congenital angular deformities are carpus valgus, can be manually reduced, and are caused by ligamentous laxity in a skeletally immature foal. In mild to moderate cases, the deformity will correct without treatment; but in moder-

ate to severe cases, progressive cases, or cases with extreme lack of development of the cuboidal bones, treatment to support the limbs is required. Foals born with straight limbs that acquire the angular deformity as they mature (usually the carpus) require assessment and usually do not improve completely with conservative management. Approximately 20% of foals present with multiple limb and joint involvement (e.g., carpus valgus plus tarsus valgus or carpus valgus with fetlock varus).[19]

Causes

The causes of ALDs are varied, complex, and multifactorial. For congenital carpal deviations, skeletal immaturity and weakness of the collateral ligaments combined with undermineralization of the cuboidal bones lead to collapse of the joint with weight bearing and spreading of the limbs to allow the head to reach the ground. The causes of the skeletal immaturity include twinning, premature birth, and dysmaturity owing to poor maternal health or nutrition. Nonreducible congenital deformities are most commonly fetlock varus and "windswept" conditions. A windswept foal has a varus deformity in one limb and a valgus deformity in the contralateral limb. Nonreducible congenital deformities may be caused by uterine malpositioning and/or may be inherited.

Developmental ALDs are considered part of the developmental orthopedic disease complex, a group of musculoskeletal diseases that occur only during growth.[4,26]

This condition may represent an abnormality of endochondral ossification of the growth plates and the cuboidal bones during growth. Factors such as age (usually 3 to 6 months), size (heavy body weight), nutrition (high-energy diets), mineral balance (low copper, low calcium with high phosphorus), and sex (males more common than females) are known to be associated with the condition. Genetic predisposition, exercise, foot care, and nutritional factors are suspected of influencing the development of the condition.

The underlying growth disturbance is asymmetric growth of the physes and cuboidal bones and, to a lesser degree, the small metacarpal/metatarsal bones. The longitudinal growth of the metaphysis of the long bones occurs at the physes and, to a lesser degree, at the epiphysis. This process of bone formation during growth is termed *endochondral ossification,* because a cartilage model is replaced by bone. A number of factors can alter or arrest endochondral ossification (see Chapters 5 and 6). Of the many factors that can influence endochondral ossification, compression trauma may be particularly important in the asymmetric growth seen in ALDs. Axial compressive forces that are within physiologic (normal) limits stimulate the growth and mineralization process. Excessive forces (nonphysiologic or abnormal compressive forces) can suppress or arrest the development of cartilage models to bone, which in turn causes a reduction in longitudinal bone growth.

It is proposed that nonphysiologic compressive forces may cause microfractures of the newly formed trabecular bone and may alter the blood supply sufficiently at the zone of provisional calcification (transition zone between cartilage and bone) to result in defective endochondral ossification.[8] An underlying abnormality in the process of endochondral ossification may be present in foals that develop ALDs and other developmental orthopedic diseases, such as osteochondrosis.[4,25] This risk factor may be partially inherited and may predispose such foals to the condition after exposure to lower environmental (nutrition) and mechanical stresses (body weight, exercise) than a normal foal. The asymmetry of the limb is noted during the most rapid growth phase for that foal, because any disturbance in growth is projected at that time.

For example, in a valgus deformity of the carpus resulting from asymmetric growth in the distal radial metaphysis, the concave side (lateral) will be under greater axial compression than the convex side (medial). In this case, there is an asymmetric axial compressive loading of the lateral aspect of the growth plate. If it is within physiologic limits, the lateral side of the growth plate will be stimulated to grow more rapidly than the medial side, and the limb will straighten on its own. However, if the compressive forces are nonphysiologic, the growth from the lateral side (concave) will be reduced or arrested, and the ALD will remain static or worsen. The more asymmetric the compressive forces, the worse the angular deformity.

For congenital ALDs, it is postulated that incomplete ossification of the cuboidal bones and/or small metacarpal bones increase the angular deformity caused by alterations in endochondral ossification by contributing to asymmetric loading from compression and collapse of the cartilage model on one side. For developmental angular carpal deformities, asymmetric compressive forces contribute to the defective endochondral ossification on the lateral side of the distal radial metaphysis. Asymmetric loading that leads to compression can be exacerbated by a severe angular deformity caused by carpal bone hypoplasia and joint laxity.[8]

Congenital Angular Limb Deformity

Congenital angular deformities of the carpus may be the caused by intrauterine malposition, overnutrition of the mare in the latter half of pregnancy, joint laxity, defective endochondral ossification (hypoplasia) of the cuboidal bones, or maldevelopment of the second and fourth metacarpal bones. Toxic chemicals and other poorly understood mechanical and endocrine influences may also have an effect.[2,8,17] Intrauterine malposition or stagnant position may cause the ALD by restricting normal movement and growth. Overweight brood mares may be prone.[15]

Foals fed a low-copper diet (7 ppm) were compared to foals fed a higher-copper diet (30 ppm); in the former group, angular limb deformities were a feature of the developmental disease.[14] Foals with hypothyroids (congenital hyperplastic goiter) show a significant delay in endochondral ossification of the cuboidal bones in utero and can be born with a chondrodystrophic phenotype that includes carpal valgus and cuboidal bone collapse. In areas with low-iodine soil, pregnant mares should have access to iodized salt blocks.[16]

Medial to lateral carpal joint laxity is present to a minor degree in normal foals, evidenced by a slight knock-kneed appearance (less than 5°) that worsens with fatigue. Normal exercise (paddock) rapidly develops the forearm muscles and carpal ligaments, improving the support to the joints. In some foals, the degree of laxity is excessive (more than 5°) and can become painful with fatigue, encouraging the foal to lay down. Excessive laxity is associated with dysmaturity, as mentioned earlier. Radiographs often demonstrate a delay in endochondral ossification for the gestational or birth age.[24] Stall confinement is recommended to limit the asymmetric loading of the bones and growth plate, which may contribute to progression of the deformity.

In ponies or miniature horses, a complete fibula and ulna may be present and is associated with severe carpus and tarsus valgus, noted at birth and worsening with growth. Surgery to release the lateral bony column is critical for arresting the deformity, because surgery to stimulate growth (periosteal elevation) alone is not successful (discussed below).[23]

Acquired Angular Limb Deformity

Foals with acquired ALDs are born with relatively straight limbs that begin to deviate within the first few weeks or months of life. Factors that are associated with the condition include an unrecognized subtle congenital ALD, a growth plate injury, excessive contralateral limb weight bearing, overnutrition, improper trimming, excessive exercise, primary asymmetric growth of the distal radial metaphysis or distal radial epiphysis, and poor conformation.[25]

Direct trauma to the distal radial physis (growth plate) can result in ALD and produce an asynchronous longitudinal growth. If the damage is severe, premature closure may occur on one side or progress across the entire growth plate.[8] This can lead to an irreversible deformity if the closure is asymmetric or a total loss in limb length if the entire growth plate is involved. The degree of alteration depends on the age of the horse at the time of injury and which growth plate is affected. The distal radial growth plate begins to decrease significantly the rate of growth after 16 months of age and contributes 75% of the limb length. The distal metacarpal/metatarsal growth plate begins to decrease significantly the rate of growth after 90 days and contributes about 5% of limb length.[9] An injury (fracture) that symmetrically involves the distal radius or distal tibial physis in a young foal has the potential to produce the most severe permanent ALD.

ALD (usually carpus varus) can occur secondary to excessive contralateral limb weight bearing in a lame foal. Rapid treatment of the primary problem to distribute limb loading more evenly is critical to prevent progression. Casts and splints can help support the collateral ligaments of the sound limb, but they do not usually produce a normal limb and have secondary complications. If progression can be arrested and the horse is a yearling or younger, surgical techniques can be used to help correct the deformity.

Overnutrition (a high-energy diet) and imbalanced nutrition may be associated with developmental ALDs. The increased body weight from overnutrition results in an increased compressive force, which, if an angular deformity is present, may lead to greater asymmetric compressive forces. Nutrient and mineral imbalances may alter the endochondral ossification process and, combined with other factors, make the cartilage more susceptible to asymmetric growth. The genetic predisposition to difficulties with the endochondral ossification process and the response to paracrine and endocrine factors may create risk. Deficiencies in trace minerals, copper in particular, has been associated with ALD deformity–endemic farms; the problems resolved after increasing copper in the diet. Commercial feeds now contain adequate amounts of copper for normal maturation.[4,25]

Signs and Diagnosis

A history should be obtained to answer questions about the foal's prematurity at birth, the age at which the deformity was noticed, the diet of the foal and mare, the course and rate of progression of the deformity, and any preceding lameness.

Foals should be evaluated on a flat, firm surface while relaxed. At the moment when the limbs are placed next to one another, an imaginary plumb line should visually bisect the limb from both the front and the side. Sites of rotation, angulation, and flexural deformity should be recorded. The degree of deformity should be estimated for each joint of origin of a deformity; the degree may be estimated with a goniometer, if available. The degree of deformity measured on the foal may be more accurate than that measured on a radiograph because radiographs

may be made under sedation or without the limb axially aligned.

All deformities should be recorded and discussed with the owner at the time of the examination. The foal should be walked and trotted to determine soundness and any other gait abnormalities that may coexist. Foals with an ADL are usually not lame, unless physitis or another unrelated condition exists, which should be investigated. Foals with carpal laxity may appear normal at rest and dramatically worsen with exercise. Joints should be palpated for effusion (possible concomitant osteochondrosis); and growth plates should be assessed for heat, pain on pressure, and swelling (indicating trauma, physitis, or a septic focus).

In carpal deformities in particular, manipulation of the distal limb can locate instability of the carpus and determine if the deformity can be reduced to normal position. Reducible deformities are treated differently from nonreducible deformities and are usually part the dysmature foal complex. Rarely, a cranial-to-caudal laxity can be appreciated with collapsed or subluxated carpal bones.[8] Conversely, the distal limb is nonreducible in deformities caused by asymmetric growth of the distal radial metaphysis and alterations of the distal radial epiphysis.

A radiographic examination of the carpus is recommended to ensure that the bone structure is normal and developed. The angle of deviation and the pivot point can be calculated from the radiographs if long plates were used and an adequate length of the long bones on either side of the joint were included in the study. A goniometer is used to draw a line that bisects the radius and one that bisects the third metacarpus; the lines are extended until they intersect. The location of intersection within the carpus and the angle at which they meet are recorded. Rarely, arthritis of the joints, significant bony malformation, or osteochondrosis is identified, altering the prognosis.

Radiographs should be obtained on long plates and should include cranio–caudal and lateral views. Typical radiographic findings for the carpus include metaphyseal flaring, asymmetric widening of the growth plate, sclerosis of the growth plate on the concave side, physeal widening on the convex side, wedging of the epiphysis, wedging of the carpal bones (particularly of the third carpal), distal displacement of the ulnar carpal bone, and distal displacement or increased angulation to the head of the lateral splint bone (the fourth metacarpal).[5] These findings do not adversely affect prognosis for most carpal deformities, including moderate to severe deformities.

Evidence of arthritis (more common with carpal varus deformities), chip fracture, traumatic growth plate injury (fracture), or septic osteomyelitis potentially decreases the prognosis for either correcting the deformity or for soundness. In neonates, the degree of mineralization (osteogenesis) depends on gestational length and fetal age. Typically, radiographs of neonates demonstrate mineralization beginning centrally in all cuboidal bones. The extent of osteogenesis in normal fetuses (70 to 340 days of gestation) to birth has been reported,[24] and a standardized skeletal ossification index is available for premature and small for gestational age foals.[1] These estimates can be used for comparison to a neonate to

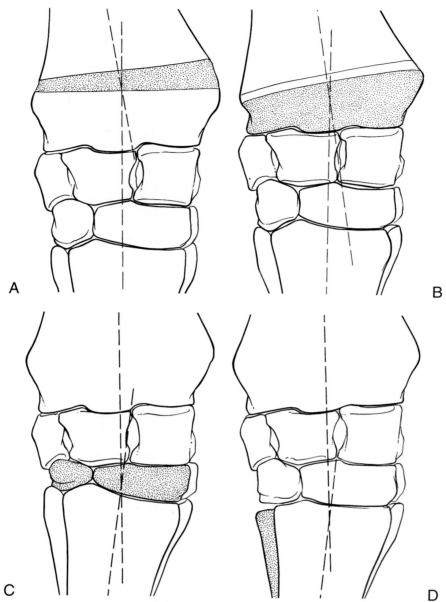

Figure 8.248 Front view of the distal radius carpus. Stippling indicates problem areas. A. The pivot point is centered over the physis, which is caused by asynchronous growth of the distal radial metaphysis. B. The pivot point is centered over the distal epiphysis of the radius, which is caused by wedging of the epiphysis. C. The pivot point is centered over the carpal joints, which is caused by wedging of the third carpal bone and hypoplasia of the fourth carpal bone. D. The pivot point is centered over the distal carpal joints, which is caused by incomplete development of the lateral small metacarpal bone. (Courtesy of T. S. Stashak.)

document delay in endochondral ossification at birth. In dysmature foals, the endochondral ossification process is delayed and the bones are undermineralized for the gestational or birth age (Fig. 8.248). Some foals with congenital carpal and tarsal angular deformity may have no evidence of osteogenesis of the cuboidal bones or proximal metacarpus on radiographs. This indicates that the cuboidal bones are composed exclusively of cartilage, which is unlikely to withstand much axial loading. In addition, asymmetric loading (angular deformity) will put the carpus at risk of developing malformations as the bones mineralize. Reestablishment of axial loading in these foals during the mineralization process (7 to 10 days of age) is critical.

The degree and components contributing to the deformity can be estimated from the degree of angulation and the location of the pivot point, respectively. A mild deformity is considered to be between 5 and 10°; a moderate deformity, between 15 and 25°; and severe deformity, greater than 25°. Today's owners and veterinarians are well educated in the signs and treatment plan; thus most foals are corrected while they still have a mild or moder-

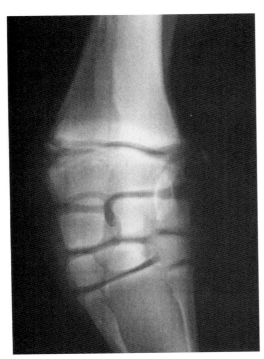

Figure 8.249 A valgus deformity. Note the irregular width of the growth plate, the wedging of the epiphysis and third carpal bone, and the hypoplasia of the fourth carpal bone and small (fourth) metacarpal bone. The lateral cortex of the diaphysis of the radius is thicker than the medial cortex. (Courtesy of T. S. Stashak.)

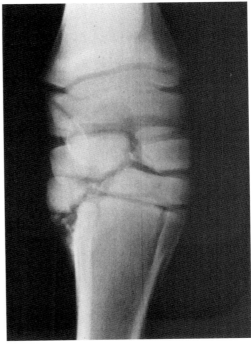

Figure 8.250 Subluxation and collapse of the fourth carpal bone. The proximal aspect of the fourth metacarpal bone is also affected. (Courtesy of T. S. Stashak.)

ate deformity. It is now uncommon to see a severe acquired carpal ALD. The location of the pivot point reveals the anatomic structures contributing to the deformity. If the point is at the physis, the physis is likely the sole or principal site of the abnormality (Fig. 8.248). Usually, the intersection is in the epiphysis or within the proximal carpal bones, indicating that the epiphysis or carpal bones, respectively, are probably contributing to the deformity (Figs. 8.248B, 8.249, and 8.250). Alterations in the development of the second and fourth metacarpal bones shift the pivot point in a distal direction (Fig. 8.248D).[5,8,21]

Treatment

Correction of the ALD is desirable for improving the conformational defect and preventing secondary degenerative changes that may result from abnormal biomechanical stresses on the deviated limb. This is particularly true of the fetlock joint, which tolerates little angular deviation without developing degenerative joint disease (DJD). Carpal deformities less than 4° are not generally associated with lameness or carpal arthritis, and treatment is optional. Rotational deformities are usually not corrected by the standard surgical procedures for ALD, and it is important that the owner be aware of this to avoid disappointment with the surgery. Careful distinction between angular and rotational deformities is necessary to estimate the final outcome of limb alignment

treatment. Correction of the angular deformity of a carpal valgus dramatically improves the appearance of a rotational deformity by pulling the limb back under the foal's body, but the degree of torsion will likely be the same. Trimming the hoof level and applying square-toe shoes may help maintain a straight breakover and improve or prevent progression of rotation.

Therapeutic options depend on the clinical syndrome. For congenital carpal angular deformity that is reducible, treatment includes stall confinement; many ALDs of the carpus will self-correct. Confinement is recommended because foals make every attempt to stay with the mares while they are on pasture. This active exercise increases the axial compressive forces to the growth plate, remodeling epiphysis, or cuboidal bones, which may result in delayed or asynchronous growth. Stall confinement helps decrease the trauma to these regions. Corrective hoof trimming (removal of the high side of the hoof wall) brings the foot back into balance.[25]

With carpus valgus, the medial side of the hoof wall is worn excessively (lower) and the lateral side of the hoof wall requires trimming to bring the hoof back into balance. Excessive trimming to correct the ALD should be avoided, because it may result in an ALD of the fetlock (see Chapter 9). Typically, these foals also have a tendency to break over the dorsomedial surface of the hoof wall. Therefore, squaring or rounding off of the toes by rasping them down to the white line helps force a break over to the central dorsal (front) part of the hoof wall.[25] Nutritional management should include good-quality alfalfa, with a free-choice mineral block and restriction of concentrates (see Chapter 5).

If the deformity does not correct within 2 or 3 weeks, if it is moderate to severe, or if the cuboidal bones are poorly mineralized on radiographs, axial alignment of the limb with tube casts or splints during the cuboidal bone mineralization process (7 to 10 days of age) is indicated. In most cases, general anesthesia is used. A combination of plaster cast or foam cast padding and fiberglass cast material is applied from the proximal radius to the distal metacarpus. The fetlock and foot are left exposed so that normal axial weight bearing can occur. This casting technique provides rigid support to the carpus without promoting osteoporosis, muscle atrophy, and tendon laxity, associated with full-limb casting techniques, particularly in foals. While the foal is anesthetized, a double layer of stockinette is applied to the limb from the foot to the elbow. Orthopedic felt is used for cast padding, and it is applied to the distal metacarpus and proximal forearm. Some clinicians like to pad the carpal region as well. With the limb placed under traction to reduce the angular deformity, two rolls of plaster material are applied in a spiral fashion from the proximal forearm to the distal metacarpus.

The limb must remain stable without applied pressure while the plaster dries. Once the plaster has cured, two to three rolls of fiberglass cast material are applied. After it is set, the stockinet is rolled over the proximal and distal ends of the cast, and each layer (inner and outer) is taped separately to the cast (Fig. 8.251). The proximal

and distal openings in the cast are covered with elastic tape to prevent any debris from entering the top or bottom of the cast. The combination of the plaster cast and fiberglass tape provides the best of both materials: The plaster casting material molds nicely to the limb, and the fiberglass tape is extremely strong and lightweight.

If casts are applied to both limbs, a sling strap can be incorporated into the proximal lateral surface of both casts. The strap fits over the withers and prevents the cast from slipping distad. This can also be done with a single limb cast. The outer strap is incorporated in the lateral surface, then runs over the back and is positioned behind the axilla of the opposite limb, and finally attaches to the proximal medial side of the cast. The attachment of the straps is best done after the foal has recovered and is standing. This allows for the best adjustment. The newer, lighter materials do not require straps.

The foal and mare should be kept in stall confinement. The cast is removed in 1 to 2 weeks, and thorough physical and radiographic examinations of the limb are then performed. Usually, maturation of the undermineralized carpal bones and stabilization of soft tissues occur in 1 to 2 weeks; only rarely will another cast have to be applied.

Alternatively, splints and braces can be used, but cast sores are common sequela.[22] Bandaging and splinting often results in more cost and labor. And slippage of the bandage causes inconsistent treatment (Fig. 8.252).

In foals with irreducible carpal ALDs (congenital or acquired), surgery to correct the deformity is usually selected. If the deformity is mild and the foal is heavy and creep fed, adjusting the diet and reducing body weight may help, but most such foals will not fully correct. Mild deformities in 2- to 3-month-old foals and moderate to severe deformities should be corrected with surgery.

Surgical Techniques

Hemicircumferential Transection of the Periosteum and Periosteal Elevation

The preferred surgical technique to correct angular deformities in foals is periosteal transection and elevation (periosteal stripping). This procedure is performed on the concave side of the metaphysis. The periosteum is hemicircumferentially transected parallel to the growth plate, and the proximal periosteum is elevated to ensure physical separation. The hemicircumferential transection and periosteal stripping stimulate endochondral ossification on that side.[3,13] Mechanical release of the periosteal cuff restraint on the growth plate has been proposed and is the mechanism for enhanced growth.

This surgery is preferred because it is simple, quick, requires little instrumentation, has a low complication rate and high success rate, and is cosmetic.[3,6] A small (1- to 2-cm) skin incision is made just proximal to the growth plate on the concave (shorter) side of the limb, just caudal to the most abaxial edge of the radius. The growth plate is assumed to the widest point of the distal radius, and the incision is extended to bone from 2 to 4 cm proximal to the growth plate. Using a hook blade, the periosteum is cut to the bone dorsally and caudally (about 3 cm), parallel to the growth plate. The hemicircumferential incision to release the periosteum is contin-

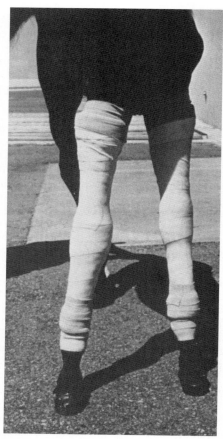

Figure 8.251 Front view of sleeve casts applied to both forelimbs. (Courtesy of T. S. Stashak.)

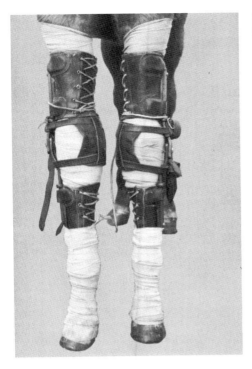
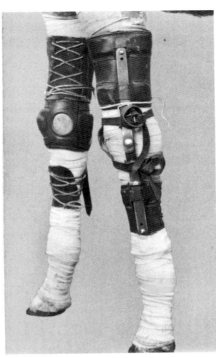

Figure 8.252 Front and side views of hinged braces used to straighten mild medial deviation of the carpi. They must be adjusted daily to avoid pressure necrosis; because they are hinged, there is little muscle atrophy. The braces can be reversed for lateral deviation. (Courtesy of T. S. Stashak.)

ued for the entire half of the distal radius. When the periosteum is transected on the lateral surface of the distal radius (as in carpus valgus), it is extended to cut the fibrous remnant of the ulna on the caudolateral border of the radius. A longitudinal incision (about 1 cm), placed centrally in the transverse incision, is created proximally to form an inverted T-incision (Fig. 8.253). Once complete, the periosteum is undermined craniad and caudad. Some surgeons prefer a cruciate patterned cut into the periosteum.

Care is taken to not enter the tendon sheath of the common digital extensor tendon (cranially) or lateral digital extensor tendon (caudally). If the sheath is entered, synovial fluid drainage from the incision can be noted and sepsis could occur in the sheath if the incision becomes infected.[12] The reflected periosteum is left open, and the subcutaneous tissue and skin are apposed in a routine manner. Light wraps are applied and maintained for 5 days; stall rest is recommended until the bandages are off.

Foals are not turned out with bandages and the bandages are not left on for long, because sores and white hair at the accessory carpal bone may produce a permanent blemish. Foals with mild deformities can be turned out, but those with more severe deformities should be confined until at least partial correction is achieved. This technique has been used successfully singularly (discussed below) or can be used in combination with temporary transphyseal bridging.

In foals with complete, intact ulnas, it is critical to remove a section of the ulna when performing the hemicircumferential transection of the periosteum (HCTP) and periosteal elevation (PE). This can be easily accomplished with an osteotome and rongeurs. At least a 1- to 2-cm segment should be removed to prevent union of the bone ends with healing. The ulna serves as a lateral

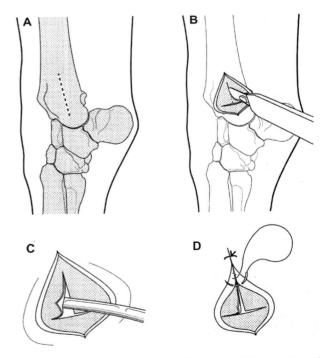

Figure 8.253 A. Incision for hemicircumferential transection of the periosteum. B. Transverse incision in the periosteum 2.5 cm proximal to the physis. A longitudinal incision is made in the periosteum to create an inverted T. C. The periosteum is elevated. D. Suture apposition of the subcutaneous tissue. Note that the incised periosteum is left open.

strap, and the stimulation of bone growth by the transection and elevation is prevented without ulna release. For ponies and miniature horses with complete ulnas and fibulas, I recommend combining HCTP and PE with ulnectomy and transphyseal bridging, because of the severity of these foals' deformities and the difficulty encountered in achieving correction.

Transphyseal Bridging

Temporary transphyseal bridging of the distal radial physis with screw and wire, staples, or a small plate can retard growth on the longer, convex side of the carpus.[10] With the physis bridged, longitudinal bone growth is arrested until the opposite (concave) side catches up. Intracarpal angular deviations are also corrected with growth retardation.[7] The current most popular technique is the screw and figure-eight wire technique, because it is more easily removed, securely opposes growth, and can be placed through smaller incisions. Staples are difficult to remove, require incisions the length of the staple, and often spring at the ends possibly permitting growth. Plates are more expensive, are difficult to remove, and require incisions the length of the plate.

Screw and wiring is an effective method to straighten carpal angular deformity if sufficient growth potential is left in the distal radial physis. This procedure can be performed in foals up to 16 to 24 months old, and some correction will be achieved because the distal radial physis retains some growth potential, although much reduced, after 16 months of age.[9] Approximately 71% of the longitudinal growth takes place within 12 months, and the most rapid longitudinal growth occurs between 0 and 8 months of age. Correction of the angulation will continue as long as the screw and wire are in place and the opposite side of the growth plate is elongating.

Transphyseal bridging allows for a greater correction of angle and is more likely to achieve correction in older animals than HCTP and PE. This technique is usually reserved for older foals that are not likely to be corrected with HCTP and PE alone (older than 5 months with a carpus ALD), for horses with severe deformities for which a rapid correction is desired (often combined with HCTP and PE), and for animals with a severe windswept deformity and malformed joints. The screw-and-wire technique is most often used for fetlock deformities, because of the earlier closure of that growth plate, the slower growth rate, and the more severe consequences of partial correction.

This surgery can be performed through a small stab incision about 3 cm proximal to the growth plate and a second stab incision in the fossa of the epiphysis distal to the growth plate. A subcutaneous tunnel is made that connects the two incisions. Alternatively, an open incision can be made that spans the growth plate. A 3.2-mm hole is drilled into the metaphysis and the epiphysis to a depth of about 40 mm and is tapped (4.5 mm). A 35-mm-long, 4.5-mm-diameter cortical bone screw is placed in the distal hole; and two preconfigured, figure-eight, ASIF (Association for the Study of Internal Fixation), 1.2-mm 18-gauge cerclage wires are threaded down the top incision and looped over the head of the distal screw

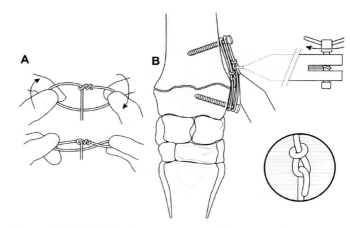

Figure 8.254 A. The free end of the cerclage wire is placed through the small loop on the other end. The wire is then twisted to form a figure eight. B. The wire is placed around the screw heads and tightened. The free end of the wire is bent distad, which facilitates easy removal through a proximally placed stab incision.

(Fig. 8.254). A similar proximal screw is placed, and the wire is tightened over its head. The twisted wire ends can lay flat at the top of the proximal screw or be bent 90° distally. The screws are tightened to provide the final tightening of the wire. The finished configuration should be a tensed figure-eight wire(s) with an eyehook relationship that is centered between the screw heads (Fig. 8.254).

The screws are placed in slight convergence for two reasons. With time and growth of the opposite side of the growth plate, the distal end of the screws will diverge. This can tilt the screw heads and loosen the wires. Also, the risk of entering the joint with the distal screw is reduced. To avoid entering the antebrachiocarpal joint with the distal screw, the carpal joints should be flexed slightly so the articular surface can be readily palpated while drilling the hole. A final craniocaudal radiograph or fluoroscopic image should be obtained.

For horses with severe rotational deformities as well as angular deformities, the screws can be offset (not directly under one another) in a manner that will provide forces to derotate the limb. I found this to be successful in three cases (Fig. 8.255).

It is important to remove the screws and wires when the limb is straight, which may not be at the same time for both forelimbs. Removal is performed under short-acting general anesthesia; a small stab incision is made directly over the screw heads. The proximal screw is easily palpated and removed. The distal screw may be more difficult; but measurements made from the radiograph will allow one to determine its general location, and it can be identified with an 18-gauge needle. The screws are removed and the wires are pulled out of the proximal hole.

For physeal stapling two reinforced vitallium staples are placed perpendicular to the longitudinal axis of the radius and perpendicular to the curvature (so they angle toward the center of bone); their legs are centered over the physis so that each is placed at an equal distance in the epiphysis and metaphysis (Fig. 8.256). A staple

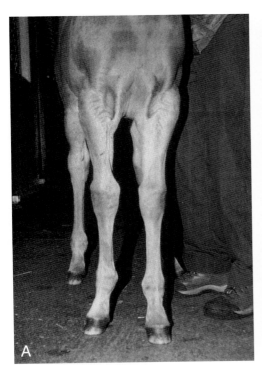 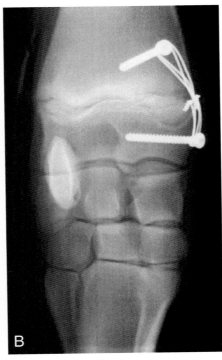

Figure 8.255 A. A 6-week-old foal with mild carpus valgus and severe outward rotational deformity. B. Postoperative view demonstrating the placement of offset screws to compress and derotate the physis.

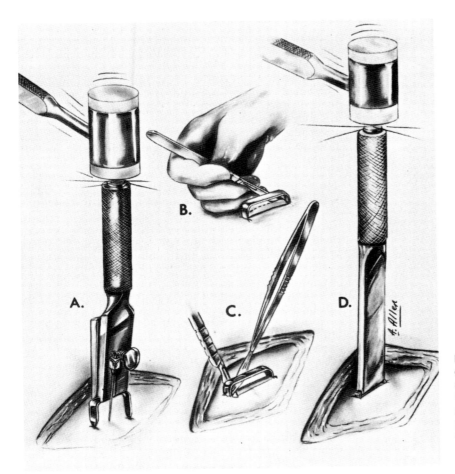

Figure 8.256 A. Insert the staple by centering it on a needle in the physis. B. Make an incision in the soft tissue under the staple. C. If desired, remove the soft tissue. D. Set the staple firmly next to bone. (Reprinted with permission from Heinze CD. Epiphyseal stapling. A surgical technique for correcting angular limb deformities. Proc Am Assoc Equine Pract 1969:59–73.)

holder holds the staples for their initial insertion. Before the staples are deeply seated, intraoperative radiographs should be taken to ensure the staples' proper placement. The carpal fascia and collateral ligament underlying the staples is incised down to bone and separated just wide enough to allow the staple to be buried. The staples are then driven down below the thick fascia with a staple driver. Care is taken not to damage the periosteum, yet it is important to seat the staple firmly in close association with bone. The fascia overlying the staple is apposed with simple interrupted synthetic absorbable sutures to cover them. The subcutaneous tissue and skin are apposed in a routine manner using simple interrupted suture patterns.

Removal of staples requires a similar incision to that which was used for their placement. Since they are buried underneath the fascia and, in some cases, the new bone growth, the staples may be difficult to identify and remove. In these cases, a 22- or 25-gauge needle is used for identification of the staples, after which they are removed with the staple remover.

Postoperative care for temporary transphyseal bridging is the same as for HCTP and PS, except bandages may be indicated for slightly longer (10 days). Owners should be instructed to assess limb straightening on a weekly basis with the foal standing squarely on a firm, level surface. Foot care and exercise is similar to HCTP and PE. Because foals requiring transphyseal bridging are typically more severely affected, stall rest may be recommended for 3 to 5 weeks to ensure partial correction.

Complications of the screw and wire technique include wire breakage, fibrosis over the screw heads, and overcorrection that produces an opposing deformity (Figs. 8.257 and 8.258). Use of two wires and minimal soft tissue dissection to the place screws minimizes the risks of wire breakage and fibrosis. Owner participation

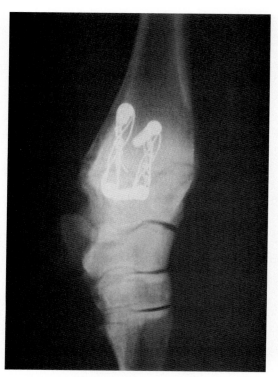

Figure 8.258 An older foal that was treated with two sets of screws and wires. (Courtesy of T. S. Stashak.)

in follow-up assessment is mandatory for successful timing of the removal of the hardware to prevent overcorrection.

The advantages of the screw-and-wire technique are immediate compression and arrest of growth; a prolonged effect; and the most dramatic effect, particularly if combined with HCTP and PE. If a foal is older, the deformity is severe, or a rapid correction is deemed important, this technique is preferable to HCTP and PE alone.

In horses with acquired ALD owing to premature closure of a small area of the growth plate from trauma, it is possible to resect the portion of the growth plate that formed a bony bridge and prevented growth to release the remaining growth plate. This "physiolysis" procedure is combined with transphyseal bridging to arrest growth on the long side of the limb, and a fat graft is placed in the resected bone segment to help prevent refusion of the growth plate during correction. This correction option can be used in foals or yearlings with this cause of angular deformity.[11]

Some foals may require HCTP and PE on several limbs and joints simultaneously. Screw-and-wire procedures can be combined with HCTP and PE or can be successful alone. The most appropriate procedure is selected on a joint by joint basis.

Prognosis

The prognosis for producing straight limbs and soundness for performance is good to excellent. Reported success is greater than 80% and is probably better

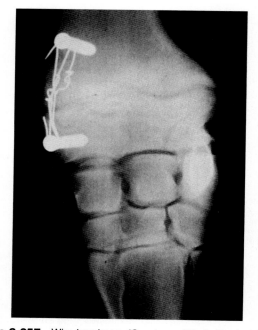

Figure 8.257 Wire breakage. (Courtesy of T. S. Stashak.)

than that today, because referral to surgery occurs earlier and mild conditions now make up a greater number of surgical cases.[3,6,10] The racing performances of 199 Thoroughbreds treated with HCTP and PE were compared with those of 1017 siblings. The treated horses had a slightly lower percentage of race starts (45 versus 55%), fewer 2-year-old starts (1.06 versus 1.72), and lower start percentile ranking numbers (33.49 versus 49.18). Starting status was significantly affected by surgery but not by anatomic site treated.[19] The reason for the lower performance in this group is not known and is not necessarily directly related to the ALD. ALD may be associated with increased risk of other developmental orthopedic diseases.

References

1. Adams R, Poulos P. A skeletal ossification index for neonatal foals. Vet Radiol 1988;29:217.
2. Auer JA, Martens RJ. Angular limb deformities in young foals. Am Assoc Equine Pract 1980;26:81.
3. Auer JA, Martens RJ. Periosteal transection and periosteal stripping for correction of angular limb deformities in foals. Am J Vet Res 1982;43(9):1530.
4. Bertone AL. Developmental Orthopedic Diseases. The Veterinarian's Practical Reference to Equine Nutrition. St. Louis: Purina Mills, Inc., 1997.
5. Bertone AL, Park RD, Turner SA. Periosteal transection and stripping for treatment of angular limb deformities in foals: Radiographic observations. J Am Vet Med Assoc 1985;187:153.
6. Bertone AL, Turner AS, Park RD. Periosteal transection and stripping for treatment of angular limb deformities in foals: Clinical observations. J Am Vet Med Assoc 1985;187:145.
7. Brauer TS, Booth TS, Riedesel E. Physeal growth retardation leads to correction of intracarpal angular deviations as well as physeal valgus deformity. Equine Vet J 1999;31:193.
8. Fretz PB. Angular limb deformities in foals. Vet Clin North Am Large Anim Pract 1980;2:125.
9. Fretz PB, Cymbaluk NK, Pharr JW. Quantitative analysis of long-bone growth in the horse. Am J Vet Res 1984;45:1602.
10. Fretz PB, Donecker JM. Surgical correction of angular limb deformities in foals: A retrospective study. J Am Vet Med Assoc 1983;183:529.
11. Gaughan EM, Bene DJ, Hoskinson JJ. Partial physiolysis with temporary transphyseal bridging for correction of physeal dysplasia and angular limb deformity in two yearling horses. Vet Compar Orthop Traumatol 1996;9:101.
12. Hawkins JF, Lescun TB. Sepsis of the common digital extensor tendon sheath secondary to hemicircumferential periosteal transection in a foal. J Am Vet Med Assoc 1997;211:331.
13. Hongaten GR, Rooker GD. The role of the periosteum in growth of long bones. J Bone Joint Surg [Br] 1979;61:218.
14. Hurtig MB, Green SL, Dobson H, et al. Defective bone and cartilage in foals fed a low-copper diet. Proc Am Assoc Equine Pract 1991;36:637.
15. Mason TA. A high incidence of congenital angular limb deformities in a group of foals. Vet Rec 1981;109:93.
16. McLaughlin BG, Doige CE. A study of ossification of carpal and tarsal bones in normal and hypothyroid foals. Can Vet J 1982;23:164.
17. McLaughlin BG, Doige CE, Fretz PB, Pharr JW. Carpal bone lesions associated with angular limb deformities. J Am Vet Med Assoc 1981;178:224–230.
18. Mitten LA, Bertone AL. Angular limb deformities in foals. J Am Vet Med Assoc 1994;204(5):717.
19. Mitten LA, Bramlage LR, Embertson RM. Racing performance after hemicircumferential periosteal transection for angular limb deformities in Thoroughbreds: 199 cases (1987–1989). J Am Vet Med Assoc 1995;207(6):746.
20. Morley PS, Townsend HGG. A survey of reproductive performance in Thoroughbred mares and morbidity, mortality and athletic potential of their foals. Equine Vet J 1997;29:290.
21. Pharr JW, Fretz PB. Radiographic findings in foals with angular limb deformities. J Am Vet Med Assoc 1981;179:812.
22. Sedrish SA, Moore RM. Diagnosis and management of incomplete ossification of the cuboidal bones in foals. Equine Pract 1997;19:16.
23. Shamis LD, Auer J. Complete ulnas and fibulas in a pony foal. J Am Vet Med Assoc 1985;186(8):802.
24. Soana S, Gnudi G, Bertoni G, et al. Anatomo-radiographic study on the osteogenesis of carpal and tarsal bones in horse fetus. Anat Histol Embryol 1998;27(5):301.
25. Stashak TS. Angular limb deformities associated with the carpus. In: Stashak TS, Ed. Adams' Lameness in Horses. 4th ed. Philadelphia: Lea & Febiger, 1987;624–641.
26. Thompson KN, Ed. St. Louis: Purina Mills, Inc. and the American Association Equine Practitioners, 1997;13:101–114.

DORSAL (ANTERIOR) DEVIATION OF THE CARPAL JOINTS (BUCKED, SPRUNG, GOAT KNEES; FLEXION DEFORMITY OF THE CARPUS)

Bucked knees is a deformity consisting of a dorsal deviation of the carpus that causes an alteration in the articulations of the bones forming the joint and results in constant partial flexion of the carpus.[5] The incidence of developmental abnormalities is reported to be 3 to 4% of all foals born; hyperflexion of the forelimbs is the most common form. In another report of congenital anomalies, 33% were "contracted foal syndrome."[1] Foals with carpal flexural deformity often cause dystocia, because their forelimbs cannot straighten out to exit the birth canal.

Causes

Several factors are involved in the cause of bucked knees. Many horses exhibit a mild dorsal deviation of both carpi, but this may not be serious, because it is often owing to a congenital condition.[5] Congenital types may be the result of the positioning of the limbs in the uterus or of a mineral or vitamin deficiency in the mare (see Chapter 5) (Fig. 8.259). An autosomal trisomy (three chromosomes) has also been identified in two foals with congenital carpal flexural deformity.[1] The authors of that study conclude that most arthrogryposis in horses is not the result of a trisomy condition, but it should be suspected when other life-threatening congenital conditions exist. The trisomies are associated with aged oocytes in otherwise cytogenetically normal mares and explains the increased incidence of carpal flexural deformities from aged mares.

Some cases of bucked knees are the result of trauma, when certain lamenesses cause inactivity of the extensor group of muscles, allowing the flexors to contract.[5] The muscles most involved are the ulnaris lateralis, flexor carpi ulnaris, and deep and/or superficial flexor tendons. Injury to the suspensory ligament, deep and/or superficial flexor tendons, or heel of the foot often causes a horse to rest the carpus in a dorsal direction. If the pain persists, the musculotendinous units contract to such a degree that the carpus cannot be straightened. In some cases, carpal injury, such as carpitis, may also cause dorsal deviation of the joint to relieve pain, which will cause contraction of the muscles and tendons. Bucked knee caused by trauma is usually unilateral.

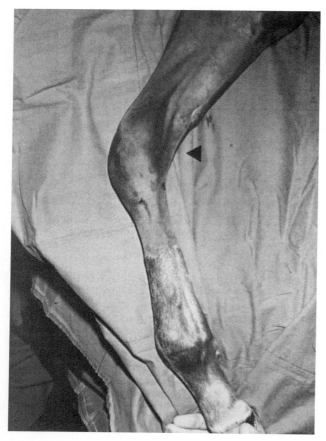

Figure 8.259 A foal with congenital bilateral flexural deformity of the carpus; neither limb can be extended. The left common digital extensor tendon is ruptured, and the right common digital extensor tendon appears inflamed. The arrow is pointing to the taut flexor tendons. (Courtesy of T. S. Stashak.)

Dorsal deviation of the carpus can also occur secondary to rupture of the common digital extensor tendon within its carpal sheath. In some horses, the opposite is probably true, and the carpal flexion deformity contributes to the rupture of the common digital extensor tendon (Figs. 8.259 and 8.260).[5]

Signs and Diagnosis

The severity of bucked knees varies considerably. In some cases, the condition is mild; but in others, it is extreme.[5] In mild cases, the bucked knees may be noted only intermittently or as a trembling at the knee. In nonreducible mild bucked knees, one or both carpi is flexed forward to some degree when the affected horse is in the normal standing position. These cases rarely cause a lameness problem and are considered a conformational abnormality. In moderate to severe cases, the condition inhibits normal movement and gait, as there is a shortening of the cranial phase of the stride. The condition may be so pronounced that the horse falls to the carpal joints while standing or walking. The carpus or carpi may be unable to support their share of weight, so damage may occur to other regions of the limb. Knuckling of the fet-

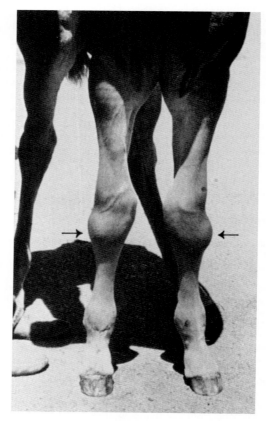

Figure 8.260 A foal with bilateral rupture of the common digital extensor tendon. Arrows point to the swellings on the dorsal lateral surfaces overlying both carpi. (Courtesy of T. S. Stashak.)

lock may also be present in this condition as a result of the shortening of the musculotendinous unit of the digital flexor tendon.

Treatment

Bucked Knees in the Foal

If the condition is not severe—i.e., the foal can put its feet flat on the ground without knuckling over to the carpus and can stand on its own—treatment often is not necessary. Many foals straighten up remarkably well by the time they are 6 months old. However, if lateral (varus) or medial (valgus) deviation of the carpal joints is present in addition to the bucked knees, corrective procedures may be necessary. If the condition is considered severe, the limbs may be put into a cast or, preferably, pulled into a polyvinyl chloride (PVC) splint. A study comparing sleeve casting and splinting revealed that more carpal hyperextension was achieved with splinting.[3]

Use of systemic administration of oxytetracycline to induce musculotendinous laxity can remarkably assist with the correction of this condition in foals, but it should always be combined with splinting to gain axial alignment while the tendons are relaxed and should always be continued for the full 3 days of treatment or recurrence rate is high. The recommended protocol is

3 g oxytetracycline administered intravenously over 30 minutes after dilution into 1 liter of a balanced electrolyte solution once daily for 3 days. Infusion should be slowed if tremors occur.

Although renal and gastrointestinal toxicities are a concern, this has not been reported in foals given the drug experimentally or in horses treated to date. The dosage is not modified based on body weight, and the same dose is given to neonates and weanlings. The response to oxytetracycline is measurable for 3 days; therefore, 6 days of laxity are anticipated from 3 days of treatment.[2,4] The response to treatment declines with age and seems to be nonexistent in mature horses. Maximal forces pulling the carpus into extension should occur during the oxytetracycline treatment.

I prefer PVC splinting, because forces can be reset as improvement occurs. The foal should be left in the cast or splint for 10 to 14 days. In many cases, it will not be necessary to reapply the cast; but if a new cast is necessary, it should not be applied until 10 to 14 days after the first cast is removed. This interval allows the foal to partially overcome the effects of disuse atrophy in the musculature.

A complete check of the horse's diet should is recommended; and the diet should be fortified, if necessary, with elements considered deficient. Foals that develop bucked knees after birth should be checked for imbalanced or excess nutrition (see Chapter 5).

Bucked Knees as a Result of Injury

When a bucked-knee condition was caused by injury to the carpus or other structures, it is necessary to direct treatment at correction of the original pathologic changes. Pathologic changes in the flexor tendons, suspensory ligament, foot, extensor tendons, or carpus are most often responsible for this type of bucked knee. If the condition is not of long duration and is corrected promptly, the musculotendinous unit will gradually stretch, and the carpus will again assume a normal position. Splinting or proximal check desmotomy may help straighten these cases.

Surgical Correction

In foals with carpal flexural deformity that is so severe that even with oxytetracycline treatment and maximal tension, flexion is still present and prevents splinting, proximal and distal check desmotomy can lengthen the flexor tendon component. This operation is most successful for bucked knees that result from trauma and is less successful for those that are congenital. The carpal bones are often deformed with congenital bucked knees, whereas the carpal bones are relatively normal with the acquired condition. Furthermore, congenital bucked knees show contraction of the deep and superficial flexor musculotendinous units and the ulnaris lateralis and flexor carpi ulnaris. The suspensory ligament can also be involved.

In my experience, desmotomy of the accessory (check) ligaments is often not adequate to straighten the limb in these severe cases, and transection of the insertions of the flexors on the accessory carpal bone (flexor ulnaris and ulnaris lateralis) improves the success. In extreme cases, flexor tendons and even the suspensory ligament may need to be transected. It is best to leave at least one flexor structure to support the fetlock, or complete fetlock breakdown is a consequence and loss of vascularity to the distal limb from overstretching of congenitally shorter neurovascular bundles can occur.

Surgical transection of the ulnaris lateralis and flexor carpi ulnaris can be performed with the horse in standing position if it is tractable, but general anesthesia is usually used in foals. Tranquilization and sedation are necessary if the operation is to be done while the horse is standing. The operative region is 2.5 to 4 cm above the accessory carpal bone on the caudal aspect of the limb.

The area is clipped, shaved, and prepared for aseptic operation. Anesthesia is accomplished by injecting a local anesthetic. If the horse is placed in recumbency, the tendons should be tensed by extending the carpus. The depression between the two tendons is located on the caudal surface of the limb about 2.5 cm above the accessory carpal bone. A 5.0-cm-long incision is made through the skin and subcutaneous tissue, and a blunt-pointed bistoury is inserted through the wound at the side of the tendon of the ulnaris lateralis muscle. Care is taken to avoid cutting the ulnar artery vein and nerve. The tendon is severed by cutting outward with the bistoury until the knife edge can be felt beneath the skin. The length of the incision allows careful identification of the structure to be severed. The limb should be extended during the cutting procedure. The bistoury is then turned, and the tendon of the flexor carpi ulnaris is severed. Do not cut too deeply, or the structures underlying the muscles may be injured.

Sutures are then placed in the incision, and the region is kept bandaged for at least 10 days. The patient should not be worked for 6 to 8 weeks. If the limb cannot be fully straightened after tenotomy, it is beneficial to place the limb in a sleeve cast from elbow to fetlock joint. This cast should be left in place 10 to 14 days. Alternatively, a bandage splint can be used.

Prognosis

A mild nonreducible bucked knee that is static from birth and not associated with lameness is considered a conformational abnormality and is not a problem for performance. For all other forms, the prognosis is guarded; and in acquired cases of carpal flexural deformity, the condition may preclude full athletic use. However, most conditions of this kind can be improved so that the horse can serve as a useful breeding animal. Breeding animals should be cytogenetically tested to be normal. The prognosis is favorable in mild, congenital forms if the nutrition of the foal has been good or is corrected. Severe congenital forms result in an unfavorable prognosis.

References

1. Buoen LC, Shang TQ, Weber AF, et al. Arthrogryposis in the foal and its possible relation to autosomal trisomy. Equine Vet J 1997; 29:60.
2. Kasper CA, Clayton HM, Wright AK, et al. Effects of high doses of oxytetracycline on metacarpophalangeal joint kinematics in neonatal foals. J Am Vet Med Assoc 1995;207:71.

3. Kelly NJ, Watrous BJ, Wagner PC. Comparison of splinting and casting on the degree of laxity induced in thoracic limbs in young horses. Equine Pract 1987;9:10.
4. Madison JB, Garber JL, Rice B, et al. Effect of oxytetracycline on metacarpophalangeal and distal interphalangeal joint angles in newborn foals. J Am Vet Med Assoc 1994;204:246.
5. Stashak TS. Dorsal anterior deviation of the carpal joints. In: Stashak TS, Ed. Adams' Lameness in Horses. 4th ed. Philadelphia: Lea & Febiger, 1987;641–643.

RUPTURE OF THE EXTENSOR CARPI RADIALIS TENDON

Rupture of the extensor carpi radialis tendon is comparatively rare. The signs of lameness are distinctive, making it easy to diagnose.[2,4]

Causes

The condition is caused by trauma. The logical conclusion is that overflexion of the limb is most apt to rupture the extensor carpi radialis tendon.[4] In most cases, the actual cause is not known.

Signs

With the resistance of the extensor carpi radialis tendon gone, the flexor tendons are able to overflex the limb. Careful observation of the gait shows that the carpus flexes considerably more in the affected limb than in the normal limb. The tendon sheath of the extensor carpi radialis is distended.[2,4] Extension is accomplished by means of the common digital extensor and the lateral digital extensor. After the rupture has been present for a short time, atrophy of the muscular portion of the extensor carpi radialis begins. Palpation over the carpus reveals the absence of the tendon on the dorsal surface of the carpus.

Treatment

If the rupture is complete and found soon after it occurs, it may be possible to bring the ends of the tendon together surgically. In this case, the limb is kept in a cast for approximately 6 weeks. In cases of longer duration, it is impossible to bring the tendon ends together. The surgeon may be able to substitute the tendon of the extensor carpi obliquus by using tendon anastomosis. With partial rupture of the extensor carpi radialis tendon, debridement of the adhesion, suturing of longitudinal splits in the tendon, and suturing of a torn tendon sheath have proven beneficial.[3,4]

Prognosis

Prognosis is unfavorable for complete rupture. In horses valuable enough to warrant surgery, either tendon anastomosis or substitution with extensor carpi obliquus may be used.[1] The prognosis is favorable for partial tears and longitudinal splitting of the extensor carpi radialis tendon and its sheath if surgery is performed.[3,4]

References
1. Adams OR. Lameness in Horses. 3rd ed. Philadelphia: Lea & Febiger, 1974.
2. Catlin JE. Rupture of the extensor carpi radialis tendon. Vet Med Small Anim Clin 1964;59:1778.
3. Mason TA. Chronic tenosynovitis of the extensor tendons and tendon sheaths of the carpal region in the horse. Equine Vet J 1977;9:186.
4. Wallace CE. Chronic tendosynovitis of the extensor carpi radialis tendon in the horse. Aust Vet 1973;48:585, 587.

RUPTURE OF THE COMMON DIGITAL EXTENSOR TENDON

Rupture of the common digital extensor tendon most frequently affects both forelimbs in young foals and is generally present at birth or develops soon after.[3,5] Affected foals may have concomitant multiple birth defects, including delayed endochondral ossification of the carpal bones and underdeveloped pectoral muscles, and they may be prognathic.[3] All this implies that the extensor rupture may be part of a complex congenital defect that may involve dysmaturity. A flexure deformity of the carpus or fetlock may also accompany the rupture. In a series of 10 cases, 4 had severe flexure deformities, 3 exhibited mild signs, and 3 had no signs of flexure deformity.[3] The flexure may represent a weakness of the extensor musculotendinous unit or be a result of the rupture and loss of extensor support to the carpus. In general, this condition is thought to be relatively uncommon; however, in one report, 10 cases were diagnosed over a 4-year period. There may be an inherited predisposition, because two mares had two successive foals in 2 years that were affected with this condition.[3,4] A higher incidence of this problem has been reported in Arabians, Quarter Horses, and Arabian–Quarter Horse crosses.[3]

Causes

This condition may be congenital, particularly if it is part of a complex congenital defect in development.[3] In some cases, however, it is difficult to determine whether the flexure deformity of the carpus results in the rupture of the common digital extensor tendon or, in fact, develops secondary to the rupture of the common digital extensor.

A common history is that the foal was shaky and buckling in the knees and then the swelling was noted. It is also postulated that rupture of the common digital extensor tendon could result from a single or repeated forced extension of the carpus against resistance. Such a situation appeared to be the case when a 24-hour-old foal was examined because of an inability to stand because of bilateral carpal flexure deformities. Physically, the carpi could not be extended (Fig. 8.260). On close observation, bilateral distension of the common digital extensor tendon sheath was evident also. At necropsy, one tendon had completely ruptured, and the other had marked inflammatory signs with a tendency toward disruption of fibers. Histopathology of the completely separated tendon indicated regions of normal tendon, immature fibrous tissue (indicating an attempt to heal), and newly torn tendon fibers with hemorrhage. Considering the foal's age and the histopathologic findings, it is reasonable to speculate that the process leading to rupture began in utero and may have become complete after birth. Possibly an inability to extend the carpus within the confines of the uterus initiated the separation of the common digital extensor tendon, and it attempted to heal. After birth, complete separation probably occurred as the foal attempted to extend the carpus against its fixed flexure deformity.[5]

Signs

A distinguishing characteristic for this condition is the presence of swelling over the dorsolateral surface of the carpus near the level of the distal carpal joint (Fig. 8.260). Foals may be able to stand normally but will frequently knuckle forward at the fetlock during progression. In foals that exhibit some degree of flexure deformity, the diagnosis of rupture of the common digital extensor tendon may go unrecognized, and a primary diagnosis of the carpal flexure deformity may be made.[3]

On palpation, fluid distension of the common digital extensor flexor tendon sheath is appreciated. The blunted ends of the extensor tendon may be palpable; this totally depends on the amount of synovial fluid present in the sheath. In cases in which an excessive amount of fluid is present, aseptic needle aspiration of the synovial fluid allows a more definitive palpation of the tendons. Flexion of the carpal joints usually does not cause a painful response, and foals are not typically lame.

Diagnosis

The diagnosis is made from the history and physical examination findings of effusion in the common digital extensor tendon sheath and palpation of the blunted ends of the separated extensor tendon. Radiographs should be taken of the carpus to rule out concomitant hypoplasia of the carpal bones.

Ultrasound of the swelling reveals fluid within the sheath and identifies the swollen tendon ends. The proximal portion is usually pulled quite proximally and the distal portion is often over the carpal joints. A gap is noted between the tendon ends. It is possible to see portions of an intact but small (possibly hypoplastic) tendon in some cases with classical clinical signs.

Treatment

In general, foals that do not have a severe flexure deformity of the carpus are treated conservatively with stall rest. The application of bandages to support the carpus and protect the dorsum of the fetlock from abrasions is recommended. Suturing of the tendon ends has been reported,[1] and surgical removal of the ruptured ends of the tendon has been recommended.[4] However, both of these procedures appear to be unnecessary for healing, and return to function usually occurs without these treatments. It is unlikely that the ruptured tendon ends reunite, but rather they adhere to the sheath; with time the limb regains function and relies more on the lateral digital extensor tendon.

Tube casts or PVC bandage splints can be used in foals exhibiting flexure deformities of the carpus, but careful monitoring is required.[2] If the flexure deformity involves the fetlock joint and is severe, carpal (inferior) check ligament desmotomy may be required to straighten the limb. After surgery, PVC bandage splints are used to support the limb in forced extension.

Prognosis

The prognosis for uncomplicated cases of rupture of the common digital extensor tendon appears to be good, and healing usually results with minimal blemish and no functional deficit. At the 4-year follow-up, one horse was moving normally and no swelling was observed in association with the previous rupture.[3] The prognosis is guarded for horses exhibiting severe carpal flexure deformity in association with rupture of the extensor tendon.[2]

References

1. Johnson JH, Lowe JE. Muscles and tendons. In: Oehme FW, Prier JE, Eds. Textbook of Large Animal Surgery. Baltimore: Williams & Wilkins, 1974;249.
2. McIlwraith CW. Tendon disorders of young horses. In: Mansmann RA, McAllister ES, Eds. Equine Medicine and Surgery. 3rd ed. Santa Barbara, CA: American Veterinary Publications, 1982.
3. Myers VS, Gordon GW. Ruptured common digital extensor tendon associated with contracted flexor tendons in foals. Am Assoc Equine Pract 1975;21:67.
4. Stevenson WL, Stevenson WG. Rupture of the common digital extensor in foals. Can J Comp Med 1942;6:197.
5. Yovich JV, Stashak TS, McIlwraith CW. Rupture of the common digital extensor tendon in foals. Cont Educ 1984;6:S373.

CONTRACTED TENDONS AND FLEXURE DEFORMITIES

See Chapter 7.

HYGROMA OF THE CARPUS

A hygroma is a swelling over the dorsal surface of the carpus, which may be lined by cells that secrete a fluid not unlike synovial fluid in color and consistency. Most commonly, it is acquired pseudobursitis resulting from trauma. Normally, there is no subcutaneous bursa in this region, but through trauma a bursa structure may form. The tendon sheath of the extensor carpi radialis or the common digital extensor may also be involved. A synovial hernia of the antebrachiocarpal or midcarpal joint capsule can occur, which causes a hygroma-like swelling that is almost indistinguishable from those caused by an acquired bursitis. However, careful physical examination and ultrasonographic evaluation reveal that the swelling on the dorsal surface of the carpus is irregular in outline and does not uniformly cover the carpus when a synovial hernia has occurred.[2] Acquired bursitis shows an evenly distributed swelling over the surface of the carpus.

Causes

Trauma is the cause in all cases. Horses that get up and down on hard ground are more commonly affected.

Hygroma also can be produced as a result of a horse pawing and hitting the carpus on a hard surface, such as a wall.[3]

Signs

Signs of hygroma of the carpus are swellings of various shapes over the dorsal surface of the carpus. The swellings vary with the structure or structures involved (Fig. 8.261). Palpation of the swelling and carpal flexion are generally not painful, and lameness is usually not observed.

Diagnosis

The diagnosis is made by needle drainage and submission of the fluid for cytologic analysis. Acute hygroma results in the formation of a serous type fluid. In chronic cases, the fluid becomes more like synovial fluid. If there is concern that a synovial fistula of the carpal joint or tendon sheath has developed, either of these structures can be injected with radio-opaque contrast material to identify the communication (Fig. 8.262).[3] Ultrasound examination may also help differentiate among the various conditions that cause swelling on the dorsal aspect of the carpus.

Treatment

Needle aspiration of the fluid, injection of a corticosteroid, followed by counterpressure with elastic band-

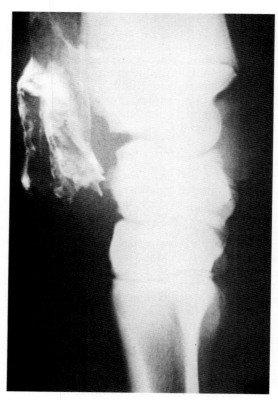

Figure 8.262 A fistulogram can reveal involvement of the tendon sheath. (Courtesy of T. S. Stashak.)

age, appears to be an effective method of treatment in some cases. The injection can be repeated. Orgotein has also been used instead of a corticosteroid. Continued pressure of the elastic bandage is used to promote adhesions between the distended skin and underlying tissues. The distended skin generally thickens, producing a permanent blemish.

Subacute and chronic cases that have not responded to the treatment described here can be treated by incisional drainage.[3,4] A 4-cm vertical incision is made in the most distal aspect of the swelling. After drainage is complete, fibrin tags are removed and the inner surface is either debrided with a large curette or chemically debrided with half-strength tincture of iodine.[3] A Penrose drain is inserted up through the distal incision and secured to the proximal limits by a through-and-through mattress suture using monofilament nylon suture. The distal incision is sutured until a 2.5-cm opening remains. One side of the Penrose drain is sutured to the distal opening to prevent the drain from being drawn up into the wound. After sterile bandaging, a PVC extension splint is applied to the palmar surface of the carpus. It should extend from the proximal forearm to the distal third of the metacarpus. Particular attention is paid to padding at the proximal and distal ends of the PVC pipe. The drain is maintained under sterile bandages for 4 to 7 days. The extension splint is maintained for 10 to 14 days. This is usually a sufficient period to allow adhesions between the two surfaces to occur. It is absolutely imperative to maintain the Penrose drain in an antiseptic environment, including the application of sterile band-

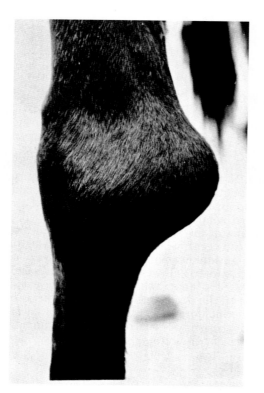

Figure 8.261 Hygroma of the carpus. The distribution of the swelling indicates a primary involvement of the midcarpal joint capsule. (Courtesy of T. S. Stashak.)

ages. Drains are two-way streets, and the risk of ascending infection is ever present. In most cases, this procedure results in cosmetic end healing.

If a cosmetic end result is not important, another treatment is to open and drain the hygroma and swab the cavity with a tincture of iodine. This causes a prolonged drainage from the lesion, which heals eventually by granulation and scar tissue formation. You must be absolutely certain that there is no communication between the hygroma and the carpal joints or tendon sheaths.

Injections of the bursal sac with Lugol iodine have also been used, as have blistering and firing of the region; these methods are not recommended.

A hygroma of long standing with a thickened synovial lining can be surgically removed under general anesthesia by en-bloc resection.[1] The hygroma is carefully dissected out after preparing the area for aseptic surgery. An elliptic incision is made over the swelling, and the mass is dissected out by using curved Mayo scissors to separate the tissues. In most cases, the bursa can be dissected completely free without puncture. However, if the bursa is punctured, it can be removed by staying outside the thickened wall. If the joint capsule is involved (e.g., a synovial hernia resembling a hygroma), the opening to it is closed with synthetic absorbable suture material. This opening is usually quite small. Subcutaneous tissue is apposed with synthetic absorbable suture material, and the skin is sutured with a noncapillary suture using simple interrupted or vertical mattress suture pattern. The operative site is handled and maintained in a manner similar to that described for more acute cases.

Prognosis

Prognosis is guarded to favorable. Old cases retain considerable swelling because of fibrous tissue that has been laid down in the inflamed region. Such cases usually have an unfavorable prognosis, because adhesions may not form after corticoid therapy, and the lesion may require surgical drainage or removal.

References

1. Jann H, Slusher SU, Courtney Q. Treatment of acquired bursitis (hygroma) by en-bloc resection. Equine Pract 1990;12:8.
2. Johnson JE, Ryan GD. Intersynovial fistula in the carpus of a horse. Cornell Vet 1975;65(1):84.
3. Stashak TS. Equine Wound Management. Philadelphia: Lea & Febiger, 1991;181–182.
4. van Veenendaal JC, Speirs VC, Harrison I. Treatment of hygromata in horses. Am Vet J 1981;57:513.

INTRAARTICULAR FRACTURES OF THE CARPUS

Intraarticular fractures associated with the carpal bones and the distal end of the radius are common injuries in racing horses, hunters, jumpers, and actively performing horses in other breeds. The carpus represents the most commonly fractured joint in the horse, most certainly the racehorse. An increased incidence of this lesion has been observed in young horses between 2 and 4 years of age. Factors such as speed, immaturity, longer limb length, position of the jockey, and distances run tend to generate tremendous concussive forces that focus on the dorsal surface of the carpal bones. From highest to lowest frequency of occurrence, the fracture can be a simple chip fracture, slab fracture, or comminuted fracture.[3,13,19,22–25,28,33,35,40–42]

Since the late 1980s more than 3392 carpal fractures have been summarized in the literature, each report emphasizing slightly different populations of horses based on breed, function (all racehorses), bone affected, and racing locale (North American, Australia, Europe, Japan). Of all fractures sustained in Thoroughbred racehorses in Japan in 1 year (1837 fractures), the carpus accounted for 33% (606 fractures).[25] For all racing breeds (Standardbred trotters and pacers, Thoroughbreds and Quarter Horses), the midcarpal joint is more commonly affected than the antebrachiocarpal (radiocarpal) joint, but the distribution between joints becomes more equal when only Thoroughbreds and Quarter Horses in the United States are considered. Standardbreds have the greatest percentages of fractures of the third carpal bone, particularly trotters.[21,28,40]

In the United States, Thoroughbreds most commonly fracture the distal aspect of the radiocarpal bone (about 35%) in the midcarpal joint and both the distolateral aspect of the radius (16%) and the proximal intermediate carpal bone in the antebrachiocarpal joint (16%). Racing Quarter Horses also most commonly fracture the distal aspect of the radiocarpal bone (34%) in the midcarpal joint but most commonly fracture the proximal intermediate carpal bone in the antebrachiocarpal joint (23%), followed by the distolateral aspect of the radius (10%).[23,34] In the racing Thoroughbreds in Japan, the most common sites of any carpal fracture are the distal radius (35%), the third carpal bone (35%), and the radiocarpal bone (29%); 87% occur as chip fractures on the dorsal surface of the bone.[25]

Slab fractures (defined as fractures that involve two articular surfaces) occur most commonly in the third carpal bone in both racing Thoroughbreds and in Standardbreds.[22,40,42] In Standardbreds, 2-year-olds were most commonly affected, and most slab fractures occurred on the dorsomedial facet (87%). In Thoroughbreds, 3-year-olds were most commonly affected and usually (59%) in the right limb.[42] Thoroughbreds also have more chip fractures in the right limb (56%), whereas Quarter Horses were equally distributed (50%).[23] Thoroughbred racehorses frequently shift to the right lead on the straightaways and are in the right lead at the end of races, which places a greater stress on that limb as the horse becomes fatigued.[2] Catastrophic fractures resulting in euthanasia occur in the third carpal bone and bones other than the distal radius and radiocarpal bone.[25]

Chip Fractures

Chip fractures (osteochondral fractures) are fragments of bone and cartilage that break off from only one articular surface. They vary in size and location and can be firmly attached, moderately loose, or free-floating (as joint mice) (Fig. 8.263). The radial, third, and intermediate carpal bones and the distal end of the radius are most commonly affected by chip fractures (Fig. 8.264). Only rarely do carpal chip fractures involve the carpometacarpal joint.

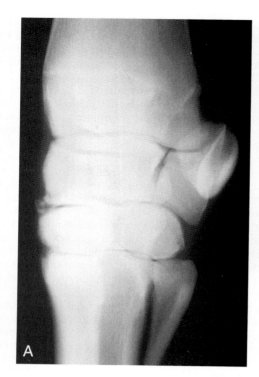

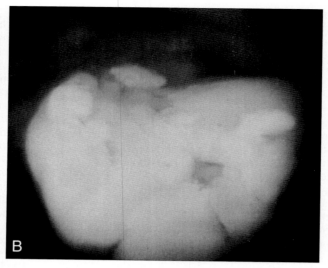

Figure 8.263 A. Fracture of the distal radiocarpal bone and proximal third carpal, two of the most commonly fractured bones in racehorses. B. Arthroscopy reveals a mildly displaced chip fracture and associated cartilage damage in the distal radiocarpal bone of a horse positioned in dorsal recumbency.

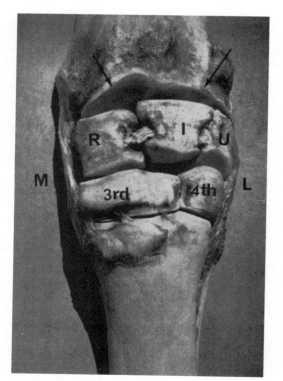

Figure 8.264 Normal left bony carpus. The joints (from proximal to distal) are the antebrachiocarpal (radiocarpal), the midcarpal (intercarpal), and the carpometacarpal. Arrows, areas where chip fractures may occur on radius; M, medial; L, lateral; R, radial carpal bone; I, intermediate carpal bone; U, ulnar carpal bone; 3rd, third carpal bone; 4th, fourth carpal bone.

Four categories of carpal chip fractures have been identified:

- Recent, complete fractures
- Fragments with synovial membrane and fibrous capsular attachments
- Chronic fractures with early bony reattachment
- Fractures with extensive bony reattachment (healed with a fibrous union)

Four grades reflect the amount of articular cartilage damage:

- *Grade 1.* Minimal loss (less than 5 mm) from the dorsal surface
- *Grade 2.* Loss of 30% of the articular surface
- *Grade 3.* Loss of 50% of the articular surface
- *Grade 4.* Significant subchondral bone loss with loss of support to the dorsal surface[23]

Slab Fractures

Slab fractures, unlike chip fractures, extend through the full thickness of the bone to involve both proximal and distal joint surfaces (Fig. 8.265).[2,22,40,42,45] They can involve any of the carpal bones; but the most commonly affected are the third, followed by the intermediate and radial carpal bones. Slab fractures usually involve the dorsal surface of the bone and vary in thickness and width. Approximately 58% of third carpal slab fractures in racing Thoroughbreds and Standardbreds are frontal plane slab fractures of the dorsomedial facet, 22% are large frontal plane slab fractures involving the intermediate and radial facets, 8% are slab fractures of the intermediate facet, and 12.4% are sagittal slab fractures.[40]

Comminuted Fractures

Comminuted fractures can involve any or all of the carpal bones, but they most frequently affect the third, radial, intermediate, and fourth carpal bones (Fig. 8.266). Comminution can accompany chip and slab fractures as well. A great degree of instability results with these fractures and the limb will usually have an angular deformity.

Oblique Fractures

Oblique fractures of the distal end of the radius are rare (see ''Fractures of the Radius'' in this chapter).

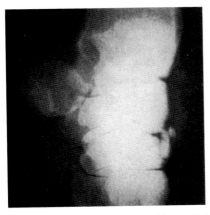

Figure 8.265   Fracture of the third carpal bone. Note that two pieces of the third bone have broken off. The large piece is a typical slab fracture. (Courtesy of T. S. Stashak.)

Causes

Trauma emanating from repeated concussion (internal axial compression cyclic failure), shear forces, or an external blow causes oblique carpal bone fractures. Biomechanically, the carpus is an unusual joint. During protraction it is freely movable in a cranial-to-caudal direction; and while in motion, the dorsal surfaces of the carpal joints open and the carpal bones become misaligned. As the foot impacts the ground, the joint spaces begin to close and, at the same time, the carpal bones begin to shift back into a more normal position to finally become locked in perfect congruity during full weight bearing. This creates a postlike position to the limb with the carpus interposed between the two long bones.[2,37] The carpus is the only joint in the horse by which vertical forces are thrust through one long bone (the large metacarpal) to the other (the radius).[36] Because of this arrangement, the carpus is susceptible to concussive trauma. The ability of the carpal bones to lock in congruity can be altered by fatigue, extreme speed, poor racing surfaces, an improper angle to the race track, and improper trimming.[2,37,47] These factors can result in an asynchronous distribution of the internal forces within the carpus. If the carpus is fully loaded (full weight bearing) when the carpal bones are slightly out of place, abnormal internal forces develop, leading to trauma.[2,37]

Greater axial loading shifts the compressive forces to the dorsal surface of the carpal bones.[29] Fatigue also creates abnormal compression on the dorsal surface of the carpal bones in two ways. First, as fatigue progresses, the soft tissue structures supporting the carpus (muscles, tendons, and ligaments) become weakened, resulting in an uncoordinated, compensatory overstriding. More specifically, as the extensor muscle groups begin to fa-

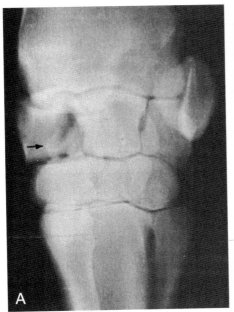 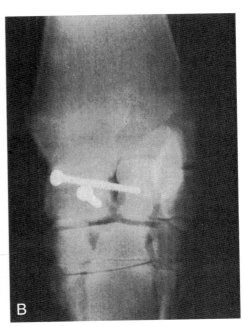

Figure 8.266   A. Comminuted fracture of the radial carpal bone (arrow). B. Two bone screws were used to repair the fracture. (Courtesy of T. S. Stashak.)

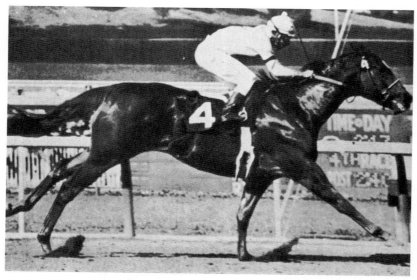

Figure 8.267 One mechanism of carpal fractures. Note the severe overextension of left carpus. (Courtesy of W. Berkley.)

tigue, the foot begins to impact before the limb is in full extension. This results in a backward, snapping, or slamming effect of the carpus rather than a smooth interlocking of the carpal bones.[2,37] As the flexor muscles begin to fatigue, the caudal support to the carpus is reduced during maximal loading and an overextension of the carpus occurs, which can be visualized in some horses at the finish line as a back-at-the-knee appearance in full load bearing (Fig. 8.267). Both result in increased trauma to the dorsal surfaces of the carpal bones.

During race training, the carpal bones undergo a process of remodeling in response to the compressive and shear stresses placed on them, in a similar manner as the cannon bone. The result is an increase in bone mineral density after 4.5 months of training, specifically in the dorsal aspect of the carpal bones (this is not identified in the palmar aspect).[12] With galloping exercise, trabecular thickening and density increase in the subchondral bone dorsally, under areas commonly affected by cartilage damage;[11] the result is greater bone stiffness in trained horses.[48] It is important to note, however, initially with exercise (6 weeks) the stiffness of the carpal subchondral bone decreases as bone resorption precedes bone deposition during remodeling[31] of the bone adjacent to the injured bone (carpal chip fractures).[27]

Studies using pressure-sensitive film have documented that constant intermediate levels of compression occur in the middle and caudal areas of the carpal bones; but at high loads, as would be expected in the load phase of a racehorse, the dorsal surfaces of the bones are intermittently exposed to high compressive loads.[29] The dorsal surfaces contain different amounts and compositions of proteoglycan in the articular cartilage and respond to exercise by increasing production of a smaller hydrodynamic size (less aggregating) proteoglycan. The result may be less compressive stiffness to the dorsal cartilage (lower aggregate modulus).[20,30,31] Thus, initially during training, carpal bone is less stiff during early remodeling but ultimately becomes stiffer and able to withstand

greater compressive stresses. Overlying the articular cartilage in the dorsal areas may be an inadequate response to intermittent high-load stresses, promoting cartilage lesions at this vulnerable site.

Faulty conformation may play a roll in high-speed performance, and it has been stated that horses that are back in the knees (calf kneed) are particularly predisposed to carpal fracture.[1,2,39] In a study measuring the degree of carpal hyperextension from radiographs and comparing a group of horses with carpal chip fracture versus horses without them, no correlation was seen to link hyperextended conformation to carpal chip fractures.[4] Intuitively, it seems that this conformation places more stress dorsally, which may stimulate more bone remodeling to handle the stresses, or it may be a difficult correlation to make without large sample sizes.

During maximal loading, stresses do become concentrated on the dorsal surface of the carpal bones. Continued repeated uneven loading leads to progressive weakening of the bone and damage to the articular surface, resulting in an articular fracture.[37] Many European-bred racehorses are slightly over in the knees, race as 3-year-olds rather than 2-year-olds, run on turf courses with subtle turns, and race in both counterclockwise and clockwise directions. These differences result in a decreased incidence of carpal chip fractures.[2]

Improper trimming and shoeing resulting in an imbalanced foot can cause unequal distribution of forces up the entire limb, affecting the carpus as well. The common practices of trimming to lower the heel and leaving the toe long also lead to abnormal, uneven compressive stresses on the carpus.

Although intraarticular fractures can occur from a single event, they probably are more often a result of continued, repeated trauma leading to an alteration in bone structure, which causes fractures (cyclic fatigue failure).[37] Continued racing or training after an intraarticular fracture may result in severe DJD of the affected joint. However, DJD does not occur in all cases, and the indication for surgery depends on the type and size of fracture sustained.

Signs

Signs of intraarticular chip fractures within the carpus are manifested by some degree of heat, pain, joint distension, and lameness. On visual examination, synovial distension of the antebrachiocarpal (radiocarpal) joint or midcarpal carpal joint is a hallmark to carpal disease. With an acute chip fracture, the synovitis is initially relatively diffuse (involving the whole joint) but eventually becomes more localized in the soft tissue over the chip fracture. This point swelling results from a localized synovitis and synovial proliferation, usually over the dorsomedial surface of the carpal joints.

With slab fractures, the swelling tends to remain diffuse and later results in an organized diffuse thickening of the joint capsule. This swelling is usually associated with the midcarpal joint and results from a slab fracture of the third carpal bone. The swelling on the dorsal surface of the carpus should be differentiated from other less common conditions, such as supracarpal bursitis and tenovaginitis of the extensor tendon sheaths.[16]

The degree of lameness depends on the extent, location, and duration of the fracture and the amount of DJD that is present. In general, most horses with acute small articular fractures of the carpus exhibit minimal signs of lameness. Horses that have sustained acute large chip fractures or slab fractures usually stand with the carpus partially flexed. At exercise, some degree of shortening of the cranial phase of the stride and decreased height of the foot flight arc is noted. Circling to the affected side usually increases the signs of lameness. Horses with more chronic fractures may exhibit minimal to moderate signs of lameness at exercise. As a rule, the earlier the problem is recognized, the easier it is to elicit pain and observe lameness.

Assessment of the degree of carpal flexion and the carpal flexion test can be valuable tools in the diagnosis of carpal lameness. Reduced, painful flexion and nonpainful flexion can be identified. Reduced, painful flexion is usually associated with acute intraarticular fractures and slab fractures. Frequently, horses with slab fractures will violently resist flexion and rear up to avoid it. Nonpainful, reduced flexion, on the other hand, can result from chronic carpitis and old healed slab fractures. Rarely will chronic intraarticular chip fractures lead to decreased flexion. The carpal flexion test is performed by holding the carpus in a flexed position for 1 minute, after which the horse is exercised at a trot. Two or three abnormal steps are normally observed. However, if more are present, there may be a problem within the carpus, particularly if there is a nodding head lameness associated with it (see Chapter 3).

Pressure palpation of the dorsal border of each carpal bone in both joints is also an important diagnostic tool. The extensor carpi radialis tendon provides a good landmark. Carpal bones medial to it include the radial and third carpal bones. Lateral to it are the intermediate carpal bone, ulnar carpal bone in the proximal row, and the lateral edge of the third carpal bone and fourth carpal bone in the distal row. All the dorsal surfaces of the carpal bones are palpated as well as the distal end of the radius. With practice, the examiner can define the fracture location (see Chapter 3).

Diagnosis

Carpal lameness can be confirmed by intrasynovial anesthesia. Between 5 and 7 mL of local anesthetic is injected into the antebrachiocarpal or midcarpal joints after withdrawal of a like amount of synovial fluid has been accomplished. The local anesthetic should not be injected if a homogenous dark red fluid is withdrawn, because of the high probability of an intraarticular fracture. The lameness is reevaluated 15 to 30 minutes after the injection. If there is any question about whether a fracture exists, it is recommended that radiographs be taken before the injection is made. Intrasynovial anesthesia in the carpus is probably most frequently used when the examiner is having a difficult time ascertaining the site of involvement or the percentage that the region contributes to the overall lameness picture (see Chapter 3). Any discoloration to the synovial fluid should be submitted for analysis and cytology. Many joints in a racehorse may have been repeatedly injected, and a reactive synovitis or brewing joint infection may appear like, and occur concurrently with, carpal fracture.

Radiographs should be taken to confirm the presence of a suspected lesion. It is recommended that six standard views be taken—dorsopalmar (DP); lateral medial (LM); dorsopalmar, lateral medial oblique (DPLMO); dorsopalmar medial lateral oblique (DPMLO); and flexed lateral medial (FLM);[46] and skyline—to assess the depth, length, and the exact location of the fractures of the third carpal bone (see Chapter 4) (Figs. 8.268A and 8.269A). In some practices, the skyline view of the proximal row of carpal bones is also routine. Most practices perform this view if any other view suggests a possible abnormality in the antebrachiocarpal joint. The dorsoproximal-dorsodistal skyline projection of the distal row of carpal bones is accurate for detecting subchondral third carpal bone sclerosis and correlates with third carpal bone density.[44] Radiographs of the contralateral carpus are indicated, because a similar chip fracture is present in about 50% of horses.[24] The exact location of the chip fractures that are not diagnosed initially by physical examination may be pinpointed by careful palpation once the radiographic examination has identified their presence.

Arthroscopy may be useful as a diagnostic tool, particularly in horses with radiographic occult lesion. In one report on horses with recurrent carpal pain without radiographic evidence of fracture, it was noted that patients may have any number of injuries. Diagnostic arthroscopic inspection of the joint revealed most had direct bone pain from crush fractures, radiographically silent fractures, or microfractures or fatigue failure of sclerotic bone.[26] Sclerosis of the third carpal bone is a progressive event in bone remodeling of the Standardbred racehorse[43] and carpal lameness is significantly associated with sclerosis. Lucency of the third carpal bone and distal radiocarpal bone are associated with lameness, and lesions are identified in bone and cartilage at arthroscopy.[8,38] Identification of carpal ligament injuries

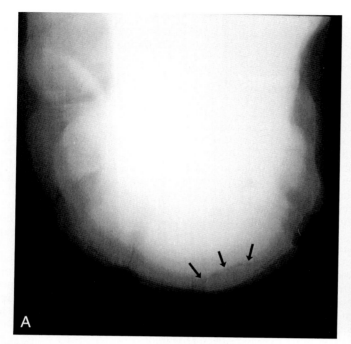 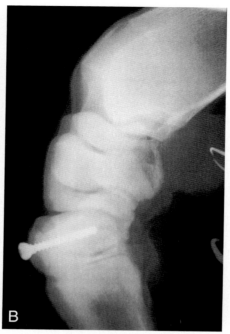

Figure 8.268 A. Skyline view indicating a slab fracture of the radial facet of the third carpal bone (arrows). B. A single 4.5-mm cortical bone screw placed in lag fashion compressed and stabilized the fracture. The proximal (trough) bone fragment was removed.

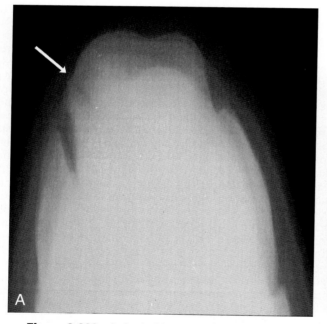 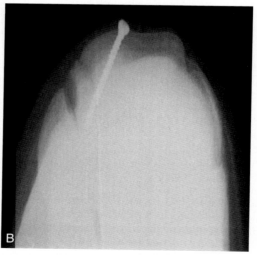

Figure 8.269 A. Sagittal fracture of the third carpal bone. B. A single 3.5-mm cortical bone screw placed in lag fashion compressed and stabilized the fracture.

at arthroscopy also explains lameness in some horses, emphasizing the importance of carpal arthroscopy as a diagnostic tool.[26] In many cases, arthroscopy offers a more accurate assessment of the condition of the carpus.[17] Injury to the palmar carpal ligaments can occur simultaneously with or independent from fracture and can cause carpal lameness. The large medial palmar intercarpal ligament connects the palmar radiocarpal bone to the palmar third and second carpal bones. Of juvenile Thoroughbreds that underwent arthroscopy of the middle carpal joints for other reasons (e.g., chip fracture), 70% had some damage to this ligament and 9% had complete ligament rupture in one study[32] and 41% had similar damage in another study.[18] Bone remodeling of the dorsodistal border of the radiocarpal bone has been associated with the severity of this injury,[32] and articular cartilage damage has been correlated with severity of ligament damage.[18]

Nuclear scintigraphic evaluation of horses with chronic carpal lameness without radiographic evidence of carpal bone fracture can assist with locating stress fracture fatigue of bone, usually the third carpal bone. In one study of lame racing Standardbreds, 43% of horses with forelimb problems had increased uptake associated with the third carpal bone, the majority of which were thought to be clinically significant. The authors believed that the scintigraphy identified early pathology associated with exercise-induced bone remodeling.[9] The third carpal bone in most racing Standardbreds has some increase in radiopharmaceutical uptake associated with stress remodeling,[43] but activity in the fracture level is usually associated with pain.

Treatment

Chip Fractures

Arthroscopic surgical removal of carpal chip fractures is the treatment of choice for most cases, particularly if return to racing performance is desired (Figs. 8.263 and 8.270). In select cases of small nondisplaced fractures or incomplete fractures, conservative management is successful. The selection of treatment depends on the physical findings, the size and shape of the chip, and its location. Other factors that should be considered are the animal's age, its sex, and its intended future use. Whether a chip fracture is painful largely depends on the duration since injury, its size and location, and the degree of displacement from the parent bone.

In general, small chip fractures firmly attached to the parent bone can be handled conservatively with some period of rest. On physical examination, these horses

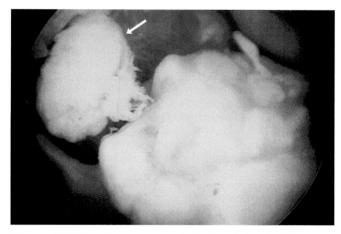

Figure 8.270 Arthroscopy reveals displaced chronic distal radiocarpal bone chip fractures. The rounded borders of the fracture and the fibrous tissue in the fracture bed indicate the chronicity of the fracture. One fragment is attached to the adjacent synovium and is not free floating (arrow).

may exhibit mild lameness or no lameness at exercise and may have minimal pain with limb manipulation and direct palpation over the fracture. Nondisplaced chip fractures of the distal end of the radius are also frequently treated this way and carry a good prognosis for return to racing if sufficient rest has been afforded.[34,45]

Surgical removal of these fractures may still be elected if it is anticipated that the convalescent time will be significantly reduced. With a small, nondisplaced fracture, 4 months of rest is anticipated for bone healing, but 2 months of rest may be all that is necessary after arthroscopic removal. In the third carpal bone, even nondisplaced fractures are best treated with surgical removal, because they may take 6 months to heal conservatively and a fibrous union may result.

Large acute chip fractures with displacement that affects the weight-bearing surface or that are floating free within the joint are best treated by surgery to prevent further degenerative changes in the form of cartilage erosion, adjacent osteolysis, osteophytosis, and "kissing" lesions on the opposite joint surfaces; not too infrequently, these chips refracture when the horse is put back into training. Most of these horses exhibit increased signs of lameness and increased pain on flexion and palpation compared to those sustaining smaller chip fractures. These chip fractures should be removed as early as practical (within 10 to 14 days).

When intraarticular steroids have recently been used and multiple fractures and cartilage damage are expected, some clinicians believe that surgery is best delayed for 30 to 45 days. During this time, the horses should be placed in stall confinement. For simple arthroscopic surgeries, the recent use of intraarticular steroids does not usually delay surgery, but different opinions exist on this issue and consideration of history reliability and sterility of injection may still warrant delay.

Conservative treatment of horses sustaining nondisplaced chip fractures usually consists of stall confinement for 6 to 12 weeks with daily hand walking beginning after 6 weeks. Free exercise can be begun at the 3rd or 4th month, and training is begun at 6 to 8 months after the injury occurred. This period is usually sufficient to allow for adequate healing of the fracture.

Nonsteroidal anti-inflammatory drugs (NSAIDs) can be used initially to reduce the acute inflammatory process. Intrasynovial or intravenous injections of sodium hyaluronate and intramuscular injections of polysulfated glycosaminoglycans may be beneficial in reducing the synovitis, the progressive cartilage destruction, and the formation of osteophytes. The intrasynovial injection of steroids is not recommended, because it delays the healing process and masks inflammatory signs. Injection of intraarticular steroid is all too often used to return the horse to racing as soon as possible. Ancillary treatments with counterirritants applied topically, pin firing, and corrective shoeing are used and may be of benefit.

The surgical approach to the fracture fragments should be carefully determined by radiographs before surgery, and an operative plan should be followed. In general, smaller fragments are removed before larger ones in a joint because distension may be difficult to maintain after removing a large fragment. The most difficult and clinical joint is performed first while the surgeon is fresh and so the most important problems can be addressed first in case the horse must be rapidly recovered.

Normally, antebrachiocarpal joint surgery is performed before midcarpal joint surgery, because subcutaneous fluids migrate toward the ground (proximal on the limb), away from the midcarpal joint. Generally, freefloating fragments are removed immediately once they are located (Fig. 8.184).

Horses are positioned in dorsal recumbency under general anesthesia to allow access to both the medial and the lateral arthroscope portals of both carpi without moving the horse and to decrease intraoperative hemorrhage (Fig. 8.271). Although other positions are used by some surgeons, they are not discussed here. After draping, the joint is flexed so that the antebrachiocarpal and midcarpal joints can be positively identified. The arthroscope portal is selected to be opposite the chip fracture, and the operative portal is placed strategically adjacent to the fragment to allow removal with rongeurs. In the carpus, the skin incisions are made in the center of the palpable divot between the extensor carpi radialis tendon and common digital extensor tendon laterally and medial to the extensor carpi radialis tendon medially. Most fractures and all of the common fractures can be removed with this approach. For unusual fractures in the palmar aspect of the joint, alternate portals can be used for access.[7]

Upon entering the joint with the arthroscope, an immediate and complete exploratory should be performed to identify expected lesions and unexpected lesions. The joint condition should be videorecorded. A probe instrument is then used to palpate lesions for looseness, cartilage depth of lesion and undermining, and softness of underlying bone. The fractures are elevated with a periosteal elevator to tear capsular attachments and then are grasped and removed with rongeurs. If chronic chip fractures are encountered an osteotome can be used to elevate the fragment from the parent bone. Abnormal bone and frayed cartilage are removed to healthy bone, and the joint is liberally lavaged to remove debris. A microfracture technique (small bone pick) can be used to penetrate the subchondral bone and enhance articular cartilage repair in larger cartilage defects.[14] A final exploratory is performed to ensure removal of all fragments and sizable debris.

If necessary, the arthroscope is inserted in the opposite side of the same joint and the process repeated. In general, the synovial membrane is not removed unless it is thought to harbor infection or is focally extremely irritated. A final videorecording is made and still photos are taken for the record. A final radiograph is taken intraoperatively to confirm complete fragment removal.

Only the skin is sutured, with one or two sutures. A sterile elastic bandage is placed intraoperatively and changed when postoperative radiographs are taken 1 to 2 days later.

Postoperatively, bandages are maintained until the skin sutures are removed at 10 days. Perioperative antibiotics are often not used, but surgeon preference varies. Pain medication usually consists of low dosages of phenylbutazone (2.2 mg/kg PO once daily). Use of intramuscular polysulfated glycosaminoglycan can begin at 6 weeks, when cartilage healing is peaking, and again before training. Sodium hyaluronate (systemic or intraarticular) can be used to treat chronic synovitis or effusion.

Postoperative care consists of box-stall rest for 6 weeks, and hand walking commences after 2 weeks. Turnout at 6 weeks and training at 12 to 16 weeks are typical. Daily passive flexion of the carpus postoperatively helps regain carpal range of motion, particularly for third carpal bone injuries that also have capsulitis. Swimming the horse helps with soft tissue convalescence. Passive joint exercises should begin after soft tissue healing is well started (at about 3 weeks) and the skin is sealed.

Complications of surgery are rare, but include joint infection (less than 0.01%), subcutaneous infection, chronic effusion of the joint, and distension of the extensor carpi radialis tendon sheath. Entering the sheath is most likely to occur during removal of large distal radius fractures. In most cases, the connection heals without blemish. Benefits of arthroscopic carpal fracture removal include short surgery time, visualization of most of the joint and sites of all common fractures, less soft tissue morbidity, shorter convalescence, increased diagnostic accuracy, and improved cosmetics. Arthrotomy is no longer used for treatment of carpal chip fractures, except under rare circumstances.

Slab Fractures

Horses with slab fractures of the carpal bone should be surgically treated as soon as practical after the injury has occurred even if corticosteroids have been injected recently. The fracture must be stabilized to minimize the

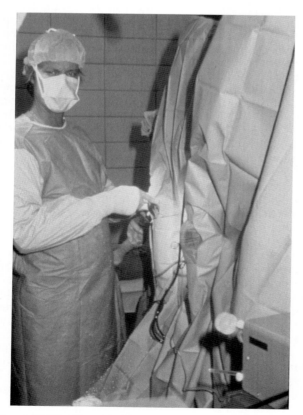

Figure 8.271 Horse positioned in dorsal recumbency and undergoing carpal arthroscopy.

chance of further articular damage and DJD. Both non-displaced and displaced fractures are best treated surgically if any expectation for return to performance is present.

Thorough evaluation of the skyline view of the region should be made to define the nature of the slab fracture (Figs. 8.268 and 8.269). This view provides the best information regarding the location of the fractures, its width, its length, and how many fracture fragments are present. The DPLMO views should be examined carefully for chip fracture off the proximal surface of the slab fracture. This fracture is located in the midcarpal joint space and is most frequently associated with displaced slab fractures of the third carpal bone. At arthroscopic surgery when this piece of bone is removed, a troughlike defect remains after screw stabilization and should be removed at surgery.

If the slab fracture is small and thin (too thin to place a screw) or is in multiple pieces or degenerative changes have progressed to the point that reduction and stabilization cannot be achieved, the dorsal fragment should be removed completely. For this procedure, the fibrous attachments on the dorsal surface of the third carpal bone are sharply incised by following the contour of the bone. Cartilage erosions elsewhere in the joint should be curetted down to subchondral bone.[2]

Larger acute slab fractures can be reattached to parent bone by interfragmentary compression using the lag screw principle. Because slab fractures of the third carpal bone occur most frequently, I will use them as an example. These fractures can be repaired through an arthrotomy or by arthroscopy.[35] Arthroscopy is recommended for fractures with concomitant chip fractures or evidence of other chronic changes in the joint, such as lucency of the distal radiocarpal bone or third carpal bone. In simple, acute frontal plane slab fractures of a clean joint, a small arthrotomy directly over the articular surface of the third carpal bone permits precise, rapid insertion of a single lag screw. The incision does not need to extend over the dorsal surface of the third carpal bone, and the screw can be inserted through a separate incision, usually lateral and proximal to the arthrotomy.

In either approach, the horse is positioned in dorsal recumbency under general anesthesia with the limb in moderate flexion to fully reduce the fracture. For arthroscopic repair, the arthroscope is placed in a lateral portal, and an exploratory is performed. In fresh displaced fractures, mobility may be limited by intraarticular displacement of the fragment. The fracture can readily be reduced by manual finger pressure from outside the joint. Needles can be placed to demarcate the medial and lateral borders of the fracture and the carpometacarpal joint directly distal to the site of screw placement.

Ideally, the screw is placed centrally in the fracture and parallel to the articular surface and carpometacarpal joint through a separate stab incision. A radiograph should be taken or fluoroscopy used to document the angle of the drill bit. The tendency is to place the screw too far medial and too proximal, close to the articular surface. This can be problematic, particularly if removal of the dorsal shelf of bone in front of the trough is elected. A 3.5-mm (less commonly a 4.5-mm) ASIF cortical bone screw (usually 30 to 40 mm long) is placed in lag fashion, and compression can be observed arthro-

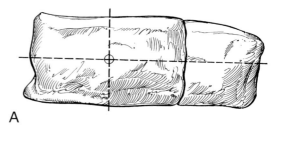

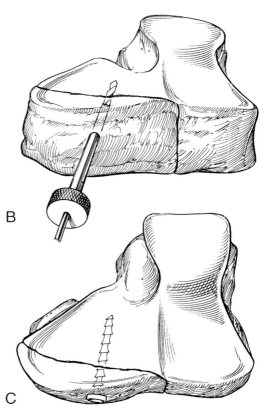

Figure 8.272 Screw placement for repair of a slab fracture of the third carpal bone. A. Proper location for the 4.5-mm drill bit used to create a gliding hole. B. A 3.2-mm drill guide is placed in the gliding hole, and a 3.2-mm drill bit is used to make the thread hole. *Note:* The drill should not penetrate the palmar cortex of the third carpal bone. C. A 4.5-mm cortical screw is used to create interfragmentary compression. (Courtesy of T. S. Stashak.)

scopically (Fig. 8.272A). Drilling is accomplished parallel to the articular surface of the third carpal bone, creating a gliding hole approximately 12-mm deep. This is usually deep enough to cross most slab fracture fragments and allows adequate thickness of bone for later countersinking. After this, a drill guide is placed in the gliding hole and a drill bit is used to make the thread hole, 20 to 25 mm deep (Fig. 8.272B). The surgeon should avoid exiting the third carpal bone at its palmar limits, since this may cause damage to the structures within the carpal canal. The gliding hole is countersunk at this time to decrease the concentrating forces that will occur at the base of the screw head. Less countersinking is necessary for a 3.5-mm screw and is an advantage, particularly for thinner fractures.

A depth gauge is used to measure the depth of the hole, and an appropriate length cortical screw is selected. It is important to ensure that the drilled hole is longer than the screw or the threads will strip. A cortical bone tap is used to create threads in the thread hole. It is also important to fully tap the thread hole, particularly for 3.5-mm screws, because in the dense bone of the third carpal bone, the screwdriver seat will strip as the screw tries to self-tap. Owing to the shallow configuration of their driver seat, 3.5-mm screws are particularly prone to this complication.

The screw is then inserted and tightened sufficiently to compress the slab fracture effectively into accurate alignment with the parent bone (Fig. 8.272C). After fracture reduction and stabilization, the rest of the joint can be surgically treated as necessary, and the fracture trough debrided (Fig. 8.268B). If a triangular piece of bone and cartilage are removed from the fracture surface, the dorsal lip of bone projecting above the fracture surface should be removed with an automated power burr.

The joint is liberally lavaged and closed with skin sutures. The incision over the screw head requires subcutaneous and skin closures. A sterile padded bandage is placed for 2 weeks. Postoperative care consists of 2 months of stall rest, 1 month of hand walking, and 3 months of turnout before training.

The disadvantages of the arthroscopic approach include distortion of the fracture, because variable magnification (i.e., the magnification changes with the distance from the scope) makes central placement of the screw difficult; fluid leakage around the fracture and lag screw owing to the disruption of the joint capsule around the fracture; and increased time for set up and manipulations.

If arthrotomy is elected, the surgery can still be performed in dorsal recumbency to minimize hemorrhage and obviate the need for a tourniquet. The arthrotomy incision (1.5 to 2 cm) is made directly over the anticipated site of the fracture on the radial facet. A small Gelpi is placed to expose the articular surface of the third carpal bone and expose the fracture. Under direct visualization, the middle of the fracture can be determined with immediate confidence. Needles (22 gauge) are placed in the carpometacarpal joint directly distal to the selected location for the screw. A separate stab incision is made to place the screw in lag fashion. Radiographic control and postoperative care are as described above. The joint capsule is closed with simple interrupted absorbable sutures, and the skin is closed routinely.

The advantages of arthrotomy are speed, precise lag screw placement, and elimination of the expense of opening arthroscopic equipment. The disadvantages are a slightly larger incision and case selection is important for reducing the risk of incisional complications.

Care should be taken to avoid ulcers on the accessory carpal bone and on the medial tuberosity of the radius. A full-limb bandage protects the joint while the animal recovers from anesthesia; and for the first 5 to 7 days after the surgery, it helps keep swelling to a minimum. The bandage is removed at 5 to 7 days and replaced with a lighter sterile elastic bandage. Perioperative antibiotics are continued for 24 hours until hemorrhage has

stopped. Phenylbutazone (2.2 mg/kg daily) is usually administered for pain.

Healing progress should be monitored by radiographs at 6, 12, and 24 weeks. The fracture should be healed by 25 weeks, when training can begin. Longer healing (8 to 9 months), however, is preferable. Use of supportive joint medication is similar as for chip fractures.

Sagittal slab fractures of the carpal bones, most commonly of the third carpal bone, are difficult to treat surgically. If they are not widely displaced, they can be treated conservatively with a 1-year course before return to racing.[13] If a lag screw can be placed (Fig. 8.269), healing can occur in 3 months, and return to racing can be rapid.

Other slab fractures can occur in any carpal bone, and the surgical principles for repair are similar to those described.[10] Without repair, DJD is expected and return to performance is unlikely.

Multiple Comminuted Fractures

Multiple comminuted carpal bone fractures occur infrequently, but generally are seen in racing and jumping horses during athletic events. Because there is a loss of internal support, a valgus or varus angulation to the limb usually occurs. Treatment should be considered for horses with breeding potential and/or sentimental value; repair requires major orthopedic surgery.[15]

The limb should be immediately stabilized until radiographs can be taken to assess the degree of damage. In cases in which a single bone has been affected with comminution, internal fixation with screws can be used (Figs. 8.266 and 8.273). One report describes two cases of comminuted fracture of the fourth carpal bone handled successfully in this manner.[45]

If several carpal bones are affected with comminution and a larger number of fragments are present, the carpus can be fused with plates and screws (Fig. 8.274). Partial carpal arthrodesis of the midcarpal joint—with either two narrow plates or one narrow plate and a T-plate—retains some degree of joint flexion. In most instances, the antebrachiocarpal joint can be spared by sta-

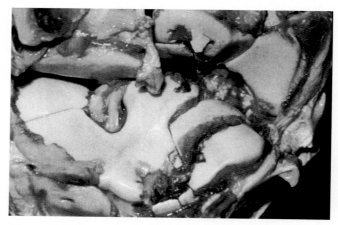

Figure 8.273 Necropsy specimen of acute fractures of the radiocarpal, intermediate carpal, and third and fourth carpal bones. This severe injury may result in elected euthanasia. Reconstruction of the bones with screws or carpal arthrodesis is an option for breeding soundness.

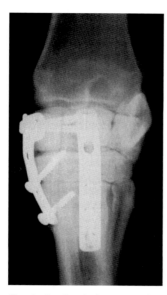

Figure 8.274   Surgical arthrodesis was performed on the midcarpal and carpometacarpal joints using a T-plate and a narrow dynamic compression plate in a horse with multiple carpal fractures. At 6 months postsurgery, the joints are completely fused and the antebrachiocarpal joint is free of arthritis. The horse had complete use of the limb and only a minimal decrease in the range of carpal joint motion.

bilizing the carpal bones in the distal row with screws and the plates. If the collateral ligament is avulsed or fractures of the radius are concurrent, then pancarpal arthrodesis with two long, broad plates is recommended. If the procedure is performed with the limb in 5 to 15° of flexion, the limb will be slightly shorter than the contralateral limb, making ambulation and standing on the fused limb easier.[5,6]

Prognosis

The prognosis for horses with chip fractures returning to racing is well supported with a large number of cases and is repeatedly good. In older studies in which chip fractures were removed by arthrotomy, 80% of 89 Thoroughbreds[19] and 76% of 220 Thoroughbreds[33] returned to performance racing, although in 210 Thoroughbreds treated similarly, horses with carpal chip fractures that were removed surgically performed inferiorly with respect to wins and wins plus places, compared with 840 control horses.[41] After arthroscopic treatment of Thoroughbred racehorses with carpal chip fractures, 68.4% returned to race 9 months later;[25] and in another study of Thoroughbreds and Quarter Horses, 68% raced at a level equal or better than before injury.[24] The severity and extent of articular cartilage damage affect the prognosis. Horses with grade 1 and 2 cartilage damage had a significantly greater chance (73%) to race at a level equal or better than preinjury compared to horses with grade 3 or 4 cartilage damage (54%).

Of Standardbred racehorses, 74% of horses in one study made at least one start after surgery. Pacers were significantly more likely to have a start than trotters.

Median earnings per start significantly decreased after surgery, and median race mark significantly increased after surgery. The majority of Standardbreds are useful racehorses after carpal arthroscopy; however, most earn less money per start and many race at a lower class.[21]

The prognosis for horses that have sustained a slab fracture of the third carpal bone that is treated by surgical excision or screw fixation is fair to good for return to athletic performance and racing. In 31 Thoroughbreds, 67.6% returned to race at least once after recovery from surgery, but these horses had a reduced claiming value.[22] In another study of 72 Thoroughbreds, 65% raced after surgery, but earnings per start declined.[42] In 61 Standardbred racehorses, 77% were able to race again, and 100% of horses that raced before sustaining a third carpal slab fracture raced again.[42] Earnings per start also declined in the Standardbreds, but not as much as for the Thoroughbreds.[42] However, a good prognosis can be given for patients that are retired for pleasure riding or breeding.[19]

For comminuted fractures, the prognosis is poor but somewhat depends on the number of carpal bones involved, the degree of displacement, and the amount of anatomic deformity. Many horses are euthanized owing to the expense of treatment and the guarded prognosis.

References

1. Adams OR. Lameness in Horses. 3rd ed. Philadelphia: Lea & Febiger, 1974;187.
2. Auer J. Diseases of the carpus. Vet Clin North Am Large Anim Pract [Special Edition: Symposium on Equine Lameness] 1980;2: 81.
3. Auer JA, Watkins JP, White NA, et al. Slab fractures of the fourth and intermediate carpal bones in five horses. J Am Vet Med Assoc 1986;88:595.
4. Barr AR. Carpal conformation in relation to carpal chip fracture. Vet Rec 1994;134:646.
5. Barr ARS, Hillyer MH, Richardson JD. Partial carpal arthrodesis for multiple carpal fractures and subluxation in a pony. Equine Vet J 1994;6:255.
6. Bertone AL, Schneiter HL, Turner AS, Shoemaker RS. Pancarpal arthrodesis for treatment of carpal collapse in the adult horse: A report of 2 cases. Vet Surg 1989;18(5):353–359.
7. Dabareiner RM, Sullins KE, Bradley W. Removal of a fracture fragment from the palmar aspect of the intermediate carpal bone in a horse. J Am Vet Med Assoc 1993;203:553.
8. Dabareiner RM, White NA, Sullins KE. Radiographic and arthroscopic findings associated with subchondral lucency of the distal radial carpal bone in 71 horses. Equine Vet J 1996;28:93.
9. Ehrlich PJ, Dohoo IR, O'Callaghan MW. Results of bone scintigraphy in racing Standardbred horses: 64 cases (1992–1994). J Am Vet Med Assoc 1999;215:982.
10. Field JR, Zaruby JF. Repair of a fracture of the fourth carpal bone in a yearling Standardbred horse. Can Vet J 1994;35:371.
11. Firth EC, Delahunt J, Wichtel JW, et al. Galloping exercise induces regional changes in bone density within the third and radial carpal bones of Thoroughbred horses. Equine Vet J 1999;31:111.
12. Firth EC, Goodship AE, Delahunt J, et al. Osteoinductive response in the dorsal aspect of the carpus of young Thoroughbreds in training occurs within months. Equine Vet J Suppl 1999;30:552.
13. Fischer AT, Stover SM. Sagittal fractures of the third carpal bone in horses: 12 cases (1977–1985). J Am Vet Med Assoc 1987;191: 106.
14. Frisbie DD, Trotter GW, Powers BE, et al. Arthroscopic subchondral bone plate microfracture technique augments healing of large chondral defects in the radial carpal bone and medial femoral condyle of horses. Vet Surg 1999;28:242.

15. Grant BD. The carpus. In: Mansmann RA, McAllister ES, Eds. Equine Medicine and Surgery. 3rd ed. Santa Barbara, CA: American Veterinary Publications, 1982;1120.

15. Grant BD. Unusual causes of "carpitis." Mod Vet Pract 1980;61: 131–134.

17. Kannegieter NJ, Burbidge HM. Correlation between radiographic and arthroscopic findings in the equine carpus. Aust Vet J 1990; 67:132.

18. Kannegieter NJ, Colgan SA. The incidence and severity of intercarpal ligament damage in the equine carpus. Aust Vet J 1993;70:89.

19. Lindsey WA, Horney FD. Equine carpal surgery. A review of 89 cases and evaluation of return to function. J Am Vet Med Assoc 1981;179:682.

20. Little CB, Ghosh P, Rose R. The effect of strenuous versus moderate exercise on the metabolism of proteoglycans in articular cartilage from different weight-bearing regions of the equine third carpal bone. Osteoarthritis Cartilage 1997;5:161.

21. Lucas JM, Ross MW, Richardson DW. Post operative performance of racing Standardbreds treated arthroscopically for carpal chip fractures: 176 cases (1986–1993). Equine Vet J 1999;31:48.

22. Martin GS, Haynes PF, McClure JR. Effect of third carpal slab fracture and repair on racing performance in Thoroughbred horses: 31 cases (1977–1984). J Am Vet Med Assoc 1988;193:107.

23. McIlwraith CW. Fractures of the carpus. In: Nixon AJ, Ed. Equine Fracture Repair. Philadelphia: WB Saunders, 1996;208.

24. McIlwraith CW, Yovich JV, Martin GS. Arthroscopic surgery for the treatment of osteochondral chip fractures in the equine carpus. J Am Vet Med Assoc 1987;191:531.

25. Mizuno Y. Fractures of the carpus in racing Thoroughbreds of the Japan Racing Association: Prevalence, location, and current modes of surgical therapy. J Equine Vet Sci 1996;16:25.

26. Moore RM, Schneider RK. Arthroscopic findings in the carpal joints of lame horses without radiographically visible abnormalities: 41 cases (1986–1991). J Am Vet Med Assoc 1995;206:1741.

27. Norrdin RW, Kawcak CE, Capwell BA, et al. Calcified cartilage morphometry and its relation to subchondral bone remodeling in equine arthrosis. Bone 1999;24:109.

28. Palmer SE. Prevalence of carpal fractures in Thoroughbred and Standardbred racehorses. J Am Vet Med Assoc 1986;188:1171.

29. Palmer JL, Bertone AL, Litsky AS. Contact area and pressure distribution changes of the equine third carpal bone during loading. Equine Vet J 1994;26:197.

30. Palmer JL, Bertone AL, Malemud CJ, et al. Site-specific proteoglycan characteristics of third carpal articular cartilage in exercised and nonexercised horses. Am J Vet Res 1995;56(12):1570.

31. Palmer JL, Bertone AL, Mansour J, et al. Biomechanical properties of third carpal articular cartilage in exercised and nonexercised horses. J Orthop Res 1995;13:854.

32. Phillips TJ, Wright IM. Observations on the anatomy and pathology of the palmar intercarpal ligaments in the middle carpal joints of Thoroughbred racehorses. Equine Vet J 1994;26:486.

33. Raidel SL, Wright JD. A retrospective evaluation of the surgical management of equine carpal injury. Aust Vet J 1996;74:198.

34. Raker CW. Orthopedic surgery-errors in surgical evaluation and management. Am Assoc Equine Pract 1973;19:205.

35. Richardson DW. Technique for arthroscopic repair of third carpal bone slab fractures in horses. J Am Vet Med Assoc 1986;188:288.

36. Roberts EJ. Carpal lameness. Proc Br Equine Vet Assoc 1964; 181.

37. Rooney JR. Biomechanics of Lameness in Horses. Baltimore: Williams & Wilkins, 1969.

38. Ross MW, Richardson DW, Beroza GA. Subchondral lucency of the third carpal bone in Standardbred racehorses: 13 cases (1982–1988). J Am Vet Med Assoc 1989;195:789.

39. Schneider RK. Incidence and location of fractures within the carpus. Am Assoc Equine Pract 1979;25:145.

40. Schneider RK, Bramlage LR, Gabel AA, et al. Incidence, location and classification of 371 third carpal bone fractures in 313 horses. Equine Vet J Suppl 1988;6:33.

41. Speirs VC, Anderson GA, Bourke JM. Assessment of prognosis for racing after carpal surgery in 210 Thoroughbreds. Equine Vet J 1986;18:187.

42. Stephens PR, Richardson DW, Spencer PA. Slab fractures of the third carpal bone in Standardbreds and Thoroughbreds: 155 cases (1977–1984). J Am Vet Med Assoc 1988;193:353.

43. Uhlhorn H, Edsell P, Sandgren B, et al. Sclerosis of the third carpal bone. A prospective study of its significance in a group of young Standardbred trotters. Acta Vet Scand 2000;41:51.

44. Uhlhorn H, Ekman S, Haglund A, et al. The accuracy of the dorsoproximal-dorsodistal projection in assessing third carpal bone sclerosis in Standardbred trotters. Vet Radiol Ultrasound 1998;39: 412.

45. Vale GT, Wagner PC, Grant BD. Surgical repair of comminuted equine fourth carpal bone fractures. Equine Pract 1982;4:6.

46. Watters JW. Radiography of the equine carpus. Comp Cont Educ Vet Pract 1981;3:248.

47. Wyburn RS, Goulden BE. Fractures of the equine carpus: A report of 57 cases. NZ Vet J 1974;22:133.

48. Young DR, Richardson DW, Markel MD, et al. Mechanical and morphometric analysis of the third carpal bone of Thoroughbreds. Am J Vet Res 1991;52:402.

LUXATIONS OF THE CARPAL JOINTS

Luxations of the carpal joints with disruption of either the lateral or medial collateral ligament are rare in the horse.[1,5-7] They can involve any one of the three carpal joints, but rupture of the medial collateral ligament appears to occur more frequently.[1,3,5] The luxation can be complete or partial. In most cases, the joint surfaces are spared; but in a small percentage of these, comminution of the carpal bones also occurs.[5,6] Multiple fractures of the carpal bones may coexist with damage to the collateral ligaments and lead to carpal collapse and carpal varus.[2,4]

Causes

Any form of severe trauma directed toward the lateral or medial surface of the carpus can result in luxation. This trauma can occur from foaling, jumping, falling, or slipping.[7] Occasionally, an avulsion fracture associated with one of the attachments of the collateral ligaments may accompany the luxation. Alterations to the vascular supply of the distal limb have also been reported with complete luxation of the carpus.

Signs

In most cases, the horse presents with a swelling and angular deformity of the affected limb and is reluctant to bear weight on it.[7] A history of severe trauma may be revealed. During movement, the horse appears obviously to be in pain, and the distal limb is abnormally mobile. This is particularly true for complete luxations and luxations associated with comminuted fractures of the carpal bones. On palpation, heat, pain, and swelling are present and some degree of instability of the distal limb is appreciated. If the carpal bones are fractured, crepitation may be felt. Horses may react quite violently to manipulation of the limb, so the examiner should be careful. The clinician may note that some of the carpal bones are displaced from their normal position.

Diagnosis

An obvious angular limb deformity of the limb coupled with an abnormal alignment of carpal bones identifies the luxated carpus. However, radiographic examination is required to define the extent of bone damage associated with the luxation. Fractured carpal bones and avulsion fractures may accompany these luxations.

Treatment

Closed reduction of the luxation with the horse under general anesthesia can be attempted.[7] If the luxation is accompanied by a medial collateral ligament rupture, the horse should be placed in lateral recumbency with the affected forelimb down. The opposite is true for a rupture of the lateral collateral ligament, for which the affected limb is placed upward. This positioning affords easier manipulation of the limb. In addition, once the luxation is reduced, gravity helps maintain the carpus in normal alignment.

Once reduced, the limb should be rotated gently in both counterclockwise and clockwise directions to assess the degree of rotational stability. If good rotational stability is present, a tube or sleeve cast, extending from the proximal radius to the distal end of the metacarpus, may be all that is needed (Fig. 8.275).[7] (See "Angular Limb Deformities Associated With the Carpus" in this chapter for more information.) If on rotation the carpus appears to be unstable, the application of a full-limb cast is advised. In most cases, immobilization of the carpus is required for about 4 weeks in foals and 6 weeks in mature horses. For foals, tube casts can be applied and left in place for the entire treatment period. On the other hand, if a full-limb cast is used, it should be removed

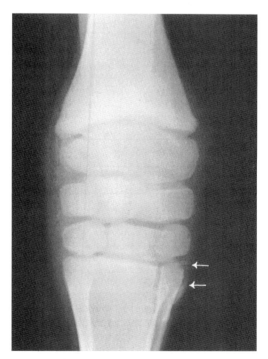

Figure 8.275 This foal was presented with a history of subluxation of the carpometacarpal joint that was noticed shortly after birth. A sleeve cast was used to treat the injury. Note the periosteitis associated with the proximal end of the second small metacarpal bone (arrows) indicating previous trauma to the attachment of the collateral ligament.

and replaced at 10- to 12-day intervals. For adults, however, a full-limb cast can be left in place for the duration of treatment. The period of 4 to 6 weeks usually provides sufficient time for the disrupted support tissues to heal in by scarring.

If multiple carpal bone fracture accompanies the luxation, complete or partial carpal arthrodesis should be performed. If the third and fourth carpal bones are unstable, an arthrodesis of the midcarpal joint—with either two narrow plates or with one narrow plate and a T-plate combined—and bone grafting will maintain some joint motion and eliminate pain (Fig. 8.274).[2] The surgeon can drill the carpometacarpal joint and use bone graft to help the fusion. A cast is necessary if the collateral ligament is not intact and medial to lateral instability is still present.[3,4]

Prognosis

The prognosis for luxation without comminuted fracture of the carpal bones appears to be good for healing of the support structures but is guarded to poor for return to previous performance. The prognosis is poor for any horse that has sustained a comminuted fracture of the carpal bones in conjunction with rupture of the collateral ligaments. Carpal arthrodesis results in a fair to good prognosis for comfort.

References

1. Auer J. Diseases of the carpus. Vet Clin North Am Large Anim Pract [Special Edition: Symposium on Equine Lameness] 1980;2:81.
2. Barr ARS, Hillyer MH, Richardson JD. Partial carpal arthrodesis for multiple carpal fractures and subluxation in a pony. Equine Vet J 1994;6:255.
3. Bertone AL. Management of orthopedic emergencies. In: Bertone JJ, Ed. Emergency Treatment of the Adult Horse. Philadelphia: WB Saunders, 1994;603–625.
4. Bertone AL, Schneiter HL, Turner AS, Shoemaker RS. Pancarpal arthrodesis for treatment of carpal collapse in the adult horse: A report of 2 cases. Vet Surg 1989;18(5):353–359.
5. Fessler JF, Amstutz HE. Fracture repair. In: Oehme FW, Prier JE, Eds. Textbook of Large Animal Surgery. Baltimore: Williams & Wilkins, 1974;306.
6. O'Connor JJ. Dollar's Veterinary Surgery. 4th ed. Chicago: Alexander Eger, 1950;830.
7. Stashak TS. Luxations of the carpal joints. In: Stashak TS, Ed. Adams' Lameness in Horses. 4th ed. Philadelphia: Lea & Febiger, 1987;657–659.

CARPAL CANAL (TUNNEL) SYNDROME

The carpal canal syndrome is a recognized condition that is associated with distal radial osteochondromas, injuries to the deep digital flexor tendon, tenosynovitis, and hyperextension injuries to the carpus.[1,4–6,8,9,11] It results from trauma or space-occupying lesions within the carpal canal. These lesions in turn compress the soft tissue structures within the nondistensible lumen of the carpal canal and result in lameness. With continued irritation to the carpal flexor retinaculum it becomes thickened causing further compression of the soft tissue structures within the carpal canal.

Causes

Trauma to the flexor tendons resulting in tendinitis, fractures of the accessory carpal bone, desmitis of the radial (superior) check ligament, and osteochondroma at the distal radius can result in compression and irritation of the soft tissue structures within the carpal canal. The resultant compression chokes the neurovascular structures at either extremity of the canal during motion, which causes a reduction in blood flow to the distal limb resulting in pain that leads to lameness.[4–6,9,11]

Signs

Horses usually present with a history of moderate, chronic, and sometimes intermittent lameness. Intermittent lameness is usually noted in horses that are rested in between exercise and for horses that have a healed accessory carpal bone fracture.

On visual observation, some degree of synovial fluid distension of the carpal canal can be seen bulging on the caudolateral aspect of the distal radius between the ulnaris lateralis and the lateral digital extensor tendon (Fig. 8.276). With severe effusion, distension of the caudomedial distal radius also occurs between the flexor carpi ulnaris and the flexor carpi radialis. Distally, a smaller fluid distended area is apparent below the carpus and between the flexor tendons and the suspensory ligament (Fig. 8.276).

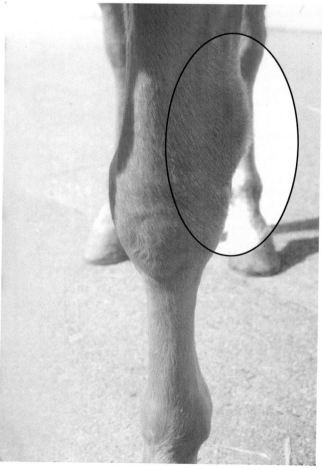

Figure 8.276 Extensive carpal sheath tenosynovitis. Note the swelling proximal to the carpus (oval).

On palpation, some degree of tenseness of the distended carpal canal can be appreciated. A reduced angle of flexion of the carpus is usually noted and rapid flexion of the carpus usually results in extreme pain, with the horse rearing to avoid manipulation. In some cases, a reduction in pulse pressure within the digital artery can be noted at the base of the proximal sesamoid. Deep palpation over the carpal canal region with the carpus held in moderate flexion allows the examiner to identify accessory carpal bone fractures and possibly osteochondromas of the distal radius.[12] Crepitation can be felt with acute fractures of the accessory carpal bone; whereas in chronic cases, an increased lateral-to-medial movement of the fractured accessory carpal bone can be perceived. Deep palpation over the caudomedial aspect of the distal radius allows the bony prominence of the osteochondroma to be felt. Palpation of these lesions usually results in considerable pain, and increased lameness is observed with exercise.

Diagnosis

A tentative diagnosis of the carpal canal syndrome can be made with physical findings of a distended carpal canal along with a decreased ability to flex the limb, painful carpal flexion, and decreased pulse pressure in the palmar digital artery. Intrasynovial anesthesia with 5 mL of anesthetic can be used to confirm the examiner's suspicion that the carpal canal syndrome is the origin of the lameness. Radiographs are required to identify osteochondromas and fractures of the accessory carpal bone as the cause and should always be performed. Ultrasound of the sheath and tendons may reveal chronic synovial proliferation, adhesions, and deep digital flexor tendinitis or tendon injury and/or desmitis of the radial check ligament.[2] If a centesis of the sheath is desired to obtain a fluid sample or to perform intrathecal anesthesia, ultrasound guidance can assist in selecting a pocket of fluid, particularly in chronic cases. Synovial fluid analysis may be normal (particularly in chronic cases), serous, or hemorrhagic (particularly in accessory carpal bone fracture); a modified transudate may be noted (in mild irritation of tendinitis or osteochondroma); or inflammation may be detected (tenosynovitis or septic tenosynovitis).

Treatment

The use of intrasynovial corticosteroids injected into the carpal canal provides only temporary relief from signs of lameness[8] and should be used only after radiographs and ultrasound have ruled out fracture or tendinitis or desmitis. Local corticosteroids are probably most beneficial for acute injuries that have an active inflammatory component and have a chance to recede to normal sheath dimensions.

In cases in which an acute fracture of the accessory carpal bone has been sustained, the use of internal fixation may preclude the development of the carpal canal syndrome.[5] Most accessory carpal bone fractures will heal successfully without internal fixation, but some sheath distension usually remains if the fracture initially caused effusion. Not all accessory carpal bone fractures cause carpal sheath effusion, but accessory carpal bone fractures that go untreated may develop carpal canal syndrome and result in chronic lameness. Because the pain is caused primarily from compression of soft tissue structures within the canal, removal of that pressure by sectioning the carpal flexor retinaculum can provide relief.

Osteochondromas located at the distal radius can be handled by surgical excision of the osteochondroma or resection of the carpal flexor retinaculum. Surgical excision is preferable and can be performed via endoscopic visualization of the sheath[3,9–11] or an incision made laterally between the ulnaris lateralis and the lateral digital extensor muscle (see "Osteochondroma Formation at the Distal Radius").[6] However, for smaller osteochondromas in which the carpal flexor retinaculum has become thickened owing to chronic irritation, resection of a portion of the carpal flexor retinaculum provides relief from pain.

Resection of the Carpal Flexor Retinaculum

For resection of the carpal flexor retinaculum, the horse is placed in lateral recumbency with the affected limb down. A 15-cm skin incision is made 5 cm caudal and parallel to the medial palmar vein over the palmaromedial aspect of the carpus (Fig. 8.276). The carpal flexor retinaculum is approached in the same plane and a 1-cm-wide elliptic piece of the tissue is removed between the medial and lateral palmar veins. Care must be taken to preserve the deeply buried palmar vein and artery. The length of the elliptic excision should be a little greater than the zone of thickening but rarely includes the entire longitudinal extent of the carpal flexor retinaculum.[7]

In most cases, the synovial sheath does not have to be entered. The subcutaneous tissues and the skin are apposed in a routine manner using a simple interrupted suture. A pressure bandage is applied and maintained for 3 weeks; sutures are removed in about 2 weeks. These horses should be confined for 6 weeks, after which light exercise can begin. Rest periods of up to 6 to 8 months may be required if the carpal canal syndrome has been associated with fracture of the accessory carpal bone. Typically, all of these horses exhibit an immediate relief from pain with a free range of nonpainful carpal flexion shortly after surgery is performed.

Prognosis

The prognosis for horses affected with carpal canal syndrome that have been treated by resecting the flexor carpal retinaculum appears to be good. A small percentage of horses that exhibit this syndrome as a result of osteochondroma formation at the distal radius may require both surgical excision of the osteochondroma as well as resection of the flexor carpal retinaculum. These cases also have a good prognosis.

References

1. Brokken TD. Acute carpal canal injury in the Thoroughbred. Am Assoc Equine Pract 1989;34:389.
2. Cauvin ER, Munroe GA, Boswell J, et al. Gross and ultrasonographic anatomy of the carpal flexor tendon sheath in horses. Vet Rec 1997;141:489.
3. Cauvin ER, Munroe GA, Boyd JS. Endoscopic examination of the carpal flexor tendon sheath in horses. Equine Vet J 1997;29:459.
4. Dyson SJ, Dik KJ. Miscellaneous conditions of tendons, tendon sheaths, and ligaments. Vet Clin North Am Equine Pract 1995;11:315.
5. Easley JE, Schneider JE. Evaluation of a surgery for repair of equine accessory carpal bone fracture. J Am Vet Med Assoc 1981;178:219.
6. Held JP, Patton CS, Shires M. Solitary osteochondroma of the radius in three horses. J Am Vet Med Assoc 1988;193:563.
7. Nixon AJ. Carpal canal syndrome. In: White NA, Moore JN, Eds. Current Practice of Equine Surgery. 2nd ed. Philadelphia: Lippincott Williams & Wilkins, 1996;461–464.
8. Radue P. Carpal tunnel syndrome due to fracture of the accessory carpal bone. Equine Pract 1981;3:8.
9. Southwood LL, Stashak TS, Fehr JE, et al. Lateral approach for endoscopic removal of solitary osteochondromas from the distal radial metaphysis in three horses. J Am Vet Med Assoc 1997;210:1166.
10. Southwood LL, Stashak TS, Kainer RA. Tenoscopic anatomy of the equine carpal flexor synovial sheath. Vet Surg 1998;27:150.
11. Squire KRE, Adams SB, Widmer WR, et al. Arthroscopic removal of a palmar radial osteochondroma causing carpal canal syndrome in a horse. J Am Vet Med Assoc 1992;201:1216.
12. Stashak TS. Carpal canal syndrome. In: Stashak TS, Ed. Adams' Lameness in Horses. 4th ed. Philadelphia: Lea & Febiger, 1987;569.

FRACTURES OF THE ACCESSORY CARPAL BONE

Fractures of the accessory carpal bone are most commonly seen in Thoroughbreds, cross-country steeplechase horses, and hunter/jumpers. Although these fractures can occur in many different planes within the accessory carpal bone, they most commonly are seen in a vertical (frontal) plane through the lateral groove formed by the long tendon of the ulnaris lateralis muscle (Fig. 8.277). The pull of the flexor muscles results in a constant distraction, and the instability with movement results in a fibrocartilaginous non-union.[2,5] This non-union may be painless and most horses will be sound with conservative treatment.[2–4,8] In some, however, a

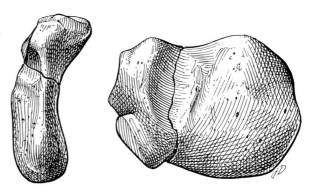

Figure 8.277 Common location for fracture of the accessory carpal bone. (Courtesy of T. S. Stashak.)

moderate to severe protracted lameness is present, which may be complicated by the carpal canal (tunnel) syndrome.[5,6,11]

Causes

The mode of trauma that induces accessory carpal bone fracture is unclear. External direct trauma from a kick or high interference is a reasonable assumption; however, most cases do not show signs of exterior trauma on the skin or hair. The possibility that an asynchronous contraction of the flexor carpi ulnaris and ulnaris lateralis muscles can cause this fracture has been proposed.[14] Also, the bowstring effect of the flexor carpi ulnaris, ulnaris lateralis, and flexor tendons, which is created when the horse lands on a partially flexed forelimb, has been incriminated.[6] The fracture may occur as a result of the bone being caught between the third metacarpal bone and the radius in a nutcracker fashion. To support this, contact lesions on the caudal aspect of the radius have been identified.[13]

Signs

Signs of lameness are usually acute. The horse may not put full weight on the limb soon after the injury; and if extensive swelling is not present, crepitation may be found in the early stages. Soon after the fracture, however, the ends are separated so that it is almost impossible to produce crepitation. The most prominent signs of the lameness are distension of the carpal sheath (Fig. 8.276) and marked pain with rapid flexion of the carpus. Weight bearing may be minimally affected, although the horse may choose to stand with the carpus slightly flexed.

Pain on carpal flexion can be severe enough to cause the horse to rear. The pain results from the fracture of the accessory carpal bone as well as the increased pressure applied to the structures within the carpal canal. Palpation of the accessory carpal bone with the limb partially flexed to reduce the tension of the ulnaris lateralis and flexor carpi ulnaris allows the examiner to perceive an abnormal lateral medial movement of the accessory carpal bone. In chronic cases, the pain resulting in lameness may be emanating entirely from carpal canal syndrome (discussed earlier in this chapter). A diagnostic feature of that syndrome is a reduced pulse pressure felt in the digital arteries with flexion of the carpus and a painful response with rapid flexion of the carpus. If the examiner suspects carpal canal syndrome, he or she can perform intrasynovial anesthesia of the carpal sheath. In most cases, a 5-mL injection of local anesthetic solution will bring about a marked improvement in lameness. Perineural anesthesia of the ulnar nerve has not been effective in blocking out these lamenesses in the limited number of cases reported.[11]

Diagnosis

Whenever the carpal sheath is distended and pain on flexion is evident, radiographs should be taken. The fracture is seen on the lateral radiograph (Fig. 8.278).

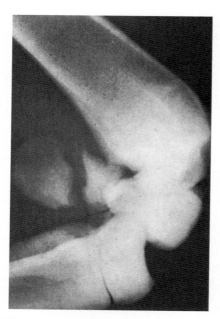

Figure 8.278 Fracture of the accessory carpal bone. Note the separation of the fragments caused by the pull of the carpal flexor tendons. (Courtesy of T. S. Stashak.)

Treatment

There are several forms of treatment that may be considered when dealing with a fracture of the accessory carpal bone. Conservative treatment consists of confining the horse to a box stall for 3 to 6 months. Eventually, a fibrocartilaginous non-union forms.[5] Horses have returned to mild, moderate, and full work with this approach.[1,2,4,11] However, a certain percentage develop carpal canal syndrome and require surgical resection of a portion of the flexor retinaculum for treatment (discussed earlier in this chapter).[6,10,11]

For the acute vertical (frontal plane) fracture of the accessory carpal bone associated with the lateral grooves of the ulnaris lateralis tendon, internal fixation using the lag screw principle can be performed and may result in bony union and soundness in a shorter recovery period.[5,12] The accessory carpal bone is approached on the palmarolateral surface of the carpus with a curved incision. A special equine C clamp is used as a drill guide.[5] This clamp improves the surgeon's ability to place the straight screws correctly in the narrow discoid-shaped accessory carpal bone. Two 4.5-mm ASIF screws are used for interfragmentary compression of the fracture (Fig. 8.279). Details are available elsewhere.[5] Good results were reported with this method when it was used on experimentally created fractures, and good radiographic healing occurred about 60 days postoperatively.[5]

Other surgical procedures include subtotal resection of the fractured accessory carpal bone (particularly in comminuted fractures)[9] and ulnar neurectomy. The removal of a fractured portion of the accessory carpal bone has been reported to be beneficial for vertical fractures that involve less than half the bone volume. A reasonably rapid return to racing soundness was observed.[13] Interesting features of this procedure are worthy of comment.

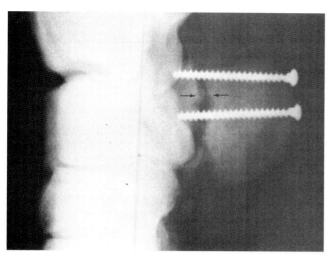

Figure 8.279 Two ASIF bone screws used to repair a fracture of the accessory carpal bone. Arrows point to the separated fracture. (Courtesy of T. S. Stashak.)

First, the carpal flexor retinaculum is incised to remove the bone, which may provide some relief from pain. Also, there may be a long-term deleterious effect on removal of the piece of fractured bone because of the loss of support from the ulnaris lateralis and flexor carpi ulnaris muscles. Carpal hyperextension and carpal arthrosis have been experimentally produced with a similar surgical technique.[7] Thus the procedure is not currently recommended.

Ulnar neurectomy has been suggested for pain relief, which allows the horse with a fractured accessory carpal bone to return to work.[11] Theoretically this neurectomy removes pain emanating from the fracture site alone and has little effect on the chronic synovitis or constriction produced by carpal canal syndrome, if it were to develop. Ulnar nerve blocks do not usually eliminate lameness in horses with accessory carpal bone fracture, so the effectiveness of neurectomy is expected to be only partial.[4] Unfortunately, the frequency of the carpal canal syndrome associated with fracture of the accessory carpal bone has not been defined, but it is consistent enough that this technique may not be of much value when used alone.

In comminuted fractures or fractures with an articular fragment at the articulation with the antebrachiocarpal joint, arthroscopic surgery or arthrotomy into the palmar pouch of the antebrachiocarpal joint can be performed to remove the articular piece. Any remaining fractures can heal conservatively.[4,8,9]

Prognosis

The prognosis for athletic function with accessory carpal bone fracture is good, but if carpal sheath distension accompanies the fracture, the prognosis is more guarded. The incidence of carpal sheath distension accompanying accessory carpal bone fracture is reported to be low.[4] Good success has been noted for experimentally created vertical fractures of the accessory carpal bone repaired acutely, or within 21 days, using interfragmentary compression.[5] The prognosis with conservative treatment is reported as good. In one study, 11 of 11 horses with accessory carpal bone fracture that was treated conservatively with stall rest were sound at the 6-month to 11-year follow-up and 7 were in competitive activity.[2] Reasonably good results can also be expected for the cases in which carpal canal syndrome develops with resection of the carpal flexor retinaculum. Rest alone may suffice in some cases in which the perceived future activity is light to moderate work or breeding status.

References

1. Adams OR. Lameness in Horses. 3rd ed. Philadelphia: Lea & Febiger, 1974.
2. Barr ARS, Sinnott MJA, Denny HR. Fractures of the accessory carpal bone in the horse. Vet Rec 1990;126:432.
3. Carson DM. The osseous repair of a horizontal fracture of the accessory carpal bone in a Thoroughbred racehorse. Equine Vet J 1990;2:173.
4. Dyson SJ. Fractures of the accessory carpal bone. Equine Vet J 1990;2:188.
5. Easley KJ, Schneider JE. Evaluation of a surgical technique for repair of equine accessory carpal bone fractures. J Am Vet Med Assoc 1981;178:219.
6. MacKay-Smith MP, Cushing LS, Leslie JA. Carpal canal syndrome in horses. J Am Vet Med Assoc 1972;160:993.
7. Manning JP, St. Clair LE. Carpal hyperextension and arthrosis in the horse. Am Assoc Equine Pract 1972;18:173.
8. McIlwraith CW. Fractures of the carpus. In: Nixon AJ, Ed. Equine Fracture Repair. Philadelphia: WB Saunders,1996;208–221.
9. Munroe GA, Cauvin E. Surgical treatment of a comminuted articular fracture of the accessory carpal bone in a Thoroughbred horse. Vet Rec 1997;141:47.
10. Nixon AJ. Carpal canal syndrome. In: White NA, Moore JN, Eds. Current Practice of Equine Surgery. 2nd ed. Philadelphia: Lippincott Williams & Wilkins, 1996;461–464.
11. Radue P. Carpal tunnel syndrome due to fracture of the accessory carpal bone. Equine Pract 1981;3:8.
12. Rijenhuizen AB, Nemeth F. Accessory carpal bone fractures in the horse. Vet Q 1994;16(Suppl 2):S101.
13. Roberts JE. Carpal lameness. Proc Br Equine Vet Assoc 1964;18.
14. Rooney JR. Biomechanics of Lameness in Horses. Baltimore: Williams & Wilkins, 1969.

Part VI

THE FOREARM (ANTEBRACHIUM)

Ted S. Stashak

OSTEOCHONDROMA FORMATION AT THE DISTAL RADIUS (SUPRACARPAL EXOSTOSES)

Osteochondroma (OC) formation at the distal end of the radius is an uncommon condition causing lameness in the horse.[5-7,11] The growth most commonly occurs in adult horses adjacent to the physis at the caudal distal aspect of the radius.[3,9,10] The cranial aspect of the radius can also (rarely) be involved (Fig. 8.280). Radiographically and histologically these new bone growths appear much like those reported for hereditary multiple exostosis. However, unlike hereditary multiple exostosis the growths appear as singular lesions or affect only a few other long bones. Hereditary multiple exostosis, on the other hand, is reported to affect numerous growing bones (see Chapter 6). Solitary OCs have also been reported in two foals. In one, the distal palmar aspect of the middle phalanx was affected, and in the other, the calcaneus was involved.[1,2]

Causes

Although a single dominant autosomal gene is responsible for the development of multiple exostosis in hu-mans and horses,[8] the genetic implications for isolated OC remains unclear. In humans, solitary OCs are not considered to be inherited.[4] It is postulated that metaplastic cartilage foci develop in the metaphysis and distal diaphysis from abnormal growth of the periosteum. As the cartilage grows it undergoes endochondral ossification similar to that occurring at the physis. When the developing exostosis is continuous with the cortex of the bone and surrounded by a cartilage cap, it is called an osteochondroma (Fig. 8.281).

Signs

Affected horses often present with a history of intermittent lameness that increases with exercise. An obvious swelling of the carpal canal sheath cranial to the ulnaris lateralis is often present (Fig. 8.282). In some cases, the swelling can be extensive (Fig. 8.283). At exercise, a moderate lameness (grade 1 to 2 out of 5) is commonly observed.[9] Palpation of the caudodistal aspect of the radius with the limb held flexed at the carpus sometimes allows the examiner to feel the bony protuberance. Deep palpation of the site is often painful, resulting in limb withdrawal from the pressure. The range of carpal flexion is usually less than normal, and considerable

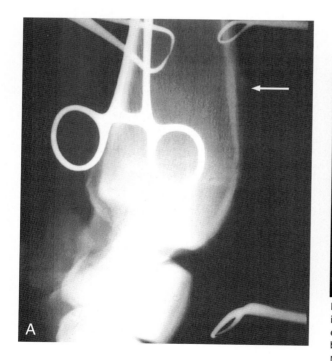

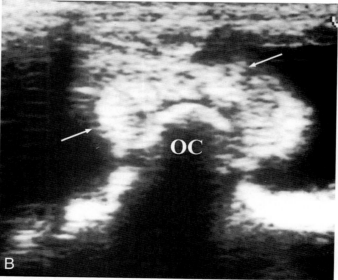

Figure 8.280 A. Lateral intraoperative view of a horse with intermittent lameness of 1-year duration that would increase with exercise, causing the cranial surface of the distal antebrachium to become swollen. Note the OC on the cranial surface of the distal radius (arrow). B. The cross-sectional ultrasound view reveals that the OC projects into the tendon of the extensor carpi radialis muscle (arrows).

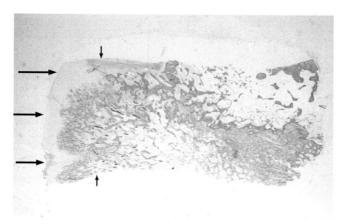

Figure 8.281   Histologic examination reveals a cartilage cap (long arrows) and an underlying bone formation extending to the base of the OC (short arrows).

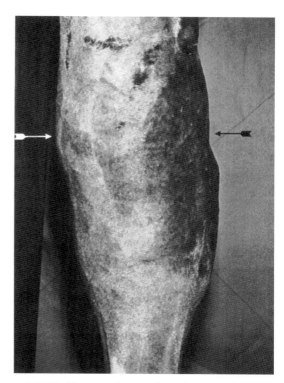

Figure 8.283   The carpal canal distension at the distal caudal radius (arrows) may be extensive with solitary OC.

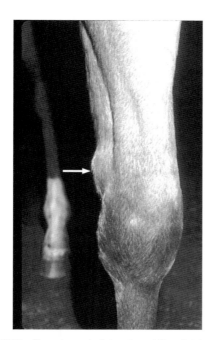

Figure 8.282   Carpal canal distension at the distal caudal radius (arrow) typically seen with OC.

pain is elicited with rapid carpal flexion. A carpal flexion test usually exacerbates the lameness.

Diagnosis

Radiography is necessary to diagnose the condition and its location. In most cases, the OC is located on the caudomedial aspect of the distal radius adjacent to the physis; however, smaller OCs have been observed on the caudolateral aspect of the distal radius as well (Fig. 8.284). Radiographically, these lesions appear as a conically shaped bony protuberance with an outer cortex and inner medullary cavity (Fig. 8.285). The size of the OC and degree of ossification are variable. Ultrasonography can also be used to determine the presence of deep digital flexor tendinitis (Fig. 8.286).[12]

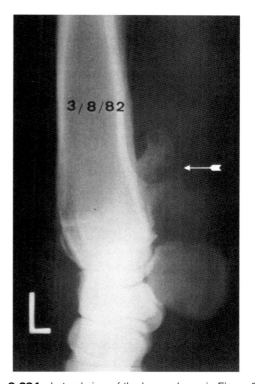

Figure 8.284   Lateral view of the horse shown in Figure 8.283.

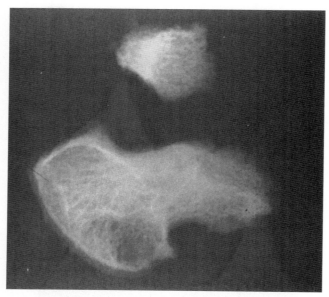

Figure 8.285 Top. Typical appearance of an osteochondroma (magnified). Bottom. Note the distinct outer cartilage cap, the cortical bone, and the medullary cavity.

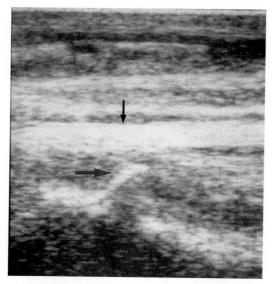

Figure 8.286 On ultrasound, the longitudinal view of the distal caudal radial metaphysis reveals a projection of bone (horizontal arrow) that is putting pressure on the deep digital flexor tendon (vertical arrow).

Treatment

Even though the instillation of corticosteroids into the tendon sheath will temporarily resolve the tenosynovitis, the clinical signs usually reoccur.[12] Presently, surgical excision of the OC is the treatment of choice and is curative in most cases. Although excision of the OCs via an open lateral or medial approach has been described,[3,6,7] an endoscopic technique is currently recommended.[9,10] Both lateral and medial endoscopic approaches have

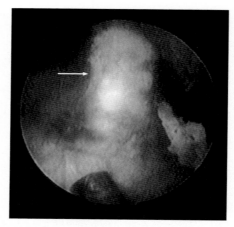

Figure 8.287 Arthroscopic view of an OC (arrow). Note the small osteotome pointing toward the base of the OC.

been described. I prefer the lateral approach because of the lower risk of injury to the medially positioned median artery, vein, and nerve; furthermore, it is technically easier to manipulate the scope and instruments without interference from the opposite limb. A brief description of the lateral endoscopic approach follows.

With the affected limb placed uppermost, the carpal sheath is distended with 20 mL sterile isotonic polyionic fluid. Next, the arthroscope is inserted into the proximal aspect of the carpal canal through a stab incision located 3.5 cm proximal to the distal radial physis between the tendons of the lateral digital extensor and ulnaris lateralis muscles. Once the arthroscope is in the carpal canal, the sheath is distended with fluid and the OC is readily identified (Fig. 8.287).

The exostosis is removed from its attachment to bone at the base with an osteotome placed through a small portal distal to the arthroscopic portal. After the OC is removed, the bone bed is curetted, the sheath is lavaged, and the portals are closed routinely.

Postsurgery, support pressure bandages are applied and maintained for 2 weeks. Stall rest is recommended for 6 weeks, with hand-walking exercise beginning after the 3rd week. In most cases, the carpal canal distension resolves without further treatment; however, sometimes intrasynovial treatment with anti-inflammatory agents are required.

Prognosis

The prognosis for surgical excision of solitary OCs is good for return to performance. In one report, two horses were free of lameness and had no apparent distension of the sheath after 1 and 2 years.[9] In another report, one horse at the 4-month follow-up was free of lameness and had no swelling in the carpal canal.[10] No lameness has been observed in two other cases at the 4- and 12-year follow-up, respectively, and the bone excision sites remained nonreactive radiographically.

References

1. Chan CC-H, Munroe GA, Callanan JJ. Congenital solitary osteochondroma affecting the tarsus in a filly foal. Equine Vet Educ 1996;8:153.

2. Easter JL, Watkins JP, Berridge B, et al. A digital osteochondroma as the cause of lameness in a foal. Vet Compar Orthop Traumatol 1998;11:44.

3. Held HP, Patton CS, Shires M. Solitary osteochondroma of the radius in three horses. J Am Vet Med Assoc 1988;193:563.

4. Jaffe HL. Tumors and Tumorous Conditions of the Bones and Joints. Philadelphia: Lea & Febiger, 1958.

5. Jansson N. Osteochondroma at the distal radial metaphysis in a horse. Pferdeheilkunde 1998;14:151–154.

6. Lee HA, Grant BD, Gallina AM. Solitary osteochondroma in a horse: A case report. J Equine Med Surg 1979;3:113.

7. Lundvall RL, Jackson LL. Periosteal new bone formation of the radius as a cause of lameness in two horses. J Am Vet Med Assoc 1976;168:612.

8. Shupe JL, Leone NC, Olson AE, Gardner EJ. Hereditary multiple exostoses: clinicopathologic features of a comparative study in horses and man. Am J Vet Res 1979;40:751.

9. Southwood LL, Stashak TS, Fehr JE, et al. Lateral approach for endoscopic removal of solitary osteochondromas from the distal radial metaphysis in three horses. J Am Vet Med Assoc 1997;210:1166.

10. Squire KRE, Adams SB, Widmer WR, et al. Arthroscopic removal of palmar radial osteochondroma causing carpal canal syndrome in a horse. J Am Vet Med Assoc 1992;201:1216.

11. Stahre L, Tufvesson G. Volar, supracarpal exostoses as causes of lameness in the horse. Nord Vet Med 1967;19:356.

12. Watkins JP. Osteochondroma. In: Auer JA, Stick JA, Eds. Equine Surgery. 2nd ed. Philadelphia: WB Saunders, 1999;840–841.

SPRAIN (DESMITIS) OF THE ACCESSORY LIGAMENT (RADIAL OR SUPERIOR CHECK LIGAMENT) OF THE SUPERFICIAL DIGITAL FLEXOR TENDON

The accessory ligament of the superficial digital flexor tendon (AL-SDFT) is a strong, fibrous band that originates from the distal caudomedial surface of the radius and joins the SDFT at that level.[4] Until recently, sprain to the AL-SDFT was poorly defined, and many conditions associated with the caudal aspect of the radius and carpus were attributed to it, including the following:[4,7]

- Lowering of the angulation of the accessory carpal bone (Fig. 8.288)
- Enthesiophyte formation at the distal caudomedial aspect of the radius (Fig. 8.289)
- Cranial displacement of the proximal end of the radius
- Alterations in the antebrachiocarpal (radiocarpal) joint capsule on its dorsal surface

With the advent of ultrasound, it was possible to define a sprain of the AL-SDFT more clearly.[2,3] The condition occurs most commonly in young adult horses with a high level of physical activity. In one report on 23 horses with abnormal ultrasonographic findings in the AL-SDFT, 11 were racehorses, 9 were sport horses, and the remaining were pleasure or instruction horses.[2]

Causes

Presumably, extreme hyperextension of the fetlock in conjunction with hyperextension of the carpus can cause a sprain of the AL-SDFT.[6,7]

Signs

Affected horses have a history of starting races and workouts quite well but are reluctant to sprint out fully.

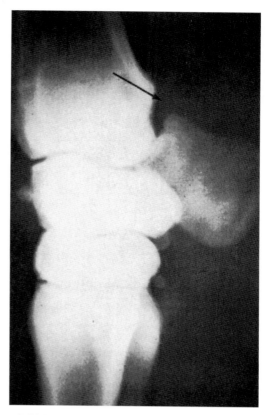

Figure 8.288 A change in the angulation of the accessory carpal bone (arrow) was once thought to be associated with sprain of the AL-SDFT.

Rarely do they attain their previous performance levels.[4,7] A visible swelling of the carpal sheath is observed in some cases. At a walk, affected horses demonstrate a gait impediment characterized by a lateral floating placement of the foot just before it contacts the ground. Furthermore, the toe and heel are placed on the ground at the same time, much like when a horse walks down an incline. In a review of 30 cases, this gait alteration was most commonly observed with radiographic lesions on the caudomedial distal aspect of the radius associated with the origin of the AL (Fig. 8.289).[4] In acute cases, the carpal sheath is frequently distended and is painful to some degree to digital palpation.[4] Simultaneous trauma to the SDFT may also occur, resulting in a painful swelling.[5]

Diagnosis

Radiographs of the caudal aspect of the distal end of the radius are usually negative in acute cases. However, in chronic cases, they may reveal enthesiophytes associated with the attachment of the AL-SDFT (Fig. 8.289). In one study, radiographs were taken of 18 horses with abnormal ultrasonographic findings of the AL-SDFT; only 4 horses had an abnormal profile at the caudal distal aspect of the radius and 14 were considered normal.[3] These findings underscore the value of an ultrasound examination for the diagnosis of desmitis of the AL-SDFT.

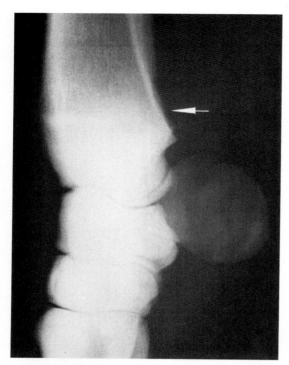

Figure 8.289 Enthesiophyte development at the distal radius (arrow) that was associated with sprain to the attachment of the AL-SDFT.

Ultrasound findings associated with injury of the AL-SDFT include thickening, hypoechoic images, and alteration in fiber pattern alignment.[3] Injury to the AL-SDFT can also be accompanied by abnormal findings involving one or more of the structures in the carpal canal, such as synovial effusion within the carpal sheath, tendinitis of the SDFT, distension and thickening of the retinaculum flexorum, tenosynovitis of the sheath of the tendon of the flexor carpi radialis muscle, and/or injury to the proximal attachment of the suspensory ligament (third interosseous muscle).

Treatment

In acute cases that exhibit carpal sheath distention, needle drainage and injection of a corticosteroid and hyaluronic acid are recommended.[2,3] Stall rest for 4 to 6 weeks is recommended, and hand-walking exercise can begin at 3 weeks. Systemic nonsteroidal anti-inflammatory drugs (NSAIDs) may be indicated for associated problems and are administered as needed. Pressure support wraps are applied and maintained for 2 to 3 weeks. After stall rest, the horse should be confined to a small run for another 6 weeks. A follow-up ultrasound examination should be done at that time to access healing. Generally, affected horses can return to performance in 4 to 6 months.[2]

Prognosis

The prognosis appears to depend on the severity of the injury, the intended use of the horse, and whether the SDFT is involved. In one study, 8 of 13 sport horses were able to return to their previous level of activity, whereas only 7 of 16 racehorses returned to racing at their previous level.[1] In another report, 6 of 8 horses suffering from an injured AL-SDFT without tendinitis returned to their previous level of performance within 4 to 6 months.[2]

References

1. Denoix JM, Guizien I, Perrot P. Injuries of the accessory ligament of the superficial digital flexor tendon (proximal check ligament) in sport and race horses. Pferdeheilkunde 1996;12:613–616.
2. Garner HE, St Clair LE, Hardenbrook HJ. Clinical and radiographic studies of the distal portion of the radius in race horses. J Am Vet Med Assoc 1966;149:1536.
3. Denoix JM, Guiizien I, Perrot P, Bousseau B. Ultrasonographic diagnosis of spontaneous injuries of the accessory ligament of the superficial digital flexor tendon (proximal check ligament) in 23 horses. Am Assoc Equine Pract 1995;41.142–143.
4. Denoix JM, Yousfi S. Spontaneous injury of the accessory ligament of the superficial digital flexor tendon (proximal check ligament): A new ultrasonographic diagnosis. J Equine Vet Sci 1996;16:191–194.
5. Johnson JH, Bartels JE. Conditions of the forelimbs. In: Catcott EJ, Smithcors JF, Eds. Equine Medicine and Surgery. 2nd ed. Wheaton, IL: American Veterinary Publications, 1972;505–562.
6. Lingard DR. Strain of the superior check ligament of the horse. J Am Vet Med Assoc 1996;148:364.
7. Manning JP, St Clair LE. Carpal hyperextension and arthrosis in the horse. Am Assoc Equine Pract 1972;18:173.

ANTEBRACHIAL FLEXOR COMPARTMENT SYNDROME

Antebrachial flexor compartment syndrome (AFCS) is an uncommon cause of lameness in horses. In one report, AFCS was believed to be the cause of progressive lameness in two horses.[7] Compartmental syndrome is a condition in which high pressure develops in a fascial space, resulting in pain caused by compression of neurovascular structures contained within. The syndrome occurs in skeletal muscles enclosed by relatively noncompliant osseofascial boundaries.[2,5] The mechanisms leading to increased intracompartmental pressure include increased fluid content of the compartment, usually from hemorrhage, and decreased compartment size, usually from external compression.[1,5]

Causes

Common causes of compartment syndrome in humans are soft tissue trauma associated with fracture, soft tissue injury alone, arterial injury, prolonged compression from a cast or bandage, and burns.[2,5] Causes for the soft tissue injury associated with AFCS in horses include slipping on ice and falling during exercise.[7]

Signs

A history of severe lameness shortly after the injury that worsens within a few hours is typical. At presentation, affected horses are usually reluctant to bear weight on the injured limb and prefer to stand with the carpus flexed and the toe on the ground. The flexor surface of the antebrachium usually appears diffusely swollen. On palpation, the regional feels firm and warm compared to the opposite limb, and digital pressure usually elicits a painful response. With time, the affected region usually feels firmer and may become cold, presumably indicating a reduction in blood flow.[7] Passive flexion and extension are also usually painful. The pulse pressure in the digital arteries may be normal or reduced on initial examination and may decrease with time. Skin sensation over the affected region and the distal limb may be diminished, but this is often difficult to interpret because of the horse's general unresponsiveness, except to deep pressure and manipulation.[7]

Diagnosis

Although intracompartmental pressures can be measured, the diagnosis of AFCS is usually made from clinical signs alone.[3,4,7] This is supported in human studies in which direct palpation of a tense compartment in the presence of supportive signs strongly indicates compartmental syndrome.[1,2,5,6] Stated another way, the determination of intracompartmental pressure may be unnecessary or may only confirm the clinical diagnosis.[1,6] Radiographs should be taken of the region to rule out a fracture of the radius.

Treatment

Mild cases have been treated successfully with NSAIDs, cold therapy followed by warm therapy, rest, and controlled exercise. Flunixin meglumine (Benamine; 1.1 mg/kg IV) is recommended initially because of its relatively immediate effect. Phenylbutazone (4.4 mg/kg PO) is given as needed. Cold treatment can be effective in reducing inflammation. It is begun as soon as possible and is most beneficial when used within the first 48 hours after injury. There are many approaches to cold therapy, but ice and water in a plastic bag (ice–water slurry) attached to limb with a light wrap appears to be effective in rapidly deep cooling the tissue. Warm therapy can begin after 48 hours and is generally continued for 6 to 10 days, depending on the case. Hand-walking exercise can begin when the lameness has resolved significantly, usually within 4 to 5 days.

Cases that do not respond to conservative treatment are candidates for a fasciotomy over the flexor muscles of the antebrachium.[7] The surgery can be done in the standing sedated horse using local anesthesia or while the horse is under general anesthesia. A 30-cm skin incision is made over the caudolateral aspect of the antebrachium to gain access to the superficial fascia overlying the ulnaris lateralis muscle. Once the fascia is exposed, it is incised for the entire length of the skin incision. The fascia readily separates, and the muscle bulges from the incision. The fascial incision is then extended proximal and distal as needed to accomplish the decompression.

Generally, an increase in the digital arterial pulse pressure is apparent immediately after the fasciotomy is complete. Suture closure of the subcutaneous tissue and skin is routine, and a bandage is placed to apply mild pressure and to protect the wound. A reduction in lameness is obvious immediately on recovery from sedation and/or

anesthesia. Hand-walking exercise can begin the day after surgery and is increased according to the horse's response to treatment.

Prognosis

The prognosis for mild cases of AFCS that are treated conservatively is generally good for return to performance within 6 to 12 weeks. However, I diagnosed a chronic fibrotic myopathy of the flexor muscles of the antebrachium in a horse that had a history consistent with a AFCS. The prognosis for horses requiring surgery also appears good. In one report on two horses with AFCS that were treated with fasciotomy, both horses returned to their intended use.[7]

References

1. Eaton RG, Green WT. Epimysiotomy and fasciotomy in the treatment of Volkmann's ischemic contracture. Orthop Clin North Am 1972;3:175–186.
2. Hargens AR, Akeson WH. Pathophysiology of the compartment syndrome. In: Mubarak SJ, Hargens AR, Eds. Compartment Syndrome and Volkmann's Contracture. Philadelphia: WB Saunders, 1981;47–70.
3. Lindsay WA, McDonnell W, Bignall W. Equine postanesthetic forelimb lameness: Intracompartmental muscle pressure changes and biochemical patterns. Am J Vet Res 1980;41:1919–1924.
4. McDonell WN, Pascoe PJ, Lindsay WA, Burgess LF. Evaluation of the wick catheter as used to measure intracompartmental muscle pressure in equine muscle. Am J Vet Res 1985;46:684–687.
5. Mubarak SJ, Hargens AR. Acute compartment syndromes. Surg Clin North Am 1983;63:539–565.
6. Owen CA. Clinical diagnosis of acute compartment syndromes. In: Mubarak SJ, Hargens AR, Eds. Compartment Syndrome and Volkmann's Contracture. Philadelphia: WB Saunders, 1981;98–105.
7. Sullins KE, Turner AS, Stashak TS. Possible antebrachial flexor compartment syndrome as a cause of lameness in two horses. Equine Vet J 1987;19:147–150.

FRACTURES OF THE RADIUS

Fractures of the radius are relatively common in the horse. In a review of 797 fractures in army horses, fracture of the radius represented 14% of all fractures.[26] In another series of 3000 fracture cases, fracture of the radius ranked fourth in frequency and represented 8% of all the fractures recorded.[11] Fractures of the diaphysis can be transverse, oblique, comminuted, complete or incomplete (including stress fractures), displaced or nondisplaced, or open or closed; they can occur anywhere along the diaphysis of the radius (Fig. 8.290).[1,8–10,22,27,28] Complete fractures can be either displaced or nondisplaced, whereas incomplete and stress fractures are nondisplaced.

Fractures involving the physis occur at the proximal and distal extremity of the radius and are classified using the Salter-Harris classification system (see Chapter 6). In a retrospective study on 47 radius fractures, comminuted fractures were most common (21 cases), followed by oblique fractures (12), transverse fractures (7), and physeal fractures (7).[22]

Complete displaced fractures of the radius are more common than nondisplaced radial fractures[4] and stress fractures. Stress fractures most commonly involve the midshaft of the radius, which is the area of peak stress

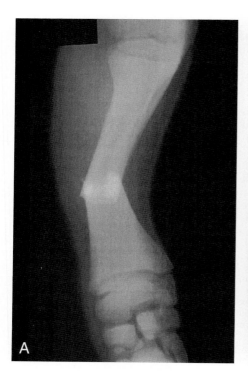
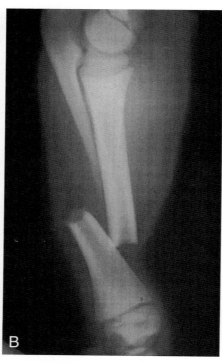

Figure 8.290 A. Cranial-caudal view of a transverse complete midshaft fracture of the radius in a foal. B. Lateral view. Note the overriding of the proximal radius in relation to the distal radius.

concentration of the bone.[6] Open fractures are not common, but they usually penetrate the medial surface of the antebrachium.[9,22,29] Contrary to this, 7 of 12 cases of radial fractures reviewed in one report were open.[1] Either the humeroradial or the antebrachiocarpal (radiocarpal) joint can be involved with oblique longitudinal and physeal fractures of the radius. Smaller articular fractures (excluding osteochondral fragments) involving the proximal and distal articulation of the radius are uncommon (Fig. 8.291).

The type of radial fracture is also related to the horse's age. In one retrospective study 14 of 21 comminuted fractures were in adult horses (older than 2 years), 8 of 12 oblique and all physeal fractures occurred in immature horses (younger than 2 years), and transverse fractures were restricted to foals (younger than 6 months of age).[22] The ulna may also be involved with displaced Salter-Harris type 1 and 2 fractures of the proximal radius (Fig. 8.292).[22]

Causes

Trauma resulting from kicks, entanglements in farm machinery or debris, and accidents involving motorized vehicles are reported to be the most common causes.[9,22,29] In one retrospective study of 48 horses with complete radius fractures, a kick by another horse was the most frequently reported cause.[22] Occasionally, a history of slipping on ice is given as the cause. Nondisplaced fractures of the radius may also occur during normal activity; it is postulated that a single event of overloading the limb is the cause.[4]

Stress fractures are believed to result from cumulative damage to the bone structure and failure of the bone to remodel adequately in response to increased athletic activity. Stress fractures of the radius are most often reported in young (3 to 5 years old) Thoroughbred racehorses in training.[17]

Signs

Complete displaced fractures of the radius are easily identified on physical examination alone. Horses present with a non-weight-bearing lameness, some degrees of swelling in the antebrachium, and instability associated with the fracture site. Crepitation may be felt, and pain may be elicited when the distal limb is manipulated. Wounds or penetration of the skin from the fracture on the distal medial side of the antebrachium is common (Fig. 8.293).

Complete or incomplete nondisplaced fracture of the radius can be more difficult to identify. Horses that present with this injury are usually lame but are willing to bear some weight on the limb. Instability and crepitation are not present. However, there is usually some swelling of the antebrachium, and pressure applied to the region is often painful.[2,4] Wounds at the site of traumatic impact are often noted on the medial distal aspect of the antebrachium.

Stress fractures are difficult to identify on physical signs alone. Horses generally present with a history of an acute onset of lameness that subsides with rest and reoccurs with exercise. Horses are often mildly lame at examination and shoulder flexion may worsen the lameness.[17] These fractures can also occur bilaterally.[17]

Diagnosis

The presence of a displaced radial fracture is confirmed on radiographic examination. Several views are

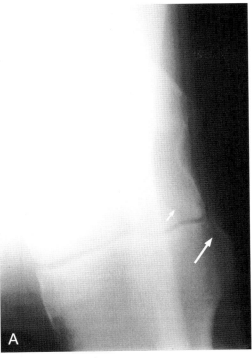
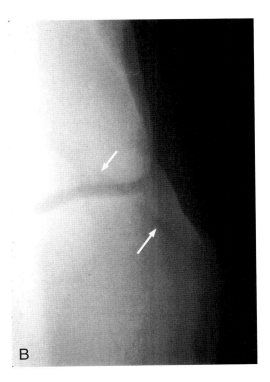
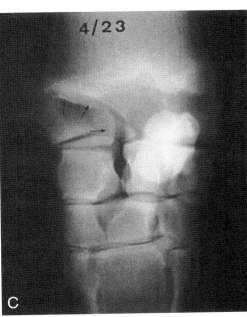

Figure 8.291   A. Cranial-caudal view showing a lateral proximal articular fracture of the radius (arrows). B. Close up of the fracture shown in panel A (arrows). C. An oblique fracture of the distal end of the radius that enters the antebrachiocarpal (radiocarpal) joint (arrows).

needed to evaluate the configuration and extent of the fracture. If surgery is contemplated, at least four views (cranial-caudal, lateral-medial, and both oblique projections) should be taken. These views determine whether surgery can be considered and help in rendering a prognosis.

Acute nondisplaced fractures may be difficult to diagnose initially on radiographic examination. If a nondisplaced fracture is suspected, the horse should be cross-tied in a stall to prevent it from lying down and repeat radiographs should be taken in 2 to 4 days.[2] This time period usually allows recognition of the fracture lines.

Alternatively, nuclear scintigraphy can be used to assist in the diagnosis (Fig. 8.294). Stress fractures are usually best diagnosed by nuclear scintigraphy, although plain radiography can be useful in some cases. A focal increased uptake of the radionuclide in the midshaft of the radius is usually found.[17]

Treatment

First Aid

The first aid management of horses sustaining a complete displaced fracture of the radius has an important

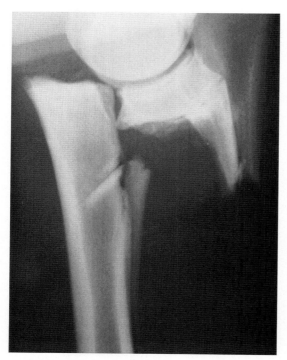

Figure 8.292 A Salter-Harris type 2 fracture of the proximal radius. Note that the ulna is also fractured.

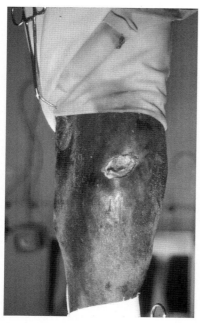

Figure 8.293 A kick wound at the distal medial antebrachium that resulted in a radial fracture.

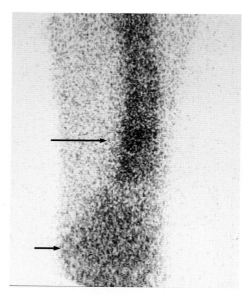

Figure 8.294 Increased uptake of the radionuclide in the radius (upper arrow) seen with a nondisplaced or stress fracture. Lower arrow, accessory carpal bone. (Courtesy of P. Steyn.)

bearing on the outcome. Wounds associated with radial fractures should be treated immediately. Wounds either from a kick or from the fracture penetrating the skin are most common on the medial surface of the antebrachium, and they usually communicate directly with the fracture (Fig. 8.295). Initial wound management in-

cludes hair removal, thorough cleansing and debridement of the wound, application of a topical antiseptic or antimicrobial, wound protection, and the systemic administration of broad-spectrum antimicrobials.

The immediate immobilization of a displaced radial fracture is mandatory. With closed displaced fractures, the application of appropriate external coaptation can prevent the fracture from becoming open. Administer a sedative to horses with unstable fractures before applying a bandage splint. Once the horse is sedated, a heavy layered cotton bandage is firmly applied from the hoof to as far proximal on the antebrachium as possible. Two splints are recommended: One is placed lateral, extending from the ground to the withers, and the other is placed caudal to the limb, extending from the ground to the olecranon process.[7] Nonelastic adhesive tape or one to two rolls of fiberglass cast material is used to affix the splints to the bandage. The portion of the lateral splint that extends proximal to the bandage should contact the brachium when the limb is in a weight-bearing position (Fig. 8.296).[29] The proximal application of the lateral splint provides counterpressure to prevent the limb from abducting with weight bearing. Generally, this approach stabilizes the limb enough to allow the patient to be transported for treatment without running the risk of further injury to the fracture site.

Displaced Fractures

Several treatments have been recommended for displaced fractures, and the rationale for the selection is based on the horse's age, size, weight, value, and temperament as well as the fracture type and configuration and economics. Treatment methods include cast application alone, transfixation pins and cast application, external coaptation with bandage splints, and internal fixation (preferred approach). The use of a cast alone or a cast with transfixation pins is generally considered for open

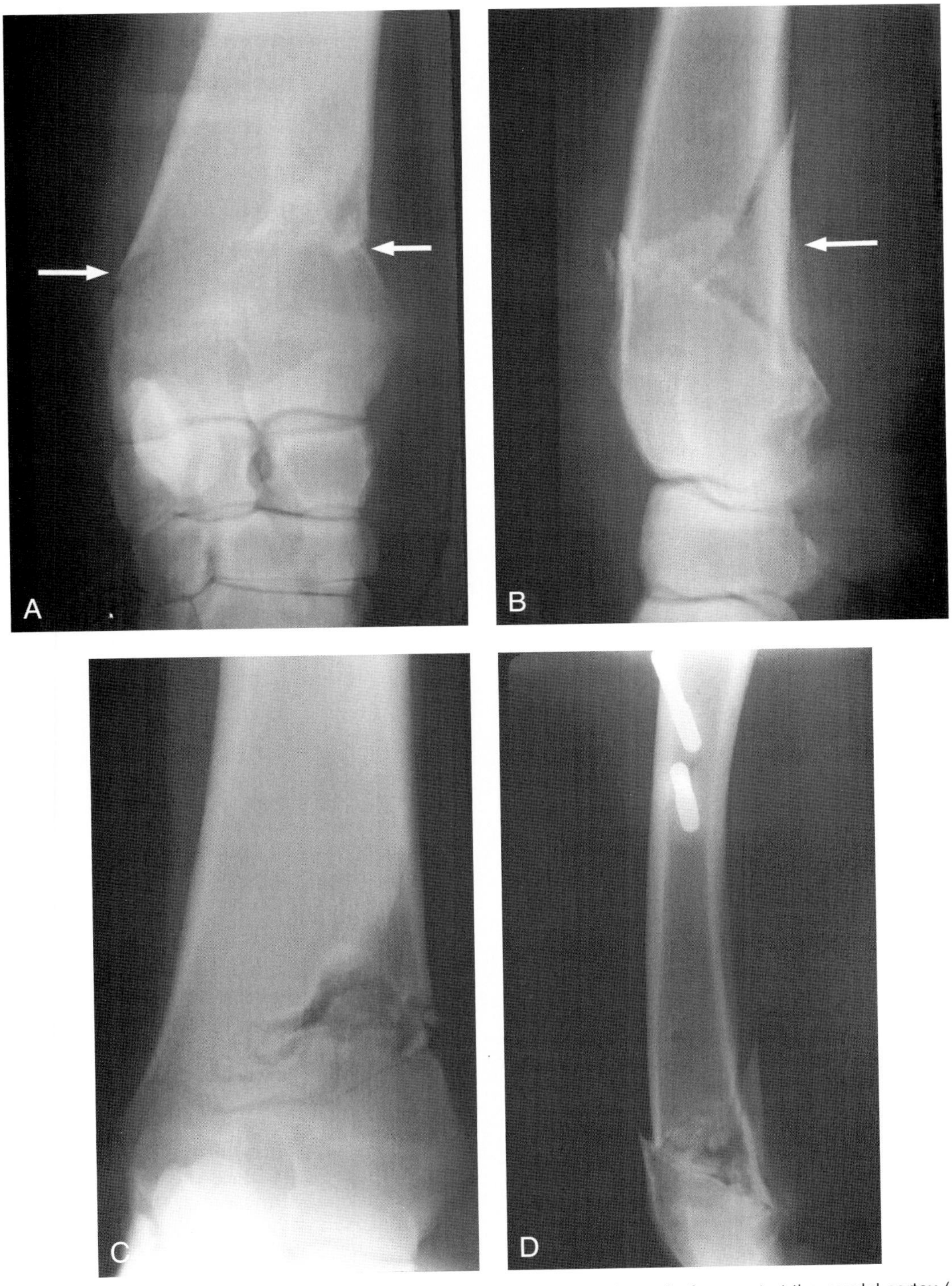

Figure 8.295   A. Cranial-caudal view of the horse shown in Figure 8.293 1 week after injury. Note the comminuted fracture of the distal radius (arrows) and the abnormal angulation of the radius at the fracture site. B. Lateral view illustrating the fracture and a large butterfly fragment at the caudal cortex (arrow). C. The limb was placed under traction to properly align the radius. D. Two transfixation pins were placed in the proximal radius, after which a full-limb cast was applied that incorporated the pins.

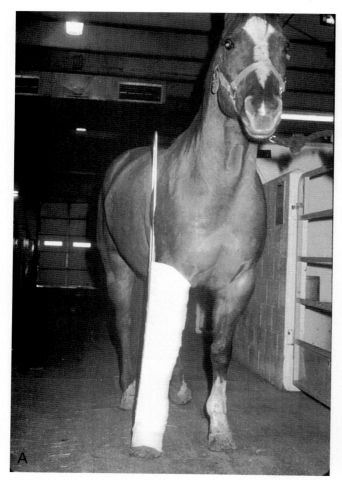

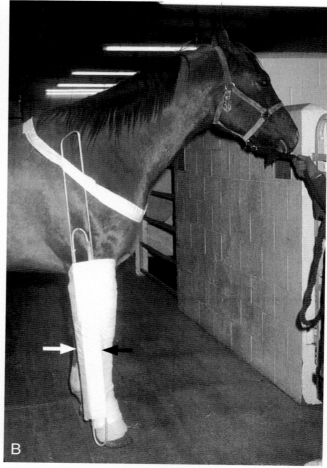

Figure 8.296 One approach to bandaging and splinting a displaced radial fracture. A. Note that the lateral splint extends from the ground to proximal to the shoulder region. The part of the lateral splint that is proximal to the bandage contacts the brachium, preventing the limb from abducting during weight bearing. B. The caudal splint was made from PVC pipe (white arrow). The portion of the lateral splint that extends proximal to the bandage is secured to the body with elastic bandage tape.

contaminated fractures when the chances of successful plate fixation is poor because of the risk of infection or when there are economic constraints.

Bandage splints have been used to treat a few horses with complete fractures of the distal radius. In one report, two horses with complete fractures (one nondisplaced, one displaced) of the distal half of the radius were treated successfully with a modified Robert-Jones bandage with the addition of light strong splints.[21] Healing occurred in 14 to 16 weeks and both horses were able to return to usefulness.

In all cases, the induction of anesthesia and recovery from anesthesia must be well thought out and controlled to protect the fracture site from further trauma. For immature horses, physical restraint alone for the induction and recovery from anesthesia is usually all that is needed. For mature horses, a splint should be in place, as described earlier, before the induction of the anesthesia. Several methods may be used, depending on the physical environment. If an anesthesia-induction stall is available, the horse may be pushed (restrained) with the affected limb against the wall until the horse begins to slump; then it is pulled into lateral recumbency before bearing excessive weight on the affected limb. This technique requires at least two people: one at the withers and the other at the tail. Alternatively, sling induction or table induction of anesthesia can also be used. With the sling, the horse is supported (suspended) until anesthesia is induced, then it is lowered and placed on the operating table or cart and transported to the operating room. If a table induction is used, the horse is first strapped to the table and then anesthesia is induced.

A quiet, controlled recovery from anesthesia is desirable for a successful outcome. For this reason, some surgeons have advocated recovery in a swimming pool or on a tilt table.[14,29] When these approaches are not available, the horse must recover from lateral recumbency to a standing position. Small doses of xylazine (50 to 100 mg) administered intravenously as needed during the recovery period will usually quiet the horse and smooth the recovery.[23] Once the horse is ready to assume a standing position, it will have to be assisted either by two people (one at the tail and one at the head) or by ropes attached to a halter on the head and to the tail and run through rings secured to the wall high in the stall. Both methods help stabilize the horse to avoid misplaced steps on the fractured limb.[23]

The application of a full-limb cast alone for displaced fractures of the radius is not acceptable in most cases because the humeroradial joint cannot be adequately immobilized. If a cast is applied, it frequently results in increased rotational forces on and movement at the fracture site. Also, the more proximal the fracture, the greater the chances that the cast will cause a pendulum (swinging) affect to the distal limb. This leads to more tissue damage and results in a failure of the fracture to heal.[9] That being said, cast application alone has been used to successfully treat some distal radial fractures when there are economic constraints. A combination of a full-limb cast and a Thomas splint has also been recommended for some uncomplicated midshaft radius fractures in young horses.[9,15]

A transfixation pin cast using positive profile, centrally threaded 0.25-inch stainless-steel pins placed transcortically is best suited for fractures in the distal third of the radius (Fig. 8.295D). Two transfixation pins are placed proximal to the fracture to support some of the horse's weight and to stabilize the fracture against torsional forces. Radiographs should be reviewed carefully before surgery to make sure no longitudinal fractures extend proximad or distad. If they do, these fracture planes must be avoided or another means of

treatment should be considered. Generally, the largest diameter (0.25-inch), centrally threaded, positive profile pins are selected. The pin holes should be predrilled with a suitable size drill bit, and the hole should be tapped before pin placement (Fig. 8.160). After the pins are placed, a limited amount of a sterile bandage material is applied over and around the pins, and casting material is applied in the same manner. This technique is of little value for proximal fractures of the radius.

Although open reduction and internal fixation with a bone plate can be used for many radial fractures, it still remains a monumental task in adult horses.[13,29] When using a single, broad, dynamic bone plate in a neonate, place it on the tension side, which is the cranial or craniolateral surface of the bone. Generally, a single-plate application is recommended only in foals less than 250 kg that have a transverse mid-diaphyseal fracture with an intact caudal cortex.[29]

In large foals and adults, two plates are used. One is placed as a tension band on the cranial surface, and the other is placed as a neutralization plate on the lateral or medial surface 90° to the other plate (Fig. 8.297).[19,22,23,29] Although lateral plate placement is technically demanding, it avoids positioning the implant subcutaneously, as is the case for a medial placed plate, and it avoids an open wound that may be present on the medial side of the limb. Plate application may have to be modi-

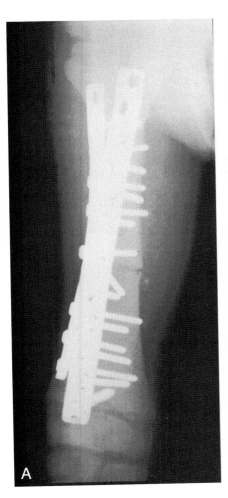
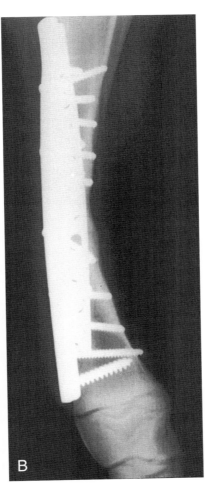

Figure 8.297 Two bone plates were used to treat the radial fracture sustained by the horse shown in Figure 8.290. One plate was placed as a tension band on the cranial surface, and the other was placed as a neutralization plate on the lateral surface. Note that the plates end at a different site on the radius and that the screws do not engage the ulna. A. Cranial-caudal view. B. Lateral view.

fied somewhat, depending on the fracture configuration. When two plates are used, their levels should be staggered, or one plate can be shorter than the other, to avoid stress concentration at one level where the bone plates end in the metaphyses (Fig. 8.297).[23,28] The plates should also span as much of the entire length of bone as possible.

It has been recommended for adult horses that one of the plates be a dynamic condylar plate, with the condylar screw placed in the smaller fracture fragment.[29] Alternatively, one of the bone plates can be a cobra head plate.[16] In foals, the physes are not bridged with a plate and screws unless this is necessary to provide stability of the fracture. Also in foals, the ulna is not engaged with screws on the caudal surface of the proximal radius; if the screws do engage the ulna, the result could be elbow dysplasia and arthritis owing to the differential growth rate of the ulna and radius.[23,25]

Because there may be considerable overriding of the bone fragments, some form of traction is needed to reduce the fracture. Reduction can usually be accomplished using manual traction on the distal limb while manipulating the fragments with a bone-reduction forceps and or bone retractors. Alternatively, traction can be applied while the horse is in dorsal recumbency using a chain around the pastern region attached to hoist. A cerclage-type device may be used in some cases to aid reduction and stabilize the fracture. One study done in ponies with cerclage devices found that the periosteal blood supply to the radius was unaffected by application of cerclage devices.[20] For comminuted fractures, the larger fragments are generally attached to the proximal and distal extent of the radius with lag screws, creating two large fragments that are then reduced.[23] In adults and large foals, 5.5-mm screws are recommended for all holes in the cranial plate, and they are also recommended for the second plate as well. To reduce costs, 5.5-mm and 4.5-mm screws can be alternated in the second plate for large foals. However, when this is done 5.5-mm screws should be used in the holes close to the fracture and at the end of the plate(s).[29]

Plate luting with antimicrobial-impregnated polymethyl methacrylate (PMMA) is recommended for all fractures of the radius, except in young foals.[24,29] In addition, cancellous bone grafts are recommended to reduce the time required for fracture healing. Grafts are generally not done in foals, because their fractures heal so rapidly.

After surgery a large cotton full-limb bandage is applied in most cases. A sleeve cast that extends to the most proximal extent of the antebrachium to the distal metacarpal region can be used for recovery from anesthesia in some cases; after recovery, the cast can be removed. Once the fracture is healed, a decision to remove the implants is made. Generally, plates are removed in all horses that are used as athletes. Plate removal is also necessary when the fixation is infected, to resolve the infection. Removal of the plates should be staged to minimize weakening of the bone owing to the stress-concentrating affect of empty screw holes.[23] Once the plate is removed, the horse should be rested in a box stall with controlled exercise until advanced bone remodeling is apparent. At least 60 days should pass before the second

plate is removed,[23] after which the horse is again rested in a box stall until healing is evident.

Nondisplaced Fractures

Horses with incomplete and nondisplaced complete fractures of the radius are candidates for conservative management.[4,18] Although some of the fractures may progress to become unstable, most heal without becoming displaced.[29] Treatment includes stall confinement, NSAIDs, and rest for prolonged periods. Stall confinement is done until substantial evidence of fracture healing is noted, which may take as long as 3 to 4 months. If the horse will tolerate it, it is initially either tied or attached to a wire that is placed high in the stall to prevent it from lying down (Fig. 8.298). This reduces the likelihood of fracture displacement from excessive forces at the fracture site while the horse attempts to get up or lay down. Low doses of phenylbutazone are used to encourage limited weight bearing on the affected limb and reduce inflammation. During the final 30 days of stall confinement, controlled hand-walking exercise is begun and gradually increased as the horse can tolerate it. Once lameness is resolved, the horse can have access to a small paddock for an additional 30 days before it is returned to intended use.

Physeal Fractures

Salter-Harris type 1 and 2 fractures of the proximal physis may be accompanied by fracture of the ulna, and sometimes the radial nerve is traumatized (Fig. 8.292). Although single-plate fixation of the ulnar fracture, with screws engaging both cortices of the radius, has been used successfully in a limited number of cases (Fig. 8.299), some clinicians recommend adding a second narrow dynamic compression plate (DCP), placed laterally with the proximal screw in the epiphysis.[29]

In small foals, transphyseal screws and wire fixation can be used in place of the lateral plate.[29] Although humeroradial joint subluxation resulting from the fixation is

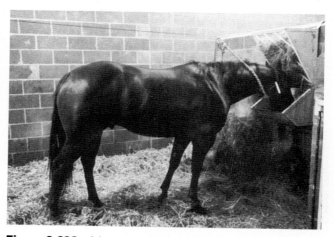

Figure 8.298 A horse being run on an overhead wire. The lead rope should be tied short enough to prevent the horse from lying down but loose enough to allow free movement along the wire's length.

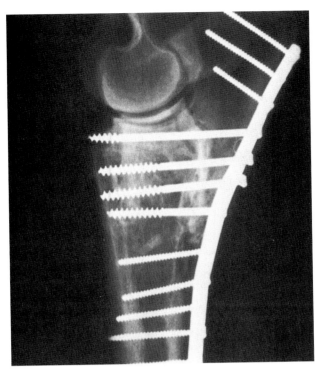

Figure 8.299 A single plate used to repair the Salter-Harris type 2 fracture shown in Figure 8.292.

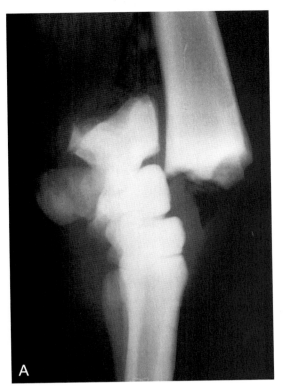

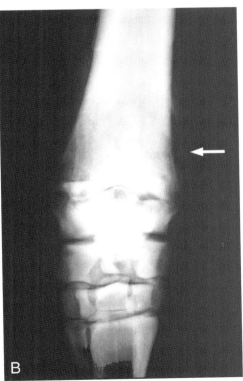

Figure 8.300 A. Lateral view of a completely displaced Salter-Harris type 2 fracture of the distal radius. Because of economic constraints, this fracture was treated with cast application alone. B. Cranial-caudal view taken at the 3-week cast change. Note the callus formation (arrow).

possible, growth from the radial physeal region is generally minimal owing to injury to the germinal cells in the growth plate. Because there is limited growth in the proximal radial physis, the ulna does not tend to displace in relationship to the radius.[29]

Nondisplaced 3 Salter-Harris type fractures are usually treated successfully with rest followed by controlled excercise.[22] However, if the fracture is displaced, recommended treatment consists of anatomic reconstruction of the joint surface with screws placed in a lag fashion in combination with tension band wiring.[12,29]

Salter-Harris type 1 fractures of the distal physis can result in medial displacement of the physis.[29] When the fracture occurs in a neonate, it is generally best treated by transphyseal bridging with or without a T-plate. Alternatively, small Steinmann pins placed transphyseal in a cruciate fashion can be used. When the fracture is healed, the implants are removed. Salter-Harris type 2 fractures of the distal physis that occur in an older horse can result in considerable displacement (Fig. 8.300A). Treatment includes cast application alone (Fig 8.300B), transphyseal application of two Steinmann pins placed in a cruciate pattern, and plate fixation using two plates with the distal screws placed in the epiphysis.

Other Fractures

Fractures involving the proximal and distal articulations of the radius are uncommon (Fig. 8.291, A and C). Displaced fractures can be treated with interfragmentary screw fixation with either cortical or cancellous screws (Fig. 8.301).[31] This ensures a rigid internal fixation and reduces the chances of the horse developing osteoarthri-

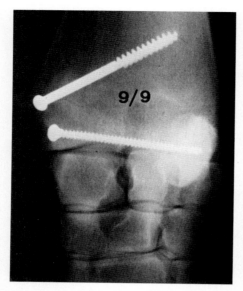

Figure 8.301 At the 4.5-month follow-up, good healing is noted for a fracture repaired with two bone screws by the principle of interfragmentary compression.

tis. Nondisplaced fractures can be treated conservatively with rest and controlled exercise. However, there is a risk of developing a subchondral bone cyst, particularly when the proximal epiphysis is involved.[30]

Prognosis

The prognosis for displaced radial fractures depends on the age and weight of the horse, its temperament, and the fracture type. In one report of 47 cases of radial fractures, successful treatment (82%) occurred only in horses less than 2 years of age.[22] Although there are a few reports of successful treatment with internal fixation of displaced radial fractures in mature horses,[3–5,10,24] generally adults that sustain displaced fractures have an unfavorable prognosis for survival no matter what treatment is selected.[9,22,29] In one report documenting the outcome in adult horses weighing more than 300 kg and presenting with radial fracture, 9 of 15 were treated with internal fixation and only 2 horses were discharged from the hospital to resume their former activities.[3] In another report, internal fixation was attempted in 6 adult horses and none survived.[22] Reasons for nonsurvival included primary implant failure, infection causing implant failure, and support limb laminitis. Comminuted fractures were associated with the highest incidence of fatal complications.

Displaced closed simple fractures of the radius in foals have a favorable prognosis. Physeal and transverse middiaphyseal fractures have an excellent prognosis. In one report two foals with Salter-Harris type 1 and 2 proximal physeal fractures and six (of seven) foals with middiaphyseal transverse fractures were treated successfully.[22] Treatment of proximal oblique fractures in three of four foals also had an excellent outcome.

Nondisplaced complete and incomplete fractures appear to have a good prognosis with conservative treatment. In three reports on four horses with nondisplaced open radial fractures, two horses resumed full work and the other two horses were able to return to light work.[1,4,8] In another report on two mature horses with complete radial fractures (one nondisplaced, one displaced) involving the distal radius, both horses responded favorably to bandage splinting and both returned to work.[21] Although no report on the outcome of stress fractures of the radius could be found, it is reasonable to expect a good outcome if the diagnosis is made, the horse is rested properly, and healing is assessed by nuclear medicine before the horse returns to work.

References

1. Alexander JT, Rooney RJ. The biomechanics, surgery and prognosis of equine fractures. Am Assoc Equine Pract 1973;18:219.
2. Auer JA. Fractures of the radius. In: Nixon AJ, Ed. Equine Fracture Repair. Philadelphia: WB Saunders, 1996;222–230.
3. Auer JA, Watkins JP. Treatment of radial fractures in adult horses: An analysis of 15 clinical cases. Equine Vet J 1987;19:103–110.
4. Barr ARS, Denny JR. Three cases of non-displaced radial fracture in horses. Vet Rec 1989;125:35–37.
5. Baxter GM, Moore JN, Budsberg SC. Repair of an open radial fracture in an adult horse. J Am Vet Med Assoc 1991;199:364–367.
6. Biewener AA, Thomason J, Goodship A, et al. Bone stress in the horse forelimb during locomotion at different gaits: A comparison of two experimental methods. J Biomechanics 1983;16:568–676.
7. Bramlage LR. Current concepts of emergency first aid treatment and transportation of equine fracture patients. Comp Cont Educ Vet Pract 1983;5S:564.
8. Dingwall JS, Duncan DB, Horney FD. Compression plating in large animal orthopedics. J Am Vet Med Assoc 1971;158:1651.
9. Fessler JF, Amstutz HE. Fracture repair. In: Oehme FW, Prier JE, Eds. Textbook of Large Animal Surgery. Baltimore: Williams & Wilkins, 1974;309.
10. Frauenfelder HC, Fessler JF. Proximal radius fracture in a horse: angle blade plate repair. Vet Surg 1981;10:96.
11. Frohner E. General Surgery. 3rd ed. Ithaca, NY: Taylor & Carpenter, 1906.
12. Gaines JD, Auer JA. Treatment of a Salter-Harris type III epiphyseal fracture in a young horse. Comp Cont Educ Vet Pract 1983;5:S102–S106.
13. Gertson KE, Brinker WO. Fracture repair in ponies using bone plates. J Am Vet Med Assoc 1969;154:900.
14. Hutchins DR, McClintock SA, Brownlow MA. Equine flotation tank design and technique. Equine Vet J 1986;18:65–67.
15. Kendrick JW. Treatment of tibial and radial fractures in large animals. Cornell Vet 1951;41:219.
16. Kirker-Head CA, Fackleman GE. Use of the cobra head bone plate for distal long bone fractures in large animals. A report of four cases. Vet Surg 1989;18:227–234.
17. Mackey VS, Trout DR, Meagher DM, Hornof WJ. Stress fractures of the humerus, radius, and tibia in horses. Clinical features and radiographic and/or scintigraphic appearance. Vet Radiol 1987;28:26–31.
18. Martin BB, Reef VB. Conservative treatment of a minimally displaced fracture of the radius of a horse. J Am Vet Med Assoc 1987;191:847–848.
19. Milne DW, Turner AS. An Atlas of Surgical Approaches to the Bones of the Horse. Philadelphia: WB Saunders, 1979;98.
20. Nyrop KA, DeBowes RM, Ferguson HR, Leipold HW et al. Vascular response to the equine radius to cerclage devices. Vet Surg 1990;19:249–253.
21. Pallaoro D. Successful treatment of complete radial fractures in aged horses using external coaptation: Two cases. Equine Pract 1998;20:16–18.

22. Sanders-Shamis M, Bramlage LR, Gable AA. Radius fractures in the horse: A retrospective study of 47 cases. Equine Vet J 1986; 18:432–437.
23. Schneider RK. Fractures of the radius. In: White NA, Moore JN, Eds. Current Practice of Equine Surgery. Philadelphia: JB Lippincott, 1990:646–652.
24. Schneider RK, Andrea R, Barnes HG. Use of antibiotic-impregnated polymethyl methacrylate for treatment of an open radial fracture in a horse. J Am Vet Med Assoc 1995;207:1454–1457.
25. Stover SM, Rick MC. Ulnar subluxation following repair of a fractured radius in a foal. Vet Surg 1985;14:27–31.
26. Trum BF. Fractures. Vet Bull Suppl Army Med Bull 1939;33:118.
27. Turner AS. Further experience with the use of dynamic compression plate in equine long bone fractures. Aust Vet J 1979;9:42.
28. Turner AS. Long bone fractures. In: 6th Surgical Forum. American College of Veterinary Surgery, Chicago, 1978.
29. Watkins JP. The radius and ulna. In: Auer JA, Stick JA, Eds. Equine Surgery. 2nd ed. Philadelphia: WB Saunders, 1999:836–841.
30. Yovich JV, Stashak TS. Subchondral osseous cyst formation after an intra-articular fracture in a filly. Equine Vet J 1989;21:72–74.
31. Zamos DT, Hunt RJ, Allen D. Repair of fractures of the distal aspect of the radius in two horses. Vet Surg 1994;23:172–176.

Part VII

THE ELBOW

Ted S. Stashak

FRACTURES OF THE ULNA

The ulna is one of the most commonly fractured long bones in the horse.[5,6,8,9,22,27,28] In one report, fractures of the ulna accounted for 5.2% of all equine fractures seen over a 30-year period.[14] Although horses of any age, size, and breed can be affected, younger horses appear to be at greater risk.[8,9,22,28] In a retrospective study of 43 horses with ulnar fractures, 79% occurred in horses younger than 2 years of age.[28] The fracture can be articular or nonarticular, simple or comminuted, open or closed, and distracted or nondistracted.[8] Ulnar fractures are classed as types 1 to 6 (Fig. 8.302).

Type 1 and 2 fractures follow the Salter-Harris classification and involve the growth plate (physis of the olecranon tuberosity) in immature horses, usually less than 12 months of age.[8] Type 1 involves the physis with separation and may include appreciable distraction of the bony epiphysis (Salter-Harris type 1) (Figs. 8.302 and 8.303). Foals less than 3 months old are predisposed to this type of fracture.[22] Type 2 fractures extend through the caudal half to two-thirds of the physis and course distad to enter the humeroradial joint adjacent to the anconeal process (Salter-Harris type 2) (Figs. 8.302 and 8.304).[4,5,8,9,19] This type of fracture occurs most commonly in weanlings and yearlings.[22] Closure of the proximal ulnar physis is not radiographically complete until 27 months; however, growth is markedly slowed between 15 and 18 months of age.[12,13,26] As the growth plate disappears, there is a reduced incidence of type 1 and 2 fractures and an increase in fractures that involve the diaphysis.

Type 3 to 6 fractures involve the diaphysis of the olecranon. The fracture can be simple or comminuted, articular or nonarticular, complete or incomplete, open or closed, and distracted or nondistracted (Figs. 8.302 and 8.305 to 8.307).[8] Most fractures in adults are articular, complete, and moderately displaced (distracted).[7–9,18,28] Fracture distraction occurs from tension produced by the triceps muscle. The degree of distraction depends on the extent and level of the fracture in the ulna. Generally, fractures distal to the level of the radiohumeral articulation (type 6) tend to be minimally displaced owing to the radioulnar interosseus ligament attachments. Fracture separation tends to be greater on the caudal cortex of the ulna because the cranial intraarticular portion of the fracture is better secured by the humeroulnar ligaments and joint capsule (Fig. 8.308).[22] Rarely, adult horses can develop radiohumeral luxation in combination with an ulnar fracture, or fracture of both the ulna and the radius.[2,7,9,16]

Causes

Type 1 and 2 fractures in juveniles may result from direct-impact trauma or from tensile overload of the triceps apparatus from sudden falls, bucking, and galloping to keep up with the mare. In adults, direct trauma to the elbow is generally the cause, and a kick by another horse is most common. Other causes include falls, penetrating wounds, and missteps made by a horse running at speed.[1,5,14,23,25]

Signs

Horses generally present with a history of being acutely non-weight-bearing lame. If the fracture is displaced (distracted) from the pull of the triceps muscle, the horse stands with the elbow dropped (dropped elbow) and the carpus flexed and is unable to weight bear on the affected limb (Fig. 8.309). In contrast, horses with nondisplaced (nondistracted) fractures may initially appear to have non-weight-bearing lameness with a dropped elbow appearance, only to have the lameness subside rapidly, allowing the horse to become progressively more weight bearing on the affected limb (Fig. 8.310). The initial non weight bearing and dropped elbow are presumably the result of pain.

Visually, the affected elbow region is swollen on the caudal surface (Fig. 8.310). The extent of the swelling and lameness generally indicate the magnitude of the injury and the complexity of the fracture. Heat, pain with pressure, and—most important—swelling are noted on

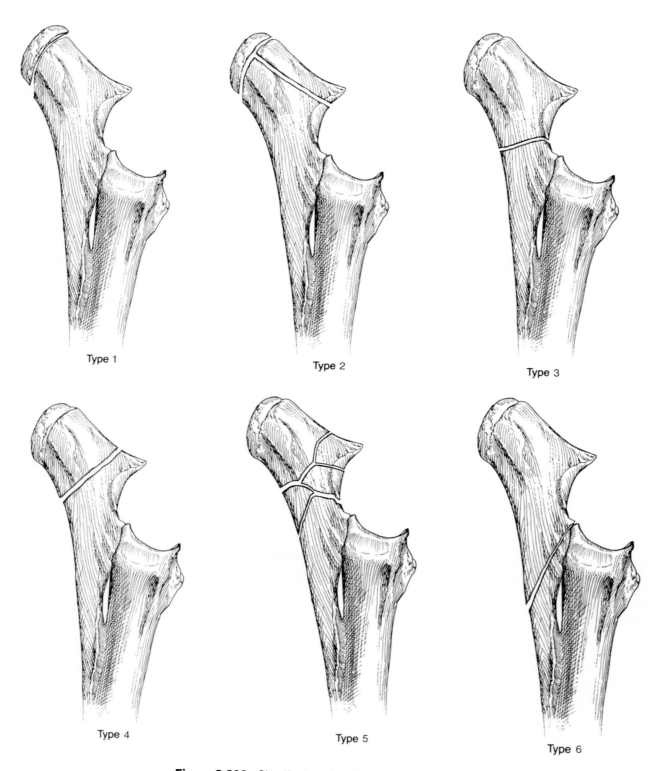

Type 1

Type 2

Type 3

Type 4

Type 5

Type 6

Figure 8.302 Classification of equine ulnar fractures.

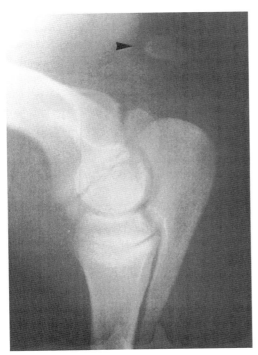

Figure 8.303   A displaced Salter-Harris type 1 fracture of the olecranon process. Note the separated epiphysis (arrow).

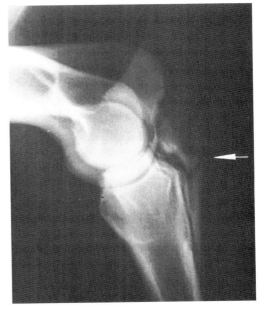

Figure 8.305   A transverse fracture of the olecranon that enters the elbow joint (arrow).

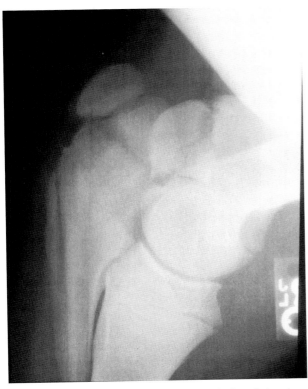

Figure 8.304   Lateral view of a minimally displaced chronic Salter-Harris type 2 fracture of the olecranon process.

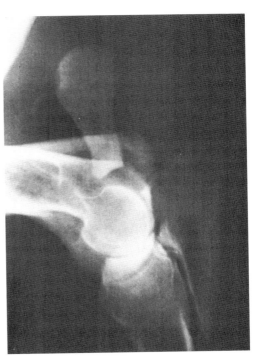

Figure 8.306   An articular fracture at the proximal end of the olecranon tuberosity.

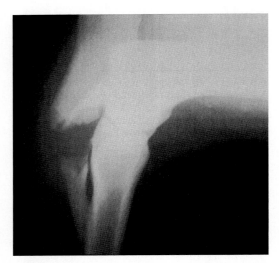

Figure 8.307   Lateral view of a nonarticular fracture of the ulna distal to the elbow joint.

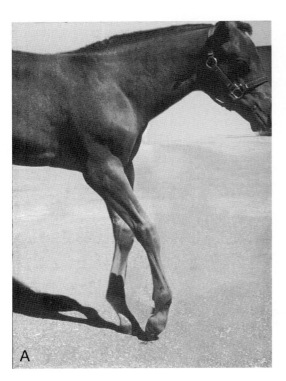

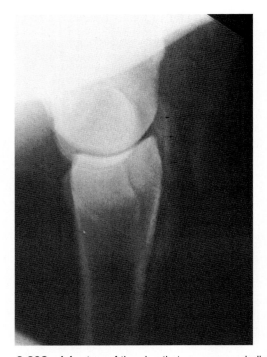

Figure 8.308   A fracture of the ulna that courses caudodistad from the elbow joint (arrows).

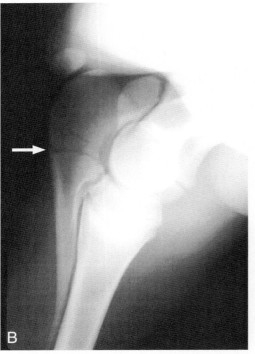

Figure 8.309   A. The dropped elbow appearance. B. Lateral view of the foal shown in panel A, revealing a comminuted minimally displaced type 3 fracture of the ulna.

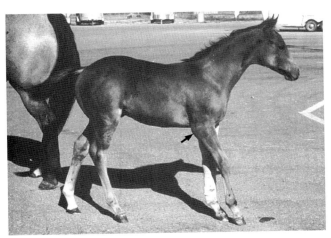

Figure 8.310 Shortly after injury, this foal was non-weight-bearing lame with a dropped elbow appearance. Just 2 days later, it was able to bear some weight on the affected right forelimb. Note the swelling in the elbow region (arrow). The diagnosis was a nondisplaced fracture of the ulna.

palpation. For nondisplaced fractures of several weeks' duration, the most localizing sign may be swelling of the elbow region (Fig. 8.311). Limb manipulation, however, usually remains painful. When the swelling is marked, fracture of the ulna must be differentiated from fracture of the distal humerus, fracture of the proximal radius, and sepsis of the elbow joint.[22] Because many olecranon fractures are caused by a kick, wounds over the fracture site are common.

Diagnosis

Diagnosis is based on appearance of the affected limb, palpation and manipulation, and radiographic examination. Although most fractures of the olecranon process can be diagnosed from the lateral view, both mediolateral and craniocaudal radiographs should be taken to identify the fracture configuration. This is important because the specific fracture configuration often dictates the repair technique to be used. In young foals, a flexed (stressed) lateral radiographic view may be needed to identify a Salter-Harris type 1 fracture of the olecranon process.[23] In some of these cases, it may also help to radiograph the opposite elbow to confirm the diagnosis and document the degree of displacement (Fig. 8.312). Since concomitant injury to radius with ulnar fractures is common in young horses, particular attention should be paid to the proximal radial physis, which may also be fractured.[23]

Treatment

Selection of treatment depends on the age of the horse and the characteristics of the fracture (classification, location, distracted or nondistracted).[3,5,20,22,25] Generally, only nondistracted or minimally distracted nonarticular (types 1 and 4) ulnar fractures (Figs. 8.307 and 8.312) and fractures involving the distal semilunar notch (type

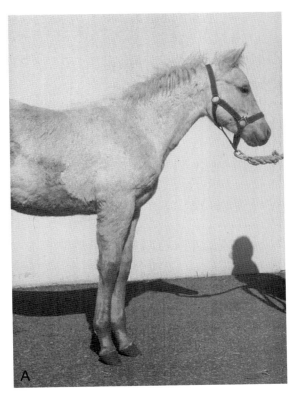
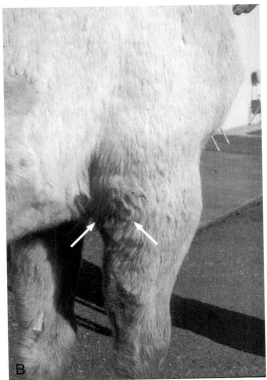

Figure 8.311 A. Although shortly after injury to the right forelimb this foal was non-weight-bearing lame, 3 weeks later it can bear weight comfortably, although the heel of the hoof is slightly higher on the right limb. B. Caudolateral view of the right forelimb reveals an obvious swelling of the caudal elbow region (arrows). Figure 8.304 for a radiographic study.

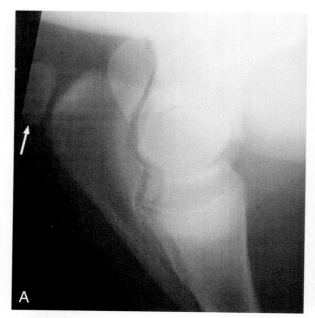

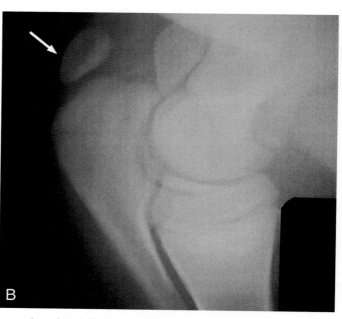

Figure 8.312 A. Lateral view of the right elbow region in a foal with non-weight-bearing lameness caused by a kick. Note the position of the epiphysis (arrow) in the unaffected limb. B. Lateral view of the left elbow region. Note the displacement (craniad and proximad) of the epiphysis (arrow).

6) of the elbow joint should be treated conservatively.[5,28] Conservative treatment usually includes bandaging and securing a splint to the caudal aspect of the limb for some time and absolute stall rest for 6 to 8 weeks (Fig. 8.313). Occasionally, for a nondisplaced or minimally displaced comminuted articular fracture that is not amenable to internal fixation or when there are economic constraints, a young horse may respond favorably to conservative treatment (Fig. 8.314). The application of a bandage with a polyvinyl chloride (PVC) pipe splint secured to the caudal aspect of the limb helps prevent further distraction of the fracture, allows the horse to bear weight on the affected limb, and generally makes the horse more comfortable. The affected limb should be radiographed periodically to check for further separation or displacement of the fracture fragments. If the fracture becomes displaced, internal fixation should be considered.

Complications associated with conservative management include contralateral forelimb angular deformity in young horses, flexure deformity of the affected limb when bandaging and splinting are not used, degenerative joint disease (DJD) of the affected elbow joint, and nonunion owing to distraction of the fracture fragments.[27,28]

Horses that have sustained comminuted, articular, or distracted fractures of the ulna and olecranon process respond best to internal fixation. In adults and large immature horses (older than 6 months), bone plate application using the tension band principle is usually best. Foals and weanlings (younger than 6 months) may be treated with a combination of screws/pins and wires, tension band wires alone, or an Arbeitsgemeinschaft fur Osteosynthesefragen/Association for the Study of Internal Fixation (AO/ASIF) hook plate.[1,4–6,10,20,21,23,24,27] Bone plates are applied to the caudal aspect of the olecranon process and ulna to counteract tension of the triceps

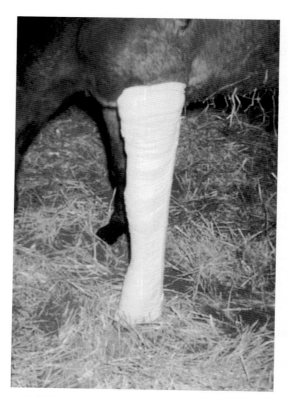

Figure 8.313 Bandaging and a PVC pipe splint applied to the caudal forelimb from the proximal antebrachium to the level of the heel bulbs.

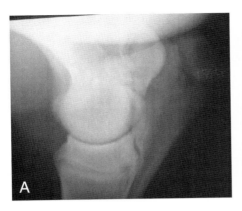
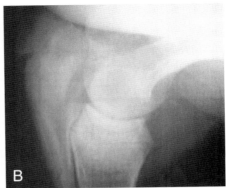
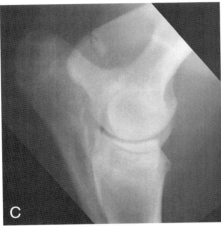

Figure 8.314 A. Lateral view identifying a comminuted, minimally displaced type 2 fracture in a horse that had sustained trauma 5 days earlier, which resulted in a non-weight-bearing lameness. The horse was treated with a bandage splint, stall rest, and low-dose nonsteroidal anti-inflammatory drugs. B. Lateral view taken at the 6-week follow-up. Note the evidence of a callus formation. C. Lateral view taken at the 1-year follow-up revealing complete healing of the fracture. No lameness was observed.

brachii muscle. The plate can be contoured to fit over the top of the olecranon tuber for proximal olecranon fractures (Fig. 8.315).[5]

For horses younger than 6 months of age, a hook plate can be used.[21] Bone screws should engage the olecranon proximal to the fracture and, in mature horses, the radius distal to the fracture. A study comparing three methods (dynamic compression plate, pins and wires, and a prototype grip system) of ulnar fixation on cadaver limbs found that the dynamic compression plate (DCP) was superior to the other methods.[13] In fact, the DCP method was twice as strong as the pins and wire technique, and the grip technique was deemed unacceptable.

The surgical approach to the ulna has been well described.[19,23,27] The horse is placed in lateral recumbency with the affected limb uppermost. A linear incision is made along the caudolateral surface of the antebrachium, with a craniolateral deviation of the incision at the proximal limits to avoid incising the skin caudally directly over the point of the elbow. The caudal aspect of the ulna is approached between the muscle bellies of the ulnaris lateralis and the ulnar head of the deep digital flexor muscles. The division between these muscles is more distinct distally and can then be extended proximally. The plane of dissection is extended to allow exposure of the fracture, and the periosteum is divided along the caudal ulna to allow precise bone plate contact.

The bone plate is contoured to fit the caudal aspect of the ulna. A narrow ASIF DCP is suitable for most horses (Fig. 8.316). If the plate has to be applied proxi-

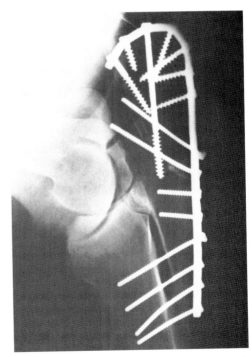

Figure 8.315 A bone plate was contoured to fit over the top of the olecranon tuberosity in the horse shown in Figure 8.306. Although good alignment of the fracture was achieved, a gap remains.

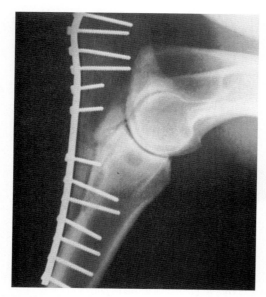

Figure 8.316 Repair of a transverse fracture of the olecranon with an ASIF bone plate. (Courtesy of A. S. Turner.)

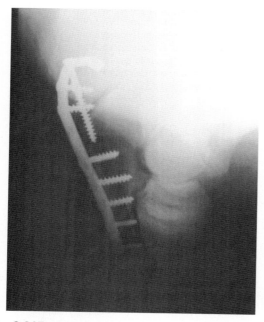

Figure 8.317 A bone plate was bent at its proximal limits to cover the top of the fractured olecranon process in a foal with a type 2 fracture. Note the screws do not penetrate the caudal cortex of the radius.

mal on the olecranon process, it may help to chisel off the caudal eminence of the process or distal fragment with an osteotome to make a flatter surface on which the bone plate can be seated.[27] If the fracture is sufficiently proximal to warrant contouring the plate over the proximal aspect of the olecranon tuber, the fibers of the triceps attachment are carefully separated on the midline with minimal abaxial reflection (Fig. 8.317). If a hook plate is used, the hook is directed through a longitudinally

oriented stab incision made in the tendon of the triceps muscle over the proximal fragment. In most cases, a narrow DCP is used; a broad DCP is reserved for large adults that are heavier than 500 kg.[22] For adults, 5.5-mm cortical screws are preferred over 4.5-mm screws.[29] In immature animals, 4.5-mm screws and occasionally 6.5-mm cancellous screws are used to provide better fixation in the soft bone of the olecranon. In adults, at least three screws proximal and four screws distal to the fracture provide ideal fixation.[22]

Fracture reduction is usually accomplished without difficulty. Interfragmental compression may be used through the plate for oblique fractures. Compression for other fractures can be applied with the initial two screws in the DCP or by a tension device applied to the distal aspect of the plate, unless the fracture is highly comminuted. Highly comminuted fractures are likely to collapse with compression and should be plated using a neutralization technique and single lag screws placed in other planes.[22] Good anatomic reduction of the fracture and anconeal process provide the best end result. The anconeal process should articulate as perfectly as possible with the humeral condyles; if it does not, a poor result can be expected.[11] In a limited number of cases, the anconeal process was removed to improve the prognosis, but the long-term effects of this are unknown.[11,22]

Screws placed below the humeroradial joint in horses younger than 2 years old engage the caudal cortex of the radius but do not have to penetrate the cranial cortex. In young horses (less than 18 months), screws should not penetrate the caudal radial cortex if possible, as continued growth of the proximal radius may lead to an abnormal development (subluxation) of the elbow joint and DJD (Fig. 8.316). Studies indicate that, although growth of the proximal radial physis is slowing at 12 months of age, it does not cease until after 18 months.[26] In fact, on average the equine radius grows another 8 mm after the animal is 12 months of age. Therefore, if screws engage the radius, the implant must be removed in many yearlings.

Comminuted fractures are reconstructed to reestablish the congruency of the articular surface and triceps function. Additional lag screws, placed lateral and medial, and (rarely) another bone plate may be required to reduce and stabilize the fracture fragments adequately.[22]

Distracted type 1 or 2 physeal fractures of the olecranon tuberosity pose a special surgical problem because they do not respond well to conservative treatment and can be difficult to treat surgically.[4,5,20] Attempts at conservative treatment have resulted in contralateral (opposite limb) angular limb deformity before weight bearing occurs in the affected limb. Internal fixation that relies on bone plates and screws has provided variable results in foals less than 3 months of age, owing to the small size of the proximal fragment.[4,20] However, a bone plate bent to cover the proximal aspect of the olecranon tuberosity was used successfully to repair these types of fractures in 5- to 8-month-old horses (Fig. 8.316B).[11,23,24] In one report, bilateral comminuted type 2 fractures were treated successfully using the bent plate technique.[25] Hook plates have also been used with a high degree of success in foals ranging from 2 weeks to 6 months of age.[21]

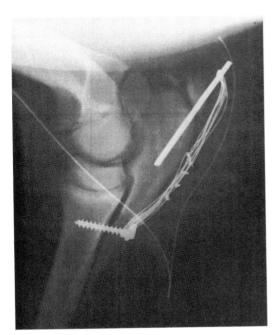

Figure 8.318 A figure-eight wire was used to create a tension band for fracture repair.

Bone screws or pins used in combination with figure-eight tension band wiring have also been used successfully.[4,17,20,23] The tension band wires are applied to the caudal surface of the olecranon and are twisted around the caudal screw head or pin proximally and fixed to the ulna distal to the fracture (Fig. 8.318). ASIF washers may be placed under the screw heads to increase the surface area of contact. This technique decreases the possibility of the apophysis of the olecranon being pulled off or split through by the pin or screw head. The surgical approach for the screw or pin tension band fixation technique is the same as previously described, and the tendon of the triceps muscle must be split longitudinally for insertion of the screws. This technique does not appear to arrest the growth of the olecranon tuberosity.[20] If bone plate application is selected, part of the long head of the triceps muscle is carefully elevated off the olecranon tuber to allow the bent plate to be placed.

Although transphyseal screw placement and screw placement only in the apophysis through the proximal bent plate have both been used, my preference, when applicable, is to place the screw(s) in the apophysis only. If the hook plate is used, the hook is directed through a stab incision made in the tendon of the triceps muscle and no dissection is needed. At the time of this writing, the use of the hook plate is the preferred approach.

Open fractures require additional care. Besides the administration of broad-spectrum antimicrobials, staged excisional wound debridement using a separate set of instruments and copious wound lavage are used before fracture repair. Lavage of the elbow joint is necessary when the fracture is intraarticular. The staged wound preparation can be done before the final preparation for surgery. If osteomyelitis becomes established, it can be difficult to resolve. However, fracture healing generally progresses, provided stabilization of the fracture is main-

tained for 8 to 10 weeks.[22] Antimicrobials are continued long term to control the infection while the fracture is healing. After healing of the fracture, the implants are removed if drainage persists. Generally, fixation failure owing to implant loosening occurs slowly with infected ulna repairs, and the results are not as devastating as sepsis in other long-bone fracture repairs.[22]

Closure is routine, and negative-pressure suction drains placed next to the plate are often employed to reduce postoperative seroma formation. A stent bandage can be applied over the surgery site to protect it. A ring of adhesive elastic bandage tape can also be sutured to the skin proximal to the elbow to provide a semipermanent attachment for a full-limb bandage. Bandaging reduces distal limb edema and swelling at the surgery site.

Recovery from anesthesia should be supervised, and manual assistance should be provided for most horses. The use of deep mats is also advised. Premature attempts to stand and inadvertent struggling are controlled by the administration of xylazine or detomidine. In most cases, horses respond remarkably well to internal fixation and frequently bear weight when returning to their stalls postoperatively. Further improvement in weight bearing is usually observed over a 7- to 10-day period. However, stall confinement is recommended until radiographic evidence of complete healing has occurred. The vacuum drain is usually removed in 12 to 48 hours. Return to full exercise typically requires 4 to 6 months.

Prognosis

The prognosis is good for nonsurgical treatment of nondisplaced, nonarticular type 1 and 4 fractures of the ulna. Nondisplaced articular fractures that are treated conservatively have a relatively good prognosis. One study evaluating the outcome of nonsurgical management of ulna fractures found that type 6 distal semilunar notch fractures responded best to conservative treatment, and 70% of patients became sound.[28]

The prognosis for displaced type 3 to 6 fractures appears good when internal fixation is used. Reports describe 68 to 76% success for management of equine ulna fractures, when narrow or broad 4.5-mm DCPs, Venable plates, or semitubular plates are applied using the tension band principle.[7,15]

The prognosis for displaced type 1 and 2 physeal fractures is based on the foal's age, the time between the injury and the repair, and the type of internal fixation selected.[20,21] Generally, foals less than 3 months are more difficult to repair with internal fixation because their bones lack the strength to hold the implants; thus implant failure may be seen. The use of the hook plate, however, has improved the outcome of these cases. One study followed 10 foals aged 2 weeks to 6 months that received a hook plate for repair of an ulna fracture. Of these foals, 7 went on to be used as athletes.[21] Another study examined 22 horses (median patient age = 4 months) in which pins and tension band wiring were used. Successful fracture healing was obtained in 18 horses (82%), and 13 were athletically sound.[17]

It has been reported that if the time interval between injury and repair is more than 5 days, problems with reduction may be encountered.[20] Horses younger than

7 months of age in which the plate screws bridge the ulna and radius should be radiographed every 4 weeks after a repair.[22] Although the inclusion of the radius in the fixation is considered undesirable, occasionally the repair requires it. If radiography identifies early humeroulnar incongruity in these horses, the bridging implant should be removed. Early removal of the implant allows most such incongruities to resolve. If the fracture is not completely healed, selective removal of the bridging screws, leaving only the screws that do not engage the radius, should be considered. Alternatively, the bridging screws can be replaced with shorter screws that do not engage the radius.[22]

References

1. Alexander JT, Rooney JR. The biomechanics, surgery and prognosis of equine fractures. Am Assoc Equine Pract 1973,18:219.
2. Arnbjerg J. Fracture of ulna in the horse: With case reports on three ponies. Nord Vet Med 1969;21:389–397.
3. Brown MP, MacCallum FJ. Anconeal process of the ulna: Separate center of ossification in the horse. Br Vet J 1974;130:434.
4. Brown MP, Norrie RD. Surgical repair of olecranon fractures in young horses. J Equine Med Surg 1978;2:545.
5. Colahan PT, Meagher DM. Repair of comminuted fracture of the proximal ulna and olecranon in young horses using tension band plating. Vet Surg 1979;8:105.
6. Denny HR. The surgical treatment of fractures of the olecranon in the horse. Equine Vet J 1976;8:20.
7. Denny HR, Barr A, Waterman A. Surgical treatment of fractures of the olecranon in the horse: A comparative review of the 25 cases. Equine Vet J 1987;19:319–325.
8. Donecker J, Bramlage L, Gabel A. Retrospective analysis of 29 fractures of the olecranon process of the equine ulna. J Am Vet Med Assoc 1984;185:183–189.
9. Easley K, Schneider J, Guffy M, Boero M. Equine ulnar fractures: A review of the twenty-five clinical cases. J Equine Vet Sci 1983; 3:5–12.
10. Fackleman GE, Nunamaker DM. Manual of Internal Fixation in the Horse. New York: Springer-Verlag, 1982;67.
11. Fessler JF, Amstutz HE. Fracture repair. In: Oehme FW, Prier JE, Eds. Textbook of Large Animal Surgery. Baltimore: Williams & Wilkins, 1974;312.
12. Getty R. Equine osteology. In: Getty R, Ed. Sisson and Grossman's The Anatomy of the Domestic Animals. 5th ed. Philadelphia: WB Saunders, 1975;255–348.
13. Hanson PD, Hartwig H, Markel MD. Comparison of three methods of ulnar fixation in horses. Vet Surg 1997;26:165–171.
14. Hertsch B, Abdin-Bey MR. Ulna fractures in horses: Retrospective analysis of 66 cases. Pferdeheilkunde 1993;9:327–339.
15. Honnas CM. Surgical treatment of selected musculoskeletal disorders of the forelimb: Ulnar fractures. In: Auer JA, Ed. Equine Surgery. Philadelphia: WB Saunders, 1992;1039–1042.
16. Levine S, Meagher D. Repair of an ulnar fracture with radial luxation. Vet Surg 1980;9:58–60.
17. Martin F, Richardson DW, Nunamaker DM, et al. Use of tension band wires in horses with fractures of the ulna: 22 cases (1980–1992). J Am Vet Med Assoc 1995;207:1085–1089.
18. McGill D, Hilbert B, Jacobs K. Internal fixation of fractures of the ulna in the horse. Aust Vet J 1982;58:101–104.
19. Milne DW, Turner AS. An Atlas of Surgical Approaches to the Bones of the Horse. Philadelphia: WB Saunders, 1979;912.
20. Monin T. Repair of physeal fractures of the tuber olecranon in the horse, using a tension band method. J Am Vet Med Assoc 1978; 172:282.
21. Murray RC, DeBowes RM, Gaughan EM, Bramlage LR. Application of a hook plate for management of equine ulnar fractures. Vet Surg 1996;25:207–212.
22. Nixon AJ. Fractures of the ulna. In: Nixon AJ, Ed. Equine Fracture Repair. Philadelphia: WB Saunders, 1996;231–241.
23. Richardson DW. Ulnar fractures. In: White HA, Moore JN, Eds. Current Practice of Equine Surgery. Philadelphia: JB Lippincott, 1990;641–646.
24. Scott EA. Tension-band fixation of equine ulnar fractures using semitubular plates. Am Assoc Equine Pract 1976;21:167.
25. Scott EA, Mattoon JS, Adams JG, et al. Surgical repair of bilateral comminuted articular ulnar fractures in a seven-month-old horse. Clinical case conference. J Am Vet Med Assoc 1998;212: 1380–1383.
26. Smith B, Auer J, Taylor T, et al. Use of orthopedic markers for quantitative determination of proximal radial and ulnar growth in foals. Am J Vet Res 1991;52:1456–1460.
27. Turner AS. Fractures of specific bones. In: Mansmann RA, McAllister EA, Eds. Equine Medicine and Surgery. 3rd ed. Santa Barbara, CA: American Veterinary, 1982;1003.
28. Wilson D, Riedesel E. Nonsurgical management of ulnar fractures in the horse. A retrospective study of 43 cases. Vet Surg 1985;14: 283–286.
29. Yovich JV, Turner AS, Smith FW. Holding power of orthopedic screws in equine third metacarpal and metatarsal bones. Part 1. Foal bone. Vet Surg 1985;14:221–229.

LUXATION AND SUBLUXATION OF THE HUMERORADIAL (ELBOW) JOINT

Although not common, subluxation and luxation of the humeroradial (elbow) joint does occur.[1–7] The elbow medial collateral ligament is most commonly involved with subluxations.[1,6] The ligament can be either partially torn or completely ruptured (Fig. 8.319). When a luxation occurs, both medial and lateral collateral ligaments are usually involved; and in most cases, they rupture (Fig. 8.320). Elbow joint luxations are also commonly associ-

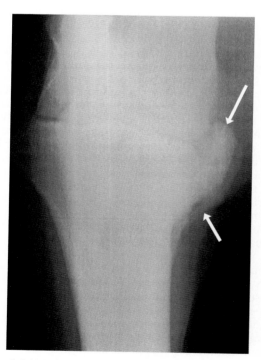

Figure 8.319 Cranial-caudal view of an injury to the elbow region that was sustained 3 months earlier. Note the extensive enthesiophyte associated with the medial collateral ligament (arrows). The elbow joint has narrowed on the medial side, and there are osteophytes at the lateral joint margin. (Courtesy of B. Graham.)

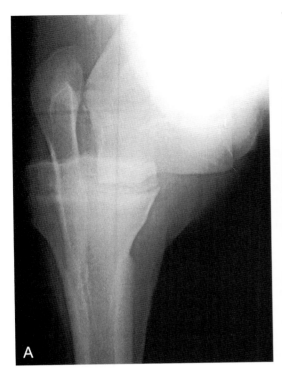
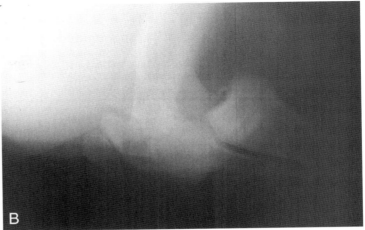
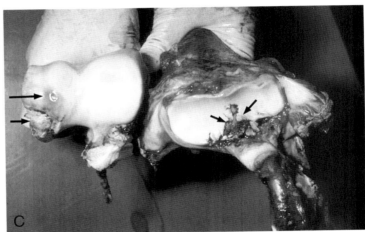

Figure 8.320   A. Cranial-caudal view of a complete luxation of the elbow. B. Lateral view of the same horse. C. Note the extensive articular cartilage damage involving the lateral condyle of the distal humerus (right arrows) and the proximal radius (left arrows). Both collateral ligaments had ruptured.

ated with a concomitant fracture of the proximal radius, a separation of the radius and ulna, and/or a fracture of the olecranon.[1-7] Occasionally, an elbow joint luxation occurs and the radius and ulna are intact.[2]

Causes

Severe limb abduction, as would occur when a foot is caught fast (e.g., under a fence) is reported as a common cause of subluxation.[1,6] In addition, elbow subluxation may occur after injury during a polo match. Luxations usually result from a fall.[2]

Signs

Subluxation of the elbow joint results in swelling in the axilla and an initial non-weight-bearing lameness. Digital pressure on the medial side of the elbow region and limb manipulation, particularly abduction, usually elicits a painful response. Limb abduction may also reveal an instability or looseness of the joint on the medial side.[1] As time passes, the swelling and localizing signs associated with the elbow region become less obvious in horses that sustain partial rupture of the medial collateral ligament. In these cases, swelling usually can be palpated on the medial side of the joint; synovial distension

or capsular thickening can be palpated laterally; and lameness remains prominent, ranging from grade 2 to grade 3 (out of 5). Upper limb flexion usually remains painful, and a flexion test often exacerbates the lameness.

Luxation of the elbow joint results in extensive swelling and pain on manipulation of the elbow region. Horses are generally unable to extend the limb to bear weight.[2] A dropped elbow appearance (the elbow of the affected limb being held lower than the contralateral elbow) may be noted.

Diagnosis

Although the clinical signs generally localize the problem to the elbow region, the definitive diagnosis is made on radiographic examination (Figs. 8.319 and 8.320). Chronic cases of subluxation may exhibit evidence of arthritis, and enthesiophytes may develop in the injured medial collateral ligament.

Treatment

Conservative management—consisting of stall rest for 9 to 12 weeks, the administration of nonsteroidal anti-inflammatory drugs (NSAIDs), and controlled exercise—has been used successfully for the treatment of some elbow joint subluxations.[1] Generally, horses that sustain a partial tear in the medial collateral ligament are expected to respond the best. However, some of these horses may go on to develop elbow joint arthritis, presumably because of joint instability (Fig. 8.319). Horses that develop arthritis after joint subluxation may benefit from intraarticular injections of an anti-inflammatory agent. It has also been suggested that a sling may be indicated for horses that completely rupture the medial collateral ligament, if their temperaments are suitable.[1] Although attempts to stabilize the elbow joint surgically in such cases appears logical, I could not find any reports in the literature describing a surgery for this condition.

Elbow joint luxation on the other hand generally requires surgery to achieve a pasture-sound horse.[2] In one horse, in which both collateral ligaments were ruptured, screws were placed laterally and medially in the epicondyles of the distal humerus and laterally and medially in the proximal tuberosities of the proximal radius close to the attachment of the collateral ligaments.[2] A prosthetic collateral ligament was then formed by placing 18-gauge wire in a figure-eight pattern around the exposed screw heads. Elbow luxations associated with fractures and/or separation of the ulna from the radius require more extensive application of orthopedic implants.

Prognosis

The prognosis for subluxation of the elbow appears to be guarded to unfavorable to return to performance, depending on the degree of injury to the medial collateral ligament.[1,6] Generally, a partial tear injury is expected to have a better prognosis, and some of these horses may be able to return to light work.

The prognosis for return to performance after complete luxation of the elbow joint is poor; however, pasture soundness may be achieved in some cases after surgical intervention. One horse that sustained elbow luxation with medial and lateral collateral ligament rupture and no associated fractures of the radius or ulna was treated surgically; it was pasture sound 14 months after surgery.[2]

References

1. Adams OR. Lameness in horses. 3rd ed. Philadelphia: Lea &Febiger, 1974.
2. Crawley GR, Grant B. Repair of elbow joint luxation without concomitant fracture in a horse. Equine Pract 1986;8:19–26.
3. Fessler JF, Amstutz HE. Ulna. In: Oehme FW, Prier JE, Eds. Textbook of Large Animal Surgery. Baltimore: Williams & Wilkins, 1974;312–316.
4. Leitch M. The upper forearm. In: Mansmann RA, McAllister ES, Eds. Equine Medicine and Surgery. Santa Barbara, CA: American Veterinary Publications, 1982;1134.
5. Levine SB, Meagher DM. Repair of an ulnar fracture with radial luxation in a horse. Vet Surg 1980;9:58.
6. O'Connor JJ. Dollar's Veterinary Surgery. 4th ed. Chicago: Alexander Eger, 1950.
7. Turner AS. Fractures of the olecranon. In: Jennings PB, Ed. The Practice of Large Animal Surgery. Vol. 2. Philadelphia: WB Saunders, 1984;800–804.

SUBCHONDRAL DEFECTS AND OSSEOUS CYSTS (CYSTLIKE LESIONS) OF THE ELBOW

Subchondral defects and subchondral osseous cysts (SOCs) of the elbow joint are uncommon. These condi-

tions, however, have been observed in a wide variety of horse breeds of all ages.[1,2,3,7] SOCs typically communicate with the joint and commonly occur on the medial side, involving either the proximal medial radius or distal medial condyle of the humerus (Fig. 8.321).[2] They can also occur bilaterally (uncommon). Subchondral defects (clefts) in the bone underlying the joint cartilage are most frequently seen on the medial joint surfaces (Fig. 8.322).

Causes

Proposed causes for subchondral defects and SOCs include osteochondrosis at a weight-bearing location in a joint and trauma.[4–7] With osteochondrosis, it is believed that cartilage retention at a central weight-bearing location in a joint results in cartilage infolding during growth and the potential for cyst development.[6] Osteochondrosis as a causal factor is supported by, for example, the condition shown in Figure 8.322, which demonstrates a defect in the subchondral bone.

Alternatively, trauma may be the initiating factor. Microfracture of subchondral trabecular bone within the epiphysis could result in resorption of bone fragments and cyst formation with collapse of the overlying cartilage.[4,5] Trauma as a possible cause is supported by one report of an SOC developing after a nondisplaced, sagittal articular fracture of the medial epiphysis of the proximal radius.[7] (See Chapter 7 for more information on SOCs.)

Signs

Horses often present with a history of an acute onset of lameness that may wax and wane with use.[1,2] On physical examination, there is usually no localizing signs other than lameness. Occasionally, the foot on the affected side will appear smaller than the contralateral foot. Palpation of the caudal aspect of the elbow joint capsule may reveal fluid distension and some thickening. Flexion and extension of the elbow region often elicits a painful response, and a flexion test usually exacerbates the lameness.[3] Horses generally present with a grade 2 to 4 lameness, and the size of the cyst or its location does not appear to influence the degree of lameness. In a small number of horses, the lameness may vary from grade 2 to grade 4 over the course of the same examination period. Intrasynovial anesthesia with a local anesthetic agent eliminates the lameness in most cases.[1,2,3]

Diagnosis

Radiographs are required to make the diagnosis. Two views should be taken to identify the lesion location (Fig. 8.321). In one study, 4 of 7 of the SOCs were located in the proximal medial radius, and 3 were located in the distal medial condyle of the humerus.[2] In another study, the SOCs were located primarily in the proximal medial radius (5 of 6), and the remaining cyst was located in the distal medial condyle of the humerus.[1] Defects in the subchondral bone were not identified.

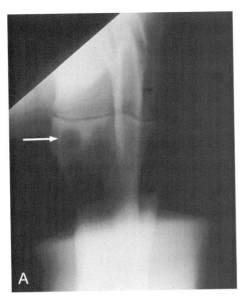

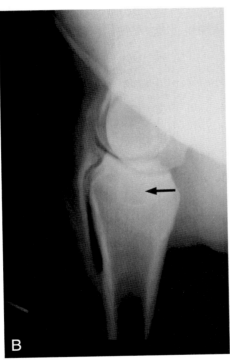

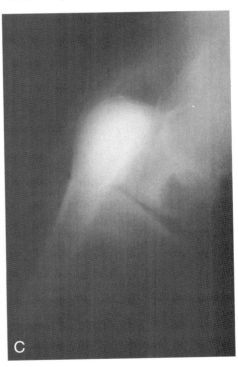

Figure 8.321 A. Cranial-caudal view revealing an SOC in the proximal medial aspect of the radius (arrow). B. Lateral view of the same horse. Note the location of the cyst in the center of the radius (arrow). C. Cranial caudal view showing an SOC in the distal medial condyle of the humerus.

Treatment

Subchondral defects are generally treated conservatively, whereas SOCs can be treated either conservatively or surgically.[1,2,7] Both subchondral defects and SOCs have been treated successfully with prolonged rest and the administration of an anti-inflammatory agent.[3,7] Rest with stall confinement and controlled exercise are recommended for at least 90 days, at which time the horse is examined to see if increased activity can be recommended or surgical intervention is advised. Intrasynovial injection of hyaluronic acid is usually given at the time of the initial examination or at 1 week after the

examination if intrasynovial anesthesia was performed. The addition of polysulfated glycosaminoglycans administered intramuscularly is optional. The administration of phenylbutazone is logical, particularly if the horse is quite lame. Generally, phenylbutazone is administered at 2.2 mg/kg PO q24h for 10 to 14 days.

Supporting the conservative approach for treating SOCs is one report in which 6 of 7 horses treated with rest and the administration of anti-inflammatory agents returned to their intended use.[2] Five of the horses returned to intense athletic performance: 4 to flat racing and 1 to barrel racing. The recommendations from this report were that nonsurgical treatment should be considered in horses without radiographic signs of DJD

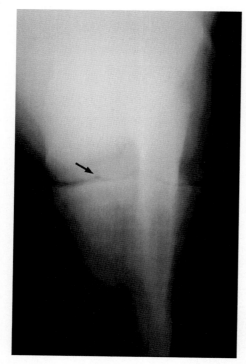

Figure 8.322 Cranial caudal view revealing a subchondral defect in the distal medial condyle of the humerus in a horse with a grade 4 lameness of 3 months' duration.

and that surgery could be considered as option if the horse remains lame at the 90-day follow-up examination.

Contrary to the recommendation for conservative treatment is another study of 6 horses with SOCs in which conservative (3 horses) and surgical (3 horses) treatments were compared.[1] The study found that surgical extraarticular enucleation of the cyst provided a better long-term success (determined by return to athletic function) with less evidence of DJD. But note that none of the horses in this study received intrasynovial injections of hyaluronic acid and that polysulfated glycosaminoglycans were not used.

The surgery is done with the horse positioned in lateral recumbency with the affected limb down. A 15-cm incision centered on the radius over the superficial transverse pectoral muscle (Fig 8.323) is used to expose the proximal medial radius. The muscle and soft tissues are dissected bluntly, and the neurovascular plexus is identified but not disturbed. After needle placement in the humeroradial joint, a radiograph is taken to confirm the location of the needle relative to the cystic lesion. The deep fascia of the flexor carpi radialis muscle is dissected, after which the muscle is retracted to expose the proximal medial aspect of the radius.

Using the needle as a guide, a 3.2-mm drill hole is made in the proximal radius parallel to the joint surface; the location of the drill bit is confirmed via radiography. Using an osteotome or air drill a 5- to 6-mm piece of bone is removed overlying the cyst (Fig. 8.324). The cystic

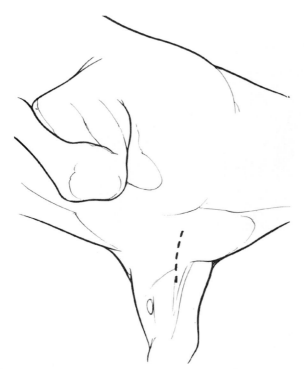

Figure 8.323 Incision location (dotted line) with the horse in lateral recumbency and the upper limb pulled caudal to expose the medial aspect of the proximal antebrachium. (Modified from Bertone AL, McIlwraith CW, Powers BE, et al. Subchondral osseous cystic lesions of the elbow of horses: Conservative versus surgical treatment. J Am Vet Med Assoc 1986;189:540–546.)

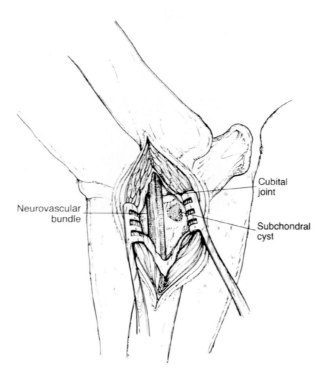

Figure 8.324 Exposure of a cyst on the proximal medial radius. (Modified from Bertone AL, McIlwraith CW, Powers BE, et al. Subchondral osseous cystic lesions of the elbow of horses: Conservative versus surgical treatment. J Am Vet Med Assoc 1986;189:540–546.)

contents are then removed with a curette. After enucleation of the cyst, forage can be performed with a 2.0-mm drill bit.

Suture closure of the wound is routine, except that the deep fascia overlying the neurovascular plexus is not closed. If it were closed, it could result in a compartmental syndrome, which could induce a neuropraxia. A stent bandage is sutured over the incision line. Recovery from anesthesia should be controlled to reduce the chance of a fracture at the site of the enucleation of the cyst in the radius.

After surgery, the horse is confined to a box stall for 2 weeks, at which time hand-walking exercise is begun and continues for the following 2 months. Box stall confinement is continued until there is radiographic evidence of marked reduction in the size of the cystic cavity.[1]

Prognosis

The prognosis appears good for conservative treatment of SOCs as long as there is no radiographic evidence of DJD. As noted earlier, in one study, 6 of 7 conservatively treated horses with SOCs returned to their intended use.[2] The use of intraarticular injections of hyaluronic acid seem to be important to the outcome. If the horse does not respond to the conservative treatment and remains lame, surgery can be considered.

The outcome of surgery done on 3 horses with SOCs resulted in 2 horses returning to their intended use and 1 sustaining a comminuted fracture of the radius during recovery from anesthesia.[1] Data are lacking for the outcome of subchondral defects, but experience with a limited number of cases is that conservative treatment can result in a favorable outcome if enough rest is given.

References

1. Bertone AL, McIlwraith CW, Powers BE, et al. Subchondral osseous cystic lesions of the elbow of horses: Conservative versus surgical treatment. J Am Vet Med Assoc 1986;189:540–546.
2. Hopen LA, Colahan PT, Turner TA, Nixon AJ. Nonsurgical treatment of cubital subchondral cyst-like lesions in horses: Seven cases (1983–1987). J Am Vet Med Assoc 1992;200:527–530.
3. Jann HW, Koblik PD, Fackelman GE. What is your diagnosis? J Am Vet Med Assoc 1986;188:1069–1070.
4. Jeffcott LB, Kold SE, Melsen F. Aspects of the pathology of stifle bone cysts in the horse. Equine Vet J 1983;15:304–311.
5. Kold SE, Hickman J, Melsen F. An experimental study of the healing process of equine chondral and osteochondral defects. Equine Vet J 1986;18:18–24.
6. Stromberg B. A review of the salient features of osteochondrosis in the horse. Equine Vet J 1979;11:211–214.
7. Yovich JV, Stashak TS. Subchondral osseous cyst formation after an intraarticular fracture in a filly. Equine Vet J 1989;21:72–74.

BURSITIS OF THE ELBOW (OLECRANON BURSITIS)

The common names for bursitis of the elbow are shoe boil and capped elbow.[1,5] Bursitis at the point of the elbow is most commonly observed in draft breeds; lighter horse breeds are affected less frequently.[1,5] Contrary to this is one report on 10 horses with olecranon bursitis; all were light horse breeds (9 Quarter Horses and 1 Pinto).[3] Although the condition primarily affects one elbow, it has been observed to occur bilaterally.[3] The characteristic movable swelling over the point of the olecranon tuberosity develops from trauma, which in turn creates an acquired (false) subcutaneous bursa. Once formed, the bursa becomes lined with a membrane that produces a synovial-like fluid.[4,7] The fluid in the bursa differs from joint synovial fluid in its viscosity and mucin clot, suggesting differences in quality or quantity of hyaluronic acid.[4] Acquired bursae are structurally identical with congenital bursae.

Chronic bursitis is characterized by the accumulation of bursal fluid and thickening of the bursal wall by fibrous tissue. Fibrous bands and septa may develop in the bursal cavity, and the subcutaneous tissues around the bursa continue to thicken.[3] Bursal enlargement usually develops as a painless swelling that does not typically interfere with function, unless it becomes greatly enlarged. In most cases, the acquired bursa is only a cosmetic blemish, unless it becomes infected. An infected bursa is painful, causes lameness, and may break open to drain. The small true bursa that underlies the insertion of the triceps brachii muscle is rarely involved.

Causes

Acquired bursitis is the result of trauma caused by the shoe on the affected limb hitting the point of the olecranon tuberosity during motion or while the horse is lying down.[1,4] Most trauma probably occurs while the horse is in sternal recumbency with the foot under the point of the elbow. American Saddlebred and Standardbred horses may hit the elbow with the foot during exercise. Trauma causes a transudative fluid to accumulate in the subcutaneous tissue; the fluid eventually becomes encapsulated by fibrous tissue, and a synovial-like membrane produces the synovial fluid.[7] Infected bursae may also develop after needle aspiration and injection of a corticosteroid.[3]

Signs

The condition is characterized by a prominent, often freely movable, swelling over the point of the elbow, which may contain fluid or may be composed primarily of fibrous tissue in the chronic stage. Lameness is usually not present, unless the bursa is greatly enlarged or infected. Infected bursae generally feel warm, and firm pressure causes pain. If the infected bursa ruptures, it is characterized by exuberant granulation, discharging sinuses, and the formation of fibrous tissue.

Diagnosis

The diagnosis can usually be made on physical findings alone. However, if the bursa appears infected, radiographs can be taken to rule out trauma or infection involving the olecranon process. If a draining tract is present, contrast material may be injected into it to identify its depth and course. Ultrasound can also be used to determine if deeper structures are involved.

Treatment

In the acute stage, the condition may resolve by preventing further trauma to the region, with the use of a shoe boil roll or a boot. In some instances, the aseptic injection of steroids may be beneficial after the fluid has been removed.[1,4,6] The lesion can be injected two to three times, at weekly intervals. If the initiating cause is removed, and the lesion is treated before extensive fibrosis occurs, it may resolve. In one report, 7 of 10 horses with the condition were treated with intrabursal steroids and none resolved.[3]

Bursal drainage followed by the injection of orgotein has been suggested as a treatment.[4] In a report of three horses with olecranon bursitis that were treated with intralesional orgotein, the bursa was reduced in all horses but none of the lesions resolved.[3] Another option is to inject the bursa with dysprosium-165. Dysprosium-165–ferric hydroxide macroaggregate is a short-lived radionuclide that has been used in humans to induce synovectomy in rheumatoid arthritis patients.[2] One horse with olecranon bursitis underwent intralesional injection with this radionuclide; the mass resolved 7 months after the second injection.[3]

Treatments for chronic bursitis have included the following:[1,3]

- Intralesional injection of 7% iodine
- Incision into the bursa and insertion of a gauze section soaked in 7% iodine (packing changed every 2 to 3 days until cavity is closed)
- Insertion of Penrose drains for 10 to 14 days to remove fluid and enhance fibrosis
- En bloc resection of the bursa

Although intralesional injection of iodine has been recommended, there is little logic for its use in the treatment of chronic bursitis in my opinion. In a study that evaluated bursal incision and packing with 7% iodine for three horses with chronic bursitis, one horse healed after 3 months and the others were subsequently treated with en bloc resection of the bursa.[3] In a report of the use of Penrose drains to treat olecranon bursitis, it was noted that the site healed with minimal fibrosis 8 weeks after implantation of the drains.[9] En bloc surgical excision appears to be the treatment of choice when the bursa is large and composed primarily of fibrous tissue.

Before surgery, the horse should be trained to be cross-tied. The surgery can be done in the standing sedated horse that is restrained in stocks.[3] Once sedated, the surrounding subcutaneous tissues are injected with 30 to 50 mL of 2% mepivacaine hydrochloride (Carbocaine). After local anesthesia, the skin is incised over the lateral portion of the mass. The incision should not be made over the caudal aspect of the elbow, so that stress on the incision during flexion and extension of the limb is reduced. Either a vertically placed fusiform or a curved incision can be used.

Once a plane of dissection is created between the subcutaneous tissue and the mass, the mass is removed en bloc. After which, excess skin is removed as needed. Interrupted suture of synthetic absorbable material is used to appose the deep and subcutaneous tissues. The skin is apposed with suture material of the surgeon's choice in an interrupted suture pattern. Before skin closure, widely placed vertical mattress sutures can be used to reduce the tension on the primary skin suture line.[8] In addition, a stent bandage, sutured in place overlying the skin suture site, is recommended to reduce tension on the primary suture site, compress the wound, and protect the surgery site.[8] After surgery, the horse is cross-tied in a stall to prevent it from lying down. One report notes that the median duration for postoperative cross-tying is 17.5 days (range 12 to 22 days).[3]

Prognosis

The prognosis for resolution of the swelling with a cosmetic outcome is guarded for the conservative approaches in which bursal drainage and injection of an agent (corticosteroid, orgotein, or radionuclide) is done. In a study of five horses with olecranon bursitis that were treated medically, only one horse treated by injection of radionuclide had a cosmetic outcome with resolution of the swelling.[3]

The prognosis for en bloc resection appears good for resolution of the olecranon bursitis with a cosmetic outcome. One report noted that the owners of four horses treated by this approach were pleased with the cosmetic result.[3] The same report revealed that incision and packing of the open wound resulted in resolution of the olecranon bursitis, but without a cosmetic outcome.

References

1. Adams OR. Lameness in Horses. 3rd ed. Philadelphia: Lea & Febiger, 1974;141.
2. English RJ, Zalutsky M, Venkatesan P, et al. Therapeutic application of dysprosium-165-FHMA in the treatment of rheumatoid knee infusions. J Nucl Med Technol 1986;14:18–20.
3. Honnas CM, Schumacher J, McClure SR, et al. Treatment of olecranon bursitis in horses: 10 cases (1986–1993). J Am Vet Med Assoc 1995;206:1022–1026.
4. McIlwraith CW. Diseases of joints, tendons, ligaments and related structures. In: Stashak TS, Ed. Adams' Lameness in Horses. 4th ed. Philadelphia: Lea & Febiger, 1987;481–485.
5. O'Conner JJ. Dollar's Veterinary Surgery. 4th ed. Chicago: Alexander Eger, 1950.
6. Ottaway CA, Worden AN. Bursa and tendon sheaths of the horse. Vet Rec 1940;52:477.
7. Shappell KK, Little CB. Special surgical procedures for equine skin. In: Auer JA, Ed. Equine Surgery. Philadelphia: WB Saunders, 1992;272–284.
8. Stashak TS. Equine Wound Management. Philadelphia: Lea & Febiger, 1991.
9. Van Veenendaal JC, Speirs VC, Harrison I. Treatment of hygromata in horses. Aust Vet J 1981;57:513–514.

Part VIII

THE HUMERUS

Ted S. Stashak

FRACTURES OF THE HUMERUS

Fractures of the humerus are relatively uncommon in horses possibly because of the short, thick configuration of this bone and the prominent surrounding heavy musculature.[1,9,16] The fracture can occur in horses of any age, breed, or sex, but most often affect foals less than 1 year of age, racing or race-training Thoroughbreds, and horses that are used for jumping or steeplechase events.[11,22,35] In a study done on 54 horses that sustained humeral fractures, the mean age for fracture occurrence was 3 years (range 1 week to 15 years), 28 horses (52%) were younger than 6 months, 4 (7.4%) were 6 months to 2 years old, 9 (17%) were between 2 and 4 years old, and 13 (24%) were between 4 and 15 years old.[11]

Humeral fractures are classified as incomplete or complete, open or closed, simple or comminuted, and nondisplaced or displaced; most are complete, closed, and displaced. Comminution occurs occasionally. Humeral fractures are also classified by location: proximal humeral head (epiphysis and metaphysis in foals), greater tubercle, deltoid tuberosity, mid-diaphyseal, distal metaphyseal and epiphyseal, and distal condylar and epicondylar.[11,15,26,34] Most fractures are reported to involve the middle third of the diaphysis and are either oblique, transverse, spiral in configuration and almost never open.[9,22] In a study done on 54 horses that sustained humeral fractures, 9 (17%) fractures involved the physis (1 proximal and 8 distal), 8 (15%) occurred in the proximal metaphysis (4 oblique and 4 transverse), 11 (20.4%) were in the distal metaphysis, 26 (48%) were in the diaphysis (2 short oblique, 4 transverse, 20 long oblique or spiral), and 1 was open.[11] In another study done on 22 horses that sustained humeral fractures, 14 fractures were spiral in configuration.[35] Uncommonly, foals will sustain multiple fractures involving the elbow region; one report noted a foal that had fractured the distal humerus, proximal radius, and the ulna.[5]

Because of the large muscular attachments to the humerus, there is often considerable overriding and displacement (the distal fragment is displaced caudad, and the proximal fragment is displaced craniad). On the other hand, it is uncommon for a proximal complete humeral fracture to become displaced to any extent because the surrounding muscles (supraspinatus, infraspinatus, subscapular, and deltoid), the biceps tendinous insertions, and the periarticular capsular attachments of the shoulder provide inherent stability to the region.[26] Incomplete stress fractures occur in two typical locations: the proximal caudal lateral cortex and the distal cranial medial cortex.[22]

Because radial nerve courses in the musculospiral groove of the humerus, it is not surprising that it may be traumatized to some degree as a result of a complete displaced diaphyseal or metaphyseal humeral fracture.[9,16,22] The damage ranges from a minor neuropraxia (alteration in the nerve conduction without direct damage to the nerve) to a complete severance of the nerve.[16] Because of the profound effect on prognosis, it is important to evaluate the degree of nerve dysfunction early in the convalescent period.

Causes

Humeral fractures frequently occur in foals, in weanlings secondary to falls or other impact injuries, and in racing breeds as either catastrophic failure during race falls or failure as a result of accumulated stress and microfracture.[9,10,19,22,28,31,35] In a study done on 54 horses that sustained humeral fractures, the causes included falls related to racing or on hard surfaces (11 horses), kicks (2), postanesthetic recovery (2), collisions with fences or another horse (3), and impact from a car (1). A total of 35 horses presented with no identifiable cause of the humeral fracture.[11] When fractures of the deltoid tuberosity or greater tubercle occur, trauma is commonly reported as the cause.[7]

The configuration of the fracture configuration seen clinically may depend on the direction of the impact sustained by the humerus. In an in vitro model, the fracture's configuration was predictable and depended on the direction from which the insult originated.[23] When the force was applied in a craniocaudal direction, the humerus fractured transversally; when the force was applied in lateral to medial direction, the humerus fractured obliquely.

Horses sustaining stress fractures of the humerus are at an increased risk for developing a complete fracture if they are not managed properly. In a study done on 34 Thoroughbred racehorses with humeral fractures, researchers found an increased risk of complete fracture in horses that returned to racing after a 2-month lay-up period.[10] The authors postulated that the humeri were predisposed to osteoporosis during the period of inactivity; therefore, when the horses returned to work, their bones may have been of a lower quality or quantity and thus more susceptible to microdamage. When bones sustain microdamage, the damaged bone is quickly resorbed by osteoclasts within 48 to 72 hours, and resorption continues for 2 to 3 weeks, further weakening the bone. The repair process is slow, and can take around 3 months. If stress is continually placed on a remodeling bone, the chance of a complete fracture is high. Examination of the periosteal callus in horses after they sustained a complete fracture supports the idea of an acute process that fits the time frame of a stress fracture occurring after a lay-up period.[10]

Signs

Horses with nondisplaced or minimally displaced proximal fractures (Salter-Harris type 1 of the epiphy-

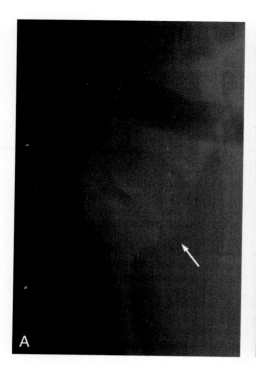 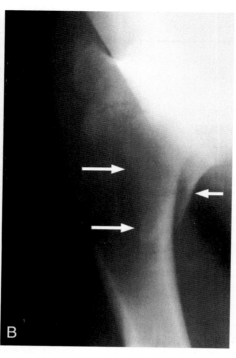

Figure 8.325 A. Lateral view of a minimally displaced Salter-Harris type 1 fracture of the proximal humerus. Note the epiphysis of the humeral head is displaced caudad (arrow). B. A moderately displaced Salter-Harris type 2 fracture of the proximal humerus (arrows). (Courtesy of G. Baxter.)

seal, greater tubercle, or deltoid tuberosity) and nondisplaced midshaft fractures often present with a history of a marked lameness that improves over a 24- to 48-hour period. Moderate swelling may be present at the site of injury for a proximal fracture or over the lateral muscles for a midshaft fracture. Pain is often present when pressure is applied over the fracture and with limb manipulation. If several days have passed, the swelling may be most prominent in a site distal to the fracture. At exercise, a moderate (grade 2 to 3 out of 5) lameness is most often seen. Radiology often provides a definitive diagnosis (Fig. 8.325).

Incomplete fractures and stress fractures resulting in lameness can be most difficult to diagnose.[21,22,28,31] Lameness and moderate swelling may be adequate in some cases to lead to a tentative diagnosis of a fracture, but the definitive diagnosis often requires nuclear imaging.[26] Follow-up radiography may identify a small amount of callus formation along the caudal cortex of the humeral metaphyseal region, particularly in some chronic cases.

Horses with complete displaced fractures often present with a history of an acute onset of a marked to nonweight-bearing lameness. Marked to moderate swelling of the muscles overlying the region is often seen, the elbow usually has a dropped elbow appearance, and the carpus and fetlock are frequently flexed in a similar manner to that seen after complete fracture of the olecranon process (Fig. 8.326). The dropped elbow may be the result of the overriding of the fracture segments, resulting in functional limb shortening, or from damage to the radial nerve.[1,11]

Limb manipulation usually causes increased pain and a greater range of motion when the limb is adducted and abducted. Crepitation is often difficult to appreciate, particularly in heavy muscled horses, because of the de-

gree of fragment displacement and the muffling effect of the swollen musculature.[16] Auscultation with a stethoscope may help identify crepitation.[1] Limited manipulation should be done, because it may result in further trauma to the radial nerve. The presence of a fracture and its configuration are confirmed by radiography (Fig. 8.327).

The evaluation of radial nerve damage is more difficult. Assessment nerve function requires electrodiagnostics: either direct nerve conduction velocity evaluation by spinal somatosensory evoked potential or muscle action evoked potential. Because there is no autonomous sensory zone for the radial nerve, peripheral skin desensitization is not a good indicator of radial nerve damage.[8] After 2 weeks, electromyography (EMG) of the antebrachial extensor muscles can be used to evaluate radial nerve damage. EMG also helps during the convalescent period for distinguishing between neurapraxia and neurotmesis in an attempt to evaluate the potential for return of radial nerve function. In one study, 4 of 40 horses treated for fractures of the humerus were destroyed because of loss of radial nerve function.[11]

Fractures of the distal epiphysis condyles, and epicondylar region are uncommon (Fig. 8.328).[26] When a horse does sustain such a fracture, it often presents with a history of marked lameness of a short duration. Swelling associated with the elbow region may be apparent, including joint effusion if the fracture is articular. Direct pressure on the affected site and limb manipulation often result in a painful response. Radiography is required to document the fracture.

Diagnosis

Radiography is used in most cases to confirm the fracture, define the configuration, and rule out secondary

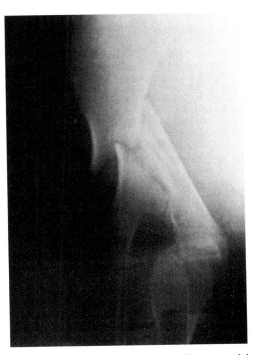

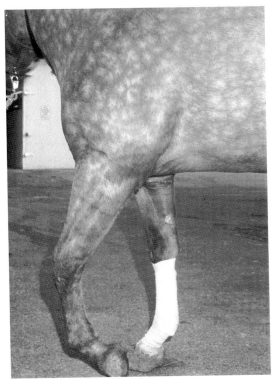

Figure 8.326 A horse that sustained a comminuted fracture of
the midhumeral region displays the dropped elbow appearance.

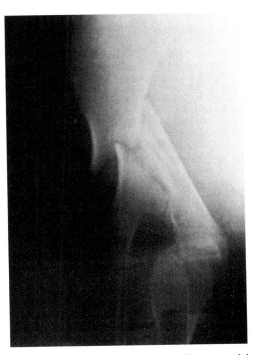

Figure 8.327 A fracture of the humerus. (Courtesy of A. S.
Turner.)

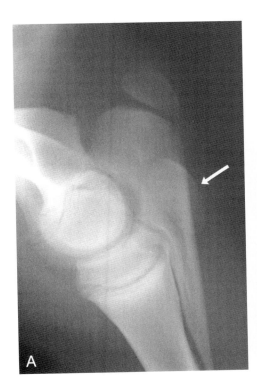

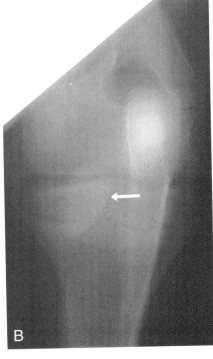

Figure 8.328 A. Lateral view of a
displaced fracture of the distal medial
epicondyle of the humerus (arrow). B.
Cranial caudal view of the same
fracture. Note that the fracture just
approximated the medial edge of the
elbow joint. (Courtesy of K. Sullins.)

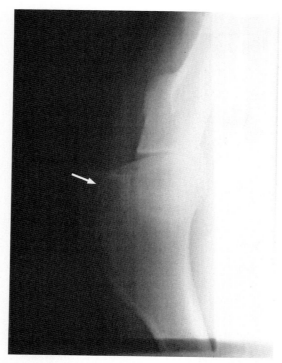

Figure 8.329 Cranial caudal oblique (skyline) view of the greater tubercle revealing a nonarticular fracture (arrow).

problems, such as fractures of the supraglenoid tubercle, ulna, and ribs. A slightly oblique medial lateral projection with the limb held in extension usually provides the information needed for epiphyseal and shaft fractures. In most cases, the study can be done in the standing sedated horse. Foals, on the other hand, can often be sedated and restrained in lateral recumbency, with affected limb down, to obtain a diagnostic lateral projection. Cranial caudal views of the distal humerus and oblique views of the proximal humerus can be obtained in most standing sedated horses and foals (Fig. 8.327). Cranial caudal views of the entire proximal humerus are, however, more difficult to obtain, and general anesthesia may be required.

Multiple radiographic views may be needed to identify fractures of the greater tubercle and deltoid tuberosity.[7] The study can usually be done in the standing horse. Oblique and skyline radiographic views of the proximal humerus are often required for visualization of the fracture (Fig. 8.329).

Treatment

Currently, three options are considered when managing a horse with a humeral fracture: nonsurgical (conservative) management with prolonged stall rest, surgical reduction followed by stabilization, and euthanasia.[9,11, 22,26,28,29] Of the two treatment approaches, nonsurgical management appears to provide a better outcome than do surgical approaches for most nonarticular incomplete or complete humeral fractures, no matter what the age of the horse.[11,35] In one report 7 of 10 horses treated nonsurgically were able to be ridden 5 to 12 months after

the diagnosis was made, and only 1 of 3 horses treated surgically (2 Rush pins, 1 lag screws) was considered sound for riding.[35] Note that 2 of the nonsurgically treated horses were lost to follow-up and were included in the group of unsuccessful cases. The age of the horses treated nonsurgically ranged from 2 to 60 months (mean = 21 ± 16.5 months). In another study, 9 of 17 horses treated conservatively were considered successful; 4 became athletically sound, and 5 were pasture sound.[11] The age of these horses ranged form 1 week to 15 years (mean = 3 years).

Euthanasia still remains a commonly selected option. In a retrospective study of 54 horses with humeral fractures, more horses were euthanized (44.4%) than were treated surgically (24%) or conservatively (32%).[11] In another report, 9 of 22 horses with humeral fractures were euthanized.[35]

Nonsurgical Management

Nonsurgical management has been used successfully to treat stress fractures, incomplete or complete nondisplaced or minimally displaced nonarticular fractures, minimally displaced Salter-Harris type 1 and 2 fractures of the proximal and distal physis (Figs. 8.325, 8.329, and 8.330), complete displaced proximal and distal transverse and oblique fractures, and complete displaced diaphyseal transverse short and spiral oblique fractures (Fig. 8.331).[6,11,22,26,35] In two reports, a better outcome using conservative treatment was obtained in horses younger than 8 months, even though the age range of horses successfully treated was 2 months to 15 years.[11,35]

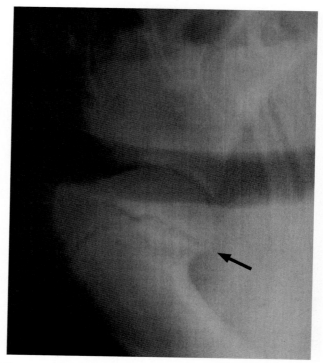

Figure 8.330 Lateral view taken at the 6-week follow-up of the foal shown in Figure 8.325A. Note the fracture has healed and the physis and metaphysis have remodeled (arrow).

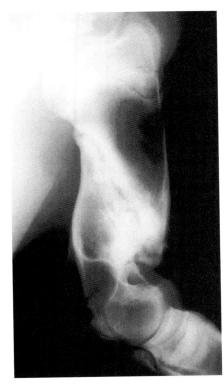

Figure 8.331 Lateral view of a healing spiral nonarticular fracture of the midhumerus taken 5 months after diagnosis. (Courtesy of G. Baxter.)

Nonsurgical management consists of stall rest, administration of nonsteroidal anti-inflammatory drugs (NSAIDs), and periodic radiographic or nuclear medical reevaluation of the fracture for healing. Stress fractures and incomplete or complete nondisplaced nonarticular fractures are best managed with the horse placed in stall confinement for 3 to 4 months.[26,28] If a horse is severely lame from a stress fracture, it should be either cross-tied or run on an overhead wire to minimize the chance of its developing a complete fracture when it attempts to get up and down.[22] This approach can also be used for incomplete or complete nondisplaced fractures. Because support limb laminitis is a concern, a horse that is tied to prevent it from lying down is probably best placed in a stall bedded with dry sand (6 inches deep).

Fracture healing is generally evaluated radiographically or with nuclear medicine (for some stress fractures) after 3 to 4 months. If healing appears adequate, the horse is allowed access to a run or small paddock for 1 month. Then, if the horse remains comfortable, it can be allowed free exercise for another 2 to 3 months. The fracture should be evaluated for healing before the horse is put back into training.

In my experience minimally displaced Salter-Harris type 1 or 2 fractures and minimally displaced greater tubercle fractures in young horses heal fairly rapidly; therefore, confinement in a stall is usually only 6 to 8 weeks to allow for adequate healing (Figs. 8.325 and 8.328). If an adequate callus has formed, the foal is allowed free exercise in a confined area for another 6 to 8 weeks. If the physical examination and radiographs indicate sufficient healing of the fracture, the foal is allowed free exercise at pasture.

Complete displaced nonarticular fractures are generally managed with stall confinement for 4 to 6 months. The longer period is often required to minimize motion and allow the fracture to heal adequately. Contraction of the heavy musculature surrounding the humerus helps stabilize the fracture while it heals. The stall should be heavily bedded to encourage recumbency. Bedding with either wood shavings or dry sand (6 inches deep) with a light straw covering (preferred) seems to work best in my experience. An apparent added benefit to the sand is that it reduces the incidence of support limb laminitis. Bandage splinting the caudal aspect of the affected limb from the elbow to the foot has been recommended to prevent the development of carpal flexural contracture and to maintain a straight limb for more support. However, the necessity of this treatment has been questioned. In one study of 10 horses with conservatively treated humeral fractures that were not splinted, the authors noted that flexural contracture of the carpus did not occur.[35] A heavy support bandage should be applied to the opposite support limb, particularly in foals, to prevent the development of an angular limb deformity breakdown of the flexor tendons.[11,35]

Although numerous complications have been reported after conservative management of humeral fractures, the complication rate and frequency have not been supported in retrospective studies. In one report, complications associated with conservative management of humeral fractures occurred in 6 of 17 horses, including sudden death (1 horse), radial nerve paralysis (1), non-union (2), support limb breakdown (1), support limb angular limb deformity (3), and persistent pain in the affected limb (1).[11] In another report, 1 of 10 horses treated conservatively developed laminitis, which resulted in euthanization.[35] In this study, the owners of the nonsurgically treated horses reported no adverse affects attributable to shortening of the humerus, such as a shortened stride or a straightened elbow joint.

Surgical Management

Various internal fixation techniques have been described for treatment of humeral fractures.[3,7,11,14,17,20–23,26,27,29,31–34] Fixation devices have included the following:

- Stacked intramedullary pins[9,11,22]
- Rush pins[17]
- Association for the Study of Internal Fixation (ASIF; Kuntscher) nails[21]
- One or more dynamic compression plates (DCPs)[1,20,22,23,26,27,29,30]
- Interlocking intramedullary nails[31–33]
- A combination of intramedullary pins and cerclage bands or wires[22]

Unfortunately the current techniques of using DCPs, intramedullary fixations, and cerclage bands or wires do not offer sufficient strength to provide adequate stability in adult horses.[9,22,23]

Intermedullary pinning, bone plating, and ASIF or interlocking intramedullary nailing or Rush pins have been used to successfully treat foals and ponies with humeral

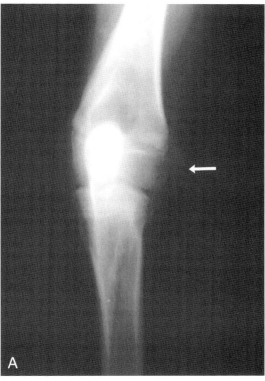

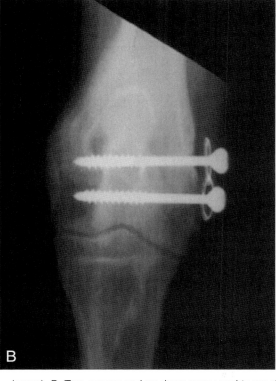

Figure 8.334 A. Cranial caudal view of a minimally displaced nonarticular epicondylar fracture of the distal medial humerus (arrow). B. Two screws and washers were used to repair the fracture.

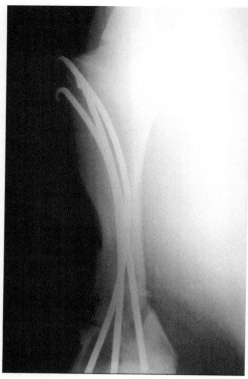

Figure 8.332 Rush pins used to treat a comminuted fracture of the humerus. (Courtesy of G. Baxter.)

eral approach is used, the brachialis muscle must be elevated, and considerable contouring of the plate is required to place the implant on the irregular lateral surface of the humerus. Usually only one plate can be applied. The cranial approach allows access to most regions of the humeral shaft and is preferred over the lateral approach.[26,27] The flat smooth cranial surface of the bone is ideal for placing the broad DCP, and it is probably the tension band side of the bone, as it is in small animals. An added benefit to the cranial approach is that a second plate, placed laterally, can be used in more mature horses to provide greater stability to the repair. Regardless of the approach, the radial nerve must be preserved.

Fracture reduction is usually maintained with bone-holding forceps, separate lag screws, or cerclage bands or wires while the plate is being contoured for application. If the plate is applied to the cranial surface, the distal screws are directed toward the medial epicondyle of the caudodistal humerus to avoid penetrating the olecranon fossa. Use of 5.5-mm cortical screws is recommended; 6.5-mm cancellous screws can be used in the soft metaphyseal bone of the proximal humerus, where the transcortex is not engaged.[26] In horses weighing more than 150 kg, a second plate can be placed on the lateral surface of the humerus, immediately caudal to the deltoid tuberosity.[26] The lateral plate is usually shorter

the horse is placed in a stall bedded with deep (6 inches) dry sand to ensure secure footing and reduce the chances of support limb breakdown and laminitis. Adding straw to the surface of the sand also appears to encourage recumbency in some horses and is, therefore, considered beneficial. Long-term maintenance of horses in partial-buoyancy floatation tanks has also been described.[18] Although the technique was successful in selected fracture cases, long-term respiratory effects were evident.

Prognosis

The prognosis for stress fracture, nondisplaced complete or incomplete fracture, and minimally displaced complete nonarticular fractures managed conservatively appears good.[11,22,28,35] To reduce the risk of complete fractures in Thoroughbred racehorses that sustain stress fractures, the horse should be cautiously reintroduced back into training after the lay-up period.[10] Gradual resumption of race training helps the skeleton to readapt to racing stresses.

The prognosis for complete displaced nonarticular fractures is guarded but appears better for horses managed conservatively rather than surgically. In one study, conservative management was used in 17 horses with a mean age of 2.2 years (range: 2 months to 14 years).[11] Of these horses, 9 (53.9%) were considered successfully healed: 4 became athletically sound, and 5 horses became pasture sound. The ages of the 4 horses that regained athletic soundness ranged from 4 months to 3 years (3 of the 4 horses were younger than 8 months old). The mean age of the 5 pasture-sound horses was 2.35 years (with a range of 3 months to 5 years). Of the pasture-sound horses, 2 were still lame in the affected limb. The others were sound in the affected limb but suffered from angular limb deformities in the contralateral limb; however, their owners considered the horses to be sound. Of the 6 horses that were considered unsuccessful, 5 were younger than 6 months of age. The distribution of fracture type in the unsuccessful group paralleled the fracture type in the successful group, suggesting that age may be a more important factor to the outcome than the fracture type. In the same study, 13 horses were treated surgically with a variety of internal fixation methods, including DCPs. Of these horses, 3 survived and became athletically sound. The horses with successful outcomes were all surgically treated with stacked pinning and were less than 2 months of age (2 were younger than 3 weeks).

In another study, conservative management was used in 10 horses, 7 of which were able to be ridden 5 to 12 months after the diagnosis was made.[35] The ages of the horses successfully treated ranged from 2 to 60 months (mean = 21 months ± 16.5 months). Note that 2 additional horses were lost to follow-up, and were put in the unsuccessful group. Of the 3 horses treated surgically, 1 became pasture sound 10 months after surgery. Horses in the surgically treated group were younger than 15 months of age (mean = 7.6 ± 6.2 months) and weighed less than 341 kg. Rush pins were used for the repair of two fractures and lag screws were used in the other case; the Rush pin–treated horses became pasture sound and could be ridden. The study concluded the best candidates for nonsurgical treatment were nonarticular humeral

fractures with minimal displacement that involve the midshaft, are spiral and oblique, and have with minimal overriding of the ends of the bone.

The limited reports on fractures involving the greater tubercle and deltoid tuberosity indicate that the prognosis is good for conservative management of nondisplaced and surgically treated displaced fractures of the greater tubercle and deltoid tuberosity.[7,12,13] Too few cases of condylar or epicondylar fracture have been reported to draw a good conclusion about the expected prognosis.

References

1. Adams OR. Lameness in Horses. 3rd ed. Philadelphia: Lea & Febiger, 1974.
2. Adams R, Turner T. Internal fixation of a greater tubercle fracture in an adolescent horse: A case report. J Equine Vet Sci 1987;7:174–176.
3. Alexander JT, Rooney JR. The biomechanics, surgery and prognosis of equine fracture. Am Assoc Equine Pract 1972;18:219.
4. Allen D, White N. Chip fracture of the greater tubercle of a horse. Comp Cont Educ Vet Pract 1984;6:39–41.
5. Auer JA, Struchen CH, Weidmann CH. Surgical management of a foal with a humerus-radius-ulna fracture. Equine Vet J 1996;28:416–420.
6. Baxter GM. What is your diagnosis? J Am Vet Med Assoc 1989;195:523–524.
7. Bleyaert H. Shoulder injuries. In: White NA, Moore JN, Eds. Current Techniques of Equine Surgery and Lameness. Philadelphia: WB Saunders, 1998;422–423.
8. Blythe LL, Kitchell RL. Electrophysiologic studies of the thoracic limb of the horse. Am J Vet Res 1982;43:1511–1524.
9. Bramlage LR. Long bone fractures. Vet Clin North Am 1983;5:285–310.
10. Carrier TK, Estberg L, Stover SM, et al. Association between long periods without high speed workouts and risk of complete humeral or pelvic fracture in Thoroughbred race horses: 54 cases (1991–1994). J Am Vet Med Assoc 1998;212:1582–1587.
11. Carter BG, Schneider RK, Hardy J, et al. Assessment and treatment of equine humeral fractures: Retrospective study of 54 cases (1972–1990). Equine Vet J 1993;25:203–207.
12. Dyson SJ. Sixteen fractures of the shoulder region in the horse. Equine Vet J 1985;17:104–110.
13. Dyson SJ, Greet TRC. Repair of a fracture of the deltoid tuberosity of the humerus in a pony. Equine Vet J 1986;18:230–232.
14. Eaton-Wells R, Richards L. Successful treatment of a proximal humeral fracture in a two-year old Thoroughbred gelding. Aust Equine Vet 1990;8:28–29.
15. Embertson RM, Bramlage LR, Herring DS, Gabel AA. Physeal fractures in the horse: Classification and incidence. Vet Surg 1986;15:223–227.
16. Fessler JF, Amstutz HE. Fracture repair. In: Oehme FW, Prier JE, Eds. Textbook of Large Animal Surgery. Baltimore: Williams & Wilkins, 1974;314.
17. Foerner JF. The use of rush pins in long bone fractures. Am Assoc Equine Pract 1977;23:223–227.
18. Herthel DJ, Hamer EJ, Martin F. An equine orthopedic trauma center: A systematic approach to long bone fracture management. Am Assoc Equine Pract 1991;37:763–766.
19. Honnas CM. Humerus fractures. In Auer JA, Ed. Equine Surgery. Philadelphia: WB Saunders, 1992;1044–1045.
20. Kelman DA. Surgical repair of a spiral fracture of a humerus in a foal. Aust Vet J 1980;10:257–259.
21. Mackey V, Trout D, Meagher D, Hornof W. Stress fractures of the humerus, radius, and tibia in horses. Vet Radiol 1987;28:26–31.
22. Markel MD. Fracture of the humerus. In: White NA, Moore JN, Eds. Current Practice of Equine Surgery. Philadelphia: JB Lippincott, 1990;652–657.
23. Markel MD, Nunamaker DM, Wheat JD, Sams AE. In-vitro comparison of three fixation methods of humeral fracture repair in adult horses. Am J Vet Res 1988;49:568–593.

24. Milne DW, Turner AS. An atlas of surgical approaches to the bones of the horse. Philadelphia: WB Saunders, 1979.
25. Nixon AJ. Arthroscopic approaches and intraarticular anatomy of the equine elbow. Vet Surg 1990;19:93–101.
26. Nixon AJ, Watkins JP. Fractures of the humerus. In: Nixon AJ, Ed. Equine Fracture Repair. Philadelphia: WB Saunders, 1996; 242–253.
27. Rakestraw PC, Nixon AJ, Kaderly RE, Ducharme NG. Cranial approach to the humerus for repair of fractures in horses and cattle. Vet Surg 1991;20:1–8.
28. Stover SM, Johnson BJ, Daft BM, et al. An association between complete and incomplete stress fractures of the humerus in racehorses. Equine Vet J 1992;24:260–263.
29. Turner AS. Fractures of the humerus. In: Jennings PB, Ed. The Practice of Large Animal Surgery. Philadelphia: WB Saunders, 1984;708–800.
30. Valdez H, Morris DL, Auer JA. Compression plating of long bone fractures in foals. J Vet Orthop 1979;1:10.
31. Watkins JP. Fractures of the humerus. In: Colahan PT, Mayhew IG, Merritt AM, Moore JN, Eds. Equine Medicine and Surgery. 4th ed. Goleta, CA: American Veterinary Publications, 1991; 1450–1451.
32. Watkins JP, Ashman RB. Intramedullary interlocking nail fixation in foals: Effects on normal growth and development of the humerus. Vet Surg 1990;19:80.
33. Watkins JP, Ashman RB. Intramedullary interlocking nail fixation in transverse humeral fractures: An in-vitro comparison with stacked pin fixation. In: Proceedings. 18th Annual Meeting of the Veterinary Orthopedic Society, Snowmass, CO, 1991;54.
34. Yovich J, Aanes W. Fracture of the greater tubercle of the humerus in a filly. J Am Vet Med Assoc 1985;187:74–75.
35. Zamos DT, Parks AH. Comparison of surgical and nonsurgical treatment of humeral fractures in horses: 22 cases (1980–1989). J Am Vet Med Assoc 1992;201:114–116.

PARALYSIS OF THE RADIAL NERVE

Paralysis of the radial nerve as a primary cause of lameness is an uncommon condition that results in the inability to extend the elbow, the carpus, and the digit. Similar dysfunction may also be observed for other conditions involving the elbow region, humerus, shoulder region, and scapula; thus differentiation can be difficult, particularly shortly after injury occurs.

The radial nerve, often the largest branch of the brachial plexus, derives its origin chiefly from the C8 and T1 nerve roots of the plexus. In 10% of horses, the C7 nerve root contributes to the radial nerve.[8] The radial nerve innervates the extensor muscles of the elbow, carpus, and digit and supplies the lateral flexor of the carpus (ulnaris lateralis). It also gives off a superficial sensory branch to the lateral cutaneous brachial nerve. Paralysis of the radial nerve inactivates these muscles and may result in some loss of sensation to the craniolateral aspect of the forearm.

Causes

In most cases, paralysis of the radial nerve is the result of trauma of the shoulder region caused by hyperextension of the forelimb or extreme abduction of the shoulder.[1,15,16] Fractures of the humerus, C7, and T1 can result in radial nerve paralysis.[11] Tumors, abscesses, and enlarged axillary lymph nodes that occur in the cranial thoracic region and along the course of the nerve and tumors of the brachial plexus and radial nerve may also result in radial nerve paralysis.[12,14] Prolonged lateral recumbency while under general anesthesia on an operating table or while on the ground

may also produce a radial-paralysis-like syndrome in the forelimb that was next to the hard surface. It is difficult to say whether the paralysis after lateral recumbency is from direct pressure or tension trauma to the radial nerve, the result of compression of the vascular supply, or from systemic hypotension leading to ischemia and anoxia of the muscles.[3,7,10,13,14,16,20] It has been shown that a radial-paralysis-like syndrome lasting 24 hours can be produced by compression of the brachial artery.[13,16,17]

Signs

The signs depend on the extent or degree and location of the paralysis. When the portion of the radial nerve that supplies the extensors of the digit is affected, the signs are characteristic. In the acute phase, the horse is unable to bear weight because of the inability to extend the elbow, carpal, and phalangeal joints. If the limb is placed under the horse and fixed in place, it can bear weight passively.[15] While the horse is standing, the shoulder is extended, the elbow is dropped (dropped elbow appearance) and extended, and the carpus and digits are flexed. The muscles of the elbow and the extensors of the carpus and digit seem relaxed, and the limb appears longer than normal. The dropped elbow appearance is not specific for radial nerve paralysis and can be seen with many other conditions associated with the elbow, humerus, and shoulder regions (Fig. 8.335). Oc-

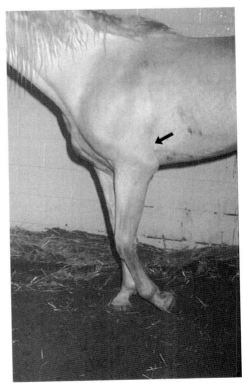

Figure 8.335 This horse presented with radial nerve paralysis as a result of a transverse fracture of the body of the scapula. Note the prominent triceps muscle atrophy (arrow) and the non-weight-bearing attitude of the left limb. The horse also had prominent atrophy of the muscles of the shoulder region.

casionally, radial nerve paralysis is accompanied by paralysis of the entire brachial plexus. In this case, the limb shows paralysis of the flexor and extensor muscles and is unable to bear weight.

With complete radial nerve paralysis, the horse is generally reluctant to move; and at a walk, the limb is dragged forward passively by the action of the proximal pectoral, biceps brachii, and coracobrachialis muscles with the dorsal surface of the hoof in contact with the ground. Owing to the physical stress associated with radial nerve paralysis, some horses may sweat profusely and have an elevated pulse and respiration.[15] Milder cases of radial nerve paralysis have milder degrees of non-weight-bearing lameness; some sign of a dropped elbow; and mild flexion of the carpal, fetlock, and phalangeal joints. At a walk, the lameness is often characterized by a lowered foot flight arch and a shortened cranial phase of the stride.[5]

Diagnosis

Because many cases of radial paralysis are the result of external trauma, the scapula, humerus, radius, and olecranon process should be examined radiographically (Figs. 8.327, 8.332, and 8.335).[12] Radial nerve paralysis needs to be further differentiated from rupture of the medial collateral ligament of the elbow; elbow arthritis; and myopathy of the biceps brachii, triceps brachii, anconeus, and extensor carpi radialis muscles.[15]

It was once believed that cutaneous sensation to the craniolateral aspect of the antebrachium would be lost if there were complete loss of nerve conduction of the radial nerve or brachial plexus. Thus if sensation was present, the lesion selectively affected the motor fibers.[15] However, studies done in horses indicate there are no areas of skin innervated only by either the radial or the axillary nerves—the ulnar, median, and musculocutaneous nerves can be related to such areas.[4]

Electrophysiologic studies can help characterize the extent of nerve damage. Electromyography can be used to determine selective denervation of the extensor muscles. Note, however, that because it takes approximately 7 days for the axon distal to the site of the damage to degenerate, electromyography done before this time has limited usefulness.[2,3] Alternatively, faradic stimulation done 7 days after clinical signs develop can be used to differentiate between neuropraxia and axonotmesis or neurotmesis.[15] Radiography, ultrasonography, and laboratory analysis of muscle enzymes may sometimes be needed to make an accurate diagnosis of radial nerve paralysis.

Treatment

Treatment consists of the administration of anti-inflammatory therapy, stall rest, the application of a bandage splint, and controlled exercise. Nonsteroidal anti-inflammatory drugs (NSAIDs) are administered in acute cases to reduce inflammation and pain. In addition, a low dose of a corticosteroid can be administered during the acute phase. Topical application of cold therapy and dimethyl sulfoxide (DMSO) may be indicated if external

swelling is obvious. The stall should be bedded deep enough to allow the horse to assume lateral recumbency comfortably. When there is a concern of support limb laminitis, the stall can be bedded with dry sand (6 inches deep) and a straw covering. A polyvinyl chloride (PVC) bandage splint applied to the caudal aspect of the limb from the proximal antebrachium to the fetlock maintains the limb in extension (Fig. 8.313). With the limb in the extended position, the horse can usually bear weight comfortably. The splint is maintained until the horse can place the limb in extension without support.

As clinical signs (neurologic function) improve, controlled exercise can be begun. The amount of exercise is dictated by the horse's capabilities. Electromyographic studies can be done at 4- to 6-week intervals to access return of nerve function. The effectiveness of direct nerve or muscle stimulation, as is done in humans, has not yet been fully evaluated in the horse, to my knowledge.

Prognosis

Electromyography has been found to have a good prognostic value in assessing the extent of the injury in a small number of cases.[5] This is also in agreement with results obtained in humans and dogs.[9,18] The outcome largely depends on the type and extent of the injury. In most cases, a guarded to poor prognosis is given,[5,6,18] but a horse with paralysis as the result of a compression or entrapment injury often sees partial or complete recovery.[19] Recovery may take a few weeks for pure neurapraxia to several months or years for axonotmesis.[6,12] Reinnervation is, however, unlikely when there is more severe nerve damage.[5]

References

1. Adams OR. Lameness in horses. 3rd ed. Philadelphia: Lea & Febiger, 1974.
2. Andrews FM, Reed SM. Diagnosis of muscle disease in the horse. Am Assoc Equine Pract 1986;98:95–100.
3. Auer JA. Equine Surgery. Philadelphia: WB Saunders, 1992;211.
4. Blythe LL, Kitchell RL. Electrophysiologic studies of the thoracic limb of the horse. Am J Vet Res 1982;43:1511–1524.
5. Cauvin E, Munroe GA, Mitsopoulos A. Peripheral neuropathy involving brachial plexus nerves in 2 horses. Equine Vet Educ 1993;5:90–94.
6. de Lahunta A. Veterinary Neuroanatomy and Clinical Neurology. 2nd ed. Philadelphia: WB Saunders, 1987.
7. Dyson S, Taylor P, Whitwell K. Femoral nerve paralysis after general anesthesia. Equine Vet J 1990;22:376–380.
8. Goshal NG. Spinal nerves. In: Getty R, Ed. Sisson and Grossman's The Anatomy of the Domestic Animals. 5th ed. Philadelphia: WB Saunders, 1975;665–688.
9. Krarup C, Sethi RS. Idiopathic brachial plexus lesion with conduction block of the ulnar nerve. Electroencephal Clin Neurophysiol 1989;72:259–267.
10. Lindsey WA, McDonell W, Bignell W. Equine postanesthetic forelimb lameness: Intracompartmental muscle pressure changes and biochemical patterns. Am J Vet Res 1980;41:1919.
11. Lopez MJ, Norberg C, Trostle S. Fracture of the 7th cervical and 1st thoracic vertebrae presenting as radial nerve paralysis in a horse. Can Vet J 1997;38:112.
12. Mayhew IG. Paresis or paralysis of one limb. In: Mayhew IG, Ed. Large Animal Neurology. A Handbook for Veterinary Clinicians. Philadelphia: Lea & Febiger, 1989;335–347.
13. Marolt I. Untersuchungen uber Funktionsstorungen des Nervus

Radialis and des Kreislaufes in der Arteria Axillaris beim Pferd. Dtsch Tierarztl Wochenschr 1962;69:181.

14. Palmer AC. Introduction to Animal Neurology. Oxford, UK: Mowbrary, 1965.

15. Rijkenhuizen ABM, Keg PR, Dik KJ. True or false radial nerve paralysis in the horse. Vet Annu 1994;34:126–133.

16. Rooney JR. Biomechanics of Lameness of Horses. Baltimore: Williams & Wilkins, 1969.

17. Rooney JR. Radial paralysis in a horse. Cornell Vet 1963;53:328.

18. Steinberg HS. A review of electromyographic and motor nerve function. Vet Clin North Am Small Anim Pract 1979;18:565–580.

19. Stewart JD, Aguayo AJ. Compression and entrapment neuropathies. In: Dyck PJ, Thomas PK, Lambert EH, et al., Eds. Peripheral Neuropathy. Vol. 2. Philadelphia: WB Saunders, 1984;1435–1457.

20. White NA, Suarez M. Change in triceps muscle intracompartmental pressure with repositioning and padding of the lowermost thoracic limb of the horse. Am J Vet Res 1986;47:2257–2260.

Part IX

THE SHOULDER

Ted S. Stashak

INFLAMMATION OF THE INTERTUBERCULAR BURSA (BICIPITAL BURSITIS)

Inflammation of the intertubercular (bicipital) bursa as a primary cause of lameness is uncommon, even though the condition can occur in horses of any age, breed, or sex.[4,8,12] Bursitis can present as a nonseptic or septic condition.[4,11,12,24] Several case studies have identified a low incidence of the problem.[7,9,10,16] In one report, the condition was responsible for lameness in 1 of 54 horses suspected of having shoulder lameness;[10] in another report, bursitis was the cause in lameness in 1 of 41 horses;[16] and another cited the problem in 1 case over a 10-year period.[7]

The bicipital bursa, which is quite extensive, is located between the bilobate tendon of origin of the biceps brachii muscle and the M-shaped tubercles at the cranio-proximal aspect of the humerus. The synovial membrane of the bursa extends around the axial and abaxial limits of the tendon and onto the margins of its cranial surface. It has been suggested, considering its embryonic development and function, that the intertubercular bursa may be more appropriately called a tendon sheath.[8] For this discussion, however, I refer to this structure as a bursa. Gliding of the biceps brachii tendon over the bicipital grooves in the humerus during movement is facilitated by this bursa. In some cases, the bursa communicates with the scapulohumeral joint.

Causes

Trauma to the cranial surface of the shoulder region is believed to be the most common cause of a primary bursitis.[4,11,12,24] A kick, blunt trauma, and/or a wound (penetrating or laceration) to the shoulder region is commonly reported. Other suggested causes include stretching or tearing of the bursa or biceps tendon during the cranial phase of the stride with the limb in full extension and a fall or slip that results in flexion of the shoulder with extension of the elbow.[21,23]

Infection, either from an open or penetrating wound or from hematogenous spread to the bursa, has also been reported.[11,20,24] At least two reports have implicated *Brucella abortus* as a cause.[7,16] Inflammation of the bicipital bursa has been noted to occur after influenza or the outbreak of other viral respiratory diseases. In one case, inflammation was seen after a long trailer ride;[1,24] it is postulated that the stress of the long trailer ride may have been associated with the development of a bacterial infection that subsequently gained access to the bursa hematogenously.

Signs

A history of trauma to the shoulder region is a common factor, although some cases will have no history or physical evidence of trauma. The signs of lameness usually have an acute onset, which is noticed during the stance and swing phases of the stride. On physical examination, swelling over the cranial aspect of the shoulder region may be evident, and a wound will not necessarily be present. In more chronic cases, generalized shoulder and pectoral muscle atrophy may be seen.[11,12,24] Pressure applied over the biceps tendon and bursal region and manipulation of the shoulder region in flexion and extension usually result in a prominent painful response (Fig. 8.336). The responses to pressure and limb manipulation should be compared to that of the contralateral unaffected limb (Fig. 8.337). In some cases, drainage from a wound is evident.[12]

At exercise a grade 3 or 4 (out of 5) lameness is generally seen, and the swing and stance phases are altered. The lameness is often characterized by a shortened cranial phase of the stride, a decrease in the height of the foot flight arc, reduced carpal flexion, and a fixed shoulder appearance during movement. The horse is often reluctant to bear full weight on the affected limb while standing.[12]

Diagnosis

If the physical examination localizes the pain that is causing the lameness to the bursal region, radiographs of the shoulder and ultrasound examination are performed. However, if the localizing signs are not obvious, confirmation of bursitis is made by centesis and local anesthe-

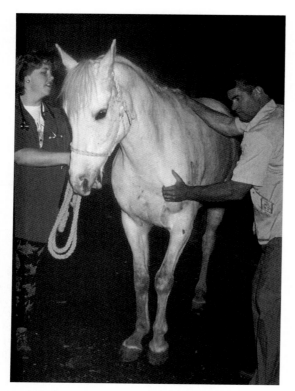

Figure 8.336 The fingers are used to grasp the shoulder and apply lateral pressure over the bicipital bursa region. Even if the horse exhibits a painful response, the reaction should be compared to that obtained on the opposite side.

sia of the bursa (see Chapter 3). A sample of synovial fluid should be taken and submitted for cytology and culture if the clinician suspects an infection (see Chapter 7).

If there has been a history of access to cattle, serum samples should be submitted for *B. abortus* titers.[7,16] Serum titers greater than 40 U/mL were reported in 42 horses with bursal or tendon sheath infections, including 2 horses with infectious bicipital bursitis.[7,16] In another report on 4 horses with septic bicipital bursitis, 1 horse had a *B. abortus* titer of 13 U/mL (no serum titers were conducted on the other 3 horses).[24] The report recommended that serum be analyzed for *B. abortus* in all horses with a suspected bicipital bursitis infection for which a wound was not the cause.

Radiographs of the shoulder region are taken to identify any osseous changes in the tubercles or bicipital groove or bursa and to rule out the possibility of fracture of the supraglenoid tuberosity or proximal humerus and ossification of the biceps tendon (Fig. 8.338).[4,11,12,15,24] Generally, only mediolateral, craniomedial-caudolateral oblique, and flexed cranioproximal-craniodistal (skyline) views can be taken in adult horses.[12,17] The skyline projection of the cranial shoulder region has proven useful for identifying lesions associated with the tubercles of the proximal humerus. Radiographic changes associated with bursitis include mottled changes in the tubercle, demineralization of the greater tubercle, osseous densities in the periarticular region, osteitis in the bicipital groove, and calcification of the bursa (Fig. 8.338).[12,15] Radio-

Figure 8.337 As the shoulder is flexed, tension is created in the tendon of the biceps brachii muscle. If the horse has bicipital bursitis or ossification of the tendon, a painful response is elicited. A flexion test can be run by holding the shoulder in a flexed position for 1 minute.

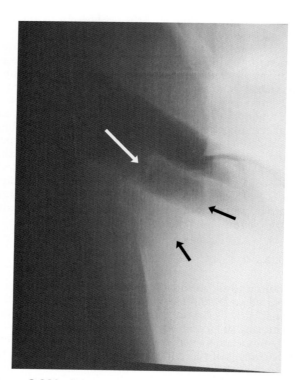

Figure 8.338 Lateral view of a horse that presented with classic signs of bicipital bursitis. Note the loss in bone density on the cranial proximal aspect of the humerus (arrows). The radiographic changes were thought to be consistent with a bone tumor.

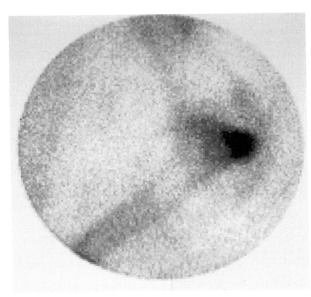

Figure 8.339 Increased uptake of the radionuclide in the greater tubercle of a horse that presented with signs of bicipital bursa pain. Both ultrasound and radiography were normal. Synoviocentesis of the bicipital bursa revealed sepsis. (Courtesy of P. Steyn.)

graphs may appear normal if the disease involves the bursa only. If a wound or draining tract is present, a sterile probe or contrast material can be placed or injected into the tract before the radiograph is taken. This may help determine if the tract communicates with the bursa or terminates adjacent to the radiographic changes seen in the bone.

Ultrasound examination of the biceps tendon, bursa, and bicipital groove can be informative, even when radiographs appear normal.[5,13,19] Ultrasound changes associated with bursitis include edema or hemorrhage in the biceps tendon or bursa, disruption of the tendon architecture with peritendinous thickening, an irregular surface of the bicipital groove, and hyperechoic material in the bicipital bursa.[6,24] Infection needs to be ruled out if hyperechoic material is seen in the bursa.[24]

Nuclear medicine may be useful in some cases to detect early infected or actively remodeling bone adjacent to the bursal region when ultrasound and radiography appear normal (Fig. 8.339).[12]

Treatment

Conservative Treatment

Noninfectious bursitis without radiographic evidence of a fracture or pathology on the cranioproximal aspect of the humerus may respond favorably to rest, parenteral administration of nonsteroidal anti-inflammatory drugs (NSAIDs), and sometimes intrasynovial injection of the bursa with corticoids and sodium hyaluronate.[1–3,8,11,14,22] Topical application of dimethyl sulfoxide (DMSO) has also been advocated.[22]

The duration of the rest generally depends on the nature of the injury, the patient's clinical response to rest,

and whether the biceps tendon was damaged. When the bursitis is acute or is secondary to a lower limb problem that is resolved, the bursal pain generally resolves quickly, usually within a matter of weeks. NSAIDs are generally administered for 10 to 14 days, and controlled (hand-walking) exercise is then begun. Exercise periods typically begin with 5 minutes twice a day, 5 days a week and increase by 2.5 minutes per week up to 20 minutes, at which time the horse is reexamined. Manipulating the limb passively through a range of motion may also be helpful.[12] Having the horse step over 1- to 2-foot-high obstacles placed 50 yards apart appears to improve the range of motion.

In chronic cases, more prolonged rest periods may be required.[25] When the tendon has been injured, rest periods of up to 3 months followed by paddock rest for another 3 months may be required to allow healing of the tendon. In these horses, controlled exercise is begun as early as possible, generally after 2 to 3 weeks of confinement, to improve range of motion and promote healing. The patient's clinical response and ultrasound findings are used to determine progress in healing.

Surgical Treatment

Bursitis that results either from a displaced fracture, from osseous changes associated with the proximocranial aspect of the humerus, or from sepsis generally requires surgery. Incisional and arthroscopic approaches to the intertubercular bursa have been used and described.[4,11,12,18] The advantages to using the arthroscope are similar to that described for other joints and tendon sheaths; and most areas of the bursa can be visualized, except for the medial aspect of the intertubercular groove.[18] If a fracture is present, the obvious objective is to remove it; if there are bone changes on the proximocranial surface of the humerus, the objective is to remove proliferative and malacic bone down to firm normal bone and then to curette and rasp the bone to smooth it.[12] Bone wax may be applied to the bleeding bone surface, if the incisional approach is used. Necrotic soft tissue and any fibrin should also be removed.

Controlled exercise as described for the conservative approach is begun at the time of suture removal in most cases. In addition, the use of therapeutic ultrasound 14 days after surgery has been advocated as an option.[12]

When infection appears to be the cause, synoviocentesis of the bursa should be done to collect fluid for culture and cytology. After this, the bursa should be drained and then lavaged with 1 to 3 liters of a sterile saline solution. In addition, the bursa can be flushed with 1 liter of a 10% DMSO solution, followed by instillation of a broad-spectrum antimicrobial into the synovial cavity. Although large needles can be used to flush the bursa, the use of an arthroscope markedly facilites the procedure. Parenteral administration of broad-spectrum antibiotics and NSAIDs is also done.

In more chronic cases that appear to be refractory to this therapy, surgical debridement and synovectomy are recommended, either through an incisional or an arthroscopic approach.[4,11,12,16,24] The application of drains and or a postoperative ingress–egress system for lavage is done according to the surgeon's preference. In some cases, the bursa is left open to drain and heal by second intention. Antimicrobial therapy is generally prolonged, lasting 3 to 4 weeks (see Chapter 7). Controlled exercise and moving the affected limb through a passive range of motion are also advocated to reduce restrictive adhesion formation.[4]

Prognosis

Acute cases of nonseptic bursitis in which fracture is not the cause often respond favorably to conservative treatment.[3,15] Conservative therapy for more chronic cases of nonseptic or septic bursitis appears less than satisfactory.[4,11,12,24] In one report on three horses with chronic nonseptic bicipital bursitis that were treated surgically, all horses became pasture sound and one could be ridden by the 6-month follow-up.[12]

For chronic septic bursitis treated conservatively, the prognosis appears poor for return to performance unless surgery is performed. In one report of six horses with chronic septic bicipital bursitis, four were treated with rest, antimicrobials, and NSAIDs. Of these, two were still lame at the 6-month follow-up, one was pasture sound, and the other could be ridden for pleasure.[24] The two horses treated surgically, including a partial synovectomy, resumed their former activity, although a subtle lameness remained in one horse. The other horse went on to be a successful racehorse.

In a report on the surgical treatment of one horse with chronic septic bursitis, the horse was considered sound by the owner 10 months after dismissal.[11] In another report, medical treatment for 9 months failed to resolve an infection in the bursa, and the horse became sound only after surgical treatment.[16] Currently, the prognosis for septic intertuberal bursitis appears better than was previously believed.[20]

References

1. Adams OR. Lameness in Horses. 3rd ed. Philadelphia: Lea & Febiger, 1974.
2. Adams SB, Blevins WE. Shoulder lameness in horses—Part 1. Comp Cont Educ Vet Pract 1989;11:64–68.
3. Adams SB, Blevins WE. Shoulder lameness in horses—Part 2. Comp Cont Educ Vet Pract 1989;11:190–195.
4. Bleyaert H. Bicipital bursitis/tenosynovitis and humeral osteitis. In: White NA, Moore JN, Eds. Current Techniques of Equine Surgery and Lameness. Philadelphia: WB Saunders, 1998;424–426.
5. Bohn A, Papageorges M, Grant BD. Ultrasonographic evaluation and surgical treatment of humeral osteitis and bicipital tenosynovitis in a horse. J Am Vet Med Assoc 1992;201:305–306.
6. Crabill MR, Chaffin MK, Schmitz DG. Ultrasonographic morphology of the bicipital tendon and bursa in clinically normal Quarter Horses. Am J Vet Res 1995;56:5–10.
7. Cosgrove JSM. Symposium on equine practice 2: Clinical aspects of equine brucellosis. Vet Rec 1961;73:1377.
8. Dyson SJ. Intertuberal (bicipital) bursitis. In: Colahan PT, Mayhew IG, Merritt AM, Moore JN, Eds. Equine Medicine and Surgery. 4th ed. Goleta, CA: American Veterinary Publications, 1991; 1456–1457.
9. Gough MR, McDiarmid. Septic intertuberal (bicipital) bursitis in a horse. Equine Vet Educ 1998;10:66–69.
10. Dyson SJ. Shoulder lameness in horses: diagnosis and differential diagnosis. Am Assoc Equine Pract 1986;32:461–480.
11. Dyson SJ. Shoulder lameness in horses: An analysis of 58 suspected cases. Equine Vet J 1986;18:230–232.
12. Grant BD, Peterson PR, Bohn A, Rantanen NW. Diagnosis and surgical treatment of traumatic bicipital bursitis in the horse. Am Assoc Equine Pract 1992;38:350–354.
13. Hamelin A, Denoix A, Bousseau B, Perrot P. Ultrasonographic examination of the proximal part of the biceps brachii in horses. Pract Vet Equine 1994;26:41–47.
14. Johnson JF, Bartels JE. Conditions of the forelimbs. In: Catcott EJ, Smithcors JF, Eds. Equine Medicine and Surgery. 2nd ed. Wheaton, IL: American Veterinary Publications, 1972;505–562.
15. Leitch M. The upper forearm. In: Mansmann RA, McAllister ES, Eds. Equine Medicine and Surgery. 3rd ed. Santa Barbara, CA: American Veterinary Publications, 1982;1131–1134.
16. Mason TA. Bicipital bursitis in a mare. Vet Rec 1980;107:330.
17. Morgan JP, Neves J, Baker T. Shoulder joint. In: Morgan JP, Neves J, Baker T, Eds. Equine Radiology. Ames: Iowa State University Press, 1991;212–219.
18. Norris Adams M, Turner TA. Endoscopy of the intertubercular bursa in horses. J Am Vet Med Assoc 1999;214:221–225.
19. Pugh CR, Johonson PJ, Crawley G, Finn ST. Ultrasonography of the equine bicipital tendon region: a case history report and review of anatomy. Vet Radiol Ultrasound 1994;35:183–188.
20. Riggs C, Rice Y, Patteson M, et al. Infection of the intertuberal (bicipital) bursa in seven horses. Proceedings. 34th BEVA Congress, 1995;46–48.
21. Rooney JR. Biomechanics of Lameness in Horses. Baltimore: Williams & Wilkins, 1969.
22. Rose RJ, Hodgson DR. Bicipital bursitis. In: Rose RJ, Hodgson DR, Eds. Manual of Equine Practice. London: WB Saunders, 1993; 109.
23. Tulleners EP, Divers TJ, Evans LH. Bilateral bicipital bursitis in a cow. J Am Vet Med Assoc 1985;186:604.
24. Vatistas NJ, Pascoe JR, Wright IM, et al. Infection of the intertubercular bursa in horses: Four cases (1978–1991). J Am Vet Med Assoc 1996;208:1434–1437.
25. Wyn-Jones G. Bicipital bursitis. In: Wyn-Jones G, Ed. Equine Lameness. Oxford, UK: Blackwell Scientific 1988;88–89.

OSSIFICATION OF THE TENDON OF THE BICEPS BRACHII MUSCLE (CALCIFYING TENDINOPATHY)

Ossification of the tendon of the biceps brachii muscle is an uncommon cause of lameness in young adult horses.[3] It can present as either a unilateral or a bilateral condition, and it can be a difficult problem to diagnose. Traumatic, developmental, and/or degenerative processes of the cranial shoulder region are thought to result in heterotopic bone formation in this tendon.

Causes

Trauma to the tendon is the most likely cause of the ossification in most cases. The tendon of the biceps brachii muscle forms two fusiform enlargements as it passes over the bicipital groove at the proximal end of the humerus. Contained within the tendon enlargements are some amount of fibrocartilage. Direct trauma to the scapulohumeral joint, extension of degenerative changes from the cranioproximal humerus, or extension of disease from the scapulohumeral joint could cause the tendon to undergo endochondral ossification (Fig. 8.340). Continued movement of the tendon in the bicipital groove could result in further damage to the bursa and adjacent bony structures, resulting in lameness.[3] Ossification of the bicipital tendon has also been associated with fracture of the supraglenoid tubercle.[1,5]

Signs

A history of chronic, low-grade, insidious lameness is most common. At presentation, a mild atrophy of the

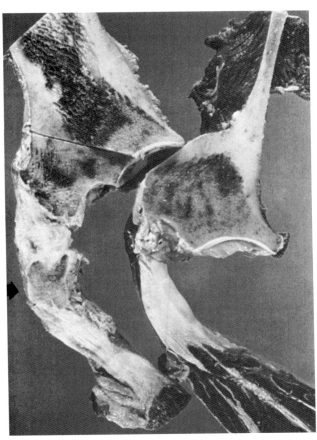

Figure 8.340 Right. The normal tendon of the biceps brachii muscle is attached to the supraglenoid tuberosity proximally. Left. Ossification is present in the tendon (arrow).

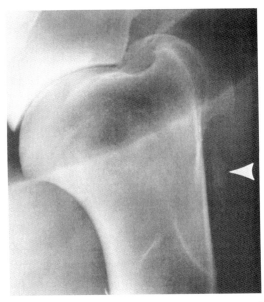

Figure 8.341 Lateral view of the shoulder revealing ossification of the tendon of the biceps brachii muscle (arrow). (Courtesy of C. W. McIlwraith.)

shoulder muscles and, in particular, the biceps brachii muscle may be present. A higher heel and a lowered toe on the hoof of the affected limb may also be evident. At exercise, a mild to moderate (grade 1 to 2) lameness is usually seen. The lameness is generally manifested by a reduction in the cranial phase of the stride, a decrease in the foot flight arc, and a reduction in the flexion of the carpus during the swing phase. Even if the condition is bilateral, one limb is usually more affected than the other. Deep palpation of the biceps tendon and muscle and manipulation of the shoulder through a range of motion usually results in a painful response (Fig. 8.337). Intrasynovial anesthesia of the bicipital bursa may be difficult because of the heterotropic bone formation and the degenerative changes associated with the bursa in the most severe cases.

Diagnosis

Radiographs are required to make a definitive diagnosis (Fig. 8.341). Ultrasound examination may also help identify other tendon and bursal pathologies associated with the heterotopic bone formation. In addition, ultrasound can identify changes in the contour of the tubercles forming the bicipital groove.

Treatment

In horses exhibiting mild to moderate lameness, the administration of anti-inflammatory agents is rational. NSAIDs administered at low doses as needed may allow the horse to be used for light work. If intrasynovial anesthesia of the bursa results in a reduction in lameness, it is logical that injection of a corticosteroid and hyaluronan would also be beneficial. Although the most effective treatment for calcifying tendinopathy in humans remains unclear,[7] treatment in horses should be aimed at removing the calcium deposits, because pain appears to be associated with the active reposition of the deposits.[2,6,7] In a report on calcifying tendinopathy of the biceps brachii resulting in lameness in a dog, the dog responded favorably to the surgical removal of the calcific mass, followed by a longitudinal suture of the transected tendon fibers.[4] To my knowledge, surgical treatment of ossification of the biceps tendon has not been described in the horse. That being said, it would be interesting to see what could be done with arthroscopy.

Prognosis

Too few cases have been reported to determine an expected prognosis.

References

1. Dyson S. Sixteen fractures of the shoulder region in the horse. Equine Vet J 1985;17:104–110.
2. Garner J, Simons B. Analysis of calcific deposits in calcifying tendonitis. Clin Orthop 1990;254:111–120.
3. Meagher DM, Pool RR, Brown MP. Bilateral ossification of the tendon of the biceps brachii muscle in the horse. J Am Vet Med Assoc 1979;174:282.

4. Muir P, Goldsmidt SE, Rothwell TLW, Bellenger CR. Calcifying tendinopathy of the biceps brachii in a dog. J Am Vet Med Assoc 1992;201:1747–1749.
5. Pankowski RL, Grant BD, Sande R, Nickels FA. Fracture of the supraglenoid tubercle: Treatment and results in five horses. Vet Surg 1986;15:33–39.
6. Resnick D. Calcium hydroxyapatite crystal deposition disease. In: Resnick D, Niwayama G, Eds. Diagnosis of Bone and Joint Disorders. 2nd ed. Philadelphia: WB Saunders, 1988;1733–1764.
7. Uhthoff HK, Sarkar K, Maynard JA. Calcifying tendonitis a new concept of its pathogenesis. Clin Orthop 1976;118:164–168.

INFLAMMATION OF THE INFRASPINATUS BURSA

Rooney described a rarely reported lameness caused by inflammation of the infraspinatus bursa.[1] The infraspinatus bursa is located between the tendon of the infraspinatus muscle and the caudal eminence of the greater tubercle of the proximal humerus.

Causes

Severe adduction of the forelimb and/or the possibility of direct trauma to this region is considered to be the cause.[1] A horse that is cast in lateral recumbency with the lower forelimb entrapped may develop the condition while struggling to become free.

Signs

The involved forelimb may be held in an abducted position, presumably in an attempt to reduce the pressure on the infraspinatus bursa. During exercise, a moderate lameness is present.[1] Adduction of the limb reportedly elicits a painful response and results in increased signs of lameness at exercise (Fig. 8.342).[1]

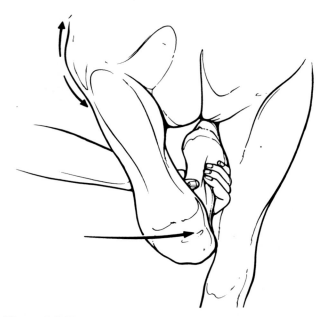

Figure 8.342 Adduction of the limb results in a painful response in horses with infraspinatus bursitis.

Treatment

In the acute stage, synoviocentesis and the administration of corticosteroids into the bursa are recommended. With sufficient stall rest (6 weeks or more) and the parenteral administration of NSAIDs, a good end result can be expected. Although this treatment can be used in chronic cases, the result is usually less gratifying, and some degree of lameness may remain.[1]

Prognosis

There are not enough data to determine the prognosis.

Reference

1. Rooney JR. Biomechanics of Lameness in the Horse. Baltimore: Williams & Wilkins, 1969;117.

OSTEOCHONDROSIS OF THE SCAPULOHUMERAL (SHOULDER) JOINT

Osteochondrosis of the scapulohumeral joint (SHJ) primarily affects young, rapidly growing horses. This is not surprising, because the primary lesion involves growing epiphyseal cartilage. The condition is most frequently diagnosed in weanlings and yearlings 6 to 12 months of age, but it has been reported in foals younger than 5 months and in horses up to 4 years of age.[3,5,7,9,11–13,15,16]

It has been suggested that the incidence of osteochondrosis is related to the rate of skeletal growth and body size; however, many affected horses appear to be normal in size for their breed and age, and some may be smaller and lighter than expected.[11] Males appear to be more commonly affected than females, and no specific breed predilection has been identified.

Although the condition is less common than osteochondritis dissecans (OCD) lesions found elsewhere, one study reported osteochondrosis of the SHJ in 54 joints of 38 young horses radiographed for shoulder problems.[13] In another study, osteochondrosis and subchondral bone cysts were observed in six of 29 horses diagnosed with SHJ problems.[5] The condition is considered the most debilitating form of OCD; and when it is diagnosed in older yearlings, the chronic manifestation of secondary degenerative joint (DJD) changes are usually present. In one study, the incidence of secondary DJD associated with osteochondrosis of the shoulder was reported in 35 of 54 joints.[13]

The primary cartilage lesion is located in the glenoid, the humeral head, or both (most common), and the disease often affects a major part of the joint surface.[13] When the caudal humeral head is involved, the lesion is similar to OCD lesions reported for many other species, except that a dissecans (dissecting) lesion is often not observed.[13] Regardless of the site of the lesion, secondary degenerative changes in the SHJ are prominent features of this disease. An exception to this is the solitary subchondral cystic lesions that are occasionally seen in the glenoid cavity; in these cases, secondary degenerative changes are not prominent.[5]

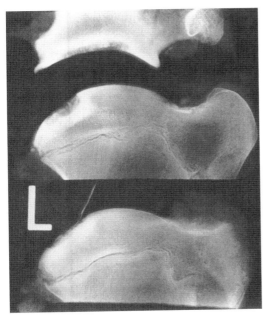

Figure 8.347   Top. Osteochondrosis in the right glenoid (cadaver specimen with the soft tissues removed). Note that the glenoid contour is abnormal and osteophytes are present at both the cranial and caudal rim. Middle. Osteochondrosis of the caudal humeral head. Note the subchondral sclerosis. Bottom. Caudal aspect of the left shoulder. Note the flattened humeral head.

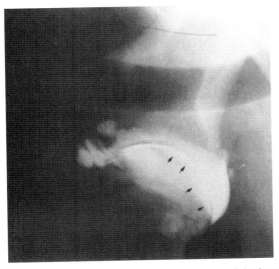

Figure 8.348   Arthrography of the shoulder joint of the horse shown in Figure 8.342 reveals OCD of the caudal margin of the humeral head. Arrows point to contrast material below the articular cartilage.

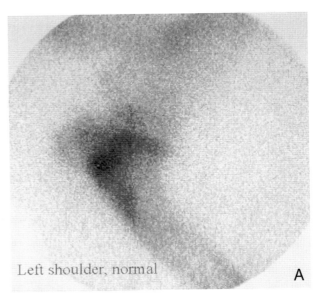

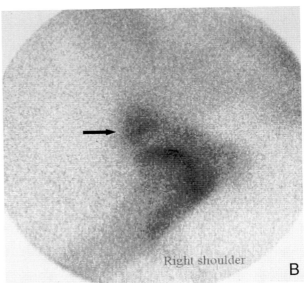

Figure 8.349   A. Scintigraphy of the left shoulder reveals normal uptake of the radionuclide. B. Scintigraphy of the right shoulder, however, reveals increased uptake of the radionuclide in the caudal aspect of the glenoid (arrow). (Courtesy of P. Steyn.)

ited usefulness in evaluating chronic injuries associated with osteochondrosis (Howard RD, McIlwraith CW, unpublished data, 1995). However, one study done on horses with subtle osteochondral lesions in the SHJ found that 4 of 6 horses had localization of the radioisotope in the humeral head: 1 had diffuse localization in the humeral head growth plate, and 3 had focal intense localization in the humeral head[4] (Fig. 8.349).

Arthroscopy may be useful for making a definitive diagnosis in cases in which the lameness is localized to the SHJ with intrasynovial anesthesia but a lesion is not identified on radiography or scintigraphy. The conclusions in one study done on 15 horses with subtle osteochondral lesions in the SHJ suggested that a combination of a physical examination, radiology, scintigraphy, and arthroscopy may be necessary to make the diagnosis.[4]

Treatment

Treatment approaches have included rest and confinement for up to 16 months with the administration of

NSAIDs (sometimes with intraarticular anti-inflammatory agents) and surgery. Rest and confinement may be considered for horses not intended for athletic performance that have mild to moderate radiographic changes.[9,13,14] Of the 17 horses treated with rest in one study, 7 horses saw a moderately successful outcome—2 were used for pleasure, 1 for racing, and 4 as brood stock.[13] Minimal radiographic changes were seen in 3 of these horses and moderate changes occurred in 2

horses. The 2 horses that had severe bilateral shoulder osteochondrosis were used for breeding. The remaining 10 horses in the study remained severely lame after the rest period, and euthanasia was recommended. All 10 had severe radiographic changes at the time of initial diagnosis.

In another report, three horses with isolated subchondral cysts in the glenoid were given 20-mg sodium hyaluronate injections into the affected SHJ. Two of the

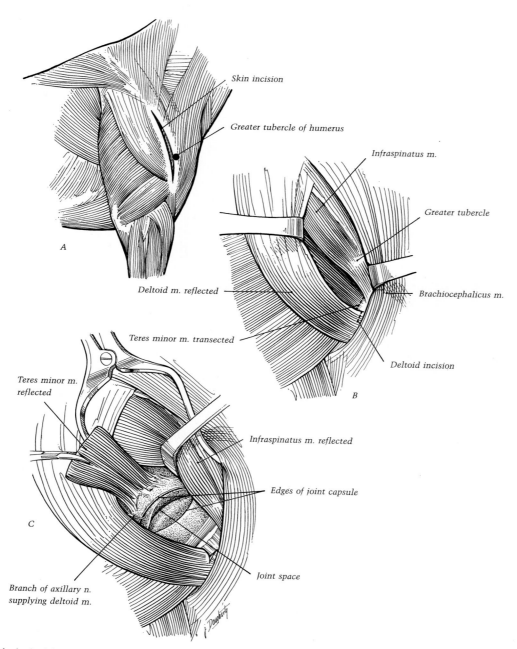

Figure 8.350 A. An incision is made just caudal to the scapular spine and greater tubercle of the humerus to separate the cranial brachiocephalicus and the caudal deltoideus. B. The brachiocephalicus and deltoideus muscles are retracted to expose the infraspinatus and teres minor muscles. Dotted lines, position for infraspinatus tenotomy; lower dotted line, partial tenotomy of the deltoideus muscle. C. The teres minor muscle is reflected proximad to expose the shoulder joint. A transverse incision is made in the joint capsule. Good exposure of the caudal aspect of the humeral head is obtained with this approach.

horses saw rapid improvement; one raced successfully despite intermittent lameness, and the other became lame after 6 months and was euthanized.[5]

Both arthrotomy and arthroscopic approaches have been described for the surgical treatment of shoulder osteochondrosis.[1–3,7,8,10,15] Surgical cases should be selected carefully, because of the generalized pathologic changes that are seen in many cases. However, surgery will benefit some horses even when secondary changes are noted.[1,3] The prognosis is poor where there are severe degenerative changes, and surgery is not recommended.

Extensive soft tissue dissection is required to make the approach for arthrotomy (Fig. 8.349). Once the arthrotomy is made, distal limb manipulation usually allows the lateral and proximal, but not the craniomedial aspects, of the joint to be explored. In two reports on three cases of shoulder osteochondrosis, a transverse infraspinatus tenotomy was used to gain access to the joint.[7,15] At the 1-year follow-up, a marked improvement in lameness was observed but slight lameness was still present after intense exercise.[7] The other horse was put in training 12 months after surgery.[15]

DeBowes et al.[3] reported on a modified surgical approach to the scapulohumeral joint through a longitudinal infraspinatus tenotomy. The technique provided adequate exposure and did not compromise the lateral support to the shoulder, which occurs with the transverse infraspinatus tenotomy. In my experience, the longitudinal infraspinatus tenotomy does not provide adequate exposure to the caudal aspect of the scapulohumeral joint.

In a report on 6 cases, a tenotomy of the insertion of the teres minor muscle was used to expose the scapulohumeral joint (Fig. 8.350).[12] The approach gives excellent access to the caudal aspect of the SHJ. Extreme adduction of the distal limb helps open the joint. Follow-up indicates good healing without loss of lateral support to the shoulder joint, and the long-term follow up has been encouraging.

Arthroscopic surgery has been used to treat these lesions and it is the preferred approach.[1,2,8,10] The advantages of arthroscopy over arthrotomy are improved visualization of the whole joint and reduced surgical morbidity; however the technique is not easy to perform and is particularly difficult in adult horses. The technique is described elsewhere.[1,2,8,10] In most instances, the cartilaginous changes extend beyond the limits of the subchondral abnormalities seen on radiographic examination. Problems associated with arthroscopic surgery in the shoulder include difficulty in arthroscope placement, difficulty with triangulation, extravasation of fluids, and difficulty reaching some lesions.

Prognosis

Generally, the prognosis with rest or surgery is considered guarded to poor, but this depends somewhat on what the horse is to be used for and the severity of the osteochondrosis lesion. Horses with mild to moderate osteochondrosis have the best prognosis; and those with severe lesions usually remain lame, but a small percentage may be used for breeding. There is concern regarding the use of these animals for breeding, however, because

there may be an associated genetic link for rapid skeletal growth and subsequent development of osteochondrosis.

In one report on the outcome of arthroscopic surgery on 11 horses (13 joints), 7 horses became athletically sound and 4 remained lame.[1] Follow-up radiographic examination on the sound horses indicated remodeling and improved contour of the glenoid and humeral head. In another study, long-term follow-up on 35 horses with osteochondrosis of the shoulder treated arthroscopically found that 16 horses were successfully treated and 19 were unable to return to athletic performance.[6]

References

1. Bertone AL, McIlwraith CW, Powers BE, Stashak TS. Arthroscopic surgery for the treatment of osteochondrosis in the equine shoulder joint. Vet Surg 1987;16:303–311.
2. Bertone AL, McIlwraith CW. Osteochondrosis of the equine shoulder: Treatment with arthroscopic surgery. Am Assoc Equine Pract 1987;33:683–688.
3. DeBowes RM, Wagner DC, Grant BD. Surgical approach to the equine scapulohumeral joint through a longitudinal infraspinatus tenotomy. Vet Surg 1982;11:125.
4. Doyle PS, White NA. Diagnostic findings and prognosis following arthroscopic treatment of subtle osteochondral lesions in the shoulder joint of horses: 15 cases (1996–1999). J Am Vet Med Assoc 2000;217:1878–1882.
5. Dyson S. Diagnostic techniques in the investigation of shoulder lameness. Equine Vet J 1986;18:25–28.
6. Dyson S. Shoulder lameness in horses: An analysis of 58 suspected cases. Equine Vet J 1986;18:29–36.
7. Mason TA, MacLean AA. Osteochondrosis dissecans of the head of the humerus in two foals. Equine Vet J 1977;9:189.
8. McIlwraith CW. Diagnostic and Surgical Arthroscopy in the Horse. 2nd ed. Philadelphia: Lea & Febiger, 1990;113–159.
9. Meagher DM, Pool R, O'Brien TR. Osteochondritis of the shoulder joint in the horse. Am Assoc Equine Pract 1977;19:247.
10. Nixon AJ. Diagnostic and surgical arthroscopy of the equine shoulder joint. Vet Surg 1987;16:44–52.
11. Nixon AJ. Osteochondrosis of the shoulder and elbow. In: White NA, Moore JN, Eds. Current Practice of Equine Surgery. Philadelphia: JB Lippincott, 1990;516–526.
12. Nixon AJ, Stashak TS, McIlwraith CW, et al. A muscle separating approach to the equine shoulder joint for the treatment of osteochondritis dissecans. Vet Surg 1984;13:247.
13. Nyack B, Morgan JP, Pool RR. Osteochondrosis of the shoulder joint of the horse. Cornell Vet 1981;71:149.
14. Rose B, Carlsen J. Results of conservative management of osteochondrosis in the horse. Am Assoc Equine Pract 1985;31:617–626.
15. Schmidt GR, Dueland R, Vaughn JT. Osteochondrosis dissecans of the equine shoulder joint. Vet Med Small Anim Clin 1975;70:542.
16. Shebitz H. Degenerative arthritis of the shoulder joint following aseptic necrosis of the humeral head in foals. Am Assoc Equine Pract 1965;11:359.
17. Tnibar MA, Auer JA, Bakkali S. Ultrasonography of the equine shoulder: Technique and normal appearance. Vet Radiol Ultrasound 1999;40:44–57.

ARTHRITIS OF THE SCAPULOHUMERAL JOINT

Arthritis of the SHJ is a relatively uncommon condition that can affect horses of a variety of breeds, ages, and uses. One report found that 3 of 29 horses with a clinical diagnosis of shoulder lameness had arthrosis.[8] Another study examined 15 horses diagnosed with subtle osteochondral changes in the SHJ that caused lameness in one limb. It found that a wide range of breeds was affected and the ages of the horses ranged from 1 to 11 years (median = 4.7 years).[5] Affected horses were also used for a variety of performance activities, including racing, show jumping, dressage, three-day eventing, field hunting, and carriage. Another report found a higher prevalence of osteoarthritis in Shetland ponies than in other breeds.[3]

Although the recognition and treatment of conditions associated with SHJ has improved, the diagnosis of specific problems related to this joint still remains a challenge.[5] As a result, some horses may require extensive diagnostic imaging, including arthroscopy, before a definitive diagnosis can be made. Unfortunately, the delay in recognition of the cause of the arthritis may increase the likelihood of the development of secondary osteoarthritis, much like what is seen with osteochondrosis in this joint.[14,17]

Arthritis of the SHJ caused by infection and osteochondrosis is not discussed in this section; instead see Chapter 7 and "Osteochondrosis of the Scapulohumeral (Shoulder) Joint" in this chapter. Large intraarticular fractures of the SHJ associated with the proximal humerus and glenoid are covered elsewhere in this chapter.

Causes

Arthritis of the SHJ can have multiple causes, some of which are believed to be developmental, others involve trauma, and the horse's age may play a role.[5,10] In one study, the fracture or cartilage lesions in horses younger than 4 years of age were thought to be the result of osteochondrosis; and cartilage fracture, fibrillation, malacia, or subchondral bone damage in horses older than 4 years of age was thought to be the result of a traumatic insult.[5] A radiographic study compared young Shetland ponies diagnosed with osteoarthritis to skeletally mature Shetland ponies without a history of lameness and to skeletally mature horses. It was found that ponies had a flattening (dysplasia) of the glenoid contour, which was believed to have made them more susceptible to the development of osteoarthritis.[3] Other causes of arthritis include intraarticular fracture and injury to the joint capsule, resulting in a synovitis and capsulitis.

Signs

A history of trauma is relatively common. In one report, 8 of 15 horses that had subtle osteochondral lesions in the SHJ had a history of a traumatic insult.[5] Mild swelling may be apparent over the shoulder region in acute cases, but muscle atrophy is less consistent and may not reflect chronicity or severity of the lameness.[6,9] Disuse atrophy of the extensor carpi radialis muscle may be apparent in the affected limb. An upright narrow foot may be observed in the affected limb. One study found a narrow upright foot in 12 of 15 horses with shoulder arthritis, suggesting that this foot conformation probably indicates shoulder problems.[5] In another study, only a small proportion (less than 5%) of horses with shoulder problems had a smaller foot on the affected limb, although a severely lame horse may have abnormal toe wear.[6,9]

Deep thumb pressure applied just cranial to the tendon of the infraspinatus muscle may elicit a painful response in young and in light-muscled mature horses (Fig. 8.345). Upper limb manipulation (flexion, extension, adduction, and abduction) may cause a painful response.[1,9]

In general, the signs of lameness are typical and the degree depends on the severity of the problem. If the lameness is moderate or severe, it will be evident at a walk and trot. At a trot, the height of the foot flight and the flexion of the carpus are decreased during the swing phase of the stride compared to the contralateral limb. The cranial phase of the stride of the lame limb is often shortened. The head and neck drop as the sound limb bears weight, but as the lame limb is advanced a prominent lifting of the head and neck occurs on the affected side.[9] In addition, the horse appears to "fix" the SHJ on the affected side.[1] Careful observation of the shoulder region during movement reveals the difference between the normal and the affected sides. The lameness grade in one study ranged from subtle and intermittent to 4 (on a scale of 5).[5] Manipulative tests and a flexion test of the upper forelimb do not always accentuate the lameness.[5,8]

Diagnostic anesthesia can assist in localizing the problem to the shoulder region.[1,5,6,9] Median, medial, cutaneous, antebrachial, and ulnar nerve blocks are used to eliminate the carpus and below as the source of lameness in most horses; and intrasynovial anesthesia of the SHJ usually localizes the problem to the joint (see Chapter 3). Improvement after intrasynovial anesthesia may be apparent in 5 minutes but may take as long as 1 hour.[9] This prolonged exposure before improvement may indicate an injury in the subchondral bone. In addition, the response to intrasynovial anesthesia can range from complete resolution of the lameness to only slight improvement.[9] In one report, intrasynovial anesthesia was used in 10 horses and 9 improved—by one grade in 2 horses and by two grades or complete resolution in the remaining horses.[5]

Diagnosis

Radiography, ultrasonography, nuclear medicine, and/or arthroscopy may be required to make a definitive diagnosis of the problem.[1,5,6] Radiography, although important in evaluating abnormalities of the shoulder joint, may be limited, because the articular cartilage and synovial membrane cannot be evaluated and subtle or delayed changes in the subchondral bone may be missed.[6,12] When a lesion is identified, radiography often underestimates the full extent of the changes involving the glenoid cavity and the humeral head. Also, because confusing air shadows may be evident for several hours after intrasynovial anesthesia, it is recommended that 6 to 8 hours should elapse after the injection and before the radiography is done.[6,7] Radiographic changes identified in one report in horses with subtle lesions in the SHJ included glenoid sclerosis, focal glenoid lysis, glenoid cysts, and alteration in the humeral head contour.[5] In another report, a flattening of the glenoid without changes in the contour of the humeral head was seen in Shetland ponies.[3] Other radiographic changes associated with arthritis include osteophyte and enthesiophyte formation.

Contrast arthrography may improve the chances of identifying a SHJ lesion.[9,14] However, general anesthesia is recommended, and the contrast material does induce a synovitis that lasts for 2 to 3 days.

The normal ultrasonographic anatomy of the shoulder region has been described.[16] Although the detection of humeral head osteochondrosis has been reported, its major value appears to be in identifying injury to the soft tissue support structures surrounding the SHJ.[1,6,16] Evaluation of the glenoid cavity with ultrasound appears to be limited.[5]

Nuclear medicine (scintigraphy) is a sensitive means of detecting increased bone metabolism and is frequently used for localizing lameness.[4,15,18] In one report, scintigraphic evaluation was used in 6 horses, 4 of which had scintigraphic abnormalities, including focal intense uptake of the radioisotope in the humeral head (3 horses) and diffuse uptake of the radioisotope of the humeral growth plate (1 horse).[5]

Arthroscopy is recognized as a valuable diagnostic technique for evaluating joints.[2,11–13] Arthroscopic abnormalities found in one study of 15 horses with subtle osteochondral lesions included clefts in the glenoid cartilage (4 horses), glenoid cysts (8), humeral head cysts (1), fibrillation of the humeral head cartilage (3), cartilage fragmentation (1), and nondisplaced fracture of the humeral head (1).[5]

Treatment

Conservative treatment may be indicated in horses that have no radiographic lesions and that respond favorably to intrasynovial anesthesia of the SHJ.[8] Treatment involves adequate rest, the administration anti-inflammatory drugs, and controlled exercise. Rest periods may be as short as a few weeks to 3 months. NSAIDs and the intrasynovial administration of a corticosteroid and sodium hyaluronate are often indicated. (For a discussion of the treatment of arthritis, see Chapter 7.)

Horses that do not respond to the conservative treatment or have radiographic or scintigraphic changes and have responded favorably to intrasynovial anesthesia are candidates for arthroscopy.[5] Localized cartilage damage is debrided down to healthy subchondral bone, and osteochondral fragments are removed if they are loose.

Prognosis

The prognosis is favorable for horses without radiographic-apparent lesions that respond favorably to intraarticular anesthesia treated conservatively. In one report of three horses treated conservatively—two with rest and intraarticular sodium hyaluronate and one with rest only—the two that received injections were able to return to full work.[8] The other horse improved but remained intermittently lame at the 1-year follow-up.

The prognosis for horses treated by arthroscopy appears good for subtle cartilage lesions. In one report of 15 horses with subtle osteochondral lesions in the SHJ, 12 horses were able to return to their previous level of performance.[5] Of the other horses, 1 was sound for light riding, 1 remained lame, and 1 was euthanatized.

References

1. Adams SB, Blevins WE. Shoulder lameness in horses—Part 1. Contin Educ 1989;11:64–70.
2. Bertone AL, McIlwraith CW, Powers BE, et al. Arthroscopic surgery for the treatment of osteochondrosis in the equine shoulder joint. Vet Surg 1987;16:303–311.
3. Boswell JC, Schramme MC, Wilson AM. A radiological study to evaluate suspected scapulohumeral joint dysplasia in Shetland ponies. Proceedings. 8th Annual ECVS Meeting, Brugge, Belgium, 1999;51–53.
4. Devous MD, Twardock AR. Techniques and applications of nuclear medicine in the diagnosis of equine lameness. J Am Vet Med Assoc 1984;184:318–325.
5. Doyle PS, White NA. Diagnostic findings and prognosis following arthroscopic treatment of subtle osteochondral lesions in the shoulder joint of horses: 15 cases (1996–1999). J Am Vet Med Assoc 2000;217:1878–1882.
6. Dyson S. Diagnostic techniques in the investigation of shoulder lameness. Equine Vet J 1986;18:25–28.
7. Dyson S. Interpreting radiographs 7: Radiology of the equine shoulder and elbow. Equine Vet J 1986;18:352–361.
8. Dyson S. Shoulder lameness in horses: An analysis of 58 suspected cases. Equine Vet J 1986;18:29–36.
9. Dyson S. Shoulder lameness in horses: Diagnosis and differential diagnosis. Am Assoc Equine Pract 1987;32:461–480.
10. Johnson JH, Bartels JE. Conditions of the forelimb. In: Catcott EJ, Smithcors JF, Eds. Equine Medicine and Surgery. 2nd ed. Wheaton, IL: American Veterinary Publications, 1972;505–562.
11. McIlwraith WC, Bertone AL. Diagnostic and surgical arthroscopy of the scapulohumeral (shoulder) joint. In: McIlwraith CW, Ed. Diagnostic and Surgical Arthroscopy in the Horse. 2nd ed. Philadelphia: Lea & Febiger 1990;196–209.
12. Moore RM, Schneider RK. Arthroscopic findings in the carpal joints of lame horses without radiographically visible abnormalities: 42 cases (1986–1991). J Am Vet Med Assoc 1995;206: 1741–1746.
13. Nixon AJ. Diagnostic and surgical arthroscopy of the equine shoulder joint. Vet Surg 1987;16:44–52.
14. Nixon AJ. Osteochondrosis of the shoulder and elbow. In: White NA, Moore JN, Eds. Current Practice of Equine Surgery. Philadelphia: JB Lippincott, 1990;516–526.
15. O'Callaghan MW. The integration of radiography and alternative imaging methods in the diagnosis of equine orthopedic disease. Vet Clin North Am Equine Pract 1991;7:339–364.
16. Tnibar MA, Auer JA, Bakkali S. Ultrasonography of the equine shoulder: Technique and normal appearance. Vet Radiol Ultrasound 1999;40:44–57.
17. Trotter GW, McIlwraith CW. Osteochondritis dissecans and subchondral cystic lesions and their relationship to osteochondrosis in the horse. J Equine Vet Sci 1981;1:157–162.
18. Williams J, Miyabayashi T, Ruggles A, et al. Scintigraphic and ultrasonographic diagnosis of soft tissue injury in the Thoroughbred horse. J Vet Med Sci 1994;56:169–172.

SUBLUXATION AND LUXATION OF THE SCAPULOHUMERAL JOINT

Luxation and subluxation of the SHJ occur uncommonly in horses. In a survey of 128 cases of suspected shoulder lameness in horses, a diagnosis was made in 51. Of theses only 2 horses had shoulder luxation.[6] Ponies appear to be at a greater risk for this condition. Of the 6 reported cases of SHJ luxation, 4 have been in ponies.[3,5,7,8,12] The head of the humerus can displace in several directions, including cranial,[9,10,12] craniolateral, lateral, craniomedial, and medial.[3,5,7] When the humerus becomes luxated, it displaces proximad owing to the contraction of the muscles surrounding the SHJ, and the direction of the luxation appears to depend on direction of the inciting injury.[5] Of the cases presented for which the direction of the luxation was documented, lateral

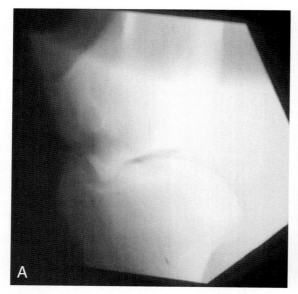
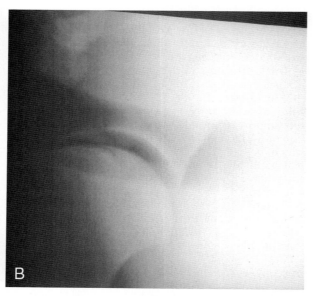

Figure 8.351   A. Stress lateral view of a subluxation of the SHJ. Note the position of the glenoid in relation to the humeral head. The glenoid extends too far cranial. B. The contralateral forelimb of the same horse. Note the position of the glenoid in relation to the humeral head.

luxation with proximal displacement was most common.[5,8,9] Because the equine SHJ is stabilized by a ball and socket articulation, the tendons from surrounding muscles, and the glenohumeral ligaments within the joint capsule, it is not surprising that luxation of the joint results in considerable damage to these structures.[3,5,11] Arthroscopic examination after closed reduction of a luxated SHJ of 2 weeks' duration revealed bony and soft tissue debris, a cartilage defect, and a tear in the joint capsule.[9] I have documented 1 case of subluxation of the SHJ (Fig. 8.351).

Causes

Luxation of the SHJ generally occurs after excessive (forceful) trauma to the shoulder region, such as may occur from a fall, when attempting to jump a fence, as a result of pulling and twisting the flexed limb while the foot is caught fast.[3,8,9,12] One report documented SHJ luxation in a septicemic foal with multiple joint laxity.[7] Luxation of the SHJ has also occurred after removal of a large supraglenoid tubercle fragment.[1,2] The cause of subluxation is unknown, but it is presumed to result from a similar but less forceful injury than that associated with luxation.

Signs

A history of trauma with an acute onset of severe lameness is common.[1,2,5,8,12] At presentation, horses typically exhibit a non-weight-bearing lameness. An abnormal stance may also be apparent, with the elbow and carpus held semiflexed and the distal limb adducted (displaced inward) or abducted (displaced outward), depending on the direction of the luxation. The distal limb is adducted when the humerus is luxated laterally, cranio-laterally, or cranially and is slightly abducted when the humerus is luxated medially. Some degree of swelling is present in the shoulder region, depending on the duration since injury.

Muscle atrophy may be most prominent in chronic cases. One report found significant muscle atrophy of the infraspinatus and supraspinatus muscles 2 weeks after luxation of the SHJ.[9] Distortion of the normal anatomic landmarks at the shoulder region may be apparent if swelling is not excessive. This anatomic distortion may aid in determining the direction of the luxation. With lateral or cranial luxation, the greater tubercle and head of the humerus may be most prominent; and with medial displacement, the lateral lip of the glenoid cavity can be felt.[9,10] Affected horses generally violently oppose upper limb manipulation.[3,8]

With the one case of SHJ subluxation that I saw, the horse had a history of lameness for 4 months' duration that worsened with exercise, and the horse was exercised regularly at a low level. During the physical examination, deep palpation of the biceps brachii and upper limb manipulation elicited a painful response. The response was compared to that found on the opposite forelimb. At exercise, a grade 1 lameness at a trot on the straightaway was observed in the affected limb. The lameness increased to grade 2+ when the horse was circled with the affected limb on the inside. Diagnostic anesthesia of the lower limb did not alter the lameness.

Diagnosis

Radiographs should be taken to confirm the diagnosis and to rule out fracture (Figs. 8.351 and 8.352). Generally, an adequate study can be obtained in the standing horse, and the mediolateral view is thought to be the most informative.[6] The addition of the craniocaudal oblique projection allows a better assessment of the di-

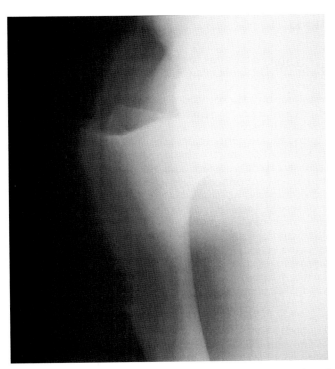

Figure 8.352 Cranial-caudal oblique view showing a luxation of the SHJ. Note that the humeral head does not articulate with the glenoid.

rection of the luxation.[4] Ultrasound examination may also be used to assess the extent of injury to the soft tissues supporting the SHJ.

Treatment

Ideally, the luxation should be corrected as soon as possible. General anesthesia is required in most cases, although there is one report of correction of a SHJ luxation using sedation in a 5-day-old foal with multiple joint laxity.[7] In all cases, the anesthetic induction should be assisted to avoid further damage to the soft tissues or joint. A sling was used to confine and support one horse with SHJ luxation before general anesthesia was induced.[9]

For foals, it is possible to pull the affected limb into extension while an assistant pushes or pulls the humeral head back into position. The foal may have to be stabilized with counterpressure applied to the chest or axilla. A mature horse can be placed in lateral or dorsal recumbency. In lateral recumbency, the body can be anchored to a fixed object and a tension-creating device attached to the radius or pastern region is used to apply traction while the operator forces the shoulder back into position. When a calving jack is used, the counterpressure (tail) portion of the jack can be placed against the sternum.[10] If the horse is placed in dorsal recumbency, a hoist can be used to apply traction, and the body weight is sufficient to provide the counterweight.[12] An audible click may be heard when the humeral head is reduced, after which it should be possible to freely manipulate the joint.[3,8]

In acute cases, reduction may be accomplished quickly. Reduction in one case of SHJ luxation was readily achieved in a pony while the affected limb was being manipulated to position the anesthetized patient.[3] In more chronic cases, reduction may require 30 minutes of gradually increasing the traction along with limb manipulation.[9] Arthroscopic examination of the SHJ after closed reduction may improve the outcome, particularly if there is evidence of bony debris within the joint on radiography.[9] A radiograph should be taken of the SHJ after the reduction is complete.

Recovery from anesthesia should be assisted in all cases. After recovery, the horse should have strict stall rest for 2 months to allow healing of the joint capsule and surrounding soft tissue structures.[3] Phenylbutazone is usually administered for 10 to 14 days to reduce inflammation and encourage ambulation of the horse. Then the horse is evaluated for suitability for free exercise and subsequent riding. Recurrence of the luxation—common in dogs—does not appear to be a problem in horses.[12]

For subluxation, stall rest is recommended for 6 weeks and phenylbutazone should be administered at a low dose for 10 days. Hand-walking exercise (5 minutes twice a day for 5 days a week) is begun after the 2nd week. The exercise period is increased by 2.5 minutes per week until the 6-week follow-up. At that time the lameness should have improved appreciably and the controlled exercise program can be accelerated. Reports of further follow-up were not available at the time of this writing.

Prognosis

The prognosis for SHJ luxation is considered good for return to soundness after closed reduction and an adequate rest period when there is no complicating fracture. All 6 reported horses with SHJ luxation treated by closed reduction returned to soundness.[1-3,5,8,9] The prognosis for larger horses may also be good. One report described shoulder luxation in a Thoroughbred filly.[9] The filly was sound for light work 8 months after closed reduction and arthroscopic examination of the joint. It has been suggested that the prognosis may be improved and more accurately predicted if arthroscopy is used after closed reduction.[3]

The prognosis for subluxation, although not well documented, seems to be favorable after an adequate rest period, as long as other complicating factors (fractures, DJD) do not exist.

References

1. Bleyaert H. Scapulohumeral joint luxations. In: White NA, Moore JN, Eds. Current Practice of Equine Surgery. Philadelphia: WB Saunders, 1998;423–424.
2. Bleyaert HB, Sullins KE, White NA. Supraglenoid tubercle fractures in horses. Comp Cont Educ Vet Pract 1994;16:531–536.
3. Colbourne CM, Yovich JV, Bolton JR. The diagnosis and successful treatment of shoulder luxation in a pony. Aust Equine Vet 1991; 9:100–102.
4. Dyson S. Interpreting radiographs 7: Radiology of the equine shoulder and elbow. Equine Vet J 1986;18:352–361.
5. Dyson S. Shoulder lameness in horses: An analysis of 58 suspected cases. Equine Vet J 1986;18:29–36.

6. Dyson S. Shoulder lameness in horses: Diagnosis ad differential diagnosis. Am Assoc Equine Pract 1986;32:461.
7. Hardy J, Marohn MA. What is your diagnosis? J Am Vet Med Assoc 1989;195:1773–1774.
8. Littlejohn A. Dislocation of the shoulder of a mare. South Afr Vet Med Assoc 1954;25:46.
9. Madison JB, Young D, Richardson D. Repair of shoulder luxation in a horse. J Am Vet Med Assoc 1991;198:455–456.
10. O'Connor JJ. Dollar's Veterinary Surgery. 4th ed. Chicago: Alexander Eger, 1950;815.
11. Sisson S. Equine syndesmology. In: Getty R, Ed. Sisson and Grossman's The Anatomy of the Domestic Animals. 5th ed. Vol 2. Philadelphia: WB Saunders, 1975;349–375.
12. Wilson RG, Reynolds WT. Scapulohumeral luxation with treatment by closed reduction in a horse. Aust Vet J 1984;61:300–301.

SUPRASCAPULAR NERVE INJURY (SWEENY)

Suprascapular nerve injury resulting in atrophy of the supraspinatus and infraspinatus muscles and shoulder joint instability can affect any age or breed of horse.[1,8,10] The condition was originally reported as most commonly affecting draft breeds and was believed to be associated with repeated trauma to the shoulder region from poorly fitted harness collars. With the decline in draft horses, the condition is most commonly seen as a result of trauma to the shoulder region. The term "Sweeny" has been defined as atrophy of the shoulder muscles in horses and is a commonly used synonym for suprascapular nerve paralysis.[3]

Causes

The cause of Sweeny is believed to be trauma to the suprascapular nerve as it passes over the cranial thin border of the scapula.[1,2,7,8,18,19,21] The suprascapular nerve originates from the C6–7 spinal segments and passes via the brachial plexus to innervate the supraspinatus and infraspinatus muscles that overly the scapula.[11] As the nerve reflects around the cranial edge of the scapula, it passes beneath a small but strong tendinous band. At this location, the nerve appears to be most susceptible to direct trauma and compression against the underlying bone.[7–9]

There is histologic evidence of chronic demyelination and remyelination at the point where the suprascapular nerve reflects over the cranial edge of the scapula in horses with no clinical evidence of muscle atrophy.[9] These findings suggest there may be chronic nerve compression caused by constriction of the small tendinous band, resulting in subclinical neuropathy. This condition is similar to suprascapular entrapment neuropathy in humans.[6] The chronic neuronal injury may make the suprascapular nerve more susceptible to acute trauma and the development of clinical signs or perhaps spontaneous development of the condition, without a traumatic insult, is possible.[7–9]

Overstretching of the suprascapular nerve, resulting in nerve injury, may occur if the limb is suddenly thrust backward.[15,17] Atrophy of the supraspinatus and infraspinatus muscles has been observed after fracture of the supraglenoid tubercle.

Signs

A history of trauma to the shoulder region is relatively common. The clinical signs depend on the extent of the nerve damage and the duration of the condition before examination. Shortly after the injury. affected horses often exhibit severe pain and are reluctant to bear weight on the affected limb. In one report of eight horses with suprascapular nerve injury, the lameness was graded 3 to 5 (out of 5) shortly after the injury occurred.[10]

As the pain subsides and the horse begins to bear weight, a pronounced lateral instability (excursion) of the shoulder joint (shoulder slip) during weight bearing is observed. This sign is usually seen within 24 hours after injury and is most apparent as the horse is walked slowly toward the examiner (Fig. 8.353).[10] The instability is the result of loss of the stabilizing function of the supraspinatus and infraspinatus muscles, which serve as the major lateral support for the shoulder.[15,17] This outward excursion of the scapula during weight bearing may cause intermittent stretching of the suprascapular nerve, leading to continued trauma and perpetuation of the paralysis.[1]

The acute lameness may be followed by complete recovery over a 2- to 3-month period or denervation atrophy of the supraspinatus and infraspinatus muscles may become evident. After injury to the nerve, muscle atrophy usually becomes apparent as early as 10 to 14 days after injury.[10,18,21] Once atrophy begins, the scapular

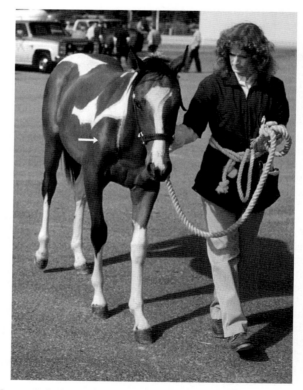

Figure 8.353 Note the lateral displacement of the shoulder (arrow) in this horse with suprascapular nerve injury of 3 weeks' duration.

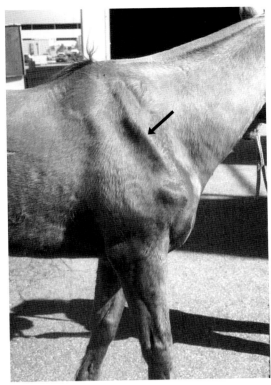

Figure 8.354 Note the prominent atrophy of the supraspinatus and infraspinatus muscles cranial and caudal to the scapular spine (arrow).

spine becomes more prominent owing to the loss of the muscles cranial and caudal to it (Fig. 8.354).

Diagnosis

A presumptive diagnosis of suprascapular nerve injury can be made from the clinical signs and the history of trauma to the region. Radiographs of the region should be obtained to rule out a fracture or DJD of the shoulder. Electromyography (EMG) confirms selective suprascapular nerve injury. For the EMG studies to be most meaningful, they should be performed at a minimum of 7 days after injury.[13,20,21] EMG findings of denervation of muscles supplied by other branches of the brachial plexus should prompt further neurologic evaluation to rule out injuries to the brachial plexus, spinal cord disease at the C6–7 segments, and other diseases (e.g., equine protozoal myelitis).[8,10]

Treatment

Both conservative and surgical treatments have been described for management of horses with suprascapular nerve injury.[1,2,4,8,9,21] Initial treatment in all cases is directed toward reducing inflammation in the region of the suprascapular nerve. Stall rest with the administration of NSAIDs and the topical application of cold hydrotherapy or ice packs and DMSO gel may resolve clinical signs.

Conservative Treatment

When conservative treatment is selected, stall rest is continued until shoulder joint stability returns. The horse is then confined to a pasture for an additional 2 to 4 months. In one study, the mean time for resolution of the gait abnormality was 7.4 months (range = 3 to 12 months) and seven of eight horses evaluated had a complete resolution of the joint instability.[10] The conclusion from this study is that stall rest appeared to be a viable alternative to surgery for the treatment of suprascapular nerve injury. The potential disadvantages of stall rest were the time required for resolution of the joint instability and the possibility that the supraspinatus and infraspinatus muscle mass may not return to normal. It was also speculated that surgical decompression may result in a faster return to athletic function and a better cosmetic result.

The use of acupuncture during the rest period may be beneficial. In one report, two horses with suprascapular nerve injury that received acupuncture became sound; muscle mass returned to normal in one horse and near normal in the other.[2] Injection of a corticosteroid into the shoulder joint may also be beneficial. In one study, six horses with suspected suprascapular nerve injury were treated successfully with intraarticular corticosteroids.[14] However, it is uncertain whether these horses had a true neurapraxia of the suprascapular nerve, SHJ inflammation that caused disuse muscle atrophy, or both. Although joint inflammation would seem to be the most likely cause, intraarticular corticosteroids may have had a local anti-inflammatory effect on the suprascapular nerve and, therefore, may be beneficial. The report also suggests that joint inflammation may be part of the overall injury in some cases, making intraarticular corticosteroids a possible benefit in acute and chronic cases.[14] Therapeutic ultrasound has also been suggested as a treatment.[4]

Surgical Treatment

In patients that continue to exhibit signs of suprascapular nerve dysfunction for 10 to 12 weeks, surgical decompression of the nerve can be considered. This time frame is based on the rate of peripheral nerve regeneration (1 mm/day) and the distance from the site of nerve injury on the cranial border of the scapula to the infraspinatus muscle (7 to 8 cm). Using these parameters, nerve function should return in 10 to 12 weeks.[18] In horses that show no improvement after 12 weeks of rest, entrapment of the suprascapular nerve by scar tissue between the overlying ligament and the cranial border of the scapula is likely. Although the time frame for reversing neurogenic muscle atrophy in a large animal is not known, in humans neurogenic muscle atrophy can be reversed if reinnervation takes place within 20 months.[16,22,23] After that time, irreversible changes within the muscle occur in humans (it is replaced by fibrous tissue).

Surgery is performed with the horse in lateral recumbency and the affected limb uppermost. A 15- to 20-cm skin incision is made beginning 8 to 10 cm above the distal end of the scapular spine and 1 cm cranial to it. The incision is continued through the subcutaneous tis-

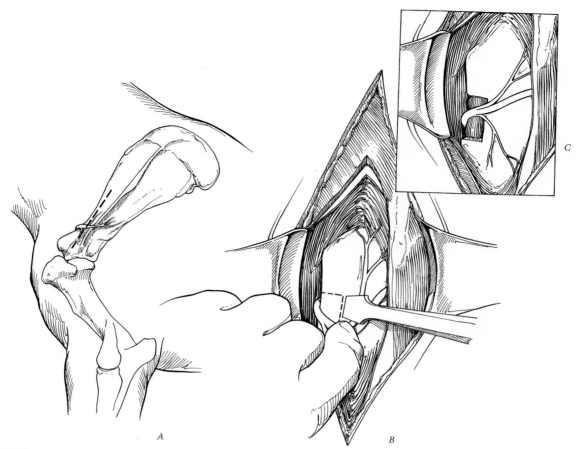

Figure 8.355 A. Location of the skin incision (dotted line), centered over the suprascapular nerve and cranial to scapular spine. B. The suprascapular nerve is identified and a small crescent-shaped piece of bone is removed from the cranial border of the scapula (dotted line). C. The bone has been removed and the tendinous band has been resected.

sue and deep fascia to expose the attachment of the supraspinatus muscle on the scapular spine (Fig. 8.355A). The scapular attachment is then incised 1 cm cranial to the scapular spine, and the supraspinatus muscle is bluntly reflected craniad out of the supraspinous fossa to expose the suprascapular nerve as it reflects over the cranial border of the scapula (Fig. 8.355B). It is important to preserve the fascia deep to the infraspinatus muscle. Leaving it attached to the scapula avoids damage to the nerve beneath it.[21]

Once the nerve is identified, the surrounding scar tissue is gently dissected from the proximal and distal limits of the nerve that is attached to the cranial border of the scapula. Careful dissection is required to identify the limits of the nerve's attachment. Then the nerve is undermined from the cranial border of the scapula. A Penrose drain is placed around the nerve to elevate it so a small crescent-shaped piece of bone on the cranial border of the scapula directly underlying the nerve can be removed (Fig. 8.355C). The bone is removed with a bone rasp, air drill and burr (my preference), small osteotome or chisel, wire saw, Kerrison Ferris-Smith rongeurs, or a combination of these instruments.[4,8,18,21,23] If an osteotome or bone chisel is used, the distal cut in the bone is made first to prevent a possible fracture of the supraglenoid tubercle. The bone edges are smoothed and rounded

with a curette and rongeur. Note that a large piece of bone is not removed, as originally described. Next, the tendinous band on the cranial and medial edge of the scapula superficial to the suprascapular nerve is severed at its distal attachment.

By removing the bone and the attachment of the tendinous band, the surgeon increases the space around the suprascapular nerve and relieves the entrapment caused by fibrous scar tissue.[21] This procedure also seems to reduce nerve tension when viewed intraoperatively, and it is thought to relieve the potential for intermittent tension on the nerve during lateral movement of the shoulder when the horse is weight bearing.

After the Penrose drain is removed, the fascia overlying the suprascapular muscle is apposed to the fascial attachments remaining on the scapular spine with simple interrupted synthetic absorbable suture. Subcutaneous tissues and skin are sutured in a routine manner, after which a stent bandage is sutured over the incision line. The use of a Penrose drain placed deep to the suprascapular muscle is optional.

Because the shoulder joint is unstable, recovery from anesthesia should be assisted in all cases until the horse is awake and appears stable. Assisted recovery decreases the forces on other stabilizing muscles of the shoulder region, in particular the attachment of biceps brachii muscle on the supraglenoid tubercle. Fractures of the supraglenoid tubercle have occurred during anesthetic recovery and in the first few weeks after surgery.[5,18,19,21]

Postoperatively, the horse is maintained on low doses of phenylbutazone for 10 to 14 days to minimize inflammation. The patient is confined to a stall until nerve function returns. The Penrose drain is usually removed in 24 hours. The stent bandage is removed in 4 to 5 days, and the skin sutures are removed in 14 days. Generally, it takes 2 to 3 months before nerve function returns and the horse regains normal function of the supraspinatus and infraspinatus muscles. Shoulder stability should be present before the horse is turned out or exercise rehabilitation is begun.[21]

Prognosis

The prognosis for return to soundness in horses with suprascapular nerve injury is favorable for both conservative and surgical treatments. In one report, seven of eight conservatively treated horses with suprascapular nerve injury were able to return to their intended use: two as brood mares and four to riding or race training.[10] The one horse that was not able to return to its intended use had a bone fragment in the shoulder joint. Although all eight horses had pronounced shoulder joint instability during weight bearing, joint stability returned within 3 to 12 months (mean = 7.4 months). Return of the supraspinatus and infraspinatus muscle mass was complete in two horses 15 and 18 months after injury and 50% complete in three horses between 5 and 12 months after injury. Two horses did not have a substantial return of muscle mass at the time of reexamination. The conclusion is that rest alone carries a good prognosis for recovery of a normal gait and return to performance; however, the recovery period may be prolonged.

A high percentage of horses that undergo surgical treatment are expected to return to performance. In one report, 18 of 20 horses with suprascapular nerve injury returned to soundness.[18] An important and severe complication associated with the surgery is the postoperative occurrence of fracture of the supraglenoid tubercle and complete subluxation of the SHJ. Both complications occur during anesthetic recovery,[12,18] and fracture may occur during postoperative stall confinement.[5,18] This complication can largely be prevented if the piece of bone is removed during surgery and the horse is assisted during recovery from anesthesia. Horses that develop severe atrophy of the supraspinatus and infraspinatus muscles may not regain normal muscle mass, and some atrophy will remain in the proximal third of the scapula.

References

1. Adams OR. Lameness in Horses. 3rd ed. Philadelphia: Lea & Febiger, 1974.
2. Adams OR, Schneider RK, Bramlage LR, et al. A surgical approach to treatment of suprascapular nerve injury in the horse. J Am Vet Med Assoc 1985;187:1016–1018.
3. Bleyaert HF. Suprascapular nerve injury. In: White NA, Morre JN, Eds. Current Techniques in Equine Surgery. Philadelphia: WB Saunders, 1998;426–428.
4. Bleyaert HF, Madison JB. Complete biceps brachii tenotomy to facilitate internal fixation of supraglenoid tubercle fracture in three horses. Vet Surg 1999;28:48–53.
5. Clein LJ. Suprascapular entrapment neuropathy. J Neurosurg 1975;43:337.
6. Clem MF, DeBowes RM. Scapular wedge resection for management of the suprascapular nerve injury. In: White NA, Morre JN, Eds. Current Practice of Equine Surgery. Philadelphia: Lippincott, 1990;171–173.
7. Duncan ID, Schneider RK. Equine suprascapular neuropathy (Sweeny): Clinical and pathologic observations. Am Assoc Equine Pract 1985;21:415–428.
8. Duncan ID, Schneider RK, Hammang JP. Subclinical entrapment neuropathy of the equine suprascapular nerve. Acta Neuropathol 1987;74:53–61.
9. Dutton DM, Honnas CM, Watkins JP. Nonsurgical treatment of suprascapular nerve injury in horses: 8 cases (1988–1998). J Am Vet Med Assoc 1999;214:1657–1659.
10. Getty R, Ed. Sisson and Grossman's The Anatomy of the Domestic Animals. 5th ed. Philadelphia: WB Saunders, 1975.
11. Honnas CM. Collateral instability of the shoulder joint. In: Auer JA, Ed. Equine Surgery. Philadelphia: WB Saunders, 1992;1050.
12. Mayhew JG, MacKay RJ. Diseases of peripheral (spinal) nerves. In: Mansmann RA, McAllister ES, Eds. Equine Medicine and Surgery. 3rd ed. Santa Barbara, CA: American Veterinary Publications, 1982;2139.
13. Miller RM, Dresher LK. Treatment of equine shoulder Sweeny with intra-articular corticosteroids. Vet Med Small Anim Clin 1977;72:1077–1079.
14. Milne DW, Turner AS. Surgical Approaches to the Bones and Joints of the Horse. Philadelphia: WB Saunders, 1979;114.
15. Rooney JR. Biomechanics of Lameness in Horses. Baltimore: Williams & Wilkins, 1969;114.
16. Rooney JR. The musculoskeletal system. In: Catcott EJ, Smithsors JF, Eds. Equine Medicine and Surgery. Wheaton, IL: American Veterinary Publications, 1972;560.
17. Schaumburg HH, Spencer PS, Thomas PJ. Disorders of Peripheral Nerves. Philadelphia: Davis, 1983.
18. Schneider JE, Adams OR, Easley KJ, et al. Scapular notch resection for suprascapular nerve decompression in 12 horses. J Am Vet Med Assoc 1985;187:1019–1020.
19. Schneider RK. Suprascapular nerve injury—Sweeny. In: Auer JA, Stick JA, Eds. Equine Surgery. 2nd ed. Philadelphia: WB Saunders, 1999;846–848.
20. Schneider RK, Bramlage LR. Suprascapular nerve injury in horses. Comp Cont Educ Vet Pract 1990;12:1783–1789.
21. Swaim SF. Peripheral nerve surgery. In: Hoerlein BF, Ed. Canine Neurology. Philadelphia: WB Saunders, 1978;296.
22. Winberg FG. Surgical treatment of suprascapular nerve entrapment—Current technique. Proceedings. 8th Annual ECVS Meeting, Brugge, Belgium, 1999;103–104.
23. Youman JR. Neurological Surgery. Philadelphia: WB Saunders, 1973.

FRACTURES OF THE SCAPULA

Fractures of the scapula are uncommon in horses.[8,9,11] This is in part because of the scapula's proximal location, its close proximity to the ribs, and the large protective muscle mass overlying the region.[1,5,10] Data collected from 29 veterinary schools in North America over a 10-year period identified 219 fractures of the scapula, which represented 1.068% of all of the fractures recorded.[1] Although scapular fractures occur in all ages and breeds of horses, young (less than 4 years) intact males seem to be more prone; of the 219 horses with scapular fractures, 31.5% were intact males.[1]

Fractures of the scapula can involve the spine, supraglenoid tubercle, body, neck, and glenoid cavity; fracture of the supraglenoid tubercle is most common (see "Fractures of the Supraglenoid Tubercle" in this chapter). Although simple scapular fractures are most common, comminuted fractures also occur. Bone sequestra may also develop after fractures of the scapular spine, particularly in horses sustaining a penetrating wound that causes a comminuted fracture.[2,6,8] As would be expected, a higher incidence of suprascapular nerve injury occurs after fractures of the neck of the scapula. Injury to the subscapularis nerve and brachial plexus is a rare complication associated with fractures of the scapula.

Causes

Scapular fractures can be caused by direct trauma, such as would occur from a kick by another horse or from running into a fixed object. Fractures of the scapula can also occur from falls during racing or jumping.[5,6] Fractures resulting from race falls at high speeds tend to be comminuted.[5] Penetrating wounds to the lateral shoulder region can also cause fractures of the scapula's spine.[5,6]

Signs

Horses frequently present with a history of trauma and with signs of lameness, ranging from mild to non-weight-bearing.[1,2,7,8] Horses with an acute fracture of the scapular spine usually exhibit focal swelling, will bear weight, and will exhibit a mild to moderate lameness at exercise. Deep palpation over the fracture site typically elicits a painful response. Evidence of penetrating wound may be present. Chronic cases of scapular spine fractures may present with a draining tract or a history of the development of a recurrent draining tract as a result of a penetrating wound and sequestration of bone fragments.[2,6]

Horses with fractures of the body or neck of the scapula usually are initially reluctant to bear weight, have difficulty advancing the affected limb, and have swelling over the fracture site. Deep palpation and limb manipulation generally elicits a painful response.[1,4,10] Crepitation may be difficult to appreciate because of the large muscle masses associated with the shoulder and the swelling, but it is apparent in some cases. Fractures of the scapular neck may also result in secondary suprascapular nerve injury and sign of paresis.

Within a few days after the fracture the swelling may migrate distad and be most prominent in the axilla and proximal antebrachium (Fig. 8.356). Horses treated with NSAIDs may be willing to bear weight, even if they have a comminuted articular fracture; however, they will still have difficulty advancing the limb (Fig. 8.356B). Chronic cases of more than 3 weeks' duration usually exhibit some degree of atrophy of the muscles in the shoulder region and proximal antebrachium (Fig. 8.357).[7] As time passes, the swelling may become more apparent in the lateral shoulder region as a result of muscle atrophy, healing soft tissues, and callus formation. At exercise, a swinging and a support limb lameness is observed. Horses sustaining these fractures should also be assessed for problems such as fractured ribs and intrathoracic trauma.[4]

Diagnosis

Radiographs of the region are needed for a definitive diagnosis. Medial to lateral, ventrodorsal, and oblique cranial to caudal projections reveal most fractures of the

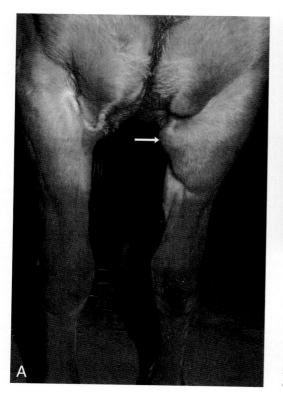
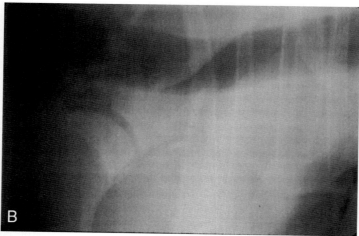

Figure 8.356 A. Note the swelling of the left axilla and proximal antebrachium (arrow) in this horse with a non-weight-bearing lameness as a result of trama sustained 3 days earlier. B. The lateral view reveals a comminuted articular fracture of the neck of the scapula.

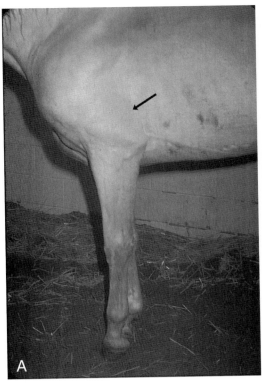

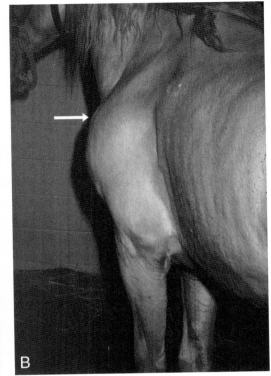

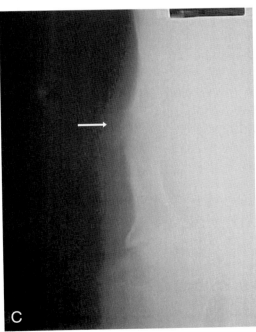

Figure 8.357 A. Note the triceps muscle atrophy (arrow) in this horse with a lameness of at least 6 weeks' duration. B. Note the prominent swelling over the lateral shoulder region (arrow). C. The oblique cranial caudal view reveals a healing transverse fracture of the body of the scapula.

scapula (Fig. 8.356B). The study can usually be done while the horse is standing. Some fractures through the body of the scapula can be difficult to image because of the superimposition of the ribs and vertebrae; in these cases, the limb will have to be protracted to obtain a diagnostic view.[7]

If the fracture is minimally displaced, it may not be apparent on the initial standing radiographic examina-

tion. Thus if a fracture is suspected, the horse should be confined to a stall; and the radiographs should be retaken 10 to 14 days later, when demineralization along the fracture line will make the fracture more obvious.[6] Some large, heavily muscled horses in severe pain may require general anesthesia before the clinician can obtain diagnostic radiographs. In these cases, be prepared to repair the fracture before allowing the horse to recover from the anesthesia so that displacement of a nondisplaced fracture is avoided.

Suprascapular nerve injury can be difficult to detect by physical examination alone in the non-weight-bearing limb. EMG can help assess nerve damage, if the injury is more than 7 days old. EMG has limited usefulness if the affected horse is examined before this time.[4]

Treatment

Conservative Treatment

Fractures of the scapular spine generally do not require surgical intervention, and most will heal by bone union. On the other hand, fractures caused by a penetrating wound may develop bone sequestra; surgery is recommended for these cases. Some minimally displaced nonarticular fractures of the scapular body and neck may also be treated conservatively with a good result.[3,7] Providing stall rest for several months, taping the shoulder to the body wall to prevent abduction of the limb, and slinging cooperative animals have been successful in cases without articular involvement.[6,7] Only horses that are able to bear weight after the injury are good candidates for the conservative approach.[10] In my experience, it has not been necessary to sling the horse to allow some of these fractures to heal (Fig. 8.357).

Surgical Treatment

Transverse fractures of the body and proximal neck can be surgically treated with internal fixation in young animals.[4,9] Administration of broad-spectrum antimicrobial agents and NSAIDs is recommended before surgery. The horse is placed in lateral recumbency with the affected limb up, and the fracture is approached with an incision made just cranial and parallel to the scapular spine. The supraspinatus and infraspinatus muscles are retracted, and the suprascapular nerve is identified and preserved. Stabilization is achieved by applying two dynamic compression plates (DCPs) cranial and caudal to the scapular spine in the angle formed by the spine and the body. This region provides thicker bone for the screw placement. The plates are placed upside down, with the convex surface facing the bone for better contact; they are staggered to avoid contact between screws. Both cortical (4.5-mm) and cancellous (3.5-mm) screws have been used,[4,9] but 5.5-mm cortical screws are recommended in foals and adults for the most stable fixation.[10]

Closure is routine; and, if necessary, a closed suction drain is used. A stent bandage can be sutured over the incision. Recovery from anesthesia should be assisted in all cases. Postoperative stall confinement is recommended for 60 to 90 days, followed by a gradual increase in exercise. Follow-up radiographs should be taken before pasture turnout to evaluate the fracture healing and state of the implants. The implants should be removed if they become loose or infected and if the horse is intended for athletic performance.[10]

Severely comminuted fractures or fractures of the distal neck and those extending into the glenoid are difficult to treat surgically with internal fixation. The configuration of the fracture and its close proximity to the shoulder joint do not permit application of orthopedic implants. Euthanasia is recommended for horses with extensive joint involvement and or with severe joint instability.[3]

Prognosis

The prognosis is good for fractures involving the scapular spine with or without surgery for removal of a sequestrum; most horses can return to performance after an adequate period of rest. Young horses with nonarticular simple or minimally comminuted fractures of the body and proximal neck have a good prognosis for soundness after application of internal fixation. At the 1-year follow-up of two horses that underwent internal fixation, complete healing and return to full function were noted.[4,9] In adults, nondisplaced fractures of the body or neck may heal satisfactorily with conservative therapy.[7] Horses with complete fractures in the distal neck, articular fractures, and severely comminuted fractures all have a poor prognosis for return to performance.[3,6]

References

1. Adams SB. Fractures of the scapula. In: Nixon A, Ed. Equine Fracture Repair. Philadelphia: WB Saunders, 1996;254–258.
2. Babinski J, Richter W. Fractures of the scapula in sporting horses. Monatshefte Veterinarmed 1990;45:93–94.
3. Bleyaert H. Shoulder injuries. In: White NA, Moore JN, Eds. Current Techniques in Equine Surgery. Philadelphia: WB Saunders, 1998;421–422.
4. Bukowiecki CF, van Fe RT, Schneiter HL. Internal fixation of comminuted transverse scapular fracture in a foal. J Am Vet Med Assoc 1989;195:781–783.
5. Denny HR. Fractures of the scapula. In: Denny HR, Ed. Treatment of Equine Fractures. London: Wright, 1989;28–33.
6. Dyson S. Sixteen fractures of the shoulder region in the horse. Equine Vet J 1985;17:104–110.
7. Dyson S. Shoulder lameness in horses—An analysis of 58 suspected cases. Equine Vet J 1986;18:29–36.
8. Fessler JF, Amstutz HE. Fracture repair. In: Oehme FW, Prier JE, Eds. Textbook of Large Animal Surgery. Baltimore: Williams & Wilkins, 1974;316–317.
9. Gobel DO, Brinker WO. Internal fixation of the equine scapula: a case report. J Equine Med Surg 1977;1:341.
10. Honnas CM. Surgical treatment of selected musculoskeletal disorders of the forelimb. In: Auer JA, Ed. Equine Surgery. Philadelphia: WB Saunders, 1992;1047–1049.
11. Leitch M. The upper forearm. In: Mansmann RA, McAllister ES, Eds. Equine Medicine and Surgery. 3rd ed. Santa Barbara, CA: American Veterinary Publications, 1982;1131.

FRACTURES OF THE SUPRAGLENOID TUBERCLE (TUBEROSITY)

Fractures of the supraglenoid tubercle (SGT), although uncommon, can occur in a variety of breeds and in horses used for a variety of purposes.[2,3,7,8,10,13] In a study done over a 10-year period, SGT fracture was observed in 8 of 24 horses with scapular fractures.[8] Another study that focused on a 9-year period found that SGT fractures were the most common fracture associated with the shoulder region: 9 of 16 horses had sustained the fracture and several breeds were affected.[5] Fractures of the SGT are often simple and intraarticular; they usually affect horses less than 2 years of age.[2,8,10] In contrast, one report of STG fractures in 9 horses found that 4 horses had comminuted fractures and 6 horses were between 3 and 13 years of age.[5]

Anatomically, the supraglenoid tubercle serves as the proximal attachment for the biceps brachii muscle and two glenohumeral ligaments, which support the SHJ.[6] The coracoid process, which is the medial projection of the tubercle, serves as an attachment for coracobrachialis muscle. The SGT and the coracoid process develop from a single center of ossification and fuse with the cranial portion of the glenoid cavity and the main body of the scapula at 10 to 12 months of age.[6] Because the fracture plane often courses along this growth plate, this fracture may result from a separation of the physis of the supraglenoid tubercle in young horses.[8,9]

Causes

Fracture of the SGT is most frequently associated with trauma to the cranial shoulder region. Because of its superficial location, it appears that the SGT is most susceptible to injury. In two reports, six of nine horses and three of five horses with SGT had a history of falling or direct trauma to the shoulder.[5,10] Overflexion of the shoulder leading to increased tension on the biceps brachii and coracobrachialis tendons that attach to the SGT has also been proposed as a mechanism for this fracture.[1,11] Fracture of the SGT has occurred in several horses with suprascapular paralysis after surgical removal of a piece of bone from the cranial border of the scapula.[2,3,12]

Signs

A history of trauma resulting in severe lameness that improves rapidly is common.[3,5,10] This rapid improvement may be the reason that the fracture is sometimes not initially diagnosed; recognition of the problem sometimes occurs only after the horse remains lame longer than expected or when muscle atrophy becomes prominent. In a report on nine cases of SGT fracture, the duration of lameness before referral ranged from 5 weeks to 18 months.[5] In another report of five cases, the duration of lameness before recognition of the problem ranged from 2 months to 1 year.[10]

In acute cases, swelling is usually apparent over the point of the shoulder, and palpation generally elicits a painful response (Fig. 8.358). Crepitation may also be appreciated. At a walk, the horse typically retains the ability to extend the SHJ, but the cranial phase of the stride is markedly shortened. A grade 3 to 4 (out of 5) lameness is common in the acute phase. Eventually, swelling over the point of the shoulder diminishes and palpation may reveal a firm nonpainful swelling over the point of the shoulder.[5] In some cases. movement of the tubercle can be perceived.

Some degree of muscle atrophy is usually apparent in chronic cases (Fig. 8.359). In one report of nine chronic cases, all horses presented with some muscle atrophy involving the muscles of the shoulder region, including the supraspinatus, infraspinatus, pectoral, and triceps.[5] Some horses may also exhibit signs of suprascapular or radial nerve paralysis. Intraarticular anesthesia of the SHJ may not improve the lameness.[5]

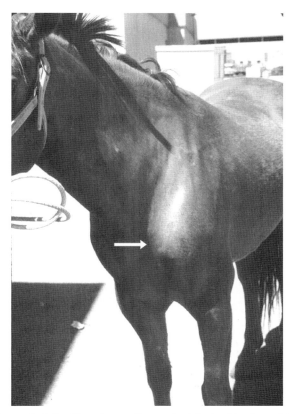

Figure 8.358   Note the swelling at the left shoulder (arrow) in this horse 5 days after it sustained a fracture of the SGT.

Diagnosis

Radiography is required to make a definitive diagnosis of the fracture (Fig. 8.360). Generally, the fracture is simple or comminuted and intraarticular (Fig. 8.361). Comminuted fractures were reported in 5 of 16 horses[5] and 5 of 19[3] horses in two studies. In another report, 1 of 5 horses had a nonarticular fracture of the SGT.[10] Calcification of the biceps tendon may also be associated with the fracture.[5] EMG studies are needed in some cases to rule out neurogenic atrophy of the affected muscles.

Treatment

Several options can be considered for management of SGT fractures. The approach depends on the nature and duration of the fracture, economics, and the expectation of performance level.

Conservative management consists of the administration of NSAIDs and 3 to 4 months of stall rest followed by 6 to 9 months of pasture turnout. Horses with nonarticular or minimally displaced intraarticular fractures respond best to this approach and may be able to return to their intended use.[3,5,10] Unfortunately, most horses with intraarticular fractures that are treated conservatively remain lame from the secondary DJD that develops from fracture fragment nonunion and incongruity of the joint surface at the fracture site. One review of the outcome of 19 horses treated conservatively found that 10

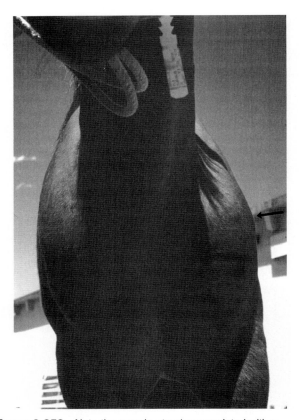

Figure 8.359 Note the muscle atrophy associated with a fracture of the SGT that had gone undiagnosed for 6 weeks. The point of the shoulder overlying the fracture appears enlarged (arrow).

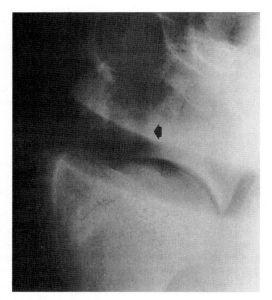

Figure 8.360 Lateral view of a displaced nonarticular fracture of the SGT.

horses were euthanatized, 7 improved (4 were pasture sound, 3 returned to performance), and 2 were lost to follow-up.[3,5,8,10]

Surgical management of horses with SGT fractures consists of either surgical removal of the fragment or internal fixation with or without transection of the biceps brachii tendon. The goal of surgery is to prevent the development of secondary DJD caused by joint incongruity.

Removal of the fragment involves dissection of the tendinous attachments of the biceps brachii and coracobrachialis muscles off the SGT. The rationale for the excision of the fragment is decreased pain created by fracture movement and prevention of further joint damage that develops from impingement of the fragment on the articular surface of the humeral head.[13] Surgical excision of the SGT appears to be best suited for chronic cases and for comminuted articular fractures.[10,12,13] In one report, four of seven horses returned to performance, including one racing Thoroughbred that had a successful career at a reduced performance level.[3] Caudal luxation of the scapula occurred in one horse.

Several methods of internal fixation, consisting of various combinations of interfragmentary compression with lag screws and tension band wires, have been used (Fig. 8.362). Cancellous bone screws placed in lag fashion across the fracture gap was reported to be unsuccessful in two horses.[8] Internal fixation using Kirschner wires in combination with cerclage wire placed in a figure eight pattern to stabilize the fracture fragment was used successfully in one case.[8] Stab incisions made through the tendon of the biceps brachii muscle to place bone screws in a lag fashion was also used successfully.[4]

The overall limited success, particularly in heavily muscled horses, associated with internal fixation has been attributed to the fact the porous bone in the scapular neck does not hold the screws adequately, fracture reduction is difficult, and fixation fails owing to the tension exerted by the biceps brachii tendon.[1–3] Partial or complete transection of the biceps tendon has been advocated to eliminate the tension on the fracture fragment and to prevent implant and bone failure. In one report, lag screws in combination with cerclage wires and partial tenotomy of the biceps brachii tendon for two-thirds of its diameter was used successfully in a 355-kg Thoroughbred.[1] Despite the clinical success, one of two 6.5-mm cancellous bone screws and one of two 1.25-mm cerclage wires failed 5 months postoperatively, suggesting that the transected tendon was still able to exert substantial tension on the fracture site. In another report, bone screws placed in lag fashion and complete tenotomy of the biceps brachii tendon was used to successfully treat SGT fractures in three horses.[2] The horses ranged in age from 8 months to 2 years, and they weighed 300 to 400 kg.

At this time, internal fixation with complete transection of the biceps brachii tendon appears to be the best approach for managing acute simple articular fractures of the SGT.

Prognosis

A good prognosis for return to performance can be expected for conservative management of horses that

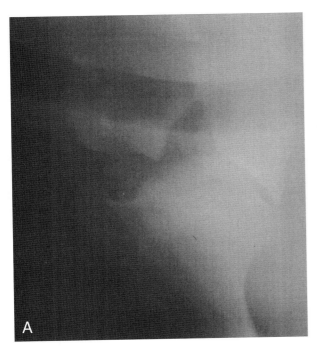

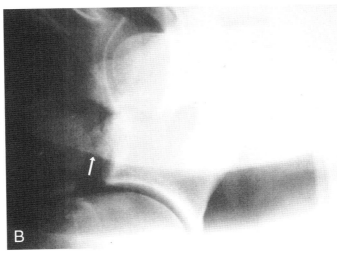

Figure 8.361   A. Lateral view revealing a large displaced articular fracture of the SGT. B. Lateral view of a chronic displaced fracture of the SGT. Note the remodeling of the fracture's edges (arrow).

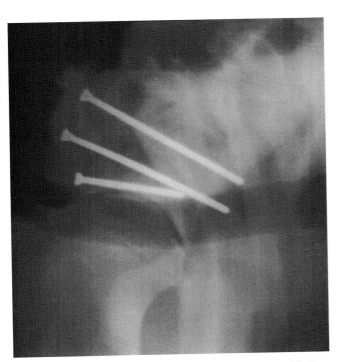

Figure 8.362   Internal fixation with lag screws was used in the horse shown in Figure 8.361. (Courtesy of G. Baxter.)

have nonarticular fractures or minimally displaced articular fractures of the SGT.[3] The prognosis for conservative management is poor to return to athletic soundness for horses that sustain simple or comminuted displaced articular fractures, but pasture soundness is possible in some.[3,5]

The prognosis after surgical excision of the fractured SGT is better than that achieved with conservative man-

agement for return to performance in horses with displaced simple or comminuted articular fractures and for chronic articular fractures.[3,5,10,13] As noted earlier, four of seven horses treated with surgical excision of the fractured tubercle returned to performance, including one racing Thoroughbred.[3]

The prognosis after internal fixation appears better than that achieved with conservative management for return to performance of horses with acute simple displaced articular fractures of the SGT.[1,3,4] Presently, the prognosis appears best if a combination of internal fixation and complete transection of the biceps brachii tendon is used for simple acute fractures. In one report, all three horses treated by this method were sound for their intended use with a good cosmetic result 6 months after surgery.[3]

References

1. Adams SB. Surgical repair of a supraglenoid tubercle fracture in a horse. J Am Vet Med Assoc 1987;191:332–334.
2. Bleyaert HF, Madison JB. Complete biceps brachii tenotomy to facilitate internal fixation of supraglenoid tubercle fractures in three horses. Vet Surg 1999;28:48–53.
3. Bleyaert HF, Sullins KE, White NA. Supraglenoid tubercle fractures in horses. Contin Educ 1994;16:531–536.
4. Dart AJ, Snyder JR. Repair of a supraglenoid tuberosity fracture in a horse. J Am Vet Med Assoc 1992;201:95–96.
5. Dyson S. Sixteen fractures of the shoulder region in the horse. Equine Vet J 1985;17:104–110.
6. Getty R. Equine osteology. In: Getty R, Ed. Sisson and Grossman's The Anatomy of the Domestic Animals. 5th ed. Philadelphia: WB Saunders, 1975;255–348.
7. Honnas CM. Fracture of the supraglenoid tubercle. In: Auer JA, Ed. Equine Surgery. Philadelphia: WB Saunders, 1992;1047–1048.
8. Leitch M. A review of treatment of tuber scapulae fractures in the horse. J Equine Med Surg 1977;1:234.
9. Myers VS, Burt JK. The radiographic location of the epiphyseal bone in equine limbs. Am Assoc Equine Pract 1966;12:21.

10. Pankowski RL, Grant BD, Sande R, Nickels FA. Fracture of the supraglenoid tubercle. Treatment and results in five horses. Vet Surg 1986;15:33–39.
11. Rooney JR. Disease of bone. In: Bone JF, Smithcors JF, Eds. Equine Medicine and Surgery. Wheaton, IL: American Veterinary Publications, 1963;407.
12. Schneider RK. Fractures of the supraglenoid tubercle. In: Auer JA, Stick JA, Eds. Equine Surgery. 2nd ed. Philadelphia: WB Saunders, 1999;844–846.
13. Wagner PC, Watrous BJ, Shires GM, Reibold TW: Resection of the supraglenoid tubercle of the scapula in a colt. Comp Cont Educ Vet Pract 1985;7:36–41.

RUPTURE OF THE SERRATUS VENTRALIS MUSCLES

Rupture of the serratus ventralis muscles is a rarely reported condition in the horse.[2,3] These muscles are large, paired, fan-shaped, and lie in the lateral thorax and cervical regions. The cervical part of each fan-shaped serratus ventralis arises from the last four cervical vertebrae; the thoracic part originates from the first eight or nine ribs. The two parts of the muscle converge to their respective insertions on the proximal cranial and caudal areas on the medial surface of the scapula and the adjacent scapular cartilage. Elastic lamellae from the dorsoscapular ligament penetrate these attachments. The contralateral muscles form a support, suspending the thorax between the forelimbs. While the horse is standing, contraction of both muscles elevates the thorax. Contraction of one muscle shifts the weight of the trunk to that side. The neck is also pulled to one side or, if both muscles are contracting, the neck is extended. During locomotion, the cervical part of the serratus ventralis pulls the dorsal border of the scapula craniad; the thoracic part then acts to pull the scapula caudad (see Chapter 1). When rupture of the serratus ventralis muscle occurs, both left and right paired muscle groups are usually involved.[2]

Causes

Dorsal impact trauma over the withers and neck can lead to rupture of the serratus ventralis muscles.[2,3] It is also reasonable to believe that a horse could sustain such an injury from jumping over a high fence or from jumping off an elevated platform.[1]

Signs and Diagnosis

After rupture of these muscles, the thorax drops between the paired scapulae and the dorsal borders of the scapulae assume a position above the thoracic spinous processes. In most instances, the croup appears higher than the withers. When examined right after the rupture occurs, these horses are in extreme pain.[1,2]

The diagnosis is made from the history and clinical signs. Radiographs should be taken of the withers region to rule out the possibility of fractures of the dorsal spinous processes.

Treatment

If treatment is attempted, the horse should be placed in a sling support for 30 to 45 days. NSAIDs should be administered if the horse is in acute pain.[1] Even after a prolonged convalescence and after healing has occurred, the withers will be lower than the scapula.

Prognosis

A poor prognosis is given if the serratus ventralis muscle is completely ruptured.[1,2]

References

1. Johnson JH, Bartels JE. Conditions of the forelimbs. In: Catcott EJ, Smithcors JF, Eds. Equine Medicine and Surgery. 2nd ed. Wheaton, IL: American Veterinary Publications, 1972;505–562.
2. Johnson JH, Lowe JE. The musculoskeletal system. In: Oehme FW, Prier JE, Eds. Textbook of Large Animal Surgery. Vol. 2. Baltimore: Williams & Wilkins, 1974;39.
3. O'Connor JJ. Dollar's Veterinary Surgery. 4th ed. Chicago: Alexander Eger, 1950.

Part X

THE TARSUS

Kenneth E. Sullins

The tarsus accounts for most hindlimb lameness in performance horses. Particularly when bilateral hindlimb lameness is present in athletes, the hocks should be suspected. However, the presence of bilateral hindlimb lameness may obscure the primary problem, particularly to horse owners. The degree of pain may be sufficiently symmetric that neither hindlimb demonstrates typical clinical signs of pain. In these horses, unilateral local anesthesia causes the problem to become more apparent. Performance horses, especially those that must work while collected, may exhibit back muscle pain owing to a functional spasm from the altered gait caused by the hindlimb pain. Occasionally, it is necessary to rest the horse and treat the back pain before a lameness examination is possible.

Excessively straight or curby conformation or angular deformity could make the tarsus the first aspect to rule out in younger horses as well. Substantial pathology can exist in the distal tarsal joints, despite an outwardly normal appearance. Conversely, the distal tarsal joints can be the cause of lameness without apparent radiographic abnormality, which can make tarsal lameness challenging to diagnose.

Tarsal lameness is usually exacerbated by hindlimb flexion (spavin test). Ideally, a digital flexion test and stifle flexion test (see Chapter 3) are performed to ascertain that component of the pain, because all the joints of the hindlimb are flexed along with the tarsus. When performing the hindlimb flexion test, some clinicians prefer to hold the foot to prevent pressure on the fetlock; others prefer to cradle the fetlock passively to prevent pressure on the metatarsal flexor structures and avoid excessive digital flexion. Consistency is the most important consideration. (See Chapter 3 for a discussion of a lameness examination.)

Tarsometatarsal (TM) or distal intertarsal (DIT) joint synovitis does not result in externally visible synovial effusion, because of tight soft tissue investment. Synovial effusion may be inferred by a release of synovial fluid for an impressive distance through a needle placed for intraarticular anesthesia (see Chapter 3). However, the ensuing intraarticular anesthesia may not completely relieve the lameness, casting doubt on the clinical significance of the increased synovial fluid. The TM and DIT joints should be anesthetized separately because they do not always communicate, and lameness may be emanating from only one of the joints.

The proximal intertarsal (PIT) joint is located within and thus communicates with the tarsocrural joint; it is alone an uncommon cause of lameness. PIT joint inflammation should be reflected in tarsocrural effusion, and persisting PIT synovitis places the more mobile tarsocrural joint at risk of osteoarthritis. However, tarsocrural effusion does not always accompany PIT disease, so radiographic signs of PIT disease without tarsocrural effusion may require a closer evaluation.

Most tarsocrural pathology is accompanied by synovial effusion (bog spavin). Synovial effusion may persist for years in successfully working horses that may not have radiographic signs of disease. Some such horses actually have no grossly apparent pathology and may remain sound. Horses that have mild, but clinically significant, disease that they have been working through eventually become more lame as osteoarthritis advances.

It is important to differentiate between tarsocrural synovial effusion and periarticular edema. Although the two may exist concurrently, they signal different situations. Congruity of the tibial tarsal bone with the distal tibia may allow weight bearing despite substantial supporting soft tissue damage. Swelling and lameness excessive for their apparent anatomic explanations should be critically evaluated for collateral ligament integrity. Ultrasound and radiographic examinations conducted while stressing the medial and lateral collateral ligaments may be necessary.

Complete evaluation of the tarsus includes radiography. A routine radiographic examination of the tarsus should include the dorsoplantar (DPl), dorsolateral, plantaromedial oblique (DLPLMO), dorsomedial, plantarolateral oblique (DMPLLO), lateral medial (LM), and flexed lateral medial (FLM) views. Some clinicians use two DPl views. In one, the beam is centered on the tibial tarsal bone; and in the other, the beam is centered on the central tarsal bone. This permits better evaluation at each level.[2] Depending on history or clinical signs, the flexed tangential or oblique flexed tangential views are required to demonstrate lesions on the caudal extremes of the trochlear ridges or margin of the tarsal canal.

Nuclear scintigraphy is sometimes useful to confirm distal tarsal joint involvement, particularly in cases in which only partial relief of lameness occurs after intraarticular analgesia of the distal tarsal joints and there are no apparent radiographic changes. MRI offers detailed anatomic imaging of the tarsus.[1] Unfortunately, its availability remains limited (see Chapter 4 for more information).

References

1. Blaik MA, Hanson RR, Kincaid SA, et al. Low-field magnetic resonance imaging of the equine tarsus: Normal anatomy. Vet Radiol 2000;41:131–141.
2. O'Brien T. Radiographic interpretation of the equine tarsus. Proc Am Assoc Equine Pract 1973;19:289.

DISTAL TARSAL SYNOVITIS AND OSTEOARTHRITIS (BONE SPAVIN)

Bone spavin (true spavin; jack spavin) is an osteoarthritis and periostitis that involves the distal intertarsal, tarsometatarsal, and occasionally the proximal intertarsal joints (Fig. 8.363). Distal tarsal osteoarthritis more accurately describes the condition (Fig. 8.364).[1,15,17,20, 22,31–33,35,42,45] Distal tarsal osteoarthritis is considered to be the most common cause of tarsal lameness.[44,48] Only 7.2% of a series of 3566 horses failed to possess radiographic indicators of osteoarthritis.[61] However, these radiographic signs did not correlate with lameness or athletic ability, a fact that may confound prepurchase examinations. Of 119 horses undergoing scintigraphy for lameness, 44% demonstrated distal tarsal activity.[41] Half of 52 horses diagnosed with distal tarsal osteoarthritis as the primary problem demonstrated uptake bilaterally. An additional 21% showed distal tarsal uptake, which was considered additional to the primary lameness.

Occult spavin, or blind spavin, has the same clinical features of osteoarthritis but lacks physical or radiographic evidence. However, scintigraphic evidence of distal tarsal inflammation may be present.[41] Occult spavin and distal tarsal osteoarthritis should be considered different stages of the same process, in which synovitis results from radiographically inapparent cartilage lesions that can be found at necropsy;[1,46] support is provided by the observation of increasing radiographic signs that correlate with the degree of physical deformity and lameness.[5] In addition, desmitis of the intratarsal ligaments can produce lameness.[1] However, despite persistent lameness, some horses fail to develop the radiographic signs of osteoarthritis.[1,20] Other horses diagnosed with blind spavin may recover completely once treated appropriately.

Distal tarsal disease is most frequently observed in mature horses that are ridden hard at a gallop and canter; horses that jump; and Western horses used for reining, roping, and cutting.[1,20] Icelandic horses may have a predisposition for the disease. In a series of 379 horses, 12% were lame in the hindlimb and 25% were lame after

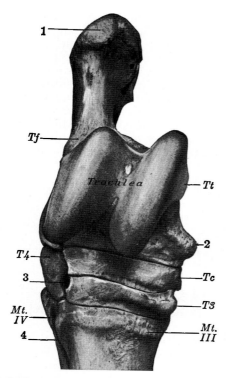

Figure 8.363   Dorsal view of the right tarsus and proximal metatarsus. The joints most commonly affected by bone spavin are the distal intertarsal joint (between Tc and T3) and the tarsometatarsal joint (between T3 and Mt. III). The proximal intertarsal joint (between Tc and the talus) communicates with the tarsocrural joint (not shown). 1, tuber calcis; Tf, fibular tarsal bone (calcaneus); T4, fourth tarsal bone; 3, vascular canal; Mt. IV, fourth metatarsal bone; 4, groove for great metatarsal artery; Tt, tibial tarsal bone (talus); 2, distal tuberosity of the talus; Tc, central tarsal bone; T3, third tarsal bone; Mt. III, third metatarsal bone. (Reprinted with permission from Sisson S, Grossman JD. The skeleton of the horse. In: Grossman JD, Ed. Anatomy of Domestic Animals. 4th ed. Philadelphia: WB Saunders, 1953;119.)

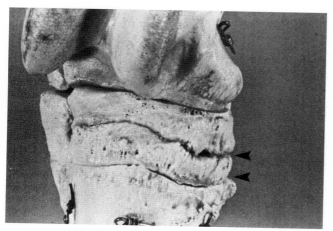

Figure 8.364   Dorsal view of the right distal tarsal joints showing bone spavin. Arrows, the medial aspects of the distal intertarsal and tarsometatarsal joints. (Courtesy of T. S. Stashak.)

hindlimb flexion.[5] Radiographically evident osteoarthritis was present in 23% of the horses, but only half of those horses were lame. In other words, twice as many horses had radiographic changes than were lame. No diagnostic anesthesia was reported.

Causes

Repeated compression and rotation of the tarsal bones and excessive tension on the attachment of the major dorsal ligaments are thought to be prominent in the development of this disease.[50,51] Rooney and Turner[47] suggest that shear owing to asynchronous movement of the tarsal bones predisposes the animal to osteoarthritis. They further suggest a difference in pathophysiology between DIT and TM disease. Horses working routinely with the hocks in a flexed position (e.g., jumpers and pulling horses) are proposed to develop DIT arthrosis, whereas horses working in a more straight-legged position (e.g., Thoroughbreds or horses short-strided owing to lameness) are proposed to be prone to TM disease. A review of distal tarsal osteoarthritis in horses that jump made no distinction between DIT and TM disease.[40] A study of Icelandic horses reports environmental factors, such as type and severity of work, do not affect the incidence and that tarsal angle and age were more important. Incidence was also related to certain sires.[4]

Conditions that disrupt the most fluid motion possible for a horse cause shear and rotation within the limb. Of 42 racing Thoroughbreds diagnosed with tarsal osteoarthritis, 85% wore shoes with elevations of the lateral or both heels, and hoof balance and flat shoes were components of the treatment in 27 horses that improved noticeably. Many of the horses in the study were affected with more than spavin.[40]

Distal tarsal osteoarthritis is commonly associated with poor conformation. Sickle hocks and cow hocks predispose a horse to osteoarthritis.[19,47] Sickle and cow hocks produce greater stress in the medial aspect of the hock joint. These two, often coexisting, malconformations and perhaps others make predisposition to osteoarthritis inheritable. Horses with narrow thin hocks are more subject to the disease than those with full well-developed hocks. However, many affected horses have none of these conformational defects.

I agree with others[39,60] that the local stresses from the type and difficulty of the work play an equal or overriding role in the pathogenesis of osteoarthritis. Furthermore, specific injury affecting the distal tarsal joints unrelated to type of work or conformation must be considered. Unilaterally affected horses in particular may fall into this category. Once acquired, treatment and outcome of injured horses may not differ from those affected from any other cause. However, horses that have not sustained articular cartilage damage tend to recover well, because their work routine may not continue to aggravate the situation.

Signs and Diagnosis

Usually there is a history of gradual onset of lameness. However, bilateral lameness may have been progressing for some time before a problem is noticed. If the horse is worked hard for several days, the lameness usually worsens and may improve with rest. Hunters may begin to jump poorly or refuse to jump at all.[39] Reining horses begin to pivot and stop poorly because of pain. In some cases, horses refuse to pivot to the affected side and exhibit their objection by laying their ears back or beginning to buck. Horses that must stop quickly often cheat by placing the greatest amount of weight on the least affected limb, which often results in a jerky slide stop because of reluctance to firmly plant the feet. The horse may feel stiff or jerky when circled to the affected side, and it may refuse to be put in the opposite lead.[39]

Lameness tends to be worse when the horse is first used; but horses with mild spavin tend to warm out of the lameness after working a short time. However, in severe cases, exercise may aggravate the lameness. Racing Thoroughbreds frequently present slightly younger (3 year olds) than other breeds and tend to have multiple problems, which are probably related to the stresses of the speed at which they work. Most of a series of 89 horses eventually diagnosed with distal tarsal osteoarthritis presented with a primary complaint other than hindlimb lameness.[40] Associated findings included fore fetlock and carpal disease, back pain, and forefoot pain. It could be argued that the high incidence of forelimb problems occurred secondarily to hindlimb pain. Only 20% of the horses with distal tarsal osteoarthritis were unaffected by other sources of lameness.

Distal tarsal osteoarthritis often causes an enlargement on the medial aspect of the hock (Fig. 8.365). The

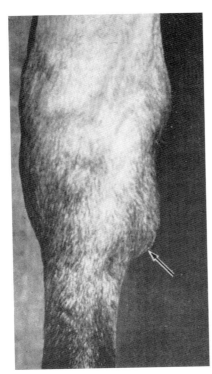

Figure 8.365 Right tarsus of a horse with bone spavin. Note the thickening on the dorsomedial aspect of the tarsus, which is caused by osteophyte and fibrous tissue production (arrow). The radiographic changes may not be as large as the external growth.

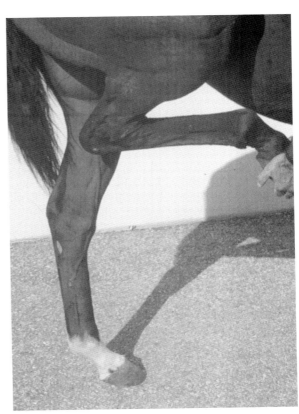

Figure 8.366 For hindlimb flexion test, the limb is flexed for 60 to 90 seconds to exacerbate lameness that may be caused by synovitis. All joints from coffin to hip are affected, and soft tissue that is stretched may also be affected. The limb should be supported either behind the fetlock or grasped at the bottom of the hoof (helpful for tall horses) and positioned with the metatarsus parallel to the ground and beneath the horse. Abduction is usually not tolerated by the horse. (Courtesy of T. S. Stashak.)

enlargement is sometimes difficult to detect visually, especially if bilateral spavin is present or if the horse normally has large boxy hocks. When standing, the horse may flex the hock periodically in a spasmodic manner. A mild to moderate hindlimb lameness (see Chapter 3) is usually observed, and it worsens after hindlimb flexion for 1 to 2 minutes (spavin test) (Fig. 8.366). The horse is often unwilling to flex the hock in its normal gait, causing a reduction in the height of the foot flight arc and a shortening of the cranial phase of the stride. The foot lands on the toe; and over time, the toe becomes too short and the heel too high. Because of the lower arc of the foot flight, some horses may drag the toe, causing it to wear on its dorsal edge. Possibly because of dorsomedial pathology associated with the distal tarsal joints, some horses swing the foot axially and land on the lateral hoof wall in a tightrope fashion, which tends to reduce dorsomedial compression of the limb.

It is advisable to conduct the flexion test on both hindlimbs for comparison or for diagnosis of bilateral osteoarthritis. I prefer to flex the least affected hindlimb first, because the more severely affected limb may retain the inflicted lameness, complicating further examination. The disease is often bilateral, and flexing the apparently unaffected limb may elicit a positive response or may cause the hindlimb gait to even out (as a result of more evenly distributed pain).

Horses that have swelling caused by periarticular changes from osteoarthritis are likely to be clinically affected, unless the joints have ankylosed; but reliance on external appearance and response to flexion test alone is ill advised (Fig. 8.365). Hindlimb lameness, positive flexion tests, reduced arc of the foot flight, reduced flexion of the hock, and wearing of the toe are all used in the diagnosis. Local infusion of the distal tarsal joints with local anesthetics is most helpful in localizing the source of the lameness (see Chapter 3). It may be expedient to evaluate the hocks first in horses displaying bilateral hindlimb lameness that are predisposed to distal tarsal lameness by their breed and line of work. Intraarticular anesthesia of the distal tarsal joints will not obscure the remainder of the lameness examination if it proves to have no effect.

Communication between a substantial percentage of TM and DIT joints has been demonstrated.[21,29,48] However, communication of the joints in an individual horse is unknown at the time of examination. Since treatment of distal tarsal inflammation may be required for a protracted period of time, it is desirable to know exactly which joints are causing pain. If there is doubt that both distal tarsal joints are involved, separate intraarticular anesthesia facilitates the design of a long-term treatment plan.

Injection of the TM and DIT joints is described in Chapter 3. Each joint typically holds 4 to 6 mL before resistance is encountered and the horse begins to object. It may be difficult to place the needle in severely degenerated joints, and diffusion of the anesthetic may be impaired as a result of obliteration of the joint spaces, which may cause an incomplete response to the intraarticular anesthesia. Observing the horse after 30 to 45 minutes may demonstrate a more positive response to the block. Some clinicians prefer specifically to block the cunean bursa in this situation. In the absence of other findings, the final diagnosis may have to be postponed, pending response to therapy.

Blocking of the caudal tibial and deep peroneal nerves is a reasonably accurate diagnostic method. However, other structures in addition to the distal tarsal joints are blocked. Furthermore, confirmation of complete analgesia is difficult, and desensitization of such a large portion of the limb occasionally alters the horse's movement. For horses that have undergone tibial and peroneal analgesia, I prefer to jog (or at least stop) them on grass for surer footing. If the blocks in and above the tarsal region follow a complete stepwise distal to proximal blocking session, it is advisable to perform the high metatarsal block using a long-acting local anesthetic, such as bupivacaine. Pain or dysesthesia from the blocks wearing off and pain from the injections render the lameness examination worthless.

Radiographs are useful for an accurate diagnosis and prognosis. The x-ray beam must be centered accurately to allow evaluation of the distal tarsal joint spaces, and some horses simply have joint surfaces that are too curved to demonstrate the typical lucency. PIT disease may be reflected more often medially. However, few adult performance horses have clean tarsal radiographs,

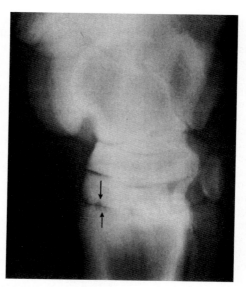

Figure 8.367 Subchondral lucency owing to distal tarsal osteoarthritis (arrows). Horses with this radiographic sign may fare better after distal tarsal arthrodesis. (Courtesy T. S. Stashak.)

and horses with significant radiographic changes may not be lame.[5,43] Radiographic evidence of osteoarthritis usually begins on the dorsomedial surfaces of the TM and DIT joints, but destructive changes often eventually involve the dorsal surface of these joints. The PIT joint is less commonly affected. However, of 60 Icelandic horses with distal tarsal osteoarthritis, the 25% that were most severely lame had PIT disease.[54]

Early radiographic changes include marginal bone lysis and cyst formation in the adjacent subchondral bone (Fig. 8.367). As the lesion progresses, irregular subchondral bone atrophy may cause the joint spaces to appear widened. As the cartilage degenerates, the joint spaces may narrow and marginal osteophytes and subchondral sclerosis develop (Figs. 8.368 to 8.370). After several months, complete ankylosis may occur (Fig. 8.368). In others cases, even after prolonged periods of time, only minimal degenerative changes are observed.[17] If ankylosis occurs, the lameness may be abolished.

A series of 4186 Warmblood and Standardbred horses revealed sufficient radiographic changes in sound horses to cause the authors to rely heavily on the clinical situation.[26] Conversely, significant lameness can emanate from radiographically normal hocks. Some horses with few radiographic signs are problematic in that the degeneration never progresses although they remain lame. Radiographic lesions usually begin on the dorsomedial aspect of the distal tarsal joints and progress dorsally. Some researchers believe that horses with cystic lucencies in their radiographs are more lame than horses without these signs. However, the degree of lameness may not be accurately reflected by any of these changes or lack thereof.

Scintigraphy generally accurately detects distal tarsal inflammation (Fig. 8.371).[57] It is most useful when the diagnosis is complicated by multiple problems or there is difficulty blocking the joints, because response to intraarticular anesthesia is definitive. Of 99 horses that

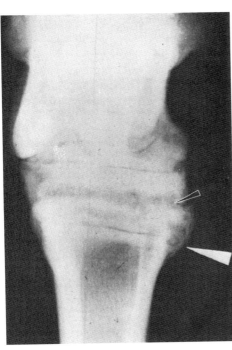

Figure 8.368 DPI view of severe distal tarsal osteoarthritis. Note the bone production on the medial aspect of the TM joint (white arrow), although the joint has not completely ankylosed. Ankylosis is more advanced in the DIT joint (black arrow), although the lucency along that joint may become more sclerotic.

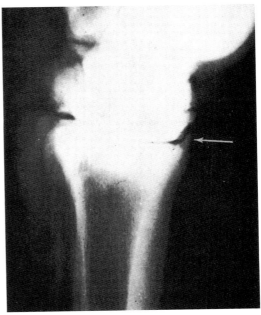

Figure 8.370 LM view of a large osteophyte (arrow) on the dorsal aspect of the proximal third metatarsal. The dorsomedial aspect of the tarsus may be typically thickened. This horse may not be lame. (Courtesy of T. S. Stashak.)

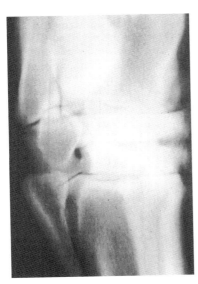

Figure 8.369 Dorsoplantar, lateromedial view demonstrating osteoarthritis involving all three of the distal tarsal joints. All the joints have lost space, although the dorsomedial aspect of the DIT joint is still healing. Because the PIT joint communicates with the tarsocrural joint above, the prognosis is relatively unfavorable.

underwent scintigraphic examinations for hindlimb lameness, 85 demonstrated distal tarsal uptake.[18] Substantiation of the diagnosis with intraarticular anesthesia and critical evaluation of the response to therapy are the most reliable diagnostic criteria.

Treatment

The goal of treatment is often affected by the radiographic signs. Horses with minimal to no distal tarsal radiographic changes may respond favorably to a period of reduced activity, corrective shoeing, and intraarticular medication. Often the lameness subsides permanently. If the history indicates that a specific injury may have occurred, more rest for soft tissue healing is warranted.

Some horses without radiographic changes have cartilage lesions that cause the synovitis to return, and the spavin eventually progresses. Once degenerative changes have begun, the goal of treatment becomes pain management until the distal joints ankylose. In this situation, extended rest beyond a limited period to allow medication to take effect is useless. Furthermore, exercise facilitates the degeneration, which may lead to subsequent ankylosis. However, in some cases, the distal tarsal joints do not ankylose. For horses with multiple problems possibly caused or aggravated by tarsal pain, more rest may be indicated.[40]

If the PIT joint is involved, control of synovitis is critical to preserving the integrity of the tarsocrural joint. Despite numerous types of therapy for treatment of distal tarsal osteoarthritis, some affected horses remain lame and resistant to all conventional methods of therapy. Unfortunately, treatment of tarsal pain in some instances remains somewhat intuitive.

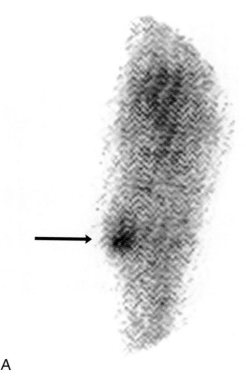

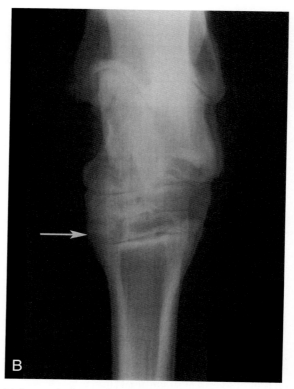

Figure 8.371 A. On scintigraphic examination, the DPI view demonstrates intense activity in the distal medial tarsus in the region of the third tarsal bone. B. DPI view showing more loss of joint space in the medial aspect of the DIT joint than in the corresponding tarsometatarsal region. Arrows, corresponding areas in the two panels.

Hoof management is aimed toward reducing the rotation and shear forces by easing breakover. My preference is to balance the foot and achieve a dorsal hoof angle 1 to 2° steeper than the pastern and to roll the toe. As much foot as possible should be removed in the process to improve stability. Particularly in show horses, wide-webbed wedged (flat) aluminum shoes help achieve the angle and support needed by a foot that tends to land unevenly. Some clinicians prefer to place a lateral extension on the shoe to minimize the axial swing of the foot.[23,39] Others believe that the presence of anything that alters the landing of the foot increases shear forces, which may be significant for racehorses.[21,40]

Anti-inflammatory therapy is required to resolve or control the pain that causes the lameness. Some horses with distal tarsal pain confirmed by intraarticular anesthesia without radiographic changes can be cured with short-acting intraarticular medication, which often consists of triamcinolone (4 mg per joint) and sodium hyaluronate, and with corrective shoeing. Shoeing can be surprisingly effective for many horses once the acute inflammation is relieved. The use of the natural balance trimming and shoeing techniques discussed in Chapter 9 have proven beneficial.

Some horses that appear to be only beginning to develop a chronic problem can be among the most difficult to treat. Ankylosis occurs faster without the influence of intraarticular corticosteroids; although cartilage degeneration is hastened, healing is impaired. Generally, the best plan is to do the minimum required to keep the horse effectively at work, because more treatment will

likely be required. A starting point includes systemic phenylbutazone (2.2 mg/kg BID), which can be continued for an extended period of time or given only when the horse will be ridden. Supporting systemic therapies include intramuscular polysulfated glycosaminoglycans, intravenous sodium hyaluronate, and oral nutraceuticals with a combination of chondroitin sulfate and glucosamine. Each horse is different and requires a unique treatment schedule. In Switzerland, a systemic treatment with an extract of a medicinal plant seems to have the same effect as phenylbutazone.[38]

If the results of systemic drugs are insufficient, intraarticular corticosteroids are indicated. Many clinicians prefer methylprednisolone acetate (80 mg per joint). The duration of effect depends on the individual. Continuing systemic therapy is important, because it maximizes the effect and reduces the frequency of intraarticular therapy. When the horse responds poorly to intraarticular steroids, a second injection in 3 to 4 weeks is often more effective. Using triamcinolone (4 mg per joint) for the first injection and scheduling a second injection with a repositol product makes sense in horses that require long-term pain control. The addition of sodium hyaluronate may increase the duration of effect.

A period of reduced (but continued) activity after medication usually improves the result. An exception would be a fit horse in work with a history of response to a specific therapy. The rest can be interpreted to allow the medication to reduce the inflammation or to facilitate conditioning of the supporting soft tissue structures.[21] Reports indicate that show horses have been rested from

5 to 14 days. For racing Thoroughbreds, 30 days' rest seems to be effective.[40] In a report on 89 Thoroughbreds, the combination of a reduced training schedule, corrective shoeing, and local and systemic anti-inflammatory drugs was more effective than any of the measures alone.

Sodium Monoiodoacetate–Induced Ankylosis

Chemically induced cartilage necrosis to induce ankylosis of the DIT and TM joints has been reported as a potential alternative to surgical arthrodesis of refractory cases of osteoarthritis.[9] Sodium monoiodoacetate (MIA) has not been approved by the Food and Drug Administration (FDA) for pharmaceutical use. For legal purchase and clinical use, an Investigational New Animal Drug number must be issued by the FDA for each specified treatment.[9] Case selection is restricted to horses with a definitive diagnosis of osteoarthritis involving the DIT and TM joints only.

Horses should be hospitalized for the procedure and should be pretreated with phenylbutazone. In my opinion, prophylactic broad-spectrum antibacterial therapy is advisable. Inflammation after injection causes severe lameness for approximately 24 hours. Tibial and peroneal nerve blocks or epidural analgesia may be considered during that period. Contrast arthrograms must be performed to confirm the location of the needle and to rule out communication of the TM or DIT joint with the PIT joint or the tarsal canal.[10] If the horse is at all recalcitrant, general anesthesia should be considered. An aseptic procedure is vital, and the needles must remain undisturbed while the radiographs are processed. If the arthrogram reveals contrast in the PIT/tarsocrural joint or in the tarsal canal or failure to fill the intended joint, the procedure is aborted. Leakage of MIA into the subcutaneous space produces noticeable inflammation, which may lead to a tissue slough. Injection under pressure increases the possibility of leakage.

Bohanon[9] reported the results of 39 horses that were injected with MIA (100 mg diluted in 2 mL sterile saline per joint). Pain was most significant during the first 18 hours after treatment; light exercise began the next day, and full exercise was resumed on the 2nd day. Horses were pretreated with phenylbutazone 12 hours before injection, and therapy continued for 5 days. Individuals were not consistently available for follow-up, but approximately 29 animals were available at each of the examinations. At the 1-, 3-, 6-, and 12-month follow-ups, 73, 70, 81, and 93% of horses, respectively, were free of lameness. Of interest is the longer-term follow-up on 25 horses, which revealed an overall rate of 80% free of lameness. A total of 16 of these 25 horses underwent radiography; 15 were considered ankylosed, 12 of which were considered to have successful outcomes. One complication experienced by 4 horses not having contrast arthrography was PIT and tarsocrural degeneration 2 to 4 years after injection.

In another report of five horses, eight TM joints were injected with 150 mg (50 mg/mL) MIA.[49] Two of the horses became sound and another one improved noticeably; the other two horses remained lame. Postinjection pain requiring phenylbutazone therapy persisted for 2 weeks in the three horses that improved. Only one of the eight joints became radiographically ankylosed (in

one of the sound horses); that joint contained a third tarsal bone fracture. The most visible degeneration and joint collapse occurred in the region of the injection at the plantarolateral aspect. However, two horses with this type of radiographic change showed improvement. It appeared that exercise is an important component of success with this treatment.

Other complications that have been observed include soft tissue necrosis at the injection site, septic arthritis, and unexplained increased lameness. I have observed open necrotic septic arthritis with osteomyelitis and tarsal collapse, which resulted in euthanasia of the horse.

In summary, the simplicity of the procedure has appeal, and notable success has been reported. The potential complications deserve attention, and horse owners should be informed of their possibility and of the experimental nature of the procedure. The fact that horses with apparently completely ankylosed distal tarsal joints may remain lame and others with incompletely ankylosed joints can become sound remains a variable.

Cunean Tenectomy

Horses that fail to respond to conservative measures require further intervention. Cunean tenectomy is technically simple and can be performed with the horse standing. Documented results are few, but one series contained positive reports from horse owners.[16] Some clinicians perform the procedure only in horses in which the lameness has improved after local anesthesia of the cunean bursa.[21] Even so, anesthetic infiltration of the cunean bursa is likely to anesthetize the adjacent joint capsules. The effectiveness of this procedure seems to depend on the early return to exercise, before the scar tissue replacement becomes restrictive. Calling the procedure into question is a report describing similar results for two groups of racing Thoroughbreds: one group was treated with cunean tenectomy in addition to other medical therapies and shoeing changes and the other group had the same measures without surgery.[40]

To perform the procedure, the area over the tendon should be clipped, shaved, and prepared for aseptic surgery. If the horse is standing, it should be heavily sedated. A local anesthetic is injected over the tendon, after which a 3- to 4-cm incision is made over the center of the longitudinal axis of the cunean tendon where it crosses the medial aspect of the hock (Figs. 8.372 and 8.373). The incision can be made vertically if desired. After the tendon is isolated (Figs. 8.374 and 8.375), a 3- to 4-cm section is removed. The skin is sutured with nonabsorbable sutures, which are removed in 10 to 14 days.

Pressure bandaging and stall rest improve the cosmetic result. Beginning when the skin has healed, Bohanon[11] describes a stepwise return to activity, consisting of hand walking, then riding over poles, and progressing to complete return to work after 6 weeks. This schedule is thought to prevent adhesion of the tendon ends to the bursal surface.

Wamberg[59] modified the cunean tenectomy to include diamond-patterned incisions into the bursal tissues and periosteum of the affected area. He believed that most of the pain came from the tissues around the bone and that the procedure denervated the area. In my hands,

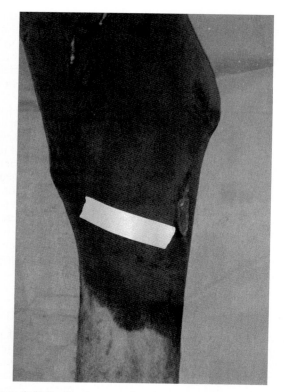

Figure 8.372 The tape overlies the cunean tendon.

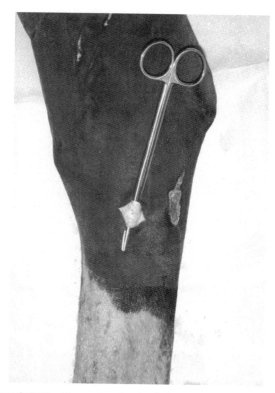

Figure 8.374 The cunean tendon is isolated with the scissors, as it is during a standing cunean tenectomy.

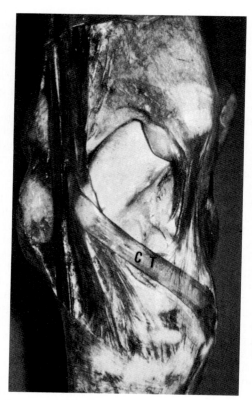

Figure 8.373 Dorsomedial view showing the dissected tarsus and the cunean tendon (CT).

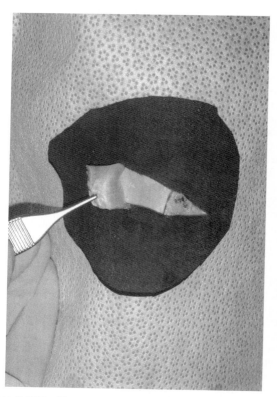

Figure 8.375 The cunean tendon has been transected and is reflected from the bursa. The surgeon removes 2 to 4 cm of the tendon.

this type of operation has been no more successful than the cunean tenectomy described earlier.

A histologic and histochemical study of bursal and tendinous tissues from horses affected with distal tarsal osteoarthritis revealed that the cunean tendons were markedly unaffected. However, the bursal tissues were inflamed and active, as evidenced by granulation response and fibrous tissue production.[8] Apparently, the tissue adjacent to the active distal tarsal synovitis is affected, but the tendon is not. These results contrasted findings from a similar study in horses unaffected with distal tarsal osteoarthritis.[12]

Surgical Arthrodesis of the Distal Tarsal Joints

A technique of surgical destruction of the joint surfaces was developed by Adams[1] that consisted of destruction of $\geq 60\%$ of the articular cartilage of the distal intertarsal and tarsometatarsal joints. The degree and duration of postoperative pain rendered the technique impractical. Further evaluation of the technique by Barber[6] again resulted in unacceptable postoperative morbidity and complications. The drilling in these procedures was done in a fan shaped, router fashion that removed substantial amounts of subchondral bone, leaving a space that resulted in instability owing to loss of joint congruity.

A single successful report of the application of internal fixation in a unilaterally severely affected breeding stallion provides food for thought.[31] Four drill paths were created from the metatarsus into the tibial tarsal bone, and 5-mm pins were driven to stabilize all three distal tarsal joints. Afterward, aggressive drilling of the joint spaces with curettage was carried out. The horse made a remarkable recovery from barely weight bearing to walking well. Although presently not advisable or necessary, this result illustrates the value of stabilization in the face of historically overly aggressive articular drilling.

More recently, techniques that create single distinct drill paths have proven to cause minimal postoperative morbidity and provide generally good outcomes.[17,24,36] These techniques include three to four drill paths with no fanning. It seems that if buttresses between the drill paths are left to maintain the structural integrity of the joints, morbidity is prevented. Drill size varies from 2.7 to 4.5 mm with similar results. A 3.2-mm drill bit is a nice compromise; it offers sufficient rigidity to drill without breaking but has just enough flexibility to follow the joint space without bypassing islands of cartilage (Fig. 8.376). Three drill paths seem to suffice (Fig. 8.377).

The success of the procedure depends on creating solid "spot welds" of bony bridging to immobilize the joints. Most surgeons consider it only a matter of time until both the TM and the DIT joints are involved, and perform arthrodesis on both regardless of diagnostic indications of the source of pain. Ideally, the drill stays within the joint space. Although minor distal penetrations will not affect the outcome, damage to the margins of the joints cause exostoses, enlargement, and potential gait compromise.[6] Some enlargement at the surgical site may occur, but the procedure should not affect the horse's movement or tarsal range of motion.

The horse is placed under stall rest until the skin sutures are removed, after 10 to 14 days; bandaging is dis-

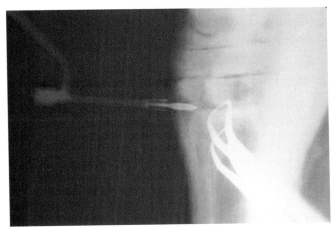

Figure 8.376 A 3.2-mm drill bit in a hand guide is used to perform the three-path technique of arthrodesis of the TM joint. (Courtesy of T. S. Stashak.)

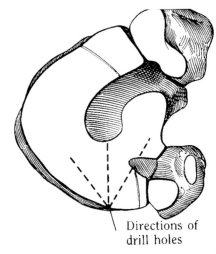

Directions of drill holes

Figure 8.377 DIT joint surface of the central tarsal bone showing the three-path technique of distal tarsal arthrodesis. The drill is inserted through a single hole and passed in three directions. A significant amount of joint surface is undisturbed, which preserves stability. (Courtesy of J. P. Sullins.)

continued after 14 days. Hand walking is allowed for an additional 2 weeks, at which time light riding is begun. Some horses, however, show a more rapid improvement. Exercise seems to be important for producing the desired fusion. Some horses take as long as 1 year for recovery and complete ankylosis of the involved joints, but most recover in 4 to 5 months, if enough of the articular surface has been destroyed and if the horse is exercised sufficiently. Systemic analgesia should be administered if required to keep the horse active.

In one report of 20 horses with distal tarsal osteoarthritis in which arthrodesis of the DIT and TM joints was performed using the three-path technique, 17 horses were sound between 3.5 and 10 months after surgery.[17] In another report, 17 of 22 horses had a successful outcome after undergoing the procedure.[24,36] In a series of 29 horses with follow-up, 66% returned to performance.

Another 14% improved but did not regain their original status. The remaining horses did not improve.[13] Subchondral bone lysis (indicating activity) tended to be associated with a better outcome, and joint narrowing was a detractor. Another study reported success in 26 of 32 horses at 6 to 9 months after surgery. Note that only one-third of those 26 horses had negative hindlimb flexion tests in the same time period. Smaller horses tended to recover faster.[56] Another report of the same three-path technique saw success in 36 of 45 horses.[7]

If the PIT joint is involved, the prognosis is less favorable,[62] but it too should be operated on, because this offers the best hope of a complete recovery. Local and systemic anti-inflammatory therapy to protect the tarsocrural joint seems logical.

One study reported a series of 30 horses treated for TM/DIT or TM/DIT/PIT disease. A variety of surgical methods, including some with internal fixation, was used. Horses with disease confined to the TM and DIT joints did better in that drilling alone was more successful in a shorter period of time (78% recovery in 3 to 6 months) compared to horses that also had PIT disease (55% recovery in 8 months). In some horses, the surgeons placed lag screws obliquely across the affected joint spaces or applied bone plates. Recovery was not hastened by the internal fixation in horses with TM and DIT disease, but the rate of success was slightly improved. The reduced success in horses with PIT disease was not improved by using implants. The horses were encouraged in typical postoperative exercise.

When failure occurred, specific reasons were not given. Of interest would be the incidence of tarsocrural osteoarthritis in horses affected with PIT disease. Because internal fixation was applied to stabilize the joint spaces for fusion, the question arises whether more rest after surgery—instead of the typical return to activity after drilling alone—would improve the results. It may have been particularly beneficial for horses affected with PIT disease that were treated with internal fixation to restrict exercise to allow the drill paths to heal without stimulating further osteoarthritis.

When bone plates are applied, 5.5-mm screws are recommended, because there is a risk of implant failure with smaller screws in adult horses.[3] In addition to drilling, cancellous bone grafting and compression of the joint spaces using a tension device were suggested. The success rate using these approaches is approximately 80% recovery within 6 to 12 months.[3]

Another method of surgical arthrodesis that has been attempted is implanting stainless-steel Bagby baskets into large drill holes between the joints.[2,53] One report noted that horses became sound after 9 months, but one horse that fractured a third tarsal bone remained lame. It appears that there is no advantage of this technique over more conventional techniques.

Intramedullary Decompression or Fenestration of the Distal Tarsal Bones

Elevated subchondral or intramedullary bone pressure has been proposed as a source of lameness in horses with osteoarthritis. Based primarily on work by Kristoffersen,[30] who described a modified drilling procedure that courses obliquely from distad to proximad through the third metatarsal bone, crossing the DIT and TM joints and entering the central tarsal bone. Multiple drill paths are created.[55] Horses treated include Standardbred racehorses, other competing breeds, pleasure horses, and ponies. Diagnostic local anesthesia was not described. Success was evaluated by telephone conversation with the owners approximately 1 year after surgery. Of the 40 horses treated, 25 had regained full working capacity, 13 were considered unsuccessful, and 2 were lost to follow-up. A later series reported 28 of 56 successful cases.[28] Although it is not possible to separate the effect of medullary decompression from immobilization owing to bone healing across the drill sites, this technique appears to be no more effective than the other techniques described.

Laser-Induced Arthrodesis of the Distal Tarsal Joints

Cartilage destruction by passing a laser fiber through the joint space has been reported. The procedure is performed using an Nd:YAG or diode (980-nm) laser and consists of a single pass through each affected joint space, using a 600-μ fiber. The power setting varied between 15 and 25 W and generated a total energy of 800 to 1000 J.[25] A vent needle is placed at another point of the joint to allow the escape of vaporized synovial fluid and/or cartilage. In one report on 24 Standardbred racehorses and Western performance horses, all improved. Stall confinement was enforced for 2 days, followed by progressive return to full activity in approximately 2 weeks. The horses were reported to become sound before fusion could have occurred, so desensitization by the heat generated during the procedure is a consideration.[25]

Extracorporeal Shock Wave Therapy

Though not new technology, extracorporeal shock wave therapy (ESWT) has recently been used as a means to treat equine soft tissue and orthopedic conditions. The principle of the procedure is that an energy wave is produced under water (invisible) by various means and is focused at the anatomic site of concern. Instruments often have radiographic or ultrasonographic means of directing the shock wave specifically at the necessary anatomy. A compressive force is created when the shock wave encounters tissue of different impedances, such as soft tissue–bone interfaces. This compression is thought to produce microfractures in the bone, which result in noticeable remodeling during the subsequent weeks. No controlled equine studies are available, but profound osseous effects have been demonstrated in rabbit femurs.[14] Note that more than one type of ESW-generating machine is available, and no objective evidence of comparative benefits is available.

A series of 74 predominantly Western horses (130 joints) were treated for distal tarsal osteoarthritis using ESWT.[34] The horses had been treated by conservative medical means and had either become nonresponsive or were response for an unacceptably short duration. The horses received 2000 pulses at 22 kV. At 90 days after treatment, 38% had improved one lameness grade and 42% had improved two lameness grades. A total of 18% became sound, all of which improved two lameness grades. Of the 15 horses that failed to improve, 8 became better after a second treatment. No radiographic differences were detectable between pretreatment studies and 90-day post-treatment evaluations. Another report relates ESWT of 1 horse with distal tarsal osteoarthritis.[52] Improvement was immediate but lasted only 90 days.

An analgesic effect of ESWT has been documented.[45] The fact that ESWT stimulated no further ankylosis in the large series of horses with distal tarsal osteoarthritis[34] causes one to more strongly consider pain relief as a significant component of the mode of action. Anecdotally, immediate but temporary relief of heel pain and other conditions has been reported in horses; some clinicians believe that analgesia may be of longer duration after multiple treatments.

Distal tarsal osteoarthritis is a condition in which pain relief alone is a benefit. Provided no soft tissue compromise occurs, soundness and continued exercise should facilitate eventual ankylosis. Recognizing the density difference between rabbit long bone and equine cuboidal bone, the induced osseous changes could eventually facilitate ankylosis. Aside from distal tarsal disease, there is cause for concern when inducing analgesia in injuries of support structures of horses.

Neurectomy of the Tibial and Deep Peroneal Nerves

The results of an improved method of partial tibial and deep peroneal neurectomy was reported in 24 Warmblood horses.[27] The horses had been affected with osteoarthritis from 2 months to 7 years. Diagnostic intraarticular or regional anesthesia was not performed. Complete tibial and peroneal neurectomy as previously reported[37] is said to have caused proprioceptive, sensory, and trophic complications and hyperextension of the tarsus (Imschoot J, unpublished data, 1988).

The surgery reported is performed with the horse in lateral recumbency, rolling the horse when the first side is completed. Using a tourniquet proximally, three 15-cm medial skin incisions are used to expose the tibial nerve and its branches into the medial and lateral plantar nerves. All the branches from the exposed nerves are transected. After rolling the horse, another incision is created between the long and lateral digital extensor muscles proximal to the tarsus to expose and resect a 3- to 4-cm segment of the deep peroneal nerve.

Postoperative care includes 2 months of stall rest with progressively increasing hand walking after the incisions have healed. Presumably because of an inability to adequately apply a pressure bandage, the lateral incisions tend to swell and organize into a firm thickening. Deficits from denervation were not observed. Results were gathered 1 to 3 years after surgery via telephone conversations with owners. Of 21 horses that were followed-up, 14 were used for dressage, riding, jumping, or eventing for 14 to 36 months. A total of 5 horses relapsed 6 to 14 months after surgery, and 2 failed to improve. Radiographic follow-up of some of the horses revealed variable stasis or progression of the osteoarthritis.

The study concluded that the convalescence was shorter than that following surgical arthrodesis, but that the surgery time was longer owing to the sizable incisions

that must be closed. A blemish usually developed at the lateral incision site.

Prognosis

The prognosis with spavin is always guarded. Horses treated medically and with corrective shoeing respond individually. Some horses that have been lame for a shorter period of time respond better. A prognosis should be withheld until an operation or other methods of therapy are used, especially when the horse shows ankylosis of either the intertarsal and/or the TM joints.

For horses not responding to conservative therapy, sodium MIA injection has been reported as 80% successful after 1 year in a group of 39 horses and 40% successful in a group of 5 horses.[9,49] This is a good rate of recovery, but the complications are serious when they occur. Surgical arthrodesis using the three-path drill technique has provided 59% return to performance, and the complications are minor. The most serious complication is lack of complete response.[13] Laser-induced ankylosis holds promise and is apparently without major complications.

References

1. Adams OR. Surgical arthrodesis for the treatment of bone spavin. J Am Vet. Med Assoc 1970;157:1480.
2. Archer RM, Schneider RK, Lindsay WA, et al. Arthrodesis of the equine distal tarsal joints by perforated stainless steel cylinders. Equine Vet J Suppl 1988;6:125–130.
3. Auer JA. Arthrodesis techniques. In: Auer JA, Stick JA, Eds. Equine Surgery. 2nd ed. Philadelphia: WB Saunders, 1999;696–704.
4. Axelsson M., Bjornsdottir S, Eksell P, et al. Risk factors associated with hindlimb lameness and degenerative joint disease in the distal tarsus of Icelandic horses. Equine Vet J 2001;33:84–90.
5. Axelsson M, Eksell P, Roneus B, et al. Relationship between hind limb lameness and radiographic signs of bone spavin in Icelandic horses in Sweden. Acta Vet Scand 1998;39:349–357.
6. Barber SM. Arthrodesis of the distal intertarsal and tarsometatarsal joints in the horse. Vet Surg 1984;13:227–235.
7. Barneveld A. Arthrodesis of the distal tarsal joint (in horses with spavin). Pferdekrankheiten 1985;29:209–219.
8. Bogner B, Bock P, Stanek C. Correlation of radiological and histological changes of the medial tendon attachment and the related subtendinous bursa of the cranial tibialis muscle in horses affected with spavin. Pferdeheilkunde 1998;14:197–204.
9. Bohanon TC. Chemical fusion of the distal tarsal joints with sodium monoiodoacetate in horses clinically affected with osteoarthrosis. Proc Am Assoc Equine Pract 1995;41:148–149.
10. Bohanon TC. Contrast arthrography of the distal intertarsal and tarsometatarsal joints in horses with bone spavin. Vet Surg 1994;23:396.
11. Bohanon TC. The tarsus. In: Auer JA, Stick JA, Eds. Equine Surgery. 2nd ed. Philadelphia: WB Saunders, 1999;848–862.
12. Burtscher WO, Bock P, Stanek C. The subtendinous bursa of the musculus tibialis cranialis—A histological study. Pferdeheilkunde 1996;12:823–829.
13. Dechant JE, Southwood LL, Baxter GM, et al. Treatment of distal tarsal osteoarthritis using a 3-drill technique in 36 horses. Proc Am Assoc Equine Pract 1999;45:160–161.
14. Delius M, Draenert K, Al Diek Y, et al. Biological effects of shock waves: In vivo effect of high energy pulses on rabbit bone. Ultrasound Med Biol 1995;21:1219–1225.
15. Dykstra RR. Bone spavin. J Am Vet Med Assoc 1913;8:143.
16. Eastman T, Bohanon T, Beeman G, et al. Owner survey on cunean tenectomy as a treatment for bone spavin in performance horses. Proc Am Assoc Equine Pract 1997;43:121.
17. Edwards GB. Surgical arthrodesis for the treatment of bone spavin in 20 horses. Equine Vet J 1982;14:117–121.

18. Ehrlich PJ, Seeherman HJ, O'Callaghan MW, et al. Results of bone scintigraphy in horses used for show jumping, hunting, or eventing: 141 cases (1988–1994). J Am Vet. Med Assoc 1998;213:1460–1467.
19. Eksell P, Axelsson M, Brostrom H, et al. Prevalence and risk factors of bone spavin in Icelandic horses in Sweden: A radiographic field study. Acta Vet Scand 1998;39:339–348.
20. Gabel AA. Lameness caused by inflammation in the distal hock. Vet Clin North Am 1980;2:101–124.
21. Gabel AA. Prevention, diagnosis and treatment of inflammation of the distal hock horse's joints. Proc Am Assoc Equine Pract 1983;28:287–298.
22. Goldberg SA. Historical facts concerning pathology of spavin. J Am Vet Med Assoc 1918;53:745.
23. Gough M, Munroe GA. Decision making in the management of bone spavin in horses. In Practice 1998;20:252–259.
24. Gustafson SB. Distal tarsal arthrodesis using 3-drill tracts for treatment of bone spavin in the equine. Unpublished manuscript, Colorado State University, 1987.
25. Hague BA, Guccione A. Clinical impression of a new technique utilizing a Nd:YAG laser to arthrodese the distal tarsal joints. Vet Surg 2000;29:464.
26. Hertsch B, Hoppner S, Leonhardt KM, et al. Radiographical examination of German Standardbred horses. Pferdeheilkunde 1997;13:97–109.
27. Imschoot J, Verschooten F, Moor AD, et al. Partial tibial neurectomy and neurectomy of the deep peroneal nerve as a treatment for bone spavin in the horse. Vlaams Diergeneesk Tijdschr 1990;59:222–224.
28. Jansson N, Sonnichesen H, Hansen E. Bone spavin in the horse: Fenestration technique. A retrospective study. Pferdeheilkunde 1995;11:97–100.
29. Kraus-Hansen AE, Jann HW, Kerr DV, et al. Arthrographic analysis of communication between the tarsometatarsal and distal intertarsal joints of the horse. Vet Surg 1992;21:139–144.
30. Kristoffersen K. Investigations of aseptic hock diseases in the horse. PhD thesis. The Royal Veterinary and Agricultural University, Copenhagen, 1981.
31. Mackay RCJ, Liddell WA. Arthrodesis in the treatment of bone spavin [Short Communication]. Equine Vet J 1972;4:34–36.
32. Manning JP. Diagnosis of occult spavin. Ill Vet 1964;7:26.
33. Martin WJ. Spavin, etiology and treatment. Am Vet Rev 1900;24:464.
34. McCarroll G, McClure S. Extracorporeal shock wave therapy for treatment of osteoarthritis of the tarsometatarsal and distal intertarsal joints. Proc Am Assoc Equine Pract 2000;46:200–202.
35. McDonough J. Hock joint lameness. Am Vet Rev 1913;43:629.
36. McIlwraith CW, Robertson JT. Arthrodesis of the distal tarsal joints. In: McIlwraith & Turner's Equine Surgery: Advanced Techniques. 2nd ed. Baltimore: Williams & Wilkins, 1998;193–197.
37. Merillat L. Veterinary Surgical Operations. Chicago: Alexander Eger, 1929.
38. Montavon S. Efficacy of a medicinal plant preparation based on Harpagophytum procumbens in cases of bone spavin of adult horses. Pract Vet Equine 1994;26:49–53.
39. Moyer W. Bone spavin: A clinical review. J Equine Med Surg 1978;2:362.
40. Moyer W, Brokken TD, Raker CW. Bone spavin in Thoroughbred race horses. Proc Am Assoc Equine Pract 1983;29:81–92.
41. Myhre GD, Boucher N, Aiken L. Incidence and correlation of scintigraphic findings to referral lameness at a private hospital. Proc Am Assoc Equine Pract 1998;44:218–221.
42. Norrie RD. Diseases of the rear legs. In: Mansmann RA, McAllister ES, Eds. Equine Medicine and Surgery. 3rd ed. Santa Barbara, CA: American Veterinary Publications, 1982;1141.
43. Novales M, Lucena R, Martin E, et al. Absence of lameness in horses with signs of pathology demonstrated by radiography. Pract Vet Equine 1997;29:41–45.
44. O'Brien T. Radiographic interpretation of the equine tarsus. Proc Am Assoc Equine Pract 1973;19:289.
45. Rompe JD, Hope C, Kullmer K, et al. Analgesic effect of extracorporeal shock-wave therapy on chronic tennis elbow. J Bone Joint Surg [Br] 1996;78:233–237.
46. Rooney JR. Biomechanics of lameness in horses. Baltimore: Williams & Wilkins, 1969.
47. Rooney JR, Turner LW. The mechanisms of horses pulling loads. J Equine Vet Sci 1985;5:355–359.
48. Sack WO, Orsini PG. Distal intertarsal and tarsometatarsal joints in the horse: Communication and injection sites. J Am Vet Med Assoc 1981;179:355–359.
49. Sammut EB, Kannegieter NJ. Use of sodium monoiodoacetate to fuse the distal hock joints in horses. Aust Vet J 1995;72:25–28.
50. Schebitz H. Spavin: Radiographic diagnosis and treatment. Proc Am Assoc Equine Pract 1965;11:207.
51. Schebitz H, Wilkins H. Bone spavin diagnosis and therapy. Munch Tierarztl Wochenschr 1967;80:385.
52. Scheuch B, Whitcomb M, Galuppo L, et al. Clinical evaluation of high-energy extracorporeal shock waves on equine orthopedic injuries. Equine Musculoskeletal High-Energy Shock Wave Therapy Symposium, Shelbyville, KY, 2001.
53. Schneider RK, Archer RM. Arthrodesis of the distal two tarsal joints in the horse using perforated stainless steel cylinders and cancellous bone graft. Vet Compar Orthop Traumatol 1991;4:21–27.
54. Sigurdsson H. Diagnosis and radiographic examination of spavin in 60 Icelandic horses. Buvisindi 1991;5:33–38.
55. Sonnichsen HV, Svalastoga E. Surgical treatment of bone spavin in the horse. Equine Pract 1985;7:6–9.
56. Stanger P, Lauk HD, Plocki KA, et al. Treatment of spavin by arthrodesis of the distal tarsal joint: Long-term results. Pferdeheilkunde 1994;10:75–79.
57. Stover SM, Hornof WJ, Richardson GL, et al. Bone scintigraphy as an aid in the diagnosis of occult distal tarsal bone trauma in three horses. J Am Vet Med Assoc 1986;188:624–628.
58. Vaughan JT. Analysis of lameness in the pelvic limb and selected cases. Proc Am Assoc Equine Pract 1965;11:223.
59. Wamberg K. A new treatment for spavin in horses. Proceedings. 15th International Veterinary Congress, 1953, 2:957.
60. Williams F, Rohe REK. Significance of genetic aspects of bone diseases in horses. Pferdeheilkunde 1996;12:345–346.
61. Winter D, Bruns E, Glodek P, Hertsch B. Genetic disposition of bone diseases in sport horses. Zuchtungskunde 1996;68:92–108.
62. Wyn-Jones G, May SA. Surgical arthrodesis for the treatment of osteoarthrosis of the proximal intertarsal, distal intertarsal and tarsometatarsal joints in 30 horses: A comparison of four different techniques. Equine Vet J 1986;18:59–64.

DISTAL TARSITIS OR OSTEOARTHRITIS IN FOALS

Foals are subject to synovitis stemming from cartilage disruption or inflammation owing to congenital or acquired deformity of the body or articular surfaces of the cuboidal bones of the distal tarsus. Unchecked, this inflammation or structural defect can lead quickly to osteoarthritis and potential permanent lameness.

Causes

Foals born with incomplete ossification of the cuboidal bones subject the tarsus to weight bearing before it is ready.[7] The result is tarsal bone wedging, generally of the dorsal portions of the bones, that leads to a curby conformation and/or valgus deformity, depending on which surface of the bone fails (Figs. 8.378 and 8.379).[1] This condition has been termed aseptic necrosis,[6] metabolic bone disease,[3] and one of several synonyms of developmental orthopedic disease (DOD).[5,10] The cause is possibly dysmaturity, but the condition has been linked to hypothyroidism and mineral or protein imbalances linked to DOD.[8] However, the dysmaturity is quite

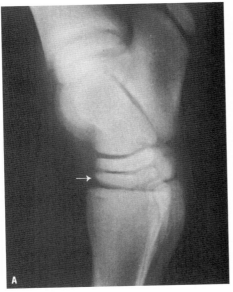
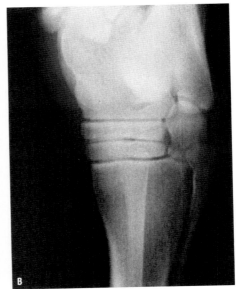
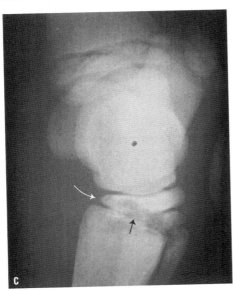

Figure 8.378 A. Lateromedial view of a neonate with delayed ossification of the distal tarsal bones demonstrating wedging of the third tarsal bone (arrow). The plantar angulation at the level of the distal tarsal joints caused a curby appearance. B. After the limb had been placed in a sleeve cast for 2 weeks, there was improved ossification of the dorsal aspect of the central and third tarsal bones. C. Oblique view of a younger foal showing wedging of the central tarsal bone (curved arrow) and complete collapse of the third tarsal bone (black arrow). Note the curby angulation of the plantar aspect of the tarsus. (Courtesy of T. S. Stashak.)

probably generalized and multisystemic, and many affected foals are weak.

Strictly speaking, endochondral ossification has failed to ossify the bones in time for normal weight bearing (Fig. 8.380). Drawing a line of demarcation between this condition and the surface defects in a group of foals apparently predisposed to osteochondritis dissecans (OCD)[10] would be difficult. The continuum of possibilities ranges from complete cuboidal bone collapse to hour-glass compression to surface defects only. All are capable of resulting in synovitis and osteoarthritis.

Signs and Diagnosis

The clinical signs in foals generally identify the condition. Foals usually present with a curby appearance (bump on the plantar surface, sometimes with an angular limb deformity) (Figs. 8.378 and 8.379). The lameness

is variable; however, the caudal or valgus deformity in the affected tarsus is suggestive. Radiographs demonstrate the osseous changes and defective endochondral ossification. Ultrasound has also been recommended as a monitoring device to evaluate cuboidal bone density.[7]

A case of plantar ligament laxity that appears quite similar to the foals described above, but with normal distal tarsal bones, was reported.[4] In addition to the curby appearance, the metatarsophalangeal joints were dropped. The foal responded well to rest and sleeve cast correction. A trailer shoe aided the distal joint laxity, which would also relieve strain on the tarsus.

Foals may also display a similar scenario when the distal tarsal bones become infected.[2] Foals with osteomyelitis are extremely lame, and the radiographs may demonstrate more aggressive bone destruction with the characteristics of sepsis. Sepsis is an entirely different situation (see Chapter 6). The prognosis is extremely poor.[2]

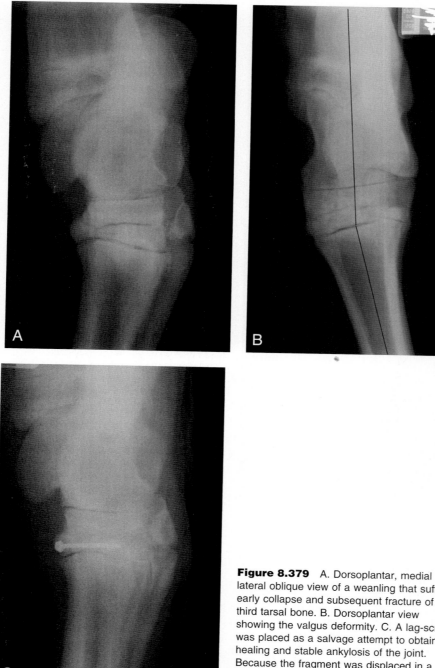

Figure 8.379 A. Dorsoplantar, medial lateral oblique view of a weanling that suffered early collapse and subsequent fracture of the third tarsal bone. B. Dorsoplantar view showing the valgus deformity. C. A lag-screw was placed as a salvage attempt to obtain healing and stable ankylosis of the joint. Because the fragment was displaced in a dorsolateral direction, two screws could not be used.

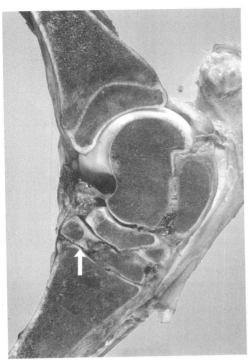

Figure 8.380 Postmortem sagittal section of a tarsus from a foal with collapse of the third tarsal bone. Note the retained cartilage core behind the fracture fragment (arrow). (Courtesy of T. S. Stashak.)

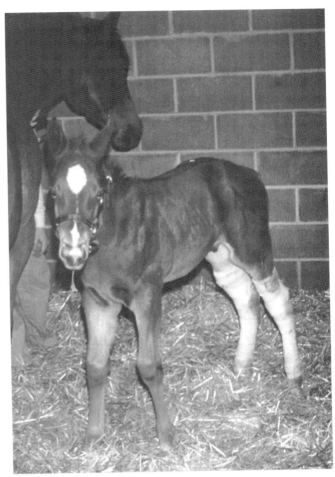

Figure 8.381 Bilateral hindlimb sleeve casts support the tarsus while normal ossification occurs. The exposed foot allows weight bearing and prevents flexor laxity.

Treatment

Most important are the recognition of the incompletely ossified cuboidal bone in foals at risk and restricting exercise until ossification is complete. If the wedging or collapse is early, supporting the limb in a sleeve cast can help (Fig. 8.381). Having the foal continue to support weight on the foot is critical for preventing overrelaxation of the suspensory apparatus, which may not be reversible. Maintaining foot balance is also important. Once a true angular deformity has occurred, correction is difficult. Because each foal is different, a schedule of postnatal maturation is not possible. The degree of ossification of the apophysis on the os calcis has been suggested as an indicator of tarsal bone maturity.[9]

Prognosis

Osteoarthritis (bone spavin) often accompanies this condition. As with adults, if the limb can maintain a reasonable alignment and the distal tarsal joints fuse, soundness may be possible. If lameness persists, most of the measures described for adults can be applied. In one study, foals with greater than 30% collapse had a much poorer prognosis than those with lesser degree.[1] In addition, other means of correcting the angular deformity when present were generally unsuccessful when the angulation was caused by the tarsal collapse.

References

1. Dutton DM, Watkins JP, Walker MA, et al. Incomplete ossification of the tarsal bones in foals: 22 cases (1988–1996). J Am Vet Med Assoc 1998;213:1590–1594.
2. Firth EC, Goedegebuure SA, Dik KJ, et al. Tarsal osteomyelitis in foals. Vet Rec 1985;116:261–266.
3. Gabel AA. Lameness caused by inflammation in the distal hock. Vet Clin North Am 1980;2:101–124.
4. Lemonnier JP. Deformation of the plant aspect of the hock in a foal. Point Vet 1993;25:155–158.
5. Lokai MD, Ford J. Disorders of endochondral ossification. Equine Pract 1981;3:48.
6. McIlwraith CW. Tarsal bone necrosis and collapse in young foals. In: Mansmann RA, McAllister ES, Eds. Equine Medicine and Surgery. 3rd ed. Santa Barbara, CA: American Veterinary Publications, 1982;1144–1145.
7. Ruohoniemi M, Hilden L, Salo L, et al. Monitoring the progression of tarsal ossification with ultrasonography and radiography in three immature foals. Vet Radiol Ultrasound 1995;36:402–410.
8. Shavers JR. Skeletal manifestations of suspected hypothyroidism in two foals. J Equine Med Surg 1979;3:269.
9. Smallwood JE, Auer JA, Martens RJ, et al. The developing equine tarsus from birth to six months of age. Equine Pract 1984;6:7–48.
10. Watrous BJ, Hultgren BD, Wagner PC. Osteochondrosis and juvenile spavin in equids. Am J Vet Res 1991;52:607–612.

DISTAL TARSITIS SYNDROME OF HARNESS-RACE HORSES (CUNEAN TENDINITIS AND BURSITIS)

Distal tarsitis syndrome involves inflammation of the cunean tendon, its bursa, and the soft tissues associated with the DIT and TM joints.[2-4] Gabel[3] states that this entity is the most common cause of hindlimb lameness in harness-racing horses. It is thought to be a reversible condition that probably affects the majority of Standardbreds sometime during their racing careers. Harness horse trainers and veterinarians alike often refer to this condition as jacks or occult or blind spavin, since no palpable swelling or pain is present and radiographs usually show no lesion. Although the condition is usually bilateral, it often manifests itself as a single hindlimb lameness that, after injection of a local anesthetic, will shift to the opposite limb.[3]

The onset of lameness most commonly occurs in the winter and spring as the 2- and 3-year-old Standardbreds are being prepared for summer races. In North America, the average date of onset is March 1; and only a few cases are diagnosed during the racing season.[3]

Causes

The causes appear to be shear stresses that result when the foot impacts the ground at a low angle and again when it pushes off during pacing or trotting. Although the shear stresses involve the entire limb, they tend to focus at the tarsus, because it is at a 90° angle. These repeated shear stresses result in the inflammation.[3] Horses that are worked too fast too soon are particularly susceptible. It is speculated that the soft tissues supporting the hock have not developed enough strength to withstand the repeated stress. The average training speed at which this condition develops is at 2.5 minutes per mile.[3] Poor training surfaces can worsen the situation.

Other factors—such as improper training and shoeing, abnormal gait, hiking, and concomitant forelimb lameness—may also play a role. Forelimb lameness may result in the horse carrying more weight on its hindlimbs, causing a cunean tarsitis. Pedal osteitis and flexor tendinitis of the forelimbs are commonly observed. Treatment of the forelimb problem often results in improvement of the condition.[3] Shoeing the hind feet with calks, grabs, trailers, or bars causes less slippage at impact and takeoff; all of which are believed to increase the stresses and incidences of this condition. It is thought that many of the interference problems seen in trotters are a result of tarsitis, which often causes the trainer to select even more severe shoeing methods.[3]

Signs and Diagnosis

At exercise, the horse will frequently carry its hind quarters to the opposite side of the jog cart from the lame limb (it may be difficult to drive), preferring to hold its head to the side of lameness. This stance may begin to interfere, slowing the horse down. A frustrating feature of this condition is that most horses look normal when trotted on a lead strap. Trainers often report a hindlimb lameness with an insidious onset that is believed to involve the stifle, back, or trochanteric bursa.[6] Although these regions are often painful, the inflammation is probably secondary to a painful hock.

Lameness diagnosis in a Standardbred racehorse in hand can be challenging. Distal tarsal lameness may be subtle, and the horses do not always show positive flexion tests. Concomitant sources of pain can cloud the picture considerably, and it may be necessary to observe the horse in the harness. Often, horses displaying the typical signs are treated empirically.

Cunean bursal anesthesia may result in partial improvement, but more significant improvement always follows intrasynovial anesthesia of the distal tarsal joints.[2] Resolution of the lameness is often seen when the distal tarsal joints are blocked first. In a significant proportion of horses, lameness in the opposite hindlimb becomes more evident after blocking the first limb. Intrasynovial anesthesia of the cunean bursae usually brings about improvement in the lameness and gait 20 minutes after the injection. A further improvement can be expected within 30 minutes after the injection (see Chapter 3).[3] Considering the condition is thought to be a synovitis/capsulitis, the blocking pattern makes sense. Cunean bursal block reaches a portion of the capsule and gradually diffuses. However, intraarticular anesthesia reaches most of the soft tissues, including those adjacent to the cunean bursa.

Radiographs are usually normal. Approximately 20% of the cases in one series had marginal lysis or osteophytes on the dorsal surface of the central and third tarsal bones, making the lateral radiographic projection more useful than in typical distal tarsal osteoarthritis cases.[2,3] Of 112 racing Standardbreds having scintigraphy for hindlimb lameness, 33% demonstrated distal tarsal inflammation.[1] True distal tarsal osteoarthritis is uncommon in harness horses but is occasionally observed in the aged trotter.[3]

Treatment

For horses without multiple problems and distal tarsal radiographic changes, anti-inflammatory therapy and a lighter training schedule are usually successful.[3,7] Restricting the horse from fast work for a few weeks decreases the inflammation, and slower workouts (4-minute miles) at longer distances (6 to 8 miles) allow the soft tissues to strengthen.[4] Severe shoeing should be eliminated and replaced with flat shoes, and ideally the horse should be exercised on soft tracks. The hoof is balanced and trimmed so that the hoof–pastern angle is straight, and the toe of the shoe is squared or rolled. Dorsiflexion of the foot compresses the dorsal aspect of the limb, intensifying distal tarsal stresses. Generally, this means that the heel should be raised. When the foot has shifted medially (lateral wall flared, medial wall steep), supporting the medial wall with a shoe slightly beyond the wall allows the hoof to grow to the shoe.[7] Although heel caulks help maintain the angle, fixing the heels to the ground accentuates undesirable shear forces within the hock. If the lameness persists or returns, the diagnosis should be reevaluated.

Injection of 100 to 130 mg methylprednisolone into the DIT and TM joints hastens the resolution of the synovitis; maximum effect begins in 4 to 7 days; some clinicians prefer to inject the TM joint only.[3] Systemic anti-inflammatory therapy improves the result; the recommendation is 2 g phenylbutazone PO per day.[5] Furthermore, the addition of 5 mL mepivacaine to increase the volume for better distribution within the joints (time to race must be considered) has been suggested; it could also serve a diagnostic function.[7] Eventual resolution of this lameness implies that no cartilage lesion is present in the majority of the cases. The addition of sodium hyaluronate to the corticosteroid may minimize any negative effect of the corticosteroid on the articular cartilage.

The rationale for cunean tenectomy has been questioned, since the removal of these structures further reduces the resistance to shear forces.[3] No significant difference in racing performance was observed between a group of 27 horses that underwent surgery and 43 horses that did not.[4] Other treatments, such as firing and Wamberg's operation, have little to recommend them.[3]

Prognosis

Determining an accurate prognosis is difficult because this condition appears to be a result of training and management problems. If the trainer will go along with rest periods, reconditioning periods, and altering shoeing methods, a good result can be expected.

References

1. Ehrlich PJ, Dohoo IR, O'Callaghan MW. Results of bone scintigraphy in racing Standardbred horses: 64 cases (1992–1994). J Am Vet Med Assoc 1999;215:982–991.
2. Gabel AA. Diagnosis, relative incidence, and probable cause of cunean tendon bursitis-tarsitis of Standardbred horses. J Am Vet Med Assoc 1979;175:1079–1085.
3. Gabel AA. Lameness caused by inflammation in the distal hock. Vet Clin North Am 1980;2:101–124.
4. Gabel AA. Treatment and prognosis for cunean tendon bursitis-tarsitis of Standardbred horses. J Am Vet Med Assoc 1979;175:1086–1088.
5. Gabel AA, Tobin T, Roy RS. Phenylbutazone in horses: A review. J Equine Med Surg 1977;1:221.
6. Harrison JC. Care and Training of the Trotter and Pacer. Columbus, OH: United States Trotting Association, 1968.
7. Moyer W. Treatment of distal tarsitis in harness horses. Proc Am Assoc Equine Pract 1989;34:413–416.

BOG SPAVIN (IDIOPATHIC SYNOVITIS, TARSOCRURAL EFFUSION)

Strictly speaking, bog spavin is a clinical sign and not a diagnosis. It is a descriptive term for synovial effusion of the tarsocrural joint. The effusion is the result of an acute or chronic low-grade synovitis, which can come from any of several causes.[2] As a primary condition, the term should be limited to situations in which the inciting cause (e.g., OCD or osteoarthritis) truly cannot be identified. The degree of lameness depends on the severity of the synovitis. Despite potential clinical insignificance, a bog becomes an important cosmetic issue in certain show situations. The dorsomedial enlargement is commonly more visible, but distension of the dorsolateral, plantarolateral, and plantaromedial joint pouches may also be

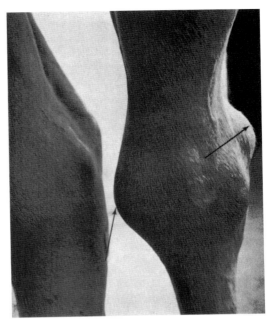

Figure 8.382 Bog spavin (tarsocrural joint effusion). Note the plantarolateral and larger dorsomedial swellings (arrows). Protrusions may also appear plantaromedially and dorsolaterally when effusion is severe. (Courtesy of T. S. Stashak.)

present or produced when the fluid is manually pushed around the joint (Fig. 8.382).

A significant proportion of affected horses do not have idiopathic synovitis (IS), but have an articular lesion that can be discovered radiographically or arthroscopically. Allowed to persist through years of work, this chronic synovitis can lead to cartilage loss and eventual osteoarthritis and a fibrotic joint capsule (Figs. 8.383 and 8.384). Truly idiopathic tarsocrural effusion is probably caused by recurring cartilage microtrauma, a result of a conformational problem such as being overly straight behind.

Causes

Clinical entities that can be diagnosed as causes of tarsocrural effusion are discussed elsewhere in this chapter. The discussion in this section is limited to situations in which a cause cannot be identified through physical or arthroscopic examination or any diagnostic imaging technique. A few individuals experience tarsocrural joint filling when they are stalled or inactive. This effusion disappears with exercise. In addition, some horses with lower hindlimb casts develop a bog spavin on the immobilized limb, presumably a result of a joint capsule sprain.

A horse that is too straight in the hock joint is predisposed to bog spavin, probably because of continuous trauma to the articular cartilage (Fig. 2.32). If a horse with straight limbs is not affected by tarsocrural IS when young, it may develop the condition after training begins. This could be owing to cartilage trauma caused by the straight conformation or it could be temporary synovitis/capsulitis typical of young horses beginning training. De-

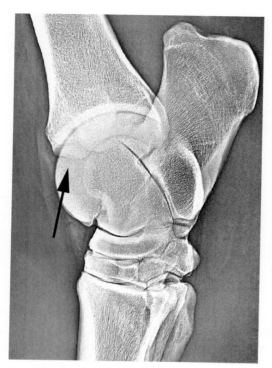

Figure 8.383 On xeroradiography, the lateromedial view reveals a small distal tibial OCD (arrow) in a mature show horse.

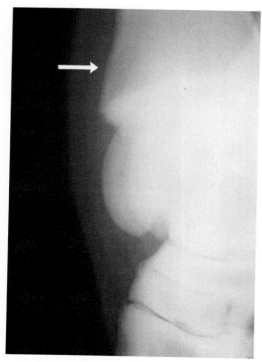

Figure 8.384 Lateromedial view of a chronic bog spavin. Note that the proximal joint capsule attachments have calcified (arrow) and the joint capsule has thickened. (Courtesy of T. S. Stashak.)

pending on the severity of the condition and the activity of the horse, these subtle cartilage lesions can worsen because of the persisting synovitis and lead to osteoarthritis. Thus IS can eventually become osteoarthritis, as can be observed in any other joint. An illustration is the report of necropsy findings Rooney[6] associated with tarsocrural effusion: articular wear lines in the distal tibia and erosive lesions on the dorsal edge of the medial and lateral grooves at the distal end of the tibia. Although frequently associated with primary pathology such as osteochondrosis, these are examples of osteoarthritis owing to chronic synovitis.

Trauma injury to the hock joint as a result of quick stops, quick turns, and other traumas cause bog spavin owing to injury of the joint capsule or tarsal ligaments. Occasionally, performance horses develop acute tarsocrural effusion and lameness approaching that of sepsis. A severe capsulitis is probably the main component. Radiographic signs being absent, horses are treated with rest and local and systemic anti-inflammatory therapy. Response to therapy can be profound and rapid. Structural damage, such as a collateral ligament sprain or a nondisplaced fracture, should be ruled out before returning the horse to work.

Deficiencies of calcium, phosphorus, vitamin A, or vitamin D, alone or in any combination, apparently can produce bog spavin. Chronic zinc intoxication has also been implicated in tarsocrural effusion.[4]

Uncommonly, horses that have had acute synovitis progressing to chronic synovitis, such as may follow septic arthritis, retain the effusion after the original cause has been resolved. The persistence appears to be the result of permanent synovial membrane changes or fibrous joint capsule distortion.

Signs and Diagnosis

By definition, the only clinical sign required is tarsocrural effusion. There are three characteristic fluctuant swellings, the largest of which is located at the dorsomedial aspect of the hock joint (Fig. 8.382). Two smaller swellings occasionally occur on either side of the surface of the hock joint at the junction of the tibial tarsal and fibular tarsal bones. However, severe effusion can produce distension of all four corners of the joint. These plantar swellings are lower (more distal) than the swellings of thorough-pin. When pressure is exerted on any one of these swellings, the other enlargements show an increase in size and an increase in the tension of the joint capsule if held. This fluctuant, moveable swelling must be differentiated from periarticular edema, which signals an extraarticular problem.

When present, lameness is the result of synovitis. The pain of synovitis is sensed by nerve endings located in the fibrous joint capsule. If the tarsocrural synovitis is severe enough to irritate those nerve endings, the horse is lame to some degree. Hindlimb flexion, specifically meant to diagnostically exacerbate that inflammation, may be required to see any lameness. If the seat of the problem is capsulitis, the response could be quite positive. More severe inflammatory situations may bring local heat, pain, and swelling. No bony changes are evident in uncomplicated bog spavin, either on palpation or on radiographs. There is one report of effusion that apparently became severe enough to rupture the fibrous joint capsule and create a synovial hernia.[3]

The presence of bog spavin is diagnostic. In most cases, the dorsomedial swelling is the largest; but in some horses, the two plantar swellings are more prominent. In some cases, the location of primary source of the synovitis may dictate the location of the largest point of effusion. The plantar swellings must be differentiated from thorough-pin, which occurs at the level of the point of the hock. The most important factor in the diagnosis is to determine the true cause, if possible.

All diagnostic capabilities should be used to rule out any correctable lesion. Even if not correctable, the prognostic value is important. Beyond radiographs and arthroscopy are CT and MRI, if available. Depending on the degree of lameness, scintigraphy may be useful.

With chronic bogs, synovial fluid changes are commonly unremarkable. Acute injuries may cause hemarthrosis or a rise in white blood cells and total protein. However, when lameness is severe, septic arthritis must be ruled out, and synovial fluid analysis is important. Synovial fluid analysis of tarsocrural effusion caused by synovitis from an adjacent or impending septic process usually reflects an elevated total protein without the expected increase in white blood cells. This situation should be monitored closely.

Treatment

Treatment is practically limited to effusions with specific causes. However, treatment can be part of a diagnostic progression. Lameness and radiographic examinations are indicated for a horse that presents with tarsocrural effusion. For an effusion of unknown origin, intraarticular therapy can be administered. Selection of the drug is influenced by the situation.

Young horses should not be treated aggressively. With the needle placed in the tarsocrural joint, as much synovial fluid as possible is removed, after which sodium hyaluronate is injected. Particularly when repeated, steroids have been known to cause cartilage exfoliation from the joint surface in young horses. A support bandage is applied to prevent return of the effusion. The joint capsule in foals can become thinned and may have difficulty regaining its normal integrity, even after the synovitis has been resolved. Activity is restricted to a stall for a few days and then to a small paddock. The bandage should be maintained for 2 to 3 weeks to allow the capsule to strengthen. If bandaging becomes difficult to maintain or the skin becomes irritated, elastic stockinet provides substantial support with minimal adhesive.

If the bog is resolved, nothing further is necessary. If the bog fails to resolve or returns, diagnostic arthroscopy is indicated. Repeat radiographs are also indicated, but often remain negative. Although OCD is the most common cause of tarsocrural effusion in young horses, systemic causes should be ruled out with bilateral tarsocrural effusion.

When no radiographic changes are present, the plan described above for young horses can be followed for adults, although a steroid would be added to the hyaluronic acid. Triamcinolone (6 mg) is a potent anti-inflammatory agent; and if the effect is positive, there is rationale for following up with a second injection of methylprednisolone 3 weeks later to produce a prolonged effect. Hyaluronic acid possibly minimizes any negative effect of steroids. If the bog returns, mature horses in work present either a simpler or a more complex situation. Without lameness, the preference would be to leave it alone. Any medical therapy is likely to produce only temporary resolution. Continuous steroid injections have an eventual negative effect, and the risk of sepsis increases with each treatment.

Intraarticular atropine has been anecdotally used to treat refractory tarsocrural effusion. There is no known pharmaceutical mechanism of action, but 4 to 6 mg has been used with noticeable success. It would be wise to purchase atropine in single-use sizes to preserve sterility. Note that there is no information about any negative effect of this drug. Because this is an off-label application of the drug, use it at your own risk.

Treatment of bog spavin caused by nutritional deficiencies is usually of no avail unless proper corrections are made in the diet. If the deficient mineral(s) and/or vitamin(s) are added to the diet, the overall nutrition regulated, and the horse freed from internal parasites, bog spavins usually disappear in 4 to 6 weeks. Nutritionally related bog spavin is most common in horses 6 months to 2 years of age. Tarsocrural effusion caused by chronic intoxication with zinc appears to respond to removal of the source of the zinc and to feeding a balanced ration supplemented with 60 g calcium carbonate per day.[4]

When irreversible synovial membrane changes have occurred, synovectomy may be useful. I resolved persistent bog spavin in one horse by synovectomy long after septic arthritis had resolved. Motorized equipment is required to do a complete job, and the caudal compartment of the tarsocrural joint should be treated as well. Intimal regeneration requires approximately 1 month, and the villi will not regenerate.[1,5] The functional significance of the loss of the villous surface area is unknown. In my experience, horses treated by synovectomy for acute septic arthritis have not demonstrated a negative clinical effect.

One reported case of synovial hernia occurring after chronic tarsocrural effusion responded favorably to surgical resection of the hernia.[3] This is a procedure that should not be taken lightly. Support bandaging and prolonged stall rest are necessary to prevent dehiscence and the creation of a much worse problem. The reported horse was under stall confinement for 3.5 months.

Prognosis

The prognosis is guarded if the cause is traumatic or nutritional. It is unfavorable if it is the result of conformation; note, however that in the majority of cases horses can continue to perform without an obvious lameness.

References

1. Doyle PS, Sullins KE, Saunders GK. Synovial regeneration in the equine carpus after arthroscopic mechanical or CO_2 laser synovectomy. Submitted for publication, 2000.

2. Gill HE. Diagnosis and treatment of hock lameness. Proc Am Assoc Equine Pract 1973;19:257.
3. Martens A, Steenhaut M, Sercu K, et al. Surgical treatment of a synovial hernia of the tarsocrural joint in a horse. Vet Surg 1997; 26:259–260.
4. Messer NT. Tibiotarsal effusion associated with chronic zinc intoxication in three horses. J Am Vet Med Assoc 1981;178:294–297.
5. Palmer JL, Bertone AL, Weisbrode SE. Histological and ultrastructural synovial membrane characteristics following surgical synovectomy. Vet Surg 1994;23:413.
6. Rooney JR. Bog spavin and tibiotarsal joint lesions in the horse. Mod Vet Pract 1973;54:43–44.

OSTEOCHONDRITIS DISSECANS OF THE TARSOCRURAL JOINT

Tarsocrural OCD is quite common in Standardbreds.[2,4,6,16,24] In 49 Standardbred horses, 61 joints were reported early.[22] A large series that included 154 racehorses contained 106 Standardbreds.[11] In addition, a recent long-term study revealed 117 joints were affected in 764 yearlings from 3 breeding years.[24] However, tarsocrural OCD is also prominent in other racing and show breeds.[1,11,15]

Horses with tarsocrural OCD usually present with joint distension (bog spavin). These animals are frequently not lame and are often seen before training. The other common scenario is the discovery of the lesion on routine radiographs taken before a sale. Horses of racing age are more likely to be presented with lameness.

Causes

See Chapter 7.

Signs and Diagnosis

Synovial effusion (bog spavin) is by far the most common presenting complaint.[9] Palpation of the tarsocrural joint capsule reveals effusion without a painful swelling. Horses with a long-standing bog may have palpable capsular thickening. However, if periarticular or regional edema or swelling beyond the tarsocrural joint are present, another problem should be suspected. Lameness may be absent or mild; severe lameness is not consistent with this diagnosis. A reduced flexion angle of the tarsus is observed in horses with excessive synovial effusion. A hindlimb flexion test may increase the lameness slightly. Horses presented after they have begun training are more likely to be lame.[11]

Affected horses without clinical signs may develop effusion after some type of incident apparently destabilizes an OCD lesion causing synovitis; among such incidents is normal training of young athletes. Synovial fluid analysis is usually unremarkable. One study demonstrated decreased viscosity that normalized with rest.[12]

A complete radiographic examination is indicated for all horses presenting with bog spavin.[25] The most commonly affected sites within the tarsocrural joint (in decreasing order of incidence) are the distal (dorsal) intermediate ridge of the tibia (Fig. 8.385), the lateral trochlear ridge of the tibiotarsal bone (Fig. 8.386), the medial malleolus of the distal tibia (Fig. 8.387), the medial trochlear ridge of the tibiotarsal bone, and proportionate combinations of these.[3,11,13,24]

The radiographic lesion can consist of a lucency, a partially ossified flap, or a larger osteochondral fragment (Fig. 8.385). All radiographic views of the both hocks should be taken, because at least one of the typically affected sites is demonstrated by each.[25] Each location has its typical appearance, but OCD also appears in other locations, so a complete evaluation must be made in every case.[14] Approximately half of affected horses have similar contralateral lesions.[6,8,26] Though less common, multiple lesions or loose bodies may also be present (Fig. 8.388).[11,20] Typical lesions can be discovered during routine radiography for sale in horses without clinical signs.[23] Some horses with tarsocrural OCD and joint effusion do not have radiographically apparent subchondral bone involvement and require arthroscopy to make the diagnosis. These lesions are apparently stable or do not disrupt the articular surface and have not caused synovitis.

The distal tibial lesion is commonly an osteochondral fragment (Fig. 8.385). Fragment size has been classified, but no correlation to clinical significance or surgical outcome was shown.[11] Lateral trochlear ridge lesions may appear as lucent defects or as partially calcified bone flaps (Fig. 8.386). Larger lesions may make up the majority of the distal lateral trochlear ridge (Fig. 8.389). Probably because of the close joint capsule contact, the frag-

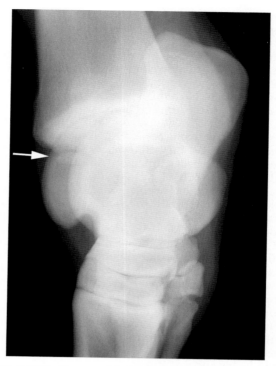

Figure 8.385 Dorsomedial plantarolateral view demonstrating OCD of the median (intermediate ridge) eminence of the distal tibia. This view reveals the typical fragment (arrow) and lesion well.

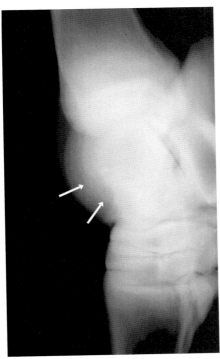

Figure 8.386   Note the osteochondral flap OCD lesion in the lateral trochlear ridge (arrows).

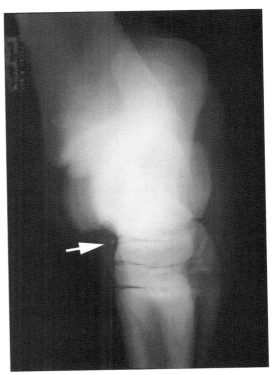

Figure 8.388   Dorsomedial, plantarolateral radiograph of a tarsus, showing a lateral trochlear ridge OCD. The fragments have become dislodged and fallen distally into the proximal intertarsal joint (arrow).

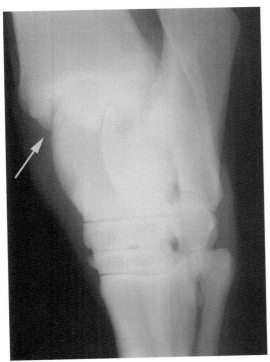

Figure 8.387   Dorsolateral, plantaromedial view of a tarsus, demonstrating a medial malleolar OCD (arrow). The lesion consists of a more abaxial lucency and a fragment adjacent to the medial trochlear ridge.

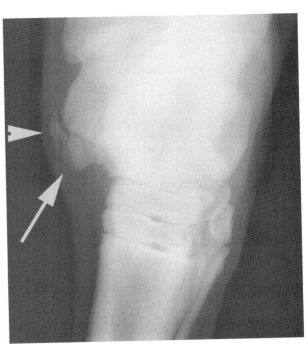

Figure 8.389   Dorsomedial, plantarolateral view of a tarsus with a large distal lateral trochlear ridge OCD lesion (arrow). An earlier fragment had dislodged, embedding in the joint capsule (arrowhead).

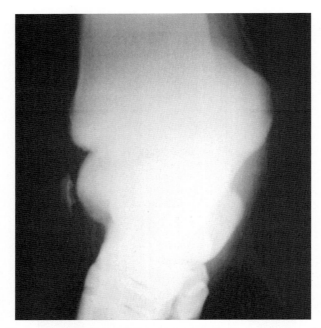

Figure 8.390 Dorsomedial, plantarolateral view of a tarsus with a large distal lateral trochlear ridge defect. A large fragment has become separated and is attached to the joint capsule.

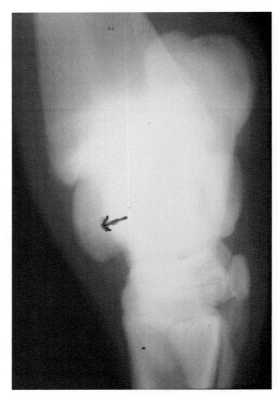

Figure 8.391 Dorsomedial, plantarolateral view of a tarsus with a subchondral cystic lesion in the lateral trochlear ridge (arrow).

ments may become displaced and lodge elsewhere in the tarsocrural or adjacent to the PIT joint (Figs. 8.389 and 8.390).[20]

Medial malleolus lesions are usually straightforward (Fig. 8.387) but should always be checked for radiographically inapparent cartilage defects.[25] Some medial malleolar lesions are axial and must be removed from the abaxial surface of the medial trochlear ridge.[25] Much of the lateral malleolus is extraarticular and is an uncommon site for OCD. However, a lateral malleolar subchondral cystic lesion accompanying distal tibial OCD has been reported.[27] Subchondral cystic lesions may also occur in the trochlear ridges (Fig. 8.391).

Radiographic findings that usually do not cause clinical signs include small buttons without osseous union to the parent bone, or dewdrop lesions (Fig. 8.392), on the distal end and a flattening of the ridge of the medial trochlear ridge (Fig. 8.393).[9,18] However, these lesions may be arthroscopically evaluated or addressed in some cases on the owner's request for the sake of future sale or if the joint is being operated on for another reason. Intracapsular osseous densities may be calcification or early fragments from OCD lesions that became embedded in the synovial membrane (Fig. 8.390). If they are extrasynovial, they are usually clinically insignificant. True distal medial trochlear ridge fractures may cause lameness,[20] and joints containing questionable findings should be evaluated if lameness is present. Synovial effusion accompanying such lesions may be the result of intraarticular lesions that are radiographically inapparent and should be investigated.

Two reports of tarsal radiographic monitoring—one on 77 Standardbred foals[16] and the other on 753 Standardbred yearlings[6]—revealed that clinically significant lesions are generally present at 1 year of age and rarely

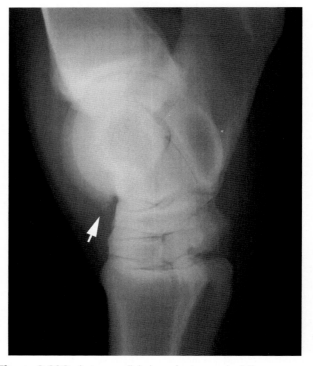

Figure 8.392 Lateromedial view of a tarsus depicting a dewdrop on the medial trochlear ridge (arrow). No treatment is indicated if there are no clinical signs.

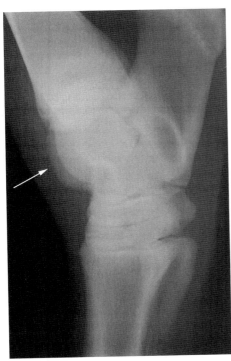

Figure 8.393 Lateromedial view of the tarsus showing a dorsal flattened area (arrow) on the medial trochlear ridge. No treatment is indicated if there are no clinical signs.

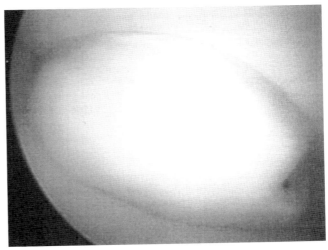

Figure 8.394 Arthroscopy reveals an OCD fragment on the distal intermediate ridge of the tibia.

appear later. Some of the affected horses had lesions by 1 to 3 months of age. However, typical lesions that were identified early in 11 foals reverted to normal by 7 to 8 months of age.[16] Usually, the lesions are discovered when examining a foal for bog. Results indicate it may be advisable to observe nondisplaced lesions in foals until the late weanling stage, when the situation allows. Control of synovitis (and exercise) is prudent in the interim.

Treatment

Horses with radiographic lesions but no clinical signs may have no immediate problem, but clinical signs can always appear during training, disrupting the schedule. After adjusting the data for problems unrelated to OCD, one report on conservative therapy without medication considered 80% of 3- to 5-year-old Warmbloods (*n* = 71) and 23% of 2- to 4-year-old Standardbreds (*n* = 75) to have been treated successfully.[13] Half of each group presented with tarsocrural effusion. Since lesion location or type was not correlated to differences in outcome, it seems that training at speed exacerbates lameness. However, it is also disappointing to find advanced osteoarthritis in experienced show and event horses that have worked with effusion all their lives, when the problem could have been prevented by early surgery (Fig. 8.383).

Even without severe lameness, the synovitis producing the joint effusion is likely to eventually lead to osteoarthritis in athletes. Studies have demonstrated better results in athletes that underwent surgical removal and debridement of the lesions than those that had no surgi-

cal treatment.[7,11,22] A retrospective study in 114 Standardbreds revealed similar racing data for surgically and conservatively treated horses.[8] Surgically treated horses had fewer total starts but equivalent earnings. Surgery produced better results than nonsurgical treatment in draft horses.[15] In another report, only 2 of 10 horses treated conservatively with intraarticular steroids and systemic supplements remained sound. No mention was made of the presenting or radiographic signs of those 2 horses.[5]

With foals, it is important to remember that some radiographically evident lesions are not actually disrupting the joint surface and will correct themselves with age.[4,19] In one series of 77 Standardbred foals, all ossification and subchondral bone abnormalities observed before 8 months of age resolved spontaneously. Distal tibial and lateral trochlear ridge fragments tended to increase in incidence at approximately the same time and remained unresolved.[4] Some foals may develop synovial effusion without radiographic signs. It is prudent to treat the synovitis to reduce the effusion and to wait and see if the situation resolves, because surgery may not be required.

Arthroscopy facilitates exploration and visualization of the tarsocrural joint and provides extensive beneficial lavage in the process (Fig. 8.394). The fact that radiographically inapparent lesions are sometimes the problem makes arthrotomy obsolete, because complete exploration is not possible. The typical dorsomedial arthroscope placement allows visualization of the entire dorsal aspect of the joint. Instrument access can be varied to reach any of the affected locations or the proximal intertarsal joint.[10] Exceptionally large fragments cannot be removed through the typical instrument portal, but the incision can be enlarged slightly or the fragment size can be reduced with an osteotome so the incision will not require conversion to an arthrotomy.

Prognosis

Some surveys of Standardbred racehorses conclude that conservatively treated horses with radiographic signs of OCD achieve performances equal to or better than normal horses.[2,21] However, no data on the incidence of clinical signs or therapy during the careers of the horses are available. Some horses eventually had surgery.[21] Long-term and individual evaluation is required to determine the effect of racing with tarsocrural OCD lesions. Statistics mean little when the mature Standardbred racehorse presents with tarsocrural osteoarthritis because of racing with OCD.

A recent survey of radiographic lesions of OCD in three yearling crops of Standardbreds (764 horses) revealed that horses with tarsocrural radiographic lesions earned less but comparable amounts to the entire group.[24] The study provides no specifics, but included horses that underwent arthroscopy. The implication is that arthroscopic surgery made no significant difference in racing success. One study revealed that horses affected with OCD were larger and more substantially built.[17] Aside from surgery not impairing athletic ability, the observation that OCD affects the best individuals may be true.[21]

Intraoperative findings of superficial cartilage fibrillation apparently had no effect on treatment outcome. However, further cartilage degeneration or erosion decreased success by 30%. Osseous densities that cannot be identified arthroscopically are unlikely to cause lameness.[20]

The prognosis for athletic activity after arthroscopic debridement of tarsocrural OCD is good.[8] In a series of 183 horses, 76.5% performed successfully after arthroscopic surgery.[11] Tarsocrural effusion resolved after surgery in 89% of racehorses and 74% of non-racehorses. However, effusion was less likely to resolve after surgery on the lateral trochlear ridge or medial malleolus. There was no correlation between resolution of effusion and athletic performance.[11] When compared to unaffected siblings, Thoroughbreds and Standardbreds that had arthroscopic removal of tarsocrural OCD fragments started at the same rate. However, affected horses were less likely to race as 2 year olds.[1] Lesion location and unilateral versus bilateral lesions had no effect on ability to start. Although the trend was present in all groups, only 2-year-old Standardbreds were significantly less likely to start a race when multiple sites within the tarsocrural joint were affected.[1,11,21]

References

1. Beard WL, Bramlage LR, Schneider RK, et al. Postoperative racing performance in Standardbreds and Thoroughbreds with osteochondrosis of the tarsocrural joint: 109 cases (1984–1990). J Am Vet Med Assoc 1994;204:1655–1659.
2. Brehm W, Staecker W. Osteochondrosis (OCD) in the tarsocrural joint of Standardbred trotters—Correlation between radiographic findings and racing performance. Proc Am Assoc Equine Pract 1999;45:164–166.
3. Canonici F, Serata V, Buldinin A, et al. 134 horses with osteochondritis dissecans of the tarso-crural joint: clinical considerations and results following arthroscopic surgery. J Equine Vet Sci 1996;16:345–348.
4. Carlsten J, Sandgren B, Dalin G. Development of osteochondrosis in the tarsocrural joint and osteochondral fragments in the fetlock joints of Standardbred trotters. I. A radiological survey. Equine Vet J 1993;16(Suppl):42–47.
5. De Moor A, Verschooten F, Desmet P, et al. Osteochondritis dissecans of the tibio-tarsal joint in the horse. Equine Vet J 1972;4:139–143.
6. Grondahl AM. The incidence of osteochondrosis in the tibiotarsal joint of Norwegian Standardbred trotters: A radiographic study. J Equine Vet Sci 1991;11:272–274.
7. Hoppe F, Philipsson J Racing performance of trotting horses with osteochondrosis of the hock. Svensk Veterinart 1984;36:285–288.
8. Laws EG, Richardson DW, Ross MW, et al. Racing performance of Standardbreds after conservative and surgical treatment for tarsocrural osteochondrosis. Equine Vet J 1993;25:199–202.
9. McIlwraith CW. Clinical aspects of osteochondrosis dissecans. Osteochondrosis dissecans of the tarsocrural joint. In: McIlwraith CW, Trotter GW, Eds. Joint Disease in the Horse. Philadelphia: WB Saunders, 1996;369–374.
10. McIlwraith CW. Diagnostic and Surgical Arthroscopy in the Horse. Philadelphia: Lea & Febiger, 1990.
11. McIlwraith CW, Foerner JJ, Davis DM. Osteochondritis dissecans of the tarsocrural joint: Results of treatment with arthroscopic surgery. Equine Vet J 1991;23:155–162.
12. Muttini A, Petrizzi L, Tinti A, et al. Synovial fluid parameters in normal and osteochondrotic hocks of horses with open physis. Boll Soc Ital Biol Sper 1994;70:337–344.
13. Peremans K, Verschooten F. Results of conservative treatment of osteochondrosis of the tibiotarsal joint in the horse. J Equine Vet Sci 1997;17:322–326.
14. Ribot X, Lions JA, Leroux D, et al. Osteochondrosis dissecans (OCD) in an unusual site. Pract Vet Equine 1998;30:235–239.
15. Riley CB, Scott WM, Caron JP, et al. Osteochondritis dissecans and subchondral cystic lesions in draft horses: A retrospective study. Can Vet J 1998;39:627–633.
16. Sandgren B. Bony fragments in the tarsocrural and metacarpo- or metatarsophalangeal joints in the Standardbred horse—A radiographic survey. Equine Vet J 1988;6(Suppl):66–70.
17. Sandgren B, Dalin G, Carlsten J. Osteochondrosis in the tarsocrural joint and osteochondral fragments in the fetlock joints in Standardbred trotters. I. Epidemiology. Equine Vet J 1993;16(Suppl):31–37.
18. Shelley J, Dyson S. Interpreting radiographs 5: Radiology of the equine hock. Equine Vet J 1984;16:488–495.
19. Smallwood JE, Auer JA, Martens RJ, et al. The developing equine tarsus from birth to six months of age. Equine Pract 1984;6:7–48.
20. Stephens PR, Richardson DW, Ross MW, et al. Osteochondral fragments within the dorsal pouch or dorsal joint capsule of the proximal intertarsal joint of the horse. Vet Surg 1989;18:151–157.
21. Storgaard Jorgensen H, Proschowsky H, Falk Ronne J, et al. The significance of routine radiographic findings with respect to subsequent racing performance and longevity in Standardbred trotters. Equine Vet J 1997;29:55–59.
22. Stromberg B, Rejno S. Osteochondrosis in the horse. I. A clinical and radiologic investigation of osteochondritis dissecans of the knee and hock joint. Acta Radiol Suppl Stockh 1978;358:139–152.
23. Torre F, Fadiga G. A radiological investigation on metacarpal/tarsal-phalangeal and tibio-tarsal joints in a selected group of Standardbred yearlings. Ippologia 1993;4:37–41.
24. Torre F, Motta M. Osteochondrosis of the tarsocrural joint and osteochondral fragments in the fetlock joints: Incidence and influence on racing performance in a selected group of Standardbred trotters. Proc Am Assoc Equine Pract 2000;46:287–294.
25. Torre F, Toniato M. Osteochondral fragments from the medial malleolus in horses: A comparison between radiographic and arthroscopic findings. Proc Am Assoc Equine Pract 1999;45:167–171.
26. Tourtoulou G, Caure S, Domaingue MC. Incidence of osteochondrosis in the Trotter foals. Pract Vet Equine 1997;29:237–244.
27. van Duin Y, Hurtig MB. Subchondral bone cysts in the distal aspect of the tibia of three horses. Can Vet J 1996;37:429–431.

ACQUIRED BONE CYSTS OF THE TARSUS

Bone cysts with no apparent relation to developmental orthopedic disease have been rarely reported in the distal tibia[1,4,5] and distal talus adjoining the PIT joint.[2]

Causes

Such lesions have been observed as a feature of septic arthritis, but these cases have no readily apparent septic basis. A consistent feature is severe aseptic synovitis, usually not seen in horses with acute or long-standing developmental orthopedic disease. A 13-month-old Standardbred that was included in one report[4] was simultaneously affected with distal tibial OCD and a lateral malleolar subchondral cystic lesion that was nonarticular and possibly does not fall into the same category as the other cases reported and described here. Other reports reveal tibial subchondral cystic lesions immediately proximal to the most proximal portion of the medial trochlear ridge of the talus.[1,5] One such case had a simultaneously accompanying cyst in the medial malleolus.[1]

Signs and Diagnosis

Affected horses or ponies ranged in age from 38 days to 13 years. Most apparent is the acute onset of significant lameness owing to synovitis of the affected joint. In adults, radiographic signs are absent during the early examinations. After rest and anti-inflammatory therapy, the condition worsens. Previously absent tarsocrural effusion appears. Subchondral bone cysts become radiographically apparent on the medial trochlear groove, the medial malleolus, or the dorsolateral aspects of the tibia.[1,4,5] Note that these subchondral cystic lesions were frequently scintigraphically apparent.[1,5] Synovial fluid analysis reflects severe aseptic inflammation or no changes.[1,5]

One report discusses a 38-day-old Thoroughbred colt that became suddenly lame and displayed tarsocrural effusion. Radiographs demonstrated a 1- to 2-cm subchondral bone cyst in the talus within the central portion of the PIT joint.[2]

Treatment

Local and systemic anti-inflammatory therapy is administered to adult horses; when the synovitis worsens and radiographic changes appear, exploratory arthroscopy is performed.[4] The surgical findings typify chronic synovitis and early osteoarthritis[4] or are negative.[1,5] None of the reported subchondral cysts could be identified arthroscopically.

In two cases, an extraarticular approach to the cysts was performed using radiographic control; the contents were debrided using a curette.[1,5] Cancellous bone was applied to one of the remaining cavities.[5] Arthroscopic surgery on a foal revealed that the PIT joint did not communicate normally with the tarsocrural joint.[2] An opening was created, and the cyst was debrided routinely. No explanation for the tarsocrural effusion was provided in the report.

Prognosis

Adult horses in which the lesions are left alone continue to be lame and cannot return to work. Two adults that underwent extraarticular debridement of the sub-chondral cysts improved shortly after surgery and became sound within 3 to 11 months.[1,5] The cyst contents may have been under pressure, which the debridement relieved. The procedure may have also relieved pain while facilitating a fibrocartilaginous filling of the defect. The benefit of cancellous bone grafting remains unproven. One study reported that a foal recovered from surgery and became sound.[2]

The probability exists that the adult and foal conditions are different. Another report of cysts unrelated to osteochondrosis in the proximal tibia described subchondral cyst formation as a degenerative change following injury and severe synovitis.[3] However, these lesions were accompanied by osteoarthritis. Despite the lack of definitive evidence of intraarticular sepsis, infection adjacent to the joint or within the cysts was not ruled out. However, the horses that improved after surgical debridement were those with acquired cysts that probably resulted from trauma. Each case must be treated individually, and the clinician should exercise caution when determining a prognosis.

References

1. Ball MA, Allen D Jr, Parks A. Surgical treatment of subchondral cyst-like lesions in the tibia of an adult pony. J Am Vet Med Assoc 1996;208:704–706.
2. Hawkins JF. Subchondral cystic lesion of the talus in a foal. Equine Pract 1998;20:8–9.
3. Textor JA, Nixon AJ, Lumsden JM, et al. Subchondral cystic lesions of the proximal extremity of the tibia in horses: 12 cases (1983–2000). J Am Vet Med Assoc 2001;218:408–413.
4. van Duin Y, Hurtig MB. Subchondral bone cysts in the distal aspect of the tibia of three horses. Can Vet J 1996;37:429–431.
5. Vits L, Adams N. Extra-articular approach to a subchondral cyst in the distal tibia of a horse. Seminar. Virginia Polytechnic Institute, Blacksburg, VA, 2001.

SLAB AND SAGITTAL FRACTURES OF THE CENTRAL AND THIRD TARSAL BONES

In a survey of 813 horses with hindlimb lameness, 59 fractures were diagnosed, of which 3 occurred in the tarsus.[20] Incidence or diagnosis of tarsal fractures is apparently increasing, because many more have been reported since that survey.[6,8,11,14,19,23] These fractures are usually the result of a racing injury. Standardbreds are overrepresented, and they seem to commonly sustain central tarsal bone fractures. The condition, however, has been reported in Thoroughbreds, Quarter Horses, Warmbloods, and one Arabian.[6,8,11,14,19,23]

Causes

The distal tarsal bones are subjected to axial compression, torsional forces, and tensile forces during exercise. The bones' main function is to absorb concussion and to neutralize the twisting forces.[17] When these bones are subjected to the great stress of racing speeds, fractures can occur.[19] One report described the normal biomechanics of the hock and concluded that asynchronous movement of the tarsal bones—which may be caused by ligament damage or rapid changes in lead—may result in fracture.[15]

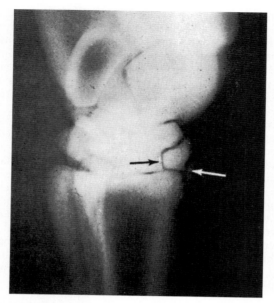

Figure 8.395 Lateromedial view of a mature horse with hourglass compression of the third tarsal bone and a slab fracture (black arrow). The concavity provides a stress riser for slab fractures in horses that work at speed. Note the osteophyte production owing to chronic synovitis (white arrow). (Courtesy of T. S. Stashak.)

A similar fracture occurs in the right tarsus in racing Greyhounds and is thought to result from an overstress mechanism.[3] The excessive medial stress that focuses on the right tarsus during counterclockwise racing is thought to cause the fracture. Although a similar mechanism has been considered in the horse,[6] it has not been substantiated in the review of 11 cases in which the right and left tarsi were almost equally affected.[19] No training effect on bone density was demonstrated after 19 weeks of progressive training in a group of Thoroughbreds compared with other horses that walked 40 minutes daily.[21] It is possible that the treadmill failed to duplicate training stresses or that the incidence of fracture is related more to conformation or a specific incident than to training.

Collapse of the dorsal or dorsolateral portion of the third tarsal bone has been described in foals; but the predisposition of this injury is thought to be a lack of bone strength related to a dysmaturity or to a metabolic or endocrine disorder.[7,9] Younger foals tend to wedge the dorsal margins of the central and third tarsal bones, whereas older (or more mature) foals may collapse the more plantar portion of the bone, producing an hourglass shape in the lateromedial or dorsoplantar, medial lateral oblique radiograph.[2,16] Once the horse is mature, the hourglass-shaped third tarsal bone tends to fracture at its narrowest point (Fig. 8.395). If the bone fragment separates completely and becomes displaced, an angular limb deformity may result.

Signs and Diagnosis

The diagnosis of central and third tarsal bone fractures can be difficult, especially when swelling is minimal and a nondisplaced slab fracture has occurred.[19] Horses typically present with a history of acute onset of lameness associated with performance. Acute cases may assume a non-weight-bearing stance when standing in a stall (Fig. 8.396). Distal tarsal fractures do not exhibit external swelling, even though they are often displaced dorsally. Because there is a communication between the PIT joint and the tarsocrural joint, tarsocrural joint effusion is usually seen with slab fractures of the central tarsal bone.[19] On palpation, heat and pain, which lead to discomfort when pressure is applied to the dorsolateral aspect of the distal row of tarsal bones, may be appreciated.[6] The acute lameness disappears rapidly, and there is usually no externally visible abnormality. However, a greater degree of lameness can be expected with extremely comminuted fractures. If bilateral fractures are present, the horse has a wide-based crabby way of moving at a jog. A marked reaction to the hock flexion test is usually observed.

The lameness may not specifically incriminate the distal tarsus. Intrasynovial anesthesia of the tarsocrural joint or PIT or DIT joints may help, but radiographic confirmation is required for a definitive diagnosis. Although the dorsoplantar and lateral medial projections are informative (Figs. 8.395 and 8.396A), the oblique projections help identify fragmentation and the specific position of the fractures.[6,8,13,19] Central tarsal fractures may be comminuted or in a more plantar location, and the dorsoplantar view should be scrutinized for a sagittal fracture (Fig. 8.397). The dorsomedial-plantarolateral 25° oblique view demonstrates the fracture line well.[5]

With localization of the source of the lameness and no definitive radiographic lesion, scintigraphy may help.[8,18] Radiographic evidence of the fracture may not appear for some time after injury if the fracture is nondisplaced.[18] Comminution or fractures in the sagittal plane may not appear in routine radiographic projection. In some cases, a projection of 5 to 10° to either side of the normal angle may reveal a fracture (Fig. 8.397). Radiographic evidence of osteoarthritis is present with a tarsal bone fracture of long duration.[1,4,9,10]

Treatment

Conservative Treatment

Recent reports indicate satisfactory results without surgery.[11,18] In one series of 25 cases, horses that recovered were restricted to the stall for 6 to 8 months. The fracture line remained radiographically visible in each of 5 horses for which follow-up films were taken; this was not correlated with a negative result. Of 12 Standardbreds with available race records, 10 horses completed at least five races after the injury; the median number of starts was 47. A total of 2 of 6 Thoroughbreds and 4 of 5 Quarter Horses returned to work. Although thickness of the fragment was not correlated to starts, earnings decreased for horses with fragments greater than 8 mm thick. The proportion of successful cases with central tarsal bone fractures (2 of 7) was significantly less than those with third tarsal bone fractures (10 of 13).[11]

Signs and Diagnosis

Intraarticular fractures cause tarsocrural effusion, and lameness is usually exacerbated by hindlimb flexion. Although usually not necessary, intraarticular local anesthesia relieves the lameness and the response to flexion. If blood is retrieved when the needle enters the joint, local anesthetic should not be injected. The hock is radiographed at that time. Radiographic examination is required to make a definitive diagnosis.

Trochlear Ridge Fractures

Trochlear ridges are affected by direct trauma; the proximal (caudal) medial is exposed when the limb is flexed, and distal lateral trochlear ridge is exposed when the limb is extended.[3] Horses are kicked while preparing to kick another horse, resulting in a fracture of the proximal medial trochlear ridge.[8,9]

The diagnosis is made based on the clinical signs and radiographic findings. Proximal medial trochlear ridge fragments appear in routine radiographic projections, but they are often superimposed on the tibia or tibial tarsal bone. The flexed lateromedial, flexed proximodistal tangential, or flexed dorsolateral to ventromedial oblique views demonstrate the lesions (Fig. 8.398). Distal lateral trochlear ridge fragments should be differentiated from OCD, which are much more common. The history, shape of the lesion, and degree of lameness are most helpful when making a differentiation.

Proximal medial trochlear ridge lesions can be removed arthroscopically using a plantar approach.[7,12] Distal lateral trochlear ridge lesions are addressed using the routine tarsal arthroscopic approach. Provided osteoarthritis has not begun or associated soft tissue injury is not limiting, the prognosis is good after fragment removal. Before any horse suffering tarsal trauma is anesthetized, the integrity of the collateral ligaments should be confirmed by physical or ultrasound examination.

Sagittal or Comminuted Fractures of the Talus

The talus can be affected by sagittal or comminuted fractures; some are completely nondisplaced (at least early on) and can be difficult to identify radiographically. The dorsoplantar radiographic projection is the most useful, but slightly oblique variations may better demonstrate the fracture line.[7]

Nondisplaced fractures can be difficult to diagnose. In a series of 11 horses with incomplete sagittal talus fractures, Standardbred racehorses were overrepresented.[4] All horses had a history of chronic hindlimb lameness that became an acute grade 2 to 4 (of 5) lameness. Tarsocrural effusion varied from absent to moderate, and hindlimb flexion was markedly positive in 6 of 7 horses in which flexion was performed. The dorsoplantar projection or one that is 10° to 20° off dorsoplantar toward dorsolateral-plantaromedial view has been described as best.[4] Xeroradiographs, digital radiographs, and/or scintigraphy may be required to make the diagnosis. Scintigraphy revealed moderate to intense uptake in the proximal aspect of the talus of all 11 horses, 6 of which had been radiographically negative. The flexed lateral scintigram is useful because it separates the proximal talus from the distal tibia (Fig. 8.399). All horses were treated conservatively with ≥1 month of stall rest and ≥1 month of small paddock turnout. Regression of the scintigraphically evident lesion was not described. A total of 7 horses returned to racing 115 to 341 days after the injury.

Displaced, noncomminuted sagittal fractures can be repaired using lag screws.[5–7] These fractures generally occur toward the medial aspect of the trochlea. Successful lag screw fixation from the lateral[6] and medial[7] approaches have been described. The medial approach provides more bone for screw purchase for compression of the fracture line. Radiographic or fluoroscopic guidance is necessary; and for displaced fractures, arthroscopic observation of reduction is advisable. With accurate re-

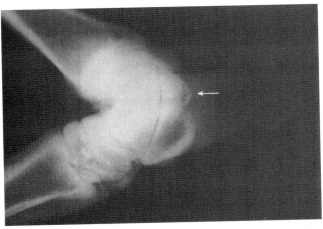

Figure 8.398 Flexed lateromedial radiograph of the tarsus of a horse with a history of lameness of 1 month. Physical examination revealed tarsocrural effusion Note the fragments from the plantar aspect of the medial trochlear ridge of the talus (arrow).

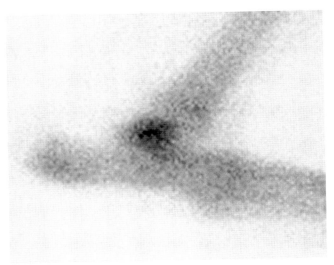

Figure 8.399 Flexed lateral scintigram of a tarsus depicting a sagittal fracture of the talus. The flexed position more clearly localizes the lesion to the talus versus the tibia. (Courtesy of M. W. Ross.)

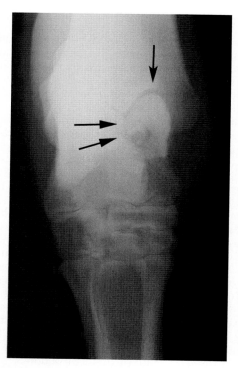

Figure 8.400 Dorsoplantar radiograph of a tarsus with a comminuted sagittal fracture of the talus (horizontal black arrows). The opening of the medial aspect of the tarsocrural joint space (vertical black arrow) indicates medial collateral instability.

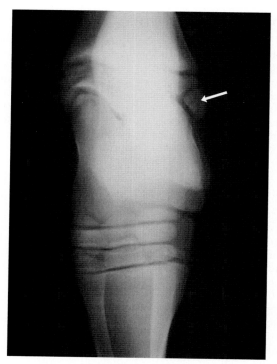

Figure 8.401 Dorsoplantar view of a fracture of the medial malleolus of the tibia (arrow). (Courtesy of T. S. Stashak).

duction and no degenerative changes, the reported outcome is good.[6,7]

Comminuted fractures are not as challenging to diagnose but are often irreparable (Fig. 8.400). Osteoarthritis and/or instability usually requires euthanization.

Fractures of the Tibial Malleoli

The tibial malleoli are fractured by direct trauma or avulsion of the collateral ligaments. The majority of horses in two reports acquired the injuries in a fall, and the lateral malleolus was most commonly affected. A kick from another horse can also result in this fracture.[5,11]

Signs and Diagnosis

Clinical signs consist of sudden onset of lameness and tarsocrural effusion. Variable amounts of periarticular swelling are present, depending on the nature and direction of the trauma. The fractures are demonstrated well in the dorsoplantar or oblique radiograph; the entire joint should be scrutinized for migrating loose bodies (Fig. 8.401). The oblique films should be evaluated to determine the total size of the fragment, which may be misleading. Concurrent collateral ligament injury is a vital consideration and is discussed more extensively later. If collateral ligament damage has occurred, general anesthesia can result in catastrophic luxation. Either a cast can be employed to protect the horse or surgery can be delayed until the soft tissue has healed. Intraarticular

sodium hyaluronate is indicated to control synovitis if effusion is present.

Treatment

The medial malleolus is affected less often than the lateral malleolus, but the fragment tends to be large enough for lag screw repair. The articular surface must be reconstructed accurately to prevent subsequent osteoarthritis; provided stability is attained, perfect reduction of the remainder of the fracture line is less important.[7] Radiographic or fluoroscopic monitoring of screw placement is important to avoid contacting the medial trochlear ridge with hardware. Return to soundness is possible, if the noted complications are avoided.[7] Much of the medial malleolus is well within the tarsocrural joint and is accessible arthroscopically for removal of smaller fragments.

The lateral malleolus is largely invested in joint capsule and collateral ligament; the intraarticular portion is limited to the actual joint surface. Many fractures affect the most dorsal portion, where the short collateral ligament attaches. When the fragments are small or comminuted, removal is indicated. More caudal lesions require direct dissection through the collateral ligament. However, the collateral ligament and some fragments may retract into the periarticular soft tissue, making removal of the fragments inadvisable and unnecessary.

Radiographic confirmation of removal or final location of fragments outside the joint is useful. My experience indicates that bone fragments may slow the healing of the collateral ligament fibers back to the fracture site, so time and ultrasonographic monitoring are important.[2] Marginally sized fragments that are repaired by internal fixation may split during the convalescent period and require removal in a second surgery. Many moderately sized fragments can be removed or left to heal on their own.[5] Stall rest of approximately 6 months with radiographic monitoring is recommended whether the horse undergoes surgery or not.

Prognosis

One study reports a 50% return to performance after surgical repair with internal fixation of lateral malleolar fractures.[3] Overall good results are reported after the removal of relatively small fragments.[11] Many of these fragments can be removed arthroscopically with minimal dissection into the joint capsule. In summary, the importance of the fragment to the integrity of the joint and the ability to repair it should be considered. The persistence of tarsocrural effusion following anti-inflammatory therapy indicates the need for arthroscopic exploration.

References

1. Baker JR, Ellis CE. A survey of post mortem findings in 480 horses 1958 to 1980: (2) disease processes not directly related to the cause of death. Equine Vet J 1981;13:47–50.
2. Berry DB, Sullins KE, Doyle PS, et al. Collateral ligament desmitis in the tarsus. Seven cases from 1994–2000. Unpublished manuscript, 2001.
3. Foerner JJ. Surgical treatment of selected musculoskeletal disorders of the rear limb. In: Auer JA, Ed. Equine Surgery. Philadelphia: WB Saunders, 1992;1055–1075.
4. Hammer EJ, Ross MW, Parente EJ. Incomplete sagittal fracture of the talus in 11 racehorses. Proc Am Assoc Equine Pract 1999; 45:162–163.
5. Jakovljevic S, Gibbs C, Yeats JJ. Traumatic fractures of the equine hock: A report of 13 cases. Equine Vet J 1982;14:62–68.
6. Meagher DM, Mackey VS. Lag screw fixation of a sagittal fracture of the talus in the horse. J Equine Vet Sci 1991;10:108–112.
7. Nixon A. Fractures of specific tarsal bones. In: Nixon A, Ed. Equine fracture Repair. Philadelphia: WB Saunders, 1996;260–267.
8. Specht TE, Moran A. What is your diagnosis? J Am Vet Med Assoc 1990;196:1307–1308.
9. Tulleners EP, Reid CF. An unusual fracture of the tarsus in two horses. J Am Vet Med Assoc 1981;178:291–294.
10. Vaughan LC, Mason BJE. A clinicopathologic study of racing accidents in horses. Dorking, UK: Adlard, 1975.
11. Wright IM. Fractures of the lateral malleolus of the tibia in 16 horses. Equine Vet J 1992;24:424–429.
12. Zamos DT, Honnas CM, Hoffman AG. Arthroscopic and intra-articular anatomy of the plantar pouch of the equine tarsocrural joint. Vet Surg 1994;23:161–166.

CONDITIONS OF THE FIBULAR TARSAL BONE (CALCANEUS): FRACTURES

Fractures of the fibular tarsal bone (calcaneus) are relatively uncommon.[10] The fractures can be simple chip fractures involving the plantar surface, or extend completely through the growth plate in foals, or extend through the body in mature horses.[9,16,21] Chip fractures involving the plantar surface can be easily missed. In some cases, however, they go on to form sequestra. Physeal fractures and fractures through the body of the bone are often open and are not difficult to diagnose because of the obvious loss of flexor support.[9,16]

The sustentaculum can also be injured, the result being either a fracture or a delayed exostosis that produces synovitis of the tarsal canal (thorough-pin).[8,12,26] The significance of the lesion is the resultant abrasion injury to the deep digital flexor tendon; and the tendon sheath may also undergo dystrophic calcification.[8] Infection sometimes complicates the situation in this location as well.[11,19,23]

Causes

In most cases, these fractures occur from external trauma, either from being kicked by another horse or from the horse kicking a solid object. The affected areas include the body or proximal epiphysis in foals and the sustentaculum tali. Penetrating wounds have also been implicated in sustentaculum injuries.

Signs and Diagnosis

Fractures of the body of the talus may be difficult to diagnose on physical examination unless an obvious swelling is present or a draining tract associated with sequestration is observed. On the other hand, fractures through the body or epiphysis are easily diagnosed because there is an obvious loss of function of the gastrocnemius muscle, and the horse assumes a dropped hock appearance.[9] The definitive diagnosis is made on radiographic examination (Fig. 8.402). The lateromedial and

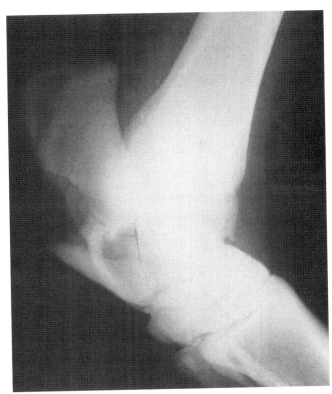

Figure 8.402   Lateromedial view of an oblique comminuted fracture of the calcaneus. (Courtesy of T. S. Stashak.)

oblique views are most important for identifying the exact location and extent of the fracture.

Lesions on the sustentaculum may appear on the lateromedial or dorsomedial-plantarolateral oblique projections. However, the gliding surface is best demonstrated in a flexed tangential (skyline) projection.[20] Contrast arthrography has been described;[5,6] however, sustentaculum lesions may be more efficiently evaluated (and treated) arthroscopically.[3] Ultrasound may help in predicting the arthroscopic findings and in providing a prognosis.[18] Some sustentacular injuries may result in a sequestrum or septic tenosynovitis and drainage.[11,19,23]

Treatment

Surgical excision of the chip fractures of the fibular tarsal bone may not be necessary unless they enter the tarsocrural joint or become sequestered and are accessible to surgical excision.[13]

Although fractures through the calcaneal tuber can be difficult to reduce and stabilize, they have been treated successfully with bone plates using the tension band principle, with the additional support of a full-limb cast.[9,21] A tension band plate is placed on the plantar aspect of the calcaneus beneath the tendon of the superficial flexor tendon to neutralize the distracting forces. The surgeons in two studies believe it is important to remove the plate to reestablish tarsal mobility.[9,21] Recovery from anesthesia is safer in a cast, which can be removed immediately if desired.

Another report on the surgical treatment of this fracture noted one case that involved a combination of internal fixation and external coaptation.[22] The treatment was successful (Fig. 8.403). Conservative approaches using casting alone have not proven to be rewarding.[10] Presumably owing to the tension from the tendon of the gastrocnemius, severely comminuted fractures of the tuber calcis fail to heal despite immobilization in a cast (Fig. 8.404).

Fractures through the growth plate in young horses are rare in my experience. An attempt to treat one open fracture resulted in osteomyelitis (Fig. 8.405). The apophysis in a foal is small and mostly cartilaginous; it is incapable of supporting the distraction by means of a single screw. Shaping the plate to cover the apophysis or using a hooked plate adds support similar to that used for olecranon fractures in foals. A cast lends further stability.

Treatment of lesions of the sustentaculum must leave a smooth surface to prevent damage to the tendon and recurrent synovitis. When a surface lesion of the bone or sepsis cannot be confirmed, intrasynovial anti-inflammatory therapy may be successful. Tonoscopy is a more accurate procedure.[3] Although successful treatment has been reported after a long delay,[24] early treatment minimizes permanent damage. The overall outcome for chronically affected horses is poor.[7,8,26] If the wound is acute and open, it is a surgical emergency. The goal of surgical therapy is debridement of the bony lesion and associated changes within the tendon sheath; septic lesions require lavage and drainage. Successes have been

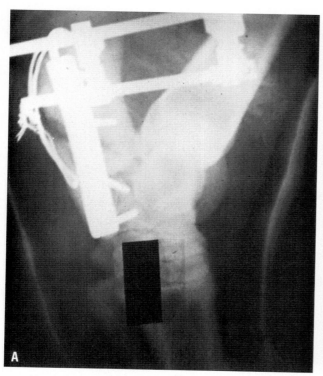

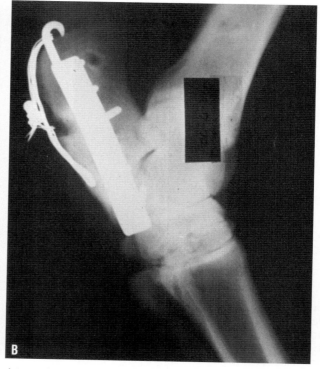

Figure 8.403 A. Lateromedial view of the horse shown in Figure 8.402. The fracture was successfully treated with a neutralization plate and tension band wire secured by an intramedullary pin. Motion was reduced by using the external fixator. B. At the 4-month follow-up, the fracture was healed (Courtesy of T. S. Stashak.)

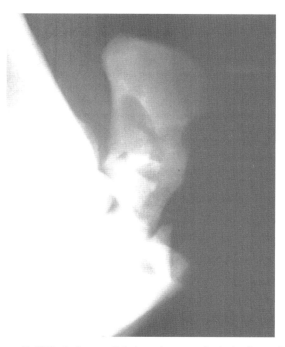

Figure 8.404 Lateromedial view of a comminuted calcaneal fracture. There is insufficient bone remaining for internal fixation. This type of traction fracture will not heal by simple immobilization in a cast. (Reprinted with permission from Sullins KE. Diseases of the tarsus. In: Colahan PT, Mayhew IG, Merritt AM, Moore JN, Eds. Equine Medicine and Surgery. Vol. 2. 5th ed. Santa Barbara, CA: American Veterinary Publications, 1999;1680.)

reported after conventional open surgery;[4,11,20,23] however, tonoscopy disrupts less tissue and is preferred when possible.[3] (See "Osteomyelitis of the Sustentaculum Tali" in this chapter.)

Prognosis

The prognosis for chip fracture of the calcaneus is considered good to guarded, depending on its location (intraarticular versus extraarticular), the size of the fragment, and whether it has become a sequestrum.

The prognosis for fractures of the growth plate and through the body is considered poor for return to full function. The outcome of fractures of the body of the calcaneus depends on the ability of the surgeon to stabilize the fragments.[9,21,22] Distraction from pull of the gastrocnemius precludes successful conservative therapy of unstable fractures.

The prognosis must be guarded to poor until proven otherwise for lesions in the tarsal canal. However, because favorable results have been reported, the attempt is worthwhile.[11,26] (See "Osteomyelitis of the Sustentaculum Tali" in this chapter.)

CONDITIONS OF THE FIBULAR TARSAL BONE (CALCANEUS): OSTEOMYELITIS AND OSTEOLYTIC LESIONS OF THE CALCANEAL TUBER

The calcaneus is exposed at the plantar aspect of the hock and subject to injury from and by kicking. Penetrat-

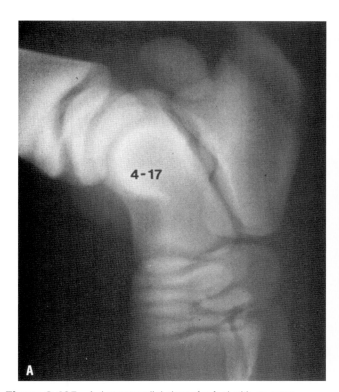

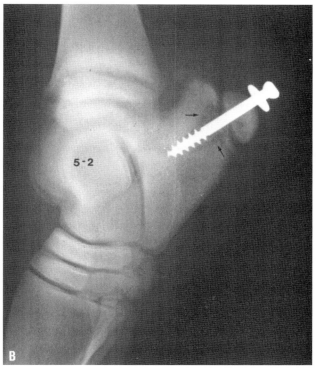

Figure 8.405 A. Lateromedial view of a foal with an open Harris-Salter type 1 fracture of the calcaneal tuber. Note that the apophysis has displaced dorsally and off the calcaneus. B. A cancellous screw was placed. However, osteomyelitis became a complication (arrows), and the screw loosened.

ing trauma is also relatively common. Of 50 horses with radiographic calcaneal lesions, 29 had osteomyelitis, including 4 foals with septic apophysitis.[15] Possibly owing to the exposure, infection and trauma tend to involve the attachments of the gastrocnemius and superficial flexor tendons.

Signs and Diagnosis

Lameness usually results at the time of the incident. Inflammation at the attachments of the gastrocnemius tendon and calcaneal bursitis can be extremely painful. Penetrating wounds are obvious, and infection leads to progressive soft tissue swelling. Radiographs are required. Although all radiographic views are useful, the single most diagnostic projection is the flexed skyline (Fig. 8.406).[15] However, some horses may be in too much pain to withstand that flexion. Also revealing is the 45° dorsomedial to plantarolateral oblique view. Radiographic signs include soft tissue swelling, osseous lysis, fragments/sequestra, and new bone production (associated more with chronic conditions).

Ultrasound may reveal disruptions of the tendons or bursa. When drainage is present, there is a high probability of a sequestrum.[15] Penetrating wounds should be evaluated completely before septic tendinitis or bursitis becomes established. Contrast radiography under aseptic conditions may be advisable.

In a study of 9 of 50 horses, chronic aseptic osseous lesions were seen on the medial, lateral, or caudolateral aspect of the calcaneus where the gastrocnemius and superficial flexor tendons insert.[15] The radiographic signs were associated with persistent lameness (Fig. 8.406).

Treatment

Septic wounds should be surgically debrided, and drainage should be established for resolution of the infectious process. Bacterial culture and sensitivity is important in these cases, because the infection tends to be well established when treatment begins. In a series of 28 horses with calcaneal osteomyelitis, a statistical difference in results of surgical or medical therapy could not be demonstrated.[14] In another study, 9 of 14 horses worsened despite appropriate therapy,[15] demonstrating that this condition tends to persist. Horses with radiographic changes limited to soft tissue developed osseous lesions within an average of 9 weeks. Sound practice still dictates that septic necrotic tissue should be removed, because the septic processes tend to progress to the tendons or bursa.[15]

Noninfected bursitis can cause significant lameness. When medical therapy fails or if there are radiographic changes, arthroscopic exploration is indicated.[1] Bursal or osseous tissue is debrided where it has been disrupted. Local and systemic anti-inflammatory therapies are indicated.

Prognosis

The prognosis is guarded. Possibly because of the continued tension of weight bearing at the attachments of the gastrocnemius and superficial flexor tendons and the compression beneath the superficial flexor on the bursal surface, affected horses tend to be lame and may remain so for long periods of time. The healing must be complete and congruent on the bursal surface or chronic bursitis will develop. Prolonged periods of severe lameness may result in laminitis in the contralateral hindlimb.

Of 26 horses treated for calcaneal osteomyelitis, 6 became sound, although 18 remained alive.[14] A total of 6 horses returned later for additional treatment for chronic osteomyelitis. Breeding soundness is a more certain goal. These relatively poor results were undoubtedly negatively influenced by the mean time of 2 months' duration of clinical signs before treatment.

Horses with aseptic bursitis also recover poorly.[1] The surface must be healed sufficiently to avert synovitis and chronic bursitis.

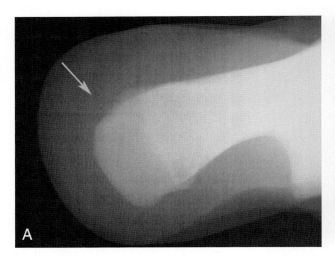 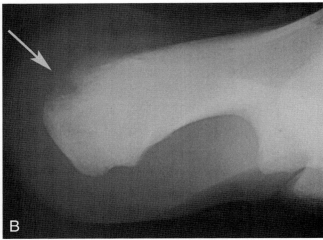

Figure 8.406 A. Skyline view of the calcaneus of a horse with a recent wound into the calcaneal bursa. Note the 2-mm focal area of lysis associated with the wound (arrow). B. The increased osteolysis (arrow) demonstrates progression of the osteomyelitis.

CONDITIONS OF THE FIBULAR TARSAL BONE (CALCANEUS): OSTEOMYELITIS OF THE SUSTENTACULUM TALI

The sustentaculum tali is the gliding fulcrum for the deep digital flexor tendon to progress distal to the hock through the tarsal sheath. When synovitis owing to sepsis or distortion of the articular surface is present, tarsal canal effusion (thorough-pin) is seen, and the horse is lame.[4,7,19,23,24]

Causes

Kick or puncture wounds generally cause the bony damage and infection.[10] A definitive diagnosis or therapy may be delayed while medical therapy is attempted. Medical therapy most often fails, and the condition worsens in the interim.[11,19]

Signs and Diagnosis

Most horses are lame at a walk or are non-weight-bearing lame. A wound may lead the way to the diagnosis, but tarsal sheath distension is obvious. Synovial fluid analysis may reveal sepsis; however, it may be difficult to obtain fluid because of fibrin deposition within the tendon sheath or the presence of an open draining wound. Radiographs often reveal osteolysis or osteophyte production at the cartilage surface of the sustentaculum tali. The flexed tangential projection is the most useful view, but some horses are too painful for that flexion. The 45° dorsomedial-plantarolateral projection is also revealing (Fig. 8.407), but all the routine radiographic views should be taken.[15,19]

Treatment

Conservative therapy is unrewarding in the majority of cases. The tarsal sheath is explored to locate and debride the damaged area. Infectious debris, adhesions, and fibrin should be removed; and the focus of the infection should be debrided to healthy tissue. The osseous lesion on the sustentaculum tali must be debrided as aggressively as necessary to remove all affected tissue, or recurrence is likely. Open exploration and drainage has been reported.[11,19] Arthroscopic debridement is also useful, because more of the tarsal sheath is visible. Power instruments are efficient for removing fibrin and adhesions and for debriding the osseous surface of the sustentaculum. Open or closed drainage is indicated while the synovial structure clears the infection.[4,7,19,23,24]

A specific culture and sensitivity is useful if possible. Long-term local and systemic broad-spectrum antibiotics and anti-inflammatory therapy are indicated. One recommendation is 4 to 6 weeks, or 2 weeks beyond resolution of signs.[11] An added benefit in many cases is a regional perfusion of antibiotics.[2,25] Antibiotic-impregnated polymethylmethacrylate (PMMA) beads are also useful, if they can be placed without causing more lameness.[2] Local steroids are contraindicated.

Deep digital flexor tenotomy (in the metatarsal region) or tenectomy within the tarsal canal was performed in two horses.[19] An extended heel shoe was necessary during convalescence, and both horses recovered to breeding soundness or were ridden lightly. The immediate effect of the procedure was relief of severe lameness and/or removal of necrotic tissue from the tendon sheath. Another report questions the necessity of tenotomy or tenectomy, which limits return to athletic soundness.[11] Severe hindlimb lameness may result in contralateral

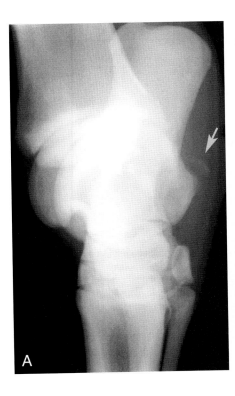
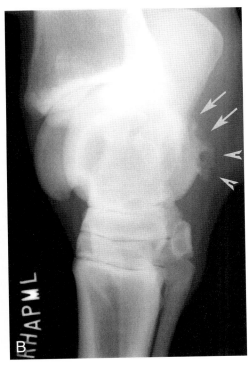

Figure 8.407 A. Dorsomedial-plantarolateral view of a horse that sustained an injury to the sustentaculum tali. At presentation, a draining tract was present and a sequestrum could be seen (arrow). B. Months after surgical debridement and healing of the wound, a large exostosis was noted on the gliding surface of the deep digital flexor tendon (arrows). The horse retained an abnormal gait that could not be changed with local analgesia, likely caused by mechanical interference from adhesions.

support limb laminitis, which is also debilitating. Each case must be evaluated individually to determine the best course. If tenotomy is considered necessary for this relatively proximal problem, deep flexor transection at the muscle–tendon junction could be considered.

Prognosis

The overall prognosis for recovery from a septic tendon sheath is fair. However, successful results can be accomplished if the debridement can be complete and infection can be controlled.[4,24] Unsuccessfully treated horses become debilitated and crippled. The outlook is improved if no radiographic changes are present (Fig. 8.407B).[7] In a series of 17 horses, 6 were considered successfully treated.[7,17,19] A like number became breeding sound, and the others were lost. In a recent series of 10 horses, 90% survival and 60% return to previous use were reported.[11] I observed one horse that retained a mechanically abnormal gait that couldn't be changed with local analgesia.

The key to success with septic tenosynovitis is early, aggressive therapy. Fibrin accumulates relatively quickly, sequestering bacteria from antibiotics; and adhesions worsen the situation. If not already affected, osteomyelitis disrupts the gliding surface and causes permanent distortion, leading to chronic lameness.

References

1. Bassage LH II, Garcia-Lopez J, Currid EM. Osteolytic lesions of the tuber calcanei in two horses. J Am Vet Med Assoc 2000;217: 710–716.
2. Baxter GM. Instrumentation and techniques for treating orthopedic infections in horses. Vet Clin North Am Equine Pract 1996;12:303–335.
3. Cauvin ER, Tapprest J, Munroe GA, et al. Endoscopic examination of the tarsal sheath of the lateral digital flexor tendon in horses. Equine Vet J 1999;31:219–227.
4. Dart AJ, Hodgson DR. Surgical management of osteomyelitis of the sustentaculum tali in a horse. Aust Vet J 1996;73:73–74.
5. Dik KJ, Keg PR. The efficacy of contrast radiography to demonstrate "false thorough-pins" in five horses. Equine Vet J 1990;22: 223–225.
6. Dik KJ, Leitch M. Soft tissue injuries of the tarsus. Vet Clin North Am Equine Pract 1995;11:235–247.
7. Dik KJ, Merkens HW. Unilateral distension of the tarsal sheath in the horse: A report of 11 cases. Equine Vet J 1987;19:307–313.
8. Edwards GB. Changes in the sustentaculum tali associated with distension of the tarsal sheath (thorough-pin). Equine Vet J 1978; 10:97–102.
9. Ferguson JG, Presnell KR. Tension band plating of a fractured equine fibular tarsal bone. Can Vet J 1976;17:314–317.
10. Fessler JF, Amstutz HE. Fracture repair. In: Oehme FW, Prier JE, Eds. Textbook of Large Animal Surgery. Baltimore: Williams & Wilkins, 1974;309.
11. Hand R, Watkins JP, Honnas CM, et al. Treatment of osteomyelitis of the sustentaculum tali and associated tenosynovitis in horses: 10 cases (1992–1998). Proc Am Assoc Equine Pract 1999;45: 158–159.
12. Hilbert BJ, Jenkinson G. Exostosis on the medial border of the calcaneus. J Am Vet Med Assoc 1984;184:1403–1404.
13. Jakovljevic S, Gibbs C, Yeats JJ. Traumatic fractures of the equine hock: a report of 13 cases. Equine Vet J 1982;14:62–68.
14. MacDonald MH, Honnas CM, Meagher DM. Osteomyelitis of the calcaneus in horses: 28 cases (1972–1987). J Am Vet Med Assoc 1989;194:1317–1323.
15. Mattoon JS, O'Brien TR. Radiographic evaluation of the calcaneus in the horse: A retrospective study. Proc Am Assoc Equine Pract 1988;34:369–379.
16. O'Brien T. Radiographic interpretation of the equine tarsus. Proc Am Assoc Equine Pract 1973;19:289.
17. Peremans K, Verschooten F, Moor AD, et al. Post-traumatic osteomyelitis of the sustentaculum tali in the horse: 4 cases. Vlaams Diergeneeskg Tijdschr 1988;57:410–417.
18. Reef VB. Equine Diagnostic Ultrasound. Philadelphia: WB Saunders, 1998.
19. Santschi EM, Adams SB, Fessler JF, et al. Treatment of lesions of the sustentaculum of the calcaneus accompanied by tarsal sheath synovitis. Proc Am Assoc Equine Pract 1993;39:249–250.
20. Santschi EM, Adams SB, Fessler JF, et al. Treatment of bacterial tarsal tenosynovitis and osteitis of the sustentaculum tali of the calcaneus in five horses. Equine Vet J 1997;29:244–247.
21. Scott EA. Surgical repair of a dislocated superficial digital flexor tendon and fractured fibular tarsal bone in a horse. J Am Vet Med Assoc 1983;183:332–333.
22. Stashak TS. Fracture of the fibular tarsal bone (calcaneus). In: Stashak TS, Ed. Adams' Lameness in Horses. 4th ed. Philadelphia: Lea & Febiger, 1987;713–714.
23. Tulleners EP, Reid CF. Osteomyelitis of the sustentaculum talus in a pony. J Am Vet Med Assoc 1981;178:290–291.
24. Welch RD, Auer JA, Watkins JP, et al. Surgical treatment of tarsal sheath effusion associated with an exostosis on the calcaneus of a horse. J Am Vet Med Assoc 1990;196:1992–1994.
25. Whitehair KJ, Bowersock TL, Blevins WE, et al. Regional limb perfusion for antibiotic treatment of experimentally induced septic arthritis. Vet Surg 1992;21:367–373.
26. Wilderjans H. New bone growth on the sustentaculum tali and medial aspect of the calcaneal bone surrounding the deep digital flexor tendon in a pony. Equine Vet Educ 1990;2:184–187.

SUBLUXATIONS AND LUXATIONS OF THE TARSAL JOINTS

Subluxations and luxations of all four tarsal joints have been reported in the literature, and avulsion fractures may occur concurrently.[1,4] Distal intertarsal luxations are rare. Furthermore, talocalcaneal luxation can occur.

Causes

A severe wrenching or twisting action that may occur from a sudden slip or fall is believed to be the cause in most cases.[1] Kicks from other horses and entrapment in fixed objects, such as fences and cattle guards, have also been implicated.[2,8] Even simply kicking a wall can result in a luxation.[5]

Signs and Diagnosis

Signs are usually quite obvious; an affected animal will present with a non-weight-bearing limb deformity associated with the tarsal joints. Usually the limb is freely moveable distal to the luxation. The exact location and extent of damage must be verified with radiographs. Luxation of the tarsocrural joint is the most severe and, in this instance, the tibia is usually displaced distad and craniad making it difficult or impossible to reduce (Fig. 8.408A). Talocalcaneal luxation is characterized by a separation between the affected joint (Fig. 8.409A).

Treatment

Reduction and immobilization with a full-limb cast will suffice in most cases of subluxation, luxation, and

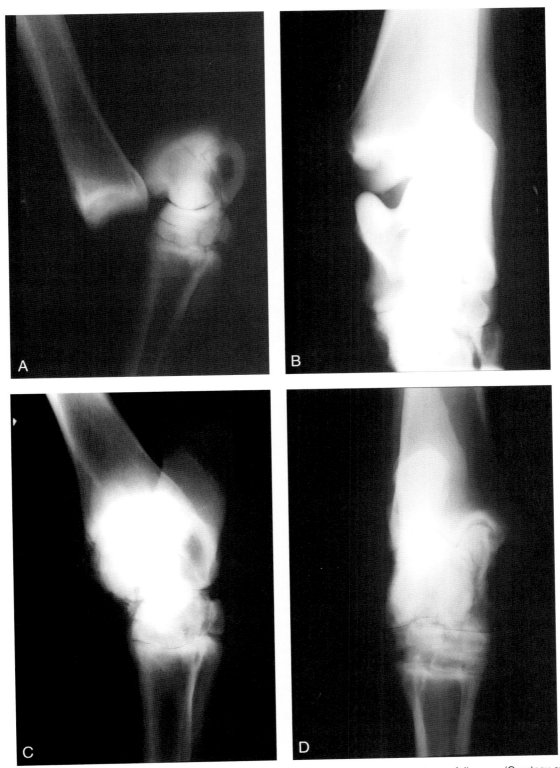

Figure 8.408   Lateromedial (A) and dorsoplantar (B) views of a tarsocrural luxation. Lateromedial (C) and dorsoplantar (D) views of the same horse at the 2-year follow-up. (Courtesy of G. W. Trotter.)

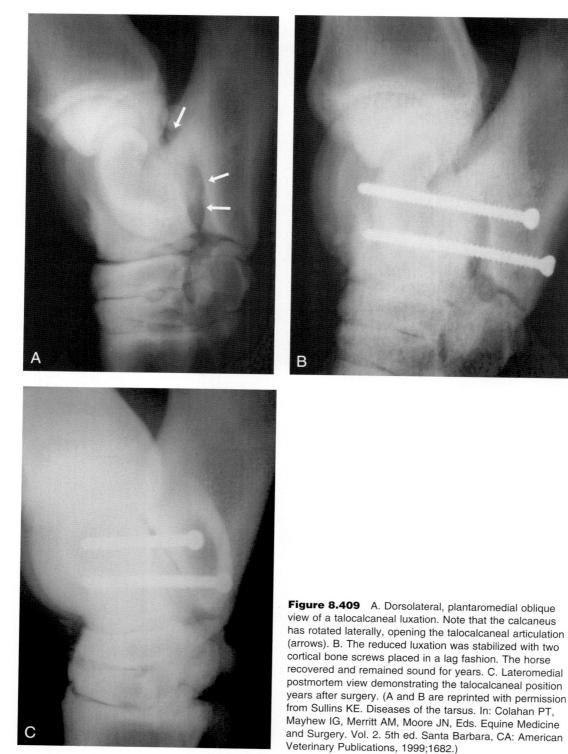

Figure 8.409   A. Dorsolateral, plantaromedial oblique view of a talocalcaneal luxation. Note that the calcaneus has rotated laterally, opening the talocalcaneal articulation (arrows). B. The reduced luxation was stabilized with two cortical bone screws placed in a lag fashion. The horse recovered and remained sound for years. C. Lateromedial postmortem view demonstrating the talocalcaneal position years after surgery. (A and B are reprinted with permission from Sullins KE. Diseases of the tarsus. In: Colahan PT, Mayhew IG, Merritt AM, Moore JN, Eds. Equine Medicine and Surgery. Vol. 2. 5th ed. Santa Barbara, CA: American Veterinary Publications, 1999;1682.)

simple fracture (Fig. 8.410).[1,5,6] Early reduction is important because some luxations cannot be reduced. Flexion can facilitate reduction.[4] A luxation that has a flat surface to buttress the proximal component is most amenable to simple cast immobilization. The cast should be applied as close to the stifle as possible to maximize immobilization of the tarsal area; it is maintained for at least 6 weeks. The principles of cast application are violated in this situation; however, the congruity of the tarsocrural joint and buttress of the distal joint surfaces seem to allow some liberal license.[5]

The luxations associated with comminuted tarsal bone fracture or oblique weight-bearing surfaces benefit more from a combination of internal fixation and casting

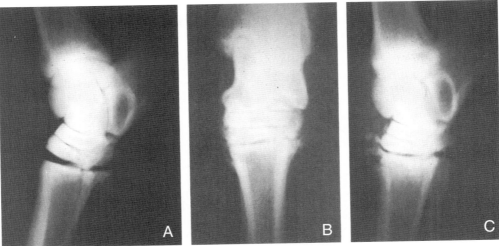

Figure 8.410 A. Lateromedial view of a dorsoplantar luxation at presentation, revealing the opening of the tarsometatarsal articulation. B. Dorsoplantar view after healing in a full-limb cast. C. Lateromedial view after healing. (Courtesy of T. S. Stashek.)

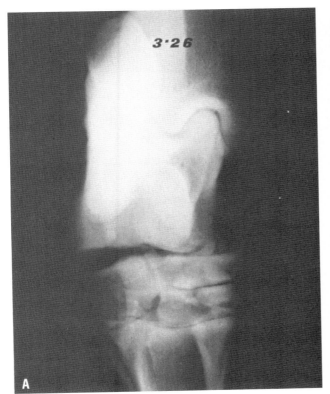
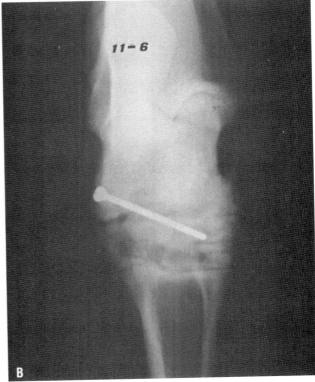

Figure 8.411 A. Dorsoplantar view of a proximal intertarsal subluxation at presentation, revealing minimal displacement. B. At the 7-month follow-up after lag screw stabilization and external coaptation in a full-limb cast, healing is evident. (Courtesy of C. W. McIlwraith.)

(Fig. 8.411).[7] Some cases require an open approach and curettage or debridement to achieve reduction. When visible, curettage of the articular cartilage from the articular surfaces of the distal tarsal bones facilitates ankylosis. The tarsocrural joint has been successfully reduced;[3,6] however, it deserves special consideration because of potential osteoarthritis (Fig. 8.408). Talocalcaneal luxation tends to be wedged apart by axial weight bearing and warrants internal fixation (Fig. 8.409).

Prognosis

It is worthwhile to attempt reduction of any tarsal luxation in which, once reduced, stability can be expected. Complications such as excessive contamination or destruction of the tarsocrural joint surfaces are examples of other important factors. The prognosis is reasonably good for simple luxation of the distal tarsal joints without fracture; however, the prognosis decreases from this point if fracture is present. Injuries restricted to nonmovable joints offer the most hope for a functional recovery. Successful reports include cast immobilization of distal tarsal[3] and tarsocrural[6] luxations reduced and placed in casts for 4 to 6 weeks. With the addition of internal fixation, talocalcaneal[7] and unstable distal tarsal[4] luxations can be successfully treated.

References

1. Fessler JF, Amstutz HE. Fracture repair. In: Oehme FW, Prier JE, Eds. Textbook of Large Animal Surgery. Baltimore: Williams & Wilkins, 1974;307–308.
2. Gross DR. Tarsal luxation and fracture in a pony. Mod Vet Pract 1964;45:68.
3. Laing JA, Caves SF, Rawlinson RJ. Successful treatment of a tarsocrural joint luxation in a pony. Aust Vet J 1992;69:200–201.
4. McIlwraith CW. Surgery of the hock, stifle, and shoulder. Vet Clin North Am 1983;5:333–362.
5. Moll HD, Slone DE, Humburg JM, et al. Traumatic tarsal luxation repaired without internal fixation in three horses and three ponies. J Am Vet Med Assoc 1987;190:297–300.
6. Reeves MJ, Trotter GW. Tarsocrural joint luxation in a horse. J Am Vet Med Assoc 1991;199:1051–1053.
7. Sullins KE. Diseases of the tarsus. In: Colahan PT, Mayhew IG, Merrit AM, Moore JN, Eds. Equine Medicine and Surgery. Vol. 2. 5th ed. Santa Barbara, CA: American Veterinary Publications, 1999; 1676.
8. Wheat JD, Rhoade EA. Luxation and fracture of the hock of the horse. J Am Vet Med Assoc 1964;145:341.

TALOCALCANEAL OSTEOARTHRITIS

Two Quarter Horses were reported to become acutely lame; one had been kicked. Tarsocrural effusion was mild, but response to hindlimb flexion was noticeable.[2] Local anesthesia was not performed, but lateral radiographs demonstrated an irregular talocalcaneal joint space with osteolytic foci and loss of joint space. Medical or surgical treatment was not attempted, and the horses remained lame. The authors speculated that surgical arthrodesis could have helped.

In the section on luxations of the tarsal joints (in this chapter) a horse that suffered a talocalcaneal luxation is described. The calcaneus was rotated away from the talus, opening the talocalcaneal articulation (Fig. 8.409). Faced with no other choice, the talocalcaneal articulation was reduced as much as possible and stabilized with lag screw fixation. From this case, it appears talocalcaneal arthrodesis is feasible.[1]

References

1. Sullins KE. Diseases of the tarsus. In: Colahan PT, Mayhew IG, Merrit AM, Moore JN, Eds. Equine Medicine and Surgery. Vol. 2. 5 ed. Santa Barbara, CA: American Veterinary, 1999;1676.
2. White NA, Turner TA. Hock lameness associated with degeneration of the talocalcaneal articulation: Report of two cases in horses. Vet Med 1980;75:678–681.

TARSOCRURAL COLLATERAL LIGAMENT DESMITIS, INSTABILITY, AND RUPTURE

Horses of any type are susceptible to collateral ligament (CL) injury. One series of cases contained a diverse population of pleasure, dressage, and eventing horses,[1] and another contained 9 Standardbred pacers.[2]

Causes

The history varies from observed incidents[1] to simply onset of lameness during training[2] to unknown.[1] The obvious injury is excessive strain in a valgus or varus direction that injures the medial or lateral collateral ligament, respectively.

Because the long collateral ligaments seem to be more prone to injury than the short collateral ligaments, it is thought that the situation arises when the limb is extended, when those ligaments are under the most tension.[5] The oblique angle of the trochlea causes lateral (outward) rotation of the talus during flexion.[5] Despite relative loosening during flexion,[5] the long medial CL is under more tension than the lateral CL. This possibly accounts the greater number of accidental injuries that predominately affect the long medial collateral ligament.[1] The long medial CL is also less substantial than the long lateral CL.[5]

Standardbred racehorses commonly injure the long lateral CL during training.[2] The long lateral CL spirals during flexion and straightens during extension, as it comes to take the load from the short lateral CLs.[5] One study theorized that cyclic stress at racing speed was responsible,[2] which could be true. Seven of the nine cases examined had histories of lameness in other limbs. Placing proportionately more weight on the hindlimb that has sustained a CL ligament injury could increase either the shear forces[3] or the varus tension on that ligament.

Signs and Diagnosis

Horses present with hindlimb lameness localized to the tarsus relatively easily. The degree of lameness varies from subtle to non weight bearing; hindlimb flexion worsens the lameness. Physical examination findings usually include tarsal swelling, characterized by edema and/or fibrosis localized over the medial or lateral collateral ligament region. Some degree of tarsocrural effusion is often present but may be obscured by the periarticular edema, of which digital pressure often elicits a painful response from the horse. Local anesthesia is usually not required to isolate the problem.

Radiographs may reveal only soft tissue swelling. However, avulsion of fragments from the origin of the affected collateral ligament on the adjacent tibial malleolus may be present (Fig. 8.412). Fragments may be intraarticular or extraarticular and buried within the substance of the ligament. Ultrasonography identifies the particular ligament involved and the degree of severity (Fig. 8.413). The long CLs seem to be more prone to this injury than the short CLs. In one study of a diverse group of horses, medial injuries were more common,[1]

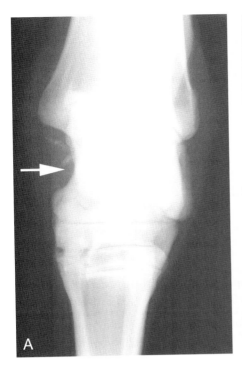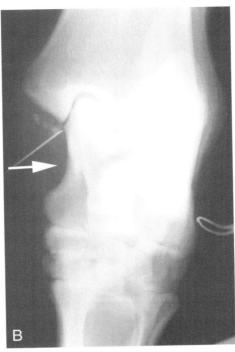

Figure 8.412 A. Dorsoplantar view of an avulsion injury of a medial collateral ligament, showing the obvious fragments from the medial malleolus. B. After anti-inflammatory therapy failed, the tarsocrural joint was explored arthroscopically. Note that the distal fragment (arrows) has been removed. The needle is placed deep within the medial collateral ligament, demonstrating that the remaining fragments will not be arthroscopically accessible.

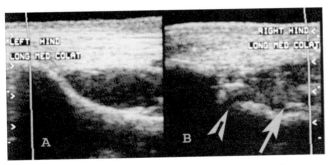

Figure 8.413 A. Ultrasound examination of the normal tarsus. B. The contralateral tarsus of a horse that had sustained a recent injury. Note that the space axial to the ligament (arrow) contains debris and hemorrhage and that an avulsed fragment lies adjacent to a cortical defect (arrowhead).

whereas Standardbred racehorses more consistently injure the lateral long collateral ligament.[2] However, horses with avulsion fractures usually seem to have short collateral ligament injury, because the location of the fragments tends to be the dorsal limit of the ligamentous attachment (see "Fractures of the Tibial Malleoli" in this chapter). Lateral collateral ligament calcification in a jumper may relate to sprain injury.[4] Scintigraphy is a further diagnostic aid for demonstrating the inflammation at the origin of the ligament and is useful when concurrent problems prevent a routine lameness examination.[2]

Treatment

For the acute injury, nonsteroidal anti-inflammatory drugs (NSAIDs) for 10 to 14 days are indicated. Cold therapy—an ice-water slurry in a plastic bag bandaged to the area for 20 minutes, three to four times a day for 48 hours—has proven beneficial. Support bandaging or splinting in the interim improves the response. Topical dimethyl sulfoxide (DMSO) and Furacin sweats once heat has diminished may provide further reduction. If joint effusion is present, intraarticular sodium hyaluronate is indicated. Further treatment consists of rest and immobilization. The duration of stall rest is defined by monitoring the sonograms of the collateral ligament, but 30 to 90 days is typical.

Horses with significant swelling or lameness should receive a cast or bandage cast. Sleeve casts that allow continued weight bearing and mobility of the fetlock usually suffice. Progressively decreasing the degree of immobilization from cast to bandage cast to bandage offers gradual increases in the stress on the ligament. Perhaps the most important characteristics of this injury are that the instability and synovitis can subtly lead to osteoarthritis and that return to work too early results in reinjury. If the affected region is continuing to swell, more immobilization is indicated.

Radiographs or lack of response to intraarticular therapy may indicate co-existing intraarticular lesions. Although arthroscopic exploration is indicated, the risk of complete luxation of the joint during recovery from general anesthesia is real. The synovitis should be controlled until the collateral ligament has healed sufficiently to withstand normal forces or a cast should be used for recovery from anesthesia.

Although persisting synovitis is an indication for surgical evaluation, some prediction of the findings can be made. Fragments in either long CL are likely to be embedded in ligamentous tissue and thus be inaccessible. Although less common, short CL injury is more exposed to the tarsocrural joint space because these liga-

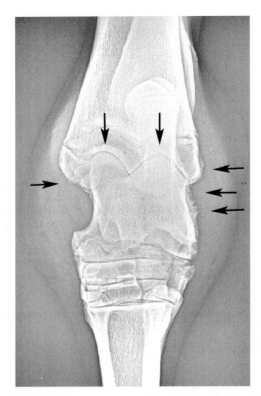

Figure 8.414 Xeroradiography of the tarsus reveals a chronic collateral ligament desmitis and instability. The dorsoplantar view demonstrates bone production at the origin and insertion of the lateral collateral ligament (three horizontal arrows). Note the osteophyte production from the resulting osteoarthritis (single horizontal arrow) and the asymmetric joint space from instability and degenerative changes (vertical arrows). Periarticular fibrosis and soft tissue thickening surround the tarsus.

ments attach on the cranial aspects of the respective malleolus (Fig. 8.412B). Concurrent radiographically inapparent articular cartilage damage must be considered.

Prognosis

In one study of seven horses, three returned to normal activity, three remained to be proven in full work, and one reinjured the ligament 2 months after reinstating gradual return to work.[1] In another study, six of nine Standardbred racehorses returned to racing (three at their previous level). However, two reinjured the limb, and three others required analgesics to train.[2] External coaptation was not used in this group of horses, and ultrasound was not available.

To summarize, this condition is one that can easily be taken too lightly. The subtle changes from the instability or joint damage sustained during the initial incident can produce osteoarthritis even before it is suspected (Fig. 8.414). Immobilization and rest periods should err on the conservative side.

References

1. Berry DB, Sullins KE, Doyle PS, et al. Collateral ligament desmitis in the tarsus. Seven cases from 1994–2000. Unpublished manuscript, 2001.

2. Boero MJ, Kneller SK, Baker GJ, et al. Clinical, radiographic, and scintigraphic findings associated with enthesitis of the lateral collateral ligaments of the tarsocrural joint in Standardbred racehorses. Equine Vet J 1988;6(Suppl):53–59.
3. Gabel AA. Lameness caused by inflammation in the distal hock. Vet Clin North Am 1980;2:101–124.
4. Moreau H, Denoix JM. Calcification of the medial collateral ligament of the hock in a jump horse. Pract Vet Equine 1994;26:219–220.
5. Updike SJ. Functional anatomy of the equine tarsocrural collateral ligaments. Am J Vet Res 1984;45:867–874.

HYPOPLASIA OF THE FUSED FIRST AND SECOND TARSAL BONES

A single case report exists of hypoplasia of the fused first and second tarsal bones. This clinically inapparent developmental deformity was seen in a Standardbred trotter. The diagnosis was made when the horse was 13 months of age, and it remained sound in race training. The patient was, however, euthanized at 2.5 years of age. The cause is unknown, but the deformity probably occurred during postnatal life, since many normal foals are born with unfused first and second tarsal bones.[1]

Reference

1. Smallwood JE, Auer JA, Martens RJ, et al. The developing equine tarsus from birth to six months of age. Equine Pract 1984;6:7–48.

IDIOPATHIC TARSOCRURAL SEPTIC ARTHRITIS

I have treated several cases of idiopathic tarsocrural septic arthritis. The affected horses were all athletes without a history of intraarticular therapy or injury. In one report of 192 horses affected with septic arthritis, 12 had no history to explain the problem.[1] The tarsocrural joint was affected in 7 of those 12 horses. The bacteria cultured were more diverse than would be expected after joint invasion. Approximately 83% of the 12 horses survived to be released from the hospital. (See Chapter 7 for more information on idiopathic septic arthritis.)

Reference

1. Schneider RK, Bramlage LR, Moore RM, et al. A retrospective study of 192 horses affected with septic arthritis/tenosynovitis. Equine Vet J 1992;24:436–442.

CURB

Curb is desmitis of the plantar ligament that originates on the plantar proximal aspect of the tuber calcis; courses laterally to the tarsal canal; and inserts on the distal part of the tuber calcis, the fourth tarsal and fourth metatarsal bones.[1,4] It is characterized by a thickening of the plantar distal aspect of the tarsus as viewed from

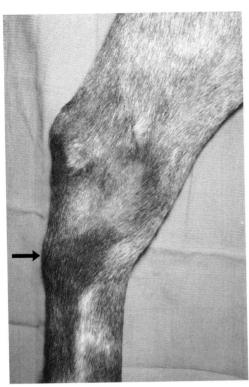

Figure 8.415 Swelling on the plantar aspect of the tarsus that can be associated with a curb (arrow). Ultrasonography revealed tendinitis of the superficial digital flexor tendon. (Courtesy of T. S. Stashak.)

the lateral side (Fig. 8.415). Other structures that occupy the same area and may produce similar swellings include the superficial digital flexor tendon and subcutaneous thickening.[4]

Causes

Plantar ligament desmitis results from excessive violent tension[8] or direct trauma. A sickle hocked (curby hocks) or cow-hocked conformation imposes exceptional stress to the plantar ligament and thus tends to produce curb. However, any horse can acquire curb from violent exertion, trauma from kicking walls or tailgates in trailers, and violent attempts to extend the hock. Conditioning may strengthen the tarsal ligaments.[8]

Foals with curby conformation are usually affected with wedging of the distal tarsal bones (described elsewhere in this chapter). However, the condition can persist into maturity and may be problematic in those individuals (Fig. 8.378A). Curby hocks were reported to be a factor reducing starts in Standardbred racehorses.[5] The incidence of curby conformation in a series of 1735 Dutch Warmblood horses was reported as 11.1%.[2] Dorsal compression of the distal tarsal bones is the predisposing factor for central and third tarsal bone fractures in athletes.

Signs and Diagnosis

Curb is indicated by an enlargement on the plantar surface of the fibular tarsal bone (Fig. 8.415). If the condition is in the acute phase, there are signs of inflammation and lameness. The horse stands with the heel elevated when the limb is at rest, and heat and swelling can be palpated in the region.[6] Swelling usually does not diminish with exercise, and exercise may actually increase lameness in acute curb. In severe cases, in which trauma is the inciting cause, periostitis on the plantar aspect of the fibular tarsal bone may result in new bone growth. If the inflammation is septic, extensive swelling and cellulitis may occur. In chronic cases, tissues surrounding the region often become infiltrated with scar tissue, and a permanent blemish results; however, lameness may not be noted. Occasionally, the proximal end of the fourth metatarsal bone is large and causes a false curb. Careful examination reveals that the swelling in this region is lateral to the plantar ligament and not on the ligament itself. This finding can be confirmed by radiologic examination, if necessary.

Presence of a swelling or thickening on the plantar aspect of the tarsus centered over the distal tarsal joints is often diagnostic. Lameness may be absent, making the point moot. Confirmation of the lesion is possible by ultrasonography[3,7] or by radiographs if bony involvement has occurred. It is important to differentiate the plantar ligament from other potentially more consequential sources of swelling, such as proximal superficial flexor tendinitis or sepsis.[4]

Treatment

Treatment for acute injury to the plantar ligament includes rest and controlled exercise, the application of cold packs for the first 48 hours after injury, and the systemic administration of anti-inflammatory agents. Rest includes stall confinement for at least 6 weeks; hand walking is often begun after 2 weeks and increased according to the horse's response. Although not reported, the application of ESWT is a reasonable consideration. Follow-up ultrasound examination is generally done between 10 and 12 weeks to assess healing.

Prognosis

If the horse has good conformation, the prognosis is favorable, providing the initial acute inflammation is controlled with corticoids. Poor conformation, however, serves as a continuing cause, and the prognosis is unfavorable. In most cases, some permanent blemish remains after recovery, even though most horses will be serviceably sound, if conformation is good. Standardbred racehorses are often successful in spite of curby conformation.[6]

References

1. Adams OR. Lameness in Horses. 3rd ed. Philadelphia: Lea & Febiger, 1974.
2. Bos H, van der Mey GJW. Comparative study of the occurrence of some visible defects in Dutch Warmblood horses. Zuchtungskunde 1986;58:66–72.
3. Dik KJ. Ultrasonography of the equine tarsus. Vet Radiol Ultrasound 1993;34:36–43.
4. Dik KJ, Leitch M. Soft tissue injuries of the tarsus. Vet Clin North Am Equine Pract 1995;11:235–247.

5. Dolvik NI, Klemetsdal G. Conformational traits of Norwegian cold-blooded trotters: Heritability and the relationship with performance. Acta Agri Scand Anim Sci 1999;49:156–162.
6. Gill HE. Diagnosis and treatment of hock lameness. Proc Am Assoc Equine Pract 1973;19:257.
7. Rantanen NW, McKinnon AO. Equine Diagnostic Ultrasonography. Baltimore: Williams & Wilkins, 1998.
8. Rooney JR. An hypothesis of the pathogenesis of curb in horses. Can Vet J 1981;22:300–301.

DISLOCATION (LUXATION) OF THE SUPERFICIAL DIGITAL FLEXOR TENDON OFF THE CALCANEAL TUBER

Dislocation of the superficial digital flexor tendon off the calcaneal tuber is occasionally seen in horses.[1] The dislocation occurs when one of the fascial attachments of the superficial digital flexor tendon to the calcaneus ruptures. Because of the severe swelling over the point of the hock, a misdiagnosis of capped hock is easy to make (Fig. 8.416). However, once the swelling decreases, dislocation is readily appreciated as a slippage of the superficial digital flexor off the point of the hock. Usually, the superficial digital flexor dislocates laterally,[1,3] although medial dislocation has been reported.[4–6] One case of division of the superficial flexor tendon and dis-

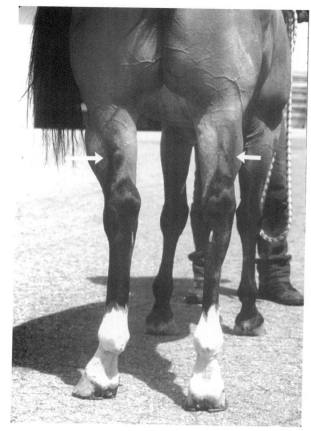

Figure 8.417 Caudal view of a bilateral luxation of the superficial digital flexor tendons (arrows). (Courtesy of T. S. Stashak.)

placement in both directions has been described.[2] Initially, affected horses appear quite lame shortly after the injury; but with time, the painful response diminishes and a partial loss of complete control of the hindlimb becomes apparent. Occasionally, the condition can occur bilaterally (Fig. 8.417).

Causes

Dislocation of the superficial flexor tendon occurs as a racing injury,[3,6] simple bucking,[4] or trauma with an accompanying fracture.[5]

Signs and Diagnosis

Shortly after the injury, the point of the hock is quite swollen, making it easy to misdiagnose it as a capped hock. As the swelling is reduced, the dislocation can be more easily appreciated (Fig. 8.416). In the acute stage, an obvious lameness is present. On palpation, the dislocation and relocation of the superficial digital flexor tendon can be appreciated. The tendon often luxates when the tarsus is flexed. With time, the lameness diminishes. The horse appears to have less control of its limb. and a periodic displacement of the superficial digital flexor tendon occurs. Although the diagnosis can be made by

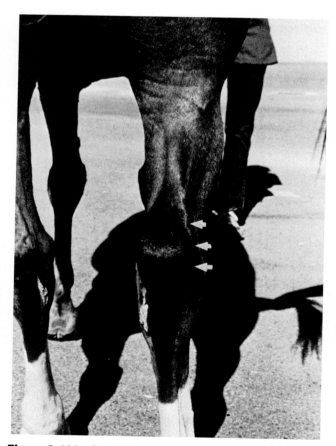

Figure 8.416 Caudal view of a horse that sustained a lateral dislocation of the superficial digital flexor tendon 4 weeks earlier. Note the swelling at the point of the hock and the margins of the tendon (arrows). (Courtesy T. S. Stashak.)

clinical signs alone, radiographs should be taken to rule out the possibility of a fracture. The severity of clinical signs depend on the degree of mobility of the superficial flexor tendon. Some horses experience only a partial tear of the attachments, and subluxation is the limit of dislocation.

Treatment

The degree of luxation and intended use of the horse dictate the treatment. When the tendon is only mildly subluxated, stall rest for 3 to 6 months often returns the horse to work. If the tendon remains on the tuber calcis, horses can often function despite the constant movement of the superficial flexor. If the luxation is severe or if athletic performance is required, surgical repair is preferred. The timing of surgery is an issue, because freshly torn tissues do not hold sutures well, and skin injury or infection may be present. However, the unaffected side of the fascia contracts, and complete reduction of the tendon becomes difficult after several days. It is difficult to maintain reduction of the tendon in a bandage or cast in the preoperative period.

Several surgical techniques have been described. All involve debridement and repair of the torn fascia.[3-6] If the tendon will not reduce with the limb in extension, releasing incisions (without complete transection) are made in the bursal surface of the unaffected side until reduction can be maintained without undue tension.[6]

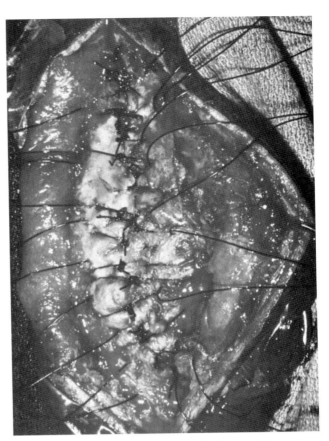

Figure 8.419   After the margins are debrided and the displaced tendon is reduced, the surgeon sutures the margins using far-near/near-far apposing sutures (tied). The preplaced mattress sutures that will anchor the polypropylene mesh are untied at this point. (Courtesy of T. S. Stashak.)

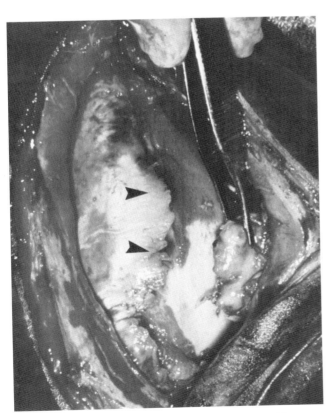

Figure 8.418   Intraoperative view of a torn superficial flexor fascia (arrowheads). The forceps hold the displaced margin of the tendon and attaching tissue. (Courtesy of T. S. Stashak.)

One report describes a single case in which sutures were the only internal supporting device.[4] Supporting the suture line with a polypropylene mesh has also been described (Figs. 8.418 to 8.420).[5-7] Strict asepsis must be maintained, because infection can reside in the nonabsorbable material. As much soft tissue as possible should cover the implant. Support of the reduced flexor tendon with two screws placed on the unaffected side has been described.[3]

All these techniques were successful in the reported cases. However, none of the reports involves a retrospective study. In practical terms, the less that can be done successfully, the better. The screw technique is a long procedure during which the patient is rolled over. The mesh technique works well, but infection can be a problem in traumatized tissue. Every case has its own aspects to be addressed.

Most clinicians immobilize the limb in a cast for at least 30 to 45 days. After this, the limb is supported in a Robert-Jones bandage, and then lesser amounts of support are used for 30 days. Hand-walking exercise can be begun 7 days after the cast is removed and continued for the next 60 days. Free exercise is begun in a confined area about 4 months postoperatively. One report described complete immobilization for only 14 days and a

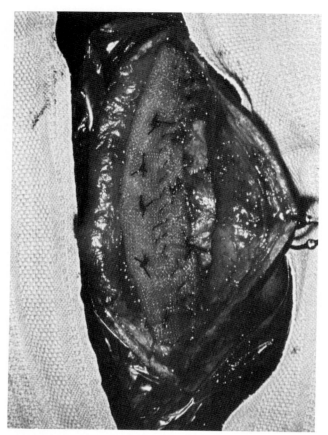

Figure 8.420 The mesh is sutured in place, and the edges are apposed by using a continuous suture. It is best to preserve at least one solid fascial layer to cover the mesh before closing the subcutaneous tissue. (Courtesy of T. S. Stashak.)

bandage splint for another week.[4] Hand walking began 21 days after surgery.

Prognosis

The prognosis for breeding soundness or light pleasure riding is good. Realistically, too few cases have been treated surgically with long-term follow-up to make an objective prognosis about athletic ability, especially because each case is a bit different. One Thoroughbred racehorse recovered and raced 51 times, and another was retired for breeding.[3] An Arabian mare became sound in hand, but work was not described.[4] In another case, the horse did not return to previous performance.[6]

Horses that have undergone surgery may not retain perfect reduction of the tendon but may still return to work. In five cases treated with surgery at the Colorado State University, three horses returned to full performance 10 months after the procedure: one to mountain riding horse, one to ranch work, and the other for pleasure. Complications associated with the other two cases were chronic infection and breakdown of the repair, a result of the horse escaping confinement and running.

References

1. Fessler JF, Amstutz HE. Fracture repair. In: Oehme FW, Prier JE, Eds. Textbook of Large Animal Surgery. Baltimore: Williams & Wilkins, 1974;249.
2. Foerner JJ. Surgical treatment of selected musculoskeletal disorders of the rear limb. In: Auer JA, Ed. Equine Surgery. Philadelphia: WB Saunders, 1992;1055–1075.
3. Meagher DM, Aldrete AV. Lateral luxation of the superficial digital flexor tendon from the calcaneal tuber in two horses. J Am Vet Med Assoc 1989;195:495–498.
4. Reiners S, Jann HW, Gillis E. Repair of medial luxation of the superficial digital flexor tendon in the pelvic limb of a filly. Equine Pract 2000;22:18–19,21.
5. Scott EA. Surgical repair of a dislocated superficial digital flexor tendon and fractured fibular tarsal bone in a horse. J Am Vet Med Assoc 1983;183:332–333.
6. Scott EA, Breuhaus B. Surgical repair of dislocated superficial digital flexor tendons in a horse. J Am Vet Med Assoc 1982;181:171.
7. Stashak TS. Luxation of the superficial digital flexor. In: Stashak TS, Ed. Adams' Lameness in Horses. 4th ed. Philadelphia: Lea & Febiger, 1987;718–220.

MEDIAL DISPLACEMENT OF THE DEEP DIGITAL FLEXOR TENDON

Medial displacement of the deep flexor from its position over the sustentaculum is a rarely diagnosed congenital anomaly. It produces no early clinical signs and is usually unobserved until the foal displays a tarsus/fetlock varus deformity owing to a bowstring effect of the deep flexor tendon along the axial surface of the distal hind-

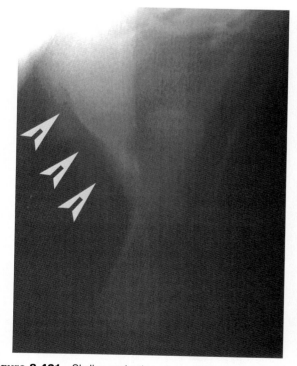

Figure 8.421 Skyline projection of a medially displaced deep flexor tendon and tarsal sheath. Note the hypoplastic sustentaculum, which failed to maintain the tarsal canal in its normal position (arrows). The result was a varus deformity of the tarsus and fetlock.

limb. Closer inspection reveals the tendon to be more misaligned than is usually seen with metatarsophalangeal varus deformity, and tracing its path proximally reveals the defect. The sustentacular defect is palpable and confirmed radiographically when compared to the contralateral hock (Fig. 8.421). The applicable view is the flexed tangential projection.

Surgical correction is the only option. The procedure consists of dissection of the tarsal sheath from the periosteal surface of the medial aspect of the sustentaculum and repositioning it in its correct position over the sustentaculum;[1] it must be supported in position. In one study, a cortical rib graft secured by bone screws was used to form the shelf. The foal was confined to a stall in a support bandage for 1 month before it was released for normal exercise.[1] I performed the only other known surgery for this condition. I used the same procedure, and the foal was maintained in a sleeve cast early postoperatively. However, the tightening of the deep flexor tendon caused a plantar-to-dorsal bowstring hyperextension of the hock. The horse became breeding sound, and the limb was straight. Given the same situation again, I would transect the deep flexor in the distal portion of the muscle tissue to relieve the tension. A third case has been reported in a yearling.[2] That horse was lame but had no angular deformity; no treatment was applied. The degree of the displacement apparently varies.

References

1. Foerner JJ. Surgical treatment of selected musculoskeletal disorders of the rear limb. In: Auer JA, Ed. Equine Surgery. Philadelphia: WB Saunders, 1992;1055–1075.
2. Lepage OM, Leveille R, Breton L, et al. Congenital dislocation of the deep digital flexor tendon associated with hypoplasia of the sustentaculum tali in a Thoroughbred colt. Vet Radiol Ultrasound 1995;36:384–386.

THOROUGH-PIN

See "Tenosynovitis" in Chapter 7.

RUPTURE OF THE PERONEUS TERTIUS

The peroneus tertius is a strong muscular band of tissue that lies between the long digital extensor and the tibialis cranialis muscle of the rear limb. It originates from the extensor fossa of the distal lateral femur and inserts distally as a tendinous band to the third metatarsal bone and laterally on the fourth metatarsal bone. It is an important part of the reciprocal apparatus, mechanically flexing the hock when the stifle joint is flexed. The muscle or tendon can rupture anywhere along its course and can result in an avulsion fracture at its origin in the extensor fossa (Fig. 8.422). When this muscle is ruptured, the stifle flexes, but the hock does not.[2]

Causes

Rupture of the peroneus tertius is usually the result of overextension of the hock joint. This may occur if the limb is entrapped and the horse struggles violently to free its limb. Rupture is also seen during the exertion of a fast start, when tremendous power is transferred to the limb, causing overextension, such as in jumping. Furthermore, it can occur after a full-limb cast is applied to the hindlimb. I have seen several ruptures in horses that barrel race.

Signs and Diagnosis

Signs of rupture of the peroneus tertius are well defined. The stifle joint flexes as the limb advances, and the hock joint is carried forward with little flexion. The

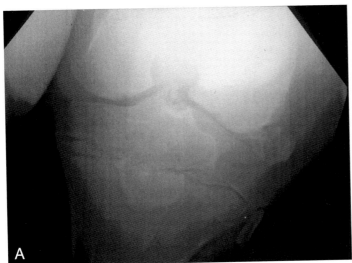
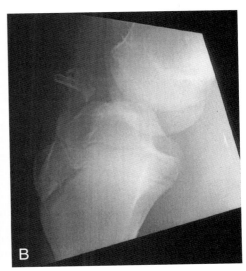

Figure 8.422 A. Craniocaudal view of an avulsion of the proximal attachment of the peroneus tertius. Note the fracture fragment associated with the avulsion. B. Lateromedial view of the same horse demonstrating avulsion of the peroneus tertius. (Courtesy of T. S. Stashak.)

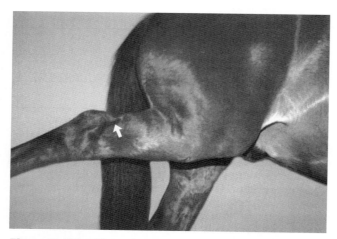

Figure 8.423 When a horse sustains a ruptured peroneus tertius, the reciprocal apparatus is not functional, allowing the clinician to extend the tarsus and fetlock while the stifle is flexed. Note the dimpling of the Achilles tendon proximal to the calcaneus (arrow).

portion of the limb below the hock tends to hang limp, giving the appearance of being fractured as it is carried forward. When the foot is put down, the horse has no trouble bearing weight and shows little pain. As the horse walks, however, there is a dimpling in the Achilles tendon. If the limb is lifted from the ground, it is easy to produce the dimpling in the Achilles tendon by extending the hock (Fig. 8.423). Note that the hock can be extended without extending the stifle, which cannot be done in the normal limb.

If the origin of the peroneus tertius fractures from the femur, femoropatellar effusion is a prominent feature. The gait deficit is similar to that described above. If the injury appears to be proximal, radiographs are advised. However, ultrasound confirmation can be obtained.[1]

Treatment

Complete rest is the best treatment. The horse should be placed in a box stall and kept quiet for at least 4 to 6 weeks. Then limited exercise should be given for the following 2 months. Most horses will heal and show normal limb action. If properly conditioned, most horses can return to normal work. Surgical intervention is not recommended. Hand leading is advisable when exercise is first begun. This helps control the horse and prevents reinjury.

Prognosis

The prognosis is guarded to favorable. When the horse is properly rested by box stall confinement, healing usually occurs. If healing is not evident at the end of 4 to 6 weeks, the prognosis is unfavorable, because the tendon may not unite. Final appraisal should not be made for at least 3 months after the injury. I saw one horse that ruptured its peroneus tertius twice. It had returned to full work after the first incident when the tendon eventually re-ruptured.

References

1. Leveille R, Lindsay WA, Biller DS. Ultrasonographic appearance of ruptured peroneus tertius in a horse. J Am Vet Med Assoc 1993; 202:1981–1982.
2. Updike SJ. Anatomy of the tarsal tendons of the equine tibialis cranialis and peroneus tertius muscles. Am J Vet Res 1984;45: 1379–1382.

RESTRICTION BY THE PERONEUS TERTIUS MUSCLE

In one report, a congenital flexure deformity of the right hock in a foal resulted from an abnormally short peroneus tertius muscle, which rendered the foal unable to walk. Tension created by the short peroneus tertius limited the hock extension to 70°. The cause was thought to be the intrauterine positioning of the foal. After resection of the peroneus tertius, the foal was able to extend its hock another 30°, and 2 months later, hock flexion and extension appeared normal.[1]

Reference

1. Trout DR, Lohse CL. Anatomy and therapeutic resection of the peroneus tertius muscle in a foal. J Am Vet Med Assoc 1981;179: 247.

COMMON CALCANEAL TENDINITIS

In one study, two horses with direct trauma to the gaskin were reported to sustain tendinitis and associated peritendinous soft tissue damage. The injury was characterized by severe lameness and local thickening of the soft tissues. Radiographic changes were absent. Ultrasound was delayed for several months but revealed little difference in thickness of the actual tendon tissue despite palpable and visual thickening. Treatment consisted of prolonged stall rest and administration of local and systemic anti-inflammatory therapy. Both horses returned to normal activity in approximately 10 months.[1]

Reference

1. Proudman CJ. Common calcaneal tendonitis in a horse. Equine Vet Educ 1992;4:277–279.

GASTROCNEMIUS TENDINITIS

Gastrocnemius tendinitis is uncommon but affects performance horses of all types. The condition is characterized by subtle to obvious lameness exacerbated by hindlimb flexion. The condition is somewhat similar to common calcaneal tendinitis,[4] but is more distal and affects the gastrocnemius individually.

Signs and Diagnosis

Some horses are perceived to have a reduced duration of weight bearing during the caudal phase of the stride. Abaxial and generalized swelling of the tendinous inser-

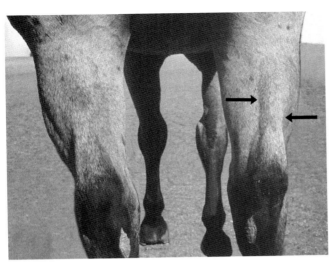

Figure 8.424 Rear view of gastrocnemius tendinitis in the right hindlimb. Note the swelling in the midgaskin region (arrows). The diagnosis was confirmed by ultrasonography. (Courtesy of T. S. Stashak.)

tion of the gastrocnemius is evident (Fig. 8.424). The firm swelling can be differentiated from thorough-pin by its location and lack of fluid distension. In some horses, however, the superficial flexor bursa may be distended, resembling a capped hock.[3] Diagnostic anesthesia of the tibial and peroneal or only the tibial nerve improves the lameness.

Radiographs generally demonstrate no lesions, but chronic cases may have a calcification at the calcaneal attachment of the gastrocnemius tendon. Ultrasound reveals enlargement, focal or diffuse hypoechoic or anechoic regions, and loss of normal fiber alignment when viewed in the longitudinal plane.[3,5] Ultrasound of the unaffected contralateral tendon is advisable for reference.[3] Associated lesions are not common, but calcaneal bursitis[1,3] or superficial flexor tendon tendinitis[4] may exist concurrently.

Treatment

Therapy consists of rest with local and systemic anti-inflammatory therapy. The recovery can be quite prolonged, so patience is important. Return to work before the ultrasonographic lesion has healed leads to reoccurrence of the lameness. Therapy that is begun in the acute stages is more successful than that begun after the horse has been lame for many weeks (Dyson SJ, personal communication, 2001). Even confined to a stall, this area is impossible to protect from normal weight bearing.

Because the problem with tendon healing is lack of an efficient blood supply, the clinician could consider surgical splitting or possibly ESWT. Neither of these methods have been reported for this condition. Anecdotally, tendons in other locations have occasionally developed excessive fibrosis after ESWT.

Prognosis

In one series, horses that had been lame up to 8 weeks were slow to recuperate. Ultrasound monitoring contin-

ued to demonstrate the persisting or enlarging focal or generalized lesions. Horses that became sound again required 9 to 12 months of healing.[2] Two horses that resumed work after 12 months became lame again, and others continued with slowly advancing exercise for at least 8 months. Another group of horses that were diagnosed much earlier after onset of signs recovered much more quickly and resumed flat racing or eventing (Dyson SJ, personal communication, 2001).

References

1. Dik KJ. Ultrasonography of the equine crus. Vet Radiol Ultrasound 1993;34:28–34.
2. Dyson SJ. Gastrocnemius tendinitis. Proceedings. 15th Bain-Fallon Memorial Lectures, 1993;63–70.
3. Dyson SJ, Kidd L. Five cases of gastrocnemius tendinitis in the horse. Equine Vet J 1992;24:351–356.
4. Proudman CJ. Common calcaneal tendonitis in a horse. Equine Vet Educ 1992;4:277–279.
5. Reef VB. Equine Diagnostic Ultrasound. Philadelphia: WB Saunders, 1998.

RUPTURE OR TEARING OF THE PROXIMAL ATTACHMENT OF THE GASTROCNEMIUS AND SUPERFICIAL DIGITAL FLEXOR MUSCLES

Rupture or tearing of the gastrocnemius and the superficial digital flexor muscles occurs infrequently in neonates and adults. The gastrocnemius and superficial digital flexor muscles make up the caudal component of the reciprocal apparatus. The two heads of the gastrocnemius originate from the medial and lateral supracondylar crests of the distal femur, and the origin of the superficial digital flexor from the supracondylar fossa is associated between and deep to that.[1] The close association of these muscles causes them to become affected similarly in most cases, although partial or complete tears of one head of the proximal attachment of the gastrocnemius muscles have been documented in adults (Stashak TS, personal communication, 2001).

Causes

It has been theorized that in adults excessive tension on the hindlimb during extension (e.g., trapping the hindlimb in extension beneath the body) causes this injury.[4] This was believed to be the case with one horse that slipped, trapping its hindlimb underneath its body, while attempting to run barrels in a muddy arena (Stashak TS, personal communication, 2001). In one study, two of three affected adults were reported to have histories of falling.[2,4] It is difficult to determine the forces involved in the causal events.

The injury in neonates is reported to accompany delivery of foals with flexure contractures, dystocia, and problems rising.[5] The overriding strength of contraction of the biceps femoris and quadriceps muscles opposing the gastrocnemius was theorized to be a factor in the foals.[5] It seems that a flexed tarsus would apply tension to the gastrocnemius and superficial flexor muscles at least as strongly as the former mechanism. One foal sustained a rupture of the gastrocnemius and superficial digital flexor muscle after jumping out of the back of a pickup (Stashak TS, personal communication, 2001).

Signs and Diagnosis

With complete rupture, the hock of the affected limb is dropped, so that there is a reduced angle to the hock joint and the hock is positioned closer to the ground than normal (Fig. 8.425). In addition, the stifle appears extended. While the horse attempts to bear weight, the hock drops further and the stifle becomes more extended, indicating loss of the reciprocal apparatus. All reported cases have been unilateral. Swelling caudal and lateral to the stifle is a consistent finding (Fig. 8.425). Foals are usually unable to rise and may be in a debilitated state with other problems, such as limb deformities. The trauma frequently causes hemorrhage owing to tearing of the caudal femoral or possibly other vessels; the hemorrhage contributes to the swelling and may be fatal.[3,5]

When there is a partial or complete tearing of one of the heads of the gastrocnemius muscle, the signs are more subtle. Swelling may be seen in the caudal thigh region (Fig. 8.426), and mild pain may be elicited with deep palpation of the muscle overlying the swollen region (Stashak TS, personal communication, 2001). At a walk,

the point of the hock may appear to drop slightly during weight bearing compared to the unaffected limb (Stashak TS, personal communication, 2001). A moderate degree of lameness (grade 2 to 3+ out of 5) is usually seen at a trot.

Radiographs are often normal, but avulsion of fragments from the caudal distal femur has been observed (Fig. 8.427).[4] Ultrasound can be used to image the injury and defects of the lateral head of the gastrocnemius and superficial digital flexor muscles.[2] The defect becomes filled with hemorrhage, which can be monitored for fibrosis during the healing process. One horse had a concurrent patellar ligament desmitis.[2]

Nuclear medicine may also be used to localize the injury to the caudal distal humeral region, and radiography may confirm the tear of the proximal attachment of the gastrocnemius (Fig. 8.428) (Stashak TS, personal communication, 2001).

Treatment

In neonates, treatment consists of supportive therapy and attempts to aid them in rising. The combination of

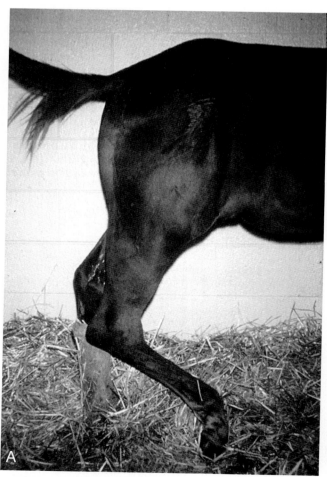 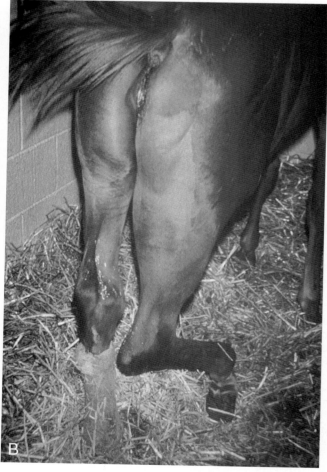

Figure 8.425   A. Note the flexed hock and extended stifle, indicating loss of the reciprocal apparatus, in a foal that ruptured the proximal attachment of the gastrocnemius and superficial digital flexor muscles when it jumped from the back of a pick-up bed. B. Note the extensive swelling in the caudal thigh region of the affected limb. (Courtesy of T. S. Stashak.)

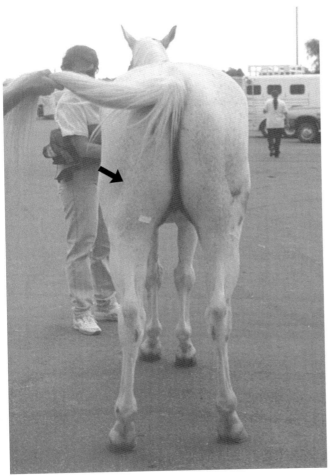

Figure 8.426 Note the swelling in the caudal thigh region in the left hindlimb (arrow) of a horse that sustained a tear of the proximal attachment of the gastrocnemius 17 days earlier. (Courtesy of T. S. Stashak.)

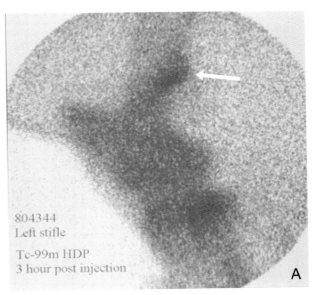

804344
Left stifle

Tc-99m HDP
3 hour post injection

A

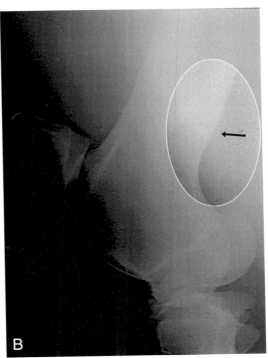

B

Figure 8.428 A. The nuclear medicine study of the horse shown in Figure 8.426 reveals increased uptake of the radionuclide in the caudal distal femur (arrow). B. Lateral view demonstrating an enthesiophyte associated with the proximal attachment of the gastrocnemius muscle (arrow). (Courtesy of T. S. Stashak.)

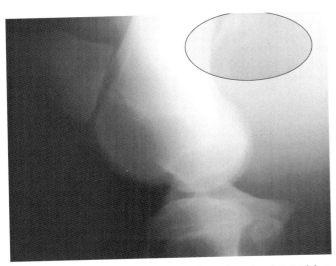

Figure 8.427 Lateral view of the stifle region, showing avulsion fractures associated with the proximal attachment of the gastrocnemius muscle (oval). (Courtesy of D. S. Biller.)

the musculoskeletal injury and debilitation often results in a decision for euthanasia.

In adults with complete rupture, the goal is to support the limb with the hock extended to facilitate fibrosis at the rupture site. Surgical therapy is not a consideration. Methods used include a Robert-Jones bandage applied to the full limb and stall confinement.[4] In one report of a weanling, a more rigid technique was used: a full-limb cast and a Thomas splint.[2] As the swelling diminishes, the casts must be replaced. In the case of the weanling, the Thomas splint and cast were replaced with a Robert-Jones bandage after 21 days.

In adults with partial or complete tears of one head of the gastrocnemius, rest, anti-inflammatory therapy, and controlled exercise appear adequate. Rest periods of 4 to 6 weeks followed by hand-walking exercise are recommended. Stepping over low (1-foot-high) obstacles is begun between the 5th and 6th weeks. The duration of hand walking and the height of the obstacles are increased according to the response to therapy and the horse's capabilities. Generally, exercise under tack is begun gradually between 3 and 4 months, and training can begin at 5 to 6 months after the injury.

Prognosis

A series of nine neonates with rupture of the gastrocnemius muscle and hemorrhage presented for necropsy. They were euthanatized because they were unable to rise and began to deteriorate physically.[5]

One of two adults managed by a Robert-Jones bandage and stall confinement survived.[4] One improved for a time but reinjured the area and deteriorated. The other recovered after 90 days of stall rest.

A weanling managed in a cast and Thomas splint was walking after 6 months and normal in pasture after 17 months.[2] Ultrasound revealed fibrosis and calcification of the injured area. Its recovery was typical of immature horses, in that flexure deformity occurred and was corrected with shoeing. Maintaining the foot in a normal position on the Thomas splint using a sleeve cast could possibly prevent that. In addition, the weanling suffered what is considered to be a traumatic femoropatellar OCD that affected both trochlear ridges and the patella.

In summary, the prognosis for neonates with rupture of the gastrocnemius and superficial digital flexor muscles appears grave. Older horses that can survive until the defect heals by fibrosis have a better possibility for recovery. The prognosis for athletic use is unknown.

It is difficult to determine the prognosis for partial or complete tears of one head because too few cases have been encountered with long-term follow-up to draw an objective opinion. Theoretically, if the injury is allowed sufficient time to heal, the horse should be able to return to performance. In one case in which long-term follow-up was available, the horse did return to full performance after 6 months of convalescence (Stashak TS, personal communication, 2001).

References

1. Kainer RA: Functional anatomy of the equine locomotor organs. In: Stashak TS, Ed. Adams' Lameness in Horses. 4th ed. Philadelphia: Lea & Febiger, 1987;57–58.
2. Lescun TB, Hawkins JF, Siems JJ. Management of rupture of the gastrocnemius and superficial digital flexor muscles with a modified Thomas splint-cast combination in a horse. J Am Vet Med Assoc 1998;213:1457–1459.
3. Pascoe RR. Death due to rupture of the origin of the gastrocnemius muscle in a filly. Aust Vet J 1975;51:107.
4. Shoemaker RS, Martin GS, Hillmann DJ, et al. Disruption of the Caudal Component of the Reciprocal Apparatus in Two Horses. Baton Rouge: School of Veterinary Medicine, Louisiana State University, 1988.
5. Sprinkle FP, Swerczek TW, Crowe MW. Gastrocnemius muscle rupture and hemorrhage in foals. Equine Pract 1985;7:10–11, 14–15,17.

RUPTURE OF THE GASTROCNEMIUS TENDON

Rupture of the gastrocnemius tendon may occur in one or both hindlimbs. It is rare for both the superficial flexor tendon and the gastrocnemius tendon (Achilles tendon) to be ruptured at the same time. The gastrocnemius tendon apparently ruptures before the superficial flexor tendon.

Causes

Trauma is the cause in all cases. Sometimes the horse is found with the condition in one or both limbs, but the specific cause is not known. Rupture of this tendon can result from strenuous efforts at stopping or from any other exertion in which great stress is applied to the hock in an attempt to extend it. Falling with the hindlimb in extension underneath the horse is such a circumstance.

Signs and Diagnosis

Signs of gastrocnemius tendon rupture are characteristic. The hock of the affected limb is dropped so that there is an excessive angle to the joint. If the condition is bilateral, the horse appears to be squatting and cannot straighten the hindlimbs. The limb can be advanced and the horse can walk, but at no time does the hock joint assume a normal angle. If the entire Achilles tendon is ruptured, the limb cannot support weight.

Treatment

Because of the persistent flexion of the hocks, the tendon ends are unable to make contact, making recovery difficult. Placing the horse in a full limb cast and slinging it so that tension on the gastrocnemius tendon and superficial flexor tendon is eased may be beneficial if used for prolonged periods (Fig. 8.429). A modified Thomas splint made from a 0.75-inch electrical conduit or a cast material may help, if the horse will tolerate it.

One study described the use of flexible carbon fiber for the repair of a ruptured gastrocnemius in a foal.[3] Because the lateral and medial insertions of the gastrocnemius tendon were torn off the tuber calcanei, a transverse hole was drilled lateral to medial to provide a site for the attachment of the carbon fiber distally. A Bunnell suture pattern was employed to attach and secure the carbon fiber to the proximal tendon. Postoperatively, the foal was placed in a full-limb cast for 60 days, after which a Robert-Jones bandage was applied. Other experiences with carbon fiber indicate another material, such as large-diameter nylon suture, would be preferable.[1,2] A locking loop or three-loop pulley suture in the tendon ends is indicated.

Prognosis

The prognosis is unfavorable because of problems inherent with immobilization of the hindlimb. There have

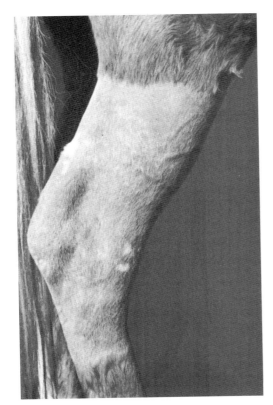

Figure 8.429 Lateral view of a gastrocnemius tendon that has healed after rupture. The limb was placed in a full-limb cast for 6 weeks. Note the thickening from fibrosis in the distal half of the gaskin. (Courtesy of J. T. Ingram.)

not been enough cases to give an accurate prognostic expectation.

References

1. Bertone AL, Stashak TS, Smith FW, et al.: A comparison of repair methods for gap healing in equine flexor tendon. Vet Surg 1990; 19:254–265.
2. Nixon AJ, Stashak TS, Smith FW, et al. Comparison of carbon fibre and nylon suture for repair of transected flexor tendons in the horse. Equine Vet J 1984;16:93–102.
3. Valdez H, Coy CH, Swanson T. Flexible carbon fiber for repair of gastrocnemius and superficial digital flexor tendons in a heifer and gastrocnemius tendon in a foal. J Am Vet Med Assoc 1982;181: 154–157.

CAPPED HOCK

See "Traumatic Bursitis" in Chapter 7.

STRINGHALT

Stringhalt is an involuntary hyperflexion of the hock when the horse moves, and the condition may affect one or both hindlimbs.[4,14] The extent of the motion may be minimal or extensive enough that the fetlock contacts the abdomen. Atrophy of the distal muscles of the hindlimb has been described.[2] Two forms of the condition occur, which are seemingly geographically predisposed.

Causes

Distributed worldwide, one form affects isolated horses and is usually unilateral. It may follow an injury to the hindlimbs.[4,14] Spontaneous recovery is rare, but improvement may be seen with rest.[4,14] The condition has been considered to involve the lateral digital extensor muscle tendon unit. Some cases are observed after trauma to this tendon, and adhesions of the tendon may form as it crosses the lateral surface of the hock joint. One series of 10 cases reported the development of stringhalt after dorsoproximal metatarsal injury to the extensor structures that healed by second intention. Most horses had suffered extensor tendon lacerations.[4] Note, however, these 10 horses represented only 19% of the total number of horses diagnosed with stringhalt during a 5-year period.

Australian stringhalt is restricted to Australia and New Zealand and commonly occurs in outbreak proportions, although sporadic incidence also occurs.[9] It is usually bilateral and occurs more frequently in the late summer and fall in years of poor pasture. During those times, affected horses are exposed to exceptionally large amounts of certain toxic weeds, including *Taraxacum officinale*, *Malva parviflora*, and *Hypochaeris radicata*, a dandelion.[3,5,12,13] The condition has also occurred in the Western Hemisphere in northern California, Washington State, and southern Chile under similar conditions.[1,6,7] However, the Washington State episode did not occur during a dry spell.

Although strongly associated with the condition, the plants mentioned have not been definitively linked as direct causes. Feeding trials using *H. radicata* failed to reproduce the condition, and *T. officinale* has been recommended for horse pastures. All exposed animals do not contract the disease.[7] An associated mycotoxin has been theorized to be present during the times at risk, while the plants themselves may not contribute directly to the situation. The incidence in Australia coincides with peak incidences of other plant-related mycotoxic diseases.[12]

The pathologic effect stems from axonopathy of the long peripheral nerves. The most noticeably affected are the recurrent laryngeal, peroneal, and tibial nerves, which account for laryngeal dysfunction and atrophy of the muscles of the gaskin.[2] The more distal portions of the axon may be affected earlier, which tends to spare the nerve cell body and favors regeneration in the time required to cover the distance of degeneration.[15] The effect on the muscle is typical of neurogenic atrophy in that type 2 fibers are more affected.

Many muscles are affected: the cricoarytenoideus dorsalis, the long and lateral digital extensors, and the gastrocnemius most notably so.[15] The pathophysiology of the hyperflexion remains unknown. A plausible theory is that the action-debilitated extensors are overridden by the comparatively minimally affected flexors: the biceps femoris and semitendinosus.[15] However, the persistence of the flexion in severely affected horses remains unexplained.

Signs and Diagnosis

The gait associated with typical Australian stringhalt has been graded.[9] Signs of the disease are quite variable;

some horses show a mild flexion of the hock during walking, whereas others show a marked jerking of the foot toward the abdomen (Fig. 8.430). The dorsal surface of the fetlock may actually hit the abdominal wall in severe cases. Some horses show these signs at each step, but in others the signs are spasmodic. In nearly all cases, the signs are exaggerated when the horse is backing. The condition is usually most noticeable after the horse has rested, but the signs may be intermittent and may disappear for some period of time. Any breed may be affected, and mild cases may not hinder the horse in use. Cold weather may cause an increase in signs, and there is usually a tendency toward decreased intensity of signs during warm weather. Most horses affected have a nervous disposition, which may play a part in the cause. Laryngeal hemiparesis results from the effect on the recurrent laryngeal nerve.

In either form, the alteration in gait is characteristic enough to make the diagnosis; but in some cases, signs may be absent at the time of examination. The condition must be differentiated from fibrotic myopathy, which produces the opposite gait, with the jerk being downward. Intermittent upward fixation of the patella and shivering should also be ruled out. Horses affected with Australian stringhalt may exhibit other muscle involvement, including laryngeal paresis.

Treatment

The classic treatment for typical North American stringhalt has been removal of the tendon and a distal portion of the lateral digital extensor muscle. Spontaneous recovery of horses affected with this disease is uncommon.[4] In one study, 1 of 4 horses treated with rest and controlled exercise recovered, 2 improved, and 1 remained the same.[4] I have seen one acute-onset string-

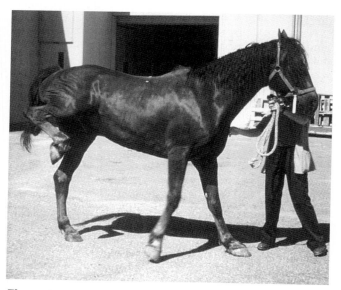

Figure 8.430 When affected by stringhalt the horse hyperflexes the limb. The downward motion of the limb is normal, but the upward (forward) motion is exaggerated. (Courtesy of T. S. Stashak.)

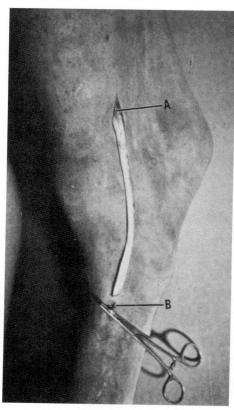

Figure 8.431 The distal end of the tendon (B) of the lateral digital extensor muscle has been transected, and the tendon has been pulled through the incision above the proximal end of the tendon sheath (A).

halt in a yearling recover after treatment with therapeutic ultrasound. In another study, 2 of 5 horses recovered completely after myotenotomy of the lateral digital flexor, another improved significantly, and 1 horse remained intermittently affected. The other horse in this series had adhesions precluding a complete myotenotomy, and it failed to improve.[4] A single horse affected with similar clinical signs responded to distal tarsal analgesia and subsequent steroid injection of those joints.[8] The hyperflexion was possibly a response to the pain of the distal tarsitis. At the Colorado State University, some benefit has been seen with the use of acupuncture in a limited number of cases.

Surgical resection can be performed in the standing position or in lateral recumbency on a surgical table. If the horse is to be left in the standing position, it should be tranquilized or sedated before preparation of the region for surgery. If the horse is placed in lateral recumbency, the affected limb should be uppermost. The region is prepared for aseptic surgery. If the standing position is selected, a local anesthetic should be injected into the muscle of the lateral digital extensor, starting about 10 cm above the lateral malleolus of the tibia. A second injection of local anesthetic should be made over the tendon below the hock joint just before it joins the long digital extensor tendon.

An incision, approximately 10 cm long, is made over the muscle of the lateral digital extensor just above the level of the point of the hock (Fig. 8.431). The muscle belly cannot be identified until several layers of fascia have been severed. Just overlying the tendon is a heavy layer of strong fascia. This is incised, and the muscle belly can be identified. An instrument is passed under the muscle belly so that it can be properly identified and tension put on it. Pulling on the muscular portion reveals movement in the distal portion just before it attaches to the long extensor. An incision, approximately 2 cm long, is then made over the distal portion of the tendon before it joins the tendon of the long extensor.

The skin and subcutaneous tissues are retracted, and a blunt-pointed bistoury is slipped under the tendon and it is severed. Rarely, there are variations in the insertion of the tendon, e.g., two tendons of insertion and insertion of the tendon on the proximal phalanx. Tension is then exerted on the proximal portion of the muscle until the tendon is pulled out. Considerable tension is sometimes required to break the adhesions that are formed around the tendon where it crosses the hock joint. If it seems as though undue force is required to pull it out, further dissection of the proximal portion of the tendon should be done to free it from the adhesions and fascia.

When the whole tendon is exposed, about 7 inches of it is pulled through the upper incision (Fig. 8.431). The tendon should be transected by removing a 7 to 10 cm of the muscle belly with it. After removal of the tendon, the fascia surrounding the muscle and the subcutaneous tissue are sutured with no. 1 synthetic absorbable suture in a simple continuous pattern. The skin incisions are closed with nonabsorbable interrupted sutures in a vertical mattress or near-far/far-near pattern.

The wounds are kept bandaged for 10 days. Opening of the upper wound sometimes occurs because of the stringhalt action of the limb; this can be prevented by applying a stent bandage or using focal pressure of a rolled 6-inch gauze directly on the suture line. It is essential that the surgery be done aseptically or septic tenosynovitis results.

Many cases show an almost immediate improvement, with complete recovery within 2 to 3 weeks. Other cases may take several months for any great improvement to occur, and still others may never show complete recovery. In cases that recur after several months or a year, an additional portion of the lateral digital extensor muscle may be removed.

An incision is made at the previous proximal incision site, extending 2 inches above the previous scar. The lateral digital extensor muscle is isolated and an additional 3 to 4 inches of the muscle is removed. This stops the sign of stringhalt in some cases. Alternatively, acupuncture can be tried before the surgery is performed to determine if more surgery will be a benefit.

For horses suffering Australian stringhalt, there is little rationale for lateral digital extensor myotenotomy, although some clinicians perform the procedure. The pathology is diffuse, and the majority of horses recover spontaneously without treatment once they are removed from pasture. Recovery can often be protracted, from several weeks to a year.

The successful use of mephenesin in one case of stringhalt was reported.[5] The drug was given in series of three injections both intravenously and intramuscularly. There was a relapse between the first and second series of injections. The drug merits further study on a significant number of cases. Other centrally acting muscle relaxants, including phenytoin[10] and baclofen,[11] appear effective; but more experience is required with these agents before their efficacy is established.

Prognosis

For North American stringhalt, the prognosis is guarded to favorable. Most horses show some improvement after surgery, but the degree of improvement is not predictable. For Australian stringhalt, the prognosis is similar. Many horses recover after removal from pasture; however, some do not recover completely.

References

1. Araya O, Krause A, Solis de Ovando M. Outbreaks of stringhalt in southern Chile. Vet Rec 1998;142:462–463.
2. Cahill JI, Goulden BE. Stringhalt—Current thoughts on aetiology and pathogenesis. Equine Vet J 1992;24:161–162.
3. Cahill JI, Goulden BE, Pearce HG. A review and some observations on stringhalt. NZ Vet 1985;33:101.
4. Crabill MR, Honnas CM, Taylor DS, et al. Stringhalt secondary to trauma to the dorsoproximal region of the metatarsus in horses: 10 cases (1986–1991). J Am Vet Med Assoc 1994;205:867–869.
5. Dixon RT, Stewart GA. Clinical and pharmacological observations in a case of equine stringhalt. Aust Vet J 1969;45:127–130.
6. Galey FD, Hullinger PJ, McCaskill J. Outbreaks of stringhalt in northern California. Vet Hum Toxicol 1991;33:176–177.
7. Gay CC, Fransen S, Richards J, et al. Hypochoeris-associated stringhalt in North America. Equine Vet J 1993;25:456–457.
8. Hebert C, Jann HW. Intra-articular corticosteroid treatment for stringhalt in a quarter horse: A case report. J Equine Vet Sci 1994;14:53–54.
9. Huntington PJ, Jeffcott LB, Friend SCE, et al. Australian stringhalt—Epidemiological, clinical and neurological. Equine Vet J 1989;21:266–273.
10. Huntington PJ, Seneque S, Slocombe RF, et al. Use of phenytoin to treat horses with Australian stringhalt. Aust Vet J 1991;68:221–224.
11. Kannegieter NJ, Malik R. The use of baclofen in the treatment of stringhalt. Aust Equine Vet 1992;10:90.
12. Pemberton DH, Caple IW. Australian stringhalt in horses. Vet Ann 1980;20:167.
13. Robertson-Smith RG, Jeffcott LB, Friend SCE, et al. An unusual incidence of neurological disease affecting horses during a drought. Aust Vet J 1985;62:6–12.
14. Seddon HO. Sudden case of stringhalt in a horse. Vet Rec 1963;75:35.
15. Slocombe RF, Huntington PJ, Friend SCE, et al. Pathological aspects of Australian stringhalt. Equine Vet J 1992;24:174–183.

SHIVERING

Shivering is an uncommon problem characterized by involuntary flexion of the limbs and elevation of the tail. The course is often progressive and worsens over a long period of time. The hindlimbs are more frequently affected, but sometimes the forelimbs may be involved.[1,3,5]

Causes

The precise cause of shivering is unknown. Some researchers have suggested that it is a peripheral nerve[4] or neuromuscular disorder subsequent to influenza, strangles, or other systemic diseases.[2] However, more recent evidence incriminates myopathy owing to polysaccharide storage disease.[6] Draft horses are reported to be more frequently affected. So many asymptomatic draft horses have some degree of glycogen storage abnormality, it is difficult to positively attribute the signs of shivers to this myopathy.[6]

Signs and Diagnosis

In mild cases, the signs may be difficult to detect, because they occur at irregular intervals, but in most cases, the signs are characteristic. Horses may randomly hyperflex any limb, but the hindlimbs are more frequently affected. Backing may cause the hyperflexion, or the horse may just drag the forelimbs reluctantly. The tail is often elevated and quivers. After a short time, the quivering ceases and the limb and tail return to a normal position. Fine body tremors may occur, but are possibly related to a more chronic debilitated state of the disease.[6] Horses may become progressively more debilitated and emaciated. Neurologic examination reveals no abnormalities. The main differential diagnosis is stringhalt.

Treatment

There is no curative treatment. Clinical signs have been reduced or controlled by feeding a high-fat, low-carbohydrate diet; and the effect is more profound when changes are made early in the progression of the disease.[7]

Prognosis

The prognosis is unfavorable because the signs usually tend to increase in severity. Dietary management instituted early may control signs indefinitely, but relapse is always possible.

References

1. Deen T. Shivering, a rare equine lameness. Equine Pract 1984;6: 19–21.
2. Mayhew IG. Large Animal Neurology. A Handbook for Veterinary Clinicians. Philadelphia: Lea & Febiger, 1989.
3. Neal FC, Ramsey FK. The nervous system. In: Catcott EJ, Smithcors JF, Eds. Equine Medicine and Surgery. 2nd ed. Santa Barbara, CA: American Veterinary Publications, 1972;486.
4. Neuman AJ. Well doc, what do you know? Draft Horse J 1990;27: 34–35.
5. Palmer AC. Introduction to Animal Neurology. 2nd ed. Oxford, UK: Blackwell Scientific, 1976.
6. Valentine BA. Polysaccharide storage myopathy in draft and draft-related horses and ponies. Equine Pract 1999;21:16–19.
7. Valentine BA, Divers TJ, Lavoie JP. Severe equine polysaccharide storage myopathy in draft horses: Clinical signs and response to dietary therapy. Proc Am Assoc Equine Pract 1996;42:294–296.

OSTEOSARCOMA OF THE DISTAL TARSUS

Osteosarcoma involving the tarsometatarsal joint has been observed in a 14-year-old gray Arabian gelding. The horse had a 10-month history of lameness and increasingly firm swelling of the left lateral proximal tarsometatarsal region. Upon presentation, the horse walked well but exhibited a grade 3 lameness at a trot. Plantarolateral swelling was present from midtarsus to proximal

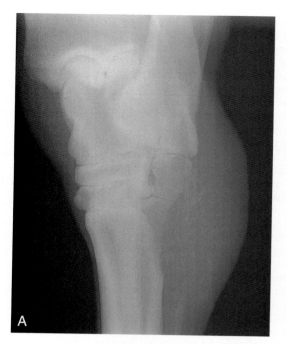
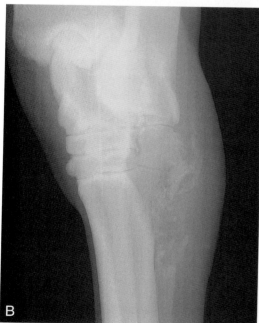

Figure 8.432 A. Dorsolateral, plantaromedial oblique view of a horse with developing swelling and lameness over a 10-month period. Note the osteolysis of the third and fourth metatarsal bones bordering the third tarsal bone. B. View taken 6 weeks after surgical debulking of the tumor mass and implanting cisplatin. Lameness improved, and tumor progression is radiographically arrested.

metatarsus. Radiographs revealed soft tissue swelling and osteolysis of the third and fourth metatarsal bones and the third tarsal bone (Fig. 8.432A). Thoracic radiographs were normal. A Tru-Cut biopsy was diagnosed as undifferentiated sarcoma.

The decision was made to debulk the tumor mass and

apply local chemotherapy. Between initial examination and readmission for surgery, the osseous defect had increased in size. The excisional biopsy report revealed telangiectatic osteosarcoma. The horse had a grade 1 lameness 1 month after surgery, and radiographs demon-strated arrested radiographic progression of the tumor and increasing osseous density in the region of the previous defect (Fig. 8.432B). Although the surgery was expected to be palliative, improvement in the early postoperative period was noticeable.

Part XI

THE TIBIA

Kenneth E. Sullins

Generally, tibial fractures occur with roughly the same frequency as fractures of other proximal long bones, although regional differences are evident.[8,19] Tibial fractures can be categorized according to type and anatomic location. Age also influences the type of fracture sustained. Because the long bones in younger horses are more elastic, they have less of a tendency to shatter and become severely comminuted, and the presence of physis provides additional sites for fractures to occur. Younger horses are not often subject to stress fractures; when they do sustain one they are virtually always injured by a traumatic incident such as a kick, being stepped on by the mare, or pivoting at speed while running in pasture. Adult athletes, on the other hand, sustain stress fractures in addition to all types of trauma-induced injuries resulting in a fracture. Each type of fracture is discussed separately.

Horses with complete displaced long bone fractures must have the affected limb immobilized for transport to a treatment facility. Without immobilization, the fragment ends self-abrade, changing their shape and making fracture somewhat inaccurate; if the fracture is articular, joint surfaces become disrupted, and good anatomic reduction of the joint surfaces cannot be achieved. Note that for the equine tibia, the fracture ends can penetrate through the skin of the medial gaskin. If the fracture is open, the hair should be clipped from around the wound and the skin cleaned and prepared with an antiseptic; then the wound is debrided and a sterile bandage is applied. This requires sedation in most patients. Broad-spectrum antimicrobials are also administered.

The tibia is difficult to immobilize adequately. Most casts and splints are applied so that the proximal end approximates the fracture site, causing the weight of the device to swing like a pendulum on the fulcrum of the fracture. Effective stabilization of a fracture requires immobilization of the joint proximal and distal to the fracture site. The stifle is impossible to completely immobilize in an adult horse. A foal can be sedated and kept down or it can even be held so further trauma is prevented.

There are two devices that are somewhat effective for immobilizing the stifle. The simpler is a temporary splint with a lateral component that extends to the hip (Fig. 8.433).[4] A padded bandage is applied to the limb and a lateral splint is affixed to the bandage with nonelastic tape. The second is a Thomas splint, which is more effec-tive but much more difficult to prepare and apply in adults (Fig. 8.434). The advantages of the Thomas splint is that mild traction is applied to stabilize the entire limb and the supports taped around the fracture further immobilize the tibia itself. A Thomas splint is easier to apply to a foal, and a shoe is not necessary for a temporary application.

The Thomas splint is a frame with a ring that fits over the thigh of the horse and extends to the foot to apply traction to the limb. The hip ring is curved medially at the distal side to position tightly against the groin, and the proximal side of the ring contacts the hip closely. The ring and upper shaft are constructed of hollow stock; the

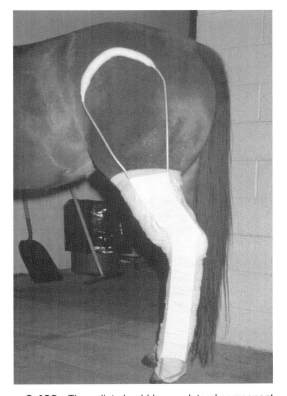

Figure 8.433 The splint should have a lateral component extending beyond the stifle to limit the motion of the tibia; if it does not, tibial instability is actually worsened. (Courtesy of T. S. Stashak.)

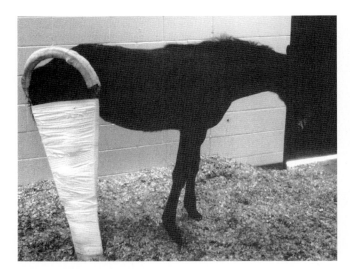

Figure 8.434 The Thomas splint places the limb in traction, and the tape supports the fracture in all directions.

size depends on the patient. Electric conduit suffices for foals, whereas galvanized pipe is required for larger horses. The distal portion of the splint is composed of a threaded rod in a size to fill the upper tube. Dual nuts are placed against the hollow tube to lock the splint in position. The most distal attachment consists of the threaded rod that is fixed to the dorsal and plantar portion of a plate fixed to the horse's shoe. The length of the splint is adjusted to apply enough traction to the affected limb. In the middle, the fracture is stabilized by applying tape hemicircumferentially around the limb and the splint. This setup offers solid stabilization of the limb without constricting the vascular supply.

If the fracture is so unstable that this arrangement is insufficient, a sleeve cast or external fixator can be added. As swelling subsides and muscles atrophy, the tension must be adjusted. If a wound exists, the bandages can be changed. For emergencies, splints can be prepared in several general sizes. For long-term application, general anesthesia is usually better than standing application. Materials should be organized, and a blacksmith should be present.

If the tibia is fractured in the distal third of the diaphysis or more distal, a cast has some effect if it is applied as proximally as possible. Although the reciprocal apparatus may be disabled, application of a full-limb cast on the hindlimb of a standing horse is difficult. To immobilize the tibia, the distal portion of the cast is not really needed, and a sleeve cast can be used (Fig. 8.381). Without the fetlock and foot included, the cast is lighter and easier to apply in the standing animal. Time is often critical, and the horse can be moved to a referral hospital sooner.

If these methods are not available, be sure that whatever is applied does not worsen the instability. Without the proper materials, leaving the affected limb alone may be a better choice.

FRACTURES OF PROXIMAL TIBIAL PHYSIS

Fracture of the proximal tibial physis has been observed in foals up to 8 months of age.[1] The injury usually occurs from direct trauma (e.g., a kick) while the limb is bearing weight,[6] from bending when the limb is somehow entrapped, or from being stepped on by the dam.[1] The forces apply pressure in a valgus direction, causing medial tension to separate the physeal cartilage. The physis opens until the lateral metaphyseal bone fractures, producing a Salter-Harris type 2 fracture.[6] The epiphysis and bone fragment becomes displaced laterally owing to the "ramp" defect left in the proximal lateral metaphysis (Fig. 8.435). The lateral metaphyseal component commonly occupies a third of the physeal surface. Uncommonly, the medial collateral ligament ruptures, which worsens the prognosis. The foal becomes acutely non weight bearing, and noticeable swelling appears around the stifle and proximal tibial regions. The proximal limb assumes a stifle valgus position.[1,6] Complete radiographs are required to define the fracture.

Conservative management can be considered for some nondisplaced fractures of the tibia, and one report notes the successful treatment of fractures of the proximal physis in one 2-week-old foal[41] and two horses.[17] For displaced fractures, the preferred treatment is internal fixation.[1,6] Because the bone surfaces rapidly become eburnated and will not fit together well, repair should be as soon as possible. Surgical techniques reported include lag screw fixation,[43] cross-pinning,[45] medial plate application,[1,6,46] and bone plates with external fixation.[47]

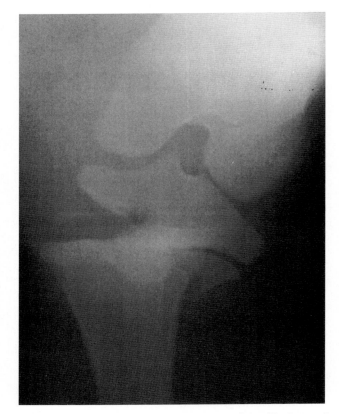

Figure 8.435 Dorsoplantar view showing a Salter-Harris type 2 fracture of the proximal tibial physis in a foal. The metaphyseal component is always lateral and usually involves approximately one-third of the distance across the physis. (Courtesy of C. W. McIlwraith.)

Most surgeons approach the proximal tibia medially to place either a dynamic compression plate (DCP) or T-plate. A screw that extends the entire length of the epiphysis is used, so as many screw threads as possible engage the epiphysis for maximum holding power (Fig. 8.436). This technique does not strictly adhere to the principles of internal fixation in that the medial cortex of the tibia is the compression side of the bone. However, this fracture tends to maintain itself in reduction by friction if the epiphysis has an adequate contact area.

Fractures in which the metaphyseal fragment occupies significantly more than the typical third of the physeal surface area are more difficult to maintain in reduction, because the proximal fragment tends to slide off laterally (Fig. 8.437). Cross-pin fixation is preferred by some surgeons for foals less than 50 kg.[21,44,45] Foals should bear some weight on the limb immediately and be walking well in 7 to 10 days;[6] complications should be suspected if this does not occur. The plate should be removed in 2 to 3 months. Angular deformity owing to the medial physeal bridging is possible, but it usually corrects after the plate is removed.

The prognosis is generally favorable, barring complications such as failure of the fixation, angular limb deformity, infection, or wound dehiscence.[1,6] The smaller the foal, the better the prognosis. The proximal physis is comparatively resilient and fracture usually does not limit normal development. The prognosis for athletic activity after successful fixation approximates 50%.[6]

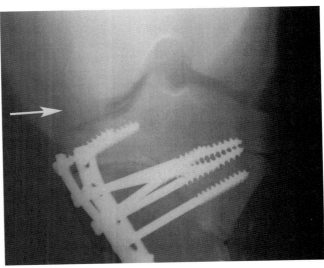

Figure 8.437   Medially stressed craniocaudal view of a Salter-Harris type 2 fracture of the proximal tibia that was repaired by internal fixation. Note that the medial collateral ligament ruptured, evidenced by the widened medial femorotibial joint space (arrow). Two plates and seven screws were used in the proximal fragment, because the metaphyseal fragment made up about 50% of the transverse length of the physis, allowing it to easily slide off.

FRACTURES OF THE DISTAL TIBIAL PHYSIS

Fractures of the distal tibial physis are less common than those of the proximal physis. Clinical signs are acute lameness, regional swelling, and pain on manipulation of the region. They may be true physeal fractures[11] or the physis may be entered by a diaphyseal fracture.[1] One instance of bilateral nondisplaced fractures extending down to the medial aspect of the physes was reported in a weanling Appaloosa that had been fed for show; conservative therapy was successful.[14]

Treatment must achieve reduction and stability of the fracture; if the tarsocrural joint is involved, the articular surfaces should be reconstructed. The distal tibial physis is comparatively thin and irregular, making it difficult to direct an implant. External coaptation, such as a cast applied as closely to the stifle as possible, may be required to augment internal fixation. Rush pins have been suggested when the entire epiphysis is intact.[13] Alternatively, Steinmann pins can be placed in a cruciate fashion (Fig. 8.438).[37] If the fracture can be reduced and there is no articular involvement, a Thomas splint can be applied to immobilize the middle to distal tibia in foals (Fig. 8.434). Some fractures simply cannot be adequately reduced or immobilized, and euthanasia is indicated.

The prognosis is generally considered fair to good if the fracture can be reduced and immobilized. However, convalescence from a long bone fracture is never simple with horses. If the fracture cannot be reduced or immobilized effectively, then euthanasia is advised.

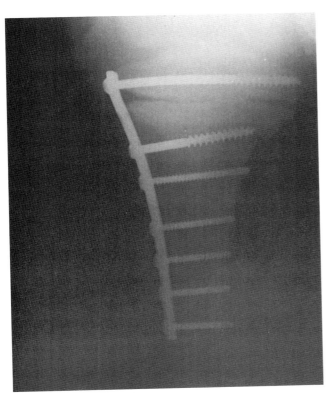

Figure 8.436   Postoperative view of the foal shown in Figure 8.435. One screw is placed as far as possible across the epiphysis, and the other screw engages the metaphyseal component of the proximal fragment. (Courtesy of C. W. McIlwraith.)

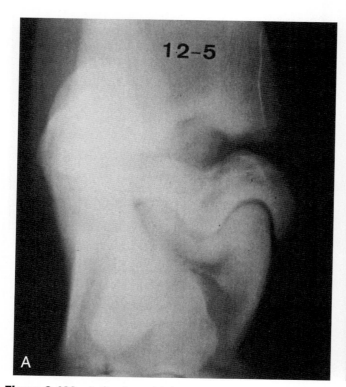

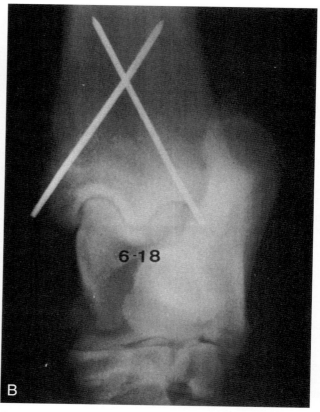

Figure 8.438 A. Craniocaudal view of a minimally displaced complete Salter-Harris type 1 fracture of distal tibia.

B. Craniocaudal view at the 7-month follow-up after repair with cross-pins and a full-limb cast. (Courtesy of T. S. Stashak.)

TIBIAL CREST FRACTURES

According to Getty,[16] the tibial crest physis is partially ossified at birth and forms a fibrocartilage union with the epiphysis during the 2nd year of life. The irregular physis remains radiographically visible until the horse is 36 to 42 months of age and may be mistaken for a fracture (Fig. 8.439).

These fractures usually occur from direct trauma (e.g., a kick) or from hitting a jump.[10] Horses may occasionally avulse the fragment owing to sudden quadriceps tension. Although affected horses frequently still have open physes, aged horses can also sustain this fracture.[35]

When the fragment remains nondisplaced, the diagnosis may be difficult. Radiographic comparison to the contralateral limb and response to direct palpation may provide the answer. When the fracture is displaced, the stifle may be dropped, and the horse may not be willing to fix the limb in extension.[1] An open wound may be present from the initial trauma, which must be taken into consideration for the timing of surgical treatment.

Traction by the patellar ligaments tends to distract the fragment, which impairs healing. However, nondisplaced or minimally displaced fractures can heal with stall rest for several weeks. Radiographic monitoring is done at 6-week intervals to document healing (Fig. 8.440), which may be expedited by internal fixation (Fig. 8.441).

Unstable, displaced, or articular fractures require internal fixation. The fragment must be reduced and stabilized in a tension band fashion, which converts the quadriceps distraction to compression.[1] The fixation may be accomplished using lag screws and plates (Fig. 8.440) or wire.[1,35] Lag screws alone and tension band wire alone have been used successfully;[15] however, the former techniques provide more stability. The recovery period is about 3 months; the implants may be left in provided lameness does not result when exercise resumes.[1] The radiographs should be examined for displaced comminuted fragments that could affect the outcome. Growth disturbance is not a factor with tibial crest fractures.

Conservative therapy can be successful in some cases, but healing is slower than for fractures that are loaded in compression. The recovery rate from surgically repaired tibial crest fractures is generally good, provided stable fixation can be accomplished. Complicating factors include failure of the fixation, infection from the wound, and disruption of the cranial tibial articular surface. The most critical point is recovery from anesthesia. In one study, two of four adults recovered; the two unsuccessful outcomes were the result of failure of the fixation.[35] Traction from the patellar ligaments is significant and tends to rotate the fragment away from the fixation. When possible, a plate on both sides of the tibial crest aligns the forces against the fixation. If only one plate is used, it should go on the craniolateral surface, which has more soft tissue cover available.[35]

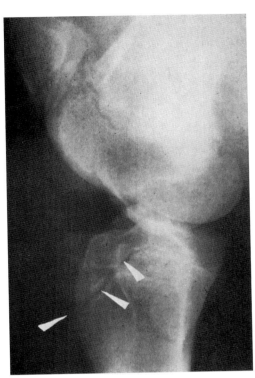

Figure 8.439 The normal physis (arrows) of the tibial tuberosity is irregular and may be mistaken for a fracture. (Courtesy of T. S. Stashak.)

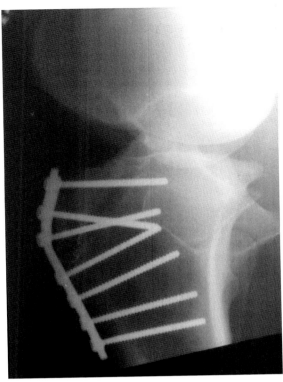

Figure 8.441 Lateromedial view of internal fixation used for an unstable tibial crest fracture. A single plate was applied to provide tension band support for the distracting forces of the patellar tendon; the screws were placed in a lag fashion. (Courtesy of T. S. Stashak.)

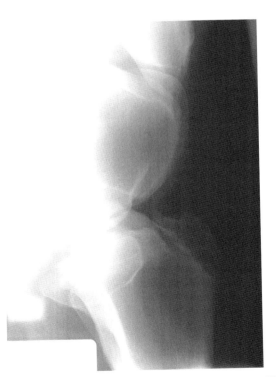

Figure 8.440 Lateromedial view of a tibial crest fracture. The lateral femoral trochlear ridge osteochondritis dissecans is not causing clinical signs. This fracture was stable at the time of diagnosis, and it successfully healed with stall rest.

TIBIAL STRESS FRACTURES

Remodeling due to cyclic fatigue of bone in horses that work at speed is thought to result in stress fractures.[38] Acute lameness may or may not abate with time, and visible or palpable swelling is often absent, making localization of the problem difficult. Tibial stress fractures in racehorses tend to have particular patterns. Typically, 2-year-olds and occasionally 3-year-olds are affected,[22,29,31] but other horses of other ages can be affected.[27] Thoroughbreds tend to develop lesions in the proximal caudal to lateral aspect of the tibia,[22,29] whereas Standardbreds and one racing Quarter Horse have been reported to develop middiaphyseal lesions on the same surfaces.[28,31]

Scintigraphy, or high-detail imaging, is often required to reveal the lesion (Fig. 8.442). To see a radiographic change, the clinician must set the beam to strike the fracture line exactly. When callus is present, imaging may be easier (Fig. 8.443).

In one series, 13 Standardbred racehorses with tibial stress fractures were managed with 8 to 16 weeks of stall rest followed by 4 to 12 weeks of pasture turnout before return to training.[31] Healing was determined by radiographic follow-up without repeating scintigraphy. Healing was evident as soon as 60 days after diagnosis. After a mean time of 9.5 months, 10 horses had returned to racing. Complications in the previously affected limbs

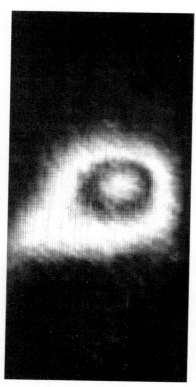

Figure 8.442 Scintigraphy reveals a tibial stress fracture. The emission from this lesion was so intense, none of the remainder of the tibia was imaged.

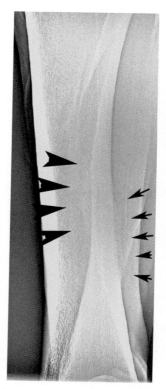

Figure 8.443 Xeroradiography demonstrates a tibial stress fracture. Note the endosteal (arrowheads) and periosteal (arrows) calluses.

were not reported, but lameness in other limbs of a few horses did occur. The potential role of persisting pain from the stress fractures is unknown. Determining the time of healing in such an obscure lesion is difficult. Racing at speed produces stresses that could cause catastrophic separation of incompletely healed stress fractures.[39]

Recently, extracorporeal shock wave therapy (ESWT) has been applied to tibial stress fractures.[33] The number of horses treated are few, precluding any conclusions. Some benefit has been observed after treating metacarpal stress fractures.[32] Note that the desensitization effect of ESWT could facilitate premature return to work with disastrous results. Complete healing should be documented before allowing the horse to return to work.

DIAPHYSEAL AND METAPHYSEAL TIBIAL FRACTURES

Most complete fractures of the tibial shaft have a spiral configuration and/or are comminuted.[6] The smaller the patient, the better the prognosis for successful treatment.[48] There are several causes of tibial fracture, although external trauma (e.g., kicking) and other stresses are frequently implicated.[3,6,7,9,12,19,30,36,42] Fractures owing to torsion combined with bending and axial compressions have been described.[30] These types of fractures resulted from falls during races and occurred spontaneously.[42] I have seen several cases in which the tibia

fractured when the horse simply pivoted while running in pasture.

Signs and Diagnosis

Incomplete or nondisplaced fractures of the tibia can be difficult to diagnose; acute lameness may abate with time. Visible or palpable swelling or pain is often absent, making localization of the problem difficult. Minimally displaced fractures may cause edema in the soft tissues overlying the thinly covered medial tibial cortex. The degree of lameness varies from severe to mild, depending on the degree of instability and duration.[19,20] Visible swelling or pain on palpation may be absent. Chronic fractures may begin to produce an externally visible callus that appears as swelling.[19]

Radiographs may have to be taken in several oblique views to demonstrate the fracture line; grid or digital enhancement is helpful. Radiographic findings may include a fracture line, but an intramedullary or extracortical callus may be the only abnormality. Nuclear scintigraphy is an invaluable imaging technique for obscure tibial lesions.[20,29]

Complete fracture of the tibia is characterized by the inability to bear weight on the affected limb, marked soft tissue swelling, angular deformity, and regional crepitation (Fig. 8.444). Craniomedial overriding of the proximal fragment coupled with valgus angulation frequently results in an open fracture because of the thin soft tissue covering the medial aspect of the tibia. Complete frac-

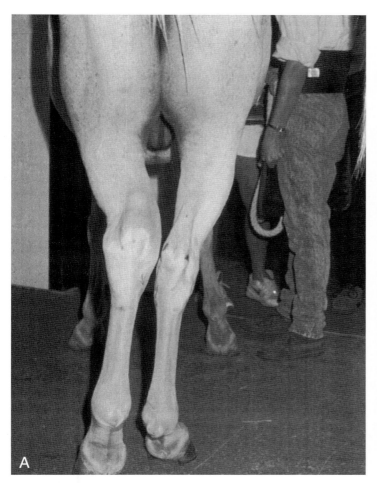

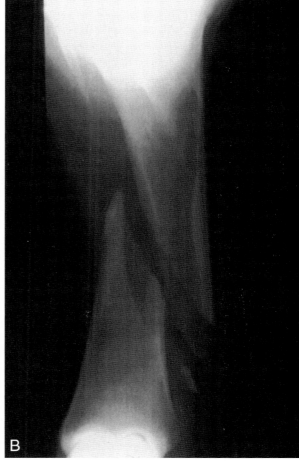

Figure 8.444   A. Caudal view of a horse with a left midshaft oblique tibial fracture. Note the valgus deviation at the point of the fracture. B. Caudocranial view of the same fracture. Although the fracture is closed, the overriding proximal fragment is at risk of puncturing the thin soft tissue covering on the medial aspect of the tibia. (Courtesy of T. S. Stashak.)

tures are unstable and are usually open as a result of severe overriding of the sharp fragments. The obvious instability, swelling, and pain make for an easy diagnosis. Radiographs are required to define the fracture configuration and formulate a treatment plan (Fig. 8.444B).

Treatment

Conservative management has been used successfully for only nondisplaced or minimally displaced tibial fractures, as long as catastrophic separation does not occur during convalescence.[19,20] Stall confinement for 3 to 6 months with radiographic and/or scintigraphic monitoring has been reported.[19,20] Horses may remain significantly lame for several weeks or become sound at a walk. Most clinicians withhold pain control to encourage the horse into taking better care of itself, avoiding the progression to a complete fracture.[19] There seems to be a high incidence of further separation of minimally displaced tibial fractures,[19] so internal fixation should be considered.[6] A bandage splint extending to the hip and putting the horse on a wire to prevent it from laying down has been recommended.[6] If the diagnosis is uncertain but believed to be a nondisplaced tibial fracture, the horse should be treated as described and radiographs should be taken at 10 days to establish a diagnosis.[6]

The effective use of external coaptation for unstable tibial fractures is difficult to achieve because the stifle cannot be adequately immobilized with a cast. Distal fractures that can self-abut to resist collapse are more amenable and can be treated with a cast and/or a Thomas splint (Fig. 8.434).[36] However, external coaptation may be considered when the fracture is too comminuted for internal fixation. Sleeve casts cause less leverage on the fracture than full-limb casts; and when reduction of the fracture is not required, they may be applied with the horse standing. Thomas splints partially immobilize the stifle and provide traction to stabilize the fracture, but they are time-consuming to prepare and usually must be custom built by a welder and a farrier.

Foals are more amenable to external coaptation, but are also more subject to fracture disease. Fracture disease refers to problems affecting the entire patient as a result of lack of complete weight bearing in the affected limb. Examples include varus deformity of the contralateral limb and forelimb flexural deformities. Unless the external coaptation is effective and achieves a quick result,

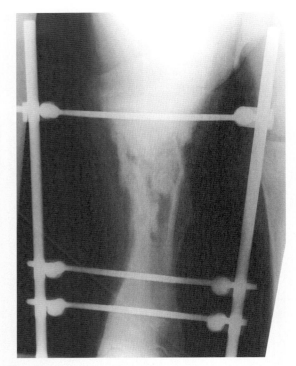

Figure 8.445 The comminuted midshaft tibial fracture sustained by the horse shown in Figure 8.434 was managed with a Thomas splint and an external fixator.

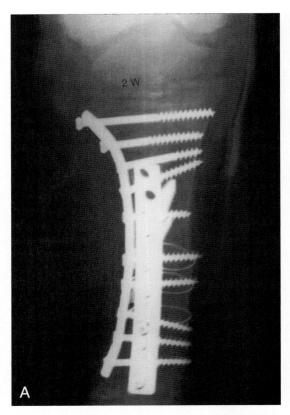

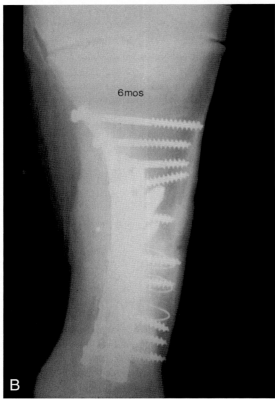

Figure 8.446 A. Craniocaudal view of a midshaft tibial fracture in a foal that was repaired with two plates. B. By the 6-month follow-up, healing of the fracture can be noted. (Courtesy of T. S. Stashak.)

the fractured limb, once healed, may turn out to be the best limb on an unsound horse. The most common complication in the adult is support limb laminitis in the contralateral or other limbs. In general, athletic function should not be expected in horses with complete tibial fractures treated by external coaptation.

Internal fixation with compression plates and screws, when applicable, is the best option.[1,6,7,9,48] Success depends on sufficient space proximal and distal to the fracture to place enough screws for adequate stability and interfragmentary compression along the fracture line. Bramlage and Hanes[7] reported the successful treatment of a tibial fracture in an adult horse. In the tibia, the tension surface is cranial and the compression surface is caudal.[18,34] With the horse in dorsal recumbency, use a cranial approach and place two plates: one craniolateral and the other craniomedial at a 90° angle to each other. Plates should extend the entire length of the bone and should not begin or end at the same point. The caudal cortex must have a buttress to prevent cycling of the plates.[5,48]

Foals occasionally require less fixation for successful repair (Figs. 8.446 and 8.447). When necessary, the fracture may be reconstructed using lag screws beside the plates to stabilize the fracture for plate application and to provide better interfragmentary compression (Fig. 8.447). A cast should not be applied for recovery, because it will change the tension forces on the bone and result in additional stresses at the fracture.[7,34] In all cases, the horse should be assisted in its recovery from anesthesia. Euthanasia is advised for adult horses that have sustained irreparable severely comminuted fractures.

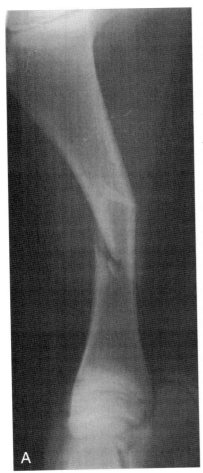
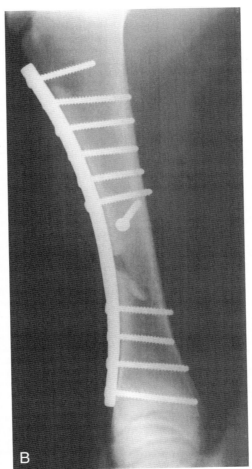
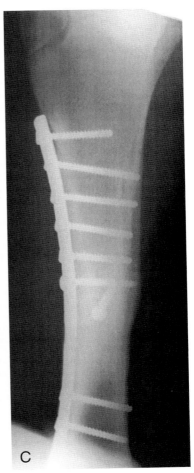

Figure 8.447 A. Lateromedial view of an oblique midshaft fracture of the tibia in a foal. B. The fracture was repaired with a single plate placed on the cranial aspect of the tibia and a single screw compressing the fracture line. Note the solid caudal buttress on the caudal aspect of the tibia. C. The healed fracture. (Courtesy of N. A. White.)

Interlocking nails have been developed to treat proximal equine long bone fractures.[23-26] Although promising in some respects, the torsional strength of the interlocking nail has not reached that of double plating. In addition, a specific fracture configuration is required. In summary, more work is needed before the technique should be applied in the clinical situation.[2]

Half-pin and transfixation pinning has also been successful in one report[3] and one foal at the author's hospital (Fig. 8.445). It is doubtful that the application is useful for adult horses. Successful experimental external fixation has been reported in foals.[40] This technique can be successfully applied only under certain circumstances, e.g., for a transverse, midshaft fracture with no proximal or distal fracture lines in a horse weighing less than 125 kg. This situation arises rarely in the clinical situation; however, one such case is reported by Bignozzi et al.[3] The authors noted that the fracture would have been more stable with double-pin fixation. The general success and lack of aftercare with internal fixation override considerations of external fixation in most situations, except when soft tissue loss has occurred. If external fixation is chosen, pin placements should be limited to the transverse plane; pins should not placed in the cranio-caudal direction. In some cases, external fixation may be used to aid stability achieved with external coaptation, such as a Thomas splint (Fig. 8.434).

Prognosis

The prognosis for a fractured tibia in an adult is guarded to poor. Nondisplaced fractures may heal with stall rest, but separation remains a possibility for several weeks. The difficulty in successfully repairing a completely separated tibial fracture in an adult is reflected in the few reports in the literature. Each case is different and has its own set of considerations.

In a series of nine foals with tibial fractures repaired by internal fixation using plates and screws, six horses obtained excellent results and two recovered.[48] However, the prognosis depends on the type of fracture sustained, its duration, and the treatment selected.

References

1. Auer JA, Watkins JP. Diseases of the tibia. In: Colahan PT, Mayhew IG, Merritt IG, Moore JN, Eds. Equine Medicine and

Surgery. Vol. 2. 5th ed. Santa Barbara, CA: American Veterinary Publications, 1999;1696–1701.

2. Auer JA, Watkins JP. Instrumentation and techniques in equine fracture fixation. Vet Clin North Am Equine Pract 1996;12: 283–302.

3. Bignozzi L, Gnudi M, Masetti L, et al. Half pin fixation in 2 cases of equine long bone fracture. Equine Vet J 1981;13:64–66.

4. Bramlage LR. First aid for the fracture patient. Proc Am Assoc Equine Pract 1982;28:97–105.

5. Bramlage LR. Long bone fractures. Vet Clin North Am Large Anim Pract 1983;5:285–310.

6. Bramlage LR. The tibia. In: Auer JA, Stick JA, Eds. Equine Surgery. Philadelphia: WB Saunders, 1999;862–867.

7. Bramlage LR, Hanes GE. Internal fixation of a tibial fracture in an adult horse. J Am Vet Med Assoc 1982;180:1090–1094.

8. Crawford WH, Fretz PB. Long bone fractures in large animals. A retrospective study. Vet Surg 1985;14:295–302.

9. Dingwall JS, Duncan DB, Horney FD. Compression plating in large animal orthopedics. J Am Vet Med Assoc 1971;158:1651–1657.

10. Dyson S. Stifle trauma in the event horse. Equine Athlete 1994;7: 1, 9–14.

11. Embertson RM, Bramlage LR, Herring DS, et al. Physeal fractures in the horse. I. Classification and incidence. Vet Surg 1986;15(3): 223–229.

12. Fessler JF, Amstutz HE. Fracture repair. In: Oehme FW, Prier JE, Eds. Textbook of Large Animal Surgery. Baltimore: Williams & Wilkins, 1974;996.

13. Foerner JJ. Surgical treatment of selected musculoskeletal disorders of the rear limb. In: Auer JA, Ed. Equine Surgery. Philadelphia: WB Saunders, 1992;1055–1075.

14. Frankeny RL, Johnson PJ, Messer NT, et al. Bilateral tibial metaphyseal stress fractures associated with physitis in a foal. J Am Vet Med Assoc 1994;205:76–78.

15. Gerring EL, Davies JV. Fracture of the tibial tuberosity in a polo pony. Equine Vet J 1982;14:158–159.

16. Getty GR. Sisson and Grossman's Anatomy of the Domestic Animals. 5th ed. Philadelphia: WB Saunders, 1975;309.

17. Harrison LJ, May SA, Richardson JD, et al. Conservative treatment of an incomplete long bone fracture of a hindlimb of four horses. Vet Rec 1991;129:133–136.

18. Hartman W, Schamhardt HC, Lammertink JL, et al. Bone strain in the equine tibia: An in vivo strain gauge analysis. Am J Vet Res 1984;45:880–884.

19. Haynes PF, Watters JW, McClure JR, et al. Incomplete tibial fractures in three horses. J Am Vet Med Assoc 1980;177:1143–1145.

20. Johnson PJ, Allhands RV, Baker GJ, et al. Incomplete linear tibial fractures in two horses. J Am Vet Med Assoc 1988;192:522–524.

21. Juswiak JS, Milton JL. Closed reduction and blind cross-pinning for repair of a proximal tibial fracture in a foal. J Am Vet Med Assoc 1985;187:743–745.

22. Mackey VS, Trout DR, Meagher DM, et al. Stress fractures of the humerus, radius, and tibia in horses. Clinical features and radiographic and/or scintigraphic appearance. Vet Radiol 1987;28: 26–31.

23. McDuffee LA, Stover SM. An in vitro biomechanical investigation of an interlocking nail for fixation of diaphyseal tibial fractures in adult horses. Am Coll Vet Sci 1993;390.

24. McDuffee LA, Stover SM, Bach JM, et al. An in vitro biomechanical investigation of an equine interlocking nail. Vet Surg 2000;29: 38–47.

25. McDuffee LA, Stover SM, Taylor KT. In vitro cyclic biomechanical properties of an interlocking equine tibial nail. Vet Surg 2000;29: 163–172.

26. McDuffee LA, Stover SM, Taylor KT, et al. An in vitro biomechanical investigation of an interlocking nail for fixation of diaphyseal tibial fractures in adult horses. Vet Surg 1994;23:219–230.

27. Nelson A. Stress fractures of the hind limb in 2 Thoroughbreds. Equine Vet Educ 1994;6:245–248.

28. Peloso JG, Watkins JP, Keele SR, et al. Bilateral stress fractures of the tibia in a racing American Quarter Horse. J Am Vet Med Assoc 1993;203:801–803.

29. Pilsworth RC, Webbon PM. The use of radionuclide bone scanning in the diagnosis of tibial "stress" fractures in the horse: a review of five cases. Equine Vet J 1988;6(Suppl):60–65.

30. Rooney JR. The mechanics of humeral and tibial fractures of the horse. Cornell Vet 1965;55:599.

31. Ruggles AJ, Moore RM, Bertone AL, et al. Tibial stress fractures in racing Standardbreds: 13 cases (1989–1993). J Am Vet Med Assoc 1996;209:634–637.

32. Scheuch B, Whitcomb M, Galuppo L, et al. Clinical evaluation of high-energy extracorporeal shock waves on equine orthopedic injuries. Proceedings. 20th Annual Meeting of the Association of Equine Sports Medicine, New Brunswick, NJ, 2000.

33. Scheuch B, Whitcomb M, Galuppo L, et al. Clinical evaluation of high-energy extracorporeal shock waves on equine orthopedic injuries. Proceedings. Equine Musculoskeletal High-Energy Shock Wave Therapy Symposium, Shelbyville, KY, 2001.

34. Schneider RK, Milne DW, Gabel AA, et al. Multidirectional in vivo strain analysis of the equine radius and tibia during dynamic loading with and without a cast. Am J Vet Res 1982;43: 1541–1550.

35. Smith BL, Auer JA, Watkins JP. Surgical repair of tibial tuberosity avulsion fractures in four horses. Vet Surg 1990;19:117–121.

36. Springstead BK. Fracture of the tibia in a horse. J Am Vet Med Assoc 1967;155:1370–1373.

37. Stashak TS. The tibia. Fractures. In: Stashak TS, Ed. Adams' Lameness in Horses. 4th ed. Philadelphia: Lea & Febiger, 1987; 726–728.

38. Stover SM, Ardans AA, Read DH, et al. Patterns of stress factors associated with complete bone fractures in racehorses. Proc Am Assoc Equine Pract 1993;39:131–132.

39. Stover SM, Johnson BJ, Daft BM, et al. An association between complete and incomplete stress fractures of the humerus in racehorses. Equine Vet J 1992;24:260–263.

40. Sullins KE, McIlwraith CW. Evaluation of 2 types of external skeletal fixation for repair of experimental tibial fractures in foals. Vet Surg 1987;16:255–264.

41. Turner AS. Fracture of specific bones. In: Mansmann RA, McAllister ES, Eds. Equine Medicine and Surgery. 3rd ed. Santa Barbara, CA: American Veterinary Publications, 1982;1018.

42. Vaughan LC, Mason BJE. A Clinicopathologic Study of Racing Accidents in Horses. Dorking Surrey, UK: Adlard & Son, 1975.

43. Wagner PC, DeBowes RM, Grant BD, et al. Cancellous bone screws for repair of proximal growth plate fractures of the tibia in foals. J Am Vet Med Assoc 1984;184:688–691.

44. Watkins JP. Fractures of the tibia. In: Nixon A, Ed. Equine Fracture Repair. Philadelphia: WB Saunders, 1996;273–283.

45. Watkins JP, Auer JA, Taylor TS. Crosspin fixation of fractures of the proximal tibia in three foals. Vet Surg 1985;14:153–159.

46. White NAD, Blackwell RB, Hoffman PE. Use of a bone plate for repair of proximal physeal fractures of the tibia in two foals. J Am Vet Med Assoc 1982;181:252–254.

47. White NA, Wheat JD. An expansion and compression technique for reducing and stabilizing proximal epiphyseal fractures of the tibia in foals. J Am Vet Med Assoc 1975;167:733–738.

48. Young DR, Richardson DW, Nunamaker DM, et al. Use of dynamic compression plates for treatment of tibial diaphyseal fractures in foals: nine cases (1980–1987). J Am Vet Med Assoc 1989; 194:1755–1760.

FRACTURE OF THE FIBULA

Obscure hindlimb lamenesses have occasionally been diagnosed as fracture of the fibula.[4,5,7] This was a common diagnosis in Standardbreds and Thoroughbreds, but it has been misused greatly. Extensive radiologic studies have revealed that what often appears to be a fracture of the fibula is merely a defect in the union of the proximal and distal segments of the bone (Fig. 8.448).[2,8,9] This defect can be demonstrated in a high percentage of horses. When radiographs are taken of the opposite fibula, the defect is usually there as well.[1]

That historical perspective notwithstanding, fracture of the fibula does occur.[6] A single case of a chronic, nonhealing proximal fibular fracture in a Standardbred racehorse was reported. The diagnosis was based on

8. Zeskov F. Fracture or congenital discontinuity of the fibula in the horse. Br Vet J 1958;114:145.
9. Zeskov F. A study of discontinuity of the fibula in the horse. Am J Vet Res 1959;78:852.

OSSIFICATION VARIATIONS OF THE TIBIAL CREST (TUBEROSITY)

In one report, a yearling Thoroughbred colt was examined and found to have bilateral shortening of the gait behind and slight unilateral hindlimb lameness.[2] Flexion of each hindlimb increased the lameness in the respective hindlimb. Radiographs revealed bilateral changes on the tibial tuberosities consisting of apparent small osseous separations on the most cranial aspect of each. The physes were also thought to be wider than normal distally. Radiographs taken after 7 weeks of stall rest demonstrated that the cranial densities had ossified to become part of the remainder of the apophysis. A previously less apparent lucency in the apophysis at the distal limit of the separate osseous density had become more radiolucent. No clinical significance could be placed on the finding.

Similar findings were reported in eight Thoroughbred horses 1 to 3 years old.[1] Unilaterally affected horses were described as moving away from the affected limb at the trot. Treatment consisted of rest of up to 3 months.

This is an interesting example of the variation in ossification patterns that may be seen in many places within immature horses. However, the tibial crest is both frequently radiographed and variable (Fig. 8.449). Lame-

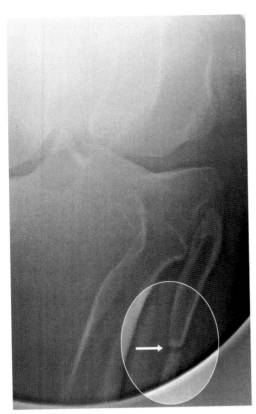

Figure 8.448 Craniocaudal view of the proximal tibia. Note the fibrous union in the fibula that is commonly mistaken for a fracture (arrow).

scintigraphic and radiographic findings; scintigraphy also revealed a probable contralateral femoral neck stress fracture. The nonunion was treated by placing an autogenous cancellous bone graft with the horse standing. The fracture ossified by 90 days after surgery, and the horse was training at 11 months. The contralateral lameness persisted, and the horse was retired.

In one study, histologically necrotic foci of fibrous tissue, islands of bone, and cartilage in the discontinuous part of the fibula were observed. Associated with these conditions were organic changes within the peroneal (fibular) and tibial nerves that were thought to contribute to a mild disorder of locomotion of the hindlimb.[3]

References

1. Banks WC. Additional studies of fibular defects in horses. J Am Vet Med Assoc 1958;133:422.
2. Delahanty DD. Defects—not fractures—of the fibula in horses. J Am Vet Med Assoc 1958;133:258.
3. Kaneko M, Kiryu K, Oikawa MA, et al. Discontinuous conditions in the fibula in the light horse. Exp Rep Equine Health Lab [Tokyo] 1975;12:1–11.
4. Lundvall RL. Fracture of the fibula in the horse. J Am Vet Med Assoc 1956;129:10.
5. Lusk ND, Rosborough JP. Fibular fracture in a filly. J Am Vet Med Assoc 1957;130:4.
6. O'Rielly JL, Bertone AL, Genovese RL. Treatment of a chronic comminuted fracture of the fibula in a horse. J Am Vet Med Assoc 1998;212:396–398.
7. A phenomenon in equine lameness [editorial]. J Am Vet Med Assoc 1957;130:51.

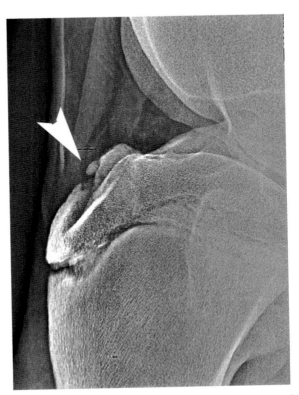

Figure 8.449 Lateromedial view demonstrating a temporarily incompletely ossified tibial crest in a yearling Standardbred filly. The fragment (arrow) eventually becomes incorporated into the remainder of the tibial crest.

ness and other potential pathology should be investigated, and the contralateral structure should always be used for comparison. Bilaterally symmetric findings are often normal variations for that animal.

References

1. Baker RH. Osteochondrosis of the tibial tuberosity of the horse. J Am Vet Med Assoc 1960;137:354–355.
2. Kold SE. Traction apophysitis in a yearling colt resembling Osgood-Schlatter disease in man. Equine Vet J 1990;22:60–61.

ENOSTOSES OF THE TIBIA

Enostoses are intramedullary osseous densities that are usually demonstrated radiographically after having been identified by scintigraphy (Fig. 8.450).[1] The cause is unknown. Affected horses have ranged in age from 3 to 10 years.

Signs and Diagnosis

The horses in which enostoses have been diagnosed were lame—and not always in the limb in which the lesion was discovered. The focal or multifocal round or irregular scintigraphic lesions may coincide with lame-

ness or may be considered incidental findings. Some lesions have been located close to the nutrient foramen.[1]

In one study, 5 of 10 horses with enostoses were affected in the tibia; other sites included the radius, humerus, and metatarsus. Of those 5, 2 horses were believed to be lame from the enostosis lesion.[1]

Treatment

Treatment consists of rest and systemic anti-inflammatory therapy. There is really no benefit to the tibia from any support or local anti-inflammatory measures.

Prognosis

The prognosis is apparently good, provided rest is allowed. Lameness resolves after 2 to 6 months. Follow-up scintigraphic examination in three horses (at 2, 6, and 9 months later, respectively) revealed normal radioisotope uptake in the affected areas.

Reference

1. Bassage LH, Ross MW. Enostosis-like lesions in the long bones of 10 horses: Scintigraphic and radiographic features. Equine Vet J 1998;30:35–42.

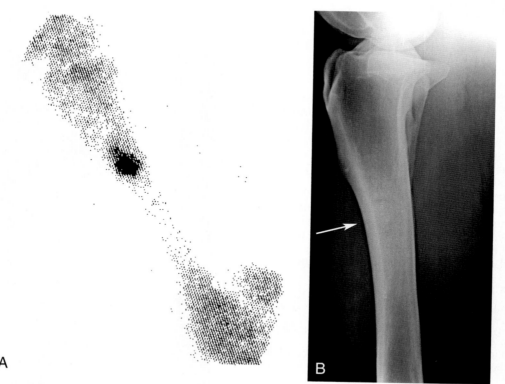

Figure 8.450 A. Scintigraphy reveals an increased uptake of enostosis in middiaphysis of the tibia. B. Radiographic appearance of the enostosis (arrow). (Courtesy of P. S. Doyle.)

Part XII

THE STIFLE

Kenneth E. Sullins

The stifle is the largest and most complex joint in the horse; therefore, it is not surprising that injury to it is an important cause of hindlimb lameness. The stifle consists of three synovial compartments: femoropatellar and medial and lateral femorotibial. The medial femorotibial and femoropatellar joint spaces frequently communicate. Fibrocartilaginous menisci separate the articular surfaces of the femoral condyles and the proximal tibia. Cruciate ligaments are positioned on the midline for cranial-caudal stability; medial and lateral collateral ligaments provide abaxial stability of femorotibial joints. Because of the complex nature of this joint, damage to one region frequently disrupts other structures, complicating the diagnosis and treatment.

Of 835 horses that presented with hindlimb and spinal conditions, Vaughan recorded 63 cases of stifle problems (8%).[20] In another report, stifle lameness occurred in 2% of 5388 specified conditions of the musculoskeletal system.[1] Of another series of 553 horses with hindlimb lameness, 795 stifles were radiographed, revealing changes in 326 horses.[17] Femoropatellar and femorotibial lesions occurred at the similar rates of 27% and 32%, respectively, and there was an overall incidence of 32% with osteoarthritis. Stifle problems are quite common in routine referral practice and are probably increasing owing to improved ability to make specific diagnoses.

Signs and Diagnosis

The evaluation of stifle lameness is made by visual observation, palpation of the joint, gait evaluation, and elimination of other types of lameness. The examiner should become acquainted with normal palpation and normal variations; asymmetry usually indicates a problem. With acute injuries, swelling may be impressive, complicating an accurate anatomic diagnosis. Acutely painful horses will usually not fix the limb in extension when walking or standing. Bruising from external trauma is common in horses that jump over fences. Local and systemic anti-inflammatory therapy may be required to reduce the swelling before a complete diagnosis can be made.[6]

Distension of the femoropatellar and the medial femorotibial joint may sometimes be seen when the horse is looked at from the side (Fig. 8.451) and cranial views, respectively. On palpation, distension and thickening of the femoropatellar joint capsule may be felt between the patellar ligaments. Comparison with the opposite stifle should be made. With some horses, both stifles can be palpated while standing behind the horse. Femoropatellar effusion that reflects a medial femorotibial joint effusion (if present at all) is less than that which occurs from a primary femoropatellar joint involvement. Some nor-

mal horses have mild femoropatellar effusion with no clinical problem. Medial and lateral femorotibial effusion may be palpated on the craniomedial and craniolateral margins of their respective joints. The proximal tibial plateau, the femoral condyles, and the cranial borders of the collateral ligaments provide landmarks for their identification. With chronicity, atrophy of the gluteal and quadriceps muscles on the affected side may be apparent (Fig. 8.452), which may be obvious or noticed only after careful comparison from the rear and side. Hindlimb flexion may induce a painful response.

Stifle lameness is fairly typical of joint pain in the hindlimb. Viewed from the side, the cranial phase of the stride is shortened, and the foot is carried closer to the ground. The toe may drag when the horse advances the limb at a trot, and toe wear may be obvious in some chronic cases (Fig. 8.453). When viewed from the rear, asymmetry in the gluteal use is observed when the horse is at trot. The duration of gluteal use is shorter, resulting

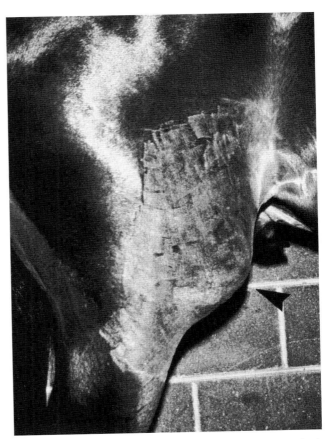

Figure 8.451 Lateral view of the stifle of a horse with marked femoropatellar effusion (arrow).

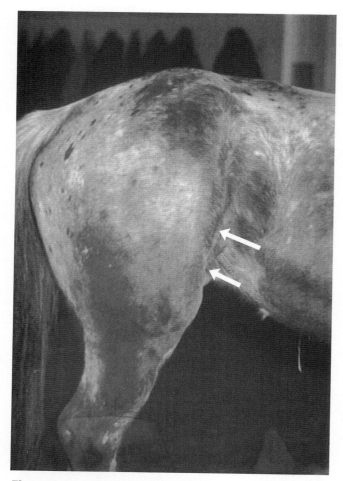

Figure 8.452 Note the atrophy of the quadriceps muscles, particularly the vastus lateralis (arrows), in a horse that sustained a stifle injury 6 months earlier. (Courtesy of T. S. Stashak.)

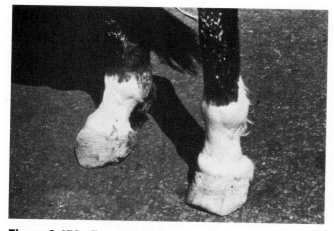

Figure 8.453 Excessive toe wear in a horse that was reluctant to raise the height of foot flight. This may be associated with stifle pain. (Courtesy of T. S. Stashak.)

in an early limb unweighting. This is frequently referred to erroneously as the hip hike; what actually occurs is that the horse takes less weight on and spends less time on the lame limb, resulting in a reduction in gluteal use that is seen as a hip roll. The degree of lameness depends on the severity of the injury; injuries that cause joint instability usually result in severe lameness. In most cases, stifle lameness cannot be definitively identified from hock pain or other sites in the hindlimb.

Flexion of the hindlimb affects the digit, hock, stifle, and hip. If the limb is held loosely around the fetlock, digital flexion is minimized. However, the source of any increased pain must be localized. The stifle flexion test can provide the examiner with some assurance that the region is involved if the horse reacts in a painful manner to flexion and the test exacerbates the lameness (see Fig. 3.73). (See Chapter 3 for a more complete description.) The cruciate ligament test consists of pushing the cranial aspect of the stifle caudally and releasing it to evaluate a painful response; excess cranial to caudal laxity indicates ligament rupture. Holding the tail may be helpful. One report on cruciate ligament injuries notes that this technique detects the problem accurately in only one of six standing horses; but all six ligament injuries could be detected when the horses were under general anesthesia.[13] Repeatedly pushing the cranial aspect of the proximal tibia caudally, while the horse bears weight on the limb, sometimes exacerbates the signs. Asymmetric pain during the process or increased lameness when the horse is moved indicates stifle injury and possible instability (see Fig. 3.75). The process should be started gradually to prevent sudden reaction by the horse and injury to the examiner.

The collateral ligaments can be examined for sprain trauma or rupture by abducting and adducting the limb. The medial collateral ligament is checked by placing the shoulder on the lateral side of the stifle and pulling the distal part of the hindlimb away from the horse (see Fig. 3.76). With a sprain, increased pain is perceived as well as increased lameness. With rupture, the horse exhibits severe pain but is quite lame anyway. To apply varus pressure to the stifle to evaluate the lateral collateral ligament signs, the horse's foot is fixed on the ground in an axial position with the examiner's foot, and the stifle is pulled laterally with a towel or a rope. The lateral collateral ligament is rarely involved. Stress radiographs are useful for detecting more subtle joint instability (Fig. 8.454). Sedation of the horse is recommended, and the examiner should take care to avoid personal injury.

Lameness can be localized to the stifle by the use of intrasynovial anesthesia. Generally, all three joints are blocked at once. In some cases, it may be desirable to block the joints separately, which more accurately determines the site of the problem for the possibility of surgical intervention. Although communication between the femoropatellar joint and medial femorotibial joint is common, communication between the femoropatellar joint and lateral femorotibial joint is rare.[16] In some horses with osteoarthritis, the femoropatellar joint communicates with both femorotibial joints.[16] None of the femorotibial joints communicates with its counterpart. Diagnostic local analgesia in the stifle is usually performed after the remainder of the limb has been ruled out as a cause of the lameness. Without effusion, the

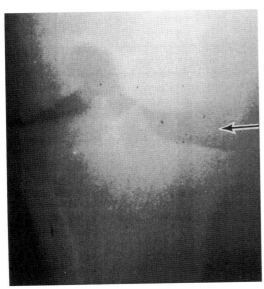

Figure 8.454 Craniocaudal view of a ruptured medial collateral ligament. Note the asymmetrically widened medial femorotibial joint space (arrow). In addition, attachment of the cranial cruciate ligament appears to have been avulsed from the medial intercondylar eminence of the tibia.

medial femorotibial joint is the logical starting point if each joint is to be blocked separately, because if there is a problem, the femoropatellar joint will usually visibly fill and the lateral femorotibial joint is not the site of a problem as often. Radiographs taken before the block (if possible without sedation that hinders the lameness examination) may provide some indication of a starting point (see Chapter 3).

A complete series of good-quality radiographs is needed to evaluate the stifle joints and provide a definitive diagnosis. A higher power machine and sedation are usually required to acquire diagnostic films. Routine survey views include caudocranial and lateromedial views. The 30° lateral craniomedial oblique separates the lateral from the medial trochlear ridge if that is needed.[18] The flexed lateromedial and caudolateral to craniomedial oblique projections provide other perspectives from which to view the femoral condyles, particularly for subchondral cyst identification. The articular surface and sagittal integrity of the patella are demonstrated best by a flexed cranioproximal-craniodistal tangential (skyline) view.[8,11] With acute trauma, the density of the tissue renders handheld radiographic units useless. Ultrasound may be more helpful for localizing accumulations of fluid, major supporting structure damage, and superficial osseous lesions.

Ultrasonography can help evaluate the soft tissue structures of the stifle.[2–5,12,15] These examinations generally provide accurate evaluation of the collateral ligaments, the menisci, and the patellar ligaments.[15] One study found a high rate of detecting obscure meniscal injuries.[4] There is mixed opinion about the value of ultrasound for imaging the cruciate ligaments.[2,12] The condylar and trochlear articular surfaces, synovial membrane, and synovial fluid can be imaged and reveal disruptions, thickening, and solid particles, respec-

tively.[14,15] Subcutaneous fluid accumulations can be differentiated between blood or serum and purulent exudate.[14]

Scintigraphy is useful for visualizing lesions in the stifle region. Many areas are difficult to block, and scintigraphy provides a guide to the problems. Osteochondrosis or subchondral cystic lesions may not have the increased vascularity to sequester the radiopharmaceutical.

MRI provides the most anatomic detail available for imaging the equine stifle.[7] Unfortunately, its availability remains limited. In a clinical trial, CT was accurate for imaging the trochlea and ridges, condyles, and proximal tibia.[19] It also accurately depicted the cruciate and collateral ligaments and menisci. Of most value was the detail in the caudal portions of the joint, including loose fragments, and the intercondylar fossa.[19]

Arthroscopy has proven invaluable for evaluating and detecting intraarticular problems of the stifle. Arthrotomy does not provide enough access for exploration, and the necessary large incision has a real risk of dehiscence. Arthroscopic access is possible for disease identified in any of the three joints of the stifle. For problems localized to the stifle but inapparent on any type of imaging, arthroscopy offers an expanded diagnostic tool.[9,10,18]

References

1. Anon R. British equine veterinary association survey of equine diseases: 1962–1963. Vet Rec 1965;77:528.
2. Cauvin ERJ, Munroe GA, Boyd JS, et al. Ultrasonographic examination of the femorotibial articulation in horses: Imaging of the cranial and caudal aspects. Equine Vet J 1996;28:285–296.
3. Denoix JM, Lacombe V. Ultrasound diagnosis of meniscal injuries in athletic horses. Vet Surg 1996;25:265.
4. Denoix JM, Lacombe V. Ultrasound diagnosis of meniscal injuries in horses. Pferdeheilkunde 1996;12:629–631.
5. Dik KJ. Ultrasonography of the equine stifle. Equine Vet Educ 1995;7:154–160.
6. Dyson SJ. Stifle trauma in the event horse. Equine Vet Educ 1994; 6:234–240.
7. Holcombe SJ, Bertone AL, Biller DS, et al. Magnetic resonance imaging of the equine stifle. Vet Radiol Ultrasound 1995;36: 119–125.
8. Jeffcott LB, Kold SE. Stifle lameness in the horse: A survey of 86 referred cases. Equine Vet J 1982;14:31–39.
9. McIlwraith CW, Robertson JT. Arthroscopic surgery of the femoropatellar joint. In: McIlwraith & Turner's Equine Surgery: Advanced Techniques. 2nd ed. Baltimore: Williams & Wilkins, 1998; 168.
10. Nickels FA, Sande R. Radiographic and arthroscopic findings in the equine stifle. Horse's joints. J Am Vet Med Assoc 1982;181: 918–924.
11. O'Brien TR, Baker TW, Koblik P. Stifle radiology: How to perform an examination and interpret the radiographs. Am Assoc Equine Pract 1986;32:531–552.
12. Penninck DG, Nyland TG, O'Brien TR, et al. Ultrasonography of the equine stifle. Vet Radiol 1990;31:293–298.
13. Prades M, Grant BD, Turner TA, et al. Injuries to the cranial cruciate ligament and associated structures: Summary of clinical, radiographic, arthroscopic and pathological findings from 10 horses. Equine Vet J 1989;21:354–357.
14. Rantanen NW, McKinnon AO. Equine Diagnostic Ultrasonography. Baltimore: Williams & Wilkins, 1998.
15. Reef VB. Equine Diagnostic Ultrasound. Philadelphia: WB Saunders, 1998.
16. Reeves MJ, Trotter GW, Kaine, RA. Anatomical and functional communications between the synovial sacs of the equine stifle joint. Equine Vet J 1991;23:215–218.

17. Samy MT, Hertsch R, Zeller R. Radiologic changes in the equine stifle joint. Equine Pract 1985;7:13–16, 21–30.
18. Stick JA, Nickels FA. The stifle. In: Auer JA, Stick JA, Eds. Equine Surgery. 2nd ed. Philadelphia: WB Saunders, 1999;867–881.
19. Tietje S. Computed tomography of the stifle region in the horse: A comparison with radiographic/ultrasonographic and arthroscopic evaluation. Pferdeheilkunde 1997;13:647–658.
20. Vaughan JT. Analysis of lameness in the pelvic limb and selected cases. Am Assoc Equine Pract 1965;11:223.

OSTEOCHONDRITIS DISSECANS OF THE STIFLE JOINTS

Pathogenesis and prevention of osteochondritis dissecans (OCD) and developmental orthopedic disease are discussed in Chapters 5 and 7. This discussion is confined to the clinical features and treatment of OCD of the stifle. The incidence of OCD in the stifle is rivaled only by that of the tarsocrural joint and is a common cause of stifle lameness.[6] In a series of 161 horses that underwent surgery, Thoroughbreds were the most commonly affected.[3] Of these horses, 78% were 2 years old or younger, and most were yearlings. Twice as many males than females presented for treatment.

Signs and Diagnosis

Femoropatellar OCD causes femoropatellar effusion (Fig. 8.451) and variable hindlimb lameness. The lesion is an osteochondral defect with cartilage separation and some degree of ossification. The lateral trochlear ridge of the femoropatellar joint is most frequently affected. Depending on the severity of synovitis, there is some effusion, and synovial fluid analysis is usually unremarkable. Subtle effusion can be compared to the contralateral stifle, but half or more of affected horses have bilateral lesions. The lameness may be so mild that joint effusion is the only presenting complaint. However, hindlimb flexion is usually positive in horses with clinically significant OCD. Other patients are extremely lame, and some youngsters may have difficulty rising from recumbency. Chronic hindlimb lameness in foals may have caused flexural deformities that could be the actual presenting complaint. The lateral trochlear ridge defect can be so severe that the patella luxates laterally.

The clinical significance of OCD lies less with the physical defect and more with the lameness and osteoarthritis owing to the resulting synovitis. (See Chapter 7 for the pathophysiology of synovitis and osteoarthritis.) Particularly with horses in active training, the clinical significance of the lesion should be confirmed by intrasynovial analgesia. The usual age at presentation varies from weanlings to 2- to 3-year-olds in training; more

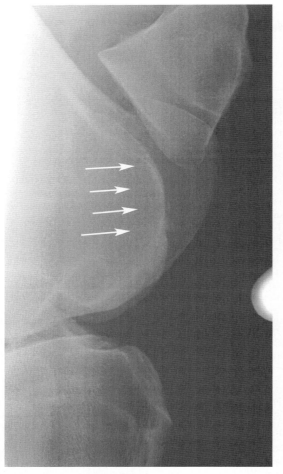

Figure 8.455 Lateromedial view of OCD of the lateral trochlear ridge. Note the subchondral limits of the lesion (arrows), which could more extensively involve cartilage. Sclerosis of subchondral bone is also present.

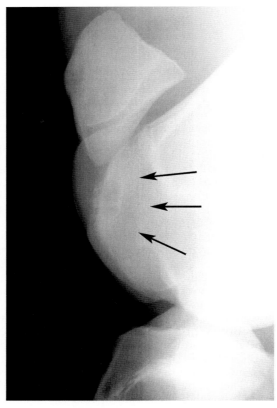

Figure 8.456 Lateromedial view of OCD of the lateral trochlear ridge. A subchondral cyst (arrows) has formed within the trochlear ridge beneath the surface fragments.

than half of a series of 161 horses were 1 year of age or younger.[3] Training presumably loosens an osteochondral fragment or disrupts a weakened cartilage area and may be required to cause the clinical signs. Horses presenting after training has begun generally have less severe lesions than weanlings or yearlings.[3] Older horses that have never undergone active training may demonstrate clinical signs from a lesion that was silent without work.

Some horses have radiographic evidence of OCD without clinical signs. Approximately half of affected horses have bilateral lesions; one limb is often more severely affected. Less commonly, horses with stifle lesions may also be affected in other joints; a complete physical examination that notes effusion in other joints is indicated.[3] In one study, femoropatellar OCD affected the lateral trochlear ridge in 161 of 252 joints; lesions may also be located on the medial trochlear ridge, the trochlear groove, and the articular surface of the patella—and in any combination.[3] The medial condylar surface surrounding subchondral cystic lesions and the caudal portions of the femoral condyles may also have OCD lesions.[4]

Lateromedial radiographs usually demonstrate a flattened defect in the proximal portion of the lateral trochlear ridge of the femur where it articulates with the distal patella (Fig. 8.455). Some degree of ossification is noted, and loose bodies may be present.[2,3,7] Less commonly, deeper ossification defects or subchondral cystic lesions occur (Figs. 8.456 and 8.457).[2,7] Caudolateral to craniomedial oblique films may provide more information about the severity of lateral trochlear ridge defects, which may extend over the lateral side of the trochlear ridge. Patellar changes may be the result of primary OCD or secondary to irritation from a severe lateral trochlear ridge lesion and may not be discovered until surgery is performed. However, severe patellar lesions can be observed in the lateromedial view, and the changes caused by osteoarthritis are more visible.

In one study, radiographically normal areas contained lesions detectable only by arthroscopy in 40% of 72 femoropatellar joints, and more than half had lesions worse than anticipated from the radiographs.[11] Young foals have normally irregular contours of the proximal trochlear ridges (Fig. 8.458).[1] Weanlings may present with femoropatellar effusion, lameness, and no radiographic changes.[2] Given a few weeks, these lesions often become radiographically evident, because the normal trochlear ridge grows around the defective area (Fig. 8.459).

The surfaces of the trochlear structures of the distal femur are readily imaged using ultrasound. The cartilage on the lateral trochlear ridge is reported to be thicker than that of the medial ridge.[10] Ultrasound can demonstrate defects in the articular surfaces of the trochlear ridges.[10] Synovial membrane proliferation and synovial effusion associated with these defects are usually not echogenic. Femoropatellar joint abnormalities that have been detected using ultrasound include excessively thick articular cartilage, partially ossified subchondral bone defects, and double echogenic lines of osteochondral flaps.[10]

In summary, a minority of horses with mild lateral trochlear ridge defects have no cartilage defect when examined during surgery (Fig. 8.460). Conversely, horses with relatively severe radiographic changes probably do have cartilage defects of the lateral ridge and possibly elsewhere in the same joint. When radiographic lesions

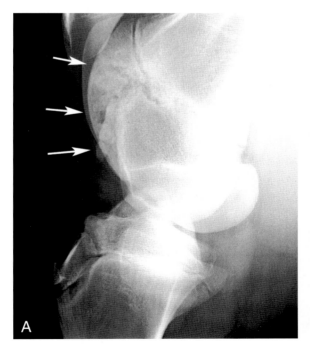

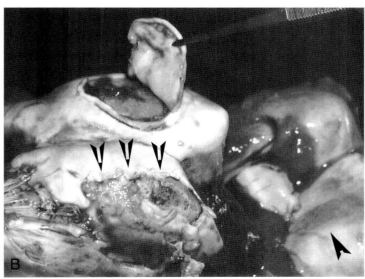

Figure 8.457   A. Lateromedial view of severe OCD. Note that most of the subchondral bone in the lateral trochlear ridge is affected (arrows). The patella luxates laterally. B. Necropsy of the horse shown in panel A reveals the hypoplastic trochlear ridge; the lesion is broad (slotted arrowheads). A radiographically inapparent cartilage flap from the medial trochlear ridge is being held in the forceps. Note that the patellar cartilage is eburnated (single arrowhead).

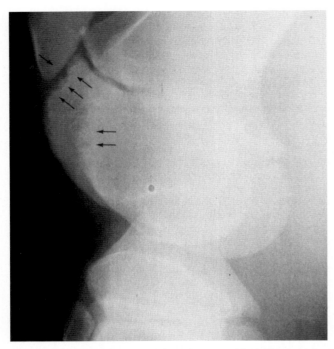

Figure 8.458 Lateromedial view of a normal foal. The irregular subchondral bone in the proximal trochlear ridges and patella (arrows) is normal. The cartilage overlying those areas is unaffected. (Courtesy of T. S. Stashak.)

are absent, lameness and synovial effusion dictate the clinical significance.

Treatment

When clinical signs are present, surgical debridement is reported to produce better results than conservative therapy.[12,13] However, foals and weanlings may be treated conservatively for a time to see if the lesion can heal.[9] Conservative therapy includes stall confinement and anti-inflammatory treatment. Stall confinement is recommended to protect the articular surface from disruption so healing can occur.[9] Intraarticular and systemic anti-inflammatory therapy to minimize the chance of degenerative changes is considered helpful.[13] Sodium hyaluronate is recommended for intraarticular treatment and polysulfated glycosaminoglycan is most often used for systemic treatment. Intraarticular steroids are inadvisable in this situation. The fluid is drained at the time of treatment, so resolution of the femoropatellar effusion can be judged. In one study, about half of 23 affected foals that were diagnosed early with OCD and treated with stall rest eventually raced.[9] The successfully treated horses tended to have less severe lesions. Sequential radiographs and clinical response to therapy are used to determine whether surgery is advisable.

Weanlings and short yearlings can present with effusion and lameness but no radiographic lesions (Fig. 8.459).[2,9] The conservative therapy just described is indi-

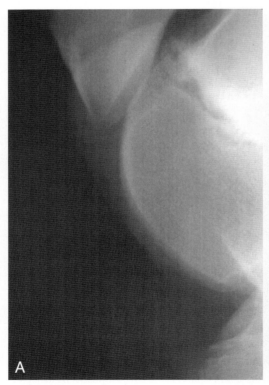
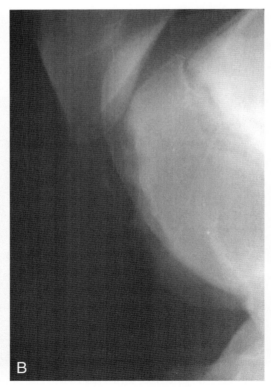

Figure 8.459 A Normal lateromedial view of a weanling that presented with femoropatellar effusion and lameness. B. At the 14-week follow-up, there is extensive OCD of the lateral trochlear ridge. The unaffected bone of the lateral trochlear ridge has grown around the defective portion, revealing the lucency.

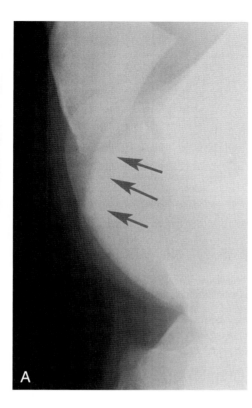

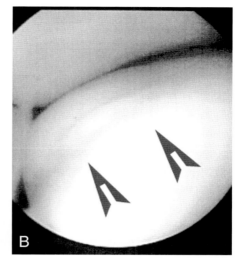

Figure 8.460 A. Lateromedial view of the lateral trochlear ridge, showing signs of OCD. The horse had mild femoropatellar effusion and a clinically significant medial condylar subchondral cystic lesion. B. Arthroscopic evaluation reveals that the cartilage contained an elevation but was intact. No debridement was performed.

cated in these cases. Subsequent radiographs may demonstrate significant trochlear ridge ossification defects, because the lesion has persisted while the surrounding trochlear ridge has ossified normally as the epiphysis has expanded.[2] Furthermore, some clinicians believe that surgical lesions in foals and weanlings may progress, suggesting that surgery be delayed until it is certain that the lesion has fully developed.[2] Medical therapy in horses without radiographic changes is diagnostic as well, because a complete response indicates there is no articular surface lesion.

In horses older than 1 year with clinical signs or when it is obvious that the lesion will not heal, arthroscopic surgery is indicated. Arthroscopy offers better visualization and access to the lesion without the inherent risk of postoperative dehiscence of a large incision.[8] The intent of surgery is removal of all loose osteochondral tissue and debridement of the lesion, leaving healthy subchondral bone to fill with fibrocartilage and resolving the synovitis (Fig. 8.461). A percentage of horses with lateral trochlear ridge lesions have apposing patellar lesions. The articular surface of the patella and the remainder of the joint must be evaluated for cartilage defects or debris that may be free in the joint (Fig. 8.462). The medial femoral condyle may also contain OCD lesions that are usually discovered when operating for a subchondral cystic lesion (SCL).[8] If necessary, the caudal portion of the femorotibial joint can also be assessed arthroscopically.[12] It is important to remove all of the debris generated during the debridement process;[5] debris can be evacuated in the process of arthroscopic power-facilitated debridement.

One report compared arthroscopy and arthrotomy for treating a series of horses affected with femoropatellar OCD.[14] Arthroscopically treated horses spent an average of 11.5 fewer days in the hospital, returned to athletic activity at a higher rate and sooner, appeared with better cosmetic results, and overcame the synovial effusion more often than horses treated by arthrotomy. The most logical explanation for the functional difference after surgery is that the lesions were not debrided as completely or other lesions were not discovered.

Prognosis

The prognosis for athletic activity after arthroscopic surgery for femoropatellar OCD is generally good. Of a series of 134 horses, only 16% had an unsuccessful outcome for reasons related to the OCD.[3] Slightly fewer patients saw success when they underwent concurrent surgery for OCD in other joints. Increased lesion size had a significantly negative effect on outcome. Defects less than 2 cm, between 2 and 4 cm, and greater than 4 cm had decreasing success rates of 78, 63, and 54%, respectively. The overall success rate of 64% was comparable to the starting rate of normal Thoroughbred horses in the same time period.[3] Outcome could not be correlated to sex, function of the horse, lesion location, unilateral versus bilateral involvement, or the presence of loose bodies.[3] For horses with apposing lateral trochlear ridge and patellar lesions, I extend the period of stall rest 90 days.

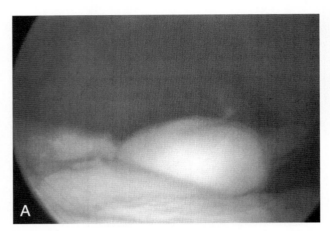

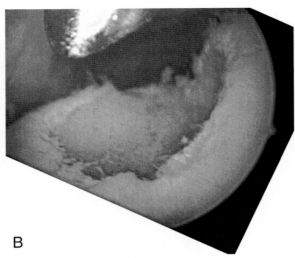

Figure 8.461 A. The femoropatellar joint shown in Figure 8.455 before arthroscopic debridement of the lateral trochlear ridge. B. After debridement, the cartilage is gone and firm subchondral bone remains. The surrounding cartilage is firmly attached to subchondral bone.

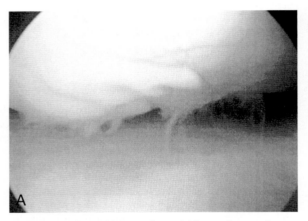

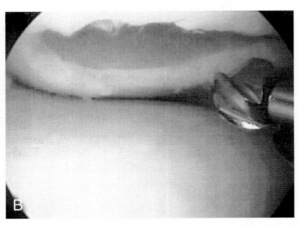

Figure 8.462 A. The articular surface of this patella contains full-thickness cartilage disruption. No radiographic evidence of this OCD lesion was present. B. After debridement to healthy subchondral bone and solid surrounding cartilage using the bur shown.

References

1. Adams WM, Thilsted JP. Radiographic appearance of the equine stifle from birth to 6 months. Vet Radiol 1985;26:126–132.
2. Dabareiner RM, Sullins KE, White NA II. Progression of femoropatellar osteochondrosis in nine young horses: Clinical, radiographic and arthroscopic findings. Vet Surg 1993;22:515–523.
3. Foland JW, McIlwraith CW, Trotter GW. Arthroscopic surgery for osteochondritis dissecans of the femoropatellar joint of the horse. Equine Vet J 1992;24:419–423.
4. Howard RD, McIlwraith CW, Trotter GW. Arthroscopic surgery for subchondral cystic lesions of the medial femoral condyle in horses: 41 cases (1988–1991). J Am Vet Med Assoc 1995;206:842–850.
5. Hurtig MB. Use of autogenous cartilage particles to create a model of naturally occurring degenerative joint disease in the horse. Equine Vet J 1988;6(Suppl):19–22.
6. Jeffcott LB, Kold SE. Stifle lameness in the horse: a survey of 86 referred cases. Equine Vet J 1982;14:31–39.
7. McIlwraith CW. Clinical aspects of osteochondrosis dissecans. Osteochondrosis dissecans of the femoropatellar joint. In: McIlwraith CW, Trotter GW, Eds. Joint Disease in the Horse. Philadelphia: WB Saunders, 1996;363–368.
8. McIlwraith CW, Robertson JT. Arthroscopic surgery of the femoropatellar joint. In: McIlwraith & Turner's Equine Surgery: Advanced Techniques. 2nd ed. Baltimore: Williams & Wilkins, 1998; 168.
9. McIntosh SC, McIlwraith CW. Natural history of femoropatellar osteochondrosis in three crops of Thoroughbreds. Equine Vet J 1993;16(Suppl):54–61.
10. Rantanen NW, McKinnon AO. Equine Diagnostic Ultrasonography. Baltimore: Williams & Wilkins, 1998.
11. Steinheimer DN, McIlwraith CW, Park RD, et al. Comparison of radiographic subchondral bone changes with arthroscopic findings in the equine femoropatellar and femorotibial joints: A retrospective study of 72 joints (50 horses). Vet Radiol Ultrasound 1995; 36:478–484.
12. Stick JA, Borg LA, Nickels FA, et al. Arthroscopic removal of an osteochondral fragment from the caudal pouch of the lateral femorotibial joint in a colt. J Am Vet Med Assoc 1992;200: 1695–1697.

13. Stromberg B, Rejno S. Osteochondrosis in the horse. I. A clinical and radiologic investigation of osteochondritis dissecans of the knee and hock joint. Acta Radiol Suppl (Stockh) 1978;358: 139–152.
14. Vatistas NJ, Wright IM, Dyson SJ. Comparison of arthroscopy and arthrotomy for the treatment of osteochondrotic lesions in the femoropatellar joint of horses. Vet Rec 1995;137:629–632.

SUBCHONDRAL CYSTIC LESIONS OF THE STIFLE

See Chapter 7 for a discussion of the cause and prevention of SCL and developmental orthopedic disease. This section is confined to the clinical features and treatment of SCL in the stifle. The medial femorotibial joint is the most commonly diagnosed location of SCL in the horse.[2,16] However, SCL also occurs in the lateral femoral condyle and in the proximal tibia.[4,8,14] Approximately half of affected horses have bilateral lesions, and one limb is usually more severely affected.

Signs and Diagnosis

The clinical signs are primarily moderate lameness in younger horses, often shortly after beginning training. These lesions are usually discovered when yearlings undergo radiographs for sale or after training has started. Older horses that have never been in active training may demonstrate clinical signs from a lesion that has been silent. The femorotibial joints do not readily exhibit synovial effusion; communication of the medial femorotibial joint with the femoropatellar joint may allow mild to moderate effusion of the femoropatellar joint to be observed, but that is an inconsistent finding.[3] Careful palpation of the femoropatellar and medial femorotibial joints of the affected limb and comparing the findings to the contralateral joints often identifies an asymmetry in distension pressure.[13]

Most SCLs are believed to begin as articular defects related to the development of orthopedic disease, but they can occur after natural or experimental articular trauma.[6,7,10,14] The clinical significance lies with the lameness and osteoarthritis owing to the resulting synovitis. Subchondral cystic lesions may be radiographically evident but cause no clinical signs. Particularly with horses in active training, the clinical significance of the lesion should be confirmed by intraarticular analgesia. Lameness is not completely eliminated by intraarticular anesthesia, because some component of the lameness is thought to originate deep within the bone. This anesthesia blocks only the synovitis, and improvement of approximately 50% is significant. After 60 minutes, again observe the horse move to see if there is any further improvement.[2] Horses with medial tibial SCL and associated osteoarthritis may not respond to the intraarticular analgesia as well as others might.[14]

A medial condylar lesion is demonstrated in the caudal to cranial radiographic projection. The flexed lateral and caudolateral to craniomedial oblique projections are also useful. The radiographic findings vary from a dimple to a deep conical or spherical osseous defect with a

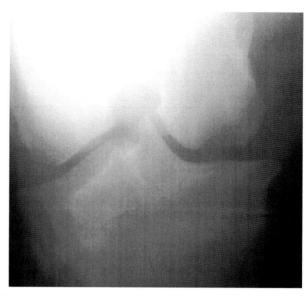

Figure 8.463 Craniocaudal view of a medial condylar SCL. The margin contains a sclerotic lining that was just developing.

sclerotic lining (Fig. 8.463).[3,17] The lesions are classified according to depth.[3,17] The sclerotic lining seems to indicate maturity of the lesion, because it is not seen in relatively new lesions.[1] Occasionally, there is a flattening of the medial condyle, which may be normal for some individuals. If lameness has been isolated to that joint, it should be compared to the opposite stifle; however, clinical signs may be the overriding factor for pursuing further diagnostics. When monitored for weeks to months, suspected lesions often progressively develop into SCL. This trend indicates the need for surgical debridement (Fig. 8.464).

In the proximal tibia, SCL may be in the medial or lateral condyle. Horses presenting with lameness before 2 years of age generally have SCL believed to result from developmental orthopedic disease that is located in the cranial aspect of the lateral tibial condyle. Patients older than 2 years of age usually have lesions that are thought to have been acquired from trauma; these SCLs are usually located in the medial tibial condyle and may be cranial or more caudally positioned.[14] Radiographically, the lesions can be identified in the craniocaudal or lateromedial projections. In one study, older horses had associated changes of osteoarthritis consisting of marginal osteophyte production, changes at the insertion of the cranial cruciate ligament, joint space narrowing, and subchondral sclerosis (Fig. 8.465).[14] Scintigraphy was needed to locate the lesion in three horses with osteoarthritis and medial tibial SCL.

The condylar surfaces can be imaged ultrasonographically.[9,11] The cartilage and subchondral bone present a consistent image from which deviations can be detected. Cartilage thickening, synovial effusion, subchondral cysts, and loose bodies can be imaged.[9,11] Scintigraphy is an inconsistent indicator of SCL,[12] but scintigraphy seems to be more important in older horses with SCL following osteoarthritis.[14]

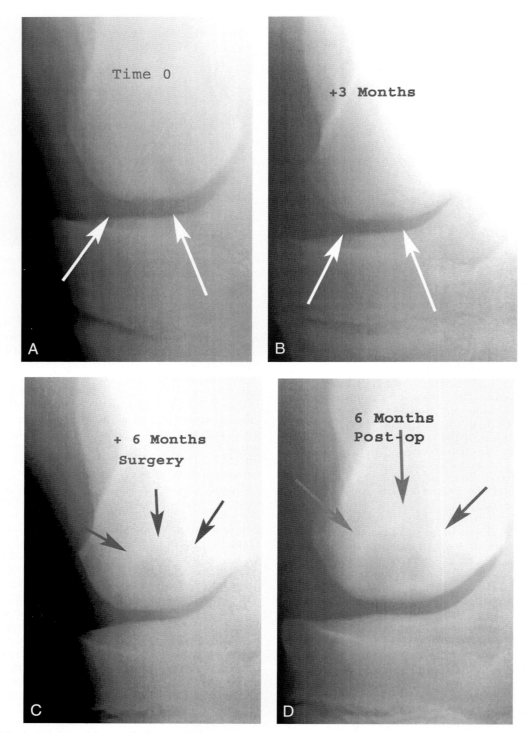

Figure 8.464   A. Craniocaudal view of slight medial condylar flattening (arrows) in a yearling Thoroughbred with lameness localized to the medial femorotibial joint. B. At the 3-month follow-up, the lesion progressed to a slight dimple (arrows). C. At the 6-month follow-up a subchondral cyst was seen (arrows), and the lesion was surgically debrided. D. By 6 months postsurgery, the cyst had a sclerotic lining and a more irregular shape.

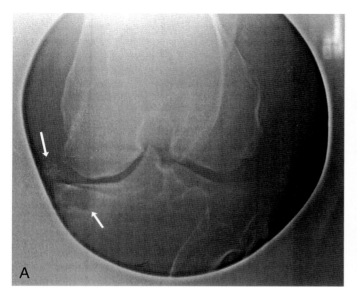

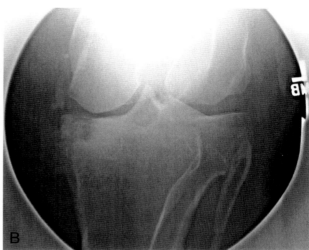

Figure 8.465 A. Coned view of a SCL in the proximal medial tibia (lower arrow) and mineralization in the soft tissue involving either the collateral ligament or the medial meniscus (upper arrow). The lesion does not seem to be extensive. B. A more centered view reveals that the lesion is extensive and involves the medial cortex. The proliferative osseous changes are thought to be the result of a fracture of the medial cortex associated with the medial border of the cyst. The soft tissue mineralization appears to be associated with the collateral ligament in this study. (Courtesy of T. S. Stashak.)

Treatment

Conservative therapy for a medial femoral condylar SCL may be effective in horses younger than 1 year old. The patient should be confined to a stall to prevent further trauma, and the lesions should be monitored radiographically. Intraarticular and systemic anti-inflammatory therapy, as described for OCD, is advisable.[1] Subchondral cystic lesions without lameness should not be treated surgically.

In one study of two horses with proximal tibial SCL believed to be developmental, one became sound and raced after medical therapy and rest.[14] Other horses with tibial SCL secondary to osteoarthritis generally do not respond favorably to medical management (Fig. 8.465).[14]

Few horses perform athletic functions with clinically evident SCL.[7] The goal of surgery is to remove the loose cartilage, the amorphous material filling the cavity, and the fibrous lining that produces inflammatory mediators (Fig. 8.466).[15] Early reports suggested drilling of the sclerotic lining to facilitate vascular ingress. However, because many of the drill paths become new SCLs, the procedure is no longer recommended.[7] Complete exploration of the joint is performed; but pathology is usually confined to the SCL, except in a few horses that have OCD adjacent to the SCL. Deep SCLs may obscure arthroscopic visualization of the depths of the lesion. In such cases, I prefer a 15-mm medial femorotibial arthrotomy to ensure that all the fibrous lining is removed, and I use a five-layer closure. The stifle can be flexed and extended for a complete examination of the medial condyle. The aftercare is identical to arthroscopically treated horses and there are no increased incisional complications, as described for the early larger arthrotomies.[17]

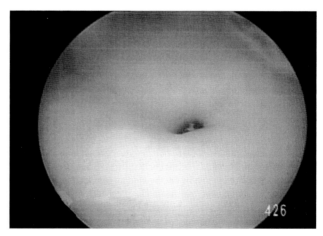

Figure 8.466 Arthroscopy reveals a medial femoral condylar cystic lesion. Note the defect in the articular surface representing the opening to the cyst. (Courtesy T. S. Stashak.)

Resolution of the lameness requires 6 to 12 months rest after surgery; bilateral cases tend toward the longer convalescent periods. The reported success rate after arthroscopic surgical debridement of SCL is 56 to 74%.[3] Success is independent of age, sex, lesion size, unilateral versus bilateral lesions, drilling of the lesion, associated OCD, and postoperative cyst enlargement. Intraoperative steroid administration reduces the incidence of postoperative enlargement of the lesion,[7] but it is not advised if an arthrotomy is performed. These success rates are not as high as previously reported for debridement via arthrotomy in 51 horses.[17] Although the exact reason is unknown, a longer period of follow-up may account for

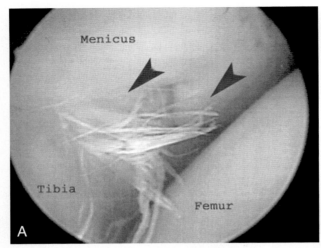
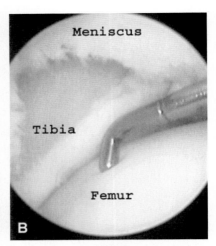

Figure 8.467 A. Arthroscopy reveals a shallow OCD lesion on the proximal tibia. A. Note the frayed cranial meniscus and meniscal ligament (arrowheads). B. After debridement, the meniscus and ligament are smooth; softened cartilage and subchondral bone have been removed from the tibial condyle.

recurrent lameness in some horses. Results have not been improved using cancellous bone grafts.[5]

By examining radiographs of unsuccessful cases, one cannot usually determine a reason for the failure. Many horses respond temporarily or permanently to intraarticular steroid therapy. In one case, a gaited horse failed to improve consistently by 17 months after undergoing surgical debridement of a medial femoral condylar subchondral cyst. I injected 80 mg methylprednisolone acetate deep within the osseous defect. At 7 months after treatment, the horse remained sound and was training.

In younger horses with proximal tibial SCL from developmental orthopedic disease, the lateral condylar lesions can be accessed arthroscopically. The lesions are located either behind or beneath the cranial ligament of the lateral meniscus. Curettage is performed routinely via a medial arthroscopic approach.[14] This area should be examined during arthroscopy if signs suggest that the lateral femorotibial joint may be involved (Fig. 8.467). Older horses with medial tibial condylar lesions can be treated using the lateral arthroscopic approach. However, some of the lesions will be located more caudally and will not be accessible.[14]

Prognosis

Horses that have subchondral bone cysts and are not lame should not be treated. For horses 1 year of age or younger, a period of stall rest and anti-inflammatory therapy is worthwhile. The success rate for treatment of horses in this category is not available. After arthroscopic surgery, 56 to 74% of horses become sound. Horses with residual lameness that were meant to work at speed may be able to function well in another line of work.

Proximal tibial SCLs, although uncommon, do not seem to respond well to treatment.[1,4] A recent report relates a positive outcome for horses under 2 years of age that have lateral tibial condylar SCLs believed to stem from developmental orthopedic disease.[14] Three of four horses that underwent surgery proceeded to perform well athletically; the other was lost to an unrelated accident. For horses with preexisting mild to moderate osteoarthritis as well as medial SCLs, debridement may allow return to work, but usually at a reduced level.[14] Severe cases or those with more caudally positioned SCLs are not good candidates for treatment.[14]

References

1. Baxter GM. Subchondral cystic lesions in horses. In: McIlwraith CW, Trotter GW, Eds. Joint Disease in the Horse. Philadelphia: WB Saunders, 1996;384–397.
2. Bramlage LR. Osteochondrosis related bone cysts. Am Assoc Equine Pract 1993;39:83–85.
3. Howard RD, McIlwraith CW, Trotter GW. Arthroscopic surgery for subchondral cystic lesions of the medial femoral condyle in horses: 41 cases (1988–1991). J Am Vet Med Assoc 1995;206:842–850.
4. Jeffcott LB, Kold SE. Clinical and radiological aspects of stifle bone cysts in the horse. Equine Vet J 1982;14:40–46.
5. Kold SE, Hickman J Results of treatment of subchondral bone cysts in the medial condyle of the equine femur with an autogenous cancellous bone graft. Equine Vet J 1984;16:414–418.
6. Kold SE, Hickman J, Melsen F. An experimental study of the healing process of equine chondral and osteochondral defects. Equine Vet J 1986;18:18–24.
7. McIlwraith CW. Subchondral bone cysts in the horse: Aetiology, diagnosis and treatment options. Equine Vet Educ 1998;10:313–317.
8. Nixon AJ. Arthroscopic debridement of cystic lesions of the proximal tibia in horses. Vet Compar Orthop Traumatol 1994;7:64.
9. Rantanen NW, McKinnon AO. Equine Diagnostic Ultrasonography. Baltimore: Williams & Wilkins, 1998.
10. Ray CS, Baxter GM, McIlwraith CW, et al. Development of subchondral cystic lesions after articular cartilage and subchondral bone damage in young horses. Equine Vet J 1996;28:225–232.
11. Reef VB. Equine Diagnostic Ultrasound. Philadelphia: WB Saunders, 1998.
12. Squire KRE, Fessler JF, Cantwell HD, et al. Enlarging bilateral femoral condylar bone cysts without scintigraphic uptake in a yearling foal. Vet Radiol 1992;33:109–113.
13. Stashak TS. Palpation of the stifle. In: Stashak TS, Ed. Adams' Lameness in Horses. 4th ed. Philadelphia: Lea & Febiger, 1987;125–126.

14. Textor JA, Nixon AJ, Lumsden JM, et al. Subchondral cystic lesions of the proximal extremity of the tibia in horses: 12 cases (1983–2000). J Am Vet Med Assoc 2001;218:408–413.

15. von Rechenberg B, Guenther H, McIlwraith CW, et al. Fibrous tissue of subchondral cystic lesions in horses produce local mediators and neutral metalloproteinases and cause bone resorption in vitro. Vet Surg 2000;29:420–429.

16. Wagner PC, Watrous BJ. Equine pediatric orthopedics: clinical, radiographic, and therapeutic aspects. 1: Osteochondrosis. Equine Pract 1990;12:32–37.

17. White NA, McIlwraith CW, Allen D. Curettage of subchondral bone cysts in medial femoral condyles of the horse. Equine Vet J 1988;6(Suppl):120–124.

INTRAARTICULAR FRACTURES OF THE FEMOROPATELLAR JOINT: FRACTURES OF THE FEMORAL TROCHLEA

One study reported chip fractures in both trochlear ridges of the distal femur of three horses.[15] One horse sustained the injury by striking a jump (stone wall) and the other two horses were injured by punctures. Sepsis is a consideration in these cases; and if it occurs, it is treated routinely. Lameness depends on the degree of periarticular inflammation, but it eventually subsides to mild. All three horses underwent routine femoropatellar arthroscopic surgery. Some degree of synovitis was encountered, but the fragments were removed routinely, and the fracture beds were debrided. All horses returned to normal work after 4 to 5 months. These lesions are not typical of OCD because of the acute onset of lameness, and complete radiographic ossification is evident, as long as the fragment is visible.

Salter-Harris type 4 fractures of the distal femur in young horses occur from direct trauma;[5,22] in one case, the horse struck a gate. Lameness is severe, and femoropatellar effusion is obvious. The fracture may involve both trochlear ridges or only one. Radiographs demonstrate the fracture in the dorsopalmar and lateromedial projections (Fig. 8.468). The tangential view may also be helpful. Acute fractures can generally be reduced, and fixation is performed using lag screws.[5,22] If necessary, screws can be placed distal to proximal through the articular surface; the screw heads are countersunk into the subchondral bone.[5,22] Although it is sometimes possible to accomplish the fixation arthroscopically, the spatial orientation can be challenging. Depending on the case, it may be more efficient to use an arthrotomy. The prognosis is reasonable for normal activity; none of the affected horses in these studies has reached training age; but they all are sound.[5,22]

INTRAARTICULAR FRACTURES OF THE FEMOROPATELLAR JOINT: FRACTURE OF THE PATELLA

Patellar fractures occur infrequently in horses. Described fracture configurations include sagittal,[2,6,8,13] transverse,[12] and comminuted;[16] fracture of the base of the patella;[23] and distal fragmentation of the patella.[14,19] When fractures do occur, they may be associated with severe soft tissue trauma involving the ligaments and joint capsule of the stifle joint.[9]

Causes

Direct trauma to the patella while the stifle joint is in a semiflexed position is a common cause. The patella is immobilized when the stifle is semiflexed, making it more susceptible to direct trauma.[4] Horses that jump can strike jumps and sustain bilateral patellar fractures,[7,13] or the fracture can occur as a result of a kick. Sudden lateral slips may cause a separation of the medial fibrocartilage.[6]

Signs and Diagnosis

Horses present with an acute onset of lameness and a significant painful swelling associated with the cranial aspect of the stifle. Significant soft tissue swelling may obscure palpation. Pain and sometimes crepitation are noted, and fragments may be palpable. Femoropatellar effusion is usually profound. Flexion of the stifle joint exacerbates the lameness and the painful response. Weight bearing may be difficult with severely comminuted patellar fractures, and the horse may stand with the limb partially flexed without locking the stifle.

Radiographs are required to document the type and extent of the fracture (Fig. 8.469). Since sagittal fractures may not be apparent on routine radiographic views, the skyline projection is required for their identification (Fig. 8.470), although small medial fragments may be obscured by the soft tissue density that is present when the hindlimb is flexed to obtain the radiograph. If the plate is placed proximal to the stifle and the beam travels distoproximad, the patella separates more completely from the trochlea, allowing better visualization.[6,16] General anesthesia makes the procedure more convenient if the horse is painful. Ultrasound is useful for identifying small fracture fragments, patellar ligament disruption, and lesions that may not be radiographically visible (e.g., medial fibrocartilage separation).[18]

Treatment

Small avulsions in which the fragments become embedded in the capsule and the patellar tendon may heal with rest and anti-inflammatory therapy. Fractures with intraarticular fragments seldom remain sound when the horse returns to work.[6,13] Fragments approximating a third or less of the patellar substance can be removed with success.[3,8,13] I prefer arthroscopic removal because visibility is improved and small fragments are less likely to be missed (Fig. 8.471).[13] The fracture usually involves the medial aspect of the patella. The fragment can be dissected from the patellar tendon with a large elevator or a motorized soft tissue resector. If the fragment is large, it can be divided with an osteotome. If surgery must be delayed because of soft tissue injury or skin trauma, intraarticular sodium hyaluronate reduces the synovitis in the interim.

Even large fragments may heal with rest if displacement is minimal; risk of osteoarthritis is real, however, with articular involvement and visible femoropatellar effusion. Large extraarticular fragments can be removed, but it may not be necessary. One consideration is

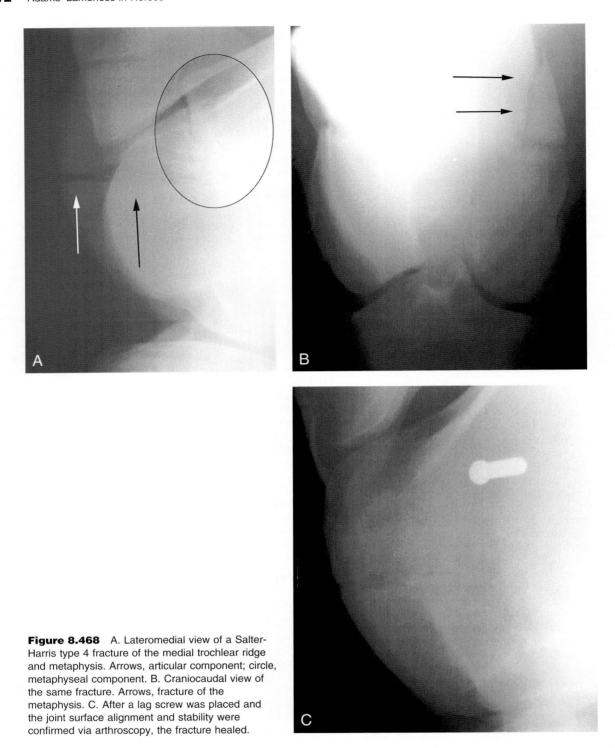

Figure 8.468   A. Lateromedial view of a Salter-Harris type 4 fracture of the medial trochlear ridge and metaphysis. Arrows, articular component; circle, metaphyseal component. B. Craniocaudal view of the same fracture. Arrows, fracture of the metaphysis. C. After a lag screw was placed and the joint surface alignment and stability were confirmed via arthroscopy, the fracture healed.

whether the healing tissue between the fragments will be as strong as the new fibrous tissue from the soft tissue attachments if the fragment is removed. Internal fixation should be considered for distracted or displaced fractures with sizable fragments. The blood supply is reported to enter from the medial direction.[16] The clinical significance of this is unknown, in that many medial fractures heal well after removal.

The successful internal fixation of transverse distracted and longitudinally displaced fractures of the patella have been reported.[1,4,12,16] Longitudinal fractures are easier to reduce and stabilize, and there is less chance of having it distract postoperatively. Transverse fractures, on the other hand, are more difficult to treat successfully because of the tendency of the proximal segment to become distracted by the pull of the quadriceps

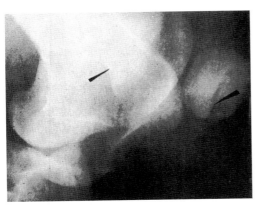

Figure 8.469 Lateromedial view of a sagittal fracture of the patella (right arrow) and a fracture of the trochlear ridge (left arrow).

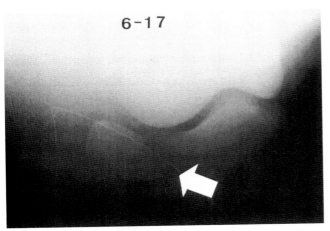

Figure 8.470. Flexed skyline of a medial sagittal fracture of the patella (arrow). (Courtesy of T. S. Stashak.)

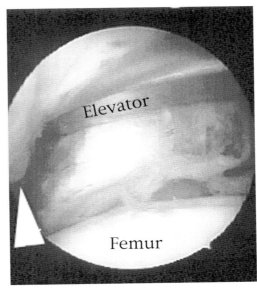

Figure 8.471 Arthroscopy reveals a medial patellar fragment. The elevator separates the patellar fragment from the soft tissue attachments. The medial trochlear ridge of the femur is also visible. Arrowhead, parent patella.

muscles. Tension band support is the best option for transverse patellar fractures.[12] In either case, failure to achieve good anatomic reduction can result in femoropatellar osteoarthritis.

Assisted recovery from anesthesia is recommended for horses that have had a large fragment removed and when internal fixation is used. Failure to have a smooth recovery may result in luxation of the remaining patella and breakdown of the repair if internal fixation is used.

Prognosis

The ultimate outcome depends on retaining an adequate, stable articular surface. Instability or persistent synovitis results in osteoarthritis. After conservative or surgical therapy, lameness may persist for some time while the synovitis resolves and any patellar ligament desmitis or enthesopathy heals.[6,17,18] If this results in continued instability, the outcome is poor.

Of a combined series of 21 horses from which medial fragments were removed, 15 returned to full work.[3,8,13] Failures occurred primarily because of preexisting osteo-

arthritis, luxation of the patella during recovery from anesthesia, and one unexplained ensuing osteoarthritis. These failures may point to the value of thorough preoperative ultrasonographic evaluation or more prolonged postoperative stall rest.

Internal fixation provides the ideal set of circumstances for a favorable outcome for displaced and distracted fractures. Recovery from anesthesia may be the most critical point in the postoperative period. Horses with severely comminuted fractures are likely to remain lame. Some of these individuals may attain breeding soundness with prolonged stall rest. However, if the quadriceps function is compromised or if severe osteoarthritis develops, euthanasia should be considered.

INTRAARTICULAR FRACTURES OF THE FEMOROPATELLAR JOINT: FRAGMENTATION OF THE DISTAL PATELLA

Fragmentation of the distal patella is an uncommon condition that often follows medial patellar desmotomy.[11,14,19–21,24] The situation seems to arise from temporary patellar instability caused by the desmotomy. Malalignment of the patella has been reported shortly after medial patellar desmotomy.[19] The characteristic lesion was experimentally reproduced in 11 of 12 horses undergoing medial patellar desmotomy.[10]

Signs and Diagnosis

The clinical signs consist of some degree of unilateral or bilateral hindlimb lameness and stiffness. Femoropatellar joint effusion is common, and palpable thickening of the joint capsule is often present. Radiographic

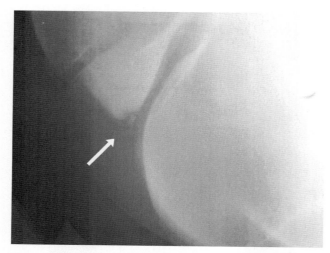

Figure 8.472 Lateromedial view of fragmentation of the apex (distal aspect) of the patella (arrow). (Courtesy of R. D. Park.)

changes include bony fragmentation, spurring (with or without an associated subchondral defect), subchondral roughening, and subchondral lysis of the distal aspect of the patella (Fig. 8.472).

Treatment

All affected horses are treated with arthroscopic surgery. The lesions at arthroscopy vary from flaking, fissuring, undermining, and fragmentation of the articular cartilage to fragmentation or lysis of the bone at the distal aspect of the patella. The subchondral bone is involved in all horses that have had previous medial patellar desmotomy. Fragments may be buried in the synovial membrane and tend to emanate from the more lateral portion of the distal patella.[14,21]

Prognosis

In one study, of the 12 horses that had a previous medial patellar desmotomy, 8 became sound for their intended use. Of the other 3 horses, 2 performed well at their intended use, but 1 was unsatisfactory.[14] Documented patellar misalignment seems to disappear with time.[19]

References

1. Aldrete AV, Meagher DM. Lag screw fixation of a patellar fracture in a horse. Vet Surg 1981;10(4):143–148.
2. Anderson BH, Turner TA, Jonson GR. What is your diagnosis? J Am Vet Med Assoc 1996;209:1847–1848.
3. Colbern GT, Moore JN. Surgical management of proximal articular fracture of the patella in a horse. J Am Vet Med Assoc 1984;185:543–545.
4. DeBowes RM, Grant BD, Chalman JA, et al. Fractured patella in a horse. Equine Pract 1980;2:49–53.
5. DeBowes RM, Grant BD, Modransky PD. Lag screw stabilization of Salter type IV femoral fracture in a young horse. J Am Vet Med Assoc 1983;182:1123–1125.
6. Dik KJ, Nemeth F. Traumatic patella fractures in the horse. Equine Vet J 1983;15:244–247.
7. Dyson SJ. Stifle trauma in the event horse. Equine Vet Educ 1994;6:234–240.
8. Fessler JF, Amstutz HE. Fracture repair. In: Oehme FW, Prier JE, Eds. Textbook of Large Animal Surgery. Baltimore: Williams & Wilkins, 1974;321.
9. Dyson S, Wright I, Kold S, et al. Clinical and radiographic features, treatment and outcome in 15 horses with fracture of the medial aspect of the patella. Equine Vet J 1992;24:264–268.
10. Gibson KT, McIlwraith CW, Park RD, et al. Production of patellar lesions by medial patellar desmotomy in normal horses. Vet Surg 1989;18:466–471.
11. Grosenbaugh DA, Honnas CM. Arthroscopic treatment of patellar lesions resulting from medial patellar desmotomy in a horse. Equine Pract 1979;17:23–25.
12. Hunt RJ, Baxter GM, Zamos DT. Tension band wiring and lag screw fixation of a transverse, comminuted fracture of a patella in a horse. J Am Vet Med Assoc 1992;200:819–820.
13. Marble GP, Sullins KE. Arthroscopic removal of patellar fracture fragments in horses: Five cases (1989–1998). J Am Vet Med Assoc 2000;216:1799–1801.
14. McIlwraith CW. Osteochondral fragmentation of the distal aspect of the patella in horses. Equine Vet J 1990;22:157–163.
15. Montesso F, Wright IM. Removal of chip fractures of the femoral trochlear ridges of three horses by arthroscopy. Vet Rec 1995;137:94–96.
16. Pankowski RL, White KK. Fractures of the patella in horses. Comp Cont Educ Pract Vet 1985;7:S566–570, S572–573.
17. Rantanen NW, McKinnon AO. Equine Diagnostic Ultrasonography. Baltimore: Williams & Wilkins, 1998.
18. Reef VB. Equine Diagnostic Ultrasound. Philadelphia: WB Saunders, 1998.
19. Riley CB, Yovich JV. Fracture of the apex of the patella after medial patellar desmotomy in a horse. Aust Vet J 1991;68:37–39.
20. Squire KRE, Blevins WE, Frederick M, et al. Radiographic changes in an equine patella following medial patellar desmotomy. Vet Radiol 1990;31:208–209.
21. Walmsley JP. Medial patellar desmotomy for upward fixation of the patella. Equine Vet Educ 1994;6:148–150.
22. Wilderjans H. New bone growth on the sustentaculum tali and medial aspect of the calcaneal bone surrounding the deep digital flexor tendon in a pony. Equine Vet Educ 1990;2:184–187.
23. Wilderjans H, Boussauw B. Treatment of basilar patellar fracture in a horse by partial patellectomy. Equine Vet Educ 1995;7:189–192.
24. Wright JD, Rose RJ. Fracture of the patella as a possible complication of medial patellar desmotomy. Aust Vet J 1989;66:189–190.

INTRAARTICULAR FRACTURES OF THE FEMOROTIBIAL JOINT

Femorotibial joint fractures are uncommon; however, they are important injuries because the ongoing synovitis and possible instability can lead to osteoarthritis and permanent lameness. Most fractures seem to occur with a compression and rotation or avulsing type of injury. These are not common sites for direct trauma.

Signs and Diagnosis

These fractures generally cause marked acute lameness, but the lesion is not readily apparent until radiographs are taken. The femorotibial joint usually remains outwardly stable, but the horse resents flexion or other manipulation. Inconsistently, femoropatellar effusion may occur. Often intraarticular analgesia is required to locate the problem. Sites that have been affected include the caudal medial femoral condyle,[2] the caudal medial tibial condyle, and the medial intercondylar eminence of the tibia (Fig. 8.473).[5,7] Also reported are Salter-Harris type 3 fractures of the lateral condyle,[3] Salter-Harris

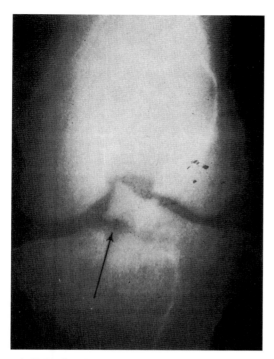

Figure 8.473 Craniocaudal view of an avulsion fracture of the medial intercondylar eminence of the tibia. Because the cranial cruciate ligament inserts at this location, it is a sprain fracture.

type 4 fractures of the distal femoral physis[3] (see Fig. 8.468), and fractures at the origin of the long digital extensor muscle or peroneus tertius muscle (Fig. 8.474).[1,4] One report noted a loose fragment in the caudal lateral femorotibial joint.[6]

Treatment

The goal of treatment is to remove or stabilize the fragment to avoid continued synovitis and osteoarthritis. The choice of treatments depends on the size and location of the fragment. The stifle is an area that is repeatedly placed under tremendous stresses during athletic activity. Salter-Harris type 3 and 4 fractures that extended through the distal femoral physis have been described.[3] In one study, a Salter-Harris type 4 fracture was repaired using an angled blade plate.[3] If the fragment cannot be securely stabilized but the articular surfaces remain adequate, removal is preferred.[2,4,5] If the articular surface must be reconstructed or if the fragment attaches important soft tissue, repair is considered.[7] Frequently, an approach must be designed and practiced to allow the surgeon access to unusual sites in the caudal portion of the joint. Some fragments are too large or too securely attached in soft tissue for arthroscopic removal (Fig. 8.475).[2]

Prognosis

The prognosis cannot be generalized for these fractures. Fragments are of different sizes and importance, so each case must be evaluated individually. In one report, a

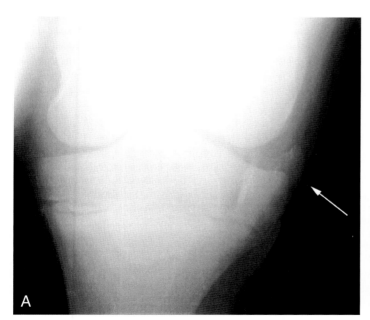

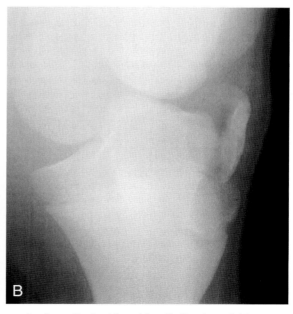

Figure 8.474 A. Craniocaudal view of an avulsion fracture of the origin of the long digital extensor muscle. Note the fragment that has been displaced distally (arrow). This should not be confused with a trochlear ridge OCD, which is typically located more proximally on the trochlear ridge. B. Craniomedial to caudolateral oblique view demonstrating the fragment positioned at the craniolateral aspect of the lateral femorotibial joint.

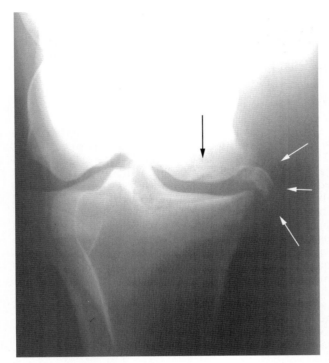

Figure 8.475 Craniocaudal view of a proximal tibial fracture that came from the medial tibial condyle caudal to the collateral ligament (white arrows); the fragment was dissected from the joint capsule and medial meniscus. Note the medial femoral condylar lesion that may have occurred at the same time (black arrow); it was debrided arthroscopically.

horse with a Salter-Harris type 3 fracture was managed conservatively and became sound for pasture; limited fracture disease self-corrected.[3] In the same study, one horse with a Salter-Harris type 4 fracture was managed conservatively and eventually raced; another horse underwent surgery for internal fixation and succumbed to complications.[3] Fragments that do not leave defects to disrupt normal joint motion or damage menisci or cartilage can be successfully removed; occasionally there is no choice.[2,5,6] Note that the stifle can remain painful after surgery for 6 to 12 months, and yet the horse can become sound. However, with any intraarticular fracture affecting a weight-bearing area, guarantees for athletic soundness cannot be made.

References

1. Blikslager AT, Bristol DG. Avulsion of the origin of the peroneus tertius tendon in a foal. J Am Vet Med Assoc 1994;204:1483–1484.
2. Dabareiner RM, Sullins KE. Fracture of the caudal medial femoral condyle in a horse. Equine Vet J 1993;25:75–77.
3. Hance SR, Bramlage LR, Schneider RK, et al. Retrospective study of 38 cases of femur fractures in horses less than one year of age. Equine Vet J 1992;24:357–363.
4. Holcombe SJ, Bertone AL. Avulsion fracture of the origin of the extensor digitorum longus muscle in a foal. J Am Vet Med Assoc 1994;204:1652–1659.
5. Mueller POE, Allen D, Watson E, et al. Arthroscopic removal of a fragment from an intercondylar eminence fracture of the tibia in a two-year-old horse. J Am Vet Med Assoc 1994;204:1793–1795.
6. Stick JA, Borg LA, Nickels FA, et al. Arthroscopic removal of an osteochondral fragment from the caudal pouch of the lateral femorotibial joint in a colt. J Am Vet Med Assoc 1992;200:1695–1697.
7. Walmsley JP. Fracture of the intercondylar eminence of the tibia treated by arthroscopic internal fixation. Equine Vet J 1997;29:148–150.

AVULSION OF THE ORIGIN OF THE PERONEUS TERTIUS AND LONG DIGITAL EXTENSOR TENDONS

These conditions are discussed elsewhere in this chapter (Figs. 8.422 and 8.474).

INTRAARTICULAR LESIONS OF THE FEMORAL CONDYLES

Cartilage lesions atypical of the OCD occur on the condylar surfaces of the distal femur.[1,4] Two groups of horses are affected. Foals are affected in the caudal condylar regions. Lesion specifics and severity varies, and some are associated with sepsis.[1] Adults generally having a history of chronic lameness may have radiographically inapparent chondral defects in the same sites as medial condylar SCLs; a few lateral condylar lesions occur as well.[4]

In one study, 20 foals with caudal femoral condylar lesions were placed into three categories based on radiographic lesions.[1] Type 1 lesions were thought to have a septic origin, whereas types 2 and 3 were nonseptic and believed to be different degrees of the same problem. Type 1 lesions had a discrete area of radiolucency within the subchondral bone of the caudal aspect of a femoral condyle and were associated with septic arthritis and osteomyelitis. Type 2 lesions had localized osseous irregularities involving less than 50% of the femoral condyle. Type 3 lesions had widespread irregularities involving a large area of the condyle, and in 5 foals with this type of lesion, there was a thin osseous fragment displaced from the condyle and free in the femorotibial joint pouch. Foals with type 1 and 3 lesions were severely lame, and foals with type 2 lesions were not as lame. The results of cytologic evaluation of the synovial fluid from foals with type 1 lesions were compatible with septic arthritis; synovial fluid from foals with type 2 and 3 lesions was not septic (Fig. 8.476).

In a study of foals with these lesions, surgical exploration and debridement were performed in 4 foals. Of these, 2 foals with type 2 lesions are currently performing athletically. The remaining 2 foals underwent surgery for type 3 lesions; both were euthanatized at surgery because of the severity of the lesions. Follow-up information was available for 5 foals that did not have surgery. Of these, 2 foals with type 1 lesions and 1 foal with a type 3 lesion were sound 1 year after diagnosis, 1 foal with a type 2 lesion had residual lameness that prevented performance, and 1 foal with a type 3 lesion was salvaged for breeding. A total of 11 foals were destroyed. Type 1 lesions represent focal epiphyseal osteomyelitis and septic arthritis. The cause of type 2 and 3 lesions is speculative, but there appeared to be a disruption or delay in endochondral ossification. In addition, lesions may be caused by osteochondrosis or may result from some vascular insult that is not currently well defined.

In another study, 11 adult horses of ages 2 to 4 years presented for hindlimb lameness of 1 to 12 months' du-

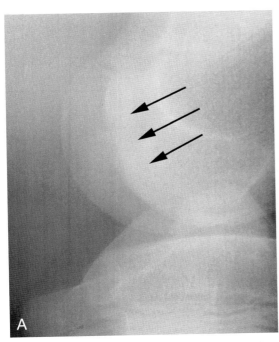
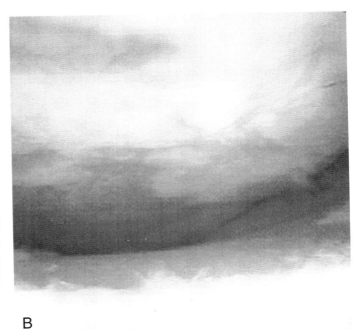

Figure 8.476 A. Lateromedial view of irregularity on the medial femoral condyle (arrows) that was noted while investigating moderate lameness after a periarticular infection. B. Arthroscopy reveals that the cartilage on the femur (upper) and tibia (lower) is eroded. The affected areas were debrided.

ration; most had been lame 3 months or longer. Although the femorotibial joints did not often show visible effusion, 2 horses with severe lesions displayed effusion. Lameness increased after hindlimb flexion and improved, but usually did not resolve, after intraarticular analgesia of all three stifle joints. Stifle radiographs were normal. In the 11 horses, 12 joints were affected in the medial femoral condyle. Based on results of the lameness examination, the joints were explored arthroscopically, which revealed cartilage defects in the central condylar regions where subchondral cystic lesions often occur. The lesions consisted of focal to generalized cartilage disruption. Cartilage was dimpled and infolded and often had sustained full-thickness damage. Overall, the lesions represented cartilage degeneration and were debrided routinely to healthy subchondral bone and surrounding cartilage. However, joints containing generalized cartilage disruption were left as found. Of the 7 horses with focal lesions, 6 recovered and returned to racing, eventing, dressage, jumping, etc. Only 1 of 4 horses with generalized cartilage disruption recovered but was soon retired from active work.

The cause of the arthropathy in adults remains speculative. The horses affected in both medial and lateral femoropatellar joints could be suspected to have suffered trauma resulting in instability. Had that been true, scintigraphy would possibly have revealed sites of enthesopathy. Also possible is chronic OCD, but that poses more questions than it answers. Full-thickness cartilage lesions involving bone have been demonstrated to cause SCLs.[2,3] Possibly the lack of radiographic findings in these horses indicates the subchondral bone resisted deeper lesion formation or perhaps the occurrence of a broader lesion prevented development of the hydraulic forces necessary to produce the bone necrosis to form the subchondral cyst. One could speculate that the adult lesions represent continuation of the type 2 lesions described in foals. However, the primarily affected areas on the condyles are different. The cause notwithstanding, the report substantiates the need for arthroscopic evaluation of many intraarticular problems localized but unremarkable on radiographs. Scintigraphy could contribute further to the understanding of the condition.

References

1. Hance SR, Schneider RK, Embertson RM, et al. Lesions of the caudal aspect of the femoral condyles in foals: 20 cases (1980–1990). J Am Vet Med Assoc 1993;202:637–646.
2. Kold SE, Hickman J, Melsen F. An experimental study of the healing process of equine chondral and osteochondral defects. Equine Vet J 1986;18:18–24.
3. Ray CS, Baxter GM, McIlwraith CW, et al. Development of subchondral cystic lesions after articular cartilage and subchondral bone damage in young horses. Equine Vet J 1996;28:225–232.
4. Schneider RK, Jenson P, Moore RM. Evaluation of cartilage lesions on the medial femoral condyle as a cause of lameness in horses: 11 cases (1988–1994). J Am Vet Med Assoc 1997;210:1649–1652.

FEMOROTIBIAL COLLATERAL LIGAMENT INJURY

Collateral ligamentous injury to the stifle is not common. When it does occur the medial collateral ligament is most commonly involved. All reported cases of femorotibial collateral ligament injury have been in adult horses,[1,6] except when associated with a Salter-Harris type 2 fracture of the proximal tibia in foals. Collateral ligament injury results in lameness from the primary injury and synovitis leading to osteoarthritis if the instability is sufficient. Injury can result in a either a desmitis or a complete rupture of the ligament. Because the stifle is so tightly supported by soft tissue structures when collateral ligament rupture occurs, other structures are usually involved. The triad of injuries seen in the stifle include the medial collateral ligament, the meniscus, and the cranial cruciate ligament.[5]

Signs and Diagnosis

The medial collateral ligament is the more commonly affected. Obvious instability with severe lameness may occur; however, localized collateral ligament injury has been reported.[6] Although lame at the walk, the overall swelling and outward appearance is localized and minimal. Lameness is exacerbated by manually stressing the medial collateral ligament in a stifle valgus direction and observing increased lameness at a walk. Of a series of seven cases of horses with soft tissue injury to the stifle, three had medial collateral ligament injury and only one of those was restricted to the collateral ligament. The others had concurrent cruciate ligament injury.[1,6] However, medial collateral regional swelling may be a feature (Fig. 8.477).

Radiographs may show that tibial or femoral fragments have also avulsed (Fig. 8.1). An abnormal opening of the medial or lateral femorotibial articulation may be seen if a medial or laterally stressed view is taken (Fig. 8.478). The medial surface is opened using pressure in a valgus direction by stabilizing the stifle and abducting the distal limb. Although not commonly necessary, the lateral surface can be stressed by fixing the horse's foot in an axial position on the floor and pulling the stifle laterally using a towel or rope. Sedation is advised. In chronic cases, radiographs may demonstrate enthesopathy.

The diagnosis may be made or confirmed by ultrasound.[2–5] Medial collateral ligament and meniscus inju-

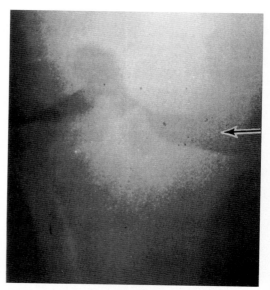

Figure 8.478 Craniocaudal view demonstrating excessive opening of the medial femorotibial joint (arrow) as a result of rupture of the medial collateral ligament. There is also a sprain fracture of the cranial cruciate ligament insertion. Major support structure disruptions in the stifle commonly affect more than one structure. (Courtesy of T. S. Stashak.)

ries have been seen without cranial cruciate injury, but avulsion of bone from the attachment of the cranial medial meniscal ligament may occur.[2] The normal medial collateral ligament is 4 to 5 mm thick with parallel fibers.[4] Injury thickens and alters its echogenicity. The degree of echolucency may reveal desmitis or rupture.[4] Chronic lesions may demonstrate bony remodeling at the origin or insertion. Collateral ligament desmitis is usually more focal than often seen in other locations. Irregular bony densities at the attachments signify enthesiophyte formation.[5]

Treatment

Stall rest is the usual method of conservative treatment, because external coaptation will not immobilize the stifle well. One report noted that surgical stabilization of a medial collateral ligament rupture was performed in an adult mare.[1] After two procedures, stability was improved but was not normal. The mare improved to the point of pasture turnout. Unfortunately, the mare fell and was euthanized before long-term follow-up was obtained. Recovery should be monitored by ultrasound, if possible, and depends on the severity of the injury to the collateral ligaments and other structures that may have been simultaneously damaged.

Prognosis

The prognosis for recovery is poor. Horses with obvious instability are usually euthanatized. Others that are restricted to a stall for 6 to 12 months may regain pasture soundness.

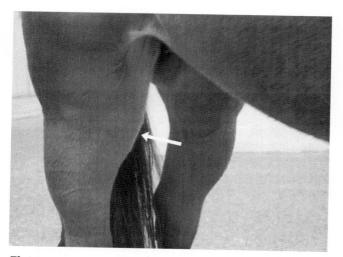

Figure 8.477 Cranial view of a horse that had sustained an injury to the medial collateral ligament 3 days earlier. Note the extensive medial swelling of the stifle region overlying the medial collateral ligament (arrow). (Courtesy of T. S. Stashak.)

References

1. Bukowiecki CF, Sanders-Shamis M, Bramlage LR. Treatment of a ruptured medial collateral ligament of the stifle in a horse. J Am Vet Med Assoc 1988;193:687–690.
2. Dik KJ. Ultrasonography of the equine stifle. Equine Vet Ed 1995; 7:154–160.
3. Penninck DG, Nyland TG, O'Brien TR, et al. Ultrasonography of the equine stifle. Vet Radiol 1990;31:293–298.
4. Rantanen NW, McKinnon AO. Equine Diagnostic Ultrasonography. Baltimore: Williams & Wilkins, 1998.
5. Reef VB. Equine Diagnostic Ultrasound. Philadelphia: WB Saunders, 1998.
6. Sanders-Shamis M, Bukowiecki CF, Biller DS. Cruciate and collateral ligament failure in the equine stifle: Seven cases (1975–1985). J Am Vet Med Assoc 1988;193:573–576.

CRANIAL OR CAUDAL CRUCIATE LIGAMENT INJURY

Cruciate ligament injury usually occurs in adults from a traumatic episode.[1,3,4,6,9] The cranial cruciate ligament (CCL) is the one most commonly ruptured and may be damaged along with the medial collateral ligament. The CCL in the horse originates from the caudomedial aspect of the lateral femoral condyle and inserts on the medial intercondylar tubercle of the tibia. It provides rotational and craniocaudal stability. Damage to the medial meniscus occurs when the cranial cruciate ligament is damaged or from the resulting instability of the femorotibial joint.

Signs and Diagnosis

The degree of lameness depends on the degree of injury and femorotibial instability. The lesion varies from simple desmitis to fiber disruption to sprain fracture (Fig. 8.473). If the ligament is sprained but not ruptured or a partial sprain fracture occurs, diagnosis can be difficult.

Femoropatellar effusion is often present. In one study, physical instability was detected via the cruciate test in only 1 of 10 standing horses and in 6 of 10 horses under general anesthesia.[6] Radiographs frequently show avulsion of a tibial fragment (Fig. 8.473 and Fig. 8.478)[6] or displacement of the femur relative to the tibia. In chronic cases, a cystic lucency may occur at the site of the injury.[10] An in vitro study in ponies demonstrated ligamentous failure only in 9 of 15 stifles, combined ligamentous tibial insertion failure in 4, and combined ligamentous and femoral insertion failure in the remaining 2 ponies.[8] The implication was that radiographs may not be useful in diagnosing CCL rupture in horses. However, clinical cases usually combine CCL rupture with medial collateral ligament (MCL) damage (Fig. 8.478), so the dynamics are evidently different. Scintigraphy may localize the injury in more obscure situations. The cruciate ligaments could not be imaged ultrasonographically in one study,[5] but were mentioned in normal horses by another.[2] The ultrasonographic image of the change may be limited to the insertion on the cranial proximal tibia.[7]

The degree of cruciate injury can be evaluated arthroscopically.[6,10] Disrupted tissue can be debrided in the hope of healing, or complete disruption can be confirmed.

Prognosis

The prognosis is quite poor when a cruciate ligament is completely ruptured. Materials currently available for reconstruction of cruciate ligaments in humans and dogs will not withstand the forces in horses. For horses that have partially ruptured cruciate ligaments, the more remaining intact ligament, the better the prognosis. Return to complete soundness after arthroscopically visible cruciate injury is uncommon.[6] A 2-year-old Standardbred colt returned to racing after removal of a fragment associated with the distal attachment of the cranial cruciate ligament and the cranial medial meniscal ligament.[4]

References

1. Baker GJ, Moustafa MAI, Boero MJ, et al. Caudal cruciate ligament function and injury in the horse. Vet Rec 1987;121:319–321.
2. Cauvin ERJ, Munroe GA, Boyd JS, et al. Ultrasonographic examination of the femorotibial articulation in horses: Imaging of the cranial and caudal aspects. Equine Vet J 1996;28:285–296.
3. Edwards RB III, Nixon AJ. Avulsion of the cranial cruciate ligament insertion in a horse. Equine Vet J 1996;28:334–336.
4. Mueller POE, Allen D, Watson E, et al. Arthroscopic removal of a fragment from an intercondylar eminence fracture of the tibia in a two-year-old horse. J Am Vet Med Assoc 1994;204:1793–1795.
5. Penninck DG, Nyland TG, O'Brien TR, et al. Ultrasonography of the equine stifle. Vet Radiol 1990;31:293–298.
6. Prades M, Grant BD, Turner TA, et al. Injuries to the cranial cruciate ligament and associated structures: Summary of clinical, radiographic, arthroscopic and pathological findings from 10 horses. Equine Vet J 1989;21:354–357.
7. Reef VB. Equine Diagnostic Ultrasound. Philadelphia: WB Saunders, 1998.
8. Rich FR, Glisson RR. In vitro mechanical properties and failure mode of the equine (pony) cranial cruciate ligament. Vet Surg 1994; 23:257–265.
9. Sanders-Shamis M, Bukowiecki CF, Biller DS. Cruciate and collateral ligament failure in the equine stifle: Seven cases (1975–1985). J Am Vet Med Assoc 1988;193:573–576.
10. Stick JA, Nickels FA, Auer JA. The stifle. Equine Surg 1999;2: 867–881.

MENISCAL INJURIES

Meniscal injuries occur from acute trauma and may progress to chronic osteoarthritis. Acute lameness may follow disruptive trauma, or subtle chronic lameness may be more difficult to localize. Osteoarthritis may occur from the instability or from the persistent synovitis. The medial meniscus is much more commonly affected than the lateral. The lateral meniscus is tightly invested by its cranial and caudal ligaments, and forces that disrupt those attachments are devastating to the horse. Of a series of 126 horses undergoing arthroscopy for stifle lameness, 7 had meniscal injury.[11] The medial meniscus was affected in 5 horses, and the lateral meniscus in 2 horses.

Signs and Diagnosis

Horses with acute injury are often extremely lame, and other soft tissue structures of the stifle are usually damaged as well.[7] Localizing the source of the lameness is not difficult in these horses. Horses with chronic injury have a more subtle lameness that often requires intraarticular analgesia for diagnosis.[11]

The diagnosis is based on localizing hindlimb lameness in the usual manner. Femoropatellar effusion is not a feature of chronic meniscal degeneration. Intraarticular anesthesia causes improvement. Radiographs may be normal, but possible changes include mineralization at the attachments of the meniscal ligaments and narrowing of the joint space. Six of seven horses in one study had proliferative new bone on the cranial aspect of the intercondylar eminence of the tibia.[11] Accurate evaluation of the femorotibial joint space requires that the horse re-main in position while the left and right caudocranial projections are taken; the x-ray tube is at the same height for both views (Fig. 8. 479). Scintigraphy may show inflammation at the attachments.

Ultrasound findings of the normal stifle have been described,[2] and meniscal injuries have been detected.[3] In a series of 49 stifles with meniscal injuries detected by ultrasound, radiographic evidence was present in only 18. Dik[4] noted that ultrasound supported radiology in most cases. The medial meniscus is often injured as part of a triad that includes the MCL and CCL.[6] Ultrasonographically evident meniscal changes are changes in size,

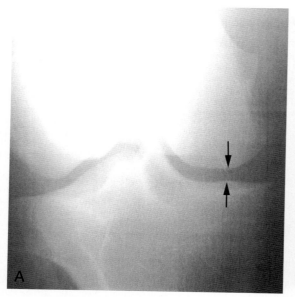
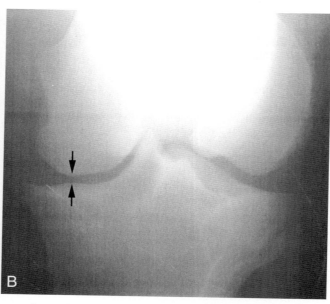

Figure 8.479   Standardized craniocaudal views of the left (A) and right (B) stifles of a horse with medial meniscal degeneration. Although there are no osseous signs of disease, the right medial femorotibial joint space is only about 50% that of the left joint (arrows).

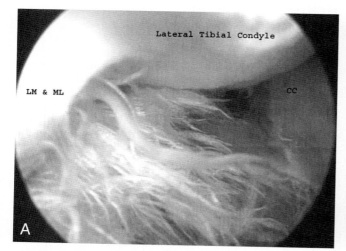
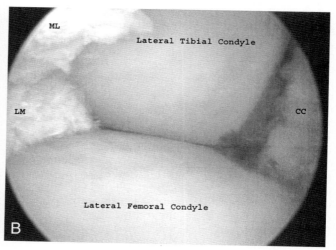

Figure 8.480   A. Arthroscopy reveals frayed fibers of the lateral meniscal ligament (ML) and meniscus (LM) in a horse in which lameness was blocked by lateral femorotibial analgesia. The cranial cruciate ligament (visible in the right background) is slightly frayed. These changes were not detected by radiography. The horse had been rested for several months while a traumatic SCL in the medial femoral condyle regressed. B. After debridement using a power synovial resector, it was evident that the cartilage was thin but intact. CC, cranial cruciate ligament.

thickness, echogenicity, and location in relation to the femur and tibial joint.[6] The normal meniscal image is that of a triangular wedge between the femur and tibia. The meniscus outwardly extrudes from between the bones if it is torn, and it is thin when collapsing. Ligament calcification or insertion desmopathy causes hyperreflectivity on ultrasound examination.[5] Echolucent pouches cranial and caudal to the collateral ligament indicate synovial effusion pushing the abaxial tissue away from the meniscus.[5]

Treatment

Therapy depends on the severity and location of the lesion. Meniscal damage accompanied by femorotibial instability or multiple injuries has a poor prognosis. Less severe lesions should be evaluated arthroscopically (Fig. 8.480). The cranial or lateral approach adequately accesses the medial meniscus, and the caudal approach has been recommended to access the lateral meniscus.[8] Fibrillation and loose meniscal tissue are debrided to stable tissue; a motorized arthroplasty unit with a new blade is useful for removing the tough elastic collagen fibers. Tears can be debrided to remove the loose edges. The menisci should be lifted with a probe to evaluate the underlying tibial surfaces for cartilage disruption.

Valdez and Adams[10] described meniscectomy through an arthrotomy in five horses with torn medial menisci. Two of the horses were treated successfully; however, the method of diagnosis was not confirmed and specific follow-up was not available. The technique has not gained widespread use and is not recommended for treatment of meniscal tears at this time.

Prognosis

If there is a rupture of one of the collateral or cruciate ligaments of the joint or damage associated with the medial meniscus, treatment is unavailing and crippling or chronic lameness results (Figs. 8.481 and 8.482). When

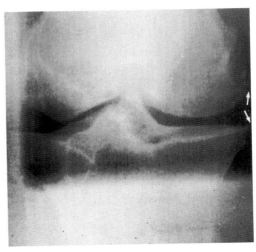

Figure 8.482 Craniocaudal view of chronic medial meniscus damage. Note the mild joint space narrowing and osteophyte production on the abaxial margins of the medial femoral and tibial condyles (arrows). (Courtesy of T. S. Stashak.)

radiographic signs of joint disease indicate a chronic process, the course may be improved by debridement. Of a series of 7 horses with cranial meniscal damage, at least 3 returned to soundness after arthroscopic surgery.[11] In a series of 29 horses with mixed meniscal and cruciate damage, 13 improved within 6 to 12 months. Of these, 8 were pasture sound and 5 were able to perform.[9] Of a series of 11 cases with predominately medial meniscus damage, 9 improved after surgery and 3 were sound.[1] Remember that many meniscal injuries involve other important support structures of the stifle.

References

1. Bertone AL, Holcombe SL. Soft tissue injuries of the equine stifle. Vet Surg 1992;21:383.
2. Cauvin ERJ, Munroe GA, Boyd JS, et al. Ultrasonographic examination of the femorotibial articulation in horses: Imaging of the cranial and caudal aspects. Equine Vet J 1996;28:285–296.
3. Denoix JM, Lacombe V. Ultrasound diagnosis of meniscal injuries in horses. Pferdeheilkunde 1996;12:629–631.
4. Dik KJ. Ultrasonography of the equine stifle. Equine Vet Educ 1995;7:154–160.
5. Rantanen NW, McKinnon AO. Equine Diagnostic Ultrasonography. Baltimore: Williams & Wilkins, 1998.
6. Reef VB. Equine Diagnostic Ultrasound. Philadelphia: WB Saunders, 1998.
7. Sanders-Shamis M, Bukowiecki CF, Biller DS. Cruciate and collateral ligament failure in the equine stifle: Seven cases (1975–1985). J Am Vet Med Assoc 1988;193:573–576.
8. Stick JA, Nickels FA. The stifle. In: Auer JA, Stick JA, Eds. Equine Surgery. 2nd ed. Philadelphia: WB Saunders, 1999;867–881.
9. Trumble TN, Baxter GM, McIlwraith CW, et al. Arthroscopic treatment of ligamentous and meniscal injuries of the femorotibial joints in 29 horses. Vet Surg 1997;26:432.
10. Valdez H, Adams OR. Surgical approach for medial meniscectomy in the horse. J Am Vet Med Assoc 1978;173:766–769.
11. Walmsley JP. Vertical tears of the cranial horn of the meniscus and its cranial ligament in the equine femorotibial joint: 7 cases and their treatment by arthroscopic surgery. Equine Vet J 1995;27: 20–25.

DESMITIS OF THE PATELLAR LIGAMENTS

Desmitis of the patellar ligaments is an infrequently reported condition. When it does occur, it is often ob-

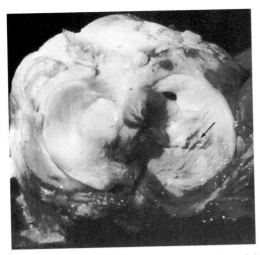

Figure 8.481 Postmortem view of the distal portion of the femorotibial joint, demonstrating the frayed and wrinkled medial meniscus (arrow). The lateral meniscus is normal. (Courtesy of T. S. Stashak.)

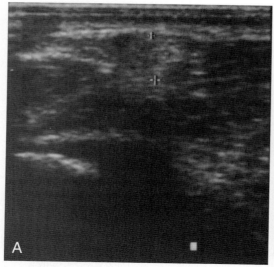

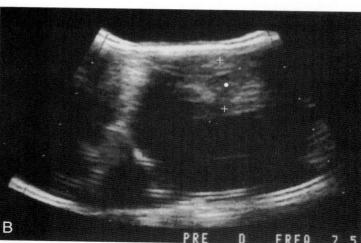

Figure 8.483 A. Ultrasound examination revealing a normal left middle patellar ligament. B. The affected right middle patellar ligament is enlarged and its central portion is hypoechogenic (large white dot). (Courtesy of T. S. Stashak.)

served in the middle patellar ligament, although any patellar ligament can be affected, and is probably caused by direct trauma (Fig. 8.483).[1,3]

Signs and Diagnosis

Affected horses are usually athletes, and many are eventers or jumpers. Direct trauma from striking a jump is a major risk factor. The degree of lameness is often related to an osseous lesion at the origin or insertion of the affected patellar tendon. These more extensive lesions are not usually challenging to locate. Identification and palpation of a swollen painful region within the ligament may be possible.

Middle patellar tendon lesions have been described as linear lucencies with fiber tearing or central hypoechoic regions similar to other desmopathies.[3] Proximal and distal enthesopathies reflect bony disruption in addition to the soft tissue lesion.[2] The medial patellar ligament is affected by upward fixation of the patella[2] and fractures from the medial aspect of the patella.[3] Extensive loss of density can be observed in animals with chronic intermittent upward fixation of the patella; after resolution, the tissue is healed, although thickened.[2] Lateral patellar ligament desmopathy has been observed concurrently with tibial tuberosity fracture.[2]

Treatment

When the injury is confined to the soft tissue, therapy consists of rest and local and systemic anti-inflammatory therapy. Smaller enthesopathies or fragments may also be treated conservatively with stall rest and time allowed to heal. Ultrasonographic monitoring of the healing process is helpful. When the ligament injury accompanies a larger or intraarticular fragment, arthroscopic removal is usually indicated. After prolonged rest and apparent soundness, synovitis and lameness tend to reoccur. It may help to remove the fragment so fibrous healing can reattach to the parent bone instead of being obstructed by the fragment.

Prognosis

The general outlook for patellar tendon injuries is good, provided adequate time is allowed the ultrasonographic lesions to resolve and the osseous lesions to heal. Continued training in spite of injury could lead to instability and osteoarthritis.

References

1. Dyson SJ. Stifle trauma in the event horse. Equine Vet Educ 1994; 6:234–240.
2. Rantanen NW, McKinnon AO. Equine Diagnostic Ultrasonography. Baltimore: Williams & Wilkins, 1998.
3. Reef VB. Equine Diagnostic Ultrasound. Philadelphia: WB Saunders, 1998.

UPWARD FIXATION OF THE PATELLA

Upward fixation of the patella (UFP) occurs when the medial patellar ligament becomes caught over the medial trochlear ridge (Fig. 8.484). If it becomes fixed in that position, the hindlimb cannot be flexed, and the horse assumes a posture in which the affected limb is extended in a caudally abducted position (Fig. 8.485). The condition may be present in only one hindlimb, but careful examination often reveals susceptibility in both hindlimbs.

Causes

UFP has generally been thought to occur in horses that have exceptionally straight hindlimbs. The femorotibial

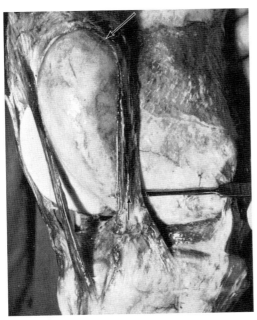

Figure 8.484 Specimen demonstrating UFP viewed from the medial aspect of the limb. Note the upward fixation of the medial patellar ligament over the medial trochlear ridge (top arrow); the bistoury is at the site for medial patellar desmotomy (bottom arrow). Note that when performing the surgery, the surgeon passes the bistoury from the cranial aspect of the stifle.

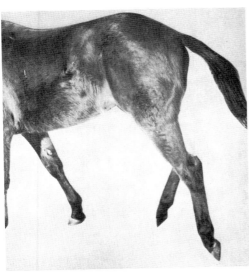

Figure 8.485 When a horse experiences UFP, the limb is locked in extension and extended caudally and a bit laterally. The digit is also fixed in the flexed position.

angle in most horses is approximately 135°; the problem occurs when the angle reaches 143 to 145°.[9] Although the exact angle of occurrence probably depends on the individual horse, it is reasonable to say that a straight-legged horse has a greater chance of reaching its individual point of injury. Furthermore, hyperextension of the limb that is exacerbated by walking a horse downhill causes the situation to occur more frequently. Body type

is strongly inherited; thus it is likely that the tendency for UFP could be congenital. Shetland ponies are particularly affected, and UFP predisposes them to coxofemoral luxation.

The condition also appears when the medial patellar ligament has reason to become long enough to reach over the medial trochlear ridge despite normal conformation. Examples of this include loss of quadriceps tone and traumatic hyperextension of the hindlimb. Once upward fixation occurs, the ligaments may be stretched, so recurrence is common. The typical presentation is a young horse beginning training, but debilitation can provide the necessary conditions. Upward fixation has also been observed in horses abruptly taken out of training and confined to a stall.

Signs and Diagnosis

With acute upward fixation of the patella, the hindlimb is locked in extension (Fig. 8.485). The stifle and hock cannot flex, but the fetlock can. The condition may temporarily relieve itself only to lock again in a few steps, or it may remain locked for several hours or even days. In other cases, there is only a catching of the patella as the horse walks, and the limb never truly locks in extension. When the medial patellar ligament releases, the hindlimb usually jerks up quickly, mimicking stringhalt from which UFP must be differentiated. This catching of the patella is most noticeable when the horse is turned in a short circle toward the affected hindlimb or walked down a slope. As the horse descends the slope, a jerky gait is noted as the result of incomplete extension of the stifle. If the stifle does go into full extension, a catch leading to a toe drag is seen in some cases.

Upon palpation, when the limb is locked in extension, the ligaments of the patella are tense, and the patella is locked above the medial trochlear ridge of the femur (Fig. 8.484). When the horse is forced to move forward with the limb locked, it drags the front of the hoof on the ground. The limb should be checked by forcing the patella upward and outward with the hand. If the limb can be manually locked in extension for one or more steps, it is predisposed to UFP. In some cases, a snapping sound may be heard when the patella is released. The examiner should take care not to be in the path when the limb releases. Lameness is not usually severe or constant, but femoropatellar synovitis and distension may occur with repeated episodes. There is reason to believe that coxofemoral strain may be associated with persistent UFP as well.[2]

Radiographs of the stifle should be taken to eliminate conditions that predispose the horse to UFP. Although uncommon, hypoplasia of the medial trochlear ridge (as occurs with OCD) facilitates the displacement.

Treatment

In the past, most horses with UFP and many others with undiagnosed hindlimb lameness underwent medial patellar desmotomy. Complications from that procedure should now deem it to be the last resort for treatment of UFP (see "Fragmentation of the Distal Patella").[3,5,6, 8,10,11] The majority of horses respond to controlled conditioning to increase quadriceps strength and tone, which tightens the medial patellar ligament.[7] However, once an affected horse drops a level of fitness, UFP may recur. Rest or confinement is contraindicated.

For a permanently fixed patella, a sideline may be applied to the affected limb so that as the limb is drawn forward the patella is pushed medially and downward, which often disengages the fixed patella. Backing the

horse may also dislodge the patellar ligament. In others, a medial patellar desmotomy is required. Fortunately, this situation is uncommon.

For the medial patellar desmotomy, the area over the middle and medial patellar ligaments is closely clipped and prepared for surgery. The horse should be sedated, and the tail wrapped to keep it from switching into the surgical sites. A local anesthetic is injected subcutaneously over the middle patellar ligament with a ⅝-inch 25-gauge needle. Then a 20-gauge 2-inch needle is inserted through this skin bleb to infiltrate the subcutaneous region over the medial patellar ligament and the medial

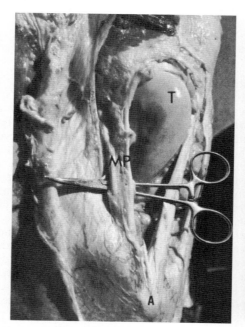
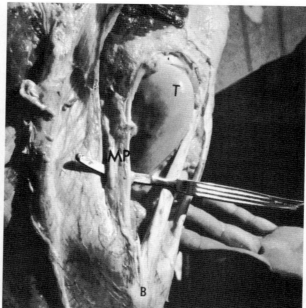
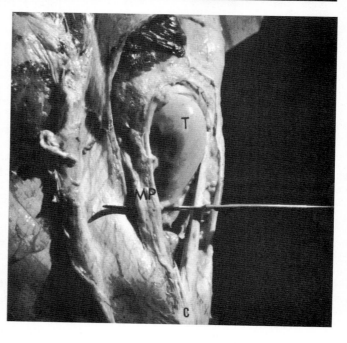

Figure 8.486 Medial patellar desmotomy. A. A curved mosquito hemostat is passed axial to the medial patellar (MP) ligament and expanded to create a path for the bistoury and to locate the caudal extent of the ligament so excessive tissue is not cut in a second effort. B. The curved bistoury is passed axial to the ligament in the path created by the hemostat. C. The bistoury rotates outwardly to expose the blade and transect the ligament. T, medial trochlea of the femur.

patellar ligament itself just above its tibial attachment. Care is used to avoid damaging the bone, or periostitis may result.

A 1-cm incision is made along the medial limit of the middle patellar ligament near its tibial attachment. A curved mosquito hemostat is inserted and dissected axial to the medial patellar ligament and is palpated subcutaneously completely caudal to the ligament. The tract is expanded by opening the hemostat and withdrawing the instrument. A Udall's teat bistoury, or other suitable blunt bistoury, is inserted along the path created, with the blade directed distally. The tip of the bistoury is palpated subcutaneously in the same position caudal to the medial patellar ligament as the hemostat was palpated (Figs. 8.484 and 8.486). The blade is rotated so that the cutting edge is against the ligament. Using a sawing action and pushing with the forefinger on the ligament from the skin surface, the medial patellar ligament is severed. All fibers of the ligament must be cut on the first attempt, because positioning after the majority of the ligament has been severed may produce a gracilis myotomy. The advantages of the large bistoury are that there is less hemorrhage and that the ligament can be cut in one stroke. A definite cavity will be felt with the forefinger when the ligament is cut. One or two sutures are used to appose the skin incision.

The horse should be kept stalled; hand walking is gradually increased over a period of 90 days. From that point a conservative conditioning program for regular work can begin.[11]

Failure of a medial patellar desmotomy to correct the problem has been reported.[4] The persisting tissue still displaces over the medial trochlear ridge. An alternative procedure was suggested in which the accessory cartilage of the patella is transected proximal to the ligamentous tissue.[4] No results have been reported.

The injection of counterirritants into the middle and medial patellar ligaments is a treatment for horses with intermittent UFP that have no palpable swelling of the femoropatellar joint capsule.[7] The injections are usually performed on the standing horse using mild sedation and nose twitch. Commonly used irritants contain iodine (hypodermin). Between 1 and 2 mL is injected in six equally distributed sites along the medial patellar ligament (total amount 6 to 12 mL). Approximately half this amount is injected into the middle patellar ligament. Most horses exhibit a slight stiffness and swelling for a few days after the injections. Daily mild exercise is recommended so there is minimal loss of muscle tone. While most horses respond well to this treatment, a few require retreatment.

The commonly held opinion about the effectiveness of counterirritant injections into the medial patellar ligament is that the ligament tightens, thereby mimicking increased tone from conditioning. A study was performed in which the tissues were harvested and evaluated histologically.[1] The majority of the (severe) inflammatory reaction and all of the drug were found in the endotenon and peritenon. Apparently, the injections follow the planes of least resistance. Within the dense collagen bundles, collagen fibers were disrupted without the same severe reaction, although there was fibrous tissue production and overall thickening. The mechanism of action

could lie in the reduced expansile ability of the fibrous medial patellar ligament. The accidental intraarticular injection of the counterirritant would likely have a disastrous result.

Prognosis

The prognosis is good for horses that respond to a conditioning program. The individual generally must be kept fit because UFP returns if quadriceps tone falls below a certain amount. For horses that do not respond to this program or that have more persisting UFP, medial patellar desmotomy is recommended. These horses must be rehabilitated carefully to prevent serious complications of the patella (see "Fragmentation of the Distal Patella").

References

1. Brown MP, Moon PD, Buergelt CD. The effects of injection of an iodine counterirritant into the patellar ligaments of ponies: Application to stifle lameness. J Equine Vet Sci 1984;4:82–87.
2. Clegg PD, Butson RJ. Treatment of a coxofemoral luxation secondary to upward fixation of the patella in a Shetland pony. Vet Rec 1996;138:134–137.
3. Gibson KT, McIlwraith CW, Park RD, et al. Production of patellar lesions by medial patellar desmotomy in normal horses. Vet Surg 1989;18:466–471.
4. Hickman J. Upward retention of the patella in the horse. Vet Rec 1964;76:1198–1199.
5. Jansson N. Treatment for upward fixation of the patella in the horse by medial patellar desmotomy: Indications and complications. Equine Pract 1996;18:24–29.
6. McIlwraith CW. Osteochondral fragmentation of the distal aspect of the patella in horses. Equine Vet J 1990;22:157–163.
7. Norrie RD. Diseases of the rear leg. In: Mansmann RA, McAllister ES, Eds. Equine Medicine and Surgery. Santa Barbara, CA: American Veterinary Publications, 1982;1137.
8. Riley CB, Yovich JV. Fracture of the apex of the patella after medial patellar desmotomy in a horse. Aust Vet J 1991;68:37–39.
9. Rooney JR. The abnormal rear leg. In: The Lame Horse. South Brunswick, NJ: Barnes, 1973;175.
10. Squire KRE, Blevins WE, Frederick M, et al. Radiographic changes in an equine patella following medial patellar desmotomy. Vet Radiol 1990;31:208–209.
11. Walmsley JP. Medial patellar desmotomy for upward fixation of the patella. Equine Vet Educ 1994;6:148–150.

DISTAL LUXATION OF THE PATELLA

McIlwraith and Warren[1] described a case of distal luxation of the patella in which it became entrapped in the cranial space between the femoral condyles (Fig. 8.487). Although the cause is unknown, it was speculated that at least partial tearing of the insertion of the quadriceps femoris muscles on the proximal patella occurred, allowing the patella to assume this abnormal position while the muscle was caught over the trochlea. Clinically, the limb was locked in flexion and the quadriceps femoris muscle was stretched over the trochlea of the femur. This position was fixed and could not be altered by manipulation. However, manipulation while under general anesthesia was successful, and the horse recovered uneventfully. No deficiency in the quadriceps femoris muscle could be appreciated, but radiographs

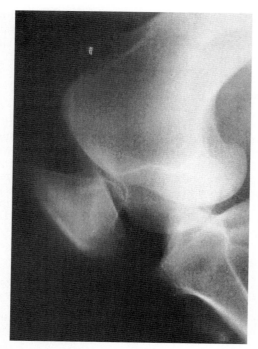

Figure 8.487 Lateromedial view of a distal luxation of the patella. (Reprinted with permission from McIlwraith CW, Warren RC. Distal luxation of the patella in a horse. J Am Vet Med Assoc 1982;181:67–69.)

some 6 months later indicated that there had been some tearing of the proximal attachment to the patella.

Reference

1. McIlwraith CW, Warren RC. Distal luxation of the patella in a horse. J Am Vet Med Assoc 1982;181:67–69.

MEDIAL AND LATERAL PATELLAR SUBLUXATION AND LUXATION (PATELLAR ECTOPIA)

Although patellar subluxation and luxation have been well documented in the literature, they are considered rare entities.[4,5,7-12,14] The condition is usually recognized shortly after birth, but may be delayed in acquired cases. Acquired patellar luxation also occurs in older horses, but it is considered even more uncommon.[11] Lateral,[2,4,6,9,11] medial,[1] unilateral, and bilateral luxations have been described, but lateral luxation is more common. The luxations can range from a mild intermittent subluxation to a complete luxation that is difficult to manually replace.

Causes

Hypoplasia of the trochlear ridges (primary bone deformation) and hypoplasia of the ligamentous support structures have been suggested as a cause.[12,14] In ponies and miniature horses, the condition is considered heritable.[7] The frequent lack of an adequate trochlear groove and lateral trochlear ridge is an obvious factor. When

the condition occurs in the mature horse, trauma is thought to be the cause. It also can occur in association with defective development of the lateral trochlear ridge caused by osteochondritis dissecans.[13]

Signs and Diagnosis

Foals with bilateral lateral luxation may not be able to stand or may stand in a crouched position. The foal is unable to extend the stifle, because the displaced patella causes the quadriceps muscle group to act as a flexor rather than function as an extensor. Signs depend on the frequency, position, and degree of displacement of the patella. If the displacement is intermittent, periods of normal ambulation occur. On palpation, some degree of patellar displacement and joint capsule distension are appreciated. When complete, patellar luxation can be difficult to replace; the intermittent patellar subluxations are usually readily replaced.

Horses with persistent lateral subluxation of the patella present much like horses with UFP.[8] The limb is held in extension, causing the patella to be placed caudolaterad. When the limb is advanced, an awkward swinging gait with typical toe dragging occurs. Because some of these animals have a fairly normal gait, the condition is often missed until serious degenerative changes within the joint have occurred.[11]

Radiographs should be taken to confirm the diagnosis and to identify the amount of degenerative changes within the joint. The skyline view is particularly beneficial for appreciating the degree of displacement. In the neonate, the irregular borders of subchondral ossification in the proximal trochlea should not be confused with degenerative changes (Fig. 8.458).

Treatment

In one reported case of bilateral congenital lateral patellar luxation in a miniature horse, the foal had overcome the crouch by 6 months of age and began to walk normally. The patellae remained luxated. Most horses are treated surgically to minimize permanent deformity of the soft tissues and osteoarthritis.

Surgical therapy takes two forms. When a sufficient femoral trochlea is present, stabilization of the patella in the correct position usually suffices. Release of the contralateral soft tissue may be required to achieve stable reduction.[4,8,11] Horses with hypoplasia of the lateral trochlear ridge and an insufficient trochlear groove require trochleoplasty.[1,3,6,9] The significant malalignment of the patellar tendons requires transposition of the tibial tuberosity as well.[1] When OCD is the cause of the hypoplasia, the cartilage surface and underlying bone are usually insufficient to sustain a trochleoplasty.[13]

Prognosis

The outlook for athletic activity without surgical correction is poor, although pasture soundness may be possible at least in miniature horses. With early surgical correction, success is reasonable. However, the horses commonly affected do not often have severe athletic demands. Horses with OCD sufficient enough to allow lateral luxation of the patella have a poor prognosis.

References

1. Arighi M, Wilson JW. Surgical correction of medial luxation of the patella in a miniature horse. Can Vet J 1993;34:499–501.
2. Burba DJ, Collier MA. What is your diagnosis? J Am Vet Med Assoc 1991;198:693–694.
3. Edinger H, Stanek C. Surgical correction of a congenital bilateral lateral stationary patellar luxation in a Shetland filly using trochleoplasty by wedge osteotomy. Pferdeheilkunde 1991;7:197–203.
4. Engelbert TA, Tate LP, Richardson DC, et al. Lateral patellar luxation in miniature horses. Vet Surg 1993;22:293–297.
5. Finocchio EJ, Guffy MM. Congenital ectopia in a foal. J Am Vet Med Assoc 1970;156:222.
6. Garlick MH, Thiemann AK. Treatment of luxating patellae. Vet Rec 1993;133:602–603.
7. Hermans WA, Kersjes AW, van der Mey GJW, Dik KJ. Investigation into the heredity of congenital lateral patellar (sub)luxation in the Shetland pony. Vet Q 1987;9:1–8.
8. Jones RD. Medial imbrication of the stifle to release lateral subluxation of the patella in a miniature horse. Equine Pract 1981;3:19.
9. Kobluk CN. Correction of patellar luxation by recession sulcoplasty in three foals. Vet Surg 1993;22:298–300.
10. Lafrance NA, Leaner DJ, O'Brien TR. Bilateral congenital lateral patellar luxation in a foal. Can Vet J 1971;12:119.
11. Leitch M, Kotlikoff M. Surgical repair of congenital lateral luxation of the patella in the foal and calf. Vet Surg 1980;9:1–4.
12. Rooney JR. Congenital lateral luxation of the patella in a horse. Cornell Vet 1971;61:670.
13. Stromberg B, Rejno S. Osteochondrosis in the horse. I. A clinical and radiologic investigation of osteochondritis dissecans of the knee and hock joint. Acta Radiol Suppl (Stockh) 1978;358:139–152.
14. Van Pelt RW, Keahey KK, Dalley JB. Congenital bilateral ectopia of the patella in the foal. Vet Med 1971;66:445.

EPIPHYSITIS

A single case report described an epiphysitis in the distal femoral physis of a growing horse that was believed to be the cause of lameness.[1] The horse also was affected with kyphosis of the cranial lumbar spine. The method of isolating the source of the lameness was not described. A complete recovery from the lameness and back problem was seen after the horse was placed on a restricted diet for 3 months.

Reference

1. Jeffcott LB, Kold SE. Stifle lameness in the horse: a survey of 86 referred cases. Equine Vet J 1982;14:31–39.

SYNOVIAL OSTEOCHONDROMA IN THE HINDLIMB

Osteochondroma is a benign tumor associated with cartilage growth centers and can be unilateral or bilateral (see Chapter 6). Young horses generally present with the problem, but since affected horses can remain clinically silent for long periods of time, older horses may also present.[3] In the hindlimb, osteochondroma has been reported in the femorotibial bursa on the proximal lateral tibia,[3] the plantar distal tibia within the tarsocrural joint,[2] within the tarsal canal on the fibular tarsal bone,[4] and on the calcaneus.[1]

Signs and Diagnosis

Synovial effusion with or without lameness is the usual presenting complaint. The location depends on which synovial structure is affected. Often the mass can be palpated percutaneously. Radiographs usually demonstrate a focal semiossified mass associated with a growth plate or ossification center. The presenting signs and radiographic findings are often sufficient to make a presumptive diagnosis. Biopsy is usually better performed as excision. The radiographic appearance indicates that trauma is unlikely to be a factor.

Treatment

Although the lesion is likely to be benign, complete excision should be accomplished. If the horse is actively competing, palliation of the synovitis could be obtained by local anti-inflammatory therapy without ill effect. That decision is made on an individual basis. Routine postoperative bandaging and exercise restriction are tailored to the affected site. Intrasynovial anti-inflammatory injections of, e.g., sodium hyaluronate, are advisable.

Prognosis

Although intrasynovial therapy is worthy of consideration, the prognosis for horses has been good following surgical excision. Each case is different, and the lesions are likely to occur in more difficult locations than have been observed in the past.

References

1. Chan CCH, Munroe GA, Callanan JJ. Congenital solitary osteochondroma affecting the tarsus in a filly foal. Equine Vet Educ 1996;8:153–156.
2. Kenzora KT, Von Matthiessen PW, Sheehan RM. A uniquely located solitary plantar tibial osteochondroma in a Thoroughbred racehorse. Equine Pract 1995;17:23–25.
3. Kirk MD. Radiographic and histologic appearance of synovial osteochondromatosis of the femorotibial bursae in a horse. A case history report. Vet Radiol 1982;23:167–170.
4. Welch RD, Auer JA, Watkins JP, et al. Surgical treatment of tarsal sheath effusion associated with an exostosis on the calcaneus of a horse. J Am Vet Med Assoc 1990;196:1992–1994.

Part XIII

THE FEMUR
Kenneth E. Sullins

FRACTURES OF THE FEMORAL DIAPHYSIS AND METAPHYSIS

Fractures of the femur are relatively common in the horse.[2,4,6,7,13] In young animals, fractures often involve the proximal or distal growth plate; and if the diaphysis is involved, the fracture is usually simple and oblique. Adults, on the other hand, usually sustain comminuted fractures of the femoral shaft. Intraarticular fractures involving the stifle joint are described elsewhere in this chapter.

Causes

Young foals frequently sustain femoral fractures during the initial handling and often during halter breaking. Occasionally, the mare steps on the foal, causing this type of injury, or the foal becomes entrapped under a fence. In a study of 38 horses less than 1 year of age, causes included falls, severe adduction, external trauma, and getting caught in a fence.[9] In the mature horse, considerable force is required to fracture the femur.

Signs and Diagnosis

The obvious sign is non-weight-bearing lameness. When viewed from the side, the affected limb may appear slightly shortened with the hock held higher than the opposite hindlimb; a dimpling of the musculature overlying the fracture may be observed (Fig. 8.488). In some cases, obvious swelling may be present.

On palpation, excessive movement of the distal limb is appreciated. In younger horses, swelling can be observed in association with the fracture site and crepitation may be apparent (Fig. 8.489). In some cases, auscultation (with a stethoscope) of crepitation over the femur can be helpful. In the mature horse, however, these sounds are often muffled because of the massive musculature and swelling (e.g., hematoma) associated with these fractures. Because of overriding, the patella often feels loose and can be manipulated easily in a lateral and medial direction. Uncommonly, clinically significant or fatal hemorrhage results, and suspected vascular compromise should be investigated.[8,17]

Young horses that have sustained proximal growth plate fractures (slipped capital epiphyses) can be difficult to diagnose; the condition must be differentiated from coxofemoral luxations. Femoral neck fractures in older horses or ponies are similar. If the fracture has overridden proximally, the hock on the affected limb will be higher than the hock on the normal limb. Frequently, affected foals can bear weight; and because of the frac-

ture location, swelling is not readily apparent in acute cases. Palpation and in some cases auscultation over the greater trochanter while the limb is being manipulated may help. If the foal is large enough, a rectal examination usually reveals crepitation when the limb is manipulated. In addition, swelling may be felt on the medial aspect of the thigh; particularly if the fracture is several days old. Fractures of the distal growth plate are usually easy to diagnose because of the displacement and swelling associated with the stifle region.

Although the clinical signs are informative, except for proximal growth plate fractures, radiographs are important for making a definitive diagnosis and defining the exact location of the fracture. Except for horses with distal growth plate fractures and distal-end femoral shaft

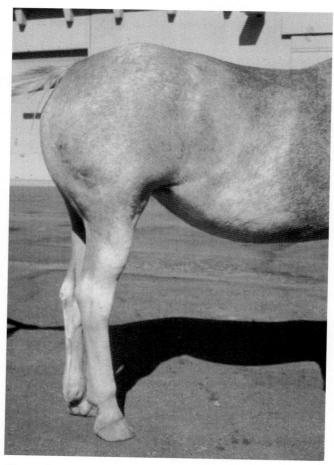

Figure 8.488 When a horse has a fractured femur, the limb is a bit shortened and the musculature of the gaskin is slightly dimpled.

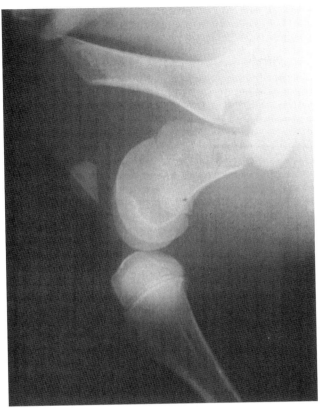

Figure 8.489 Lateromedial view of a closed oblique midshaft fracture of the femur. (Courtesy of T. S. Stashak.)

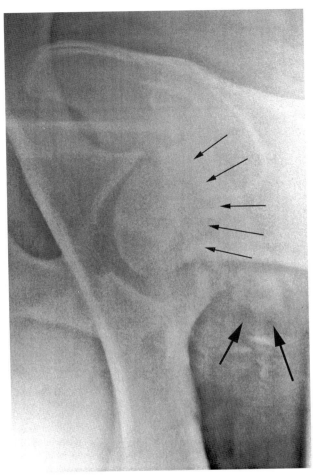

Figure 8.490 Standing dorsoventral view of a fracture of the proximal femur while the limb is held in abduction. Small arrows, fracture line; large arrows, fragments.

fractures, a recumbent position is required to take the radiographs. Most handheld x-ray units cannot penetrate the massive musculature overlying the femur in the adult horse. With the proper equipment, a standing oblique view of the coxofemoral region can be taken in smaller horses (Fig. 8.490). Digital enhancement of the radiographs often precludes the need for a grid technique.

In a series of 38 foals with femoral fractures, 26 had fractures of the femoral diaphysis and 18 sustained fractures involving two-thirds of the length of the diaphysis.[8] A total of 12 foals had distal physeal fractures, and the most common fracture configuration was a Salter-Harris type 2. In another series of foals treated during the same time period 25 sustained fractures of the capital femoral physis, neck, or greater trochanter.[11]

Treatment

Treatment of femoral shaft fractures depends on the age of the animal and the type and location of the fracture. Generally, euthanasia should be performed for adults and yearlings that have sustained femoral shaft fractures, unless exceptional circumstances exist.

Diaphyseal fractures have been treated with stall rest in foals weighing up to approximately 200 kg.[13]

Compression plating is the treatment of choice for foals that have sustained diaphyseal fractures when athletic soundness is desired. Of 15 foals with diaphyseal fractures that were plated, 14 patients required two plates for the repair.[8] One plate was placed laterally and the other cranially. However, single-plate application has occasionally been used.[1,8] More distal fractures can be repaired using angled blade plates or dynamic condylar screw plates.[8] When there are no complications, the plates are not removed.

Fractures that have no caudal cortical buttress are at risk of receiving an unstable repair and should be given a poor prognosis.[8] Because traction on the distal limb is generally useless, toggling and locally applied distraction devices are necessary to reduce the fracture. Negative pressure suction drains should be applied until drainage stops (usually 4 to 5 days).[8,22] Inability to control seroma formation is related to an increase in infection rates.[8]

Intramedullary pinning using the stacked pin technique or a single 0.5-inch pin has been used successfully in young foals with femoral diaphyseal fractures.[20] However, problems with pin migration should be ex-

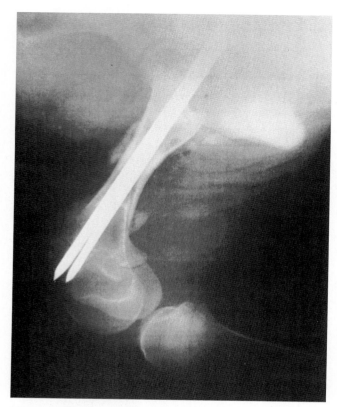

Figure 8.491 Repair of the fracture shown in Figure 8.489, using a stacked pin technique. There must be enough pins to prevent rotational instability. (Courtesy of T. S. Stashak.)

pected. One report in experimental fractures in (65- to 140-kg) donkeys noted some success; however, the study was performed in adult donkeys.[21] Controlled relatively atraumatic fractures produced in adult bone do not simulate clinical fractures in foals. This pinning technique is most useful when used in young, sedate foals (Fig. 8.491).

Interlocking nails have been investigated for repair of diaphyseal femoral fractures. The work to date has generally demonstrated that double-plate fixation provides more rotational stability.[14,16]

Bone screw fixation provides good stabilization of capital or femoral neck fractures if the screws can be properly placed and interfragmentary compression is added.[5,18] In one report, a nondisplaced fracture of the proximal femoral growth plate was treated successfully by direct pinning with Knowles pins and intraoperative radiographic monitoring.[23] Repair of displaced fractures of the proximal femoral physis requires open reduction to reposition the head and the neck before pinning (Fig. 8.492).[23] Femoral head ostectomy was described for three ponies and six horses; one pony and two horses survived. Although a permanent lameness resulted, the pain was relieved and the animals were sound for reproductive purposes.[19] A device for repairing femoral neck fractures was investigated, but further reports have not been made.[10]

Distal physeal fractures are difficult to repair because there is little space for an adequate number of screws to be placed distal to the fracture; thus many are not treated.[8] Options for stabilizing distal physeal fractures include an angled blade plate,[8] condylar buttress plate,[15] cobra-head and dynamic compression plate (DCP),[12] and cross-pins or Rush pins. One Salter-Harris type 2 fracture was repaired using an angled blade plate.[8] Rush pins or cruciate placement of Steinmann pins can also be considered (Fig. 8.493). Use of a condylar buttress plate in the successful repair of a Salter-Harris type 2 fracture in a yearling Pony of America has been reported.[15] The plate was not removed. A minimally displaced Salter-Harris type 4 fracture in a yearling that was treated conservatively healed to allow the horse to reach racing status.[8] A more displaced Salter-Harris type 4 fracture in a yearling was successfully treated by lag screw repair.[3]

Prognosis

The prognosis for fracture of the femur largely depends on the age of the horse, the location and type of fracture, and the horse's intended use. Generally, femoral fractures in horses older than yearlings carry a poor prognosis for a successful outcome. A much better prognosis can be expected in young animals with nondisplaced fractures or simple oblique midshaft fractures that are stabilized by internal fixation.[8] In a series of 17 surgically repaired diaphyseal fractures, 9 healed.[1,8] Of those, 6 were considered to have no sign of previous fracture.[8] The mean age for successfully treated foals was 2 months compared to 4 months for unsuccessfully treated foals.[8] Of 4 foals with oblique midshaft femoral fractures treated by stall rest alone, 3 horses became sound for breeding, but fracture disease associated with prolonged non weight bearing presented problems during the healing period.[13]

Proximal and distal growth plate fractures have a guarded prognosis for athletic function, but breeding status is possible. A single successful report of lag screw repair of a proximal growth plate fracture in a 2-month-old Arabian foal included removal of the screws after 10 months.[18] Another report describes the successful repair of a femoral neck fracture in an adult pony.[5] Pin fixation of a nondisplaced femoral capital fracture was also successful.[23]

In a series of 25 horses (aged 11 days to 12 months) with proximal growth plate fractures that also sustained proximal physeal fractures, 21 were destroyed because of a poor prognosis as a result of duration and osteoarthritis.[10] In another study, surgical repair was attempted in 2 foals using stacked intramedullary pins and in 1 foal using a lag screw and plate fixation. The 2 patients repaired with pins were euthanatized within 2 weeks owing to failure of the repair. The foal with the lag screw fixation became breeding sound. Nonsurgical treatment of displaced capital fractures results in osteoarthritis. For slipped capital epiphyses, femoral head ostectomy may be considered as a salvage procedure for breeding.

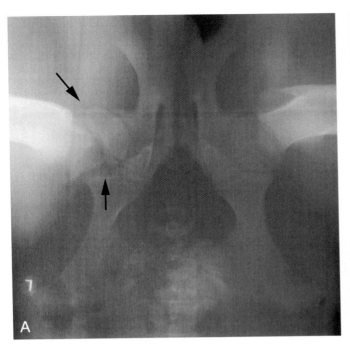 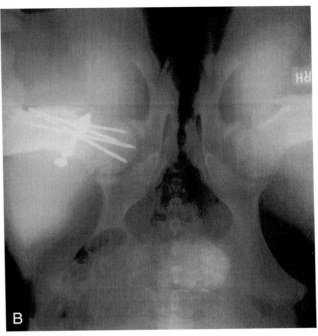

Figure 8.492   A. Ventrodorsal view of a proximal physeal fracture of the femur in which the femoral head has separated from the femoral neck (arrows). The acetabulum is intact, an important consideration when determining treatment. B. The fracture was repaired by using intramedullary pins. The pins must diverge to maintain reduction, and an additional pin in the more cranial aspect of the epiphysis would have been good. The screws were used to replace the greater trochanter, which was removed to approach the coxofemoral joint.

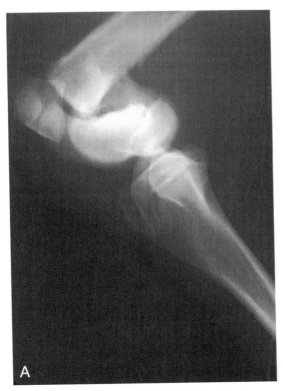 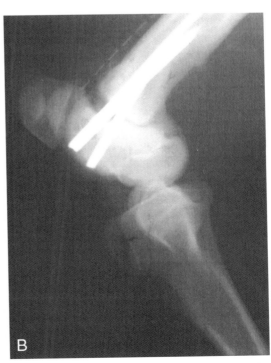

Figure 8.493   A. A Salter-Harris type 2 fracture involving the distal femur. B. The fracture was stabilized with Steinmann pins placed in a cruciate fashion. This fracture healed successfully, and the pins were removed 3 months postoperatively. (Courtesy of T. S. Stashak.)

References

1. Boulton CH, Dallman MJ. Equine femoral fracture repair: A case report. J Equine Vet Sci 1983;3:60–64.
2. Clayton-Jones DC. The repair of equine fractures. Vet Rec 1975; 97:193.
3. DeBowes RM, Grant BD, Modransky PD. Lag screw stabilization of Salter type IV femoral fracture in a young horse. J Am Vet Med Assoc 1983;182:1123–1125.
4. Denny HR. The surgical treatment of equine fractures. Vet Rec 1978;102:273–277.
5. Denny HR, Watkins PE, Waterman A. Fracture of the femoral neck in a Shetland pony. Equine Vet J 1983;15:283–284.
6. Fessler JF, Amstutz HE. Fracture repair. In: Oehme FW, Prier JE, Eds. Textbook of Large Animal Surgery. Baltimore: Williams & Wilkins, 1974;321.
7. Hance SR, Bramlage LR, Embertson RM, et al. Retrospective study of femoral fractures in foals. Vet Surg 1992;21:391.
8. Hance SR, Bramlage LR, Schneider RK, et al. Retrospective study of 38 cases of femur fractures in horses less than one year of age. Equine Vet J 1992;24:357–363.
9. Held JP, Patton CS, Shires M. Solitary osteochondroma of the radius in three horses. J Am Vet Med Assoc 1988;193:563–564.
10. Hunt DA, Snyder JR, Morgan JP, et al. Evaluation of an interfragmentary compression system for the repair of equine femoral capital physeal fractures. Vet Surg 1990;19:107–116.
11. Hunt DA, Snyder JR, Morgan JP, et al. Femoral capital physeal fractures in 25 foals. Vet Surg 1990;19:41–49.
12. Kirker-Head CA, Fackelman GE. Use of the cobra head bone plate for distal long bone fractures in large animals. A report of four cases. Vet Surg 1989;18:227–234.
13. McCann ME, Hunt RJ Conservative management of femoral diaphyseal fractures in four foals. Cornell Vet 1993;83:125–132.
14. McClure SR, Watkins JP, Ashman RB. In vivo evaluation of intramedullary interlocking nail fixation of transverse femoral osteotomies in foals. Vet Surg 1998;27:29–36.
15. Orsini JA, Buonanno AM, Richardson DW, et al. Condylar buttress plate fixation of femoral fracture in a colt. J Am Vet Med Assoc 1990;197:1184–1186.
16. Radcliffe RM, Lopez MJ, Turner TA, et al. An in vitro biomechanical comparison of interlocking nail constructs and double plating for fixation of diaphyseal femur fractures in immature horses. Vet Surg 2001;30:179–190.
17. Rose PL, Watkins JP, Auer JA. Femoral fracture repair complicated by vascular injury in a foal. J Am Vet Med Assoc 1984;185:795–797.
18. Smyth GB, Taylor EG. Stabilization of a proximal femoral physeal fracture in a filly by use of cancellous bone screws. J Am Vet Med Assoc 1992;201:895–898.
19. Squire KRE, Fessler JF, Toombs JP, et al. Femoral head ostectomy in horses and cattle. Vet Surg 1991;20:453–458.
20. Stick JA, Derksen FJ. Intramedullary pinning of a fractured femur in a foal. J Am Vet Med Assoc 1980;176:627–629.
21. Taneja AK, Singh J, Behl SM, et al. Repair techniques for femoral fractures in horses. Equine Pract 1986;8:35–40.
22. Turner AS. Surgical repair of a fractured femur in a foal: A case report. J Equine Med Surg 1977;1:180.
23. Turner AS, Milne DW, Hohn RB, et al. Surgical repair of fractured capital femoral epiphysis in three foals. J Am Vet Med Assoc 1979; 175:1198–1202.

FIBROTIC AND OSSIFYING MYOPATHY

Fibrotic and ossifying myopathy is a fibrosis or ossification of the muscle tissue in the crus that often results in adhesions between the semitendinosus, semimembranosus, gracilis, or biceps femoris muscles (Fig. 8.494). The significance is that most of these adhesions limit the action of the semitendinosus muscle, causing an abnormal gait characterized by a slapping down (Fig. 8.495). If the semitendinosus is more affected, the slap is from cranial to caudal. If the gracilis is more affected, the slap

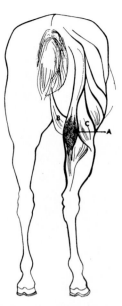

Figure 8.494   The muscles in the gaskin of a horse affected with fibrotic myopathy. A, semitendinosus; B, semimembranosus; c, biceps femoris.

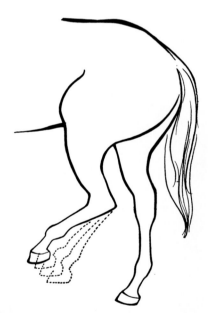

Figure 8.495   Characteristic action of the hindlimb of a horse affected with fibrotic myopathy. The limb jerks backward and downward (dotted lines) during the last 3 to 5 inches of the stride, resulting in a slapping of the foot on the ground. If the gracilis muscle is affected, the swing of the hindlimb is lateral to medial instead.

is from lateral to medial. The character of the gait of semitendinosus-affected horses has been described in detail.[3] The affected hindlimb approaches the ground more vertically than normal and strikes it toe first, making more of a slap than the normal heel-toe manner of landing. Rarely, the condition occurs in the forelimb.[1]

A congenital form of fibrotic myopathy-type syndrome has been reported.[2] Foals are born with an alteration in their gait characteristic of fibrotic myopathy in the hindlimb. On palpation, a tightening of the semitendinosus muscle is appreciated but no firm thickening of the muscle typical of fibrotic myopathy is palpated. Because no fibrous thickening of the muscle is present, congenital restrictive myopathy may be a more appropriate description of this entity.

Causes

The cause of the fibrosis is always trauma, which takes several forms. Involved muscles may be injured during sliding stops in rodeo work, from slipping and getting the hindlimb caught on the underside of a horse trailer, from resisting a sideline, from catching a foot in a halter, from intramuscular injections, or from being kicked.[2] The lesions are usually unilateral, but a case of bilateral fibrotic myopathy resulting from a trailer accident has been reported.[2] In some cases, the exact cause of the injury is not known, since clinical signs are often missed during the initial inflammatory stage. When the injury heals and adhesions form between the involved muscles, the adhesions cause lameness. Ossification is believed to be a more severe progression from the fibrosis.

The cause of the congenital form is unknown, although parturient muscle trauma has been described to cause rupture of the gastrocnemius muscle.[5] It is conceivable that similar trauma could also affect the semitendinosus under different stresses at birth or shortly after.

Three cases of fibrotic myopathy accompanied by neurogenic atrophy of the affected muscles have been reported.[7] All three horses underwent necropsy where peripheral nerve and muscle degeneration were discovered. One horse had a fracture of the greater trochanter and accompanying sciatic nerve impingement. No gross lesions were found in the other two horses.

Signs and Diagnosis

The signs are the result of adhesions between the semitendinosus muscle and the semimembranosus muscle medially and between the semitendinosus and the biceps femoris muscle laterally (Fig. 8.494). These adhesions partially inhibit the normal action of the muscles. In the cranial phase of the stride, the foot of the affected hindlimb is suddenly pulled caudally 3 to 5 inches just before contacting the ground (Fig. 8.495). Usually, the lameness is most noticeable when the horse walks. The cranial phase of the stride is shortened, so consequently the caudal phase is lengthened. This abnormal gait, which is easily identified, may result from either fibrotic or ossifying myopathy. An area of firmness can be palpated over the affected muscles on the caudal surface of the affected limb at the level of the stifle joint and immediately above it (Fig. 8.496). Occasionally, the lesion is deep and difficult to palpate or it is in the medial gaskin affecting the gracilis. If the gracilis is affected, the slap motion is more lateral to medial.

The diagnosis is based on the altered gait and on palpation of a hardened area on the caudal surface of the

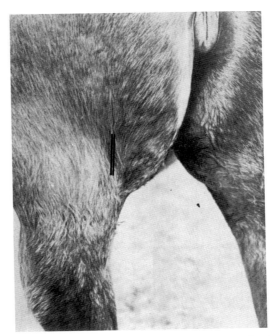

Figure 8.496 The area most commonly affected by fibrotic myopathy is indicated with double lines. This is also the line of incision for directly approaching the mass for removal.

limb at the level of the stifle joint. In making the diagnosis, stringhalt should also be considered. In stringhalt, the limb is pulled toward the abdomen, whereas in fibrotic myopathy, the foot is pulled toward the ground in a caudal direction just before the foot contacts the ground. In fibrotic myopathy, the limb is limited in the cranial phase of the stride by adhesions and by lack of elasticity in the affected area of the muscle belly, causing the limb to be pulled caudally before the full length of stride is reached.

Treatment

There are two approaches to surgical correction of fibrotic myopathy. Adams[1] described complete removal of the affected fibrotic muscle tissue. Bramlage et al.[2] described a semitendinosus tenotomy to release that muscle. The latter technique is less invasive and is expected to be effective if the problem is unaffected by other muscles.

To completely remove the affected fibrotic muscle tissue, the horse is positioned in lateral recumbency with the affected limb up. The area of the crus caudal to the stifle is aseptically prepared. A vertical incision at least 10 cm long is made over the caudal aspect of the semitendinosus tendon (Fig. 8.496). The tendon is identified, and the adhesions from the semimembranosus and the biceps femoris muscles are removed. The belly of the fibrotic semitendinosus muscle (or affected muscles) is isolated, and a 4-inch portion is removed. The part removed should include 4 cm of tendon and 4 cm of muscle

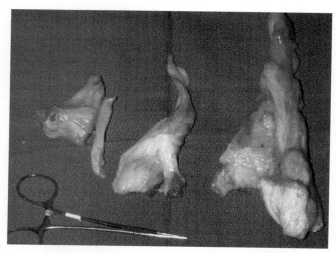

Figure 8.497 Fibrotic portions of the three muscles that were dissected from the gaskin region of a horse with fibrotic myopathy.

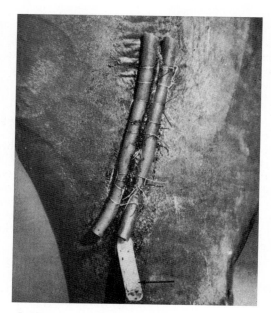

Figure 8.498 After dissection of the fibrotic mass from the muscles of the gaskin, the skin is closed with this technique. The quills support the sutures under tension, and the drain (arrow) prevents accumulation of fluid in the dead space. The drain is removed when the drainage subsides, and the quills are left in place for 2 weeks. Despite these measures, many incisions at least partially dehisce.

belly when possible (Fig. 8.497). After removal, the remaining muscle contracts immediately, and a large cavity results. If ossifying myopathy is present, the skin should be reflected and the bony cover over the semitendinosus muscle dissected free.

All layers are closed separately, using synthetic absorbable material. A Penrose drain is placed to allow drainage. Tension sutures in the skin are advisable (Fig. 8.498). The drain is removed in approximately 7 days. Hand walking is started when the skin has healed, and

normal exercise is allowed after 6 weeks. The gait has been reported to improve completely if the semitendinosus is singly affected, but some degree of improvement occurs if adhesions to other muscles are present.[4]

To perform the semitendinosus tenotomy,[2] the horse is positioned in lateral recumbency with the affected limb down. The area surrounding and caudal to the stifle is aseptically prepared. The affected limb should be extended to facilitate the procedure. The tibial insertion of the semitendinosus tendon is palpated caudomedial to the proximal end of the tibia. An 8-cm incision is created over the tendon to expose it. The tendon is then isolated with a hemostat and transected. Adhesions at the caudal border of the tibia should also be transected. All layers are closed separately using synthetic absorbable material. Tension sutures in the skin and the placement of a stent bandage overlying the incision are advisable. Hand walking is started when the skin has healed, and normal exercise is allowed after 6 weeks.

Prognosis

With partial myectomy, some relief is evident in all cases. After healing, some horses develop characteristic, but less pronounced, signs, although limb function is nearly normal and signs are noticeable only at the walk. Occasionally, it takes 3 to 7 days for the maximum benefits of surgical correction to become evident. One report cites a 50% frequency of complications after the partial myectomy of the semitendinosus (e.g., wound dehiscence, disfigurement, scar formation, and recurrence of lameness).[6]

The prognosis for tenotomy of the semitendinosus appears to be at least equivalent to the myectomy procedure, although only four cases have been reported. The defect is smaller and leaves less dead space for recurrence. It may take a few days to several weeks in some cases to appreciate the full benefit of the procedure. The results described for younger horses affected with the congenital form were good.[2]

The prognosis for successful surgery in horses affected by neurogenic atrophy of the muscles is poor. If the muscle mass appears abnormal, nerve conduction studies or electromyography (EMG) is advisable.

References

1. Adams OR. Fibrotic myopathy in the hindlegs of horses. J Am Vet Med Assoc 1961;139:1089.
2. Bramlage LR., Reed SM, Embertson RM. Semitendinosus tenotomy for treatment of fibrotic myopathy in the horse. J Am Vet Med Assoc 1985;186:565–567.
3. Clayton HM. Cinematographic analysis of the gait of lame horses V: Fibrotic myopathy. Equine Vet Sci 1988;8:297–301.
4. Gomez-Villamandos R, Santisteban J, Ruiz I, et al. Tenotomy of the tibial insertion of the semitendinosus muscle of two horses with fibrotic myopathy. Vet Rec 1995;136:67–68.
5. Sprinkle FP, Swerczek TW, Crowe MW. Gastrocnemius muscle rupture and hemorrhage in foals. Equine Pract 1985;7:10–17.
6. Turner AS, Trotter GW. Fibrotic myopathy in the horse. J Am Vet Med Assoc 1984;184:335–338.
7. Valentine BA, Rousselle SD, Sams AE, et al.: Denervation atrophy in three horses with fibrotic myopathy. J Am Vet Med Assoc 1994; 205:332–336.

RUPTURED QUADRICEPS

Ruptured quadriceps muscle is a rare condition that causes the horse to present with a dropped stifle. A single case was observed in a nursing foal and was of unknown cause. The patella was prominent owing to the cranial position of the stifle without the quadriceps attachment (Stashak TS, personal communication, 2001). An additional case was reported in the literature.[1]

Reference

1. Nicoletti JLM, Hussni CA, Thomassian A, et al. Rupture of the quadriceps femoris muscle in a horse. Ars Vet 1989;5:117–119.

FEMORAL NERVE PARALYSIS (CRURAL PARALYSIS)

Paralysis of the femoral nerve affects the quadriceps femoris group of muscles. This muscle group is composed of the rectus femoris muscle, the vastus lateralis muscle, the vastus medialis muscle, and the vastus intermedius muscle. This large muscular mass covers the front and sides of the femur, inserts onto the patella, and extends and fixes the stifle.

Causes

Femoral nerve paralysis may arise from trauma or from unknown causes and may be associated with rhabdomyolysis. Injury to the nerve may occur from overstretching of the limb during exertion, kicking, slipping, or while the horse is tied in a recumbent position. It has also been reported as a complication of general anesthesia.[1]

Hemorrhagic neuritis was described in one horse that was euthanatized because of femoral paralysis.[1] Normal horses compared at necropsy had no such lesions. The affected horse also had myoglobinuria and lesions of rhabdomyolysis. Postmortem studies revealed that the femoral nerves were placed in tension by extending the hindlimbs behind the horse, whereas lifting the horse by the hindlimbs did not place tension on the femoral nerves.[1] The potential roles or the interaction of femoral paralysis and rhabdomyolysis warrants further investigation.

Signs and Diagnosis

The horse assumes a crouched position with the fetlocks flexed and the toes on the ground; it is not able to bear weight on the affected limb. The horse has difficulty advancing the limb but can do so because the hock can be sufficiently flexed to pull the limb forward. Because the horse cannot bear weight on the limb, compensation must be made in the gait. After the condition has been present for some time, atrophy of the quadriceps muscles occurs, causing these muscles to lose their normal softness and become more like tendinous structures (Fig.

8.499). If rhabdomyolysis is present, the horse is in more pain and is less willing to attempt to stand.

These signs are characteristic and are used for diagnosis. The condition should be differentiated from lateral (true) luxation of the patella, rupture of the quadriceps femoris muscles, avulsion of the tibial crest, and distal luxation of the patella. Any of these conditions could cause a similar syndrome; however, all of these conditions are rare. Lateral luxation of the patella can be diagnosed by palpation of the displaced patella; rupture of the quadriceps femoris muscle can also be palpated. A radiologic examination can determine avulsion of the tibial crest where the patellar ligaments insert. EMG of the quadriceps femoris muscles—conducted 5 days after the first signs of femoral nerve paralysis are noted—provides a definitive diagnosis.

Treatment

No treatment is known. If the condition is the result of injury of the femoral nerve, the animal should be stalled until improvement has occurred. If rhabdomyolysis is present, intensive care and support is indicated for that, and repeated attempts to use the muscles should be discouraged.

Prognosis

The prognosis is guarded to unfavorable. In a report of two cases of postanesthetic femoral paralysis, one had concurrent rhabdomyolysis and was euthanatized. The other responded to supportive therapy and was standing well 7 days after the onset.[1] The prognosis should be withheld until sufficient time has elapsed to determine if any function will return.

Reference

1. Dyson S, Taylor P, Whitwell K. Femoral nerve paralysis after general anesthesia. Equine Vet J. 1988;20:376–380.

CALCINOSIS CIRCUMSCRIPTA

Calcinosis circumscripta in the horse is a calcified mass commonly located on the lateral aspect of the gaskin adjacent to the stifle. The condition has also been observed to occur over the carpus,[4] tarsus,[2] shoulder, tarsus, and pectoral region.[5] A review of 18 reported cases of calcinosis circumscripta revealed that 16 were adjacent to the stifle and all were in young male horses.[3] In another report, the age range at presentation for the condition was from 1 to 13 years.[5] The condition has not been reported in foals younger than 6 months of age.

Causes

The cause is unknown. The description of the lesion best fits that of dystrophic calcinosis characterized by calcinosis circumscripta. Tumor calcinosis implies a metabolic derangement in calcium–phosphorus metabolism, leading to hyperphosphatemia and resulting accumulation of deposits of calcium phosphate.[6] Although few

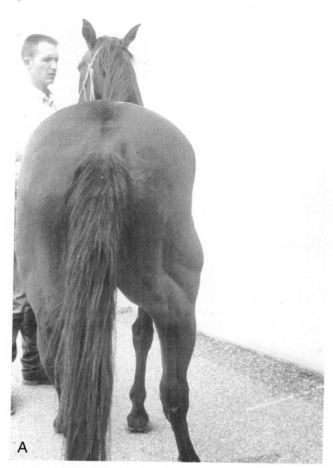

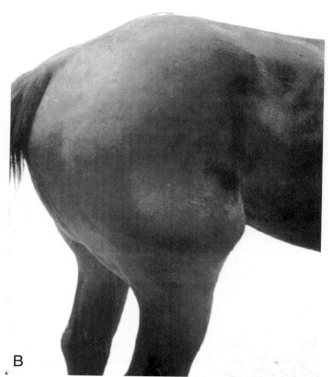

Figure 8.499 Lateral (A) and rear (B) views of the extensive muscle atrophy of the quadriceps muscle group, which was due to neurogenic atrophy, which was confirmed by EMG. (Courtesy of T. S. Stashak.)

studies have investigated the serum chemistries of affected horses, hyperphosphatemia has not been a reported feature of the condition in horses.

Signs and Diagnosis

Because clinical signs of lameness seldom occur, horses could carry the lesion for years before presentation to a hospital. The masses are generally 3 to 12 cm in diameter. The skin is freely moveable over the density because it lies beneath the superficial and deep fascia. It is often attached to the joint capsule of the lateral femorotibial joint.

Once dissected free, the lesions are encapsulated in a tough white fibrous capsule.[3] The interior is composed of loculations of finely granular, gritty, white pastelike material.[2] Histologically, the granules are surrounded by a granulomatous inflammatory reaction.[2] Although it is difficult to make a broad comparison, the lesion in humans is believed to be secondary to collagen necrosis.[7]

Treatment

The only treatment is surgical excision. However, the lesions seldom cause a clinical problem. The location is one that tends to dehisce after surgery, and postoperative complications must be taken seriously. One report in horses describes three of four cases that dehisced postoperatively, and one horse was lost to septic arthritis.[3] If surgery is performed, a tension-relieving closure using mattress sutures and a sutured stent bandage is advised. In addition, a circumferential adherent surgical drape helps prevent swelling.

Prognosis

The prognosis is good for soundness and future use. Clinical problems or lameness is uncommon. The prognosis after surgery must be guarded, depending on the size of the lesion, owing to the potential for incisional complications.[1]

References

1. Bertoni G, Gnudi G, Pezzoli G. Two cases of calcinosis circumscripta in the horse. Ann Facolta Med Vet Univ Parma 1993;13:201–210.
2. Dodd DC, Raker CW. Tumoral calcinosis (calcinosis circumscripta) in the horse. J Am Vet Med Assoc 1970;157:968–972.
3. Goulden BE. Tumoral calcinosis in the horse. NZ Vet J 1980;28:217–219.

4. Grant BD, Wagner PC. Unusual causes of carpitis. Mod Vet Pract 1980;61:131–134.
5. Hutchins DR. Tumoral calcinosis in the horse. Aust Vet J 1972;48: 200–202.
6. Stone WC, Wilson DA, Dubielzig RR, et al. The pathologic mineralization of soft tissue: Calcinosis circumscripta in horses. Comp Cont Educ Pract Vet 1990;12:1643–1649.
7. Thomson SW, Sullivan DJ. Calcifying collagenolysis (tumoral calcinosis). Br J Radiol 1966;39:526–532.

TROCHANTERIC BURSITIS (TROCHANTERIC LAMENESS, WHIRLBONE LAMENESS)

Trochanteric bursitis, most common in Standardbreds, is an inflammation of the bursa beneath the tendon of the middle gluteus muscle as it passes over the greater trochanter of the femur. The tendon of the middle gluteus muscle also may be involved, as well as the cartilage over the trochanter major. The deep portion of the gluteus medius muscle has a strong, flat tendon that passes over the convexity of the trochanter before it inserts into the crest. The trochanter is covered with cartilage and the trochanteric bursa is interposed between it and the tendon.

Causes

Lameness is caused by bruising as a result of the horse falling on the affected side, by straining the tendon during racing or training, or by a direct kick on the trochanter. It also has been found after an attack of distemper. In most cases, osteoarthritis also exists in the affected hindlimb, and hock lameness produces the bursitis.

Trochanteric bursitis occurs in horses racing on small tracks, where the turns are close together, and in horses working on their hindlimbs that are frequently exercised in soft, deep arenas. Short heels and long toes in the hindfeet seem to predispose the horse to this lameness.

Signs and Diagnosis

Pain may be evident when pressure is applied over the great trochanter. Careful interpretation is required, because some horses naturally tend to shy away when pressure is applied over the hip joint. At rest, the limb may remain flexed; as the horse moves, weight may be placed on the inside of the foot so that the inside wall of the foot wears more than the outside wall. This can be best seen when observing the horse from behind; the foot is carried inward and the horse sets the foot down on a line between the forelimbs. The horse tends to travel dog fashion, since the hindquarters move toward the sound side because the stride of the affected limb is shorter than that of the sound side. After the condition has been present for some time, atrophy of the gluteal muscles occurs. In cases for which the cause was a severe trauma, such as a direct kick, the cartilage or the bone of the trochanter may be fractured, causing persistent lameness.

The foregoing symptoms should be used in diagnosis. The condition is difficult to differentiate from inflammation of the coxofemoral joint. The lameness, which is not common, may be confused with spavin lameness. A lameness of unknown cause is sometimes ascribed to trochanteric bursitis. Injection of a local anesthetic into the bursa helps differentiate the condition from coxofemoral joint arthritis. Nuclear scintigraphy should identify the area as inflamed (see Chapter 4).

Treatment

Rest and anti-inflammatory treatment appear to help in some cases. Injection of the bursa with corticoids appears to be the most effective method of treatment. Other treatments consist of injections of Lugol's solution of iodine into or around the bursa as a counterirritant. Hot packs applied to the affected area in the acute stages relieve some pain. Phenylbutazone given orally for 3 to 4 weeks is also logical. When the cartilage or bone has been damaged with fracture or periostitis, treatment is difficult. Although surgery may be indicated in these cases, no reports could be found regarding the use of surgery.

Prognosis

The prognosis is guarded to unfavorable. If the horse responds to therapy within 4 to 6 weeks, it may again become sound. However, if the injury is more severe, the lameness may remain indefinitely or may recur when the horse is put back into training.

Part XIV

THE COXOFEMORAL JOINT

Dean A. Hendrickson

PARTIAL TEAR AND RUPTURE OF THE ACCESSORY (ROUND) LIGAMENT OF THE COXOFEMORAL (HIP) JOINT

A partial tear or rupture of the accessory ligament of the coxofemoral joint is a rare condition that can affect any age or breed of horse. When it does occur, it can represent a diagnostic and therapeutic challenge.

The hip joint of the horse has several ligaments which hold it together. The largest and strongest is the accessory ligament, which is unique to the horse and donkey among domestic species.[2] The ligament begins as a detachment from the prepubic tendon and passes through the acetabular notch to insert on the humeral head. A smaller shorter ligament rises from the pubic groove and attaches to the fovea in the head of the femur adjacent to the accessory ligament. This smaller ligament appears to play only a small role in joint stability. Occasionally, a partial tear or complete rupture of the accessory ligament can occur without resulting in a coxofemoral luxation. In this case, the head of the femur has a greater range of motion than is normal, resulting in degenerative changes in the joint and lameness.

Etiology

Trauma is the etiology of the partial tear or rupture of the accessory ligament. The same stresses/injury that cause luxation of the coxofemoral joint can cause injury to the accessory ligament without resulting in a joint luxation.

Signs

A history of trauma or acute onset of lameness is common. Although the history indicates a problem, the diagnosis may be delayed particularly if the ligament is only partially torn.[5]

Signs of accessory ligament rupture are very similar to those of luxation. The notable exception is that the hindlimbs are the same length.[1] Signs that characterize accessory ligament rupture are toe-out, stifle-out, and hock-in appearance of the affected hindlimb. This same appearance is also present in luxation of the coxofemoral joint, but the limbs are uneven in length (Fig. 8.500). If the condition is chronic, atrophy of the gluteal muscles on the affected side is usually apparent. Direct firm intermittent pressure applied over the greater trochanter will usually result in a painful response. Limb manipulation and flexion of the hip joint are also painful. Crepitation over the joint may be present because of the excessive motion of the femur allowed by rupture of the ligament or because of osteoarthritic changes that occur.[1] Comparison of the limbs will show that they are equal in length when the ligament is ruptured and luxation has not occurred. Although the signs often localize the problem to the hip region, intrasynovial anesthesia may be required in some to prove the joint is affected. For information regarding the technique for intrasynovial anesthesia of the hip joint the reader is referred to Chapter 3.

Signs associated with a partial tear of the accessory ligament are less clear than those seen with complete rupture of the ligament. Varying degrees of gluteal muscle atrophy will be observed, particularly in chronic cases. Limb manipulation, particularly hip abduction and flexion of the joint, is usually resented, but crepitation is not felt. Intermittent firm pressure applied externally to the greater trochanter usually elicits a painful response.[1] Lameness is moderate to severe, but the hock-in and stifle- and toe-out appearance is generally not observed. Intrasynovial anesthesia of the coxofemoral joint will be required in some cases to localize the problem to the hip joint.

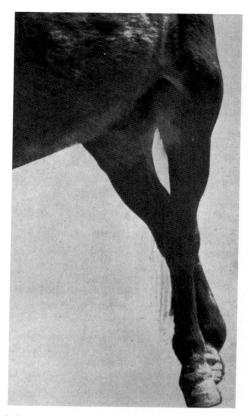

Figure 8.500 Rupture of the accessory ligament of the coxofemoral joint. The stifle-out, toe-out, hock-in attitude of the limb typifies rupture of the round ligament. This same attitude is also present when the joint has luxated. When the round ligament ruptures, but the joint does not luxate, the limbs are the same length.

Diagnosis

Diagnosis for complete rupture of the accessory ligament is based on the signs of stifle-out, toe-out, and hock-in appearance with equal length of the limbs. If the horse is anesthetized and laid on its back, a radiograph of the joint can be taken. If the condition is long standing, radiography will reveal severe degenerative (DJD) changes. Otherwise, the abnormal position of the femoral head in the acetabulum can be identified.[1]

Diagnostic approaches used to identify a partial tear of the accessory ligament may include scintigraphy, radiography, and arthroscopy. Although not diagnostic for a partial tear, scintigraphy will show a mild to moderate radionucleotide accumulation in the affected hip, particularly if degenerative joint changes (DJD) are present.[4,5] Lateral and dorsoventral scans are recommended. Radiography may identify changes associated with DJD of the hip joint. However, in acute cases the study may appear normal. Arthroscopy of the coxofemoral joint, although challenging, has been used to diagnose partial and complete ruptures of the accessory ligament.[3,5]

Treatment

There is no effective treatment for complete rupture of the accessory ligament of the hip joint. Affected horses remain lame. However, arthroscopy of the hip joint has been used successfully for debridement of partial tears of the accessory ligament and to perform a synovectomy.[3,5]

Prognosis

Prognosis is poor for complete rupture of the accessory ligament no matter what the treatment. However, the response to debridement of partial tears and synovectomy has been favorable in a limited number of cases, resulting in a lasting improvement in the lameness.[5]

References

1. Adams OR. Lameness in Horses. 3rd ed. Philadelphia: Lea & Febiger, 1974;301–303.
2. Dyce JM, Sack WO, Wensing CHG. Textbook of Veterinary Anatomy. Philadelphia: WB Saunders, 1987;576.
3. Honnas CM, Zamos DT, Ford TS. Arthroscopy of the coxofemoral joint of foals. Vet Surg 1993;22:115–121.
4. Lamb CR, Morris EA. Coxofemoral arthrosis in an aged mare. Equine Vet J 1987;19:350–352.
5. Nixon AJ. Coxofemoral joint arthroscopy. In: White NA, Moore JN, Eds. Current Techniques in Equine Surgery and Lameness. 2nd ed. Philadelphia: WB Saunders, 1998;448–451.

COXOFEMORAL LUXATION (DISLOCATION OF THE HIP JOINT)

Luxation of the coxofemoral joint is an uncommon condition. When it does occur, young horses and ponies are most frequently affected.[4,6,15,18–20] In horses, the ilium tends to fracture before luxation of the hip occurs. This is probably due in part to the fact that the hip is surrounded by strong supportive soft tissue structures. The accessory ligament, which is attached to the femoral head, provides the primary stability.[9] Additionally, the acetabulum is surrounded by a fibrocartilaginous cotyloid ligament that further stabilizes the head of the femur in the joint. Also, the heavy musculature surrounding the hip joint provides further stability to the joint.

Etiology

In most cases, trauma is the etiology. Both the accessory and the smaller ligament must rupture for a luxation to occur. Violent overextension and falling on the point of the stifle with the femur in a vertical position occasionally produces fracture and/or luxation of the coxofemoral joint. A tethered horse that catches its foot in a rope or a halter may dislocate the hip in the struggle to free itself (Fig. 8.501). The hip may also become dislocated if the horse fights a sideline or as a result of a similar trauma. Because the acetabulum is deep and the head of the femur is large, excessive trauma is necessary to dislocate this joint. Also, because of the deep acetabulum in the horse, fractures of the dorsal rim occur frequently with luxation.[10] Additionally, abnormalities of the coxofemoral joint associated with absence or tearing of the accessory ligament of the head of the femur can predis-

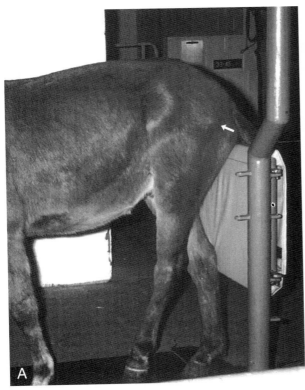

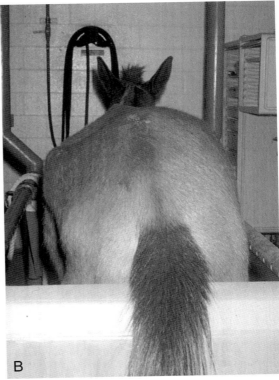

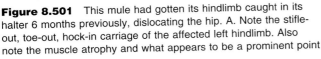

Figure 8.501   This mule had gotten its hindlimb caught in its halter 6 months previously, dislocating the hip. A. Note the stifle-out, toe-out, hock-in carriage of the affected left hindlimb. Also note the muscle atrophy and what appears to be a prominent point of the hip (arrow). B. Rear view of the mule. Note the extensive gluteal muscle atrophy of the affected region. (Courtesy of T. S. Stashak.)

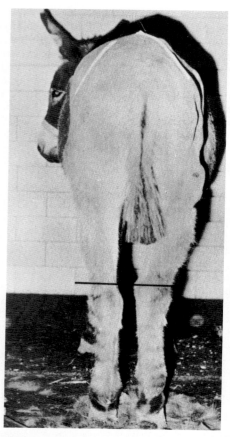

Figure 8.502 Dorsal luxation of the right coxofemoral joint in a burro. Notice the shortening of the right hindlimb, as shown by the point of the right hock being higher than the point of the left hock.

pose to subluxation and luxation with or without associated trauma.[1,2,10,12] Coxofemoral luxations may also be complicated by upward patellar fixation[4,5,14] or can occur secondary to external immobilization of the tarsus with a cast.[22] The secondary luxation is believed to occur as a result of the violent contraction of the quadriceps muscles trying to flex the limb while the stifle is locked in extension. The net result is that the head of the femur luxates out of the acetabulum rather than the stifle flexing. In cases where upward fixation of the patella precedes the luxation, the patella becomes unfixed at the time of the luxation.

Signs

A history of trauma resulting in a severe non-weight-bearing lameness is common. The femur is usually displaced upward and forward (craniodorsad) when the hip luxates (Fig. 8.502). Signs that usually accompany dislocation are a limb that appears to dangle somewhat because of shortening and the point of the hock on the affected side will be higher than that of the opposite limb. The toe and stifle turn outward and the hock turns inward (Fig. 8.500). At exercise, the horse will generally have a limited cranial stride, because of a pronounced shortening of the limb, and more prominence of the

greater trochanter of the femur. Soft tissue swelling may make this prominence difficult to determine in early stages. Crepitation of the joint, as a result of the femur rubbing on the shaft of the ilium, may cause one to think the pelvis is fractured. A rectal examination should be done to eliminate such a possibility. By placing the hand on the caudal aspect of the greater trochanter and pushing forward, one may be able to move the femur farther than is normal when dislocation has occurred.

Diagnosis

Radiography confirms the diagnosis (Fig. 8.503) and rules out pelvic fractures or a physeal fracture of the femoral head.[13,16]

Treatment

Treatment of this condition depends on several factors. If the acetabular rim has fractured, the region is further destabilized, making maintenance of the luxation reduction unlikely. If the luxation is chronic, the acetabulum fills rapidly with granulation tissue, which can prevent a successful reduction. Barring these complications the luxation can possibly be reduced while the horse is under general anesthesia.

In horses with an acute luxation that have not fractured the dorsal rim of the acetabulum, while the horse is under general anesthesia the luxation can be reduced by direct traction and manipulation if good muscle relaxation is obtained.[10,17] Traction can be applied either by using a hoist with the horse placed in dorsal recumbency or with a calf jack if lateral recumbency is selected. Traction combined with external rotation and adduction of the limb, followed by internal rotation as the traction is reduced, will complete the reduction.

Reduction can be appreciated when the hip clicks into place. Closed reduction is often difficult, and when it is successful, the reduction may fail within a few days.[4,15] In one case, an Ehmer sling was used after the second closed reduction in a pony, which improved the outcome.[6]

Several surgical approaches have been described for those cases that continue to reluxate or cannot be reduced. They include open reduction, transposition of the greater trochanter (Fig. 8.504), femoral head and neck resection (Fig. 8.505), toggle pinning, or augmentation of the lateral joint capsule with synthetic sutures attached to screws.[3,8,19] One report described the use of an experimental joint prosthesis to determine the usefulness in ponies. The implants, which were made for humans, did not work well in the ponies.[23]

To perform open reduction, the horse should be anesthetized and the area over the greater trochanter prepared for surgical procedure. An incision 8-inches long should be made cranial to the greater trochanter, and the muscles divided by blunt dissection. Traction should be placed on the foot, using a block and tackle or a calf puller, and the limb pulled downward until the head of the femur rests in the acetabulum. This can be determined by exploring with the fingers while palpating the head of the femur and the acetabulum through the incision. This operation should be done soon after the dislo-

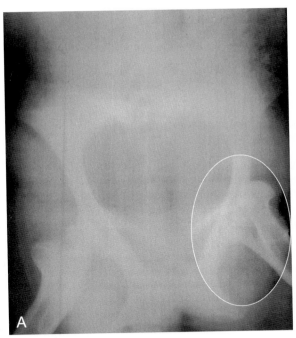 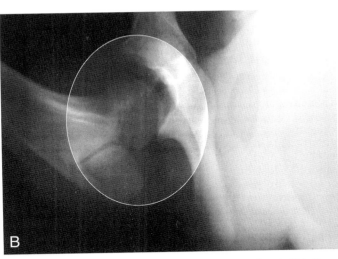

Figure 8.503   Ventral dorsal radiographic views. A. Horse with a hip luxation. Note the head of the femur on the left side is cranial to the acetabulum (oval). B. An example of a hip subluxation. Note the head of the femur is not "seated" in the acetabulum (oval). (B is provided courtesy of T. S. Stashak.)

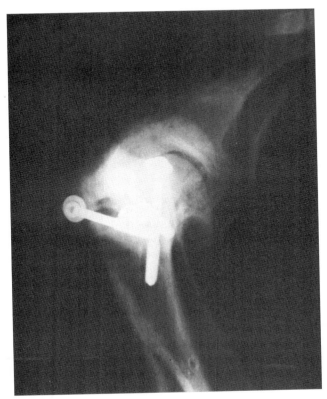 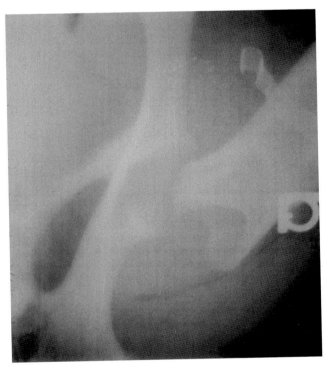

Figure 8.504   The greater trochanter was transposed to a more lateral distal position on the femur to prevent reluxation of the head of the femur. This technique has been used successfully in a calf. (Courtesy of T. S. Stashak.)

Figure 8.505   Ventral dorsal radiograph of a miniature horse after femoral head and neck excision.

cation occurs; otherwise contraction of the muscles will make it very difficult to reduce the dislocation. In some cases, muscles may be severed to facilitate relocation of the head of the femur.

If the dorsal rim of the acetabulum is fractured in association with coxofemoral luxation, simple reduction of the femur is futile. In young animals, excision of the femoral head and neck and dorsal rim of the fractured acetabulum should be considered and will aid in the development of a pseudoarthrosis.[10,11,17,21]

Prognosis

Prognosis is guarded to unfavorable. In horses, there is a better chance of the head of the femur remaining in the acetabulum if it remains in place for approximately 3 months. Horses may return to complete soundness after the head of the femur is replaced, but this is the exception. Most horses, however, can be made sound enough for breeding purposes. If the animal is valuable, surgical correction is advisable and should be done; otherwise, destruction may be necessary.

References

1. Adams OR. J Am Vet Med Assoc 1957;130:515.
2. Adams OR. Lameness in Horses. 3rd ed. Philadelphia: Lea & Febiger, 1974;299–301.
3. Adams OR. Lameness in Horses. 3rd ed. Philadelphia: Lea & Febiger, 1974;301–303.
4. Bennett D, Campbell JR, Rawlinson JR. Coxofemoral luxation complicated by upward fixation of the patella in the pony. Equine Vet J 1977;9:192–194.
5. Blackford JT, Blackford LAW. Coxofemoral joint luxation. In: Auer JA, Ed. Equine Surgery. Philadelphia: WB Saunders, 1992; 1056.
6. Clegg PD, Butson RJ. Treatment of a coxofemoral luxation secondary to upward fixation of the patella in a Shetland pony. Vet Rec 1996;138:134–137.
7. Davidson PJ. Coxofemoral subluxation in a Welsh pony. Vet Rec 1967;80(14):141–144.
8. Ducharme NG. Pelvic fracture and coxofemoral luxation. In: Nixon AJ, Ed. Equine Fracture Repair. Philadelphia: WB Saunders, 1996;295–298.
9. Dyce KM, Sack WO, Wensing CJG. The hindlimb of the horse: The hip joint. In: Textbook of Veterinary Anatomy. Philadelphia: WB Saunders, 1987;576.
10. Fessler JF, Amstutz HE. Fracture repair. In: Oehme FW, Prier JE, Eds. Textbook of Large Animal Surgery. Baltimore: Williams & Wilkins, 1974;325.
11. Field JR, McLaughlin R, Davies M. Surgical repair of coxofemoral luxation in a miniature horse. Can Vet J, 1992, 33:404–405.
12. Jogi P, Narberg I. Malformation in the hip joint of a Standardbred horse. Vet Rec 1962;74:421.
13. Lewis RE, Heinze CD. Radiographic examination of the equine pelvis: Technique. J Am Vet Med Assoc 1970;159:1387–1390.
14. Mackay-Smith MP. J Am Vet Med Assoc 1961;145(3):248–251.
15. Malark JA, Nixon AJ, Haughland MA, et al. Equine coxofemoral luxations: 17 cases (1975–1990). Cornell Vet 1992;82:79–90.
16. May SA, Patterson LJ, Peacock PJ, et al. Radiographic technique for the pelvis in the standing Horse. Equine Vet J 1991;23:312–314.
17. Nyack B, Willard MJ, Stott J, et al. Non-surgical repair of coxofemoral luxation in a Quarterhorse filly. Equine Pract 1982;6:11.
18. Platt D, Wright IM, Houlton JEF. Treatment of chronic coxofemoral luxation in a Shetland pony by excision arthroplasty of the femoral head: A case report. Br Vet J 1990;146:374–379.
19. Richardson DW. Coxofemoral luxations. In: Auer JA, Stick JA, Eds. Equine Surgery. 2nd ed. Philadelphia: WB Saunders, 1999; 885–886.
20. Rothenbacher H, Hokanson JF. Coxofemoral joint luxation in a Quarterhorse. J Am Vet Med Assoc 1965;147:148.
21. Squire KRE, Fessler JF, Toombs JP, et al. Femoral head ostectomy in horse and cattle. Vet Surg 1991;20:453–458.
22. Trotter GW, Auer JA, Warwick A, et al. Coxofemoral luxation in two foals wearing hindlimb casts. J Am Vet Med Assoc 1986;189:56.
23. Von Recum AF, Parchinski TJ, Lunceford EM, et al. Experimental coxofemoral replacement hemiarthroplasty in the pony. Vet Surg 1980;9:116–120.

OSTEOCHONDROSIS OF THE COXOFEMORAL JOINT

While subchondral cystic lesions have been described in many locations in the horse, the lesion has been reported once in the coxofemoral joint.[4]

Etiology

The etiology is assumed to be the same as for other osteochondrosis lesions. The reader is referred to Chapter 7 for more information on the etiology of osteochondrosis.

Signs

In the reported case, the horse had a stiff stilted hindlimb gait, with a low foot-flight arc and a shorted cranial phase of stride. The horse was reluctant to circle in either direction, and circling exacerbated dragging of the hind feet. Crepitus could not be elicited.[4]

Diagnosis

Diagnosis of coxofemoral disease can be achieved with intraarticular local anesthetic, although horses with a large muscle mass make the approach very difficult. Definitive diagnosis is achieved via radiography. Radiographs are generally obtained under general anesthesia.[2] A technique for radiographs of the pelvis in the standing horse has been described.[3]

Treatment

Diagnostic and operative arthroscopy has been described in the coxofemoral joint of horses. The technique is more easily performed in foals and weanlings, but can be accomplished in older horses with proper equipment.[1,5] Surgical debridement of the affected cartilage and subchondral bone would be the treatment of choice. In severe cases, a femoral head ostectomy may provide a salvage procedure for breeding soundness.[6]

Prognosis

Except in young animals in which arthroscopic debridement is successful, prognosis should be considered poor for athletic function.

References

1. Honnas CM, Zamos DT, Ford TS. Arthroscopy of the coxofemoral joint of foals. Vet Surg 1993;22:115–121.

2. Lewis RE, Heinze CD. Radiographic examination of the equine pelvis: Technique. J Am Vet Med Assoc 1971;159:1387–1390.
3. May SA, Patterson LJ, Peacock PJ, et al. Radiographic technique for the pelvis in the standing horse. Equine Vet J 1991;23:312–314.
4. Nixon AJ, Adams RM, Teigland MB. Subchondral cystic lesions (osteochondrosis) of the femoral heads in a horse. J Am Vet Med Assoc 1988;192:301–362.
5. Nixon AJ. Diagnostic and operative arthroscopy of the coxofemoral joint in horses. Vet Surg 1994;23:377–385.
6. Squire DRE, Fessler JF, Toombs JP, et al. Femoral head ostectomy in horses and cattle. Vet Surg 1991;20:453–458.

OSTEOARTHRITIS OF THE COXOFEMORAL JOINT

Osteoarthritis of the coxofemoral joint is rare.

Etiology

Any of the previously described disease processes of the coxofemoral joint can lead to osteoarthritis. Reported cases of coxofemoral joint arthritis have identified idiopathic infection,[1] a proposed hereditary basis,[2] abnormal development of the coxofemoral joint,[3–5] and trauma as etiologic agents of osteoarthritis.

Signs

The most common gait abnormality is a low arc of flight and a reduced cranial phase of stride. In horses with bilateral disease, the hindlimbs are often carried very straight with a shift of weight onto the thoracic limbs. In cases of septic arthritis, it is only possible in young foals to palpate joint swelling.

Diagnosis

The most definitive diagnosis for septic arthritis is synovial fluid analysis. Injection of local anesthetic into the coxofemoral joint can be used to localize pain to the hip. Radiographs in long-standing cases of either septic or nonseptic arthritis will often show evidence of bone remodeling (Fig. 8.506). Nuclear scintigraphy can be helpful in diagnosing cases of septic or nonseptic arthritis.

Treatment

Treatment for septic arthritis is as for other joints, including systemic antimicrobials, joint lavage, and local antimicrobial therapy. Treatment for nonseptic arthritis is palliative with the use of nonsteroidal anti-inflammatory drugs or intraarticular medications such as sodium hyaluronate, polysulfated glycosaminoglycans, or corticosteroids (refer to Chapter 7 for more information on treatment).

Prognosis

There are no long-term reports on the prognosis for septic or nonseptic arthritis of the coxofemoral joint. In

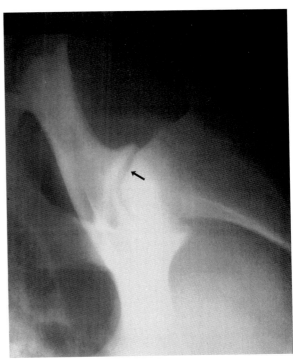

Figure 8.506 Ventral dorsal radiograph of the coxofemoral joint, showing mild osteophyte production and an altered contour of the femoral head (arrow). (Courtesy of T. S. Stashak.)

general, intraarticular therapy is difficult to achieve, and the prognosis is thought to be poor.

References

1. Clegg PD. Idiopathic infective arthritis of the coxofemoral joint in a mature horse. Vet Rec 1995;137:460–464.
2. Haakenstad LH. Undersokelser over den pathologiske hofteleddluksasjon hos hest med hensyn til lidelsens vesen og etiologiske forhold. Nord Vet Med 1953;5:884–896.
3. Jogi P, Norbery I. Malformation of the hip-joint in a Standardbred horse. Vet Rec 1962;74:421–422.
4. Speirs VC, Wrigley R. A case of bilateral hip dysplasia in a foal. Equine Vet J 1979;11:202–204.
5. Trent AM. Bilateral degenerative coxofemoral joint disease in a foal. J Am Vet Med Assoc 1985;186:284–287.

HIP DYSPLASIA

Hip dysplasia is an uncommonly reported disease in the horse.[1–4] In cases of bilateral disease, the hindlimbs are usually carried straight with a shift of weight forward onto the forelimbs. The animals will often have difficulty ambulating and if allowed to survive will often get osteoarthritis of the coxofemoral joint. Unilateral disease in ponies or miniature horses can be treated by femoral head and neck resection.

References

1. Haakenstad LH. Undersokelser over den pathologiske hofteleddluksasjon hos hest med hensyn til lidelsens vesen og etiologiske forhold. Nord Vet Med 1953;5:884–896.
2. Jogi P, Norbery I. Malformation of the hip-joint in a Standardbred horse. Vet Rec 1962;74:421–422.
3. Speirs VC, Wrigley R. A case of bilateral hip dysplasia in a foal. Equine Vet J 1979;11:202–204.
4. Trent AM. Bilateral degenerative coxofemoral joint disease in a foal. J Am Vet Med Assoc 1985;186:284–287.

Part XV

THE PELVIS

Dean A. Hendrickson

THROMBOSIS OF THE CAUDAL AORTA OR ILIAC ARTERIES

Thrombus formation in the caudal aorta, iliac arteries, or femoral artery occasionally causes lameness in horses. Such thrombi presumably cause lameness of the hindlimb as a result of circulatory interference (Fig. 8.507). Thrombus formation has also been recorded in the brachial artery of the forelimb, causing lameness of that limb. Thrombophlebitis of the external iliac vein has also been reported.[6]

Etiology

It is commonly thought that the thrombi are caused by larval forms of *Strongylus vulgaris*, which cause damage to the intima of the arteries and subsequent thrombus formation. On the basis of the findings in 38 cases, Azzie believes that *Strongylus* species are not involved in aortic/iliac thrombosis.[1] However, one should consider that larvae could damage the intima of these vessels and then be resorbed. Any damage, however slight, to the intima of these vessels could cause platelet adhesion and clot formation. Azzie proposes that trauma to the aorta and/or iliac arteries from other causes and possible hormonal factors should be considered.

Mayhew considered the possibility of disseminated intravascular coagulopathy, since fibrin-split products and decreased fibrinogen levels were reported in one case.[5] However, it is hard to explain why the coagulopathy would only be manifested locally and not in other organs as well.

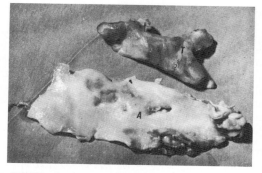

Figure 8.507 Portion of aorta (A) and its enclosed thrombus (T). The bifurcation of the thrombus on the right shows how it had occluded not only the aorta but also the iliac division. The horse afflicted with this thrombus was able to move only a few steps before incoordination and pain began. The limbs were cold and the condition was diagnosed by rectal examination, which revealed very weak pulsation in the iliac arteries.

Signs

Signs vary with the size of the thrombus and the amount of occlusion of the blood vessel. Signs also vary in the time of their appearance after exercise. If the thrombus is small and the occlusion of the vessel is not great, the horse may be exercised vigorously before lameness occurs; however, in most cases the lameness occurs shortly after exercise begins and may be confused with azoturia. While at rest, the blood supply to the muscles may be adequate to prevent lameness, but some horses will be lame even when walking.

When lameness appears, profuse sweating, pain, and anxiety occur if the horse is forced to continue the exercise. The affected limb will be cooler than the opposite member, and pulsation of the femoral artery will be less than that in the opposite limb unless both limbs are involved. An outstanding characteristic of this lameness is its intermittent character; it appears with exercise and disappears with rest. If the thrombosis is bilateral in the aorta, the horse may have difficulty in supporting its hindquarters.

The veins on the affected limb will be indistinct, while the veins on the normal limb will stand out. Another sign that may be evident if the condition is unilateral is that the affected limb will not sweat, while the opposite normal limb does.

Diagnosis

The diagnosis is established by rectal examination of the aorta and the iliac arteries. If there is a noticeable decrease of pulsation in the iliacs of the affected side or if there is fremitus in these arteries, thrombosis should be suspected. In some cases, the thrombosis may actually be palpated.[1–6,9] The femoral artery pulsation on the inside of the thigh may be compared in both limbs; this is helpful in the diagnosis. The affected limb or limbs will feel cool while in azoturia, the quadriceps muscles become hard, and urine is coffee colored. Ultrasound can be used to document the size and extent of the thrombus and its location.[2,4,7,10]

Treatment

Two cases successfully treated with sodium gluconate appear in the literature.[3,9] Both authors stress giving the drug slowly intravenously in a dosage of 500 to 600 mg/kg body weight. Alarming signs may occur during injection, and the rate must be slow (2 hours and 30 minutes to administer the dosage in 1500 mL of a 20% solution of sodium gluconate). These reports are encouraging and the methods merit trial, since other treatments are usually unsuccessful. In addition, the horse should be wormed with thiabendazole at the rate of 4 g/100 lb (4 g/45.4 kg) body weight once weekly for 3 weeks. This will aid in destroying migrating *Strongylus* larvae. The drug ivermectin may also be considered. In one report, treatment with heparin and long-term prophylaxis with Marcoumar showed clinical improvement but no change in the ultrasonographic findings.[8] Surgical removal of the thrombi with a thrombectomy catheter has been described in 2 horses, with complete reversal of the disease in 1 horse and return to limited function in the second horse.[2]

In the absence of treatment, the vessels may, in time, be able to establish collateral circulation that will overcome the effects of the thrombus. However, some horses become progressively worse and destruction is necessary.

Prognosis

Prognosis is always guarded, and unfavorable if there is bilateral involvement or if the horse seems to be getting progressively worse.

References

1. Azzie MAJ. Aortic iliac thrombosis of thoroughbred horses. Equine Vet J 1969;1(3):113.
2. Brama PAJ, Rijkenhuizen ABM, van Swieten HA, et al. Thrombosis of the aorta and the caudal arteries in the horse; additional diagnostics and a new surgical treatment. Vet Q 1996;18(Suppl 2):S85–S89.
3. Branscomb BL. Treatment of arterial thrombosis in a horse with sodium gluconate. J Am Vet Med Assoc 1968;152(11):1643.
4. Edwards GB, Allen WE. Aorto-iliac thrombosis in five horses: Clinical course of the disease and use of real time ultrasonography to confirm diagnosis. Equine Vet J 1987;20:384–391.
5. Mayhew IG, Kryger MD. Aortic-iliac-femoral thrombosis. Vet Med Small Anim Clin 1975;70:1281.
6. Miller RM. Thrombophlebitis of the external iliac vein in a horse. Vet Med Small Anim Clin 1970;65:153.
7. Reef VB, Roby DAW, Richardson DW, et al. Use of ultrasonography for the detection of aortic-iliac thrombosis in horses. J Am Vet Med Assoc 1987;190:286–288.
8. Thiébaud G, Hermann M, Flückiger M. Thrombose der aorta und der arteriae iliacae internae überprüfung der wirksamkeit einer langzeittherapie mit Marcoumar® an hand von gerinnungstests und ultraschalluntersuchungen. Pferdeheilkunde 1989;5:147–151.
9. Tillotson PJ. Treatment of aortic thrombosis in a horse. J Am Vet Med Assoc 1966;149(6):766.
10. Tithof PK, Rebhun WC, Dietze AE. Ultrasonographic diagnosis of aorto-iliac thrombosis. Cornell Vet 1985;75(4):540–544.

FRACTURES OF THE PELVIS

Fractures of the pelvis in horses are relatively uncommon, ranging from 0.9 to 4.4% of all equine lameness cases.[1,3,6] They are most commonly found in the wing and shaft of the ilium, but fractures of the tuber coxae, symphysis pubis, obturator foramen, acetabulum, and ischium also occur (Fig. 8.508).

Fractures through the wing of the ilium are usually seen in older horses (more than 6 years of age) as a sequel to the accidents that occur while jumping at high speeds, whereas fractures of the pubic bone, acetabulum, and ischium are more frequently observed in young horses.

Etiology

Trauma is the etiology in all cases. Horses that slip and fall on their sides may fracture the pelvis. Horses can also fracture the ilium by fighting a sideline or struggling while the hindlimbs are tied in a casting harness. The coxofemoral articulation of horses is rarely dislocated because of the strong formation of the hip joint; the ilium or acetabulum usually fractures instead. Acetabular fractures frequently result when the horse slips or "splits" (spread-eagles). Stress fractures of the pelvis were shown to have a high prevalence in a sample of Thoroughbred racehorses that had died for other reasons, suggesting that stress fractures of the pelvis should be considered in cases of hindlimb lameness when other areas are ruled out.[2,5]

Signs

Signs of fracture of the pelvis are variable because of the different sites of fractures.[3,4,6,7,10,12–17] However, horses are frequently presented with a history of trauma or a fall that resulted in a unilateral lameness with eventual muscle atrophy over the affected site. If the tuber coxae is fractured, very little lameness will be present, but when the horse is observed from behind, the hip on the fractured side will be flatter than the hip on the opposite side (knocked-down hip; Fig. 8.509). In some cases, the fractured pieces of bone become sequestra causing a draining tract and must be removed surgically (Fig. 8.510). In severe cases of fracture of the tuber coxae, the skin may be broken and the fractured ilium may protrude through the skin at the site of the tuber coxae.

If the shaft of the ilium is broken, it may break in front of, behind, or through the acetabulum. If there is overriding of the fragments, the limb of the affected side will appear shorter than the opposite limb. The horse will be very lame, often refusing to place the foot of the affected limb on the ground. The lameness will closely resemble hip-joint lameness when the horse walks, especially if the fracture has occurred through the acetabulum. The cranial phase of the stride will be short, and the horse will evidence pain as its weight passes onto the affected limb.

If the fracture occurs through the symphysis pubis or through the obturator foramen, the horse will often appear to be lame in both hindlimbs, walking with a hesitating gait that is short in the cranial phase of the stride. Also, swelling of the vulva or vagina from edema and hemorrhage may be observed in fillies or mares.[16]

With the exception of fracture of the tuber coxae, if the fracture is acute, limb manipulation on the affected side will cause pain, and crepitation may be felt or heard. As time passes, these signs will be reduced.

Diagnosis

The diagnosis is dependent on physical signs and examination by rectal palpation. The most accurate method of diagnosis is to move the horse while one hand is held in the rectum. Crepitation will be detected as the horse moves and often the site of fracture can be pinpointed. In some fractures of the ilium, large hematomas that are easily palpable will be present. In other cases, one of the iliac arteries may be severed by the fractured

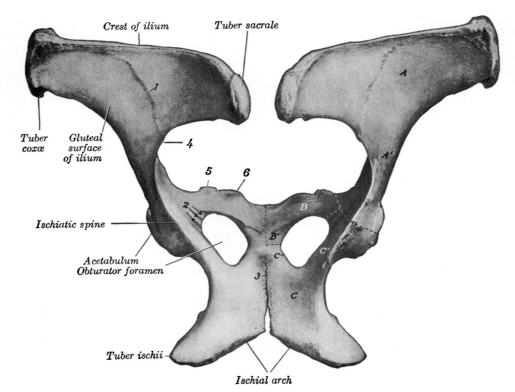

Figure 8.508   Ossa coxarum of the horse; dorsal view. A, wing of ilium; B, acetabular branch of pubis; B′, symphyseal branch of pubis; C, body of ischium; C′, acetabular branch (or shaft of ischium); C″, symphyseal branch of ischium; 1, gluteal line; 2, grooves for obturator nerve and vessels; 3, symphysis pelvis; 4, greater sciatic notch; 5, iliopectineal eminence; 6, pubic tubercle. Dotted lines indicate primitive separation of three bones, which are potential fracture sites. (Reprinted with permission from Sisson S. Equine osteology. In: Grossman JD, Ed. Anatomy of Domestic Animals. 4th ed. Philadelphia: WB Saunders, 1953.)

ilium and the horse will die shortly after injury because of internal hemorrhage. Fractures of the symphysis pubis and obturator foramen may have no hematomas, so they should be detected by movement of bone fragments on rectal palpation. Grasping the tuber coxae and attempting to move it while keeping one hand in the rectum is helpful in distorting the pelvis and producing crepitation if fracture is present. A vaginal examination should be performed on mares, for this can be most helpful in identifying fractures of the pubis and ischium.[16] Crepitation will not be obvious in all cases, so careful and continued examination is necessary for an accurate diagnosis. Separation of the sacroiliac junction and sacral fracture must be included in the differential diagnosis.[4,6,7,12–18]

If a radiographic examination can be performed, the most diagnostic study is done while the horse is under general anesthesia and placed in dorsal recumbency. Lateral radiographs are of very little value except for the identification of sacral fractures. One of the pitfalls of this pursuit of a diagnosis is the development of a more complete fracture and displacement while the horse is recovering from anesthesia. Displacement of sharp fractures may also result in laceration of large vessels (e.g., iliac arteries) associated with the pelvic region. May et al.[8] described a radiographic technique for the pelvis in the standing horse. The major benefit of this technique is obviating the need for general anesthesia and subsequent recovery.

Scintigraphy can be a useful adjuvant to diagnosing pelvic fractures. Standard scintigraphy can be misleading with the large muscle mass and proximity to the urinary bladder. Probe point counting, although more time consuming, has been shown to be very accurate in the diagnosis of pelvic fractures. Scintigraphy is the best diagnostic technique for horses with suspected stress fractures. Scintigraphy can also be used for follow-up examination to determine if bone remodeling activity has subsided.[9]

Transcutaneous ultrasonography using a 3.5-MHz probe has been shown to be beneficial in diagnosing fractures of the ilium. It is possible that using ultrasonography transrectally would be of benefit in diagnosing other pelvic fractures.[11]

Treatment

At present, no surgical methods have been devised for correcting fractures of the pelvis of horses. The best treatment appears to be to place the horse in a box stall and limit its movement. Healing of the pelvis, however, sometimes does not take place until a year after the original injury. So, if the horse is valued highly by the owner, it should not be destroyed until a year has passed, provided the horse is not suffering great pain. Close confinement will be necessary for long periods, and the maximum space requirement will be a small paddock.

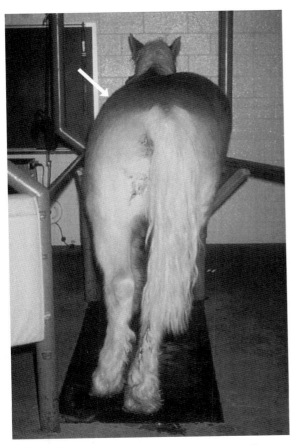

Figure 8.509 Photograph of a horse with the left tuber coxae "knocked down" (arrow).

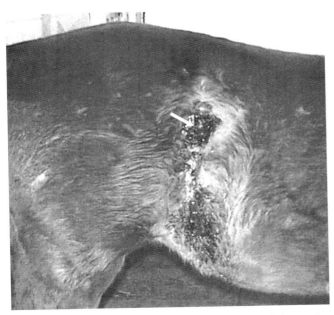

Figure 8.510 Photograph of a horse showing a draining tract caused by trauma and subsequent sequestration of the tuber coxae.

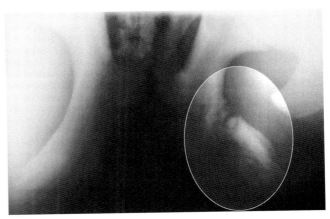

Figure 8.511 Ventral dorsal radiograph of a horse with a fracture and sequestrum of the tuber coxae.

Preferably, the horse should be box-stalled for 3 months or more. Surgical removal of a bone fragment from a fracture of the tuber coxae or tuber ischii will be necessary if the fragments become sequestra (Fig. 8.511). In some cases, it may be beneficial to sling the horse initially for a period of 6 to 8 weeks.

Prognosis

Although the prognosis is guarded in all cases, it is somewhat dependent on the location of the fracture and the animal's age. Generally, young animals with a good bony union heal more rapidly than older horses. In one report on 19 cases, 7 of 11 horses (64%) that were allowed to survive had a positive outcome for either breeding or performance.[7] Fractures through the tuber coxae, tuber ischii, and tuber sacrale offer a better prognosis for return to soundness. Sequestrum may develop, requiring surgical excision. Fractures through the wing of the ilium and the body of the ischium offer a reasonably good prognosis, whereas fractures through the body of the pubis, shaft of the ilium, and acetabulum are attendant with a poor prognosis. Fractures through the acetabulum frequently result in degenerative joint disease of the coxofemoral joint (coxitis). Other complications to consider are lacerations of major vessels, leading to death, and the development of a large callus with displacement of the fracture such that the pelvic canal diameter is reduced to the point that brood mare status may be out of the question.

References

1. British Equine Veterinary Association. Survey of equine disease 1962–1963. Vet Rec 1965;77:528.
2. Carrier TK, Estberg L, Stover SM, et al. Association between long periods without high-speed workouts and risk of complete humeral or pelvic fracture in Thoroughbred racehorses: 54 cases (1991–1994). J Am Vet Med Assoc 1998;212:1582–1587.
3. Cochran D. Lameness of the hip joint. Am Vet Rev 1913;43:491.
4. Ducharme NG. Pelvic fracture and coxofemoral luxation. In: Nixon AJ, Ed. Equine Fracture Repair. Philadelphia: WB Saunders,1996;295–298.
5. Haussler KK, Stover SM. Stress fractures of the vertebral lamina and pelvis in Thoroughbred racehorses. Equine Vet J 1998;30:374–381.

6. Jeffcott LB. Pelvic lameness in the horse. Equine Pract 1982;4:21.
7. Little C, Hilbert B. Pelvic fractures in horses: 19 cases (1974–1984). J Am Vet Med Assoc 1987;190:1203–1206.
8. May SA, Patterson LJ, Peacock PJ, et al. Radiographic technique for the pelvis in the standing horse. Equine Vet J 1991;23:312–314.
9. Pilsworth RC, Holmes MA, Sheperd M. An improved method for the scintigraphic detection of acute bone damage to the equine pelvis by probe point counting. Vet Rec 1993;133:490–495.
10. Pilsworth RC, Sheperd M, Herinckx BMB, et al. Fracture of the wing of the ilium, adjacent to the sacroiliac joint, in Thoroughbred racehorses. Equine Vet J 1994;26:94–99.
11. Reef VB. Diagnosis of pelvic fractures in horses using ultrasonography. Vet Radiol 1992;33:121.
12. Richardson DW. The femur and pelvis. In: Auer JA, Stick J, Eds. Equine Surgery. 2nd ed. Philadelphia: WB Saunders, 1999; 881–886.
13. Rutkowski JA, Richardson DW. The diagnosis and treatment of pelvic fractures in horses. Proc Am Assoc Equine Pract 1987;33: 701–705.
14. Rutkowski JA, Richardson DW. A retrospective study of 100 pelvic fractures in horses. Equine Vet J 1989;21:256–259.
15. Shepherd MC, Pilsworth RC, Hopes R, et al. Clinical signs, diagnosis, management and outcome of complete and incomplete fracture to the ilium: A review of 20 cases. Proc Am Assoc Equine Pract 1994;40:1777–1806.
16. Stashak TS. Fractures of the pelvis. In: Stashak TS, Ed. Adams' Lameness in Horses. 4th ed. Philadelphia: Lea & Febiger, 1987; 752–753.
17. Vaughan JT. Analysis of lameness in the pelvic limb and selected cases. Proc Am Assoc Equine Pract 1965;11:223.
18. Wheat JO. Lameness' of the hip. Proc Am Assoc Equine Pract 1973;19:301–302.

LESIONS OF THE ISCHIAL TUBEROSITY

Lameness associated with the ischial tuberosity (Tuber ischii) or avulsion of the origin of the semitendinosus muscle is not a common cause of lameness in horses.

Etiology

The most common cause appears to be use-related trauma; however, the condition may be present with other diseases of the pelvic region (e.g., sacroiliac sprain). In some horses, a history of slipping with the hindlimb getting caught underneath a fixed object may be revealed.

Signs

A history of poor performance is often given. In most cases no changes in the contour of the tuber ischii region will be seen. However, horses that have a history of slipping and getting the affected hindlimb caught underneath a fixed object may exhibit evidence of fibrosis at the proximal attachment (origin) of the semitendinosus muscle. This is most often seen in chronic cases (Fig. 8.512). In some cases pain may be elicited when pressure is applied over the tuber ischii. At exercise, a moderate to severe lameness, with a shortened cranial phase of stride and positive upper limb flexion, may be present.

Diagnosis

Lameness of the lower limb is ruled out with diagnostic anesthesia. Scintigraphy is more sensitive than radiog-

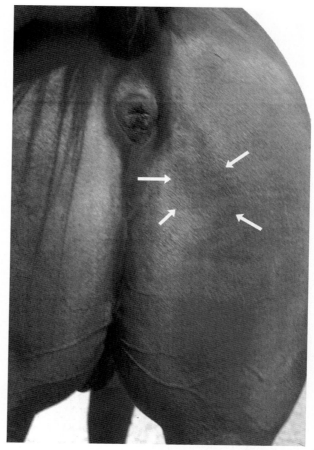

Figure 8.512 Photograph of a horse with fibrosis of the origin of the semitendinosus muscle and deviation of the anus to the right side. The fibrosis resulted in a visual depression in the muscle (arrows). This horse sustained the injury from slipping and getting its hindlimb caught underneath a trailer 3 months ago. (Courtesy of T. S. Stashak.)

raphy in localizing the source of lameness to the ischial tuberosity, especially in those cases without visual evidence of trauma (Fig. 8.513).

Treatment

The treatment of choice for injury to the tuber ischii or avulsion of the semitendinosus origin is box stall confinement until healing of the avulsion has occurred. This should be followed by controlled exercise beginning 2 to 4 weeks postinjury and for at least 3 months. Adding obstacles for the horse to step over can be done to improve the range of motion in the affected hindlimb. Follow-up scintigraphy may also be done to determine when complete healing has occurred.

Prognosis

Prognosis for return to function is good.

Reference

1. Geissbuhler U, Busato A, Ueltschi G. Abnormal bone scan findings of the equine ischial tuberosity and third trochanter. Vet Radiol Ultrasound 1998;39:572–577.

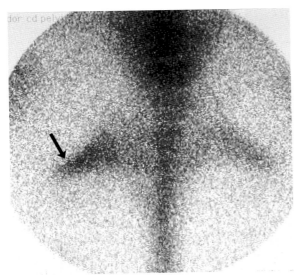

Figure 8.513 Nuclear scintigraphy of the caudal pelvis, showing increased uptake of radiopharmaceutical in the tuber ischii (arrow). (Courtesy of T. S. Stashak.)

SUBLUXATION OF THE SACROILIAC JOINT (SACROILIAC STRAIN)

Injury to the sacroiliac joint of the horse is a common finding. The sacroiliac joint in the horse is a diarthrosis formed between the articular surfaces of the sacrum and the ilium (Figs. 8.514 and 8.515).[16] The surfaces are not smooth in the adult, but are marked by reciprocal eminences and depressions covered by a thin layer of cartilage. The joint cavity is only a cleft and is often crossed by fibrous bands. The joint capsule is very close fitting and is attached around the margins of the articular surfaces. The joint is reinforced by a ventral sacroiliac ligament that surrounds the joint (see Figs. 8.514 and 8.515). This is a very strong ligament above, where it occupies the angle between the ilium and the wing of the sacrum, and it consists chiefly of nearly vertical fibers. Movement in the joint is inappreciable in the adult, with

stability, not mobility, being desirable. In addition to the ventral sacroiliac ligament, there is a dorsal sacroiliac ligament, which is a strong band attached to the tuber sacrale and the summits of the sacral spines. There is also a lateral sacroiliac ligament, which is attached in front to the tuber sacrale and adjacent part of the medial border of the ilium above the greater sciatic notch and below to the lateral border of the sacrum. It blends above with the dorsal sacroiliac ligament, below with the sacrosciatic ligament, and behind with the coccygeal fascia. The sacral surface is primarily covered by hyaline cartilage, while the iliac surface is covered by fibrocartilage. There has been deterioration of the cartilage noted with the increasing age of horses.[3-5] Because the sacroiliac joint is not meant to be mobile, stresses that produce motion may produce subluxation. Once the continuity of the joint is disturbed, there may be chronic pain resulting from the partial displacement and instability. Reflex muscular spasm will usually be present until healing by scar tissue is sufficient to prevent any mobility in the joint. Ligament injury heals by scar tissue and therefore is subject to reinjury.

Etiology

Falls, slipping, and any other trauma that causes twisting or high stress to the sacroiliac joint can cause the lameness.[12,13,15] Rooney feels that sacroiliac arthrosis and subluxation results from repeated trauma rather than a single event and is probably an important underrated entity in harness-race horses.[14] Others that are at high risk are horses that work primarily at gaits other than a gallop (draft, carriage, and endurance horses).[2] In a postmortem study of thoroughbred racehorses that had either died or were euthanatized, 2 of 36 horses had acute sacroiliac joint injury.[6] One horse had flipped over backwards and sustained a skull fracture and had an avulsion fracture of the S1–S4 lateral sacral crest at the insertion of the dorsal sacroiliac ligament. Another horse had obvious laxity of the sacroiliac joint bilaterally. Degenerative arthritic changes were noted in the sacroiliac articulation in all specimens.

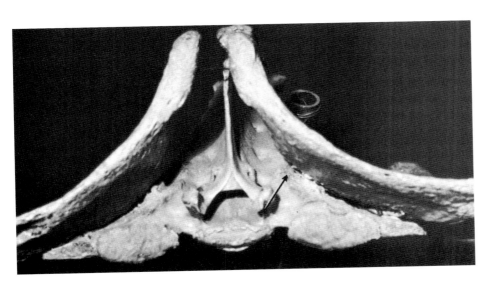

Figure 8.514 Skeletal model of the sacroiliac joint. Arrow points between the sacrum and ilium. (Reprinted with permission from Adams OR. Subluxation of the sacroiliac joint in horses. Proc Am Assoc Equine Pract 1969:191.)

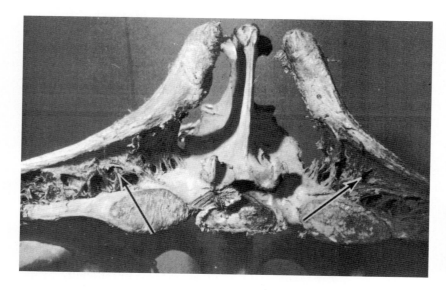

Figure 8.515 Skeletal model of the sacroiliac joint. Arrows point to dried and separated ventral sacroiliac ligament. (Reprinted with permission from Adams OR. Subluxation of the sacroiliac joint in horses. Proc Am Assoc Equine Pract 1969:191.)

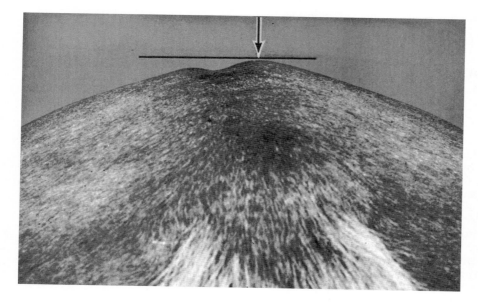

Figure 8.516 Arrow points to upward displacement of tuber sacrale. The view is over the rump of the horse, looking forward. This area may move when the horse is walking and may show unilateral or bilateral displacement in subluxation of the sacroiliac joint.

Signs

A typical history is of chronic intermittent lameness that "waxes and wanes with use." The lameness is often most prominent when the horse has been worked hard. The clinical signs of subluxation of the sacroiliac joint are highly variable.[1,2,7,8,11–15] Usually stiffness and pain in the hindquarters are shown, with considerable variation in the signs. Pain may be elicited with intermittent firm downward pressure on the tuber coxae causing rotation of the pelvis and movement of the sacroiliac joint.[1] There is often some surrounding muscular pain caused by spasm of the surrounding muscles in their attempt to reestablish the rigidity of the sacroiliac joint. The condition is most often chronic, and the tuber sacrale may become prominent either unilaterally or bilaterally depending on whether one or both sides are involved (Figs. 8.516 and 8.517). The prominence of one or both of the tuber sacrale (hunter's bumps) is due to subluxation of

one or both sacroiliac joints. It is important to recognize that fracture of the wing of the ilium adjacent to the sacroiliac joint may cause signs of lameness similar to that of sacroiliac disease. Crepitation can sometimes be produced by applying finger and thumb pressure over the sacroiliac region, causing the horse to exhibit lordosis.

Rooney describes two acute cases in which the horses went down and were destroyed.[12–13] He also describes shortening of the stride, limitation in hindlimb joint movement, and reluctance to jump. The lameness may be unilateral or bilateral depending on whether one or both sides are involved. The common complaint in the hunter-jumper horse is that the horse is stiff and refuses to jump, or does a poor job of it. Apparently, the lameness with subluxation of the sacroiliac joint is caused by inflammation resulting from instability of the joint(s) and sympathetic muscular spasm. Dissimilarity or protrusion of the tuber sacrale, either unilaterally or bilater-

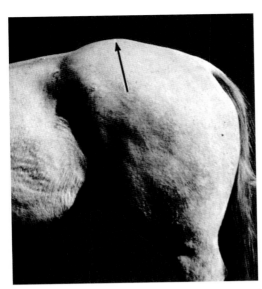

Figure 8.517 Side view showing location of tuber sacrale (arrow). This point should be closely observed when a horse walks for signs of movement and, in old cases, for signs of unilateral or bilateral displacement. (Reprinted with permission from Adams OR. Subluxation of the sacroiliac joint in horses. Proc Am Assoc Equine Pract 1969:191–207.)

ally, may be present in a horse not now affected with the condition (see Fig. 8.516). This can happen if a previous lesion has healed solidly and no motion is now present in the joint(s).

Clinical signs of sacroiliac arthrosis are most clearly seen in the harness-race horse at the trotting and pacing gaits and are rarely seen at the walk.[2] It is best to observe the horse after a fast workout. Characteristic signs include the affected pelvic limb's staying on the ground too long and then suddenly being jerked forward.[11] Normally, the hind feet impact the ground before the fore feet; however, with sacroiliac luxation, the fore feet hit first because subprotraction of the hindlimb is delayed. A hiking or jerking motion of the hip is commonly observed early on when the horse is exercised in circles. Later, hiking occurs when the horse is trotted in a straight line.

Rooney suggests that the Gaenslen's test, used by human orthopedic surgeons, may be helpful in the identification of sacroiliac arthrosis.[15] It is performed like a spavin test, except that the limb opposite the affected limb is flexed for 1.5 to 2 minutes; then the horse is trotted off and observed for stiffness and abnormal rolling of the croup of the affected side.

Rectal examination findings of sacroiliac subluxation will not be diagnostic unless enough motion is present in the joint to produce some crepitation. Crepitation in the pelvis is difficult to pinpoint because of bone conduction. The rectal examination should be done while the horse is walking slowly and while pressure is put on the tuber coxae in an effort to produce rotation of the pelvis and crepitation.

Rocking the horse back and forth, causing the horse to shift its weight from one hindlimb to the other, often produces the crepitation necessary for diagnosis of the

condition. The hand in the rectum should be held on the bottom of the sacrum as close to the sacroiliac junction as possible. When the horse is walking, movement of one or both tuber sacrale may be noticeable. In inactive cases, nonmovable displacement (hunter's bumps) will be present unilaterally or bilaterally.

Diagnosis

Prior to the advent of nuclear scintigraphy, the diagnosis of sacroiliac subluxation was dependent upon elimination of other causes of pain. In some cases of sacroiliac subluxation, there may be slight motion of one or both tuber sacrale during walking. Close observation should be made at this point. Whenever there is unevenness or excessive prominence (hunter's bumps) of the tuber sacrale, one should consider that at least at one time there has been movement and subluxation of this joint (see Fig. 8.516). Nuclear scintigraphic imaging of the pelvis from the dorsal view has been reported as being extremely accurate in confirming or ruling out cases of sacroiliac dislocation.[17,18] Increased uptake of the radionucleotide indicates disruption and remodeling of the articulation (Fig. 8.518). Scintigraphy can also be used to determine when bone remodeling has diminished.

Although radiographic studies require special equipment, they can be informative. Slight rotation of the pelvis or sacrum can be identified along with widening of the sacroiliac joint space, and in some, degenerative changes can be observed.[7]

Treatment

Patience, as with any type of ligamentous disruption, is very important in treating subluxation of the sacroiliac

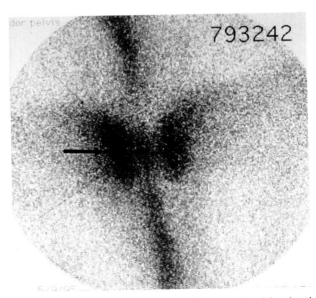

Figure 8.518 Nuclear scintigraphy of the dorsal pelvis, showing increased uptake of radiopharmaceutical in the left sacroiliac joint (arrow). (Courtesy of T. S. Stashak.)

joint. Complete rest, preferably in a box stall for at least 45 days, is recommended. Hand walking for 5 minutes 2 times a day for up to 5 days a week is begun during the third or fourth week of confinement. The horse can be backed up for 10 steps when it is taken out of confinement before hard walking is begun and backed up 10 steps before it is put back into confinement. Backing the horse is believed to create movement that may improve alignment and healing of the sacroiliac region. During controlled exercise the horse is encouraged to step over obstacles, which at first are low in height and increase in height as time passes. The obstacles are often placed 40 to 50 yards apart. Exercise is usually increased by 2.5 minutes/week up to a maximum of 20 minutes 2 times a day, 5 days a week. After 45 days the horse is allowed access to a small run if lameness has improved. Generally, the patient is reevaluated in 90 days and the decision for increasing exercise is made at this time. It usually takes 8 to 10 months of rest and controlled exercise before horses are ready to return to training and performance. Complementary therapy including acupuncture, chiropractic manipulation, and massage therapy can be considered, especially to reduce muscle spasm. Phenylbutazone may need to be administered for 14 to 21 days, depending on the degree of lameness and pain on manipulation. Intravenous administration of sodium hyaluronate 1 treatment/week for 4 weeks, followed by monthly administration, has also been recommended.

Prognosis

Prognosis is always guarded, and in those cases in which there had been repeated injury and extensive injury and/or weakening of the ligamentous attachments, healing might never occur. Prognosis is more favorable for horses that have convalesced successfully and appear healed, exhibiting no painful lameness. However, in a study of Standardbred Trotters, horses that had asymmetry of the sacroiliac region had lower earnings, lower number of races, and slower race times than normal horses. It was suggested that Trotters with asymmetry are less likely to become successful racehorses.[2] A healed injury of this type is probably more subject to reinjury and damage than is the normal sacroiliac joint, and owners should be cautioned to avert such injury if at all possible.

References

1. Adams OR. Subluxation of the sacroiliac joint in horses. Proc Am Assoc Equine Pract 1969;15:191.
2. Dalin G, Magnusson LE, Thafvelin BC. Retrospective study of hindquarter asymmetry in Standardbred Trotters and its correlation with performance. Equine Vet J 1985;17:292–296.
3. Dalin G, Jeffcott LB. Sacroiliac joint of the horse: 1. Gross morphology. Anat Histol Embryol 1986;15:80–94.
4. Dalin G, Jeffcott LB. Sacroiliac joint of the horse: 2. Morphometric features. Anat Histol Embryol 1986;15:97–107.
5. Dalin G, Jeffcott LB. Sacroiliac joint of the horse: 3. Histological appearance. Anat Histol Embryol 1986;15:108–121.
6. Haussler KK, Stover SM, Willis NH. Pathologic changes in the lumbosacral vertebrae and pelvis in Thoroughbred racehorses. Am J Vet Res 1999;60:143–163.
7. Jeffcott LB. Pelvic lameness in the horse. Equine Pract 1982;4:21.
8. Jeffcott LB, Dalin G, Ekman S, et al. Sacroiliac lesions as a cause of chronic poor performance in competitive horses. Equine Vet J 1985;17:111–118.
9. Pilsworth RC, Sheperd M, Herinckx BMB, et al. Fracture of the wing of the ilium, adjacent to the sacroiliac joint, in Thoroughbred racehorses. Equine Vet J 1994;26:94–99.
10. Roberts EJ. Resection of thoracic or lumbar spinous processes for the relief of pain responsible for lameness and some other locomotor disorders of horses. Proc Am Assoc Equine Pract 1968;14:13.
11. Rooney JR. Biomechanics of Lameness in Horses. Baltimore: Williams & Wilkins, 1969;90–95.
12. Rooney JR. Sacroiliac luxation in the horse. Proc Am Assoc Equine Pract 1969;15:193.
13. Rooney JR. Sacroiliac luxation in the horse. Equine Vet J 1969;1(6):287.
14. Rooney JR. Sacroiliac arthrosis and stifle lameness. Mod Vet Pract 1977;58:138.
15. Rooney JR. The horse's back: Biomechanics of lameness. Equine Pract 1982;4:17.
16. Sisson S. In: Getty GR, Ed. Sisson and Grossman's The Anatomy of the Domestic Animals. 5th Ed. Philadelphia: WB Saunders, 1975;362–363.
17. Steckel RR. The role of scintigraphy in the lameness evaluation. Vet Clin North Am Equine Pract 1991;7:207–239.
18. Tucker RL, Schneider RK, Sondhof AH, et al. Bone scintigraphy in the diagnosis of sacroiliac injury in twelve horses. Equine Vet J 1998;30:390–395.

THE SACRAL-COCCYGEAL REGION

Injuries of the sacral and coccygeal region have rarely been documented. Injury can result in lameness, gait abnormalities, dysfunction in micturition, and defecation.

Etiology

The most common history on presentation is that of trauma from a sudden fall.[1-3] In a report of 10 cases, 4 of 10 had a history of acute onset following a fall or sitting down after pulling back against a rope.[1]

Signs

Presenting signs will vary with the extent of the trauma. In one report of 10 horses, 2 of 10 had trouble defecating and micturating, 5 of 10 had distortion of the pelvis and tail, 8 of 10 had gait and lameness abnormalities, 10 of 10 showed pain on digital pressure, and 3 of 10 had increased pain with hind leg flexion.[1] Manual elevation of the tail will often cause discomfort for the horse.

Diagnosis

Diagnostics that have been used in these cases have included physical examination, radiographs, scintigraphy, and electromyography. Radiographs were beneficial in 7 of 8 cases, whereas scintigraphy was beneficial in all 4 cases that it was used on. A caudal epidural contrast study was performed in one horse and confirmed compression of the region.[1]

Treatment

Caudal epidural steroid administration, which is commonly used in humans, has been used to successfully treat this condition. Methylprednisolone acetate at a dose of 200 mg diluted in distilled water to a volume of 20 mL has been prescribed. With continued pain on palpation, the treatment can be repeated in 2 to 3 weeks.[1] Surgery may be indicated in cases of comminuted fractures or with severe fracture displacement.[2,3]

Prognosis

Improvement was seen in 5 of 7 horses in one study with medical treatment with mixed results to surgical intervention.[1]

References

1. Grant BD, Cannon JH, Rantanen NW, et al. Medical and surgical treatment of sacral-coccygeal pathology. Proc Am Assoc Equine Pract 1998;44:213–215.
2. Collatos C, Allen D, Chambers J, et al. Surgical treatment of sacral fracture in a horse. J Am Vet Med Assoc 1997;198:877–879.
3. Nixon A. Equine Fracture Repair. Philadelphia: WB Saunders, 1996; 310–311.

Part XVI

THE THORACOLUMBAR SPINE

Dean A. Hendrickson

ASSOCIATED BACK PROBLEMS

There is little doubt that back problems associated with the thoracolumbar spine are an important cause of altered performance in horses. Two surveys carried out in the United Kingdom indicate the incidences of back problems ranging from 0.9% in general practice to 94% in a specialty referral practice.[1,11] A higher incidence of thoracolumbar problems has also been noted in competitive jumpers (show and eventing) and dressage horses.[11] In a postmortem study involving 36 Thoroughbred racehorses that had died or been euthanatized, there was impingement of the dorsal spinous processes in 92% of the horses and impingement of the transverse processes in 97%.[7]

Although a wide range of problems can affect the thoracolumbar spine, they can be separated into three major categories: 1) congenital deformities of the spine, 2) soft tissue injury, and 3) bony problems associated with the vertebra. Congenital deformities of the thoracolumbar spine include abnormalities in the curvature (scoliosis or lordosis) and vertebral fusion (synostosis). Soft tissue problems include sprained muscles, strained ligaments, disc disease, diskospondylitis, and skin lesions from sitfast and warbles underneath the saddle area. Bone damage includes ossifying spondylosis, spondylosis deformans, overriding of the dorsal spinous processes, arthrosis of the articular processes, and fractures of the dorsal spinous processes, articular processes, neural arch, and vertebral bodies.[4,6,8,10,12,13,24,25] Fractures that frequently result in myelopathy will be covered under "Wobbler Syndrome" in this chapter.

Although there is an acute awareness that back problems exist and the back is frequently examined as a site of lameness, it is still difficult to obtain a definitive diagnosis. The diagnosis is difficult because of the variable clinical picture, variable temperament of the horse, the inability to directly palpate and manipulate the thoracolumbar vertebrae, and the expensive equipment required to achieve images of this region. To add to the confusion, sensitive skin (thin-skinned) horses and "cold-backed" horses persistently resent palpation of the back, which may be incorrectly interpreted as a back problem. "Cold-backed" horses that show a persistent hypersensitivity over the back and hip and stiffen the back when the rider first mounts the horse rarely have radiographic changes. After the initial stiffness is gone, no effect in performance is noted. The question of whether the reaction resulted from pain or guarding because of previous injury or simply the horse's temperament is unknown. The possibility of peripheral nerve lesions such as those seen in humans has not been explored or evaluated in the horse.[13] It is important that other sources of lameness, such as hindlimb lameness, be ruled out before a diagnosis of primary back soreness is made.

Etiology

Although there are many causes of back injury (direct trauma, poor-fitting saddles, improper seating of the rider, twisting and wrenching of the spine), there appears to be a correlation between the horse's conformation, sex, what it is used for, and breed as to the type of injury that is sustained.[11–13]

Generally, horses that are short-backed with limited flexibility are more prone to vertebral lesions, whereas horses with long flexible backs are affected more frequently with muscular and ligament strain. Mares are more frequently affected with ossifying spondylosis, and overriding of the dorsal spinous processes is more frequently observed in geldings.[12] Where sacroiliac strain is most prevalent in horses jumping at speeds, bone damage to the thoracolumbar spine is more frequent in competitive jumpers. Musculoligamentous strain occurs with about equal frequency no matter what type of jumping is involved.[11] Thoroughbred racehorses are more frequently affected with soft tissue injury than with lesions to the vertebrae. Also, bone damage to the thoracolumbar spine is most likely to be centered around the midpoint of the back, while soft tissue injury is more frequently just caudal to the withers and over the loin.[12] Stress fractures of the vertebra most likely occur more frequently than previously observed. In one study, 18 of 36 specimens had incomplete fractures and focal periosteal proliferation of the lamina stemming from vertebral stress fractures.[7] The fractures occurred most commonly near the junction of the cranial articular process and the spinous process.

Osteoarthritis of the articular processes has been noted in horses. In a review of 36 Thoroughbred horses, 97% of the horses showed variable degrees of osteoarthritis, which should be considered as a possible source of back pain.[7]

Rooney feels that spondylosis deformans results from excessive dorsiflexion that occurs when the horse's back muscles fatigue. This in turn leads to tearing of the ventral and ventrolateral aspects of the anulus fibrosus, compressing the intervertebral joint and eventually leading to impingement of the dorsal spinous processes.[22] In the most advanced cases, fusion occurs between the intervertebral joints.

Signs

Horses with chronic thoracolumbar problems frequently present with a history of loss of performance indicated by stiffness, inability to stride out, lack of enthusiasm for work, and lack of fluidity and timing when jumping.[3,10,12,14,16] Owners will often relate a loss of "suppleness" in the back. Horses that have sustained recent acute trauma to the vertebral column exhibit rather precise signs of back pain that are usually easy to localize. In those with fracture, stiffness, malalignment of the vertebral column, and a neurologic deficiency may be a part of the history.

On visual examination, the horse should be viewed from the side to gain an appreciation for the dorsoventral curvature (lordosis or kyphosis) of the spine and the alignment of the summits of the dorsal spinous processes. An elevation or swelling may indicate trauma to the soft tissue or dorsal spinous processes from the saddle if it is located over the withers or from a fall if it is located in the caudal, thoracic, or lumbar region (Fig. 8.519). Atrophy of the dorsal musculature should also be noted. The sacroiliac and sacrococcygeal regions are best viewed from behind while the horse is standing square on all four limbs. The alignment of the sacrococcygeal region and typical signs of hunter's bumps should be

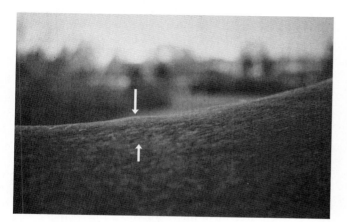

Figure 8.519   Photograph of the caudal thoracic spine of a horse showing focal muscle atrophy (lower arrow) and elevation of the dorsal spinous processes (upper arrow). (Courtesy of T. S. Stashak.)

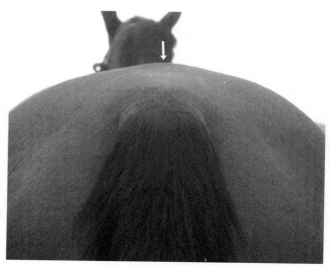

Figure 8.520   Photograph of a horse showing malalignment of the sacrococcygeal region. Note the pelvis is asymmetric and there is a proximal displacement of the tuber sacrale (hunter's bump) on the right side, indicating a subluxation of the sacroiliac joint (arrow). Also note the tail head is rotated clockwise. This horse presented with a history of poor performance as a jumper. (Courtesy of T. S. Stashak.)

noted (refer to sacroiliac subluxation [Fig. 8.520]). The lateral curvature of the thoracolumbar spine is best appreciated from above while the animal is standing square on all four limbs and the head and neck are held straight. Abnormal curvature of the thoracolumbar spine may indicate vertebral injury, malformation, or muscle spasms (spastic scoliosis) (Fig. 8.521). Epaxial muscle atrophy may be seen in some horses with chronic severe back pain.

On palpation, sensitive (thin-skinned) horses or "cold-backed" horses will frequently withdraw rapidly when palpated over the thoracolumbar spine. This is often misconstrued as a sign of back soreness emanating from the spine or musculoligamentous support structures when, in fact, it is more likely a sign of skin sensitivity. The open hand with fingers extended should be used to evaluate back pain. Hands are gently run along the dorsal epaxial muscles from the withers to the base of the tail. Asymmetry should be noted. The pressure is increased after each passage. A positive sign of back pain is elicited when the horse cringes and the muscle firmness (spasm) is evidenced over the site of the lesion. The muscle response of the horse is one of guarding to prevent movement of the affected region. Some horses will exhibit a more dramatic response and grunt, kick, or rear when pressure is applied. In any case, this sign should be repeatable and the intensity should not decrease with subsequent palpation. The dorsal spinous processes are palpated; they should be evenly spaced, axially aligned, and about the same height except for the elevations associated with the withers and the depression associated with the lumbosacral junction.

Lateral flexion of the back is assessed by running a ballpoint pen down from the longissimus dorsi muscle to the lateral thoracic and paralumbar regions. This is done on both sides. Horses with back problems often

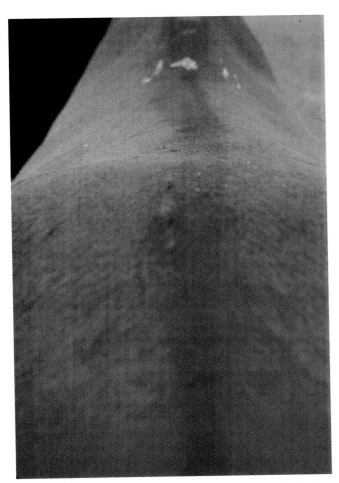

Figure 8.521 Dorsal view of the horse in Figure 8.520 showing abnormal curvature of the spine. It is important when making this assessment that the horse is standing square and the head and neck are in axial alignment with the body. (Courtesy of T. S. Stashak.)

exhibit less expressive (reduced) lateral flexion and guard against it by splinting the musculature. Extension (elevation) of the back is checked by running a ballpoint pen over each croup. Again, reluctance to flex is often indicative of a problem. Usually, the most affected side shows the least amount of movement. Horses with very sore backs may be reluctant to fully flex their neck from side to side and consequently are reluctant to eat off the ground. A rectal examination is usually performed to evaluate the sublumbar muscles. Although rectal examinations are rarely informative for thoracolumbar problems, they can be beneficial in identifying problems associated with the sacroiliac, sacral, and sacrococcygeal regions.

At exercise a stiffness of the back is usually appreciated, particularly when the horse is turned sharply to one side or the other. A shortening of the stride with decreased hock flexion and a tendency to drag the toes may also be evident. Signs like these make it difficult to make a distinction between back soreness and hock and stifle lameness. If the pain is quite severe, horses may exhibit a wide straddling hindlimb gait.[14] Horses may

also exhibit a reduction in the normal truncal sway (side-to-side movement of the trunk), which is best observed from the rear while the horse is walking. On backing, the horse may be reluctant at first to raise its head. When moving backward it may do so in a rather awkwardly flexed position.

Lunging the horse at a trot for 10 to 15 minutes may exacerbate the condition. Prior to exercise a blood sample should be taken to obtain baseline data on serum muscle enzymes, aminoaspartate transferase, and creatinine kinase. While lunging, the horse with thoracolumbar problems will often show exaggerated contraction of the longissimus dorsi muscle. Some may elevate their heads higher than normal and may be reluctant to stride out or change leads. Although not definitive for back pains, some horses will switch their tails incessantly. After exercise, another blood sample is taken immediately and 18 to 24 hours later. Active muscle damage is identified by a 2- to 5-fold increase in muscle enzymes as compared to resting levels.

Diagnosis

Because a lot of the signs associated with thoracolumbar pain are nonspecific, other conditions considered in the differential diagnosis should be ruled out. They include problems associated with the pelvis, stifle, and hock joints primarily, but compressive myelopathy, bad-fitting saddles, and temperament problems should also be considered. Muscle damage can be identified by a 2- to 5-fold increase in serum enzymes.

Nuclear scintigraphy has provided perhaps the most important single major advance in the diagnosis of primary back disease. It is a very sensitive technique but is not very specific. It can be performed on the standing horse while under sedation. Commonly identified lesions include impinging dorsal spinous processes, while less commonly found are fractured vertebra and ribs.[19,23] Other conditions include arthritis of thoracolumbar articular facets, pathologic nondisplaced fracture of the dorsal spinous process, vertebral osteomyelitis, and diskospondylitis. A ciprofloxacin scan can be performed to definitively diagnose osteomyelitis or a diskospondylitis (see "Vertebral Osteomyelitis and Diskospondylitis" in this chapter).

Radiographs will often be necessary to accurately diagnose the condition, whereas scintigraphy can show the location of the disease process.[19] Radiographic examination of the thoracolumbar spine, although difficult, is most valuable for the identification of vertebral lesions (Figs. 8.522 and 8.523). However, a negative radiographic examination does not mean the thoracolumbar spine is not involved. Powerful equipment is required to radiograph the horse's vertebral column and up to 150 KV and 500 MAS may be required for large horses.[12] Although equipment is now available to examine the thoracolumbar spine in the standing horse, better films are usually obtained while the horse is under general anesthesia (Fig. 8.524). For radiographic evaluation of the iliac regions it is necessary to place the horse on its back under general anesthesia so that the ventral dorsal view can be taken.

Various soft tissue injuries can be diagnosed with ultrasound examination. Areas that can be imaged include

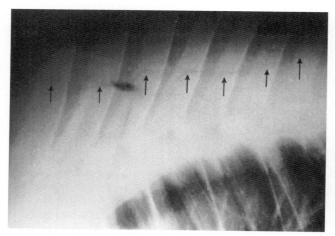

Figure 8.522 Lateral radiograph of the withers of a horse, indicating fracture of the dorsal spinous processes of T4 through T10 (arrows).

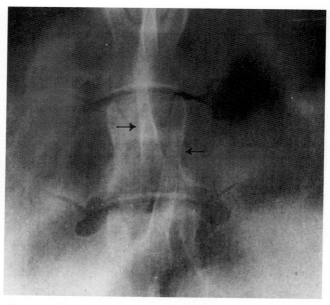

Figure 8.524 Dorsal ventral radiograph of the lumbar spine. Note two spinous processes (arrows) are displaced to opposite sides, indicating fracture of the spinous processes. (Courtesy of T. S. Stashak.)

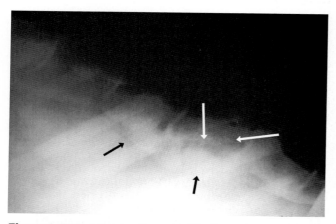

Figure 8.523 Lateral radiograph of the horse shown in Figure 8.519, revealing a spondylopathy of the caudal thoracic vertebrae. Proliferative bone is attempting to bridge the intervertebral space (black arrows). Note the indistinct collapsed intervertebral space (white arrows). (Courtesy of T. S. Stashak.)

Definitive diagnosis of back pain is difficult at best, and in many cases, multiple structures are involved. It is important to look at the entire horse and rule out other causes of lameness, such as forelimb or hindlimb lameness, that may be contributing to the back soreness. In some cases, direct infiltration of a local anesthetic can be used to confirm the location of the disease process (e.g., impingement of the dorsal spinous processes).

Treatment

Anti-inflammatories and long-term parenteral administration of analgesics have been utilized. Early reports suggested that prolonged rest of up to 6 months appears to be the most beneficial treatment independent of other adjunctive therapies.[11–13] Controlled exercise, including having the horse step over obstacles, should be done during the rest period.

The surgical resection of the dorsal summits of the spinous processes for the alleviation of chronic overriding has been successfully applied for this specific condition (see "Overlapping . . . of the Thoracic and/or Lumbar Dorsal Spinous Processes" in this chapter).[12] Prolonged antimicrobial therapy and, in some cases, surgical curettage may be required for the treatment of vertebral osteomyelitis and diskospondylitis (see "Vertebral Osteomyelitis and Diskospondylitis" in this chapter).

Alternative therapies including chiropractic manipulation and acupuncture have become popular modalities in the treatment of equine back disease. Stimulation of acupuncture points with saline and low-powered infrared laser in two separate studies on horses with chronic back pain showed improvement in 13 of 15 and 10 of 14 horses, respectively.[17,18] Many acupuncture techniques have been described, including dry needling,

supraspinous ligament, spinous processes, articular processes, transverse processes, intervertebral discs, and the lumbosacral joint.[5]

Thermography has been used to diagnose neuromuscular disease in 53 of 53 cases. In this report, it was suggested that animals with chronic back pain generally have cold regions rather than "hot" spots and cautions the user that thermography involves more than just looking for areas of increased temperature.[26] Thermography should be considered in horses with training problems, lameness, or back pain. One author has seen a high incidence of abnormal thermographic signs of back-related neuromuscular disease in horses with training and behavioral faults that have not shown overt lameness.[26] In general, thermography should be considered for any cases of locomotion abnormalities that are not candidates for nerve blocks and that fail to be diagnosed by other clinical examinations.

electroacupuncture, acupuncture using hypodermic needles, laser acupuncture, and injection acupuncture. Herbal medicine has been used in combination with acupuncture for treatment of severe back injury. Acupuncture has also been used to treat muscular atrophy.[15,20,27,28] The reader is directed to the listed references for more information on the techniques used in equine acupuncture. Unwanted side effects of acupuncture therapy include abscessation at the site of needle puncture. At this time, even with the lack of hard scientific evidence, the use of acupuncture should be considered in the treatment of equine back disease. Chiropractic treatments are based upon the principle that joint dysfunction affects the normal neurologic balance found in healthy individuals and current spinal research no longer supports the "bone out of place" theory.[9] It is important to realize that treatment by the use of chiropractics should be performed by someone with the proper training and skills and that early involvement of a chiropractor may lead to a greater success when dealing with back pain. It is also important to realize that many disease processes including fractures, infections, neoplasia, metabolic disorders, and impinged spinous processes are not candidates for chiropractic manipulation. As a manipulative technique there are potential side effects associated with improperly applied technique, such as torn ligaments and injured muscles.

Physical therapy as a treatment for equine musculoskeletal disease has been sorely overlooked. Physiotherapy should not be considered as a stand-alone procedure but should be considered as an extension to normal veterinary care. There are many facets of physiotherapy including machine use, such as magnetic field therapy devices, Faradaic muscle stimulators, therapeutic ultrasound, and lasers, to name a few. Swimming has also been recommended. Massage is perhaps the earliest form of physiotherapy.[2,21] It is important to consider that with all of the modalities available for physiotherapy, the operator must take the time to understand the characteristics of each modality, as well as the best time to apply them. Without this knowledge, the end result may not be as good as possible and may even be detrimental. As with all therapeutic modalities, negative side effects can occur if the person applying them does not fully understand the potential ramifications. Physiotherapy is also very beneficial in rehabilitating horses from surgical intervention.

Prognosis

Jeffcott reported a 57% recovery rate irrespective of the diagnosis and treatment in a series of 190 horses that were presented for back problems and were available for clinical follow-up. However, the prognosis is more realistically dependent on the type of injury sustained.[13] A good prognosis can be expected for most cases in which a soft tissue injury involving the support structures has been sustained. In one report a good recovery was observed in 73% of the cases with a recurrence rate of only 27%.[13] The poorest prognosis is expected with spondylosis in which a 91% recurrence rate of back pain has been reported.[13] Of course a very poor prognosis is given for cases sustaining fracture of the vertebral column as well.

References

1. British equine veterinary association survey of equine disease 1962–1963. Vet Rec 1965;77:528.
2. Bromiley MW. Physical therapy for the equine back. Vet Clin North Am Equine Pract 1999;15(1):223–246.
3. Cauvin E. Assessment of back pain in horses. Equine Pract 1997;19:522–533.
4. Crowhurst RC. Symposium on back problems. Equine Vet J 1975;7:66.
5. Denoix JM. Ultrasonographic evaluation of back lesions. Vet Clin North Am Equine Pract 1999;15(1):131–159.
6. Haussler KK, Stover SM. Stress fractures of the vertebral lamina and pelvis in Thoroughbred racehorses. Equine Vet J 1998;30:374–381.
7. Haussler KK, Stover SM, Willits NH. Pathologic changes in the lumbosacral vertebrae and pelvis in Thoroughbred racehorses. Am J Vet Res 1999;60:143–163.
8. Haussler KK. Osseous spinal pathology. Vet Clin North Am Equine Pract 1999;15(1):103–111.
9. Haussler KK. Chiropractic evaluation and management. Vet Clin North Am Equine Pract 1999;15(1):195–210.
10. Jeffcott LB. Diagnosis of back problems in the horse. Comp Cont Educ Pract Vet 1981;3:134.
11. Jeffcott LB. Disorders of the thoracolumbar spine of the horse: A survey of 443 cases. Equine Vet J 1980;12:197.
12. Jeffcott LB. Guidelines for the diagnosis and treatment of back problems in horses. Proc Am Assoc Equine Pract 1980;26:381.
13. Jeffcott LB. Back problems in the horses: A look at past, present, and future progress. Equine Vet J 1979;11:129.
14. Jeffcott LB, et al. Effects of induced back pain on gait and performance of Trotting horses. Equine Vet J 1982;14:129.
15. Klide AM, Martin BB. Methods of stimulating acupuncture points for treatment of chronic back pain in horses. J Am Vet Med Assoc 1989;195:1375–1379.
16. Licka T, Peham C. An objective method for evaluating the flexibility of the back of standing horses. Equine Vet J 1998;30:412–415.
17. Martin BB, Klide AM. Treatment of chronic back pain in horses: Stimulation of acupuncture points with a low powered infrared laser. Vet Surg 1987;16:106–110.
18. Martin BB, Klide AM. Use of acupuncture for the treatment of chronic back pain in horses; Stimulation of acupuncture points with saline solution injections. J Am Vet Med Assoc 1987;190:1177–1180.
19. Nowak N. Die klinische, röntgenologische und szintigraphische Untersuchung bei den sogenannten Rückenproblemen des Pferdes. Pferdeheilkunde 1988;4:193–198.
20. Ridgeway K. Acupuncture as a treatment modality for back problems. Vet Clin North Am Equine Pract 1999;15(1):211–221.
21. Ridgeway K, Harman J. Equine back rehabilitation. Vet Clin North Am Equine Pract 1999;15(1):263–280.
22. Rooney JR. The horse's back: Biomechanics of lameness. Equine Pract 1982;4:17.
23. Steckel RR. The role of scintigraphy in the lameness evaluation. Vet Clin North Am Equine Pract 1991;7:207–239.
24. Townsend HGG, Leach DH. Relationship between intervertebral joint morphology and mobility in the equine thoracolumbar spine. Equine Vet J 1984;16:461–465.
25. Townsend HGG, Leach DH, Doige CE, et al. Relationship between spinal biomechanics and pathological changes in the equine thoracolumbar spine. Equine Vet J 1986;18:107–112.
26. von Schweinitz DG. Thermographic diagnostics in equine back pain. Vet Clin North Am Equine Pract 1999;15(1):161–178.
27. Xie H, Asquith RL, Kivipelto J. A review of the use of acupuncture for treatment of equine back pain. J Equine Vet Sci 1996;16:285–290.
28. Xie H, Liu H, Foster M. Equine back pain: A traditional Chinese medical review. Equine Pract 1997;19(6):6–12.

OVERLAPPING OR CROWDING OF THORACIC AND/OR LUMBAR DORSAL SPINOUS PROCESSES

Overlapping or crowding of the dorsal spinous processes is one of the most common causes of back soreness in horses. In one report this condition was one of the most common vertebral (bone associated) causes of back pain in a series of 443 cases.[8] In another study of Thoroughbred racehorses, impingement of the dorsal spinous processes was seen in 92% of horses that had been euthanatized.[4]

Etiology

Horses may have suffered an injury to the back, or impingement may be secondary to exercise. This condition may be due to such mishaps as going over backward, falling, or struggling in a casting harness. Signs may not be evident until 2 to 3 years after the injury.[2,5] It has been suggested that overlapping or impingement of the dorsal spinous processes can occur secondary to spondylosis deformans.[12] In this condition, tearing of the ventral and ventrolateral support structures of the anulus fibrosus causes the intervertebral joint to become impacted, which causes a tilting of the dorsal spinous processes toward each other. The most common site for the impingement is the midback region, where the weight of the rider is most focused and the interspinous spaces are the most narrow. In one study, the condition was more common in Thoroughbred horses, which have been found to have narrower interspinous spaces.[8]

Signs

Historically, changes in behavior and temperament are common. The horse often resents saddling and grooming. Bucking and lying down after saddling may occur. As the cinch is tightened, the horse may groan and exhibit other signs of discomfort. There may be a reluctance to lift the feet for cleaning or shoeing. Horses may also be presented for loss of performance and increased stiffness in the back or an abnormal hindlimb gait.[14] Pressure along the back may cause signs of pain in some cases. Many other variations may result.[10,11] The condition appears to be most prevalent in hunters and jumpers, and it is common for the horse to refuse jumps. In long-standing cases, there may be atrophy of the longissimus dorsi muscles. It is not uncommon for other vertebral abnormalities to be present.

Diagnosis

Palpation along the back may reveal irregularities in the size of the summits of the spinous processes of the thoracic or lumbar vertebrae. Deep digital palpation is necessary in most cases to reveal these changes. Examination should begin forward at the withers and work backward.[4] One will have to differentiate resentment shown by some horses to this examination from distress resulting from other back conditions. Tests of the spine to show loss of flexibility are useful. (Refer to "Examination of the Back" in Chapter 3.) A horse with overlapping of the spinous processes will show little or no movement from these tests. If satisfactory radiographs of the dorsal processes can be obtained, they will greatly aid

the diagnosis (Fig. 8.525). Nuclear scintigraphy is also of great help in diagnosing overriding dorsal spinous processes and may require oblique views to differentiate between vertebral body disease and dorsal process disease (Fig. 8.526).[9,13] It is important to recognize that the dorsal spinous processes at the withers region have a unique radiographic and scintigraphic appearance, and the normal anatomy must be completely understood before diagnosing overriding of the spinous processes. Ultrasonography can be very helpful in diagnosing spinous process abnormalities but requires a good understanding of normal anatomy to determine abnormal changes.[1]

Jeffcott found that direct infiltration of local anesthetic solution between and around the overlapping dor-

Figure 8.525 Radiograph of impingement of the dorsal spinous processes.

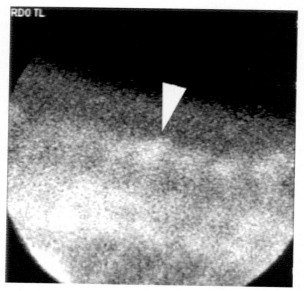

Figure 8.526 Nuclear scintigraphy of impingement of the dorsal spinous processes.

sal spinous processes would alleviate the pain and was helpful in the diagnosis.[8]

The above signs are by no means specific and may be similar to those seen with other conditions involving the back region. The diagnosis is best established with history, physical examination including manipulation and palpation findings, and evidence of impingement on radiography. A positive radiographic examination will show diminished space between, and possibly overlapping of, the affected dorsal spinous processes.

Jeffcott, however, found that the radiographic changes associated with overlapping of the dorsal spinous processes were not always related to clinical signs and that many horses exhibiting these radiographic findings performed satisfactorily. In one review, 34% of horses with functionally normal thoracolumbar specimens and 33% of horses with a history of thoracolumbar disease had radiographic evidence of dorsal spinous process impingement.[14] In another group of horses, 92% of the specimens had impingement of the dorsal spinous processes.[2]

Treatment

Conservative therapies include rest, nonsteroidal anti-inflammatory drugs (NSAIDs), local injections of anti-inflammatory agents, acupuncture, and physiotherapy. Horses that are rested will often improve during the rest period but become sore again shortly after reinstating exercise. Systemic therapy with NSAIDs will help horses with very minor lesions but will not cure more severe lesions. Injections of corticosteroids between affected spinous processes, combined with nonsteroidal systemic therapy, can be quite helpful in reducing or removing pain. Based on the bone involvement, chiropractic manipulations are thought to be at least potentially contraindicated in this disease process.[3]

Although Jeffcott could not identify a clear-cut advantage to surgery over conservative treatment (rest), most horses treated surgically were the most severely affected and tended to make better progress, returning to full work earlier.[6] Therefore, surgery should be relegated for the most severely involved cases.

Surgical treatment will give satisfactory results in most cases if the diagnosis is accurate.[7,10,11] The summit of the affected spinous process is removed through an incision on either side of the midline. If there is pressure between as many as three spinous processes, removal of the center one will usually relieve the symptoms. The supraspinous ligament is dissected free of the processes but not severed. The operative field is crowded by the longissimus dorsi muscle, making complete exposure of the process difficult. Only enough of the process is removed to relieve pressure between processes. A bone saw or wire saw can be used for cutting. For a detailed description of the surgical procedure, the reader is referred to the original discussions.[7,11]

Aftercare consists of 2 to 3 months in a box stall and 1 month of hand walking before beginning riding. Some cases do not show full benefit for several months.

Prognosis

The prognosis is guarded. Diagnosis is sometimes difficult because of the size of the x-ray machine required for adequate radiographs and the fact that not all horses with radiographic signs of overriding of the dorsal spinous processes show clinical signs. Because of this the clinical significance of this finding should be closely scrutinized before judgment is made regarding the treatment. Nuclear scintigraphy can be used to follow horses with mild cases to determine if full resolution of the disease has occurred.

References

1. Denoix JM. Ultrasonographic evaluation of back lesions. Vet Clin North Am Equine Pract 1999;15(1):131–159.
2. Haussler KK. Osseous spinal pathology. Vet Clin North Am Equine Pract 1999;15(1):103–111.
3. Haussler KK. Chiropractic evaluation and management. Vet Clin North Am Equine Pract 1999;15(1):195–210.
4. Haussler KK, Stover SM, Willits NH. Pathologic changes in the lumbosacral vertebrae and pelvis in Thoroughbred racehorses. Am J Vet Res 1999;60:143–153.
5. Jeffcott LB. The diagnosis of diseases of the horse's back. Equine Vet J 1975;7:69–78.
6. Jeffcott LB. Back problems in the horse: A look at past, present, and future progress. Equine Vet J 1979;11:129.
7. Jeffcott LB, Hickman J. The treatment of horses with chronic back pain by resecting the summits of the impinging dorsal spinous processes. Equine Vet J 1975;7:115.
8. Jeffcott LB. Disorders of the thoracolumbar spine of the horse: A survey of 443 cases. Equine Vet J 1980;12:197.
9. Nowak N. Die klinische, röntgenologische und szintigraphische Untersuchung bei den sogenannten Rückenproblemen des Pferdes. Pferdeheilkunde 1988;4:193–198.
10. Roberts EJ. Amputation of a lumbar spinous process in the horse. Proc Am Assoc Equine Pract 1968;14:115–117.
11. Roberts EJ. Resection of thoracic or lumbar spinous processes for the relief of pain responsible for lameness and some other locomotor disorders of horses. Proc Am Assoc Equine Pract 1968;14:13–30.
12. Rooney JR. The horse's back: Biomechanics of lameness. Equine Pract 1982;4:17.
13. Steckel RR. The role of scintigraphy in the lameness evaluation. Vet Clin North Am Equine Pract 1991;7:207–239.
14. Townsend HGG, Leach DH, Doige CE, et al. Relationship between spinal biomechanics and pathological changes in the equine thoracolumbar spine. Equine Vet J 1986; 18:107–112.

VERTEBRAL BODY OSTEOMYELITIS AND DISKOSPONDYLITIS

Vertebral body osteomyelitis and diskospondylitis are infrequently diagnosed diseases in the horse.

Etiology

Vertebral body osteomyelitis is most commonly seen in young animals regardless of the species.[4] This may be due to poor transfer of passive immunity, increased blood supply to the bone, and sharp loops of metaphyseal vessels, leading to increased bacterial sequestration. Other sources of infection should be investigated because the vertebrae are usually secondarily involved. Trauma has also been proposed in the etiology of diskospondylitis in the horse, especially of the cervical vertebrae.[1–3]

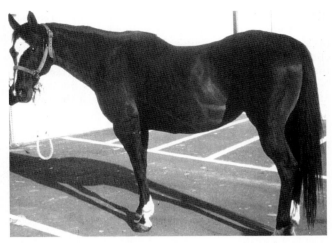

Figure 8.527 This horse presented with a history of sustaining a sacral fracture 5 months ago. Two months after the injury, the owner noticed that the horse appeared to have increased back pain and was reluctant to eat off the ground. This photograph shows the horse at presentation exhibiting atrophy of epaxial muscles, a splinted caudal abdomen. This is as far as the horse would allow us to flex its neck to one side or the other. (Courtesy of T. S. Stashak.)

Cases involving the thoracic and lumbar vertebrae following trauma have also been seen at Colorado State University (CSU) (Stashak TS, personal communication, 2001). However, it is still widely considered that the infections are caused by hematogenous spread and the primary site of infection should be identified.

Signs

The signs will vary depending on what portion of the vertebral column is affected.[1-3] Signs compatible with spinal cord compression, fever, back or neck pain, and stiffness may be the earliest signs with osteomyelitis if the vertebral body is involved (Stashak TS, personal communication, 2001; and Ref. 4). Meningitis may occur in later stages of the disease process. If a dorsal spinous process is involved, the signs can be more localized.

Signs of weight loss, back or neck pain, fever, stiffness, and ataxia may all be notable with cases of diskospondylitis. Atrophy of the epaxial muscle in the thoracolumbar region may be evident in some horses suffering from chronic diskospondylitis in this region (Stashak TS, personal communication, 2001) (Fig. 8.527). Some horses are so affected that they are reluctant to eat off the ground. Lateral neck flexion can be markedly obtunded as well. The abdomen may also be held rigid as though intraabdominal pain was present. Blood analysis may reveal a leukocytosis and elevated fibrinogen.

Diagnosis

Osteomyelitis and diskospondylitis can occur in any region of the vertebral column. Nuclear scintigraphy, especially with the emergence of ciprofloxacin scans, allows early diagnosis of both osteomyelitis and diskospondylitis (Fig. 8.528, A and B).[1,2] Radiographic examination of the thoracolumbar spine, although difficult, is most valuable for the identification of vertebral lesions (Fig. 8.529). However, a negative radiographic examination does not indicate that the thoracolumbar spine is not involved. Radiographic changes may not occur for 2 to 8 weeks after the onset of signs.[2] Ultrasonography can also be helpful in identifying a perivertebral abscess (Fig. 8.530).

Treatment

Successful treatment depends on early detection and accurate identification of the bacteria involved. Bone or

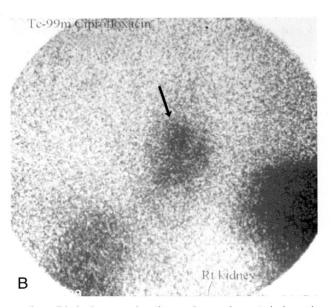

Figure 8.528 A. Nuclear scintigraphy of the horse in Figure 8.527. Note the marked increased uptake of the radionuclide in the caudal thoracic vertebrae. B. Nuclear scintigraphy with ciprofloxacin of this horse indicating an increased uptake of the radionuclide in the same location as the previous study (arrow). This indicates the lesion is septic and confirms a diagnosis of diskospondylitis. (Courtesy of T. S. Stashak.)

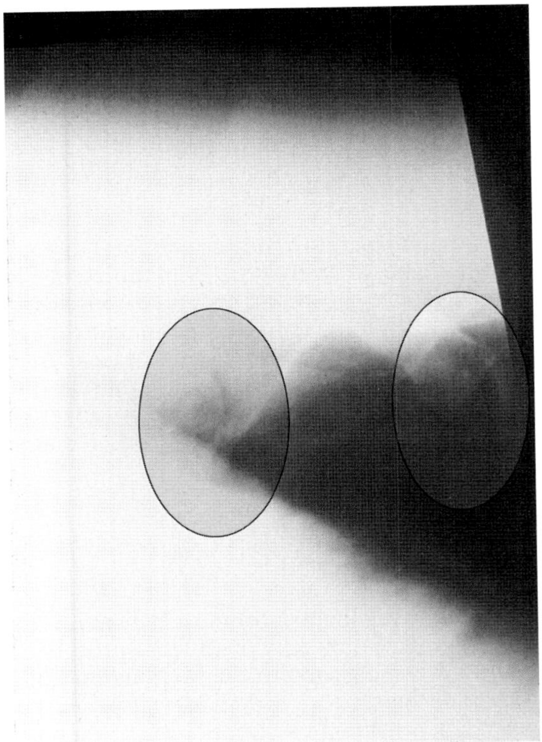

Figure 8.529   Lateral radiograph of the horse in Figure 8.528. Note the collapsed intervertebral space and the vertebral lysis (left oval) associated with the affected caudal thoracic vertebrae. Also note the normal intervertebral space caudal to the affected region (right oval). (Courtesy of T. S. Stashak.)

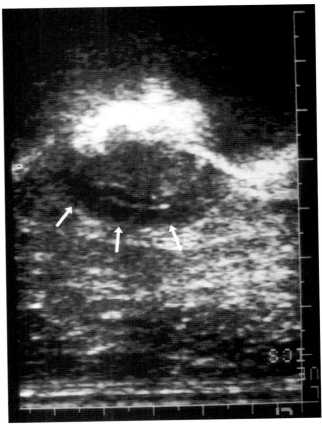

Figure 8.530   Ultrasound examination of the caudal thoracic region of the horse illustrated in Figure 8.529. Note the circumscribed perivertebral abscess (arrows). Needle aspiration of the abscess was accomplished by using ultrasound guidance. (Courtesy of T. S. Stashak.)

disc biopsies and subsequent culture and sensitivity should be performed in all cases, and appropriate antibiotic therapy should be instituted. Ultrasound needle aspiration can be performed on a perivertebral abscess (see Fig. 8.530). Long-term therapy may be indicated.[1-4] Antimicrobial therapy (4 to 6 months) will generally be required for the successful treatment of vertebral osteomyelitis and diskospondilitis. Nuclear scintigraphy with ciprofloxacin can be used to determine effectiveness of therapy and continued use of antibiotics. Vertebral curettage should be performed in cases where access to the lesion is possible.

Prognosis

Prognosis is guarded unless early detection and early institution of appropriate therapy occurs. With respect to diskospondylitis, 1 of 5 cases in one report[1] and 1 of 1 in another report[3] returned to normal after therapy. The outcome in a limited number of cases treated at CSU with prolonged antimicrobial therapy appears good for pasture soundness. However, none of the cases have been able to return to riding performance at the time of this writing. Two of 5 horses with vertebral body osteomyelitis returned to normal after long-term therapy.[4]

References

1. Adams SB, Steckel R, Blevins W. Diskospondylitis in five horses. J Am Vet Med Assoc 1985;186:270–272.
2. Carpenter E, Gibbons D, Stashak T, et al. Diskospondylitis in an adult horse diagnosed using ciprofloxacin nuclear scintigraphy. Unpublished data.
3. Hillyer MH, Innes JF, Patteson MW, et al. Diskospondylitis in an adult horse. Vet Rec 1996;139:519–521.
4. Markel MD, Madigan JE, Lichtensteiger CA, et al. Vertebral body osteomyelitis in the horse. J Am Vet Med Assoc 1986;188:632–634.

Part XVII

MUSCLE PROBLEMS

Dean A. Hendrickson

MYOSITIS OF THE PSOAS AND LONGISSIMUS DORSI MUSCLES

The muscular support of the equine spine is provided by numerous muscles and allows both stability and flexibility. The various muscles are used to a greater or lesser extent based upon use and fitness of the horse. The pain in the loin (lumbar) region often causes the owner to think the horse has "kidney trouble."

Etiology

The pain associated with muscle disease may be caused by acute rhabdomyolysis, recurrent exertional rhabdomyolysis, and polysaccharide storage myopathy.[5,7] Pain may be due to persistent muscle contraction secondary to a skeletal disorder. Consequently, a full examination should be performed to rule out other causes of pain before looking entirely to the muscles. The psoas muscles are very important in the driving action of the hindlimbs and are subject to injury when the horse is improperly trained. Muscle atrophy could be caused by neurogenic atrophy, myogenic atrophy, or immune-mediated myositis. The most common cause of neurogenic atrophy in horses is equine motor neuron disease or equine protozoal myelitis. Blunt trauma can also damage motor nerves. Myogenic atrophy is most commonly associated with severe rhabdomyolysis but can occur after muscle trauma.

Signs

Typical signs of muscle disease include atrophy, focal swelling, pain on palpation, generally enlarged muscles, poor performance, behavioral change, difficulty accepting saddle, lameness, and shortened stride.[4] Often, horses will not use the hindlimbs properly for propulsion, and the hindlimb gait will appear stiffened bilaterally. The abdomen may be held rigid as though intraabdominal pain was present. Serum muscle enzymes aminoaspartate transferase (APT) and creatine kinase (CK) will be elevated in the active stage.[4]

Diagnosis

Diagnostic tests to determine the presence of muscle disease include physical examination, thermography,[8] ultrasound,[2] measurement of plasma/serum enzymes, and muscle biopsy.[7] Many horses with back pain will respond to palpation of the epaxial musculature. The muscle soreness may be secondary to other disease processes, making a full physical examination critical in rul-

ing out other abnormalities such as vertebral disease and other limb lameness. Transrectal palpation can be performed to evaluate the psoas group of muscles. With muscle disease, it is important to examine the other muscles of the body, since primary muscle disease of the back is usually a component of generalized muscle disease. Muscle biopsy is rarely used in the early stages of the disease process and is best used after other diagnostic tests have been performed.[7]

Treatment

Once a definitive diagnosis of muscle disease is identified, therapy is determined by the disease process occurring. The reader is directed to the sections on nutrition and diseases of muscle for particular treatment regimens in Chapter 5. Chiropractic manipulations, acupuncture, and physiotherapy can be beneficial to treat the horses, and perhaps prevent reinjury.[1,3,5,6]

Prognosis

Prognosis can be guarded in some cases where a diagnosis cannot be found or where generalized muscle disease is present. However, many horses return to full use.

References

1. Bromiley MW. Physical therapy for the equine back. Vet Clin North Am Equine Pract 1999;15(1):223–246.
2. Denoix JMD. Ultrasonographic evaluation of back lesions. Vet Clin North Am Equine Pract 1999;15(1):131–160.
3. Haussler KK. Chiropractic evaluation and management. Vet Clin North Am Equine Pract 1999;15(1):195–210.
4. Hodgson DR. Myopathies in the athletic horse. Comp Cont Educ Pract Vet 1985;7:S551–S555.
5. Ridgway K. Acupuncture as a treatment modality for back problems. Vet Clin North Am Equine Pract 1999;15(1):211–222.
6. Ridgway K, Harman J. Equine back rehabilitation. Vet Clin North Am Equine Pract 1999;15(1):263–280.
7. Valberg SJ. Spinal Muscle Pathology. Vet Clin North Am Equine Pract 1999;15(1):87–96.
8. von Schweinitz DG. Thermographic diagnostics in equine back pain. Vet Clin North Am Equine Pract 1999;15(1):161–178.

MUSCULAR DYSTROPHY

Muscular dystrophy has been observed in the horse, yet it is an uncommon disease. It has been reported in the semitendinosus muscle,[1-3] the gluteal muscle,[2,3] trunk muscles,[3] and the masseter muscle[1]. Muscular dystrophy differs from simple atrophy in that the muscle completely disappears.

Etiology

The etiology of muscular dystrophy is unknown.

Signs

In early stages of the disease, the animal may be unable to rise, or it may have an abnormal gait. In later stages, complete loss of the muscular tissue is obvious. In some of the cases observed, the horse affected with dystrophy of the right masseter showed only bone to palpation on the affected side. The semitendinosus on the left hindlimb was completely absent. In another case, the semitendinosus on the right hindlimb was completely

absent. Bilateral dystrophy of both masseter muscles has also been observed. Dystrophy leaves a deformity in the limb and a deep grooving where the muscle was.

Treatment

No treatment is known for muscular dystrophy.

Prognosis

Prognosis is unfavorable.

References

1. Cecil RL, Loeb RF. A Textbook of Medicine. 11th Ed. Philadelphia: WB Saunders, 1963;1451.
2. Sarli G, Salda D, Marcato PS. Dystrophy-like myopathy in a foal. Vet Rec 1994;135:156–160.
3. Shirakawa T, Ide M, Taniyama H, et al. Muscular dystrophy-like disease in a Thoroughbred foal. J Compar Pathol 1989;100:287–294.

Part XVIII

WOBBLER SYNDROME

A. J. Nixon

Many diseases of the spinal cord produce locomotor disorders that appear clinically similar. Signs can vary from lameness and poor performance to overt neurologic abnormalities. Traditionally the collective term "wobbler" has been applied to all horses with signs of ataxia, weakness, and spasticity, but recently more emphasis has been directed toward establishing a neuroanatomic and etiologic diagnosis, since this provides a more accurate prognosis and determines appropriate treatment.

The more common causes of ataxic paresis in the horse are cervical vertebral malformation, equine protozoal myeloencephalitis, equine degenerative myeloencephalopathy, equine herpes virus type 1 (EHV-1) myeloencephalitis, and vertebral trauma. Vertebral osteomyelitis, neoplasia, fibrocartilaginous infarcts, intervertebral disc protrusion, Sudan grass toxicosis, equine infectious anemia, and spinal nematodiasis are seen less frequently.

CERVICAL VERTEBRAL MALFORMATION

Cervical vertebral malformation (CVM) is one of the most common causes of the "wobbler" syndrome in young, rapidly growing horses younger than 4 years of age.[57,62,64,65,68] This category includes not only malformation of the bones and joints of the cervical vertebrae, but also malarticulations and degenerative changes of joints. It is most prevalent in Thoroughbred and Quarter horse males, but all breeds and both sexes are affected.[29,57,62,76]

Two subdivisions of CVM have been described.[57,62,76,96] Cervical static stenosis (CSS) is a narrowing of the vertebral canal that persists throughout the range of neck movements.[76,89] Cervical vertebral instability (CVI), on the other hand, results in a dynamic stenosis, compressing the spinal cord only when the neck is flexed. In the neutral and extended positions, the narrowing of the vertebral canal is largely relieved. Vertebral instability occurs predominantly in the midcervical vertebrae, whereas the static stenoses are largely confined to the caudal neck.[62,68,74,76]

Pathogenesis

Cervical vertebral instability occurs most frequently in horses 6 to 12 months of age. The midcervical (C3–C4 to C5–C6) vertebrae are involved and exhibit several types of malformation. Narrowing of the vertebral canal at the cranial or caudal orifice is common and produces a vertebral canal that appears to undulate from vertebra to vertebra (Fig. 8.531). Developmental defects within the physes and epiphyseal end plates with "mushrooming" of the metaphyses produce an uneven vertebral canal with the potential to subluxate and compress the spinal cord on flexion. Malformation and asymmetry of the articular facets are often present, and osteochondritis dissecans (OCD) lesions occur frequently in these joints (Fig. 8.532). Reduced growth of the caudal physis in the more cranial of the two adjacent vertebrae at an affected articulation results in a short vertebral body, compared with the dorsal lamina, and partial flexion (kyphosis)

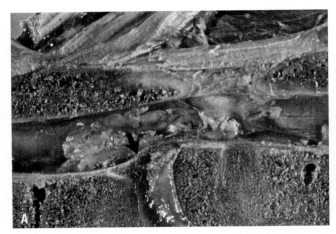

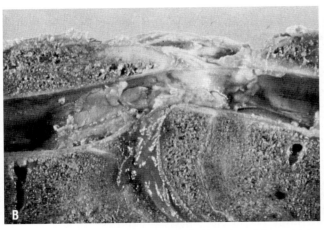

Figure 8.531 Cervical vertebral instability at C3–C4. A. Neutral position. The caudal orifice of the cranial vertebra is narrower than normal because of "mushrooming" of the metaphysis and epiphysis (arrow). B. Flexed position. Subluxation of the caudal vertebra in relation to the cranially adjacent vertebra with narrowing of the vertebral canal.

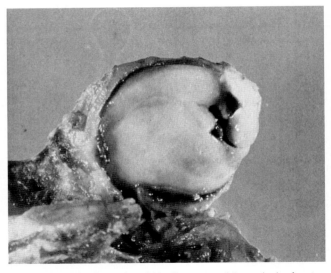

Figure 8.532 Osteochondritis dissecans of the articular facet joint. Same case as in Figure 8.531.

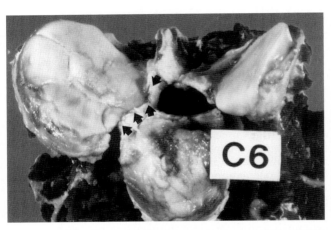

Figure 8.533 Cervical static stenosis due to a severely arthritic facet joint from the C5–C6 junction of a 2-year-old Thoroughbred. Periarticular osteophytes and joint capsule fibrosis have encroached on the vertebral canal and lateral foramen (arrows).

of the articulation in the standing animal. The fibrous intervertebral disc firmly unites adjacent vertebrae, which promotes dorsal subluxation of the caudal vertebra at the affected junction on flexion. The result is compression of the spinal cord between the cranial end of one vertebra and the dorsal lamina of the cranially adjacent vertebra (see 8.531B). While cartilage defects from OCD of the articular facets are commonly observed at sites of spinal cord compression and other noncompressed articulations in the cervical vertebrae, these facet lesions are not pathognomonic for spinal cord compression.

Cervical static stenosis (CSS) typically occurs in slightly older horses, most being 1 to 4 years of age. The less mobile caudal cervical vertebrae (C5–C6, C6–C7) are affected almost exclusively.[62,67,74] Bony abnormalities involve the articular facets and the dorsal laminae rather than the vertebral bodies. Degenerative joint disease (DJD), possibly precipitated by OCD, is manifest as cartilage erosion, periarticular osteophytosis, subchondral bone sclerosis, and joint capsule hypertrophy and distension (Fig. 8.533). In addition to osteochondrosis of the facet joints, trauma to the immature cartilage surfaces of the facet may result in degenerative joint disease. Associated with the degenerative joint disease of the articular facets are further growth and occasionally massive enlargement of the perimeter of the facets from osteophyte development. Compounding this enlargement are hypertrophy and fibrosis of the synovial membrane and joint capsule (Fig. 8.533). Encroachment on the vertebral canal and lateral foramina can occur from either or both of these tissues.[57,64] Subsequent compression of the spinal cord, in addition to the cervical spinal nerves, results in clinical disease. Changes in the joint capsules, including fibrosis and fibrovascular proliferation, extend axially to blend imperceptibly with the ligamentum flavum, which frequently contains areas of hemorrhage, fibrovascular proliferation, and occasionally foci of fibrocartilage.[73] Proliferation of these soft tissues is thought to result from the DJD of the facet joint. Osteosclerosis of the dorsal laminae is common and results from increased tension on the lamina by the ligamentum flavum. Increased fibrocartilage and later endochondral ossification at the insertion of the ligamentum flavum on the dorsal lamina possibly result from tension and stretching of the ligamentum flavum.

Etiology

The precise cause of the bone and joint developmental abnormalities that result in CVM are not clearly defined. Many factors probably contribute to modify the normal development of the cervical vertebra. These include nutrition, genetics, biomechanical forces (possibly due to conformation), and exercise (including the possibility of traumatic incidents).[15,77] Cervical vertebral malformation is one clinical entity in the group of developmental orthopedic diseases that include physitis, contracted tendons, OCD, malformation of cuboidal bones of the carpus and tarsus, and juvenile arthritis.

Although initial reports proposed that CVM may be inherited,[19-21,28] subsequent reports found no heritable mechanism.[15,43,87,90] A genetic study of wobbler matings of horses with CVM revealed that none of the offspring were clinical wobblers; however, the offspring had an extraordinarily high incidence of contracted tendons, OCD, and physitis.[97] One of the early studies implicated a genetic propensity for rapid growth and superior performance,[19] but another survey found no evidence that CVM was genetically predetermined.[29]

Dietary factors, particularly trace minerals, are clearly important in the pathogenesis of developmental orthopedic diseases.[46] Feeding trials suggest copper deficiency is a major determinant of aberrant endochondral ossification.[35,45] Postmortem examination of copper-deficient animals showed an extraordinarily high incidence of osteochondrosis of the vertebral articulations.[75] Other complicating dietary factors, such as elevated caloric and protein intake, are undoubtedly involved in developmental orthopedic diseases, including CVM.[2,57,68] Marginally low levels of trace minerals may be of particular metabolic importance under circumstances of maximum need, as during rapid growth.[81] Young horses with CVM are frequently reported to have a large body size for their age. The interplay of dietary components and genetics in the etiology of developmental orthopedic diseases and CVM is still under investigation.

Signs

Many horses are large for their age and breed and present with a history of an acute traumatic incident that initiated the signs of ataxia and weakness. Some horses become neurologically stable while others improve and then deteriorate presumably because of repeated spinal cord trauma associated with excessive vertebral movement.

Horses appear physically normal, although cutaneous abrasions can be seen and, rarely, vertebral malalignment can be so pronounced as to be visible and palpable externally. Pain on palpation and a reluctance to turn the neck to either side is a frequent finding. Distended joints, especially the hock and stifle, can occasionally be seen, possibly indicating other sites of OCD.

Incoordination, weakness, spasticity, and dysmetria are the major gait changes. One or both hindlimbs are initially affected, followed by progression to the forelimbs. Slight asymmetry in signs is common and may be marked. Extraordinarily severe forelimb signs are usually associated with severe C6–C7 or C7–T1 malformation with pressure on the cervical intumescence and exiting nerve roots. With synovial cysts or lateral foraminal stenosis, signs of pectoral and shoulder muscle atrophy have been seen; however, this is considered uncharacteristic for CVM.

Diagnosis

The radiographic and myelographic examinations are often the most definitive and valuable diagnostic methods in differentiating animals with CVM from those with spinal cord disease resulting in similar clinical signs. The interpretation of plain cervical radiographs can be difficult, and the presence of obvious bone change does not necessarily indicate a compressive spinal cord lesion. Myelography is the best means of positively demonstrating spinal cord compression.[74] However, a tentative diagnosis can generally be obtained from plain cervical radiographs, based on narrowing of the vertebral canal, degenerative joint disease of the facet joints, or malalignment of the vertebrae. Plain radiographs of the midcervical region should be analyzed for evidence of malalignment associated with metaphyseal and epiphyseal flaring, disparate length of the vertebral body and dorsal lamina, and malformation and OCD of the articular facets (Fig. 8.534).

Measuring the vertebral canal diameter on plain radiographs has been advocated as a more objective measure of canal stenosis and spinal cord compression.[57,62,83,93] The value for minimal flexed diameter and minimal dural space diameter can be obtained at the time of myelography and compared to normal values. Horses with values less than normal minimums are almost certain to have vertebral canal stenosis. When the vertebral canal diameter on plain radiographs is being assessed, magnification artifacts can be minimized by using a ratio of the absolute minimum sagittal diameter to the sagittal width of the vertebral body (Fig. 8.534).[83] This sagittal ratio value corrects for inherent magnification by providing a ratio of the two measurements, thereby increasing the sensitivity of measuring the vertebra on plane radiographs. Ranges of ratio values have been derived for C4 to C7 and are presented in Table 8.1.[82] Using a combination of corrected sagittal ratio data and scores for

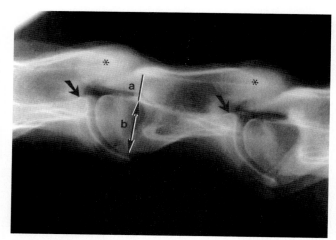

Figure 8.534 Radiograph of the C3–C4 and C4–C5 intervertebral junctions, showing sites for measurements of the (a) conventional minimum sagittal diameter of the vertebral canal and (b) sagittal width of the vertebral body. Bony indicators of vertebral instability also include kyphotic angulation of the C3–C4 articulation, caudal metaphyseal flaring or "ski-jump" (arrows), and caudal overhang of the dorsal laminae (asterisks). The ratio of a/b is derived and compared to values in Table 8.1 to determine the "likelihood ratio" or predictive index of spinal cord compression.

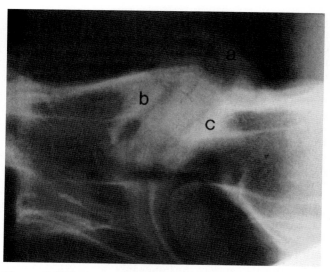

Figure 8.535 Lateral radiograph of the caudal cervical vertebrae of a horse with cervical static stenosis. Degenerative joint disease is apparent with osteophytosis (a) and subchondral bone sclerosis (b). Osteosclerosis of the dorsal lamina is also evident (c).

Table 8.1 SAGITTAL RATIO DATA FROM THE MINIMUM SAGITTAL DIAMETER AND SAGITTAL VERTEBRAL WIDTH (SEE FIG. 8.534) FOR C4 THROUGH C7[a]

Vertebral Sites	Sagittal Ratio	Likelihood Ratio
C4	>0.560	0.04
	0.531–0.560	0.13
	0.501–0.530	1.72
	<0.501	28.6
C5	>0.560	0.04
	0.531–0.560	0.16
	0.501–0.530	2.31
	<0.501	26.1
C6	>0.560	0.03
	0.531–0.560	0.24
	0.501–0.530	1.63
	<0.501	41.5
C7	>0.580	0.04
	0.551–0.580	0.39
	0.521–0.550	1.26
	<0.521	39.0

[a] Modified from Rush MB, et al. Comp Cont Educ Pract Vet 1995;17: 419–426 and Nixon AJ. Nervous system: Cervical vertebral malformation and malarticulation. In: Colahan PT, Mayhew IG, Merritt AM, Moore JN. Equine Medicine and Surgery. 5th ed. Philadelphia: CV Mosby, 1999; 956–972. The statistical likelihood that the sagittal ratio is abnormal, indicating cervical stenotic myelopathy, is provided by the likelihood ratio. Higher values indicate likely abnormalities.

metaphyseal-epiphyseal flaring (ski-jump), caudal extension of the dorsal lamina, angular deviations, abnormal ossification patterns, and degenerative osteoarthritis, a final score can be developed to provide a sensitive and specific indication for cervical stenotic myelopathy.[56,62]

The caudal cervical vertebrae should also be examined for additional radiographic features consistent with the cervical stenotic form of CVM. Signs of degenerative osteoarthritis, such as osteophytes, subchondral bone sclerosis, and narrowed, irregular, or obliterated joint spaces, can be significant (Fig. 8.535).[72] Sclerosis and increased dorsoventral thickness of the dorsal laminae are also common findings in the static stenotic form of CVM.

Positive contrast myelography is necessary to confirm the diagnosis, particularly if surgery is being contemplated. Accurate assessment of the number of affected intervertebral junctions and the severity of each lesion is important in defining the likelihood of recovery following surgery. Techniques for myelography in horses are described in the literature.[5,61,69,72,74] Only water-soluble, nonionic contrast agents are suitable for use in equine myelography. Iohexol is currently the most popular contrast agent. The procedure should be performed with the animal under general anesthesia to allow for flexed and ventrodorsal views of the cervical vertebrae (Fig. 8.536). It should be noted that obliteration of the ventral contrast column occurs over the intervertebral disc spaces on a normal flexed myelogram. The dorsal contrast column of a normal myelogram remains uniformly wide over the vertebral junction from the first to the sixth cervical vertebrae but is narrowed beneath the laminae of C7 and T1.[62,68,69] Only narrowing of both dorsal and ventral contrast columns is considered a focal compressive lesion, and a 50% narrowing of the contrast column has been described as being sufficient to indicate significant compression.[57,74]

Myelography of the caudal cervical spine often reveals narrowing of the vertebral canal at levels where plain radiographs previously indicated DJD of the articular

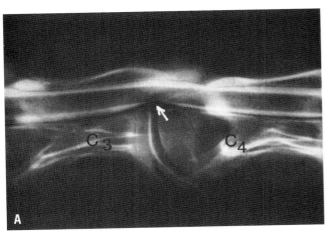
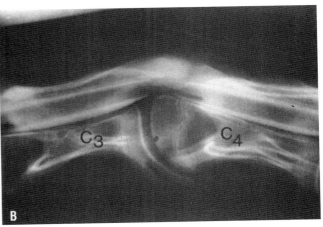

Figure 8.536 Myelogram of a horse with cervical vertebral instability. A. Neutrally positioned, the ventral contrast column narrows normally as it crosses the C3–C4 intervertebral disc space (arrow). The dorsal contrast column expands in width at this

level. B. With flexion, the cranial end of the C4 vertebra has subluxated dorsally, compressing the spinal cord and narrowing both dorsal and ventral contrast columns.

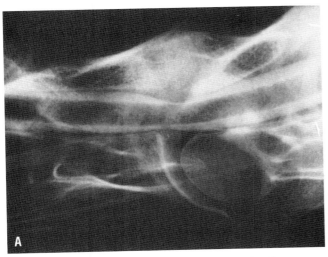
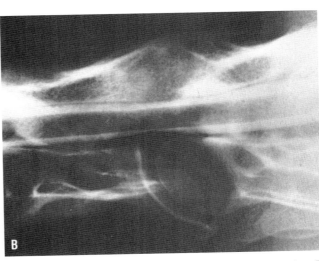

Figure 8.537 Myelogram of a horse with cervical static stenosis. Compression arises predominantly from the ligamentum flavum and joint capsules. A. Neutrally positioned, the dorsal and

ventral contrast columns are narrowed at the vertebral junction. B. With flexion, partial relief of the dorsal compression has occurred.

facets or thickening of the dorsal laminae. The compression is directed to the dorsal or lateral aspects of the spinal cord. Compression predominantly due to the joint capsules and ligamentum flavum will frequently be partially relieved when the neck is flexed (Fig. 8.537). With advancing disease, articular facet proliferation increases, the dorsal laminae become increasingly dense and thick, and vertebral ankylosis progresses to the point where dorsal spinal cord compression is constant (Fig. 8.538); hence, this form of CVM is termed "cervical static stenosis." It occurs most frequently at C6–C7, occasionally at C5–C6, and rarely at C7–T1. Interpretation of the myelogram becomes increasingly difficult when the degree of contrast column narrowing approaches 50%. It is critical that the narrowed areas of the dorsal and ventral contrast columns are diametrically opposed.

Ancillary Testing

Cerebrospinal Fluid (CSF) Studies

The technique for collecting CSF has been described elsewhere.[54,59] Lumbosacral and, occasionally, cisternal CSF samples are routinely analyzed. CFS from horses with CVM is relatively normal.[13,57,59,76] The most consistent changes are slight xanthochromia and an elevated protein content (70 to 130 mg/dL). CFS changes with other neurologic diseases in the differential diagnosis of CVM are described later.

Laboratory Studies

Complete blood counts from horses with CVM are rarely abnormal but can reflect endogenous corticoste-

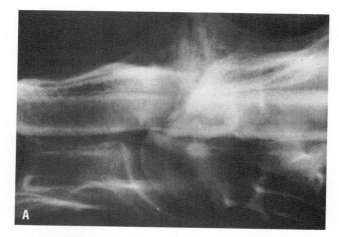

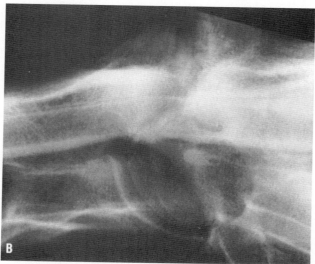

Figure 8.538 Myelogram of a horse with cervical static stenosis. Vertebral bony changes have resulted in persistent compression of the spinal cord. A. Neutrally positioned, there is marked narrowing of the dorsal and ventral contrast columns. B. With flexion, no relief of compression occurs.

roid release or exogenous corticosteroid therapy. Blood chemical and enzyme analyses are often normal but may indicate and reflect the severity of self-inflicted trauma in severely affected horses. Paired serum samples and CSF are routinely submitted for EHV-1 laboratory tests, particularly where signs of cervical myelopathy exist but a myelogram was normal.

Electromyography

The use of the electromyogram (EMG) in horses with signs of cervical spinal cord disease is directed toward the detection of diseases other than CVM. Occasionally, vertebral malformations, articular osteophytes, joint capsule proliferations, or synovial cysts exert sufficient pressure on the exiting nerve roots that lower motor neuron signs detectable with EMG are produced.

Treatment

Medical therapy aimed at treating the inflammation within the spinal cord has been used for many years.

Although palliative, stabilization of signs for extended periods is not uncommon, but permanent improvement is rare. Dexamethasone and other corticosteroids are used frequently. The dangers of corticosteroid-induced laminitis, especially following large doses of dexamethasone, must be explained to the client before use. Dimethyl sulfoxide (DMSO) frequently is given in conjunction with, or in lieu of, corticosteroids; the usual dose is 1 g/kg given slowly intravenously, at a maximum concentration of 20%. The beneficial effects of DMSO are largely because of its diuretic, vasodilatory, anti-inflammatory, and membrane-stabilizing capabilities, in addition to its potential to scavenge superoxide radicals.[16,80] Additionally, it increases cellular resistance to hypoxia and ischemia. Diuretics, such as furosemide, can be given but rarely result in clinical improvement. Phenylbutazone appears to be beneficial, especially when arthritic conditions of the vertebral articulations are present. The response to therapy depends on the dose used and the duration and severity of ataxia being treated. Return of clinical signs can be expected after drug administration is stopped. Stall rest, combined with anti-inflammatory therapy, is recommended to minimize further damage to the spinal cord.

Surgical intervention in cases of cervical vertebral malformation has improved the otherwise poor prognosis formerly given to this condition. Stabilization by interbody fusion of cervical vertebrae is indicated for horses having cervical vertebral instability. The technique is a modification of the Cloward method used for stabilizing human cervical vertebrae, and improvement has been reported in 90% of horses.[98,99,100] Since cervical static stenosis causes persistent compression directed to the dorsal and lateral aspects of the spinal cord, subtotal dorsal laminectomy is the procedure of choice. Several descriptions of laminectomy appear in the literature.[66,68,89,98]

Ventral stabilization by interbody fusion involves removing a major portion of the intervertebral disc and associated vertebral epiphyses.[99] A slightly oversized stainless-steel basket is then tamped into the hole to provide immediate stabilization and promote eventual bony union of the two vertebrae. Horses are positioned in dorsal recumbency with a brace beneath the neck acting as a fulcrum to extend the cervical spine at the intervertebral junction to be fused. A 30-cm ventral midline skin incision exposes the sternothyrohyoid and omohyoid muscles, which are divided longitudinally to expose the trachea. After division of the deep cervical fascia, the trachea is retracted to the left, and the right carotid artery and vagosympathetic trunk are retracted to the right. The ventral crest of the cranial vertebra of the unstable intervertebral junction is cleared of insertions of the longus colli muscles and removed with an osteotome to create a level surface for the drill guide. An 18-mm drill guide centered over the caudal physis of the cranial vertebra is placed (Fig. 8.539), and a hole is drilled to a premeasured depth. If this guide hole centers on the intervertebral disc, then a larger drill guide is placed and a 25-mm hole is made with a large twist drill. If the guide hole is not centered correctly, then adjustments are made in placing the 25-mm drill guide. The drillings (cancellous bone and disc material) from the guide hole and 25-mm hole are packed into the open cylinder of the

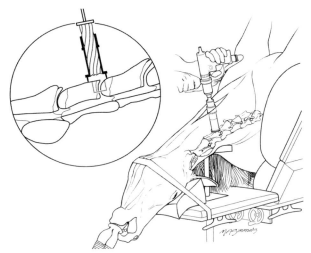

Figure 8.539 Intervertebral fusion using a modified Cloward ventral interbody fusion technique. A 25-mm drill removes most of the disc and vertebral epiphysis, allowing stabilization by inserting a stainless-steel cylinder. (Reprinted with permission from Nixon AJ. Surgical management of equine cervical vertebral malformations. Prog Vet Neurol 1991;2:183–195.)

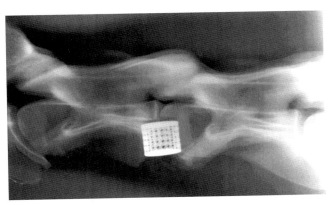

Figure 8.540 Standing lateral radiograph of a horse 14 days after intervertebral fusion. The implant is seated into the soft vertebral bone and is held in place by collapse of the bone around the implant. (Reprinted with permission from Nixon AJ. Surgical management of equine cervical vertebral malformations. Prog Vet Neurol 1991;2:183–195.)

stainless-steel basket. After cleaning debris from the drill hole, the stainless-steel basket is tamped into place until it is seated well into the vertebral bone (Fig. 8.540). If more than one space is being fused, then a plastic spinal plate is secured over the hole with cancellous bone screws.

The longus colli muscles are reapposed over the exposed interspace with sutures. A suction drain is placed between these muscles and the trachea and exteriorized from the skin ventral to the jugular vein. The sternothyrohyoid muscles, subcutaneous tissue, and skin are sutured, and a stent bandage is applied over the wound. Antibiotics and phenylbutazone are continued for 3 to 5 days after surgery, and the drain and stent bandage are removed in 4 to 5 days. Most horses are confined to a stall for 12 weeks following surgery and then turned out to pasture. Results of cervical fusion are encouraging.[65,98,99] Most horses improve neurologically over a period of 15 months, and many return to useful activity.

Dorsal laminectomy is indicated to remove compression originating from the dorsal laminae and ligamentum flavum.[67] It also provides access to the inner aspects of the neural canal for removing encroaching joint capsules, malformed articular facets, and periarticular new bone growth.[66] Because of the complexity and incidence of postoperative fractures of the vertebral pedicle following dorsal laminectomy, however, vertebral fusion has been evaluated and found to be equally effective in providing decompression of cervical static stenosis cases involving the caudal cervical vertebra. Intervertebral fusion of the caudal cervical region is less complex but still requires a deep dissection to adequately expose the ventral surface of these vertebrae.[37,64] As for ventral stabilization for decompression of caudal cervical spinal cord compression in the horse, experimental studies have shown that articular facets and soft tissues atrophy after cervical fusion.[17] Similar atrophy occurs after fusion of caudal cervical vertebrae with static stenosis. Regression of bony enlargements, thickened lamina, and synovial capsule and ligamentum flavum overgrowth gradually decompresses the spinal cord. Seven of eight horses in a preliminary report improved at least one grade within 10 months.[37] The major disadvantage to fusion when static compression is present is the slow rate of bone remodeling that follows fusion. A horse with the majority of compression because of soft tissues, such as the synovial capsule, is a better candidate for intervertebral fusion, since these tissues atrophy quicker than bone can remodel (Fig. 8.541A); however, significant bone remodelling occurs during the postoperative phase, and marked decompression is frequently evident within 6 months of surgery (Fig. 8.541B).

The long-term effectiveness of fusion for cervical static stenosis appears to be quite satisfactory. Although recovery of neurologic dysfunction is slow, complete resolution of deficits has been evident in 7 of 13 horses beyond 2 years evaluated by the author, and several have raced or entered other competitive events. None developed fatal complications due to the surgery. Published data, however, describe fatal complications in 4 of 5 horses where interbody fusion was used to treat cervical static stenosis at C6–C7, indicating the need for caution in recommending surgery.[84]

Prognosis

The prognosis for horses with confirmed CVM depends on the degree of neurologic deficit, the length of time the animal is affected, the intended use, and whether surgery is performed. Generally, horses that are only mildly affected for a short duration have the best prognosis following surgical treatment. Without surgery, some horses become sufficiently stable neurologically to successfully breed. In most cases, however, the disease is progressive. For surgically treated horses intended for breeding, the prognosis is fair to good. The prognosis for return to athletic function is guarded, but this is dependent on the duration and degree of neurologic deficit and whether the surgery completely decompresses the spinal cord.

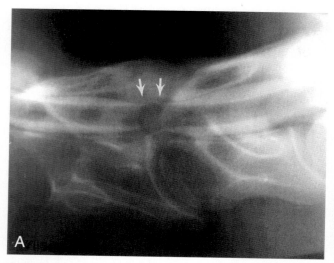
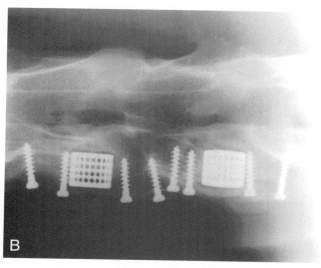

Figure 8.541 A. A myelogram from a 3-year-old horse with cervical static stenosis at C6–C7. A significant soft tissue component is compressing the spinal cord from a dorsal direction (arrows). B. Four-month postoperative radiograph showing progressive bony union of C5–C6 and C6–C7 in a 2-year-old Thoroughbred. The dorsal facet joints have atrophied and regressed from the vertebral canal.

EQUINE PROTOZOAL MYELOENCEPHALITIS

Equine protozoal myeloencephalitis (EPM) has become a prominent and serious equine neurologic disease in North, Central, and South America. Sporadic cases have also been documented in most regions of the world in horses imported from the Americas, often months to years after their arrival. The incidence rates in North America have been estimated as high as 35%.[36] Because the clinical signs of EPM vary, it must be included in the differential diagnosis of any ataxic horse on the American continent. Many breeds, particularly Thoroughbreds and Standardbreds, are affected at racetracks, and many other breeds show sporadic incidence.

Etiopathogenesis

Equine protozoal myeloencephalitis is a focal to multifocal, asymmetric, nonsuppurative inflammatory disorder of the white and gray matter of the spinal cord and brain stem.[6,27] The disease was first reported in Kentucky in 1964[79] and was originally ascribed to an organism that resembled *Toxoplasma gondii*.[47] The definitive host is the opossum.[30] The organism has now been categorized and named *Sarcocystis neurona*.[26] The disease has also been produced in foals by feeding *Sarcocystis* sporocysts isolated from opossums.[31] This has led to an interest in the development of a vaccine for the prevention of EPM.

Signs

Clinical signs of EPM can mimic many neurologic diseases, largely due to widely varying anatomic target regions throughout the central nervous system (CNS). The predominant signs include ataxia and paresis because of the involvement of white or gray matter. Lesions in the white matter of the cervical spinal cord result in ataxia of all four limbs, making it difficult to differentiate from cervical compressive myelopathies. Lesions in the gray matter of the spinal cord, particularly in the cervical or lumbosacral intumescence, can cause lower motor neuron signs of the affected forelimbs or hindlimbs, such as paresis and muscle atrophy. Gray matter involvement is frequently asymmetric, resulting in a disease syndrome that mimics lameness. Muscle atrophy is common in gluteal, quadriceps, infraspinatus and supraspinatus, and longissimus muscle groups. Brain stem and cerebral signs occur in less than 10% of affected horses.[52] Signs include head tilt, nasal deviation, dysphagia, and, occasionally, seizures or personality changes.

Clinical signs can appear suddenly. Gait abnormalities can be acute or more insidious. Progress can be quite rapid and recurrence of ataxia is common. Clinical symptoms often attributed to specific musculoskeletal lameness, such as toe dragging, difficulty in maintaining a specific limb lead, and even upward fixation of the patella, may be due to EPM. Complete lameness and a neurologic examination, including the use of serologic testing, are important for differentiating EPM from other causes of neurologic disease and, more importantly, from other musculoskeletal causes of lameness. Moreover, EPM can occur in horses already suffering ataxia due to cervical vertebral malformation, and the differentiation of the more important of the two specific causes of spinal dysfunction is difficult.

Diagnosis

There is still no definitive antemortem diagnostic test for EPM, despite major improvements in serologic tests. The diagnosis is generally based on a combination of the clinical signs, ruling out other disease causes for ataxic paresis, the presence of CSF antibodies against *Sarco-*

cystis neurona, and the response to appropriate treatment for EPM. The Western blot test for Sarcocystis neurona antibodies in the CSF is the most sensitive test, but a positive result does not necessarily mean the ataxic horse has clinical signs attributable to EPM.[8] Reasons for false positives include previous infection with the infectious organism Sarcocystis neurona, transfer of previously antigen-primed lymphocytes to the CNS, existing quiescent Sarcocystis species in the CNS not necessarily causing disease, blood or plasma contaminated CSF tap, and laboratory error. Because of the concern associated with blood contamination of CSF samples, the atlantooccipital site may be preferable to a lumbosacral tap for retrieving CSF. This necessitates general anesthesia, compared to lumbosacral taps, most of which can be done standing. Nevertheless, the use of the Western blot test for analysis of antibodies in CSF provides significant evidence for incriminating EPM as a cause of neurologic disease. Analysis of serum levels of antibodies against Sarcocystis neurona are generally of limited value because of the high prevalence of antibodies in most adult horses in many parts of northern America. A serum-positive test simply means previous exposure to the infectious organism. It does not indicate active CNS involvement. Analysis of CSF samples is clearly advantageous, and the most significant result is a negative antibody titer in the CSF. This eliminates EPM as the cause of this specific neurologic deficit. To a lesser extent, a negative serum level of EPM is also useful information in the workup of a lameness case. Collecting CSF from clinically normal horses for the purpose of EPM testing is generally meaningless.

Various tests have been devised to correct for blood contamination of CSF samples, thereby differentiating between serum-contaminated positive EPM titers and a true CSF-derived antibody titer. The albumin quotient and IgG indices have been developed to indicate blood contamination. More recently, quantitation of red blood cells in the CSF have been used to indicate blood contamination.[60] Additionally, other tests have been devised specifically looking for the DNA of the infectious organism. This includes the polymerase chain reaction (PCR), where a strongly positive PCR suggests that the DNA from Sarcocystis neurona is present in the CSF. This assay can be falsely negative, however, because the DNA is confined to the neural tissue and capillaries, and either is not in the CSF or is present in minute amounts.

Routine CSF analysis reveals approximately half of the horses with clinical signs associated with EPM have elevated protein concentrations in the CSF. Additionally, the CSF is often xanthochromatic.

Treatment

Treatment is based on the use of antiprotozoal drugs that act by inhibiting folic acid synthesis. Additionally, use of anti-inflammatory, antioxidant, and immunomodulatory treatments is helpful. Current recommendations include the use of pyrimethamine at 1 mg/kg once daily, in combination with sulfadiazine or trimethoprim-sulfadiazine given orally at 20 to 25 mg/kg twice daily. Treatment generally should be for a minimum of 90 days, and ideally should be continued until the CSF anal-

ysis for Sarcocystis antibodies is negative on Western blot. Relapses are relatively common, particularly in horses that have had clinical signs for an extended duration. Many horses are treated for at least 4 weeks beyond the resolution of clinical signs. Current treatment with folic acid inhibitors can affect mammalian cells, as well as the protozoa, when administered for extended periods. Pyrimethamine and sulfonamides can cause bone marrow suppression, which manifests as macrocytic anemia and neutropenia in 10 to 20% of treated horses. Fetuses and neonates are also susceptible to the toxic effects of these drugs. Therefore, appropriate client education is important if pregnant or nursing mares are to be treated. All treated horses should be monitored with white blood cell counts every 4 weeks and antiprotozoal therapy should be reduced or discontinued if leukopenia develops. If supplementation is necessary, such as in pregnant mares, then folinic acid at 0.1 to 0.3 mg/kg orally once daily should be instituted. Additionally, access to green hay or a pasture should be provided. Pyrimethamine has the greatest in vitro activity against Sarcocystic neurona, followed by trimethoprim, with the sulfonamides having no in vitro activity when used alone. The pyrimethamine concentration in CSF is unlikely to exceed 0.1 mg/mL in horses, suggesting that it should be used in combination with a sulfonamide.[22] Approximately 70% of horses treated with a combination of pyrimethamine and sulfonamides respond to therapy, and treatment should continue for at least 3 to 6 months.[22] The relapse rate after treatment is unknown; however, most horses treated for 3 months or less have positive CSF antibody results on Western blot.

Diclazuril (Clinacox, Schering-Plough Animal Health), a newer antiprotozoal drug used in the poultry industry, has been evaluated for treatment of EPM in horses. It is currently not approved for use in horses. Preliminary results of a trial using diclazuril at 2.5 g/450 kg orally for 21 to 28 days indicated approximately 60% of the horses had improved neurologic deficits.[7] Exacerbation of clinical signs can occur, resulting from the death of large numbers of Sarcocystis organisms; however, this is not unique to the use of diclazuril. Absorption of diclazuril from the gastrointestinal tract of horses is reported to be good, with a plasma half-life of 50 hours.[7] An intravenous formulation of the drug has also been tested, given daily for a 5-day course.

The antiprotozoal agent toltrazuril (Baycox, Bayer, Inc., Canada) has also been evaluated for the treatment of EPM. This anticoccidial drug has been used in avian species and ruminants. An oral daily dose of either 5 or 10 mg/kg for 1 month has been the most common regimen. Currently, the drug can only be imported for single case administration and only with approval through the FDA. Anecdotal reports suggest noticeable clinical improvement in horses on toltrazuril after failure to respond to diclazuril and the pyrimethamine/sulfonamide combinations.

Lastly, the antiprotozoal agent nitazoxanide, which is used in humans to treat protozoal and helminth infections, has been evaluated in a limited number of horses. Oral nitazoxanide at 25 mg/kg once daily for 5 days, followed by 50 mg/kg once daily for 23 days, improved the clinical status of 86% of horses.[94] Serious side effects are rare.[94] Nitazoxanide is thought to be protozoicidal, which may be a distinct advantage for treating EPM in the horse. Other than pyrimethamine and the sulfonamide groups, none of these products is licensed for use in the horse. Moreover, three of the four described antiprotozoal regimens, including pyrimethamine and the sulfonamides, result in improvement in approximately 70% of EPM cases.[22] Information is still being collated concerning relapse rates.

Other supportive therapy, including anti-inflammatory agents (such as DMSO and nonsteroidal anti-inflammatory drugs), may be helpful, particularly in the early phases of treatment. Immunostimulants may enhance nonspecific cell-mediated immunity and may be of some value in treating EPM. Levamisole, 1 to 2 mg/kg given orally once daily for 7 to 14 days, killed *Propionibacterium acne*, and mycobacterial cell wall extracts have all been used as immunostimulants.[22]

Prevention

Access of opossums to horse feed, water, stables, and pastures should be prevented as best as possible. Birds, insects, and rodents might act as mechanical vectors for oocysts and should not be allowed access to horse feeds. Intermittent use of antiprotozoal agents may be useful, given that a lapse time of 2 to 4 weeks is required for the ingested sporocysts to develop into merozoites and enter the CNS.[22]

A vaccine has recently been approved for use in horses (conditional licensing, Fort Dodge Animal Health, Kansas). Two particular surface antigens of *Sarcocystis neurona* are thought to be virulence factors, and specific vaccination may have merit. Naturally occurring circulating antibody, however, appears to have little effect in preventing the disease.

EQUINE DEGENERATIVE MYELOENCEPHALOPATHY

Equine degenerative myeloencephalopathy (EDM) is a diffuse degenerative disease of the spinal cord and brain stem occurring in young horses and zebras.[41,58] The cause of the disease is thought to involve nutritional and hereditary factors. Deficiency of vitamin E is a definitive cause, and many affected animals have low serum vitamin E levels. However, certain family lines seem to be predisposed to the disease, particularly in areas that have low vitamin E and selenium levels in pastures.[9] Studies of the interaction of low alpha-tocopherol levels in growing foals that are predisposed through some heritable mechanism showed that low plasma concentration of vitamin E is a factor in the weanling and yearling age group.[53]

Signs and Diagnosis

Clinical signs include symmetric ataxia, weakness, and spasticity and usually begin before 6 months of age. Individual animals are usually involved, although whole groups of weanlings and yearlings can be affected on one farm. Signs are generally progressive and resemble those seen in cases of CVM, although greater variation be-

tween thoracic and pelvic limb involvement is common. Onset of clinical signs is often abrupt and can rapidly progress. Some yearlings become recumbent and others remain stable for several months. In chronic cases, hyporeflexia of the neck and trunk region is common.[41] Normal radiographic and myelographic findings, often coupled with normal hematology, serum chemistry and CSF values, and low EHV_1 titers, lead to a tentative diagnosis of EDM. Serum vitamin E levels are a useful diagnostic test early in the disease. Infected horses frequently have less than 1 mg/mL in serum, although yearlings in the later phases of the disease may have normal vitamin E levels (1.5 mg/mL).

Treatment

Treating individual animals includes supplementation of vitamin E at 1.5 mg/kg per day in the feed. Affected horses may also be treated with 1000 to 3000 IU as a daily intramuscular injection for up to 1 week, followed by 6000 IU given in the feed for the following months or even years. Early recognition of the disease and treatment can be effective. Follow-up evaluation of serum vitamin E levels should be done to assess the progress of treatment. The heritable nature of this disease should also be discussed with the owners of affected stock. A definitive diagnosis cannot be established without a postmortem examination. Since the disease usually progresses despite supportive therapy, many horses with EDM are euthanatized.

EQUINE HERPES VIRUS TYPE 1 (EHV-1)

Of the eight EHVs that have been identified in horses, only EHV-1, EHV-3, and EHV-4 cause obvious clinical syndromes.[70] Importantly, only EHV-1 results in neurologic signs. EHV-1 produces four major disease syndromes in the horse, one being CNS signs due to myeloencephalitis. Although neurologic symptoms are a much less common sequela to EHV-1 infection than rhinopneumonitis, abortion, or birth of weak foals, morbidity reportedly can be as high as 100%.[41] The cause of the myeloencephalitis is believed to be an arterial vasculitis of the CNS, with the symptoms resulting from secondary ischemic infarction and areas of hemorrhage.

Signs and Diagnosis

Peracute onset of paresis and ataxia, particularly severe in the hindlimbs, is occasionally preceded by other symptoms of EHV-1 infection, such as fever, cough, and serous nasal discharge. Urinary incontinence with bladder distension, penile flaccidity, and decreased tail and anal sphincter tone are very common. Recumbency may ensue within 24 hours, but most horses rapidly stabilize soon after the onset of signs. Most horses that remain standing improve slowly and recover completely. Even recumbent horses have been known to recover with nursing care and the use of a sling.

Definitive diagnosis depends on showing a rising antibody titer between acute and convalescent serum samples. CSF antibody titers can also be evaluated but are rarely elevated. CSF is often xanthochromic with normal cell numbers but marked protein elevations. The exact pathogenesis has not been fully determined. Evidence currently favors an immune-mediated disease of the CNS microvasculature, precipitated by viral antigen.[50] Direct viral effects, however, have not been ruled out. The virus is rarely isolated, nor are inclusion bodies seen in the spinal cord or brain from affected animals.

Treatment

Treatment consists of supportive care, with attention to rectal evacuation, bladder decompression, and control of secondary bacterial cystitis and respiratory diseases. Corticosteroids may be beneficial.

The use of EHV-1 vaccines, either modified live or inactivated, does not necessarily prevent the development of EHV-1 myeloencephalitis; however, the general recommendation has been to continue the use of vaccination to minimize the incidence of viremia in horses. The vaccination of horses in the face of an outbreak of EHV-1 myeloencephalitis may not necessarily prevent viremia and the spread of the disease.[40]

EQUINE MOTOR NEURON DISEASE

Equine motor neuron disease, probably similar to Lou Gehrig's disease in humans, was first described in 1990.[12] The disease incidence is increasing, as awareness of the symptoms becomes more widespread. The syndrome occurs in most countries and is characterized by the loss of lower motor neurons of the brain stem and spinal cord. The disease appears to be slightly more common in older horses, with one study showing a peak incidence at 16 years of age. In most cases, the horses have had little or no access to green grass.[23]

Signs

Many horses exhibit weight loss despite reasonable nutritional planes, with muscle tremors and periods of increased voluntary recumbency. Affected horses frequently shift weight between the hindlimbs and occasionally have an abnormally low head carriage. A short stiff gait is apparent, and many horses have a raised tail head.[24] Clinical signs can stabilize several months after onset, although marked muscle wasting develops and further progression is common.

Diagnosis and Treatment

The diagnosis can be difficult. Characteristic clinical stance and muscle trembling are important, coupled with low serum vitamin E concentrations. Electromyographic studies are consistently abnormal in affected animals. A biopsy taken of coccygeal muscle confirms the presence of neurogenic muscle atrophy, and further antemortem confirmation can be provided by performing a biopsy of the ventral branch of the spinal accessory nerve. Degeneration of myelinated axons is present in both acute and chronic cases. The etiology of equine motor neuron disease may involve low serum vitamin E levels; treatment with vitamin E injections may improve early cases but is rarely curative.

SORGHUM SP. TOXICOSIS (SUDAN GRASS)

Sorghum sp. toxicosis produces clinical signs of urinary incontinence, ataxia, and paresis and results from pasturing horses on hybrid sorghum or Sudan grasses.[1] Initial signs of urinary incontinence, with scalding of the pelvic limbs and cystitis, are followed by ataxia and paresis of the pelvic and thoracic limbs. Degeneration of white matter tracts of the spinal cord is believed to be a result of chronic low-level cyanide toxicosis. Treatment is unsuccessful once signs are prominent. Early cases usually recover when removed from the toxic pasture.

VERTEBRAL OSTEOMYELITIS AND EPIDURAL EMPYEMA

Bacterial osteomyelitis of the vertebrae occasionally compresses the spinal cord by the forming epidural empyema or pathologic fractures. Most cases occur as a rare sequela to bacterial septicemia, and foals are predominantly affected. Direct penetrating wounds to the vertebrae or neural canal are also rarely involved. Bacteria involved include *Actinobacillus equuli*, *Escherichia coli*, *Streptococcus spp.*, *Staphylococcus spp.*, *Salmonella spp.*, and *Rhodococcus equi*.[41] Adult horses can be affected by the same organisms, and *Mycobacterium bovis* and *Brucella abortus* have also been isolated.[18,44]

Signs and Diagnosis

Neurologic signs are often preceded by other septic conditions, such as diarrhea, umbilical abscess, polyarthritis, or pulmonary abscess. In foals, bacteremia frequently results in seeding of the vertebral bodies adjacent to the physeal growth plates. As the septic focus develops, symptoms include neck stiffness and pain on lateral bending and some sensitivity to palpation. Enlargement of the lesion results in destruction of the epiphyseal and metaphyseal bone and eventual penetration of the disc and/or adjacent vertebra (Fig. 8.542). Neurologic symptoms develop when the abscess penetrates into the epidural space, causing compression of the spinal cord. Acute onset of ataxia, weakness, and spasticity is seen and, at times, is profoundly asymmetric due to a lateralized location within the vertebra. Heat, pain, and swelling of the affected site may be detected.

Diagnosis is generally achieved by plain radiography and myelography (see Fig. 8.529). Computed tomography may also be helpful to establish the diagnosis and, occasionally, to guide needle centesis for culture confirmation of the organism (Fig. 8.543). Ultrasonography may also be helpful in identifying a perivertebral abscess

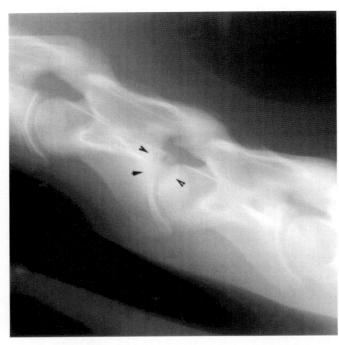

Figure 8.542 Vertebral osteomyelitis of C4 and C5 in a 5-month-old Thoroughbred foal. The lytic lesion involves primarily the caudal epiphysis of C4 but has expanded into the adjacent disc and cranial epiphysis of C5 (arrows). The foal had marked neck stiffness and pain but minimal signs of spinal cord compression.

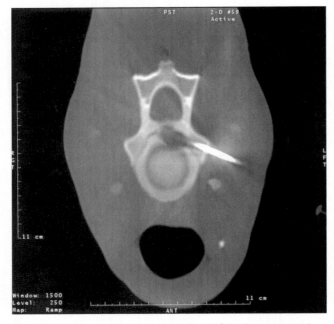

Figure 8.543 Vertebral osteomyelitis of C4 using computed tomography-guided biopsy for culture and sensitivity and for histologic confirmation of bacterial osteomyelitis.

(see Fig. 8.530). Similarly, nuclear scintigraphy and, more specifically, a ciprofloxacin scan may help isolate the site of early osteomyelitis in the vertebral bodies (for more information about a ciprofloxacin scan, see "Vertebral Body Osteomyelitis and Diskospondylitis" in Part 17, "The Thoracolumbar Spine," in this chapter) (see Fig. 8.528). Since the infection usually extends only to the epidural space, it is not surprising that CSF analyses may be within normal limits. In some there may be an indication of compression with xanthochromia and mild elevation of protein and mononuclear cells. Only rarely will there be an indication of infection. In these, the fluid should be submitted for aerobic and anaerobic culture. If the vertebral body is involved, then direct needle biopsy may be helpful. This sample should be submitted for Gram stain, culture and sensitivity, and cytology.

Treatment

Treatment involves appropriate long-term antibiotic therapy. Surgical exploration for culture, curettage, and drainage is often indicated, especially when neurologic status is poor or deteriorating. The prognosis is guarded; however, if adequate drainage and long-term antibiotic (3 to 6 months) therapy can be maintained, then resolution is possible.

SPINAL NEMATODIASIS

Migrating parasites occasionally penetrate the spinal cord and cause variable neurologic deficits, depending on the number, size, and species of parasite involved, and their location within the spinal cord. *Strongylus vulgaris, Halicephalobus (Micronema) deletrix, Draschia megastoma, Setaria spp.,* and *Hypoderma spp.* have all been reported in the CNS of horses.[3,33,39,48,49,56,92]

Clinical signs often mimic other causes of ataxia and limb paresis in the horse. Strong support for a diagnosis of spinal nematodiasis can be obtained when eosinophils are present in the CSF, although eosinophils are occasionally present with EPM.

Treatment with larvicidal anthelmintics, particularly fenbendazole (60 mg/kg, once), diethylcarbamazine citrate, and organophosphates, have been described.[40,56] The use of ivermectin (0.2 mg/kg) may not be suitable for treatment of parasites in the CNS since it does not cross the blood-brain barrier with enough efficiency to develop effective concentrations.

VERTEBRAL FRACTURES

Vertebral fractures with or without associated spinal cord injury are common occurrences, especially among foals and weanlings. Of 125 horses destroyed due to fractures occurring at race meetings in Britain, nearly one-quarter of these involved fractures of the vertebrae.[95] Approximately one-half of these were fractures of the cervical vertebrae. Other cases described in the literature are also predominantly of the cervical vertebrae.[4,32,34,38,42,51,71,88,95]

Cervical Fractures

Cervical fractures are more common in foals and often involve separation of an epiphysis from the remainder of a vertebral body. Lesions of the occipitoatlantoaxial region, especially of the dens, have been most frequently reported in the literature.[4,34,38,51,78,88] Separation of the dens allows the axis to displace ventrad and compress the spinal cord (Fig. 8.544). If cord damage is severe, then death can occur immediately; however, most foals exhibit ataxia and paresis or paralysis of all limbs and frequently recumbency with an inability to raise the head and neck. Sensory deficits can be marked, and crepitation and neck swelling are frequently seen. The diagnosis is confirmed by radiography.

Hyperflexion and hyperextension injuries of the second to sixth cervical vertebrae are often caused by falls and frequently result in separating a vertebral epiphyseal end plate from the vertebral body. This is often complicated by tearing of the joint capsules with a dislocation or fracture of the dorsal articular facets. This combination allows vertebral subluxation or angulation with spinal cord contusion (Fig. 8.545). Trauma to the middle cervical or caudal cervical vertebrae results in ataxia and tetraparesis and occasionally recumbency. The cervical musculature usually retains innervation, and skin sensation is intact. Swelling, angulation, and splinting of the neck are common.

In foals or adults, many combinations of vertebral body and articular process fracture and luxation are seen. Unfortunately there is little consistency in neurologic signs resulting from them. Multiple fractures of a vertebra resulting in tetraplegia in one horse paradoxically can result in few if any neurologic signs in others (Fig. 8.546). It may be that a radiograph taken at the time of examination reveals little of the vertebral dynamics that occurred at the time of injury.

For most animals, diuretic, anti-inflammatory, and analgesic agents are immediately indicated. Dexamethasone at 0.1 to 0.2 mg/kg may be given intravenously

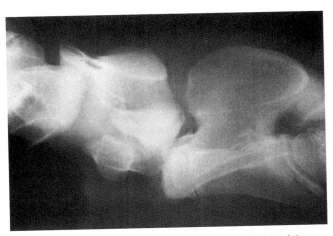

Figure 8.544 Fracture of the axis through the physis of the dens, allowing the axis to displace ventrad and compress the spinal cord.

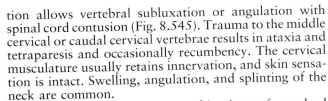
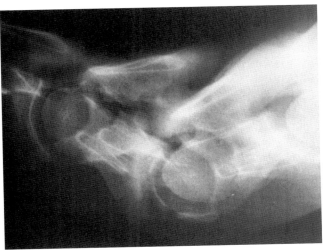

Figure 8.546 Multiple fractures of the fifth cervical vertebra associated with minimal neurologic signs. Paradoxically, cases with similar radiographic features are often tetraplegic.

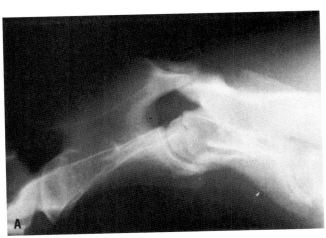

Figure 8.545 Separation of the cranial epiphyseal end plate of C3 with tearing of the joint capsules dorsally and subsequent

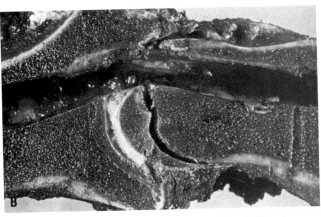

vertebral malalignment with spinal cord contusion. A. Standing cervical radiograph. B. Necropsy specimen.

and repeated every 8 hours depending on the response. Hyperosmolar diuretics such as 20% Mannitol (1 to 2 g/kg IV) or glycerol in water given orally at (1 g/kg/ tid) are suggested. In addition, sedation with acetyl promazine, chloral hydrate, or diazepam may help reduce struggling and further damage to the spinal cord. Analgesia should be provided with phenylbutazone (6 mg/kg IV). DMSO (1 g/kg) administered intravenously as a 20% solution in 5% dextrose and water may be useful; however, experimental studies in other species are contradictory. Greater dilutions (10%) of DMSO result in less intravascular hemolysis. Continued evaluation of the response to therapy is mandatory. Deteriorating clinical status usually indicates repeated spinal cord trauma, due to vertebral instability or progressive hemorrhage, or self-perpetuating vascular reactions within the cord triggered by the initial traumatic incident. Surgical treatment is indicated when progressive deterioration is apparent, and radiographs demonstrate a lesion amenable to stabilization or decompression.

External manipulation with external or internal fixation may be required. Surgical fusion and/or decompression may also be indicated but are infrequently employed. Many nondisplaced fractures of the vertebral arch and articular processes do not compress the cord directly but result in an epidural hematoma that compresses the cord acutely over a wide region. Many of these horses have progressively deteriorating neurologic signs and need immediate decompression to prevent the extensive vascular compromise to the spinal cord that is implicated in progressive myelomalacia.[10,25,85] Some horses fail to respond to surgery because of an inability to arrest this self-perpetuating vascular cascade.

Careful manipulation under general anesthesia may reduce some fracture-luxations and better align other multiple vertebral fractures. This, in conjunction with a neck cast, is certainly preferable to conservatively treating a steadily deteriorating animal. Fiberglass neck casts have been used successfully in the repair of upper cervical fracture luxations.[86]

Surgical repairs of fracture-luxations of the dens have been described. Pins were used successfully to stabilize a fractured dens with luxation of the axis in a foal.[71] A ventral approach for atlantoaxial fusion with lag screws and a cancellous bone graft has also been used for a similar case (Fig. 8.547).

An adult horse with tearing of the left joint capsule at C2–C3 and lateral luxation with torticollis was successfully repaired by open reduction and lag screw fixation between the involved articular facets.[78] In some instances, horses with fractures of the midcervical vertebrae remain neurologically stable or slowly improve and may be best managed medically; however, healing of such fractures often results in residual vertebral malalignment and, on occasion, delayed recurrence of neurologic signs due to a progressive bony callus formation within the vertebral canal. If neurologic deficits do not improve or continue to deteriorate, then surgical stabilization is warranted. There are several descriptions of ventral plating in the literature for the surgical repair of middle cervical fractures.[63] Despite the soft vertebral bone, ventral plating and the use of cancellous screws can be effective for maintaining the alignment of frac-

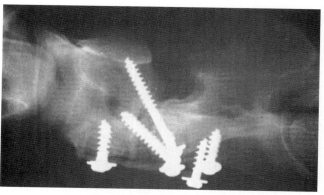

Figure 8.547 Postoperative radiograph following repair of case in Figure 8.544. A ventral approach with dens removal and lag screw fixation has realigned the atlas and axis. A neck cast provides external support.

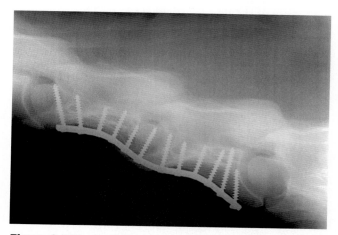

Figure 8.548 Application of a ventral plate to stabilize fractures of C4 and C5. The 6.5-mm cancellous screws engage the dorsal cortex of the vertebral body and must be inserted with care.

tured midcervical vertebrae (Fig. 8.548). The full length of the associated pair of vertebrae should be included in the plate fixation. The 6.5-mm cancellous screws should also engage both ventral and dorsal cortices of the vertebral body. Careful drilling and conservative measurement of screw length is vital to prevent screw penetration of the vertebral venous sinuses and the dura mater. Recovery from neurologic deficit can result, however—horses that are already recumbent at the time of surgery are poor candidates for surgical fracture realignment and plate fixation.

Thoracolumbar Fractures

Fractures of the dorsal spinous processes of the thoracic vertebrae are relatively common sequelae to a backward fall. No neurologic signs result, and the fractures usually heal without complication.

Thoracolumbar vertebral body fractures are not common. When they do occur, the cranial thoracic (T1 to

T3), midthoracic (T9 to T16), and lumbar vertebrae (L1 to L6) are predisposed sites.[42] Jumping accidents, race falls, electrocution, lightning strikes, and tetanus have all caused fracture of the thoracolumbar spine. Sudden onset of ataxia and paraparesis or paraplegia is common. Vertebral fracture displacement often anatomically or physiologically severs the cord. Reflexes of the pelvic limbs and perineal region are maintained and, although rare in the horse, the Schiff-Sherrington phenomenon with extensor rigidity of the thoracic limbs is occasionally seen. The prognosis is poor. Some nondisplaced fractures with hemorrhage and edema produce signs of ataxia and paresis, but these horses can stabilize and, with stall rest, eventually recover. Even the totally paraplegic case with intact deep pain sensation should be given the benefit of 24 hours of intensive medical therapy before a decision on euthanasia is made. A rectal examination may reveal evidence of a fracture of the lumbar vertebrae. The diagnosis of fracture displacement can be substantiated by radiography. Medical treatment options are similar to cervical fractures.

Sacral and Coccygeal Fractures

Sacral and sacrococcygeal fractures usually result from a horse falling backward and impacting on these bones. Clinical signs due to compression of the cauda equina occur soon after and depend on the vertebrae affected.[63,101] Fractures of the sacrum may result in gait disturbances, fecal and urinary incontinence, and atrophy of the gluteal muscles (Fig. 8.549). Neuritis of the cauda equina produces similar signs and needs to be considered in the differential diagnosis. More caudal sacral and sacrococcygeal fractures produce loss of motor tone in the tail, relaxation of bladder and anal sphincters, loss of sensation, and, occasionally, hyperesthesia in the perineal area. Radiography and rectal examination are used to diagnose the site of fracture. Electromyography of the tail, gluteal, and perineal regions after 1 week will aid in the diagnosis, prognosis, and determination of response to treatment. Positive contrast epidurography and vertebral venography of the sacrococcygeal area are sometimes useful to determine the extent of compression, especially if surgical decompression is being considered. Medical treatment with anti-inflammatory agents and analgesics, combined with rectal evacuation and urinary bladder catheterization, are usually indicated. If improvement is not seen within a week, then the prognosis for complete recovery is poor. Surgical decompression and stabilization of the sacrococcygeal region is possible; however, access to the dorsal aspect of the cranial sacrum is limited by the tuber sacrale.[11]

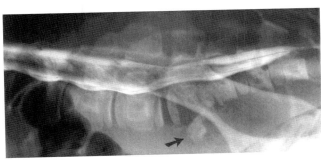

Figure 8.549 Myelographic examination of a foal with a burst fracture of the first sacral vertebra and ventral compression of the cauda equina has developed (arrow).

References

1. Adams LG, Dollahite JW, Romane WM, et al. Cystitis and ataxia associated with sorghum ingestion by horses. J Am Vet Med Assoc 1969;155:518.
2. Alitalo I, Karkkainen M. Osteochondrotic changes in the vertebrae of four ataxic horses suffering from cervical vertebral malformation. Nord Vet Med 1983;35:468–478.
3. Alstad AD, Berg IE, Samuel C. Disseminated *Micronema deletrix* infection in the horse. J Am Vet Med Assoc 1979;174:264.
4. Baker GJ. Comminuted fracture of the axis. Equine Vet J 1970; 2:37.
5. Beech J. Metrizamide myelography in the horse. J Am Vet Rad Soc 1979;20:22.
6. Beech J, Dodd DC. Toxoplasma-like encephalomyelitis in the horse. J Vet Pathol 1974;11:87.
7. Bentz BB, et al. Preliminary report on diclazuril and equine protozoal myeloencephalitis. In: Proceedings. 8th International Conference, Equine Infectious Diseases, Dubai, United Arab Emirates, 1998;138.
8. Bernard WB. Equine protozoal myelitis-laboratory tests and interpretations. In: Proceedings. International Equine Neurology Conference, Cornell University, Ithaca, NY, 1997;7–11.
9. Blythe LL, Craig AM. Equine degenerative myeloencephalopathy. I. Clinical signs and pathogenesis. Comp Cont Educ Pract Vet 1992;13:1215–1221.
10. Braund KG. Acute spinal cord traumatic compression. In: Bojrab MJ, Ed. Pathophysiology in Small Animal Surgery. Philadelphia: Lea & Febiger, 1981;220.
11. Collatos C, Allen D, Chambers J, Henry M. Surgical treatment of sacral fracture in a horse. J Am Vet Med Assoc 1991;198: 877–879.
12. Cummings JF, de Lahunta A, George C, et al. Equine motor neuron disease: A preliminary report. Cornell Vet 1990;80:357–379.
13. deLahunta A. Veterinary Neuroanatomy and Clinical Neurology. 2nd ed. Philadelphia: WB Saunders, 1983.
14. deLahunta A. Diagnosis of equine neurologic problems. Cornell Vet 1978;68(Suppl 6):122.
15. De Lahunta A, Hedhammar A, Wu FM, Krook L. Overnutrition and skeletal disease: An experimental study in growing Great Dane dogs. Part VII. Cervical vertebrae and spinal cord. Cornell Vet 1974;64(Suppl 5):58.
16. De La Torre JC, Johnson CM, Goode DJ, Mullan S. Pharmacologic treatment and evaluation of permanent experimental spinal cord trauma. Neurology 1975;25:508.
17. DeBowes RM, Grant BD, Bagby GW, et al. Cervical vertebral interbody fusion in the horse: A comparative study of bovine xenografts and autografts supported by stainless steel baskets. Am J Vet Res 1984;45:191–199.
18. Denny HR. A review of brucellosis in the horse. Equine Vet J 1973;5:121.
19. Dimock WW. "Wobbles," a hereditary disease in horses. J Hered 1950;41:319–323.
20. Dimock WW. Incoordination of horses (wobbles). Bull Kentucky Agric Exp Station 1950;553:1.
21. Dimock WW, Errington BJ. Incoordination of Equidae: Wobblers. J Am Vet Med Assoc 1939;95:261.
22. Divers TJ, Berman DD, deLahunta A. Equine protozoal myeloencephalitis: Recent advances in diagnosis and treatment. Vet Med [The Veterinary CE Advisor Supplement] February 2000: 3–18.
23. Divers TJ, Mohammed HO, Cummings JF, et al. Equine motor neuron disease: Findings in 28 horses and proposal of a pathophysiological mechanism for the disease. Equine Vet J 1994;26: 409–415.
24. Divers TJ, et al. Equine motor neuron diseases: A new cause of weakness, trembling and weight loss. Comp Cont Educ Pract Vet 1992;14:1222–1226.

25. Docker TB, Kindt GW, Kempe LG. Pathological findings in acute experimental spinal cord trauma. J Neurosurg 1971;35:700.

26. Dubey JP, Davis SW, Speer CA, et al. Sarcocystis neurona n. sp. [Protozoa: Apicomplexa], the etiologic agent of equine protozoal myeloencephalitis. J Parasitol 1991;77:212–218.

27. Dubey JP, Davis GW, Koestner A, Kiryu K. Equine encephalomyelitis due to a protozoan parasite resembling Toxoplasma gondii. J Am Vet Med Assoc 1974;165:249.

28. Errington BJ. Causes of "wobbles." Army Med Bull [Vet Bull Suppl] 1938;32:152.

29. Falco MJ, Whitwell K, Palmer AC. An investigation into the genetics of "wobbler" disease in Thoroughbred horses in Britain. Equine Vet J 1976;8:165–169.

30. Fenger CF, et al. Identification of opossums [Didelphis virginiana] as the putative definitive host of Sarcocystis neurona. J Parasitol 1995;81:916–919.

31. Fenger CK, et al. Experimental induction of equine protozoal myeloencephalitis in horses using Sarcocystis sporocysts from the opossum. Vet Parasitol 1997;68:199–213.

32. Fessler JF, Amstutz HE. Fracture repair. In: Oehme FW, Prier JE, Eds. Textbook of Large Animal Surgery. Baltimore: Williams & Wilkins, 1974;328.

33. Frauenfelder HC, Kazacos KR, Lichtenfels JR. Cerebrospinal nematodiasis caused by a filariid in a horse. J Am Vet Med Assoc 1980;177:359.

34. Funk KA, Erickson ED. A case of atlanto-axial subluxation in a horse. Can Vet J 1968;9:120.

35. Gabel AA, et al. Comparison of incidence and severity of developmental orthopedic disease on 17 farms before and after adjustment of ration. Proc Am Assoc Equine Pract 1987;33:163–170.

36. Granstrom DE. Equine protozoal myeloencephalitis testing: Review of 1993 and 1994. Proc Am Assoc Equine Pract 1995;41:218–219.

37. Grant BD, et al. Ventral stabilization for decompression of caudal cervical spinal cord compression in the horse. Proc Am Assoc Equine Pract 1985;31:75–90.

38. Guffy MM, Cofpman JR, Strafuss AC. Atlantoaxial luxation in a foal. J Am Vet Med Assoc 1969;155:754.

39. Hadlow WJ, Ward JK, Krinsky WL. Intracranial myiasis by Hypoderma bovis (Linnaeus) in a horse. Cornell Vet 1977;67:272.

40. Hahn CN, Mayhew IG, MacKay RJ. Nervous system: Diseases of multiple or unknown sites. In: Colahan PT, Mayhew IG, Merritt AM, Moore JN, Eds. Equine Medicine and Surgery. 5th ed. Philadelphia: CV Mosby, 1999;884–903.

41. Hahn CN, Mayhew IG, MacKay RJ. Nervous system: Diseases of the spinal cord. In: Colahan PT, Mayhew IG, Merritt AM, Moore JN, Eds. Equine Medicine and Surgery. 5th ed. Philadelphia: CV Mosby, 1999;945–956.

42. Jeffcott LB, Whitwell KE. Fractures of the thoracolumbar spine of the horse. Proc Am Assoc Equine Pract 1976;22:91.

43. Jones TC, Doll ER, Brown RG. The pathology of equine incoordination (ataxia or "wobbles") of foals. In: Proceedings. 91st American Veterinary Medical Association, 1954;139.

44. Kelly WR, et al. Vertebral osteomyelitis in a horse associated with Mycobacterium tuberculosis var. bovis (M. bovis). J Am Vet Radiol Soc 1972;13:59.

45. Knight DA, Weisbrode SE, Schmall LM, et al. The effects of copper supplementation on the prevalence of cartilage lesions in foals. Equine Vet J 1990;122:426–432.

46. Knight DA, et al. Correlation of dietary mineral to incidence and severity of metabolic bone disease in Ohio and Kentucky. Proc Am Assoc Equine Pract 1985;31:445–461.

47. Kusick PK, et al. Toxoplasmosis in two horses. J Am Vet Med Assoc 1974;164:77–80.

48. Lester G. Parasitic encephalomyelitis in horses. Comp Cont Educ Pract Vet 1992;14:1624–1630.

49. Little PB. Cerebrospinal nematodiasis of Equidae. J Am Vet Med Assoc 1972;160:1407.

50. Little PB, Thorsen J. Disseminated necrotizing myeloencephalitis: A herpes associated neurological disease of horses. J Vet Pathol 1976;13:161.

51. Lundvall RL. Ataxia of colts as a result of injuries. Norden News 1969;Summer:6.

52. MacKay RJ. Equine protozoal myeloencephalitis. Vet Clin North Am Equine Pract 1997;13:79–96.

53. Mayhew IG. Measurements of the accuracy of clinical diagnoses of equine neurologic disease. J Vet Internal Med 1991;5:332–334.

54. Mayhew IG. Collection of cerebrospinal fluid from the horse. Cornell Vet 1975;65:500.

55. Mayhew IG, Donawick WJ, Green SL, et al. Diagnosis and prediction of cervical vertebral malformation in Thoroughbred foals based on semi-quantitative radiographic indicators. Equine Vet J 1993;25:435–440.

56. Mayhew IG, Lichtenfels JR, Greiner EC, et al. Migration of a spiruroid nematode through the brain of a horse. J Am Vet Med Assoc 1982;180:1306.

57. Mayhew IG, deLahunta A, Whitlock RH, et al. Spinal cord disease in the horse. Cornell Vet 1978;68(Suppl. 6):1–207.

58. Mayhew IG, deLahunta A, Whitlock RH, Geary JC. Equine degenerative myeloencephalopathy. J Am Vet Med Assoc 1977;170:195–201.

59. Mayhew IG, Mackay RJ. The nervous system. In: Mansmann RA, McAllister ES, Eds. Equine Medicine and Surgery. 3rd ed. Santa Barbara, CA: American Veterinary Publications, 1982;1214.

60. Miller MM, Sweeney CR, Russell GE, et al. Effects of blood contamination of cerebrospinal fluid on Western blot analysis for detection of antibodies against Sarcocystis neurona and on albumin quotient and immunoglobulin G index in horses. J Am Vet Med Assoc 1999;215:67–71.

61. Neuwirth L. Equine myelography. Comp Cont Educ Pract Vet 1992;14:72–78.

62. Nixon AJ. Nervous system: Cervical vertebral malformation and malarticulation. In: Colahan PT, Mayhew IG, Merritt AM, Moore JN, Eds. Equine Medicine and Surgery. 5th ed. Philadelphia: CV Mosby, 1999;956–972.

63. Nixon AJ. Fractures of the vertebrae. In: Nixon AJ, Ed. Equine Fracture Repair. Philadelphia: WB Saunders, 1996;299–312.

64. Nixon AJ. Surgical management of equine cervical vertebral malformations. Prog Vet Neurol 1991;2:183–195.

65. Nixon AJ, Stashak TS. Surgical therapy for spinal cord disease in the horse. Proc Am Assoc Equine Pract 1985;31:61–74.

66. Nixon AJ, Stashak TS. Dorsal laminectomy in the horse I: Review of the literature and description of a new procedure. J Vet Surg 1983;12:172.

67. Nixon AJ, Stashak TS, Ingram JT. Dorsal laminectomy in the horse III: Results in horses with cervical vertebral malformation. J Vet Surg 1983;12:184.

68. Nixon AJ, Stashak TS, Ingram JT. Diagnosis of cervical vertebral malformation in the horse. Proc Am Assoc Equine Pract 1982;28:253–266.

69. Nyland TG, et al. Metrizamide myelography in the horse: Clinical, radiographic and pathologic changes. Am J Vet Res 1980;41:204–211.

70. Ostlund EN. The equine herpes viruses. Vet Clin North Am Equine Pract 1993;9:283–294.

71. Owen R, Maxie LL. Repair of fractured dens of the axis in a foal. J Am Vet Med Assoc 1978;173:854.

72. Pappageorges M, et al. Radiographic and myelographic examination of the cervical vertebral column in 306 ataxic horses. Vet Radiol 1987;28:53–59.

73. Powers BE, et al. Pathology of the vertebral column of horses with cervical static stenosis. Vet Pathol 1986;23:392–399.

74. Rantanen NW, et al. Ataxia and paresis in horses. Part II. Radiographic and myelographic examination of the cervical vertebral column. Comp Cont Educ Pract Vet 1981;3:S161–S171.

75. Reed SM, et al. The relationship of cervical vertebral malformation to developmental orthopedic disease. Proc Am Assoc Equine Pract 1987;33:139–142.

76. Reed SM, et al. Ataxia and paresis in horses, Part I: Differential diagnosis. Comp Cont Educ Pract Vet 1981;3:S88.

77. Reiland S. Morphology of osteochondrosis and sequelae in pigs. Acta Radiol Suppl 1978;358:45.

78. Robinson PA, Currall JHS. Surgical repair of a cervical fracture-dislocation in a mature horse. NZ Vet J 1981;29:28.

79. Rooney JR, et al. Focal myelitis-encephalitis in horses. Cornell Vet 1970;60:494–501.
80. Rucker NC, Lumb WV, Scott RJ. Combined pharmacologic and surgical treatments for acute spinal cord trauma. Am J Vet Res 1981;42:1138.
81. Ruff SJ, et al. A comparison of growth rates of normal Thoroughbred foals and foals diagnosed with cervical vertebral malformation. J Equine Vet Sci 1993;13:596–599.
82. Rush Moore B, et al. Diagnosis of equine protozoal myeloencephalitis and cervical stenotic myelopathy. Comp Cont Educ Pract Vet 1995;17:419–426.
83. Rush Moore B, et al. Assessment of vertebral canal diameter and bony malformations of the cervical part of the spine in horses with cervical stenotic myelopathy. Am J Vet Res 1994;55:5–13.
84. Rush Moore B, et al. Surgical treatment of cervical stenotic myelopathy in horses: 73 cases (1983–1992). J Am Vet Med Assoc 1993;203:108–112.
85. Sandier AN, Tator CH. Review of the effect of spinal cord trauma on the vessels and blood flow in the spinal cord. J Neurosurg 1976;45:638.
86. Schneider JE. Immobilizing cervical vertebral fractures. Proc Am Assoc Equine Pract 1981;27:253.
87. Schulz LC, et al. Zur Pathogenese der spinalen ataxie des pferdes. Spondylarthrosis. Pathologisch-anatomische untersuchungen. Dtsch Tiererztl Wschr 1965;72:502.
88. Slone DE, Bergfeld WA, Walker TL. Surgical decompression for traumatic atlantoaxial subluxation in a weanling filly. J Am Vet Med Assoc 1979;174:1234.
89. Stashak TS. The nervous system: Specific procedures. In: Jennings PB, ed. Practice of Large Animal Surgery. Philadelphia: WB Saunders, 1984;1023.
90. Steel JD, Whittem JH., Hutchins DR. Equine sensory ataxia ("wobbles"). Aust Vet J 1959;35:442.
91. Stromberg B. A review of the salient features of osteochondrosis in the horse. Equine Vet J 1979;11:211.
92. Swanstrom OG, Rising JL, Carlton WW. Spinal nematodiasis in a horse. J Am Vet Med Assoc 1969;155:748.
93. Tomizawa N, Nishimura R, Sasaki N, et al. Efficacy of the new radiographic measurement method for cervical vertebral instability in wobbling foals. J Vet Med Sci 1994;56:1119–1122.
94. Vatistas N, et al. Initial experiences with the use of nitazoxanide in the treatment of equine protozoal myeloencephalitis in northern California. Equine Pract 1999;21:18–21.
95. Vaughan LC, Mason BJE. A clinico-pathological study of racing accidents in horses. Surg Dept, Royal Vet College, North Mymms, Hatfield, Herts, England, 1976.
96. Wagner PC. Diseases of the spine. In: Mansmann RA, McAllister ES, Eds. Equine Medicine and Surgery. 3rd ed. Santa Barbara, CA: American Veterinary Publications, 1982;1145.
97. Wagner PC, et al. A study of the heritability of cervical vertebral malformation in horses. Proc Am Assoc Equine Pract 1985;31: 1985.
98. Wagner PC, et al. Ataxia and paresis in horses, Part III: Surgical treatment of cervical spinal cord compression. Comp Cont Educ Pract Vet 1981;3:S192.
99. Wagner PC, et al. Evaluation of cervical spinal fusion as a treatment in the equine "wobbler" syndrome. J Vet Surg 1979;8:84.
100. Wagner PC, et al. Surgical stabilization of the equine cervical spine. J Vet Surg 1979;8:7.
101. Wagner PC, et al. Traumatic injury of the cauda equina in the horse: A case report. J. Equine Med Surg 1977;1:282.

Trimming and Shoeing for Balance and Soundness*

TED S. STASHAK, CHERRY HILL, RICHARD KLIMESH, AND GENE OVNICEK

Since the hoof capsule is malleable, the manner in which it is trimmed and shod can have a marked effect on performance and soundness of the equine athlete. Hoof imbalance, characterized by improper toe and heel length, inappropriate hoof angle, and mediolateral hoof imbalance, is common.[4,12,16,30,37,48,52] Although some horses can tolerate these imbalances, others cannot and may enter a cycle that results in lameness.

Trimming and shoeing can be categorized as preventive, corrective, or therapeutic. *Preventive* trimming and shoeing is characterized by balance, support, and protection; and the goals are long-term soundness for performance. *Corrective* trimming and shoeing consists of alterations in the hoof and or shoe to affect stance or stride and breakover. Properly employed corrective farriery does not force a limb into an abnormal position; it allows the hoof and limb to attain a desirable configuration, achieve more normal movement, and enhance breakover. *Therapeutic* trimming and shoeing is designed to protect or support an injured hoof or limb or to prevent or encourage a particular movement until healing can take place. For example, heel elevation may be used to reduce the tension on the deep digital flexor tendon, which in turn reduces the pressure on the navicular bone in horses suffering from navicular syndrome.

A lateral radiograph of the hoof, with markers in place, is commonly taken to identify the proper location for breakover when corrective or therapeutic farriery is being employed (Fig. 8.47). Even though some lamenesses may not be affected by shoeing, preventive trimming and shoeing should be a part of the routine hoof care program for every performance horse.

SHOEING PROCEDURE

Good shoeing is an art and a science. For farriers to do their best work, a proper area should be provided, and well-mannered (tractable) horses should be presented (Fig. 9.1). There should be a place to tie horses safely at a height above the withers, and the area should be well lighted, uncluttered, and level. A concrete slab covered with a rubber mat is ideal. Shade and shelter should be provided for summer as well as for winter work. Access to electrical outlets for power tools is essential. It is the horse owner's responsibility to present the farrier with a cooperative horse that has been trained to have its limbs handled and its hooves worked on.

Before removing the old shoes, the farrier should discuss with the trainer, owner, and/or veterinarian any problems or concerns regarding the horse's hooves or the horse's way of moving. If the horse is a regular client, the farrier should have records related to the horse's previous shoeings.

The horse's movement should be evaluated at a walk and at a trot in a straight line so that the farrier can watch (from the front, rear, and side) the manner in which the horse picks up its hooves, moves them, and puts them down. From the side view, the hoof should land flat or slightly heel first but generally not toe first. From the front and rear view, the hooves should land flat. A hoof that does not land properly when it is time for a reset may indicate that the hoof was not correctly shod in the first place, the hoof has grown out of balance since the last shoeing, the horse is compensating for pain, or the horse's conformation is such that the hoof does not land flat. The way a hoof lands differs with each gait and from forelimb to hindlimb. Most horses require shoeing every 5 to 8 weeks, partly because the hoof wall at the toe grows faster than that at the heels, which causes the hoof to become imbalanced.

After removing the old shoes, each hoof and shoe are examined for clues to wear patterns (see display "How to Remove a Shoe" and Figs. 9.2 to 9.9). The hoof angle can be determined by using a hoof gauge, and the length of the untrimmed hoof can be measured with dividers or a ruler. The balance, shape, and symmetry of the hoof are assessed, and any tendencies to form flares or dishes are noted. Hoof symmetry and size are evaluated by comparing one hoof to the other.

HOW TO REMOVE A SHOE

Assemble the necessary tools for removing a shoe: the clinch cutter, hammer, pull-offs, and crease nail puller (Fig. 9.2).

Using the chisel end of the clinch cutter, open the clinches by tapping the spine of the clinch cutter with the hammer (Fig. 9.3).

The "clinch" is the end of the nail that is folded over; this needs to be opened so that the nails can be pulled through the hoof wall without breaking off large hunks of the hoof (Fig. 9.4).

If the shoe is creased, use the crease nail puller to extract each nail individually, which allows the shoe to come off (Fig. 9.5).

Nails with protruding heads can be pulled out by using the pull-offs (Fig. 9.6).

If the nails cannot be pulled out individually, remove the shoe with the pull-offs. After the clinches have been opened, grab the shoe heel and pry toward the center of the frog. Do the same with the other shoe heel (Fig. 9.7A).

When both heels are loose, grab one side of the shoe at the toe and pry toward the center of the frog. Repeat around the shoe until it is removed (Fig. 9.7B). Never pry toward the outside of the hoof, or you risk ripping big pieces out of the hoof wall. As the nail heads protrude while the shoe is loosened, pull them out with the pull-offs.

Pull out any nails that may remain in the hoof (Fig. 9.8).

To protect the hoof until the shoe is replaced, either wrap the hoof edges with tape (Fig. 9.9A), or, if the horse has a tender sole, tape a cloth over the bottom of the hoof (Fig. 9.9B) or use a protective boot. If the shoes are being pulled to let the horse go barefoot, a qualified farrier should trim the hoof to minimize breakage and ensure balance.

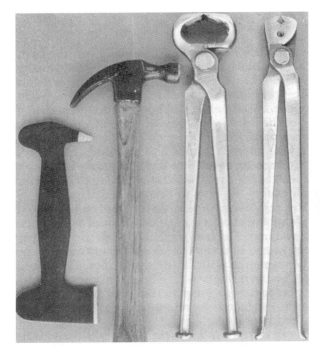

Figure 9.2 Tools for removing a shoe (from left): clinch cutter, hammer, pull-offs, crease nail puller. (Reprinted with permission from Hill C, Klimesh R. Maximum Hoof Power. North Pomfret, VT: Trafalgar Square Publishing, 2000.)

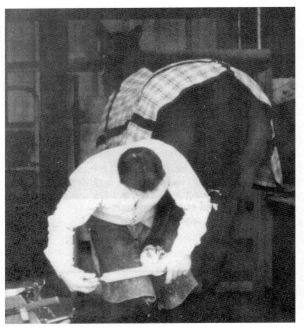

Figure 9.1 A good work area for shoeing. (Reprinted with permission from Hill C, Klimesh R. Maximum Hoof Power. North Pomfret, VT: Trafalgar Square Publishing, 2000.)

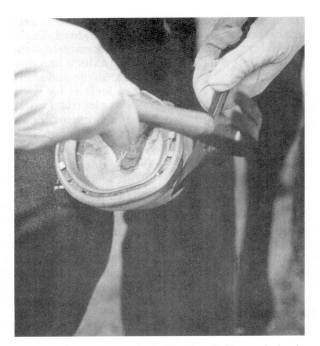

Figure 9.3 Opening the clinch. (Reprinted with permission from Hill C, Klimesh R. Maximum Hoof Power. North Pomfret, VT: Trafalgar Square Publishing, 2000.)

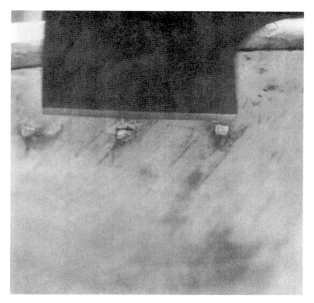

Figure 9.4   A clinch cutter in position. (Reprinted with permission from Hill C, Klimesh R. Maximum Hoof Power. North Pomfret, VT: Trafalgar Square Publishing, 2000.)

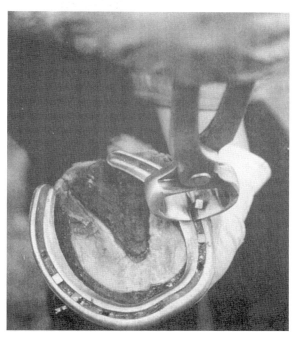

Figure 9.6   Using pull-offs to remove nails. (Reprinted with permission from Hill C, Klimesh R. Maximum Hoof Power. North Pomfret, VT: Trafalgar Square Publishing, 2000.)

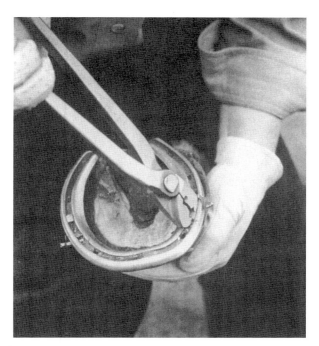

Figure 9.5   Using a crease nail puller to remove nails. (Reprinted with permission from Hill C, Klimesh R. Maximum Hoof Power. North Pomfret, VT: Trafalgar Square Publishing, 2000.)

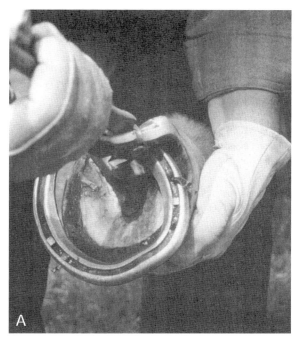

Figure 9.7   Using pull-offs to remove the shoe. A. Prying the shoe heel toward the center of the frog. (Reprinted with permission from Hill C, Klimesh R. Maximum Hoof Power. North Pomfret, VT: Trafalgar Square Publishing, 2000.)

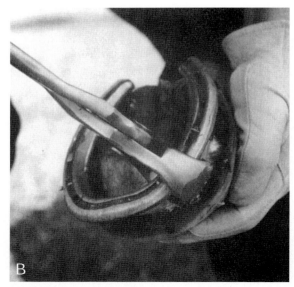

Figure 9.7 *(continued)*   B. Prying the side of the shoe toward the center of the frog. (Reprinted with permission from Hill C, Klimesh R. Maximum Hoof Power. North Pomfret, VT: Trafalgar Square Publishing, 2000.)

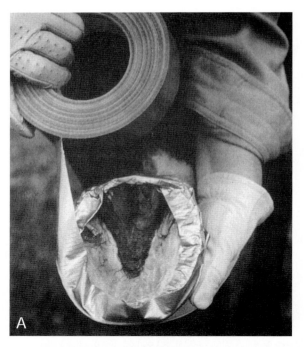

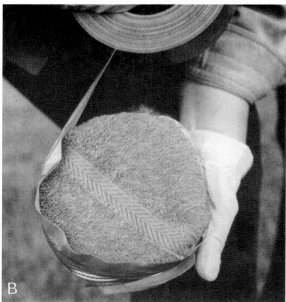

Figure 9.9   Protecting the hoof until the shoe is replaced. A. Taping the hoof. B. Taping a cloth to the bottom of the sole. (Reprinted with permission from Hill C, Klimesh R. Maximum Hoof Power. North Pomfret, VT: Trafalgar Square Publishing, 2000.)

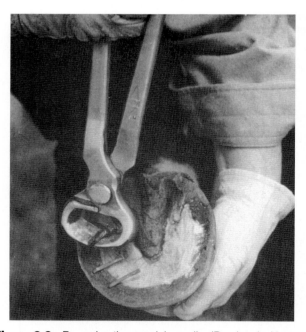

Figure 9.8   Removing the remaining nails. (Reprinted with permission from Hill C, Klimesh R. Maximum Hoof Power. North Pomfret, VT: Trafalgar Square Publishing, 2000.)

Next, the sole is pared (if necessary), the hoof wall is nipped or rasped, and any excess frog is trimmed. The outside of the hoof wall is rasped (dressed) if it has flares or dishes. Once trimming is completed, the hoof angle and length are measured, and the levelness of the hoof wall is evaluated (Figs. 9.10 to 9.19) Shoes of the proper size and type for the horse are then selected.

The farrier should shape the shoe to fit a prepared hoof, not the other way around. When the farrier is satisfied with the shape of the shoe and the way it seats on the hoof wall, he or she begins nailing. Usually, two nails are driven, the sharp tips are wrung off or bent over, and the hoof is set down to see how the shoe is positioned. The shoe is adjusted if necessary, and the remain-

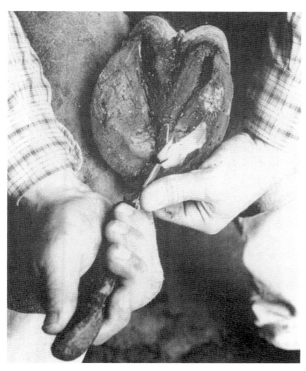

Figure 9.10 Trimming the sole. (Reprinted with permission from Hill C, Klimesh R. Maximum Hoof Power. North Pomfret, VT: Trafalgar Square Publishing, 2000.)

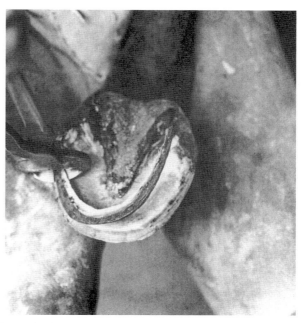

Figure 9.12 Nipping the hoof wall. (Reprinted with permission from Hill C, Klimesh R. Maximum Hoof Power. North Pomfret, VT: Trafalgar Square Publishing, 2000.)

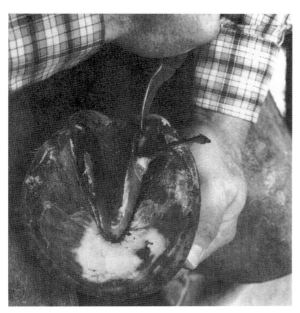

Figure 9.11 Trimming the frog. (Reprinted with permission from Hill C, Klimesh R. Maximum Hoof Power. North Pomfret, VT: Trafalgar Square Publishing, 2000.)

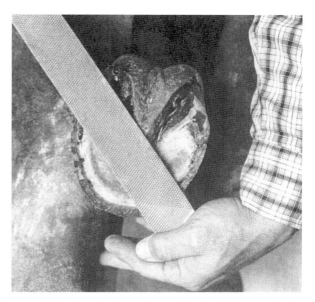

Figure 9.13 Rasping the bottom of the hoof. (Reprinted with permission from Hill C, Klimesh R. Maximum Hoof Power. North Pomfret, VT: Trafalgar Square Publishing, 2000.)

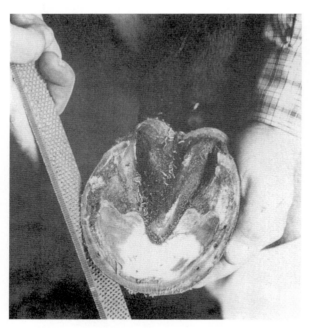

Figure 9.14   Shaping the hoof. (Reprinted with permission from Hill C, Klimesh R. Maximum Hoof Power. North Pomfret, VT: Trafalgar Square Publishing, 2000.)

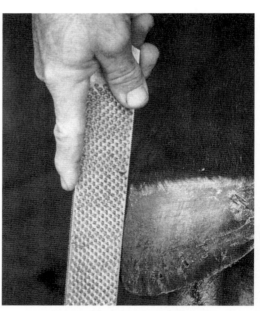

Figure 9.16   Checking for dish. (Reprinted with permission from Hill C, Klimesh R. Maximum Hoof Power. North Pomfret, VT: Trafalgar Square Publishing, 2000.)

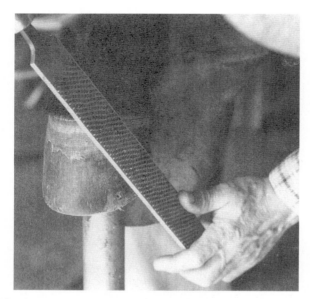

Figure 9.15   Dressing a flare. (Reprinted with permission from Hill C, Klimesh R. Maximum Hoof Power. North Pomfret, VT: Trafalgar Square Publishing, 2000.)

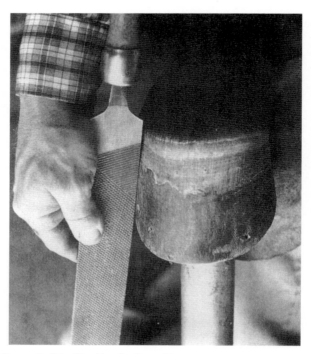

Figure 9.17   Checking for flare. (Reprinted with permission from Hill C, Klimesh R. Maximum Hoof Power. North Pomfret, VT: Trafalgar Square Publishing, 2000.)

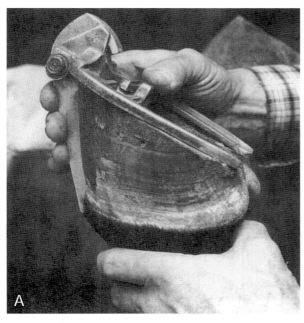

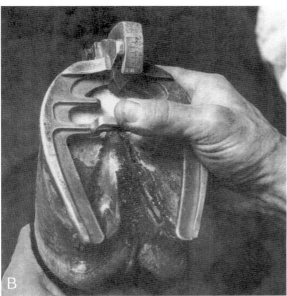

Figure 9.18   Measuring the hoof angle. A. Placing the hoof gauge. B. Reading the gauge. (Reprinted with permission from Hill C, Klimesh R. Maximum Hoof Power. North Pomfret, VT: Trafalgar Square Publishing, 2000.)

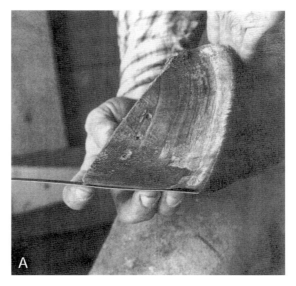

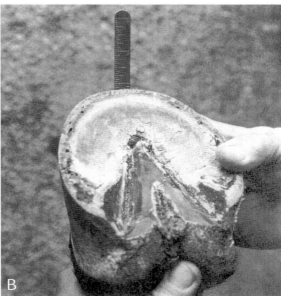

Figure 9.19   Measuring the toe length. A. Placing the ruler. B. Reading the ruler. (Reprinted with permission from Hill C, Klimesh R. Maximum Hoof Power. North Pomfret, VT: Trafalgar Square Publishing, 2000.)

ing nails are driven and wrung off or bent over. After the nails have been driven, the clinches are set or tightened and filed or cut to a short, consistent length. The clinches are then folded flat against the hoof wall and filed smooth (Figs. 9.20 to 9.24).

A hoof sealer can be applied to prevent the hoof from drying out, especially if the outer surface of the hoof wall required rasping. Wax or another substance is used to fill all nail holes, which prevents mud, urine, and water from invading and weakening the hoof (Fig. 9.25).

Principles of Preventive Shoeing

Preventive trimming and shoeing should be a part of the routine hoof care program for every horse. The balance, support, and protection afforded by preventive shoeing contribute to a horse's comfort during movement.

Balance

Balance as it applies to horseshoeing is three-dimensional and may be defined as an equal weight or force around the center of gravity of the horse's limb. Ideally, the limb's center of gravity is identical with that of the foot.[13]

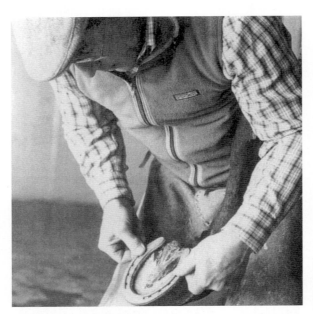

Figure 9.20   Positioning the shoe on the hoof. (Reprinted with permission from Hill C, Klimesh R. Maximum Hoof Power. North Pomfret, VT: Trafalgar Square Publishing, 2000.)

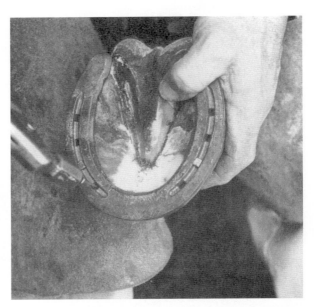

Figure 9.22   Driving the nails. (Reprinted with permission from Hill C, Klimesh R. Maximum Hoof Power. North Pomfret, VT: Trafalgar Square Publishing, 2000.)

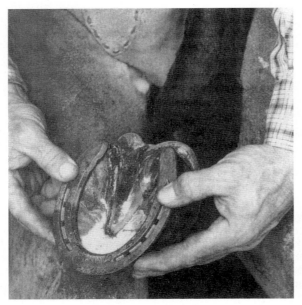

Figure 9.21   Checking the shoe's fit. (Reprinted with permission from Hill C, Klimesh R. Maximum Hoof Power. North Pomfret, VT: Trafalgar Square Publishing, 2000.)

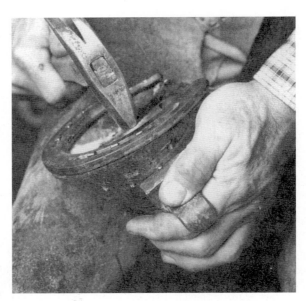

Figure 9.23   Setting the clinches. (Reprinted with permission from Hill C, Klimesh R. Maximum Hoof Power. North Pomfret, VT: Trafalgar Square Publishing, 2000.)

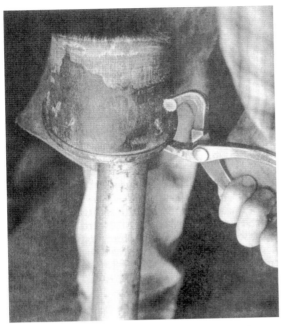

Figure 9.24   Folding the clinches flat. (Reprinted with permission from Hill C, Klimesh R. Maximum Hoof Power. North Pomfret, VT: Trafalgar Square Publishing, 2000.)

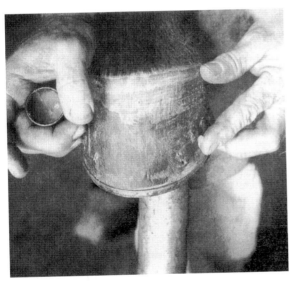

Figure 9.25   Filling the nail holes. (Reprinted with permission from Hill C, Klimesh R. Maximum Hoof Power. North Pomfret, VT: Trafalgar Square Publishing, 2000.)

STATIC VERSUS DYNAMIC BALANCE

Static (geometric) balance refers to a geometric equilibrium of the limb and the hoof in the standing position[13] (see display "Shoeing Quality Control Checklist"). Generally, when the ground surface of the hoof is perpendicular to the axis of the limb (when viewed from the front, the medial and lateral hoof walls are equal in length, and the coronet is parallel to the ground), the hoof is in static balance.

SHOEING QUALITY CONTROL CHECKLIST
Hoof Preparation
Balance
Static versus dynamic
Toe-heel tubule alignment
Dorsal-palmar (plantar)
Medial-lateral
Length
Levelness
Sole
Frog
Shape
Symmetry of hoof pairs
Shoe Preparation
Selection
Fit
Hoof expansions
Heel support
Contact with wall
Sole pressure
Nails
Heads
Placement
Pattern
Clinches
Details

Dynamic (functional) balance refers to the placement of the foot on (flat, level) ground during movement.[13] When a hoof is in dynamic balance, it lands flat.[4,13] This does not mean there is equal weight distributed on the bottom of the foot, however, since more weight is normally placed on the caudomedial side of the hoof during the stance phase.[1,37] For a hoof to be dynamically balanced for efficient motion and symmetric strides, the trimming and shoeing must take conformation and other factors into consideration. Achieving dynamic balance, especially when working on a gait abnormality, often involves trial and error. The more the conformation deviates from standard guidelines, the less likely static and dynamic trimming techniques will produce similar results.

TOE-HEEL TUBULE ALIGNMENT

The angle of the hoof at the heel should be parallel to the angle at the toe. When the heel angle is 5° less than the toe angle, the hoof is said to have underrun heels (Fig. 9.26). In such a case, the horn tubules at the heel may be crushed and collapsed forward and may be more nearly parallel than perpendicular to the ground surface. Rarely is the heel angle steeper than the toe angle, but it may appear that way if the toe is allowed to grow out with a dish.

DORSAL-PALMAR/PLANTAR BALANCE

Dorsal-palmar/plantar (DP) balance refers to the hoof angle (relationship between the dorsal wall of the hoof and the ground) and the alignment of the hoof angle and the pastern angle. Hoof angle is measured at the toe with a hoof protractor (Fig. 9.18). For years, textbooks cited

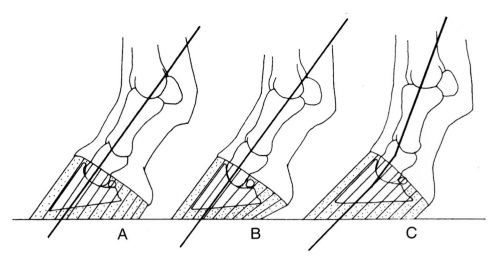

Figure 9.26 Toe-heel tubule alignment. A. Normal: tubules parallel from toe to heel. B. Underrun heel: tubules not parallel. C. Low heels: tubules parallel. (Reprinted with permission from Hill C, Klimesh R. Maximum Hoof Power. North Pomfret, VT: Trafalgar Square Publishing, 2000.)

45 to 50° as normal for the fore hoof angle and 50 to 55° for a hind hoof angle. But observations by farriers indicate that normal forelimb pastern and hoof angles for domestic riding horses range from 53 to 58° and normal hindlimb pastern and hoof angles range from 55 to 60°, with the angles of an occasional normal horse falling outside these ranges.[24] One study found that the mean forelimb hoof angle was 53.8° (range: 48 to 55°) and the hindlimb mean hoof angle was 54.8° (range: 49 to 60°), with an occasional steeper angle being observed in the fore hooves than in the hind hooves.[14]

It is interesting to note that the dorsal hoof angles in wild horses were found to depend on the terrain. They ranged from 57 to 68° in soft, sandy environments; 54 to 62° in packed sod; and 51 to 57° in gravel and hard rock.[41]

Each horse has its own ideal hoof angle. The angle of the hoof is considered correct when the hoof and pastern are in alignment; i.e., the dorsal surface of the hoof is parallel to an imaginary line (axis) passing through the center of the long pastern bone (proximal phalanx) (Fig. 9.27). The goal is to align the dorsal surface of the coffin bone with the long pastern bone axis. The hoof wall can be used as a guide only when it has no flares or distortions, particularly in the area just below the coronary band.[40] The hoof wall should be straight all the way to the ground. If there are no flares or distortions in the normal hoof, the dorsal surfaces of the hoof wall and coffin bone are parallel.

This alignment is best viewed from the side of the horse with the horse standing squarely on a hard, level surface with the cannon bone vertical. An imaginary line through the center of the long pastern bone is used for the pastern angle; it needs to be remembered that the pastern joint is invariably slightly overextended regardless of hoof angle.[1] Using the irregular surface formed by hair and skin at the dorsal (front) surface of the pastern can result in inaccurate alignment.

Because more lamenesses are associated with low heels (and low hoof angle) than with steep heels (and higher hoof angles) and because the hoof angle gets progressively lower during the 5- to 8-week shoeing cycle (because the toes grows faster than the heels), it is usually better for the horse to be shod a little on the steep side than at too low an angle. When a farrier uses the natural balance trimming and shoeing approach described later in this chapter, the toes do not have a tendency to grow faster than the heels; therefore, the horse is not shod with a slightly steeper angle. To a large degree the proper hoof angle is determined by reading the bottom of the foot when natural balance trimming and shoeing is used.

In many horses, the appreciation of hoof and pastern alignment may be unclear. Weight bearing and the position of the limb under the body can skew judgment; furthermore, the farrier must be able to recognize a subtle hoof deformity in the upper hoof wall and know how it affects the overall lateral picture. In these cases, reading the bottom of the foot to determine balance is often helpful.

If the hoof angle is too low in relation to the pastern angle, the centerline will be broken back near the vicinity of the coronary band (Fig. 9.28). The lower the hoof angle, the higher the pastern angle and the more broken back the hoof-pastern axis. Decreasing the hoof angle increases the tension on the deep digital flexor tendon and the navicular ligaments, making the horse more susceptible to developing navicular syndrome and superficial digital flexor tendon strain.[18,32] Horses trimmed with a broken-backward hoof-pastern axis and observed for approximately 1 year develop typical signs of navicular syndrome. Low hoof angles have also been shown to increase (prolong) the time for breakover (the interval between heel off and toe off) in both forelimbs and hindlimbs.[14,16] In addition, low hind hoof angles result in significant increases in overreach distances and overreach duration.[16] Furthermore, raising the toe (lowering

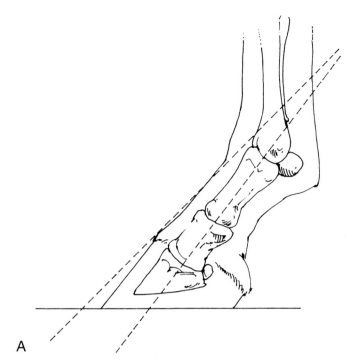

A

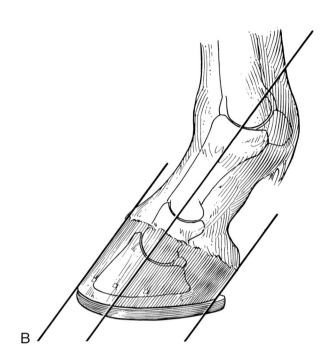

B

Figure 9.27 A. The pastern angle is represented by a line through the center of the long pastern bone, not a line at the dorsal surface of the pastern. (Reprinted with permission from Hill

C, Klimesh R. Maximum Hoof Power. North Pomfret, VT: Trafalgar Square Publishing, 2000.) B. Side view showing lines indicating the correct hoof-pastern axis.

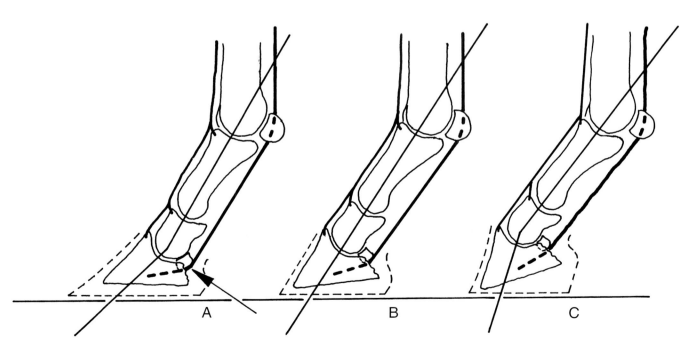

A   B   C

Figure 9.28 A. Broken back axis resulting in excess pressure on the navicular region (arrow). B. Straight axis. Note: It is normal for the bottom of the coffin bone to be 5 to 7° above the horizontal.

C. Broken forward axis. (Reprinted with permission from Hill C, Klimesh R. Maximum Hoof Power. North Pomfret, VT: Trafalgar Square Publishing, 2000.)

the hoof angle) in normal horses impedes blood flow in the lateral part of the hoof.[18] The blood flow returns to normal, however, when the toe is returned to its normal position. A low hoof angle on the rear limbs is often associated with sore hocks and a sore back.

Lateral radiographs of the hindfeet may reveal a coffin bone that is parallel to the ground surface or one whose tip (dorsal limit) is elevated compared with the heel region (Fig. 9.29). In these cases, lowering the toe and leaving the heels alone may suffice to reestablish the nor-

mal position of the coffin bone (3° higher at the heels). In others, a 3° wedge pad may be required. Radiographic examination has also shown that decreasing the hoof angle extends the coffin and pastern joints slightly and flexes the fetlock joint very slightly.[10]

If the hoof angle is too high in relation to the pastern angle, the line will be broken forward. The higher the hoof angle, the lower the pastern angle and the more broken forward the hoof-pastern axis. Increasing the hoof angle decreases the strain on the deep digital flexor

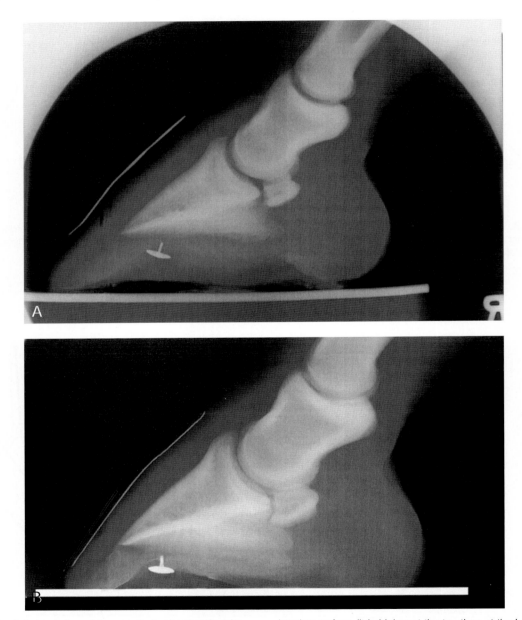

Figure 9.29 A. Lateral view of the rear limb, showing that the solar margin of the distal phalanx is parallel to the weight-bearing surface and that the dorsal surface of the hoof wall appears straight and parallel to the distal phalanx. Because there is sufficient hoof wall and sole at the toe, it can be trimmed to reestablish a normal 3° elevation of the distal phalanx at the heel in relation to the toe. B. Lateral view of the rear limb, showing that the solar margin of the distal phalanx is not parallel to the weight-bearing surface (it is higher at the toe than at the heel). The dorsal hoof appears distorted (protrudes outward), as does the dorsal surface of the distal phalanx, and phalangeal alignment is poor (broken backward). There may be sufficient hoof wall and sole at the toe to trim the hoof to reestablish a normal 3° elevation of the distal phalanx at the heel in relation to the toe; if not, a 3° wedge pad can be applied.

tendon and may decrease the breakover time.[1] Extremely high hoof angles (60° or more) result in excessive coffin joint flexion and a clubfoot appearance. Problems associated with high hoof angles include coffin joint arthritis, extensor process injury, pedal osteitis, and increased strain on the suspensory ligament and the superficial digital flexor tendon.[4,19] In a study done on walking ponies, elevating the heels significantly decreased the strain on the deep digital flexor tendon by 0.1% and the inferior check ligament by 1.0% but increased the strain on the superficial digital flexor tendon by 0.2% and the suspensory ligament by 0.3%.[4] These findings, however, were not corroborated in an in vitro study.[49]

A study that documented the effects of lengthening or shortening the toe by 1 cm while maintaining the same heel length found that elongation of the toe resulted in a more acute angle of the dorsal hoof wall and an elongation of the bearing surface of the hoof. At the same time, the angle between the solar surface of the coffin bone and the bearing surface of the hoof became more acute.[14] Lowering the heels and leaving the toe the same length had the same effect.

MEDIAL-LATERAL BALANCE

Medial-lateral (ML) balance refers to the relationship between the medial (inside) wall of the hoof and the lateral (outside) wall of the hoof. Determining ML balance is one of the most challenging aspects of farriery and relies as much on art as it does on science. The goal is to trim the hoof in such a way that the ground surface of the hoof is centered beneath the limb. This allows the hoof structure to bear the weight of the limb evenly. Altering the relative lengths of the sides of the hoof shifts the position of the hoof beneath the limb. Lowering the lateral wall tends to position the hoof more toward the midline of the horse, whereas lowering the medial wall tends to position the hoof away from the midline of the horse.

Repositioning the limb by trimming, however, may have undesirable consequences. One study evaluating the effects of ML balance showed that elevation of the medial heel in sound horses increased the peak force and impulse on that side of the foot.[5] Problems associated with inappropriate ML hoof balance that lead to disproportionate forces applied to the hoof wall include laterally distorted hooves; chronic heel soreness; sheared heels; quarter, heel, and bar cracks; thrush; side bones; navicular syndrome; and chronic metacarpophalangeal (fetlock) joint synovitis.[2,38]

There are many methods for determining ML balance, none of which works for all horses. Considerations affecting the approach used to achieve ML balance include the farrier's or veterinarian's experience, the age of the horse, the degree of abnormality, the accompanying problems, and the horse's use.

One method of achieving static ML balance is to trim the hoof so that the coronet is parallel to level ground (Fig. 9.30). This works with relatively straight limbs. But if a hoof has remodeled over time to accommodate for limb deviations, this trimming method may put uneven stress on the limb. A similar method is to trim the hoof so that the plane of the ground surface is perpendicular to the cannon bone. A T-bar or similar device can be

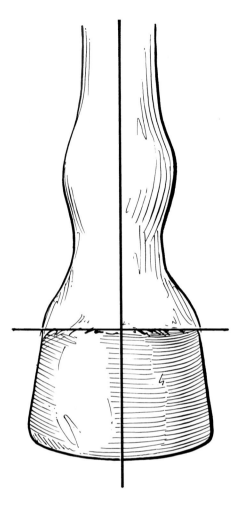

Figure 9.30   The hoof is said to be in ML balance when an imaginary line through the coronet is parallel to the ground surface and perpendicular to a line that bisects the limb axis when viewed from the front.

used to make this determination. This method is also suitable for normally conformed limbs. A third method is to trim the hoof so that its ground surface is perpendicular to the midline of the horse. This can be checked by picking up the forelimb. With the horse's knee flexed and the metacarpus (cannon) lightly resting in the hand, the farrier sights across the ground surface of the hoof. This approach works well on horses whose limbs deviate from the ideal and often results in dynamic ML balance.

New thoughts on ML balance exist. The junction between the exfoliating and nonexfoliating sole (sole plane) is used as a guide and reference for the bottom of the coffin bone (P-3). The sole plane is found by removing the exfoliating chalky material next to the ground that crumbles or flakes when pared with the hoof knife. The exfoliating chalky material will have a white appearance compared with the nonexfoliating waxlike tissue beneath this chalky outer layer. The nonexfoliating tissue is that sole material found distal to the peripheral border of P-3. If this structure is not overtrimmed, it will be the same depth from the distal extent of P-3 to the ground, once the exfoliating material has been removed. When the sole plane is determined, the outer hoof wall is prepared to an equal depth or height to the sole plane on each side of the foot. The medial and lateral toe wall must be prepared equal to each other. The heels behind the widest point of the foot must be trimmed so that each side is the same distance to the ground, in vertical depth.

Trimming the sole more on one side of the foot than the other, when trying to establish ML balance, is believed to cause P-3 to settle or move distally in the area where the nonexfoliating sole has been thinned more than the rest of the foot. This results in an immediate response by the foot to protect itself from harm. The horse responds by having a short stride or avoids pain by landing on one side of the foot or toe first. Thinning the sole also can cause lamina strain and equal or unequal P-3 displacement, depending on which side of the sole has been thinned the most. Excessive trimming of the sole or unequal trimming may also result in laminar tearing.

It is generally agreed that the hoof is in dynamic balance when the medial and lateral walls strike the ground at the same time. If a hoof is landing on the lateral wall first, that side is assumed to be longer and should be trimmed shorter to allow a flat landing. Shoe wear, however, must be considered before the hoof is trimmed. Turner[51] described a protocol of using a combination of hoof measurements and radiographs to develop a graphic record of hoof shape, cornet displacement relative to the solar margin, and frog dimensions. If one side of the hoof was longer, treatment involved making the hoof wall length equal.

If a horse lands on its lateral toe, it often loads on its medial heel. This diagonal imbalance can cause jamming of the coronary band at the medial heel, resulting in proximal displacement of the heel and toe regions and lamness.[42] Synovial effusion of the phalangeal and fetlock joints may also be seen with this condition. In addition, since the toe contacts the ground first, its forward motion is stopped while the remaining part of the hoof rotates around this point of contact until the heel contacts the ground. This results in torque to the hoof, which continues up the limb. These rotational forces may be responsible for undue stress to the phalanges, fetlock, and suspensory apparatus during the load phase of the stride.[48] Treatment for the hoof distortion and lameness involves lowering the parts of the hoof that contact (toe) and load (heel). The finished solar surface is not necessarily flat. A flat shoe is then applied to the foot, and gaps may be apparent at the lowered regions.[42]

Snow et al.[48] used hoof and support measurements, radiographs, and slow-motion video analysis of horses on a treadmill to document the point of contact and point of load impact and to evaluate the torque being applied to the upper limb.[48] Treatment involved trimming the feet, soaking the feet in hot water for 15 minutes, applying moist bandages and a Lily pad, giving phenylbutazone, and using bedded stall confinement for 12 to 24 hours. After this period, the feet were reevaluated and balanced. In some cases, high-motion video analysis was used to document that foot balance was achieved. In the small number of cases reported, a high

degree of success was obtained in correcting the hoof distortion and lameness.

Unfortunately, some horses are conformed so that it is impossible to achieve a flat landing. Overzealous trimming should be avoided because lameness could result from the attempt to make a sound horse's apparently unbalanced hooves conform to an "ideal." It is important to realize that the way the hoof contacts the ground differs with each gait. A hoof that does not land flat at the walk may land flat at the trot or canter.[1] Landing flat is only one guideline to achieving balance.

Many hooves, especially hind hooves, cannot be balanced dynamically by trimming the medial and lateral sides to be equal in length. Examining the shoe for wear can help determine a plan for trimming that will result in even wear on both branches of the shoe (Figs. 9.31 and 9.32). Usually, if the side of the hoof (shoe) that shows the least amount of shoe wear is trimmed shorter, the subsequent wear on the shoe will be equal. This rule may not apply for a horse that is lame or has an unusual way of moving, so it is wise not to rely on just one guideline when attempting something as complex as balancing the equine limb. It is valuable to record the trimming

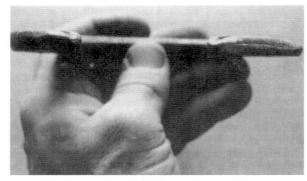

Figure 9.31 Examining the shoe for wear. (Reprinted with permission from Hill C, Klimesh R. Maximum Hoof Power. North Pomfret, VT: Trafalgar Square Publishing, 2000.)

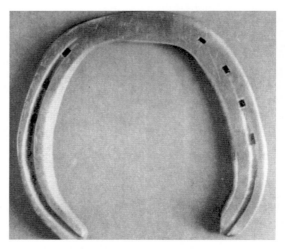

Figure 9.32 Uneven shoe wear. The right crease has been completely worn away. (Reprinted with permission from Hill C, Klimesh R. Maximum Hoof Power. North Pomfret, VT: Trafalgar Square Publishing, 2000.)

approach and to label and save the used shoes so that changes in the wear pattern can be recorded and future trimming can be adjusted accordingly. If the hoof wall is worn too short to balance by trimming alone, wedge pads, shims, or custom shoes can be used to achieve balance until the hoof grows.

Using the natural balance trimming principles for ML balance for the forefeet will also work for the hindfeet. A noticeable difference between forelimbs and hindlimbs is that uneven shoe wear may occur from one side to the other in horses with sore backs, hocks, and stifles. Reducing the breakover to its natural position and preparing the foot equally to the sole plane, from one side to the other, will give surprisingly good results with basic shoes and wedge pads with impression material. Uneven shoe wear from side to side can also be caused by the way a horse pivots and turns when confined to a pen. In this case, the uneven wear is not caused by pain.

Length

The length of the hoof is measured at the center of the toe from the point where the soft coronet (periople) meets the hard hoof wall (stratum externum) to the ground surface. The toe length determines the length of the lever that the limb must break or pivot over. Long toes create a longer lever arm, a delayed breakover, and increased tension on the palmar/plantar soft tissue support structures. Extreme toe length may cause a prominent flare of the distal border of the hoof wall and tearing of the lamina.[4] In cases in which the entire hoof wall is too long, the heels often contract and the walls narrow, causing the foot to become hoof bound. In chronic cases, the sole flattens and lameness usually develops.

Hoof length can also alter limb kinematics. In a study on seven normal horses, three hoof heights were evaluated: shoe only, shoe plus a 2.5-cm pad, and shoe plus a 5.0-cm pad. The weight of the pad and shoe combinations did not vary more than 1 g. Video analysis revealed that the swing-phase maximum height that occurred shortly after lift off was significantly increased from 19.5 cm with a normal hoof length to 21.3 cm with a 2.5-cm pad length and 21.7 cm with a 5.0-cm pad.[3] Short feet may be associated with slow hoof growth or poor hoof durability. Excessive trimming of the hoof wall can also predispose the sole and frog and the underlying corium to bruising.[4,34]

The appropriate toe length of a freshly trimmed hoof ready for shoeing varies according to the horse's size, body weight, and breed. For example, the toe length of a small 360- to 400-kg Arabian might be 7.6 cm (3 inches), that of a medium 425- to 475-kg Quarter Horse might be 8.25 cm (3.3 inches), and that of a large 525- to 575-kg Warmblood might be 8.9 cm (3.6 inches).[4] If a horse is to be barefoot, the hoof is left 0.25 inch longer than if it is to be shod. One must keep in mind that the optimum length of the hoof wall is really dictated by the optimum thickness of the sole. In a study done in wild horses, toe lengths ranged from 6.7 cm (2.5 inches) to 8.3 cm (3.25 inches).[41]

Levelness

The entire bottom of the hoof wall should be level so that it makes perfect (even) contact with a smooth ground surface or a flat shoe (Fig. 9.33). Any unevenness will cause the hoof to bear weight unevenly. In some cases, a farrier may purposely remove a portion of the hoof wall at the ground surface to relieve a crack, flare, or displaced coronet.[35,38,42] In most instances, however, the hoof wall should be level.

Sole

The natural sole is slightly cupped from side to side as well as from front to rear. At the time of trimming, the sole is pared evenly to a concave shape down to the sole plane. If the sole is trimmed excessively, it will cause

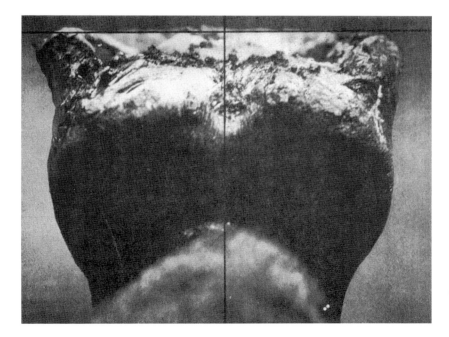

Figure 9.33 An imaginary line bisecting the limb longitudinally and a transverse line across the heels should give two 90° angles at their intersection. If the transverse line is tilted either way, the foot is off level.

the horse to be sore when it walks on gravel. If the sole is left too thick, however, it can reduce hoof expansion during weight bearing and may inhibit the natural springing action of the hoof capsule, which has an important shock-absorbing function. Also, a thick sole may prevent the farrier from trimming the toe sufficiently to attain DP balance. Excessive trimming of the sole can weaken the bars.

Frog

The frog should be smoothly pared, with no loose or overgrown tissue that could trap dirt and manure and harbor microorganisms. The clefts of the frog at the heels should be trimmed out so that the hoof can self-clean. It is not necessary or desirable for the frog to bear weight when the horse stands on level ground. Contrary to this is the concept is that the frog is designed to bear weight, since the proprioceptive (sensory) receptors are found in the frog buttress. Also, the lip that forms at the sides of the frog is designed to trap and hold dirt in the frog commissure, which in turn provides support.

Shape

The inside wall of the hoof is generally steeper than the outside wall. The wall at the toe is thicker than at the quarters. The entire hoof wall from the coronary band to the ground should be straight, i.e., without dips or bulges. Flares and dishes tend to be self-perpetuating. If there are any dishes (concavity in the hoof wall at the toe) or flares (concavity in the sides of the hoof), the wall should be rasped straight. This encourages the growth of a normal hoof shape.

To evaluate shape, the farrier finds the normal center of the bottom of the foot, most recently referred to as Duckett's dot. On the average riding horse, Duckett's dot is located $\frac{3}{8}$ to $\frac{3}{4}$ inch back from the tip of the trimmed frog.[13] A line drawn from the dot vertically through the foot would intersect the center of the coffin bone and the articulation of the extensor process. The dot is considered the external landmark for the foot vertical center axis. Once the horse's hoof has been trimmed and shaped, the distance from the dot to the toe should equal that from the dot to the outermost border of the medial wall (Fig. 9.34). The distance from the dot to the lateral wall is usually greater.

Symmetry of Hoof Pairs

Generally, the toe length of a hoof should be equal to that of its counterpart. Variation in hoof angle, however, often occurs in paired limbs because of individual limb conformation. In some horses, the difference should be minimized through trimming and shoeing; but in many animals, the mismatched hooves should be allowed to be different. Dynamic balance may indicate which path the farrier should choose: The hooves will be trimmed and shod differently so that they move the same.

There is a normal difference in shape and hoof angle between forefeet and hindfeet. The forefeet are usually larger, rounder, and wider at the heels and have flatter soles than the hindfeet. Hindfeet are commonly one shoe size smaller, are more pointed at the toe, and have a more concave sole and higher hoof angle.

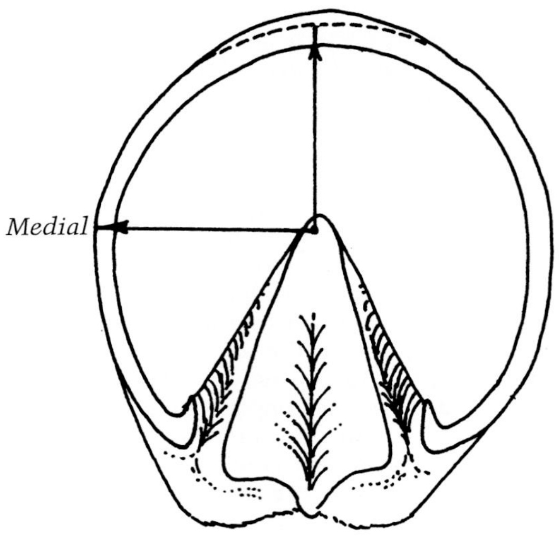

Figure 9.34 Duckett's dot. (Reprinted by permission from Hill C, Klimesh R. Maximum Hoof Power. North Pomfret, VT: Trafalgar Square Publishing, 2000.)

NATURAL BALANCE TRIMMING AND SHOEING

A recent trend in hoof trimming and shoeing is referred to as natural balance trimming and shoeing. Wild horse hooves have served as a blueprint for this technique.[40,41] In its most extreme form, the walls of the hooves bear weight at only four points: the heels and at both lateral and medial pillars (the junction of the toe and the quarters). To accomplish this with trimming, the sole and wall at the toe are rasped at an angle to the ground surface. This creates a wider, rounder toe; and a more dorsal breakover occurs. Theoretically, natural balance improves or eases the mechanics of breakover by reducing the leverage force. Taking the quarters out of contact with the ground is also believed to reduce leverage forces that occur during turning, and it is thought to offer more support to P-3 via the frog apex. This approach also redistributes the hoof mass one-third dorsal and two-thirds palmar/plantar to the widest part of the foot, which causes the frog, bars, and sole to contribute support to the palmar/plantar aspect of the foot.[40,41] In a study done on unshod horses maintained on pasture for 6 weeks, this natural balance pattern developed normally as a result of uneven wear on the solar surface and bearing hoof wall. When the same horses were placed on concrete, however, the four-point pattern disappeared in 7 days.[25]

The natural balance trimming procedure should be used *only on horses that are going to be left barefoot*. This procedure is not used when applying shoes. The technique is as follows:

1. Clean loose debris and dirt from the bottom of the foot. It is not necessary to remove the hard-packed dirt deep in the commissures of the frog. The hard-packed dirt is believed to be necessary for proper weight distribution to the caudal portion of the foot.
2. Remove the loose pieces of frog, bars, and sole material that can be easily removed with a hoof knife or hoof pick.

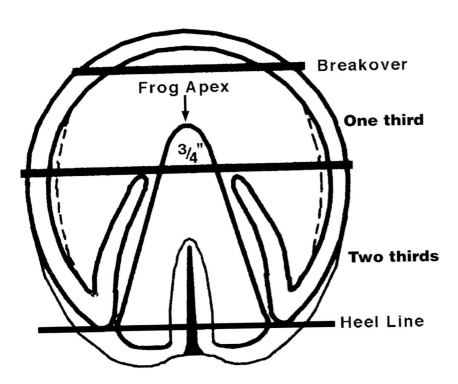

Figure 9.35 Bottom of a horse's foot. The line ¾ inch behind the apex of the frog represents the widest part of the foot (TL). The topline is where breakover should be and is approximately one-third of the total length of the bottom of the foot. The distance between the heel line to TL is approximately two-thirds the total length. (Modified from Ovnicek G. New Hope for Soundness: Seen Through the Window of Wild Horse Hoof Patterns. Columbia Falls, MT: Equine Digital Support System, 1997.)

3. Identify the true tip (apex) of the frog. This is done by removing excess frog at its apex until one can clearly see where it attaches to the sole. The widest part (also the center) of the foot is generally ¾ inch behind the true apex of the frog (Fig. 9.35). The true apex of the frog is used to determine the position of the breakover (rocker) at the toe and will identify how much exfoliating sole is present and where and how much, if any, should be removed.

4. To create breakover, measure ahead of the true frog apex *approximately* 1 inch for foot sizes 00 to 0, 1¼ inches for foot sizes 1 to small 2, or 1½ inches for foot sizes 2 to 3. A raised area of the sole is generally seen in this location; this is the sole callus ridge (Fig. 8.44B). This solar structure is designed to support P-3 by suspension and ground contact. It can be closer to the frog than 1¼ inches. The back edge of the raised area (sole callus) is where the natural breakover is for that foot (Fig. 9.35). When exfoliating the sole area ahead of the frog apex, be extra careful that the sole callus is not destroyed. Nippers or a rasp can be used to rocker the toe ahead of the back edge of the sole callus at a 15 to 20° angle (Fig. 9.36).

5. Using a rasp or nippers, trim the heels back by conservatively following the nonexfoliating sole through the quarters and along the sole plane. Leave a small spike or raised portion of the hoof wall at the heel buttress (Fig. 9.36). *Be sure not to invade any sensitive nonexfoliating sole.*

6. If the feet have a poor wall connection on the ground surface, severe flares, and flat soles, simply remove the wall, in a "dubbed" fashion, back to the lamina around the complete ground surface of the hoof wall. Do not try to rocker the toe and do not trim the sole or frog.

7. Using a rasp or nippers, remove (lower) the medial and lateral hoof wall by following close to the sole plane in the quarters. This will create a gradual arc pattern between the toe impression mark and the heel impression mark on each side of the foot (Fig. 9.36). There should also be a rounded hoof wall edge around the outside of the hoof wall, leaving the high point of the wall at the lamina.

8. Remove the flares from the front and around the outer edge of the hoof wall to prevent chipping and to give the hoof a smoother, more natural look.

Special attention should be given to trimming the hoof wall level with the toe callus at the junction of the rocker (ML toe callus or toe pillars). The toe pillars serve as ground contact points that should be left strong in the sole lamina region. These pillars should also be allowed to share the weight bearing of the dorsal portion of the hoof capsule and provide a point for breakover. Little to no sole, frog, and bars are ever removed.

Generally within a few months, the foot will normally produce a cupped sole and the heels will start to spread. The frog will develop fully and healthfully if poor hoof quality has preceded this procedure.

Shoe Selection and Preparation

The size of the shoe should be appropriate for the size of the horse and its hoof. The shoe should be strong enough to support the horse's weight but not unnecessarily heavy, or it may negatively affect the horse's stride and agility. One study evaluated the effect of increasing shoe weight and hoof length in normal horses trotting on a treadmill. The fore hooves were shod with three different combinations of steel shoes and pads: normal weighted shoe plus a 0.3-cm pad, double-weighted shoe

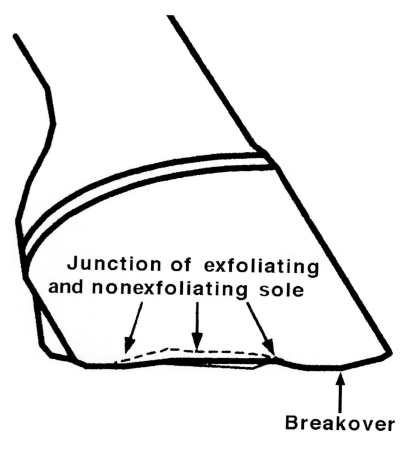

Figure 9.36   Side view of the foot, showing that the heel and toe are longer than the slightly arched quarters. Also note that the toe on the weight-bearing surface is beveled at 15 to 20° upward (dorsal) to ease breakover. (Modified from Ovnicek G. New Hope for Soundness: Seen Through the Window of Wild Horse Hoof Patterns. Columbia Falls, MT: Equine Digital Support System, 1997.)

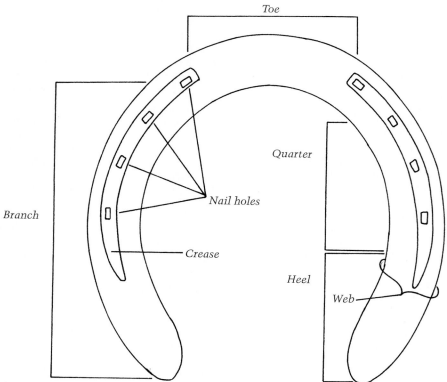

Figure 9.37   Parts of a shoe. (Reprinted with permission from Hill C, Klimesh R. Maximum Hoof Power. North Pomfret, VT: Trafalgar Square Publishing, 2000.)

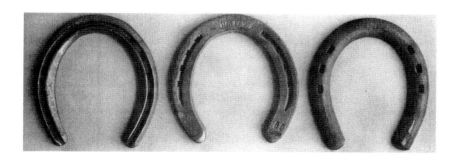

Figure 9.38 Left to right: rim shoe, plain shoe, half-round shoe. (Reprinted with permission from Hill C, Klimesh R. Maximum Hoof Power. North Pomfret, VT: Trafalgar Square Publishing, 2000.)

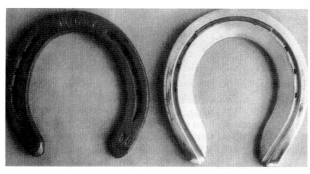

Figure 9.39 Left to right: plain steel shoe, wide-web aluminum shoe. (Reprinted with permission from Hill C, Klimesh R. Maximum Hoof Power. North Pomfret, VT: Trafalgar Square Publishing, 2000.)

plus a 0.3-cm pad, and double-weighted shoe plus a 2.5-cm pad. It was found that adding weight to the shoes of hooves of the same length increased the maximum height of the shoe, the height of the foot flight arc throughout most of the swing phase, and the flexion of the fetlock joint. Adding length (2.5-cm pads) to the hooves of horses shod with double-weighted shoes increased the shoe height, the height of the foot flight arc above that seen with the weighted shoe alone, flexion of the fetlock joint, and breakover.[6]

Shoes should provide adequate protection and traction. Furthermore, the nail heads should be protected from wear by setting them in either a crease or a hole stamped in the shoe (Fig. 9.37).

Hot versus cold shoeing refers to the way the farrier makes, shapes, or applies shoes. "Hot shoeing" means that the farrier makes the shoes from scratch in a forge, modifies keg shoes in a forge, or fits a hot shoe to the hoof. "Cold shoeing" means the farrier shapes and applies the shoe without heating it up. Many farriers use a combination of hot and cold shoeing techniques.

Steel, the material most commonly used in making horseshoes, is a combination of iron and other elements, mainly carbon (see display "Horseshoe Materials, Types, and Sizes" and Fig. 9.38). Steel is graded by the amount of carbon it contains; the higher the carbon content, the harder the steel. Mild (low-carbon) steel is used for horseshoes because it is easily shaped and yet durable enough to last for one or more shoeing periods. A high-carbon steel, such as used for springs or tools, would last longer but would be more difficult to shape and would have less traction on hard surfaces. All but the largest sizes of mild steel horseshoes can be shaped while

cold to fit the hoof. Large shoes used for Warmbloods and draft horses must be heated in a forge to be shaped.

HORSESHOE MATERIALS, TYPES, AND SIZES

Materials

Steel
Aluminum
Titanium
Plastic
Plastic or rubber over a steel or aluminum core

Types

Plain Flat shoe with a crease (also called a fuller or swedge) on the ground surface of the shoe in the area of the nail heads (Figs. 9.38 and 9.39)
Stamped Flat shoe without a crease but with pockets stamped in the shoe for the nail heads; also called a punched shoe
Rim Shoe with a crease around the entire ground surface for traction and for recessing the nail heads (Fig. 9.38)
Training plate Light, thin steel shoe
Polo A light, thin, steel rim shoe with a higher inside rim; stronger than a training plate (Fig. 9.40)
Barrel racing Light, thin, steel rim shoe with a higher outside rim
Toed and heeled Steel shoe with a bar protruding across the ground surface of the toe and a square protrusion (called a calk) at each heel to provide traction in soft footing
Half-round Shoe that is flat on the hoof surface and round on the ground surface, with stamped nail holes (Fig. 9.38)
Racing plate Very light, thin, aluminum shoe, usually with a steel wear insert at the toe, available in a wide variety of styles
Wedge Steel or aluminum shoe thicker at the heels than at the toe; also called swelled heel (Fig. 9.41)
Wide web Formed from wider steel (Fig. 9.39)

Sizes

Until recently, there were no standard shoe sizes. For example, a shoe with a 14-inch circumference (from heel to heel) could be one of eight sizes (ranging from 1 to 12), depending on the company that makes it.

Recently, the Farrier Industry Association developed a chart that categorizes most available steel, aluminum, and plastic horseshoes according to their circumference from heel to heel. Horseshoe companies are beginning to size shoes by the inch, according to this chart.

Aluminum, which is lighter than steel, is also used for horseshoes (see display "Horseshoe Materials, Types,

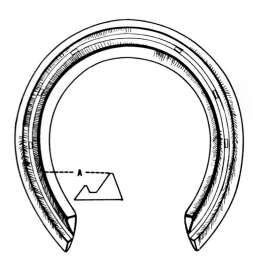

Figure 9.40 Ground surface view of a polo shoe. The low outside rim facilitates breakover in any direction. Inset. Cross-section of the web. A, the inside rim.

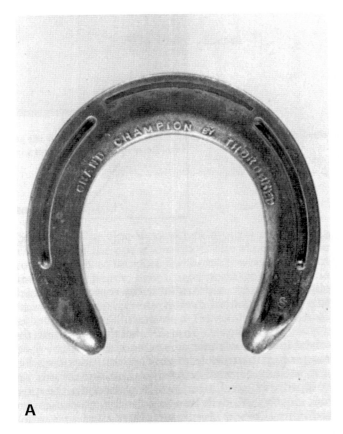

A

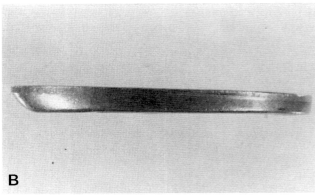

B

Figure 9.41 Top view (A) and side view (B) of an aluminum wedge shoe. Note the toe of the shoe (panel B, right) is thinner than the heels.

and Sizes" and Figs. 9.39 to 9.41). Because of this weight advantage, aluminum is the material from which most Thoroughbred racing shoes, or "plates," are made. By using aluminum, shoe manufacturers can make the shoe wider for support or thicker to alter DP balance without increasing the weight significantly. Being softer than steel, however, aluminum does not wear as long; thus many aluminum shoes are equipped with steel inserts at the toes where the most wear occurs. Some manufacturers are producing shoes made of aluminum alloys. They wear much longer than aluminum shoes; if they are heated for shaping or forming clips, however, the wear is often greatly reduced.

Because aluminum shoes bend or spring more easily than steel shoes, they often cannot provide the support that a horse needs. This is especially true for larger horses or jumpers that produce a great deal of force on landing and turning.

Another drawback of aluminum horseshoes is that in the presence of moisture, galvanic corrosion occurs between the steel nails and the aluminum. This reaction corrodes the hoof surface of the shoe and affects the hoof itself. Evidence of this corrosion is seen as a pasty white substance between the shoe and hoof when the shoe is removed.

Titanium is a corrosion-resistant element that was, until recently, considered a strategic material, so civilian access to and research with titanium have been limited. Horseshoes made of titanium alloys, usually aluminum and magnesium, have the strength of steel and are almost as light as aluminum. They have not gained wide popularity, primarily because they must be worked and shaped hot and, when heated, titanium gives off toxic fumes. Also, because of its hardness, titanium is extremely slippery on concrete or pavement.

Attempts have been made for years to develop a successful *plastic* horseshoe. The main drawback of nail-on plastic shoes is that the inherent flexibility of the material does not provide sufficient support for a horse's hoof.

Furthermore, the slippery surface of the plastic encourages the hoof to spread over the edges of the shoe.

Plastic horseshoes that are glued to the hoof wall by means of a cuff or series of tabs are valuable for therapeutic applications. They are used when the wall is too damaged or weak to hold nails securely and on foal hooves that are too thin walled to nail safely. Because their application is relatively atraumatic, glue-on shoes can be used on laminitic horses and other horses that are in extreme pain. The Dalric shoe is one that is designed for foals. It is prefitted with a number of extensions and supports to address a wide variety of postnatal problems.[26]

Several types of horseshoes are available that combine a *core of steel or aluminum with an outer shell of plastic or rubber*. These shoes give more support to the hoof than does plastic alone, and many can be shaped like a conventional steel shoe. The supposed advantage of these shoes is their ability to absorb shock. There is a scarcity of independent research, however, concerning the effectiveness of shock-absorbing hoof wear and of the effects of shock on the equine limb.

Horseshoes are either individually hand forged by the farrier or mass-produced in a factory. At one time, factory-made shoes were transported in wooden kegs; therefore the term "keg shoe" refers to a ready-made commercial shoe. When keg shoes were lacking in both quality and variety, it was worth the farrier's time to hand forge the shoes that were used. Today, keg shoes are available in many shapes, materials, thickness, widths, and qualities. Many top farriers seldom find it necessary to make a shoe from bar stock; others enjoy the forge work so much that they hand make all the shoes they apply.

It is common, however, for farriers to modify keg shoes to suit particular purposes. The most common modifications are repositioning the nail holes, adding a bar, altering the shape of the toe (rolled, rocker, square), altering the heel shape and length (trailers, extended heels, spooned heels), and forging or attaching clips.

Fit

A shoe should follow the natural shape of the properly prepared hoof, being neither too wide nor too narrow, too short nor too long. When it is viewed from above with the foot on the ground, between $\frac{1}{16}$ and $\frac{1}{8}$ inch of the edge of the properly fitted shoe should be visible from the quarters back to the heels (Fig. 9.42). This indicates that the shoe has adequate allowance for heel growth and expansion.

Hoof Expansion

A shoe is fitted full to accommodate heel movement and the normal increase in hoof width during the 5- to 8-week shoeing period. As the horse's weight descends with each step on the foot, it causes movement (expansion) at the heels (Fig. 9.43). As the weight is lifted, be-

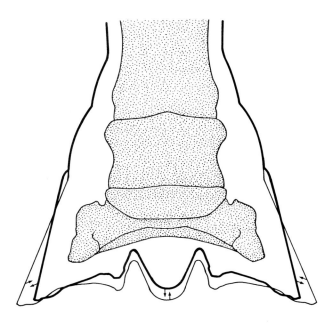

Figure 9.43 During weight bearing, the frog and sole are forced downward, causing expansion of the hoof wall. During non-weight bearing, the reverse occurs.

fore breakover, the heels return (contract) to their original position. These events are evidenced by the grooves worn in the hoof surface of the shoe. A study using strain gauges concluded that conventional nailed-on iron shoes restrict the flexion and spreading of the hoof wall at the ground surface but have little effect on the degree of expansion of the heels.[21] In another study, shoeing was found to impair the natural viscous dampening by the hoof at impact.[22] Frog pressure has been shown to have a variable effect on heel expansion.[20]

Because the hoof is cone shaped, as it grows longer, its base becomes wider, while the steel shoe that is nailed to it retains its original size. Therefore, it is necessary to start with a shoe that is wider than the hoof, so that at the end of the shoeing cycle the shoe still supports the heel area, which has grown since the shoe was applied.

Too little expansion room allows the hoof wall to spread over the edge of the shoe as it grows, resulting in lack of support and hoof wall and sole damage (Fig. 9.44). Too much expansion room increases the chance that the shoe will be lost by the horse stepping on it. Upright hooves need less expansion room than flatter, spread-out hooves that have more sloping walls.

Heel Support

Enough shoe should extend beyond the heels so that the limb is adequately supported. Generally, the heels of the shoe should be below the midline of the cannon bone when the cannon is vertical (Fig. 9.45). Another guide is that the length of the shoe should be equal to or greater than twice the toe length of the prepared hoof (Fig. 9.46). Short shoeing (using a shoe that is too small) does not provide ample support and can result in underrun heels (Fig. 9.47).

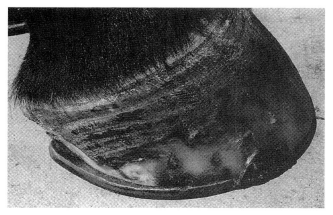

Figure 9.42 Good shoe fit. (Reprinted with permission from Hill C, Klimesh R. Maximum Hoof Power. North Pomfret, VT: Trafalgar Square Publishing, 2000.)

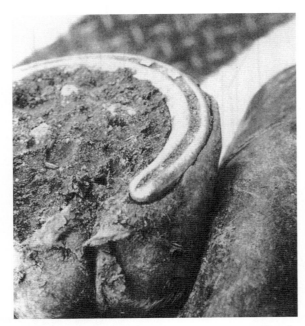

Figure 9.44 This horse is well overdue for shoeing. Note the hoof spread over the shoe from quarter to heel. (Reprinted with permission from Hill C, Klimesh R. Maximum Hoof Power. North Pomfret, VT: Trafalgar Square Publishing, 2000.)

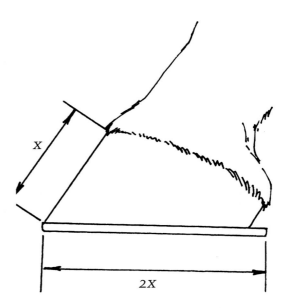

Figure 9.46 A shoe length guide. (Reprinted with permission from Hill C, Klimesh R. Maximum Hoof Power. North Pomfret, VT: Trafalgar Square Publishing, 2000.)

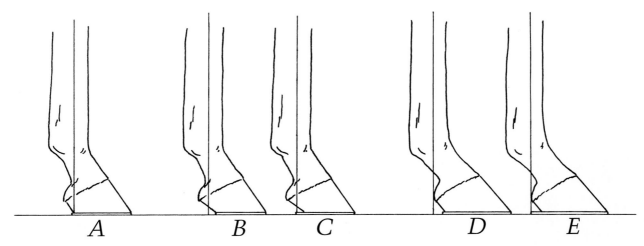

Figure 9.45 Heel support. A. In the ideal situation, the hoof is in DP balance, the heels are not underrun, and there is proper heel support. Note that the shoe extends just slightly behind the heel. B. In this case of short shoeing, the hoof is in DP balance, but the toe-heel alignment is not parallel, the heel is underrun, and thus the hoof is inadequately supported. C. A longer shoe applied to hoof B provides proper support. D. In this case of short shoeing, the hoof is in DP balance and the toe-heel alignment is parallel, but the low hoof-pastern angle results in a hoof that is well ahead of the limb and thus is inadequately supported. E. A longer shoe applied to hoof D provides proper support. (Reprinted with permission from Hill C, Klimesh R. Maximum Hoof Power. North Pomfret, VT: Trafalgar Square Publishing, 2000.)

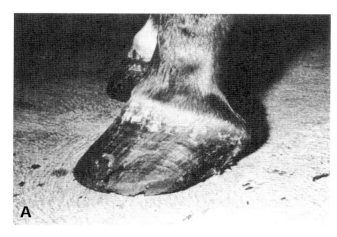

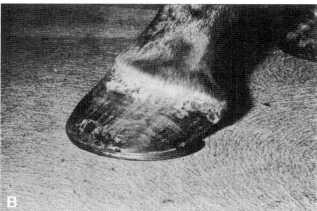

Figure 9.47   A. Before trimming and shoeing, this horse has a long toe and underrun heels. B. The same horse after the toe was rasped shorter and lower and the heel was left higher. Note that the shoe is fit well back on the foot to expand past the heel. (Reprinted with permission from Hill C, Klimesh R. Maximum Hoof Power. North Pomfret, VT: Trafalgar Square Publishing, 2000.)

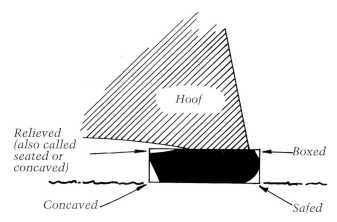

Figure 9.48   Modifications made to shoe edges. (Reprinted with permission from Hill C, Klimesh R. Maximum Hoof Power. North Pomfret, VT: Trafalgar Square Publishing, 2000.)

Contact With the Wall

Unless some of the hoof wall is missing because of hoof damage or has been purposely removed to treat a crack or a persistent flare or other abnormality, the shoe should contact the hoof wall completely. The corner of a business card should not fit between the hoof and the shoe at any point around the outside perimeter of the hoof. Hot fitting a shoe properly (heating the shoe and pressing it onto the prepared hoof) scorches the high spots on the hoof, indicating the areas that need to be removed with a rasp. If the shoe is very hot, it will melt the hoof horn and provide a perfect match between shoe and hoof. When a shoe is cold fitted, the farrier must be skilled with a rasp to be sure that the hoof and shoe meet all the way around.

Sole Pressure

Although the shoe should be in contact with the entire hoof wall, it should not contact more than $\frac{1}{8}$ inch of the sole. If a horse has very flat soles, the inner edge of the hoof surface of the shoe needs to be relieved to avoid creating unwanted sole pressure (Figs. 9.48 and 9.49).

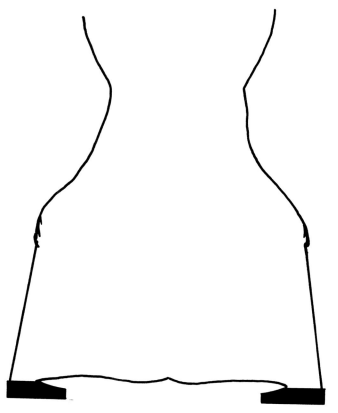

Figure 9.49   The hoof surface of the shoe is relieved to prevent sole pressure. (Reprinted with permission from Hill C, Klimesh R. Maximum Hoof Power. North Pomfret, VT: Trafalgar Square Publishing, 2000.)

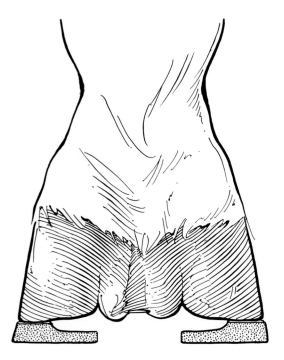

Figure 9.50   A wide-web shoe with a concave solar surface protects the sole without applying pressure to it.

This is especially important when the horse is shod with wide-web shoes (Fig. 9.50). Sole pressure can disrupt blood flow and lead to lameness, abscesses, and corns.

Nails

Heads

The nail head should seat tightly in the crease or stamped hole and should protrude below the shoe about $\frac{1}{16}$ inch.

Placement

The nail should enter the hoof within the white line. If the nail enters outside the white line, the clinches are likely to be too low, and the shoe may not be secure (Fig. 9.51). If the nail enters too far inside the white line, sensitive structures may be invaded. The tip of the nail is beveled so that it travels in a curved path in dense horn tissue and exits the hoof wall. If the nail is angled to the center of the hoof or placed inside the white line, the soft tissue there may not provide enough resistance to curve the nail outward, and the nail will not exit the hoof wall. The bevel is on the same side as the pattern on the nail head (Fig. 9.52). The nail is placed with the bevel toward the inside of the hoof so that the nail, when driven, curves away from the bevel. Six to eight nails are used; generally, nails are not placed behind the widest portion of the hoof wall, and those nail holes in the shoe are left empty.

Pattern

The height of the nail farthest back on the shoe should be approximately one-third the distance from the ground

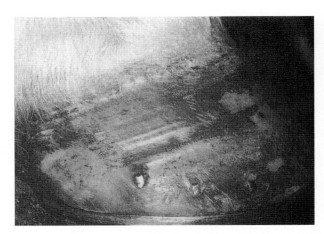

Figure 9.51   Low clinches. (Reprinted with permission from Hill C, Klimesh R. Maximum Hoof Power. North Pomfret, VT: Trafalgar Square Publishing, 2000.)

to the coronary band. The nail pattern is affected by the quality of the hoof, the skill of the farrier, and the quality and design of the shoes and nails being used. Ideally, the nail pattern should form a straight line (Fig. 9.53), and the two nails in the toe should be at equal heights when viewed from the front.

Clinches

The clinches should be "square," i.e., only as long as they are wide. Such clinches open easily, allowing the shoe to come off if it gets caught on something. Rectangular clinches, which are longer than they are wide, usually hold the shoe on so securely that, if the shoe gets caught on a fence or the horse steps on it, large portions of the hoof may be ripped off along with the nails and the shoe. Clinches should be uniform and set flush with the hoof wall and should not be set into a groove filed in the hoof wall. They should feel smooth to the touch.

Details

The hoof wall should be smooth and, unless it is necessary to remove a flare, never rasped above the clinches. The edge of the hoof wall and the edge of the shoe should be smooth. Old nail holes should be filled with wax or other appropriate substance to prevent moisture, mud, and other contaminants from entering the hoof (Fig. 9.25).

Any exposed edges of the shoe should be rounded with a rasp or grinder to decrease the chance that the shoe will come off if stepped on (Fig. 9.48). This also removes any burrs or steel slivers that may injure a person handling the feet.

Natural Balance Shoeing

The following procedure is used when applying Natural Balance Shoes, World Race Plates, or modified keg shoes. For optimum results, it is important for the shoe to comply with the natural balance principles of support, protection, and breakover position. The procedure for natural balance shoeing is as follows:

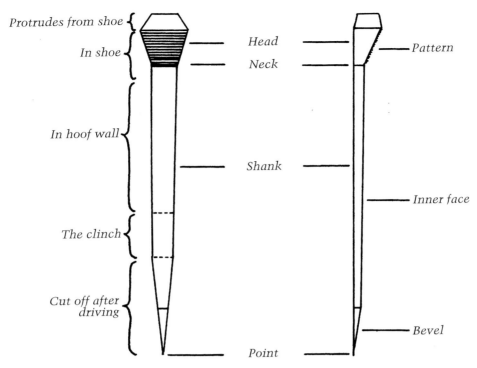

Protrudes from shoe {
In shoe {
Head
Neck

In hoof wall {
Shank

The clinch {

Cut off after driving {

Point

Pattern
Inner face
Bevel

Figure 9.52 Parts of a nail. (Reprinted with permission from Hill C, Klimesh R. Maximum Hoof Power. North Pomfret, VT: Trafalgar Square Publishing, 2000.)

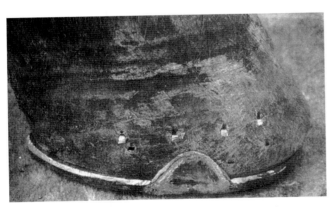

Figure 9.53 Clinches showing good size, height, and pattern (nail holes have not yet been filled). Note the squared-toe shoe. (Reprinted with permission from Hill C, Klimesh R. Maximum Hoof Power. North Pomfret, VT: Trafalgar Square Publishing, 2000.)

1. Clean and remove only excess sole and frog material to get a clear view of the sole plane (the junction between the exfoliating and nonexfoliating sole) and the true apex of the frog.
2. Start at the widest part of the foot and trim the wall flat toward the heel, not dipped in the quarters. Prepare the foot so that the trimmed heel terminates close to the widest part of the frog. This generally requires removing the heel so that the hoof wall is about $\frac{1}{16}$ to $\frac{1}{8}$ inch—no more than $\frac{1}{4}$ inch—from the nonexfoliating sole at the deepest part of the quarters. Each side should be prepared so that the nonexfoliating sole depths to the ground surface of the wall are the same. Do not make contact with the sensitive sole tissue at the heel.
3. From the widest part of the foot, trim toward the toe to the level of the sole plane. The wall at the toe should be trimmed to equal depths into the toe sole callus at the medial and lateral toe quarters to ensure balance; excessive rasping into the toe sole callus should be avoided. The flattened sole callus should be level with the hoof wall and no more than $\frac{1}{8}$ to $\frac{1}{4}$ inch wide (Fig. 9.54). Using this approach will allow sufficient sole clearance under the inner edge of the shoe to ensure that there is no sole pressure from the shoe at this point. Hot seating the shoe will also ensure clearance between the shoe and sole. If too much of the toe sole callus is removed, sole pressure and pain will result when the shoe is applied.

The distance from the frog apex to the inside border of the Natural Balance Shoe should be approximately $\frac{1}{8}$ to $\frac{1}{4}$ inch for small shoes, $\frac{1}{4}$ to $\frac{3}{8}$ inch for medium shoes, and $\frac{3}{8}$ to $\frac{1}{2}$ inch for large shoes (see Fig. 8.46). If World Race Plates or modified keg shoes are used, the distance between the breakover and the tip of the frog should be approximately 1 inch for small feet and $1\frac{1}{2}$ inches for large feet (Fig. 9.54). All shoes should extend to the palmar/plantar (caudal) end of the frog, which usually means most shoes extend beyond the buttress of the heels.

When finishing the foot, remove only the flares that are obvious; then undercut the remaining hoof left over the shoe. This will give the appearance of the naturally

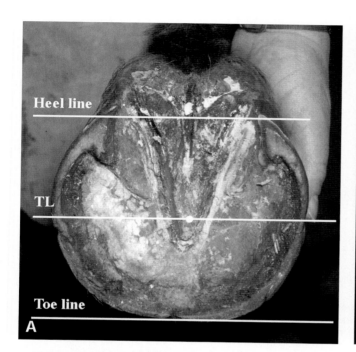

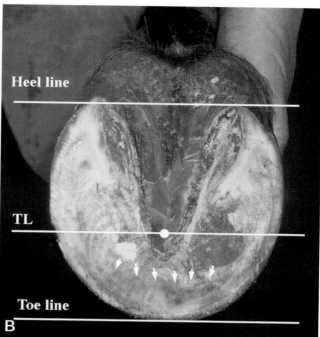

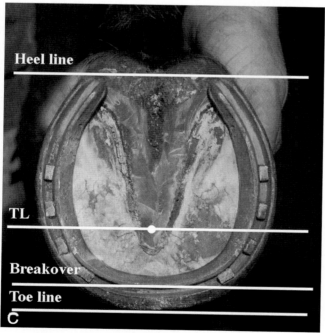

Figure 9.54 A. The foot before trimming. The widest part of the foot (TL) is located approximately ¾ inch behind the frog apex. The distances from TL to the heel line and TL to the toe line are about equal. B. The foot after trimming. The distance from TL to the heel line is approximately two-thirds the length of the bottom of the foot, and distance from TL to the toe line is approximately one-third the length. Arrows indicate toe callus. C. The foot with a modified keg shoe (the front rim was ground off to create a bevel). Note that the breakover occurs at the back (palmar/plantar) rim of the shoe and the heel of the shoe extends slightly beyond the heel buttress.

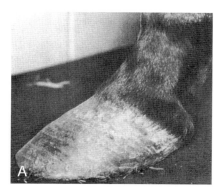

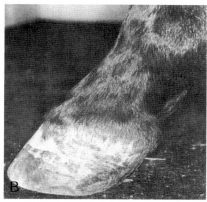

Figure 9.55 Neglect. A. Before trimming. B. After trimming. (Reprinted with permission from Hill C, Klimesh R. Maximum Hoof Power. North Pomfret, VT: Trafalgar Square Publishing, 2000.)

worn bare foot. For extreme flares, rasp only from the midregion of the dorsal hoof wall to the ground. Do not rasp completely through the wall at the ground level. *Do not rasp the dorsal hoof wall from the center of the toe back to the shoe.*

COMMON HOOF PROBLEMS AND TREATMENT

Neglect

Failing to provide regular, competent hoof care is a main cause of hoof problems. Neglect includes allowing the bare hoof to wear too short or to grow so long that it breaks off; leaving the shoe on so long that the hoof grows over the shoe or becomes unbalanced (Figs. 9.44 and 9.55); overfeeding or underfeeding; and failing to examine the hoof regularly for imbedded rocks, nails, and other foreign objects.

Hoof Damage

Broken hooves can alter hoof balance and cause lameness (Fig. 9.56). It is not uncommon, however, for flared hooves to break, even though the horse remains sound. Similarly, a horse can rip off a shoe and portions of the hoof wall and be reshod routinely. When a large section of hoof wall is missing, hoof repair may be necessary.

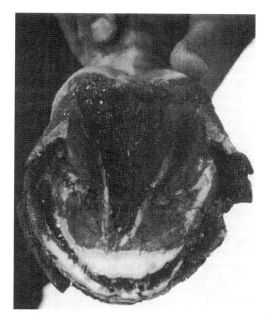

Figure 9.56 A broken and separated hoof. (Reprinted with permission from Hill C, Klimesh R. Maximum Hoof Power. North Pomfret, VT: Trafalgar Square Publishing, 2000.)

Hoof repair materials have similar properties to natural hoof horn and adhere to the hoof wall for months, allowing new growth to replace the damaged area. If the injury extends to the sensitive tissues, an antibiotic-impregnated hoof repair material can be applied to the defect without fear of thermal injury or infection.[54] Furthermore, hoof repair materials can be used to build up the low side of a hoof, replace missing sections of the wall, or build up thin walls so a shoe can be nailed on. The prosthetic hoof can be trimmed and shaped like a normal hoof and is strong enough to secure a nail-on shoe.

If the hoof wall is too weak or damaged to secure a shoe with nails or if the horse is in too much pain to allow nails to be driven into the hoof, glue-on shoes are a good alternative.[26] These shoes are available from several sources and come in many configurations for a variety of applications, from foal treatment to racing shoes to founder treatment. One type of glue-on shoe consists of a cuff to which a steel or aluminum shoe is riveted; the cuff is glued or taped to the hoof. Another type has a steel shoe bonded to a braided fabric cuff, which is glued to the hoof wall. Other types have plastic tabs around the shoe that are glued onto the surface of the hoof wall (see "Resources" in this chapter).

Poor Hoof Quality

Good-quality hoof horn is dry, hard, and tough—not brittle, spongy, or soft. Poor nutrition, faulty metabolism, unhealthy environment, improper management, disease, some drugs, and trauma can all affect hoof quality.

In some cases, poor hoof quality is caused by poor nutrition. In others, the problem lies with a horse's inability to synthesize essential nutrients. A horse's ration should provide adequate amounts of the essential amino acid DL-methionine, biotin (a component of the vitamin B complex), and other nutrients. It may be necessary to use a supplement to meet a horse's nutritional requirements (see "Resources" in this chapter). One study found that dietary biotin supplements improved equine hoof horn growth rate and hardness. Greater growth rates and hardness were achieved at a daily dose of 15 mg rather than at 7.5 mg of biotin.[9] Generally, if nutrition is adequate, genetics, poor management practices, or both may cause poor-quality hooves.

Historically, advice for improving hoof quality has ranged from prescribing hoof dressings and packing to standing a horse in the mud around its overflowing water trough. Contrary to what is often believed, many hooves crack and peel from *too much* moisture or repeated wet-dry episodes rather than not enough moisture. Current recommendations include providing the horse with adequate exercise (which provides moisture internally via the blood) and maintaining the external moisture at a constant, relatively dry level.

In a normal hoof, the outer hoof layer is dense and tough, with a moisture content of 15 to 20%. The inner layer averages a moisture content of about 45%. The two layers are joined together by interlocking sheaves of epidermal (insensitive) laminae (from the outer layer) and blood-rich dermal (sensitive) laminae (from the inner layer). Blood and lymph vessels in the dermal laminae provide adequate moisture for the inner layer. Moisture diffuses outward from the moist, sensitive laminae toward the dry, hard outer wall. When blood circulates freely to and from the hoof, the dynamic balance of moisture is operating at an optimum level. When there is a lack of exercise or a disease of the hoof (e.g., laminitis or navicular syndrome), an imbalance in the hoof, or an ill-fitting shoe, circulation may be interrupted to the point at which moisture is no longer provided through blood flow. A hoof that is too dry is inflexible and is an inefficient shock absorber. It also tends to contract and tighten around the sensitive inner structures. If a horse is getting adequate exercise, the moisture level of the inner layer generally remains constant.

A hoof that is kept too soft (e.g., when a horse is in a wet environment or hooves are regularly covered with hoof dressing) contains too much moisture in the external hoof wall. The soft wall cannot oppose the pressure from the inner structures of the foot, and the hoof spreads out and flattens. Excess moisture weakens the hoof material; soft, punky hoof walls often peel and separate, resulting in the lack of a solid hoof wall to bear the horse's weight or to hold a nailed-on shoe.

Too much moisture can also make a horse's soles soft and susceptible to sole bruises and abscesses. The condition of the hooves worsens during hot, humid weather, especially when horses are turned out at night. In such a situation, horses walk around in dew-laden pastures and then are either left out where the sun will dry the hooves or are put in a stall where the bedding dries them. Horses that repeatedly walk through mud and then stand in the sun experience a similar decay in hoof quality. In both cases, the hoof is going through a stressful moisture-related expansion-contraction that damages the hoof structures. Mud has the effect of drawing out moisture and oils and tightening pores, much like a poultice. In the process of drying out, the outer layer of the hoof

wall will attempt to bend or warp but cannot do so because of the hold the inner layer has on it. Instead, it develops cracks and checks to relieve the stresses from the shearing forces of the opposition of the layers. The cracks may then become packed with more mud and dirt so that they cannot close and thus continue to get larger and spread upward.

Because excess moisture can be so damaging to a hoof, some discourage the application of any grease or oil to the hoof. Because the hoof has two natural protective layers, dressings may not be able to penetrate the hoof anyway. A waxy covering, the periople, is located at the coronary band and is visible as an inch-wide strip that encircles the top of the hoof. The protective, varnish-like outer layer of the hoof wall, the stratum externum, is composed of hard horn. Both coatings retard moisture movement from either direction, from the outside environment into the hoof and from the inner layer of the hoof to the outside.

Hoof dressing is warranted when the bulbs of the heels begin to crack. To restore their pliability, a product containing animal grease, such as lanolin or fish oil, can be applied daily until the desired result has been achieved. A hoof sealer, which penetrates better than a dressing, is often beneficial in stabilizing hoof moisture content if the horse is in particularly wet or dry conditions. An in vitro study documenting the ability of commercial hoof wall products to maintain hoof wall hydration found that oil-, pine tar-, and petroleum-based products maintained the highest percent wall hydration, whereas products that contain alcohol, ketones, toluene, and acetate maintained the lowest percent wall hydration.[45]

A horse with low-quality hoof horn requires at least 1 year for new growth from the coronary band to reach the ground. In the meantime, the farrier can try to minimize trauma to the weak hooves by using fewer nails, thinner nails, clips, hand-forged shoes with strategically placed nail holes, acrylics to build up thin walls, and/or glue-on shoes.

Poor Hoof Shape

The hoof capsule is plastic-like and adapts its shape in response to the stresses that are placed on it. The higher its moisture content, the more plastic it is. Fortunately, many deformed hooves can be re-formed. Every time the hoof is trimmed, its shape should be evaluated and adjusted to ensure it is growing in the proper manner. When a hoof is being actively re-formed, the change in shape during one trimming may be dramatic (Fig. 9.57). Even for normal feet, however, the hoof must be shaped and the shoe must be carefully adjusted with each shoeing. Whether this is done or not is often the difference between a good farrier and a fast farrier.

Flares in the side walls of the hoof can result from a ML imbalance, a genetically or nutritionally weak hoof structure, a too-high moisture content in the hoof, or (most likely) a combination of these factors. A flare on only one side of the hoof is usually caused by ML imbalance. If the hoof wall flares out on both sides, it is usually a combination of hoof conformation and high moisture.

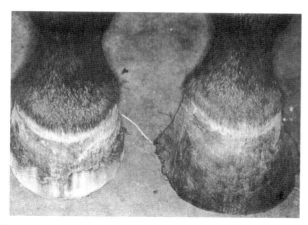

Figure 9.57   The hoof shape can be altered quite dramatically in just one trimming. (Reprinted with permission from Hill C, Klimesh R. Maximum Hoof Power. North Pomfret, VT: Trafalgar Square Publishing, 2000.)

Contracted Heels

Contraction of one or both heels of a hoof can be caused by long-toe–low-heel configuration; nonuse of the foot (such as when the limb is injured and non-weight bearing for a period of time or when the horse's exercise is restricted); or physical restriction of the hoof by horseshoe nails, clips, bandaging, or a cast. Identification of contracted heels can be made by the following methods. The width of the heels 4 inches from the buttresses should equal or exceed the width of the trimmed hoof 1 inch back from the toe (Fig. 9.58). If the heel measurement is less than toe measurement, the heels are said to be contracted. Alternatively, if the frog width is less than 67% of the frog length, it is contracted.[51] Some horses, however, have a congenital or adapted hoof shape that fits the definition of contracted heels, but the hoof is balanced by other criteria, and the animal is sound. In these cases, it is not advisable to try to spread the heels.

As a hoof deviates toward a long-toe–low-heel configuration, the hoof elongates from toe to heel, and the heels generally move closer together. One study that evaluated the effects of toe angle on hoof growth and contraction over a period of 126 days found that hooves trimmed to the long-toe–low-heel configuration were 7% smaller in width than they had been at day 0.[23] In addition, when a horse's weight rotates over the long toe in a prolonged breakover, the heels of the hoof are drawn inward. To allow such a hoof to function more normally and to encourage the heels to spread, the farrier should balance the hoof and use a squared-toe shoe, which provides adequate heel support.

When a horse lacks exercise, the blood flow in the hoof is decreased, causing a drop in the moisture content of the hoof capsule. In the idle horse, the lack of pressure pushing outward from the descending weight of the horse during movement and the increased inward-curling force from the drying outer hoof wall cause the hoof capsule to contract at the heels. This contraction can compress the sensitive inner structures of the hoof and result in lameness or soreness.

The treatment is to increase the exercise level of the horse and retard the evaporation of internal moisture

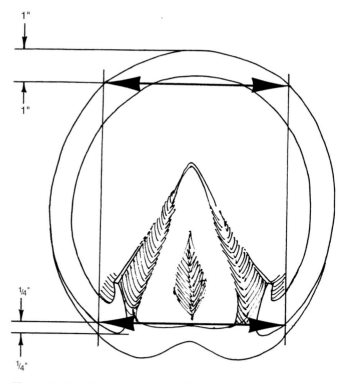

Figure 9.58   One method of identifying contracted heels. (Reprinted with permission from Hill C, Klimesh R. Maximum Hoof Power. North Pomfret, VT: Trafalgar Square Publishing, 2000.)

by application of a hoof sealer (see "Resources" in this chapter). In some instances, a shoe with slippered heels may be applied until the hoof regains its shape (Fig. 9.59). The heel portion of the bearing surface of this shoe is sloped outward to spread the hoof physically as the horse's weight descends. If the horse cannot be exercised, the moisture content of the hoof may need to be increased by wet bandages or by placing the horse in a stall with damp sand or sawdust. Other, more dramatic mechanical devices have been used to spread the heels of a contracted hoof physically; but these are futile if the cause of the contraction is not removed. Increasing frog pressure alone has been shown to have a variable effect on hoof expansion.[20]

Studies indicating there are proprioceptive (sensory) receptors located in the buttress of the frog support the idea that frog contact or pressure is important. This information, combined with the fact that wild horses land heel first, seems to indicate that the rear portion of the frog is important for sensory perception. Domestic horses appear to benefit if heel-first landing can be attained, when the frog buttress makes primary ground contact. Frog buttress contact should not be confused with hoof wall contact or frog-only loading. The ideal sequence is for the foot to land heel first enough to allow the frog buttress to make contact with the ground only before the foot is fully loaded. Feet that are prepared using the natural balance approach load the back portion of the foot equally when the foot is flat on the ground. One of us (G.O.) has had good results expanding the heels of horses suffering from contracted heels. The technique follows.

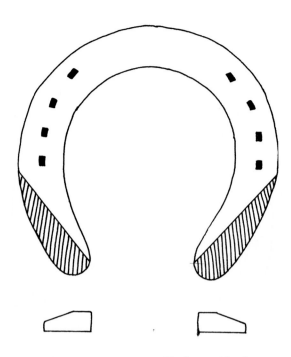

Figure 9.59 A shoe with slippered heels.

Hoof preparation is the same as described previously for natural balance trimming except that the quarters are not lowered to form an arch and the heel and toe pillars are not left long for selective contact and weight bearing. A one-third dorsal (forward) and two-thirds palmar/plantar (backward) relationship with the widest part of the foot—located ¾ of an inch behind the true apex of the frog—is established (Fig. 9.35). Two-part impression material is then applied to the sulci and on the surface of the frog. A hard impression (firm plastic) pad is secured to the bottom of the foot with duct tape, and the horse is allowed to bear weight. The plastic plate and weight bearing flattens the two-part impression material (Fig. 8.50A). The impression material is then rasped lightly so no projections exist.

After the application of the impression material, a Natural Balance Shoe is fitted so it extends palmar/plantar to the frog buttress. The pad should extend beyond the heels of the shoe ¼ to ⅜ inch. A wedge-shaped insert should always be used, attached to the pad as far to the rear as possible. The attached frog insert should be short and extend dorsal (forward) only about half the length of the frog. The portion of the wedge frog insert that extends beyond the heel of the shoe should be thicker than the heel of the shoe (about ⅛ inch or slightly more). When heel rails are used with the Equine Digit Support System, the frog insert must be raised until it extends about ⅛ inch beyond the height of the heels and about ¼ inch behind the heel rails (Fig. 8.50B). The frog inserts available with the Equine Digit Support System work best. The available selection of sizes makes it easy to choose the appropriate one for each horse. The inserts attach easily to the Equine Digit Support System pad, and adjustments can be made without removing the shoe. When conventional wedges or flat pads are used,

the insert must be riveted to the pad and cannot be changed without removing the shoe. Both approaches work well, however, once the support to the back of the pad is appropriate for the horse. Rail height selection is based on heel-first contact. Proper heel landing should not be excessive and could be interpreted as intermittent flat landing. Three of five strides at a walk should be noticeably recognized as landing heel first.

When the hoof must be in a cast or restrictive shoe for a long period, the heels usually contract. A similar contraction may result from consistently shoeing with the nails too far back toward the heels. Factory-made shoes have nail holes that are behind the widest part of the hoof. These nails are usually omitted unless they are specifically used to restrict the expansion of a bilaterally flared hoof. In most cases, the hoof will return to normal when the restriction is removed, the hoof is balanced, and the horse resumes regular exercise.

Long-Toe–Low-Heel and Underrun Heels

When proper DP hoof balance is not maintained by trimming or shoeing, the hoof attains an abnormal long-toe–low-heel configuration, which can result in excess stress to flexor tendons and ligaments, heel soreness, hoof cracks, contracted heels, and development of the navicular syndrome (caudal heel pain).[4,37,52] A relationship between a long-toe–low-heel configuration and ossification of the collateral cartilages has also been identified.[46]

The long-toe–low-heel configuration can occur in several ways: A horse with poor-quality hoof horn is left barefoot; the hooves are not trimmed regularly and grow a long toe; the horse receives poor trimming and shoeing; or the horse is overdue for shoeing.

If the heel is trimmed too short, the toe is left too long, and a shoe is placed on the hoof, the hoof angle is fixed at a too-low angle at the outset, and it becomes worse as the hoof grows. Furthermore, if a shoe is left too long on a properly balanced hoof, the heels will expand over the shoe and the horn at the heels will be crushed while the toe continues to grow longer but is prevented from wear by the shoe.

The long-toe–low-heel configuration places excess stress on the deep digital flexor tendon and navicular region. This stress can cause underrun heels, an often irreversible condition in which the angle of the hoof horn at the heels is lower than the toe angle by 5° or more.

To trim a hoof with low heels, the farrier trims the toe of the hoof wall as short as is practical, tapering off toward the quarters. The heels are taken down only enough to get a good bearing surface of healthy horn, which can usually be accomplished with the rasp alone, minimizing the risk of trimming them too much.

Underrun heels should be trimmed short enough, however, so that the support for the hoof is more rearward. Leaving underrun heels long in an attempt to align the hoof-pastern axis only forces the heels to grow farther forward underneath the limb (Fig. 9.60) and creates an open invitation for lost shoes. After trimming the heels very short, the farrier can align the hoof-pastern axis by elevating the heels with wedge-heel shoes or

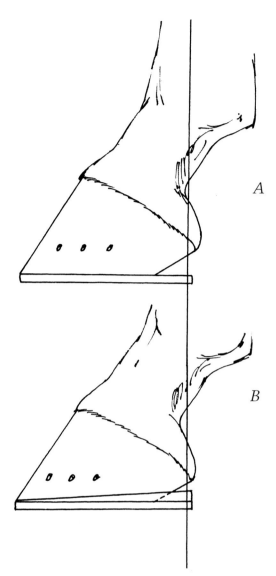

Figure 9.60 Although both shoe setups provide adequate support, the one shown in panel B will more likely correct underrun heels and result in fewer lost shoes. (Reprinted with permission from Hill C, Klimesh R. Maximum Hoof Power. North Pomfret, VT: Trafalgar Square Publishing, 2000.)

wedge pads (degree pads) (Fig. 9.60). An alternative is to rebuild the heels to a normal length and angle with a prosthetic hoof material (see "Resources" in this chapter). The hoof can then be shod in a normal manner.[36,47]

In the natural balance approach, the same procedures used for contracted heels are applied to horses with underrun heels. The key points are to get the breakover close to the frog apex—1 to $1\frac{1}{2}$ inches—and to follow the sole callus guidelines previously discussed. Prepare the heels of the foot close to the nonexfoliating sole in the quarters. For severe cases, use two-part impression material and frog buttress support, whenever possible, to start the treatment. Using this approach, one of us (G.O.) has achieved good results.

Navicular Syndrome

Navicular syndrome is a chronic forelimb lameness involving the navicular bone and associated structures. Not all lameness associated with the heel region of the hoof, however, should be attributed to navicular syndrome. Factors thought to predispose a horse to navicular problems include poor conformation, improper or irregular shoeing, and stress to the navicular region. A common error that can lead to navicular syndrome is associated with the false economy of stretching the intervals between shoeing. As a hoof grows past its optimum reset time, the toe gets too long and the heel too low, resulting in a broken back axis. Increased pressure between the deep flexor tendon and the navicular bone may cause the heel pain associated with navicular syndrome (Fig. 9.28).

The egg bar shoe (discussed later in this chapter) has proved beneficial in the treatment of some cases of the navicular syndrome. It is a noninvasive, inexpensive treatment with virtually no negative side effects or risks. In addition, the egg bar shoe has positive effects on hoof conformation. Some horses show dramatic clinical improvement 3 to 6 weeks after egg bar shoes are applied. Some underrun hooves, however, have gone past a critical horn-tubule angle and have reached the point of no return. Although these hooves are not likely to show a reversal of the underrun heel condition, the horse may be usable and comfortable working in egg bar shoes for many years.

Full pads may be recommended for some horses with navicular syndrome, particularly those that have thin, painful soles or those that have grade 3/4 pain over the central third of the frog. Pads may also be recommended for horses pastured on rocky terrain. In addition, hooves with wide open, low heels may incur navicular pain or heel soreness from the direct concussion to the frog and heel region. Full pads are used to protect this area. Care must be taken, however, because the pad may sometimes transmit concussion to the navicular region. A straight bar or full-support shoe may be more effective in providing protection for this type of navicular problem. Presently, we are using the natural balance trimming and shoeing procedures described previously for this problem. (Refer to Chapter 8 for more information.)

Wry Hoof

A wry hoof (diagonal ML imbalance) is a deformation that is usually, but not always, associated with sheared heels. The entire hoof wall, when viewed from the front, appears to sweep off to one side. When a hoof is wry to the inside, the medial wall flares inward and the outer wall curls in underneath the hoof. A wry hoof is caused primarily by a ML imbalance. This imbalance can be the result of improper trimming; from pain in the limb, which causes the horse to land more heavily on one side of the hoof; or from the way in which the hoof is worn as the horse turns in a habitual way in a stall or pen.

To return a wry hoof to a normal configuration, the flare is dressed off (Fig. 9.61), and the hoof is shod with a bar shoe that is centered beneath the limb. This means

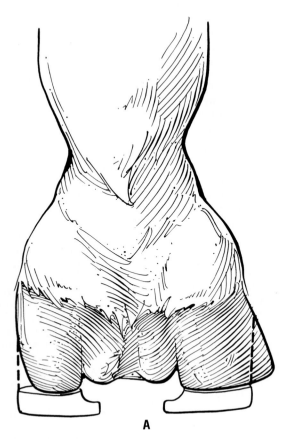
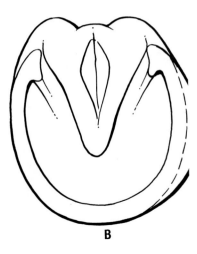

Figure 9.61 Placing a shoe on a wry foot. A. The shoe is placed where the foot should be. B. The flared hoof wall will be rasped off (dotted line).

that the shoe extends beyond the turned-under hoof wall by as much as ¼ to ⅜ inch and is shod close to the wall on the flared side. In cases in which the coronet band has become displaced proximally, the hoof may be floated to relieve pressure, or the foot may be soaked in water and placed in a moist bandage until the hoof settles.[42,48] Refer to sheared heels for more information.

The remaining hooves should be checked closely for balance. This should be done because abnormalities affecting the shape of one hoof often affect other hooves, usually those on the diagonal limb.

Sheared Heels and Quarters

ML imbalance can lead to sheared heels and cracks.[38] On a straight limb, lines from the coronet to the ground on the medial and lateral sides of the hoof are the same lengths, and the coronet forms a smooth line around the top of the hoof. The hoof strikes the ground flat (both sides simultaneously) at a walk.

When one side of the hoof becomes too short through wear or trimming, uneven stress is placed on the entire hoof structure. When a disproportionate amount of weight is borne by one side of the hoof, the entire side of the hoof wall can be displaced upward, actually shear-

ing the heels between the bulbs (Fig. 9.62). Grasping a heel of a sheared hoof in each hand, one can sometimes move the heels independently. Some horses' hoof structure adapts to this sheared configuration over many years, making a return to normal impossible and, sometimes, undesirable. If imbalanced during the formative years, a hoof may be permanently fixed into that abnormal balance, which then becomes "normal" for that horse. A recent development of sheared heels, often causing soreness and lameness, can usually be remedied by therapeutic shoeing methods.

If a small area of the hoof wall is allowed to be too long (such as when the shoe does not fit flat on the hoof) or if a small area of the hoof is growing fast, focal pressure is directed up the hoof wall, which can cause a section of the coronet to be displaced upward (and may result in a crack in the hoof wall). A coronet displacement often goes undetected and can be the cause of subtle lameness.

The treatment for sheared heels is to allow the displaced hoof wall to drop down to its original position. The hoof is trimmed in balance as if it were not sheared, and a bar shoe is fit to the hoof. Before the bar shoe is applied, the ground surface of the displaced heel is further trimmed ("floated") so that it will not bear on the shoe. There should be a gap of ¼ to ½ inch between the

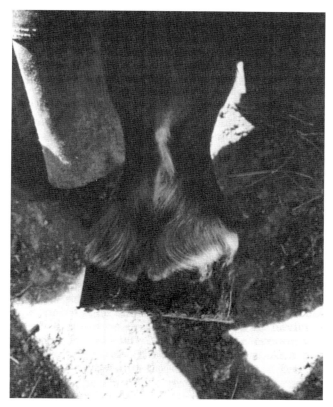

Figure 9.62 Back view of a horse with sheared heels. Note that the medial coronet of the heel and quarter region are higher than the lateral side. The medial hoof wall is also straighter than the lateral side. (Reprinted with permission from Hill C, Klimesh R. Maximum Hoof Power. North Pomfret, VT: Trafalgar Square Publishing, 2000.)

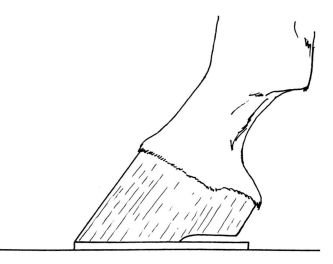

Figure 9.63 Floating a heel. (Reprinted with permission from Hill C, Klimesh R. Maximum Hoof Power. North Pomfret, VT: Trafalgar Square Publishing, 2000.)

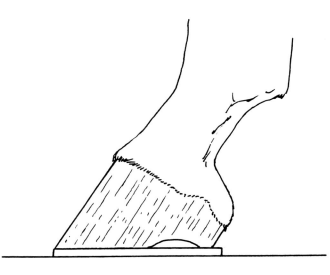

Figure 9.64 Treating a displaced coronet. (Reprinted with permission from Hill C, Klimesh R. Maximum Hoof Power. North Pomfret, VT: Trafalgar Square Publishing, 2000.)

shoe and the hoof, tapering to meet at midquarter (Fig. 9.63). Supporting the frog buttress as previously described has also proven beneficial in the treatment of sheared heels and quarters. Whatever the approach used, some hooves will remodel in one or two shoeings. Other long-standing cases may never return to normal.

The treatment for a displaced coronet is similar to that for sheared heels. Below the site of the displacement (following the horn tubules to the ground surface), the hoof wall is sculpted out to parallel the bulge at the coronet (Fig. 9.64), which allows the displaced portion of the hoof wall to descend to the shoe and the coronet to assume its normal position. This re-forming of the hoof can be facilitated (after trimming in the aforementioned manner) by leaving the shoes off of the affected hooves and keeping the horse in a stall with a base of damp sand or a deep layer of dampened coarse sawdust for several days. The hoof will re-form (and deform) more readily with a greater moisture content, and this footing will support the entire ground surface of the hoof, allowing the hoof wall to settle down to a normal level. The hooves may also be encouraged in this remodeling by soaking the foot in warm water for 15 minutes, wrapping it with moist bandages for 12 to 24 hours, and periodically rasping the ground surface of the hoof at the site of displacement as it settles[48] (refer to Chapter 8 for more information).

Using the natural balance trimming and shoeing approach (described earlier) will also help prevent the development of sheared heels and quarters.

Cracks

Cracks are separations or breaks in the hoof wall. Vertical cracks between the tubules of the hoof horn are referred to by their location, such as toe cracks, quarter cracks, and heel cracks. Cracks that originate at the coronet are called sand (incomplete) cracks (Fig. 9.65), whereas those that start at the ground surface are called grass cracks.

A horizontal crack in the hoof wall is called a "blowout" (Fig. 9.66). Blowouts are caused either by an injury

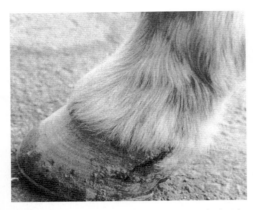

Figure 9.65 Sand crack. (Reprinted with permission from Hill C, Klimesh R. Maximum Hoof Power. North Pomfret, VT: Trafalgar Square Publishing, 2000.)

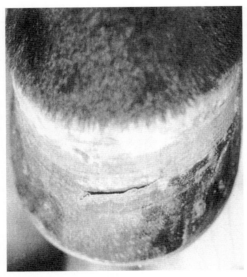

Figure 9.66 A blowout crack that has grown down from its initial site near the coronary band. (Reprinted with permission from Hill C, Klimesh R. Maximum Hoof Power. North Pomfret, VT: Trafalgar Square Publishing, 2000.)

to the coronary band or by a blow to the hoof wall. A blowout usually does not result in lameness and many times goes unnoticed until the farrier spots it. Once they occur, these cracks seldom increase in size horizontally and usually require no treatment. Because the hoof is weaker at this site, however, a blowout can set the stage for a vertical crack if the hoof is further undermined by excess moisture or is not in ML balance.

Since cracks do not "heal" back together, the hoof wall must be replaced primarily by new growth from the coronary band, just as a damaged fingernail must grow out. This will take 9 to 12 months. For optimum hoof growth, a ration containing nutrients necessary for healthy hoof horn can be fed (see "Resources" in this chapter).

Sand cracks can result from an injury to the coronet or from an infection in the white line ("gravel") that breaks out at the coronet. Sometimes, a horse bumps the

coronet when loading or unloading from a trailer, or the horse might strike the coronet during fast work or an uncoordinated movement. These cracks can also develop with ML and diagonal imbalances.[42,48]

A wet environment containing sand or gravel can soften a horse's hooves and allow particles to be forced up into the white line. If infection results, it can travel upward through the laminae and break out at the coronet, possibly causing a crack. Cracks often appear at the site of a displaced coronet.

The first step in dealing with sand cracks is to determine the cause and remove it. This, accompanied by trimming and shoeing to balance the hoof, may be all that is necessary to stabilize the hoof as it replaces the damaged horn (Fig. 9.67). Severe cracks can be held immobile by a variety of methods until the hoof grows out. Such methods include nailing or screwing across the crack; drilling holes on either side and lacing the crack up like a boot; fastening brass metal plates on both sides of the crack with 22-gauge stainless-steel wire placed in a horizontal mattress suture pattern; using an adjustable steel hose clamp; and patching the crack together with plastic, high-resin fiberglass tape or using a fiberglass tape held in place with screws[7,11,35,57] (Fig.9.68).

In a study of 24 horses with 38 hoof wall cracks that were repaired with the stainless-steel hose clamp method, only one failure was recognized.[7] To apply this method, the hose clamp is cut so the offset tension device remains. The clamp is then secured to the hoof wall with standard 8- × 3/8-inch sheet metal screws, after which the clamp is tightened by twisting the offset tension device. Once compression is achieved, the band is secured with another screw placed closer to the crack, and the tension device is removed. An advantage to this method is that it is simple to apply, it is versatile, and compression can be applied directly to stabilize the crack.

There are several high-tech hoof repair materials developed specifically to bond to the hoof wall. Some of these materials mimic the consistency of the hoof wall so that, once applied, they can be nailed into, trimmed, and rasped along with the hoof wall as it grows down. The prosthetic materials can be used to fill the crack completely or to form a patch across the crack (see "Resources" in this chapter). This material can also be impregnated with antibiotics for repair of chronic nonhealing hoof cracks that result from low-grade infection and for hoof defects that extend to the sensitive tissues.[54]

Before a crack is stabilized, it must be thoroughly debrided so that dirt, loose hoof horn, and bacteria are removed. If there is any evidence of moisture, the crack is treated until it is completely dry. It has generally been accepted that applying any type of patching material over a moist crack or exposed sensitive tissue has the potential of trapping bacteria and providing a perfect environment for an infection to develop. The addition of an antibiotic (e.g., metronidazole) to the hoof repair material, however, has allowed earlier application of the acrylic to hoof defects.[54] The antibiotic elutes out of the acrylic in therapeutic concentrations to prevent and/or treat infection.

Chronic or severe cracks toward the heel of the hoof are sometimes dealt with by removing the section of the hoof wall behind the crack (Fig. 9.67). A full-support shoe then supports the hoof until new hoof grows down. A similar but less involved approach is to apply a full-

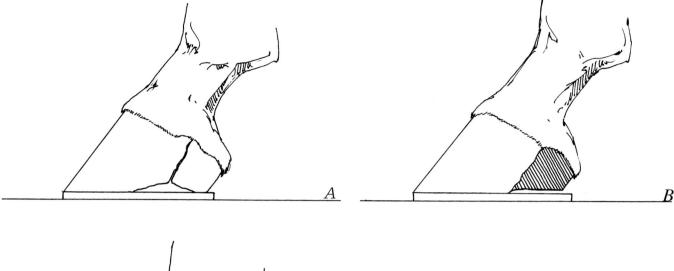

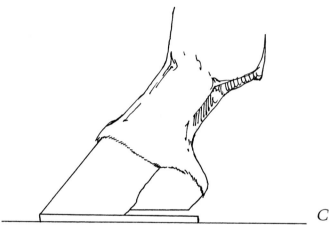

Figure 9.67   Treating a crack. A. Relieving. B. Resecting. C. Floating. (Reprinted with permission from Hill C, Klimesh R. Maximum Hoof Power. North Pomfret, VT: Trafalgar Square Publishing, 2000.)

support shoe and "float" the portion of the hoof behind the crack. "Floating" means to trim that portion of the hoof about ¼ inch shorter so that it will not contact the shoe (Fig. 9.67). By eliminating weight bearing behind the crack, movement of the two halves of the crack is minimized, and the hoof often grows down intact. A horse that is very active or in work, however, is likely to need to have the crack more securely stabilized.

Grass cracks (beginning at the ground) most often appear in unshod hooves that have been allowed to grow too long. Often, all that is needed to control these cracks is a good trimming. More severe cracks may require shoes for several months until new hoof tissue can grow down and replace the cracked horn. To help toe cracks grow out, the hoof angle must be kept up where it belongs, and a squared-toe shoe must be applied to minimize the prying effect of breakover.

Surface cracks are tiny fissures that cover some portion of the hoof wall. They are most often caused by a change in hoof moisture, such as when a horse on wet pasture is put in a stall with dry bedding or when a horse that has been standing in mud then stands in the sun. Surface cracks are remedied by stabilizing the horse's moisture balance, minimizing the exposure to wetness, and using a hoof sealer. Thick hoof dressings may fill the cracks and improve the exterior appearance of a hoof, but a hoof sealer is more beneficial to long-term hoof health (see "Resources" in this chapter). One of us (G.O.) suggests that leaving the sole and frog intact and the wall trimmed to the level of the sole is natural and, therefore, can help in the maintenance of horses with hoof cracks.

Bruises, Corns, and Abscesses

When the hoof is trimmed, the outer wall should be long enough so that it, not the sole, is the primary weight-bearing structure. Pressure on the perimeter of the sole inside the white line can cause pain and can compress the blood vessels beneath the sole. If the wall is trimmed too short, if the sole is very flat, or if a barefoot horse has worn its hooves so short that the soles are flat or protruding below the hoof wall, the sole is likely to be bruised (Fig. 9.69). Horses in muddy pens, whether shod or barefoot, often bruise their soles when the temperature drops and the lumpy mud freezes hard.

One of us (G.O.) suggests that leaving the sole and frog intact and the wall trimmed to the level of the sole is natural and, therefore, can help in the maintenance of horses with bruises, corns, and some abscesses.

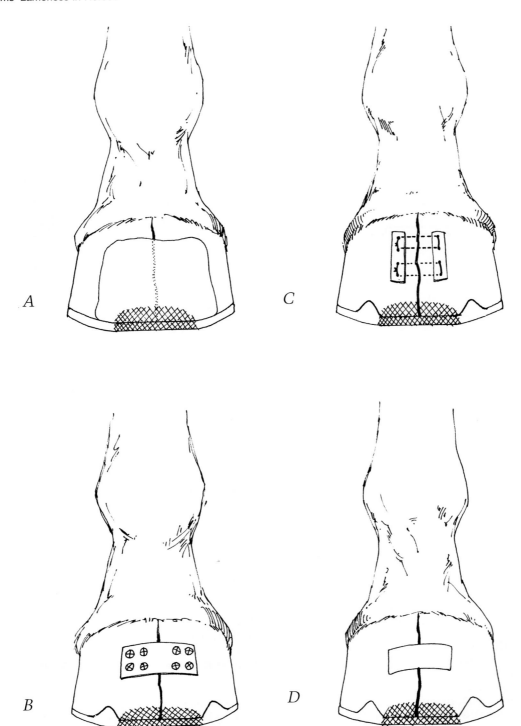

Figure 9.68 Stabilizing a crack. A. Acrylic patch. B. Screwed-on plate. C. Laced patch. D. Glued-on patch. Cross-hatched areas indicate a squared toe. (Reprinted with permission from Hill C, Klimesh R. Maximum Hoof Power. North Pomfret, VT: Trafalgar Square Publishing, 2000.)

Normally, the healthy sole has a concave shape like a shallow bowl and is about ¼ inch thick on a saddle horse. A properly trimmed sole gives or feels springy only under very heavy thumb pressure. If the sole gives to moderate pressure, it may be too short to protect the inner structures adequately from bruising, especially on rocky or frozen ground. A thin-soled horse may lack confidence of movement and be "off." Bruising may develop into an abscess, which can cause some degree of lameness. If a thin sole is the result of recent trimming,

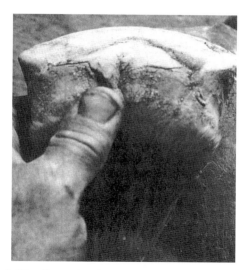

Figure 9.69 Excess hoof wall wear resulting in sole pressure. (Reprinted with permission from Hill C, Klimesh R. Maximum Hoof Power. North Pomfret, VT: Trafalgar Square Publishing, 2000.)

the horse, even when shod, may be sore when walked over gravel or rough ground that contacts the sole. Usually in 1 or 2 weeks, the sole thickens enough for the horse to be comfortable.

Generally, do not remove any sole beyond that which crumbles with a light pull of the knife; there are exceptions, however. In some horses, for whatever reason, the sole is thick and firm and will not crumble with a light pull of the knife. Such is the case in horses that are sole bound, that live in very dry climates and have limited exercise, or that live in extremely cold climates. In these cases, strenuous hoof knife work may be required to trim the sole and balance the hoof.

Corns are bruises or abscesses that occur inside the buttress where the hoof wall curves to join the bars. This site is actually referred to as the seat of corn. Corns are usually caused by pressure from a horseshoe or from a stone wedged between the shoe and the hoof. When the hoof is trimmed, the seat of corn should be pared below the level of the hoof wall to prevent contact with the shoe. If a shoe is left on too long and the hoof overgrows the shoe, the heels often collapse, and pressure is put on the seat of corn, resulting in a bruise or abscess. A corn can cause some degree of lameness. Trimming to remove pressure on the corn may be all that is required. If the corn is infected, it is treated as an abscess.

Full pads are often used to protect a bruised sole while it heals. If a pad is applied over a sole bruise that is on the verge of abscess, however, it will tend to fester the abscess quickly. The horse may exhibit great pain a day or so after the pad has been applied, necessitating the removal of the pad. Once the abscess has been treated and has dried out, a pad can be reapplied, if necessary, for protection.

Hot Nail

A horseshoe nail driven into the hoof wall that puts pressure on the sensitive inner structures without actu-

ally piercing them is referred to as a close nail (Fig. 9.70). A close nail may cause the horse immediate discomfort or may go unnoticed for many days or until the horse is put into work. Usually, the offending nail can be located by the use of a hoof tester or by judicious tapping with a hammer at the location of each nail. Removal of the close nail often returns the horse to soundness because the sensitive structures have not been invaded.

A nail that is driven into the sensitive structures of the hoof is called a hot nail. A hot nail usually causes the horse to exhibit immediate pain unless the horse is under sedation. If the animal is normally fractious when being shod, the response to a hot nail may go unnoticed. On removing a hot nail, blood is likely to be seen in the nail hole and on the nail itself. The hole should be flushed with an antiseptic such as povidone iodine (Betadine) and plugged to prevent contamination. A nail should not be placed in the hole. The horse should be current on tetanus vaccination and should be observed for several days for continuing or developing lameness.

If an abscess develops, a veterinarian should be contacted. Usually, the shoe is removed and the hoof is soaked in a hot water-Epsom salt solution twice daily for 2 to 3 days. When the veterinarian determines that the infection has cleared, the shoe can be replaced.

Thrush

Anaerobic bacteria (*Spherophorus necrophorus*) that thrive in the warm, dark recesses of the hoof cause thrush. The bacteria's foul-smelling black exudate is most commonly found in the clefts of the frog; if left untreated, it can invade sensitive tissues, especially deep in the central cleft, and cause lameness. Thrush also inhabits separations and cracks in the hoof wall, especially if the horse is in a moist environment. Cleanliness is the best prevention and the first step of any treatment program. Sugardyne is effective for treating thrush: A thin paste is made from white sugar and a povidone iodine (Betadine) solution or ointment and spread on the cleaned areas daily until the problem is resolved. Commercial preparations for treating thrush are available and are effective in different degrees. Severe cases of thrush can be treated with a CVP gasket pad (see section on pads in this chapter).

White Line Disease

When an area of separation occurs in the hoof wall, it provides a moist, dark environment, ideal for the growth of horn-digesting organisms. Soil and manure may be forced up into the interlaminar space as the white line deteriorates. If left unchecked, this situation can progress to white line disease and result in lameness.

White line disease, sometimes incorrectly called seedy toe, is most likely caused by invasion of the inner horn by bacteria, fungus (onychomycosis), or yeast, which results in some degree of damage to the structural integrity of the hoof. There seems to be a greater occurrence of the condition in hot, humid climates. The area of an affected hoof is characteristically filled with a white cheesy material and air pockets that are often packed

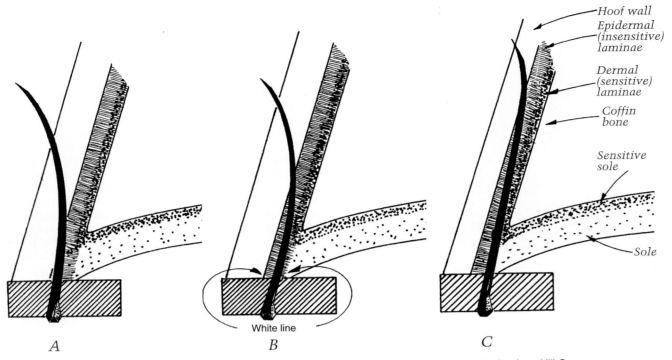

Hoof wall
Epidermal
(insensitive)
laminae
Dermal
(sensitive)
laminae
Coffin
bone

Sensitive
sole

Sole

White line

A   *B*   *C*

Figure 9.70 Nail path. A. Good nail. B. Close nail. C. Hot nail. (Reprinted with permission from Hill C, Klimesh R. Maximum Hoof Power. North Pomfret, VT: Trafalgar Square Publishing, 2000.)

with debris. The disease starts at ground level and, if not controlled, can work its way up to the coronary band.

An affected horse may show symptoms similar to those of laminitis: lameness, heat, sole tending to be flat, slow horn growth, tenderness when nailing, and pain over the sole when hoof testers are applied. There may be areas of the hoof wall that, when tapped, give a hollow sound. Depending on the extent of the damage, lameness can result from mechanical loss of horn support. In severe cases, the destruction of the laminae may allow a rotation of the coffin bone to occur.

Any separation in the white line should be considered a seed for white line disease. A separation is often found between the heel and the quarter in the white line. The cavity may be ¼ inch deep or extend halfway up the hoof wall. The space is usually filled with a white chalky substance or thrush's foul-smelling, tarlike residue. These heel caves can be treated by digging out as much of the decomposed horn as possible and packing the hole by use of the CVP method (see section on pads later in this chapter). If the hole is deep, the treatment materials may need to be layered. A shoe is applied to protect the packing and to prevent further contamination. The horse should be kept in a dry environment, and the shoes should be reset regularly, at which time the packing is replaced. The hoof deterioration can usually be prevented from spreading with this treatment, and the hoof grows down solid. If the area of separation is large or extends for a distance along the white line, this treatment is used in conjunction with the application of a CVP gasket pad.

Treatment of severe cases of white line disease involves resection of the undermined hoof wall and the

topical application of an antiseptic, such as Merthiolate,[31] or the application of antibiotic-impregnated hoof repair material. One study documented a high degree of success using 1 g metronidazole powder added to 1 ounce hoof acrylic.[54] An added benefit to this approach is that the authors of this study were able to rebuild the weight-bearing hoof wall to prevent further disruption of the hoof wall-coffin bone attachments.

Canker

Canker (chronic hypertropic pododermatitis) is a rare condition that is most commonly diagnosed in horses in the semitropical climate of the southern United States.[53] It may involve one or more feet and localized inflammation; pain resulting in lameness is common. The exact cause of canker is unknown; affected horses, however, often have a history of being on damp moist pastures in year-round warm climates. The causative agents are thought to be *Fusobacterium necrophorum* and one or more *Bacteroides* spp.[55]

The diagnosis is made on physical examination. A moist exudative pododermatitis with characteristic hypertrophic filamentous fronds is seen. Histologic examination confirms the diagnosis. Occasionally, a gram-negative filamentous coccobacillus can be seen microscopically in the affected epithelieum.[55]

Treatment is difficult and recurrence is common. Surgical debridement, the topical application of antimicrobials, and bandaging appear to be important. It is recommended that general anesthesia be used for problematic cases. Debridement should be deep enough to remove

CORRECTIVE AND THERAPEUTIC TRIMMING AND SHOEING TECHNIQUES

Corrective trimming and shoeing alters the hoof, affecting stance or stride, including breakover. Therapeutic shoeing is an important part of some lameness treatments. Corrective and therapeutic shoeing techniques aim to restore DP balance, ML balance, shape, and hoof integrity as well as to provide additional support, protection, and traction, if necessary. Furthermore, corrective shoeing techniques can sometimes help in resolving movement abnormalities.

The implementation of corrective and therapeutic shoeing techniques should be a team effort between an experienced farrier, an equine veterinarian, and the horse owner. A shoeing prescription can be made to document the recommended approach to trimming and shoeing and for record-keeping purposes (Fig. 9.73).

Dorsal-Palmar Balance

The most common DP imbalance is a long-toe–low-heel configuration, often accompanied by underrun heels. When trimming a hoof with low heels, the toe of the hoof wall is trimmed as short as practical, tapering off toward the quarters. The heels are taken down only enough to get a good bearing surface of healthy horn; this can often be accomplished more precisely with the rasp alone, minimizing the risk of trimming too much. Trimming underrun heels extends the base of support of the hoof rearward; leaving underrun heels long in an attempt to align the hoof-pastern angle only forces the heels to grow farther forward underneath the limb (Fig. 9.45).

Horses that have low heels and a broken-back hoof-pastern axis often benefit from the application of wedge-heel shoes or wedge pads (degree pads) applied between the hoof and a flat shoe. Wedge-heel shoes are thicker in the heel than in the toe (Fig. 9.60). Wedge pads are thick on one end and taper to quite thin at the other end (Fig. 9.74). Depending on how much the heels of the hoof need to be elevated, the farrier can use a single wedge pad of the appropriate thickness or a stack of several pads.

Wedge pads not only can realign hoof-pastern angles but also can prevent direct pressure on the navicular region. The thicker wedge pads are often stiff enough across the heels to protect the frog and thus the navicular region from direct ground pressure, provided that there is no undue pressure on the frog from its excess length or from improper hoof packing. Wedge pads are available as full coverage pads or as bar pads, which have an open center to permit the sole to respire normally. The open center, however, collects debris, which can be difficult to clean out. Horses with bone spavin (arthritis of the distal tarsal joints) may get some relief from wedge heels or wedge pads with a squared or rocker-toe shoe.

A less common DP imbalance is a short-toe–long-heel configuration. It is important to determine the cause of the long heel before attempting to lower the hoof to align with the pastern. Damage to the hoof or limb structures can be caused by trimming the heels too much and trying to force the heels down. The short-toe–long-heel con-figuration often occurs to a hoof that has been non-weight bearing for a period of time because of an injury; it can also be the result of a flexural deformity (contracted muscle-tendon unit) associated with the deep digital flexor tendon. To prevent the overly long heel horn from deforming, trim the heels down within ⅛ inch of the nonexfoliating sole in the quarters behind the widest part of the foot and then elevate the heels by using wedge pads or an elevated heel shoe to allow the hoof to bear weight evenly. One of the most important parts of the treatment procedure is to bring breakover back to its natural position, which is closer to the frog apex on feet that are more upright than those that are deemed normal. Although this trimming and shoeing procedure is helpful, the underlying cause must be addressed for a satisfactory outcome. Desmotomy of the carpal check ligament may be required.

A half-shoe can be used for a short-toe–long-heel condition that results from toe dragging, pawing, or other causes of excessive toe wear. This shoe can be made from the front half of a training plate that covers the toe and leaves the heel bare. The ends of the half-shoe are tapered, or set into the hoof, so that there is no abrupt step where the shoe makes the transition to the heels of the hoof. This shoe protects the toe of the hoof but allows the heels of the hoof to wear down as they grow.

Hoof Shape

If the hoof has a flare, the flare should be dressed off and that side of the wall should be shortened (lowered). The quarter where the flare was located should be sculpted out with a rasp so that the hoof at that region bears no weight. This removes the bending forces on the horn tubules and results in the new hoof horn growing down straighter.

Many horses have "pancake" hooves that tend to spread out and become flat. The treatment for these hooves includes stabilizing the moisture content by keeping them in a dry environment and applying a hoof sealer to minimize the absorption of external moisture. The flares should be dressed off to about half the thickness of the hoof wall, and a shoe should be applied with side clips located across the widest part of the flared hoof (Fig. 9.75). (Use a bar or open shoe that is strong enough to withstand the spreading forces of the hoof.) The straighter the hoof wall becomes, the stronger it will be. Once the shape of the hoof is restored and the moisture content stabilized, the hoof can often be shod with a regular shoe with no clips.

Often, the hoof is not flared symmetrically but distorted across the diagonal of the hoof base, such as a medial toe flare with a lateral heel flare. Along with this, the opposing points (the medial heel and lateral toe) are pulled inward. Trimming the hoof into balance may prevent further distortion of the hoof, but a shoe is usually required to re-form the hoof to a more functional, symmetric shape. The shoe is applied with clips across the longest diagonal. These clips contain the hoof as it grows down, encouraging expansion across the narrow diagonal and resulting in a more symmetric hoof (Fig. 9.75).

A flare at the front of the hoof wall is called a dish. Most hooves dish to some degree, and as part of the

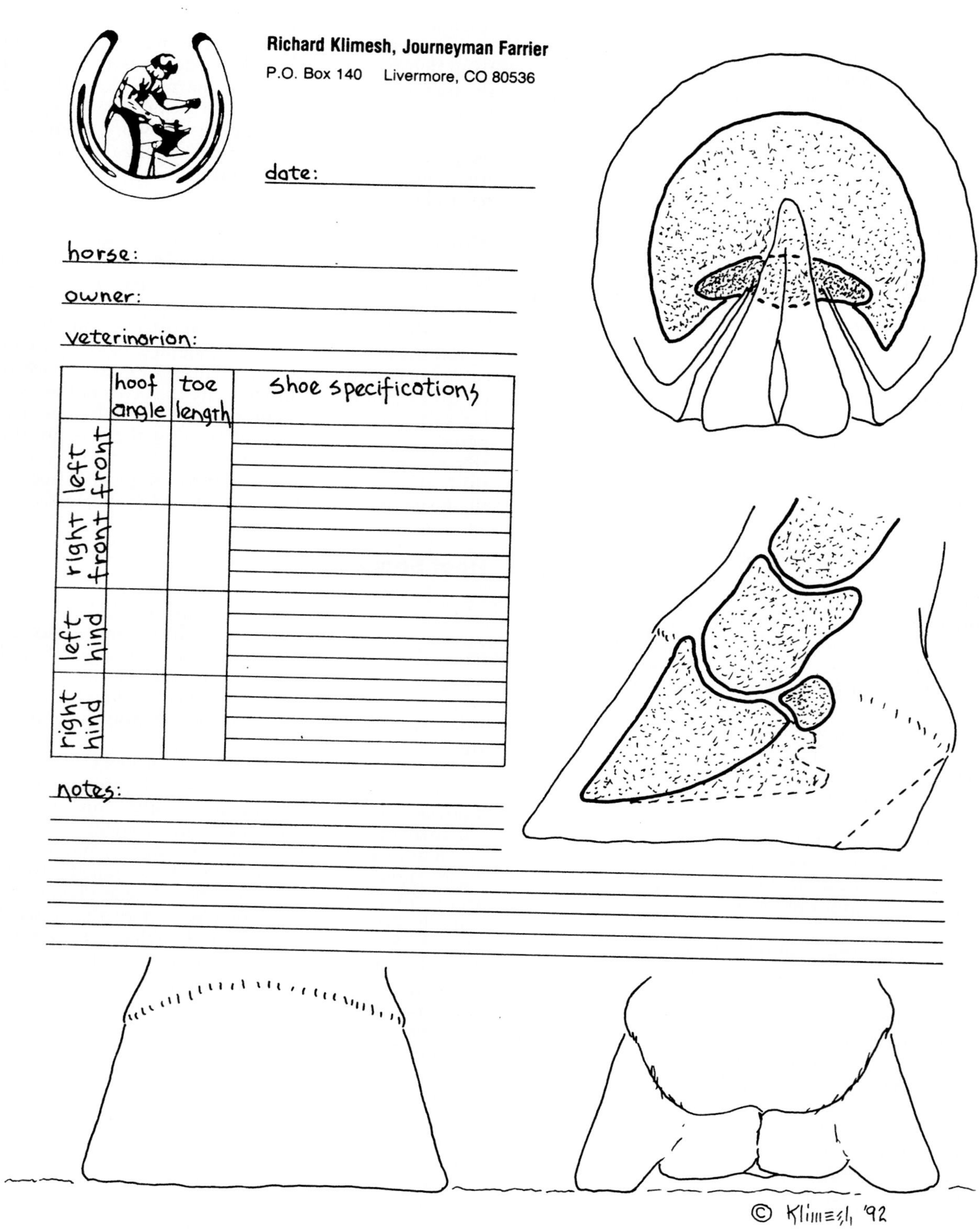

Richard Klimesh, Journeyman Farrier
P.O. Box 140   Livermore, CO 80536

date: _____

horse: _____

owner: _____

veterinarian: _____

	hoof angle	toe length	Shoe specifications
left front			
right front			
left hind			
right hind			

notes: _____

© Klimesh '92

Figure 9.73 Shoeing prescription form.

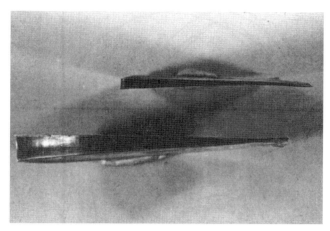

Figure 9.74   Plastic wedge pads. (Reprinted with permission from Hill C, Klimesh R. Maximum Hoof Power. North Pomfret, VT: Trafalgar Square Publishing, 2000.)

regular trimming process this dish should be dressed so that the hoof wall at the toe is straight from the coronet to the ground. If this is not done, the dish will cause the breakover point of the hoof and the entire base of support to be too far forward. Laying a straightedge such as a rasp against the hoof wall allows the farrier to easily identify the presence of any dish (Fig. 9.16).

A dished toe is sometimes the result of shortening (contraction) of the deep digital flexor muscle-tendon unit. This contraction exerts constant pull on the coffin bone within the hoof capsule, which causes the hoof wall to bend away from the coffin bone, creating the dish. The treatment is to elevate the angle of the hoof by trimming or using a wedge pad or shoe. This often lessens the pull on the coffin bone enough to allow the deep digital flexor muscle-tendon unit to relax. Then the hoof may be lowered over several trimming periods back to its normal angle. If the problem persists, a carpal check ligament desmotomy may be done to correct the problem.

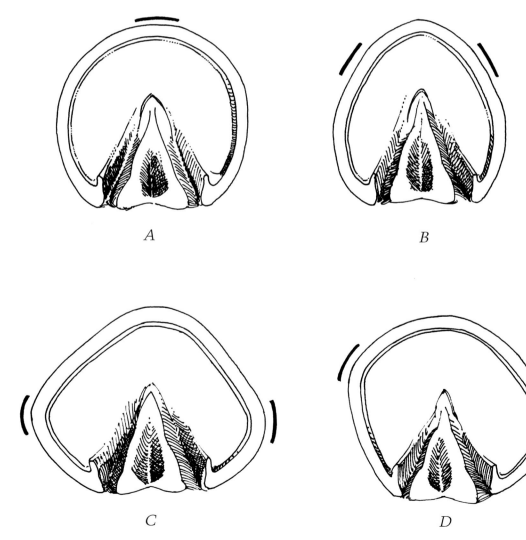

A

B

C

D

Figure 9.75   Clip positions. A. Toe clip. B. Forward-placed side clip. C. Rearward-placed side clip. D. Asymmetric side clips.

(Reprinted with permission from Hill C, Klimesh R. Maximum Hoof Power. North Pomfret, VT: Trafalgar Square Publishing, 2000.)

A clubfoot or even just a normally steep hoof might develop a dish if the heels are lowered too much in an attempt to "balance" the foot. These types of hooves are better maintained at a relatively steep angle of 60 to 65°. Enhancing the breakover is also important.

As with flares, an increase in hoof moisture allows the hoof wall to dish more easily, so it is best to keep the hooves dry, with a hoof sealer, if necessary.

Additional Support

Extended-Heel Shoes

Extended heel shoes are used to lengthen the base of support for the limb. In a properly trimmed hoof, the length of the support base (shoe) is commonly twice the toe length (Fig. 9.46). In an ideally conformed hoof, the amount of shoe extended past the heel of the hoof is ⅛ to ¼ inch, enough to allow for the normal forward migration of the shoe over the 5- to 8-week shoeing period. Hooves with some degree of underrun heels require longer shoes to achieve the necessary support.

The shape of extended-heel shoes when applied to the forefeet usually follows the shape of an egg bar shoe, and in fact, they are called "open egg bars." On the hindfeet, the extended heels can be bent straight back to form a true extended-heel shoe or bent out 45° to form bilateral trailers (Fig. 9.76). Bilateral trailers widen as well as lengthen the support base, adding stability to the foot and limb. The clefts of the frogs of hooves with shoes with outward-bent heels can be cleaned more easily than those with open egg bar shoes (Fig. 9.77); unfortunately, these shoes further prevent the natural rotation that occurs during the impact phase of the stride. The danger of using these shoes on the front is that the trailers are likely to be stepped on. Generally, the extended-heel shoe is an excellent support shoe and performance enhancer when used on the hindfeet of horses engaged in strenuous athletic activities, such as dressage and jumping.

Egg Bar Shoe

A shoe with extended branches that curve inward and connect to each other at the heels is an egg bar (Fig. 9.78). Egg bar shoes provide a large, stable base that extends behind the heels. This longer base supports the heels in soft footing, prevents the hoof from rocking back, and takes some stress off the flexor support structures, the navicular region, and the coffin joint.

Egg bar shoes can be used to treat many conditions, including navicular syndrome, caudal heel pain, sheared heels and quarters, contracted heels, collapsed and underrun heels, and flat soles. A flat-soled hoof ("dead hoof") is one that lands with a thud; it is not conformed to transmit resilient energy. Such a hoof shod with an egg bar shoe may, over time, begin to develop a more cupped (concave) sole, a desirable configuration that creates a trampoline-like contraction and expansion, allowing the hoof to spring off the ground.

By virtue of the shape of the bar and the extra amount of material in an egg bar shoe, the horse's weight is spread out over a larger area of ground, providing a larger base of support than does a conventional shoe. This is particularly important for horses that have a disproportionate relationship between their body weight and the circumference of their hooves (heavy horses, small hooves).

The egg bar shoe is especially beneficial for horses whose heels have collapsed forward and inward, resulting in an underrun hoof, often with a flat sole. If the heel tubules are already angled forward, the condition may be irreversible. This shoe may also help horses

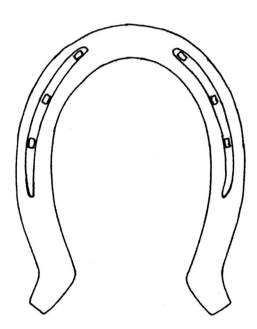

Figure 9.77 Shoe with trailers.

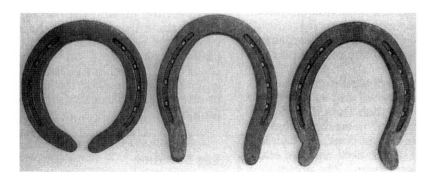

Figure 9.76 Left to right: open egg bar shoe, extended heel shoe, extended heel shoe with bilateral trailers. (Reprinted with permission from Hill C, Klimesh R. Maximum Hoof Power. North Pomfret, VT: Trafalgar Square Publishing, 2000.)

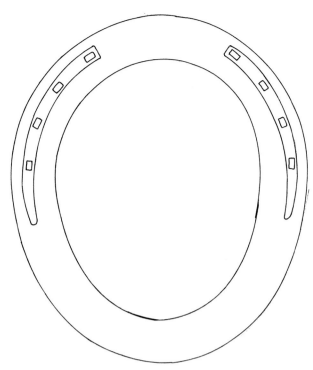

Figure 9.78 Egg bar shoe. (Reprinted with permission from Hill C, Klimesh R. Maximum Hoof Power. North Pomfret, VT: Trafalgar Square Publishing, 2000.)

whose hooves are flared outward on the sides with the heels collapsed forward.

The weight of a horse with underrun heels or a long-toe–low-heel configuration is concentrated at the back of the hoof or even behind the hoof, which causes excess flexor support stress. In soft or deep footing, the larger ground surface of an egg bar "catches" the horse's weight as it descends down the limb, thereby reducing the pressure on the flexors, navicular region, and coffin joint. The egg bar also extends the base of support and effectively redirects the horse's weight forward toward the center of the hoof. This creates a more desirable, upright hoof-pastern axis.

Because the bar of an egg bar is located behind the frog, the heel bulbs are protected. The egg bar shoe not only prevents the heels from sinking down into soft footings but also protects the bulbs from the direct trauma of striking the ground.

The hoof must be trimmed properly before an egg bar shoe is applied. If the toe is left long, it will impede breakover, which defeats the purpose of the shoe. Modifying the toe of the shoe, by rockering or squaring it, can ease breakover. The egg bar shoe should be fitted wide from the broadest part of the foot toward the rear. The length of this shoe depends on the configuration of the hoof. It may be short enough to resemble a straight bar shoe, or it may extend to the back of the heel bulbs, forming a true egg shape.

Because the egg bar shoe consists of more material than a standard shoe, the action of the horse may be affected by the additional weight. The hoof may reach a higher arc in its flight, and the knees and hocks may

exhibit a greater degree of flexion. During extension, the slight increase in weight at the end of the limb may result in a slight exaggeration of the horse throwing the foot forward. If this is the case and the action is undesirable, an aluminum egg bar, which is much lighter, is appropriate.

Depending on the circumstances, the horse wearing bar shoes may require different management. A bar shoe tends to collect and retain bedding, mud, or manure, so the hooves must be cleaned regularly. Horses wearing egg bars should not be turned out in deep or muddy footing.

The egg bar shoe is used in a wide variety of therapeutic applications and on horses involved in performing show jumping, hunting, dressage, cutting, reining, pleasure riding, and trail riding. In addition to potentially increasing the useful life of a horse, this shoe encourages the development of a more correct, functionally sound hoof. Recognition of the value of egg bar shoes has prompted several manufacturers to add both steel and aluminum egg bar shoes to their product lines.

Full-Support Shoes

A full-support shoe is an egg bar shoe with a frog support plate (Fig. 9.79). It is often called a "heart bar/egg bar." The plate of the full-support shoe contacts a large portion of the frog, whereas the tip of a true heart bar may contact only a small area of the frog (the size of a dime). Full-support shoes are available commercially or can be made by a qualified farrier. The full-support shoe is used to treat hooves with flat or dropped soles and hooves with weak or underrun heels. A portion of

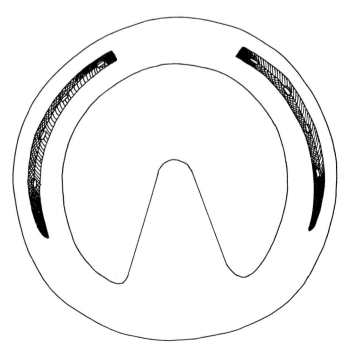

Figure 9.79 Full-support shoe. (Reprinted with permission from Hill C, Klimesh R. Maximum Hoof Power. North Pomfret, VT: Trafalgar Square Publishing, 2000.)

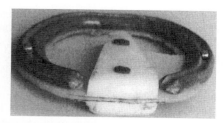

Figure 9.80   Frog support pad. (Photo courtesy of Richard Klimesh.)

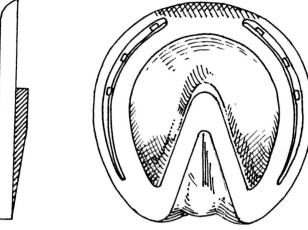

Figure 9.81   Heart bar shoe.

the horse's weight is carried by the frog plate, which allows the heels of the hoof to grow down without being crushed.

This shoe is also useful in the treatment of hooves that have had a portion of the hoof wall removed (as in a heel resection for a crack) or injured (as in a heel avulsion). Contrasted with an egg bar shoe, which is used to support a hoof that has had the heel "floated" to allow a displaced heel to descend to the shoe, the full-support shoe is used when it is desirable to stabilize the hoof capsule while the hoof grows new horn.

A heel resection exposes a portion of the full-support (or egg bar) shoe, and the risk of the horse stepping it off is increased. To prevent the hindfoot from stepping off a front shoe, heel shields or wide clips can be welded around the exposed portion of the front shoe.

A full-support shoe is fitted in the same manner as an egg bar shoe, described previously. The frog plate should follow the shape of the frog and support it completely from ½ inch back from the tip of the trimmed frog. When the shoe is set on the prepared hoof, the frog plate should just contact the frog. The frog support plate should not extend beyond the boundaries of the frog, or circulation within the hoof might be impaired. If the frog is recessed below the level of the hoof wall, shims of the appropriate size and shape can be attached to the frog plate to achieve contact.

The configuration of the full-support shoe makes it difficult to keep the sole clean, especially if the horse is in mud, gravel, or dirty bedding. If the hoof wall is of poor quality or the horse is in undesirable footing, a full pad may need to be used with the full-support shoe.

In lieu of a full-support shoe, a full-support pad can be used. This type of pad is available commercially or can be fabricated by a farrier. It might be difficult to fit the pad properly to the frog, however, because the opaque pad surface prevents direct observation of frog contact. To function properly, the ground surface of the pad must be supported beneath the frog either by a frog plate on the shoe or by the addition of a frog-shaped shim (the thickness of the shoe) on the pad itself (Fig. 9.80).

Heart Bar Shoe

The heart bar shoe has a V-shaped bar that contacts the frog (Fig. 9.81). In laminitis cases, the heart bar shoe is used to support the coffin bone via the frog. The rigid heart bar is welded in place and applies a fixed amount of support (see the section on focal versus diffuse in this chapter). The adjustable heart bar shoe has a screw that

varies the amount of support provided to the frog. Both types can be used with a full pad if a frog-shaped shim is fixed to the hoof surface of the pad to transfer the support to the frog and prevent any pressure from being applied to the sole. The location of the tip of support is approximately ⅜ inch back from the apex of the trimmed frog. Ideally, the location is determined from radiographs, by measuring the length of the coffin bone and coming back from the tip of the coffin bone 33% of its length.

There is some debate as to whether the entire frog plate should contact the frog (diffuse support) or just a small, dime-sized area at the tip of the plate (focal support). Successes and failures have occurred with both methods. The focal support method requires accurate measurement and placement of the heart bar tip and optimum amount support (pressure). This in not an easy shoe to build and apply correctly and can be misapplied. The diffuse support method is more forgiving in that the amount of support pressure is less critical.

In some laminitis cases, it is necessary to remove portions of the hoof wall, usually at the toe but sometimes at one or both quarters as well. This resection relieves pressure between the hoof wall and the coffin bone, allows the hoof wall and coffin bone to become reoriented, and removes the dead tissue (laminar wedge) that impedes the proper growth of new hoof tissue. If resection is confined to the toe, there is usually sufficient hoof wall remaining to support the attachment of a heart bar shoe by nails or glue. Side clips are often placed just behind the resected area to prevent the weakened wall from spreading and to help secure the shoe to the hoof.

If the hoof wall is too weak or shelly to attach nails and if glue-on shoes are not available, the shoe can be secured by using one or more T-bars or goosenecks (Fig. 9.82). The base of the T-bar is welded to the edge of the shoe, and the crossbar is attached to solid horn high up on the hoof wall. When the exposed laminae have dried and cornified sufficiently, a prosthetic hoof material can be used to rebuild the hoof to its normal shape. A shoe can then be attached to the rebuilt hoof by glue or nails.

Other Bar Shoes

A bar can be placed anywhere across the branches of the shoe to protect the hoof from ground contact and

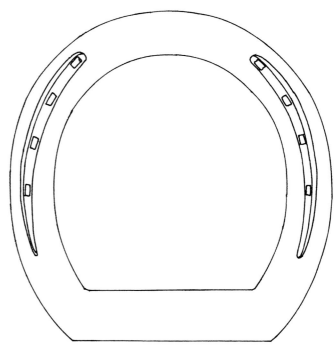

Figure 9.83   Straight bar shoe. (Reprinted with permission from Hill C, Klimesh R. Maximum Hoof Power. North Pomfret, VT: Trafalgar Square Publishing, 2000.)

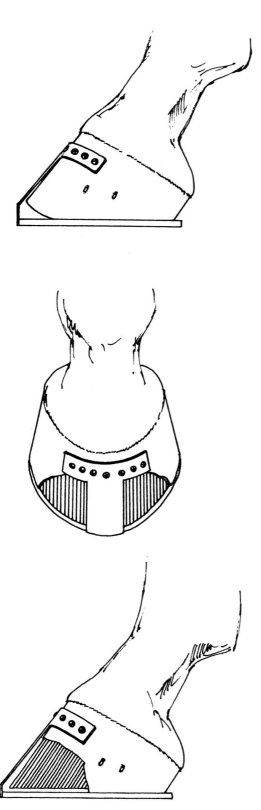

Figure 9.82   Gooseneck.

trauma. A straight bar connects the heels of the shoe and protects the frog (Fig. 9.83). If the frog is prominent or the heels low, the bar can be set away from the frog and is called a drop bar. A crossbar can go diagonally across the shoe or straight across to protect the sole or the navicular region of the frog. The V-bar shoe extends from the heels over the frog to connect to the toe of the shoe (Fig. 9.84). It can be used in conjunction with a frog support pad for a laminitic hoof to protect the tender sole region just ahead of the frog. A wide bar bisecting a straight bar shoe is used for the same purpose and is called a phi bar. If a pad is used, it must be riveted to the central bar in front of the frog to hold the pad away from the sole.

A bar crossing the hoof should not contact the sole at any point because it could impair circulation within the foot or cause bruises and abscesses. When a bar is used to protect the hoof, debris (e.g., bedding, manure, rocks, and dirt) must be kept from accumulating because this can put pressure on the hoof during weight bearing, defeating the purpose of the bar. A full pad may be helpful (see the section on pads in this chapter); however, careful attention must be paid to the amount of packing used so excess pressure is not applied to the sole.

A therapeutic bar shoe that is used to elevate the heel of the hoof significantly is called a Patten shoe (Fig. 9.85). The Patten shoe may be used on a horse convalescing from a lacerated flexor tendon and/or contraction of the flexor muscle-tendon unit. This shoe can be forged from one piece of steel or fabricated from a standard shoe with the addition of the heel elevation bar, either by bolts or by welding. Many variations of this shoe are in use; some can be adjusted for elevation while on the

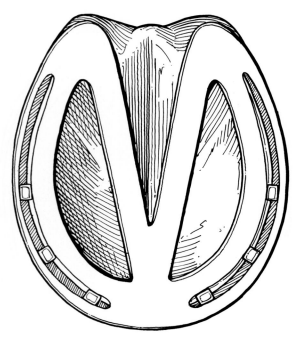

Figure 9.84   The V-bar shoe provides good protection to the frog region.

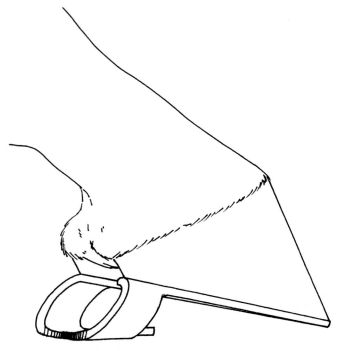

Figure 9.85   Patten shoe.

horse, but most have to be removed, adjusted, and reset onto the hoof.

Contiguous Clip Shoe

The Klimesh contiguous clip shoe can be used to treat fractures of the coffin bone (Fig. 9.86). The shoe is made by first fitting a straight bar or egg bar shoe (depending on the hoof configuration) to the trimmed hoof. The shoe should have a deep crease for the nail heads, such as a rim shoe, to facilitate removal of the nails individually at time of reset. It may be advisable to use a rocker or squared toe to minimize the pull of the deep digital flexor tendon on the coffin bone during breakover. The shoe is fit close around the entire perimeter of the hoof wall with no allowance for normal expansion.

A series of tall clips (16-gauge uncoated steel) are welded around the outer perimeter of the shoe. The shoe is nailed to the hoof with four nails, and the clips are bent in with a hammer to within $\frac{1}{6}$ inch of touching the hoof wall. A hard-setting acrylic is then applied between the clips and the hoof wall (see "Resources" in this chapter). This effectively immobilizes the hoof capsule and the coffin bone inside. Depending on the configuration of the hoof and the management of the horse's environment, it may be advisable to use a full pad or treatment plate to prevent trauma to the coffin bone through the bottom of the hoof.

The shoe can be easily removed by pulling the four nails with a crease nail puller and gently prying the clips away from the hoof wall with a clinch cutter. The hoof capsule usually has contracted to some degree during the 6-week shoeing period, which facilitates removal of the shoe. At time of reset, the bar of the shoe may need to be cut and rewelded to accommodate the smaller size of the hoof. When lameness is no longer evident and radiography indicates satisfactory healing, the hoof can be shod with a bar shoe and two side clips to stabilize the hoof and prevent refracture (refer to Chapter 8 for more information; see "Resources" in this chapter).

Continuous Rim-Type Shoe

A continuous rim-type shoe can be used as an alternative to the contiguous clip shoe for the treatment of coffin bone fractures. Although the design is simple, the construction is tedious and technically demanding.[39] The foot is trimmed so it lands flat, and the hoof wall is rasped lightly to remove bulges and wall flares to improve the fit of the rim. A full bar shoe is constructed to fit the foot exactly, except at the toe where it should extend approximately $\frac{1}{8}$ inch beyond the weight-bearing surface.

The rim is constructed from 16-gauge sheet metal or an equivalent thickness of aluminum plate. To create a precise fit for the rim, a template of aluminum foil is made and then molded to the entire hoof wall and then smoothed. Generally, the height of the rim is $1\frac{1}{2}$ to 2 inches at the toe.

Protection

Pads

There are four main reasons to use hoof pads: to protect the sole, to reduce concussion, to change the angle of the hoof, and to prevent snow and debris from balling up in the bottom of the hoof ("snowballing"). Wedge pads were discussed in the section on balance. The other three functions of pads all relate to protection.

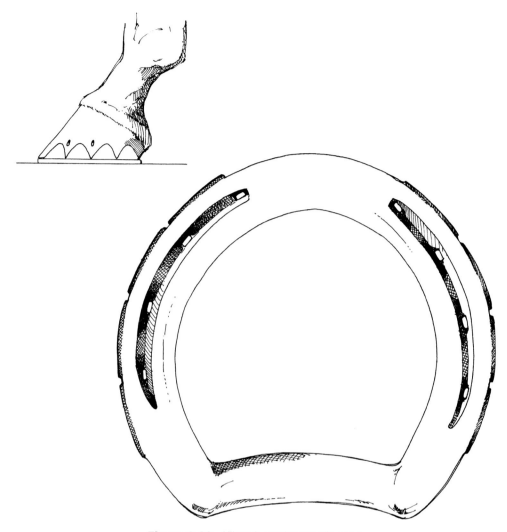

Figure 9.86   Klimesh contiguous clip shoe.

A full pad is a protective material covering the entire bottom of the horse's foot. It is installed between the hoof and the shoe with or without hoof packing. Full pads may be made of leather, plastic, or other synthetic materials. Side clips are often used with pads to help maintain the position of the pad and shoe on the hoof and to decrease the stress on the nails. Horses that have flat or thin soles may benefit from wearing full pads. Even horses that have normally concave soles, if worked regularly on gravel or rocky terrain, may require full pads to prevent bruising.

Hoof Packing

Opinions differ on whether to pack the space between the pad and the hoof and what materials to use for packing. Although tradition calls for pine tar with oakum, using this mixture has drawbacks. Oakum is a loose, stringy hemp fiber that retains water, breaks down over time, and shifts beneath the pad, often working out between the heels. Another option is silicone, which is either squirted into the sole space with a caulking gun

after the shoe and pad are in place or mixed with a catalyst to speed curing and applied to the sole before the shoe and pad are nailed on. There are several drawbacks, however, to using silicone. It tends to concentrate moisture and heat against the sole, and too much silicone puts pressure on the sole and prevents the sole from descending as part of its normal shock-absorbing function. Also, silicone allows sand and mud to accumulate between the pad and the sole, causing sole pressure.

A relatively new product for packing appears to improve circulation to the foot and thus has been helpful in restoring contracted heels and degenerative frogs to their natural state. The packing material is a two-part impression material, similar to that used for dental impressions. Application instructions are simple. Mix equal parts of material (1 part base with 1 part catalyst) and apply to the bottom of the foot, taping a hard impression pad over it until the material cures. After the impression material cures, the impression pad is removed and the two-part impression material is trimmed to fill only the area around the frog sulcus in cases of laminitis. In all other applications, the impression material is left in its complete molded form. The impression material is lightly rasped, and a pad and shoe are applied. This impression material/packing approach has been helpful in treating cases of laminitis, quarter cracks, and navicular syndrome.

Commercial hoof packing preparations are available. They are associated with different degrees of success (see "Resources" in this chapter).

CVP Method

An excellent alternative for packing is the Klimesh CVP gasket pad technique. CVP is an acronym for the three main ingredients: copper sulfate powder, Venice turpentine, and polypropylene (poly) hoof felt. Poly felt, which does not readily absorb water, was developed specifically as a hoof packing material. The copper sulfate and Venice turpentine combine to make a medicated adhesive that binds the poly felt to the sole, forming a gasket between the pad and the hoof. This gasket protects the hoof wall and sole from the invasion of sand, dirt, mud, water, and other foreign matter for the entire 5- to 8-week shoeing period.

The Venice turpentine is spread onto either the hoof or the poly felt, and the copper sulfate is lightly sprinkled over it; or the two are stirred together to form a light green mixture (approximately 3 tablespoons copper sulfate to 1 pint Venice turpentine), which is then spread onto the hoof or felt. The copper sulfate migrates into fissures in the hoof wall and sole, preventing the growth of undesirable organisms and eliminating the foul odor often associated with the use of full pads.

The CVP packing forms a barrier that prevents excess moisture from baths, creeks, or muddy pens from softening the hoof. If too much copper sulfate is used, however, the hoof tissues may dry out and become flaky. After the hoof is trimmed and ready for the pad and shoe, the commissures of the frog are filled with appropriately sized pieces of poly felt, which is lightly coated with the CV mixture. If the frog is recessed below the level of the hoof, pieces of CVP are placed on the back half of the frog to build up the area between the heels to the level of the trimmed hoof wall. This prevents mud and debris from getting between the pad and the sole.

If the sole has an extreme cup to it, CVP is used to fill the area level with the wall. The packing should not bulge out the center of the pad when it is applied to the hoof. As the horse moves, the CVP packing will be compressed and conform to the contours of the sole and frog. If the horse loses a shoe, often the CVP gasket will remain adhered to the sole, providing sole protection until the pad and shoe can be replaced.

Pad Uses

Full pads are often used to protect a bruised sole while it heals. If a pad is applied over a sole bruise that may abscess, however, it tends to fester the abscess quickly. The horse may exhibit great pain after the pad has been on for a short period, necessitating the removal of the pad. Once the abscess has been treated and has dried out (see the section on treatment plates), a pad can be applied again, if necessary, for protection.

For many years, full pads were used in the treatment of acutely laminitic horses, with the belief that the pads provided protection for the horse's sore feet. The pressure transferred to the sole by a pad and packing, however, may compromise blood flow and lead to further degeneration of structures within the hoof. In addition, if sole abscesses develop, pads may increase the pressure of the abscesses on the sensitive sole, making treatment more difficult. Many horses with chronic founder, however, have benefited from the application of a hard plastic pad and minimal packing of hoof felt and Venice turpentine.

In cases in which injury or surgery results in a partial loss of the hoof wall, a full pad can keep the sole free from debris and decrease the amount of bandaging material needed. Full pads may be prescribed for horses that have navicular syndrome, particularly those that are the most painful to hoof testers over the central third of the frog. Hooves with wide-open, low heels are sometimes believed to have incurred navicular syndrome or heel soreness from the direct concussion to the frog and heel regions. In some cases, full pads used to protect this area may actually transmit the concussion to the navicular region. A straight bar or V-bar shoe might be more effective in providing protection for this type of navicular problem.

Along with the use of full pads comes an interruption in hoof moisture balance. When a full pad covers the sole of a hoof, outward moisture migration via the sole is halted, and the hoof structures can become softened and weakened. In addition, full pads tend to trap moisture from slush, mud, snow, and normal hoof respiration next to the hoof structures, causing sole deterioration and providing a suitable environment for growth of bacteria, fungus, and yeast (see the section on CVP method). Some experts believe that horses tend to develop an even thinner sole from wearing pads full time, thus becoming dependent on pads. Some horses with weak soles have developed a thick normal sole with the use of full pads and the CVP method.

Traction is decreased with a full flat pad; the cup of the bare sole and the frog are covered; therefore, the grip of the shoe is all that remains. Some full-support pads have an artificial frog built onto the ground surface, which helps compensate for traction loss. The added weight of a pad and packing can exaggerate a horse's action and travel.

There are many pads on the market that claim to protect the horse by reducing concussion. The effectiveness of shock-absorbing pads is largely undocumented and widely debated. A properly shod healthy foot provides all the shock absorption necessary for normal work by transferring the energy of the hoof's impact to the shock-absorbing structures: the hoof wall, the laminae, the frog, and the digital cushion. If the hoof structures are abnormal or the work is excessive, concussion-reducing pads are sometimes prescribed. Success depends on the type of pad used, the horse's conformation, the degree of hoof pain, the footing, and other management factors. One study that assessed the homotypic variations in shoe characteristics of Thoroughbred racehorses found that bonded rim pads were the most common (20.8% of horses) and were more frequently found on older (above 2 years) than younger (2-year-old) horses.[28]

A wide variety of concussion-reducing pads are available as full pads and rim pads. The pad's material must have the ability to absorb the force of concussion quickly and release it slowly. With repeated compression and expansion, the pad may become permanently compressed, shift sideways, or become cut by the hoof wall. The result may be loose clinches, premature wearing of the nail holes, loose or lost shoes, and possible weakened or split hoof walls.

Snowballing can be stressful to the support structures of a horse's limb, whether the horse is standing or moving. The barefoot horse is the best equipped for shedding snow and ice from its hooves; but if shoeing is needed for traction or protection, several antisnowballing pads are available. Full flat pads, full pads with a convex bubble in the center, and tube-type rim pads all work with varying degrees of success, depending on installation, hoof shape, temperature, and type of snow. Of these, the tube-type pads are by far the best for antisnowballing.

Some breed and performance associations have rules specifically related to the use of hoof pads at horse competitions. It is the horse owner's and exhibitor's responsibility to know and abide by the pertinent regulations.

Wide-Web Shoes

Wide-web shoes are used to protect the perimeter of the sole and to provide more ground contact and a more stable support for the hoof. These shoes have gained popularity with increase in the population of the larger Warmblood horses. Because of their extra width, these shoes are more resistant to deforming under the weight of a horse. Their increased surface area is thought to dissipate some of the shock of impact.

One drawback to increased ground surface contact is a decrease in traction. When used on performance horses, wide-web shoes often require some sort of traction device (see the section on traction). When a wide-web shoe is used on a hoof with a flat sole, it is necessary to relieve or concave the inner hoof surface of the shoe or to apply a rim pad between the shoe and the hoof wall to prevent pressure from being applied to the sole (Fig. 9.50). On some commercial wide-web shoes, the nail holes are placed proportionately farther inward on the web. Care must be taken when applying these shoes to thin-walled hooves to avoid driving a close or hot nail. This is less of a problem with hand-forged wide-webbed shoes because the farrier can take the wall thickness into account when placing the nail holes.

Treatment Plate

A treatment plate, or hospital plate, is used to protect the sole or frog and to provide regular access to these areas for inspection and medication. These shoes are useful in treating feet with a dropped sole, protruding coffin bones, sole abscesses, and puncture wounds to the sole or frog. Although a hard plastic pad or metal plate can simply be taped to the bottom of the shoe to serve this purpose, if treatment extends over more than a few days, a treatment plate that bolts on to the bottom of the shoe will be more economical in terms of both time and money. Treatment plates can be custom-made by a farrier and are available commercially. If positive protection is required but access for treatment is not necessary, a steel plate can be permanently welded to cover the center of the shoe and used with CVP packing.

Gait Defects

Breakover Alterations

Breakover is the phase of the stride between stance and swing (see Chapter 2). It is the moment when the hoof prepares to leave the ground. It starts when the heel lifts and the hoof begins to pivot at the toe and ends when the toe leaves the ground. The deep and superficial digital flexor tendons (assisted by the suspensory ligament) are still stretched just before the beginning of breakover to counteract the downward pressure of the weight of the horse's body.

The ideal hoof breaks over near the center of the toe. The location of breakover is different for fore and hind hooves. The coffin bone and hoof of a forefoot are usually round with sloping hoof walls and wide areas of support on each side of the hoof. This configuration encourages breakover to occur at the center of the toe. For this reason, front shoes usually show the most wear at the toe (Fig. 9.87).

Hind hooves are more pointed and triangular in shape and have straighter walls with less lateral support than front hooves. The hindfeet are the horse's means to push, pivot, and change direction, so they perform a wide variety of ML movements. Also, most horses are conformed and travel in a slightly toed-out configuration in the hindlimbs. This allows the hip and stifle to move freely forward (and slightly to the outside) without being hindered by the flank and coupling. Therefore, hind hooves (and shoes) often do not break over at the center of the toe but slightly to the inside of center. Instead of showing wear from breakover at one particular point the way front shoes do, hind shoes usually show wear more evenly from sliding as they hit the ground.

The point of breakover should not be forced to occur at a point that is unnatural for the individual horse. A hoof can be encouraged, however, to break over in a position that contributes to balanced movement. If a horse's hooves are balanced, the horse is most likely breaking over at its ideal spot.

Provided that a horse's hoof is aligned with the pastern, some correlations can be drawn between angles and

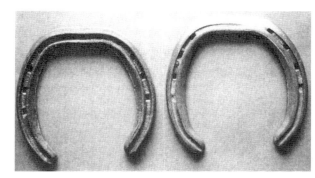

Figure 9.87 Left: new squared-toe shoe. Right: wear from breakover on a squared-toe right front shoe. (Reprinted with permission from Hill C, Klimesh R. Maximum Hoof Power. North Pomfret, VT: Trafalgar Square Publishing, 2000.)

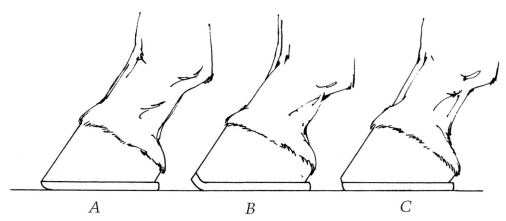

Figure 9.88 Modified shoes. A. Rolled-toe shoe. B. Rocker-toe shoe. C. Squared-toe shoe. (Reprinted with permission from Hill C, Klimesh R. Maximum Hoof Power. North Pomfret, VT: Trafalgar Square Publishing, 2000.)

breakover. Hooves with longer or lower pasterns (53° or lower) tend to be on the ground for a longer period of time than those with shorter or more upright pasterns (56° or higher).

The length and the position of the hoof's base of support in relation to the cannon and fetlock determine how much time and effort it takes to break over. A hoof is in the proper position to support a horse's weight if the bulbs of the heels are approximately underneath the midpoint of the cannon bone (when standing) and the heels of the hoof only slightly ahead of the bulbs (Fig. 9.45A). Hooves that are small or have underrun heels (and are not shod to counteract this) sink more at the heels during loading and thus experience more stress, require more effort to lift, and have a delayed breakover.

Hoof wall dishes or extra length at the toe, if not removed, increases flexor support stresses and delays breakover. If a dish is not rasped to result in a straight hoof wall from the coronary band to the ground, the shoe is likely to be applied ahead of the optimum point of breakover.

Several modifications to standard shoes and several specialized shoes can specifically affect breakover (Fig. 9.88).

Squared-toe shoe. The toe of the shoe is squared and set back from the toe of the hoof to facilitate easy breakover. The toe of the hoof is usually rounded with the rasp to prevent chipping. Used on the hindlimbs, squared-toe shoes may help prevent the stepping off of front shoes (Figs. 9.89 and 9.90).

Roller-toe shoe. The hoof surface of the shoe is flat. The ground surface of the shoe has a rounded toe much like a naturally worn shoe.

Rocker-toe shoe. The entire toe of the shoe is bent upward. This requires that the toe of the hoof be rasped or cut to fit the shoe. The hoof is encouraged to break over specifically at the point of the rocker location.

Roller-motion shoe. Combining the rocker toe with swelled heels results in a roller-motion shoe (Fig. 9.91).

Half-round shoe. The ground surface of the outside and inside edges of the entire shoe is round. A half-round

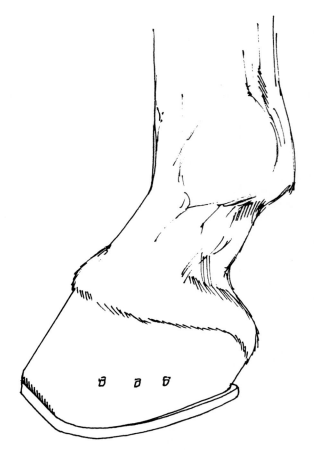

Figure 9.89 Squared-toe shoe. (Reprinted with permission from Hill C, Klimesh R. Maximum Hoof Power. North Pomfret, VT: Trafalgar Square Publishing, 2000.)

shoe allows a horse to break over more easily in any direction (Fig. 9.38).

Although squared-, roller-, and rocker-toe shoes are designed to affect breakover, one controlled study in sound trotting horses did not identify a shortened dura-

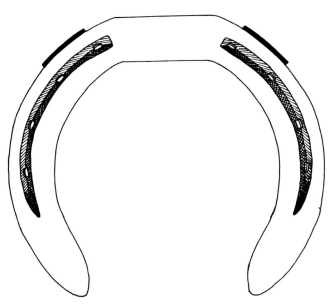

Figure 9.90 Squared-toe shoe with forward-placed side clips. (Reprinted with permission from Hill C, Klimesh R. Maximum Hoof Power. North Pomfret, VT: Trafalgar Square Publishing, 2000.)

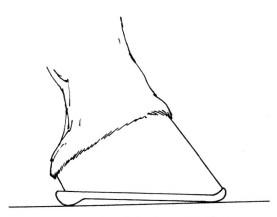

Figure 9.91 Full roller-motion shoe.

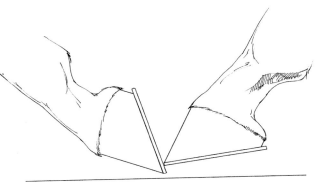

Figure 9.92 Forging. (Reprinted with permission from Hill C, Klimesh R. Maximum Hoof Power. North Pomfret, VT: Trafalgar Square Publishing, 2000.)

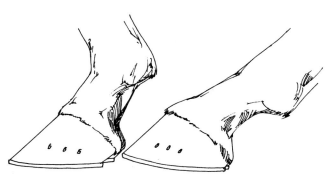

Figure 9.93 Overreaching, showing the moment a shoe might be grabbed when the front foot is greatly delayed in breakover. (Reprinted with permission from Hill C, Klimesh R. Maximum Hoof Power. North Pomfret, VT: Trafalgar Square Publishing, 2000.)

tion of breakover with these shoes compared with a plain steel shoe.[17] (See "Natural Balance Trimming and Shoeing" in this chapter for further information.)

Forging and Overreaching Solutions

Forging is a gait defect commonly heard when a horse is trotting (Fig. 9.92). It occurs when a hindfoot (or hind shoe) contacts a forefoot (or front shoe) on the same side. Overreaching (Fig. 9.93) is a related gait defect with more serious consequences of an injury to the forelimb (heel bulb, coronary band, fetlock, or flexor tendon) or a pulled shoe.

Assuming management and training related factors have been evaluated and modified if required (see Chapter 2), shoeing may be able to help eliminate the problem of persistent forging or overreaching. Most corrective shoeing is based on restoring a horse's normal hoof configuration and balance.

There are no absolutes when it comes to corrective shoeing for forging or overreaching. Although most experts agree how to modify the forefeet of a horse that forges or overreaches, the opinions are varied for treatment of the hindfeet. Often, just balancing the front hooves and easing their breakover eliminate forging. This balancing is often accomplished by shortening the toe or raising the hoof angle to align the hoof-pastern axis. Breakover can be eased with a modified (squared, rolled, rocker, or roller-motion) shoe.

The DP balance of the rear hooves should be evaluated and, if necessary, adjusted. Putting a modified toe shoe, such as a squared-toe shoe, on the hindfeet of a horse whose chest and hindquarters are relatively equal in width might also eliminate forging. Why would this work, since the breakover of both the forelimbs and hindlimbs have been made easier? In the case of a horse with pointed hind hooves, sometimes squaring the front hooves and leaving the hind hooves pointed results in a break in the synchronization of the movement of the diagonal pairs of limbs. Squaring the hind toes may smooth out and equalize the movement. A pointed hind toe tends to hit and perhaps grab a front shoe more easily than would a squared hind toe. Using half-round shoes on the hind hooves may also be helpful.

To prevent pulled shoes caused by overreaching, many farriers remove the sharp outer edges of the shoes.

Chamfering the outer edge of the hoof surface of the shoe is called "boxing," and rounding the outer edge of the ground surface of the shoe is called "safeing." These procedures make it less likely that a front shoe will be stepped off if contacted by a hind shoe (Fig. 9.48).

Trailers have been touted as an aid to encourage a hoof to stop sooner on landing if the hoof is meeting the ground heel first or flat. If the thinking is based on a larger surface area providing additional drag or friction, it is faulty, as the opposite is true with smooth trailers. A smooth trailer increases the surface area of the shoe and actually provides less traction. A calk or sticker on the trailer would contact the ground sooner and create additional drag, but the trailer just provides a place for the calk to be placed. It is the calk that is doing the stopping, not the trailer. This is where the confusion may have originated.

Even if trailers on the hinds did encourage a slightly quicker stop to the hoof's motion as it lands, would it prevent forging or overreaching? According to some slow-motion videos, the answer is no. The moment when contact between the toe of the hind hoof and the front shoe would occur is before the hind shoe (and its smooth trailer) actually touches the ground. Trailers do offer a greater measure of support for the flexor tendons than do normal shoes. Exaggerated trailers, however, can be dangerous to people and other horses in the event of a kick. Egg bar shoes are a safer alternative for providing such an extension and support.

Interference Adjustments

"Interference" refers to a regularly occurring abnormal sideways (axial) limb swing that results in a physical contact with the opposite limb. Why a horse interferes is usually due to a variety of interrelated factors (see Chapter 2), including conformation, soundness, age, conditioning, training, rider proficiency, and farriery. In some cases, finding a solution requires the owner, farrier, and perhaps veterinarian to work together during a period of trial and error.

First, a farrier should examine the horse's shoes for signs of imbalance. Shoe wear, which is related to the hoof landing, loading, and taking off, is valuable information for assessing a foot flight problem. The torque, or twisting force, that the deviating foot experiences and expresses in flight is a direct result of the impact of loading and the release of that force during breakover. If a hoof lands unbalanced, it usually sends the energy upward and forward in an unbalanced fashion, and the flight of the limb or hoof will show a resulting deviation.

Examining the shoe for wear can help determine a plan for trimming that will result in more even wear on both branches of the shoe. Signs of unequal shoe wear include a rounding of one area of the shoe, nail heads worn more in one area of the shoe, and a thinning of the shoe in one region. Usually, if the side of the hoof that shows the least amount of shoe wear is trimmed shorter, the subsequent wear on the shoe will be equal. This rule is excepted by a horse that is lame or has an unusual way of going, so it is wise not to rely on just one guideline when attempting something as complex as balancing the equine limb. An examination of the hoof

itself can show imbalance, such as in the self-perpetuating condition referred to as sheared heels. If one heel is higher than the other, as the horse repeatedly lands with unequal impact, it tends to force the heel even higher.

If the hoof is obviously unbalanced, alternations in trimming and shoeing should come first. Otherwise, conscientious corrections to all riding, conditioning, and training deficiencies should be made before turning to farriery for additional solutions. Shoeing alterations should be approached conservatively and monitored closely. One of the most serious misconceptions surrounding corrective farriery is the notion that crooked limbs should be made to point forward. Although there can be merit to this in the developing young horse, forcing a foot to conform to an ideal on a horse over 1 year of age may result in excessive stress to joint alignment and function.

When farrier corrections are warranted, they can affect the breakover, flight, landing, or weight bearing of the hoof. Some interference problems require experimentation over a period of several shoeings before a pattern begins to emerge and the solution materializes. Unfortunately, some horses continue to interfere despite the best management, riding, training, and farrier care.

In the opinion of one of us (G.O.), gait faults, forging, and overreach problems all stem from hoof imbalance when the limb conformation appears reasonably normal. This can be easily assessed by looking at the bottom of the foot and mapping out the percentage of hoof ground surface ahead at the widest part of the foot compared with the amount that is behind the widest part of the foot. The widest part of the foot is generally identified by a line drawn across the foot about ¾ inch behind the frog apex. The dorsal projections of the bars will generally terminate at this same line (Fig. 9.35). If there is more hoof mass ahead of the widest part of the foot than behind, using the heel of the shoe as the rear bearing point, the horse probably is experiencing one or all of the above gait fault problems, including toe-first landing.

An overwhelming number of these problems can be resolved by following the natural balance trimming and shoeing guidelines. When the farrier is finished, approximately one-third of the ground surface of the shoe should be ahead of the widest part of the foot to the point of breakover (rolled-toe shoe is usually best), and two-thirds should be to the rear of the widest part of the foot (Fig. 9.54).

Breakover

A squared- or rocker-toe shoe can encourage the breakover to occur at a point other than the natural one, if desired. Often, it is necessary to experiment during several shoeing periods to find the optimum breakover to help an interfering horse. Although it is better to encourage breakover to occur at the desired point rather than to prevent it from occurring at an undesirable point, in some therapeutic instances, toe extensions are used to alter the point of breakover. A toe extension is a metal piece forged or welded to a particular portion of the shoe to inhibit breakover at that point (Fig. 9.94). Toe extensions are used on the inside of a base-narrow toed-out horse to help the horse break over centrally. The

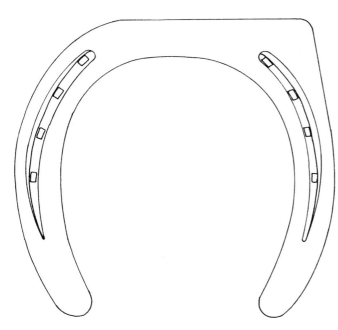

Figure 9.94 Toe extension shoe.

extension is added from the center of the toe of the shoe to approximately the second nail hole.

Half-round shoes allow breakover in any direction, so they are inappropriate when trying to redirect the breakover, but they do allow a horse to find its natural breakover point relatively easily.

Foot Flight

To affect the natural flight of a hoof as little as possible, it is best to use the lightest shoe that still provides adequate support for the hoof. Increasing the weight of the shoe has been shown to increase the height of the foot flight arc in trotting horses.[6] If the foot flight pattern of the front feet needs to be widened, lowering the outside wall, reducing inside flares, and possibly adding a calk on the inside may work. If the foot flight pattern of the hind feet of a cow-hocked horse needs to be widened, lowering the outside wall, adding a trailer on the outside, and adding a calk on the inside may work. If the foot flight pattern of the hindfeet of a base-narrow or bow-legged horse needs to be widened, lowering the inside wall, reducing inside flares, and adding a calk or a trailer on the outside may work. Bear in mind, however, that by lowering one side of a hoof that is in balance to affect foot flight or by using calks on only one branch of a shoe, the limb support structures experience uneven stresses, which may cause worse problems than interfering. One study showed that elevation of the medial heel in sound horses increased the peak force and impulse on that side of the foot.[5]

Undesirable torque in flight is usually due to an imbalanced foot or misaligned limb. Joint rotation, such as is seen in the bow-legged or knock-kneed horse, increases as speed or extension within a gait increases. Sometimes, the foot flight pattern can be improved by applying the shoes so they are in line with the horse's body regardless of how the hooves point.

Some Standardbred farriers use side-weighted shoes to control knee torque and alter foot flight. These shoes are more appropriate for high-speed or high-action horses than for horses moving at normal gaits. Weight affects forelimbs and hindlimbs differently. Added weight on a forefoot tends to move the limb away from the weighted side. Added weight on a hindfoot tends to pull the limb toward the weighted side.

Landing

Encouraging a hoof to land in a balanced fashion begins with trimming the hoof level and shoeing it to land flat or slightly heel first. If alterations to landing are desired, they are usually accomplished by altering the balance of the hoof. Trailers or calks on one heel of a shoe are sometimes used to turn the hoof on landing; but, as previously mentioned, unilateral calks are considered by many experts to be dangerous because of the uneven stresses they put on the structures of the limb.

Weight Bearing

Ideally during the loading phase of the stride, the horse's weight is borne over the center of the hoof. If a horse shows a dynamic imbalance in weight bearing, an attempt to move the hoof under the center of the limb can be made by raising or lowering the pertinent side of the hoof. Lowering the lateral (outer) wall moves the hoof toward the midline, whereas lowering the medial (inner) wall often moves the hoof away from the midline. Often, a farrier approaches the situation by placing the shoe on the hoof so that the shoe is under the center of the limb, although the hoof may be slightly off to one side. In this case, the shoe would fit close on one side of the hoof and extend beyond the hoof on the other side (Fig. 9.95).

Traction

Most barefoot horses have good traction in a variety of situations, especially horses with naturally balanced hooves, dense hoof horns, and well-cupped soles (Fig. 9.96). Such a hoof is able to grip most surfaces without hoof damage, and the naturally concave sole sheds mud and slush well. In contrast, the hoof with an long-toe–low-heel configuration, brittle or pithy horn, and a flat sole does not always provide adequate traction. Shod horses often require added traction, depending on the season and footing. Horses wearing certain therapeutic shoes may need added traction for security.

A study assessing the homotypic variations of shoe characteristics of 201 Thoroughbred racehorses found that toe grabs were present on 86.7% of front shoes and 90.5% of hind shoes and that rim shoes (Fig. 9.97) were present on 15.9% of front shoes and 2% of hind shoes. Heel traction devices were less common on front hooves (2.5%) than on rear hooves (6%).[28]

Traction Principles

Using traction devices (see display "Types of Shoes and Devices That Affect Traction" and Figs. 9.97 to

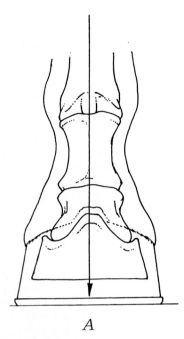

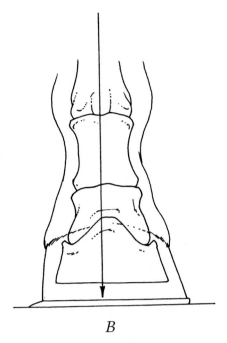

Figure 9.95   Base of support centered under the limb. A. Centered hoof. B. Offset hoof. (Reprinted with permission from Hill

C, Klimesh R. Maximum Hoof Power. North Pomfret, VT: Trafalgar Square Publishing, 2000.)

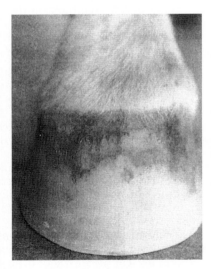

Figure 9.96   A properly trimmed bare hoof. Note the mild proximal displacement of the coronet. (Reprinted with permission from Hill C, Klimesh R. Maximum Hoof Power. North Pomfret, VT: Trafalgar Square Publishing, 2000.)

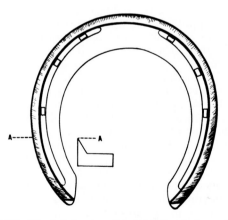

Figure 9.97   The full-rim shoe has a full rim on the outside edge of the web to increase traction, especially among Standardbreds. Inset. Cross section of the web with rim (A) on the outside.

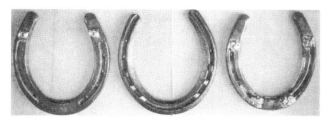

Figure 9.98   Left to right: studs, ice nails, borium. (Reprinted with permission from Hill C, Klimesh R. Maximum Hoof Power. North Pomfret, VT: Trafalgar Square Publishing, 2000.)

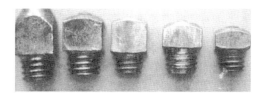

Figure 9.99   An assortment of screw-in studs. (Reprinted with permission from Hill C, Klimesh R. Maximum Hoof Power. North Pomfret, VT: Trafalgar Square Publishing, 2000.)

9.98) unwisely can be dangerous. Adhering to the following principles minimizes risk:

- Determine the activity level of the horse.
- Take into account the normal footing.
- Select the appropriate type of traction device.
- Apply traction devices slowly and carefully because of the added torque and stresses that may develop.
- Use traction devices on both forefeet and hindfeet and on both sides of the shoe to prevent uneven torque.
- Gradually build up the traction to the optimum level.
- Closely monitor the horse for signs of lameness.
- Realize that a small degree of slide on landing is natural and desirable because it dissipates some shock that would otherwise be transmitted to the horse's limb.

It is advisable to use clips whenever calks, ice nails, or borium spots or smears are applied. Adding traction devices essentially stops the shoe, but the horse's body mass (including the hoof that is attached to the shoe) is still moving forward. Once the nails become loose and movement begins, the hoof wall can split and break. Clips help keep the shoe from shifting and loosening and take much of the strain off the nails.

Usually, quarter clips (so-called because they are applied at the quarters of the hoof) are used; however, a single toe clip is sometimes used on each front shoe. Quarter clips are applied somewhere between the toe and the quarter on both branches of the shoe.

A hoof (or foot) normally goes through a certain amount of slide and often some degree of rotation as it lands and takes off again. If a horse is deprived of this normal motion (suddenly or excessively), the forces are taken up by the joints, soft tissue support structures, and tendons. Injuries from excessive or inappropriate traction can show up immediately or after long-term use. One study evaluating the effect of $\frac{1}{4}$-inch calks placed in a balanced manner found that the devices changed the

TYPES OF SHOES AND DEVICES THAT AFFECT TRACTION

Standard keg shoe   Plain steel shoes, whether creased or punched for the nail heads, usually provide adequate traction for most situations.

Aluminum shoe   Aluminum shoes may have a slightly better grab than steel shoes because they are softer but wear out faster. Wear can be extended by inserting a steel wear plate at the toe or borium to the ground surface. Aluminum racing plates with toe grabs or heel stickers can be used successfully in some situations.

Rim shoe   The nail crease that is on the ground surface of most keg shoes is called the swedge. When swedging extends the entire length of the shoe, it is termed a full-swedged or rim shoe (Fig. 9.97). Lighter variations of the rim shoe are the polo shoe, which is full swedged with a higher inside rim, and the barrel-racing shoe, which has a higher outside rim. Rim shoes provide added traction because the rims, until they are worn down, grab the ground. Also, the dirt that packs into the swedge provides more traction against the ground than does a flat steel shoe.

Toed and heeled shoes   Keg shoes are available with permanent calks forged at the heels or at the toe and heels. In soft footing, such as warm winter conditions, these sink into semifrozen ground or soft ice and give good traction. On hard ice or rocks, however, these shoes are not as effective.

Borium   Borium (tungsten carbide) or other hard-surfacing materials can be applied to the ground surface of the horse's normal shoe in smears, beads, or points (Fig. 9.98).

Nails   Commercial frost or mud nails with ribbed or specially hardened heads can be substituted for regular horseshoe nails to provide added traction. One at each midpoint nail position may be all that is necessary. The treated or pointed heads resist wear and dig into hard ground or ice (Fig. 9.98).

Calks   Calks are projections added to the ground surface of the shoe for providing traction. They can be permanent or removable. Threaded studs (removable) have bullet-shaped or blocky heads and range in height from 11/16 inch for show jumpers to $\frac{1}{4}$- to $\frac{1}{2}$-inch road calks (Fig. 9.99). Although removable studs offer the advantage of applying the right amount of traction for a particular footing, the sudden change may not allow a horse to adapt to its new traction. Permanent calks are driven or forged into the shoe or brazed or welded onto the shoe (Fig. 9.98). Because of their permanence, a horse can become thoroughly familiar and confident with the new traction, but the amount of traction provided cannot be changed between shoeings to accommodate different footings.

Toe grabs   Toe grabs are devices formed by steel inserts in the toe of the shoe that extend toward the ground surface. The grab can be low (4 mm), regular (6 mm), or high (8 mm).

forces placed on fetlock and phalangeal joint surfaces and on the tendon and ligament structures in the lower limb during the stance phase. The authors hypothesized that the change in forces would increase the chances of injury to these sites.[50]

Another study, in which the effects of toe grabs in racehorses euthanized because of injuries sustained while racing or training were evaluated, found that the risk of fatal musculoskeletal injury, suspensory apparatus failure, and cannon bone condylar fracture increases as the height of the toe grab increases. In fact, the odds of a horse shod with regular toe grabs suffering a fatal musculoskeletal injury, suspensory apparatus failure, and cannon bone condylar fracture was 3.5, 15.6, and 17.1 times greater, respectively, than horses shod without toe grabs. The study also found that rim shoes might be a safe alternative to toe grabs for increasing traction on racing surfaces.[27,29] Both toe grabs and heel calks have been implicated in sole bruising.[34]

Requiring a horse to work on precarious footing without adequate traction can result in muscle strain (e.g., in the gluteals and hamstrings) caused by constant slipping. Therefore, optimum traction but no extra traction is the goal in most cases.

Traction should be used bilaterally. Borium spots or smears, ice nails, and calks should always be applied on both sides of a shoe (and on both shoes of a pair of limbs) to prevent uneven torque or twist on landing or take-off (Fig. 9.98). There are a few instances, however, when the judicious application of only one traction device on a shoe or two different devices on the same shoe might be warranted, such as for correcting a travel defect. Borium and ice nails are generally used for horses traveling at a slow to moderate speed on slippery footing. Customarily, ice nails are applied at the third nail hole position, at the midpoint of each side of the shoe. This results in the safest grab with minimal torque. Borium is usually added just ahead of both toe nails and just behind each heel nail. Because horses that require calks often are moving at a high rate of speed, the goal is a secure landing, so calks are usually placed behind the heel nail. The horse should be monitored for signs of lameness and swelling. When a horse realizes that its hooves are going to stick rather than land, slide, and twist, it will be able to adjust its balance and movement accordingly. As traction is increased, it is important to stay within an individual horse's limits of tolerance. Again, the goal is optimum traction, not maximum traction.

The warning signs of excessive traction are lameness, swelling, heat, a reluctance to work, a shortened stride, and a bad attitude. All of these can indicate that a horse is trying to protect itself.

Proper Limb Development in Foals

Foal hoof management should be designed in light of the foal's present configuration and its anticipated adult conformation. Since most foals are born with crooked limbs, they should be examined by a veterinarian a day or so after birth to determine whether the limb deviations are normal or whether they require close observation or treatment. Carpal (distal radius) valgus, fetlock (distal metacarpus or metatarsus) valgus, and varus angular limb deformities are common.

In most horses, these limb deviations self-correct through natural forces applied to the growth centers (physes). Partial correction of carpal valgus to within 5 to 7° of a straight limb is expected by about 4 months of age (Fig. 9.100). Then a plateau is reached at which there is very little correction until 8 to 10 months of age, when a growth spurt occurs in the lateral aspect of the distal radial physis, which brings about straightening before the growth plate closes (Figs. 9.101).[8] Therefore, it is normal for a weanling to have a mild degree of carpus valgus. Weanlings that are perfectly straight often develop carpus varus after the final growth spurt occurs.[8] Foals with greater than 15° of carpal angular limb deformity (ALD) and 8° of fetlock ALD usually require immediate attention; however, the majority of foals do not fall into this category.

Articular ALDs associated with immaturity of the cuboidal bones and ligamentous laxity must be differentiated from ALDs associated with the distal radial physis. Articular ALDs are generally reversible if they are treated in the first few weeks of life. After 3 to 4 weeks of age, however, ossification of the malformed cuboidal bones has begun, and the deformation may be permanent[8] (refer to Chapter 8 for more information).

External rotational limb deformities (torsion of the limb around its long axis) are common in young foals with narrow chests. Generally, these deformities originate high in the limb, resulting in the carpus and fetlock joints facing outward. These limb deformities usually improve with age; as the chest broadens, the humerus and elbow joint are forced outward, resulting in a derotational effect. As the limb undergoes internal rotation, the carpus and fetlock assume a more normal frontal position.[8] No treatment is generally indicated with this condition.

Rotational deformities that develop distal to the carpus with the fetlock rotated inward or outward do not correct naturally. These deformities tend to be inherited and thus should be selected against in breeding programs.[8]

Some ALDs cause an apparent rotational deformity. For example, a carpus valgus gives the appearance that the distal limb is rotated externally (outward), and a fetlock varus appears to create an internal rotation of the phalanges.[8] Once the ALD (the primary problem) is corrected, the rotational deformity is no longer apparent.

A foal is born with soft feathers of horn on the bottom of its hooves. These wear off by the end of a normal first day. The texture of the hoof itself is cornified, yet soft and waxy. It is generally that way the first week and gradually hardens to more durable hoof horn. The last bit of neonate (baby) hoof will have grown down to ground level by about 6 months of age.

Physeal (growth plate) closure has an important bearing on the timing of corrective treatments (refer to Chapter 8). As noted, many foals born with crooked limbs straighten without any specific treatment, and those that do not can most often be corrected with proper veterinary care and management.

It has been suggested that foals should spend the first few hours and even weeks on a firm dirt surface and be encouraged to move around, following their mothers for several hours a day. The idea behind this is to stimulate proprioceptive (sensory) receptors in the frog that control muscle movement. It is postulated that this early muscle response may help straighten and strengthen the limbs early in a foal's life.

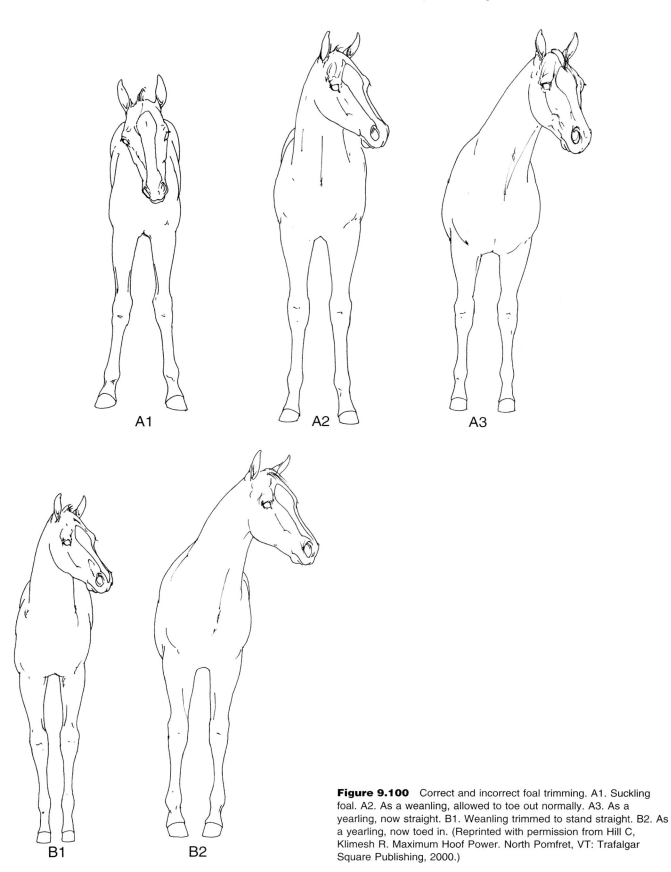

Figure 9.100   Correct and incorrect foal trimming. A1. Suckling foal. A2. As a weanling, allowed to toe out normally. A3. As a yearling, now straight. B1. Weanling trimmed to stand straight. B2. As a yearling, now toed in. (Reprinted with permission from Hill C, Klimesh R. Maximum Hoof Power. North Pomfret, VT: Trafalgar Square Publishing, 2000.)

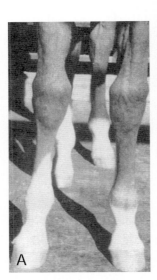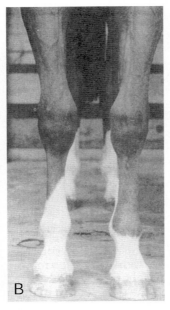

Figure 9.101 A. Weanling foal at 4 months. B. Same horse at 10 months. (Reprinted with permission from Hill C, Klimesh R. Maximum Hoof Power. North Pomfret, VT: Trafalgar Square Publishing, 2000.)

A regular program of farrier care should begin when the foal is about 1 month of age. Overly enthusiastic rasping or radical trimming, however, can do more harm than good with the very young foal. Therefore, it is essential that the farrier and veterinarian confer. A foal with a mild to moderate carpal valgus deformity, kept level and balanced through the growing months, will stand relatively straight as a yearling. Advances in glue-on shoe technology allow corrective shoes to be applied to foals only a few weeks of age (see "Resources" in this chapter).

Incorrect "Corrective" Trimming

Some age-old corrective trimming principles are no longer employed on foals. One procedure to correct a toed-out horse is to rotate the hoof capsule inward by lowering the outside hoof wall to make it shorter than the inside wall. In addition, a half-shoe is applied to the inside wall to rotate the hoof farther inward. This has the effect of moving the limb in under the horse's body and shifting more of the weight to the outside of the limb. Lowering the outside hoof wall of toed-out foals before 3 months of age, however, can interrupt the normal developmental pattern and result in a varus deformity of the fetlock region (Fig. 9.100). The growth plates of the fetlock region have remodeled according to the alteration in weight bearing caused by the trimming.

Impatience to "correct" a normally carpus valgus fetlock-rotated-out foal by lowering the outside hoof wall can also result in sheared heels and quarters. Such a problem is not likely to occur if the hoof is kept in ML balance and the foal's own development is allowed to correct the carpus valgus. Therefore, it is important not to lower the outside wall on such foals that are under 3 months of age. Squaring the toe of the hoof may help restore ML balance. Because a carpus valgus foal tends

to break over medial of the hoof center, squaring the toe encourages a more central breakover.

Regular Farrier Care

Besides assessing a foal's hooves in relation to its limbs when it is standing, a farrier evaluates the foal's hoof wear patterns. In most cases, rasping required to balance a hoof should be done conservatively and with close monitoring of the natural wear. By squaring the toe, a hoof can be encouraged to break over at the center. By checking for evenness and symmetry, the farrier can evaluate the natural tendency of the fetlock, pastern, and hoof to align with the cannon. With the foal's forelimb flexed at the knee, the farrier lets the extensor surface of the cannon rest in the palm of the hand. The fetlock and hoof are allowed to fall into their normal axis at rest. The farrier can then evaluate the heels for evenness, the relationship of the hoof to the limb, and the symmetry of the frog in relation to the hoof.

Trimming and maintenance should consist of keeping the wall trimmed away from the sole of the foot, as the wall that the foal was born with was never intended to bear weight. The frog bearing the majority of the weight will keep the forces centered under the bone column and palmar/plantar so ML and DP forces are reduced. If help is needed to straighten severe deformities, lateral extensions may be of use when applied for short periods of time.

TEAMWORK

A horse's health and soundness are a result of a team effort. The horse owner is responsible for coordinating the efforts of the other team members: manager, trainer, instructor, rider, veterinarian, and farrier.

The farrier's primary role is to trim and shoe the horse as naturally as possible, keeping the principles of balance in mind. The farrier's goals should be long-term soundness and optimum performance. In addition, the farrier can assist the veterinarian, to the extent of his or her experience, in the treatment of some hoof and limb problems. It is important that the veterinarian and farrier have an opportunity to interact. The combination of their knowledge and experience usually benefits the horse.

Whenever a hoof injury involves sensitive tissue (hot nail, puncture, abscess, bleeding crack, coronary wound), it is important that a veterinarian be involved in the treatment. Although the farrier may perform the actual work (paring an abscess, relieving or resecting a crack, treating a hot nail), it should be done under a veterinarian's supervision.

Farrier Publications

American Farriers Journal
   Official journal of the American Farriers Association
   P.O. Box 624, Brookfield, WI 53008-0624
   E-mail: info@lesspub.com
   Web site: www.lesspub.com/afj/
Anvil
   Practical articles on horseshoeing and blacksmithing
   P.O. Box 1810, Georgetown, CA 95634-1810
   E-mail: anvil@anvilmag.com
   Web site: www.anvilmag.com/

European Farriers Journal
Bimonthly international magazine
16 rue d'Opprebais, B 1360 Malèves-Sainte-Marie, Belgium
Phone: +32-0-10-88-88-98
E-mail: Info@farriersjournal.com
Web site: www.farriersjournal.com
Hoofcare and Lameness Quarterly Report
Practical articles and research on farrier science
P.O. Box 6600, Gloucester, MA 01930
E-mail: franjurga@aol.com
Web site: www.hoofcare.com/

Farrier Organizations

American Farriers Association
4059 Iron Works Pike, Lexington, KY 40511
Phone: 606-233-7411
E-mail: farriers@aol.com
Web site: www.americanfarriers.org
Brotherhood of Working Farriers Association
14013 East Highway 136, LaFayette, GA 30728
Phone: 706-397-8047
E-mail: farrierhdq@aol.com
Web site: www.bwfa.net/
Guild of Professional Farriers
P.O. Box 684, Locust, NC 28097
Phone: 301-898-6990
E-mail: theguild@horseshoes.com
Web site: www.horseshoes.com/theguild/

Resources

Centaur Forge, Ltd.
Farrier books and tools, shoe size comparison chart, studs, hoof boots, hoof sealer, pads
P.O. Box 340, Burlington, WI 53105
Phone: 414-763-9175
E-mail: centforge1@aol.com
Web site: www.centaurforge.com
Equilox International
Equilox, prosthetic hoof repair material
PO Box 428A, Pine Island, MN 55963
Phone: 800-551-4394
E-mail: equilox123@aol.com
Web site: www.equilox.com
Equine Digit Support System, Inc.
506 Highway 115, Penrose, CO 81240
Phone: 719-372-7463
E-mail: edss@ris.net
Web site: www.hopeforsoundness.com/
Web site: www.edsshoofcare.com
Hawthorne Products, Inc.
Hoof packing
16828 North State Road 167, North Dunkirk, IN 47336
Phone: 765-768-6585 or 800-548-5658
E-mail: drhobso@ibm.net
Web site: www.hawthorne-products.com/
Kentucky Blacksmith
Glue-on shoes, foal extensions, Lily pads
P.O. Box 1086, 747 Mt. Eden Road, Shelbyville, KY 40065
Phone: 502-633-3598 or 888-458-7463
E-mail: kyblacksmith@worldnet.att.net
Web site: www.kyblacksmith.com/
Level-It
Material for hoof leveling, balancing, and repair
10235 West Sample Road, Suite 207, Coral Springs, FL 33065
Phone: 800-408-2900
E-mail: llevel-it@aol.com
Web site: www.horseshoes.com/supplies
Life Data Labs, Inc.
Farrier's Formula
P.O. Box 490, Cherokee, AL 35616
Phone: 800-624-1873
E-mail: msgravlee@lifedatalabs.com
Web site: http://www.lifedatalabs.com

Mustad Hoofcare
Glue-on shoes
P.O. Box 7315, Bloomfield, CT 06002
Phone: 203-726-1927
E-mail: info@mustadinc.com
Web site: www.mustadinc.com
Richard Klimesh
Welding clips with a wire-feed welder, videos, Klimesh contiguous clip shoe, heel shields
P.O. Box 140, Livermore, CO 80536
Phone: 970-221-2948
E-mail: rklimesh@horsekeeping.com
Web site: www.horsekeeping.com
Sound Horse Technologies
P.O. Box 689, Unionville, PA 19375
Phone: 800-801-2654 or 610-347-0453
Fax: 610-347-1822

References

1. Balch O. The effects of changes in hoof angle, mediolateral balance and toe length on kinetic and temporal parameters of horses walking, trotting, and cantering on a high-speed treadmill. PhD Thesis, College of Veterinary Medicine, Pullman, WA, 1991.
2. Balch O, et al. Degenerative joint disease in the fetlock managed by balanced shoeing: A case report. Equine Pract 1985;7:35.
3. Balch O, et al. Effects of increasing hoof length on limb kinematics of trotting horses. Proc Am Assoc Equine Pract 1994;40:43.
4. Balch O, et al. Hoof balance and lameness: Improper toe length, hoof angle, and mediolateral balance. Compendium1995;17:1275.
5. Balch O, et al. Locomotor effects of hoof angle and mediolateral balance of horses exercising on a high speed treadmill: Preliminary results. Proc Am Assoc Equine Pract 1992;38:687.
6. Balch O, et al. Weight and length induced changes in limb kinematics in trotting horses. Proc Am Assoc Equine Pract 1996;42:218.
7. Blackford JT, et al. Adjustable tension band stabilization of hoof wall cracks in horses. Proc Am Assoc Equine Pract 1991;37:497.
8. Bramlage LR, et al. Observations on the evaluation and selection of foal limb deformities for surgical treatment. Proc Am Assoc Equine Pract 1990;36:273.
9. Buffa EA, et al. Effect of dietary biotin supplement on equine hoof horn growth rate and hardness. Equine Vet J 1992;24:472.
10. Bushe T, et al. The effect of hoof angle on coffin, pastern and fetlock joint angles. Proc Am Assoc Equine Pract 1987;33:729.
11. Butler JL. The repair of hoof defects using fiberglass and screws. Proc Am Assoc Equine Pract 1976;22:235.
12. Butler KD. The prevention of lameness by physiologically-sound shoeing. Proc Am Assoc Equine Pract 1986;32:465.
13. Butler KD. What every practitioner should know about hoof balance. Proc Am Assoc Equine Pract 1994;40:133.
14. Clayton HM. Comparison of the stride of trotting horses trimmed with a normal and a broken-back hoof axis. Proc Am Assoc Equine Pract 1987;33:289.
15. Clayton HM. The effect of an acute hoof wall angulation in the stride kinematics of trotting horses. Equine Vet J 1990;9(Suppl):86.
16. Clayton HM. The effect of an acute angulation of the hind hooves on diagonal synchrony of trotting horses. Equine Vet J 1990;9(Suppl):91.
17. Clayton HM, et al. Effect of three shoe types on duration of breakover in sound trotting horses. J Equine Vet Sci 1991;11:129–132.
18. Colles CM. Concepts of blood flow in the etiology and treatment of navicular disease. Proc Am Assoc Equine Pract 1983;29:265.
19. Colles CM. Interpreting radiographs. 1. The foot. Equine Vet J 1983;15:297.
20. Colles CM. The relationship of frog pressure to heel expansion. Equine Vet J 1989;21:13.
21. Colles CM. A technique for assessing hoof function in the horse. Equine Vet J 1989;21:17.
22. Dyhre-Poulsen P, et al. Equine hoof function investigated by pressure transducers inside the hoof and accelerometers mounted on the first phalanx. Equine Vet J 1994;26:362.
23. Glade MJ, et al. Effect of toe angle on hoof growth and contraction in the horse. J Equine Vet Sci 1985;5:45.

24. Hill C, Klimesh R. Maximum Hoof Power. North Pomfret, VT: Trafalgar Square Publishing, 2000.
25. Hood DM, et al. Effects of ground surface on solar load distribution. Proc Am Assoc Equine Pract 1997;43:360.
26. Juell AA. The glue-on industry. Am Farriers J 1989;15:10–15.
27. Kane AJ, et al. Horseshoe characteristics as possible risk factors for fatal musculoskeletal injury in Thoroughbred racehorses. Am J Vet Res 1996;57:1147.
28. Kane AJ, et al. Postmortem evaluation of homotypic variation in shoe characteristics of 201 Thoroughbred racehorses. Am J Vet Res 1996;57:1141.
29. Kane AJ, et al. Toe grabs and rim shoes as possible risk factors for catastrophic injury of Thoroughbred racehorses. Proc Am Assoc Equine Pract 1996;42:286.
30. Kobluk C, et al. The effect of conformation and shoeing: A cohort study of 95 Thoroughbred racehorses. Proc Am Assoc Equine Pract 1989;35:259.
31. Lieberman RJ. Don't call it "white line disease." Mod Horse Breeding 1994;Dec:46.
32. Lockner F, et al. In vivo and in vitro measurement of tendon strain in the horse. Am J Vet Res 1980;41:1927.
33. Madison JB, et al. Oxytetracycline decreases fetlock angle in newborn foals. Proc Am Assoc Equine Pract 1992;38:745.
34. Moyer W. Chronic subsolar bruising. Proc Am Assoc Equine Pract 1988;34:333.
35. Moyer W. Management of proximal incomplete quarter cracks in Standardbred racehorses. Proc Am Assoc Equine Pract 1988;34:329.
36. Moyer W. Preliminary experience and uses of composite hoof wall repair. Proc Am Assoc Equine Pract 1991;37:681.
37. Moyer W, et al. Lameness caused by improper shoeing. J Am Vet Med Assoc 1975;166:47.
38. Moyer W, et al. Sheared heels: Diagnosis and treatment. J Am Vet Med Assoc 1975;166:53.
39. Moyer W, et al. Treatment of distal phalanx fractures in racehorses using a continuous rim-type shoe. Proc Am Assoc Equine Pract 1988;34:325.
40. Ovnicek G. New Hope for Soundness: Seen Through the Window of Wild Horse Hoof Patterns. Columbia Falls, MT: Equine Digital Support System, 1997.
41. Ovnicek G, et al. Wild horse hoof patterns offer a formula for preventing and treating lameness. Proc Am Assoc Equine Pract 1995;41:258.
42. Page B, et al. Diagonal imbalance of the equine foot: A cause of lameness. Proc Am Assoc Equine Pract 1992;38:413.
43. Painter HJ, et al. Use of polyvinylchloride pipe to create hoof extensions in foals. Proc Am Assoc Equine Pract 1996;42:216.
44. Redden RF. A method of treating club feet. Proc Am Assoc Equine Pract 1988;34:321.
45. Robertson IP, et al. Ability of commercial hoof wall products to maintain hydration of the equine hoof wall. Proc Am Assoc Equine Pract 1996;42:208.
46. Ruohoniemi M, et al. Relationship between ossification of the cartilages of the foot and conformation and radiographic measurements of the front feet in Finnhorses. Equine Vet J 1997;29:44.
47. Sigafoos R. Composite reconstruction of equine underrun heels. Proc Am Assoc Equine Pract 1991;37:673.
48. Snow VE, et al. Specific parameters used to evaluate hoof balance and support. Proc Am Assoc Equine Pract 1991;37:299.
49. Thompson KN, et al. The effect of toe angle on tendon, ligament and hoof wall strains in vitro. J Equine Vet Sci 1993;13:51.
50. Thompson KN, et al. Metacarpophalangeal and phalangeal joint kinematics in horses shod with hoof caulks. J Equine Vet Sci 1994;14:319.
51. Turner T. The use of hoof measurements for the objective assessment of hoof balance. Proc Am Assoc Equine Pract 1992;38:389.
52. Turner T, et al. Hoof abnormalities and their relationship to lameness. Proc Am Assoc Equine Pract 1988;34:293.
53. Turner T, et al. Treatment of equine canker. Proc Am Assoc Equine Pract 1988;34:307.
54. Turner TA, et al. Use of antibiotic-impregnated hoof repair material for the treatment of hoof wall separation: A promising new treatment. Proc Am Assoc Equine Pract 1996;42:205.
55. Wilson DG, et al. Equine canker: Prospective and retrospective study. Abst Vet Surg 1985;14:70.
56. Wright AK, et al. Effect of high dose oxytetracycline on renal parameters in neonatal foals. Proc Am Assoc Equine Pract 1992;38:297.
57. Young RL, et al. Hoof repair using high-resin fiberglass tape. Proc Am Assoc Equine Pract 1989;35:451.

INDEX

Numbers in *italics* denote figures; numbers followed by "t" denote tables.

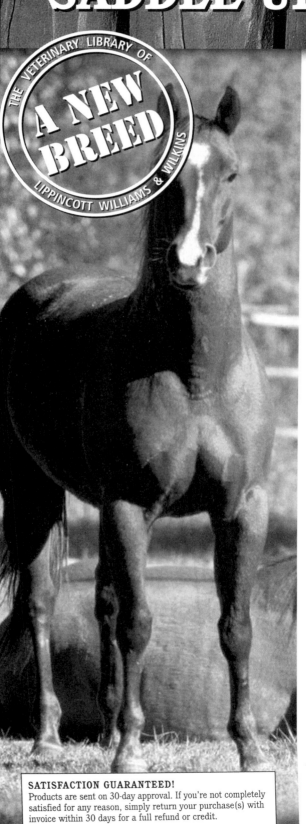
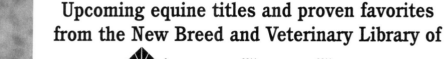
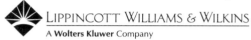
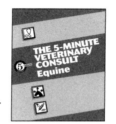
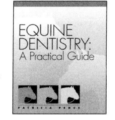